CLINICAL ANATOMY BY REGIONS

Clinical Anatomy By Regions

EIGHTH EDITION

Richard S. Snell, M.R.C.S., L.R.C.P., MB, BS, MD, PhD

Emeritus Professor of Anatomy
George Washington University
School of Medicine and Health Sciences
Washington, D.C.
Formerly
Associate Professor of Anatomy and Medicine, Yale University Medical School;
Lecturer in Anatomy, King's College, University of London;
and Visiting Professor of Anatomy, Harvard Medical School

Wolters Kluwer | Lippincott Williams & Wilkins
Health

Philadelphia • Baltimore • New York • London
Buenos Aires • Hong Kong • Sydney • Tokyo

Acquisitions Editor: Crystal Taylor
Managing Editor: Kelly Horvath
Marketing Manager: Valerie Sanders
Production Editor: Julie Montalbano
Designer: Doug Smock
Compositor: Maryland Composition, Inc.

351 West Camden Street
Baltimore, MD 21201

530 Walnut Street
Philadelphia, PA 19106

The publisher is not responsible (as a matter of product liability, negligence, or otherwise) for any injury resulting from any material contained herein. This publication contains information relating to general principles of medical care that should not be construed as specific instructions for individual patients. Manufacturers' product information and package inserts should be reviewed for current information, including contraindications, dosages, and precautions.

Printed in China

Seventh Edition, 2004

Library of Congress Cataloging-in-Publication Data

Snell, Richard S.
Clinical anatomy by regions / Richard S. Snell. —8th ed.
p. ; cm.
Rev. ed. of: Clinical anatomy. 7th ed. c2004.
Includes bibliographical references and index.
ISBN-13: 978-0-7817-6404-9
ISBN-10: 0-7817-6404-1
1. Human anatomy. I. Snell, Richard S. Clinical anatomy. II. Title.
[DNLM: 1. Anatomy. QS 4 S671c 2007]
QM23.2.S55 2007
611—dc22

2006023959

The publishers have made every effort to trace the copyright holders for borrowed material. If they have inadvertently overlooked any, they will be pleased to make the necessary arrangements at the first opportunity.

To purchase additional copies of this book, call our customer service department at **(800) 638-3030** or fax orders to **(301) 223-2320.** International customers should call **(301) 223-2300.**

Visit Lippincott Williams & Wilkins on the Internet: http://www.LWW.com. Lippincott Williams & Wilkins customer service representatives are available from 8:30 am to 6:00 pm, EST.

08 09 10 11
2 3 4 5 6 7 8 9 10

PREFACE

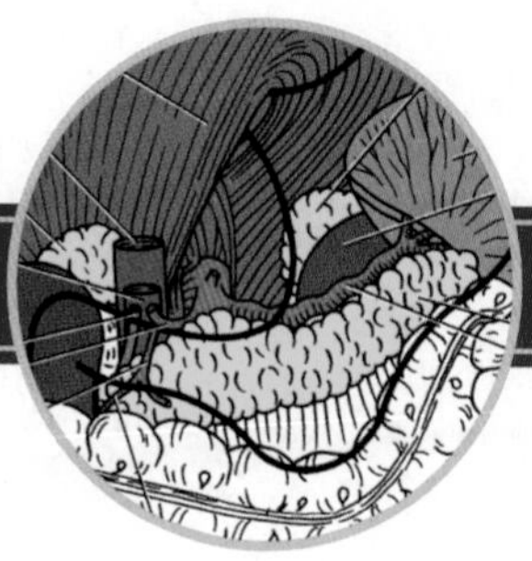

Each patient that you examine in your clinic with medical problems is composed of gross anatomic structures, which may or may not exhibit functional deficits. All students must therefore enter medicine with a basic knowledge of anatomy that is clinically relevant.

The explosion in the knowledge of medical disease and the technological advances associated with the diagnosis and treatment of diseases have dictated a complete restructuring of the curriculum for medical students, dental students, allied health students, and nursing students. In the United States, students in many schools are now being offered programs in gross anatomy in which only part of the body is dissected, and this is supplemented by the use of prosected specimens, plastinated specimens, and computer imagery.

To assist in the necessary curriculum changes, in the eighth edition, great efforts have been made to weed out unnecessary material and streamline the text. The following changes have been introduced:

1. All the line illustrations have been recolored and the label print upgraded.
2. All the surface anatomy illustrations are in color.
3. The anatomy of common medical procedures has been further expanded and again includes sections on complications caused by an ignorance of normal anatomy.
4. The computed tomography (CT) scans, magnetic resonance imaging (MRI) studies, and sonograms have been upgraded as the technology has advanced.
5. Tables have been used wherever possible to reduce the size of the text. This includes reference tables at the end of the text that give important dimensions and capacities of various anatomic structures.
6. The clinical problems section at the end of each chapter has been reviewed and, when necessary, brought up to date.

Each chapter of *Clinical Anatomy* is constructed in a similar manner. This gives students ready access to material and facilitates moving from one part of the book to another. Each chapter is divided into the following categories:

1. **Clinical Example:** A short case report that dramatizes the relevance of anatomy in medicine introduces each chapter.
2. **Clinical Objectives:** This section focuses the student on the material that is most important to learn and understand in each chapter. It emphasizes the basic structures in the area being studied so that, once mastered, the student is easily able to build up his or her knowledge base. This section also points out structures on which examiners have repeatedly asked questions.
3. **Basic Clinical Anatomy:** This section provides basic information on gross anatomic structures that are of clinical importance. Numerous examples of normal radiographs, CT scans, MRI studies, and sonograms are also provided. Labeled photographs of cross-sectional anatomy of the head, neck, and trunk are included to stimulate students to think in terms of three-dimensional anatomy, which is so important in the interpretation of imaging studies.
4. **Surface Anatomy:** This section provides surface landmarks of important anatomic structures, many of which are located some distance beneath the skin. This section is important because most practicing medical personnel seldom explore tissues to any depth beneath the skin. Photographs of living subjects have been used extensively.
5. **Clinical Problem Solving:** Examples of clinical cases are given at the end of each chapter. Each is followed by multiple-choice questions. Answers to the problems are given at the end of the section.
6. **Review Questions:** The purpose of the questions is threefold: to focus attention on areas of importance, to enable students to assess their areas of weakness, and to provide a form of self-evaluation for questions asked under examination conditions. Some of the questions are centered around a clinical problem that requires an anatomic answer. Solutions to the problems are provided at the end of the section.

To assist in the quick understanding of anatomic facts, the book is heavily illustrated. Most figures have been kept simple, and color has been used extensively. Illustrations summarizing the nerve and blood supply of regions have been retained, as have overviews of the distribution of cranial nerves.

R.S.S.

ACKNOWLEDGMENTS

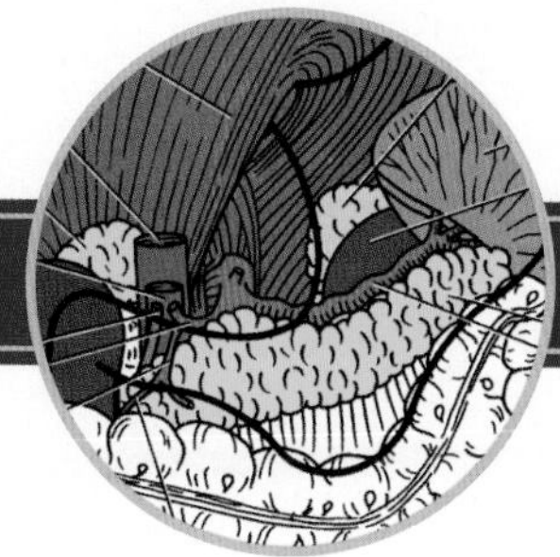

I am greatly indebted to many faculty members of the Department of Radiology at the George Washington University School of Medicine and Health Sciences for the loan of the radiographs, computed tomography (CT) scans, and magnetic resonance imaging (MRI) that have been reproduced in different sections of this book. I am also grateful to Dr. Carol Lee, Dr. Gordon Sze, and Dr. Robert Smith of the Department of Radiology at Yale University Medical Center for supplying examples of mammograms, CT scans of the vertebral column, and MRIs of the limbs. My special thanks are owed to Dr. Michael Remetz of the Department of Cardiology at Yale for providing examples of coronary arteriograms.

My special thanks are owed to Larry Clark, who, as a senior technician in the Department of Anatomy at George Washington University, greatly assisted me in the preparation of anatomic specimens for photography and for the preparation of plastinated specimens of many different organs. His enthusiasm for the many projects was contagious and greatly helped in the final production of outstanding specimens, many of which are illustrated in the text.

I wish also to express my sincere thanks to Terry Dolan, Virginia Childs, Myra Feldman, and Ira Grunther for preparation of the artwork.

Finally, I wish to express my deep gratitude to the staff of Lippincott Williams & Wilkins for their great help and support in the preparation of this new edition.

CONTENTS

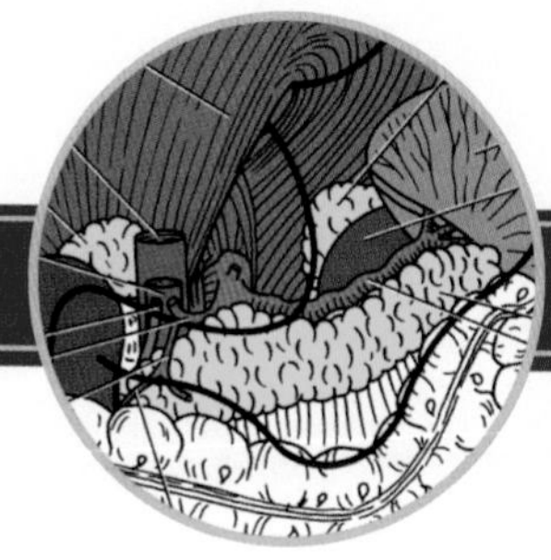

	Preface	vii
	Acknowledgments	ix
CHAPTER 1	Introduction	1
CHAPTER 2	The Thorax: Part I—The Thoracic Wall	45
CHAPTER 3	The Thorax: Part II—The Thoracic Cavity	77
CHAPTER 4	The Abdomen: Part I—The Abdominal Wall	145
CHAPTER 5	The Abdomen: Part II—The Abdominal Cavity	201
CHAPTER 6	The Pelvis: Part I—The Pelvic Walls	307
CHAPTER 7	The Pelvis: Part II—The Pelvic Cavity	337
CHAPTER 8	The Perineum	387
CHAPTER 9	The Upper Limb	425
CHAPTER 10	The Lower Limb	549
CHAPTER 11	The Head and Neck	667
CHAPTER 12	The Back	851
	Appendix	899
	Index	901

CHAPTER 1

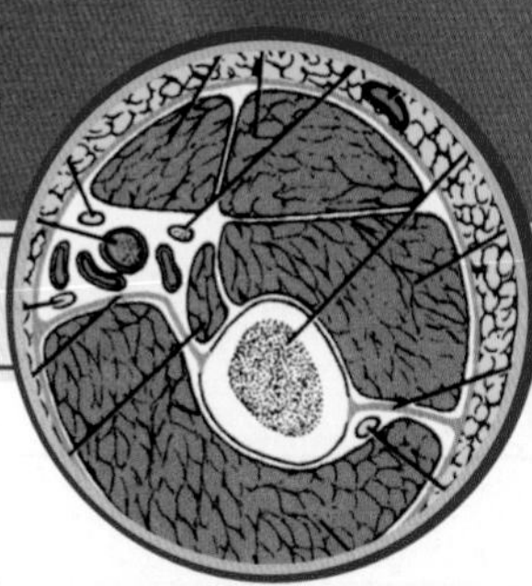

INTRODUCTION

A 65-year-old man was admitted to the emergency department complaining of the sudden onset of a severe crushing pain over the front of the chest spreading down the left arm and up into the neck and jaw. On questioning, he said that he had had several attacks of pain before and that they had always occurred when he was climbing stairs or digging in the garden. Previously, he found that the discomfort disappeared with rest after about 5 minutes. On this occasion, the pain was more severe and had occurred spontaneously while he was sitting in a chair; the pain had not disappeared.

The initial episodes of pain were angina, a form of cardiac pain that occurs on exertion and disappears on rest; it is caused by narrowing of the coronary arteries so that the cardiac muscle has insufficient blood. The patient has now experienced myocardial infarction, in which the coronary blood flow is suddenly reduced or stopped and the cardiac muscle degenerates or dies. Myocardial infarction is the major cause of death in industrialized nations. Clearly, knowledge of the blood supply to the heart and the arrangement of the coronary arteries is of paramount importance in making the diagnosis and treating this patient.

CHAPTER OUTLINE

Basic Anatomy 2
Descriptive Anatomic Terms 2
Terms Related to Position 2
Terms Related to Movement 3
Basic Structures 4
Skin 4
Fasciae 8
Muscle 8
Joints 12
Ligaments 17
Bursae 17
Synovial Sheath 17
Blood Vessels 18
Lymphatic System 20
Nervous System 21
Mucous Membranes 30
Serous Membranes 30
Bone 32
Cartilage 35
Effects of Sex, Race, and Age on Structure 36
Radiographic Anatomy 36
Clinical Problem Solving 40
Answers to Clinical Problems 42
Review Questions 42
Answers to Review Questions 43

CHAPTER OBJECTIVES

- It is essential that students understand the terms used for describing the structure and function of different regions of gross anatomy. Without these terms, it is impossible to describe in a meaningful way the composition of the body. Moreover, the physician needs these terms so that anatomic abnormalities found on clinical examination of a patient can be accurately recorded.
- This chapter also introduces some of the basic structures that compose the body, such as skin, fascia, muscles, bones, and blood vessels.

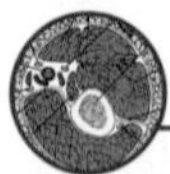

Basic Anatomy

Anatomy is the science of the structure and function of the body.

Clinical anatomy is the study of the macroscopic structure and function of the body as it relates to the practice of medicine and other health sciences.

Basic anatomy is the study of the minimal amount of anatomy consistent with the understanding of the overall structure and function of the body.

Descriptive Anatomic Terms

It is important for medical personnel to have a sound knowledge and understanding of the basic anatomic terms. With the aid of a medical dictionary, you will find that understanding anatomic terminology greatly assists you in the learning process.

The accurate use of anatomic terms by medical personnel enables them to communicate with their colleagues both nationally and internationally. Without anatomic terms, one cannot accurately discuss or record the abnormal functions of joints, the actions of muscles, the alteration of position of organs, or the exact location of swellings or tumors.

Terms Related to Position

All descriptions of the human body are based on the assumption that the person is standing erect, with the upper limbs by the sides and the face and palms of the hands directed forward (Fig. 1-1). This is the so-called **anatomic position.** The various parts of the body are then described in relation to certain imaginary planes.

Median Sagittal Plane

This is a vertical plane passing through the center of the body, dividing it into equal right and left halves (Fig. 1-1). Planes situated to one or the other side of the median plane and parallel to it are termed **paramedian.** A structure situated nearer to the median plane of the body than another is said to be **medial** to the other. Similarly, a structure that lies farther away from the median plane than another is said to be **lateral** to the other.

Coronal Planes

These planes are imaginary vertical planes at right angles to the median plane (Fig. 1-1).

Horizontal, or Transverse, Planes

These planes are at right angles to both the median and the coronal planes (Fig. 1-1).

The terms **anterior** and **posterior** are used to indicate the front and back of the body, respectively (Fig. 1-1). To describe the relationship of two structures, one is said to be anterior or posterior to the other insofar as it is closer to the anterior or posterior body surface.

In describing the hand, the terms **palmar** and **dorsal surfaces** are used in place of anterior and posterior, and in describing the foot, the terms **plantar** and **dorsal surfaces** are used instead of lower and upper surfaces (Fig. 1-1). The terms **proximal** and **distal** describe the relative distances from the roots of the limbs; for example, the arm is proximal to the forearm and the hand is distal to the forearm.

The terms **superficial** and **deep** denote the relative distances of structures from the surface of the body, and the terms **superior** and **inferior** denote levels relatively high or low with reference to the upper and lower ends of the body.

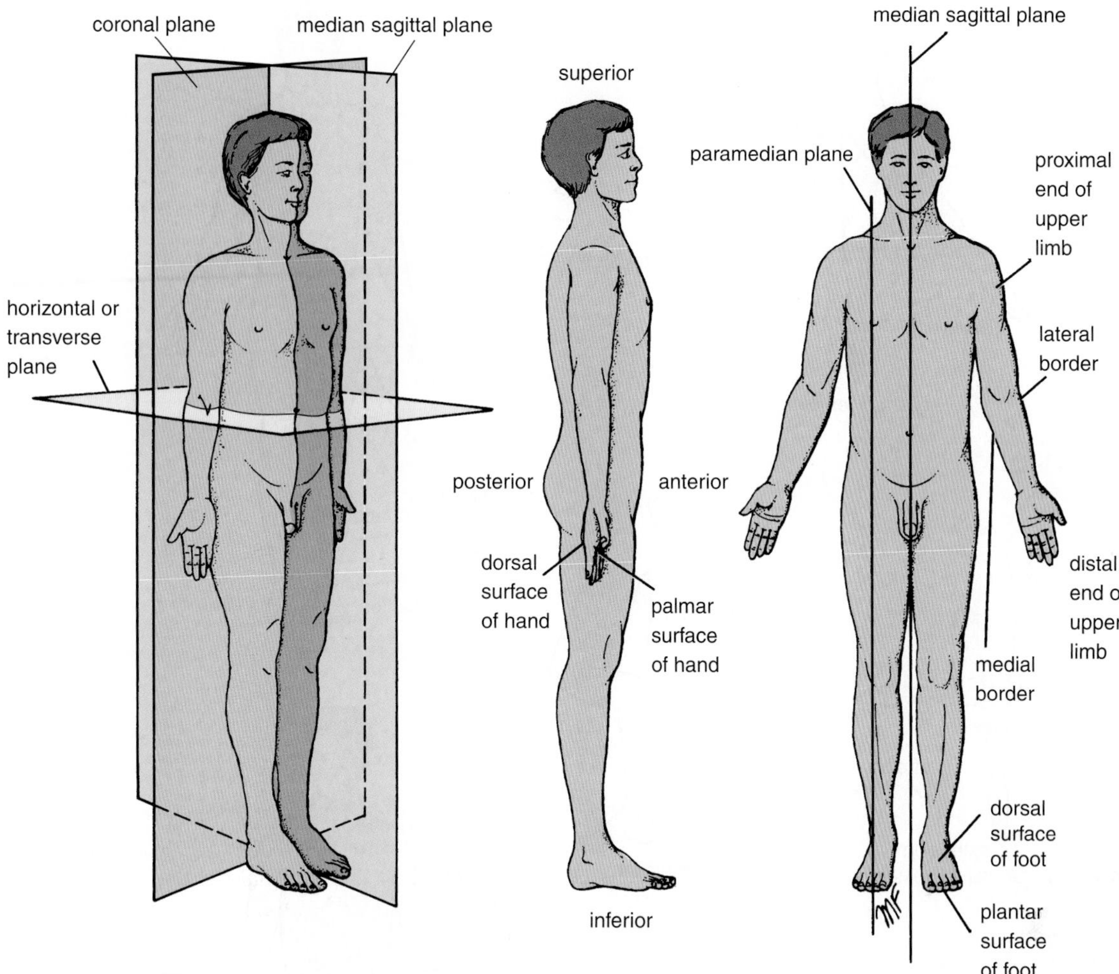

Figure 1-1 Anatomic terms used in relation to position. Note that the subjects are standing in the anatomic position.

The terms **internal** and **external** are used to describe the relative distance of a structure from the center of an organ or cavity; for example, the internal carotid artery is found inside the cranial cavity and the external carotid artery is found outside the cranial cavity.

The term **ipsilateral** refers to the same side of the body; for example, the left hand and left foot are ipsilateral. **Contralateral** refers to opposite sides of the body; for example, the left biceps brachii muscle and the right rectus femoris muscle are contralateral.

The **supine** position of the body is lying on the back. The **prone** position is lying face downward.

Terms Related to Movement

A site where two or more bones come together is known as a **joint.** Some joints have no movement (sutures of the skull), some have only slight movement (superior tibiofibular joint), and some are freely movable (shoulder joint).

Flexion is a movement that takes place in a sagittal plane. For example, flexion of the elbow joint approximates the anterior surface of the forearm to the anterior surface of the arm. It is usually an anterior movement, but it is occasionally posterior, as in the case of the knee joint (Fig. 1-2). **Extension** means straightening the joint and usually takes place in a posterior direction (Fig. 1-2). **Lateral flexion** is a movement of the trunk in the coronal plane (Fig. 1-3).

Abduction is a movement of a limb away from the midline of the body in the coronal plane (Fig. 1-2).

Adduction is a movement of a limb toward the body in the coronal plane (Fig. 1-2). In the fingers and toes, abduction is applied to the spreading of these structures and adduction is applied to the drawing together of these structures (Fig. 1-3). The movements of the thumb (Fig. 1-3), which are a little more complicated, are described on page 517.

Rotation is the term applied to the movement of a part of the body around its long axis. **Medial rotation** is the movement that results in the anterior surface of the part facing medially. **Lateral rotation** is the movement that results in the anterior surface of the part facing laterally.

Pronation of the forearm is a medial rotation of the forearm in such a manner that the palm of the hand faces posteriorly (Fig. 1-3). **Supination of the forearm** is a lateral

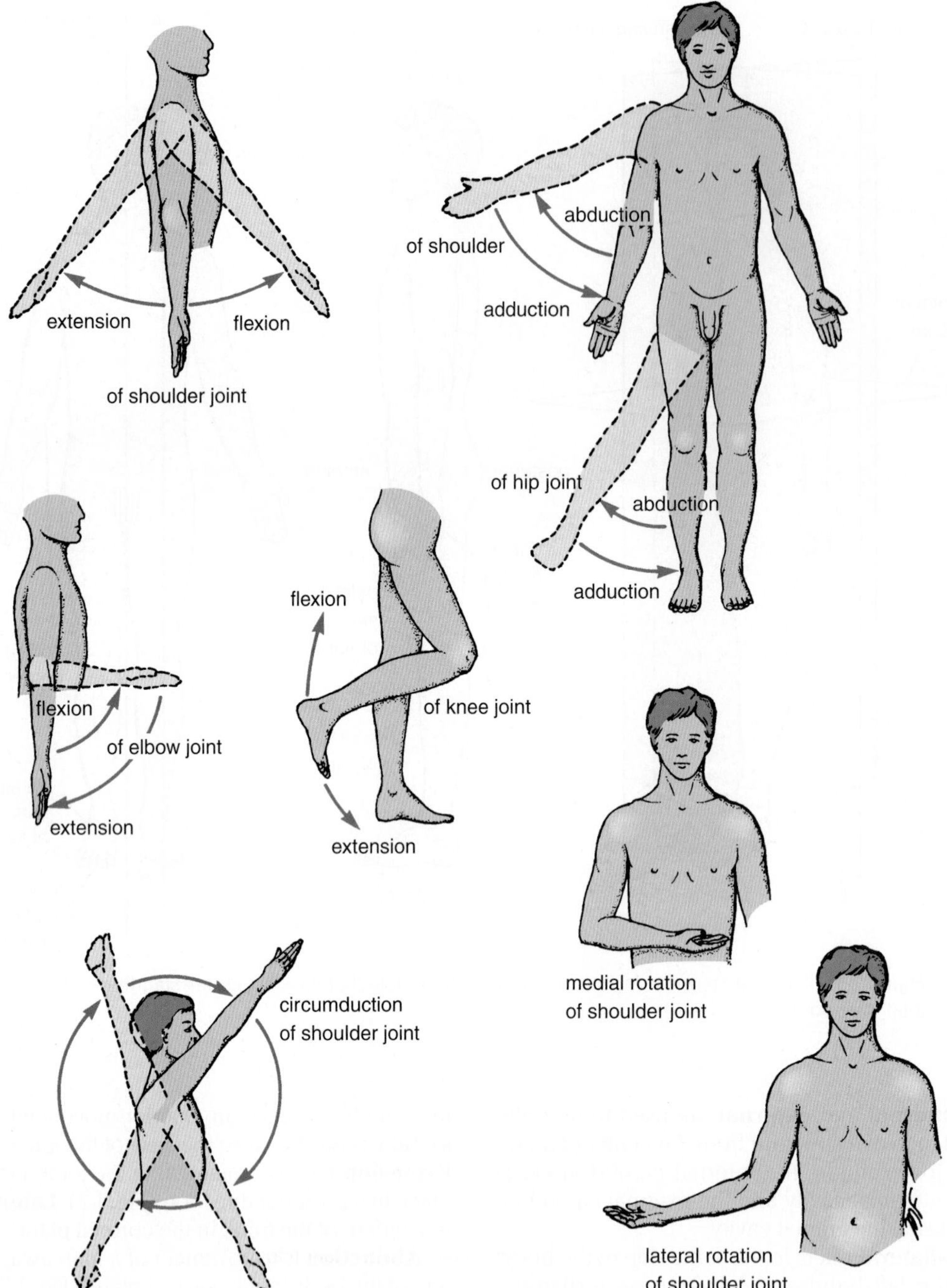

Figure 1-2 Some anatomic terms used in relation to movement. Note the difference between flexion of the elbow and that of the knee.

rotation of the forearm from the pronated position so that the palm of the hand comes to face anteriorly (Fig. 1-3).

Circumduction is the combination in sequence of the movements of flexion, extension, abduction, and adduction (Fig. 1-2).

Protraction is to move forward; **retraction** is to move backward (used to describe the forward and backward movement of the jaw at the temporomandibular joints).

Inversion is the movement of the foot so that the sole faces in a medial direction (Fig. 1-3). **Eversion** is the opposite movement of the foot so that the sole faces in a lateral direction (Fig. 1-3).

Basic Structures

Skin

The skin is divided into two parts: the superficial part, the **epidermis,** and the deep part, the **dermis** (Fig. 1-4). The epidermis is a stratified epithelium whose cells become flattened as

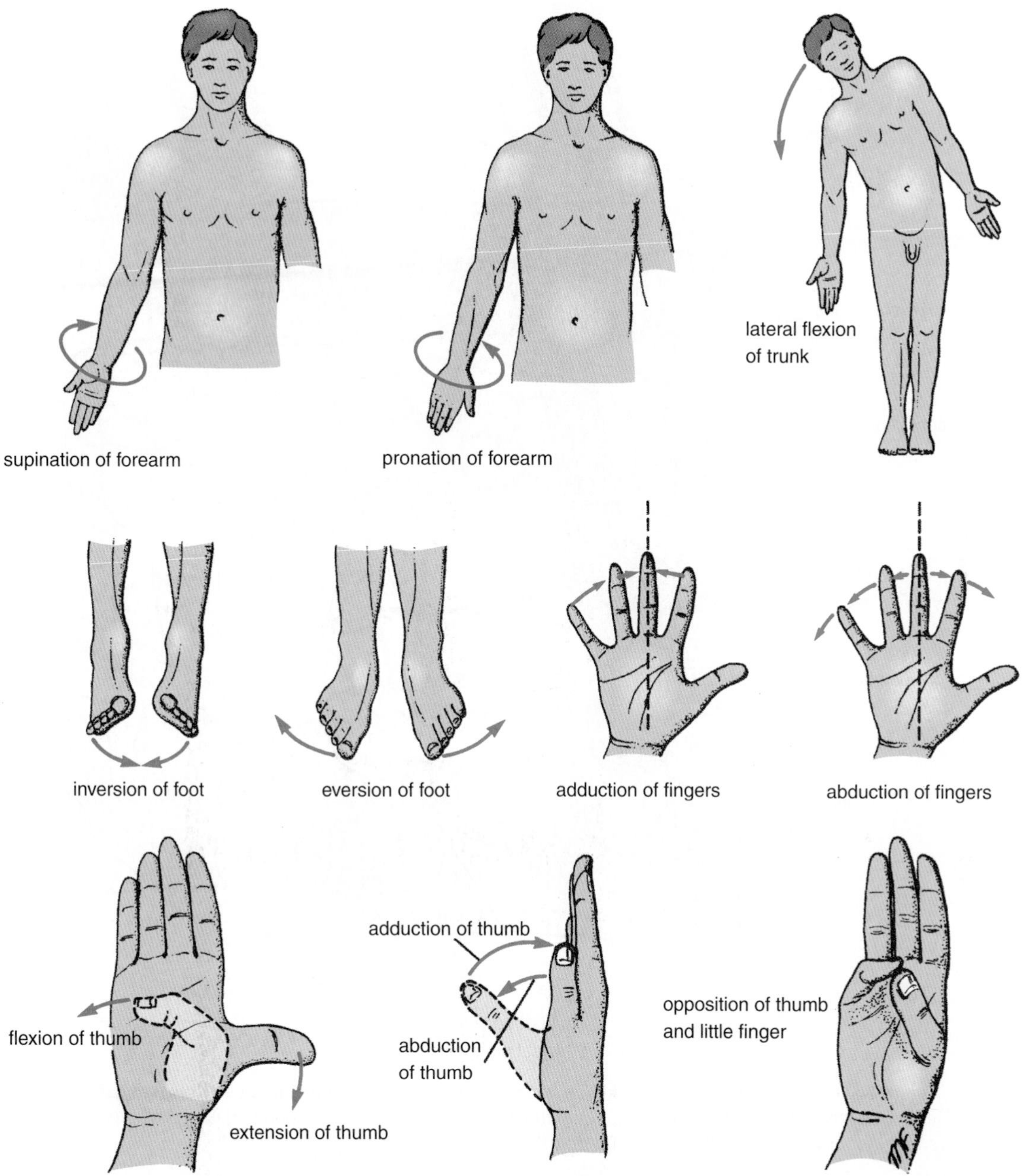

Figure 1-3 Additional anatomic terms used in relation to movement.

they mature and rise to the surface. On the palms of the hands and the soles of the feet, the epidermis is extremely thick, to withstand the wear and tear that occurs in these regions. In other areas of the body, for example, on the anterior surface of the arm and forearm, it is thin. The dermis is composed of dense connective tissue containing many blood vessels, lymphatic vessels, and nerves. It shows considerable variation in thickness in different parts of the body, tending to be thinner on the anterior than on the posterior surface. It is thinner in women than in men. The dermis of the skin is connected to the underlying deep fascia or bones by the **superficial fascia,** otherwise known as **subcutaneous tissue.**

The skin over joints always folds in the same place, the **skin creases** (Fig. 1-5). At these sites, the skin is thinner than elsewhere and is firmly tethered to underlying structures by strong bands of fibrous tissue.

The appendages of the skin are the **nails, hair follicles, sebaceous glands,** and **sweat glands.**

The **nails** are keratinized plates on the dorsal surfaces of the tips of the fingers and toes. The proximal edge of the plate is the **root of the nail** (Fig. 1-5). With the exception of the distal edge of the plate, the nail is surrounded and overlapped by folds of skin known as **nail folds.** The surface of skin covered by the nail is the **nail bed** (Fig. 1-5).

Hairs grow out of **follicles,** which are invaginations of the epidermis into the dermis (Fig. 1-4). The follicles lie obliquely to the skin surface, and their expanded extremities, called **hair bulbs,** penetrate to the deeper part of the

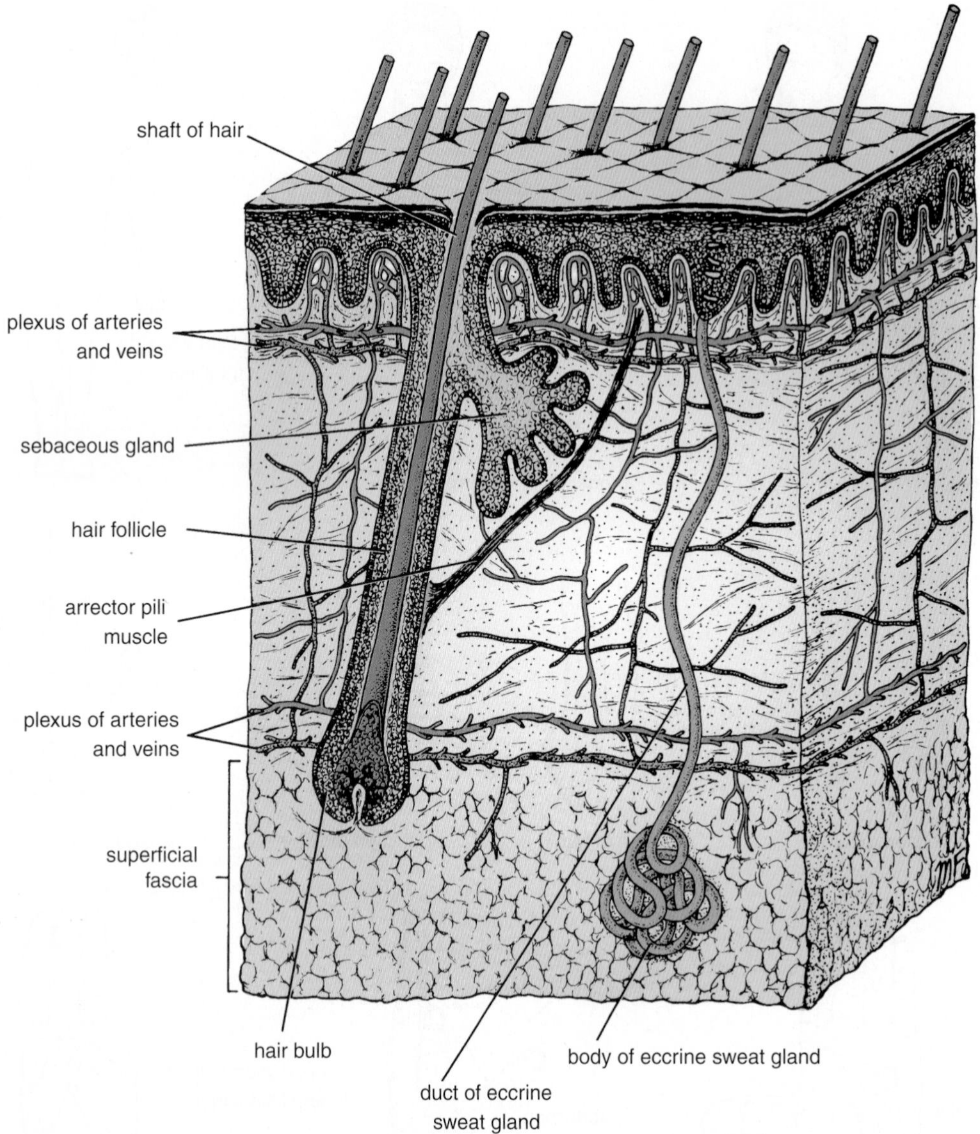

Figure 1-4 General structure of the skin and its relationship to the superficial fascia. Note that hair follicles extend down into the deeper part of the dermis or even into the superficial fascia, whereas sweat glands extend deeply into the superficial fascia.

dermis. Each hair bulb is concave at its end, and the concavity is occupied by vascular connective tissue called **hair papilla.** A band of smooth muscle, the **arrector pili,** connects the undersurface of the follicle to the superficial part of the dermis (Fig. 1-4). The muscle is innervated by sympathetic nerve fibers, and its contraction causes the hair to move into a more vertical position; it also compresses the sebaceous gland and causes it to extrude some of its secretion. The pull of the muscle also causes dimpling of the skin surface, so-called **gooseflesh.** Hairs are distributed in various numbers over the whole surface of the body, except on the lips, the palms of the hands, the sides of the fingers, the glans penis and clitoris, the labia minora and the internal surface of the labia majora, and the soles and sides of the feet and the sides of the toes.

Sebaceous glands pour their secretion, the sebum, onto the shafts of the hairs as they pass up through the necks of the follicles. They are situated on the sloping undersurface of the follicles and lie within the dermis (Fig. 1-4). **Sebum** is an oily material that helps preserve the flexibility of the emerging hair. It also oils the surface epidermis around the mouth of the follicle.

Sweat glands are long, spiral, tubular glands distributed over the surface of the body, except on the red margins of the lips, the nail beds, and the glans penis and clitoris (Fig. 1-4). These glands extend through the full thickness of the dermis, and their extremities may lie in the superficial fascia. The sweat glands are therefore the most deeply penetrating structures of all the epidermal appendages.

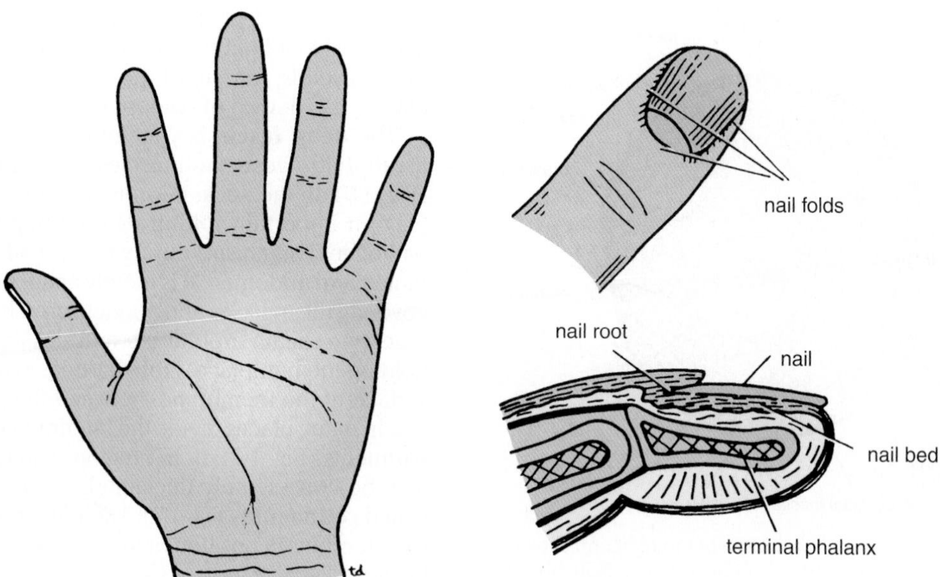

Figure 1-5 The various skin creases on the palmar surface of the hand and the anterior surface of the wrist joint. The relationship of the nail to other structures of the finger is also shown.

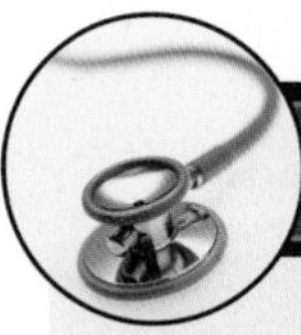

CLINICAL NOTES

Skin Infections

The nail folds, hair follicles, and sebaceous glands are common sites for entrance into the underlying tissues of pathogenic organisms such as ***Staphylococcus aureus.*** Infection occurring between the nail and the nail fold is called a **paronychia.** Infection of the hair follicle and sebaceous gland is responsible for the common **boil.** A **carbuncle** is a staphylococcal infection of the superficial fascia. It frequently occurs in the nape of the neck and usually starts as an infection of a hair follicle or a group of hair follicles.

Sebaceous Cyst

A **sebaceous cyst** is caused by obstruction of the mouth of a sebaceous duct and may be caused by damage from a comb or by infection. It occurs most frequently on the scalp.

Shock

A patient who is in a state of **shock** is pale and exhibits gooseflesh as a result of overactivity of the sympathetic system, which causes vasoconstriction of the dermal arterioles and contraction of the arrector pili muscles.

Skin Burns

The depth of a **burn** determines the method and rate of healing. A partial-skin-thickness burn heals from the cells of the hair follicles, sebaceous glands, and sweat glands as well as from the cells at the edge of the burn. A burn that extends deeper than the sweat glands heals slowly and from the edges only, and considerable contracture will be caused by fibrous tissue. To speed up healing and reduce the incidence of contracture, a deep burn should be grafted.

Skin Grafting

Skin grafting is of two main types: split-thickness grafting and full-thickness grafting. In a split-thickness graft the greater part of the epidermis, including the tips of the dermal papillae, is removed from the donor site and placed on the recipient site. This leaves at the donor site for repair purposes the epidermal cells on the sides of the dermal papillae and the cells of the hair follicles and sweat glands.

A full-thickness skin graft includes both the epidermis and dermis and, to survive, requires rapid establishment of a new circulation within it at the recipient site. The donor site is usually covered with a split-thickness graft. In certain circumstances the full-thickness graft is made in the form of a pedicle graft, in which a flap of full-thickness skin is turned and stitched in position at the recipient site, leaving the base of the flap with its blood supply intact at the donor site. Later, when the new blood supply to the graft has been established, the base of the graft is cut across.

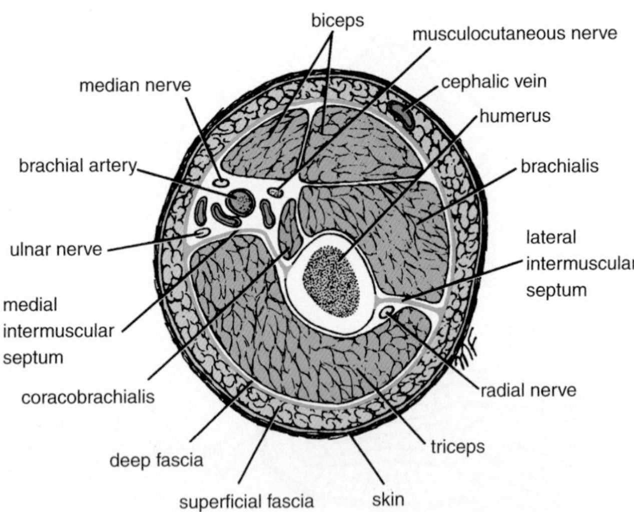

Figure 1-6 Section through the middle of the right arm showing the arrangement of the superficial and deep fascia. Note how the fibrous septa extend between groups of muscles, dividing the arm into fascial compartments.

Fasciae

The fasciae of the body can be divided into two types—**superficial** and **deep**—and lie between the skin and the underlying muscles and bones.

The **superficial fascia,** or subcutaneous tissue, is a mixture of loose areolar and adipose tissue that unites the dermis of the skin to the underlying deep fascia (Fig. 1-6). In the scalp, the back of the neck, the palms of the hands, and the soles of the feet, it contains numerous bundles of collagen fibers that hold the skin firmly to the deeper structures. In the eyelids, auricle of the ear, penis and scrotum, and clitoris, it is devoid of adipose tissue.

The **deep fascia** is a membranous layer of connective tissue that invests the muscles and other deep structures (Fig. 1-6). In the neck, it forms well-defined layers that may play an important role in determining the path taken by pathogenic organisms during the spread of infection. In the thorax and abdomen, it is merely a thin film of areolar tissue covering the muscles and aponeuroses. In the limbs, it forms a definite sheath around the muscles and other structures, holding them in place. Fibrous septa extend from the deep surface of the membrane, between the groups of muscles, and in many places divide the interior of the limbs into compartments (Fig. 1-6). In the region of joints, the deep fascia may be considerably thickened to form restraining bands called **retinacula** (Fig. 1-7). Their function is to hold underlying tendons in position or to serve as pulleys around which the tendons may move.

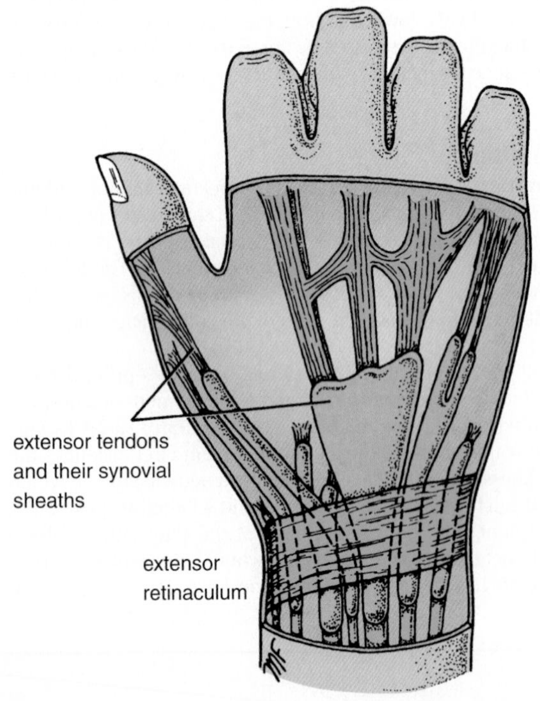

Figure 1-7 Extensor retinaculum on the posterior surface of the wrist holding the underlying tendons of the extensor muscles in position.

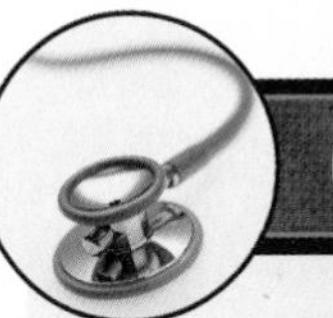

CLINICAL NOTES

Fasciae and Infection

A knowledge of the arrangement of the deep fasciae often helps explain the path taken by an infection when it spreads from its primary site. In the neck, for example, the various fascial planes explain how infection can extend from the region of the floor of the mouth to the larynx.

Muscle

The three types of muscle are skeletal, smooth, and cardiac.

Skeletal Muscle

Skeletal muscles produce the movements of the skeleton; they are sometimes called **voluntary muscles** and are made up of striped muscle fibers. A skeletal muscle has two or more attachments. The attachment that moves the least is referred to as the **origin,** and the one that moves the most, the **insertion** (Fig. 1-8). Under varying circumstances the degree of mobility of the attachments may be reversed; therefore, the terms *origin* and *insertion* are interchangeable.

The fleshy part of the muscle is referred to as its **belly** (Fig. 1-8). The ends of a muscle are attached to bones, cartilage, or ligaments by cords of fibrous tissue called **tendons** (Fig. 1-9). Occasionally, flattened muscles are attached by a thin but strong sheet of fibrous tissue called an **aponeurosis** (Fig. 1-9). A **raphe** is an interdigitation of the tendinous ends of fibers of flat muscles (Fig. 1-9).

Internal Structure of Skeletal Muscle

The muscle fibers are bound together with delicate areolar tissue, which is condensed on the surface to form a fibrous envelope, the **epimysium.** The individual fibers of a muscle are arranged either parallel or oblique to the long axis of the

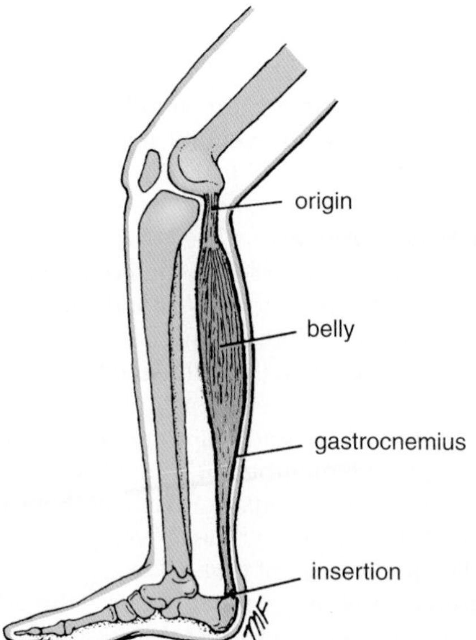

Figure 1-8 Origin, insertion, and belly of the gastrocnemius muscle.

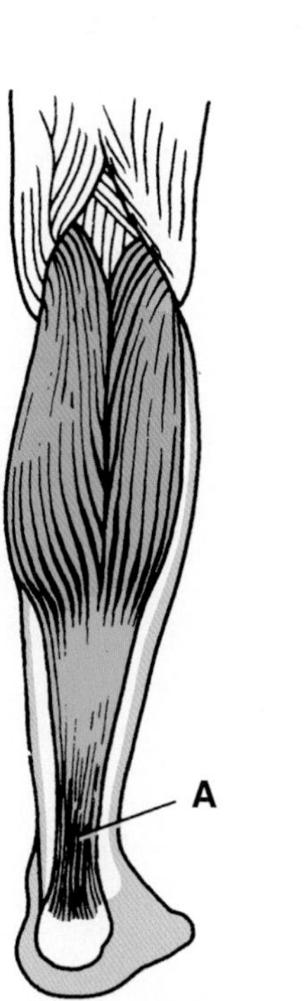

common tendon for the insertion of the gastrocnemius and soleus muscles

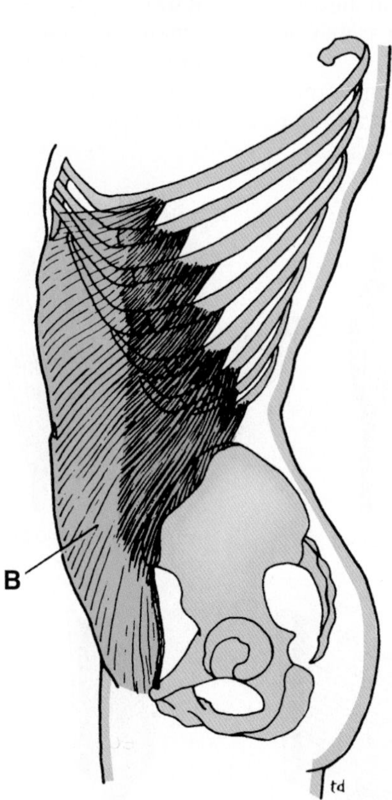

external oblique aponeurosis

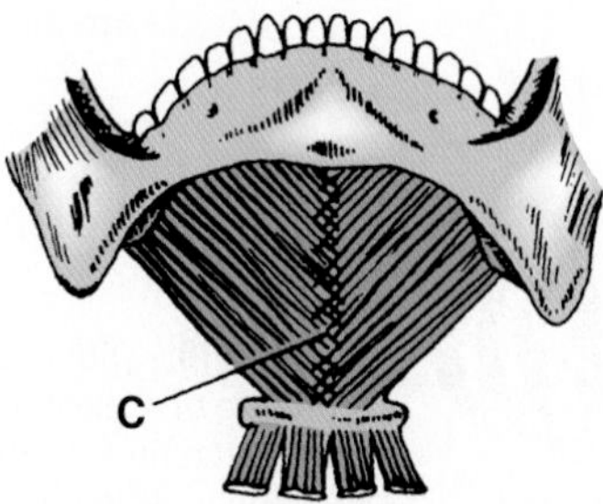

raphe of mylohyoid muscles

Figure 1-9 Examples of (**A**) a tendon, (**B**) an aponeurosis, and (**C**) a raphe.

muscle (Fig. 1-10). Because a muscle shortens by one third to one half its resting length when it contracts, it follows that muscles whose fibers run parallel to the line of pull will bring about a greater degree of movement compared with those whose fibers run obliquely. Examples of muscles with parallel fiber arrangements (Fig. 1-10) are the sternocleidomastoid, the rectus abdominis, and the sartorius.

Muscles whose fibers run obliquely to the line of pull are referred to as **pennate muscles** (they resemble a feather) (Fig. 1-10). A **unipennate muscle** is one in which the tendon lies along one side of the muscle and the muscle fibers pass obliquely to it (e.g., extensor digitorum longus). A **bipennate muscle** is one in which the tendon lies in the center of the muscle and the muscle fibers pass to it from two sides (e.g., rectus femoris). A **multipennate muscle** may be arranged as a series of bipennate muscles lying alongside one another (e.g., acromial fibers of the deltoid) or may have the tendon lying within its center and the muscle fibers passing to it from all sides, converging as they go (e.g., tibialis anterior).

For a given volume of muscle substance, pennate muscles have many more fibers compared to muscles with parallel fiber arrangements and are therefore more powerful; in other words, range of movement has been sacrificed for strength.

Skeletal Muscle Action

All movements are the result of the coordinated action of many muscles. However, to understand a muscle's action it is necessary to study it individually.

A muscle may work in the following four ways:

- **Prime mover:** A muscle is a prime mover when it is the chief muscle or member of a chief group of muscles responsible for a particular movement. For example, the quadriceps femoris is a prime mover in the movement of extending the knee joint (Fig. 1-11).
- **Antagonist:** Any muscle that opposes the action of the prime mover is an antagonist. For example, the biceps femoris opposes the action of the quadriceps femoris when the knee joint is extended (Fig. 1-11). Before a prime mover can contract, the antagonist muscle must be equally relaxed; this is brought about by nervous reflex inhibition.

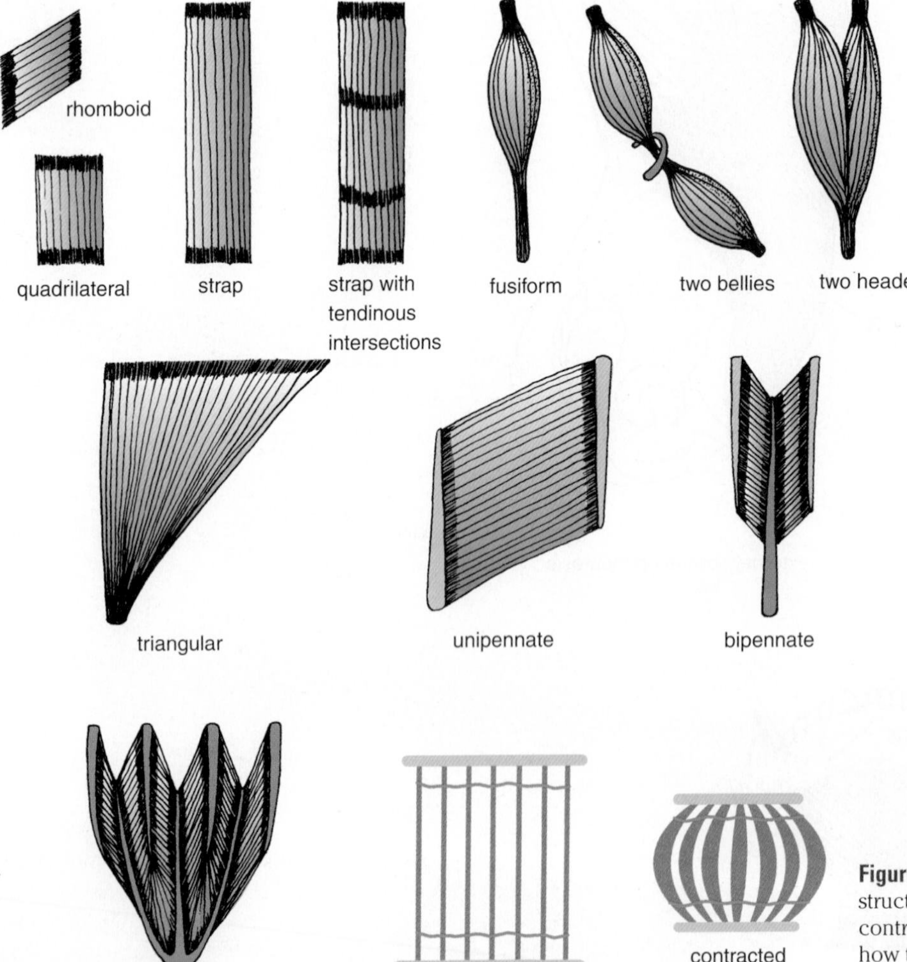

Figure 1-10 Different forms of the internal structure of skeletal muscle. A relaxed and a contracted muscle are also shown; note how the muscle fibers, on contraction, shorten by one third to one half of their resting length. Note also how the muscle swells.

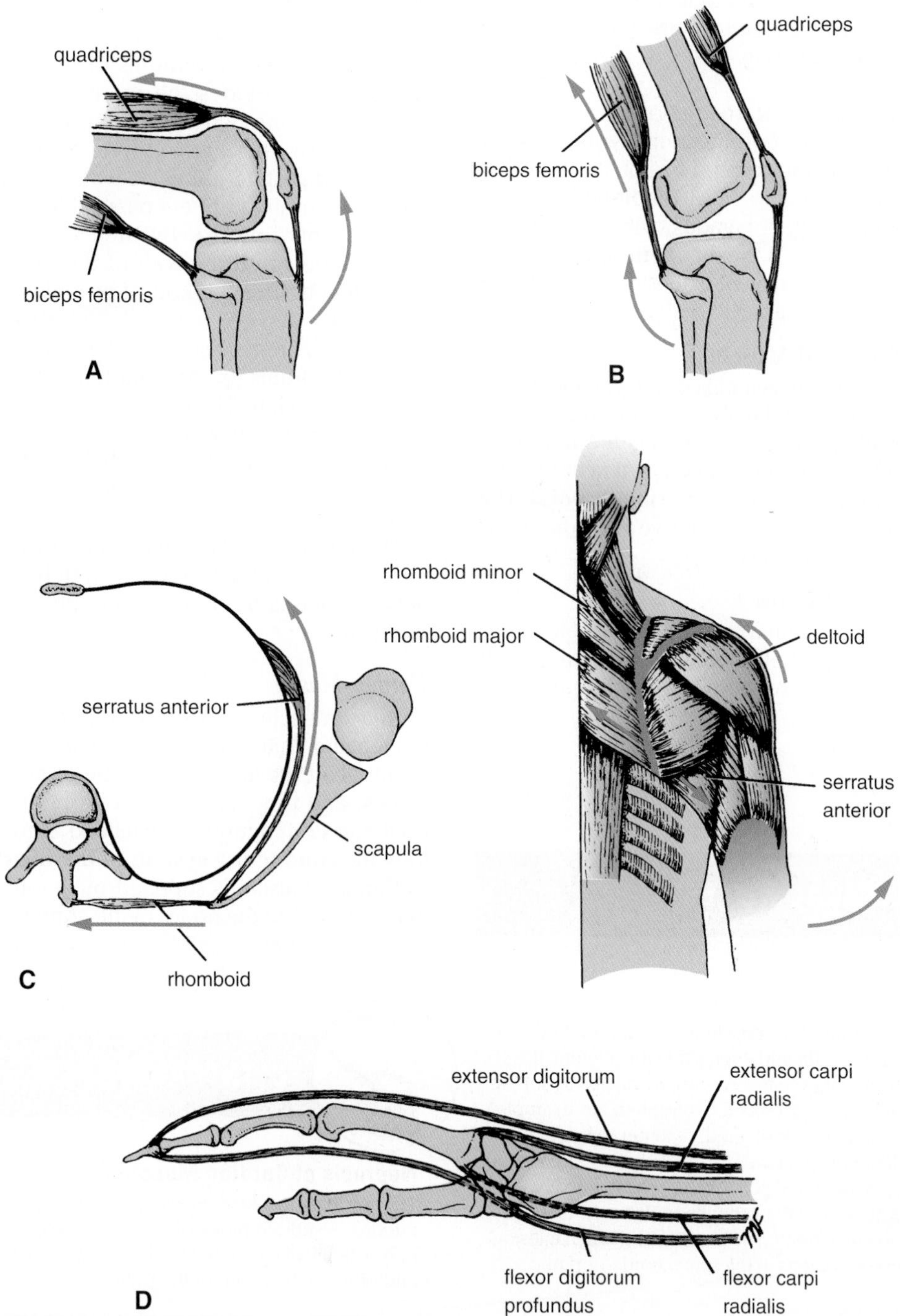

Figure 1-11 Different types of muscle action. **A.** Quadriceps femoris extending the knee as a prime mover, and biceps femoris acting as an antagonist. **B.** Biceps femoris flexing the knee as a prime mover, and quadriceps acting as an antagonist. **C.** Muscles around shoulder girdle fixing the scapula so that movement of abduction can take place at the shoulder joint. **D.** Flexor and extensor muscles of the carpus acting as synergists and stabilizing the carpus so that long flexor and extensor tendons can flex and extend the fingers.

- **Fixator:** A fixator contracts isometrically (i.e., contraction increases the tone but does not in itself produce movement) to stabilize the origin of the prime mover so that it can act efficiently. For example, the muscles attaching the shoulder girdle to the trunk contract as fixators to allow the deltoid to act on the shoulder joint (Fig. 1-11).
- **Synergist:** In many locations in the body the prime mover muscle crosses several joints before it reaches the joint at which its main action takes place. To prevent unwanted movements in an intermediate joint, groups of muscles called synergists contract and stabilize the intermediate joints. For example, the flexor and extensor

muscles of the carpus contract to fix the wrist joint, and this allows the long flexor and extensor muscles of the fingers to work efficiently (Fig. 1-11).

These terms are applied to the action of a particular muscle during a particular movement; many muscles can act as a prime mover, an antagonist, a fixator, or a synergist, depending on the movement to be accomplished.

Muscles can even contract paradoxically, for example, when the biceps brachii, a flexor of the elbow joint, contracts and controls the rate of extension of the elbow when the triceps brachii contracts.

Nerve Supply of Skeletal Muscle

The nerve trunk to a muscle is a mixed nerve, about 60% is motor and 40% is sensory, and it also contains some sympathetic autonomic fibers. The nerve enters the muscle at about the midpoint on its deep surface, often near the margin; the place of entrance is known as the **motor point.** This arrangement allows the muscle to move with minimum interference with the nerve trunk.

Naming of Skeletal Muscles

Individual muscles are named according to their shape, size, number of heads or bellies, position, depth, attachments, or actions. Some examples of muscle names are shown in Table 1-1.

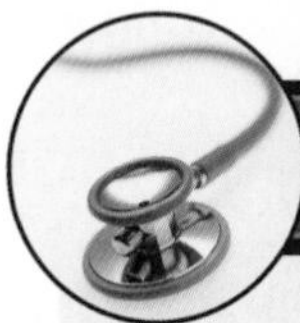

CLINICAL NOTES

Muscle Tone

Determination of the **tone** of a muscle is an important clinical examination. If a muscle is **flaccid,** then either the afferent, the efferent, or both neurons involved in the reflex arc necessary for the production of muscle tone have been interrupted. For example, if the nerve trunk to a muscle is severed, both neurons will have been interrupted. If poliomyelitis has involved the motor anterior horn cells at a level in the spinal cord that innervates the muscle, the efferent motor neurons will not function. If, conversely, the muscle is found to be hypertonic, the possibility exists of a lesion involving higher motor neurons in the spinal cord or brain.

Muscle Attachments

The importance of knowing the main attachments of all the major muscles of the body need not be emphasized. Only with such knowledge is it possible to understand the normal and abnormal actions of individual muscles or muscle groups. How can one even attempt to analyze, for example, the abnormal gait of a patient without this information?

Muscle Shape and Form

The general shape and form of muscles should also be noted, since a paralyzed muscle or one that is not used (such as occurs when a limb is immobilized in a cast) quickly atrophies and changes shape. In the case of the limbs, it is always worth remembering that a muscle on the opposite side of the body can be used for comparison.

Smooth Muscle

Smooth muscle consists of long, spindle-shaped cells closely arranged in bundles or sheets. In the tubes of the body it provides the motive power for propelling the contents through the lumen. In the digestive system it also causes the ingested food to be thoroughly mixed with the digestive juices. A wave of contraction of the circularly arranged fibers passes along the tube, milking the contents onward. By their contraction, the longitudinal fibers pull the wall of the tube proximally over the contents. This method of propulsion is referred to as **peristalsis.**

In storage organs such as the urinary bladder and the uterus, the fibers are irregularly arranged and interlaced with one another. Their contraction is slow and sustained and brings about expulsion of the contents of the organs. In the walls of the blood vessels the smooth muscle fibers are arranged circularly and serve to modify the caliber of the lumen.

Depending on the organ, smooth muscle fibers may be made to contract by local stretching of the fibers, by nerve impulses from autonomic nerves, or by hormonal stimulation.

Cardiac Muscle

Cardiac muscle consists of striated muscle fibers that branch and unite with each other. It forms the myocardium of the heart. Its fibers tend to be arranged in whorls and spirals, and they have the property of spontaneous and rhythmic contraction. Specialized cardiac muscle fibers form the **conducting system of the heart.**

Cardiac muscle is supplied by autonomic nerve fibers that terminate in the nodes of the conducting system and in the myocardium.

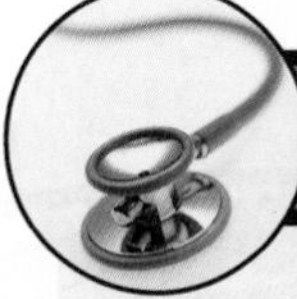

CLINICAL NOTES

Necrosis of Cardiac Muscle

The cardiac muscle receives its blood supply from the coronary arteries. A sudden block of one of the large branches of a coronary artery will inevitably lead to necrosis of the cardiac muscle and often to the death of the patient.

Joints

A site where two or more bones come together, whether or not movement occurs between them, is called a **joint.** Joints are classified according to the tissues that lie between the bones: fibrous joints, cartilaginous joints, and synovial joints.

Fibrous Joints

The articulating surfaces of the bones are joined by fibrous tissue (Fig. 1-12), and thus very little movement is possible. The sutures of the vault of the skull and the inferior tibiofibular joints are examples of fibrous joints.

Table 1-1 Naming of Skeletal Muscles[a]

Name	Shape	Size	Number of Heads or Bellies	Position	Depth	Attachments	Actions
Deltoid	Triangular						
Teres	Round						
Rectus	Straight						
Major		Large					
Latissimus		Broadest					
Longissimus		Longest					
Biceps			Two heads				
Quadriceps			Four heads				
Digastric			Two bellies				
Pectoralis				Of the chest			
Supraspinatus				Above spine of scapula			
Brachii				Of the arm			
Profundus					Deep		
Superficialis					Superficial		
Externus					External		
Sternocleidomastoid						From sternum and clavicle to mastoid process	
Coracobrachialis						From coracoid process to arm	
Extensor							Extend
Flexor							Flex
Constrictor							Constrict

[a] These names are commonly used in combination, for example, flexor pollicis longus (long flexor of the thumb).

Cartilaginous Joints

Cartilaginous joints can be divided into two types: primary and secondary. A **primary cartilaginous joint** is one in which the bones are united by a plate or bar of hyaline cartilage. Thus, the union between the **epiphysis** and the **diaphysis** of a growing bone and that between the first rib and the manubrium sterni are examples of such a joint. No movement is possible.

A **secondary cartilaginous joint** is one in which the bones are united by a plate of fibrocartilage and the articular surfaces of the bones are covered by a thin layer of hyaline cartilage. Examples are the joints between the vertebral bodies (Fig. 1-12) and the **symphysis pubis.** A small amount of movement is possible.

Synovial Joints

The articular surfaces of the bones are covered by a thin layer of hyaline cartilage separated by a joint cavity (Fig. 1-12). This arrangement permits a great degree of freedom of movement. The cavity of the joint is lined by **synovial membrane,** which extends from the margins of one articular surface to those of the other. The synovial membrane is protected on the outside by a tough fibrous membrane referred to as the **capsule** of the joint. The articular surfaces are lubricated by a viscous fluid called **synovial fluid,** which is produced by the synovial membrane. In certain synovial joints, for example, in the knee joint, discs or wedges of fibrocartilage are interposed between the articular surfaces of the bones. These are referred to as **articular discs.**

Fatty pads are found in some synovial joints lying between the synovial membrane and the fibrous capsule or bone. Examples are found in the hip (Fig. 1-12) and knee joints.

The degree of movement in a synovial joint is limited by the shape of the bones participating in the joint, the coming together of adjacent anatomic structures (e.g., the thigh against the anterior abdominal wall on flexing the hip joint), and the presence of fibrous **ligaments** uniting the bones. Most ligaments lie outside the joint capsule, but in the knee some important ligaments, the **cruciate ligaments,** lie within the capsule (Fig. 1-13).

Synovial joints can be classified according to the arrangement of the articular surfaces and the types of movement that are possible.

- **Plane joints:** In plane joints, the apposed articular surfaces are flat or almost flat, and this permits the bones to slide on one another. Examples of these joints are the sternoclavicular and acromioclavicular joints (Fig. 1-14).
- **Hinge joints:** Hinge joints resemble the hinge on a door, so that flexion and extension movements are possible. Examples of these joints are the elbow, knee, and ankle joints (Fig. 1-14).

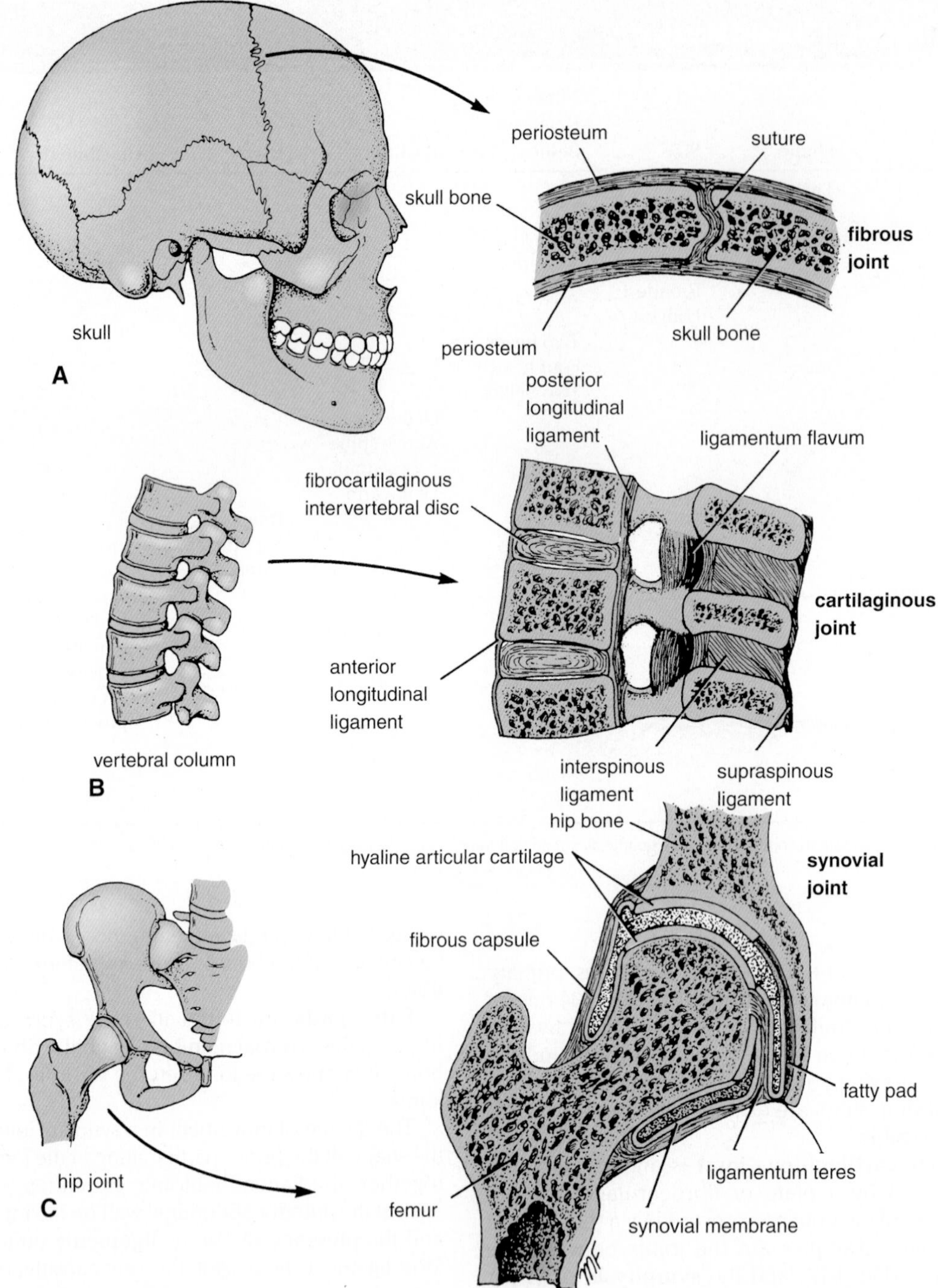

Figure 1-12 Examples of three types of joints. **A.** Fibrous joint (coronal suture of skull). **B.** Cartilaginous joint (joint between two lumbar vertebral bodies). **C.** Synovial joint (hip joint).

- **Pivot joints:** In pivot joints, a central bony pivot is surrounded by a bony–ligamentous ring (Fig. 1-14), and rotation is the only movement possible. The atlantoaxial and superior radioulnar joints are good examples.
- **Condyloid joints:** Condyloid joints have two distinct convex surfaces that articulate with two concave surfaces. The movements of flexion, extension, abduction, and adduction are possible together with a small amount of rotation. The metacarpophalangeal joints or knuckle joints are good examples (Fig. 1-14).
- **Ellipsoid joints:** In ellipsoid joints, an elliptical convex articular surface fits into an elliptical concave articular surface. The movements of flexion, extension, abduction, and adduction can take place, but rotation is impossible. The wrist joint is a good example (Fig. 1-14).

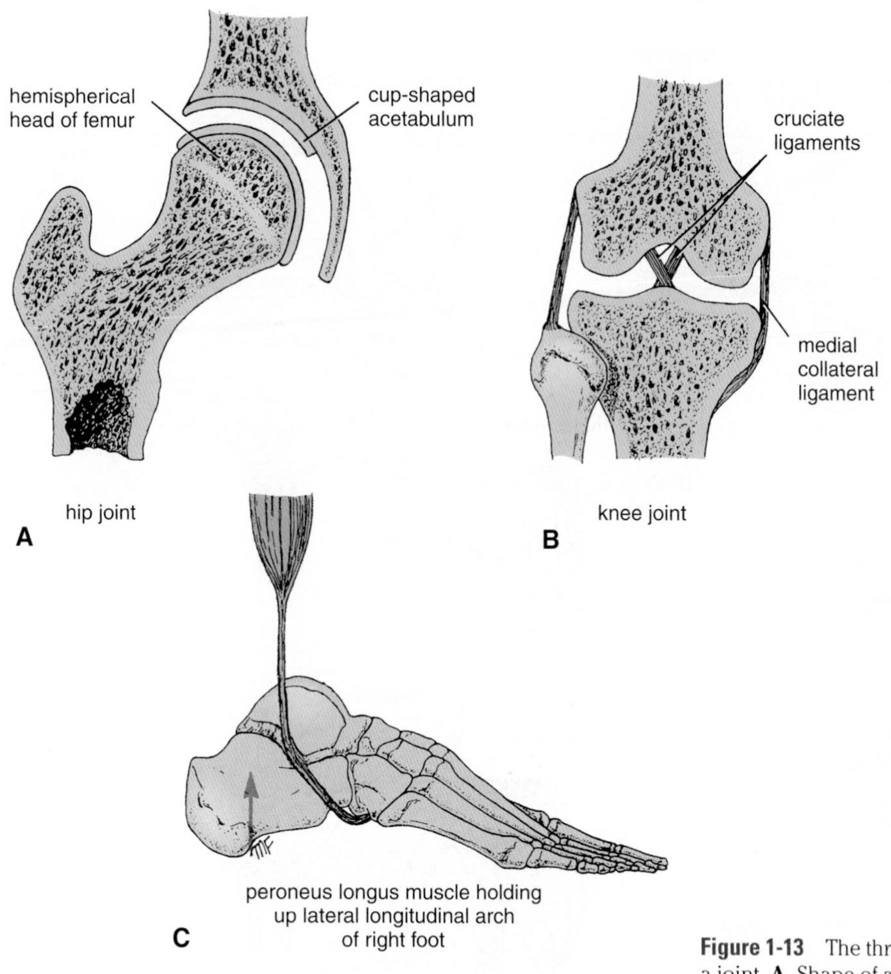

Figure 1-13 The three main factors responsible for stabilizing a joint. **A.** Shape of articular surfaces. **B.** Ligaments. **C.** Muscle tone.

- **Saddle joints:** In saddle joints, the articular surfaces are reciprocally concavoconvex and resemble a saddle on a horse's back. These joints permit flexion, extension, abduction, adduction, and rotation. The best example of this type of joint is the carpometacarpal joint of the thumb (Fig. 1-14).
- **Ball-and-socket joints:** In ball-and-socket joints, a ball-shaped head of one bone fits into a socketlike concavity of another. This arrangement permits free movements, including flexion, extension, abduction, adduction, medial rotation, lateral rotation, and circumduction. The shoulder and hip joints are good examples of this type of joint (Fig. 1-14).

Stability of Joints

The stability of a joint depends on three main factors: the shape, size, and arrangement of the articular surfaces; the ligaments; and the tone of the muscles around the joint.

Articular Surfaces

The ball-and-socket arrangement of the hip joint (Fig. 1-13) and the mortise arrangement of the ankle joint are good examples of how bone shape plays an important role in joint stability. Other examples of joints, however, in which the shape of the bones contributes little or nothing to the stability include the acromioclavicular joint, the calcaneocuboid joint, and the knee joint.

Ligaments

Fibrous ligaments prevent excessive movement in a joint (Fig. 1-13), but if the stress is continued for an excessively long period, then fibrous ligaments stretch. For example, the ligaments of the joints between the bones forming the arches of the feet will not by themselves support the weight of the body. Should the tone of the muscles that normally support the arches become impaired by fatigue, then the ligaments will stretch and the arches will collapse, producing flat feet.

Elastic ligaments, conversely, return to their original length after stretching. The elastic ligaments of the auditory ossicles play an active part in supporting the joints and assisting in the return of the bones to their original position after movement.

Muscle Tone

In most joints, muscle tone is the major factor controlling stability. For example, the muscle tone of the short muscles around the shoulder joint keeps the hemispherical head of the humerus in the shallow glenoid cavity of the scapula. Without the action of these muscles, very little force would

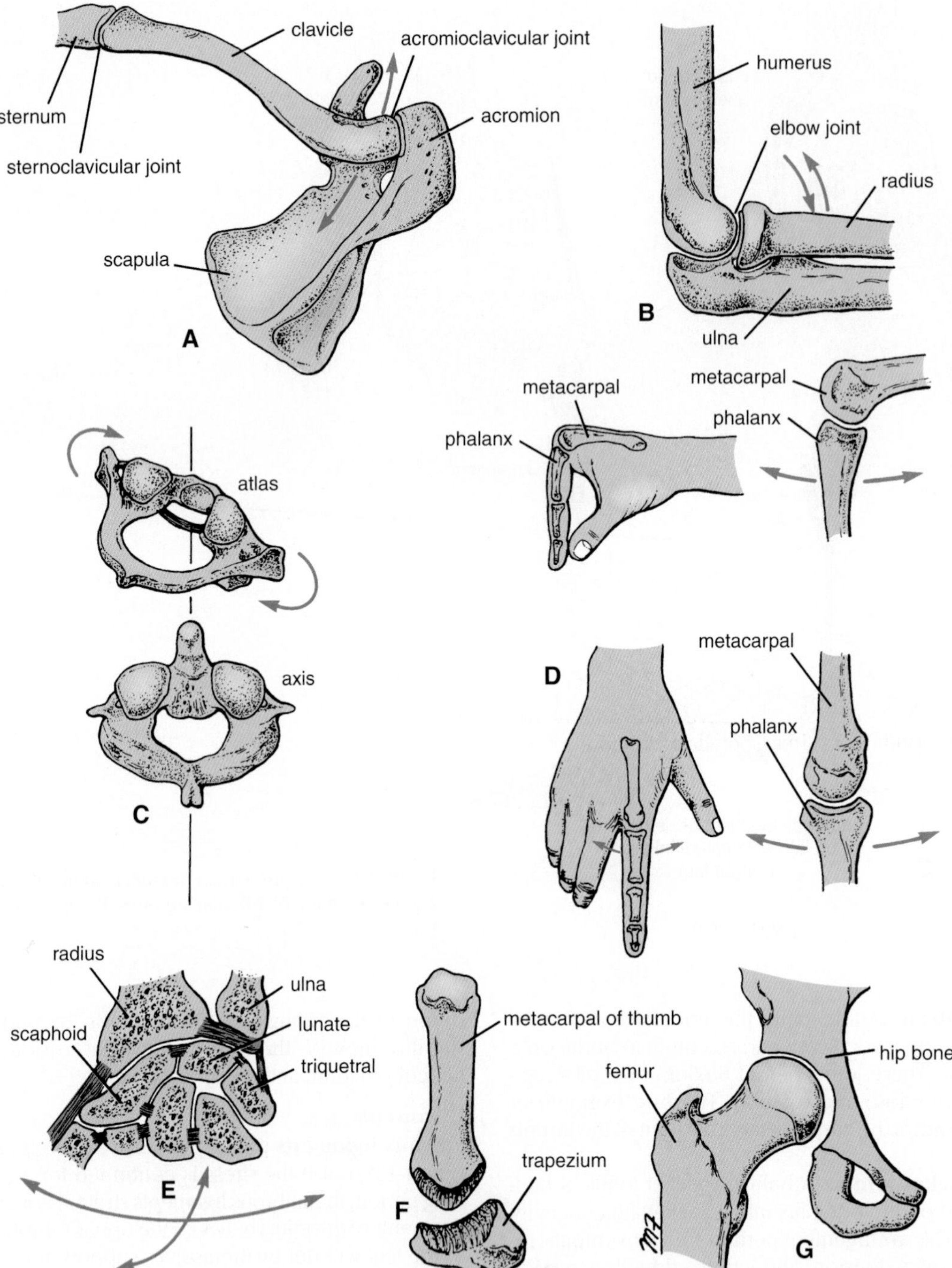

Figure 1-14 Examples of different types of synovial joints. **A.** Plane joints (sternoclavicular and acromioclavicular joints). **B.** Hinge joint (elbow joint). **C.** Pivot joint (atlantoaxial joint). **D.** Condyloid joint (metacarpophalangeal joint). **E.** Ellipsoid joint (wrist joint). **F.** Saddle joint (carpometacarpal joint of the thumb). **G.** Ball-and-socket joint (hip joint).

be required to dislocate this joint. The knee joint is very unstable without the tonic activity of the quadriceps femoris muscle. The joints between the small bones forming the arches of the feet are largely supported by the tone of the muscles of the leg, whose tendons are inserted into the bones of the feet (Fig. 1-13).

Nerve Supply of Joints

The capsule and ligaments receive an abundant sensory nerve supply. A sensory nerve supplying a joint also supplies the muscles moving the joint and the skin overlying the insertions of these muscles, a fact that has been codified as **Hilton's law.**

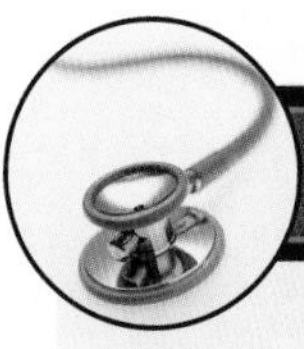

CLINICAL NOTES

Examination of Joints

When examining a patient, the clinician should assess the normal range of movement of all joints. When the bones of a joint are no longer in their normal anatomic relationship with one another, then the joint is said to be **dislocated.** Some joints are particularly susceptible to dislocation because of lack of support by ligaments, the poor shape of the articular surfaces, or the absence of adequate muscular support. The shoulder joint, temporomandibular joint, and acromioclavicular joints are good examples. Dislocation of the hip is usually congenital, being caused by inadequate development of the socket that normally holds the head of the femur firmly in position.

The presence of cartilaginous discs within joints, especially weightbearing joints, as in the case of the knee, makes them particularly susceptible to injury in sports. During a rapid movement the disc loses its normal relationship to the bones and becomes crushed between the weightbearing surfaces.

In certain diseases of the nervous system (e.g., **syringomyelia**), the sensation of pain in a joint is lost. This means that the warning sensations of pain felt when a joint moves beyond the normal range of movement are not experienced. This phenomenon results in the destruction of the joint.

Knowledge of the classification of joints is of great value because, for example, certain diseases affect only certain types of joints. **Gonococcal arthritis** affects large synovial joints such as the ankle, elbow, or wrist, whereas **tuberculous arthritis** also affects synovial joints and may start in the synovial membrane or in the bone.

Remember that more than one joint may receive the same nerve supply. For example, the hip and knee joints are both supplied by the obturator nerve. Thus, a patient with disease limited to one of these joints may experience pain in both.

Ligaments

A ligament is a cord or band of connective tissue uniting two structures. Commonly found in association with joints, ligaments are of two types. Most are composed of dense bundles of collagen fibers and are unstretchable under normal conditions (e.g., the iliofemoral ligament of the hip joint and the collateral ligaments of the elbow joint). The second type is composed largely of elastic tissue and can therefore regain its original length after stretching (e.g., the ligamentum flavum of the vertebral column and the calcaneonavicular ligament of the foot).

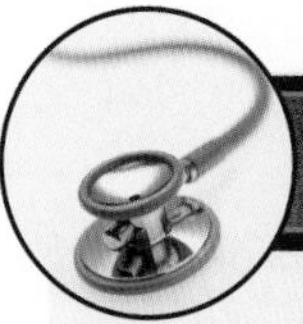

CLINICAL NOTES

Damage to Ligaments

Joint ligaments are very prone to excessive stretching and even tearing and rupture. If possible, the apposing damaged surfaces of the ligament are brought together by positioning and immobilizing the joint. In severe injuries, surgical approximation of the cut ends may be required. The blood clot at the damaged site is invaded by blood vessels and fibroblasts. The fibroblasts lay down new collagen and elastic fibers, which become oriented along the lines of mechanical stress.

Bursae

A bursa is a lubricating device consisting of a closed fibrous sac lined with a delicate smooth membrane. Its walls are separated by a film of viscous fluid. Bursae are found wherever tendons rub against bones, ligaments, or other tendons. They are commonly found close to joints where the skin rubs against underlying bony structures, for example, the prepatellar bursa (Fig. 1-15). Occasionally, the cavity of a bursa communicates with the cavity of a synovial joint. For example, the suprapatellar bursa communicates with the knee joint (Fig. 1-15) and the subscapularis bursa communicates with the shoulder joint.

Synovial Sheath

A synovial sheath is a tubular bursa that surrounds a tendon. The tendon invaginates the bursa from one side so that the tendon becomes suspended within the bursa by a **mesotendon** (Fig. 1-15). The mesotendon enables blood vessels to enter the tendon along its course. In certain situations, when the range of movement is extensive, the mesotendon disappears or remains in the form of narrow threads, the **vincula** (e.g., the long flexor tendons of the fingers and toes).

Synovial sheaths occur where tendons pass under ligaments and retinacula and through osseofibrous tunnels. Their function is to reduce friction between the tendon and its surrounding structures.

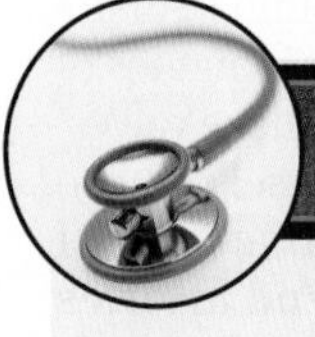

CLINICAL NOTES

Trauma and Infection of Bursae and Synovial Sheaths

Bursae and synovial sheaths are commonly the site of traumatic or infectious disease. For example, the extensor tendon sheaths of the hand may become inflamed after excessive or unaccustomed use; an inflammation of the prepatellar bursa may occur as the result of trauma from repeated kneeling on a hard surface.

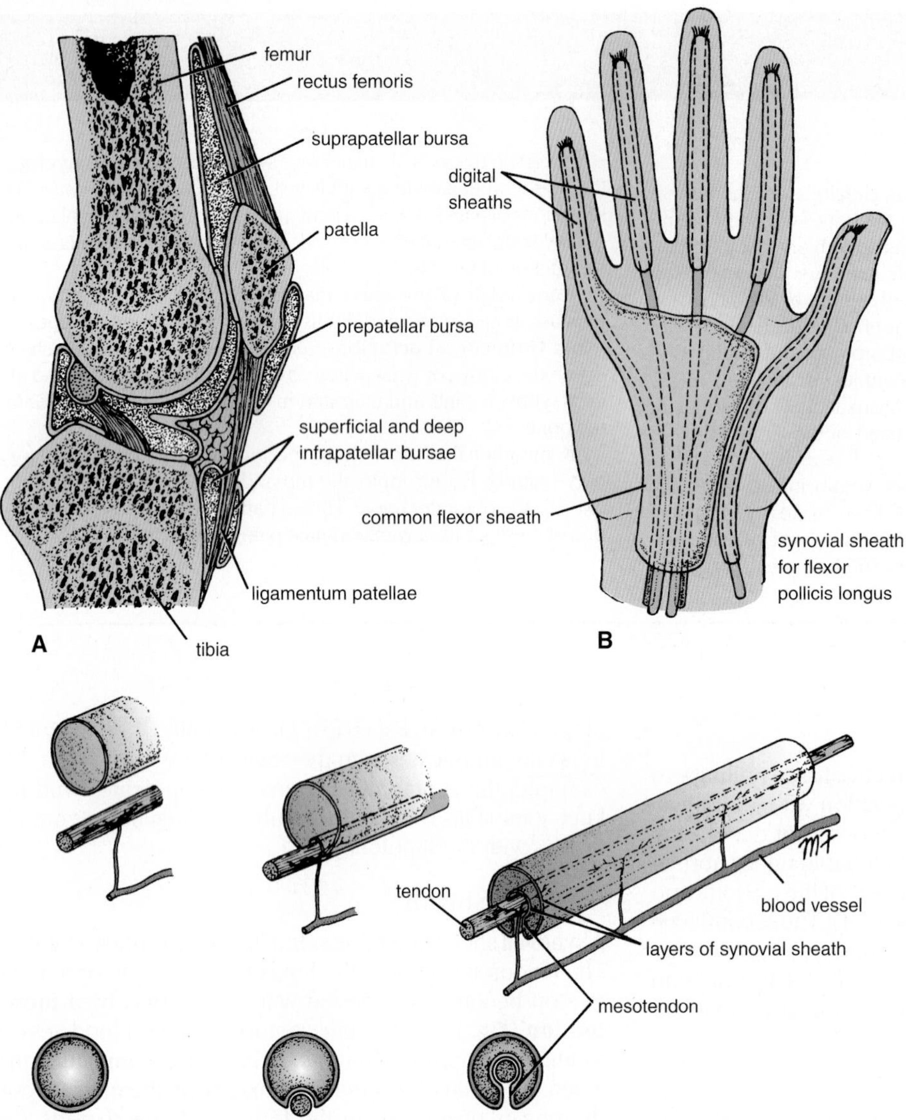

Figure 1-15 **A.** Four bursae related to the front of the knee joint. Note that the suprapatellar bursa communicates with the cavity of the joint. **B.** Synovial sheaths around the long tendons of the fingers. **C.** How tendon indents synovial sheath during development, and how blood vessels reach the tendon through the mesotendon.

Blood Vessels

Blood vessels are of three types: arteries, veins, and capillaries (Fig. 1-16).

Arteries transport blood from the heart and distribute it to the various tissues of the body by means of their **branches** (Figs. 1-16 and 1-17). The smallest arteries, <0.1 mm in diameter, are referred to as **arterioles.** The joining of branches of arteries is called an **anastomosis.** Arteries do not have valves.

Anatomic end arteries (Fig. 1-17) are vessels whose terminal branches do not anastomose with branches of arteries supplying adjacent areas. **Functional end arteries** are vessels whose terminal branches do anastomose with those of adjacent arteries, but the caliber of the anastomosis is insufficient to keep the tissue alive should one of the arteries become blocked.

Veins are vessels that transport blood back to the heart; many of them possess valves. The smallest veins are called **venules** (Fig. 1-17). The smaller veins, or **tributaries,** unite to form larger veins, which commonly join with one another to form **venous plexuses.** Medium-size deep arteries are often accompanied by two veins, one on each side, called **venae comitantes.**

Veins leaving the gastrointestinal tract do not go directly to the heart but converge on the **portal vein;** this vein enters the liver and breaks up again into veins of diminishing size, which ultimately join capillary-like vessels, termed **sinusoids,** in the liver (Fig. 1-17). A **portal system** is thus a system of vessels interposed between two capillary beds.

Capillaries are microscopic vessels in the form of a network connecting the arterioles to the venules (Fig. 1-17).

Sinusoids resemble capillaries in that they are thin-walled blood vessels, but they have an irregular cross diameter and are wider than capillaries. They are found in the bone marrow, the spleen, the liver, and some endocrine glands. In some areas of the body, principally the tips of the fingers and toes, direct connections occur between the arteries and veins without the intervention of capillaries. The sites of such connections are referred to as **arteriovenous anastomoses** (Fig. 1-17).

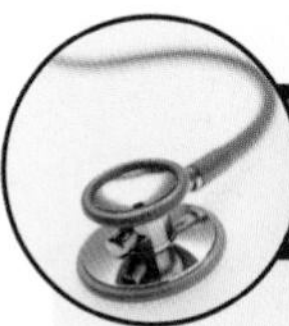

CLINICAL NOTES

Diseases of Blood Vessels

Diseases of blood vessels are common. The surface anatomy of the main arteries, especially those of the limbs, is discussed in the appropriate sections of this book. The **collateral circulation** of most large arteries should be understood, and a distinction should be made between anatomic end arteries and functional end arteries.

All large arteries that cross over a joint are liable to be kinked during movements of the joint. However, the distal flow of blood is not interrupted because an adequate anastomosis is usually between branches of the artery that arise both proximal and distal to the joint. The alternative blood channels, which dilate under these circumstances, form the collateral circulation. Knowledge of the existence and position of such a circulation may be of vital importance should it be necessary to tie off a large artery that has been damaged by trauma or disease.

Coronary arteries are functional end arteries, and if they become blocked by disease (coronary arterial occlusion is common), the cardiac muscle normally supplied by that artery will receive insufficient blood and undergo necrosis. Blockage of a large coronary artery results in the death of the patient. (See the clinical example at the beginning of this chapter.)

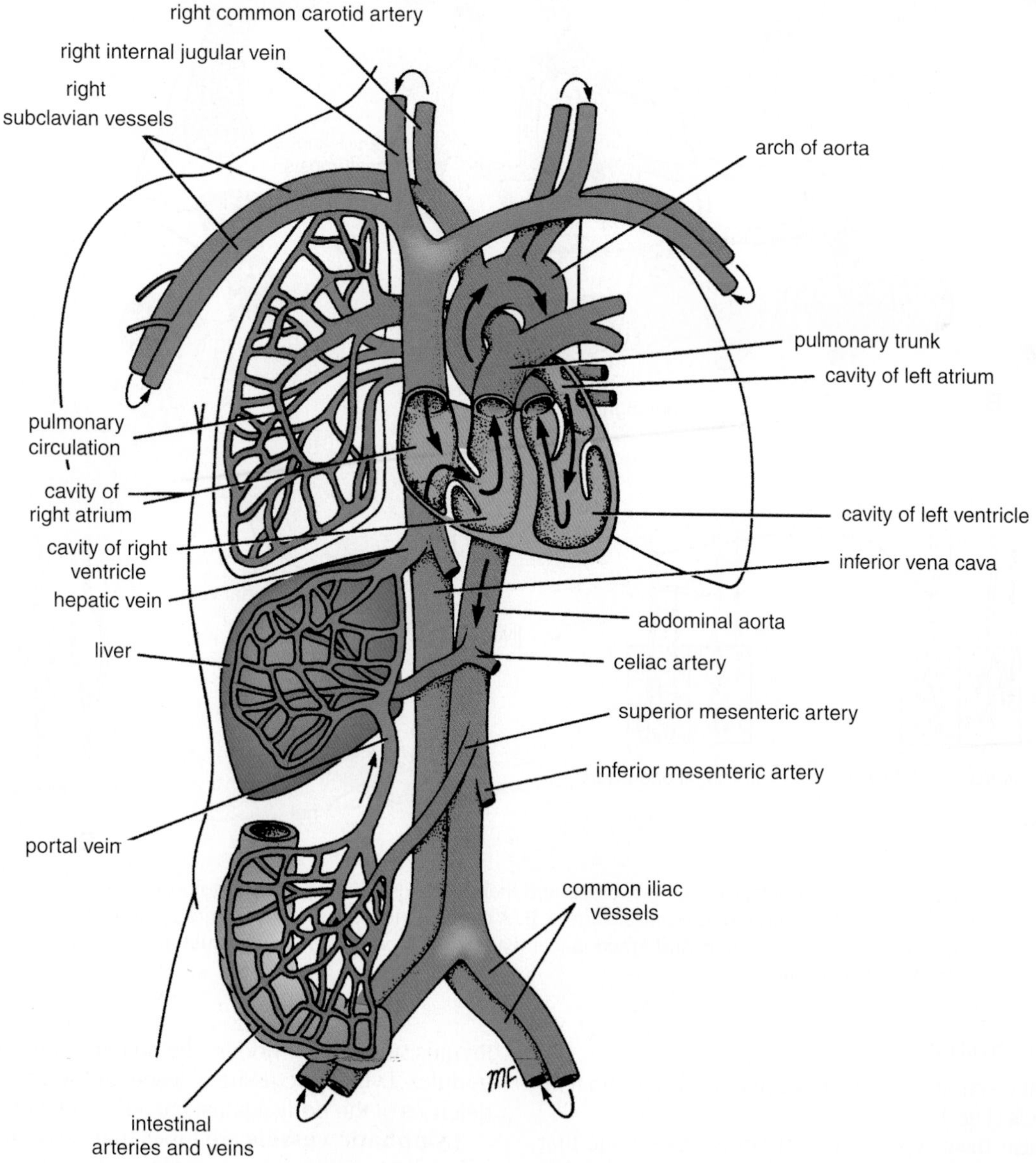

Figure 1-16 General plan of the blood vascular system.

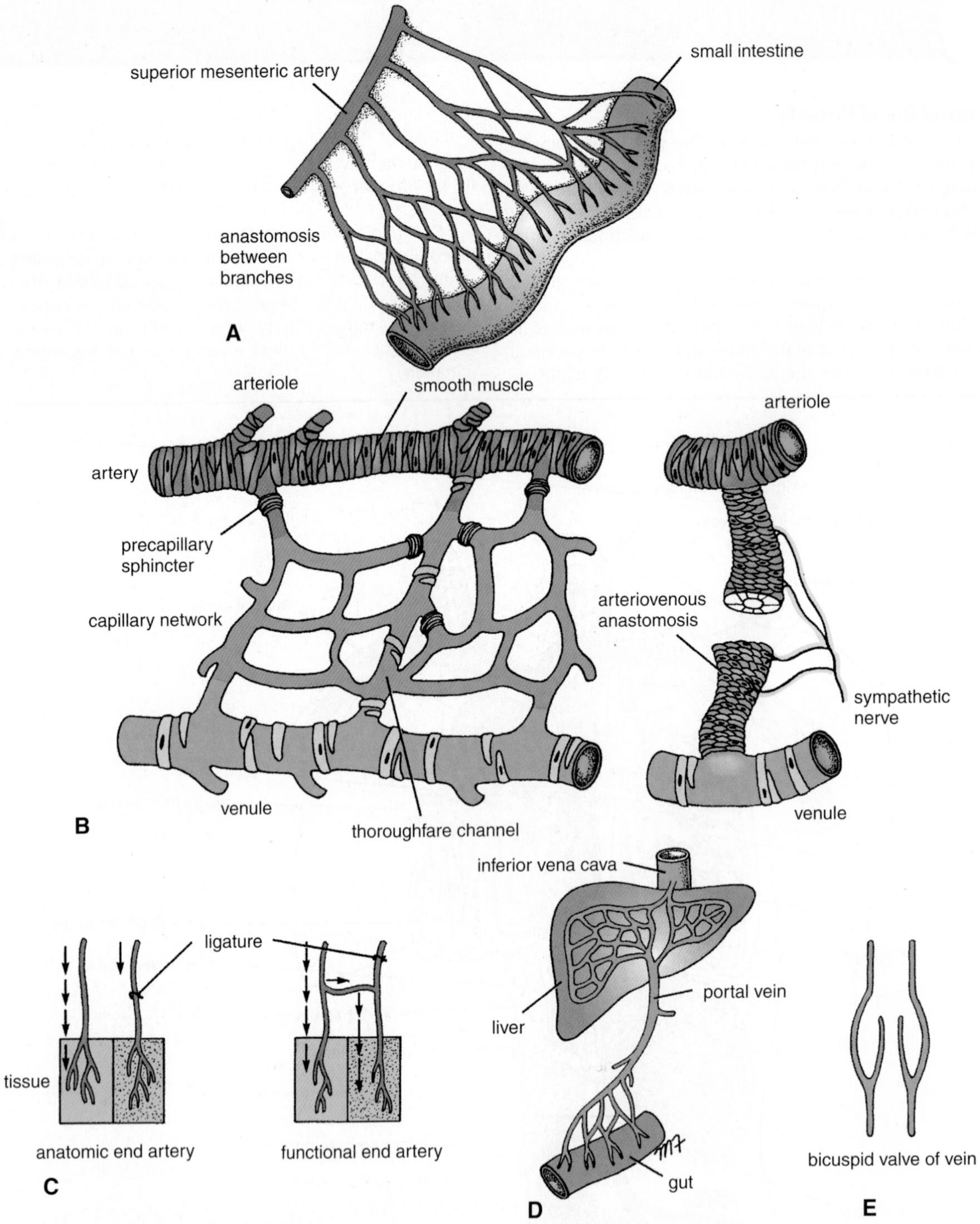

Figure 1-17 Different types of blood vessels and their methods of union. **A.** Anastomosis between the branches of the superior mesenteric artery. **B.** A capillary network and an arteriovenous anastomosis. **C.** Anatomic end artery and functional end artery. **D.** A portal system. **E.** Structure of the bicuspid valve in a vein.

Lymphatic System

The lymphatic system consists of lymphatic tissues and lymphatic vessels (Fig. 1-18).

Lymphatic tissues are a type of connective tissue that contains large numbers of lymphocytes. Lymphatic tissue is organized into the following organs or structures: the thymus, the lymph nodes, the spleen, and the lymphatic nodules. Lymphatic tissue is essential for the immunologic defenses of the body against bacteria and viruses.

Lymphatic vessels are tubes that assist the cardiovascular system in the removal of tissue fluid from the tissue spaces of the body; the vessels then return the fluid to the blood. The lymphatic system is essentially a drainage system, and there is no circulation. Lymphatic vessels are found in all tissues and organs of the body except the central nervous system, the eyeball, the internal ear, the epidermis of the skin, the cartilage, and the bone.

Lymph is the name given to tissue fluid once it has entered a lymphatic vessel. **Lymph capillaries** are a network of fine vessels that drain lymph from the tissues. The capillaries are in turn drained by small lymph vessels, which unite to form large lymph vessels. Lymph vessels have a beaded appearance because of the presence of numerous valves along their course.

Before lymph is returned to the bloodstream, it passes through at least one **lymph node** and often through several. The lymph vessels that carry lymph to a lymph node are referred to as **afferent** vessels (Fig. 1-18); those that transport it away from a node are **efferent** vessels. The lymph reaches the bloodstream at the root of the neck by large lymph vessels called the **right lymphatic duct** and the **thoracic duct** (Fig. 1-18).

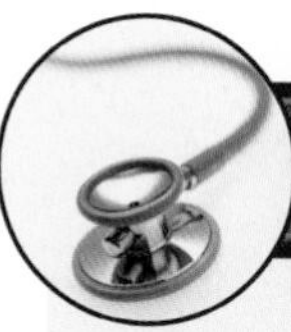

CLINICAL NOTES

Disease of the Lymphatic System

The lymphatic system is often deemphasized by anatomists on the grounds that it is difficult to see on a cadaver. However, it is of vital importance to medical personnel, since lymph nodes may swell as the result of metastases, or primary tumor. For this reason, the lymphatic drainage of all major organs of the body, including the skin, should be known.

A patient may complain of a swelling produced by the enlargement of a lymph node. A physician must know the areas of the body that drain lymph to a particular node if he or she is to be able to find the primary site of the disease. Often the patient ignores the primary disease, which may be a small, painless cancer of the skin.

Conversely, the patient may complain of a painful ulcer of the tongue, for example, and the physician must know the lymph drainage of the tongue to be able to determine whether the disease has spread beyond the limits of the tongue.

Nervous System

The nervous system is divided into two main parts: the **central nervous system,** which consists of the brain and spinal cord, and the **peripheral nervous system,** which consists of 12 pairs of cranial nerves and 31 pairs of spinal nerves and their associated ganglia.

Functionally, the nervous system can be further divided into the **somatic nervous system,** which controls voluntary activities, and the **autonomic nervous system,** which controls involuntary activities.

The nervous system, together with the endocrine system, controls and integrates the activities of the different parts of the body.

Central Nervous System

The central nervous system is composed of large numbers of nerve cells and their processes, supported by specialized tissue called **neuroglia. Neuron** is the term given to the nerve cell and all its processes. The nerve cell has two types of processes, called **dendrites** and an **axon.** Dendrites are the short processes of the cell body; the axon is the longest process of the cell body (Fig. 1-19).

The interior of the central nervous system is organized into gray and white matter. **Gray matter** consists of nerve cells embedded in neuroglia. **White matter** consists of nerve fibers (axons) embedded in neuroglia.

Peripheral Nervous System

The peripheral nervous system consists of the cranial and spinal nerves and their associated ganglia. On dissection, the cranial and spinal nerves are seen as grayish white cords. They are made up of bundles of nerve fibers (axons) supported by delicate areolar tissue.

Cranial Nerves

There are 12 pairs of cranial nerves that leave the brain and pass through foramina in the skull. All the nerves are distributed in the head and neck except the Xth (vagus), which also supplies structures in the thorax and abdomen. The cranial nerves are described in Chapter 11.

Spinal Nerves

A total of 31 pairs of spinal nerves leave the spinal cord and pass through intervertebral foramina in the vertebral column (Figs. 1-20 and 1-21). The spinal nerves are named according to the region of the vertebral column with which they are associated: 8 **cervical,** 12 **thoracic,** 5 **lumbar,** 5 **sacral,** and 1 **coccygeal.** Note that there are eight cervical nerves and only seven cervical vertebrae and that there is one coccygeal nerve and four coccygeal vertebrae.

During development, the spinal cord grows in length more slowly than the vertebral column. In the adult, when growth ceases, the lower end of the spinal cord reaches inferiorly only as far as the lower border of the first lumbar vertebra. To accommodate for this disproportionate growth in length, the length of the roots increases progressively from above downward. In the upper cervical region, the spinal nerve roots are short and run almost horizontally, but the roots of the lumbar and sacral nerves below the level of the termination of the cord form a vertical bundle of nerves that resembles a horse's tail and is called the **cauda equina** (Fig. 1-20).

Each spinal nerve is connected to the spinal cord by two roots: the **anterior root** and the **posterior root** (Figs. 1-19 and 1-21). The anterior root consists of bundles of nerve fibers carrying nerve impulses away from the central nervous system (Fig. 1-21). Such nerve fibers are called **efferent** fibers. Those efferent fibers that go to skeletal muscle and cause them to contract are called **motor fibers.** Their cells of origin lie in the anterior gray horn of the spinal cord.

The posterior root consists of bundles of nerve fibers that carry impulses to the central nervous system and are called **afferent** fibers (Fig. 1-19). Because these fibers are concerned with conveying information about sensations of

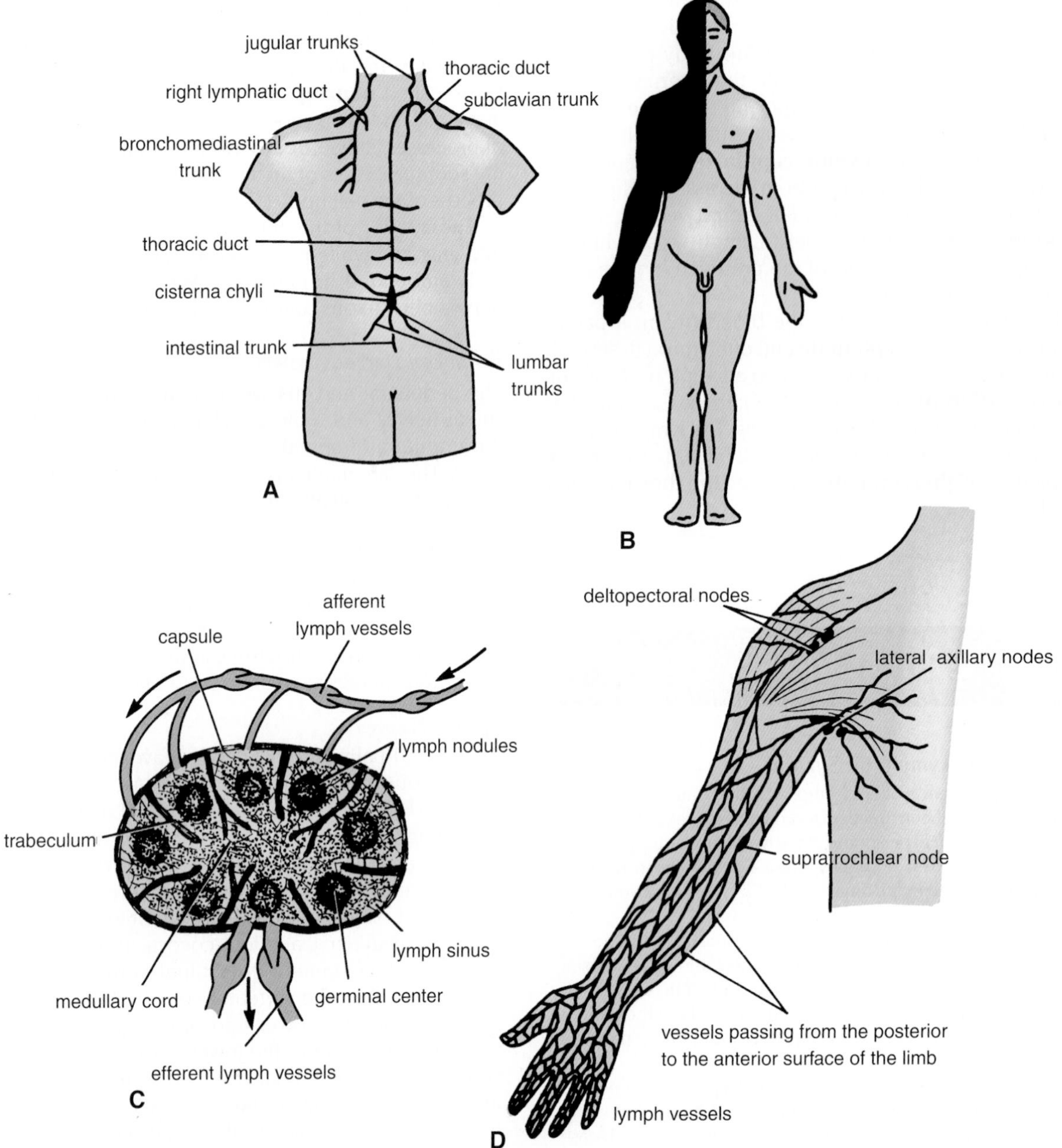

Figure 1-18 **A.** The thoracic duct and right lymphatic duct and their main tributaries. **B.** The areas of body drained into thoracic duct (*clear*) and right lymphatic duct (*black*). **C.** General structure of a lymph node. **D.** Lymph vessels and nodes of the upper limb.

touch, pain, temperature, and vibrations, they are called **sensory fibers.** The cell bodies of these nerve fibers are situated in a swelling on the posterior root called the **posterior root ganglion** (Figs. 1-19 and 1-21).

At each intervertebral foramen, the anterior and posterior roots unite to form a spinal nerve (Fig. 1-21). Here, the motor and sensory fibers become mixed together, so that a spinal nerve is made up of a mixture of motor and sensory fibers (Fig. 1-19). On emerging from the foramen, the spinal nerve divides into a large **anterior ramus** and a smaller **posterior ramus.** The posterior ramus passes posteriorly around the vertebral column to supply the muscles and skin of the back (Figs. 1-19 and 1-21). The anterior ramus continues anteriorly to supply the muscles and skin over the anterolateral body wall and all the muscles and skin of the limbs.

In addition to the anterior and posterior rami, spinal nerves give a small **meningeal branch** that supplies the vertebrae and the coverings of the spinal cord (the meninges). Thoracic spinal nerves also have branches, called **rami communicantes,** that are associated with the sympathetic part of the autonomic nervous system (see below).

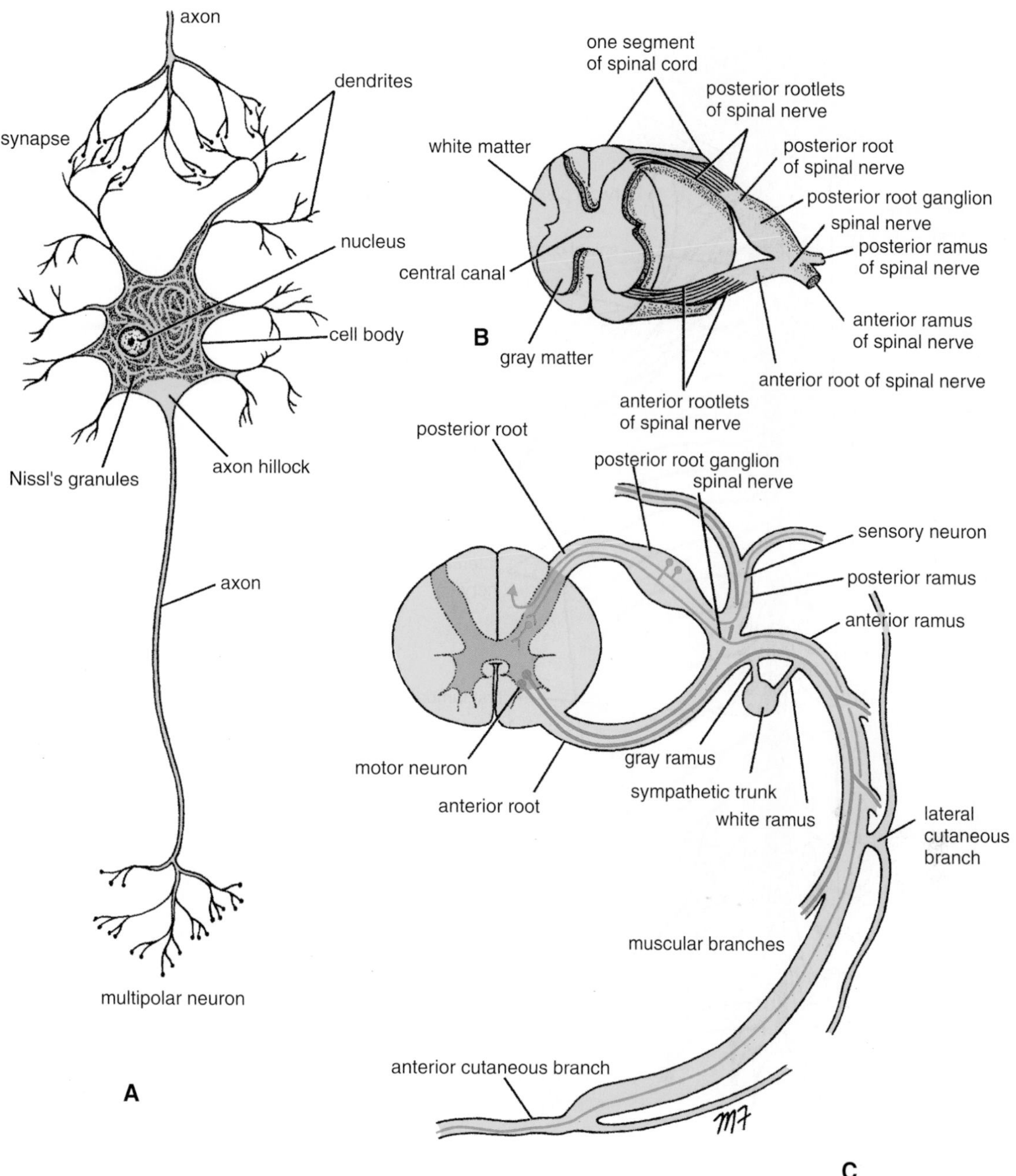

Figure 1-19 **A.** Multipolar motor neuron with connector neuron synapsing with it. **B.** Section through thoracic segment of spinal cord with spinal roots and posterior root ganglion. **C.** Cross section of thoracic segment of spinal cord showing roots, spinal nerve, and anterior and posterior rami and their branches.

Plexuses

At the root of the limbs, the anterior rami join one another to form complicated nerve plexuses (Fig. 1-20). The **cervical** and **brachial plexuses** are found at the root of the upper limbs, and the **lumbar** and **sacral plexuses** are found at the root of the lower limbs.

The classic division of the nervous system into central and peripheral parts is purely artificial and one of descriptive convenience because the processes of the neurons pass freely between the two. For example, a motor neuron located in the anterior gray horn of the first thoracic segment of the spinal cord gives rise to an axon that passes through the anterior root of the first thoracic nerve (Fig. 1-22), passes through the brachial plexus, travels down the arm and forearm in the ulnar nerve, and finally reaches the motor end plates on several muscle fibers of a small muscle of the hand—a total distance of about 3 ft (90 cm).

To take another example: Consider the sensation of touch felt on the lateral side of the little toe. This area of skin

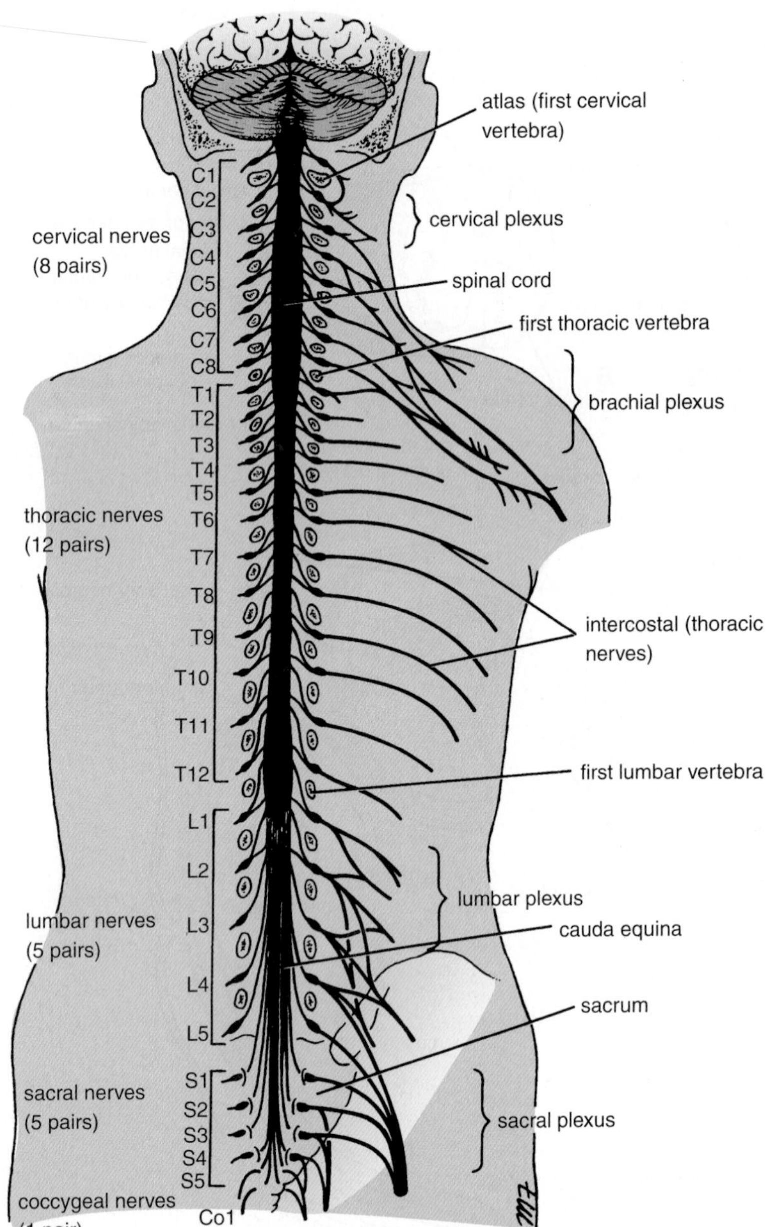

Figure 1-20 Brain, spinal cord, spinal nerves, and plexuses of limbs.

is supplied by the first sacral segment of the spinal cord (S1). The fine terminal branches of the sensory axon, called **dendrites,** leave the sensory organs of the skin and unite to form the axon of the sensory nerve. The axon passes up the leg in the sural nerve (Fig. 1-22) and then in the tibial and sciatic nerves to the lumbosacral plexus. It then passes through the posterior root of the first sacral nerve to reach the cell body in the posterior root ganglion of the first sacral nerve. The central axon now enters the posterior white column of the spinal cord and passes up to the nucleus gracilis in the medulla oblongata—a total distance of about 5 ft (1.5 m). Thus, a single neuron extends from the little toe to the inside of the skull.

Both these examples illustrate the great length of a single neuron.

Autonomic Nervous System

The autonomic nervous system is the part of the nervous system concerned with the innervation of involuntary structures such as the heart, smooth muscle, and glands throughout the body and is distributed throughout the central and peripheral nervous system. The autonomic system may be divided into two parts—the **sympathetic** and the **parasympathetic**—and both parts have afferent and efferent nerve fibers.

The activities of the sympathetic part of the autonomic system prepare the body for an emergency. It accelerates the heart rate, causes constriction of the peripheral blood vessels, and raises the blood pressure. The sympathetic part of the autonomic system brings about a redistribution of the blood so that it leaves the areas of the skin and intestine and becomes available to the brain, heart, and skeletal muscle.

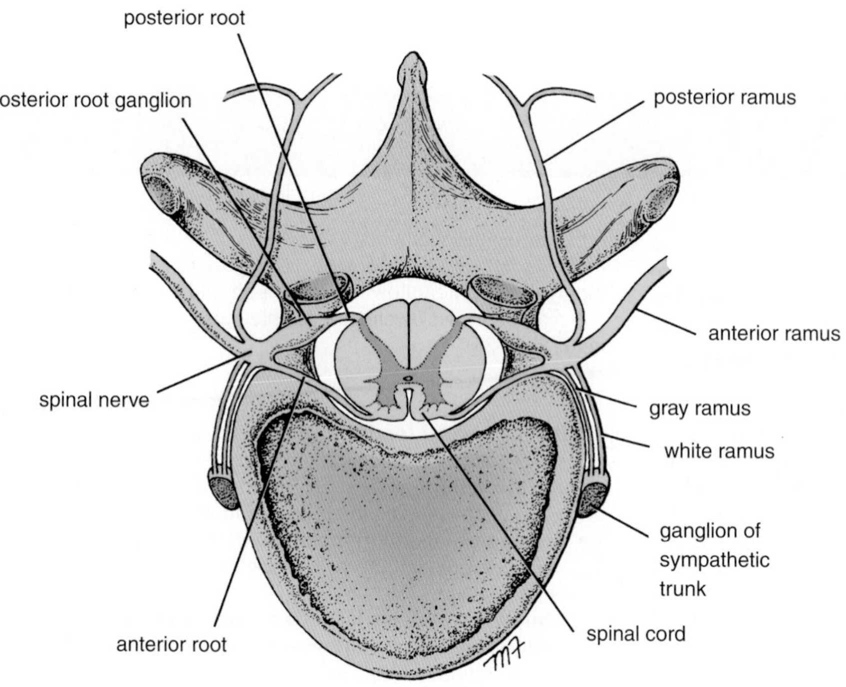

Figure 1-21 The association between spinal cord, spinal nerves, and sympathetic trunks.

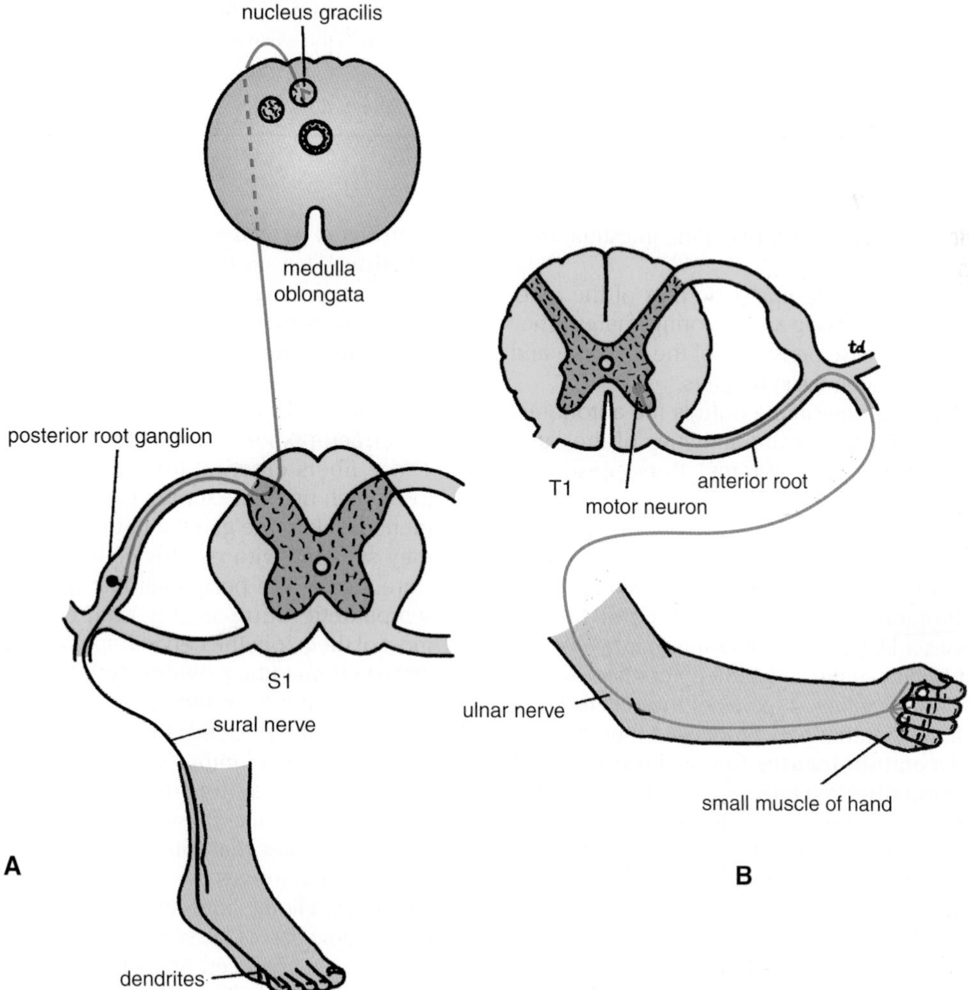

Figure 1-22 Two neurons that pass from the central to the peripheral nervous system. **A.** Afferent neuron that extends from the little toe to the brain. **B.** Efferent neuron that extends from the anterior gray horn of the first thoracic segment of spinal cord to the small muscle of the hand.

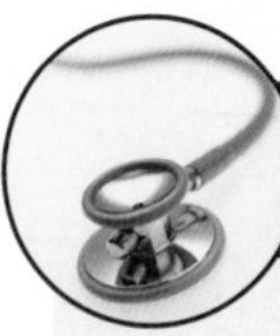

CLINICAL NOTES

Segmental Innervation of the Skin

The area of skin supplied by a single spinal nerve, and therefore a single segment of the spinal cord, is called a **dermatome.** On the trunk, adjacent dermatomes overlap considerably; to produce a region of complete anesthesia, at least three contiguous spinal nerves must be sectioned. Dermatomal charts for the anterior and posterior surfaces of the body are shown in Figures 1-23 and 1-24.

In the limbs, arrangement of the dermatomes is more complicated because of the embryologic changes that take place as the limbs grow out from the body wall.

A physician should have a working knowledge of the segmental (dermatomal) innervation of skin, because with the help of a pin or a piece of cotton he or she can determine whether the sensory function of a particular spinal nerve or segment of the spinal cord is functioning normally.

Segmental Innervation of Muscle

Skeletal muscle also receives a segmental innervation. Most of these muscles are innervated by two, three, or four spinal nerves and therefore by the same number of segments of the spinal cord. To paralyze a muscle completely, it is thus necessary to section several spinal nerves or to destroy several segments of the spinal cord.

Learning the segmental innervation of all the muscles of the body is an impossible task. Nevertheless, the segmental innervation of the following muscles should be known because they can be tested by eliciting simple muscle reflexes in the patient (Fig. 1-25):

- **Biceps brachii tendon reflex:** C5 and **6** (flexion of the elbow joint by tapping the biceps tendon)
- **Triceps tendon reflex:** C6, **7**, and **8** (extension of the elbow joint by tapping the triceps tendon)
- **Brachioradialis tendon reflex:** C5, **6**, and 7 (supination of the radioulnar joints by tapping the insertion of the brachioradialis tendon)
- **Abdominal superficial reflexes (contraction of underlying abdominal muscles by stroking the skin):** Upper abdominal skin T6 to 7, middle abdominal skin T8 to 9, and lower abdominal skin T10 to 12
- **Patellar tendon reflex (knee jerk):** L2, **3**, and **4** (extension of the knee joint on tapping the patellar tendon)
- **Achilles tendon reflex (ankle jerk):** **S1** and S2 (plantar flexion of the ankle joint on tapping the Achilles tendon)

At the same time, it inhibits peristalsis of the intestinal tract and closes the sphincters.

The activities of the parasympathetic part of the autonomic system aim at conserving and restoring energy. They slow the heart rate, increase peristalsis of the intestine and glandular activity, and open the sphincters.

The hypothalamus of the brain controls the autonomic nervous system and integrates the activities of the autonomic and neuroendocrine systems, thus preserving homeostasis in the body.

Sympathetic System

Efferent Fibers The gray matter of the spinal cord, from the first thoracic segment to the second lumbar segment, possesses a lateral horn, or column, in which are located the cell bodies of the sympathetic connector neurons (Fig. 1-26). The myelinated axons of these cells leave the spinal cord in the anterior nerve roots and then pass via the **white rami communicantes** to the **paravertebral ganglia** of the **sympathetic trunk** (Figs. 1-21, 1-26, and 1-27). The connector cell fibers are called preganglionic as they pass to a peripheral ganglion. Once the preganglionic fibers reach the ganglia in the sympathetic trunk, they may pass to the following destinations:

1. They may terminate in the ganglion they have entered by synapsing with an excitor cell in the ganglion (Fig. 1-26). A **synapse** can be defined as the site where two neurons come into close proximity but not into anatomic continuity. The gap between the two neurons is bridged by a neurotransmitter substance, **acetylcholine.** The axons of the excitor neurons leave the ganglion and are nonmyelinated. These postganglionic nerve fibers now pass to the thoracic spinal nerves as **gray rami communicantes** and are distributed in the branches of the spinal nerves to supply the smooth muscle in the walls of blood vessels, the sweat glands, and the arrector pili muscles of the skin.
2. Those fibers entering the ganglia of the sympathetic trunk high up in the thorax may travel up in the sympathetic trunk to the ganglia in the cervical region, where they synapse with excitor cells (Figs. 1-26 and 1-27). Here, again, the postganglionic nerve fibers leave the sympathetic trunk as gray rami communicantes, and most of them join the cervical spinal nerves. Many of the preganglionic fibers entering the lower part of the sympathetic trunk from the lower thoracic and upper two lumbar segments of the spinal cord travel down to ganglia in the lower lumbar and sacral regions, where they synapse with excitor cells (Fig. 1-27). The postganglionic fibers leave the sympathetic trunk as gray rami communicantes that join the lumbar, sacral, and coccygeal spinal nerves.
3. The preganglionic fibers may pass through the ganglia on the thoracic part of the sympathetic trunk without synapsing. These myelinated fibers form the three **splanchnic nerves** (Fig. 1-27). The **greater splanchnic nerve** arises from the fifth to the ninth thoracic ganglia, pierces the diaphragm, and synapses with excitor cells in the ganglia of the celiac plexus. The **lesser splanchnic nerve** arises

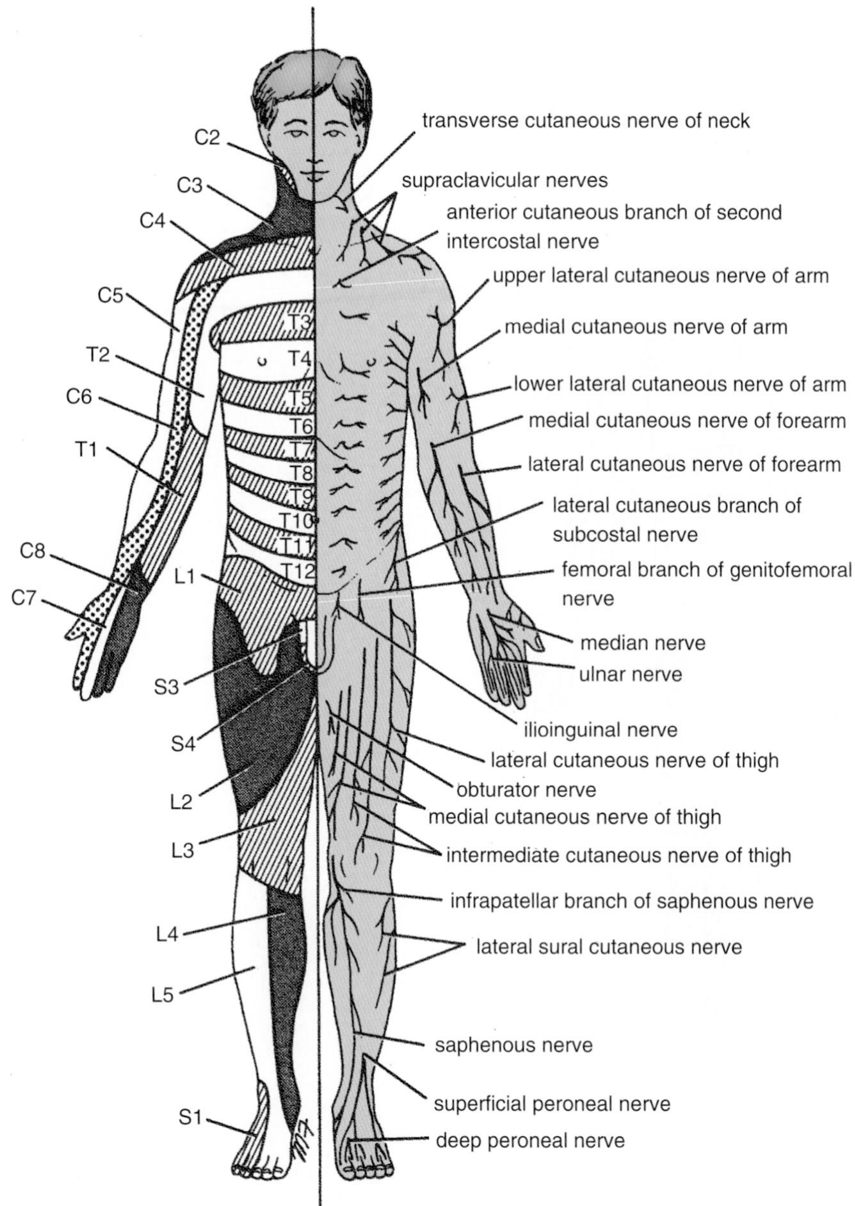

Figure 1-23 Dermatomes and distribution of cutaneous nerves on the anterior aspect of the body.

from the 10th and 11th ganglia, pierces the diaphragm, and synapses with excitor cells in the ganglia of the lower part of the celiac plexus. The **lowest splanchnic nerve** (when present) arises from the 12th thoracic ganglion, pierces the diaphragm, and synapses with excitor cells in the ganglia of the renal plexus. Splanchnic nerves are therefore composed of preganglionic fibers. The postganglionic fibers arise from the excitor cells in the peripheral plexuses previously noted and are distributed to the smooth muscle and glands of the viscera. A few preganglionic fibers traveling in the greater splanchnic nerve end directly on the cells of the suprarenal medulla. These medullary cells may be regarded as modified sympathetic excitor cells.

Sympathetic trunks are two ganglionated nerve trunks that extend the whole length of the vertebral column (Fig. 1-27). There are 3 ganglia in each trunk of the neck, 11 or 12 ganglia in the thorax, 4 or 5 ganglia in the lumbar region, and 4 or 5 ganglia in the pelvis. The two trunks lie close to the vertebral column and end below by joining together to form a single ganglion, the **ganglion impar.**

Afferent Fibers The afferent myelinated nerve fibers travel from the viscera through the sympathetic ganglia without synapsing (Fig. 1-26). They enter the spinal nerve via the white rami communicantes and reach their cell bodies in the posterior root ganglion of the corresponding spinal nerve. The central axons then enter the spinal cord

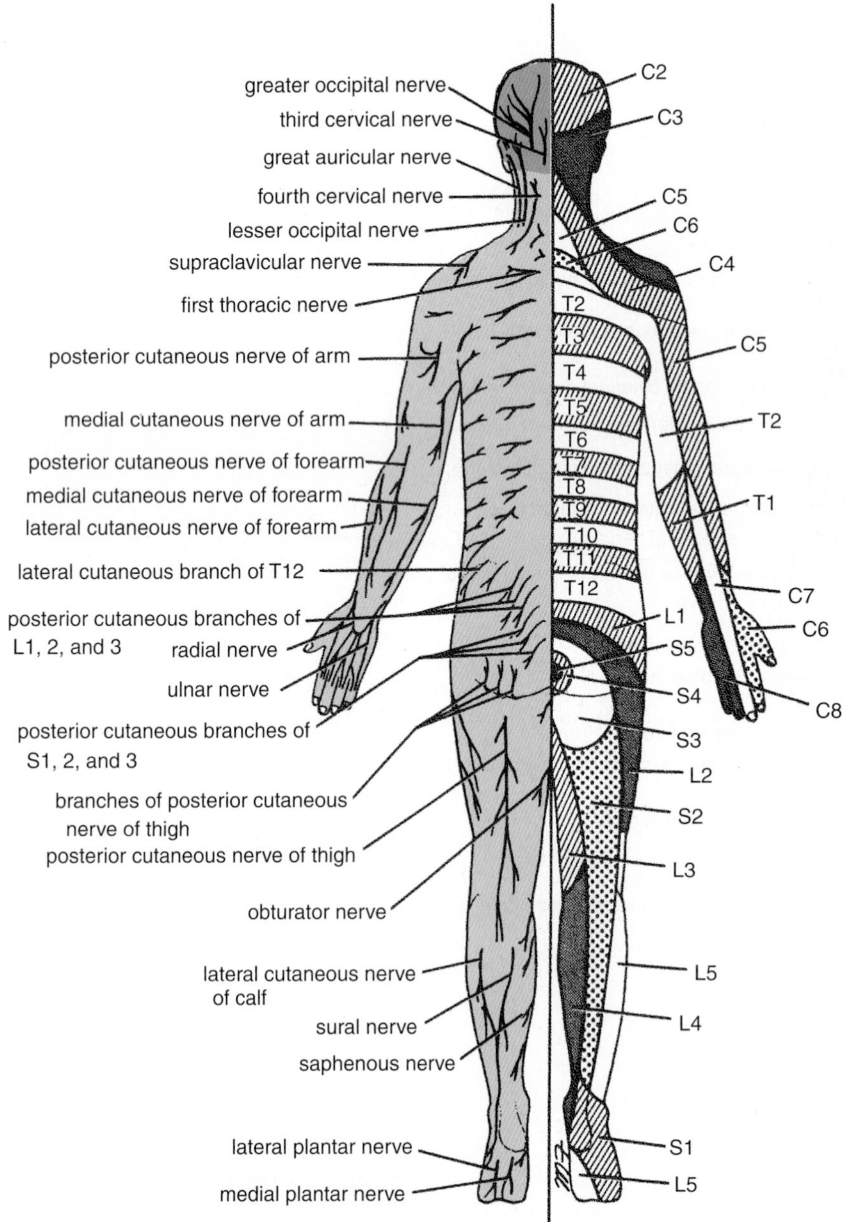

Figure 1-24 Dermatomes and distribution of cutaneous nerves on the posterior aspect of the body.

and may form the afferent component of a local reflex arc. Others may pass up to higher autonomic centers in the brain.

Parasympathetic System

Efferent Fibers The connector cells of this part of the system are located in the brain and the sacral segments of the spinal cord (Fig. 1-27). Those in the brain form parts of the nuclei of origin of cranial nerves III, VII, IX, and X, and the axons emerge from the brain contained in the corresponding cranial nerves.

The sacral connector cells are found in the gray matter of the second, third, and fourth sacral segments of the cord. These cells are not sufficiently numerous to form a lateral gray horn, as do the sympathetic connector cells in the thoracolumbar region. The myelinated axons leave the spinal cord in the anterior nerve roots of the corresponding spinal nerves. They then leave the sacral nerves and form the **pelvic splanchnic nerves.**

All the efferent fibers described so far are preganglionic, and they synapse with excitor cells in peripheral ganglia, which are usually situated close to the viscera they innervate. The cranial preganglionic fibers relay in the **ciliary, pterygopalatine, submandibular,** and **otic ganglia** (Fig. 1-27). The preganglionic fibers in the pelvic splanchnic nerves relay in ganglia in the hypogastric

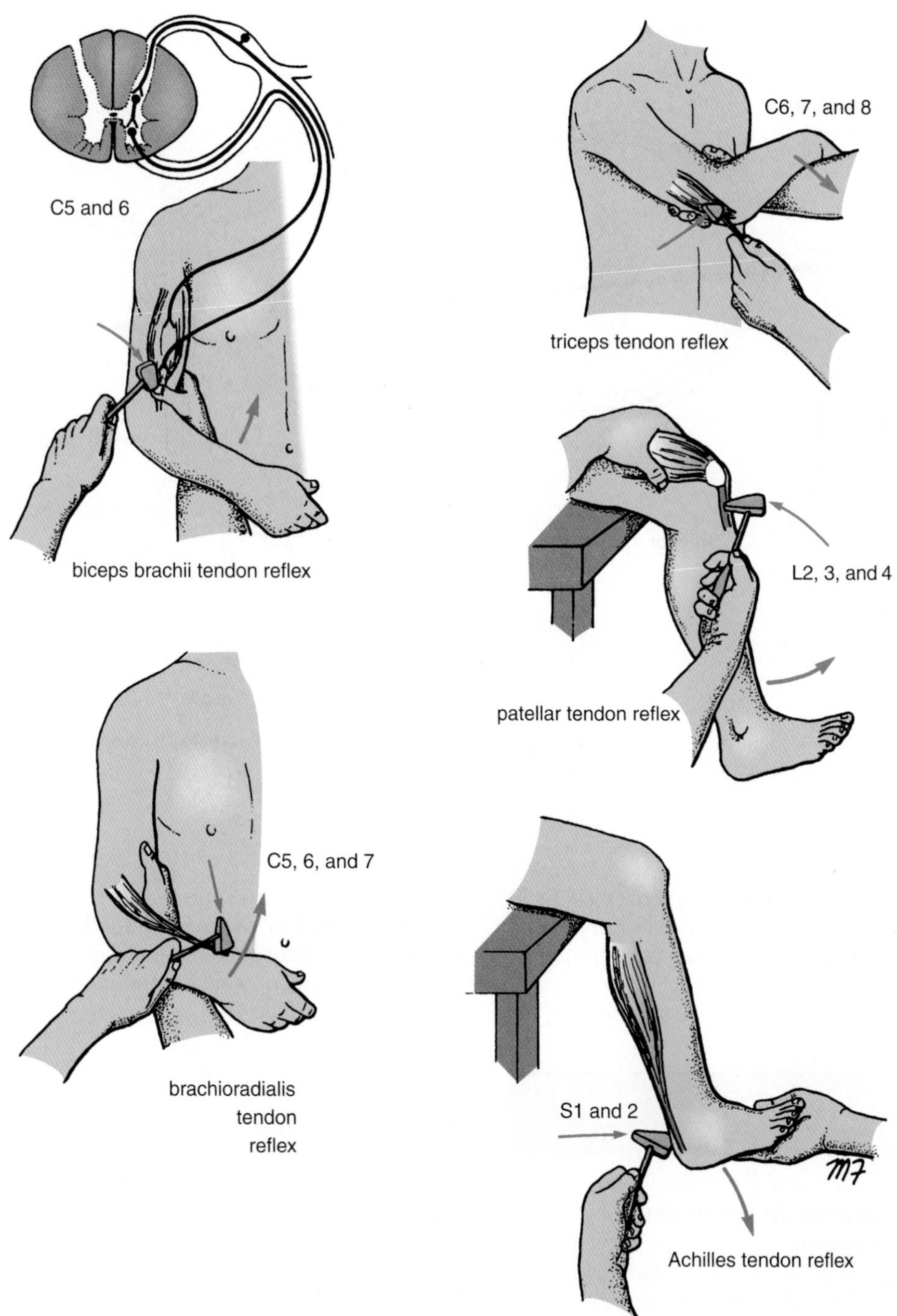

Figure 1-25 Some important tendon reflexes used in medical practice.

plexuses or in the walls of the viscera. Characteristically, the postganglionic fibers are nonmyelinated and are relatively short compared with sympathetic postganglionic fibers.

Afferent Fibers The afferent myelinated fibers travel from the viscera to their cell bodies located either in the sensory ganglia of the cranial nerves or in the posterior root ganglia of the sacrospinal nerves. The central axons then enter the central nervous system and take part in the formation of local reflex arcs, or pass to higher centers of the autonomic nervous system.

The afferent component of the autonomic system is identical to the afferent component of somatic nerves and forms part of the general afferent segment of the entire nervous system. The nerve endings in the autonomic afferent component may not be activated by such sensations as heat or

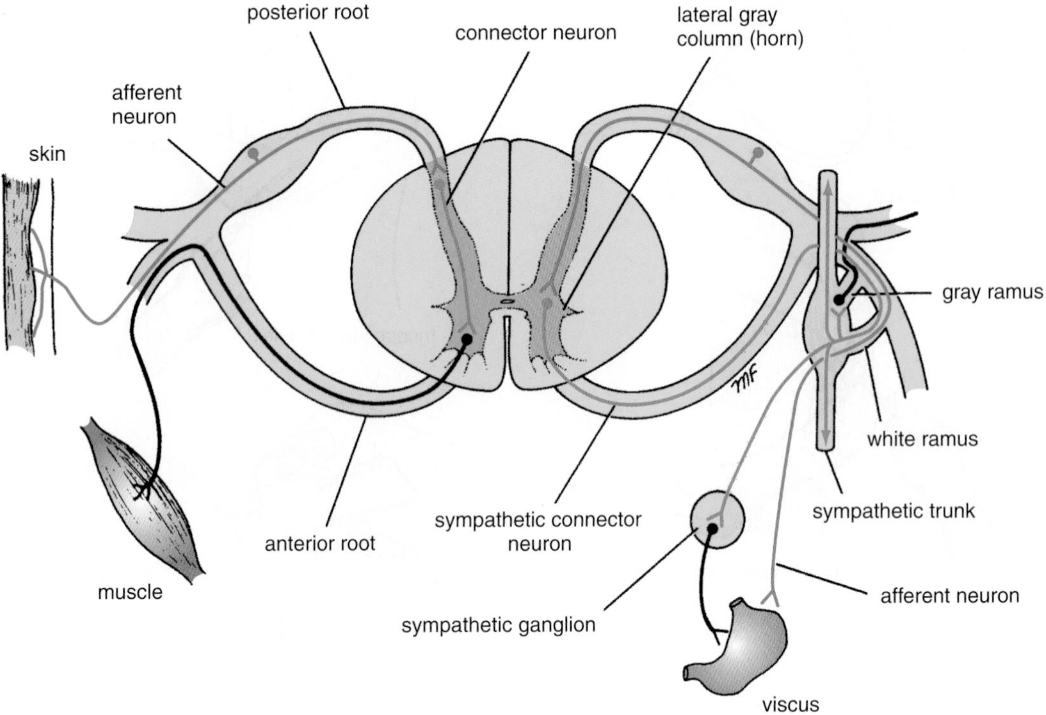

Figure 1-26 General arrangement of somatic part of nervous system (*left*) compared to autonomic part of nervous system (*right*).

touch but instead by stretch or lack of oxygen. Once the afferent fibers gain entrance to the spinal cord or brain, they are thought to travel alongside, or are mixed with, the somatic afferent fibers.

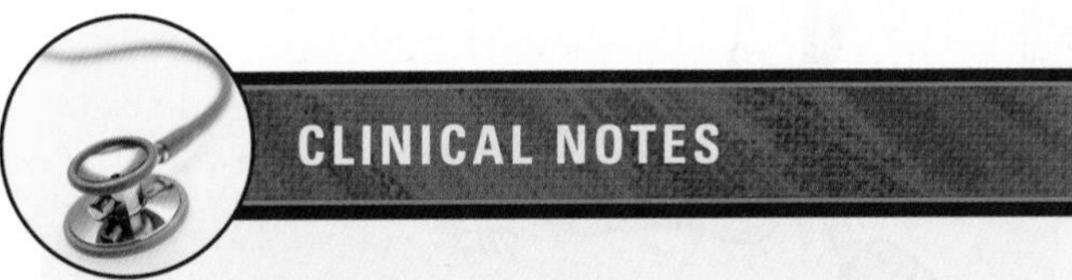

Clinical Modification of the Activities of the Autonomic Nervous System

Many drugs and surgical procedures that can modify the activity of the autonomic nervous system are available. For example, drugs can be administered to lower the blood pressure by blocking sympathetic nerve endings and causing vasodilatation of peripheral blood vessels. In patients with severe arterial disease affecting the main arteries of the lower limb, the limb can sometimes be saved by sectioning the sympathetic innervation to the blood vessels. This produces a vasodilatation and enables an adequate amount of blood to flow through the collateral circulation, thus bypassing the obstruction.

Mucous Membranes

Mucous membrane is the name given to the lining of organs or passages that communicate with the surface of the body. A mucous membrane consists essentially of a layer of epithelium supported by a layer of connective tissue, the **lamina propria.** Smooth muscle, called the **muscularis mucosa,** is sometimes present in the connective tissue. A mucous membrane may or may not secrete mucus on its surface.

Serous Membranes

Serous membranes line the cavities of the trunk and are reflected onto the mobile viscera lying within these cavities (Fig. 1-28). They consist of a smooth layer of mesothelium supported by a thin layer of connective tissue. The serous membrane lining the wall of the cavity is referred to as the **parietal layer,** and that covering the viscera is called the **visceral layer.** The narrow, slitlike interval that separates these layers forms the **pleural, pericardial,** and **peritoneal cavities** and contains a small amount of serous liquid, the **serous exudate.** The serous exudate lubricates the surfaces of the membranes and allows the two layers to slide readily on each other.

The mesenteries, omenta, and serous ligaments are described in other chapters of this book.

The parietal layer of a serous membrane is developed from the somatopleure (inner cell layer of mesoderm) and is richly supplied by spinal nerves. It is therefore sensitive to all common sensations such as touch and pain. The visceral layer is developed from the splanchnopleure (inner cell layer of mesoderm) and is supplied by autonomic nerves. It is insensitive to touch and temperature but very sensitive to stretch.

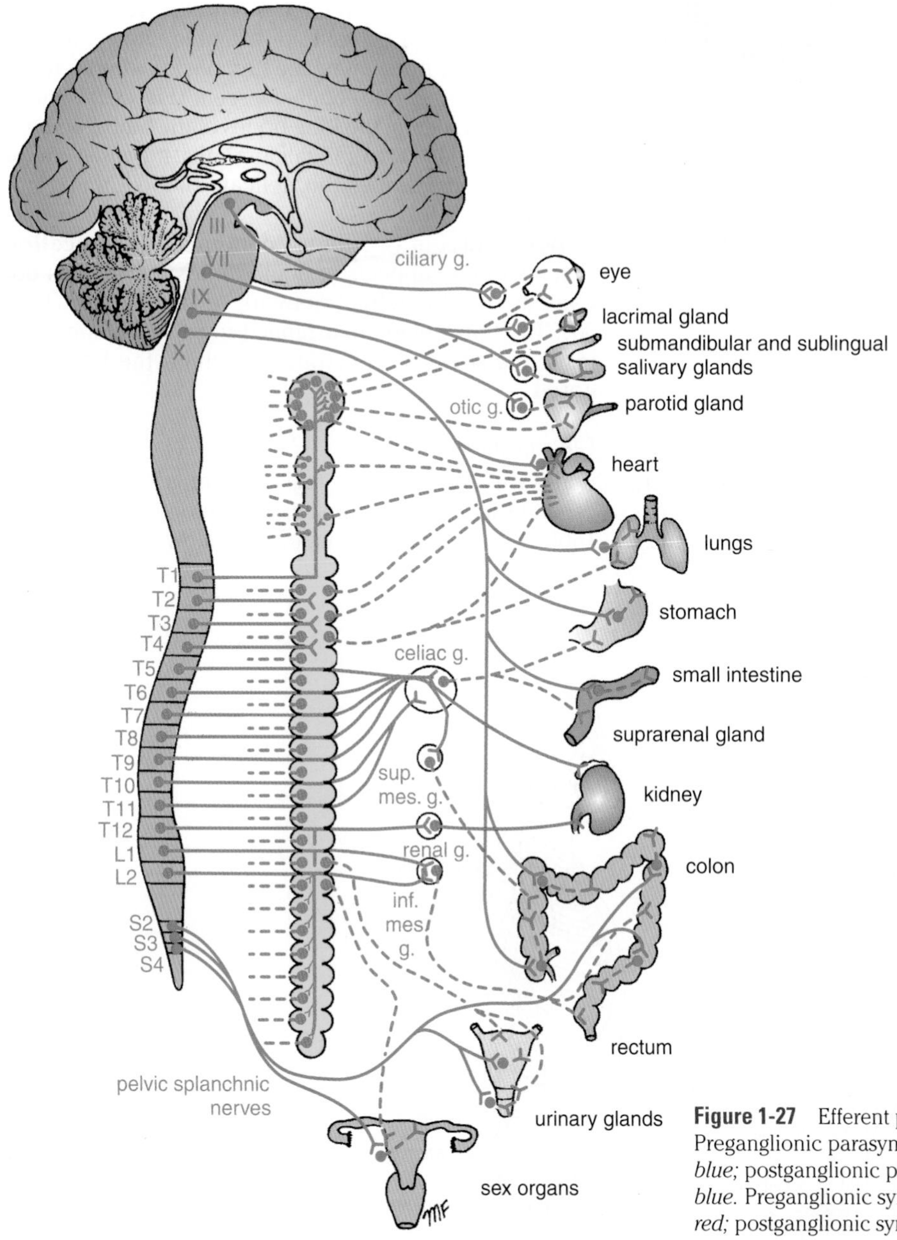

Figure 1-27 Efferent part of autonomic nervous system. Preganglionic parasympathetic fibers are shown in *solid blue;* postganglionic parasympathetic fibers, in *interrupted blue.* Preganglionic sympathetic fibers are shown in *solid red;* postganglionic sympathetic fibers, in *interrupted red.*

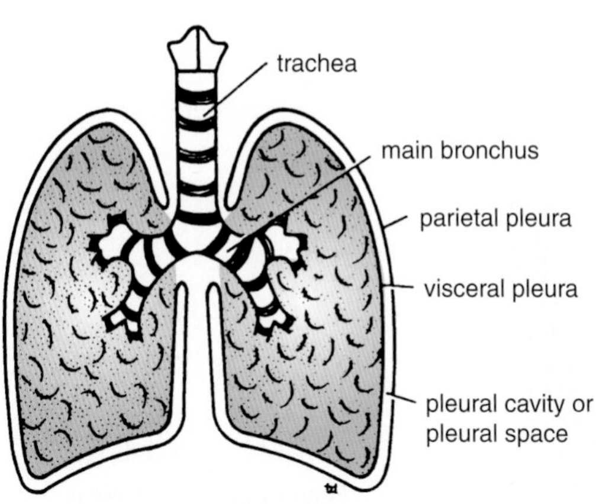

Figure 1-28 Arrangement of pleura within the thoracic cavity. Note that under normal conditions the pleural cavity is a slitlike space; the parietal and visceral layers of pleura are separated by a small amount of serous fluid.

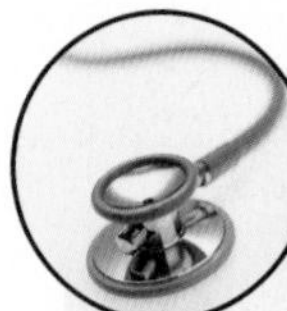

CLINICAL NOTES

Mucous and Serous Membranes and Inflammatory Disease

Mucous and serous membranes are common sites for inflammatory disease. For example, rhinitis, or the common cold, is an inflammation of the nasal mucous membrane, and pleurisy is an inflammation of the visceral and parietal layers of the pleura.

Bone

Bone is a living tissue capable of changing its structure as the result of the stresses to which it is subjected. Like other connective tissues, bone consists of cells, fibers, and matrix. It is hard because of the calcification of its extracellular matrix and possesses a degree of elasticity because of the presence of organic fibers. Bone has a protective function; the skull and vertebral column, for example, protect the brain and spinal cord from injury; the sternum and ribs protect the thoracic and upper abdominal viscera (Fig. 1-29). It serves as a lever, as seen in the long bones of the limbs, and as an important storage area for calcium salts. It houses and protects within its cavities the delicate blood-forming bone marrow.

Bone exists in two forms: **compact** and **cancellous.** Compact bone appears as a solid mass; cancellous bone consists of a branching network of **trabeculae** (Fig. 1-30). The trabeculae are arranged in such a manner as to resist the stresses and strains to which the bone is exposed.

Classification of Bones

Bones may be classified regionally or according to their general shape. The regional classification is summarized in Table 1-2. Bones are grouped as follows based on their

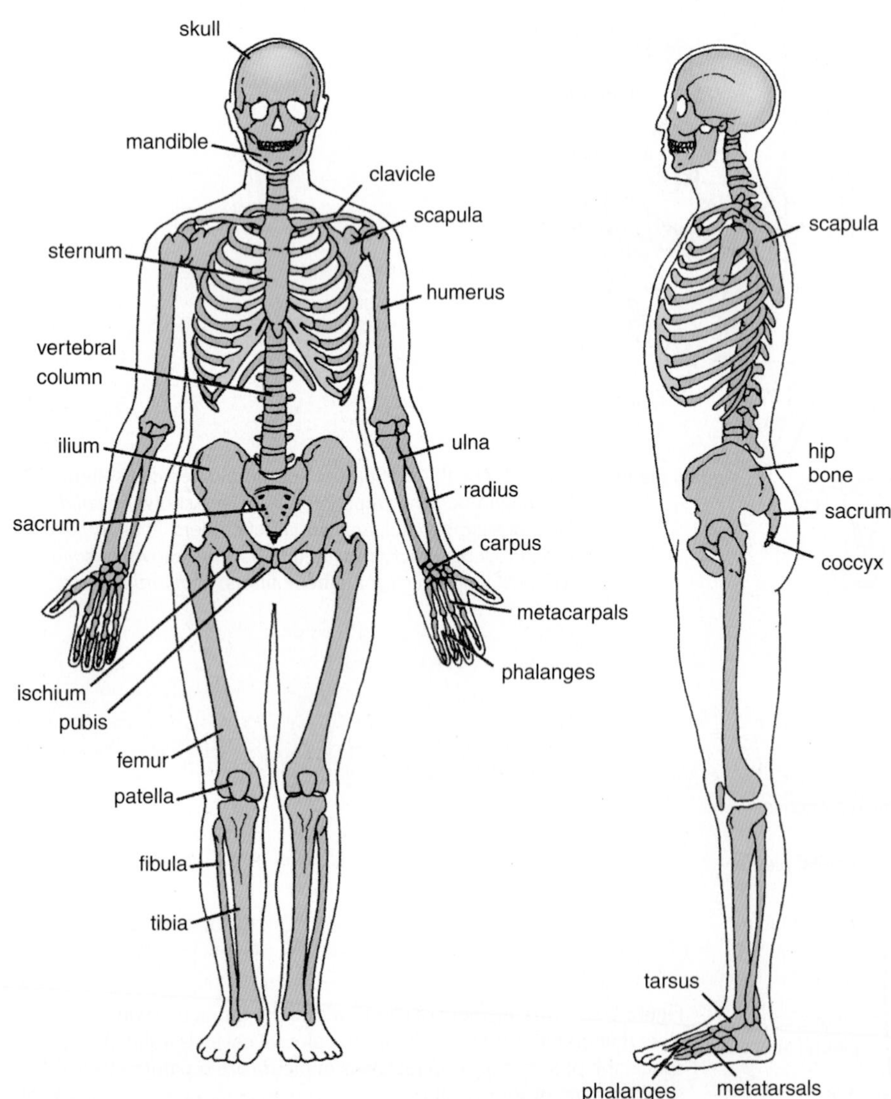

Figure 1-29 The skeleton. **A.** Anterior view. **B.** Lateral view.

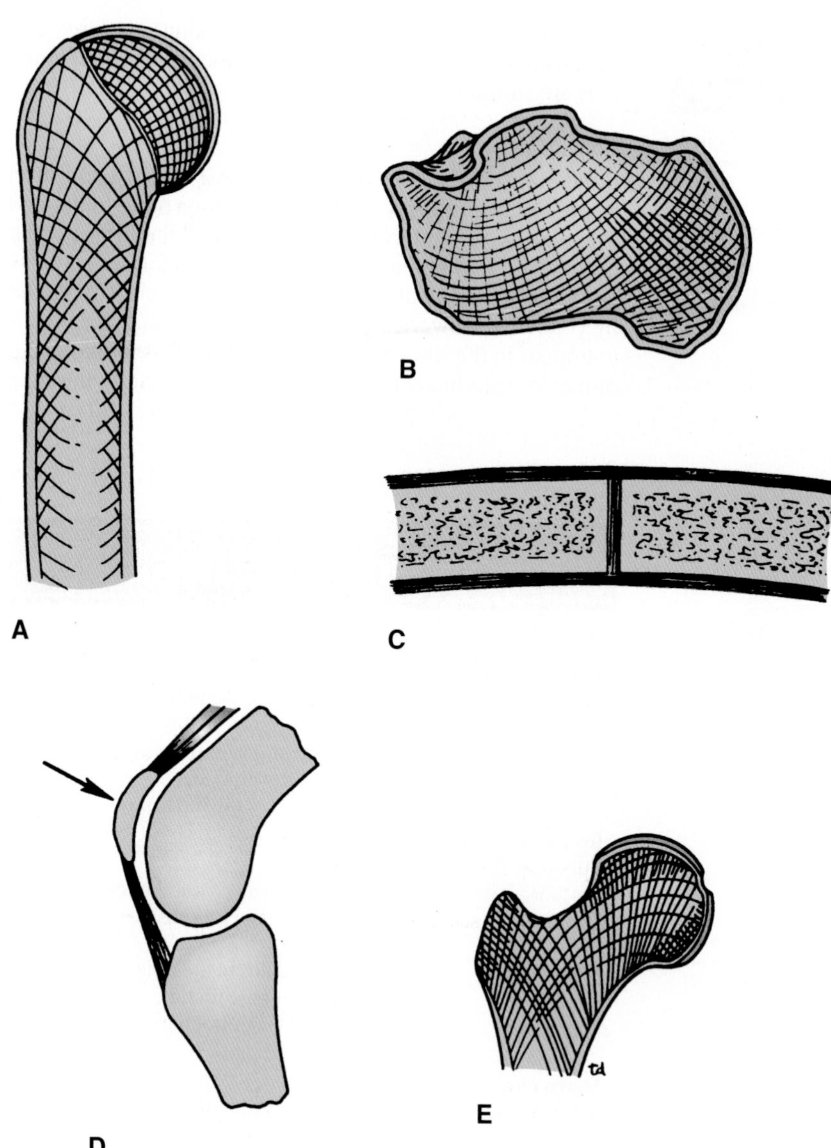

Figure 1-30 Sections of different types of bones. **A.** Long bone (humerus). **B.** Irregular bone (calcaneum). **C.** Flat bone (two parietal bones separated by the sagittal suture). **D.** Sesamoid bone (patella). **E.** Note arrangement of trabeculae to act as struts to resist both compression and tension forces in the upper end of the femur.

general shape: long bones, short bones, flat bones, irregular bones, and sesamoid bones.

Long Bones

Long bones are found in the limbs (e.g., the humerus, femur, metacarpals, metatarsals, and phalanges). Their length is greater than their breadth. They have a tubular shaft, the **diaphysis,** and usually an **epiphysis** at each end. During the growing phase, the diaphysis is separated from the epiphysis by an **epiphyseal cartilage.** The part of the diaphysis that lies adjacent to the epiphyseal cartilage is called the **metaphysis.** The shaft has a central **marrow cavity** containing **bone marrow.** The outer part of the shaft is composed of compact bone that is covered by a connective tissue sheath, the **periosteum.**

The ends of long bones are composed of cancellous bone surrounded by a thin layer of compact bone. The articular surfaces of the ends of the bones are covered by hyaline cartilage.

Short Bones

Short bones are found in the hand and foot (e.g., the scaphoid, lunate, talus, and calcaneum). They are roughly cuboidal in shape and are composed of cancellous bone surrounded by a thin layer of compact bone. Short bones are covered with periosteum, and the articular surfaces are covered by hyaline cartilage.

Flat Bones

Flat bones are found in the vault of the skull (e.g., the frontal and parietal bones). They are composed of thin inner and outer layers of compact bone, the **tables,** separated by a layer of cancellous bone, the **diploë.** The scapulae, although irregular, are included in this group.

Irregular Bones

Irregular bones include those not assigned to the previous groups (e.g., the bones of the skull, the vertebrae, and the pelvic bones). They are composed of a thin shell of

Table 1-2 Regional Classification of Bones

Region of Skeleton	Number of Bones
Axial skeleton	
Skull	
Cranium	8
Face	14
Auditory ossicles	6
Hyoid	1
Vertebrae (including sacrum and coccyx)	26
Sternum	1
Ribs	24
Appendicular skeleton	
Shoulder girdles	
Clavicle	2
Scapula	2
Upper extremities	
Humerus	2
Radius	2
Ulna	2
Carpals	16
Metacarpals	10
Phalanges	28
Pelvic girdle	
Hip bone	2
Lower extremities	
Femur	2
Patella	2
Fibula	2
Tibia	2
Tarsals	14
Metatarsals	10
Phalanges	28
	206

compact bone with an interior made up of cancellous bone.

Sesamoid Bones

Sesamoid bones are small nodules of bone that are found in certain tendons where they rub over bony surfaces. The greater part of a sesamoid bone is buried in the tendon, and the free surface is covered with cartilage. The largest sesamoid bone is the patella, which is located in the tendon of the quadriceps femoris. Other examples are found in the tendons of the flexor pollicis brevis and flexor hallucis brevis. The function of a sesamoid bone is to reduce friction on the tendon; it can also alter the direction of pull of a tendon.

Surface Markings of Bones

The surfaces of bones show various markings or irregularities. Where bands of fascia, ligaments, tendons, or aponeuroses are attached to bone, the surface is raised or roughened. These roughenings are not present at birth. They appear at puberty and become progressively more obvious during adult life. The pull of these fibrous structures causes the periosteum to be raised and new bone to be deposited beneath.

In certain situations, the surface markings are large and are given special names. Some of the more important markings are summarized in Table 1-3.

Bone Marrow

Bone marrow occupies the marrow cavity in long and short bones and the interstices of the cancellous bone in flat and irregular bones. At birth, the marrow of all the bones of the body is red and hematopoietic. This blood-forming activity gradually lessens with age, and the red marrow is replaced by yellow marrow. At 7 years of age, yellow marrow begins to appear in the distal bones of the limbs. This replacement of marrow gradually moves proximally, so that by the time

Table 1-3 Surface Markings of Bones

Bone Marking	Example
Linear elevation	
Line	Superior nuchal line of the occipital bone
Ridge	The medial and lateral supracondylar ridges of the humerus
Crest	The iliac crest of the hip bone
Rounded elevation	
Tubercle	Pubic tubercle
Protuberance	External occipital protuberance
Tuberosity	Greater and lesser tuberosities of the humerus
Malleolus	Medial malleolus of the tibia, lateral malleolus of the fibula
Trochanter	Greater and lesser trochanters of the femur
Sharp elevation	
Spine or spinous process	Ischial spine, spine of vertebra
Styloid process	Styloid process of temporal bone
Expanded ends for articulation	
Head	Head of humerus, head of femur
Condyle (knucklelike process)	Medial and lateral condyles of femur
Epicondyle (a prominence situated just above condyle)	Medial and lateral epicondyles of femur
Small flat area for articulation	
Facet	Facet on head of rib for articulation with vertebral body
Depressions	
Notch	Greater sciatic notch of hip bone
Groove or sulcus	Bicipital groove of humerus
Fossa	Olecranon fossa of humerus, acetabular fossa of hip bone
Openings	
Fissure	Superior orbital fissure
Foramen	Infraorbital foramen of the maxilla
Canal	Carotid canal of temporal bone
Meatus	External acoustic meatus of temporal bone

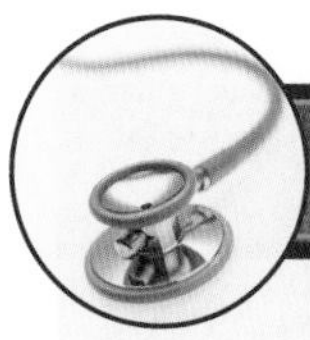

CLINICAL NOTES

Bone Fractures

Immediately after a **fracture,** the patient suffers severe local pain and is not able to use the injured part. Deformity may be visible if the bone fragments have been displaced relative to each other. The degree of deformity and the directions taken by the bony fragments depend not only on the mechanism of injury but also on the pull of the muscles attached to the fragments. Ligamentous attachments also influence the deformity. In certain situations—for example, the ilium—fractures result in no deformity because the inner and outer surfaces of the bone are splinted by the extensive origins of muscles. In contrast, a fracture of the neck of the femur produces considerable displacement. The strong muscles of the thigh pull the distal fragment upward so that the leg is shortened. The very strong lateral rotators rotate the distal fragment laterally so that the foot points laterally.

Fracture of a bone is accompanied by a considerable hemorrhage of blood between the bone ends and into the surrounding soft tissue. The blood vessels and the fibroblasts and osteoblasts from the periosteum and endosteum take part in the repair process.

the person becomes an adult, red marrow is restricted to the bones of the skull, the vertebral column, the thoracic cage, the girdle bones, and the head of the humerus and femur.

All bone surfaces, other than the articulating surfaces, are covered by a thick layer of fibrous tissue called the **periosteum.** The periosteum has an abundant vascular supply, and the cells on its deeper surface are osteogenic. The periosteum is particularly well united to bone at sites where muscles, tendons, and ligaments are attached to bone. Bundles of collagen fibers known as Sharpey's fibers extend from the periosteum into the underlying bone. The periosteum receives a rich nerve supply and is very sensitive.

Development of Bone

Bone is developed by two processes: membranous and endochondral. In the first process the bone is developed directly from a connective tissue membrane; in the second, a cartilaginous model is first laid down and is later replaced by bone. For details of the cellular changes involved, a textbook of histology or embryology should be consulted.

The bones of the vault of the skull are developed rapidly by the membranous method in the embryo, and this serves to protect the underlying developing brain. At birth, small areas of membrane persist between the bones. This is important clinically because it allows the bones a certain amount of mobility, so that the skull can undergo molding during its descent through the female genital passages.

The long bones of the limbs are developed by endochondral ossification, which is a slow process that is not completed until the 18th to 20th year or even later. The center of bone formation found in the shaft of the bone is referred to as the **diaphysis;** the centers at the ends of the bone, as the **epiphyses.** The plate of cartilage at each end, lying between the epiphysis and diaphysis in a growing bone, is called the **epiphyseal plate.** The **metaphysis** is the part of the diaphysis that abuts onto the epiphyseal plate.

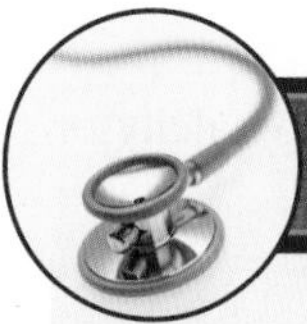

CLINICAL NOTES

Rickets

Rickets is a defective mineralization of the cartilage matrix in growing bones. This produces a condition in which the cartilage cells continue to grow, resulting in excess cartilage and a widening of the epiphyseal plates. The poorly mineralized cartilaginous matrix and the osteoid matrix are soft, and they bend under the stress of bearing weight. The resulting deformities include enlarged costochondral junctions, bowing of the long bones of the lower limbs, and bossing of the frontal bones of the skull. Deformities of the pelvis may also occur.

Epiphyseal Plate Disorders

Epiphyseal plate disorders affect only children and adolescents. The epiphyseal plate is the part of a growing bone concerned primarily with growth in length. Trauma, infection, diet, exercise, and endocrine disorders can disturb the growth of the hyaline cartilaginous plate, leading to deformity and loss of function. In the femur, for example, the proximal epiphysis can slip because of mechanical stress or excessive loads. The length of the limbs can increase excessively because of increased vascularity in the region of the epiphyseal plate secondary to infection or in the presence of tumors. Shortening of a limb can follow trauma to the epiphyseal plate resulting from a diminished blood supply to the cartilage.

Cartilage

Cartilage is a form of connective tissue in which the cells and fibers are embedded in a gel-like matrix, the latter being responsible for its firmness and resilience. Except on the exposed surfaces in joints, a fibrous membrane called the **perichondrium** covers the cartilage. There are three types of cartilage:

- **Hyaline cartilage** has a high proportion of amorphous matrix that has the same refractive index as the fibers embedded in it. Throughout childhood and adolescence, it plays an important part in the growth in length of long bones (epiphyseal plates are composed of hyaline cartilage). It has a great resistance to wear and covers the articular surfaces of nearly all synovial joints. Hyaline cartilage is incapable of repair when fractured; the defect is filled with fibrous tissue.
- **Fibrocartilage** has many collagen fibers embedded in a small amount of matrix and is found in the discs within

joints (e.g., the temporomandibular joint, sternoclavicular joint, and knee joint) and on the articular surfaces of the clavicle and mandible. Fibrocartilage, if damaged, repairs itself slowly in a manner similar to fibrous tissue elsewhere. Joint discs have a poor blood supply and therefore do not repair themselves when damaged.
- **Elastic cartilage** possesses large numbers of elastic fibers embedded in matrix. As would be expected, it is flexible and is found in the auricle of the ear, the external auditory meatus, the auditory tube, and the epiglottis. Elastic cartilage, if damaged, repairs itself with fibrous tissue.

Hyaline cartilage and fibrocartilage tend to calcify or even ossify in later life.

Effects of Sex, Race, and Age on Structure

Descriptive anatomy tends to concentrate on a fixed descriptive form. Medical personnel must always remember that sexual and racial differences exist and that the body's structure and function change as a person grows and ages.

The adult male tends to be taller than the adult female and to have longer legs; his bones are bigger and heavier and his muscles are larger. He has less subcutaneous fat, which makes his appearance more angular. His larynx is larger and his vocal cords are longer so that his voice is deeper. He has a beard and coarse body hair. He possesses axillary and pubic hair, the latter extending to the region of the umbilicus.

The adult female tends to be shorter than the adult male and to have smaller bones and less bulky muscles. She has more subcutaneous fat and fat accumulations in the breasts, buttocks, and thighs, giving her a more rounded appearance. Her head hair is finer and her skin is smoother in appearance. She has axillary and pubic hair, but the latter does not extend up to the umbilicus. The adult female has larger breasts and a wider pelvis than the male. She has a wider carrying angle at the elbow, which results in a greater lateral deviation of the forearm on the arm.

Until the age of approximately 10 years, boys and girls grow at about the same rate. Around 12 years, boys often start to grow faster than girls, so that most males reach a greater adult height than females.

Puberty begins between ages 10 and 14 in girls and between 12 and 15 in boys. In the girl at puberty, the breasts enlarge and the pelvis broadens. At the same time, a boy's penis, testes, and scrotum enlarge; in both sexes, axillary and pubic hair appear.

Racial differences may be seen in the color of the skin, hair, and eyes and in the shape and size of the eyes, nose, and lips. Africans and Scandinavians tend to be tall, as a result of long legs, whereas Asians tend to be short, with short legs. The heads of central Europeans and Asians also tend to be round and broad.

After birth and during childhood, the bodily functions become progressively more efficient, reaching their maximum degree of efficiency during young adulthood. During late adulthood and old age, many bodily functions become less efficient.

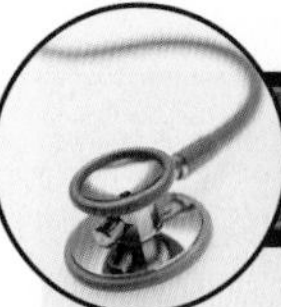

CLINICAL NOTES

Clinical Significance of Age on Structure

The fact that the structure and function of the human body change with age may seem obvious, but it is often overlooked. A few examples of such changes are given here:

1. In the infant, the bones of the skull are more resilient than in the adult, and for this reason fractures of the skull are much more common in the adult than in the young child.
2. The liver is relatively much larger in the child than in the adult. In the infant, the lower margin of the liver extends inferiorly to a lower level than in the adult. This is an important consideration when making a diagnosis of hepatic enlargement.
3. The urinary bladder in the child cannot be accommodated entirely in the pelvis because of the small size of the pelvic cavity and thus is found in the lower part of the abdominal cavity. As the child grows, the pelvis enlarges and the bladder sinks down to become a true pelvic organ.
4. At birth, all bone marrow is of the red variety. With advancing age, the red marrow recedes up the bones of the limbs so that in the adult it is largely confined to the bones of the head, thorax, and abdomen.
5. Lymphatic tissues reach their maximum degree of development at puberty and thereafter atrophy, so the volume of lymphatic tissue in older persons is considerably reduced.

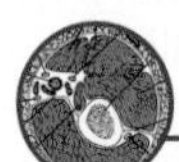

Radiographic Anatomy

As a medical professional, you will be frequently called on to study normal and abnormal anatomy as seen on radiographs. Familiarity with normal radiographic anatomy permits one to recognize abnormalities quickly, such as fractures and tumors.

The most common form of radiographic anatomy is studied on a **radiograph** (x-ray film), which provides a two-dimensional image of the interior of the body (Fig. 1-31). To produce such a radiograph, a single barrage of x-rays is passed through the body and exposes the film. Tissues of differing densities show up as images of differing densities on the radiograph (or fluorescent screen). A tissue that is relatively dense absorbs (stops) more x-rays than tissues that are less dense. A very dense tissue is said to be **radiopaque,** but a less dense tissue is said to be **radiolucent.** Bone is very dense and fat is moderately dense; other soft tissues are less dense.

Unfortunately, an ordinary radiograph shows the images of the different organs superimposed onto a flat sheet of film. This overlap of organs and tissues often makes it difficult to visualize them. This problem is overcome to some extent by taking films at right angles to one another or by making stereoscopic films.

Computed tomography (CT) scanning or **computerized axial tomography** (CAT) scanning permits the study

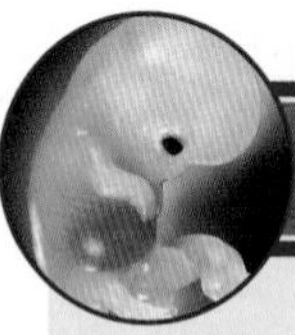

EMBRYOLOGIC NOTES

Embryology and Clinical Anatomy

Embryology provides a basis for understanding anatomy and an explanation of many of the congenital anomalies that are seen in clinical medicine. A very brief overview of the development of the embryo follows.

Once the ovum has been fertilized by the spermatozoon, a single cell is formed, called the **zygote.** This undergoes a rapid succession of mitotic divisions with the formation of smaller cells. The centrally placed cells are called the **inner cell mass** and ultimately form the tissues of the embryo. The outer cells, called the **outer cell mass,** form the trophoblast, which plays an important role in the formation of the **placenta** and the **fetal membranes.**

The cells that form the embryo become defined in the form of a bilaminar **embryonic disc,** composed of two germ layers. The upper layer is called the **ectoderm** and the lower layer, the **entoderm.** As growth proceeds, the embryonic disc becomes pear shaped, and a narrow streak appears on its dorsal surface formed of ectoderm, called the **primitive streak.** The further proliferation of the cells of the primitive streak forms a layer of cells that will extend between the ectoderm and the entoderm to form the third germ layer, called the **mesoderm.**

Ectoderm

Further thickening of the ectoderm gives rise to a plate of cells on the dorsal surface of the embryo called the **neural plate.** This plate sinks beneath the surface of the embryo to form the **neural tube,** which ultimately gives rise to the **central nervous system.** The remainder of the ectoderm forms the **cornea, retina,** and **lens** of the **eye** and the **membranous labyrinth** of the **inner ear.** The ectoderm also forms the **epidermis** of the **skin;** the **nails** and **hair;** the **epithelial cells** of the **sebaceous, sweat,** and **mammary glands;** the **mucous membrane** lining the **mouth, nasal cavities,** and **paranasal sinuses;** the **enamel** of the **teeth;** the **pituitary gland** and the **alveoli** and **ducts** of the **parotid salivary glands;** the mucous membrane of the lower half of the **anal canal;** and the terminal parts of the **genital tract** and the **male urinary tract.**

Entoderm

The entoderm eventually gives origin to the following structures: the **epithelial lining** of the **alimentary tract** from the **mouth cavity** down to halfway along the anal canal and the **epithelium** of the glands that develop from it—namely, the **thyroid, parathyroid, thymus, liver,** and **pancreas**—and the epithelial linings of the **respiratory tract, pharyngotympanic tube** and **middle ear, urinary bladder,** parts of the female and male **urethras, greater vestibular glands, prostate gland, bulbourethral glands,** and **vagina.**

Mesoderm

The mesoderm becomes differentiated into the paraxial, intermediate, and lateral mesoderms. The **paraxial mesoderm** is situated initially on either side of the midline of the embryo. It becomes segmented and forms the **bones, cartilage,** and **ligaments** of the **vertebral column** and part of the base of the **skull.** The lateral cells form the **skeletal muscles** of their own segment, and some of the cells migrate beneath the ectoderm and take part in the formation of the **dermis** and **subcutaneous tissues** of the skin.

The **intermediate mesoderm** is a column of cells on either side of the embryo that is connected medially to the paraxial mesoderm and laterally to the lateral mesoderm. It gives rise to portions of the **urogenital system.**

The **lateral mesoderm** splits into a **somatic layer** and a **splanchnic layer** associated with the ectoderm and the entoderm, respectively. It encloses a cavity within the embryo called the **intraembryonic coelom.** The coelom eventually forms the **pericardial, pleural,** and **peritoneal cavities.**

The embryonic mesoderm, in addition, gives origin to **smooth, voluntary,** and **cardiac muscle;** all forms of **connective tissue,** including cartilage and bone; **blood vessel walls** and **blood cells; lymph vessel walls** and **lymphoid tissue;** the **synovial membranes** of **joints** and **bursae;** and the **suprarenal cortex.**

When appropriate, a more detailed account of the development of different organs is given in the chapters to follow.

---

of tissue slices so that tissues with minor differences in density can be recognized. CT scanning relies on the same physics as conventional x-rays but combines it with computer technology. A source of x-rays moves in an arc around the part of the body being studied and sends out a beam of x-rays. The x-rays, having passed through the region of the body, are collected by a special x-ray detector. Here, the x-rays are converted into electronic impulses that produce readings of the density of the tissue in a 1-cm slice of the body. From these readings, the computer is able to assemble a picture of the body called a **CT scan,** which can be viewed on a fluorescent screen and then photographed for later examination (Fig. 1-32). The procedure is safe and quick, lasts only a few seconds for each slice, and for most patients requires no sedation.

The technique of **magnetic resonance imaging** (MRI) uses the magnetic properties of the hydrogen nucleus excited by radiofrequency radiation transmitted by a coil surrounding the body part. The excited hydrogen nuclei emit a signal that is detected as induced electric currents in a receiver coil. MRI is absolutely safe to the patient, and because it provides better differentiation between different soft tissues, its use can be more revealing than a CT scan. The reason for this is that some tissues contain more hydrogen in the form of water than do other tissues (Fig. 1-33).

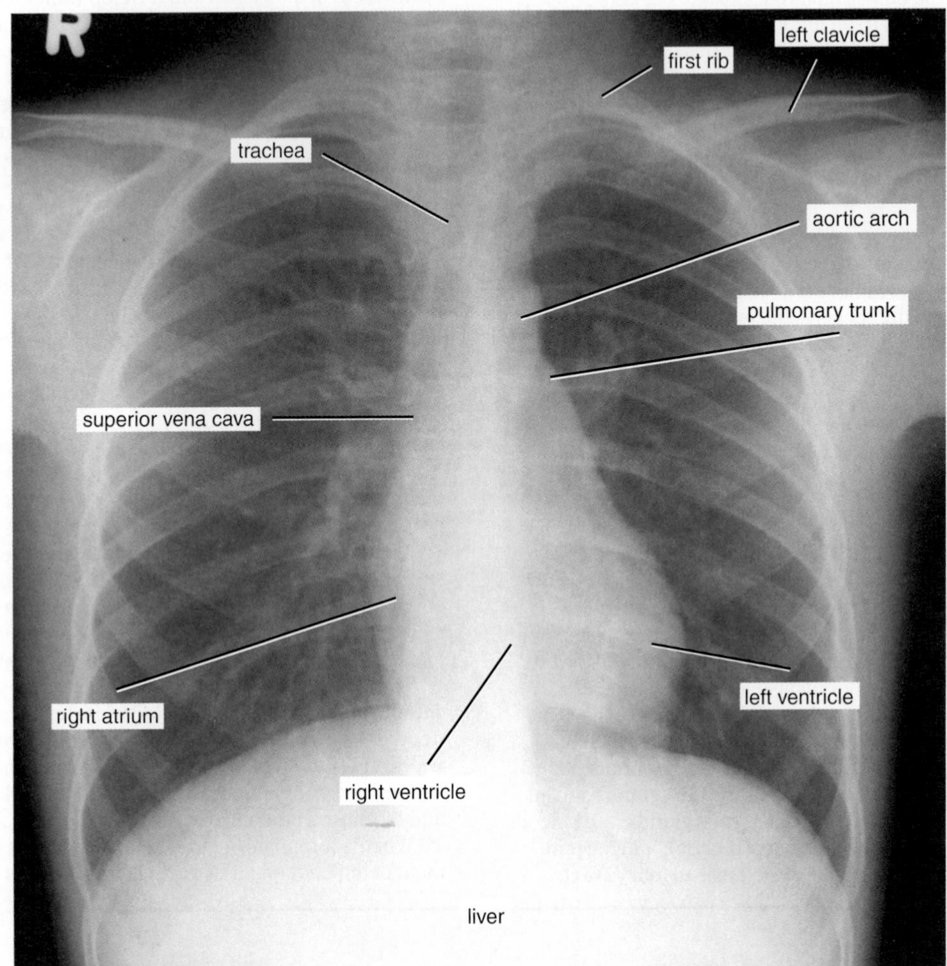

Figure 1-31 Posteroanterior radiograph of the thorax.

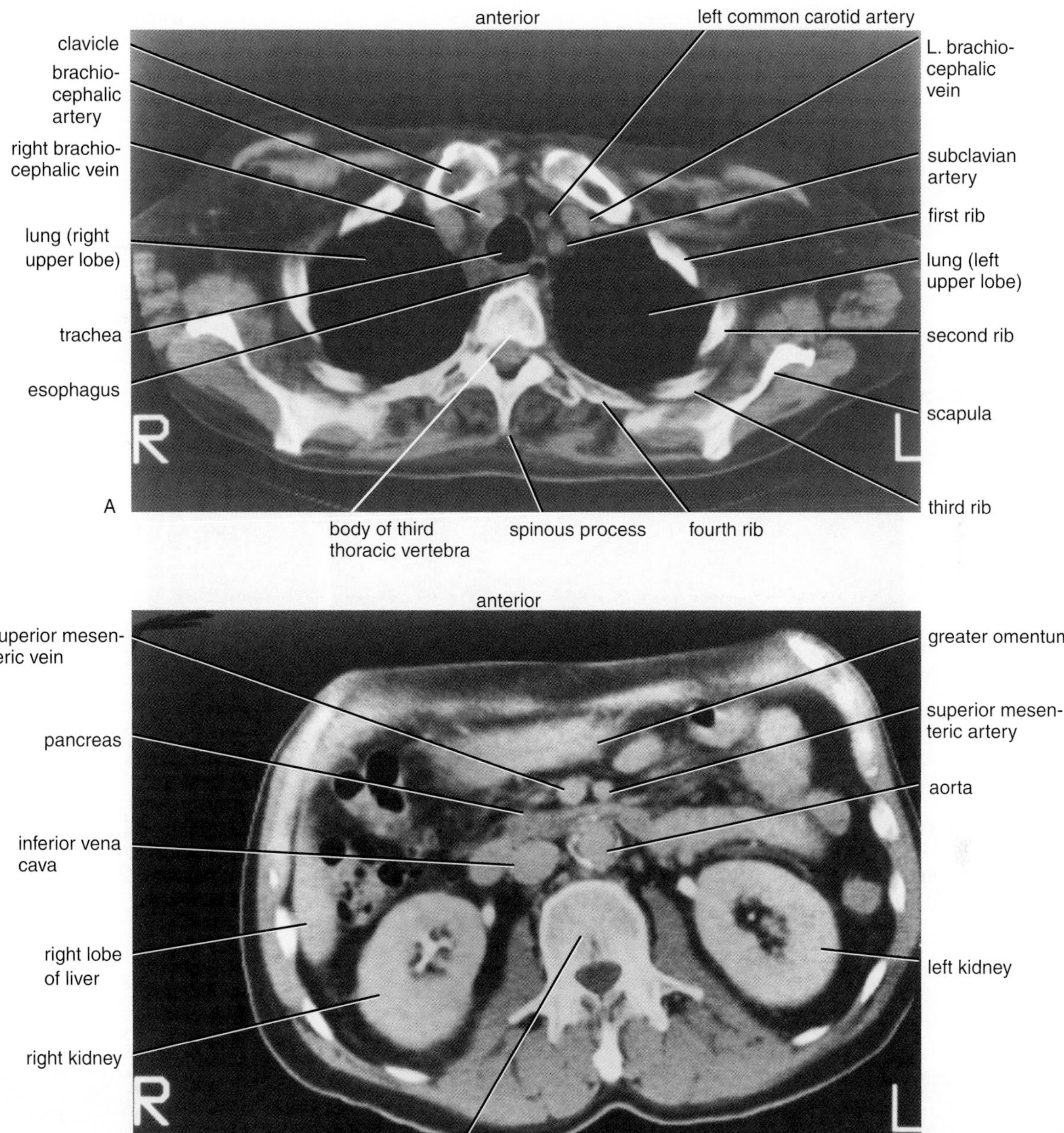

Figure 1-32 Computed tomography (CT) scans. **A.** The upper thorax at the level of the third thoracic vertebra. **B.** The upper abdomen at the level of the second lumbar vertebra. All CT scans are viewed from below. Thus, the right side of the body appears on the left side of the figure.

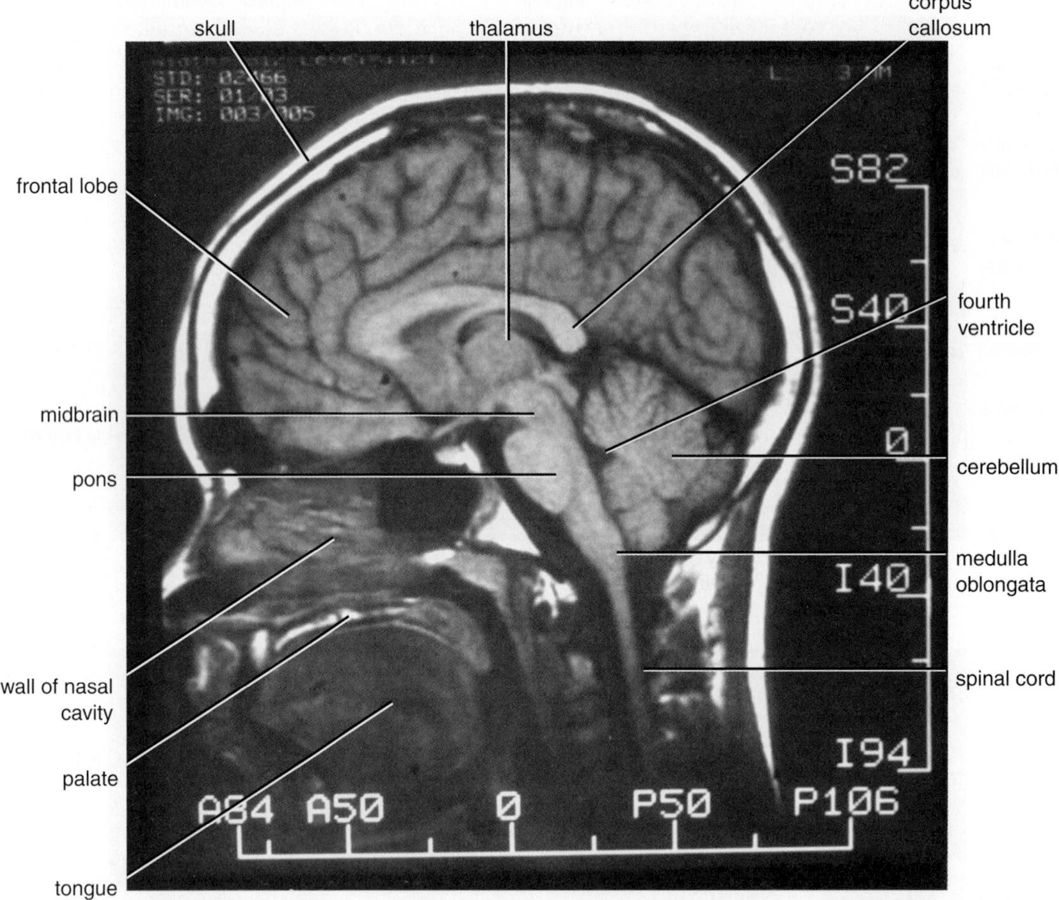

Figure 1-33 Magnetic resonance imaging study of the head in a sagittal plane showing different parts of the brain.

CLINICAL PROBLEM SOLVING

Study the following case histories and select the *best* answer to the questions following them.

A 45-year-old patient has a small, firm, mobile tumor on the dorsum of the right foot just proximal to the base of the big toe and superficial to the bones and the long extensor tendon but deep to the superficial fascia.

1. The following information concerning the tumor is correct except which?
   (a) It is situated on the upper surface of the foot close to the root of the big toe.
   (b) It is not attached to the first metatarsal bone.
   (c) It lies superficial to the deep fascia.
   (d) It lies superficial to the tendon of the extensor hallucis longus muscle.
   (e) It is attached to the capsule of the metatarsophalangeal joint of the big toe.

A 31-year-old woman has a history of poliomyelitis affecting the anterior horn cells of the lower thoracic and lumbar segments of the spinal cord on the left side. On examination, she has severe right lateral flexion deformity of the vertebral column.

2. The following statements are true about this case except which?
   (a) The virus of poliomyelitis attacks and destroys the motor anterior horn cells of the spinal cord.
   (b) The disease resulted in the paralysis of the muscles that normally laterally flex the vertebral column on the left side.
   (c) The muscles on the right side of the vertebral column are unapposed.
   (d) The right lateral flexion deformity is caused by the slow degeneration of the sensory nerve fibers originating from the vertebral muscles on the right side.

A 20-year-old woman severely sprains her left ankle while playing tennis. When she tries to move the foot so that the sole faces medially, she experiences severe pain.

3. What is the correct anatomic term for the movement of the foot that produces the pain?
   (a) Pronation
   (b) Inversion
   (c) Supination
   (d) Eversion

A 25-year-old man has a deep-seated abscess in the posterior part of the neck.

4. The following statements are correct concerning the abscess except which?
   (a) The abscess probably lies deep to the deep fascia.
   (b) The deep fascia determines the direction of spread of the abscess.
   (c) The abscess would be incised through a vertical skin incision.
   (d) The lines of cleavage are important when considering the direction of skin incisions.
   (e) The abscess would be incised through a horizontal skin incision.

A 40-year-old workman received a severe burn on the anterior aspect of his right forearm. The area of the burn exceeded 4 in.^{2} (10 cm^2). The greater part of the burn was superficial and extended only into the superficial part of the dermis.

5. In the superficially burned area, the epidermis cells would regenerate from the following sites except
   (a) the hair follicles.
   (b) the sebaceous glands.
   (c) the margins of the burn.
   (d) the deepest ends of the sweat glands.
6. In a small area the burn penetrated as far as the superficial fascia; in this region, the epidermal cells would regenerate from the following sites except
   (a) the ends of the sweat glands that lie in the superficial fascia.
   (b) the margins of the burn.
   (c) the sebaceous glands.

In a 63-year-old man, an MRI of the lower thoracic region of the vertebral column reveals the presence of a tumor pressing on the lumbar segments of the spinal cord. He has a loss of sensation in the skin over the anterior surface of the left thigh and is unable to extend his left knee joint. Examination reveals that the muscles of the front of the left thigh have atrophied and have no tone and that the left knee jerk is absent.

7. The following statements concerning this patient are correct except which?
   (a) The tumor is interrupting the normal function of the efferent motor fibers of the spinal cord on the left side.
   (b) The quadriceps femoris muscles on the front of the left thigh are atrophied.
   (c) The loss of skin sensation is confined to the dermatomes L1, 2, 3, and 4.
   (d) The absence of the left knee jerk is because of involvement of the first lumbar spinal segment.
   (e) The loss of muscle tone is caused by interruption of a nervous reflex arc.

A woman recently took up employment in a factory. She is a machinist, and for 6 hours a day she has to move a lever repeatedly, which requires that she extend and flex her right wrist joint. At the end of the second week of her employment, she began to experience pain over the posterior surface of her wrist and noticed a swelling in the area.

8. The following statements concerning this patient are correct except which?
   (a) Extension of the wrist joint is brought about by several muscles that include the extensor digitorum muscle.
   (b) The wrist joint is diseased.
   (c) Repeated unaccustomed movements of tendons through their synovial sheaths can produce traumatic inflammation of the sheaths.
   (d) The diagnosis is traumatic tenosynovitis of the long tendons of the extensor digitorum muscle.

A 19-year-old boy was suspected of having leukemia. It was decided to confirm the diagnosis by performing a bone marrow biopsy.

9. The following statements concerning this procedure are correct except which?
   (a) The biopsy was taken from the lower end of the tibia.
   (b) Red bone marrow specimens can be obtained from the sternum or the iliac crests.
   (c) At birth, the marrow of all bones of the body is red and hematopoietic.
   (d) The blood-forming activity of bone marrow in many long bones gradually lessens with age, and the red marrow is gradually replaced by yellow marrow.

A 22-year-old woman had a severe infection under the lateral edge of the nail of her right index finger. On examination, a series of red lines were seen to extend up the back of the hand and around to the front of the forearm and arm, up to the armpit.

10. The following statements concerning this patient are probably correct except which?
    (a) Palpation of the right armpit revealed the presence of several tender enlarged lymph nodes (lymphadenitis).
    (b) The red lines were caused by the superficial lymphatic vessels in the arm, which were red and inflamed (lymphangitis) and could be seen through the skin.
    (c) Lymph from the right arm entered the bloodstream through the thoracic duct.
    (d) Infected lymph entered the lymphatic capillaries from the tissue spaces.

ANSWERS TO CLINICAL PROBLEMS

1. E. The tumor is mobile and not fixed to the joint capsule. The tumor is a neurofibroma of a digital nerve.
2. D
3. B
4. C. If possible, skin incisions in the neck are made in a horizontal direction to conform with the lines of cleavage.
5. D
6. C
7. D. The patellar tendon reflex (knee jerk) involves L2, 3, and 4 segments of the spinal cord.
8. B
9. A. In a 19-year-old boy, the bone marrow at the lower end of the tibia is yellow.
10. C. Lymph from the right upper limb enters the bloodstream through the right lymphatic duct.

REVIEW QUESTIONS

Completion Questions

Select the phrase that *best* completes each statement.

1. A patient who is standing in the anatomic position is
   (a). facing laterally.
   (b) has the palms of the hands directed medially.
   (c) has the ankles several inches apart.
   (d) is standing on his or her toes.
   (e) has the upper limbs by the sides of the trunk.
2. A patient is performing the movement of flexion of the hip joint when she
   (a) moves the lower limb away from the midline in the coronal plane.
   (b) moves the lower limb posteriorly in the paramedian plane.
   (c) moves the lower limb anteriorly in the paramedian plane.
   (d) rotates the lower limb so that the anterior surface faces medially.
   (e) moves the lower limb toward the median sagittal plane.

Matching Questions

Match each structure listed below with a structure or occurrence with which it is most closely associated. Each lettered answer may be used more than once.

3. Superficial fascia
4. Deep fascia
5. Skeletal muscle
   (a) Divides up interior of limbs into compartments
   (b) Adipose tissue
   (c) Tendon spindles
   (d) None of the above

For each joint listed below, indicate with which type of movement it is associated.

6. Sternoclavicular joint
7. Superior radioulnar joint
8. Ankle joint
   (a) Flexion
   (b) Gliding
   (c) Both A and B
   (d) Neither A nor B

For each joint listed below, give the most appropriate classification.

9. Joints between vertebral bodies
10. Inferior tibiofibular joint
11. Sutures between bones of vault of skull
12. Wrist joint
    (a) Synovial joint
    (b) Cartilaginous
    (c) Fibrous
    (d) None of the above

For each type of synovial joint listed below, give an appropriate example from the list of joints.

13. Hinge joint
14. Condyloid joint
15. Ball-and-socket joint
16. Saddle joint
    (a) Metacarpophalangeal joint of index finger
    (b) Shoulder joint
    (c) Wrist joint
    (d) Carpometacarpal joint of the thumb
    (e) None of the above

For each type of muscle action listed below, select the most appropriate definition.

17. Prime mover
18. Fixator
19. Synergist
20. Antagonist
    (a) A muscle that contracts isometrically to stabilize the origin of another muscle
    (b) A muscle that opposes the action of a flexor muscle
    (c) A muscle that is chiefly responsible for a particular movement
    (d) A muscle that prevents unwanted movements in an intermediate joint so that another muscle can cross that joint and act primarily on a distal joint
    (e) A muscle that opposes the action of a prime mover

For each type of blood vessel listed below, select an appropriate definition.

21. Arteriole
22. Portal vein
23. Anatomic end artery
24. Venule
    (a) A vessel that connects two capillary beds
    (b) A vessel whose terminal branches do not anastomose with branches or arteries supplying adjacent areas
    (c) A vessel that connects large veins to capillaries
    (d) An artery <0.1 mm in diameter
    (e) A thin-walled vessel that has an irregular cross diameter

For each of the lymphatic structures listed below, select an appropriate structure or function.

25. Lymph capillary
26. Thoracic duct
27. Right lymphatic duct
28. Lymph node
    (a) Present in the central nervous system
    (b) Drains lymph directly from the tissues
    (c) Contains lymphatic tissue and has both afferent and efferent vessels
    (d) Drains lymph from the right side of the head and neck, the right upper limb, and the right side of the thorax
    (e) Drains lymph from the right side of the abdomen

Multiple-Choice Questions

Directions: Read the case histories and select the *best* answer to the question following them.

The surgical notes of a patient state that she had a right infraumbilical paramedian incision through the skin of the anterior abdominal wall.

29. Where exactly was this incision made?
    (a) In the midline below the umbilicus
    (b) In the midline above the umbilicus
    (c) To the right of the midline above the umbilicus
    (d) To the right of the midline below the umbilicus
    (e) Just below the xiphoid process in the midline

After an attack of pericapsulitis of the left shoulder joint, a patient finds that a particular movement of the joint is restricted.

30. Which of the joint movements is restricted and by how much?
    (a) Abduction is limited to 30°.
    (b) Lateral rotation is limited to 45°.
    (c) Medial rotation is limited to 55°.
    (d) Flexion is limited to 90°.
    (e) Extension is limited to 45°.

ANSWERS TO REVIEW QUESTIONS

1. E
2. C
3. B
4. A
5. C
6. B
7. D
8. A
9. B
10. C
11. C
12. A
13. E
14. A
15. B
16. D
17. C
18. A
19. D
20. E
21. D
22. A
23. B
24. C
25. B
26. E
27. D
28. C
29. D
30. A

CHAPTER 2

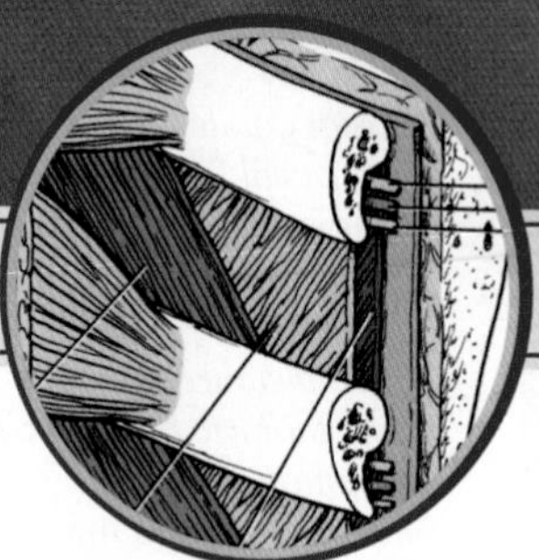

THE THORAX: PART I—THE THORACIC WALL

A 20-year-old woman was the innocent victim of a street shoot-out involving drugs. On examination, the patient showed signs of severe hemorrhage and was in a state of shock. Her pulse was rapid and her blood pressure was dangerously low. There was a small entrance wound about 1 cm across in the fourth left intercostal space about 3 cm from the lateral margin of the sternum. There was no exit wound. The left side of her chest was dull on percussion, and breath sounds were absent on that side of the chest. A chest tube was immediately introduced through the chest wall. Because of the massive amounts of blood pouring out of the tube, it was decided to enter the chest (thoracotomy). The physician carefully counted the ribs to find the fourth intercostal space and cut the layers of tissue to enter the pleural space (cavity). She was particularly careful to avoid important anatomic structures.

The incision was made in the fourth left intercostal space along a line that extended from the lateral margin of the sternum to the anterior axillary line. The following structures were incised: skin, subcutaneous tissue, pectoral muscles and serratus anterior muscle, external intercostal muscle and anterior intercostal membrane, internal intercostal muscle, innermost intercostal muscle, endothoracic fascia, and parietal pleura. The internal thoracic artery, which descends just lateral to the sternum and the intercostal vessels and nerve, must be avoided as the knife cuts through the layers of tissue to enter the chest. The cause of the hemorrhage was perforation of the left atrium of the heart by the bullet. A physician must have a knowledge of chest wall anatomy to make a reasoned diagnosis and institute treatment.

CHAPTER OUTLINE

Basic Anatomy 46
Structure of the Thoracic Wall 46
Sternum 46
Ribs 47
Costal Cartilages 51
Intercostal Spaces 52
Intercostal Muscles 52
Intercostal Arteries and Veins 53
Intercostal Nerves 55
Suprapleural Membrane 57
Endothoracic Fascia 57
Diaphragm 57
Internal Thoracic Artery 63
Internal Thoracic Vein 62
Levatores Costarum 63
Serratus Posterior Superior Muscle 63
Serratus Posterior Inferior Muscle 63
Radiographic Anatomy 63
Surface Anatomy 64
Anterior Chest Wall 64
Ribs 65
Diaphragm 65
Nipple 66
Apex Beat of the Heart 66
Axillary Folds 66
Posterior Chest Wall 66
Lines of Orientation 68
Trachea 68
Lungs 68
Pleura 72
Heart 72
Thoracic Blood Vessels 73
Mammary Gland 73
Clinical Problem Solving 73
Answers to Clinical Problems 74
Review Questions 75
Answers to Review Questions 76

CHAPTER OBJECTIVES

- An understanding of the structure of the chest wall and the diaphragm is essential if one is to understand the normal movements of the chest wall in the process of aeration of the lungs.
- Contained within the protective thoracic cage are the important life-sustaining organs—lungs, heart, and major blood vessels. In addition, the lower part of the cage overlaps the upper abdominal organs, such as the liver, stomach, and spleen, and offers them considerable protection. Although the chest wall is strong, blunt or penetrating wounds can injure the soft organs beneath it. This is especially so in an era in which automobile accidents, stab wounds, and gunshot wounds are commonplace.
- Because of the clinical importance of the chest wall, examiners tend to focus on this area. Questions concerning the ribs and their movements; the diaphragm, its attachments, and its function; and the contents of an intercostal space have been asked many times.

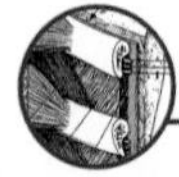

Basic Anatomy

The thorax (or chest) is the region of the body between the neck and the abdomen. It is flattened in front and behind but rounded at the sides. The framework of the walls of the thorax, which is referred to as the **thoracic cage,** is formed by the vertebral column behind, the ribs and intercostal spaces on either side, and the sternum and costal cartilages in front. Superiorly the thorax communicates with the neck, and inferiorly it is separated from the abdomen by the diaphragm. The thoracic cage protects the lungs and heart and affords attachment for the muscles of the thorax, upper extremity, abdomen, and back.

The cavity of the thorax can be divided into a median partition, called the **mediastinum,** and the laterally placed pleurae and lungs. The lungs are covered by a thin membrane called the **visceral pleura,** which passes from each lung at its root (i.e., where the main air passages and blood vessels enter) to the inner surface of the chest wall, where it is called the **parietal pleura.** In this manner, two membranous sacs called the **pleural cavities** are formed, one on each side of the thorax, between the lungs and the thoracic walls.

Structure of the Thoracic Wall

The thoracic wall is covered on the outside by skin and by muscles attaching the shoulder girdle to the trunk. It is lined with parietal pleura.

The thoracic wall is formed posteriorly by the thoracic part of the vertebral column; anteriorly by the sternum and costal cartilages (Fig. 2-1); laterally by the ribs and intercostal spaces; superiorly by the suprapleural membrane; and inferiorly by the diaphragm, which separates the thoracic cavity from the abdominal cavity.

Sternum

The sternum lies in the midline of the anterior chest wall. It is a flat bone that can be divided into three parts: manubrium sterni, body of the sternum, and xiphoid process.

The **manubrium** is the upper part of the sternum. It articulates with the body of the sternum at the manubriosternal joint, and it also articulates with the clavicles and with the first costal cartilage and the upper part of the second costal cartilages on each side (Fig. 2-1). It lies opposite the third and fourth thoracic vertebrae.

The **body of the sternum** articulates above with the manubrium at the **manubriosternal joint** and below with the xiphoid process at the **xiphisternal joint.** On each side it articulates with the second to the seventh costal cartilages (Fig. 2-1).

The **xiphoid process** (Fig. 2-1) is a thin plate of cartilage that becomes ossified at its proximal end during adult life. No ribs or costal cartilages are attached to it.

The **sternal angle** (angle of Louis), formed by the articulation of the manubrium with the body of the sternum, can be recognized by the presence of a transverse ridge on the anterior aspect of the sternum (Fig. 2-2). The transverse ridge lies at the level of the second costal cartilage, the point from which all costal cartilages and ribs are counted. The sternal angle lies opposite the intervertebral disc between the fourth and fifth thoracic vertebrae.

The **xiphisternal joint** lies opposite the body of the ninth thoracic vertebra (Fig. 2-2).

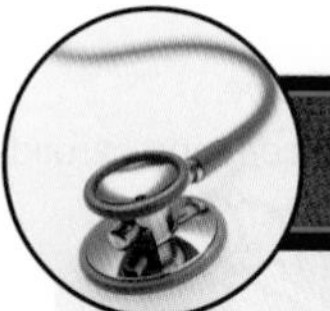

CLINICAL NOTES

Sternum and Marrow Biopsy

Since the sternum possesses red hematopoietic marrow throughout life, it is a common site for **marrow biopsy.** Under a local anesthetic, a wide-bore needle is introduced into the marrow cavity through the anterior surface of the bone. The sternum may also be split at operation to allow the surgeon to gain easy access to the heart, great vessels, and thymus.

Ribs

There are 12 pairs of ribs, all of which are attached posteriorly to the thoracic vertebrae (Figs. 2-1, 2-3, 2-4, and 2-5). The ribs are divided into three categories:

True ribs: The upper seven pairs are attached anteriorly to the sternum by their costal cartilages.

False ribs: The 8th, 9th, and 10th pairs of ribs are attached anteriorly to each other and to the 7th rib by

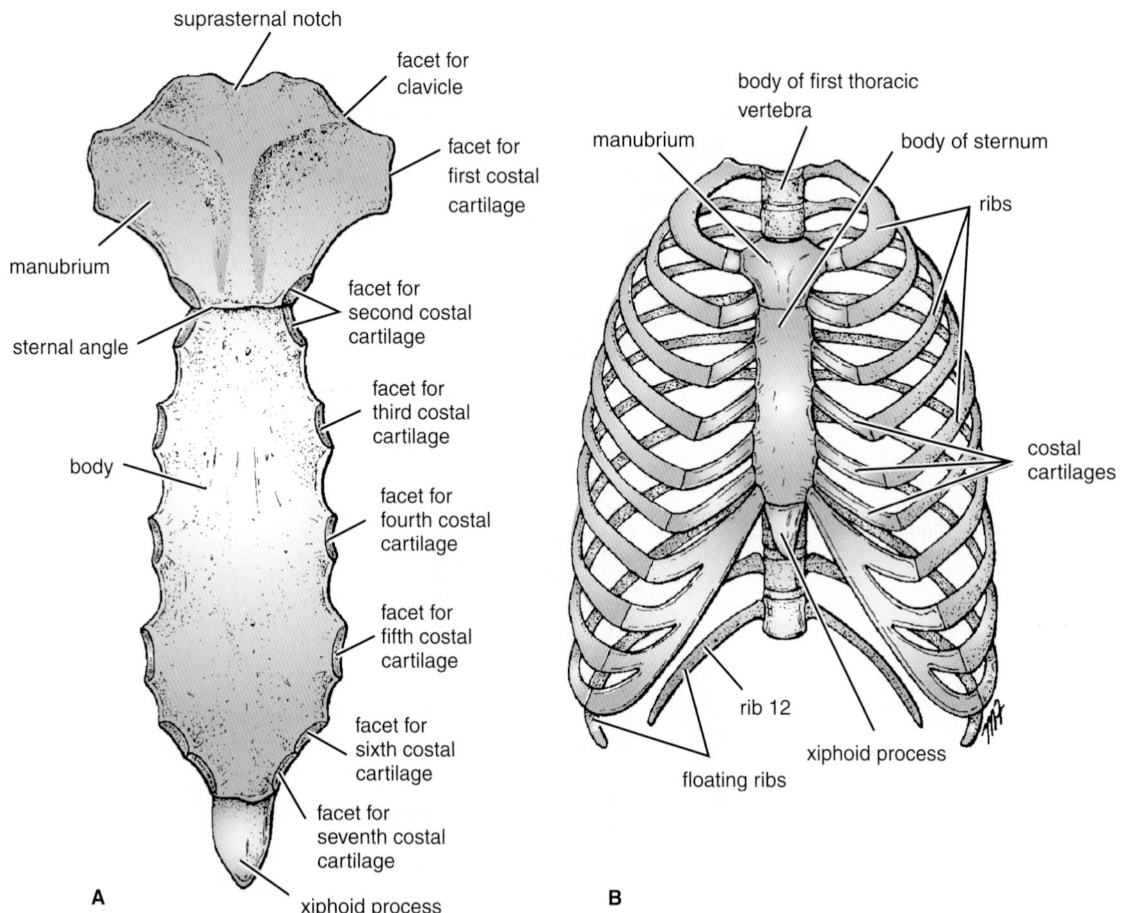

Figure 2-1 **A.** Anterior view of the sternum. **B.** Sternum, ribs, and costal cartilages forming the thoracic skeleton.

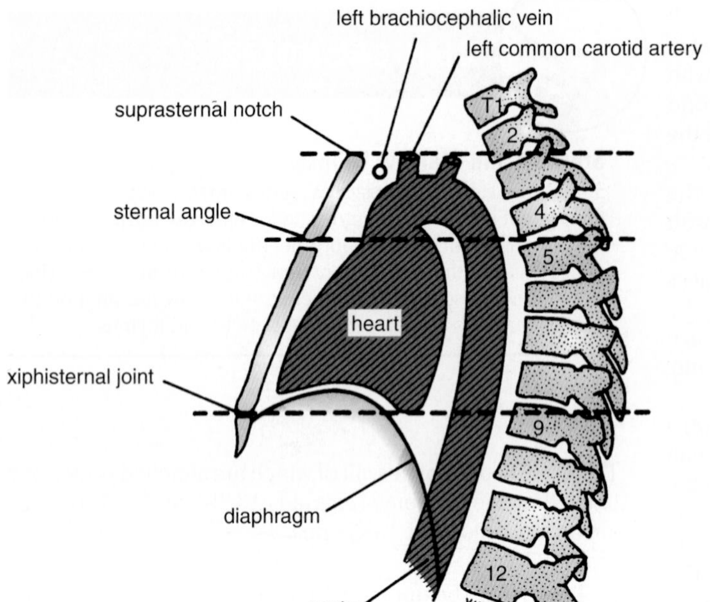

Figure 2-2 Lateral view of the thorax showing the relationship of the surface markings to the vertebral levels.

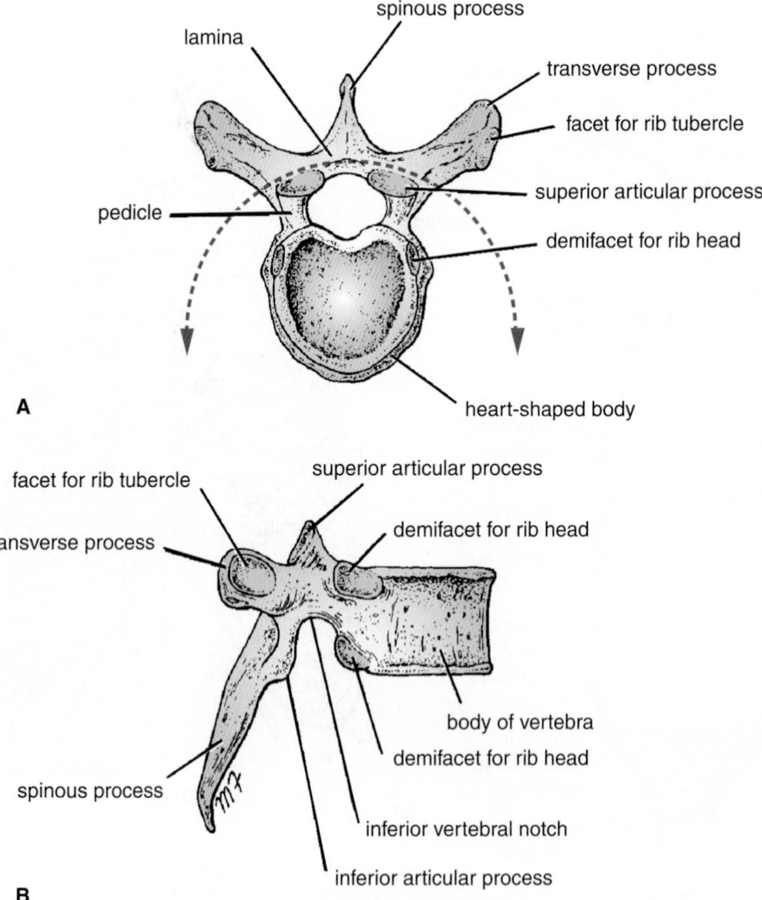

Figure 2-3 Thoracic vertebra. **A.** Superior surface. **B.** Lateral surface.

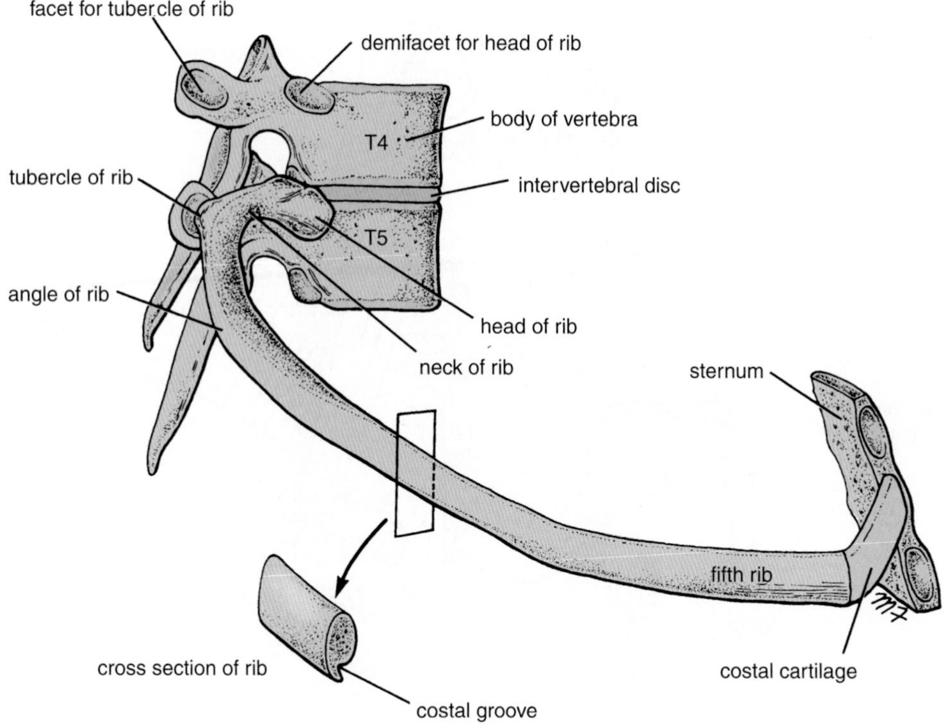

Figure 2-4 Fifth right rib as it articulates with the vertebral column posteriorly and the sternum anteriorly. Note that the rib head articulates with the vertebral body of its own number and that of the vertebra immediately above. Note also the presence of the costal groove along the inferior border of the rib.

means of their costal cartilages and small synovial joints.

Floating ribs: The 11th and 12th pairs have no anterior attachment.

Typical Rib

A typical rib is a long, twisted, flat bone having a rounded, smooth superior border and a sharp, thin inferior border (Figs. 2-4 and 2-5). The inferior border overhangs and forms the **costal groove,** which accommodates the intercostal vessels and nerve. The anterior end of each rib is attached to the corresponding costal cartilage (Fig. 2-4).

A rib has a **head, neck, tubercle, shaft,** and **angle** (Figs. 2-4 and 2-5). The **head** has two facets for articulation with the numerically corresponding vertebral body and that of the vertebra immediately above (Fig. 2-4). The **neck** is a constricted portion situated between the head and the

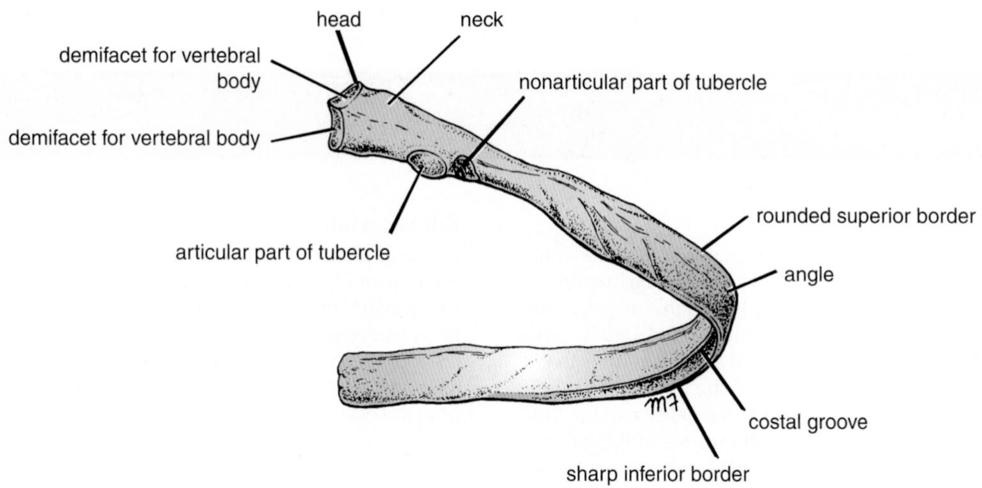

Figure 2-5 Fifth right rib, as seen from the posterior aspect.

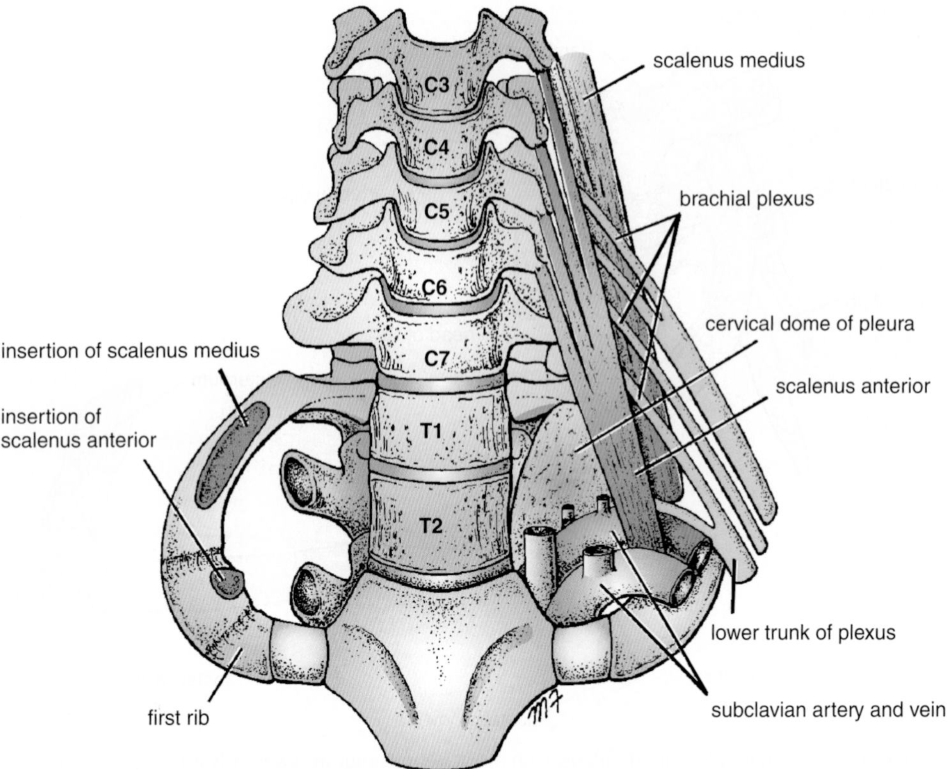

Figure 2-6 Thoracic outlet showing the cervical dome of pleura on the left side of the body and its relationship to the inner border of the first rib. Note also the presence of brachial plexus and subclavian vessels. (Anatomists often refer to the thoracic outlet as the thoracic inlet.)

tubercle. The **tubercle** is a prominence on the outer surface of the rib at the junction of the neck with the shaft. It has a facet for articulation with the transverse process of the numerically corresponding vertebra (Fig. 2-4). The shaft is thin and flattened and twisted on its long axis. Its inferior border has the costal groove. The angle is where the shaft of the rib bends sharply forward.

Atypical Rib

The first rib is important clinically because of its close relationship to the lower nerves of the brachial plexus and the main vessels to the arm, namely, the subclavian artery and vein (Fig. 2-6). This rib is small and flattened from above downward. The scalenus anterior muscle is attached to its upper surface and inner border. Anterior to the scalenus anterior, the subclavian vein crosses the rib; posterior to the muscle attachment, the subclavian artery and the lower trunk of the brachial plexus cross the rib and lie in contact with the bone.

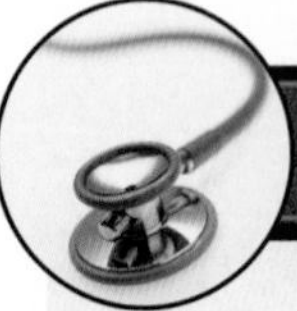

CLINICAL NOTES

Cervical Rib

A cervical rib (i.e., a rib arising from the anterior tubercle of the transverse process of the seventh cervical vertebra) occurs in about 0.5% of humans (Fig. 2-7). It may have a free anterior end, may be connected to the first rib by a fibrous band, or may articulate with the first rib. The importance of a cervical rib is that it can cause pressure on the lower trunk of the brachial plexus in some patients, producing pain down the medial side of the forearm and hand and wasting of the small muscles of the hand. It can also exert pressure on the overlying subclavian artery and interfere with the circulation of the upper limb.

Rib Excision

Rib excision is commonly performed by thoracic surgeons wishing to gain entrance to the thoracic cavity. A longitudinal incision is made through the periosteum on the outer surface of the rib and a segment of the rib is removed. A second longitudinal incision is then made through the bed of the rib, which is the inner covering of periosteum. After the operation, the rib regenerates from the osteogenetic layer of the periosteum.

Costal Cartilages

Costal cartilages are bars of cartilage connecting the upper seven ribs to the lateral edge of the sternum and the 8th, 9th, and 10th ribs to the cartilage immediately above. The cartilages of the 11th and 12th ribs end in the abdominal musculature (Fig. 2-1).

The costal cartilages contribute significantly to the elasticity and mobility of the thoracic walls. In old age, the costal cartilages tend to lose some of their flexibility as the result of superficial calcification.

Joints of the Chest Wall

Joints of the Sternum

The **manubriosternal joint** is a cartilaginous joint between the manubrium and the body of the sternum. A small amount of angular movement is possible during respiration. The **xiphisternal joint** is a cartilaginous joint between the xiphoid process (cartilage) and the body of the sternum. The xiphoid process usually fuses with the body of the sternum during middle age.

Joints of the Ribs

Joints of the Heads of the Ribs

The first rib and the three lowest ribs have a single synovial joint with their corresponding vertebral body. For the second to the ninth ribs, the head articulates by means of a synovial joint with the corresponding vertebral body and that of the vertebra above it (Fig. 2-4). There is a strong **intraarticular ligament** that connects the head to the intervertebral disc.

Joints of the Tubercles of the Ribs

The tubercle of a rib articulates by means of a synovial joint with the transverse process of the corresponding vertebra (Fig. 2-4). (This joint is absent on the 11th and 12th ribs.)

Joints of the Ribs and Costal Cartilages

These joints are cartilaginous joints. No movement is possible.

Joints of the Costal Cartilages with the Sternum

The first costal cartilages articulate with the manubrium, by cartilaginous joints that permit no movement (Fig. 2-1). The 2nd to the 7th costal cartilages articulate with the lateral border of the sternum by synovial joints. In addition, the 6th, 7th, 8th, 9th, and 10th costal cartilages articulate with one another along their borders by small synovial joints. The cartilages of the 11th and 12th ribs are embedded in the abdominal musculature.

Movements of the Ribs and Costal Cartilages

The 1st ribs and their costal cartilages are fixed to the manubrium and are immobile. The raising and lowering of the ribs during respiration are accompanied by movements in both the joints of the head and the tubercle, permitting the neck of each rib to rotate around its own axis.

Openings of the Thorax

The chest cavity communicates with the root of the neck through an opening called the **thoracic outlet.** It is called an outlet because important vessels and nerves emerge from the thorax here to enter the neck and upper limbs. The opening is bounded posteriorly by the first thoracic vertebra, laterally by the medial borders of the first ribs and their costal cartilages, and anteriorly by the superior border of the manubrium sterni. The opening is obliquely placed facing upward and forward. Through this small opening pass the esophagus and trachea and many vessels and nerves. Because of the obliquity of the opening, the apices of the lung and pleurae project upward into the neck.

The thoracic cavity communicates with the abdomen through a large opening. The opening is bounded posteriorly by the 12th thoracic vertebra, laterally by the curving costal margin, and anteriorly by the xiphisternal joint. Through this large opening, which is closed by the diaphragm, pass the esophagus and many large vessels and nerves, all of which pierce the diaphragm.

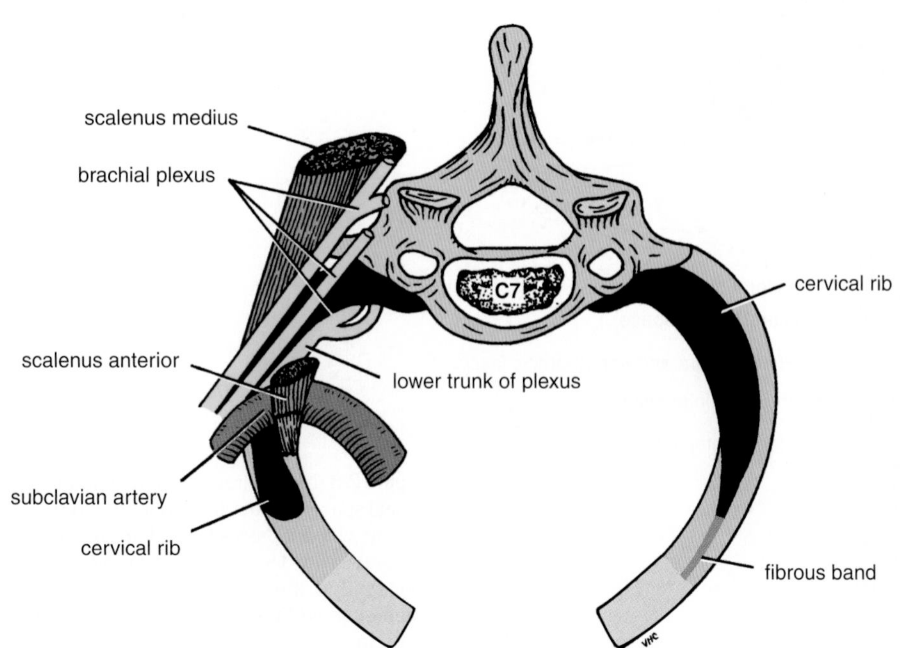

Figure 2-7 Thoracic outlet as seen from above. Note the presence of the cervical ribs (*black*) on both sides. On the right side of the thorax, the rib is almost complete and articulates anteriorly with the first rib. On the left side of the thorax, the rib is rudimentary but is continued forward as a fibrous band that is attached to the first costal cartilage. Note that the cervical rib may exert pressure on the lower trunk of the brachial plexus and may kink the subclavian artery.

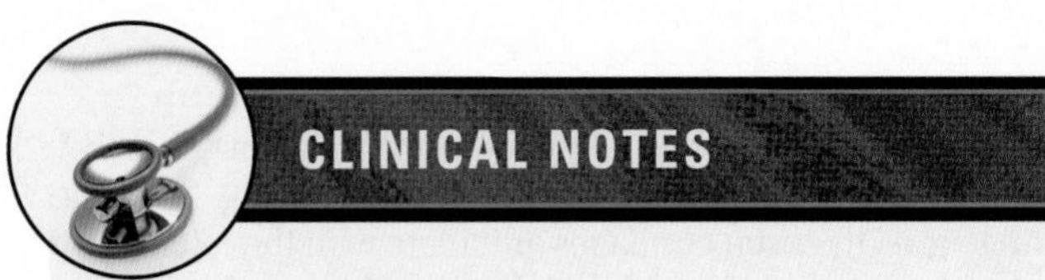

The Thoracic Outlet Syndrome

The brachial plexus of nerves (C5, 6, 7, and 8 and T1) and the subclavian artery and vein are closely related to the upper surface of the first rib and the clavicle as they enter the upper limb (see Fig. 2-6). It is here that the nerves or blood vessels may be compressed between the bones. Most of the symptoms are caused by pressure on the lower trunk of the plexus producing pain down the medial side of the forearm and hand and wasting of the small muscles of the hand. Pressure on the blood vessels may compromise the circulation of the upper limb.

Intercostal Spaces

The spaces between the ribs contain three muscles of respiration: the external intercostal, the internal intercostal, and the innermost intercostal muscle. The innermost intercostal muscle is lined internally by the **endothoracic fascia,** which is lined internally by the parietal pleura. The intercostal nerves and blood vessels run between the intermediate and deepest layers of muscles (Fig. 2-8). They are arranged in the following order from above downward: intercostal vein, intercostal artery, and intercostal nerve (i.e., VAN).

Intercostal Muscles

The **external intercostal muscle** forms the most superficial layer. Its fibers are directed downward and forward from the inferior border of the rib above to the superior

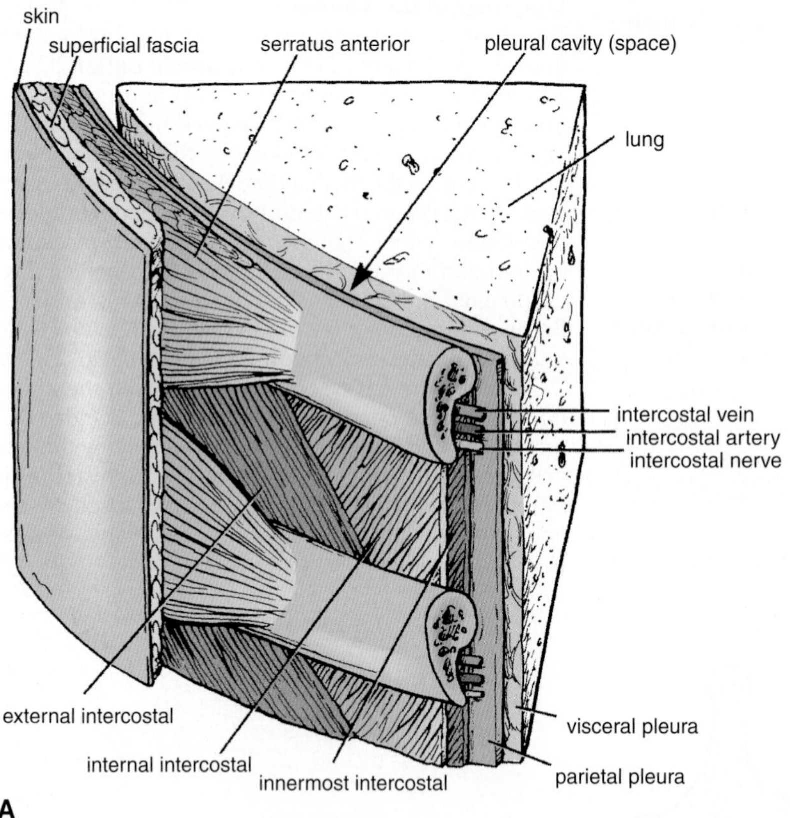

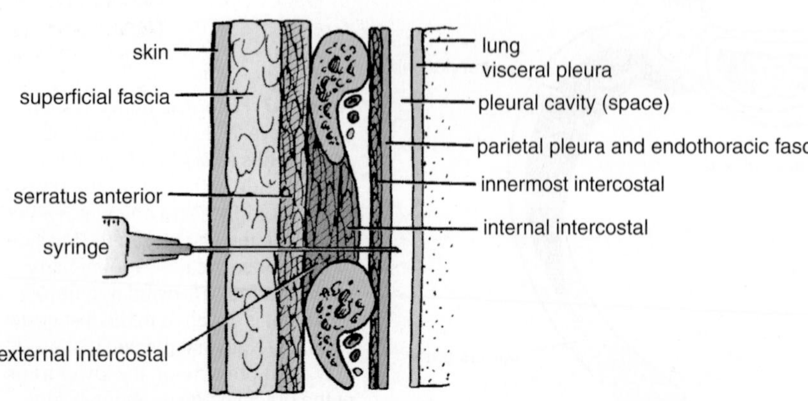

Figure 2-8 **A.** Section through an intercostal space. **B.** Structures penetrated by a needle when it passes from skin surface to pleural cavity. Depending on the site of penetration, the pectoral muscles will be pierced in addition to the serratus anterior muscle.

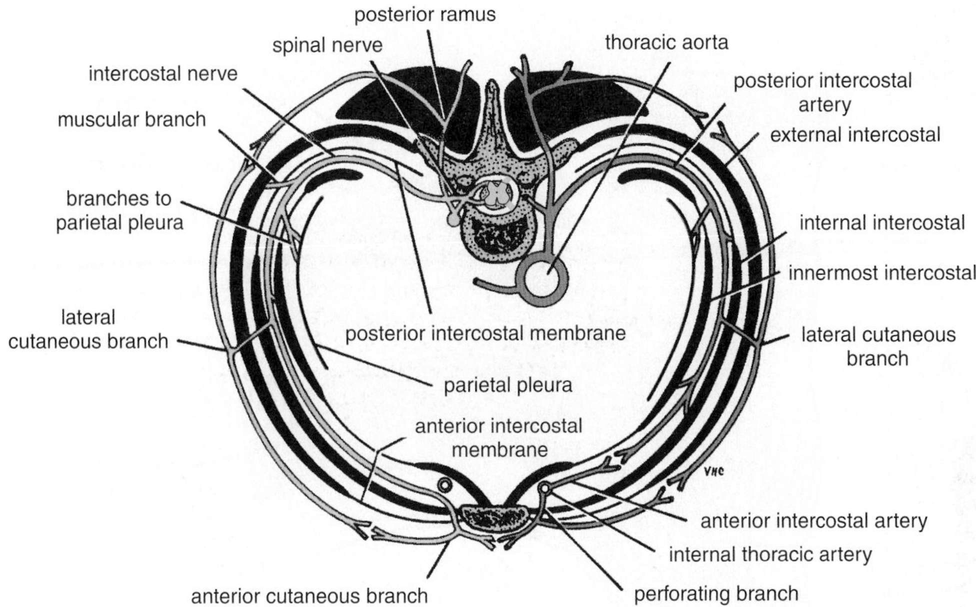

Figure 2-9 Cross section of the thorax showing distribution of a typical intercostal nerve and a posterior and an anterior intercostal artery.

border of the rib below (Fig. 2-8). The muscle extends forward to the costal cartilage where it is replaced by an aponeurosis, the **anterior (external) intercostal membrane** (Fig. 2-9).

The **internal intercostal muscle** forms the intermediate layer. Its fibers are directed downward and backward from the subcostal groove of the rib above to the upper border of the rib below (Fig. 2-8). The muscle extends backward from the sternum in front to the angles of the ribs behind, where the muscle is replaced by an aponeurosis, the **posterior (internal) intercostal membrane** (Fig. 2-9).

The **innermost intercostal muscle** forms the deepest layer and corresponds to the transversus abdominis muscle in the anterior abdominal wall. It is an incomplete muscle layer and crosses more than one intercostal space within the ribs. It is related internally to fascia (endothoracic fascia) and parietal pleura and externally to the intercostal nerves and vessels. The innermost intercostal muscle can be divided into three portions (Fig. 2-9), which are more or less separate from one another.

Action

When the intercostal muscles contract, they all tend to pull the ribs nearer to one another. If the 1st rib is fixed by the contraction of the muscles in the root of the neck, namely, the scaleni muscles, the intercostal muscles raise the 2nd to the 12th ribs toward the first rib, as in inspiration. If, conversely, the 12th rib is fixed by the quadratus lumborum muscle and the oblique muscles of the abdomen, the 1st to the 11th ribs will be lowered by the contraction of the intercostal muscles, as in expiration. In addition, the tone of the intercostal muscles during the different phases of respiration serves to strengthen the tissues of the intercostal spaces, thus preventing the sucking in or the blowing out of the tissues with changes in intrathoracic pressure. For further details concerning the action of these muscles, see **mechanics of respiration** on page 100.

Nerve Supply

The intercostal muscles are supplied by the corresponding intercostal nerves.

The intercostal nerves and blood vessels (the neurovascular bundle), as in the abdominal wall, run between the middle and innermost layers of muscles (Figs. 2-8 and 2-9). They are arranged in the following order from above downward: intercostal vein, intercostal artery, and intercostal nerve (i.e., VAN).

Intercostal Arteries and Veins

Each intercostal space contains a large single posterior intercostal artery and two small anterior intercostal arteries.

- The **posterior intercostal arteries** of the first two spaces are branches from the superior intercostal artery, a branch of the costocervical trunk of the subclavian artery. The posterior intercostal arteries of the lower nine spaces are branches of the descending thoracic aorta (Figs. 2-9 and 2-10).
- The **anterior intercostal arteries** of the first six spaces are branches of the internal thoracic artery (Figs. 2-9 and 2-10), which arises from the first part of the subclavian artery. The anterior intercostal arteries of the lower spaces are branches of the musculophrenic artery, one of the terminal branches of the internal thoracic artery.

Each intercostal artery gives off branches to the muscles, skin, and parietal pleura. In the region of the breast in the female, the branches to the superficial structures are particularly large.

The corresponding **posterior intercostal veins** drain backward into the azygos or hemiazygos veins (Figs. 2-10 and 2-11), and the **anterior intercostal veins** drain forward into the internal thoracic and musculophrenic veins.

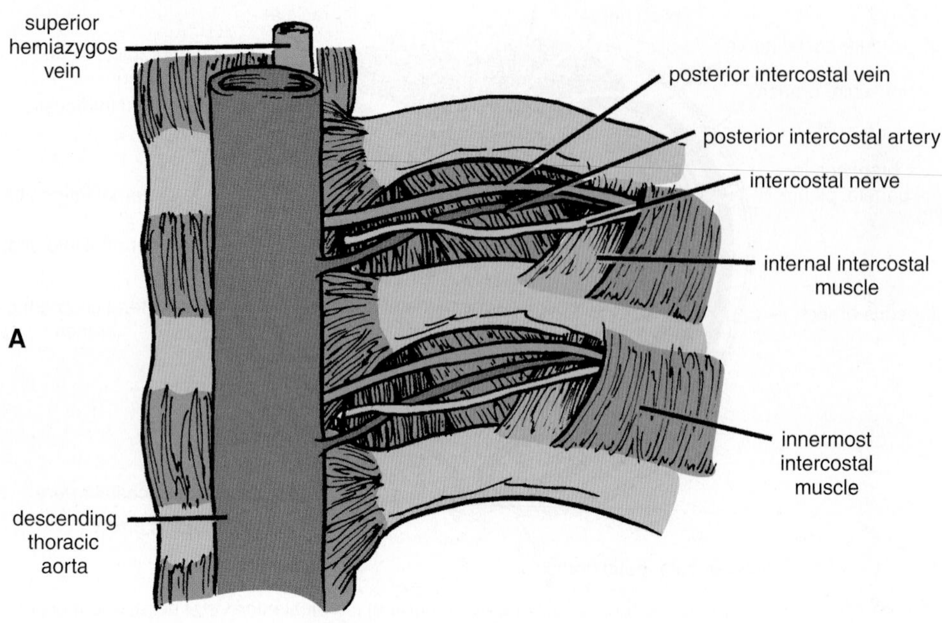

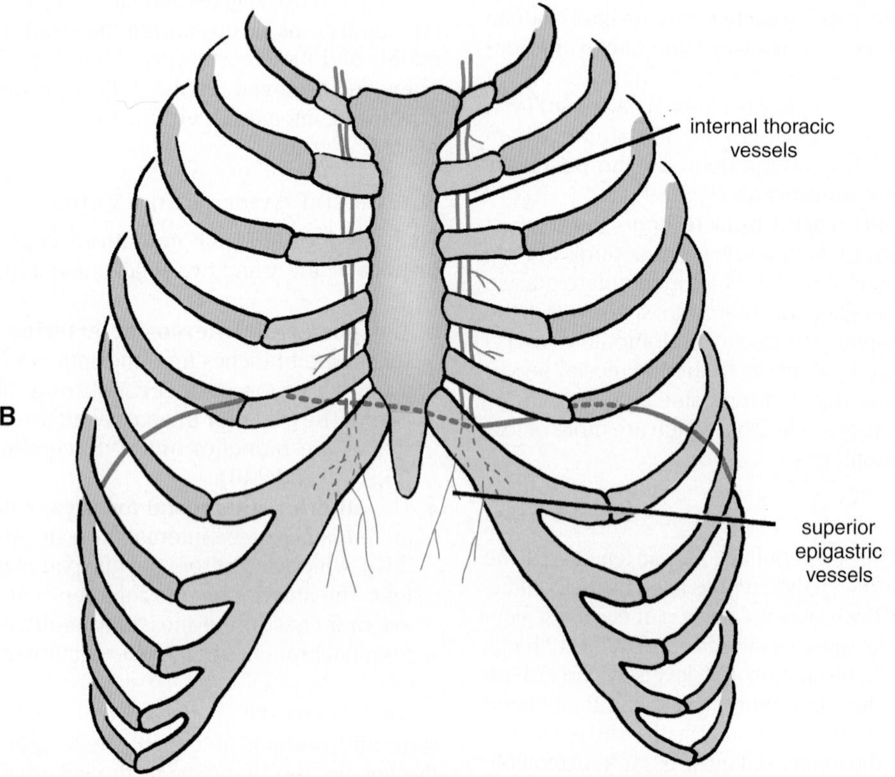

Figure 2-10 **A.** Internal view of the posterior end of two typical intercostal spaces; the posterior intercostal membrane has been removed for clarity. **B.** Anterior view of the chest showing the courses of the internal thoracic vessels. These vessels descend about one fingerbreadth from the lateral margin of the sternum.

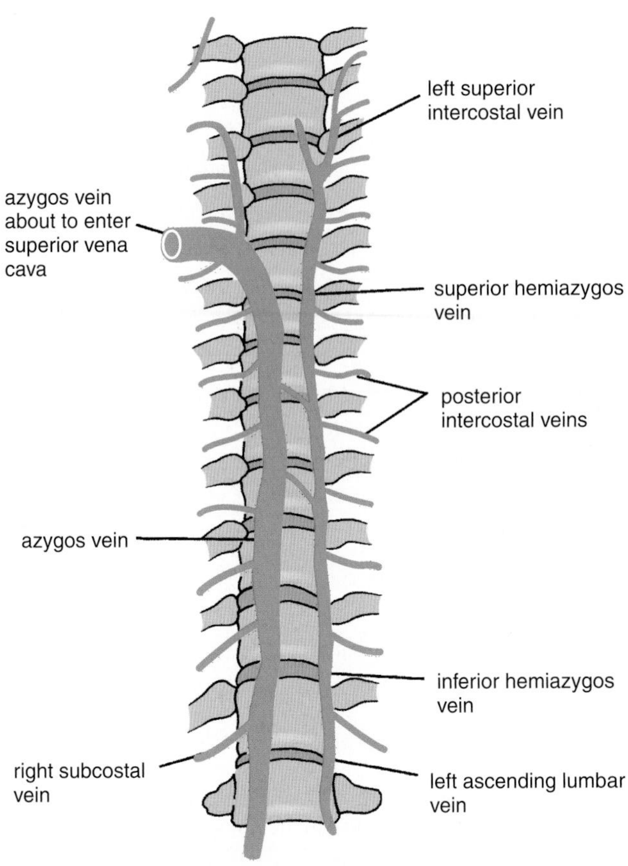

Figure 2-11 The common arrangement of the azygos vein, the superior hemiazygos (accessory hemiazygos) vein, and the inferior hemiazygos (hemiazygos) vein.

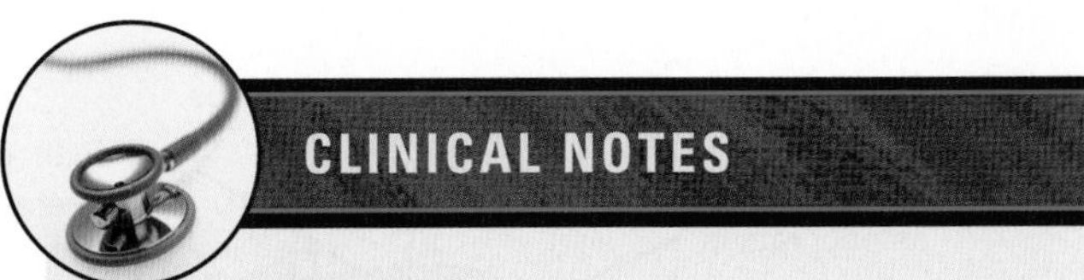

Skin Innervation of the Chest Wall and Referred Pain

Above the level of the sternal angle, the cutaneous innervation of the anterior chest wall is derived from the **supraclavicular nerves** (C3 and 4). Below this level, the anterior and lateral cutaneous branches of the intercostal nerves supply oblique bands of skin in regular sequence. The skin on the posterior surface of the chest wall is supplied by the posterior rami of the spinal nerves. The arrangement of the dermatomes is shown in Figures 1-23 and 1-24.

An intercostal nerve not only supplies areas of skin, but also supplies the ribs, costal cartilages, intercostal muscles, and parietal pleura lining the intercostal space. Furthermore, the 7th to 11th intercostal nerves leave the thoracic wall and enter the anterior abdominal wall so that they, in addition, supply dermatomes on the anterior abdominal wall, muscles of the anterior abdominal wall, and parietal peritoneum. This latter fact is of great clinical importance because it means that disease in the thoracic wall may be revealed as pain in a dermatome that extends across the costal margin into the anterior abdominal wall. For example, a pulmonary thromboembolism or a pneumonia with pleurisy involving the costal parietal pleura could give rise to abdominal pain and tenderness and rigidity of the abdominal musculature. The abdominal pain in these instances is called **referred pain.**

Herpes Zoster

Herpes zoster, or shingles, is a relatively common condition caused by the reactivation of the latent varicella-zoster virus in a patient who has previously had chickenpox. The lesion is seen as an inflammation and degeneration of the sensory neuron in a cranial or spinal nerve with the formation of vesicles with inflammation of the skin. In the thorax the first symptom is a band of dermatomal pain in the distribution of the sensory neuron in a thoracic spinal nerve, followed in a few days by a skin eruption. The condition occurs most frequently in patients older than 50 years.

Intercostal Nerves

The intercostal nerves are the anterior rami of the first 11 thoracic spinal nerves (Fig. 2-12). The anterior ramus of the 12th thoracic nerve lies in the abdomen and runs forward in the abdominal wall as the **subcostal nerve.**

Each intercostal nerve enters an intercostal space between the parietal pleura and the posterior intercostal membrane (Figs. 2-8 and 2-9). It then runs forward inferiorly to the intercostal vessels in the subcostal groove of the corresponding rib, between the innermost intercostal and internal intercostal muscle. The first six nerves are distributed within their intercostal spaces. The seventh to ninth intercostal nerves leave the anterior ends of their intercostal spaces by passing deep to the costal cartilages, to enter the anterior abdominal wall. The 10th and 11th nerves, since the corresponding ribs are floating, pass directly into the abdominal wall.

Branches

See Figures 2-9 and 2-12.

- **Rami communicantes** connect the intercostal nerve to a ganglion of the sympathetic trunk (see Fig. 1-26). The gray ramus joins the nerve medial at the point at which the white ramus leaves it.
- The **collateral branch** runs forward inferiorly to the main nerve on the upper border of the rib below.
- The **lateral cutaneous branch** reaches the skin on the side of the chest. It divides into an anterior and a posterior branch.
- The **anterior cutaneous branch,** which is the terminal portion of the main trunk, reaches the skin near the midline. It divides into a medial and a lateral branch.
- **Muscular branches** run to the intercostal muscles.
- **Pleural sensory branches** go to the parietal pleura.
- **Peritoneal sensory branches** (7th to 11th intercostal nerves only) run to the parietal peritoneum.

The **first intercostal nerve** is joined to the brachial plexus by a large branch that is equivalent to the lateral cutaneous branch of typical intercostal nerves. The remainder of the first intercostal nerve is small, and there is no anterior cutaneous branch.

The **second intercostal nerve** is joined to the medial cutaneous nerve of the arm by a branch called the **intercostobrachial nerve,** which is equivalent to the

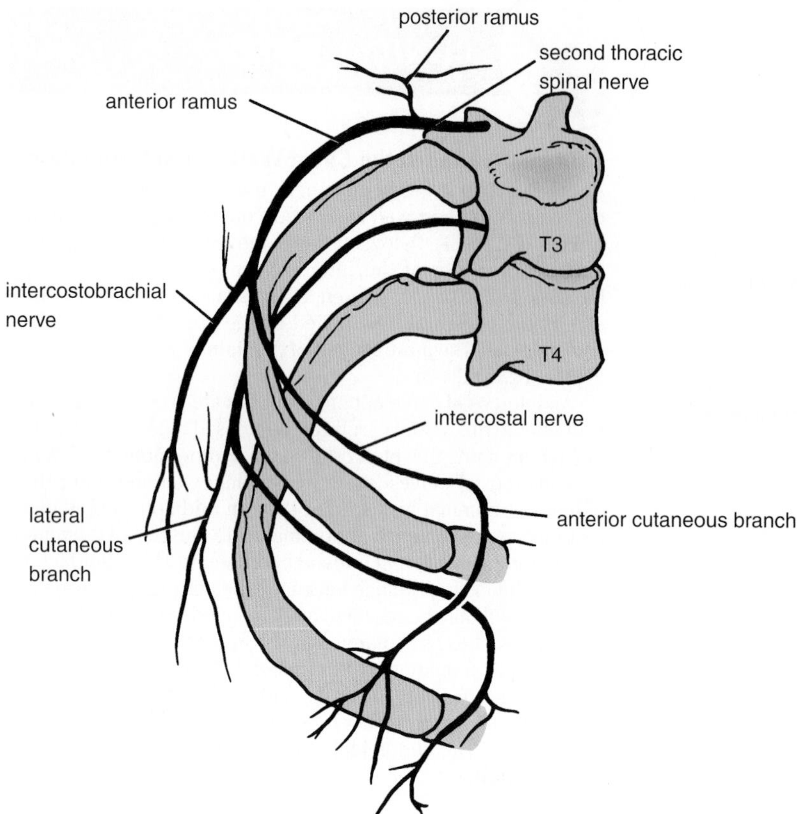

Figure 2-12 The distribution of two intercostal nerves relative to the rib cage.

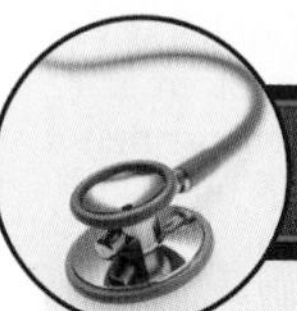

CLINICAL NOTES

Intercostal Nerve Block

Area of Anesthesia

The skin and the parietal pleura cover the outer and inner surfaces of each intercostal space, respectively; the 7th to 11th intercostal nerves supply the skin and the parietal peritoneum covering the outer and inner surfaces of the abdominal wall, respectively. Therefore, an intercostal nerve block will also anesthetize these areas. In addition, the periosteum of the adjacent ribs is anesthetized.

Indications

Intercostal nerve block is indicated for repair of lacerations of the thoracic and abdominal walls, for relief of pain in rib fractures, and to allow pain-free respiratory movements.

Procedure

To produce analgesia of the anterior and lateral thoracic and abdominal walls, the intercostal nerve should be blocked before the lateral cutaneous branch arises at the midaxillary line. The ribs may be identified by counting down from the 2nd (opposite sternal angle) or up from the 12th. The needle is directed toward the rib near the lower border (Fig. 2-8), and the tip comes to rest near the subcostal groove, where the local anesthetic is infiltrated around the nerve. Remember that the order of structures lying in the neurovascular bundle from above downward is intercostal vein, artery, and nerve and that these structures are situated between the posterior intercostal membrane of the internal intercostal muscle and the parietal pleura. Furthermore, laterally the nerve lies between the internal intercostal muscle and the innermost intercostal muscle.

Anatomy of Complications

Complications include pneumothorax and hemorrhage.

Pneumothorax can occur if the needle point misses the subcostal groove and penetrates too deeply through the parietal pleura.

Hemorrhage is caused by the puncture of the intercostal blood vessels. This is a common complication, so aspiration should always be performed before injecting the anesthetic. A small hematoma may result.

lateral cutaneous branch of other nerves. The second intercostal nerve therefore supplies the skin of the armpit and the upper medial side of the arm. **In coronary artery disease, pain is referred along this nerve to the medial side of the arm.**

With the exceptions noted, the first six intercostal nerves therefore supply the skin and the parietal pleura covering the outer and inner surfaces of each intercostal space, respectively, and the intercostal muscles of each intercostal space and the levatores costarum and serratus posterior muscles.

In addition, the 7th to the 11th intercostal nerves supply the skin and the parietal peritoneum covering the outer and inner surfaces of the abdominal wall, respectively, and the anterior abdominal muscles, which include the external oblique, internal oblique, transversus abdominis, and rectus abdominis muscles.

Suprapleural Membrane

Superiorly, the thorax opens into the root of the neck by a narrow aperture, the **thoracic outlet** (see page 51). The outlet transmits structures that pass between the thorax and the neck (esophagus, trachea, blood vessels, etc.) and for the most part lie close to the midline. On either side of these structures the outlet is closed by a dense fascial layer called the **suprapleural membrane** (Fig. 2-13). This tent-shaped fibrous sheet is attached laterally to the medial border of the first rib and costal cartilage. It is attached at its apex to the tip of the transverse process of the seventh cervical vertebra and medially to the fascia investing the structures passing from the thorax into the neck. It protects the underlying cervical pleura and resists the changes in intrathoracic pressure occurring during respiratory movements.

Endothoracic Fascia

The endothoracic fascia is a thin layer of loose connective tissue that separates the parietal pleura from the thoracic wall. The suprapleural membrane is a thickening of this fascia.

Diaphragm

The diaphragm is a thin muscular and tendinous septum that separates the chest cavity above from the abdominal cavity below (Fig. 2-16). It is pierced by the structures that pass between the chest and the abdomen.

The diaphragm is the most important muscle of respiration. It is dome shaped and consists of a peripheral muscular part, which arises from the margins of the thoracic opening, and a centrally placed tendon (Fig. 2-16). The origin of the diaphragm can be divided into three parts:

- A **sternal part** arising from the posterior surface of the xiphoid process (Fig. 2-2)
- A **costal part** arising from the deep surfaces of the lower six ribs and their costal cartilages (Fig. 2-16)
- A **vertebral part** arising by vertical columns or crura and from the arcuate ligaments

The **right crus** arises from the sides of the bodies of the first three lumbar vertebrae and the intervertebral discs; the **left crus** arises from the sides of the bodies of the first

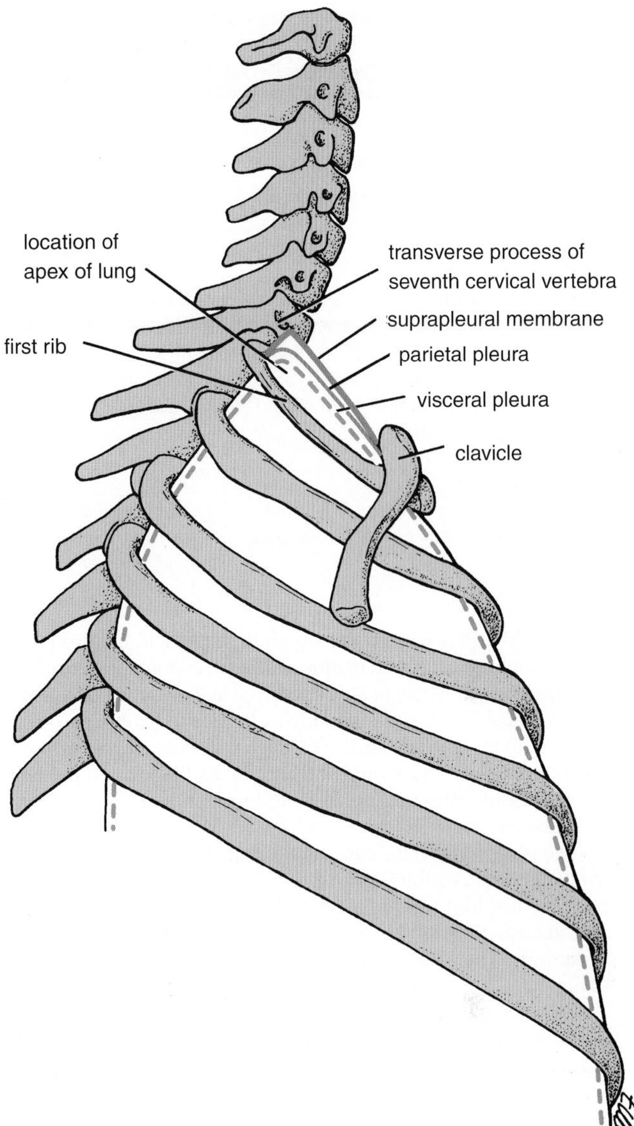

Figure 2-13 Lateral view of the upper opening of the thoracic cage showing how the apex of the lung projects superiorly into the root of the neck. The apex of the lung is covered with visceral and parietal layers of pleura and is protected by the suprapleural membrane, which is a thickening of the endothoracic fascia.

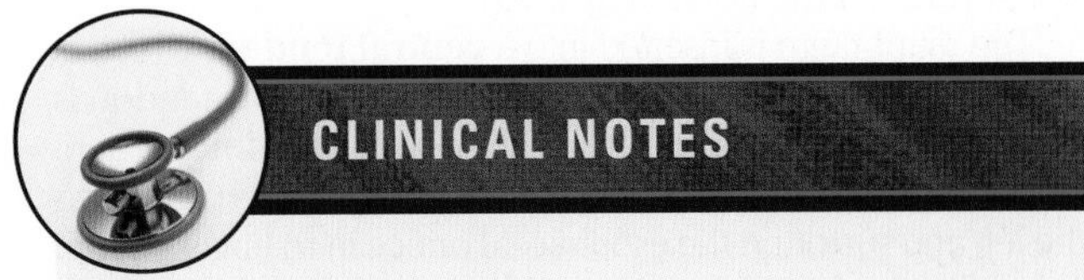

Thoracic Cage Distortion

The shape of the thorax can be distorted by congenital anomalies of the vertebral column or by the ribs. Destructive disease of the vertebral column that produces lateral flexion or scoliosis results in marked distortion of the thoracic cage.

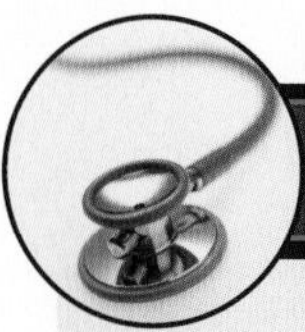

CLINICAL NOTES

Traumatic Injury to the Thorax

Traumatic injury to the thorax is common, especially as a result of automobile accidents.

Fractured Sternum

The sternum is a resilient structure that is held in position by relatively pliable costal cartilages and bendable ribs. For these reasons, fracture of the sternum is not common; however, it does occur in high-speed motor vehicle accidents. Remember that the heart lies posterior to the sternum and may be severely contused by the sternum on impact.

Rib Contusion

Bruising of a rib, secondary to trauma, is the most common rib injury. In this painful condition, a small hemorrhage occurs beneath the periosteum.

Rib Fractures

Fractures of the ribs are common chest injuries. In children, the ribs are highly elastic, and fractures in this age group are therefore rare. Unfortunately, the pliable chest wall in the young can be easily compressed so that the underlying lungs and heart may be injured. With increasing age, the rib cage becomes more rigid, owing to the deposit of calcium in the costal cartilages, and the ribs become brittle. The ribs then tend to break at their weakest part, their angles.

The ribs prone to fracture are those that are exposed or relatively fixed. Ribs 5 through 10 are the most commonly fractured ribs. The first four ribs are protected by the clavicle and pectoral muscles anteriorly and by the scapula and its associated muscles posteriorly. The 11th and 12th ribs float and move with the force of impact.

Because the rib is sandwiched between the skin externally and the delicate pleura internally, it is not surprising that the jagged ends of a fractured rib may penetrate the lungs and present as a **pneumothorax.**

Severe localized pain is usually the most important symptom of a fractured rib. The periosteum of each rib is innervated by the intercostal nerves above and below the rib. To encourage the patient to breathe adequately, it may be necessary to relieve the pain by performing an intercostal nerve block.

Flail Chest

In severe crush injuries, a number of ribs may break. If limited to one side, the fractures may occur near the rib angles and anteriorly near the costochondral junctions. This causes flail chest, in which a section of the chest wall is disconnected to the rest of the thoracic wall. If the fractures occur on either side of the sternum, the sternum may be flail. In either case, the stability of the chest wall is lost, and the flail segment is sucked in during inspiration and driven out during expiration, producing paradoxical and ineffective respiratory movements.

Traumatic Injury to the Back of the Chest

The posterior wall of the chest in the midline is formed by the vertebral column. In severe posterior chest injuries the possibility of a vertebral fracture with associated injury to the spinal cord should be considered. Remember also the presence of the scapula, which overlies the upper seven ribs. This bone is covered with muscles and is fractured only in cases of severe trauma.

Traumatic Injury to the Abdominal Viscera and the Chest

When the anatomy of the thorax is reviewed, it is important to remember that the upper abdominal organs—namely, the liver, stomach, and spleen—may be injured by trauma to the rib cage. In fact, any injury to the chest below the level of the nipple line may involve abdominal organs as well as chest organs.

---

two lumbar vertebrae and the intervertebral disc (Fig. 2-16). Lateral to the crura the diaphragm arises from the **medial** and **lateral arcuate ligaments** (Fig. 2-16). The medial arcuate ligament extends from the side of the body of the second lumbar vertebra to the tip of the transverse process of the first lumbar vertebra. The lateral arcuate ligament extends from the tip of the transverse process of the first lumbar vertebra to the lower border of the 12th rib. The medial borders of the two crura are connected by a **median arcuate ligament,** which crosses over the anterior surface of the aorta (Fig. 2-16).

The diaphragm is inserted into a **central tendon,** which is shaped like three leaves. The superior surface of the tendon is partially fused with the inferior surface of the fibrous pericardium. Some of the muscle fibers of the right crus pass up to the left and surround the esophageal orifice in a slinglike loop. These fibers appear to act as a sphincter and possibly assist in the prevention of regurgitation of the stomach contents into the thoracic part of the esophagus (Fig. 2-16).

Shape of the Diaphragm

As seen from in front, the diaphragm curves up into **right and left domes,** or cupulae. The right dome reaches as high as the upper border of the fifth rib, and the left dome may reach the lower border of the fifth rib. (The right dome lies at a higher level, because of the large size of the right lobe of the liver.) The central tendon lies at the level of the xiphisternal joint. The domes support the right and left lungs, whereas the central tendon supports the heart. The levels of the diaphragm vary with the phase of respiration, the posture, and the degree of distention of the abdominal viscera. The diaphragm is lower when a person is sitting or standing; it is higher in the supine position and after a large meal.

When seen from the side, the diaphragm has the appearance of an inverted J, the long limb extending up from the vertebral column and the short limb extending forward to the xiphoid process (Fig. 2-2).

Nerve Supply of the Diaphragm

Motor nerve supply: The right and left phrenic nerves (C3, 4, 5)

Sensory nerve supply: The parietal pleura and peritoneum covering the central surfaces of the diaphragm are from the phrenic nerve and the periphery of the diaphragm is from the lower six intercostal nerves.

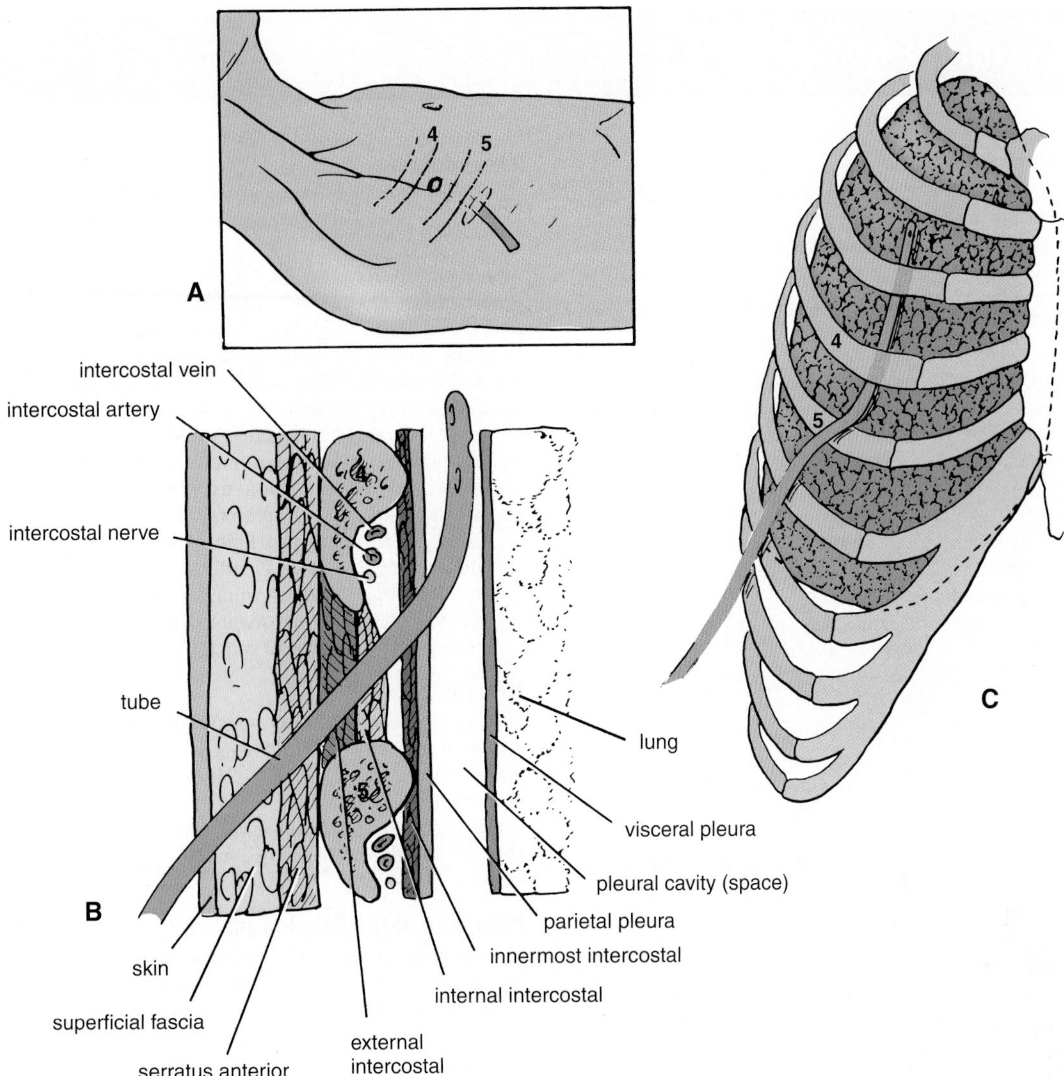

Figure 2-14 Tube thoracostomy. **A.** The site for insertion of the tube at the anterior axillary line. The skin incision is usually made over the intercostal space one below the space to be pierced. **B.** The various layers of tissue penetrated by the scalpel and later the tube as they pass through the chest wall to enter the pleural cavity (space). The incision through the intercostal space is kept close to the upper border of the rib to avoid injuring the intercostal vessels and nerve. **C.** The tube advancing superiorly and posteriorly in the pleural space.

Action of the Diaphragm

On contraction, the diaphragm pulls down its central tendon and increases the vertical diameter of the thorax.

Functions of the Diaphragm

- **Muscle of inspiration:** On contraction, the diaphragm pulls its central tendon down and increases the vertical diameter of the thorax. The diaphragm is the most important muscle used in inspiration.
- **Muscle of abdominal straining:** The contraction of the diaphragm assists the contraction of the muscles of the anterior abdominal wall in raising the intra-abdominal pressure for micturition, defecation, and parturition. This mechanism is further aided by the person taking a deep breath and closing the glottis of the larynx. The diaphragm is unable to rise because of the air trapped in the respiratory tract. Now and again, air is allowed to escape, producing a grunting sound.
- **Weight-lifting muscle:** In a person taking a deep breath and holding it (fixing the diaphragm), the diaphragm assists the muscles of the anterior abdominal wall in raising the intra-abdominal pressure to such an extent that it helps support the vertebral column and prevent flexion. This greatly assists the postvertebral muscles in the lifting of heavy weights. Needless to say, it is important to have adequate sphincteric control of the bladder and anal canal under these circumstances.
- **Thoracoabdominal pump:** The descent of the diaphragm decreases the intrathoracic pressure and at the same time increases the intra-abdominal pressure. This pressure change compresses the blood in the inferior vena cava and forces it upward into the right atrium of the heart. Lymph

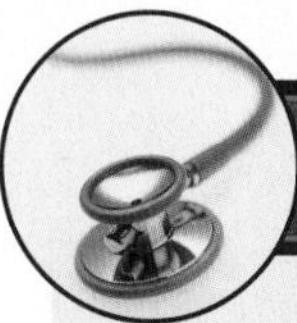

CLINICAL NOTES

Needle Thoracostomy

A needle thoracostomy is necessary in patients with tension pneumothorax (air in the pleural cavity under pressure) or to drain fluid (blood or pus) away from the pleural cavity to allow the lung to re-expand. It may also be necessary to withdraw a sample of pleural fluid for microbiologic examination.

Anterior Approach

For the anterior approach, the patient is in the supine position. The sternal angle is identified, and then the second costal cartilage, the second rib, and the second intercostal space are found in the midclavicular line.

Lateral Approach

For the lateral approach, the patient is lying on the lateral side. The second intercostal space is identified as above, but the anterior axillary line is used.

The skin is prepared in the usual way, and a local anesthetic is introduced along the course of the needle above the upper border of the third rib. The thoracostomy needle will pierce the following structures as it passes through the chest wall (Fig. 2-8): (a) skin, (b) superficial fascia (in the anterior approach the pectoral muscles are then penetrated), (c) serratus anterior muscle, (d) external intercostal muscle, (e) internal intercostal muscle, (f) innermost intercostal muscle, (g) endothoracic fascia, and (h) parietal pleura.

The needle should be kept close to the upper border of the third rib to avoid injuring the intercostal vessels and nerve in the subcostal groove.

Tube Thoracostomy

The preferred insertion site for a tube thoracostomy is the fourth or fifth intercostal space at the anterior axillary line (Fig. 2-14). The tube is introduced through a small incision. The neurovascular bundle changes its relationship to the ribs as it passes forward in the intercostal space. In the most posterior part of the space, the bundle lies in the middle of the intercostal space. As the bundle passes forward to the rib angle, it becomes closely related to the lower border of the rib above and maintains that position as it courses forward.

The introduction of a thoracostomy tube or needle through the lower intercostal spaces is possible provided that the presence of the domes of the diaphragm is remembered as they curve upward into the rib cage as far as the fifth rib (higher on the right). Avoid damaging the diaphragm and entering the peritoneal cavity and injuring the liver, spleen, or stomach.

Thoracotomy

In patients with penetrating chest wounds with uncontrolled intrathoracic hemorrhage, thoracotomy may be a life-saving procedure. After preparing the skin in the usual way, the physician makes an incision over the fourth or fifth intercostal space, extending from the lateral margin of the sternum to the anterior axillary line (Fig. 2-15). Whether to make a right or left incision depends on the site of the injury. For access to the heart and aorta, the chest should be entered from the left side. The following tissues will be incised (Fig. 2-14): (a) skin, (b) subcutaneous tissue, (c) serratus anterior and pectoral muscles, (d) external intercostal muscle and anterior intercostal membrane, (e) internal intercostal muscle, (f) innermost intercostal muscle, (g) endothoracic fascia, and (h) parietal pleura.

Avoid the **internal thoracic artery,** which runs vertically downward behind the costal cartilages about a fingerbreadth lateral to the margin of the sternum, and the **intercostal vessels** and **nerve,** which extend forward in the subcostal groove in the upper part of the intercostal space (Fig. 2-14).

Hiccup

Hiccup is the involuntary spasmodic contraction of the diaphragm accompanied by the approximation of the vocal folds and closure of the glottis of the larynx. It is a common condition in normal individuals and occurs after eating or drinking as a result of gastric irritation of the vagus nerve endings. It may, however, be a symptom of disease such as pleurisy, peritonitis, pericarditis, or uremia.

Paralysis of the Diaphragm

A single dome of the diaphragm may be paralyzed by crushing or sectioning of the phrenic nerve in the neck. This may be necessary in the treatment of certain forms of lung tuberculosis, when the physician wishes to rest the lower lobe of the lung on one side. Occasionally, the contribution from the fifth cervical spinal nerve joins the phrenic nerve late as a branch from the nerve to the subclavius muscle. This is known as the **accessory phrenic nerve.** To obtain complete paralysis under these circumstances, the nerve to the subclavius muscle must also be sectioned.

Penetrating Injuries of the Diaphragm

Penetrating injuries can result from stab or bullet wounds to the chest or abdomen. Any penetrating wound to the chest below the level of the nipples should be suspected of causing damage to the diaphragm until proved otherwise. The arching domes of the diaphragm can reach the level of the fifth rib (the right dome can reach a higher level).

---

within the abdominal lymph vessels is also compressed, and its passage upward within the thoracic duct is aided by the negative intrathoracic pressure. The presence of valves within the thoracic duct prevents backflow.

Openings in the Diaphragm

The diaphragm has three main openings:

- The **aortic opening** lies anterior to the body of the 12th thoracic vertebra between the crura (Fig. 2-16). It transmits the aorta, the thoracic duct, and the azygos vein.
- The **esophageal opening** lies at the level of the 10th thoracic vertebra in a sling of muscle fibers derived from the right crus (Fig. 2-16). It transmits the esophagus, the right and left vagus nerves, the esophageal branches of the left gastric vessels, and the lymphatics from the lower third of the esophagus.
- The **caval opening** lies at the level of the eighth thoracic vertebra in the central tendon (Fig. 2-16). It transmits the inferior vena cava and terminal branches of the right phrenic nerve.

In addition to these openings, the sympathetic splanchnic nerves pierce the crura; the sympathetic trunks pass posterior to the medial arcuate ligament on each side; and the superior epigastric vessels pass between the sternal and costal origins of the diaphragm on each side (Fig. 2-16).

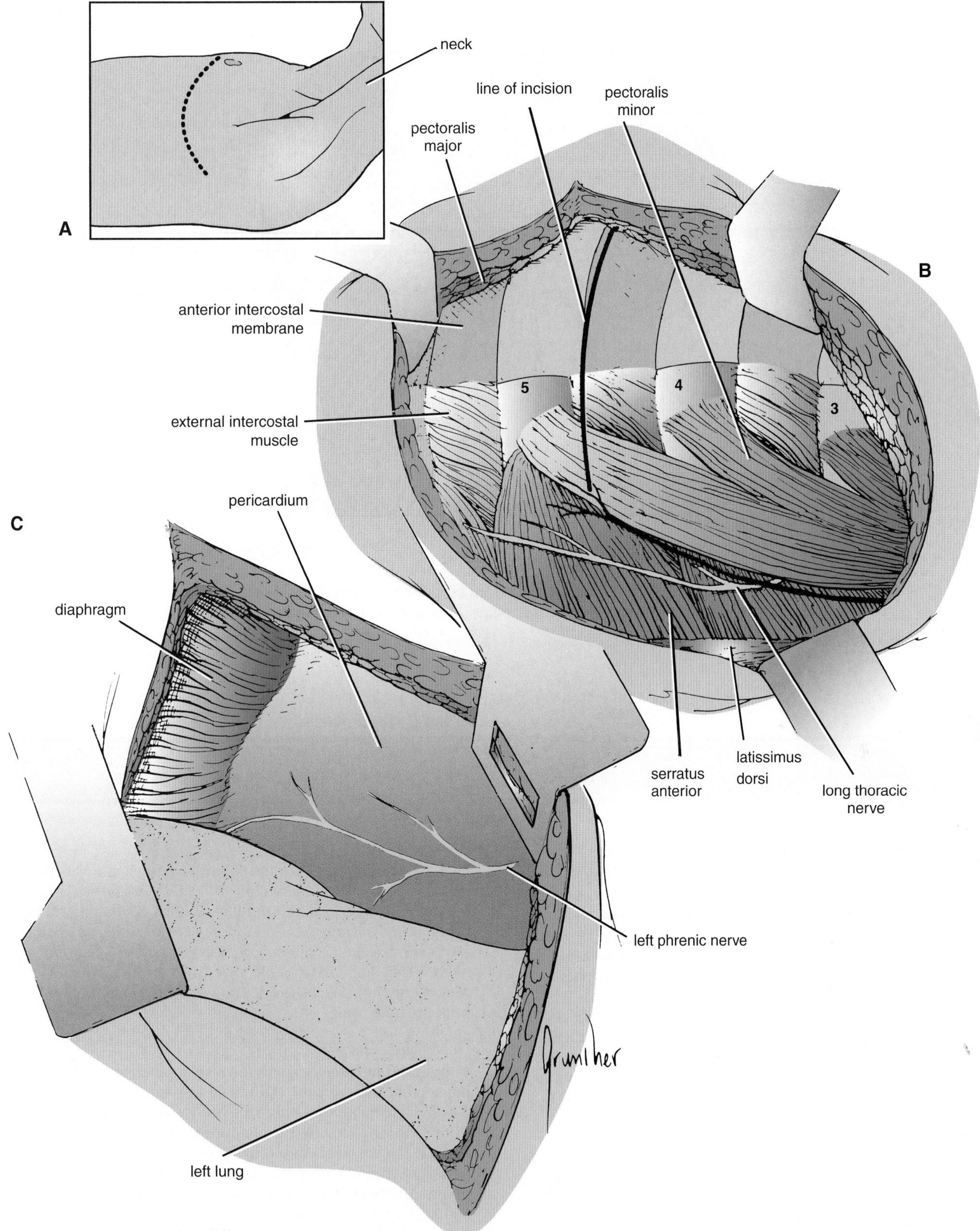

Figure 2-15 Left thoracotomy. **A.** Site of skin incision over fourth or fifth intercostal space. **B.** The exposed ribs and associated muscles. The line of incision through the intercostal space should be placed close to the upper border of the rib to avoid injuring the intercostal vessels and nerve. **C.** The pleural space opened and the left side of the mediastinum exposed. The left phrenic nerve descends over the pericardium beneath the mediastinal pleura. The collapsed left lung must be pushed out of the way to visualize the mediastinum.

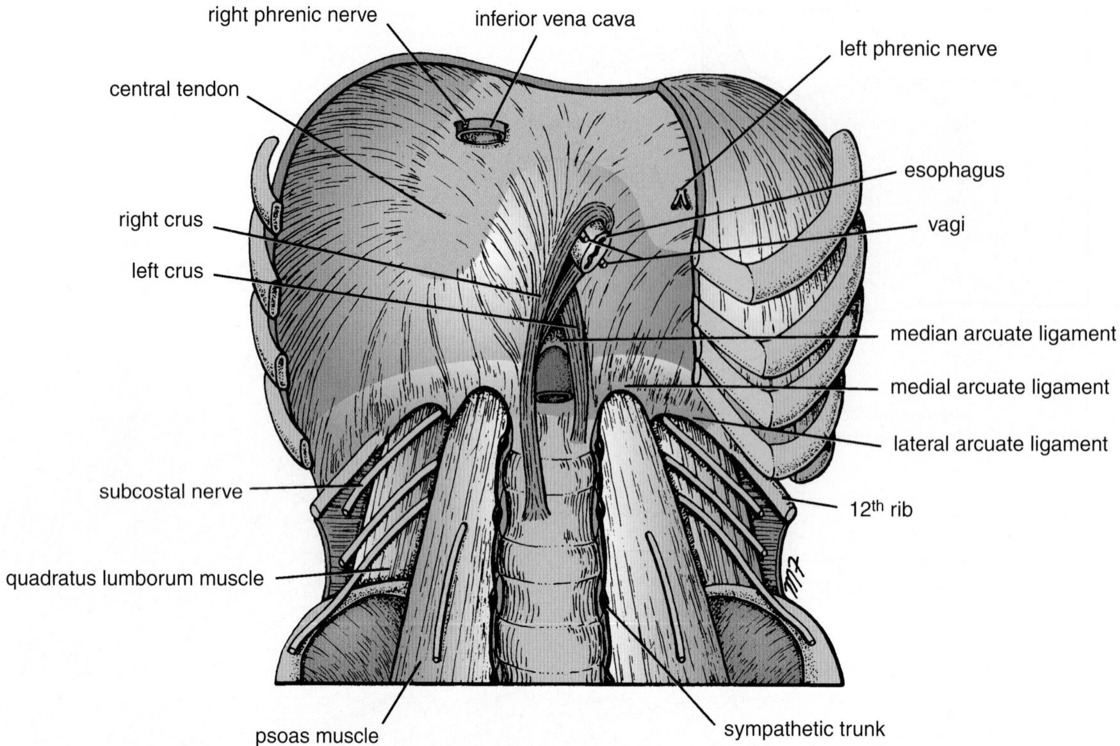

Figure 2-16 Diaphragm as seen from below. The anterior portion of the right side has been removed. Note the sternal, costal, and vertebral origins of the muscle and the important structures that pass through it.

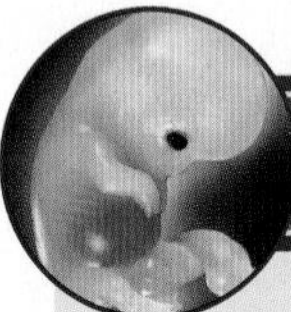

EMBRYOLOGIC NOTES

Development of the Diaphragm

The diaphragm is formed from the following structures: (a) the **septum transversum,** which forms the muscle and central tendon; (b) the two **pleuroperitoneal membranes,** which are largely responsible for the peripheral areas of the diaphragmatic pleura and peritoneum that cover its upper and lower surfaces, respectively; and (c) the dorsal mesentery of the esophagus, in which the crura develop.

The septum transversum is a mass of mesoderm that is formed in the neck by the fusion of the myotomes of the third, fourth, and fifth cervical segments. With the descent of the heart from the neck to the thorax, the septum is pushed caudally, pulling its nerve supply with it; thus, its motor nerve supply is derived from the third, fourth, and fifth cervical nerves, which are contained within the phrenic nerve.

The pleuroperitoneal membranes grow medially from the body wall on each side until they fuse with the septum transversum anterior to the esophagus and with the dorsal mesentery posterior to the esophagus. During the process of fusion, the mesoderm of the septum transversum extends into the other parts, forming all the muscles of the diaphragm.

The motor nerve supply to the entire muscle of the diaphragm is the phrenic nerve. The central pleura on the upper surface of the diaphragm and the peritoneum on the lower surface are also formed from the septum transversum, which explains their sensory innervation from the phrenic nerve. The sensory innervation of the peripheral parts of the pleura and peritoneum covering the peripheral areas of the upper and lower surfaces of the diaphragm is from the lower six thoracic nerves. This is understandable, since the peripheral pleura and peritoneum from the pleuroperitoneal membranes are derived from the body wall.

Diaphragmatic Herniae

Congenital herniae occur as the result of incomplete fusion of the septum transversum, the dorsal mesentery, and the pleuroperitoneal membranes from the body wall. The herniae occur at the following sites: (a) the pleuroperitoneal canal (more common on the left side; caused by failure of fusion of the septum transversum with the pleuroperitoneal membrane), (b) the opening between the xiphoid and costal origins of the diaphragm, and (c) the esophageal hiatus.

Acquired herniae may occur in middle-aged people with weak musculature around the esophageal opening in the diaphragm. These herniae may be either sliding or paraesophageal (Fig. 2-17).

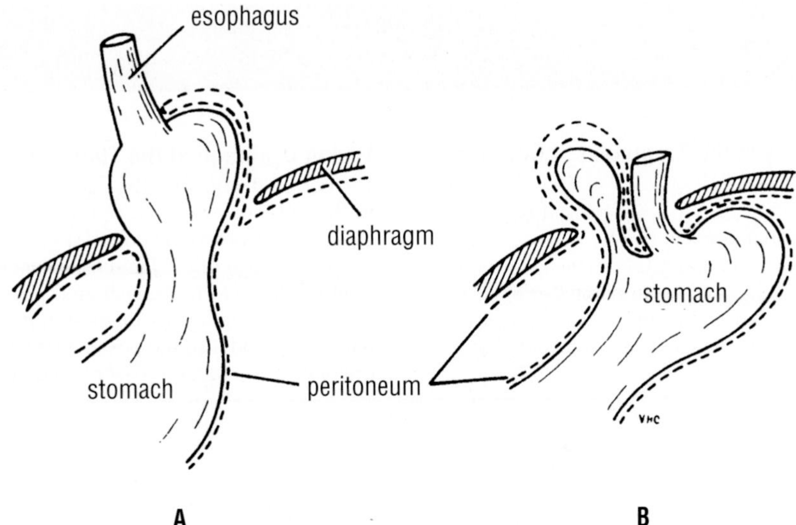

Figure 2-17 **A.** Sliding esophageal hernia. **B.** Paraesophageal hernia.

Internal Thoracic Artery

The internal thoracic artery supplies the anterior wall of the body from the clavicle to the umbilicus. It is a branch of the first part of the subclavian artery in the neck. It descends vertically on the pleura behind the costal cartilages, a fingerbreadth lateral to the sternum, and ends in the sixth intercostal space by dividing into the superior epigastric and musculophrenic arteries (Figs. 2-9 and 2-10).

Branches

- Two **anterior intercostal arteries** for the upper six intercostal spaces
- **Perforating arteries,** which accompany the terminal branches of the corresponding intercostal nerves
- The **pericardiacophrenic artery,** which accompanies the phrenic nerve and supplies the pericardium
- **Mediastinal arteries** to the contents of the anterior mediastinum (e.g., the thymus)
- The **superior epigastric artery,** which enters the rectus sheath of the anterior abdominal wall and supplies the rectus muscle as far as the umbilicus
- The **musculophrenic artery,** which runs around the costal margin of the diaphragm and supplies the lower intercostal spaces and the diaphragm

Internal Thoracic Vein

The internal thoracic vein accompanies the internal thoracic artery and drains into the brachiocephalic vein on each side.

Levatores Costarum

There are 12 pairs of muscles. Each levator costa is triangular in shape and arises by its apex from the tip of the transverse process and is inserted into the rib below.

- **Action:** Each raises the rib below and is therefore an inspiratory muscle.
- **Nerve supply:** Posterior rami of thoracic spinal nerves

Serratus Posterior Superior Muscle

The serratus posterior superior is a thin, flat muscle that arises from the lower cervical and upper thoracic spines. Its fibers pass downward and laterally and are inserted into the upper ribs.

- **Action:** It elevates the ribs and is therefore an inspiratory muscle.
- **Nerve supply:** Intercostal nerves

Serratus Posterior Inferior Muscle

The serratus posterior inferior is a thin, flat muscle that arises from the upper lumbar and lower thoracic spines. Its fibers pass upward and laterally and are inserted into the lower ribs.

- **Action:** It depresses the ribs and is therefore an expiratory muscle.
- **Nerve supply:** Intercostal nerves

A summary of the muscles of the thorax, their nerve supply, and their actions is given in Table 2-1.

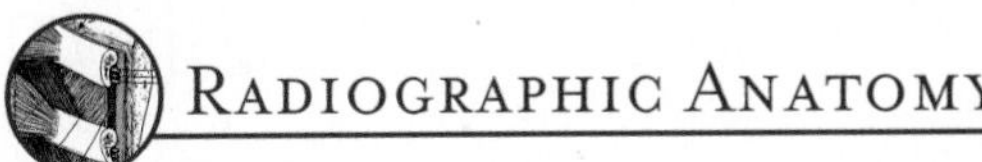

Radiographic Anatomy

This is fully described on page 131.

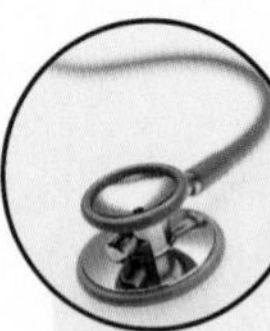

CLINICAL NOTES

Internal Thoracic Artery in the Treatment of Coronary Artery Disease

In patients with occlusive coronary disease caused by atherosclerosis, the diseased arterial segment can be bypassed by inserting a graft. The graft most commonly used is the great saphenous vein of the leg (see page 572). In some patients, the myocardium can be revascularized by surgically mobilizing one of the internal thoracic arteries and joining its distal cut end to a coronary artery.

Lymph Drainage of the Thoracic Wall

The **lymph drainage** of the skin of the anterior chest wall passes to the anterior axillary lymph nodes; that from the posterior chest wall passes to the posterior axillary nodes (Fig. 2-18). The lymph drainage of the intercostal spaces passes forward to the internal thoracic nodes, situated along the internal thoracic artery, and posteriorly to the posterior intercostal nodes and the para-aortic nodes in the posterior mediastinum. The lymphatic drainage of the breast is described on page 427.

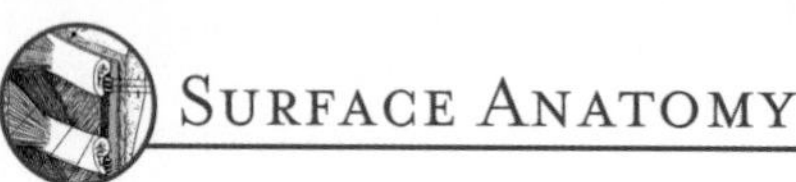

SURFACE ANATOMY

Anterior Chest Wall

The **suprasternal notch** is the superior margin of the manubrium sterni and is easily felt between the prominent medial ends of the clavicles in the midline (Figs. 2-19 and 2-20). It lies opposite the lower border of the body of the second thoracic vertebra (Fig. 2-2).

The **sternal angle (angle of Louis)** is the angle made between the manubrium and body of the sternum (Figs. 2-19 and 2-20). It lies opposite the intervertebral disc between the fourth and fifth thoracic vertebrae (Fig. 2-2). The position of the sternal angle can easily be felt and is often seen as a transverse ridge. The finger moved to the right or to the left will pass directly onto the second costal cartilage and then the second rib. All ribs may be counted from this point. Occasionally in a very muscular male, the ribs and intercostal spaces are often obscured by large pectoral muscles. In these cases, it may be easier to count up from the 12th rib.

The **xiphisternal joint** is the joint between the xiphoid process of the sternum and the body of the sternum (Fig. 2-21). It lies opposite the body of the ninth thoracic vertebra (Fig. 2-2).

The **subcostal angle** is situated at the inferior end of the sternum, between the sternal attachments of the seventh costal cartilages (Fig. 2-21).

The **costal margin** is the lower boundary of the thorax and is formed by the cartilages of the 7th, 8th, 9th, and 10th ribs and the ends of the 11th and 12th cartilages (Figs. 2-19 and 2-20). The lowest part of the costal margin is formed by the 10th rib and lies at the level of the third lumbar vertebra.

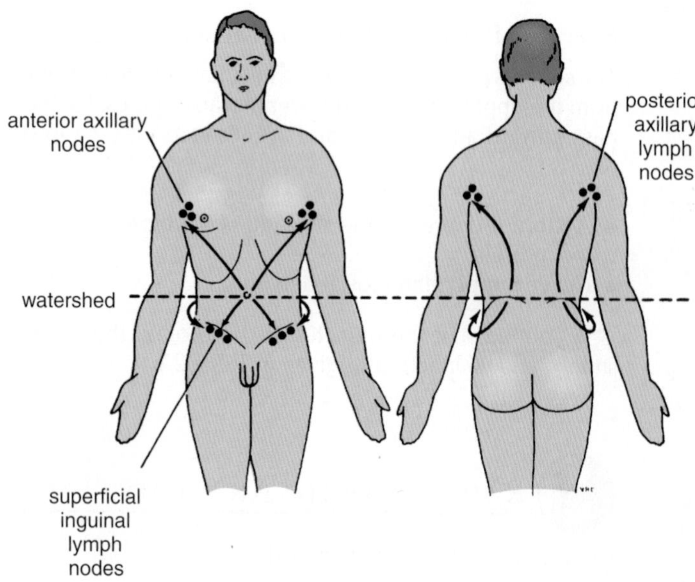

Figure 2-18 Lymph drainage of the skin of the thorax and abdomen. Note that levels of the umbilicus anteriorly and iliac crests posteriorly may be regarded as watersheds for lymph flow.

Table 2-1 Muscles of the Thorax

Name of Muscle	Origin	Insertion	Nerve Supply	Action
External intercostal muscle (11) (fibers pass downward and forward)	Inferior border of rib	Superior border of rib below	Intercostal nerves	With first rib fixed, they raise ribs during inspiration and thus increase anteroposterior and transverse diameters of thorax
Internal intercostal muscle (11) (fibers pass downward and backward)	Inferior border of rib	Superior border of rib below	Intercostal nerves	With last rib fixed by abdominal muscles, they lower ribs during expiration
Innermost intercostal muscle (incomplete layer)	Adjacent ribs	Adjacent ribs	Intercostal nerves	Assists external and internal intercostal muscles
Diaphragm (most important muscle of respiration)	Xiphoid process; lower six costal cartilages, first three lumbar vertebrae	Central tendon	Phrenic nerve	Very important muscle of inspiration; increases vertical diameter of thorax by pulling central tendon downward; assists in raising lower ribs Also used in abdominal straining and weight lifting
Levatores costarum (12)	Tip of transverse process of C7 and T1–11 vertebrae	Rib below	Posterior rami of thoracic spinal nerves	Raises ribs and therefore inspiratory muscles
Serratus posterior superior	Lower cervical and upper thoracic spines	Upper ribs	Intercostal nerves	Raises ribs and therefore inspiratory muscles
Serratus posterior inferior	Upper lumbar and lower thoracic spines	Lower ribs	Intercostal nerves	Depresses ribs and therefore expiratory muscles

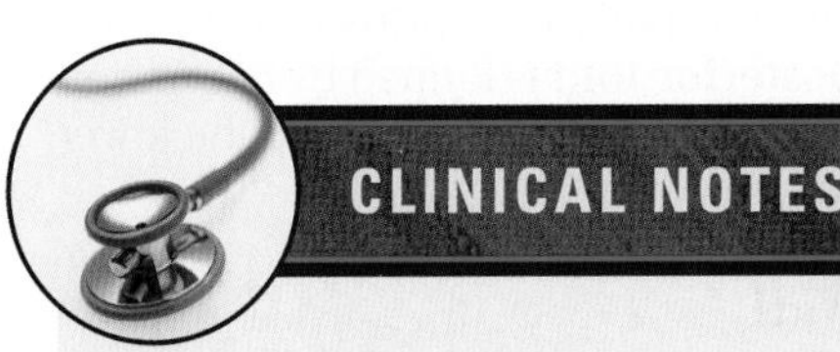

Anatomic and Physiologic Changes in the Thorax with Aging

Certain anatomic and physiologic changes take place in the thorax with advancing years:

- The **rib cage** becomes more rigid and loses its elasticity as the result of calcification and even ossification of the costal cartilages; this also alters their usual radiographic appearance.
- The stooped posture **(kyphosis),** so often seen in the old because of degeneration of the intervertebral discs, decreases the chest capacity.
- **Disuse atrophy** of the thoracic and abdominal muscles can result in poor respiratory movements.
- **Degeneration of the elastic tissue** in the lungs and bronchi results in impairment of the movement of expiration.

These changes, when severe, diminish the efficiency of respiratory movements and impair the ability of the individual to withstand respiratory disease.

The **clavicle** is subcutaneous throughout its entire length and can be easily palpated (Figs. 2-19 and 2-20). It articulates at its lateral extremity with the acromion process of the scapula.

Ribs

The first rib lies deep to the clavicle and cannot be palpated. The lateral surfaces of the remaining ribs can be felt by pressing the fingers upward into the axilla and drawing them downward over the lateral surface of the chest wall. The 12th rib can be used to identify a particular rib by counting from below. However, in some individuals, the 12th rib is very short and difficult to feel. For this reason, an alternative method may be used to identify ribs by first palpating the sternal angle and the second costal cartilage.

Diaphragm

The central tendon of the diaphragm lies directly behind the xiphisternal joint. In the midrespiratory position the summit of the right dome of the diaphragm arches upward as far as the upper border of the fifth rib in the midclavicular line, but the left dome only reaches as far as the lower border of the fifth rib.

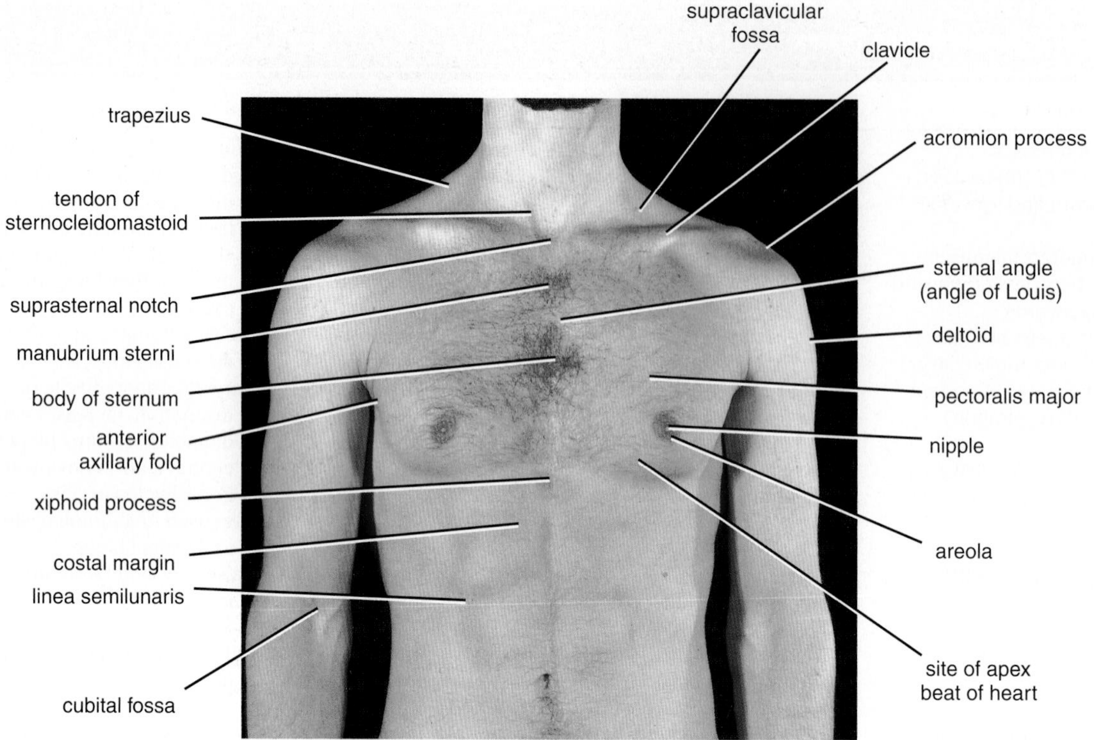

Figure 2-19 Anterior view of the thorax of a 27-year-old man.

Nipple

In the male, the nipple usually lies in the fourth intercostal space about 4 in. (10 cm) from the midline. In the female, its position is not constant.

Apex Beat of the Heart

The apex of the heart is formed by the lower portion of the left ventricle. The apex beat is caused by the apex of the heart being thrust forward against the thoracic wall as the heart contracts. (The heart is thrust forward with each ventricular contraction because of the ejection of blood from the left ventricle into the aorta; the force of the blood in the aorta tends to cause the curved aorta to straighten slightly, thus pushing the heart forward.) The apex beat can usually be felt by placing the flat of the hand on the chest wall over the heart. After the area of cardiac pulsation has been determined, the apex beat is accurately localized by placing two fingers over the intercostal spaces and moving them until the point of maximum pulsation is found. The apex beat is normally found in the fifth left intercostal space 3.5 in. (9 cm) from the midline. Should you have difficulty in finding the apex beat, have the patient lean forward in the sitting position.

In a female with pendulous breasts, the examining fingers should gently raise the left breast from below as the intercostal spaces are palpated.

Axillary Folds

The **anterior fold** is formed by the lower border of the pectoralis major muscle (Figs. 2-19 and 2-20). This can be made to stand out by asking the patient to press a hand hard against the hip. The **posterior fold** is formed by the tendon of the latissimus dorsi muscle as it passes around the lower border of the teres major muscle.

Posterior Chest Wall

The **spinous processes** of the **thoracic vertebrae** can be palpated in the midline posteriorly (Fig. 2-22). The index finger should be placed on the skin in the midline on the posterior surface of the neck and drawn downward in the nuchal groove. The first spinous process to be felt is that of the seventh cervical vertebrae **(vertebra prominens).** Below this level are the overlapping spines of the thoracic vertebrae. The spines of C1 to 6 vertebrae are covered by a large ligament, the ligamentum nuchae. It should be noted that the tip of a spinous process of a thoracic vertebra lies posterior to the body of the next vertebra below.

The **scapula** (shoulder blade) is flat and triangular in shape and is located on the upper part of the posterior surface of the thorax. The **superior angle** lies opposite the spine of the second thoracic vertebra (Figs. 2-20 and 2-22). The **spine of the scapula** is subcutaneous, and the root of the spine lies on a level with the spine of the third thoracic vertebra (Figs. 2-21 and 2-22). The **inferior angle** lies on a level with the spine of the seventh thoracic vertebra (Figs. 2-20 and 2-22).

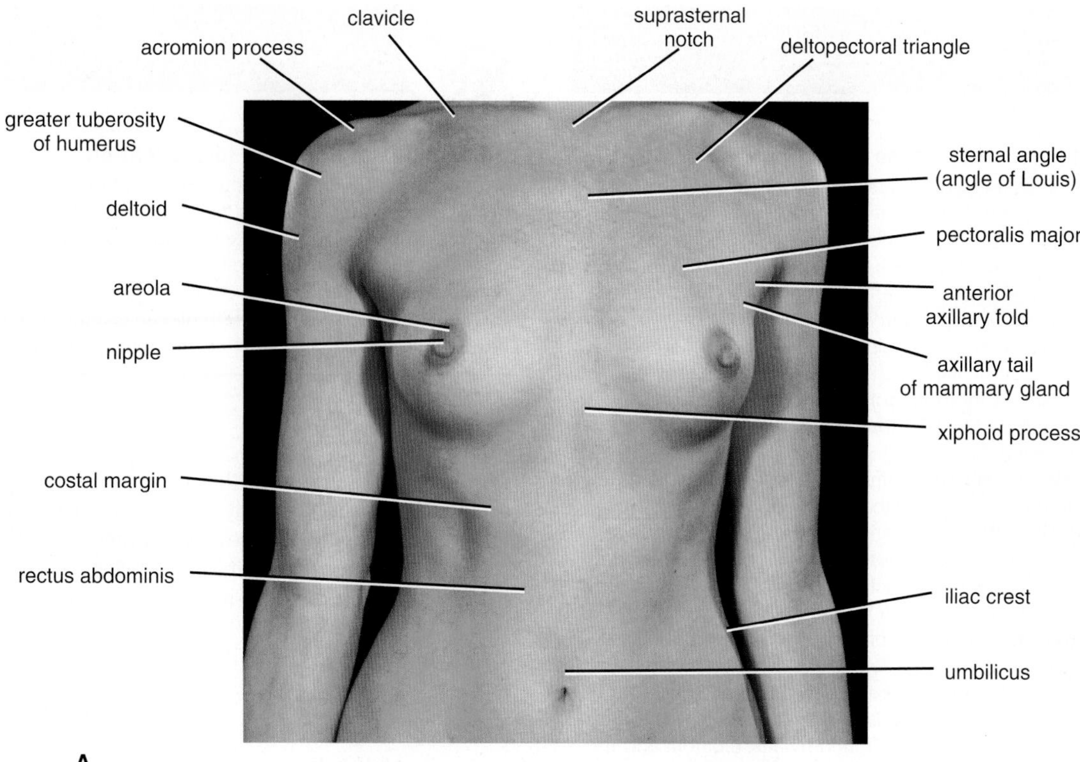

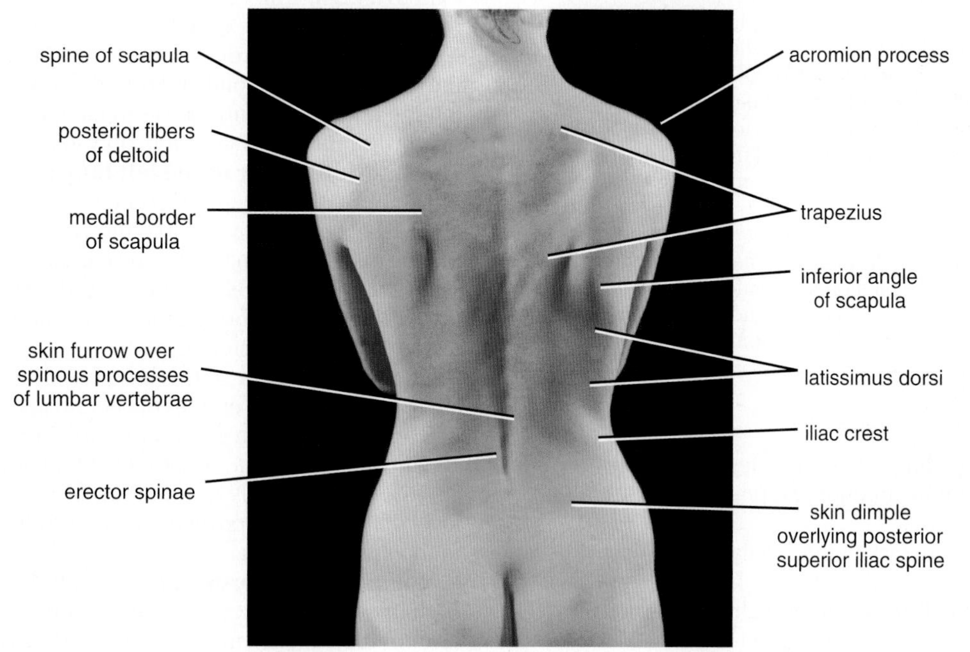

Figure 2-20 **A.** Anterior view of the thorax and abdomen of a 29-year-old woman. **B.** Posterior view of the thorax of a 29-year-old woman.

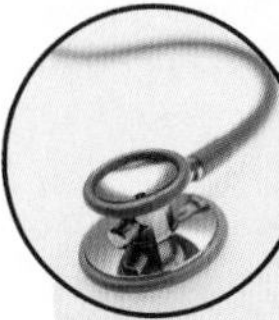

CLINICAL NOTES

Clinical Examination of the Chest

As medical personnel, you will be examining the chest to detect evidence of disease. Your examination consists of inspection, palpation, percussion, and auscultation.

Inspection shows the configuration of the chest, the range of respiratory movement, and any inequalities on the two sides. The type and rate of respiration are also noted.

Palpation enables the physician to confirm the impressions gained by inspection, especially of the respiratory movements of the chest wall. Abnormal protuberances or recession of part of the chest wall is noted. Abnormal pulsations are felt and tender areas detected.

Percussion is a sharp tapping of the chest wall with the fingers. This produces vibrations that extend through the tissues of the thorax. Air-containing organs such as the lungs produce a resonant note; conversely, a more solid viscus such as the heart produces a dull note. With practice, it is possible to distinguish the lungs from the heart or liver by percussion.

Auscultation enables the physician to listen to the breath sounds as the air enters and leaves the respiratory passages. Should the alveoli or bronchi be diseased and filled with fluid, the nature of the breath sounds will be altered. The rate and rhythm of the heart can be confirmed by auscultation, and the various sounds produced by the heart and its valves during the different phases of the cardiac cycle can be heard. It may be possible to detect friction sounds produced by the rubbing together of diseased layers of pleura or pericardium.

To make these examinations, the physician must be familiar with the normal structure of the thorax and must have a mental image of the normal position of the lungs and heart in relation to identifiable surface landmarks. Furthermore, it is essential that the physician be able to relate any abnormal findings to easily identifiable bony landmarks so that he or she can accurately record and communicate them to colleagues.

Since the thoracic wall actively participates in the movements of respiration, many bony landmarks change their levels with each phase of respiration. In practice, to simplify matters, the levels given are those usually found at about midway between full inspiration and full expiration.

Lines of Orientation

Several imaginary lines are sometimes used to describe surface locations on the anterior and posterior chest walls.

- **Midsternal line:** Lies in the median plane over the sternum (Fig. 2-21)
- **Midclavicular line:** Runs vertically downward from the midpoint of the clavicle (Fig. 2-21)
- **Anterior axillary line:** Runs vertically downward from the anterior axillary fold (Fig. 2-21)
- **Posterior axillary line:** Runs vertically downward from the posterior axillary fold
- **Midaxillary line:** Runs vertically downward from a point situated midway between the anterior and posterior axillary folds
- **Scapular line:** Runs vertically downward on the posterior wall of the thorax (Fig. 2-22), passing through the inferior angle of the scapula (arms at the sides)

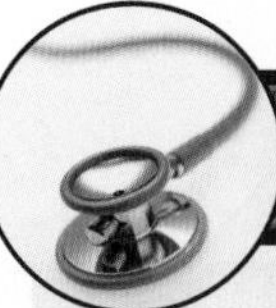

CLINICAL NOTES

Rib and Costal Cartilage Identification

When one is examining the chest from in front, the **sternal angle** is an important landmark. Its position can easily be felt and often be seen by the presence of a transverse ridge. The finger moved to the right or to the left passes directly onto the second costal cartilage and then the second rib. All other ribs can be counted from this point. The 12th rib can usually be felt from behind, but in some obese persons this may prove difficult.

Trachea

The trachea extends from the lower border of the cricoid cartilage (opposite the body of the sixth cervical vertebra) in the neck to the level of the sternal angle in the thorax (Fig. 2-23). It commences in the midline and ends just to the right of the midline by dividing into the right and left principal bronchi. At the root of the neck it may be palpated in the midline in the suprasternal notch.

Lungs

The **apex of the lung** projects into the neck. It can be mapped out on the anterior surface of the body by drawing a curved line, convex upward, from the sternoclavicular joint to a point 1 in. (2.5 cm) above the junction of the medial and intermediate thirds of the clavicle (Fig. 2-23).

The **anterior border of the right lung** begins behind the sternoclavicular joint and runs downward, almost reaching the midline behind the sternal angle. It then continues downward until it reaches the xiphisternal joint (Fig. 2-23). The **anterior border of the left lung** has a similar course, but at the level of the fourth costal cartilage it deviates laterally and extends for a variable distance beyond the lateral margin of the sternum to form the **cardiac notch** (Fig. 2-23). This notch is produced by the heart displacing the lung to the left. The anterior border then turns sharply downward to the level of the xiphisternal joint.

The **lower border of the lung** in midinspiration follows a curving line, which crosses the 6th rib in the midclavicular line and the 8th rib in the midaxillary line, and reaches the 10th rib adjacent to the vertebral column posteriorly (Figs. 2-23, 2-24, and 2-25). It is important to understand that the level of the inferior border of the lung changes during inspiration and expiration.

The **posterior border of the lung** extends downward from the spinous process of the 7th cervical vertebra to the level of the 10th thoracic vertebra and lies about 1.5 in. (4 cm) from the midline (Fig. 2-24).

The **oblique fissure** of the lung can be indicated on the surface by a line drawn from the root of the spine of the scapula obliquely downward, laterally and anteriorly, following the course of the sixth rib to the sixth costochondral junction. In the left lung the upper lobe lies above and anterior to this line; the lower lobe lies below and posterior to it (Figs. 2-23 and 2-24).

In the right lung is an additional fissure, the **horizontal fissure,** which may be represented by a line drawn

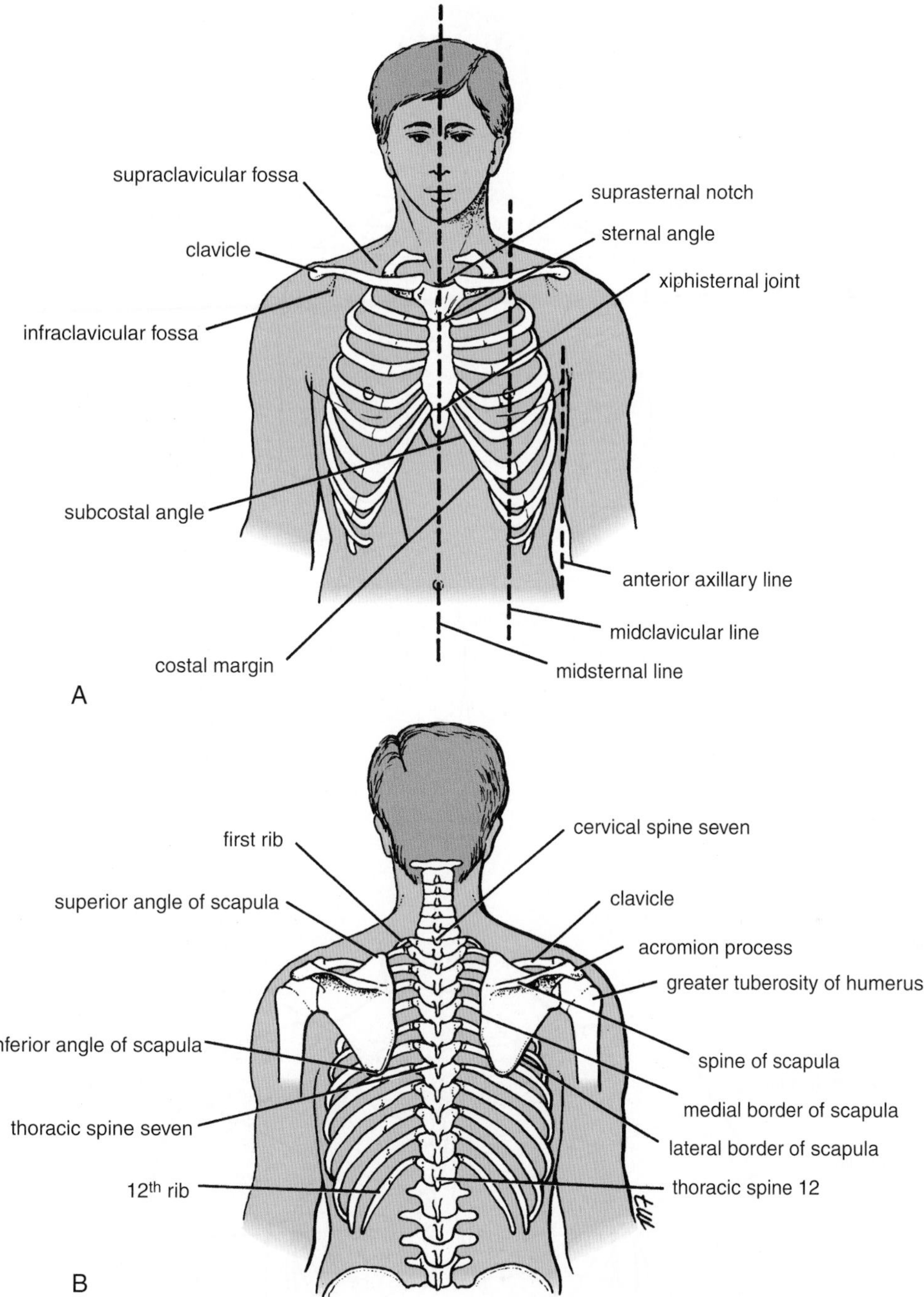

Figure 2-21 Surface landmarks of anterior **(A)** and posterior **(B)** thoracic walls.

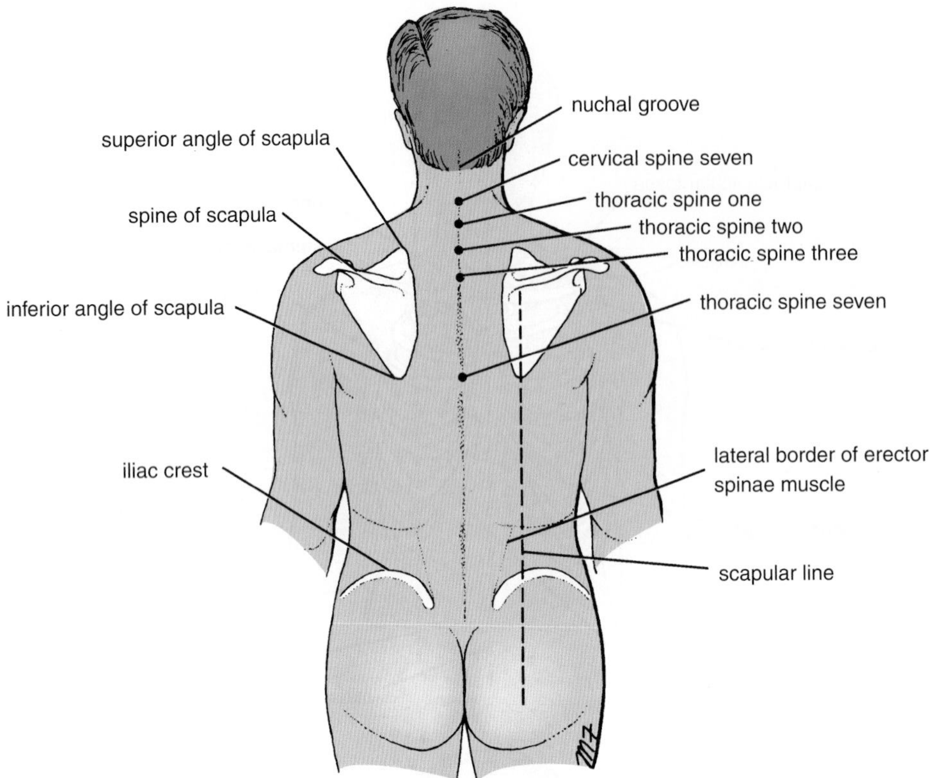

Figure 2-22 Surface landmarks of the posterior thoracic wall.

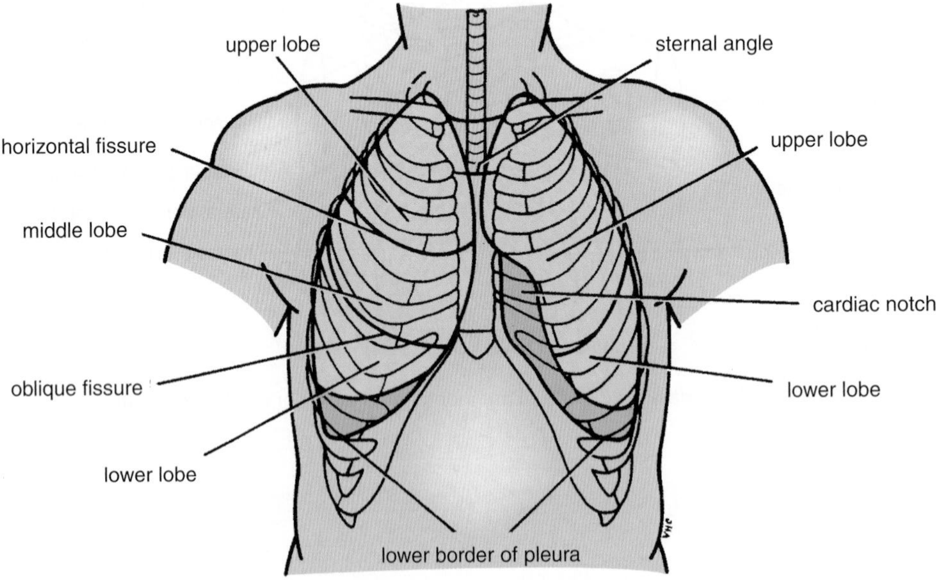

Figure 2-23 Surface markings of lungs and parietal pleura on the anterior thoracic wall.

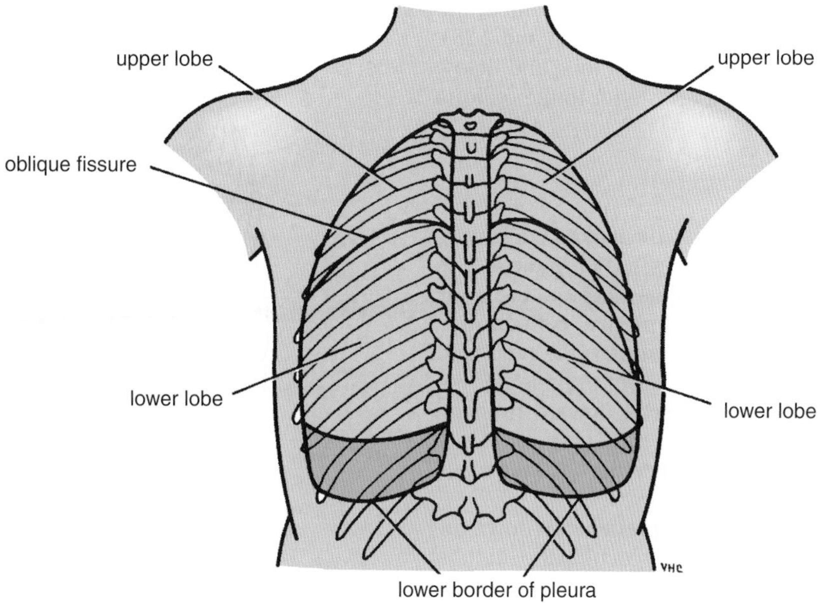

Figure 2-24 Surface markings of the lungs and parietal pleura on the posterior thoracic wall.

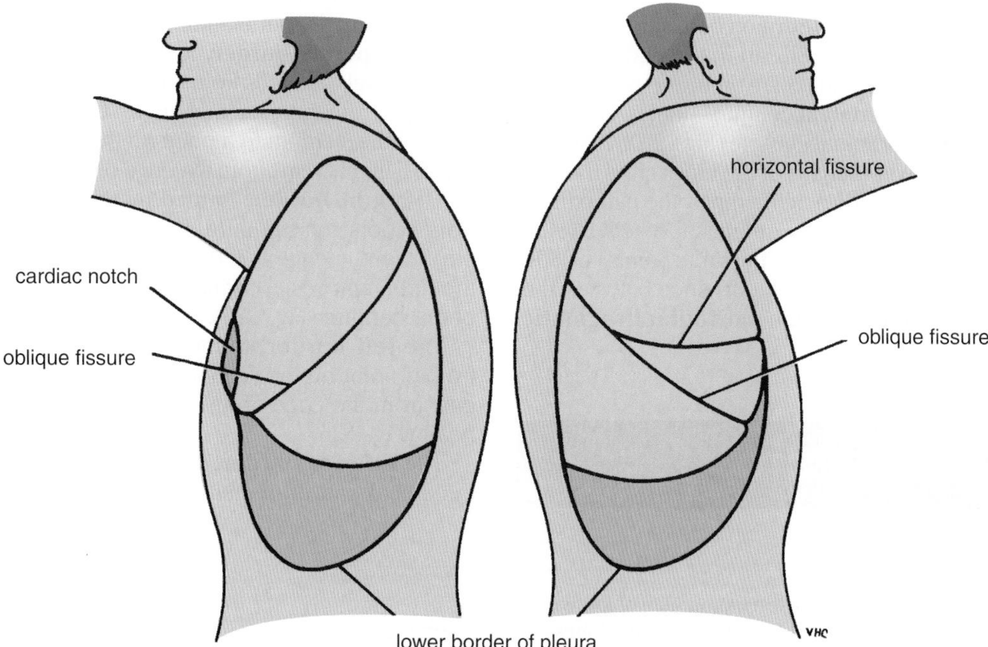

Figure 2-25 Surface markings of the lungs and parietal pleura on the lateral thoracic walls.

horizontally along the fourth costal cartilage to meet the oblique fissure in the midaxillary line (Figs. 2-23 and 2-25). Above the horizontal fissure lies the upper lobe and below it lies the middle lobe; below and posterior to the oblique fissure lies the lower lobe.

Pleura

The boundaries of the pleural sac can be marked out as lines on the surface of the body. The lines, which indicate the limits of the parietal pleura where it lies close to the body surface, are referred to as the **lines of pleural reflection.**

The **cervical pleura** bulges upward into the neck and has a surface marking identical to that of the apex of the lung. A curved line may be drawn, convex upward, from the sternoclavicular joint to a point 1 in. (2.5 cm) above the junction of the medial and intermediate thirds of the clavicle (Fig. 2-23).

The **anterior border of the right pleura** runs down behind the sternoclavicular joint, almost reaching the midline behind the sternal angle. It then continues downward until it reaches the xiphisternal joint. The **anterior border of the left pleura** has a similar course, but at the level of the fourth costal cartilage it deviates laterally and extends to the lateral margin of the sternum to form the cardiac notch. (Note that the pleural cardiac notch is not as large as the cardiac notch of the lung.) It then turns sharply downward to the xiphisternal joint (Fig. 2-23).

The **lower border of the pleura** on both sides follows a curved line, which crosses the 8th rib in the midclavicular line and the 10th rib in the midaxillary line, and reaches the 12th rib adjacent to the vertebral column—that is, at the lateral border of the erector spinae muscle (Figs. 2-23, 2-24, and 2-25). Note that the lower margins of the lungs cross the 6th, 8th, and 10th ribs at the midclavicular lines, the midaxillary lines, and the sides of the vertebral column, respectively; the lower margins of the pleura cross, at the same points, the 8th, 10th, and 12th ribs, respectively. The distance between the two borders corresponds to the **costodiaphragmatic recess.** (See page 84.)

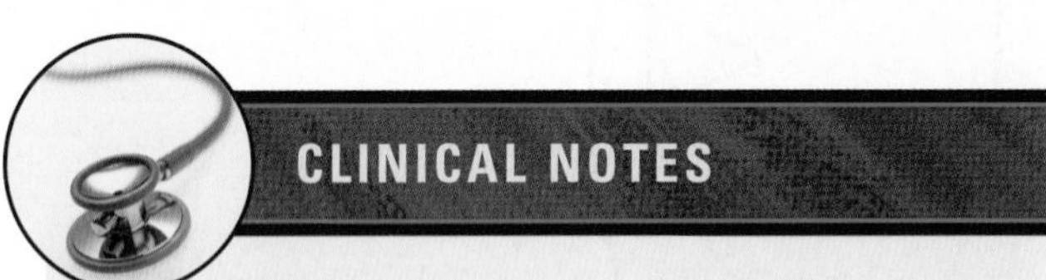

Pleural Reflections

It is hardly necessary to emphasize the importance of knowing the surface markings of the pleural reflections and the lobes of the lungs. When listening to the breath sounds of the respiratory tract, it should be possible to have a mental image of the structures that lie beneath the stethoscope.

The **cervical dome of the pleura** and the **apex of the lungs** extend up into the neck so that at their highest point they lie about 1 in. (2.5 cm) above the clavicle (Figs. 2-6, 2-13, and 2-23). Consequently, they are vulnerable to stab wounds in the root of the neck or to damage by an anesthetist's needle when a nerve block of the lower trunk of the brachial plexus is being performed.

Remember also that the **lower limit of the pleural reflection,** as seen from the back, may be damaged during a nephrectomy. The pleura crosses the 12th rib and may be damaged during removal of the kidney through an incision in the loin.

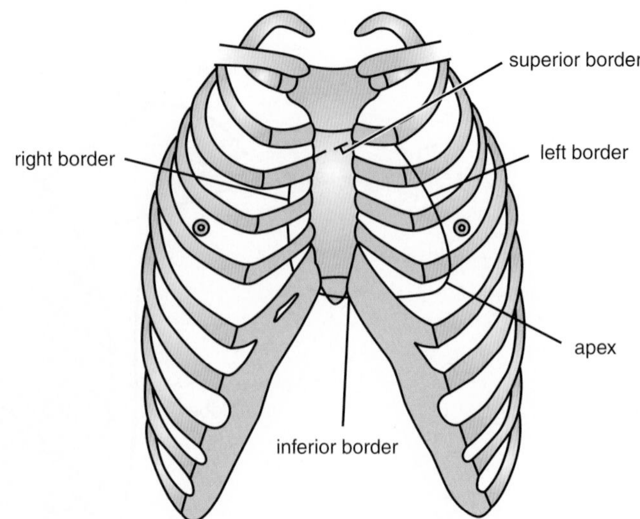

Figure 2-26 Surface markings of the heart.

Heart

For practical purposes, the heart may be considered to have both an apex and four borders.

The **apex,** formed by the left ventricle, corresponds to the apex beat and is found in the fifth left intercostal space 3.5 in. (9 cm) from the midline (Fig. 2-26).

The **superior border,** formed by the roots of the great blood vessels, extends from a point on the second left costal cartilage (remember sternal angle) 0.5 in. (1.3 cm) from the edge of the sternum to a point on the third right costal cartilage 0.5 in. (1.3 cm) from the edge of the sternum (Fig. 2-26).

The **right border,** formed by the right atrium, extends from a point on the third right costal cartilage 0.5 in. (1.3 cm) from the edge of the sternum downward to a point on the sixth right costal cartilage 0.5 in. (1.3 cm) from the edge of the sternum (Fig. 2-26).

The **left border,** formed by the left ventricle, extends from a point on the second left costal cartilage 0.5 in. (1.3 cm) from the edge of the sternum to the apex beat of the heart (Fig. 2-26).

The **inferior border,** formed by the right ventricle and the apical part of the left ventricle, extends from the sixth

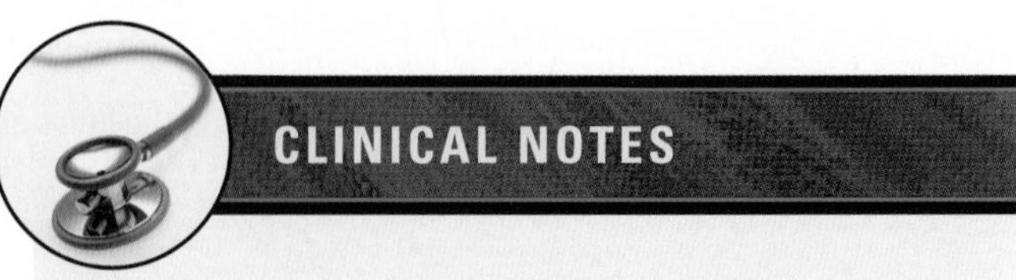

Position and Enlargement of the Heart

The surface markings of the heart and the position of the apex beat may enable a physician to determine whether the heart has shifted its position in relation to the chest wall or whether the heart is enlarged by disease. The apex beat can often be seen and almost always can be felt. The position of the margins of the heart can be determined by percussion.

right costal cartilage 0.5 in. (1.3 cm) from the sternum to the apex beat (Fig. 2-26).

Thoracic Blood Vessels

The **arch of the aorta** and the roots of the **brachiocephalic** and **left common carotid arteries** lie behind the manubrium sterni (Fig. 2-2).

The **superior vena cava** and the terminal parts of the **right** and **left brachiocephalic veins** also lie behind the manubrium sterni.

The **internal thoracic vessels** run vertically downward, posterior to the costal cartilages, 0.5 in. (1.3 cm) lateral to the edge of the sternum (Figs. 2-9 and 2-10), as far as the sixth intercostal space.

The intercostal vessels and nerve ("vein, artery, nerve"—VAN—is the order from above downward) are situated 72 immediately below their corresponding ribs (Fig. 2-8).

Mammary Gland

The mammary gland lies in the superficial fascia covering the anterior chest wall (Fig. 2-20). In the child and in men, it is rudimentary. In the female after puberty, it enlarges and assumes its hemispherical shape. In the young adult female, it overlies the second to the sixth ribs and their costal cartilages and extends from the lateral margin of the sternum to the midaxillary line. Its upper lateral edge extends around the lower border of the pectoralis major and enters the axilla. In middle-aged multiparous women, the breasts may be large and pendulous. In older women past menopause, the adipose tissue of the breast may become reduced in amount and the hemispherical shape lost; the breasts then become smaller, and the overlying skin is wrinkled.

The structure of the mammary gland is described fully on page 427.

CLINICAL PROBLEM SOLVING

Study the following case histories and select the best answer to the questions following them.

On percussing the anterior chest wall of a patient, you find the right margin of the heart to lie 2 in. (5 cm) to the right of the edge of the sternum.

1. Which chamber of the heart is likely to be enlarged?
   (a) The left ventricle
   (b) The left atrium
   (c) The right ventricle
   (d) The right atrium

A 31-year-old soldier received a shrapnel wound in the neck during the Persian Gulf War. Recently, during a physical examination, it was noticed that when he blew his nose or sneezed, the skin above the right clavicle bulged upward.

2. The upward bulging of the skin could be explained by
   (a) injury to the cervical pleura.
   (b) damage to the suprapleural membrane.
   (c) damage to the deep fascia in the root of the neck.
   (d) ununited fracture of the first rib.

A 52-year-old woman was admitted to the hospital with a diagnosis of right-sided pleurisy with pneumonia. It was decided to remove a sample of pleural fluid from her pleural cavity. The resident inserted the needle close to the lower border of the eighth rib in the anterior axillary line. The next morning he was surprised to hear that the patient had complained of altered skin sensation extending from the point where the needle was inserted downward and forward to the midline of the abdominal wall above the umbilicus.

3. The altered skin sensation in this patient after the needle thoracostomy could be explained by which of the following?
   (a) The needle was inserted too low down in the intercostal space.
   (b) The needle was inserted too close to the lower border of the eighth rib and damaged the eighth intercostal nerve.
   (c) The needle had impaled the eighth rib.
   (d) The needle had penetrated too deeply and pierced the lung.

A 68-year-old man complained of a swelling in the skin on the back of the chest. He had noticed it for the last 3 years and was concerned because it was rapidly enlarging. On examination, a hard lump was found in the skin in the right scapula line opposite the seventh thoracic vertebra. A biopsy revealed that the lump was malignant.

4. Because of the rapid increase in size of the tumor, which of the following lymph nodes were examined for metastases?
   (a) Superficial inguinal nodes
   (b) Anterior axillary nodes
   (c) Posterior axillary nodes
   (d) External iliac nodes
   (e) Deep cervical nodes

A 65-year-old man and a 10-year-old boy were involved in a severe automobile accident. In both patients the thorax had been badly crushed. Radiographic examination revealed that the man had five fractured ribs but the boy had no fractures.

5. What is the most likely explanation for this difference in medical findings?
   (a) The patients were in different seats in the vehicle.
   (b) The boy was wearing his seat belt and the man was not.
   (c) The chest wall of a child is very elastic, and fractures of ribs in children are rare.
   (d) The man anticipated the impact and tensed his muscles, including those of the shoulder girdle and abdomen.

On examination of a posteroanterior chest radiograph of an 18-year-old woman, it was seen that the left dome of the diaphragm was higher than the right dome and reached to the upper border of the fourth rib.

6. The position of the left dome of the diaphragm could be explained by one of the following conditions except which?
   (a) The left lung could be collapsed.
   (b) There is a collection of blood under the diaphragm on the left side.
   (c) There is an amebic abscess in the left lobe of the liver.
   (d) The left dome of the diaphragm is normally higher than the right dome.
   (e) There is a peritoneal abscess beneath the diaphragm on the left side.

A 43-year-old man was involved in a violent quarrel with his wife over another woman. In a fit of rage, the wife picked up a carving knife and lunged forward at her husband, striking his anterior neck over the left clavicle. The husband collapsed on the kitchen floor, bleeding profusely from the wound. The distraught wife called an ambulance.

7. On examination in the emergency department of the hospital, the following conditions were found except which?
   (a) A wound was seen about 1 in. (2.5 cm) wide over the left clavicle.
   (b) Auscultation revealed diminished breath sounds over the left hemithorax.
   (c) The trachea was deflected to the left.
   (d) The left upper limb was lying stationary on the table, and active movement of the small muscles of the left hand was absent.
   (e) The patient was insensitive to pin prick along the lateral side of the left arm, forearm, and hand.

A 72-year-old man complaining of burning pain on the right side of his chest was seen by his physician. On examination the patient indicated that the pain passed forward over the right sixth intercostal space from the posterior axillary line forward as far as the midline over the sternum. The physician noted that there were several watery blebs on the skin in the painful area.

8. The following statements are correct except which?
   (a) This patient has herpes zoster.
   (b) A virus descends along the cutaneous nerves, causing dermatomal pain and the eruption of vesicles.
   (c) The sixth right intercostal nerve was involved.
   (d) The condition was confined to the anterior cutaneous branch of the sixth intercostal nerve.

An 18-year-old woman was thrown from a horse while attempting to jump a fence. She landed heavily on the ground, striking the lower part of her chest on the left side. On examination in the emergency department she was conscious but breathless. The lower left side of her chest was badly bruised, and the 9th and 10th ribs were extremely tender to touch. She had severe tachycardia, and her systolic blood pressure was low.

9. The following statements are possibly correct except which?
   (a) There was evidence of tenderness and muscle spasm in the left upper quadrant of the anterior abdominal wall.
   (b) A posteroanterior radiograph of the chest revealed fractures of the left 9th and 10th ribs near their angles.
   (c) The blunt trauma to the ribs had resulted in a tear of the underlying spleen.
   (d) The presence of blood in the peritoneal cavity had irritated the parietal peritoneum, producing reflex spasm of the upper abdominal muscles.
   (e) The muscles of the anterior abdominal wall are not supplied by thoracic spinal nerves.

ANSWERS TO CLINICAL PROBLEMS

1. D
2. B. The suprapleural membrane prevents the cervical dome of the pleura from bulging up into the neck.
3. B
4. C
5. C
6. D
7. E. The lower trunk of the brachial plexus was cut by the knife. This would explain the loss of movement of the small muscles of the left hand. It would also explain the loss of skin sensation that occurred in the C8 and T1 dermatomes on the medial, not on the lateral, side of the left forearm and hand. The knife had also pierced the left dome of the cervical pleura, causing a left pneumothorax with left-sided diminished breath sounds and a deflection of the trachea to the left.
8. D. The skin over the sixth intercostal space is innervated by the lateral cutaneous branch as well as the anterior cutaneous branch of the sixth intercostal nerve.
9. E. The 7th to the 11th intercostal nerves supply the muscles of the anterior abdominal wall.

REVIEW QUESTIONS

Multiple-Choice Questions

Select the best answer for each question.

1. The following statements concerning structures in the intercostal space are correct except which?
   (a) The anterior intercostal arteries of the upper six intercostal spaces are branches of the internal thoracic artery.
   (b) The intercostal nerves travel forward in an intercostal space between the internal intercostal and innermost intercostal muscles.
   (c) The intercostal blood vessels and nerves are positioned in the order of vein, nerve, and artery from superior to inferior in a subcostal groove.
   (d) The lower five intercostal nerves supply sensory innervation to the skin of the lateral thoracic and anterior abdominal walls.
   (e) The posterior intercostal veins drain backward into the azygos and hemiazygos veins.
2. The following statements concerning the diaphragm are correct except which?
   (a) The right crus provides a muscular sling around the esophagus and possibly prevents regurgitation of stomach contents into the esophagus.
   (b) On contraction, the diaphragm raises the intra-abdominal pressure and assists in the return of the venous blood to the right atrium of the heart.
   (c) The level of the diaphragm is higher in the recumbent position than in the standing position.
   (d) On contraction, the central tendon descends, reducing the intrathoracic pressure.
   (e) The esophagus passes through the diaphragm at the level of the eighth thoracic vertebra.
3. The following statements concerning the intercostal nerves are correct except which?
   (a) They provide motor innervation to the peripheral parts of the diaphragm.
   (b) They provide motor innervation to the intercostal muscles.
   (c) They provide sensory innervation to the costal parietal pleura.
   (d) They contain sympathetic fibers to innervate the vascular smooth muscle.
   (e) The 7th to the 11th intercostal nerves provide sensory innervation to the parietal peritoneum.
4. To pass a needle into the pleural space (cavity) in the midaxillary line, the following structures will have to be pierced except which?
   (a) Internal intercostal muscle
   (b) Levatores costarum
   (c) External intercostal muscle
   (d) Parietal pleura
   (e) Innermost intercostal muscle
5. The following statements concerning the thoracic outlet (anatomic inlet) are true except which?
   (a) The manubrium sterni form the anterior border.
   (b) On each side, the lower trunk of the brachial plexus and the subclavian artery emerge through the outlet and pass laterally over the surface of the first rib.
   (c) The body of the seventh cervical vertebra forms the posterior boundary.
   (d) The first ribs form the lateral boundaries.
   (e) The esophagus and trachea pass through the outlet.
6. The following statements concerning the thoracic wall are correct except which?
   (a) The trachea bifurcates opposite the manubriosternal joint (angle of Louis) in the midrespiratory position.
   (b) The arch of the aorta lies behind the body of the sternum.
   (c) The apex beat of the heart can normally be felt in the left intercostal space about 3.5 in. (9 cm) from the midline.
   (d) The lower margin of the right lung on full inspiration could extend down in the midclavicular line to the eighth costal cartilage.
   (e) All intercostal nerves are derived from the anterior rami of thoracic spinal nerves.

Completion Questions

Select the phrase that best completes each statement.

7. Clinicians define the thoracic outlet as
   (a) the lower opening in the thoracic cage.
   (b) the gap between the crura of the diaphragm.
   (c) the esophageal opening in the diaphragm.
   (d) the upper opening in the thoracic cage.
   (e) the gap between the sternal and costal origins of the diaphragm.
8. The costal margin is formed by
   (a) the 6th, 8th, and 10th ribs.
   (b) the inner margins of the 1st ribs.
   (c) the edge of the xiphoid process.
   (d) the costal cartilages of the 7th, 8th, 9th, and 10th ribs.
   (e) the costal cartilages of the 7th to the 10th ribs and the ends of the cartilages of the 11th and 12th ribs.
9. The lower margin of the left lung in midrespiration crosses
   (a) the 6th, 8th, and 10th ribs.
   (b) the 7th, 8th, and 9th ribs.
   (c) the 10th, 11th, and 12th ribs.
   (d) the 8th rib only.
   (e) the 6th, 11th, and 12th ribs.
10. The suprapleural membrane is attached laterally to the margins of
   (a) the 1st rib.
   (b) the 6th, 8th, and 10th ribs.
   (c) the manubriosternal junction.
   (d) the 2nd rib.
   (e) the xiphoid cartilage.

11. The mammary gland in the young adult female overlies
    (a) the 1st to the 5th ribs.
    (b) the 2nd to the 6th ribs.
    (c) the 1st and 2nd ribs.
    (d) the 2nd and 3rd ribs.
    (e) the 4th to the 6th ribs.
12. The parietal pleura
    (a) is sensitive only to the sensation of stretch.
    (b) is separated from the pleural space by endothoracic fascia.
    (c) is sensitive to the sensations of pain and touch.
    (d) receives its sensory innervation from the autonomic nervous system.
    (e) is formed from splanchnopleuric mesoderm.

Fill-in-the-Blank Questions

Fill in the blank with the best answer.

13. The thoracic duct passes through the ________ opening in the diaphragm.
14. The superior epigastric artery passes through the ________ opening in the diaphragm.
15. The right phrenic nerve passes through the ________ opening in the diaphragm.
16. The left vagus nerve passes through the ________ opening in the diaphragm.
    (a) aortic
    (b) esophageal
    (c) caval
    (d) none of the above
17. The aortic opening in the diaphragm lies at the level of the ________ thoracic vertebra.
18. The xiphisternal joint lies at the level of the ________ thoracic vertebra.
19. The caval opening in the diaphragm lies at the level of the ________ thoracic vertebra.
    (a) 10th
    (b) 12th
    (c) 8th
    (d) 9th
    (e) 7th

Multiple-Choice Questions

Read the case history and select the best answer to the question following it.

A 35-year-old man complaining of severe pain in the lower part of his left chest was seen by his physician. The patient had been coughing for the last 4 days and was producing blood-stained sputum. He had an increased respiratory rate and had a pyrexia of 104°F. On examination, the patient was found to have fluid in the left pleural space.

20. With the patient in the standing position, the pleural fluid would most likely gravitate down to the
    (a) oblique fissure.
    (b) cardiac notch.
    (c) costomediastinal recess.
    (d) horizontal fissure.
    (e) costodiaphragmatic recess.

ANSWERS TO REVIEW QUESTIONS

1. C. The order from superior to inferior is intercostal vein, artery, and nerve.
2. E. The esophagus passes through the diaphragm at the level of the 10th thoracic vertebra.
3. A. They provide sensory innervation to the pleura and peritoneum covering the peripheral parts of the diaphragm.
4. B. The levator costarum is located on the back away from the area involved.
5. C. The body of the first thoracic vertebra forms the posterior boundary.
6. B. The arch of the aorta lies behind the manubrium sterni.
7. D
8. E
9. A
10. A
11. B
12. C
13. A
14. D. The superior epigastric artery enters the anterior abdominal wall between the sternal and the costal origins of the diaphragm.
15. C
16. B
17. B
18. D
19. C
20. E. This patient started his illness with an upper respiratory infection, which he ignored. Now he has left-sided pneumonia complicated by pleurisy. With pleurisy, the inflammatory exudate may remain at the site of the pneumonia. If the pleural fluid is excessive and the patient assumes the upright position, the fluid may gravitate downward to the lowest part of the pleural space—namely, the costodiaphragmatic recess.

CHAPTER 3

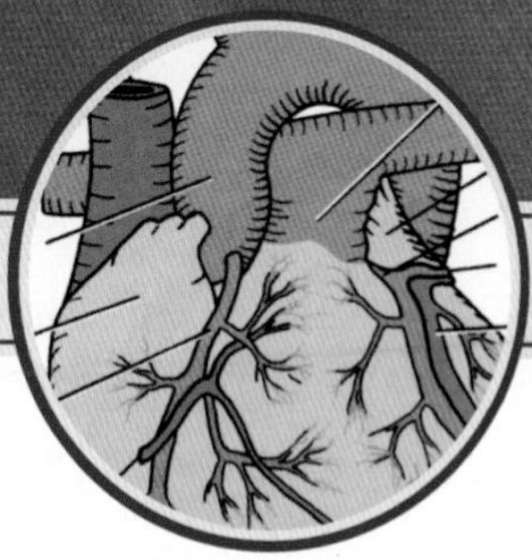

THE THORAX: PART II—THE THORACIC CAVITY

A 54-year-old woman complaining of a sudden excruciating knifelike pain in the front of the chest was seen by a physician. During the course of the examination, she said that she could also feel the pain in her back between the shoulder blades. On close questioning she said she felt no pain down the arms or in the neck. Her blood pressure was 200/110 mm Hg in the right arm and 120/80 mm Hg in the left arm.

The evaluation of chest pain is one of the most common problems facing an emergency physician. The cause can vary from the simple to one of life-threatening proportions. The severe nature of the pain and its radiation through to the back made a preliminary diagnosis of aortic dissection a strong possibility. Myocardial infarction commonly results in referred pain down the inner side of the arm or up into the neck.

Pain impulses originating in a diseased descending thoracic aorta pass to the central nervous system along sympathetic nerves and are then referred along the somatic spinal nerves to the skin of the anterior and posterior chest walls. In this patient the aortic dissection had partially blocked the origin of the left subclavian artery, which would explain the lower blood pressure recorded in the left arm.

CHAPTER OUTLINE

Basic Anatomy 78
Chest Cavity 78
Mediastinum 80
Superior Mediastinum 80
Inferior Mediastinum 80
Pleurae 80
Nerve Supply of the Pleura 84
Trachea 87
Nerve Supply of the Trachea 87
Principal Bronchi 88
Lungs 89
Lobes and Fissures 92
Bronchopulmonary Segments 94
Blood Supply of the Lungs 96
Lymph Drainage of the Lungs 98
Nerve Supply of the Lungs 98
The Mechanics of Respiration 100
Pericardium 103
Fibrous Pericardium 103
Serous Pericardium 103
Pericardial Sinuses 104
Nerve Supply of the Pericardium 104
Heart 105
Surfaces of the Heart 105
Borders of the Heart 107
Chambers of the Heart 107
Structure of the Heart 111
Conducting System of the Heart 111
Arterial Supply of the Heart 113
Venous Drainage of the Heart 116
Nerve Supply of the Heart 116
Action of the Heart 117
Large Veins of the Thorax 123
Brachiocephalic Veins 123
Superior Vena Cava 123
Azygos Veins 123
Inferior Vena Cava 123
Pulmonary Veins 123
Large Arteries of the Thorax 123
Aorta 123
Lymph Nodes and Vessels of the Thorax 126
Thoracic Wall 126
Mediastinum 126
Thoracic Duct 126
Right Lymphatic Duct 127
Nerves of the Thorax 127
Vagus Nerves 127
Phrenic Nerves 127
Thoracic Part of the Sympathetic Trunk 127
Esophagus 128
Blood Supply of the Esophagus 128
Lymph Drainage of the Esophagus 128
Nerve Supply of the Esophagus 128
Thymus 129
Blood Supply 129
Cross-Sectional Anatomy of the Thorax 131
Radiographic Anatomy 131
Posteroanterior Radiograph 131
Right Oblique Radiograph 134
Left Oblique Radiograph 135
Bronchography and Contrast Visualization of the Esophagus 135
Coronary Angiography 136
CT Scanning of the Thorax 137
Clinical Problem Solving 140
Answers to Clinical Problems 142
Review Questions 142
Answers to Review Questions 144

CHAPTER OBJECTIVES

- To understand the general arrangement of the thoracic viscera and their relationship to one another and to the chest wall.
- To be able to define what is meant by the term **mediastinum** and to learn the arrangement of the pleura relative to the lungs. This information is fundamental to the comprehension of the function and disease of the lungs.
- Appreciating that the heart and the lungs are enveloped in serous membranes that provide a lubricating mechanism for these mobile viscera and being able to distinguish between such terms as **thoracic cavity, pleural cavity** (pleural space), **pericardial cavity,** and **costodiaphragmatic recess.**
- To learn the structure of the heart, including its conducting system and the arrangement of the different chambers and valves, which is basic to understanding the physiologic and pathologic features of the heart. The critical nature of the blood supply to the heart and the end arteries and myocardial infarction is emphasized.
- To understand that the largest blood vessels in the body are located within the thoracic cavity, namely, the aorta, the pulmonary arteries, the venae cavae, and the pulmonary veins. Trauma to the chest wall can result in disruption of these vessels, with consequent rapid hemorrhage and death. Because these vessels are hidden from view within the thorax, the diagnosis of major blood vessel injury is often delayed, with disastrous consequences to the patient.

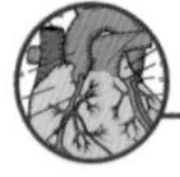

Basic Anatomy

Chest Cavity

The chest cavity is bounded by the chest wall and below by the diaphragm. It extends upward into the root of the neck about one fingerbreadth above the clavicle on each side (see Fig. 3-5). The diaphragm, which is a very thin muscle, is the only structure (apart from the pleura and peritoneum) that separates the chest from the abdominal viscera. The chest cavity can be divided into a median partition, called the mediastinum, and the laterally placed pleurae and lungs (Figs. 3-1, 3-2, and 3-3).

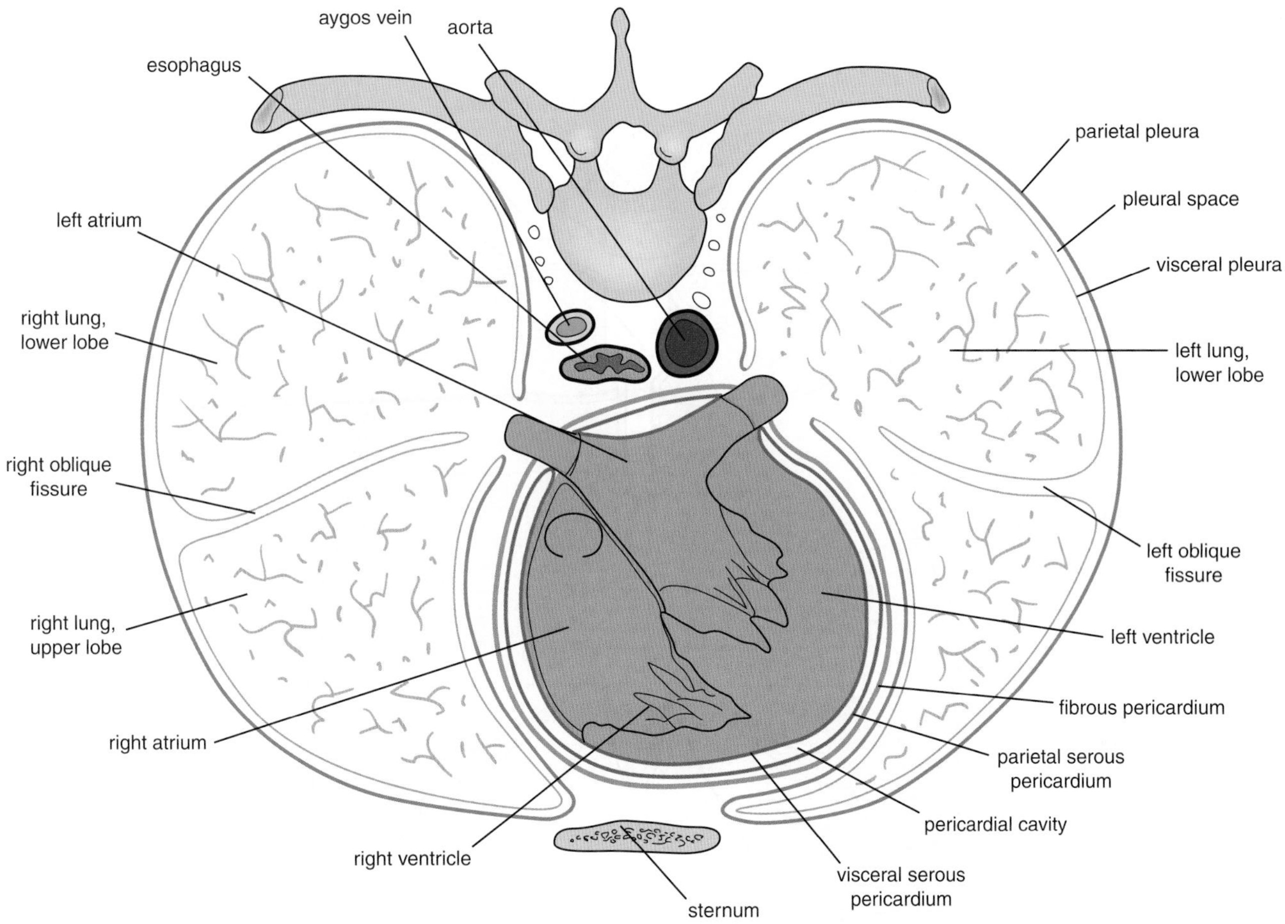

Figure 3-1 Cross section of the thorax at the level of the eighth thoracic vertebra. Note the arrangement of the pleura and pleural cavity (space) and the fibrous and serous pericardia.

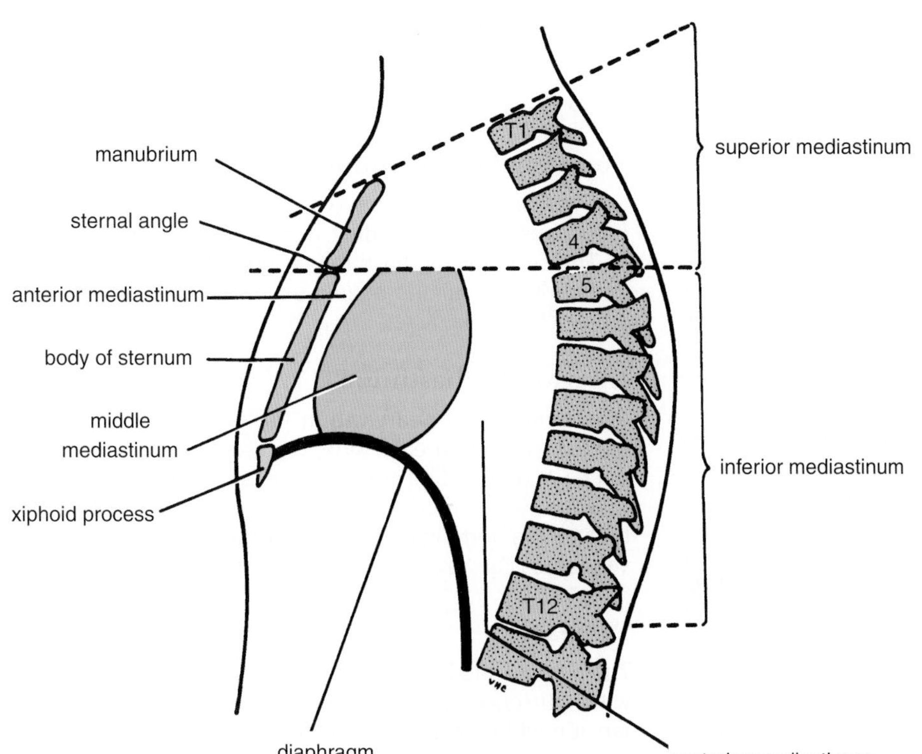

Figure 3-2 Subdivisions of the mediastinum.

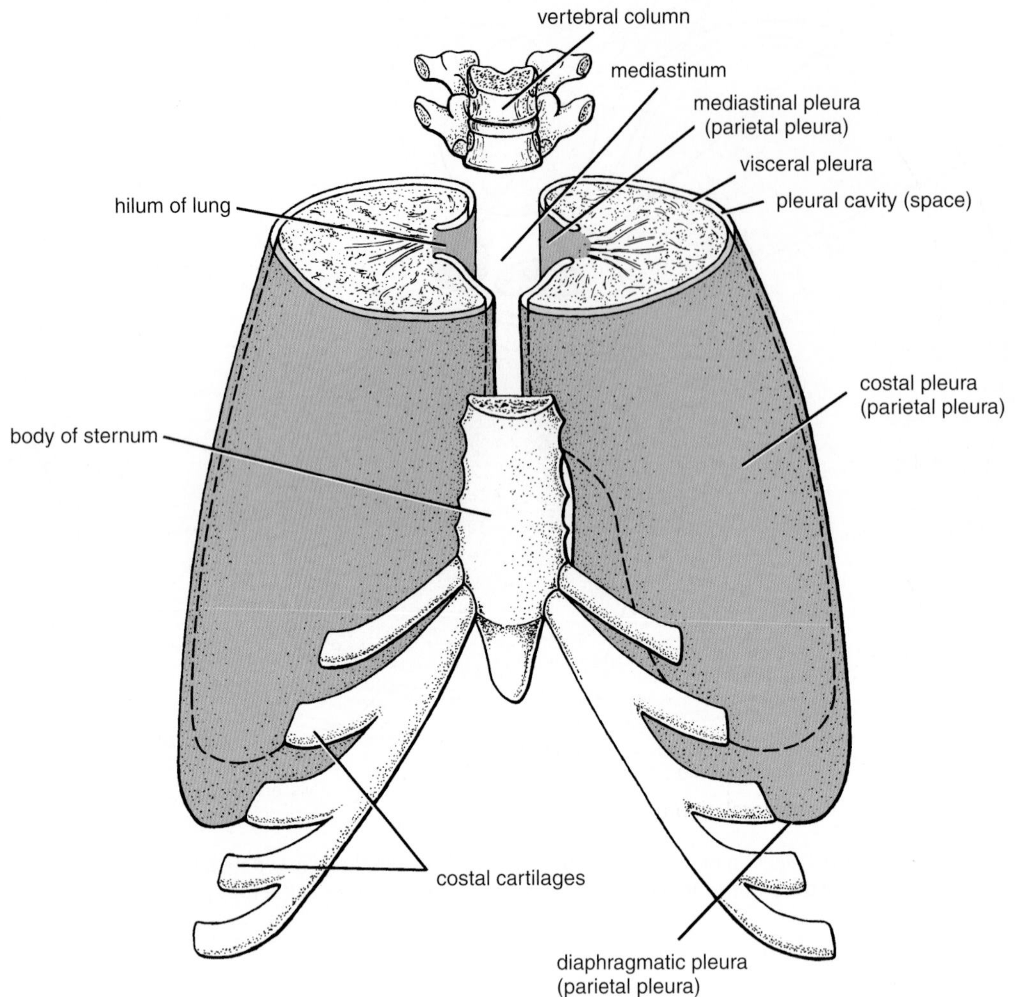

Figure 3-3 Pleurae from above and in front. Note the position of the mediastinum and hilum of each lung.

Mediastinum

The mediastinum, though thick, is a movable partition that extends superiorly to the thoracic outlet and the root of the neck and inferiorly to the diaphragm. It extends anteriorly to the sternum and posteriorly to the vertebral column. It contains the remains of the thymus, the heart and large blood vessels, the trachea and esophagus, the thoracic duct and lymph nodes, the vagus and phrenic nerves, and the sympathetic trunks.

The mediastinum is divided into **superior** and **inferior mediastina** by an imaginary plane passing from the sternal angle anteriorly to the lower border of the body of the fourth thoracic vertebra posteriorly (Fig. 3-2). The inferior mediastinum is further subdivided into the **middle mediastinum,** which consists of the pericardium and heart; the **anterior mediastinum,** which is a space between the pericardium and the sternum; and the **posterior mediastinum,** which lies between the pericardium and the vertebral column.

For purposes of orientation, it is convenient to remember that the major mediastinal structures are arranged in the following order from anterior to posterior.

Superior Mediastinum

(a) Thymus, (b) large veins, (c) large arteries, (d) trachea, (e) esophagus and thoracic duct, and (f) sympathetic trunks

The superior mediastinum is bounded in front by the manubrium sterni and behind by the first four thoracic vertebrae (Fig. 3-2).

Inferior Mediastinum

(a) Thymus, (b) heart within the pericardium with the phrenic nerves on each side, (c) esophagus and thoracic duct, (d) descending aorta, and (e) sympathetic trunks

The inferior mediastinum is bounded in front by the body of the sternum and behind by the lower eight thoracic vertebrae (Fig. 3-2).

Pleurae

The pleurae and lungs lie on either side of the mediastinum within the chest cavity (Fig. 3-3). Before discussing the pleurae, it might be helpful to look at the illustrations of the development of the lungs in Figure 3-4.

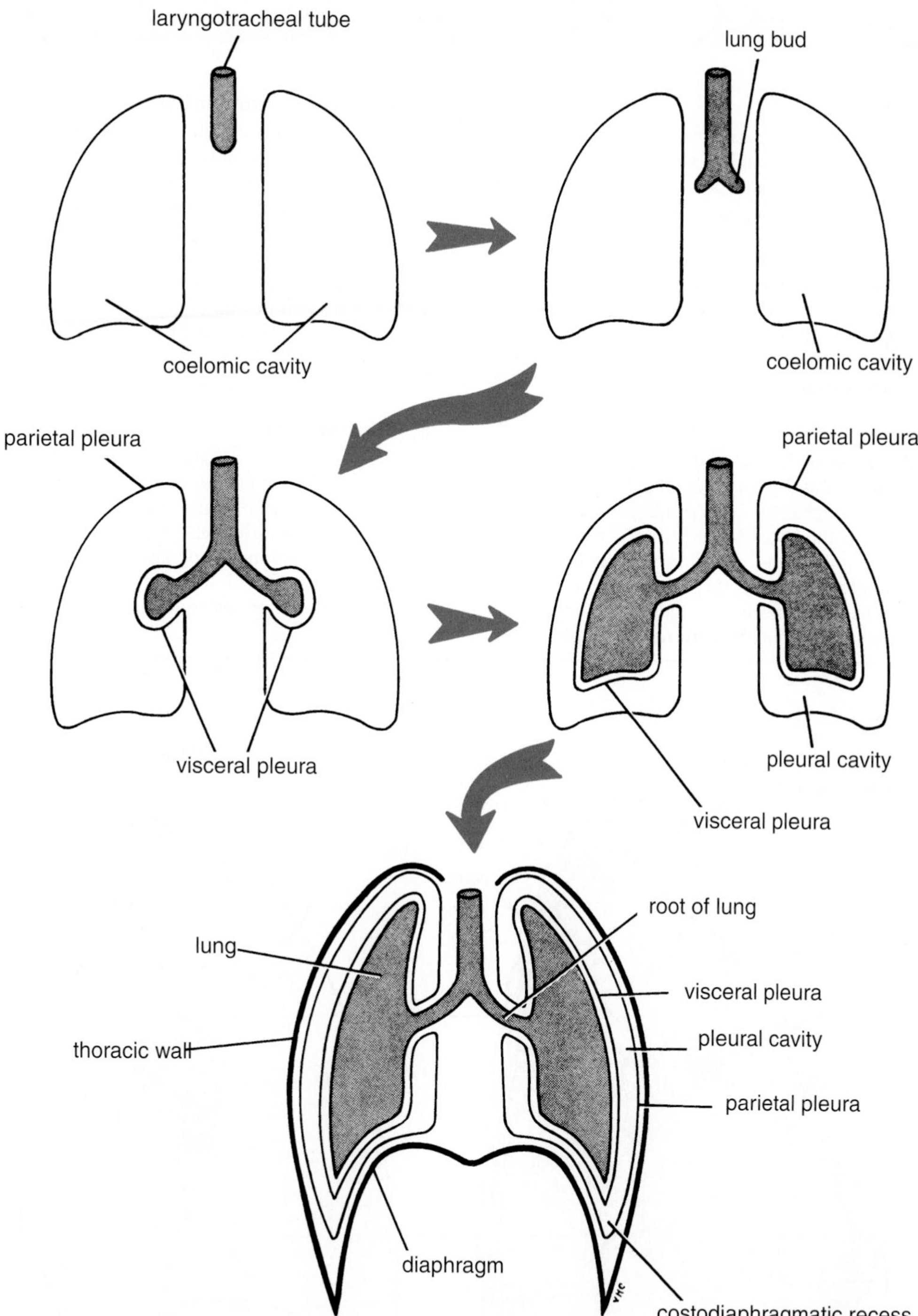

Figure 3-4 Formation of the lungs. Note that each lung bud invaginates the wall of the coelomic cavity and then grows to fill a greater part of the cavity. Note also that the lung is covered with visceral pleura and the thoracic wall is lined with parietal pleura. The original coelomic cavity is reduced to a slitlike space called the pleural cavity as a result of the growth of the lung.

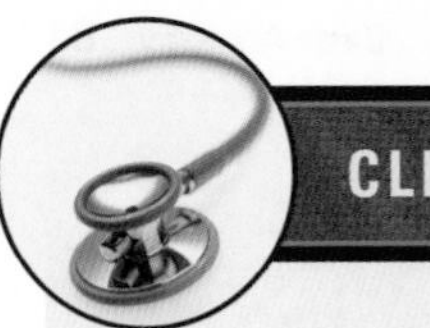

CLINICAL NOTES

Deflection of Mediastinum

In the cadaver, the mediastinum, as the result of the hardening effect of the preserving fluids, is an inflexible, fixed structure. In the living, it is very mobile; the lungs, heart, and large arteries are in rhythmic pulsation, and the esophagus distends as each bolus of food passes through it.

If air enters the pleural cavity (a condition called **pneumothorax),** the lung on that side immediately collapses and the mediastinum is displaced to the opposite side. This condition reveals itself by the patient's being breathless and in a state of shock; on examination, the trachea and the heart are found to be displaced to the opposite side.

Mediastinitis

The structures that make up the mediastinum are embedded in loose connective tissue that is continuous with that of the root of the neck. Thus, it is possible for a deep infection of the neck to spread readily into the thorax, producing a mediastinitis. Penetrating wounds of the chest involving the esophagus may produce a mediastinitis. In esophageal perforations, air escapes into the connective tissue spaces and ascends beneath the fascia to the root of the neck, producing **subcutaneous emphysema.**

Mediastinal Tumors or Cysts

Because many vital structures are crowded together within the mediastinum, their functions can be interfered with by an enlarging tumor or organ. A tumor of the left lung can rapidly spread to involve the mediastinal lymph nodes, which on enlargement may compress the left recurrent laryngeal nerve, producing paralysis of the left vocal fold. An expanding cyst or tumor can partially occlude the superior vena cava, causing severe congestion of the veins of the upper part of the body. Other pressure effects can be seen on the sympathetic trunks, phrenic nerves, and sometimes the trachea, main bronchi, and esophagus.

Mediastinoscopy

Mediastinoscopy is a diagnostic procedure whereby specimens of tracheobronchial lymph nodes are obtained without opening the pleural cavities. A small incision is made in the midline in the neck just above the suprasternal notch, and the superior mediastinum is explored down to the region of the bifurcation of the trachea. The procedure can be used to determine the diagnosis and degree of spread of carcinoma of the bronchus.

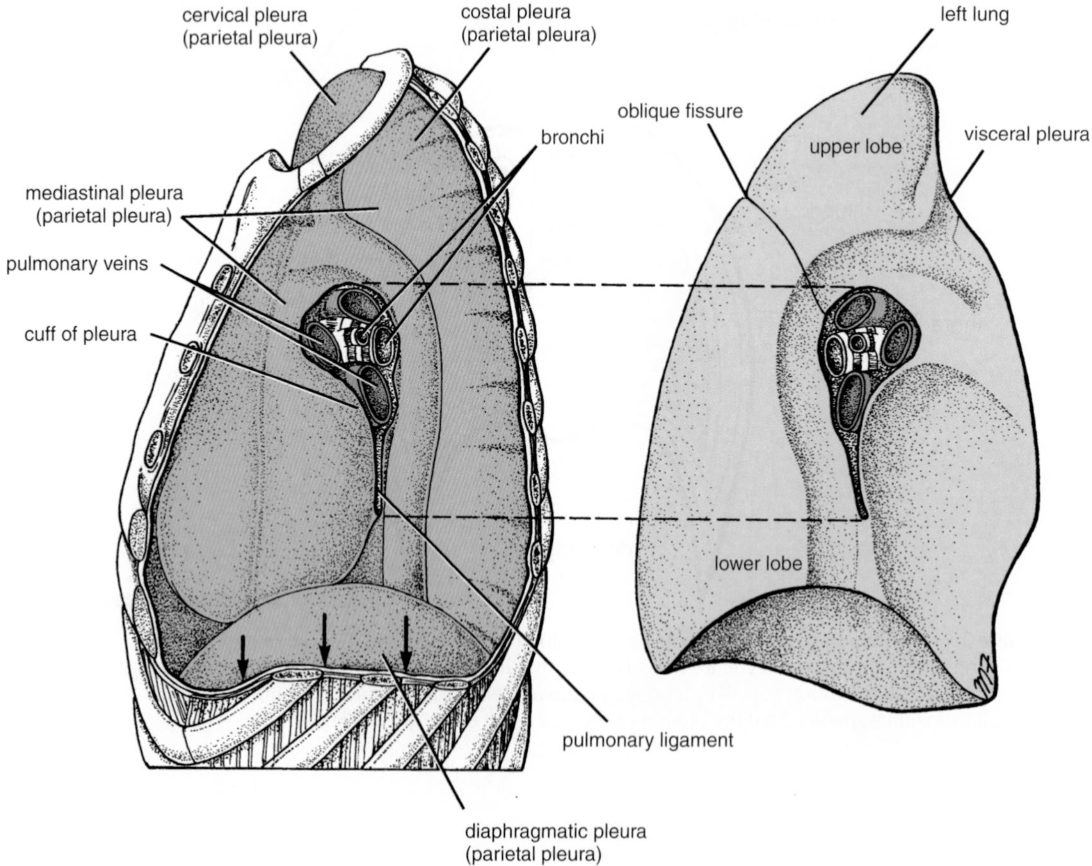

Figure 3-5 Different areas of the parietal pleura. Note the cuff of pleura (*dotted lines*) that surrounds structures entering and leaving the hilum of the left lung. It is here that the parietal and visceral layers of pleura become continuous. Arrows indicate the position of the costodiaphragmatic recess.

Each pleura has two parts: a **parietal layer,** which lines the thoracic wall, covers the thoracic surface of the diaphragm and the lateral aspect of the mediastinum, and extends into the root of the neck to line the undersurface of the suprapleural membrane at the thoracic outlet; and a **visceral layer,** which completely covers the outer surfaces of the lungs and extends into the depths of the interlobar fissures (Figs. 3-1, 3-3, 3-4, 3-5, and 3-6).

The two layers become continuous with one another by means of a cuff of pleura that surrounds the structures entering and leaving the lung at the hilum of each lung (Figs. 3-3, 3-4, and 3-5). To allow for movement of the pulmonary vessels and large bronchi during respiration, the pleural cuff hangs down as a loose fold called the **pulmonary ligament** (Fig. 3-5).

The parietal and visceral layers of pleura are separated from one another by a slitlike space, the **pleural cavity** (Figs. 3-3 and 3-4). (Clinicians are increasingly using the term **pleural space** instead of the anatomic term **pleural cavity.** This is probably to avoid the confusion between

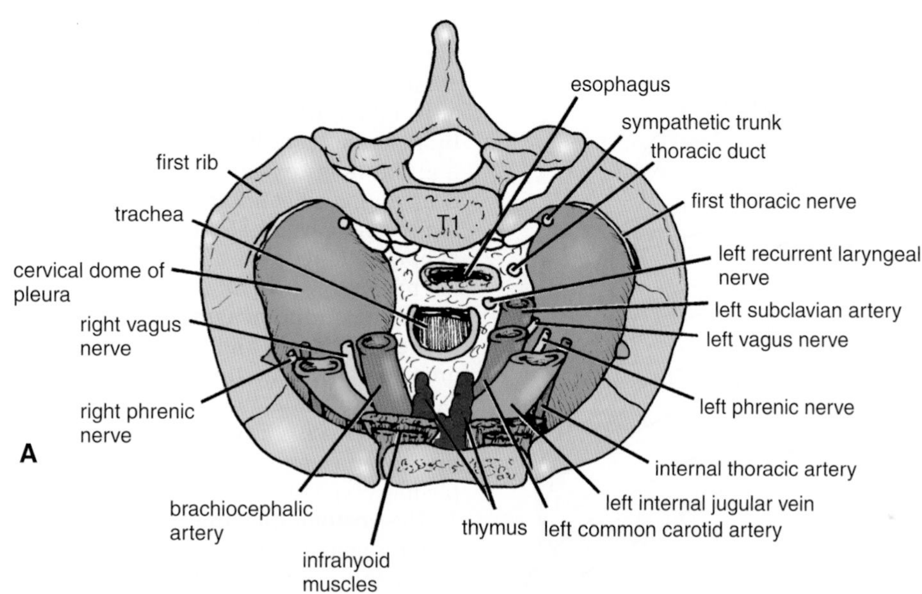

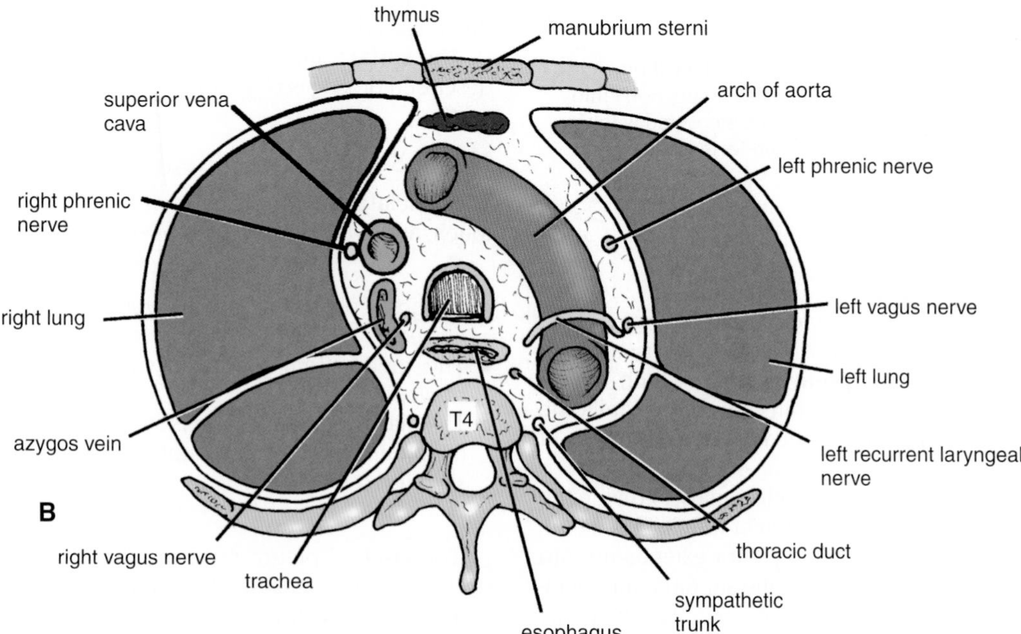

Figure 3-6 Cross section of the thorax. **A.** At the inlet, as seen from above. **B.** At the fourth thoracic vertebra, as seen from below.

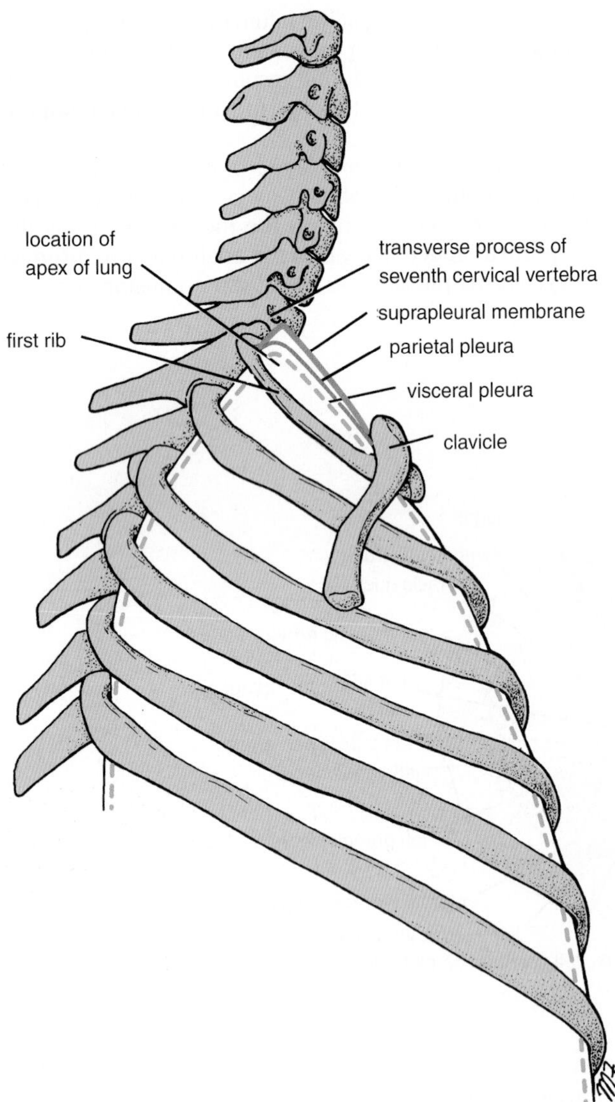

Figure 3-7 Lateral view of the upper opening of the thoracic cage showing how the apex of the lung projects superiorly into the root of the neck. Note that the lung apex is covered with visceral and parietal layers of pleura and is protected by the suprapleural membrane.

the pleural cavity [slitlike] space and the larger chest cavity.) The pleural cavity normally contains a small amount of tissue fluid, the **pleural fluid,** which covers the surfaces of the pleura as a thin film and permits the two layers to move on each other with the minimum of friction.

For purposes of description, it is customary to divide the parietal pleura according to the region in which it lies or the surface that it covers. The cervical pleura extends up into the neck, lining the undersurface of the suprapleural membrane (Fig. 3-7). It reaches a level 1 to 1.5 in. (2.5 to 4 cm) above the medial third of the clavicle.

The **costal pleura** lines the inner surfaces of the ribs, the costal cartilages, the intercostal spaces, the sides of the vertebral bodies, and the back of the sternum (Fig. 3-3).

The **diaphragmatic pleura** covers the thoracic surface of the diaphragm (Figs. 3-3 and 3-5). In quiet respiration, the costal and diaphragmatic pleurae are in apposition to each other below the lower border of the lung. In deep inspiration, the margins of the base of the lung descend, and the costal and diaphragmatic pleurae separate. This lower area of the pleural cavity into which the lung expands on inspiration is referred to as the **costodiaphragmatic recess** (Figs. 3-4 and 3-5).

The **mediastinal pleura** covers and forms the lateral boundary of the mediastinum (Figs. 3-3 and 3-5). At the hilum of the lung, it is reflected as a cuff around the vessels and bronchi and here becomes continuous with the visceral pleura. It is thus seen that each lung lies free except at its hilum, where it is attached to the blood vessels and bronchi that constitute the **lung root.** During full inspiration the lungs expand and fill the pleural cavities. However, during quiet inspiration the lungs do not fully occupy the pleural cavities at four sites: the right and left costodiaphragmatic recesses and the right and left costomediastinal recesses.

The **costodiaphragmatic recesses** are slitlike spaces between the costal and diaphragmatic parietal pleurae that are separated only by a capillary layer of pleural fluid. During inspiration, the lower margins of the lungs descend into the recesses. During expiration, the lower margins of the lungs ascend so that the costal and diaphragmatic pleurae come together again.

The **costomediastinal recesses** are situated along the anterior margins of the pleura. They are slitlike spaces between the costal and the mediastinal parietal pleurae, which are separated by a capillary layer of pleural fluid. During inspiration and expiration, the anterior borders of the lungs slide in and out of the recesses.

The surface markings of the lungs and pleurae were described on pages 68 and 72.

Nerve Supply of the Pleura

The parietal pleura (Fig. 3-8) is sensitive to pain, temperature, touch, and pressure and is supplied as follows:

- The costal pleura is segmentally supplied by the intercostal nerves.
- The mediastinal pleura is supplied by the phrenic nerve.
- The diaphragmatic pleura is supplied over the domes by the phrenic nerve and around the periphery by the lower six intercostal nerves.

The visceral pleura covering the lungs is sensitive to stretch but is insensitive to common sensations such as pain and touch. It receives an autonomic nerve supply from the pulmonary plexus (Fig. 3-8).

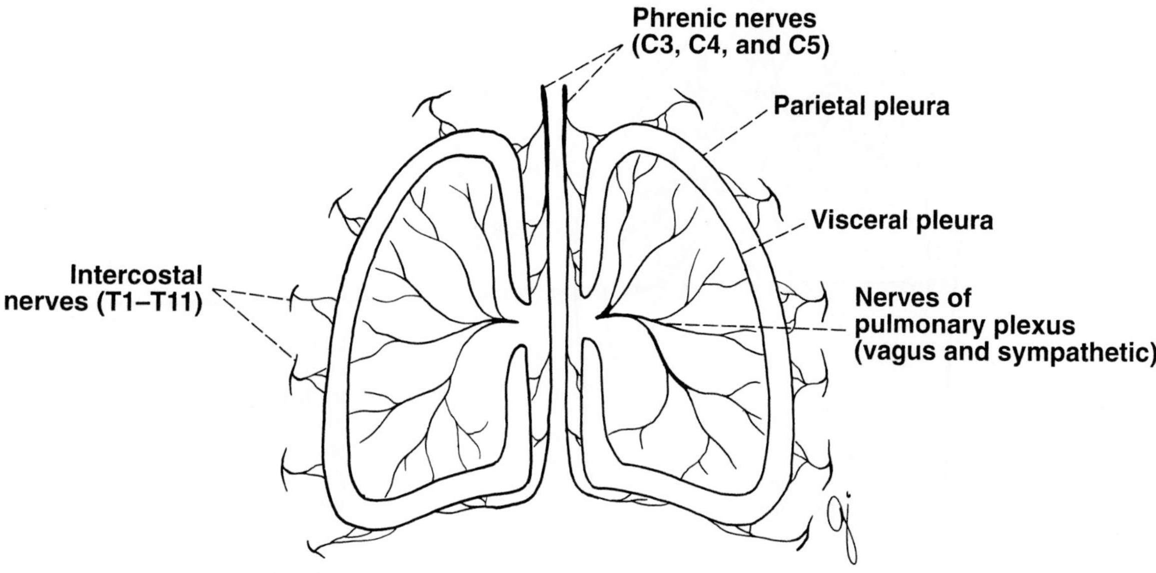

Figure 3-8 Diagram showing the innervation of the parietal and visceral layers of pleura.

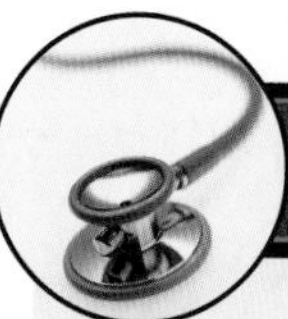

CLINICAL NOTES

Pleural Fluid

The pleural space normally contains 5 to 10 mL of clear fluid, which lubricates the apposing surfaces of the visceral and parietal pleurae during respiratory movements. The formation of the fluid results from hydrostatic and osmotic pressures. Since the hydrostatic pressures are greater in the capillaries of the parietal pleura than in the capillaries of the visceral pleura (pulmonary circulation), the pleural fluid is normally absorbed into the capillaries of the visceral pleura. Any condition that increases the production of the fluid (e.g., inflammation, malignancy, congestive heart disease) or impairs the drainage of the fluid (e.g., collapsed lung) results in the abnormal accumulation of fluid, called a **pleural effusion.** The presence of 300 mL of fluid in the costodiaphragmatic recess in an adult is sufficient to enable its clinical detection. The clinical signs include decreased lung expansion on the side of the effusion, with decreased breath sounds and dullness on percussion over the effusion.

Pleurisy

Inflammation of the pleura **(pleuritis** or **pleurisy),** secondary to inflammation of the lung (e.g., **pneumonia),** results in the pleural surfaces becoming coated with inflammatory exudate, causing the surfaces to be roughened. This roughening produces friction, and a **pleural rub** can be heard with the stethoscope on inspiration and expiration. Often the exudate becomes invaded by fibroblasts, which lay down collagen and bind the visceral pleura to the parietal pleura, forming **pleural adhesions.**

Pneumothorax, Empyema, and Pleural Effusion

As the result of disease or injury (stab or gunshot wounds), air can enter the pleural cavity from the lungs or through the chest wall (pneumothorax). In the old treatment of tuberculosis, air was purposely injected into the pleural cavity to collapse and rest the lung. This was known as **artificial pneumothorax.** A **spontaneous pneumothorax** is a condition in which air enters the pleural cavity suddenly without its cause being immediately apparent. After investigation, it is usually found that air has entered from a diseased lung and a bulla (bleb) has ruptured.

Stab wounds of the thoracic wall may pierce the parietal pleura so that the pleural cavity is open to the outside air. This condition is called **open pneumothorax.** Each time the patient inspires, it is possible to hear air under atmospheric pressure being sucked into the pleural cavity. Sometimes the clothing and the layers of the thoracic wall combine to form a valve so that air enters on inspiration but cannot exit through the wound. In these circumstances, the air pressure builds up on the wounded side and pushes the mediastinum toward the opposite side. In this situation, a collapsed lung is on the injured side and the opposite lung is compressed by the deflected mediastinum. This dangerous condition is called a **tension pneumothorax.**

Air in the pleural cavity associated with serous fluid is known as **hydropneumothorax,** associated with pus as **pyopneumothorax,** and associated with blood as **hemopneumothorax.** A collection of pus (without air) in the pleural cavity is called an **empyema.** The presence of serous fluid in the pleural cavity is referred to as a **pleural effusion** (Fig. 3-9). Fluid (serous, blood, or pus) can be drained from the pleural cavity through a wide-bore needle, as described on page 60.

In hemopneumothorax, blood enters the pleural cavity. It can be caused by stab or bullet wounds to the chest wall, resulting in bleeding from blood vessels in the chest wall, from vessels in the chest cavity, or from a lacerated lung.

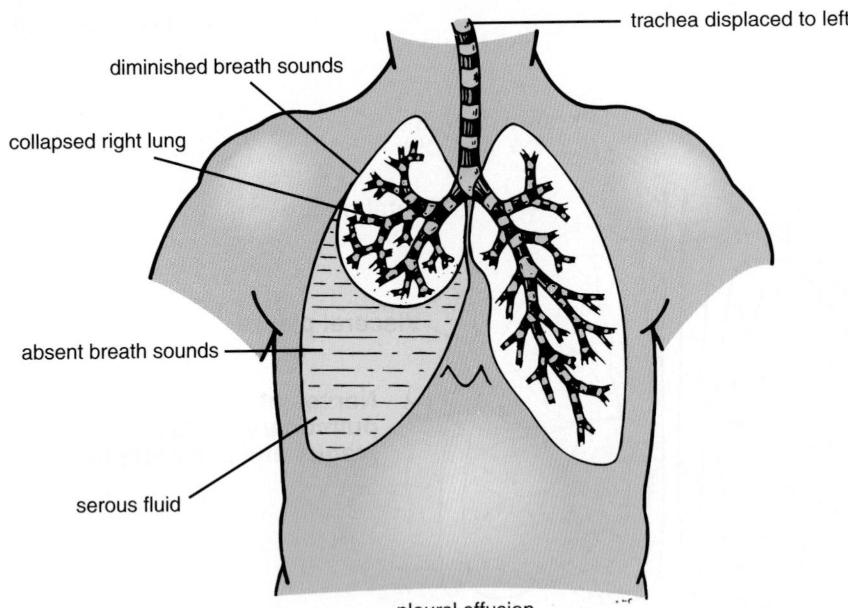

Figure 3-9 Case of right-sided pleural effusion. The mediastinum is displaced to the left, the right lung is compressed, and the bronchi are narrowed. Auscultation would reveal only faint breath sounds over the compressed lung and absent breath sounds over fluid in the pleural cavity.

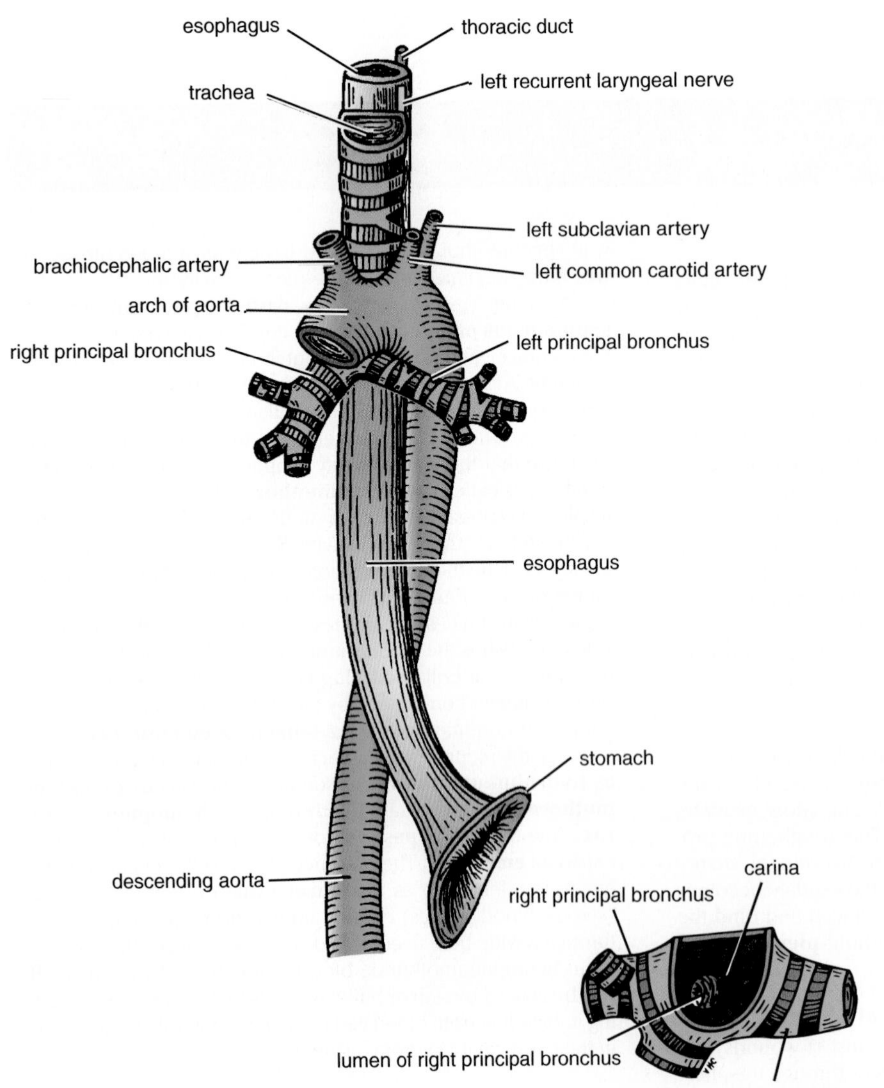

Figure 3-10 Thoracic part of the trachea. Note that the right principal bronchus is wider and has a more direct continuation of the trachea than the left. Bifurcation of the trachea viewed from above is also shown.

Trachea

The trachea is a mobile cartilaginous and membranous tube (Fig. 3-10). It begins in the neck as a continuation of the larynx at the lower border of the cricoid cartilage at the level of the sixth cervical vertebra. It descends in the midline of the neck. In the thorax the trachea ends below at the **carina** by dividing into right and left principal (main) bronchi at the level of the sternal angle (opposite the disc between the fourth and fifth thoracic vertebrae). During expiration the bifurcation rises by about one vertebral level, and during deep inspiration may be lowered as far as the sixth thoracic vertebra.

In adults the trachea is about 4½ in. (11.25 cm) long and 1 in. (2.5 cm) in diameter (Fig. 3-10). The fibroelastic tube is kept patent by the presence of U-shaped bars (rings) of hyaline cartilage embedded in its wall. The posterior free ends of the cartilage are connected by smooth muscle, the **trachealis muscle.**

The relations of the trachea in the neck are described on page 810.

The relations of the trachea in the superior mediastinum of the thorax are as follows:

- **Anteriorly:** The sternum, the thymus, the left brachiocephalic vein, the origins of the brachiocephalic and left common carotid arteries, and the arch of the aorta (Figs. 3-6A, 3-10, and 3-31)
- **Posteriorly:** The esophagus and the left recurrent laryngeal nerve (Fig. 3-6A)
- **Right side:** The azygos vein, the right vagus nerve, and the pleura (Figs. 3-6, 3-16A, and 3-17)
- **Left side:** The arch of the aorta, the left common carotid and left subclavian arteries, the left vagus and left phrenic nerves, and the pleura (Figs. 3-6, 3-16B, and 3-18)

Blood Supply of the Trachea

The upper two thirds are supplied by the inferior thyroid arteries and the lower third is supplied by the bronchial arteries.

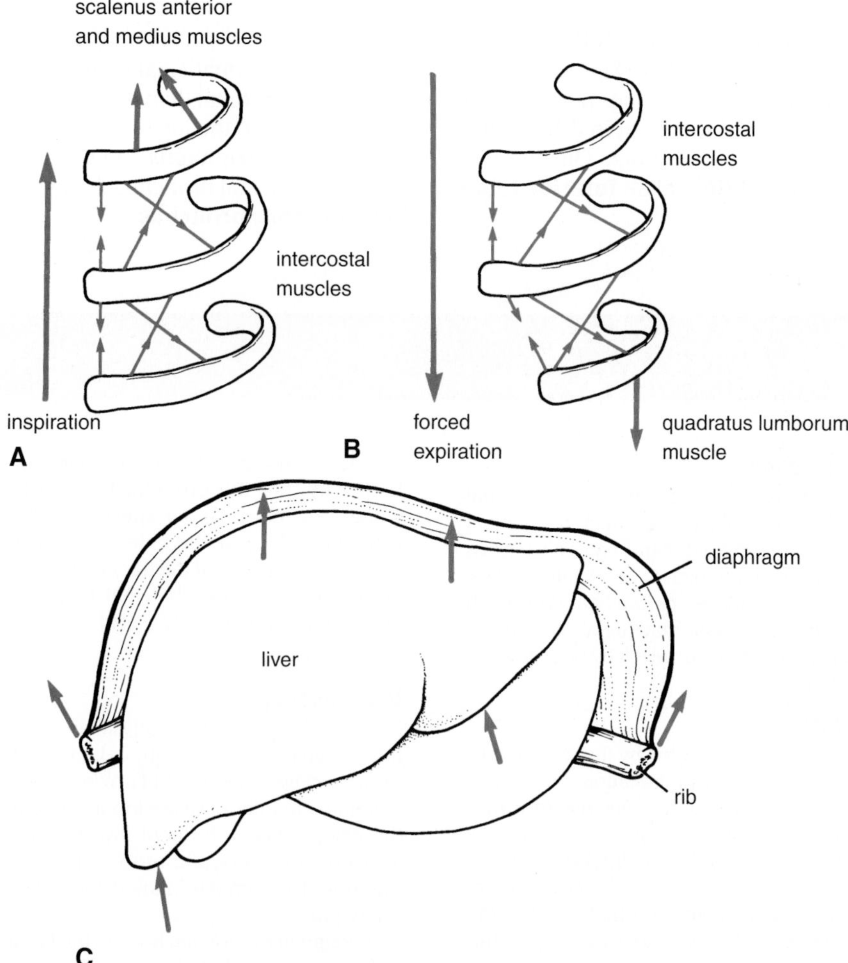

Figure 3-11 **A.** How the intercostal muscles raise the ribs during inspiration. Note that the scaleni muscles fix the first rib or, in forced inspiration, raise the first rib. **B.** How the intercostal muscles can be used in forced expiration, provided that the 12th rib is fixed or is made to descend by the abdominal muscles. **C.** How the liver provides the platform that enables the diaphragm to raise the lower ribs.

Lymph Drainage of the Trachea

The lymph drains into the pretracheal and paratracheal lymph nodes and the deep cervical nodes.

Nerve Supply of the Trachea

The sensory nerve supply is from the vagi and the recurrent laryngeal nerves. Sympathetic nerves supply the trachealis muscle.

The Bronchi

The trachea bifurcates behind the arch of the aorta into the **right and left principal (primary, or main) bronchi** (Figs. 3-10, 3-19, and 3-20). The bronchi divide dichotomously, giving rise to several million terminal bronchioles that terminate in one or more respiratory bronchioles. Each respiratory bronchiole divides into 2 to 11 alveolar ducts that enter the alveolar sacs. The alveoli arise from the walls of the sacs as diverticula (see page 94).

Principal Bronchi

The right principal (main) bronchus (Fig. 3-12) is wider, shorter, and more vertical than the left (Figs. 3-10, 3-19, and 3-20) and is about 1 in. (2.5 cm) long. Before entering the hilum of the right lung, the principal bronchus gives off the **superior lobar bronchus.** On entering the hilum, it divides into a **middle** and an **inferior lobar bronchus.**

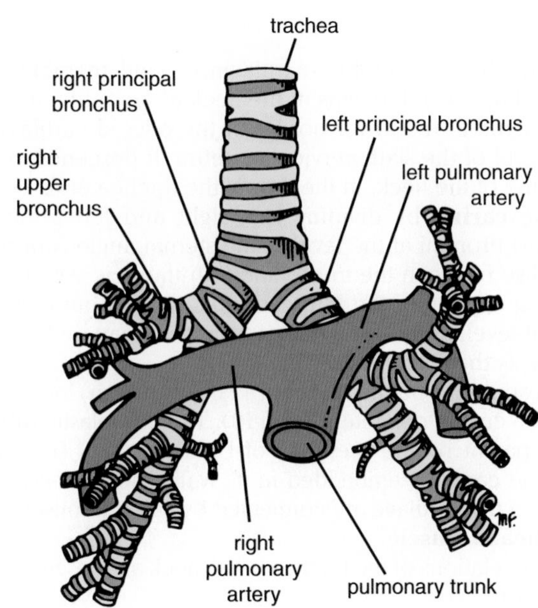

Figure 3-12 Relationship of the pulmonary arteries to the bronchial tree.

The left principal (main) bronchus is narrower, longer, and more horizontal than the right and is about 2 in. (5 cm) long. It passes to the left below the arch of the aorta and **in front of the esophagus.** On entering the hilum of the left lung, the principal bronchus divides into a **superior** and an **inferior lobar bronchus.**

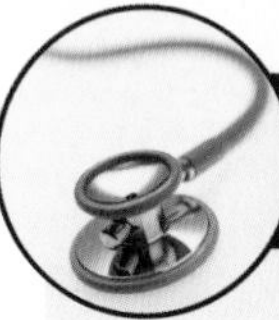

CLINICAL NOTES

Compression of the Trachea

The trachea is a membranous tube kept patent under normal conditions by U-shaped bars of cartilage. In the neck, a unilateral or bilateral enlargement of the thyroid gland can cause gross displacement or compression of the trachea. A dilatation of the aortic arch (aneurysm) can compress the trachea. With each cardiac systole the pulsating aneurysm may tug at the trachea and left bronchus, a clinical sign that can be felt by palpating the trachea in the suprasternal notch.

Tracheitis or Bronchitis

The mucosa lining the trachea is innervated by the recurrent laryngeal nerve and, in the region of its bifurcation, by the pulmonary plexus. A tracheitis or bronchitis gives rise to a raw, burning sensation felt deep to the sternum instead of actual pain. Many thoracic and abdominal viscera, when diseased, give rise to discomfort that is felt in the midline (see page 280). It seems that organs possessing a sensory innervation that is not under normal conditions directly relayed to consciousness display this phenomenon. The afferent fibers from these organs traveling to the central nervous system accompany autonomic nerves.

Inhaled Foreign Bodies

Inhalation of foreign bodies into the lower respiratory tract is common, especially in children. Pins, screws, nuts, bolts, peanuts, and parts of chicken bones and toys have all found their way into the bronchi. Parts of teeth may be inhaled while a patient is under anesthesia during a difficult dental extraction. Because the right bronchus is the wider and more direct continuation of the trachea (Figs. 3-19 and 3-20), foreign bodies tend to enter the right instead of the left bronchus. From there, they usually pass into the middle or lower lobe bronchi.

Bronchoscopy

Bronchoscopy enables a physician to examine the interior of the trachea; its bifurcation, called the **carina;** and the main bronchi (Figs. 3-13 and 3-14). With experience, it is possible to examine the interior of the lobar bronchi and the beginning of the first segmental bronchi. By means of this procedure, it is also possible to obtain biopsy specimens of mucous membrane and to remove inhaled foreign bodies (even an open safety pin).

Lodgment of a foreign body in the larynx or edema of the mucous membrane of the larynx secondary to infection or trauma may require immediate relief to prevent asphyxiation. A method commonly used to relieve complete obstruction is tracheostomy (see page 813).

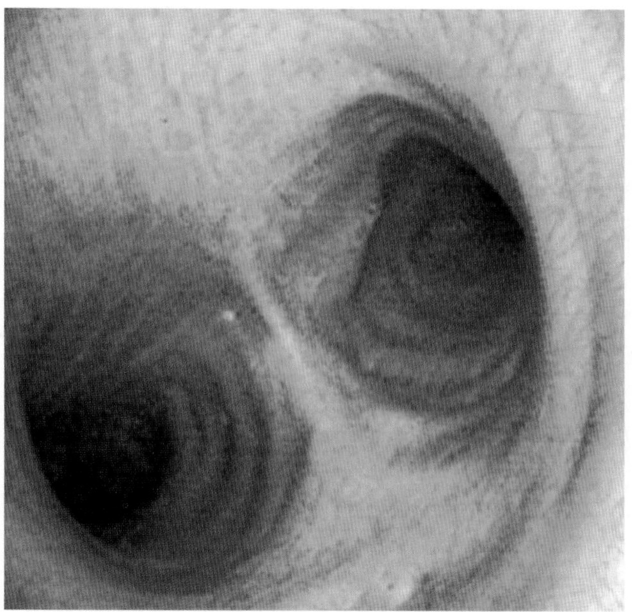

Figure 3-13 The bifurcation of the trachea as seen through an operating bronchoscope. Note the ridge of the carina in the center and the opening into the right main bronchus on the right, which is a more direct continuation of the trachea. (Courtesy of E.D. Andersen.)

Figure 3-14 The interior of the left main bronchus as seen through an operating bronchoscope. The openings into the left upper lobe bronchus and its division and the left lower lobe bronchus are indicated. (Courtesy of E.D. Andersen.)

Lungs

During life, the right and left lungs are soft and spongy and very elastic. If the thoracic cavity were opened, the lungs would immediately shrink to one third or less in volume. In the child, they are pink, but with age, they become dark and mottled because of the inhalation of dust particles that become trapped in the phagocytes of the lung. This is especially well seen in city dwellers and coal miners. The lungs are situated so that one lies on each side of the mediastinum. They are therefore separated from each other by the heart and great vessels and other structures in the mediastinum. Each lung is conical, covered with visceral

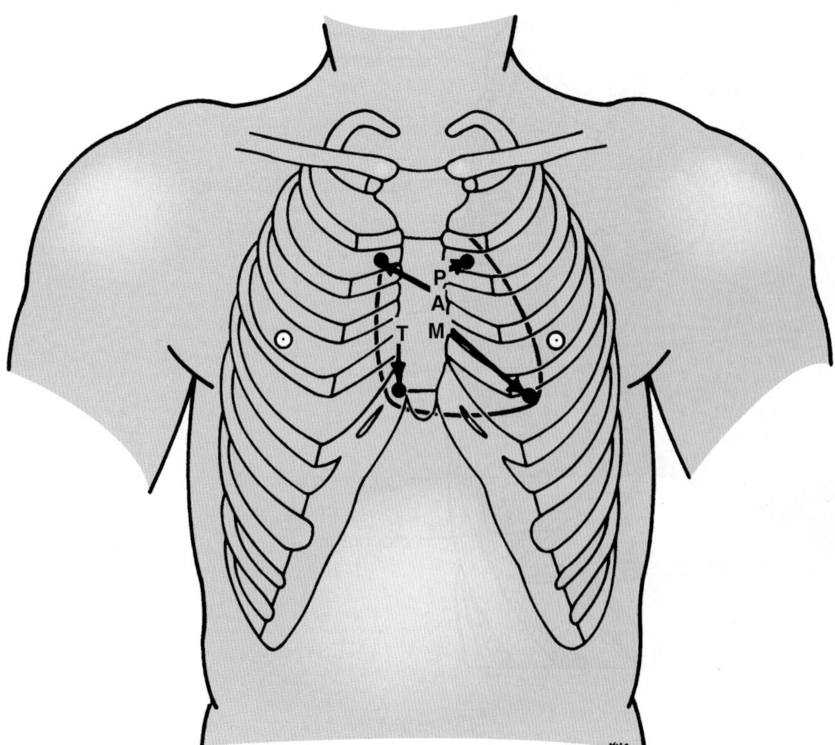

Figure 3-15 Position of the heart valves. P, pulmonary valve; A, aortic valve; M, mitral valve; T, tricuspid valve. Arrows indicate position where valves may be heard with least interference.

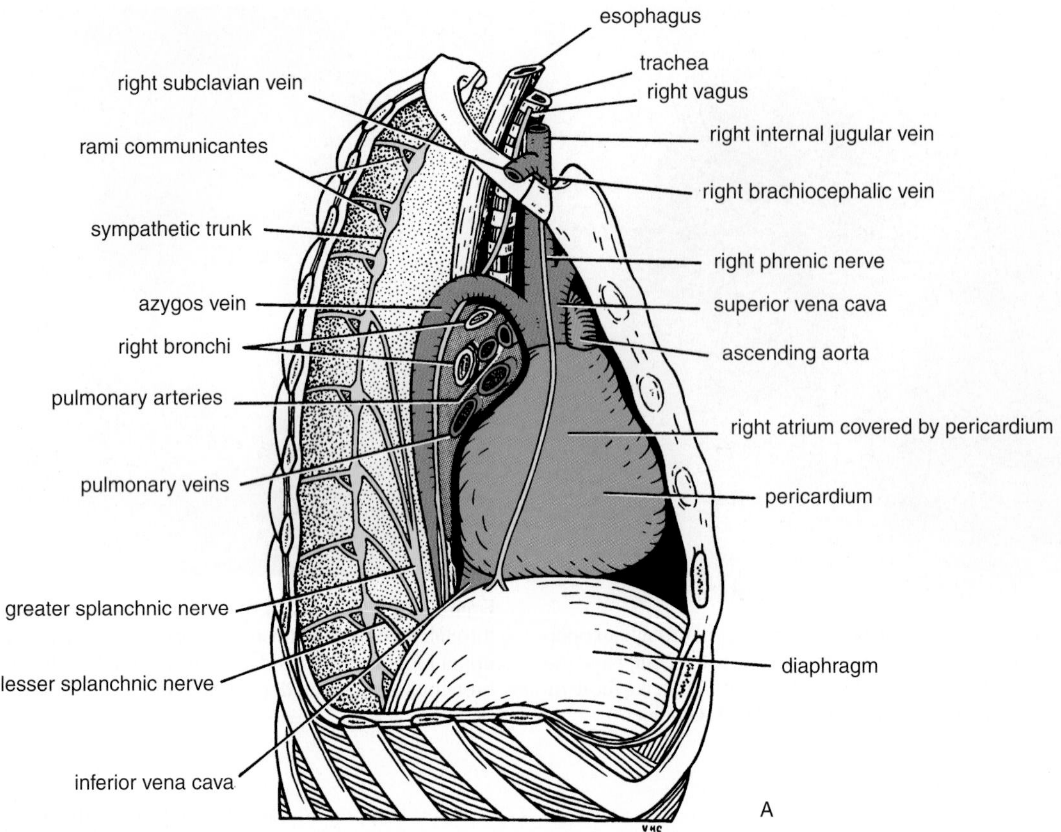

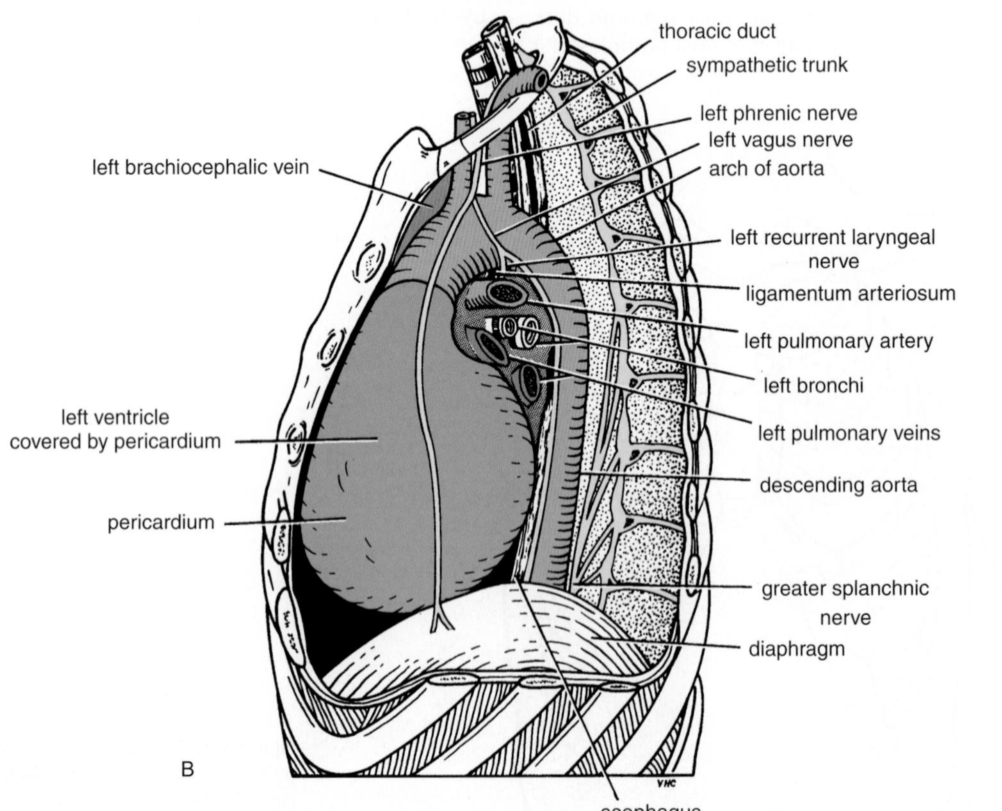

Figure 3-16 **A.** Right side of the mediastinum. **B.** Left side of the mediastinum.

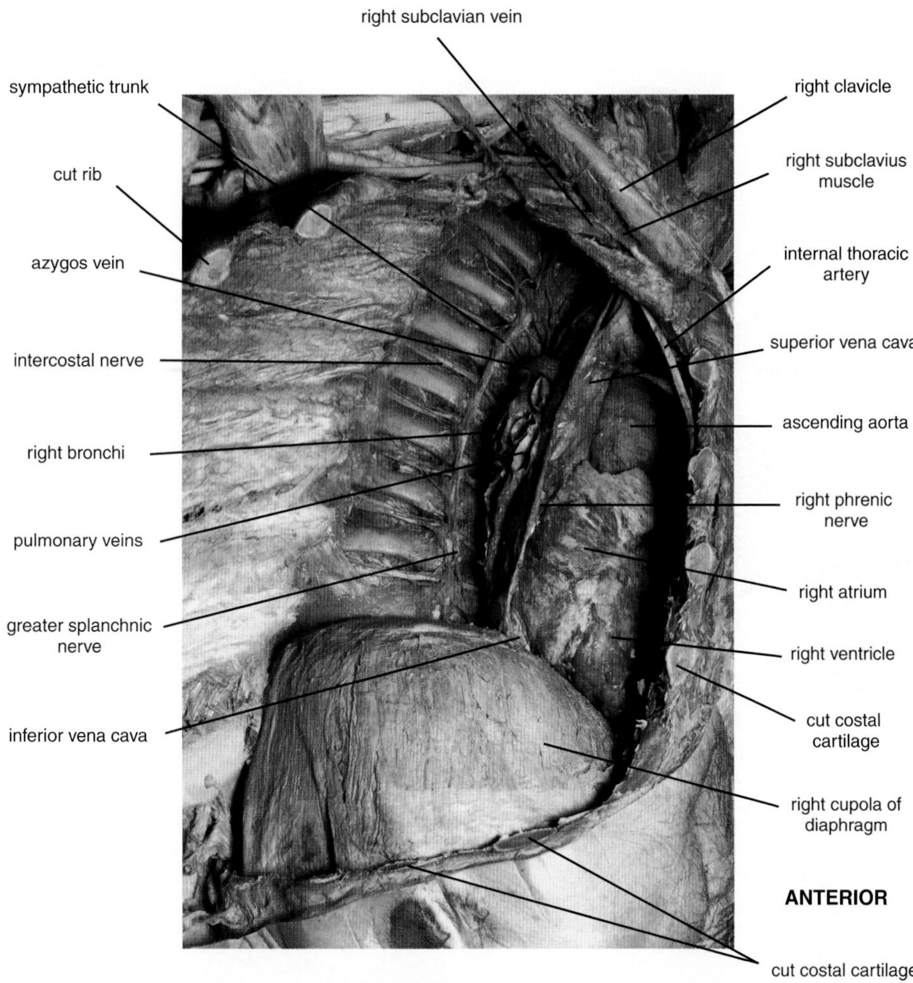

Figure 3-17 Dissection of the right side of the mediastinum; the right lung and the pericardium have been removed. The costal parietal pleura has also been removed.

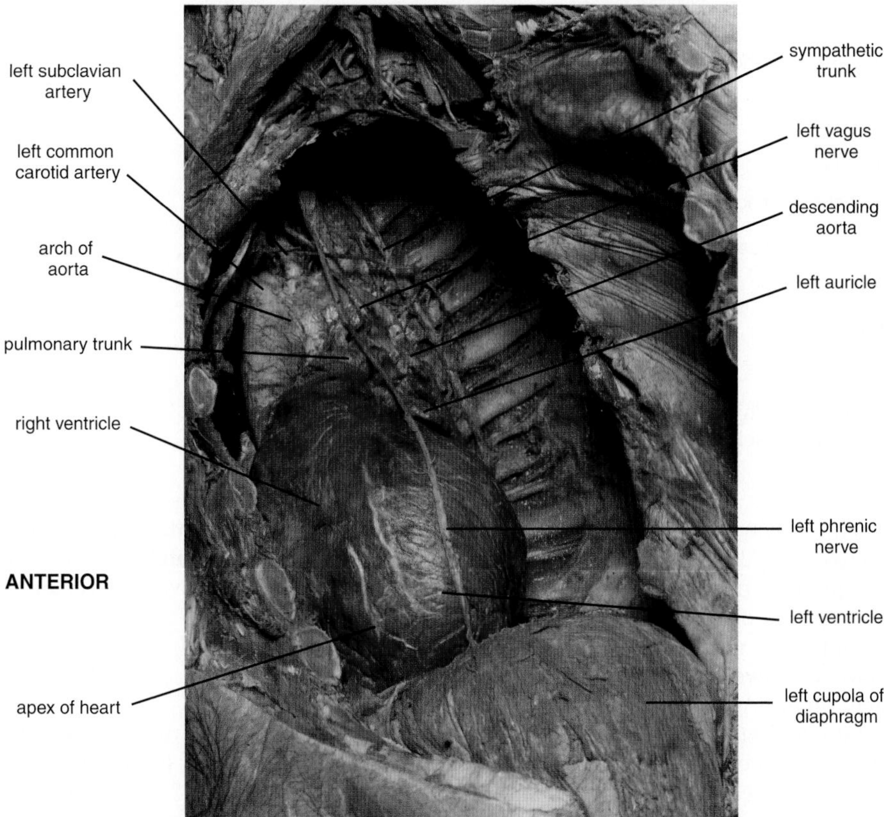

Figure 3-18 Dissection of the left side of the mediastinum; the left lung and the pericardium have been removed. The costal parietal pleura has also been removed.

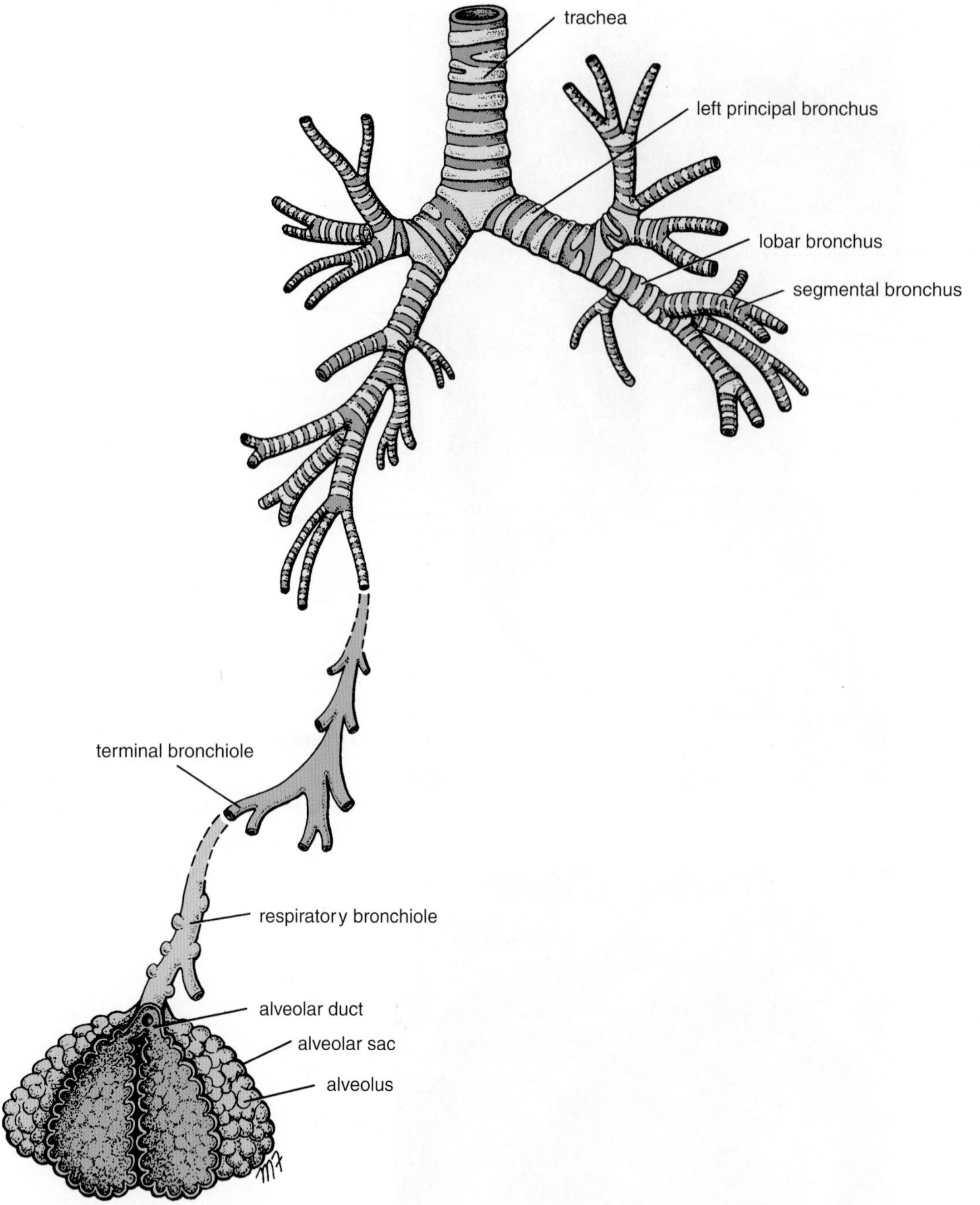

Figure 3-19 Trachea, bronchi, bronchioles, alveolar ducts, alveolar sacs, and alveoli. Note the path taken by inspired air from the trachea to the alveoli.

pleura, and suspended free in its own pleural cavity, being attached to the mediastinum only by its root (Fig. 3-4).

Each lung has a blunt **apex,** which projects upward into the neck for about 1 in. (2.5 cm) above the clavicle; a concave **base** that sits on the diaphragm; a convex **costal surface,** which corresponds to the concave chest wall; and a concave **mediastinal surface,** which is molded to the pericardium and other mediastinal structures (Figs. 3-21 and 3-22). At about the middle of this surface is the **hilum,** a depression in which the bronchi, vessels, and nerves that form the **root** enter and leave the lung.

The **anterior border** is thin and overlaps the heart; it is here on the left lung that the **cardiac notch** is found. The posterior border is thick and lies beside the vertebral column.

Lobes and Fissures

Right Lung

The right lung is slightly larger than the left and is divided by the oblique and horizontal fissures into three lobes: the **upper, middle,** and **lower lobes** (Fig. 3-21). The **oblique fissure** runs from the inferior border upward and backward

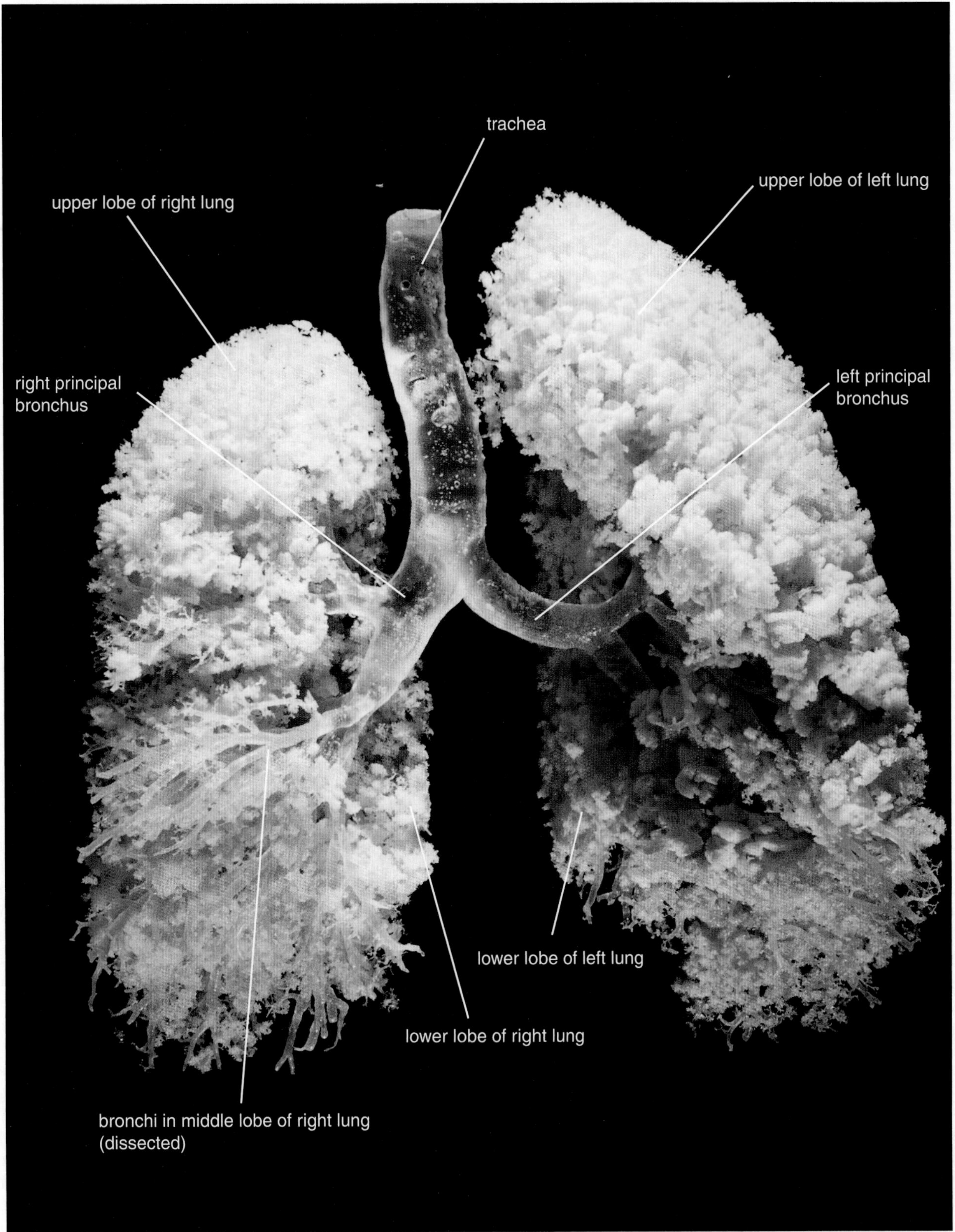

Figure 3-20 A plastinized specimen of an adult trachea, principal bronchi, and lung; some of the lung tissue has been dissected to reveal the larger bronchi. Note that the right main bronchus is wider and a more direct continuation of the trachea than the left main bronchus.

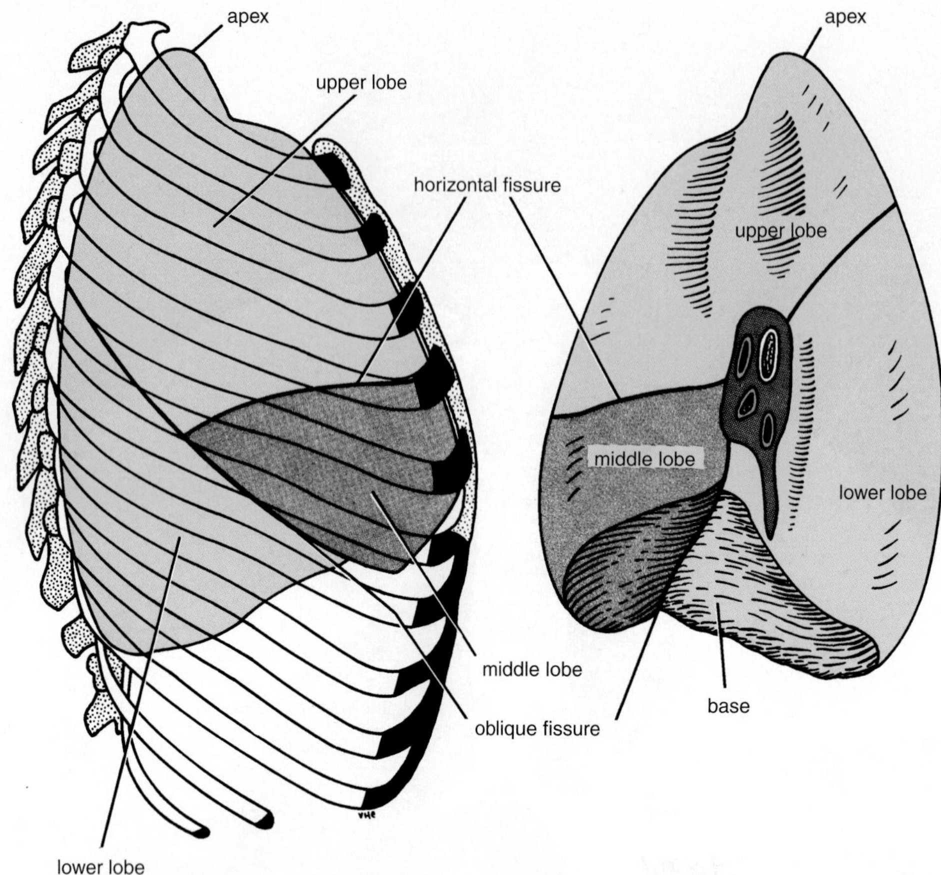

Figure 3-21 Lateral and medial surfaces of the right lung.

across the medial and costal surfaces until it cuts the posterior border about 2.5 in. (6.25 cm) below the apex. The **horizontal fissure** runs horizontally across the costal surface at the level of the fourth costal cartilage to meet the oblique fissure in the midaxillary line. The middle lobe is thus a small triangular lobe bounded by the horizontal and oblique fissures.

Left Lung

The left lung is divided by a similar oblique fissure into two lobes: the **upper** and **lower lobes** (Fig. 3-22). There is no horizontal fissure in the left lung.

Bronchopulmonary Segments

The bronchopulmonary segments are the anatomic, functional, and surgical units of the lungs. Each lobar (secondary) bronchus, which passes to a lobe of the lung, gives off branches called **segmental (tertiary) bronchi** (Fig. 3-19). Each segmental bronchus passes to a structurally and functionally independent unit of a lung lobe called a **bronchopulmonary segment,** which is surrounded by connective tissue (Fig. 3-23). The segmental bronchus is accompanied by a branch of the pulmonary artery, but the tributaries of the pulmonary veins run in the connective tissue between adjacent bronchopulmonary segments. Each segment has its own lymphatic vessels and autonomic nerve supply.

On entering a bronchopulmonary segment, each segmental bronchus divides repeatedly (Fig. 3-23). As the bronchi become smaller, the U-shaped bars of cartilage found in the trachea are gradually replaced by irregular plates of cartilage, which become smaller and fewer in number. The smallest bronchi divide and give rise to **bronchioles,** which are less than 1 mm in diameter (Fig. 3-23). Bronchioles possess no cartilage in their walls and are lined with columnar ciliated epithelium. The submucosa possesses a complete layer of circularly arranged smooth muscle fibers.

The bronchioles then divide and give rise to **terminal bronchioles** (Fig. 3-23), which show delicate outpouchings from their walls. Gaseous exchange between blood and air takes place in the walls of these outpouchings, which explains the name **respiratory bronchiole.** The diameter of a respiratory bronchiole is about 0.5 mm. The respiratory bronchioles end by branching into **alveolar ducts,** which lead into tubular passages with numerous thin-walled outpouchings called **alveolar sacs.** The alveolar sacs consist of several alveoli opening into a single chamber (Figs. 3-23 and 3-24). Each alveolus is surrounded by a rich network of blood capillaries. Gaseous exchange takes place between the air in the alveolar lumen through the alveolar wall into the blood within the surrounding capillaries.

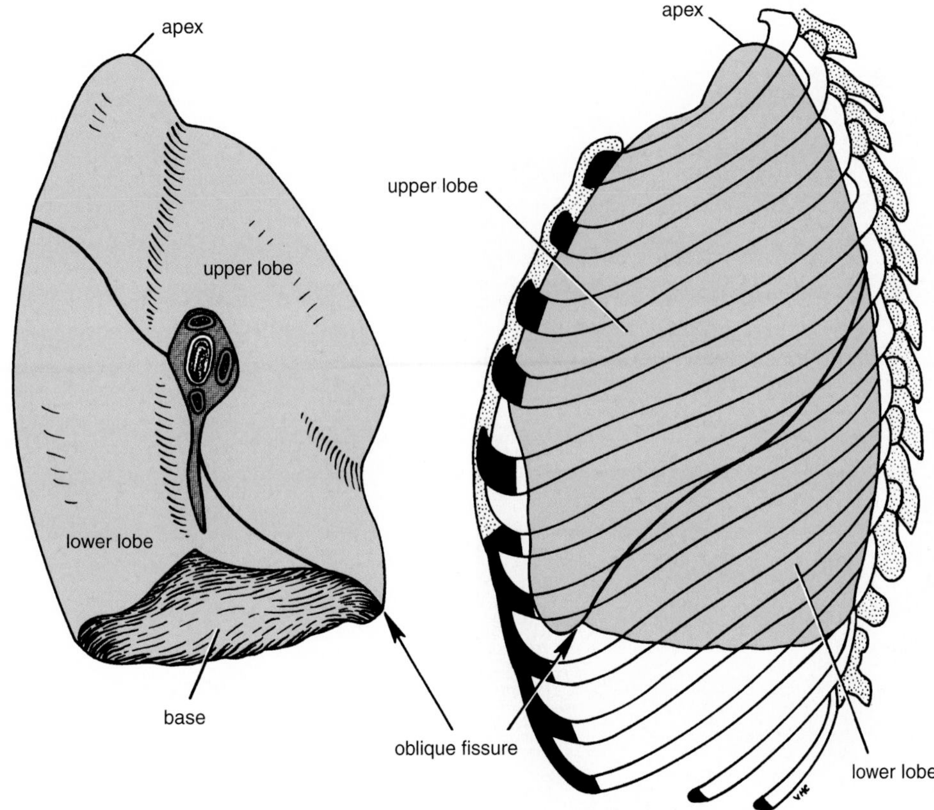

Figure 3-22 Lateral and medial surfaces of the left lung.

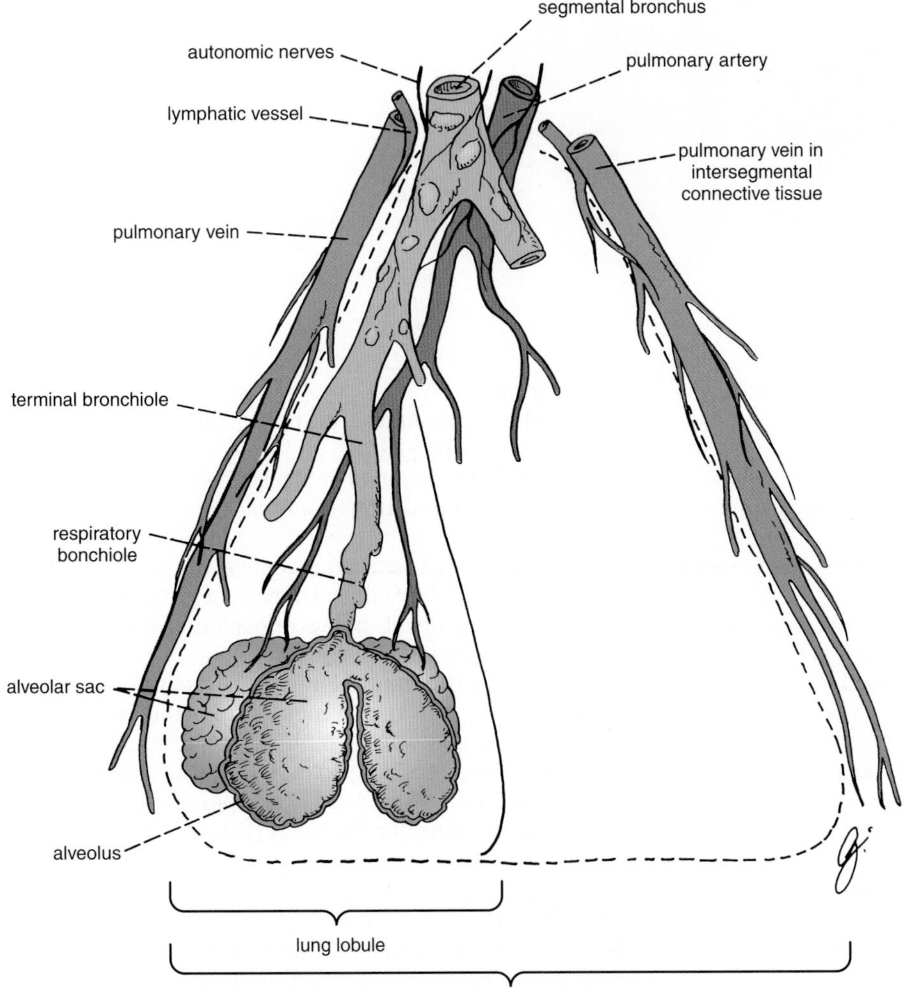

Figure 3-23 A bronchopulmonary segment and a lung lobule. Note that the pulmonary veins lie within the connective tissue septa that separate adjacent segments.

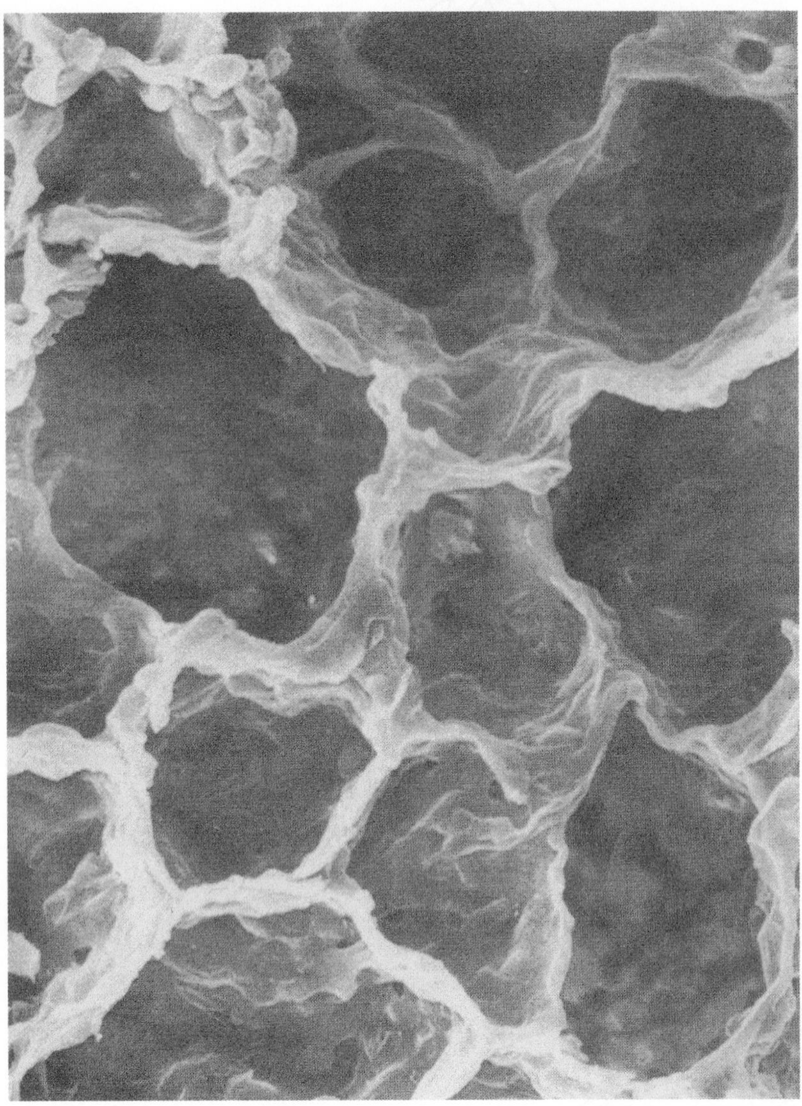

Figure 3-24 Scanning electron micrograph of the lung showing numerous alveolar sacs. The alveoli are the depressions, or alcoves, along the walls of the alveolar sac. (Courtesy of Dr. M. Koering.)

The main characteristics of a bronchopulmonary segment may be summarized as follows:

- It is a subdivision of a lung lobe.
- It is pyramid shaped, with its apex toward the lung root.
- It is surrounded by connective tissue.
- It has a segmental bronchus, a segmental artery, lymph vessels, and autonomic nerves.
- The segmental vein lies in the connective tissue between adjacent bronchopulmonary segments.
- Because it is a structural unit, a diseased segment can be removed surgically.

The main bronchopulmonary segments (Figs. 3-25 and 3-26) are as follows:

- **Right lung**
  Superior lobe: Apical, posterior, anterior
  Middle lobe: Lateral, medial
  Inferior lobe: Superior (apical), medial basal, anterior basal, lateral basal, posterior basal
- **Left lung**
  Superior lobe: Apical, posterior, anterior, superior lingular, inferior lingular
  Inferior lobe: Superior (apical), medial basal, anterior basal, lateral basal, posterior basal

Although the general arrangement of the bronchopulmonary segments is of clinical importance, it is unnecessary to memorize the details unless one intends to specialize in pulmonary medicine or surgery.

The **root of the lung** is formed of structures that are entering or leaving the lung. It is made up of the bronchi, pulmonary artery and veins, lymph vessels, bronchial vessels, and nerves. The root is surrounded by a tubular sheath of pleura, which joins the mediastinal parietal pleura to the visceral pleura covering the lungs (Figs. 3-5, 3-16, 3-17, and 3-18).

Blood Supply of the Lungs

The bronchi, the connective tissue of the lung, and the visceral pleura receive their blood supply from the bronchial

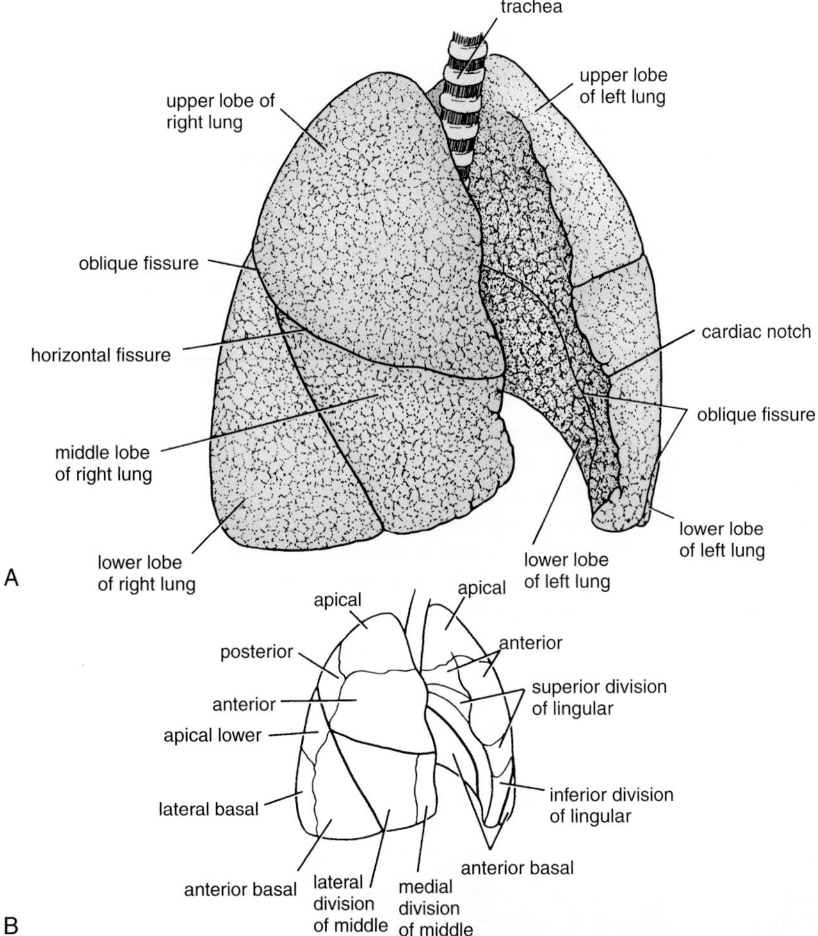

Figure 3-25 Lungs viewed from the right. **A.** Lobes. **B.** Bronchopulmonary segments.

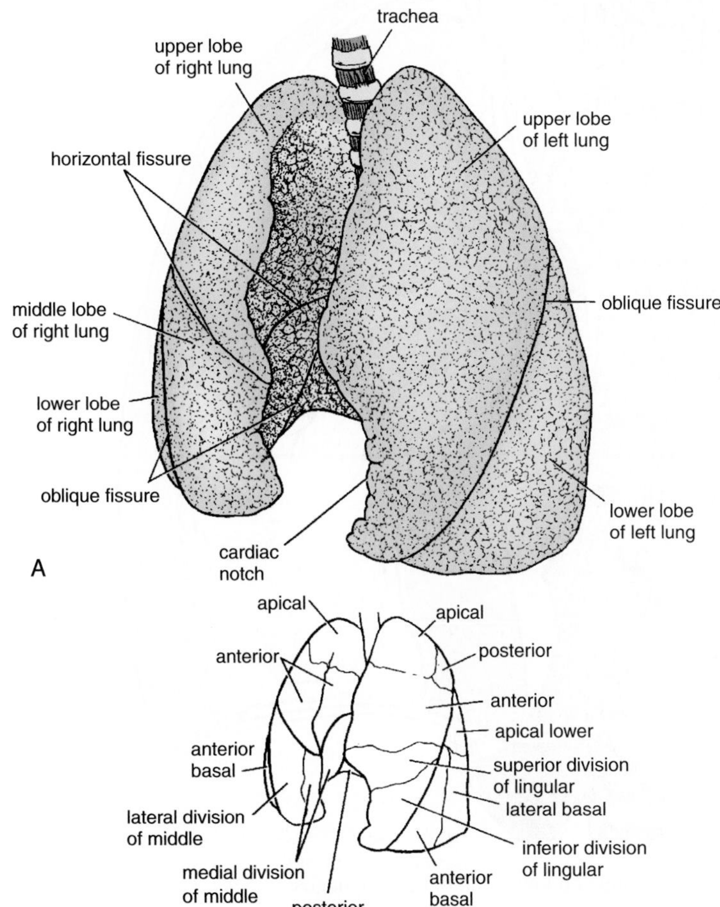

Figure 3-26 Lungs viewed from the left. **A.** Lobes. **B.** Bronchopulmonary segments.

arteries, which are branches of the descending aorta. The bronchial veins (which communicate with the pulmonary veins) drain into the azygos and hemiazygos veins.

The alveoli receive deoxygenated blood from the terminal branches of the pulmonary arteries. The oxygenated blood leaving the alveolar capillaries drains into the tributaries of the pulmonary veins, which follow the intersegmental connective tissue septa to the lung root. Two pulmonary veins leave each lung root (Fig. 3-16) to empty into the left atrium of the heart.

Lymph Drainage of the Lungs

The lymph vessels originate in superficial and deep plexuses (Fig. 3-27); they are not present in the alveolar walls. The **superficial (subpleural) plexus** lies beneath the visceral pleura and drains over the surface of the lung toward the hilum, where the lymph vessels enter the **bronchopulmonary nodes.** The **deep plexus** travels along the bronchi and pulmonary vessels toward the hilum of the lung, passing through **pulmonary nodes** located within the lung substance; the lymph then enters the bronchopulmonary nodes in the hilum of the lung. All the lymph from the lung leaves the hilum and drains into the **tracheobronchial nodes** and then into the **bronchomediastinal lymph trunks.**

Nerve Supply of the Lungs

At the root of each lung is a **pulmonary plexus** composed of efferent and afferent autonomic nerve fibers. The plexus is formed from branches of the sympathetic trunk and receives parasympathetic fibers from the vagus nerve.

The sympathetic efferent fibers produce bronchodilatation and vasoconstriction. The parasympathetic efferent fibers produce bronchoconstriction, vasodilatation, and increased glandular secretion.

Afferent impulses derived from the bronchial mucous membrane and from stretch receptors in the alveolar walls pass to the central nervous system in both sympathetic and parasympathetic nerves.

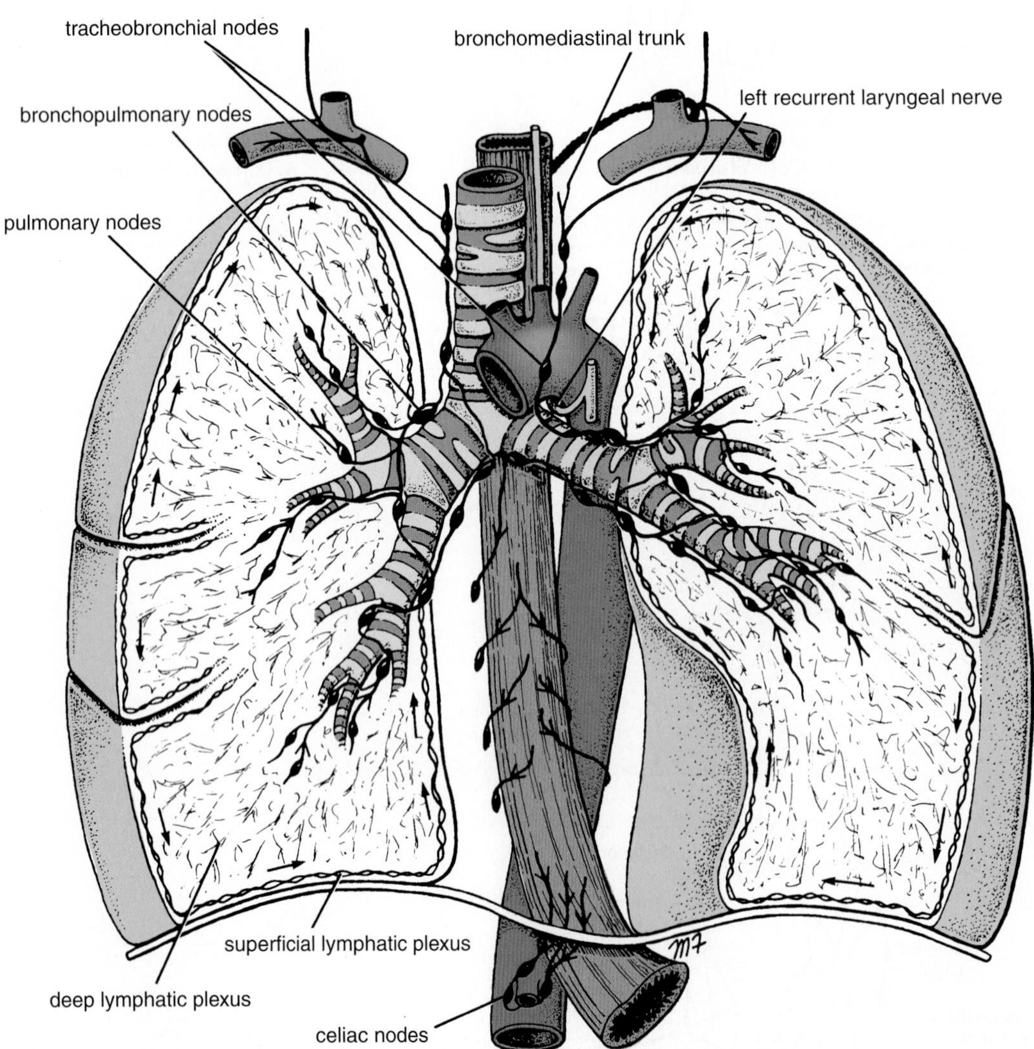

Figure 3-27 Lymph drainage of the lung and lower end of the esophagus.

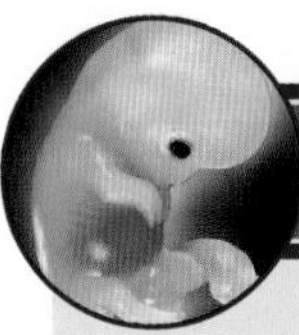

EMBRYOLOGIC NOTES

Development of the Lungs and Pleura

A longitudinal groove develops in the entodermal lining of the floor of the pharynx. This groove is known as the **laryngotracheal groove.** The lining of the larynx, trachea, and bronchi and the epithelium of the alveoli develop from this groove. The margins of the groove fuse and form the **laryngotracheal tube** (Fig. 3-28). The fusion process starts distally so that the lumen becomes separated from the developing esophagus. Just behind the developing tongue, a small opening persists that will become the permanent opening into the larynx. The laryngotracheal tube grows caudally into the splanchnic mesoderm and will eventually lie anterior to the esophagus. The tube divides distally into the right and left **lung buds.** Cartilage develops in the mesenchyme surrounding the tube, and the upper part of the tube becomes the **larynx,** whereas the lower part becomes the **trachea.**

Each lung bud consists of an entodermal tube surrounded by splanchnic mesoderm; from this, all the tissues of the corresponding lung are derived. Each bud grows laterally and projects into the pleural part of the embryonic coelom (Fig. 3-28). The lung bud divides into three lobes and then into two, corresponding to the number of **main bronchi** and **lobes** found in the fully developed lung. Each main bronchus then divides repeatedly in a dichotomous manner, until eventually the **terminal bronchioles** and **alveoli** are formed. The division of the terminal bronchioles, with the formation of additional bronchioles and alveoli, continues for some time after birth.

Each lung will receive a covering of **visceral pleura** derived from the splanchnic mesoderm. The **parietal pleura** will be formed from somatic mesoderm. By the seventh month, the capillary loops connected with the pulmonary circulation have become sufficiently well developed to support life, should premature birth take place. With the onset of respiration at birth, the lungs expand and the alveoli become dilated. However, it is only after 3 or 4 days of postnatal life that the alveoli in the periphery of each lung become fully expanded.

Congenital Anomalies

Esophageal Atresia and Tracheoesophageal Fistula

If the margins of the laryngotracheal groove fail to fuse adequately, an abnormal opening may be left between the laryngotracheal tube and the esophagus. If the tracheoesophageal septum formed by the fusion of the margins of the laryngotracheal groove should be deviated posteriorly, the lumen of the esophagus would be much reduced in diameter. The different types of atresia, with and without fistula, are shown in Figure 3-29. Obstruction of the esophagus prevents the child from swallowing saliva and milk, and this leads to aspiration into the larynx and trachea, which usually results in pneumonia. With early diagnosis, it is often possible to correct this serious anomaly surgically.

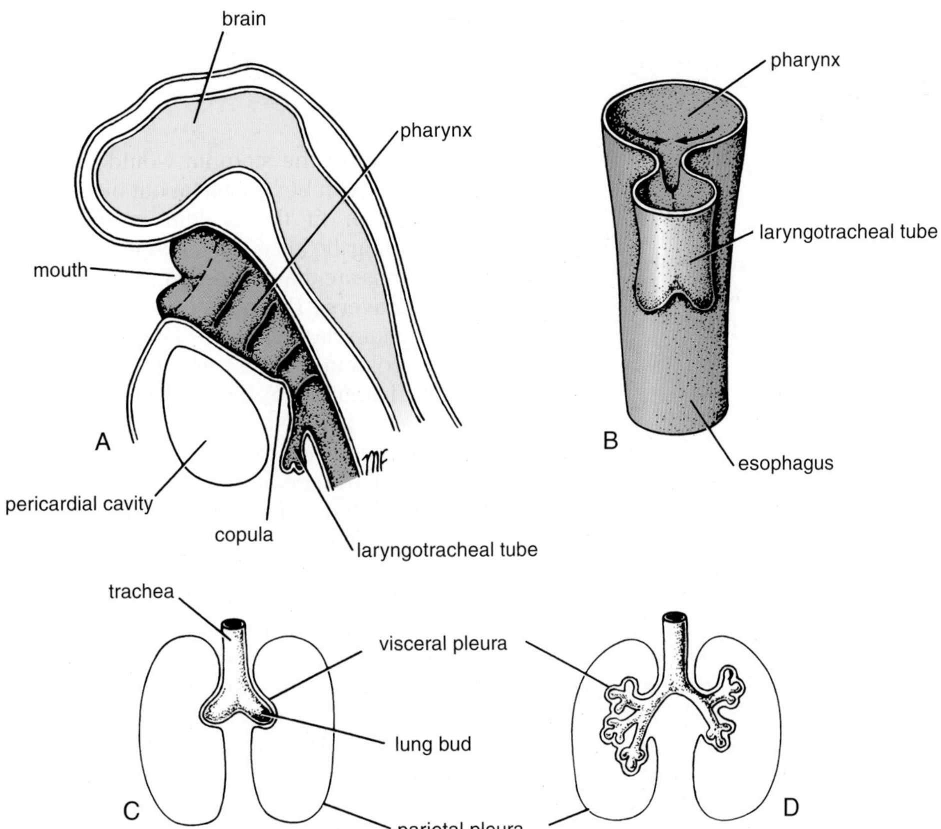

Figure 3-28 The development of the lungs. **A.** The laryngotracheal groove and tube have been formed. **B.** The margins of the laryngotracheal groove fuse to form the laryngotracheal tube. **C.** The lung buds invaginate the wall of the intraembryonic coelom. **D.** The lung buds divide to form the main bronchi.

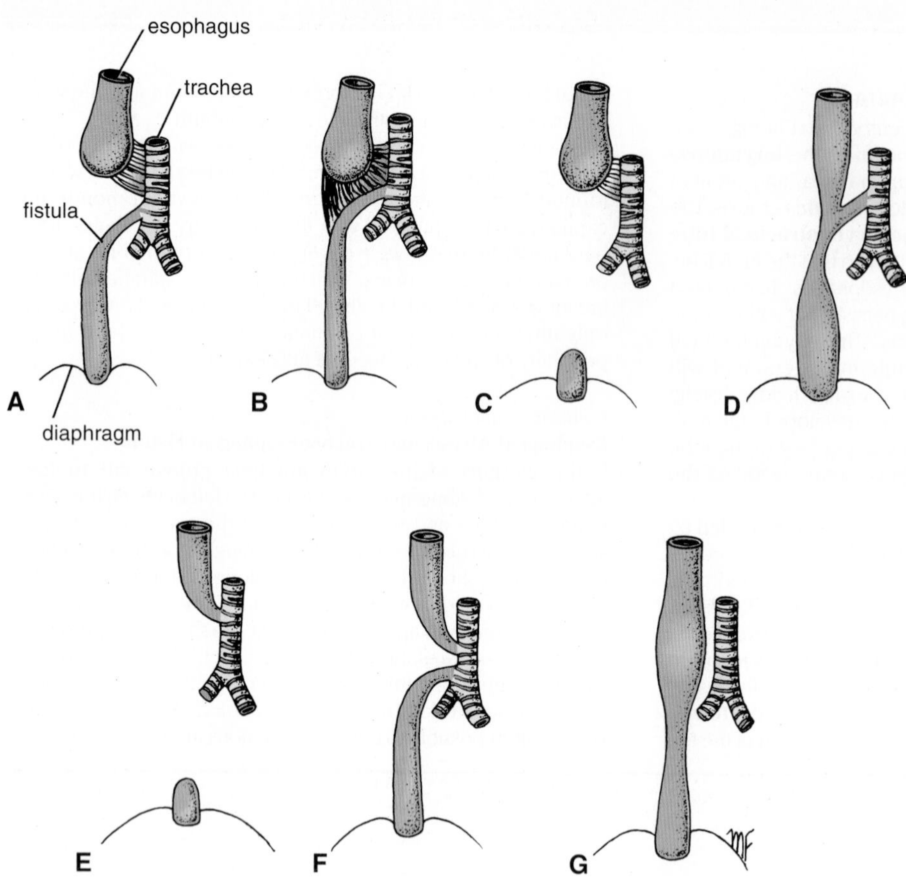

Figure 3-29 Different types of esophageal atresia and tracheoesophageal fistula. **A.** Complete blockage of the esophagus with a tracheoesophageal fistula. **B.** Similar to type A, but the two parts of the esophagus are joined together by fibrous tissue. **C.** Complete blockage of the esophagus; the distal end is rudimentary. **D.** A tracheoesophageal fistula with narrowing of the esophagus. **E.** An esophagotracheal fistula; the esophagus is not connected with the distal end, which is rudimentary. **F.** Separate esophagotracheal and tracheoesophageal fistulas. **G.** Narrowing of the esophagus without a fistula. In most cases, the lower esophageal segment communicates with the trachea, and types A and B occur more commonly.

The Mechanics of Respiration

Respiration consists of two phases—inspiration and expiration—which are accomplished by the alternate increase and decrease of the capacity of the thoracic cavity. The rate varies between 16 and 20 per minute in normal resting patients and is faster in children and slower in the elderly.

Inspiration

Quiet Inspiration

Compare the thoracic cavity to a box with a single entrance at the top, which is a tube called the trachea (Fig. 3-30). The capacity of the box can be increased by elongating all its diameters, and this results in air under atmospheric pressure entering the box through the tube.

Consider now the three diameters of the thoracic cavity and how they may be increased (Fig. 3-30).

Vertical Diameter Theoretically, the roof could be raised and the floor lowered. The roof is formed by the suprapleural membrane and is fixed. Conversely, the floor is formed by the mobile diaphragm. When the diaphragm contracts, the domes become flattened and the level of the diaphragm is lowered (Fig. 3-30).

Anteroposterior Diameter If the downward-sloping ribs were raised at their sternal ends, the anteroposterior diameter of the thoracic cavity would be increased and the lower end of the sternum would be thrust forward (Fig. 3-30). This can be brought about by fixing the first rib by the contraction of the scaleni muscles of the neck and contracting the intercostal muscles (Fig. 3-11). By this means, all the ribs are drawn together and raised toward the first rib.

Transverse Diameter The ribs articulate in front with the sternum via their costal cartilages and behind with the vertebral column. Because the ribs curve downward as well as forward around the chest wall, they resemble bucket handles (Fig. 3-30). It therefore follows that if the ribs are raised (like bucket handles), the transverse diameter of the thoracic cavity will be increased. As described previously, this can be accomplished by fixing the first rib and raising the other ribs to it by contracting the intercostal muscles (Fig. 3-11).

An additional factor that must not be overlooked is the effect of the descent of the diaphragm on the abdominal viscera and the tone of the muscles of the anterior abdominal wall. As the diaphragm descends on inspiration, intra-abdominal pressure rises. This rise in pressure is accommodated by the reciprocal relaxation of the abdominal wall musculature. However, a point is reached when no further abdominal relaxation is possible, and the liver and other upper abdominal viscera act as a platform that resists further diaphragmatic descent. On further contraction, the diaphragm will now have its central tendon supported from below, and its shortening muscle fibers will assist the intercostal muscles in raising the lower ribs (Fig. 3-11).

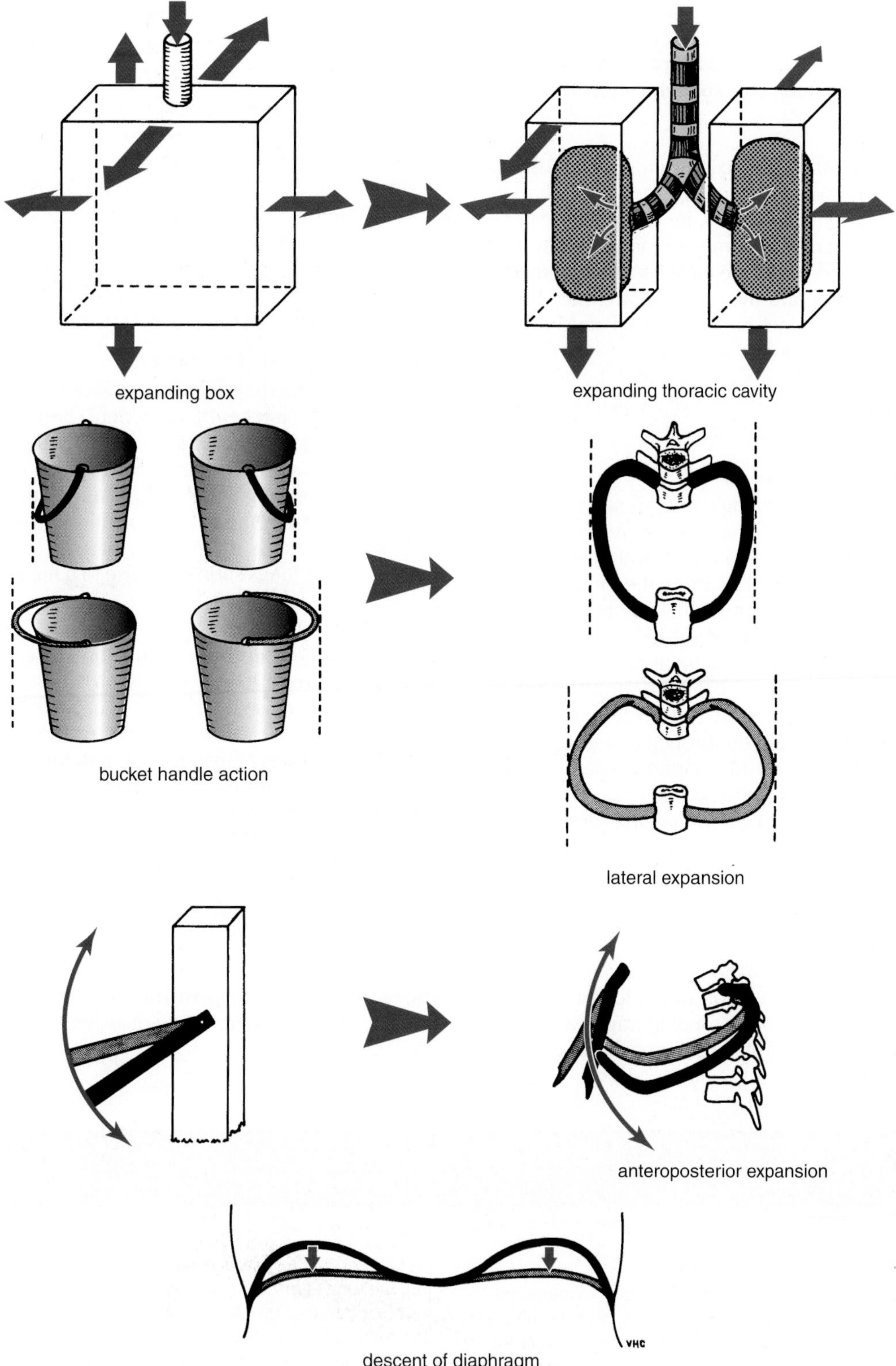

Figure 3-30 The different ways in which the capacity of the thoracic cavity is increased during inspiration.

Apart from the diaphragm and the intercostals, other less important muscles also contract on inspiration and assist in elevating the ribs, namely, the **levatores costarum muscles** and the **serratus posterior superior muscles.**

Forced Inspiration

In deep forced inspiration, a maximum increase in the capacity of the thoracic cavity occurs. Every muscle that can raise the ribs is brought into action, including the scalenus anterior and medius and the sternocleidomastoid. In respiratory distress the action of all the muscles already engaged becomes more violent, and the scapulae are fixed by the trapezius, levator scapulae, and rhomboid muscles, enabling the serratus anterior and pectoralis minor to pull up the ribs. If the upper limbs can be supported by grasping a chair back or table, the sternal origin of the pectoralis major muscles can also assist the process.

Lung Changes on Inspiration

In inspiration, the root of the lung descends and the level of the bifurcation of the trachea may be lowered by as much as two vertebrae. The bronchi elongate and dilate and the alveolar capillaries dilate, thus assisting the pulmonary circulation. Air is drawn into the bronchial tree as the result of the positive atmospheric pressure exerted through the upper part of the respiratory tract and the negative pressure on the outer surface of the lungs brought about by the increased capacity of the thoracic cavity. With expansion of the lungs, the elastic tissue in the bronchial walls and connective tissue are stretched. As the diaphragm descends, the costodiaphragmatic recess of the pleural cavity opens, and the expanding sharp lower edges of the lungs descend to a lower level.

Expiration

Quiet Expiration

Quiet expiration is largely a passive phenomenon and is brought about by the elastic recoil of the lungs, the relaxation of the intercostal muscles and diaphragm, and an increase in tone of the muscles of the anterior abdominal wall, which forces the relaxing diaphragm upward. The **serratus posterior inferior muscles** play a minor role in pulling down the lower ribs.

Forced Expiration

Forced expiration is an active process brought about by the forcible contraction of the musculature of the anterior abdominal wall. The quadratus lumborum also contracts and pulls down the 12th ribs. It is conceivable that under these circumstances some of the intercostal muscles may contract, pull the ribs together, and depress them to the lowered 12th rib (Fig. 3-11). The serratus posterior inferior and the latissimus dorsi muscles may also play a minor role.

Lung Changes on Expiration

In expiration, the roots of the lungs ascend along with the bifurcation of the trachea. The bronchi shorten and contract. The elastic tissue of the lungs recoils, and the lungs become reduced in size. With the upward movement of the diaphragm, increasing areas of the diaphragmatic and costal parietal pleura come into apposition, and the costodiaphragmatic recess becomes reduced in size. The lower margins of the lungs shrink and rise to a higher level.

Types of Respiration

In babies and young children, the ribs are nearly horizontal. Thus, babies have to rely mainly on the descent of the diaphragm to increase their thoracic capacity on inspiration. Because this is accompanied by a marked inward and outward excursion of the anterior abdominal wall, which is easily seen, respiration at this age is referred to as the **abdominal type of respiration.**

After the second year of life, the ribs become more oblique, and the adult form of respiration is established.

In the adult a sexual difference exists in the type of respiratory movements. The female tends to rely mainly on the movements of the ribs rather than on the descent of the diaphragm on inspiration. This is referred to as the **thoracic type of respiration.** The male uses both the thoracic and abdominal forms of respiration, but mainly the abdominal form.

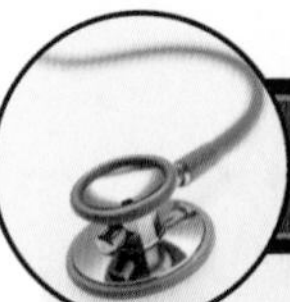

CLINICAL NOTES

Physical Examination of the Lungs

For physical examination of the patient, it is helpful to remember that the upper lobes of the lungs are most easily examined from the front of the chest and the lower lobes from the back. In the axillae, areas of all lobes can be examined.

Trauma to the Lungs

A physician must always remember that the apex of the lung projects up into the neck (1 in. [2.5 cm] above the clavicle) and can be damaged by stab or bullet wounds in this area.

Although the lungs are well protected by the bony thoracic cage, a splinter from a fractured rib can nevertheless penetrate the lung, and air can escape into the pleural cavity, causing a pneumothorax and collapse of the lung. It can also find its way into the lung connective tissue. From there, the air moves under the visceral pleura until it reaches the lung root. It then passes into the mediastinum and up to the neck. Here, it may distend the subcutaneous tissue, a condition known as **subcutaneous emphysema.**

The changes in the position of the thoracic and upper abdominal viscera and the level of the diaphragm during different phases of respiration relative to the chest wall are of considerable clinical importance. A penetrating wound in the lower part of the chest may or may not damage abdominal viscera, depending on the phase of respiration at the time of injury.

(continues)

Clinical Notes, *continued*

Pain and Lung Disease

Lung tissue and the visceral pleura are devoid of pain-sensitive nerve endings, so that pain in the chest is always the result of conditions affecting the surrounding structures. In tuberculosis or pneumonia, for example, pain may never be experienced.

Once lung disease crosses the visceral pleura and the pleural cavity to involve the parietal pleura, pain becomes a prominent feature. Lobar pneumonia with pleurisy, for example, produces a severe tearing pain, accentuated by inspiring deeply or coughing. Because the lower part of the costal parietal pleura receives its sensory innervation from the lower five intercostal nerves, which also innervate the skin of the anterior abdominal wall, pleurisy in this area commonly produces pain that is referred to the abdomen. This has sometimes resulted in a mistaken diagnosis of an acute abdominal lesion.

In a similar manner, pleurisy of the central part of the diaphragmatic pleura, which receives sensory innervation from the phrenic nerve (C3, 4, and 5), can lead to referred pain over the shoulder because the skin of this region is supplied by the supraclavicular nerves (C3 and 4).

Surgical Access to the Lungs

Surgical access to the lung or mediastinum is commonly undertaken through an intercostal space (see page 60). Special rib retractors that allow the ribs to be widely separated are used. The costal cartilages are sufficiently elastic to permit considerable bending. Good exposure of the lungs is obtained by this method.

Segmental Resection of the Lung

A localized chronic lesion such as that of tuberculosis or a benign neoplasm may require surgical removal. If it is restricted to a bronchopulmonary segment, it is possible carefully to dissect out a particular segment and remove it, leaving the surrounding lung intact. Segmental resection requires that the radiologist and thoracic surgeon have a sound knowledge of the bronchopulmonary segments and that they cooperate fully to localize the lesion accurately before operation.

Bronchogenic Carcinoma

Bronchogenic carcinoma accounts for about one third of all cancer deaths in men and is becoming increasingly common in women. It commences in most patients in the mucous membrane lining the larger bronchi and is therefore situated close to the hilum of the lung. The neoplasm rapidly spreads to the tracheobronchial and bronchomediastinal nodes and may involve the recurrent laryngeal nerves, leading to hoarseness of the voice. Lymphatic spread via the bronchomediastinal trunks may result in early involvement in the lower deep cervical nodes just above the level of the clavicle. Hematogenous spread to bones and the brain commonly occurs.

Conditions That Decrease Respiratory Efficiency

Constriction of the Bronchi (Bronchial Asthma)

One of the problems associated with bronchial asthma is the spasm of the smooth muscle in the wall of the bronchioles. This particularly reduces the diameter of the bronchioles during expiration, usually causing the asthmatic patient to experience great difficulty in expiring, although inspiration is accomplished normally. The lungs consequently become greatly distended and the thoracic cage becomes permanently enlarged, forming the so-called **barrel chest.** In addition, the air flow through the bronchioles is further impeded by the presence of excess mucus, which the patient is unable to clear because an effective cough cannot be produced.

Loss of Lung Elasticity

Many diseases of the lungs, such as **emphysema** and **pulmonary fibrosis,** destroy the elasticity of the lungs, and thus the lungs are unable to recoil adequately, causing incomplete expiration. The respiratory muscles in these patients have to assist in expiration, which no longer is a passive phenomenon.

Loss of Lung Distensibility

Diseases such as **silicosis, asbestosis, cancer,** and **pneumonia** interfere with the process of expanding the lung in inspiration. A decrease in the compliance of the lungs and the chest wall then occurs, and a greater effort has to be undertaken by the inspiratory muscles to inflate the lungs.

Postural Drainage

Excessive accumulation of bronchial secretions in a lobe or segment of a lung can seriously interfere with the normal flow of air into the alveoli. Furthermore, the stagnation of such secretions is often quickly followed by infection. To aid in the normal drainage of a bronchial segment, a physiotherapist often alters the position of the patient so that gravity assists in the process of drainage. Sound knowledge of the bronchial tree is necessary to determine the optimum position of the patient for good postural drainage.

Pericardium

The pericardium is a fibroserous sac that encloses the heart and the roots of the great vessels. Its function is to restrict excessive movements of the heart as a whole and to serve as a lubricated container in which the different parts of the heart can contract. The pericardium lies within the middle mediastinum (Figs. 3-2, 3-31, 3-32, and 3-33), posterior to the body of the sternum and the second to the sixth costal cartilages and anterior to the fifth to the eighth thoracic vertebrae.

Fibrous Pericardium

The fibrous pericardium is the strong fibrous part of the sac. It is firmly attached below to the central tendon of the diaphragm. It fuses with the outer coats of the great blood vessels passing through it (Fig. 3-32)—namely, the aorta, the pulmonary trunk, the superior and inferior venae cavae, and the pulmonary veins (Fig. 3-33). The fibrous pericardium is attached in front to the sternum by the **sternopericardial ligaments.**

Serous Pericardium

The serous pericardium lines the fibrous pericardium and coats the heart. It is divided into parietal and visceral layers (Fig. 3-32).

The **parietal layer** lines the fibrous pericardium and is reflected around the roots of the great vessels to become

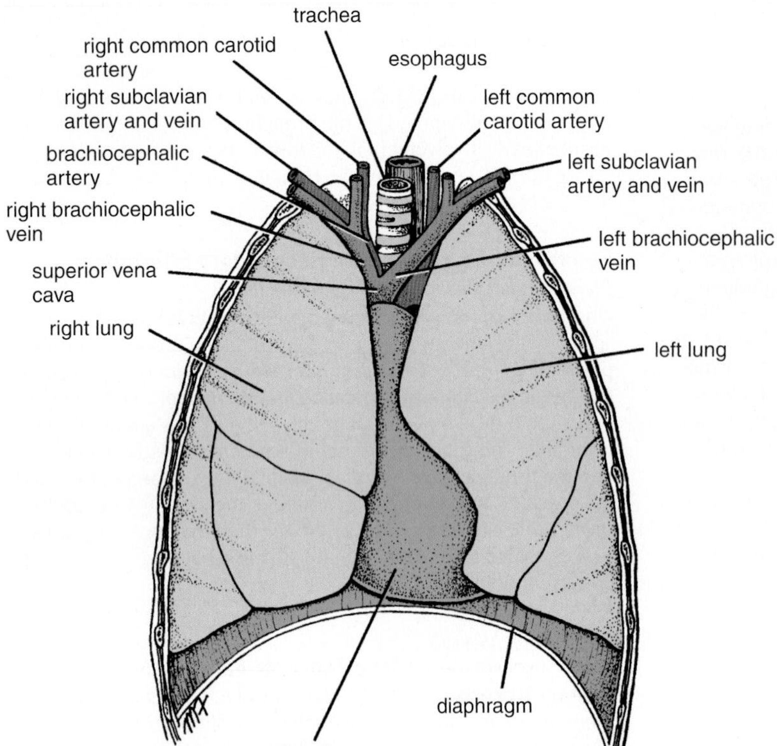

Figure 3-31 The pericardium and the lungs exposed from in front.

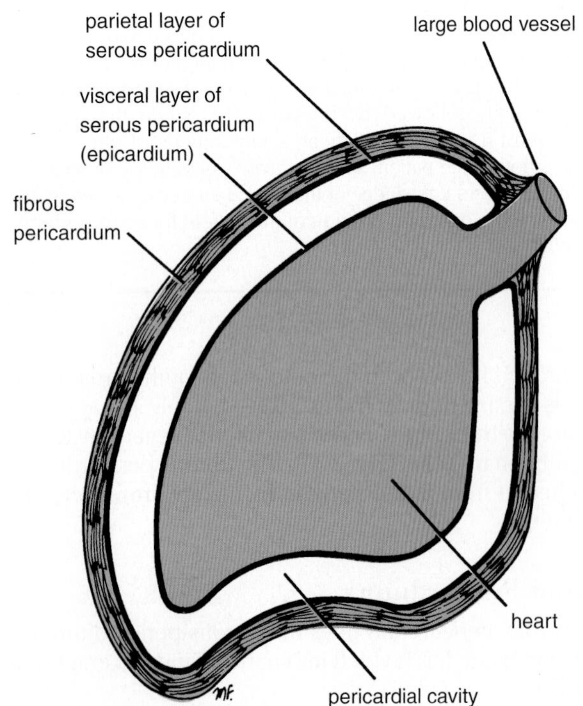

Figure 3-32 Different layers of the pericardium.

continuous with the visceral layer of serous pericardium that closely covers the heart (Fig. 3-33).

The **visceral layer** is closely applied to the heart and is often called the **epicardium.** The slitlike space between the parietal and visceral layers is referred to as the **pericardial cavity** (Fig. 3-32). Normally, the cavity contains a small amount of tissue fluid (about 50 mL), the **pericardial fluid,** which acts as a lubricant to facilitate movements of the heart.

Pericardial Sinuses

On the posterior surface of the heart, the reflection of the serous pericardium around the large veins forms a recess called the **oblique sinus** (Fig. 3-33). Also on the posterior surface of the heart is the **transverse sinus,** which is a short passage that lies between the reflection of serous pericardium around the aorta and pulmonary trunk and the reflection around the large veins (Fig. 3-33). The pericardial sinuses form as a consequence of the way the heart bends during development (see page 118). They have no clinical significance.

Nerve Supply of the Pericardium

The fibrous pericardium and the parietal layer of the serous pericardium are supplied by the phrenic nerves. The visceral layer of the serous pericardium is innervated by branches of the sympathetic trunks and the vagus nerves.

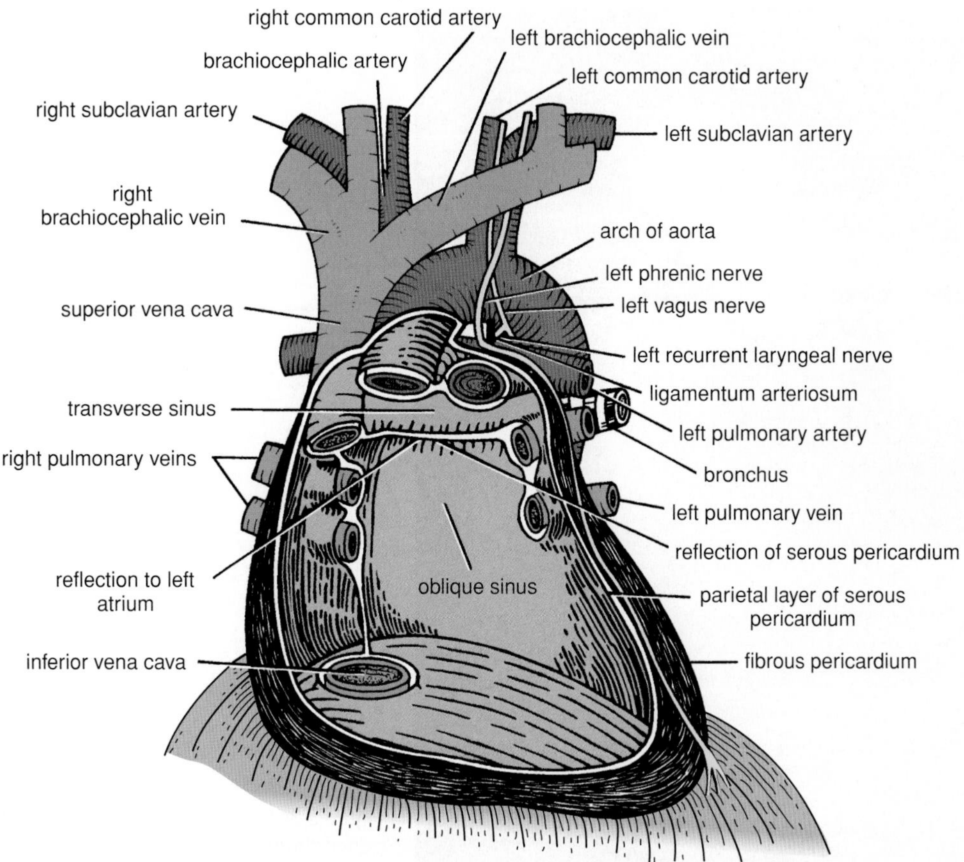

Figure 3-33 The great blood vessels and the interior of the pericardium.

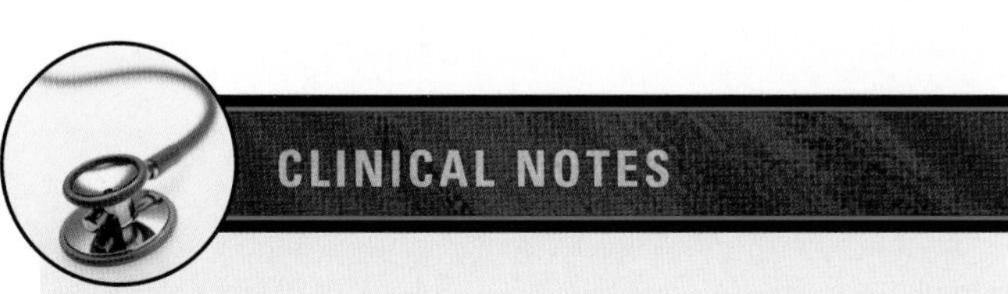

Pericarditis

In inflammation of the serous pericardium, called pericarditis, pericardial fluid may accumulate excessively, which can compress the thin-walled atria and interfere with the filling of the heart during diastole. This compression of the heart is called **cardiac tamponade.**

Cardiac tamponade can also occur secondary to stab or gunshot wounds when the chambers of the heart have been penetrated. The blood escapes into the pericardial cavity and can restrict the filling of the heart.

Roughening of the visceral and parietal layers of serous pericardium by inflammatory exudate in acute pericarditis produces **pericardial friction rub,** which can be felt on palpation and heard through a stethoscope.

Pericardial fluid can be aspirated from the pericardial cavity should excessive amounts accumulate in pericarditis. This process is called **paracentesis.** The needle can be introduced to the left of the xiphoid process in an upward and backward direction at an angle of 45° to the skin. When paracentesis is performed at this site, the pleura and lung are not damaged because of the presence of the cardiac notch in this area.

Heart

The heart is a hollow muscular organ that is somewhat pyramid shaped and lies within the pericardium in the mediastinum (Figs. 3-34 and 3-35). It is connected at its base to the great blood vessels but otherwise lies free within the pericardium.

Surfaces of the Heart

The heart has three surfaces: sternocostal (anterior), diaphragmatic (inferior), and a base (posterior). It also has an apex, which is directed downward, forward, and to the left.

The **sternocostal surface** is formed mainly by the right atrium and the right ventricle, which are separated from each other by the vertical atrioventricular groove (Fig. 3-35). The right border is formed by the right atrium; the left border, by the left ventricle and part of the left auricle. The right ventricle is separated from the left ventricle by the anterior interventricular groove.

The **diaphragmatic surface** of the heart is formed mainly by the right and left ventricles separated by the posterior interventricular groove. The inferior surface of the right atrium, into which the inferior vena cava opens, also forms part of this surface.

The **base of the heart,** or the posterior surface, is formed mainly by the left atrium, into which open the four

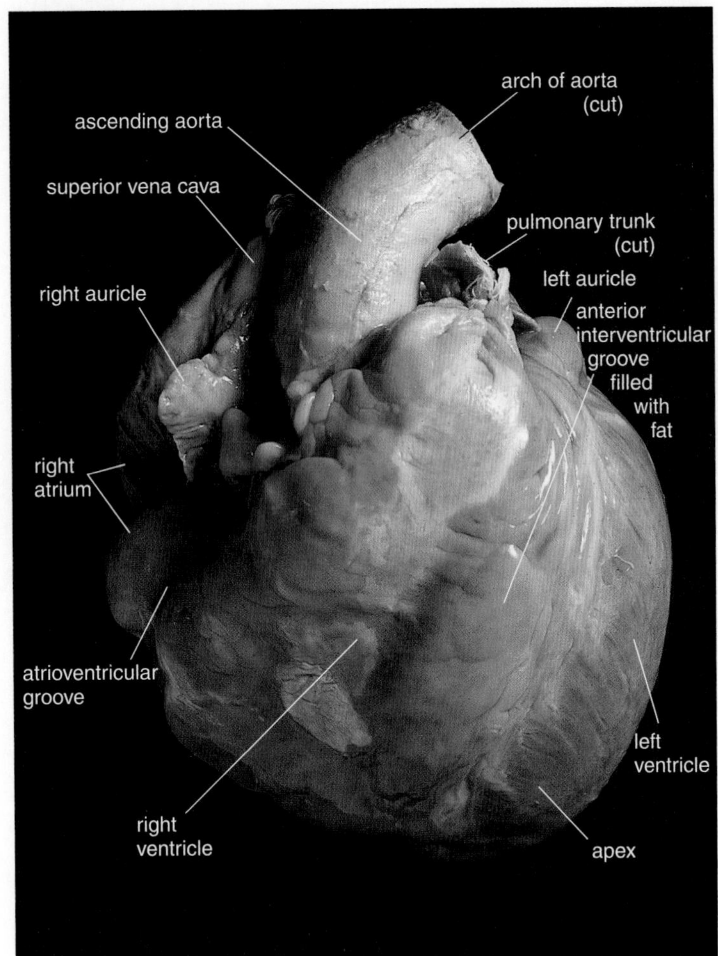

Figure 3-34 The anterior surface of the heart; the fibrous pericardium and the parietal serous pericardium have been removed. Note the presence of fat beneath the visceral serous pericardium in the atrioventricular and interventricular grooves. The coronary arteries are embedded in this fat.

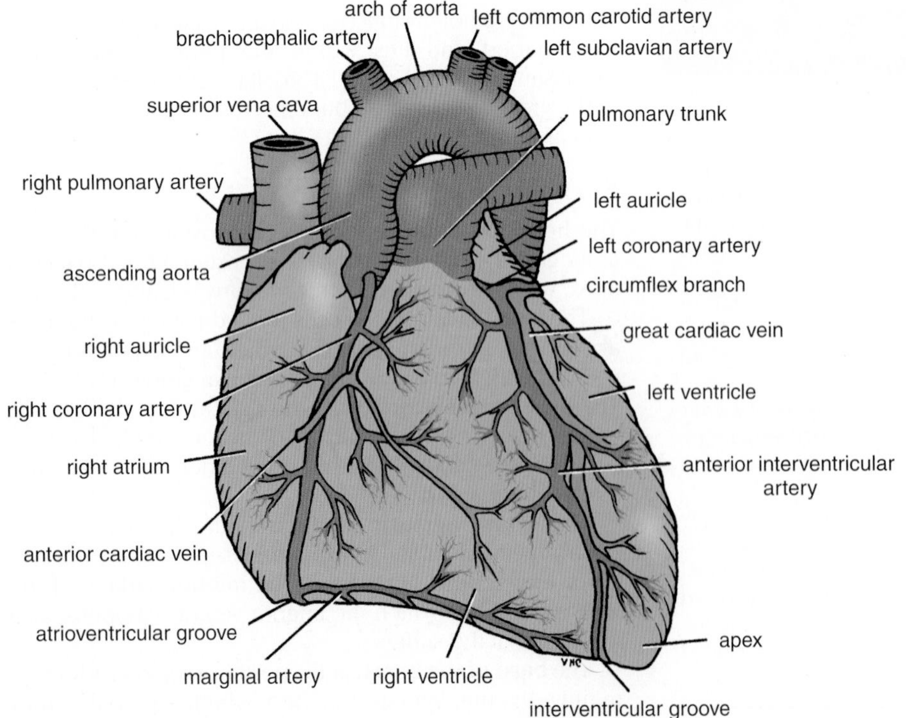

Figure 3-35 The anterior surface of the heart and the great blood vessels. Note the course of the coronary arteries and the cardiac veins.

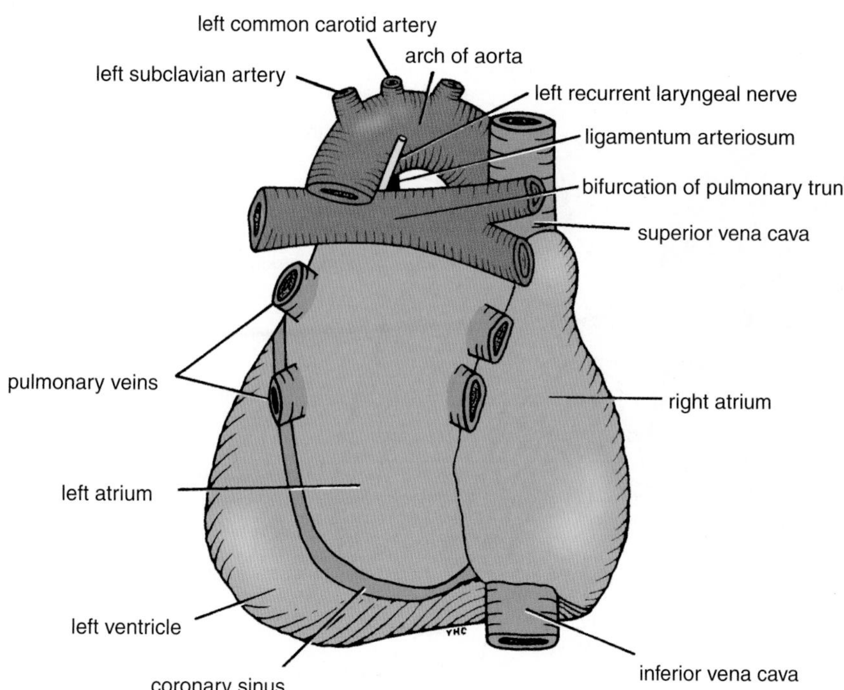

Figure 3-36 The posterior surface, or the base, of the heart.

pulmonary veins (Fig. 3-36). The base of the heart lies opposite the apex.

The **apex of the heart,** formed by the left ventricle, is directed downward, forward, and to the left (Fig. 3-35). It lies at the level of the fifth left intercostal space, 3.5 in. (9 cm) from the midline. In the region of the apex, the apex beat can usually be seen and palpated in the living patient.

Note that the base of the heart is called the base because the heart is pyramid shaped; the base lies opposite the apex. The heart does not rest on its base; it rests on its diaphragmatic (inferior) surface.

Borders of the Heart

The right border is formed by the right atrium; the left border, by the left auricle; and below, by the left ventricle (Fig. 3-35). The lower border is formed mainly by the right ventricle but also by the right atrium; the apex is formed by the left ventricle. These borders are important to recognize when examining a radiograph of the heart.

Chambers of the Heart

The heart is divided by vertical septa into four chambers: the right and left atria and the right and left ventricles. The right atrium lies anterior to the left atrium, and the right ventricle lies anterior to the left ventricle.

The walls of the heart are composed of cardiac muscle, the **myocardium;** covered externally with serous pericardium, the **epicardium;** and lined internally with a layer of endothelium, the **endocardium.**

Right Atrium

The right atrium consists of a main cavity and a small outpouching, the auricle (Figs. 3-35 and 3-37). On the outside of the heart at the junction between the right atrium and the right auricle is a vertical groove, the **sulcus terminalis,** which on the inside forms a ridge, the **crista terminalis.** The main part of the atrium that lies posterior to the ridge is smooth walled and is derived embryologically from the sinus venosus. The part of the atrium in front of the ridge is roughened or trabeculated by bundles of muscle fibers, the **musculi pectinati,** which run from the crista terminalis to the auricle. This anterior part is derived embryologically from the primitive atrium.

Openings into the Right Atrium

The **superior vena cava** (Fig. 3-37) opens into the upper part of the right atrium; it has no valve. It returns the blood to the heart from the upper half of the body. The **inferior vena cava** (larger than the superior vena cava) opens into the lower part of the right atrium; it is guarded by a rudimentary, nonfunctioning valve. It returns the blood to the heart from the lower half of the body.

The **coronary sinus,** which drains most of the blood from the heart wall (Fig. 3-37), opens into the right atrium between the inferior vena cava and the atrioventricular orifice. It is guarded by a rudimentary, nonfunctioning valve.

The **right atrioventricular orifice** lies anterior to the inferior vena caval opening and is guarded by the tricuspid valve (Fig. 3-37).

Many small orifices of small veins also drain the wall of the heart and open directly into the right atrium.

Fetal Remnants

In addition to the rudimentary valve of the inferior vena cava are the **fossa ovalis** and **anulus ovalis.** These latter structures lie on the **atrial septum,** which separates the right atrium from the left atrium (Fig. 3-37). The fossa ovalis is a shallow depression, which is the site of the **foramen**

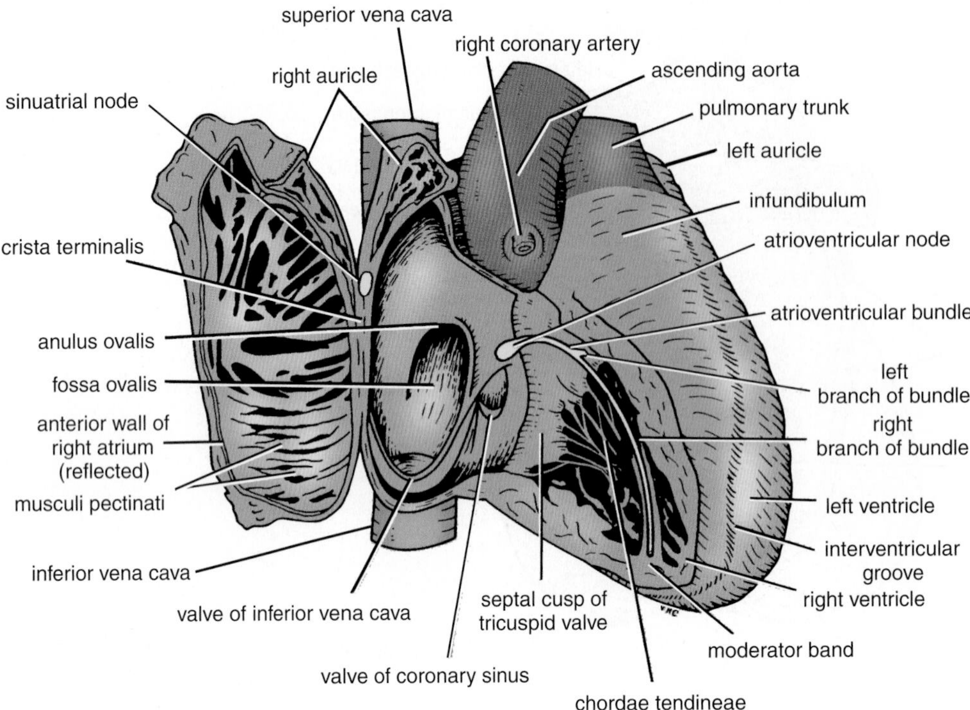

Figure 3-37 Interior of the right atrium and the right ventricle. Note the positions of the sinuatrial node and the atrioventricular node and bundle.

ovale in the fetus (Fig. 3-38). The anulus ovalis forms the upper margin of the fossa. The floor of the fossa represents the persistent septum primum of the heart of the embryo, and the anulus is formed from the lower edge of the septum secundum (Fig. 3-38).

Right Ventricle

The right ventricle communicates with the right atrium through the atrioventricular orifice and with the pulmonary trunk through the pulmonary orifice (Fig. 3-37). As the cavity approaches the pulmonary orifice it becomes funnel shaped, at which point it is referred to as the **infundibulum.**

The walls of the right ventricle are much thicker than those of the right atrium and show several internal projecting ridges formed of muscle bundles. The projecting ridges give the ventricular wall a spongelike appearance and are known as **trabeculae carneae.** The trabeculae carneae are composed of three types. The first type comprises the **papillary muscles,** which project inward, being attached by their bases to the ventricular wall; their apices are connected by fibrous chords (the **chordae tendineae**) to the cusps of the tricuspid valve (Fig. 3-37). The second type is attached at the ends to the ventricular wall, being free in the middle. One of these, the **moderator band,** crosses the ventricular cavity from the septal to the anterior wall. It conveys the right branch of the atrioventricular bundle, which is part of the conducting system of the heart. The third type is simply composed of prominent ridges.

The **tricuspid valve** guards the atrioventricular orifice (Figs. 3-37 and 3-39) and consists of three cusps formed by a fold of endocardium with some connective tissue enclosed: **anterior, septal,** and **inferior** (posterior) cusps. The anterior cusp lies anteriorly, the septal cusp lies against the ventricular septum, and the inferior or posterior cusp lies inferiorly. The bases of the cusps are attached to the fibrous ring of the skeleton of the heart (see below), whereas their free edges and ventricular surfaces are attached to the **chordae tendineae.** The chordae tendineae connect the cusps to the **papillary muscles.** When the ventricle contracts, the papillary muscles contract and prevent the cusps from being forced into the atrium and turning inside out as the intraventricular pressure rises. To assist in this process, the chordae tendineae of one papillary muscle are connected to the adjacent parts of two cusps.

The **pulmonary valve** guards the pulmonary orifice (Fig. 3-39A) and consists of three semilunar cusps formed by folds of endocardium with some connective tissue enclosed. The curved lower margins and sides of each cusp are attached to the arterial wall. The open mouths of the cusps are directed upward into the pulmonary trunk. No chordae or papillary muscles are associated with these valve cusps; the attachments of the sides of the cusps to the arterial wall prevent the cusps from prolapsing into the ventricle. At the root of the pulmonary trunk are three dilatations called the **sinuses,** and one is situated external to each cusp (see **aortic valve**).

The three semilunar cusps are arranged with one posterior (left cusp) and two anterior (anterior and right cusps).

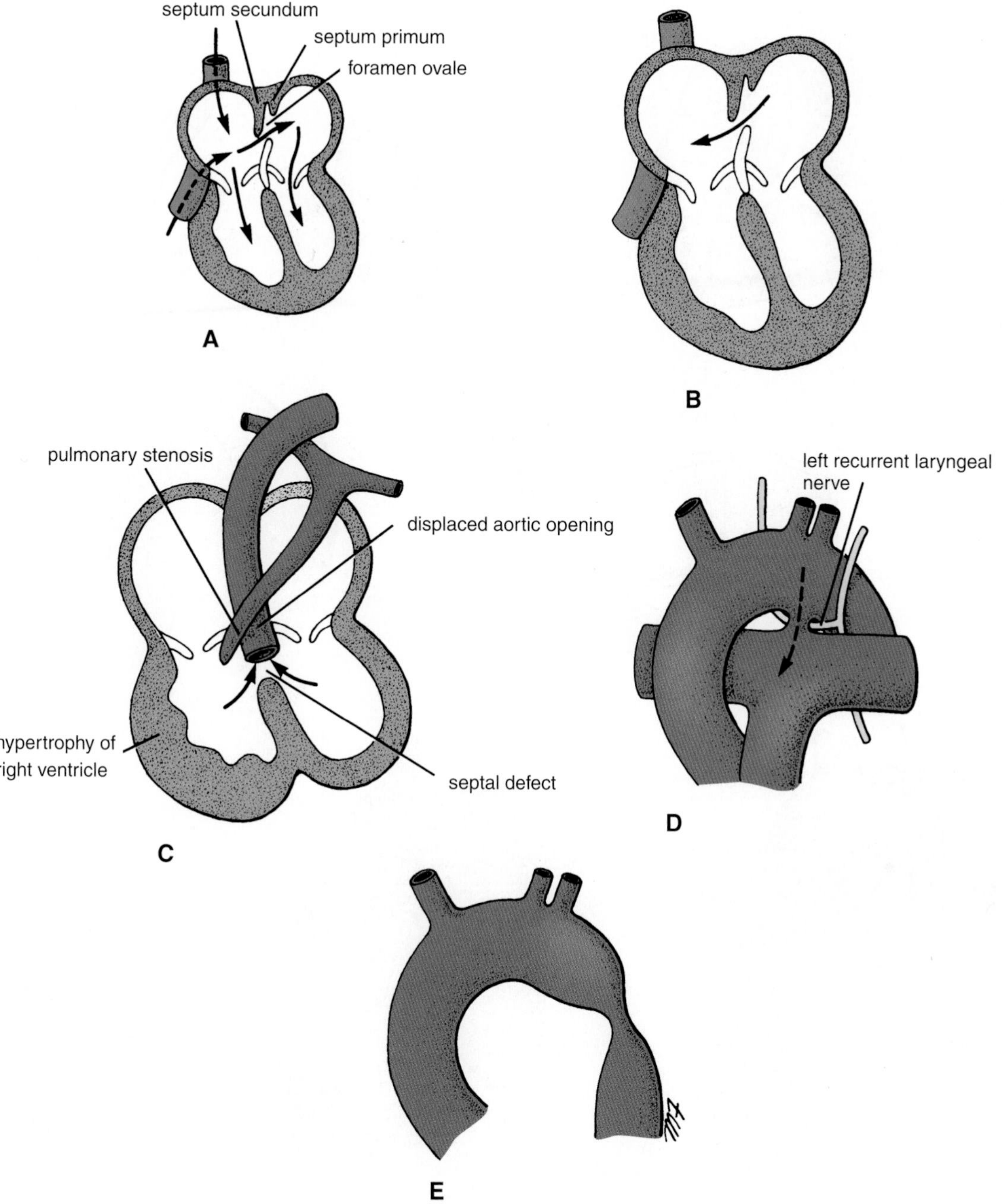

Figure 3-38 **A.** Normal fetal heart. **B.** Atrial septal defect. **C.** Tetralogy of Fallot. **D.** Patent ductus arteriosus (note the close relationship to the left recurrent laryngeal nerve). **E.** Coarctation of the aorta.

(The cusps of the pulmonary and aortic valves are named according to their position in the fetus before the heart has rotated to the left. This, unfortunately, causes a great deal of unnecessary confusion.) During ventricular systole, the cusps of the valve are pressed against the wall of the pulmonary trunk by the out-rushing blood. During diastole, blood flows back toward the heart and enters the sinuses; the valve cusps fill, come into apposition in the center of the lumen, and close the pulmonary orifice.

Left Atrium

Similar to the right atrium, the left atrium consists of a main cavity and a left auricle. The left atrium is situated behind the right atrium and forms the greater part of the base or the posterior surface of the heart (Fig. 3-36). Behind it lies the oblique sinus of the serous pericardium, and the fibrous pericardium separates it from the esophagus (Figs. 3-33 and 3-40).

The interior of the left atrium is smooth, but the left auricle possesses muscular ridges as in the right auricle.

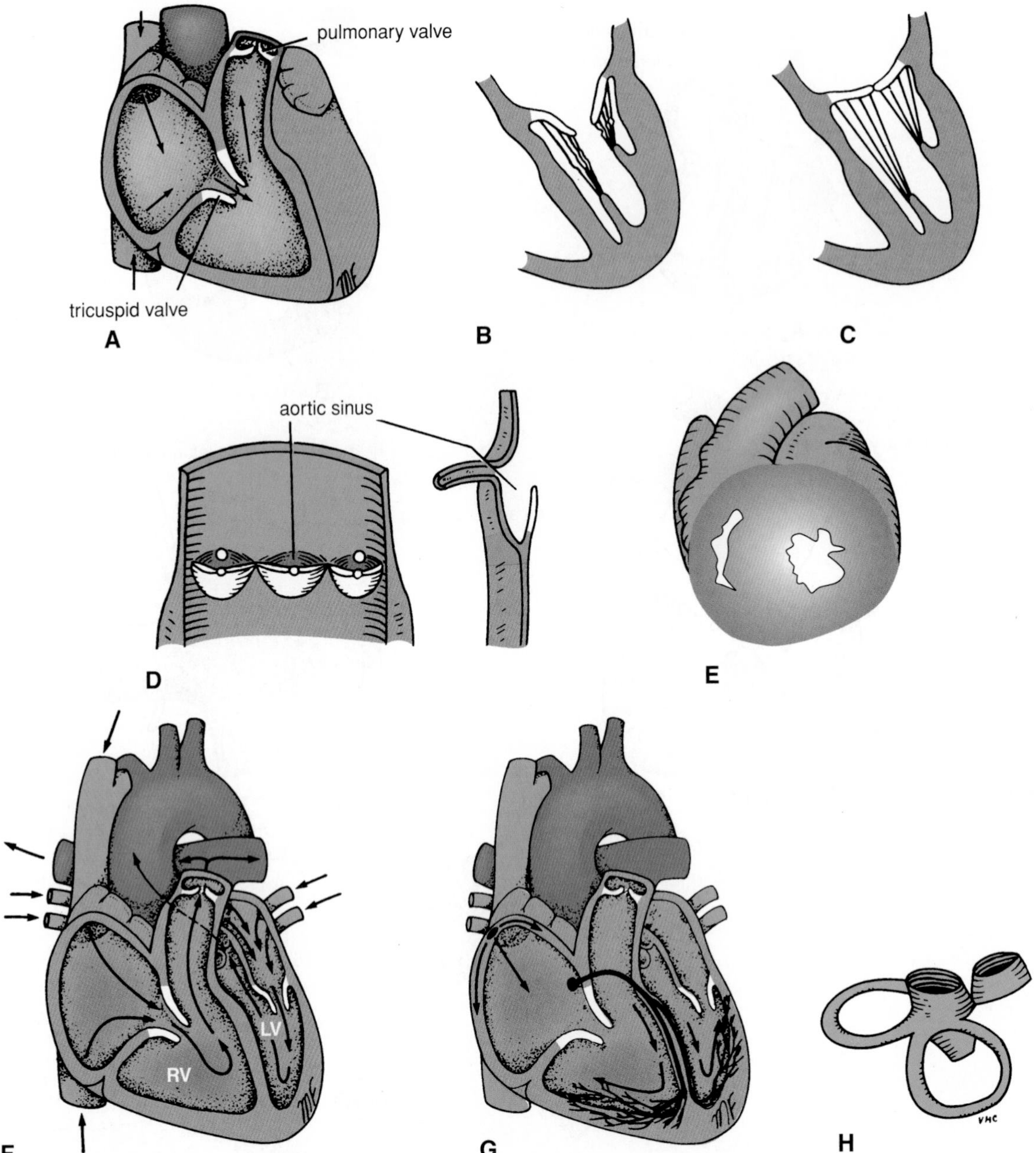

Figure 3-39 **A.** Position of the tricuspid and pulmonary valves. **B.** Mitral cusps with valve open. **C.** Mitral cusps with valve closed. **D.** Semilunar cusps of the aortic valve. **E.** Cross section of the ventricles of the heart. **F.** Path taken by the blood through the heart. **G.** Path taken by the cardiac impulse from the sinuatrial node to the Purkinje network. **H.** Fibrous skeleton of the heart.

Openings into the Left Atrium

The four pulmonary veins, two from each lung, open through the posterior wall (Fig. 3-36) and have no valves. The left atrioventricular orifice is guarded by the mitral valve.

Left Ventricle

The left ventricle communicates with the left atrium through the atrioventricular orifice and with the aorta through the aortic orifice. The walls of the left ventricle (Fig. 3-39) are three times thicker than those of the right ventricle. (The left intraventricular blood pressure is six times higher than that inside the right ventricle.) In cross section, the left ventricle is circular; the right is crescentic because of the bulging of the ventricular septum into the cavity of the right ventricle (Fig. 3-39). There are well-developed trabeculae carneae, two large papillary muscles, but no moderator band. The part of the ventricle below the aortic orifice is called the **aortic vestibule.**

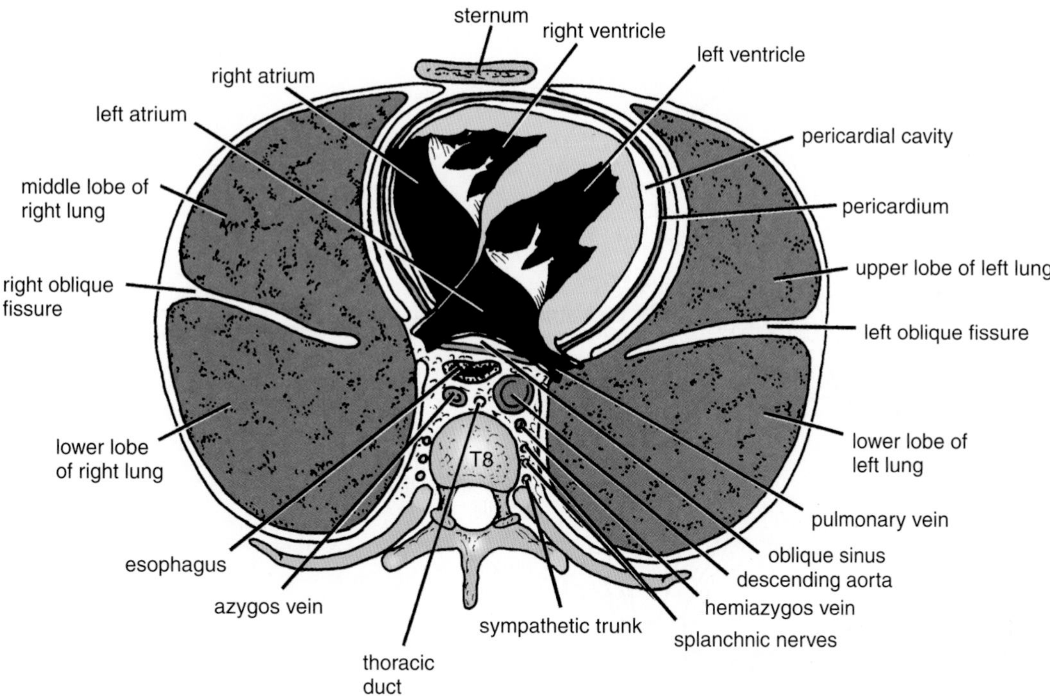

Figure 3-40 Cross section of the thorax at the eighth thoracic vertebra, as seen from below. (Note that all computed tomography scans and magnetic resonance imaging studies are viewed from below.)

The **mitral valve** guards the atrioventricular orifice (Fig. 3-39). It consists of two cusps, one anterior and one posterior, which have a structure similar to that of the cusps of the tricuspid valve. The anterior cusp is the larger and intervenes between the atrioventricular and the aortic orifices. The attachment of the chordae tendineae to the cusps and the papillary muscles is similar to that of the tricuspid valve.

The **aortic valve** guards the aortic orifice and is precisely similar in structure to the pulmonary valve (Fig. 3-39). One cusp is situated on the anterior wall (right cusp) and two are located on the posterior wall (left and posterior cusps). Behind each cusp the aortic wall bulges to form an **aortic sinus.** The anterior aortic sinus gives origin to the right coronary artery, and the left posterior sinus gives origin to the left coronary artery.

Structure of the Heart

The walls of the heart are composed of a thick layer of cardiac muscle, the myocardium, covered externally by the epicardium and lined internally by the endocardium. The atrial portion of the heart has relatively thin walls and is divided by the **atrial (interatrial) septum** into the right and left atria. The septum runs from the anterior wall of the heart backward and to the right. The ventricular portion of the heart has thick walls and is divided by the **ventricular (interventricular) septum** into the right and left ventricles. The septum is placed obliquely, with one surface facing forward and to the right and the other facing backward and to the left. Its position is indicated on the surface of the heart by the anterior and posterior interventricular grooves. The lower part of the septum is thick and formed of muscle. The smaller upper part of the septum is thin and membranous and attached to the fibrous skeleton.

The so-called **skeleton of the heart** (Fig. 3-39) consists of fibrous rings that surround the atrioventricular, pulmonary, and aortic orifices and are continuous with the membranous upper part of the ventricular septum. The fibrous rings around the atrioventricular orifices separate the muscular walls of the atria from those of the ventricles but provide attachment for the muscle fibers. The fibrous rings support the bases of the valve cusps and prevent the valves from stretching and becoming incompetent. The skeleton of the heart forms the basis of electrical discontinuity between the atria and the ventricles.

Conducting System of the Heart

The normal heart contracts rhythmically at about 70 to 90 beats per minute in the resting adult. The rhythmic contractile process originates spontaneously in the conducting system and the impulse travels to different regions of the heart, so the atria contract first and together, to be followed later by the contractions of both ventricles together. The slight delay in the passage of the impulse from the atria to the ventricles allows time for the atria to empty their blood into the ventricles before the ventricles contract.

The conducting system of the heart consists of specialized cardiac muscle present in the **sinuatrial node,** the **atrioventricular node,** the **atrioventricular bundle** and its right and left terminal branches, and the subendocardial plexus of **Purkinje fibers** (specialized cardiac muscle fibers that form the conducting system of the heart).

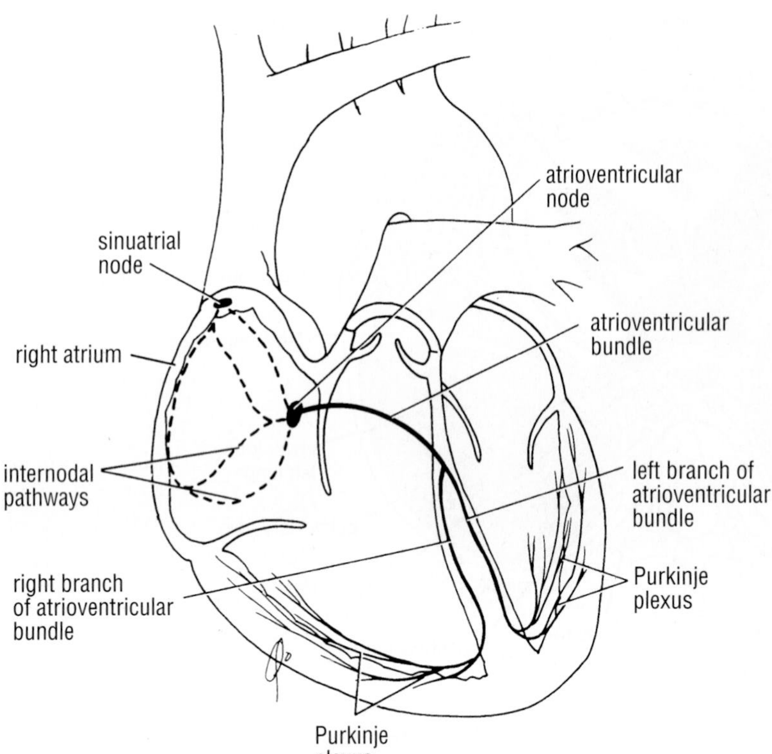

Figure 3-41 The conducting system of the heart. Note the internodal pathways.

Sinuatrial Node

The sinuatrial node is located in the wall of the right atrium in the upper part of the sulcus terminalis just to the right of the opening of the superior vena cava (Figs. 3-37 and 3-39). The node spontaneously gives origin to rhythmic electrical impulses that spread in all directions through the cardiac muscle of the atria and cause the muscle to contract.

Atrioventricular Node

The atrioventricular node is strategically placed on the lower part of the atrial septum just above the attachment of the septal cusp of the tricuspid valve (Figs. 3-37 and 3-39). From it, the cardiac impulse is conducted to the ventricles by the atrioventricular bundle. The atrioventricular node is stimulated by the excitation wave as it passes through the atrial myocardium.

The speed of conduction of the cardiac impulse through the atrioventricular node (about 0.11 seconds) allows sufficient time for the atria to empty their blood into the ventricles before the ventricles start to contract.

Atrioventricular Bundle

The atrioventricular bundle (bundle of His) is the only pathway of cardiac muscle that connects the myocardium of the atria and the myocardium of the ventricles and is thus the only route along which the cardiac impulse can travel from the atria to the ventricles (Fig. 3-41). The bundle descends through the fibrous skeleton of the heart.

The atrioventricular bundle then descends behind the septal cusp of the tricuspid valve to reach the inferior border of the membranous part of the ventricular septum. At the upper border of the muscular part of the septum it divides into two branches, one for each ventricle. The right bundle branch (RBB) passes down on the right side of the ventricular septum to reach the moderator band, where it crosses to the anterior wall of the right ventricle. Here it becomes continuous with the fibers of the Purkinje plexus (Fig. 3-41).

The left bundle branch (LBB) pierces the septum and passes down on its left side beneath the endocardium. It usually divides into two branches (anterior and posterior), which eventually become continuous with the fibers of the Purkinje plexus of the left ventricle.

It is thus seen that the conducting system of the heart is responsible not only for generating rhythmic cardiac impulses, but also for conducting these impulses rapidly throughout the myocardium of the heart so that the different chambers contract in a coordinated and efficient manner.

The activities of the conducting system can be influenced by the autonomic nerve supply to the heart. The parasympathetic nerves slow the rhythm and diminish the rate of conduction of the impulse; the sympathetic nerves have the opposite effect.

*Internodal Conduction Paths**

Impulses from the sinuatrial node have been shown to travel to the atrioventricular node more rapidly than they can travel by passing along the ordinary myocardium. This phenomenon has been explained by the description of special pathways in the atrial wall (Fig. 3-41), which have a structure consisting of a mixture of Purkinje fibers and ordinary car-

*The occurrence of specialized internodal pathways has been dismissed by some researchers, who claim that it is the packaging and arrangement of ordinary atrial myocardial fibers that are responsible for the more rapid conduction.

diac muscle cells. The **anterior internodal pathway** leaves the anterior end of the sinuatrial node and passes anterior to the superior vena caval opening. It descends on the atrial septum and ends in the atrioventricular node. The **middle internodal pathway** leaves the posterior end of the sinuatrial node and passes posterior to the superior vena caval opening. It descends on the atrial septum to the atrioventricular node. The **posterior internodal pathway** leaves the posterior part of the sinuatrial node and descends through the crista terminalis and the valve of the inferior vena cava to the atrioventricular node.

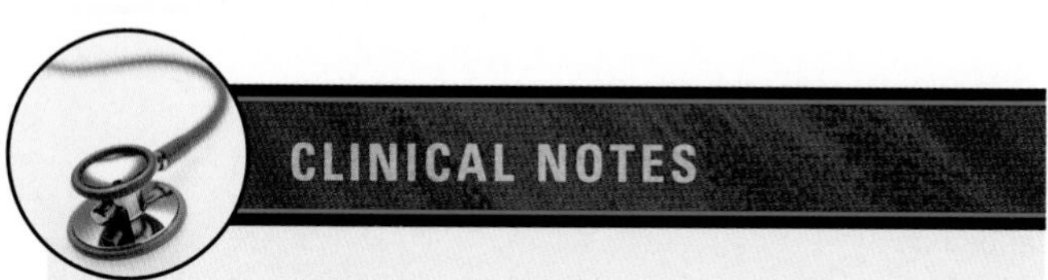

Failure of the Conduction System of the Heart

The sinuatrial node is the spontaneous source of the cardiac impulse. The atrioventricular node is responsible for picking up the cardiac impulse from the atria. The atrioventricular bundle is the only route by which the cardiac impulse can spread from the atria to the ventricles. Failure of the bundle to conduct the normal impulses results in alteration in the rhythmic contraction of the ventricles (arrhythmias) or, if complete bundle block occurs, complete dissociation between the atria and ventricular rates of contraction. The common cause of defective conduction through the bundle or its branches is atherosclerosis of the coronary arteries, which results in a diminished blood supply to the conducting system.

Arterial Supply of the Heart

The arterial supply of the heart is provided by the right and left coronary arteries, which arise from the ascending aorta immediately above the aortic valve (Fig. 3-42). The coronary arteries and their major branches are distributed over the surface of the heart, lying within subepicardial connective tissue.

The **right coronary artery** arises from the anterior aortic sinus of the ascending aorta and runs forward between the pulmonary trunk and the right auricle (Fig. 3-35). It descends almost vertically in the right atrioventricular groove, and at the inferior border of the heart it continues posteriorly along the atrioventricular groove to anastomose with the left coronary artery in the posterior interventricular groove. The following branches from the right coronary artery supply the right atrium and right ventricle and parts of the left atrium and left ventricle and the atrioventricular septum.

Branches

1. The **right conus artery** supplies the anterior surface of the pulmonary conus (infundibulum of the right ventricle) and the upper part of the anterior wall of the right ventricle.
2. The **anterior ventricular branches** are two or three in number and supply the anterior surface of the right ventricle. The **marginal branch** is the largest and runs along the lower margin of the costal surface to reach the apex.
3. The **posterior ventricular branches** are usually two in number and supply the diaphragmatic surface of the right ventricle.
4. The **posterior interventricular (descending) artery** runs toward the apex in the posterior interventricular groove. It gives off branches to the right and left ventricles, including its inferior wall. It supplies branches to the posterior part of the ventricular septum but not to the apical part, which receives its supply from the anterior interventricular branch of the left coronary artery. A large septal branch supplies the **atrioventricular node.** In 10% of individuals the posterior interventricular artery is replaced by a branch from the left coronary artery.
5. The **atrial branches** supply the anterior and lateral surfaces of the right atrium. One branch supplies the posterior surface of both the right and left atria. The **artery of the sinuatrial node** supplies the node and the right and left atria; in 35% of individuals it arises from the left coronary artery.

The **left coronary artery,** which is usually larger than the right coronary artery, supplies the major part of the heart, including the greater part of the left atrium, left ventricle, and ventricular septum. It arises from the left posterior aortic sinus of the ascending aorta and passes forward between the pulmonary trunk and the left auricle (Fig. 3-35). It then enters the atrioventricular groove and divides into an anterior interventricular branch and a circumflex branch.

Branches

1. The **anterior interventricular (descending) branch** runs downward in the anterior interventricular groove to the apex of the heart (Fig. 3-42). In most individuals it then passes around the apex of the heart to enter the posterior interventricular groove and anastomoses with the terminal branches of the right coronary artery. In one third of individuals it ends at the apex of the heart. The anterior interventricular branch supplies the right and left ventricles with numerous branches that also supply the anterior part of the ventricular septum. One of these ventricular branches **(left diagonal artery)** may arise directly from the trunk of the left coronary artery. A small **left conus artery** supplies the pulmonary conus.
2. The **circumflex artery** is the same size as the anterior interventricular artery (Fig. 3-42). It winds around the left margin of the heart in the atrioventricular groove. A **left marginal artery** is a large branch that supplies the left margin of the left ventricle down to the apex. **Anterior ventricular** and **posterior ventricular branches** supply the left ventricle. **Atrial branches** supply the left atrium.

Variations in the Coronary Arteries

Variations in the blood supply to the heart do occur, and the most common variations affect the blood supply to the diaphragmatic surface of both ventricles. Here the origin, size, and distribution of the posterior interventricular artery are variable (Fig. 3-43). In **right dominance,** the posterior interventricular artery is a large branch of the right coronary artery. Right dominance is present in most individuals (90%). In **left dominance,** the posterior interventricular

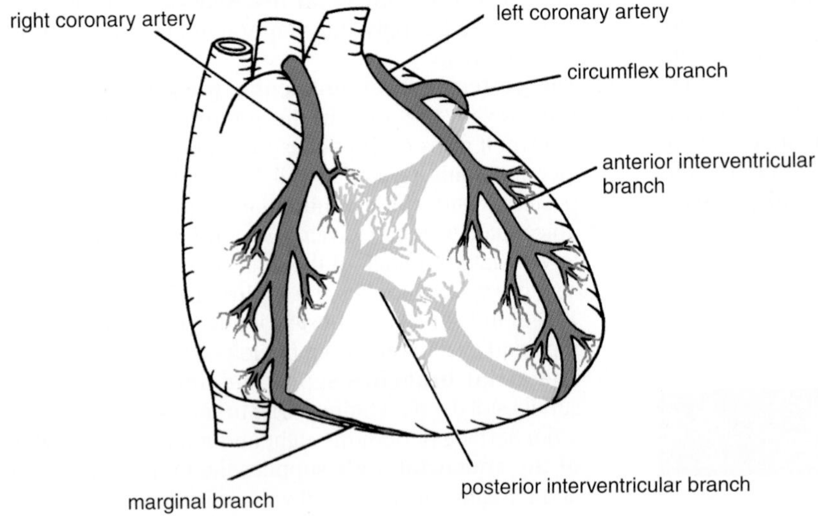

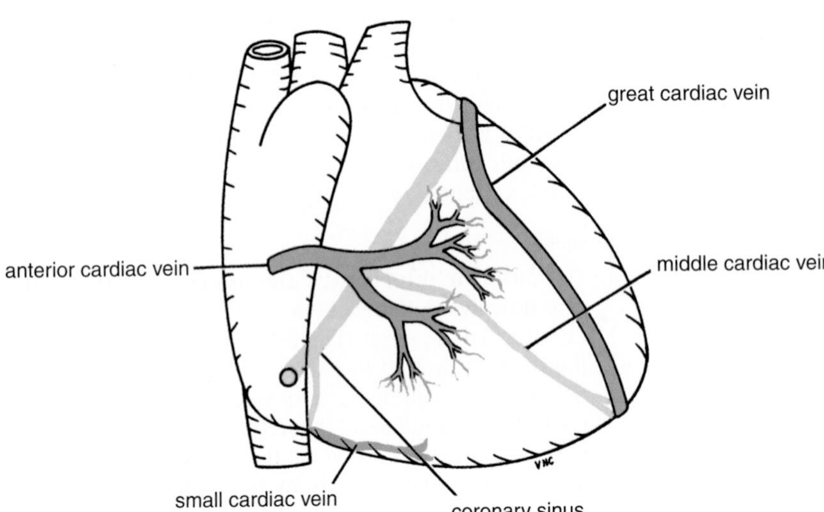

Figure 3-42 Coronary arteries and veins.

artery is a branch of the circumflex branch of the left coronary artery (10%).

Coronary Artery Anastomoses

Anastomoses between the terminal branches of the right and left coronary arteries (collateral circulation) exist, but they are usually **not large enough** to provide an adequate blood supply to the cardiac muscle should one of the large branches become blocked by disease. A sudden block of one of the larger branches of either coronary artery usually leads to myocardial death (myocardial infarction), although sometimes the collateral circulation is enough to sustain the muscle.

Summary of the Overall Arterial Supply to the Heart in Most Individuals

The **right coronary artery** supplies all of the right ventricle (except for the small area to the right of the anterior interventricular groove), the variable part of the diaphragmatic surface of the left ventricle, the posteroinferior third of the ventricular septum, the right atrium and part of the left atrium, and the sinuatrial node and the atrioventricular node and bundle. The LBB also receives small branches.

The **left coronary artery** supplies most of the left ventricle, a small area of the right ventricle to the right of the interventricular groove, the anterior two thirds of the ventricular septum, most of the left atrium, the RBB, and the LBB.

Arterial Supply to the Conducting System

The sinuatrial node is usually supplied by the right but sometimes by the left coronary artery. The atrioventricular node and the atrioventricular bundle are supplied by the right coronary artery. The RBB of the atrioventricular bundle is supplied by the left coronary artery; the LBB is supplied by the right and left coronary arteries (Fig. 3-43).

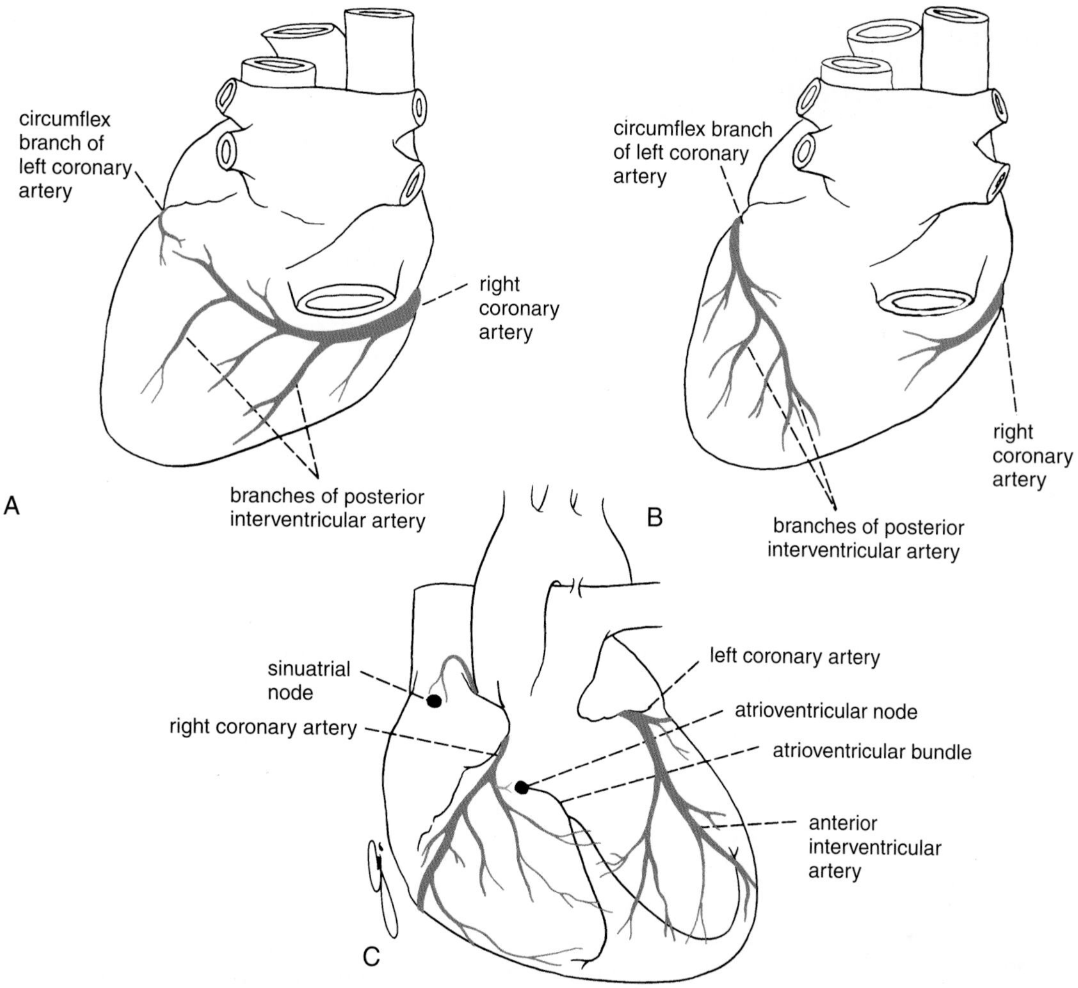

Figure 3-43 **A.** Posterior view of the heart showing the origin and distribution of the posterior interventricular artery in the right dominance. **B.** Posterior view of the heart showing the origin and distribution of the posterior interventricular artery in the left dominance. **C.** Anterior view of the heart showing the relationship of the blood supply to the conducting system.

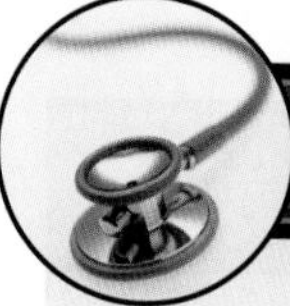

CLINICAL NOTES

Coronary Artery Disease

The myocardium receives its blood supply through the right and left coronary arteries. Although the coronary arteries have numerous anastomoses at the arteriolar level, they are essentially **functional end arteries.** A sudden block of one of the large branches of either coronary artery will usually lead to necrosis of the cardiac muscle (myocardial infarction) in that vascular area, and often the patient dies. Most cases of coronary artery blockage are caused by an acute thrombosis on top of a chronic atherosclerotic narrowing of the lumen.

Arteriosclerotic disease of the coronary arteries may present in three ways, depending on the rate of narrowing of the lumina of the arteries: (1) General degeneration and fibrosis of the myocardium occur over many years and are caused by a gradual narrowing of the coronary arteries. (2) **Angina pectoris** is cardiac pain that occurs on exertion and is relieved by rest. In this condition, the coronary arteries are so narrowed that myocardial ischemia occurs on exertion but not at rest. (3) **Myocardial infarction** occurs when coronary flow is suddenly reduced or stopped and the cardiac muscle undergoes necrosis. Myocardial infarction is the major cause of death in industrialized nations.

Table 3-1 shows the different coronary arteries that supply the different areas of the myocardium. This information can be helpful when attempting to correlate the site of myocardial infarction, the artery involved, and the electrocardiographic signature.

Because coronary bypass surgery, coronary angioplasty, and coronary artery stenting are now commonly accepted methods of treating coronary artery disease, it is incumbent on the student to be prepared to interpret still- and motion-picture angiograms that have been carried out before treatment. For this reason, a working knowledge of the origin, course, and distribution of the coronary arteries should be memorized.

Table 3-1 Coronary Artery Lesions, Infarct Location, and ECG Signature

Coronary Artery	Infarct Location	ECG Signature
Proximal LAD	Large anterior wall	ST elevation: I, L, V1–V6
More distal LAD	Anteroapical	ST elevation: V2–V4
	Inferior wall if wraparound LAD	ST elevation: II, III, F
Distal LAD	Anteroseptal	ST elevation: V1–V3
Early obtuse, marginal	High lateral wall	ST elevation: I, L, V4–V6
More distal marginal branch, circumflex	Small lateral wall	ST elevation: I, L, or V4–V6, or no abnormality
Circumflex	Posterolateral	ST elevation: V4–V6; ST depression: V1–V2
Distal RCA	Small inferior wall	ST elevation: II, III, F; ST depression: I, L
Proximal RCA	Large inferior wall and posterior wall	ST elevation: II, III, F; ST depression: I, L, V1–V3
	Some lateral wall	ST elevation: V5–V6
RCA	Right ventricular	ST elevation: V2R–V4R; some ST elevation: V1; or ST depression: V2, V3
	Usually inferior	ST elevation: II, III, F

ECG, electrocardiographic; LAD, left anterior descending (interventricular); RCA, right coronary artery.

Venous Drainage of the Heart

Most blood from the heart wall drains into the right atrium through the coronary sinus (Fig. 3-42), which lies in the posterior part of the atrioventricular groove and is a continuation of the **great cardiac vein.** It opens into the right atrium to the left of the inferior vena cava. The **small** and **middle cardiac veins** are tributaries of the coronary sinus. The remainder of the blood is returned to the right atrium by the **anterior cardiac vein** (Fig. 3-42) and by small veins that open directly into the heart chambers.

Nerve Supply of the Heart

The heart is innervated by sympathetic and parasympathetic fibers of the autonomic nervous system via the **cardiac plexuses** situated below the arch of the aorta. The sympathetic supply arises from the cervical and upper thoracic portions of the sympathetic trunks, and the parasympathetic supply comes from the vagus nerves.

The postganglionic sympathetic fibers terminate on the sinuatrial and atrioventricular nodes, on cardiac muscle fibers, and on the coronary arteries. Activation of these nerves results in cardiac acceleration, increased force of contraction of the cardiac muscle, and dilatation of the coronary arteries.

The postganglionic parasympathetic fibers terminate on the sinuatrial and atrioventricular nodes and on the coronary arteries. Activation of the parasympathetic nerves results in a reduction in the rate and force of contraction of the heart and a constriction of the coronary arteries.

Afferent fibers running with the sympathetic nerves carry nervous impulses that normally do not reach consciousness. However, should the blood supply to the myocardium become impaired, pain impulses reach consciousness via this pathway. Afferent fibers running with the vagus nerves take part in cardiovascular reflexes.

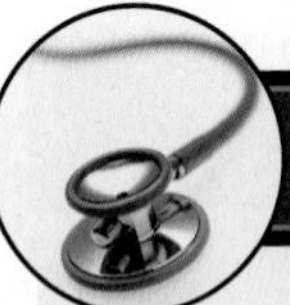

CLINICAL NOTES

Cardiac Pain

Pain originating in the heart as the result of acute myocardial ischemia is assumed to be caused by oxygen deficiency and the accumulation of metabolites, which stimulate the sensory nerve endings in the myocardium. The afferent nerve fibers ascend to the central nervous system through the cardiac branches of the sympathetic trunk and enter the spinal cord through the posterior roots of the upper four thoracic nerves. The nature of the pain varies considerably, from a severe crushing pain to nothing more than a mild discomfort.

The pain is not felt in the heart, but is referred to the skin areas supplied by the corresponding spinal nerves. The skin areas supplied by the upper four intercostal nerves and by the intercostobrachial nerve (T2) are therefore affected. The intercostobrachial nerve communicates with the medial cutaneous nerve of the arm and is distributed to skin on the medial side of the upper part of the arm. A certain amount of spread of nervous information must occur within the central nervous system, for the pain is sometimes felt in the neck and the jaw.

Myocardial infarction involving the inferior wall or diaphragmatic surface of the heart often gives rise to discomfort in the epigastrium. One must assume that the afferent pain fibers from the heart ascend in the sympathetic nerves and enter the spinal cord in the posterior roots of the seventh, eighth, and ninth thoracic spinal nerves and give rise to referred pain in the T7, T8, and T9 thoracic dermatomes in the epigastrium.

Because the heart and the thoracic part of the esophagus probably have similar afferent pain pathways, it is not surprising that painful acute esophagitis can mimic the pain of myocardial infarction.

Action of the Heart

The heart is a muscular pump. The series of changes that take place within it as it fills with blood and empties is referred to as the **cardiac cycle.** The normal heart beats 70 to 90 times per minute in the resting adult and 130 to 150 times per minute in the newborn child.

Blood is continuously returning to the heart; during ventricular systole (contraction), when the atrioventricular valves are closed, the blood is temporarily accommodated in the large veins and atria. Once ventricular diastole (relaxation) occurs, the atrioventricular valves open, and blood passively flows from the atria to the ventricles (Fig. 3-39). When the ventricles are nearly full, atrial systole occurs and forces the remainder of the blood in the atria into the ventricles. The sinuatrial node initiates the wave of contraction in the atria, which commences around the openings of the large veins and milks the blood toward the ventricles. By this means, blood does not reflux into the veins.

The cardiac impulse, having reached the atrioventricular node, is conducted to the papillary muscles by the atrioventricular bundle and its branches (Fig. 3-39). The papillary muscles then begin to contract and take up the slack of the chordae tendineae. Meanwhile, the ventricles start contracting and the atrioventricular valves close. The spread of the cardiac impulse along the atrioventricular bundle (Fig. 3-39) and its terminal branches, including the Purkinje fibers, ensures that myocardial contraction occurs at almost the same time throughout the ventricles.

Once the intraventricular blood pressure exceeds that present in the large arteries (aorta and pulmonary trunk), the semilunar valve cusps are pushed aside, and the blood is ejected from the heart. At the conclusion of ventricular systole, blood begins to move back toward the ventricles and immediately fills the pockets of the semilunar valves. The cusps float into apposition and completely close the aortic and pulmonary orifices.

Surface Anatomy of the Heart Valves

The surface projection of the heart was described on page 72. The surface markings of the heart valves are as follows (Fig. 3-15):

- The **tricuspid valve** lies behind the right half of the sternum opposite the fourth intercostal space.
- The **mitral valve** lies behind the left half of the sternum opposite the fourth costal cartilage.
- The **pulmonary valve** lies behind the medial end of the third left costal cartilage and the adjoining part of the sternum.
- The **aortic valve** lies behind the left half of the sternum opposite the third intercostal space.

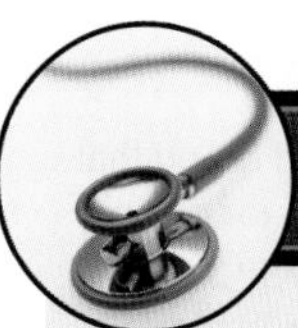

CLINICAL NOTES

Auscultation of the Heart Valves

On listening to the heart with a stethoscope, one can hear two sounds: **lūb-dŭp.** The first sound is produced by the contraction of the ventricles and the closure of the tricuspid and mitral valves. The second sound is produced by the sharp closure of the aortic and pulmonary valves. It is important for a physician to know where to place the stethoscope on the chest wall so that he or she will be able to hear sounds produced at each valve with the minimum of distraction or interference.

- The **tricuspid valve** is best heard over the right half of the lower end of the body of the sternum (Fig. 3-15).
- The **mitral valve** is best heard over the apex beat, that is, at the level of the fifth left intercostal space, 3.5 in. (9 cm) from the midline (Fig. 3-15).
- The **pulmonary valve** is heard with least interference over the medial end of the second left intercostal space (Fig. 3-15).
- The **aortic valve** is best heard over the medial end of the second right intercostal space (Fig. 3-15).

Valvular Disease of the Heart

Inflammation of a valve can cause the edges of the valve cusps to stick together. Later, fibrous thickening occurs, followed by loss of flexibility and shrinkage. Narrowing (stenosis) and valvular incompetence (regurgitation) result, and the heart ceases to function as an efficient pump. In rheumatic disease of the mitral valve, for example, not only do the cusps undergo fibrosis and shrink, but also the chordae tendineae shorten, preventing closure of the cusps during ventricular systole.

Valvular Heart Murmurs

Apart from the sounds of the valves closing, **lūb-dŭp,** the blood passes through the normal heart silently. Should the valve orifices become narrowed or the valve cusps distorted and shrunken by disease, however, a rippling effect would be set up, leading to turbulence and vibrations that are heard as heart murmurs.

Traumatic Asphyxia

The sudden caving in of the anterior chest wall associated with fractures of the sternum and ribs causes a dramatic rise in intrathoracic pressure. Apart from the immediate evidence of respiratory distress, the anatomy of the venous system plays a significant role in the production of the characteristic vascular signs of traumatic asphyxia. The thinness of the walls of the thoracic veins and the right atrium causes their collapse under the raised intrathoracic pressure, and venous blood is dammed back in the veins of the neck and head. This produces venous congestion; bulging of the eyes, which become injected; and swelling of the lips and tongue, which become cyanotic. The skin of the face, neck, and shoulders becomes purple.

The Anatomy of Cardiopulmonary Resuscitation

Cardiopulmonary resuscitation (CPR), achieved by compression of the chest, was originally believed to succeed because of the compression of the heart between the sternum and the ver-

(continues)

Clinical Notes, *continued*

tebral column. Now it is recognized that the blood flows in CPR because the whole thoracic cage is the pump; the heart functions merely as a conduit for blood. An extrathoracic pressure gradient is created by external chest compressions. The pressure in all chambers and locations within the chest cavity is the same. With compression, blood is forced out of the thoracic cage. The blood preferentially flows out the arterial side of the circulation and back down the venous side because the venous valves in the internal jugular system prevent a useless oscillatory movement. With the release of compression, blood enters the thoracic cage, preferentially down the venous side of the systemic circulation.

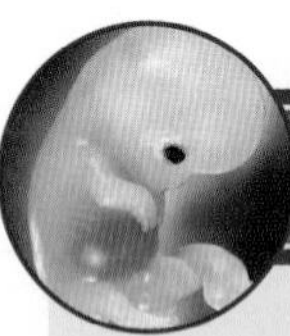

EMBRYOLOGIC NOTES

Development of the Heart

Formation of the Heart Tube

Clusters of cells arise in the mesenchyme at the cephalic end of the embryonic disc, cephalic to the site of the developing mouth and the nervous system. These clusters of cells form a plexus of endothelial blood vessels that fuse to form the **right** and **left endocardial heart tubes.** These, too, soon fuse to form a single **median endocardial tube.** As the head fold of the embryo develops, the endocardial tube and the pericardial cavity rotate on a transverse axis through almost 180°, so that they come to lie ventral to (in front of) the esophagus and caudal to the developing mouth.

The heart tube starts to bulge into the pericardial cavity (Fig. 3-44). Meanwhile, the endocardial tube becomes surrounded by a thick layer of mesenchyme, which will differentiate into the **myocardium** and the **visceral layer of the serous pericardium.** The primitive heart has been established, and the cephalic end is the arterial end and the caudal end is the venous end. The arterial end of the primitive heart is continuous beyond the pericardium with a large vessel, the **aortic sac** (Fig. 3-45). The heart begins to beat during the third week.

Further Development of the Heart Tube

The heart tube then undergoes differential expansion so that several dilatations, separated by grooves, result. From the arterial to the venous end, these dilatations are called the **bulbus cordis,** the **ventricle,** the **atrium,** and the **right** and **left horns of the sinus venosus.** The bulbus cordis and ventricular parts of the tube now elongate more rapidly than the remainder of the tube, and since the arterial and venous ends are fixed by the pericardium, the tube begins to bend (Fig. 3-46). The bend soon becomes U-shaped and then forms a compound S-shape, with the atrium lying posterior to the ventricle; thus, the venous and arterial ends are brought close together as they are in the adult. The passage between the atrium and the ventricle narrows to form the **atrioventricular canal.** As these changes are taking place, a gradual migration of the heart tube occurs so that the heart passes from the neck region to what will become the thoracic region.

Development of the Atria

The primitive atrium becomes divided into two—the right and left atria—in the following manner (Fig. 3-47). First, the atrioventricular canal widens transversely. The canal then becomes divided into right and left halves by the appearance of ventral and dorsal atrioventricular cushions, which fuse to form the **septum intermedium.** Meanwhile, another septum, the **septum primum,** develops from the roof of the primitive atrium and grows down to fuse with the septum intermedium. Before fusion occurs, the opening between the lower edge of the septum primum and septum intermedium is referred to as the **foramen primum.** The atrium now is divided into right and left parts. Before complete obliteration of the foramen primum has taken place, degenerative changes occur in the central portion of the septum primum; a foramen appears, the **foramen secundum,** so that the right and left atrial chambers again communicate. Another, thicker, septum (the **septum secundum)** grows down from the atrial roof on the right side of the septum primum. The lower edge of the septum secundum overlaps the foramen secundum in the septum primum but does not reach the floor of the atrium and does not fuse with the septum intermedium. The space between the free margin of the septum secundum and the septum primum is now known as the **foramen ovale** (Fig. 3-47).

Before birth, the foramen ovale allows oxygenated blood that has entered the right atrium from the inferior vena cava to pass into the left atrium. However, the lower part of the septum primum serves as a flaplike valve to prevent blood from moving from the left atrium into the right atrium. At birth, owing to raised blood pressure in the left atrium, the septum primum is pressed against the septum secundum and fuses with it, and the foramen ovale is closed. The two atria thus are separated from each other. The lower edge of the septum secundum seen in the right atrium becomes the **anulus ovalis,** and the depression below this is called the **fossa ovalis.** The **right** and **left auricular appendages** later develop as small diverticula from the right and left atria, respectively.

Development of the Ventricles

A muscular partition projects upward from the floor of the primitive ventricle to form the **ventricular septum** (Fig. 3-47). The space bounded by the crescentic upper edge of the septum and the endocardial cushions forms the **interventricular foramen.** Meanwhile, spiral subendocardial thickenings, the **bulbar ridges,** appear in the distal part of the bulbus cordis. The bulbar ridges then grow and fuse to form a **spiral aorticopulmonary septum** (Fig. 3-48). The interventricular foramen closes as the result of proliferation of the bulbar ridges and the fused endocardial cushions (septum intermedium). This newly formed tissue grows down and fuses with the upper edge of the muscular ventricular septum to form the **membranous part of the septum** (Fig. 3-47). The closure of the interventricular foramen not only shuts off the path of communication between the right and left ventricles, but also ensures that the right ventricular cavity communicates with the pulmonary trunk and the left ventricular cavity communicates with the aorta. In addition, the right atrioventricular opening now connects exclusively with the right ventricular cavity and the left atrioventricular opening, with the left ventricular cavity.

(continues)

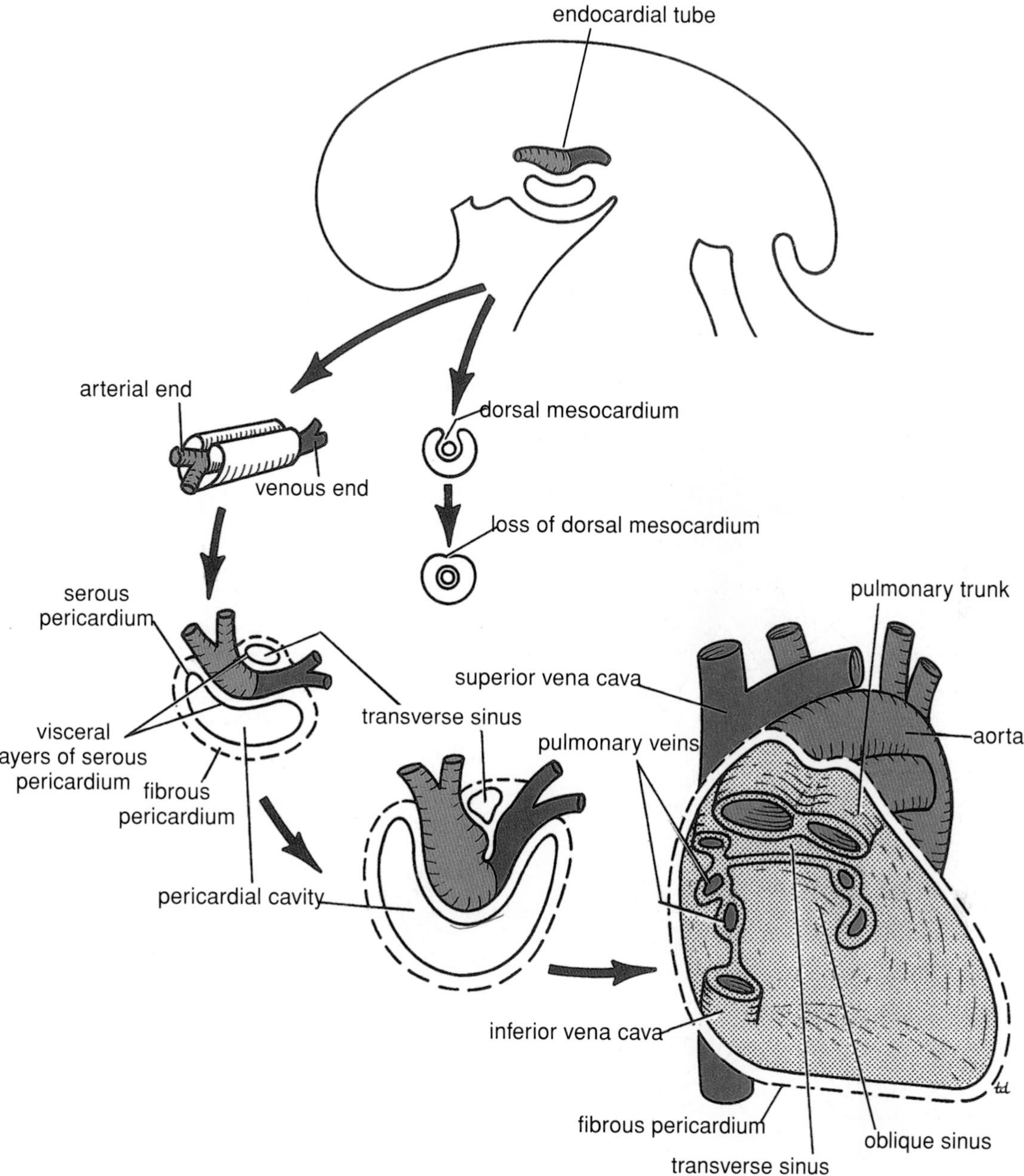

Figure 3-44 The development of the endocardial tube in relation to the pericardial cavity.

Embryologic Notes, *continued*

Development of the Roots and Proximal Portions of the Aorta and Pulmonary Trunk

The distal part of the bulbus cordis is known as the **truncus arteriosus** (Fig. 3-45). It is divided by the spiral aorticopulmonary septum to form the roots and proximal portions of the aorta and pulmonary trunk (Fig. 3-48). With the establishment of right and left ventricles, the proximal portion of the bulbus cordis becomes incorporated into the right ventricle as the definitive **conus arteriosus** or **infundibulum,** and into the left ventricle as the **aortic vestibule.** Just distal to the aortic valves, the two **coronary arteries** arise as outgrowths from the developing aorta.

Development of the Cardiac Valves

Semilunar Valves of the Aorta and Pulmonary Arteries

After the formation of the aorticopulmonary septum, three swellings appear at the orifices of both the aorta and the pulmonary artery. Each swelling consists of a covering of endothelium over loose connective tissue. Gradually, the swellings

(continues)

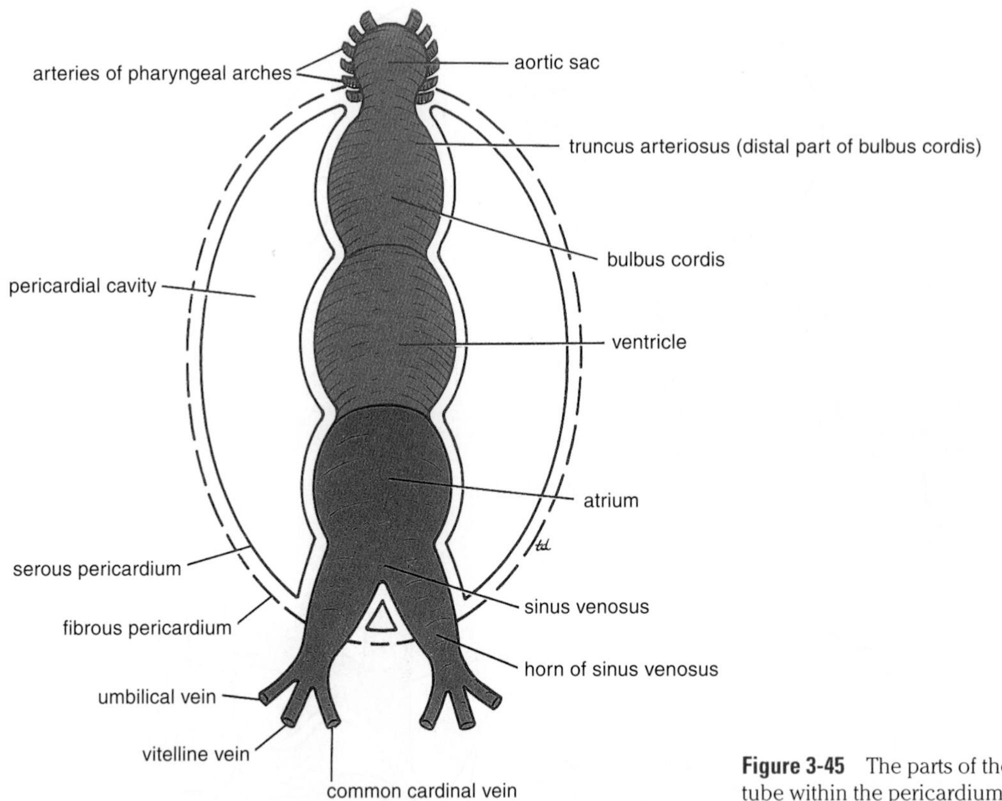

Figure 3-45 The parts of the endocardial heart tube within the pericardium.

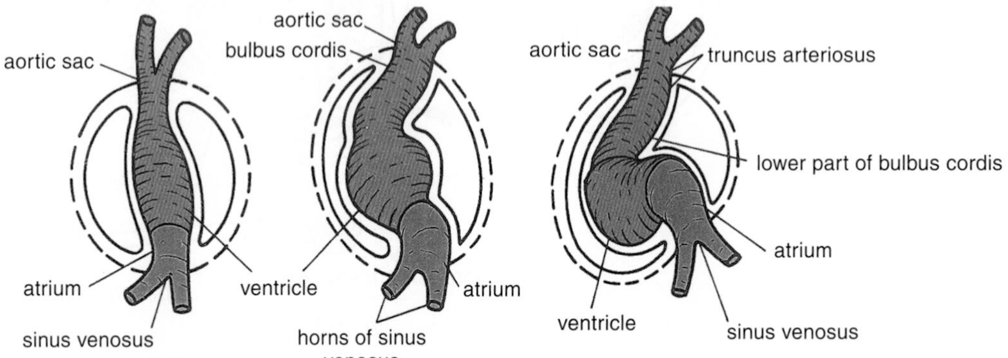

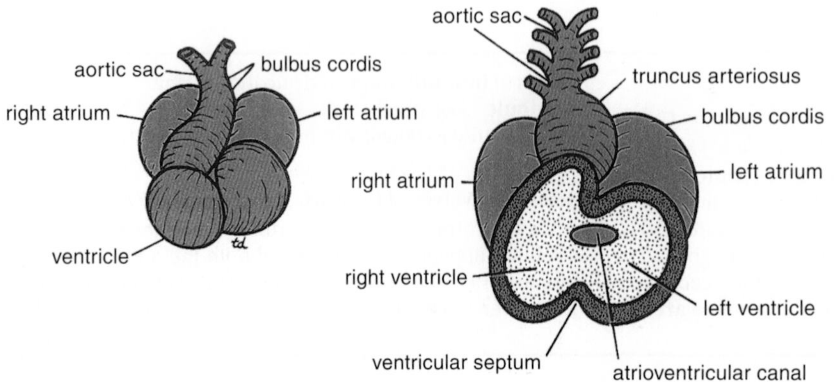

Figure 3-46 The bending of the heart tube within the pericardial cavity. The interior of the developing ventricles is shown at the bottom right.

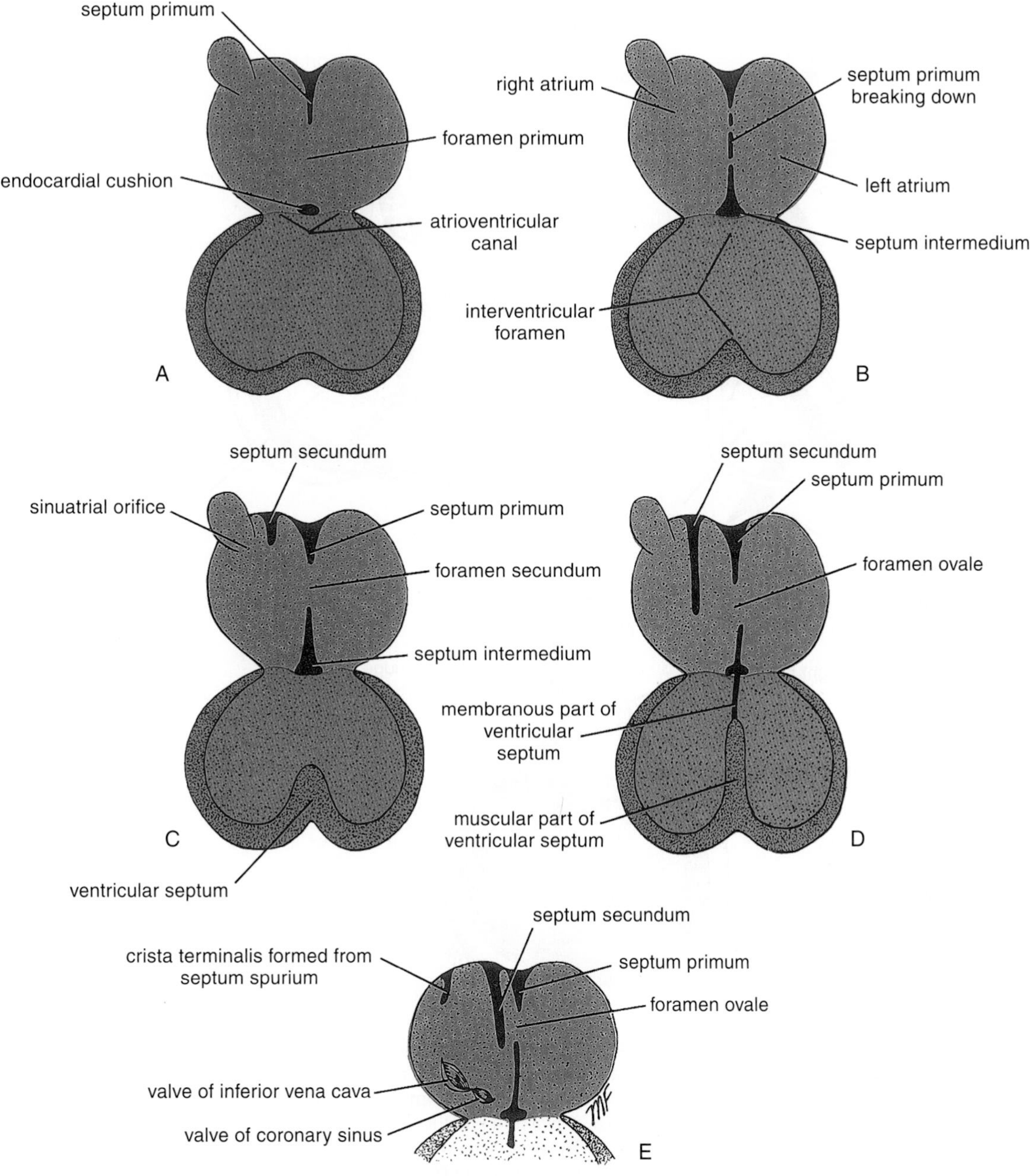

Figure 3-47 The division of the primitive atrium into the right and left atria by the appearance of the septa. The sinuatrial orifice and the fate of the venous valves are shown, as is the appearance of the ventricular septum.

Embryologic Notes, *continued*

become excavated on their upper surfaces to form the semilunar valves.

Atrioventricular Valves

After the formation of the septum intermedium, the atrioventricular canal becomes divided into right and left atrioventricular orifices. Raised folds of endocardium appear at the margins of these orifices. These folds are invaded by mesenchymal tissue that later becomes hollowed out from the ventricular side. Three valvular cusps are formed about the right atrioventricular orifice and constitute the **tricuspid valve;** two cusps are formed about the left atrioventricular orifice to become the **mitral valve.** The newly formed cusps enlarge, and their mesenchymal core becomes differentiated into fibrous tissue. The cusps remain attached at intervals to the ventricular wall by muscular strands. Later, the muscular strands become differentiated into **papillary muscles** and **chordae tendineae.**

(continues)

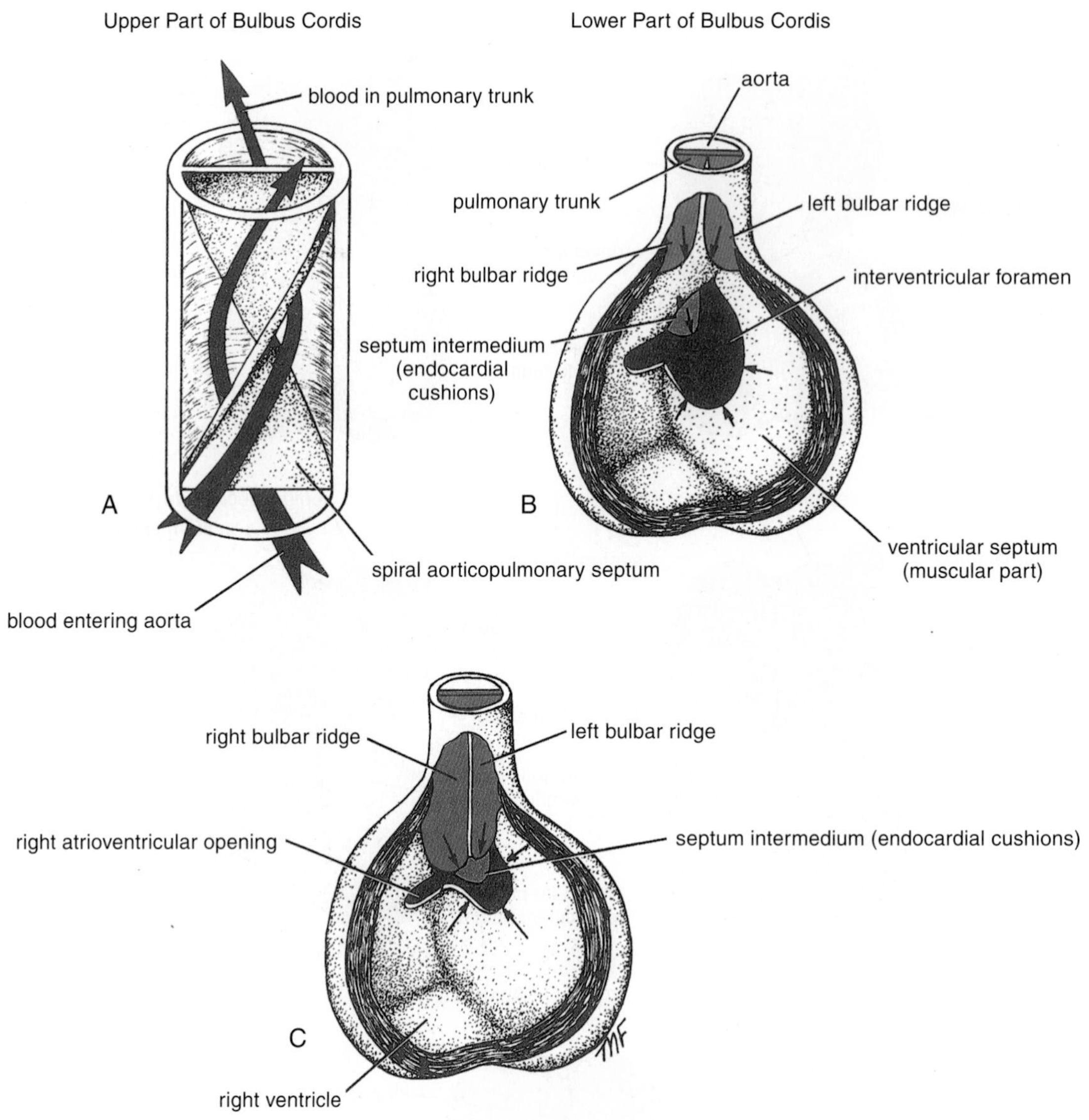

Figure 3-48 The division of the bulbus cordis by the spiral aorticopulmonary septum into the aorta and pulmonary trunk. **A.** The spiral septum in the truncus arteriosus (upper part of the bulbus cordis). **B.** The lower part of the bulbus cordis showing the formation of the spiral septum by fusion of the bulbar ridges (*red*), which then grow down and join the septum intermedium (*blue*) and the muscular part of the ventricular septum. **C.** The area of the ventricular septum that is formed from the fused bulbar ridges (*red*) and the septum intermedium (*blue*) is called the membranous part of the ventricular septum.

Embryologic Notes, *continued*

Congenital Anomalies of the Heart

Atrial Septal Defects

After birth, the foramen ovale becomes completely closed as the result of the fusion of the septum primum with the septum secundum. In 25% of hearts, a small opening persists, but this is usually of such a minor nature that it has no clinical significance. Occasionally, the opening is much larger and results in oxygenated blood from the left atrium passing over into the right atrium (Fig. 3-38).

Ventricular Septal Defects

The ventricular septum is formed in a complicated manner and is complete only when the membranous part fuses with the muscular part. Ventricular septal defects are less frequent than atrial septal defects. They are found in the membranous part of the septum and can measure 1 to 2 cm in diameter. Blood under high pressure passes through the defect from left to right, causing enlargement of the right ventricle. Large defects are serious and can shorten life if surgery is not performed.

(continues)

Embryologic Notes, *continued*

Tetralogy of Fallot

Normally, the bulbus cordis becomes divided into the aorta and pulmonary trunk by the formation of the spiral aorticopulmonary septum. This septum is formed by the fusion of the bulbar ridges. If the bulbar ridges fail to fuse correctly, unequal division of the bulbus cordis may occur, with consequent narrowing of the pulmonary trunk resulting in interference with the right ventricular outflow.

This congenital anomaly is responsible for about 9% of all congenital heart disease (Fig. 3-38). The anatomic abnormalities include large ventricular septal defect; stenosis of the pulmonary trunk, which can occur at the infundibulum of the right ventricle or at the pulmonary valve; exit of the aorta immediately above the ventricular septal defect (instead of from the left ventricular cavity only); and severe hypertrophy of the right ventricle, because of the high blood pressure in the right ventricle. The defects cause congenital cyanosis and considerably limit activity; patients with severe untreated abnormalities die. Once the diagnosis has been made, most children can be successfully treated surgically.

Most children find that assuming the squatting position after physical activity relieves their breathlessness. This happens because squatting reduces the venous return by compressing the abdominal veins and increasing the systemic arterial resistance by kinking the femoral and popliteal arteries in the legs; both these mechanisms tend to decrease the right to left shunt through the ventricular septal defect and improve the pulmonary circulation.

Large Veins of the Thorax

Brachiocephalic Veins

The **right brachiocephalic vein** is formed at the root of the neck by the union of the right subclavian and the right internal jugular veins (Figs. 3-16 and 3-49). The **left brachiocephalic vein** has a similar origin (Figs. 3-31 and 3-33). It passes obliquely downward and to the right behind the manubrium sterni and in front of the large branches of the aortic arch. It joins the right brachiocephalic vein to form the superior vena cava (Fig. 3-49).

Superior Vena Cava

The superior vena cava contains all the venous blood from the head and neck and both upper limbs and is formed by the union of the two brachiocephalic veins (Figs. 3-33 and 3-49). It passes downward to end in the right atrium of the heart (Fig. 3-30). The vena azygos joins the posterior aspect of the superior vena cava just before it enters the pericardium (Figs. 3-16 and 3-49).

Azygos Veins

The azygos veins consist of the main azygos vein, the inferior hemiazygos vein, and the superior hemiazygos vein. They drain blood from the posterior parts of the intercostal spaces, the posterior abdominal wall, the pericardium, the diaphragm, the bronchi, and the esophagus (Fig. 3-49).

Azygos Vein

The origin of the azygos vein is variable. It is often formed by the union of the **right ascending lumbar vein** and the **right subcostal vein.** It ascends through the aortic opening in the diaphragm on the right side of the aorta to the level of the fifth thoracic vertebra (Fig. 3-49). Here it arches forward above the root of the right lung to empty into the posterior surface of the superior vena cava (Fig. 3-16).

The azygos vein has numerous tributaries, including the **eight lower right intercostal veins,** the **right superior intercostal vein,** the **superior** and **inferior hemiazygos veins,** and numerous **mediastinal veins.**

Inferior Hemiazygos Vein

The inferior hemiazygos vein is often formed by the union of the left ascending lumbar vein and the left subcostal vein. It ascends through the left crus of the diaphragm and, at about the level of the eighth thoracic vertebra, turns to the right and joins the azygos vein (see Fig. 2-11). It receives as tributaries some **lower left intercostal veins** and **mediastinal veins.**

Superior Hemiazygos Vein

The superior hemiazygos vein is formed by the union of the fourth to the eighth intercostal veins. It joins the azygos vein at the level of the seventh thoracic vertebra (see Fig. 2-11).

Inferior Vena Cava

The inferior vena cava pierces the central tendon of the diaphragm opposite the eighth thoracic vertebra and almost immediately enters the lowest part of the right atrium (Figs. 3-16, 3-37, and 3-49).

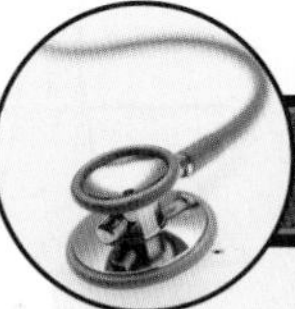

CLINICAL NOTES

Azygos Veins and Caval Obstruction

In obstruction of the superior or inferior venae cavae, the azygos veins provide an alternative pathway for the return of venous blood to the right atrium of the heart. This is possible because these veins and their tributaries connect the superior and inferior venae cavae.

Pulmonary Veins

Two pulmonary veins leave each lung carrying oxygenated blood to the left atrium of the heart (Figs. 3-16, 3-36, and 3-40).

Large Arteries of the Thorax

Aorta

The aorta is the main arterial trunk that delivers oxygenated blood from the left ventricle of the heart to the tissues of the

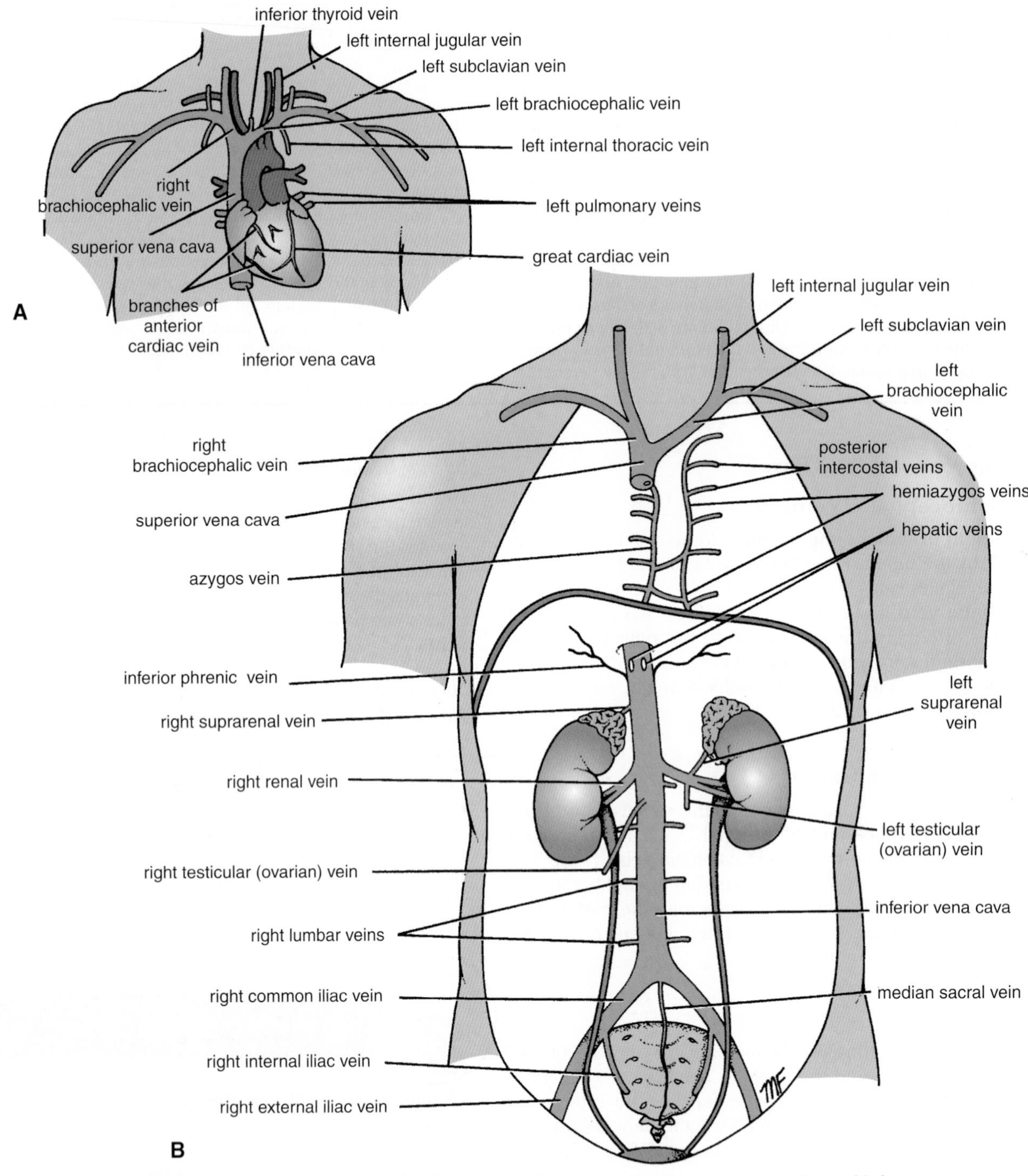

Figure 3-49 **A.** Major veins entering the heart. **B.** Major veins draining into the superior and inferior venae cavae.

body. It is divided for purposes of description into the following parts: ascending aorta, arch of the aorta, descending thoracic aorta, and abdominal aorta.

Ascending Aorta

The ascending aorta begins at the base of the left ventricle and runs upward and forward to come to lie behind the right half of the sternum at the level of the sternal angle, where it becomes continuous with the arch of the aorta (Fig. 3-35). The ascending aorta lies within the fibrous pericardium (Fig. 3-33) and is enclosed with the pulmonary trunk in a sheath of serous pericardium. At its root it possesses three bulges, the **sinuses of the aorta,** one behind each aortic valve cusp.

Branches

The **right coronary artery** arises from the anterior aortic sinus, and the **left coronary artery** arises from the left posterior aortic sinus (Figs. 3-35 and 3-42). The further course of these important arteries is described on pages 113 to 114.

Arch of the Aorta

The arch of the aorta is a continuation of the ascending aorta (Fig. 3-35). It lies behind the manubrium sterni and arches upward, backward, and to the left in front of the trachea (its main direction is backward). It then passes downward to the left of the trachea and, at the level of the sternal angle, becomes continuous with the descending aorta.

Branches

The **brachiocephalic artery** arises from the convex surface of the aortic arch (Figs. 3-35 and 3-50). It passes upward and to the right of the trachea and divides into the right subclavian and right common carotid arteries behind the right sternoclavicular joint.

The **left common carotid artery** arises from the convex surface of the aortic arch on the left side of the brachiocephalic artery (Figs. 3-35 and 3-50). It runs upward and to the left of the trachea and enters the neck behind the left sternoclavicular joint.

The **left subclavian artery** arises from the aortic arch behind the left common carotid artery (Figs. 3-35, 3-36, and 3-50). It runs upward along the left side of the trachea and the esophagus to enter the root of the neck (Fig. 3-16). It arches over the apex of the left lung.

Descending Thoracic Aorta

The descending thoracic aorta lies in the posterior mediastinum and begins as a continuation of the arch of the aorta on the left side of the lower border of the body of the fourth thoracic vertebra (i.e., opposite the sternal angle). It runs downward in the posterior mediastinum, inclining forward and medially to reach the anterior surface of the vertebral column (Figs. 3-16 and 3-50). At the level of the 12th

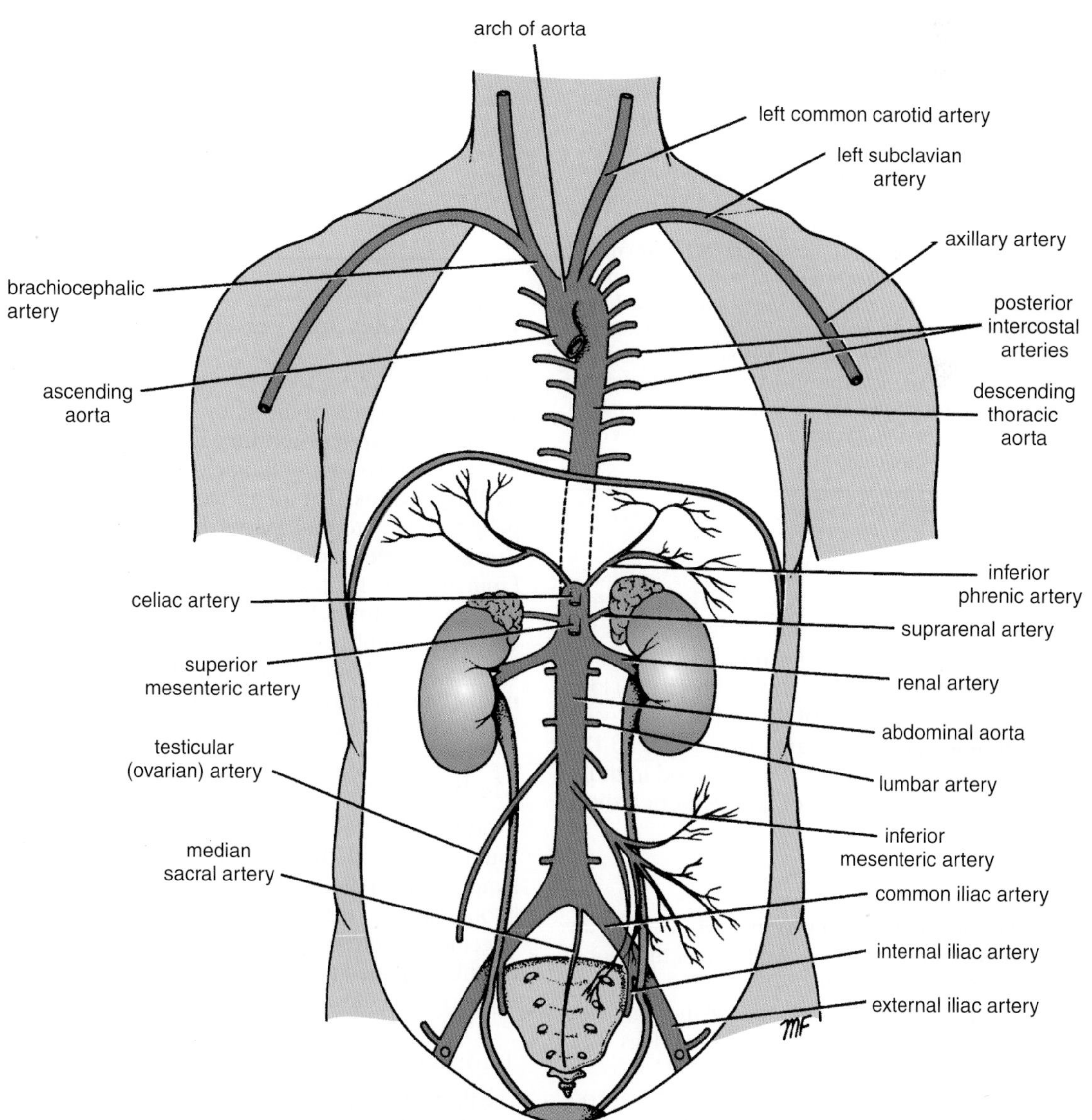

Figure 3-50 Major branches of the aorta.

thoracic vertebra, it passes behind the diaphragm (through the aortic opening) in the midline and becomes continuous with the abdominal aorta.

Branches

Posterior intercostal arteries are given off to the lower nine intercostal spaces on each side (Fig. 3-50). **Subcostal arteries** are given off on each side and run along the lower border of the 12th rib to enter the abdominal wall.

Pericardial, esophageal, and **bronchial arteries** are small branches that are distributed to these organs.

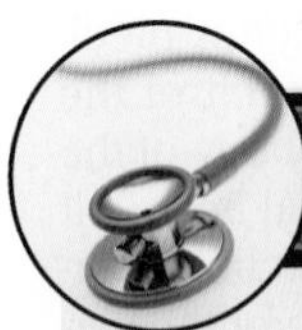

CLINICAL NOTES

Aneurysm and Coarctation of the Aorta

The arch of the aorta lies behind the manubrium sterni. A gross dilatation of the aorta (aneurysm) may show itself as a pulsatile swelling in the suprasternal notch.

Coarctation of the aorta is a congenital narrowing of the aorta just proximal, opposite, or distal to the site of attachment of the ligamentum arteriosum. This condition is believed to result from an unusual quantity of ductus arteriosus muscle tissue in the wall of the aorta. When the ductus arteriosus contracts, the ductal muscle in the aortic wall also contracts, and the aortic lumen becomes narrowed. Later, when fibrosis takes place, the aortic wall also is involved, and permanent narrowing occurs.

Clinically, the cardinal sign of aortic coarctation is absent or diminished pulses in the femoral arteries of both lower limbs. To compensate for the diminished volume of blood reaching the lower part of the body, an enormous collateral circulation develops, with dilatation of the internal thoracic, subclavian, and posterior intercostal arteries. The dilated intercostal arteries erode the lower borders of the ribs, producing characteristic notching, which is seen on radiographic examination. The condition should be treated surgically.

Pulmonary Trunk

The pulmonary trunk conveys deoxygenated blood from the right ventricle of the heart to the lungs. It leaves the upper part of the right ventricle and runs upward, backward, and to the left (Fig. 3-35). It is about 2 in. (5 cm) long and terminates in the concavity of the aortic arch by dividing into right and left pulmonary arteries (Fig. 3-12). Together with the ascending aorta, it is enclosed in the fibrous pericardium and a sheath of serous pericardium (Fig. 3-33).

Branches

The **right pulmonary artery** runs to the right behind the ascending aorta and superior vena cava to enter the root of the right lung (Figs. 3-12, 3-16, and 3-35).

The **left pulmonary artery** runs to the left in front of the descending aorta to enter the root of the left lung (Figs. 3-12, 3-16, and 3-35).

The **ligamentum arteriosum** is a fibrous band that connects the bifurcation of the pulmonary trunk to the lower concave surface of the aortic arch (Figs. 3-16 and 3-36). The ligamentum arteriosum is the remains of the ductus arteriosus, which in the fetus conducts blood from the pulmonary trunk to the aorta, thus bypassing the lungs. The left recurrent laryngeal nerve hooks around the lower border of this structure (Figs. 3-16 and 3-36). After birth, the ductus closes. Should it remain patent, aortic blood will enter the pulmonary circulation, producing pulmonary hypertension and hypertrophy of the right ventricle (Fig. 3-38). Surgical ligation of the ductus is then necessary.

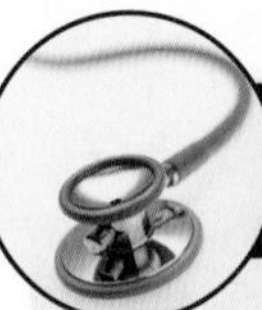

CLINICAL NOTES

Patent Ductus Arteriosus

The ductus arteriosus represents the distal portion of the sixth left aortic arch and connects the left pulmonary artery to the beginning of the descending aorta (Fig. 3-38D). During fetal life, blood passes through it from the pulmonary artery to the aorta, thus bypassing the lungs. After birth, it normally constricts, later closes, and becomes the **ligamentum arteriosum.**

Failure of the ductus arteriosus to close may occur as an isolated congenital abnormality or may be associated with congenital heart disease. A persistent patent ductus arteriosus results in high-pressure aortic blood passing into the pulmonary artery, which raises the pressure in the pulmonary circulation. A patent ductus arteriosus is life threatening and should be ligated and divided surgically.

Lymph Nodes and Vessels of the Thorax

Thoracic Wall

The lymph vessels of the skin of the anterior thoracic wall drain to the **anterior axillary nodes.** The lymph vessels of the skin of the posterior thoracic wall drain to the **posterior axillary nodes.** The deep lymph vessels of the anterior parts of the intercostal spaces drain forward to the **internal thoracic nodes** along the internal thoracic blood vessels. From here, the lymph passes to the thoracic duct on the left side and the bronchomediastinal trunk on the right side. The deep lymph vessels of the posterior parts of the intercostal spaces drain backward to the **posterior intercostal nodes** lying near the heads of the ribs. From here, the lymph enters the thoracic duct.

Mediastinum

In addition to the nodes draining the lungs, other nodes are found scattered through the mediastinum. They drain lymph from mediastinal structures and empty into the bronchomediastinal trunks and thoracic duct. Disease and enlargement of these nodes may exert pressure on important neighboring mediastinal structures, such as the trachea and superior vena cava.

Thoracic Duct

The thoracic duct begins below in the abdomen as a dilated sac, the **cisterna chyli.** It ascends through the aortic opening in the diaphragm, on the right side of the descending aorta. It gradually crosses the median plane behind the esophagus and reaches the left border of the esophagus (Fig. 3-6B) at the level of the lower border of the body of the fourth thoracic vertebra (sternal angle). It then runs upward along the left edge of the esophagus to enter the root of the neck (Fig. 3-6B). Here, it bends laterally behind the carotid sheath and in front of the vertebral vessels. It turns downward in front of the left phrenic nerve and crosses the subclavian artery to enter the beginning of the left brachiocephalic vein.

At the root of the neck, the thoracic duct receives the **left jugular, subclavian,** and **bronchomediastinal lymph trunks,** although they may drain directly into the adjacent large veins.

The thoracic duct thus conveys to the blood all lymph from the lower limbs, pelvic cavity, abdominal cavity, left side of the thorax, and left side of the head, neck, and left arm (see Fig 1-21).

Right Lymphatic Duct

The right jugular, subclavian, and bronchomediastinal trunks, which drain the right side of the head and neck, the right upper limb, and the right side of the thorax, respectively, may join to form the right lymphatic duct. This common duct, if present, is about 0.5 in. (1.3 cm) long and opens into the beginning of the right brachiocephalic vein. Alternatively, the trunks open independently into the great veins at the root of the neck.

Nerves of the Thorax

Vagus Nerves

The **right vagus nerve** descends in the thorax, first lying posterolateral to the brachiocephalic artery (Fig. 3-6), then lateral to the trachea and medial to the terminal part of the azygos vein (Fig. 3-16). It passes **behind** the root of the right lung and assists in the formation of the **pulmonary plexus.** On leaving the plexus, the vagus passes onto the posterior surface of the esophagus and takes part in the formation of the **esophageal plexus.** It then passes through the esophageal opening of the diaphragm behind the esophagus to reach the posterior surface of the stomach.

The **left vagus nerve** descends in the thorax between the left common carotid and the left subclavian arteries (Figs. 3-6 and 3-16). It then crosses the left side of the aortic arch and is itself crossed by the left phrenic nerve. The vagus then turns backward **behind** the root of the left lung and assists in the formation of the **pulmonary plexus.** On leaving the plexus, the vagus passes onto the anterior surface of the esophagus and takes part in the formation of the **esophageal plexus.** It then passes through the esophageal opening in the diaphragm in front of the esophagus to reach the anterior surface of the stomach.

Branches

Both vagi supply the lungs and esophagus. The right vagus gives off cardiac branches, and the left vagus gives origin to the left recurrent laryngeal nerve. (The right recurrent laryngeal nerve arises from the right vagus in the neck and hooks around the subclavian artery and ascends between the trachea and esophagus.)

The **left recurrent laryngeal nerve** arises from the left vagus trunk as the nerve crosses the arch of the aorta (Figs. 3-16 and 3-36). It hooks around the ligamentum arteriosum and ascends in the groove between the trachea and the esophagus on the left side (Fig. 3-6). It supplies all the muscles acting on the left vocal cord (except the cricothyroid muscle, a tensor of the cord, which is supplied by the external laryngeal branch of the vagus).

Phrenic Nerves

The phrenic nerves arise from the neck from the anterior rami of the third, fourth, and fifth cervical nerves (see page 771).

The **right phrenic nerve** descends in the thorax along the right side of the right brachiocephalic vein and the superior vena cava (Figs. 3-6 and 3-16). It passes **in front** of the root of the right lung and runs along the right side of the pericardium, which separates the nerve from the right atrium. It then descends on the right side of the inferior vena cava to the diaphragm. Its terminal branches pass through the caval opening in the diaphragm to supply the central part of the peritoneum on its underaspect.

The **left phrenic nerve** descends in the thorax along the left side of the left subclavian artery. It crosses the left side of the aortic arch (Fig. 3-16) and here crosses the left side of the left vagus nerve. It passes **in front** of the root of the left lung and then descends over the left surface of the pericardium, which separates the nerve from the left ventricle. On reaching the diaphragm, the terminal branches pierce the muscle and supply the central part of the peritoneum on its underaspect.

The phrenic nerves possess efferent and afferent fibers. The efferent fibers are the **sole nerve supply** to the muscle of the diaphragm.

The afferent fibers carry sensation to the central nervous system from the peritoneum covering the central region of the undersurface of the diaphragm, the pleura covering the central region of the upper surface of the diaphragm, and the pericardium and mediastinal parietal pleura.

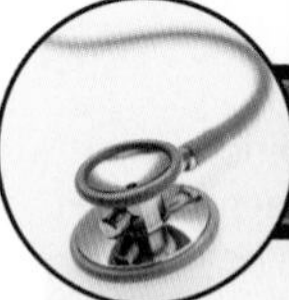

CLINICAL NOTES

Paralysis of the Diaphragm

The phrenic nerve may be paralyzed because of pressure from malignant tumors in the mediastinum. Surgical crushing or sectioning of the phrenic nerve in the neck, producing paralysis of the diaphragm on one side, was once used as part of the treatment of lung tuberculosis, especially of the lower lobes. The immobile dome of the diaphragm rests the lung.

Thoracic Part of the Sympathetic Trunk

The thoracic part of the sympathetic trunk is continuous above with the cervical and below with the lumbar parts of the sympathetic trunk. It is the most laterally placed structure in the mediastinum and runs downward on the heads of the ribs (Fig. 3-16). It leaves the thorax on the side of the body of the 12th thoracic vertebra by passing behind the medial arcuate ligament.

The sympathetic trunk has 12 (often only 11) segmentally arranged ganglia, each with **white** and **gray ramus communicans** passing to the corresponding spinal nerve. The first ganglion is often fused with the inferior cervical ganglion to form the **stellate ganglion.**

Branches

1. Gray rami communicantes go to all the thoracic spinal nerves. The postganglionic fibers are distributed through the branches of the spinal nerves to the blood vessels, sweat glands, and arrector pili muscles of the skin.
2. The first five ganglia give postganglionic fibers to the heart, aorta, lungs, and esophagus.
3. The lower eight ganglia mainly give preganglionic fibers, which are grouped together to form the splanchnic nerves (Fig. 3-16) and supply the abdominal viscera. They enter the abdomen by piercing the crura of the diaphragm. The **greater splanchnic nerve** arises from ganglia 5 to 9, the **lesser splanchnic nerve** arises from ganglia 10 and 11, and the **lowest splanchnic nerve** arises from ganglion 12. For details of the distribution of these nerves in the abdomen, see page 279.

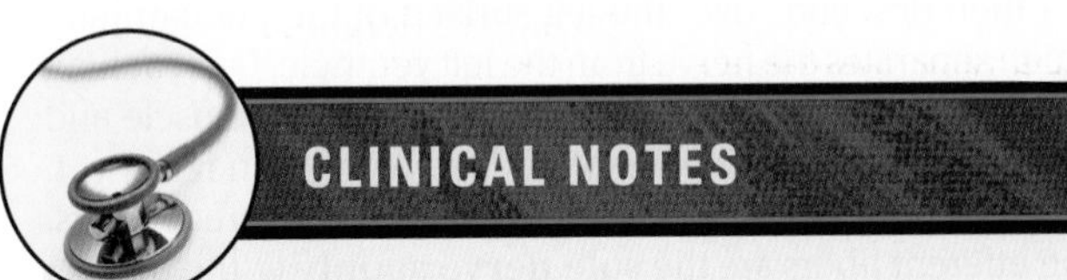

Sympathetic Trunk in the Treatment of Raynaud Disease

Preganglionic sympathectomy of the second and third thoracic ganglia can be performed to increase the blood flow to the fingers for such conditions as Raynaud disease. The sympathectomy causes vasodilatation of the arterioles in the upper limb.

Spinal Anesthesia and the Sympathetic Nervous System

A high spinal anesthetic may block the preganglionic sympathetic fibers passing out from the lower thoracic segments of the spinal cord. This produces temporary vasodilatation below this level, with a consequent fall in blood pressure.

Esophagus

The esophagus is a tubular structure about 10 in. (25 cm) long that is continuous above with the laryngeal part of the pharynx opposite the sixth cervical vertebra. It passes through the diaphragm at the level of the 10th thoracic vertebra to join the stomach (Fig. 3-10).

In the neck, the esophagus lies in front of the vertebral column; laterally, it is related to the lobes of the thyroid gland; and anteriorly, it is in contact with the trachea and the recurrent laryngeal nerves (see page 795).

In the thorax, it passes downward and to the left through the superior and then the posterior mediastinum. At the level of the sternal angle, the aortic arch pushes the esophagus over to the midline (Fig. 3-6).

The relations of the thoracic part of the esophagus from above downward are as follows:

- **Anteriorly:** The trachea and the left recurrent laryngeal nerve; the left principal bronchus, which constricts it; and the pericardium, which separates the esophagus from the left atrium (Figs. 3-6 and 3-40)
- **Posteriorly:** The bodies of the thoracic vertebrae; the thoracic duct; the azygos veins; the right posterior intercostal arteries; and, at its lower end, the descending thoracic aorta (Figs. 3-6 and 3-40)
- **Right side:** The mediastinal pleura and the terminal part of the azygos vein (Fig. 3-16)
- **Left side:** The left subclavian artery, the aortic arch, the thoracic duct, and the mediastinal pleura (Fig. 3-16)

Inferiorly to the level of the roots of the lungs, the vagus nerves leave the pulmonary plexus and join with sympathetic nerves to form the **esophageal plexus.** The left vagus lies anterior to the esophagus and the right vagus lies posterior. At the opening in the diaphragm, the esophagus is accompanied by the two vagi, branches of the left gastric blood vessels, and lymphatic vessels. Fibers from the right crus of the diaphragm pass around the esophagus in the form of a sling.

In the abdomen, the esophagus descends for about 0.5 in. (1.3 cm) and then enters the stomach. It is related to the left lobe of the liver anteriorly and to the left crus of the diaphragm posteriorly.

Blood Supply of the Esophagus

The upper third of the esophagus is supplied by the inferior thyroid artery, the middle third by branches from the descending thoracic aorta, and the lower third by branches from the left gastric artery. The veins from the upper third drain into the inferior thyroid veins, from the middle third into the azygos veins, and from the lower third into the left gastric vein, a tributary of the portal vein.

Lymph Drainage of the Esophagus

Lymph vessels from the upper third of the esophagus drain into the deep cervical nodes, from the middle third into the superior and posterior mediastinal nodes, and from the lower third into nodes along the left gastric blood vessels and the celiac nodes (Fig. 3-27).

Nerve Supply of the Esophagus

The esophagus is supplied by parasympathetic and sympathetic efferent and afferent fibers via the vagi and sympathetic trunks. In the lower part of its thoracic course, the esophagus is surrounded by the esophageal nerve plexus.

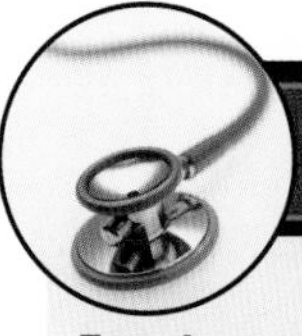

CLINICAL NOTES

Esophageal Constrictions

The esophagus has three anatomic and physiologic constrictions. The first is where the pharynx joins the upper end, the second is where the aortic arch and the left bronchus cross its anterior surface, and the third occurs where the esophagus passes through the diaphragm into the stomach. These constrictions are of considerable clinical importance because they are sites where swallowed foreign bodies can lodge or through which it may be difficult to pass an **esophagoscope.** Because a slight delay in the passage of food or fluid occurs at these levels, strictures develop here after the drinking of caustic fluids. Those constrictions are also the common sites of carcinoma of the esophagus. It is useful to remember that their respective distances from the upper incisor teeth are 6 in. (15 cm), 10 in. (25 cm), and 16 in. (41 cm), respectively (Fig. 3-51).

Portal–Systemic Venous Anastomosis

At the lower third of the esophagus is an important portal–systemic venous anastomosis. (For other portal–systemic anastomoses, see page 246). Here, the esophageal tributaries of the azygos veins (systemic veins) anastomose with the esophageal tributaries of the left gastric vein (which drains into the portal vein). Should the portal vein become obstructed, as, for example, in **cirrhosis of the liver, portal hypertension** develops, resulting in the dilatation and varicosity of the portal–systemic anastomoses. Varicosed esophageal veins may rupture during the passage of food, causing **hematemesis** (vomiting of blood), which may be fatal.

Carcinoma of the Lower Third of the Esophagus

The lymph drainage of the lower third of the esophagus descends through the esophageal opening in the diaphragm and ends in the celiac nodes around the celiac artery (Fig. 3-27). A malignant tumor of this area of the esophagus would therefore tend to spread below the diaphragm along this route. Consequently, surgical removal of the lesion would include not only the primary lesion, but also the celiac lymph nodes and all regions that drain into these nodes, namely, the stomach, the upper half of the duodenum, the spleen, and the omenta. Restoration of continuity of the gut is accomplished by performing an esophagojejunostomy.

The Esophagus and the Left Atrium of the Heart

The close relationship between the anterior wall of the esophagus and the posterior wall of the left atrium has already been emphasized. A barium swallow may help a physician assess the size of the left atrium in cases of left-sided heart failure, in which the left atrium becomes distended because of back pressure of venous blood.

Thymus

The thymus is a flattened, bilobed structure (Fig. 3-6) lying between the sternum and the pericardium in the anterior mediastinum. In the newborn infant, it reaches its largest size relative to the size of the body, at which time it may extend up through the superior mediastinum in front of the great vessels into the root of the neck. The thymus continues to grow until puberty but thereafter undergoes involution. It has a pink, lobulated appearance and is the site for development of T (thymic) lymphocytes.

Blood Supply

The blood supply of the thymus is from the inferior thyroid and internal thoracic arteries.

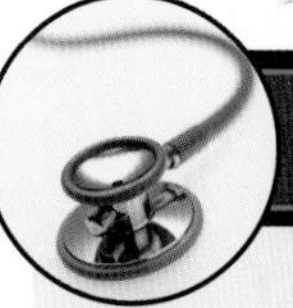

CLINICAL NOTES

Chest Pain

The presenting symptom of chest pain is a common problem in clinical practice. Unfortunately, chest pain is a symptom common to many conditions and may be caused by disease in the thoracic and abdominal walls or in many different thoracic and abdominal viscera. The severity of the pain is often unrelated to the seriousness of the cause. Myocardial pain may mimic esophagitis, musculoskeletal chest wall pain, and other non–life-threatening causes. Unless the physician is astute, a patient may be discharged with a more serious condition than the symptoms indicate. **It is not good enough to have a correct diagnosis only 99% of the time with chest pain.** An understanding of chest pain helps the physician in the systematic consideration of the differential diagnosis.

Somatic Chest Pain

Pain arising from the chest or abdominal walls is intense and discretely localized. Somatic pain arises in sensory nerve endings in these structures and is conducted to the central nervous system by segmental spinal nerves.

Visceral Chest Pain

Visceral pain is diffuse and poorly localized. It is conducted to the central nervous system along afferent autonomic nerves. Most visceral pain fibers ascend to the spinal cord along sympathetic nerves and enter the cord through the posterior nerve roots of segmental spinal nerves. Some pain fibers from the pharynx and upper part of the esophagus and the trachea enter the central nervous system through the parasympathetic nerves via the glossopharyngeal and vagus nerves.

(continues)

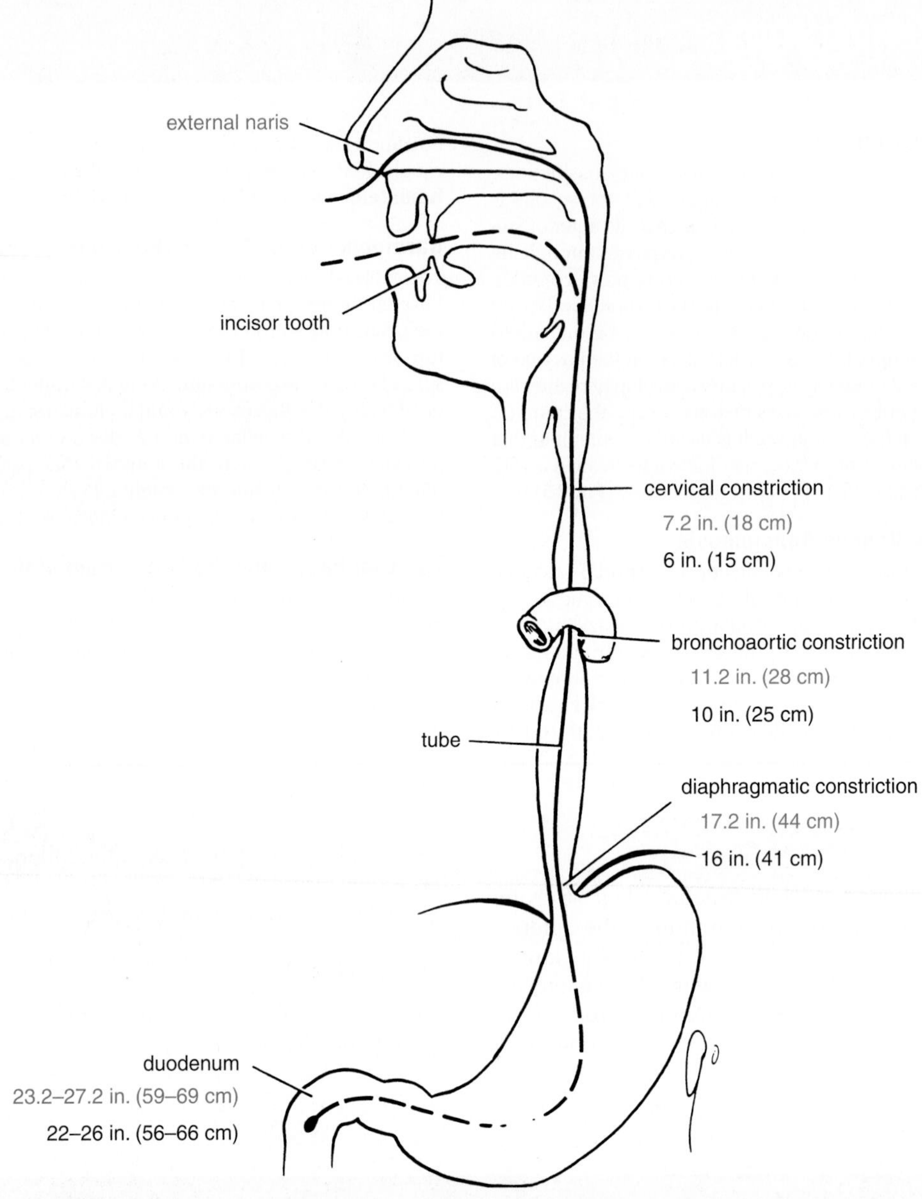

Figure 3-51 The approximate respective distances from the incisor teeth (*black*) and the nostrils (*red*) to the normal three constrictions of the esophagus. To assist in the passage of a tube to the duodenum, the distances to the first part of the duodenum are also included.

Clinical Notes, *continued*

Referred Chest Pain

Referred chest pain is the feeling of pain at a location other than the site of origin of the stimulus, but in an area supplied by the same or adjacent segments of the spinal cord. Both somatic and visceral structures can produce referred pain.

Thoracic Dermatomes

To understand chest pain, a working knowledge of the thoracic dermatomes is essential (see pages 27 and 28).

Pain and Lung Disease

For a full discussion, see page 103.

Cardiac Pain

For a full discussion, see page 116.

Cross-Sectional Anatomy of the Thorax

To assist in the interpretation of CT scans of the thorax, study the labeled cross sections of the thorax shown in Figure 3-52. The sections have been photographed on their inferior surfaces (see Figs. 3-53 and 3-54 for CT scans).

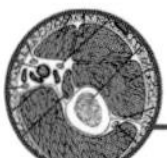

Radiographic Anatomy

Only the more important features seen on standard posteroanterior and oblique lateral radiographs of the chest are discussed here.

Posteroanterior Radiograph

A posteroanterior radiograph is taken with the anterior wall of the patient's chest touching the cassette holder and with the x-rays traversing the thorax from the posterior to the anterior aspect (Figs. 3-55 and 3-56). First check to make sure that the radiograph is a true posteroanterior radiograph and is not slightly oblique. Look at the sternal ends of both clavicles; they should be equidistant from the vertebral spines.

Now examine the following in a systematic order:

1. **Superficial soft tissues.** The nipples in both sexes and the breasts in the female may be seen superimposed on

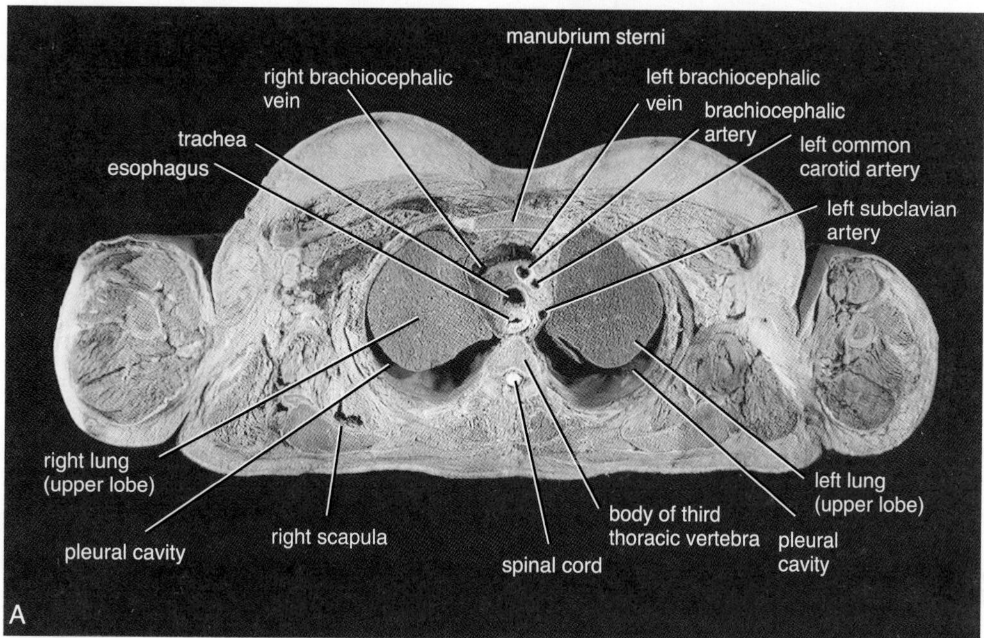

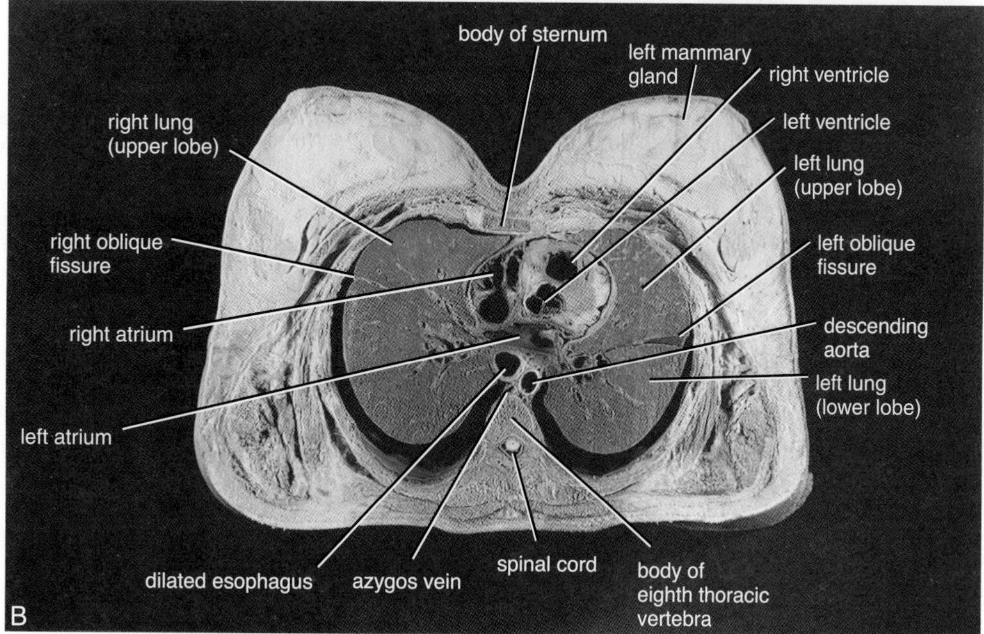

Figure 3-52 Cross sections of the thorax viewed from below. **A.** At the level of the body of the third thoracic vertebra. **B.** At the level of the eighth thoracic vertebra. Note that in the living, the pleural cavity is only a potential space. The large space seen here is an artifact and results from the embalming process.

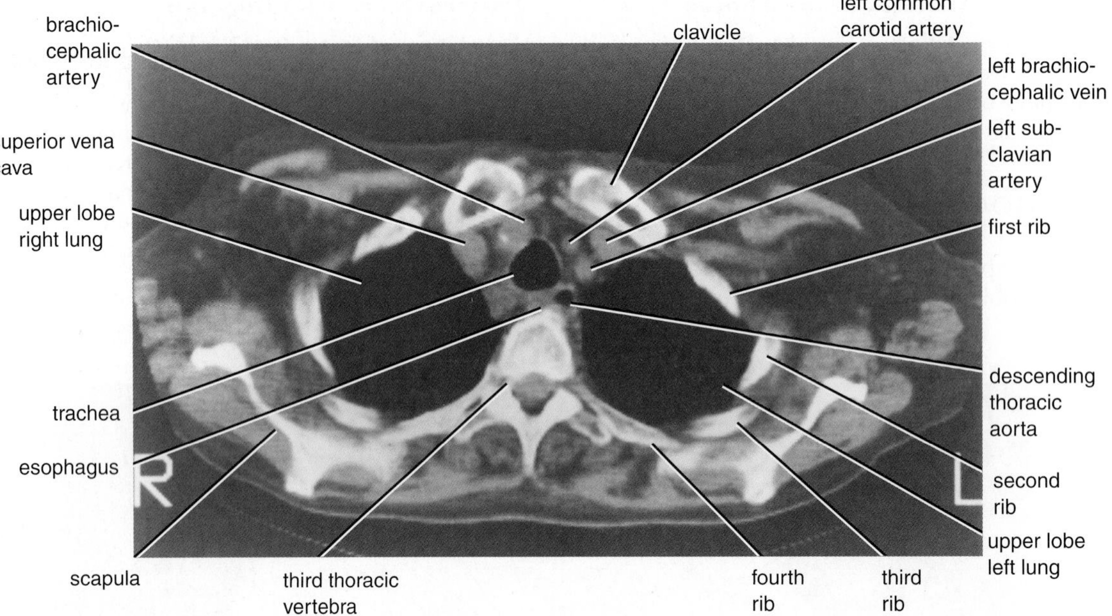

Figure 3-53 Computed tomography scan of the upper part of the thorax at the level of the third thoracic vertebra. The section is viewed from below.

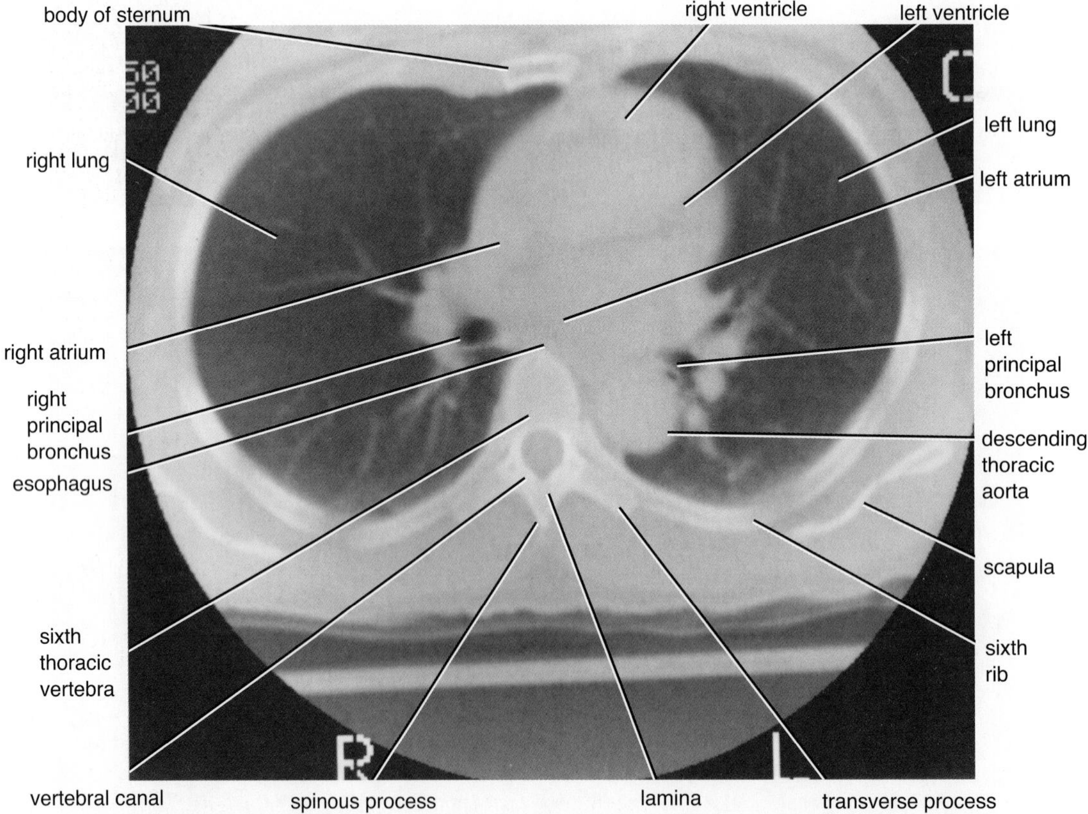

Figure 3-54 Computed tomography scan of the middle part of the thorax at the level of the sixth thoracic vertebra. The section is viewed from below.

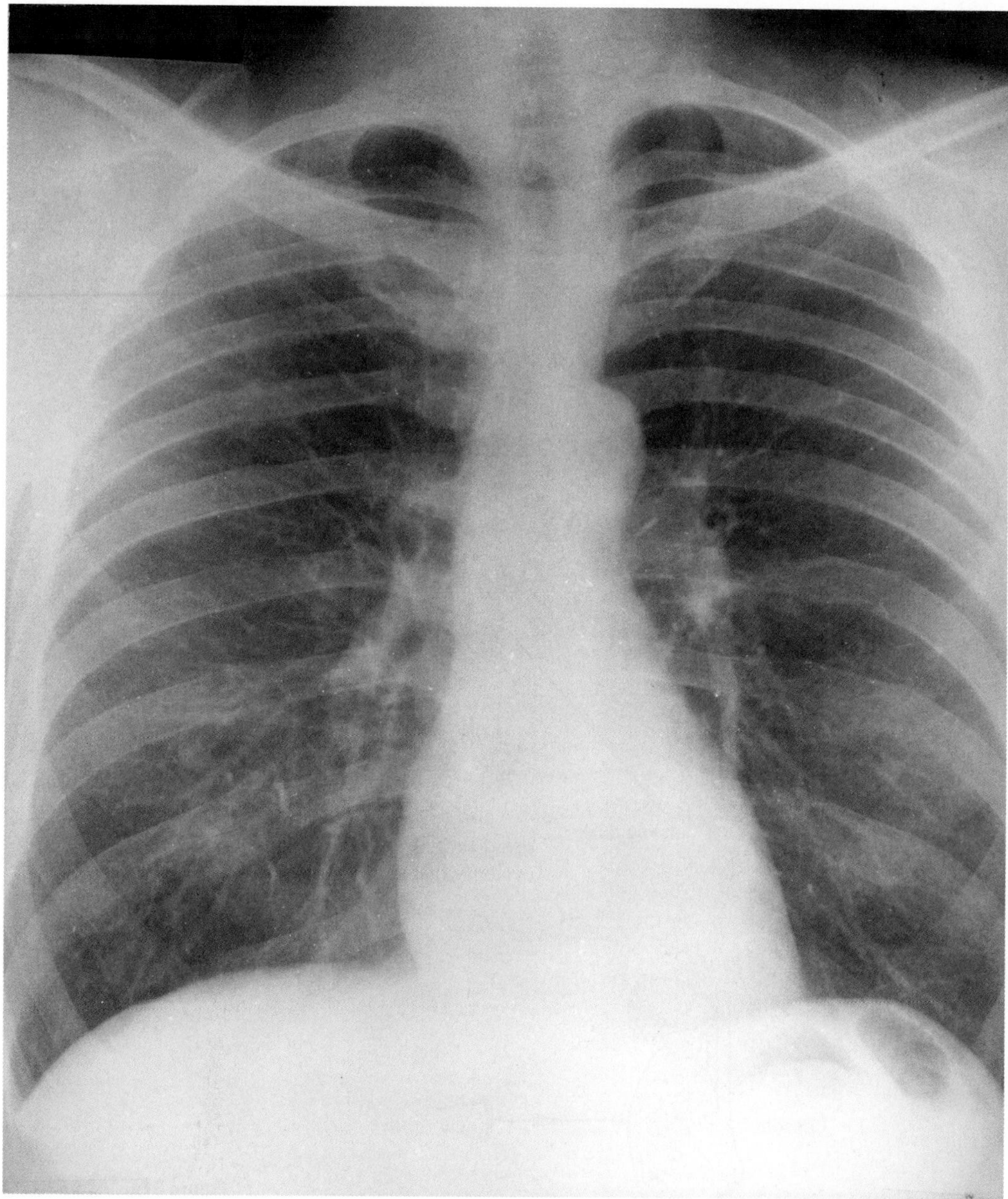

Figure 3-55 Posteroanterior radiograph of the chest of a normal adult man.

the lung fields. The pectoralis major may also cast a soft shadow.

2. **Bones.** The thoracic vertebrae are imperfectly seen. The costotransverse joints and each rib should be examined in order from above downward and compared to the fellows of the opposite side (Fig. 3-55). The costal cartilages are not usually seen, but if calcified, they will be visible. The clavicles are clearly seen crossing the upper part of each lung field. The medial borders of the scapulae may overlap the periphery of each lung field.
3. **Diaphragm.** The diaphragm casts dome-shaped shadows on each side; the one on the right is slightly higher than the one on the left. Note the costophrenic angle, where the diaphragm meets the thoracic wall (Fig. 3-55). Beneath the right dome is the homogeneous, dense shadow of the liver, and beneath the left dome a gas bubble may be seen in the fundus of the stomach.
4. **Trachea.** The radiotranslucent, air-filled shadow of the trachea is seen in the midline of the neck as a dark area (Fig. 3-55). This is superimposed on the lower cervical and upper thoracic vertebrae.
5. **Lungs.** Looking first at the lung roots, one sees relatively dense shadows caused by the presence of the blood-filled pulmonary and bronchial vessels, the large bronchi, and the lymph nodes (Fig. 3-55). The lung fields, by virtue of the air they contain, readily permit the passage of x-rays. For this reason, the lungs are more translucent on full inspiration than on expiration. The pulmonary blood vessels are seen as a series of shadows radiating from the lung root. When seen end on, they

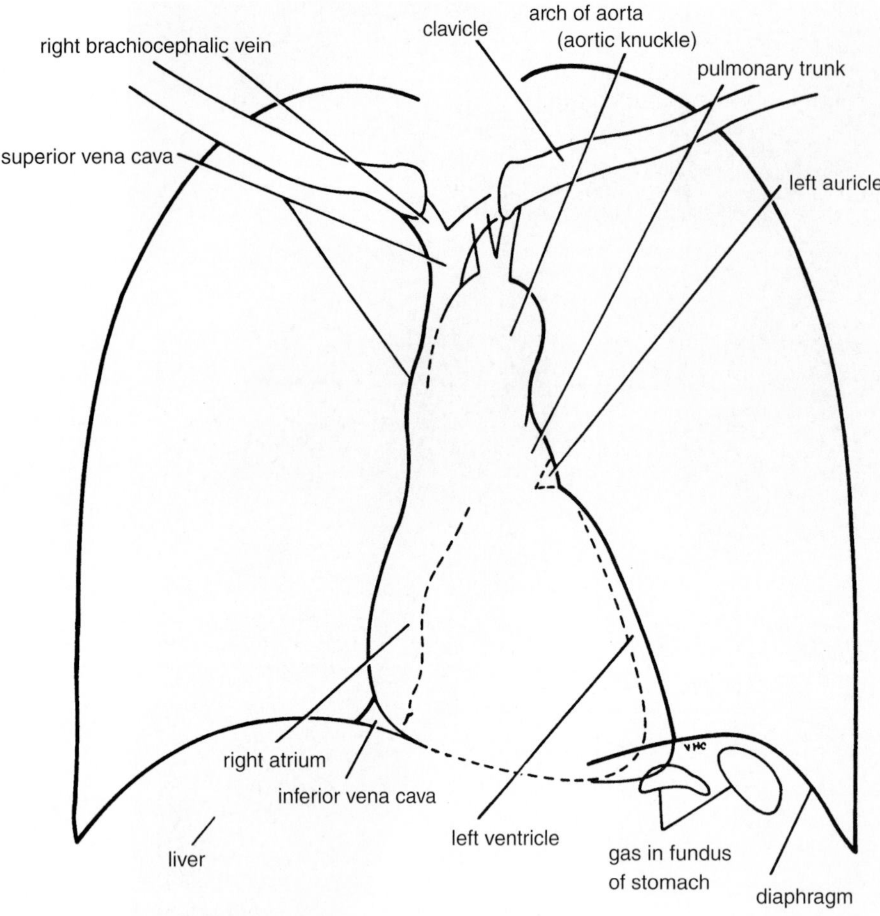

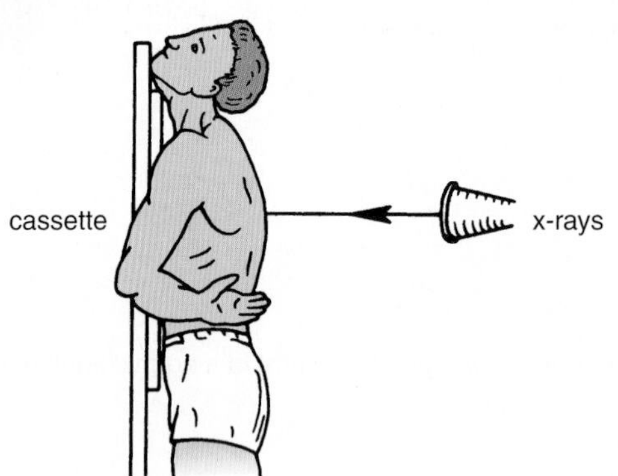

Figure 3-56 Main features observable in the posteroanterior radiograph of the chest shown in Figure 3-55. Note the position of the patient in relation to the x-ray source and cassette holder.

appear as small, round, white shadows. The large bronchi, if seen end on, also cast similar round shadows. The smaller bronchi are not seen.

6. **Mediastinum.** The shadow is produced by the various structures within the mediastinum, superimposed one on the other (Figs. 3-49 and 3-55). Note the outline of the heart and great vessels. The transverse diameter of the heart should not exceed half the width of the thoracic cage. Remember that on deep inspiration, when the diaphragm descends, the vertical length of the heart increases and the transverse diameter is narrowed. In infants, the heart is always wider and more globular in shape than in adults.

The right border of the mediastinal shadow from above downward consists of the right brachiocephalic vein, the superior vena cava, the right atrium, and sometimes the inferior vena cava (Figs. 3-55 and 3-56). The left border consists of a prominence, the **aortic knuckle,** caused by the aortic arch; below this are the left margin of the pulmonary trunk, the left auricle, and the left ventricle (Figs. 3-55 and 3-56). The inferior border of the mediastinal shadow (lower border of the heart) blends with the diaphragm and liver. Note the **cardiophrenic angles.**

Right Oblique Radiograph

A right oblique radiograph is obtained by rotating the patient so that the right anterior chest wall is touching the cassette holder and the x-rays traverse the thorax from posterior to anterior in an oblique direction (Figs. 3-57 and 3-58). The

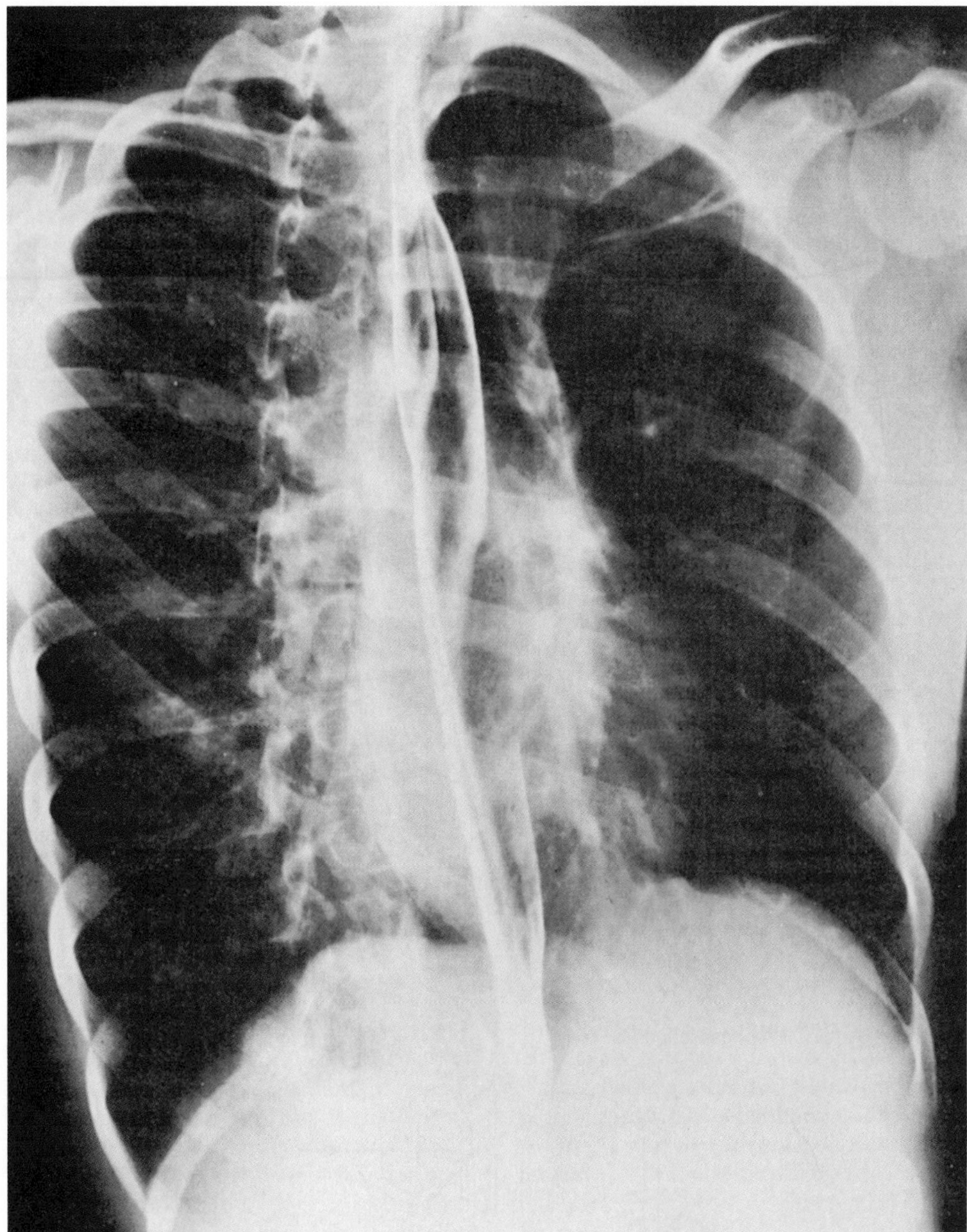

Figure 3-57 Right oblique radiograph of the chest of a normal adult man after a barium swallow.

heart shadow is largely made up by the right ventricle. A small part of the posterior border is formed by the right atrium. For further details of structures seen on this view, see Figures 3-57 and 3-58.

Left Oblique Radiograph

A left oblique radiograph is obtained by rotation of the patient so that the left anterior chest wall is touching the cassette holder and the x-rays traverse the thorax from posterior to anterior in an oblique direction. The heart shadow is largely made up of the right ventricle anteriorly and the left ventricle posteriorly. Above the heart, the aortic arch and the pulmonary trunk may be seen.

An example of a left lateral radiograph of the chest is shown in Figures 3-59 and 3-60.

Bronchography and Contrast Visualization of the Esophagus

Bronchography is a special study of the bronchial tree by means of the introduction of iodized oil or other contrast medium into a particular bronchus or bronchi, usually under fluoroscopic control. The contrast media are nonirritating and sufficiently radiopaque to allow good visualization of the bronchi (Fig. 3-61). After the radiographic examination is completed, the patient is asked to cough and expectorate the contrast medium.

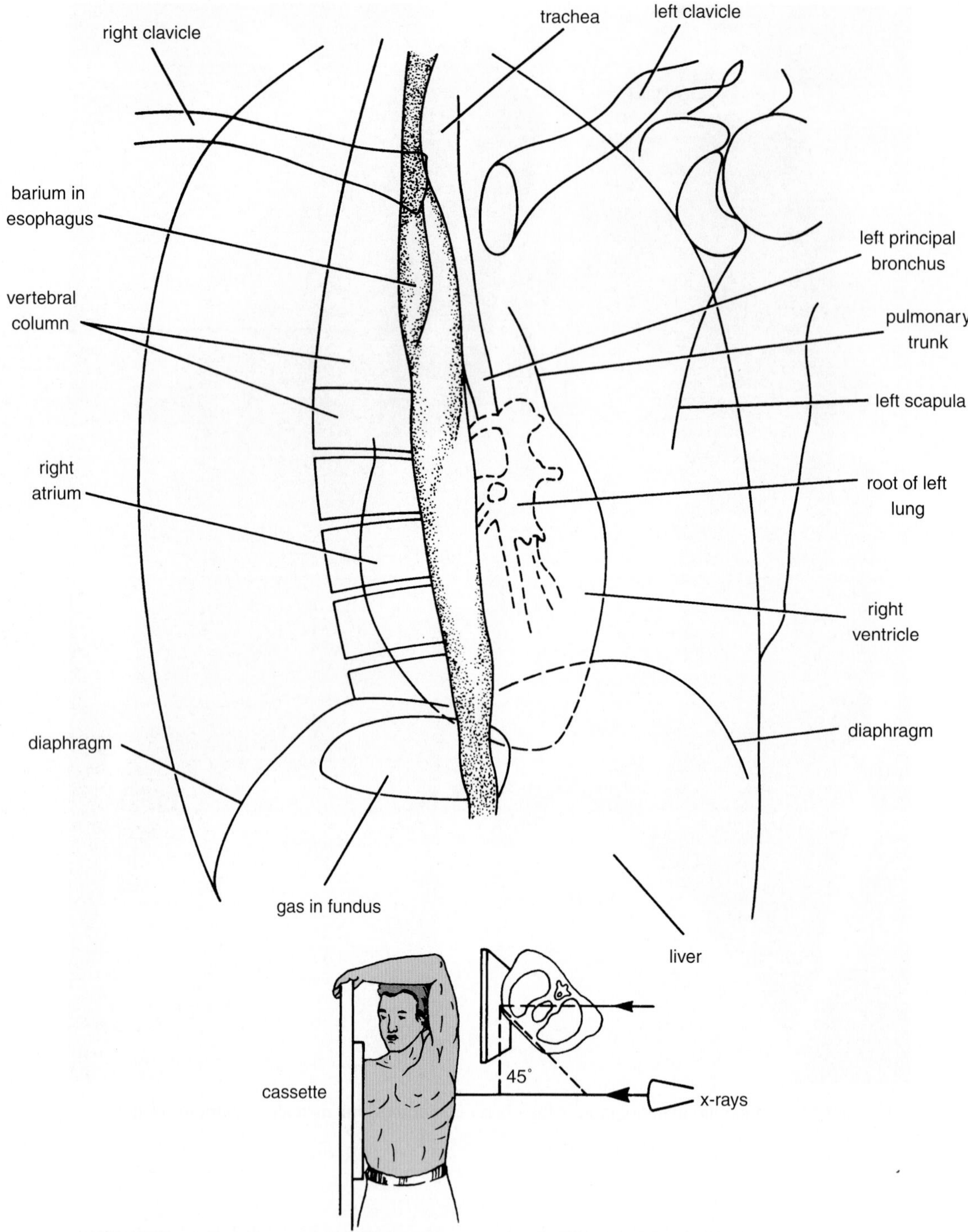

Figure 3-58 Main features observable in the right oblique radiograph of the chest shown in Figure 3-57. Note the position of the patient in relation to the x-ray source and cassette holder.

Contrast visualization of the esophagus (Figs. 3-57 and 3-59) is accomplished by giving the patient a creamy paste of barium sulfate and water to swallow. The aortic arch and the left bronchus cause a smooth indentation on the anterior border of the barium-filled esophagus. This procedure can also be used to outline the posterior border of the left atrium in a right oblique view. An enlarged left atrium causes a smooth indentation of the anterior border of the barium-filled esophagus.

Coronary Angiography

The coronary arteries can be visualized by the introduction of radiopaque material into their lumen. Under fluoroscopic control, a long narrow catheter is passed into the ascending aorta via the femoral artery in the leg. The tip of the catheter is carefully guided into the orifice of a coronary artery and a small amount of radiopaque material is injected to reveal the lumen of the artery and its branches. The information can be recorded on radiographs (Fig. 3-62)

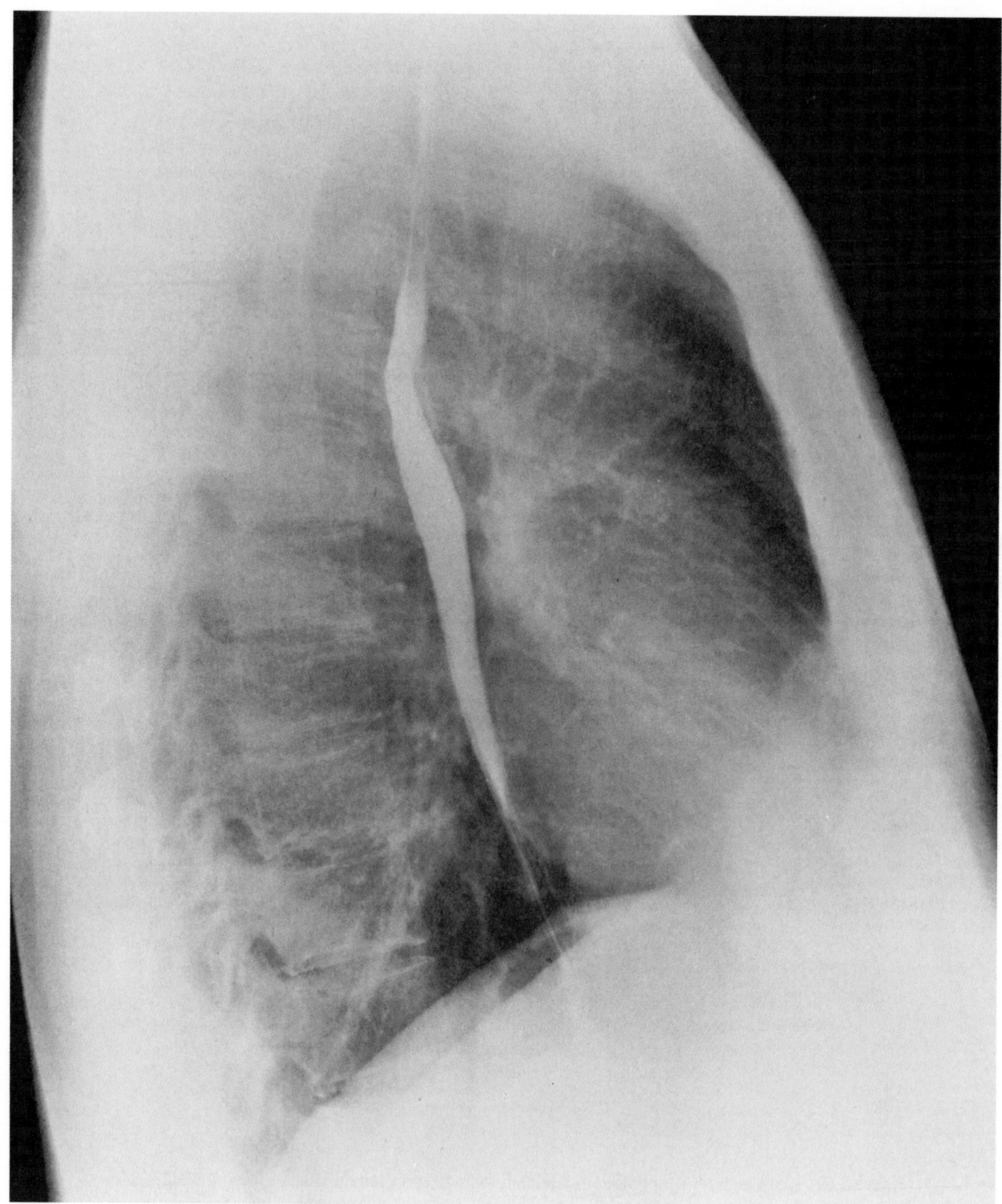

Figure 3-59 Left lateral radiograph of the chest of a normal adult man after a barium swallow.

or by cineradiography. Using this technique, pathologic narrowing or blockage of a coronary artery can be identified.

CT Scanning of the Thorax

CT scanning relies on the same physics as conventional x-rays but combines it with computer technology. A source of x-rays moves in an arc around the thorax and sends out a beam of x-rays. The beams of x-rays, having passed through the thoracic wall and the thoracic viscera, are converted into electronic impulses that produce readings of the density of the tissue in a 1-cm slice of the body. From these readings, the computer assembles a picture of the thorax called a CT scan, which can be viewed on a fluorescent screen and then photographed (Figs. 3-53 and 3-54).

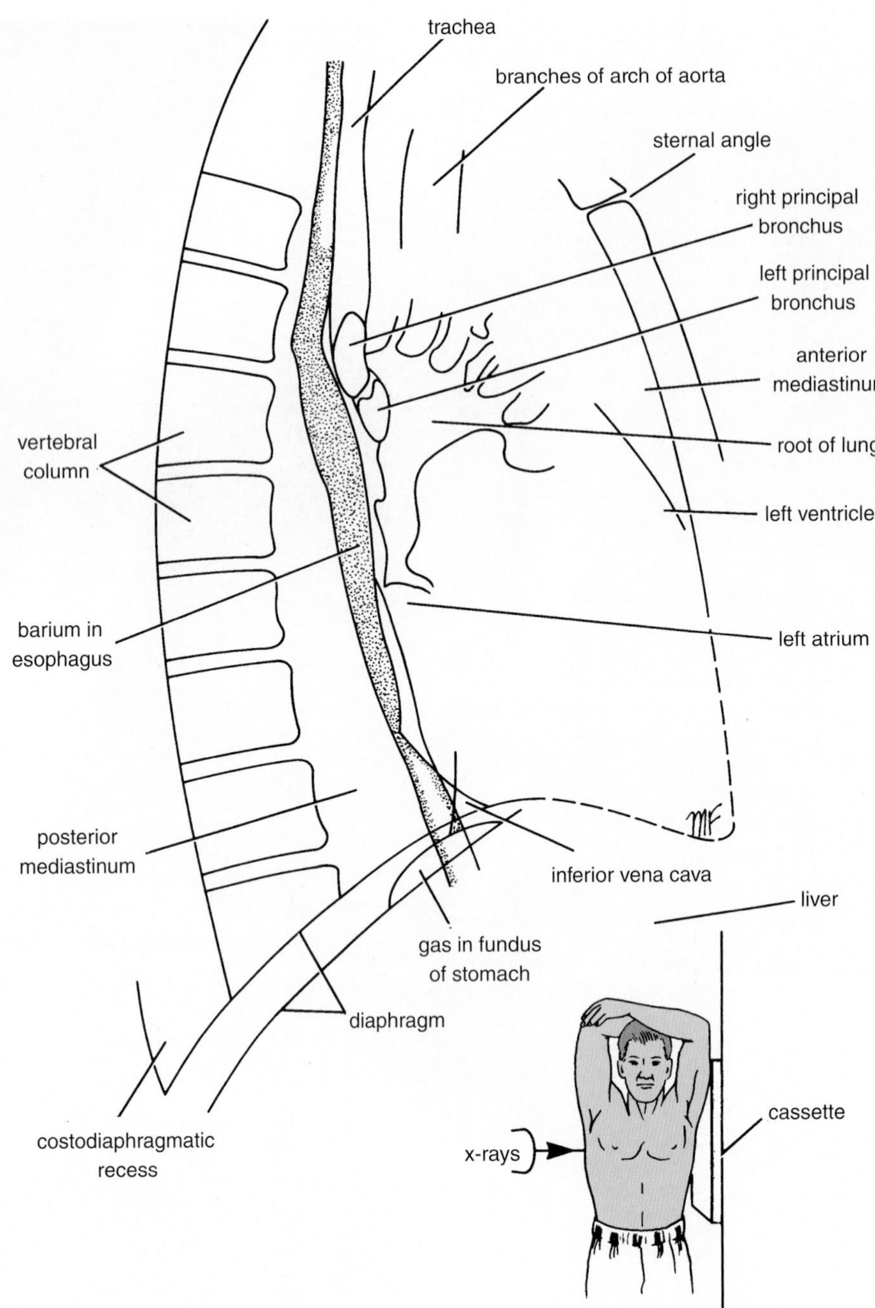

Figure 3-60 Main features observable in a left lateral radiograph of the chest shown in Figure 3-59. Note the position of the patient in relation to the x-ray source and cassette holder.

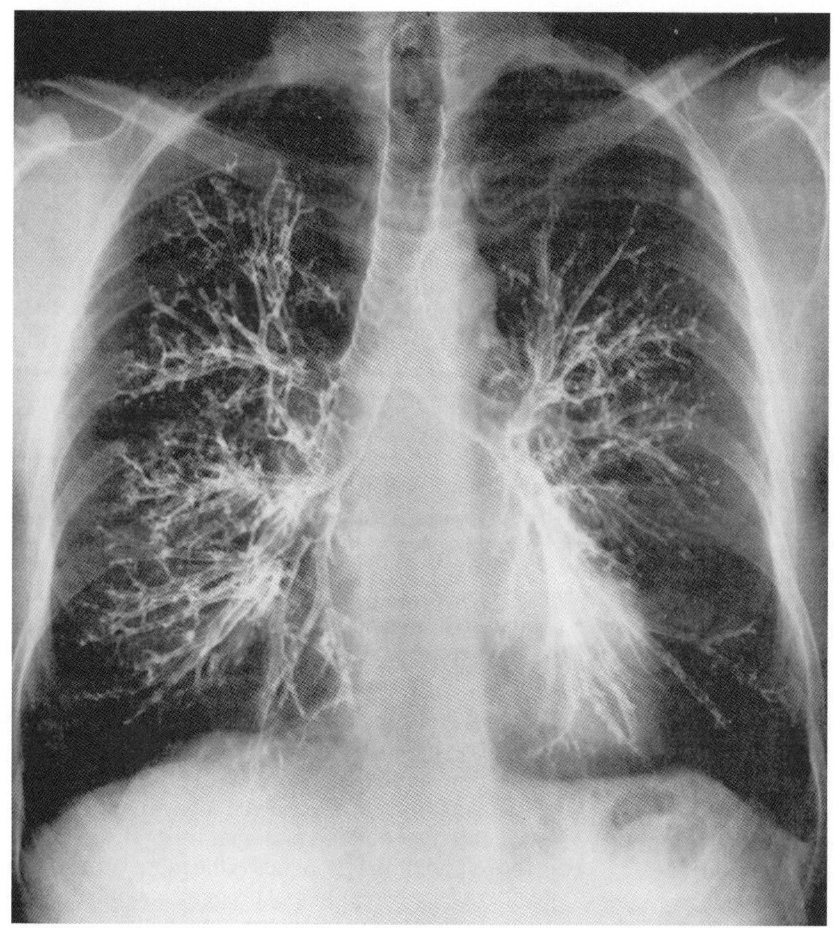

Figure 3-61 Posteroanterior bronchogram of the chest.

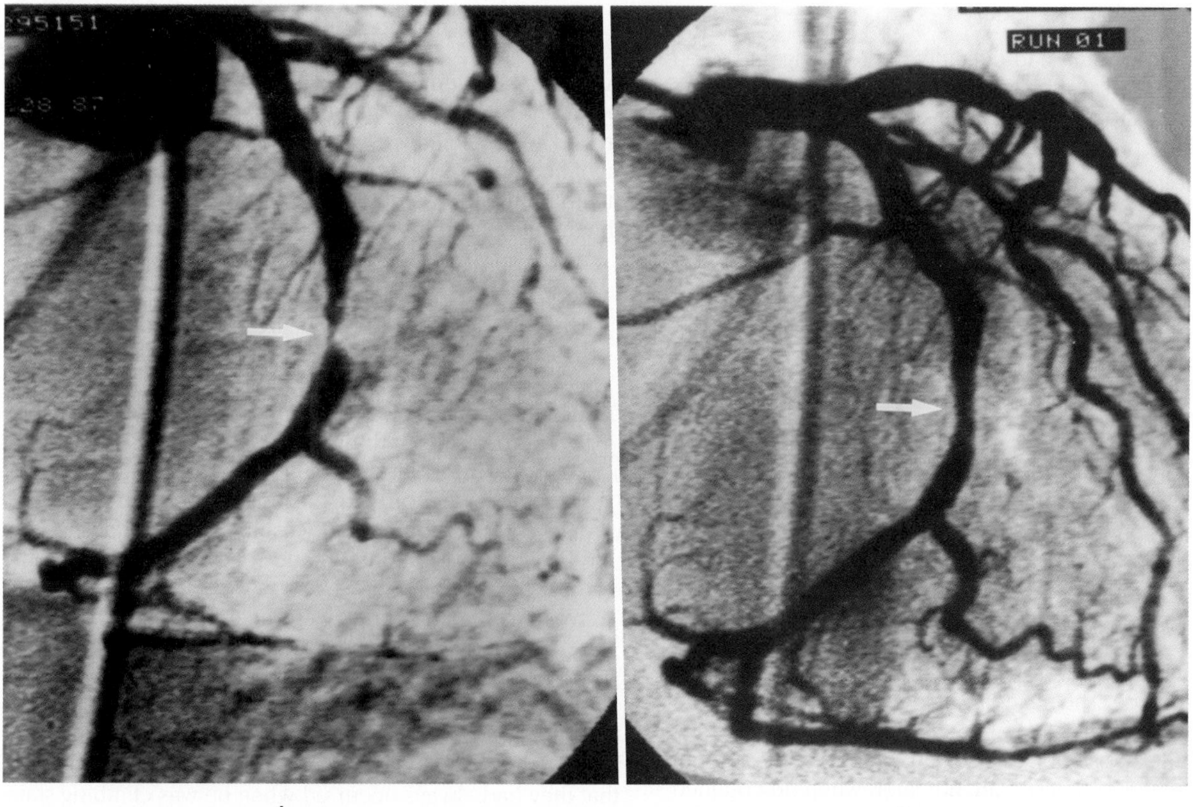

Figure 3-62 Coronary angiograms. **A.** An area of extreme narrowing of the circumflex branch of the left coronary artery (*white arrow*). **B.** The same artery after percutaneous transluminal coronary angioplasty. Inflation of the luminal balloon has dramatically improved the area of stenosis (*white arrow*).

CLINICAL PROBLEM SOLVING

Study the following case histories and select the best answer to the question following them.

A 55-year-old man states that he has noticed an alteration in his voice. He has lost 40 lb (18 kg) and has a persistent cough with blood-stained sputum. He smokes 50 cigarettes a day. On examination, the left vocal fold is immobile and lies in the adducted position. A posteroanterior chest radiograph reveals a large mass in the upper lobe of the left lung with an increase in width of the mediastinal shadow on the left side.

1. The symptoms and signs displayed by this patient can be explained by the following statements except which?
   (a) This patient has advanced carcinoma of the bronchus in the upper lobe of the left lung, which was seen as a mass on the chest radiograph.
   (b) The carcinoma has metastasized to the bronchomediastinal lymph nodes, causing their enlargement and producing a widening of the mediastinal shadow seen on the chest radiograph.
   (c) The enlarged lymph nodes had pressed on the left recurrent laryngeal nerve.
   (d) Partial injury to the recurrent laryngeal nerve resulted in paralysis of the abductor muscles of the vocal cords, leaving the adductor muscles unopposed.
   (e) The enlarged lymph nodes pressed on the left recurrent nerve as it ascended to the neck anterior to the arch of the aorta.

A 35-year-old woman had difficulty in breathing and sleeping at night. She says she falls asleep only to wake up with a choking sensation. She finds that she has to sleep propped up in bed on pillows with her neck flexed to the right.

2. The following statements concerning this case are correct except which?
   (a) Veins in the skin at the root of the neck are congested.
   (b) The U-shaped cartilaginous rings in the wall of the trachea prevent it from being kinked or compressed.
   (c) The left lobe of the thyroid gland is larger than the right lobe.
   (d) On falling asleep, the patient tends to flex her neck laterally over the enlarged left thyroid lobe.
   (e) The enlarged thyroid gland extends down the neck into the superior mediastinum.
   (f) The brachiocephalic veins in the superior mediastinum were partially obstructed by the enlarged thyroid gland.

A 15-year-old boy was rescued from a lake after falling through thin ice. The next day, he developed a severe cold, and 3 days later his general condition deteriorated. He became febrile and started to cough up blood-stained sputum. At first, he had no chest pain, but later, when he coughed, he experienced severe pain over the right fifth intercostal space in the midclavicular line.

3. The following statements would explain the patient's signs and symptoms except which?
   (a) The patient had developed lobar pneumonia and pleurisy in the right lung.
   (b) Disease of the lung does not cause pain until the parietal pleura is involved.
   (c) The pneumonia was located in the right middle lobe.
   (d) The visceral pleura is innervated by autonomic nerves that contain pain fibers.
   (e) Pain associated with the pleurisy was accentuated when movement of the visceral and parietal pleurae occurred, for example, on deep inspiration or coughing.

A 2-year-old boy was playing with his toy car when his babysitter noticed that a small metal nut was missing from the car. Two days later the child developed a cough and became febrile.

4. This child's illness could be explained by the following statements except which?
   (a) The child had inhaled the nut.
   (b) The metal nut could easily be seen on posteroanterior and right oblique radiographs.
   (c) The left principal bronchus is the more vertical and wider of the two principal bronchi, and inhaled foreign bodies tend to become lodged in it.
   (d) The nut was successfully removed through a bronchoscope.
   (e) Children who are teething tend to suck on hard toys.

A 23-year-old woman was examined in the emergency department because of the sudden onset of respiratory distress. The physician was listening to breath sounds over the right hemithorax and was concerned when no sounds were heard on the front of the chest at the level of the 10th rib in the midclavicular line.

5. The following comments concerning this patient are correct except which?
   (a) In a healthy individual, the lower border of the right lung in the midclavicular line in the midrespiratory position is at the level of the sixth rib.
   (b) The parietal pleura in the midclavicular line crosses the 10th rib.
   (c) The costodiaphragmatic recess is situated between the lower border of the lung and the parietal pleura.
   (d) The lung on extreme inspiration could descend in the costodiaphragmatic recess only as far as the eighth rib.
   (e) No breath sounds were heard because the stethoscope was located over the liver.

A 61-year-old man was seen in the emergency department complaining of a feeling of pressure within his chest. On questioning, he said that he had several attacks before and that they had always occurred when he was climbing stairs or digging in the garden. He found that the discomfort disappeared with rest after about 5 minutes. The reason he came to the emergency department was that the chest discomfort had occurred with much less exertion.

6. The following comments concerning this case are correct except which?
   (a) The diagnosis is a classic case of angina pectoris.
   (b) The sudden change in history, that is, pain caused by less exertion, should cause the physician concern that the patient now has unstable angina or an actual myocardial infarction.
   (c) The afferent pain fibers from the heart ascend to the central nervous system through the cardiac branches of the sympathetic trunk to enter the spinal cord.
   (d) The afferent pain fibers enter the spinal cord via the posterior roots of the 10th to the 12th thoracic nerves.
   (e) Pain is referred to dermatomes supplied by the upper four intercostal nerves and the intercostal brachial nerve.

A 55-year-old woman has severe aortic incompetence, with the blood returning to the cavity of the left ventricle during ventricular diastole.

7. To hear the aortic valve with the least interference from the other heart sounds, the best place to place your stethoscope on the chest wall is
   (a) the right half of the lower end of the body of the sternum.
   (b) the medial end of the second right intercostal space.
   (c) the medial end of the second left intercostal space.
   (d) the apex of the heart.
   (e) the fifth left intercostal space 3.5 in. (9 cm) from the midline.

A 33-year-old woman was jogging across the park at 11 p.m. when she was attacked by a gang of youths. After she was brutally mugged and raped, one of the youths decided to stab her in the heart to keep her silent. Later in the emergency department she was unconscious and in extremely poor shape. A small wound about 0.5 in. in diameter was present in the left fifth intercostal space about 0.5 in. from the lateral sternal margin. Her carotid pulse was rapid and weak, and her neck veins were distended. No evidence of a left-sided pneumothorax existed. A diagnosis of cardiac tamponade was made.

8. The following observations are in agreement with the diagnosis except which?
   (a) The tip of the knife had pierced the pericardium.
   (b) The knife had pierced the anterior wall of the left ventricle.
   (c) The blood in the pericardial cavity was under right ventricular pressure.
   (d) The blood in the pericardial cavity pressed on the thin-walled atria and large veins as they traversed the pericardium to enter the heart.
   (e) The backed-up venous blood caused congestion of the veins seen in the neck.
   (f) The poor venous return severely compromised the cardiac output.
   (g) A left-sided pneumothorax did not occur because the knife passed through the cardiac notch.

A 36-year-old woman with a known history of emphysema (dilatation of alveoli and destruction of alveolar walls with a tendency to form cystic spaces) suddenly experiences a severe pain in the left side of her chest, is breathless, and is obviously in a state of shock.

9. Examination of this patient reveals the following findings except which?
   (a) The trachea is displaced to the right in the suprasternal notch.
   (b) The apex beat of the heart can be felt in the fifth left intercostal space just lateral to the sternum.
   (c) The right lung is collapsed.
   (d) The air pressure in the left pleural cavity is at atmospheric pressure.
   (e) The air has entered the left pleural cavity as the result of rupture of one of the emphysematous cysts of the left lung (left-sided pneumothorax).
   (f) The elastic recoil of the lung tissue caused the lung to collapse.

A wife was told that her husband was suffering from cancer of the lower end of the esophagus. The physician told her that to save his life, the surgeon would have to remove the lower part of the esophagus, the stomach, the spleen, and the upper part of the duodenum. The wife could not understand why such a drastic operation was required to remove such a small tumor.

10. The following statements explain this extensive operation except which?
   (a) Carcinoma of the esophagus tends to spread via the lymphatic vessels.
   (b) The lymphatic vessels descend through the aortic opening in the diaphragm to enter the celiac lymph nodes.
   (c) The tumor of the esophagus and an area of normal adjacent esophagus have to be removed.
   (d) The lymphatic vessels and nodes that drain the diseased area have to be removed.
   (e) Because of the risk that retrograde spread had occurred, the other organs draining into the lymph nodes also have to be removed.

A 50-year-old man with chronic alcoholism was told by his physician that he had cirrhosis of the liver with portal hypertension.

11. The following statements explain why the patient recently vomited a cupful of blood except which?
   (a) The lower third of the esophagus is the site of a portal–systemic anastomosis.
   (b) At the lower third of the esophagus the esophageal veins of the left gastric vein anastomose with the esophageal veins of the inferior vena cava.
   (c) In cirrhosis of the liver, the portal circulation through the liver is obstructed by fibrous tissue, producing portal hypertension.
   (d) Many of the dilated veins that lie within the mucous membrane and submucosa are easily damaged by swallowed food.
   (e) Copious hemorrhage from these veins is difficult to treat and is often terminal.

A 5-year-old boy was seen in the emergency department after an attack of breathlessness during which he had lost consciousness. The mother said that her child had had several attacks before and sometimes his skin had become bluish. Recently, she had noticed that he breathed more easily when he was playing in a squatting position; he also seemed to sleep more easily with his knees drawn up. An extensive workup, including angiography, demonstrated that the patient had severe congenital heart disease.

12. The following observations in this patient are consistent with the diagnosis of tetralogy of Fallot except which?
    (a) The child was thinner and shorter than normal.
    (b) His lips, fingers, and toes were cyanotic.
    (c) A systolic murmur was present down the left border of the sternum.
    (d) The heart was considerably enlarged to the left.
    (e) Pulmonary stenosis impairs the pulmonary circulation so that a right to left shunt occurs and the arterial blood is poorly oxygenated.
    (f) A large ventricular septal defect was present.
    (g) The aortic opening into the heart was common to both ventricles.

ANSWERS TO CLINICAL PROBLEMS

1. E. The left recurrent laryngeal nerve ascends to the neck by passing under the arch of the aorta; it ascends in the groove between the trachea and the esophagus.
2. B. The trachea is a mobile, fibroelastic tube that can be kinked or compressed despite the presence of the cartilaginous rings.
3. D. Lung tissue and the visceral pleura are not innervated with pain fibers. The costal parietal pleura is innervated by the intercostal nerves, which have pain endings in the pleura.
4. C. The right principal (main) bronchus is the more vertical and wider of the two principal bronchi and for this reason an inhaled foreign body passes down the trachea and tends to enter the right main bronchus, where it was lodged in this patient.
5. B. The parietal pleura in the midclavicular line only extends down as far as the eighth rib.
6. D. The afferent pain fibers from the heart enter the spinal cord via the posterior nerve roots of the upper four thoracic spinal nerves.
7. B
8. B. The knife had pierced the anterior wall of the right ventricle.
9. C. The left lung collapsed immediately when air entered the left pleural cavity because the air pressures within the bronchial tree and in the pleural cavity were then equal.
10. B. The lymphatic vessels draining the esophagus accompany the left gastric blood vessels through the esophageal opening in the diaphragm to reach the celiac nodes.
11. B. The esophageal veins of the azygos system of veins anastomose with the esophageal veins of the left gastric vein.
12. D. Because of the pulmonary stenosis and the ventricular septal defect, right ventricular hypertrophy is causing the heart to enlarge to the right.

REVIEW QUESTIONS

Multiple-Choice Questions

Select the best answer for each question.

1. The following statements concerning the trachea are true except which?
    (a) It lies anterior to the esophagus in the superior mediastinum.
    (b) In deep inspiration, the carina may descend as far as the level of the sixth thoracic vertebra.
    (c) The left principal bronchus is wider than the right principal bronchus.
    (d) The arch of the aorta lies on its anterior and left sides in the superior mediastinum.
    (e) The sensory innervation of the mucous membrane lining the trachea is derived from branches of the vagi and the recurrent laryngeal nerves.
2. The following statements concerning the root of the right lung are true except which?
    (a) The right phrenic nerve passes anterior to the lung root.
    (b) The azygos vein arches over the superior margin of the lung root.
    (c) The right pulmonary artery lies posterior to the principal bronchus.
    (d) The right vagus nerve passes posterior to the lung root.
    (e) The vessels and nerves forming the lung root are enclosed by a cuff of pleura.
3. The following statements concerning the right lung are true except which?
    (a) It possesses a horizontal and an oblique fissure.
    (b) Its covering of visceral pleura is sensitive to pain and temperature.
    (c) The lymph from the substance of the lung reaches the hilum by the superficial and deep lymphatic plexuses.
    (d) The pulmonary ligament permits the vessels and

nerves of the lung root to move during the movements of respiration.
(e) The bronchial veins drain into the azygos and hemiazygos veins.

4. The anterior surface of the heart is formed by the following structures except which?
(a) Right ventricle
(b) Right atrium
(c) Left ventricle
(d) Left atrium
(e) Right auricle

5. In a posteroanterior radiograph of the thorax, the following structures form the left margin of the heart shadow except which?
(a) Left auricle
(b) Pulmonary trunk
(c) Arch of aorta
(d) Left ventricle
(e) Superior vena cava

6. All of the following statements concerning the esophagus are correct except which?
(a) It receives an arterial blood supply from both the descending thoracic aorta and the left gastric artery.
(b) It is constricted by the presence of the left principal bronchus.
(c) It crosses from right to left posterior to the descending aorta.
(d) It pierces the diaphragm, with the left vagus on its anterior surface and the right vagus on its posterior surface.
(e) It joins the stomach about 16 in. (41 cm) from the incisor teeth.

7. All of the following statements concerning the mediastinum are correct except which?
(a) The mediastinum forms a partition between the two pleural spaces (cavities).
(b) The mediastinal pleura demarcates the lateral boundaries of the mediastinum.
(c) The heart occupies the middle mediastinum.
(d) Should air enter the left pleural cavity, the structures forming the mediastinum are deflected to the right.
(e) The anterior boundary of the mediastinum extends to a lower level than the posterior boundary.

8. All of the following statements regarding the conducting system of the heart are true except which?
(a) The impulse for cardiac contraction spontaneously begins in the sinuatrial node.
(b) The atrioventricular bundle is the sole pathway for conduction of the waves of contraction between the atria and the ventricles.
(c) The sinuatrial node is frequently supplied by the right and left coronary arteries.
(d) The sympathetic nerves to the heart slow the rate of discharge from the sinuatrial node.
(e) The atrioventricular bundle descends behind the septal cusp of the tricuspid valve.

9. All of the following statements regarding the mechanics of inspiration are true except which?
(a) The diaphragm is the most important muscle of inspiration.
(b) The suprapleural membrane can be raised.
(c) The sternum moves anteriorly.
(d) The ribs are raised superiorly.
(e) The tone of the muscles of the anterior abdominal wall is diminished.

10. The following statements concerning the lungs are correct except which?
(a) Inhaled foreign bodies most frequently enter the right lung.
(b) The left lung is in direct contact with the arch of the aorta and the descending thoracic aorta.
(c) There are no lymph nodes within the lungs.
(d) The structure of the lungs receives its blood supply from the bronchial arteries.
(e) The costodiaphragmatic recesses are lined with parietal pleura.

11. The following statements concerning the blood supply to the heart are correct except which?
(a) The coronary arteries are branches of the ascending aorta.
(b) The right coronary artery supplies both the right atrium and the right ventricle.
(c) The circumflex branch of the left coronary artery descends in the anterior interventricular groove and passes around the apex of the heart.
(d) Arrhythmias (abnormal heart beats) can occur after occlusion of a coronary artery.
(e) Coronary arteries can be classified as functional end arteries.

12. The following statements concerning the bronchopulmonary segments are correct except which?
(a) The veins are intersegmental.
(b) The segments are separated by connective tissue septa.
(c) The arteries are intrasegmental.
(d) Each segment is supplied by a secondary bronchus.
(e) Each pyramid-shaped segment has its base pointing toward the lung surface.

Completion Questions

Match each structure listed below with the region in which it is found. Each lettered answer may be used more than once.

13. Coronary sinus (opening)
14. Moderator band
15. Anulus ovalis
16. Right pulmonary veins (openings)
(a) Left atrium
(b) Right ventricle
(c) Right atrium
(d) Left ventricle
(e) Right auricle

Multiple-Choice Questions

Read the case histories and select the best answer to the question following them.

On performing a routine examination of a 7-year-old girl, a pediatrician heard a continuous machinery-like murmur in the second left intercostal space. The murmur occupied both systole and diastole. The child was not cyanotic, the heart was of normal size, and there was no clubbing of the fingers.

Radiographic examination of the chest revealed slight enlargement of the left atrium, left ventricle, and pulmonary trunk. A diagnosis of patent ductus arteriosus was made.

17. Based on the clinical history and the diagnosis, the following statements concerning the case are correct except which?
    (a) The patent ductus represents the distal portion of the sixth left aortic arch artery.
    (b) The ductus connects the right pulmonary artery to the descending thoracic aorta.
    (c) The ductus in fetal life is the normal bypass of blood to the aorta from the pulmonary trunk.
    (d) At birth, the ductus arteriosus normally constricts in response to a rise in arterial oxygen.
    (e) The ductus arteriosus closes to become the ligamentum arteriosum.
18. The presence of a patent ductus presents the following physiologic and pathologic consequences except which?
    (a) Aortic blood passes into the pulmonary artery, producing the machinery-like murmur.
    (b) The shunting of blood occurs only during systole as the result of the higher blood pressure in the aorta and the lower blood pressure in the pulmonary artery.
    (c) The left ventricle shows hypertrophy because of the leak from the aorta.
    (d) The pulmonary trunk becomes enlarged and the right ventricle hypertrophied owing to the raised pressure in the pulmonary circulation.
    (e) Because of the risk of bacterial infection of the wall of the pulmonary artery (bacterial endarteritis) caused by the pulmonary hypertension, the patent ductus should be ligated and divided surgically.

A 12-year-old boy was examined by a pediatrician and found to have absent femoral pulses in both femoral arteries. The blood pressure in both upper limbs was higher than in both lower limbs. The diagnosis was coarctation of the aorta.

19. The following statements about this case are correct except which?
    (a) The aorta is narrowed just proximal to the site of origin of the left common carotid artery.
    (b) There is no femoral pulse because the small aortic pulse wave does not reach the femoral arteries.
    (c) The high blood pressure in the arteries of the upper limbs and the cerebral circulation is an attempt by the heart to force blood through the narrowed aorta.
    (d) To compensate for the diminished blood flow into the lower limbs, the internal thoracic, subclavian, and posterior intercostal arteries become dilated.
    (e) The raised blood pressure proximal to the aortic narrowing may later result in cerebral hemorrhage and heart failure.

ANSWERS TO REVIEW QUESTIONS

1. C. The right principal bronchus is wider than the left. This is clearly seen in the normal posteroanterior bronchogram shown in Figure 3-54.
2. C. The right pulmonary artery lies anterior to the principal bronchus.
3. B. The visceral pleura is innervated by sympathetic and vagal afferent fibers via the pulmonary plexus and is not sensitive to pain and temperature, but it is sensitive to the sensation of stretch.
4. D. The left atrium lies behind the heart.
5. E
6. C. The esophagus crosses from right to left anterior to the descending aorta.
7. E. The anterior boundary of the mediastinum extends down to the xiphisternal joint anteriorly—that is, to the level of the ninth thoracic vertebral body. The posterior boundary extends down farther, to the level of the 12th thoracic vertebra.
8. D. The sympathetic nerves to the heart increase the rate of discharge from the sinuatrial node.
9. B. The suprapleural membrane is composed of fibrous tissue and is attached to the transverse process of the seventh cervical vertebra; it cannot be raised during inspiration.
10. C
11. C. The circumflex branch of the left coronary artery winds around the left margin of the heart in the atrioventricular groove.
12. D. Each segment of the lung is supplied by a segmental bronchus.
13. C
14. B
15. C
16. A
17. B. The ductus arteriosus represents the distal portion of the sixth left aortic arch artery and connects the left pulmonary artery at its origin from the pulmonary trunk to the junction of the aortic arch and the descending thoracic aorta.
18. B. The machinery-like murmur occurs during both systole and diastole and is caused by the shunting of blood from the aorta to the pulmonary artery owing to the higher blood pressure in the aorta during both phases of the cardiac cycle.
19. A

CHAPTER 4

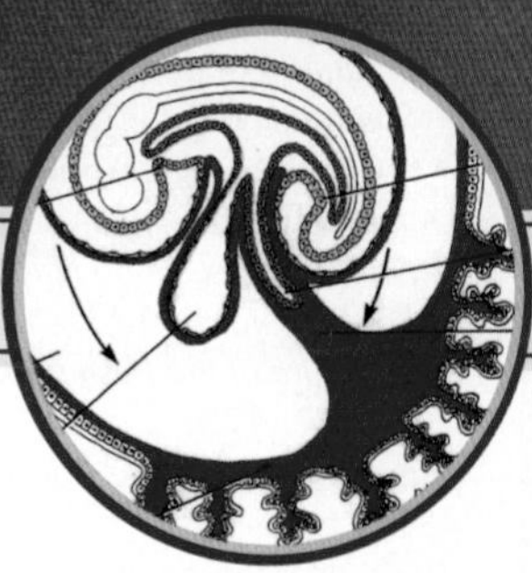

THE ABDOMEN: PART I—THE ABDOMINAL WALL

A 26-year-old man complaining of a painful swelling in the right groin was seen by his physician; he had vomited four times in the previous 3 hours. On examination, he was dehydrated and his abdomen was moderately distended. A large, tense swelling, which was very tender on palpation, was seen in the left groin and extended down into the scrotum. An attempt to gently push the contents of the swelling back into the abdomen was impossible. A diagnosis of a right complete, irreducible, indirect inguinal hernia was made. The vomiting and abdominal distention were secondary to the intestinal obstruction caused by the herniation of some bowel loops into the hernial sac.

An indirect inguinal hernia is caused by a congenital persistence of a sac formed from the lining of the abdomen. This sac has a narrow neck, and its cavity remains in free communication with the abdominal cavity. Hernias of the abdominal wall are common. It is necessary to know the anatomy of the abdomen in the region of the groin before one can make a diagnosis or understand the different hernial types that can exist. Moreover, without this knowledge it is impossible to appreciate the complications that can occur or to plan treatment. A hernia may start as a simple swelling, but it can end as a life-threatening problem.

CHAPTER OUTLINE

Basic Anatomy 146
Structure of the Anterior Abdominal Wall 146
Inguinal Canal 163
Spermatic Cord 164
Coverings of the Spermatic Cord 165
Scrotum, Testis, and Epididymides 167
Labia Majora 173
Structure of the Posterior Abdominal Wall 173
Fascial Lining of the Abdominal Walls 177
Peritoneal Lining of the Abdominal Walls 177
Radiographic Anatomy 191
Surface Anatomy 191
Surface Landmarks of the Abdominal Wall 191
Xiphoid Process 191
Costal Margin 191
Iliac Crest 191
Pubic Tubercle 191
Symphysis Pubis 191
Inguinal Ligament 191
Superficial Inguinal Ring 191
Scrotum 191
Linea Alba 191
Umbilicus 191
Rectus Abdominis 191
Tendinous Intersections of the Rectus Abdominis 191
Linea Semilunaris 192
Abdominal Lines and Planes 192
Vertical Lines 192
Transpyloric Plane 192
Subcostal Plane 192
Intercristal Plane 192
Intertubercular Plane 192
Abdominal Quadrants 192
Surface Landmarks of the Abdominal Viscera 192
Liver 192
Gallbladder 192
Spleen 192
Pancreas 192
Kidneys 192
Stomach 193
Duodenum (First Part) 193
Cecum 193
Appendix 195
Ascending Colon 195
Transverse Colon 195
Descending Colon 195
Urinary Bladder and Pregnant Uterus 195
Aorta 195
External Iliac Artery 195
Clinical Problem Solving 195
Answers to Clinical Problems 197
Review Questions 197
Answers to Review Questions 199

CHAPTER OBJECTIVES

- Acute abdominal pain, abdominal swellings, and blunt and penetrating trauma to the abdominal wall are common problems facing the physician. The problems are complicated by the fact that the abdomen contains multiple organ systems, and knowing the spatial relationships of these organs to one another and to the anterior abdominal wall is essential before an accurate and complete diagnosis can be made.
- The abdominal wall is a flexible structure through which the physician can often feel diseased organs that lie within the abdominal cavity. An intact abdominal wall is essential for the support of the abdominal contents. A defect or malfunction of the wall can allow the abdominal contents to bulge forward and form a hernia. The abdominal wall provides the surgeon with a site for access to deep-lying diseased structures.
- For the above reasons, the anatomy of the anterior abdominal wall must be learned in detail. Because of its great clinical importance, examiners ask many questions in this area.

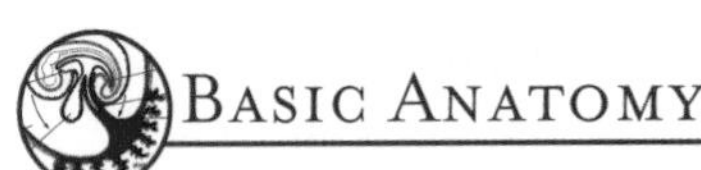

BASIC ANATOMY

The abdomen is the region of the trunk that lies between the diaphragm above and the inlet of the pelvis below.

Structure of the Anterior Abdominal Wall

The anterior abdominal wall is made up of skin, superficial fascia, deep fascia, muscles, extraperitoneal fascia, and parietal peritoneum.

Skin

The skin is loosely attached to the underlying structures except at the umbilicus, where it is tethered to the scar tissue. The natural **lines of cleavage** in the skin are constant and run downward and forward almost horizontally around the trunk. The **umbilicus** is a scar representing the site of attachment of the umbilical cord in the fetus; it is situated in the linea alba (see below).

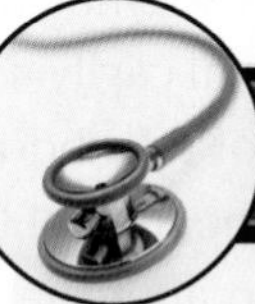

CLINICAL NOTES

Surgical Incisions

If possible, all surgical incisions should be made in the lines of cleavage where the bundles of collagen fibers in the dermis run in parallel rows. An incision along a cleavage line will heal as a narrow scar, whereas one that crosses the lines will heal as wide or heaped-up scars.

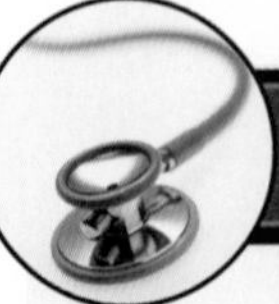

CLINICAL NOTES

Infection of the Umbilicus

In the adult, the umbilicus often receives scant attention in the shower and is consequently a common site of infection.

Nerve Supply

The cutaneous nerve supply to the anterior abdominal wall is derived from the anterior rami of the lower six thoracic and the first lumbar nerves (see Fig. 4-16). The thoracic nerves are the lower five intercostal and the subcostal nerves; the first lumbar nerve is represented by the iliohypogastric and the ilioinguinal nerves.

The dermatome of T7 is located in the epigastrium over the xiphoid process. The dermatome of T10 includes the umbilicus, and that of L1 lies just above the inguinal ligament and the symphysis pubis. The dermatomes and distribution of cutaneous nerves are shown in Figure 4-16.

Blood Supply

Arteries

The skin near the midline is supplied by branches of the superior and the inferior epigastric arteries. The skin of the flanks is supplied by branches of the intercostal, the lumbar, and the deep circumflex iliac arteries (see Fig. 4-15). In addition, the skin in the inguinal region is supplied by the superficial epigastric, the superficial circumflex iliac, and the superficial external pudendal arteries, branches of the femoral artery.

Veins

The venous drainage passes above mainly into the axillary vein via the lateral thoracic vein and below into the femoral vein via the superficial epigastric and the great saphenous veins (see Fig. 4-18).

Superficial Fascia

The superficial fascia is divided into a superficial **fatty layer** (fascia of Camper) and a deep **membranous layer (Scarpa's fascia)** (Fig. 4-1). The fatty layer is continuous with the superficial fat over the rest of the body and may be extremely thick (3 in. [8 cm] or more in obese patients). The membranous layer is thin and fades out laterally and above,

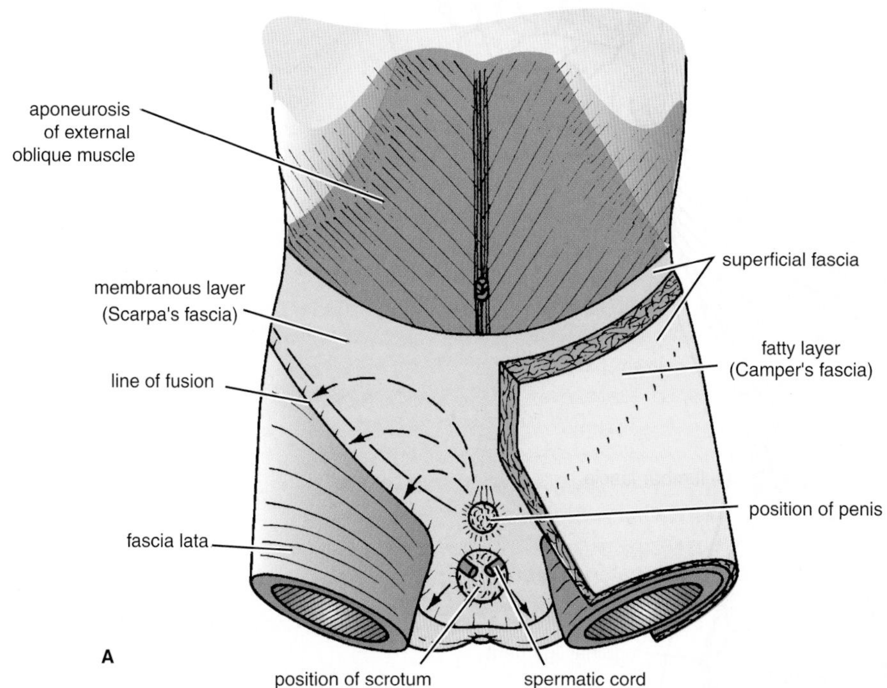

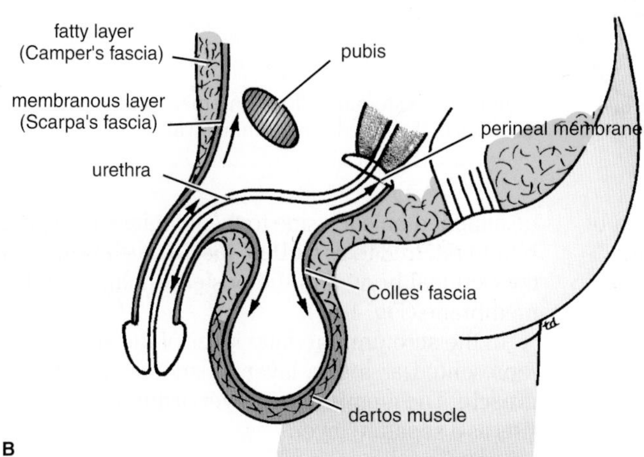

Figure 4-1 **A.** Arrangement of the fatty layer and the membranous layer of the superficial fascia in the lower part of the anterior abdominal wall. Note the line of fusion between the membranous layer and the deep fascia of the thigh (fascia lata). **B.** Note the attachment of the membranous layer to the posterior margin of the perineal membrane. Arrows indicate paths taken by urine in cases of ruptured urethra.

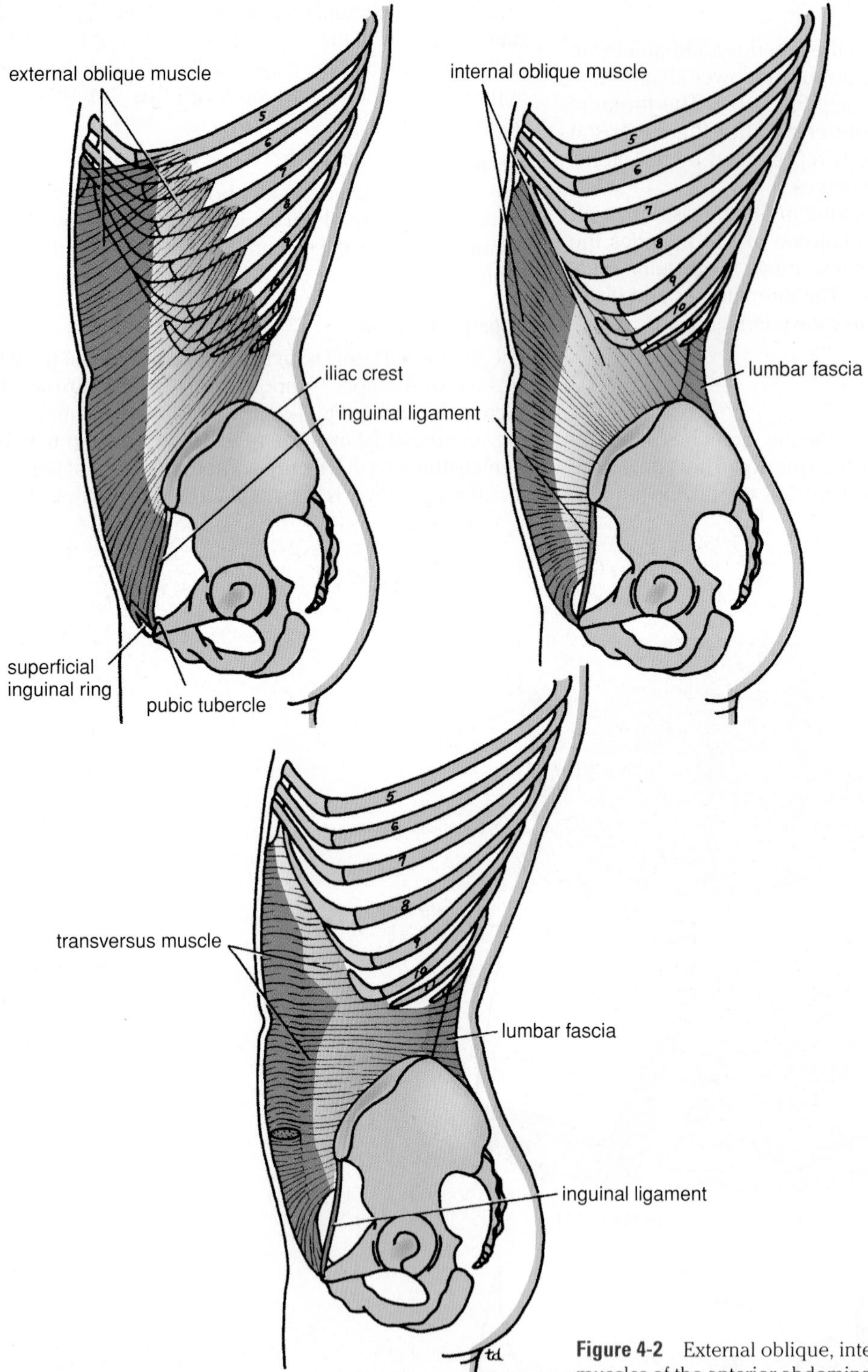

Figure 4-2 External oblique, internal oblique, and transversus muscles of the anterior abdominal wall.

where it becomes continuous with the superficial fascia of the back and the thorax, respectively. Inferiorly, the membranous layer passes onto the front of the thigh, where it fuses with the deep fascia one fingerbreadth below the inguinal ligament. In the midline inferiorly, the membranous layer of fascia is not attached to the pubis but forms a tubular sheath for the penis (or clitoris). Below in the perineum, it enters the wall of the scrotum (or labia majora). From there it passes to be attached on each side to the margins of the pubic arch; it is here referred to as **Colles' fascia.** Posteriorly, it fuses with the perineal body and the posterior margin of the perineal membrane (Fig. 4-1B).

In the scrotum, the fatty layer of the superficial fascia is represented as a thin layer of smooth muscle, the **dartos muscle**. The membranous layer of the superficial fascia persists as a separate layer.

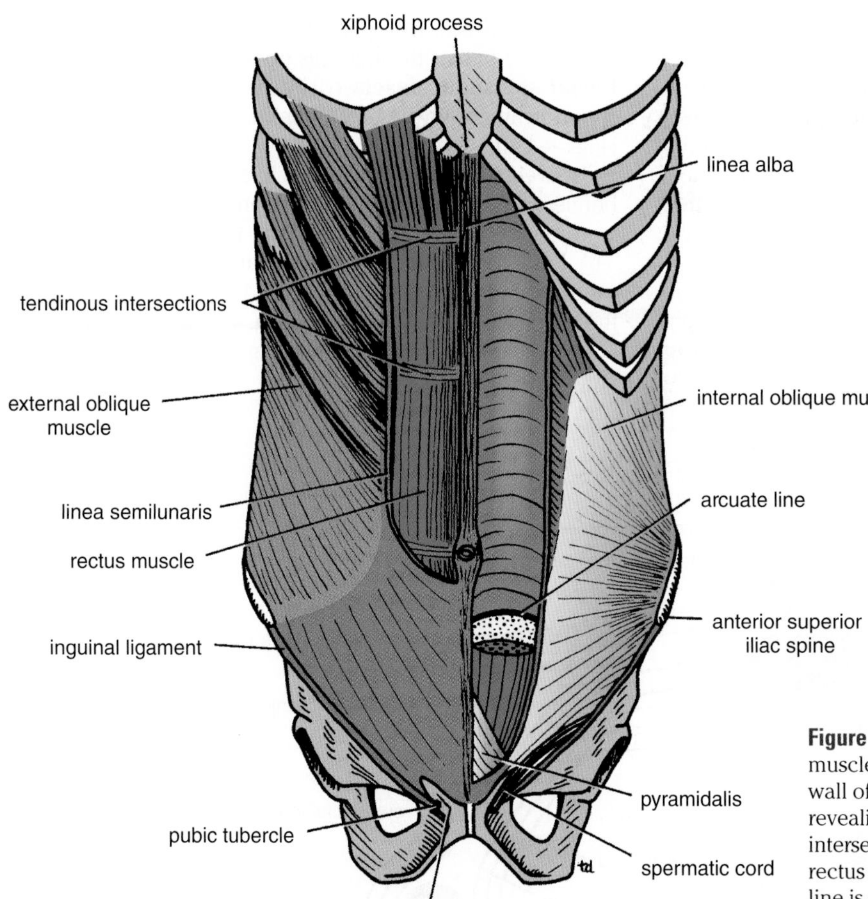

Figure 4-3 Anterior view of the rectus abdominis muscle and the rectus sheath. **Left:** The anterior wall of the sheath has been partly removed, revealing the rectus muscle with its tendinous intersections. **Right:** The posterior wall of the rectus sheath is shown. The edge of the arcuate line is shown at the level of the anterior superior iliac spine.

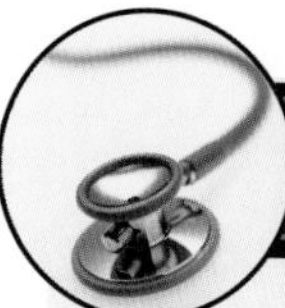

CLINICAL NOTES

Membranous Layer of Superficial Fascia and the Extravasation of Urine

The membranous layer of the superficial fascia is important clinically because beneath it is a potential closed space that does not open into the thigh but is continuous with the superficial perineal pouch via the penis and scrotum. Rupture of the penile urethra may be followed by extravasation of urine into the scrotum, perineum, and penis and then up into the lower part of the anterior abdominal wall deep to the membranous layer of fascia. The urine is excluded from the thigh because of the attachment of the fascia to the fascia lata (Fig. 4-1).

When closing abdominal wounds it is usual for a surgeon to put in a continuous suture uniting the divided membranous layer of superficial fascia. This strengthens the healing wound, prevents stretching of the skin scar, and makes for a more cosmetically acceptable result.

Deep Fascia

The deep fascia in the anterior abdominal wall is merely a thin layer of connective tissue covering the muscles; it lies immediately deep to the membranous layer of superficial fascia.

Muscles of the Anterior Abdominal Wall

The muscles of the anterior abdominal wall consist of three broad thin sheets that are aponeurotic in front; from exterior to interior they are the external oblique, internal oblique, and transversus (Fig. 4-2). On either side of the midline anteriorly is, in addition, a wide vertical muscle, the rectus abdominis (Fig. 4-3). As the aponeuroses of the three sheets pass forward, they enclose the rectus abdominis to form the rectus sheath. The lower part of the rectus sheath might contain a small muscle called the pyramidalis.

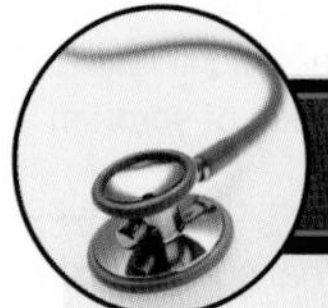

CLINICAL NOTES

General Appearances of the Abdominal Wall

The normal abdominal wall is soft and pliable and undergoes inward and outward excursion with respiration. The contour is subject to considerable variation and depends on the tone of its muscles and the amount of fat in the subcutaneous tissue. Well-developed muscles or an abundance of fat can prove to be a severe obstacle to the palpation of the abdominal viscera.

External Oblique

The external oblique muscle is a broad, thin, muscular sheet that arises from the outer surfaces of the lower eight ribs and fans out to be inserted into the xiphoid process, the linea alba, the pubic crest, the pubic tubercle, and the anterior half of the iliac crest (Fig. 4-2). Most of the fibers are inserted by means of a broad aponeurosis. Note that the most posterior fibers passing down to the iliac crest form a posterior free border.

A triangular-shaped defect in the external oblique aponeurosis lies immediately above and medial to the pubic tubercle. This is known as the **superficial inguinal ring** (Figs. 4-2 and 4-3). The spermatic cord (or round ligament of the uterus) passes through this opening and carries the **external spermatic fascia** (or the external covering of the round ligament of the uterus) from the margins of the ring (Figs. 4-4 and 4-5).

Between the anterior superior iliac spine and the pubic tubercle, the lower border of the aponeurosis is folded backward on itself, forming the **inguinal ligament** (Figs. 4-2 and 4-6). From the medial end of the ligament, the **lacunar ligament** extends backward and upward to the pectineal line on the superior ramus of the pubis (Fig. 4-6). Its sharp, free crescentic edge forms the medial margin of the **femoral ring**

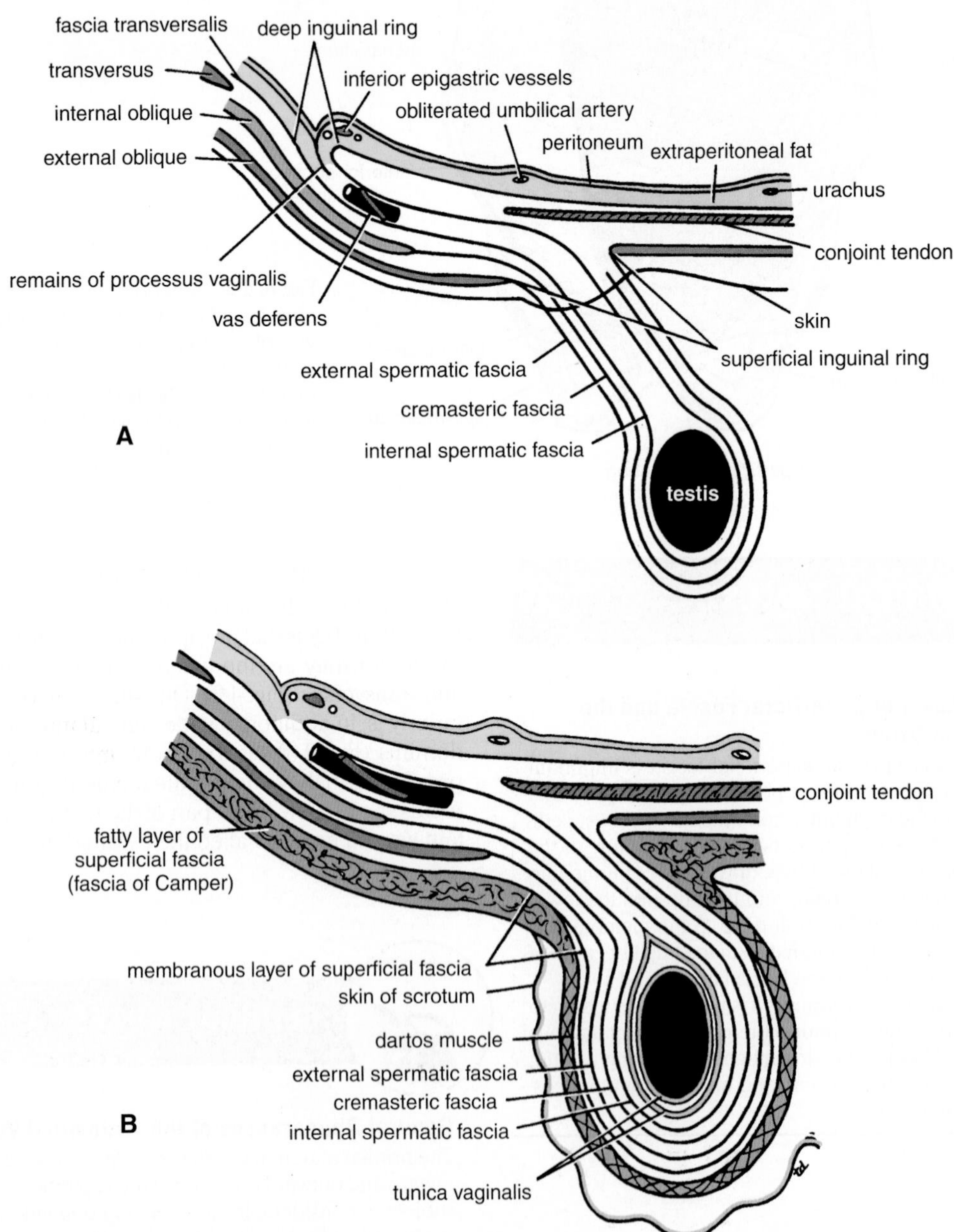

Figure 4-4 **A.** Continuity of the different layers of the anterior abdominal wall with coverings of the spermatic cord. **B.** The skin and superficial fascia of the abdominal wall and scrotum have been included, and the tunica vaginalis is shown.

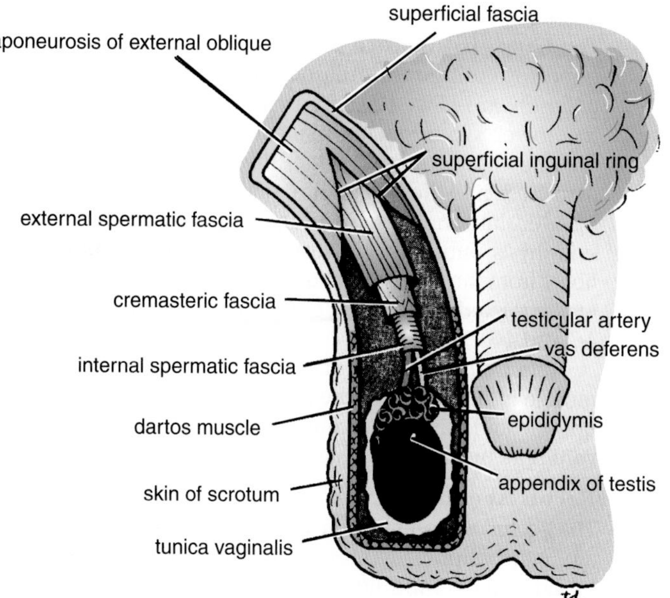

Figure 4-5 Scrotum dissected from in front. Note the spermatic cord and its coverings.

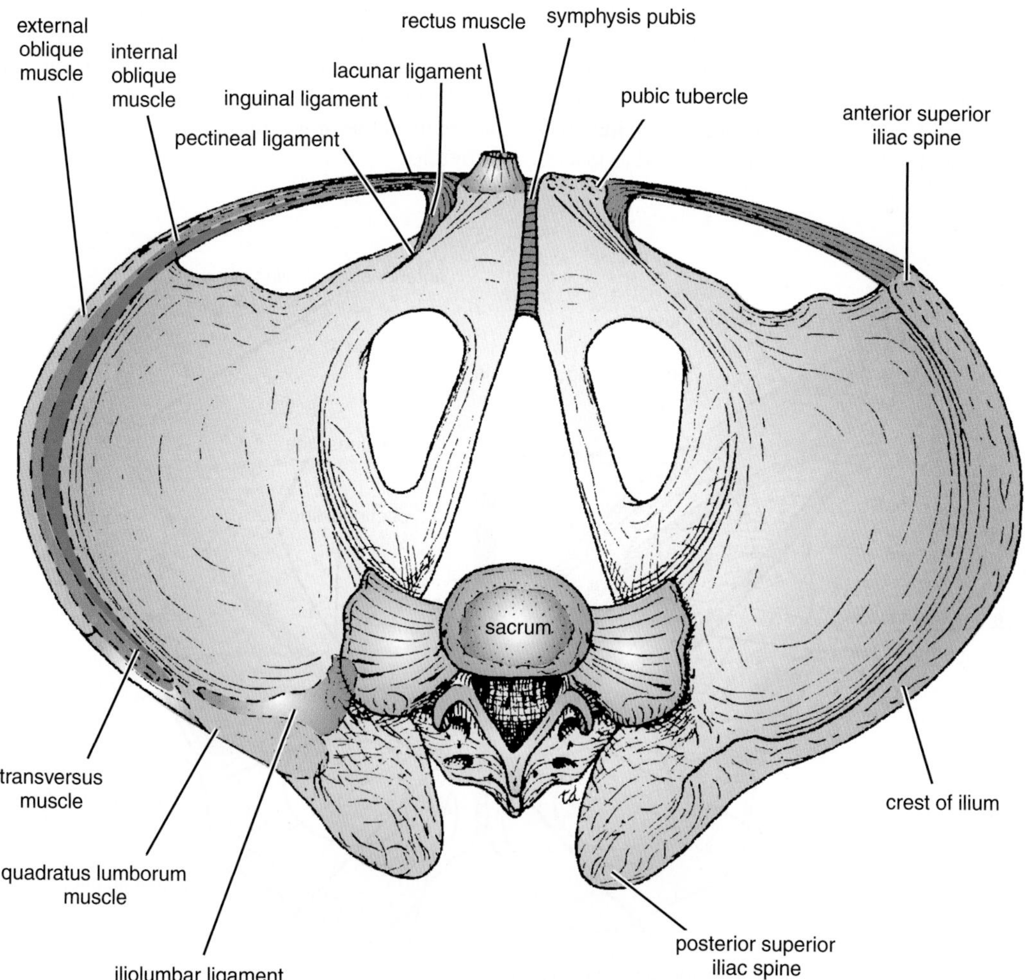

Figure 4-6 Bony pelvis viewed from above. Note the attachments of the inguinal, lacunar, and pectineal ligaments.

(see page 579). On reaching the pectineal line, the lacunar ligament becomes continuous with a thickening of the periosteum called the **pectineal ligament** (Fig. 4-6).

The lateral part of the posterior edge of the inguinal ligament gives origin to part of the internal oblique and transversus abdominis muscles. To the inferior rounded border of the inguinal ligament is attached the deep fascia of the thigh, the **fascia lata** (Fig. 4-1).

Internal Oblique

The internal oblique muscle is also a broad, thin, muscular sheet that lies deep to the external oblique; most of its fibers run at right angles to those of the external oblique (Fig. 4-2). It arises from the lumbar fascia, the anterior two thirds of the iliac crest, and the lateral two thirds of the inguinal ligament. The muscle fibers radiate as they pass upward and forward. The muscle is inserted into the lower borders of the lower three ribs and their costal cartilages, the xiphoid process, the linea alba, and the symphysis pubis. The internal oblique has a lower free border that arches over the spermatic cord (or round ligament of the uterus) and then descends behind it to be attached to the pubic crest and the pectineal line. Near their insertion, the lowest tendinous fibers are joined by similar fibers from the transversus abdominis to form the conjoint tendon (Figs. 4-7 and 4-8). The **conjoint tendon** is attached medially to the linea alba, but it has a lateral free border.

As the spermatic cord (or round ligament of the uterus) passes under the lower border of the internal oblique, it carries with it some of the muscle fibers that are called the **cremaster muscle** (Figs. 4-7 and 4-8). The **cremasteric fascia** is the term used to describe the cremaster muscle and its fascia.

Transversus

The transversus muscle is a thin sheet of muscle that lies deep to the internal oblique, and its fibers run horizontally forward (Fig. 4-2). It arises from the deep surface of the lower six costal cartilages (interdigitating with the diaphragm), the lumbar fascia, the anterior two thirds of the iliac crest, and the lateral third of the inguinal ligament. It is inserted into the xiphoid process, the linea alba, and the symphysis pubis. The lowest tendinous fibers join similar fibers from the internal oblique to form the conjoint tendon, which is fixed to the pubic crest and the pectineal line (Figs. 4-7 and 4-8).

Note that the posterior border of the external oblique muscle is free, whereas the posterior borders of the internal oblique and transversus muscles are attached to the lumbar vertebrae by the lumbar fascia (Figs. 4-2 and 4-9).

Rectus Abdominis

The rectus abdominis is a long strap muscle that extends along the whole length of the anterior abdominal wall. It is broader above and lies close to the midline, being separated from its fellow by the linea alba.

The rectus abdominis muscle arises by two heads, from the front of the symphysis pubis and from the pubic crest (Figs. 4-6 and 4-10). It is inserted into the fifth, sixth, and seventh costal cartilages and the xiphoid process (Fig. 4-3). When it contracts, its lateral margin forms a curved ridge that can be palpated and often seen and is termed the **linea semilunaris** (Figs. 4-3, 4-11, and 4-12). This extends from the tip of the ninth costal cartilage to the pubic tubercle.

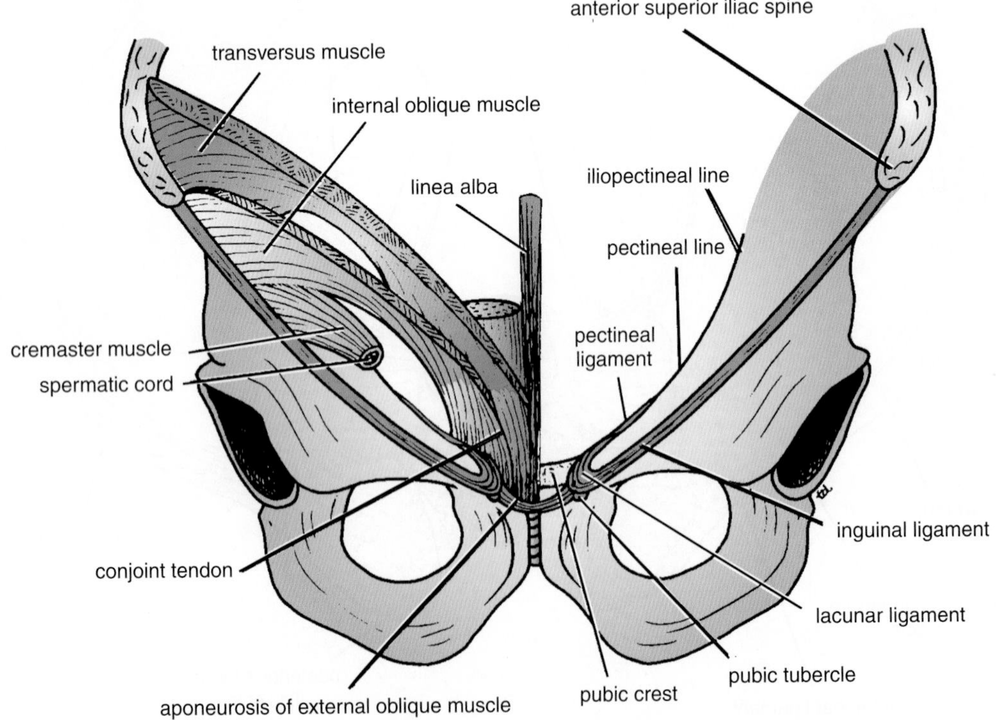

Figure 4-7 Anterior view of the pelvis showing the attachment of the conjoint tendon to the pubic crest and the adjoining part of the pectineal line.

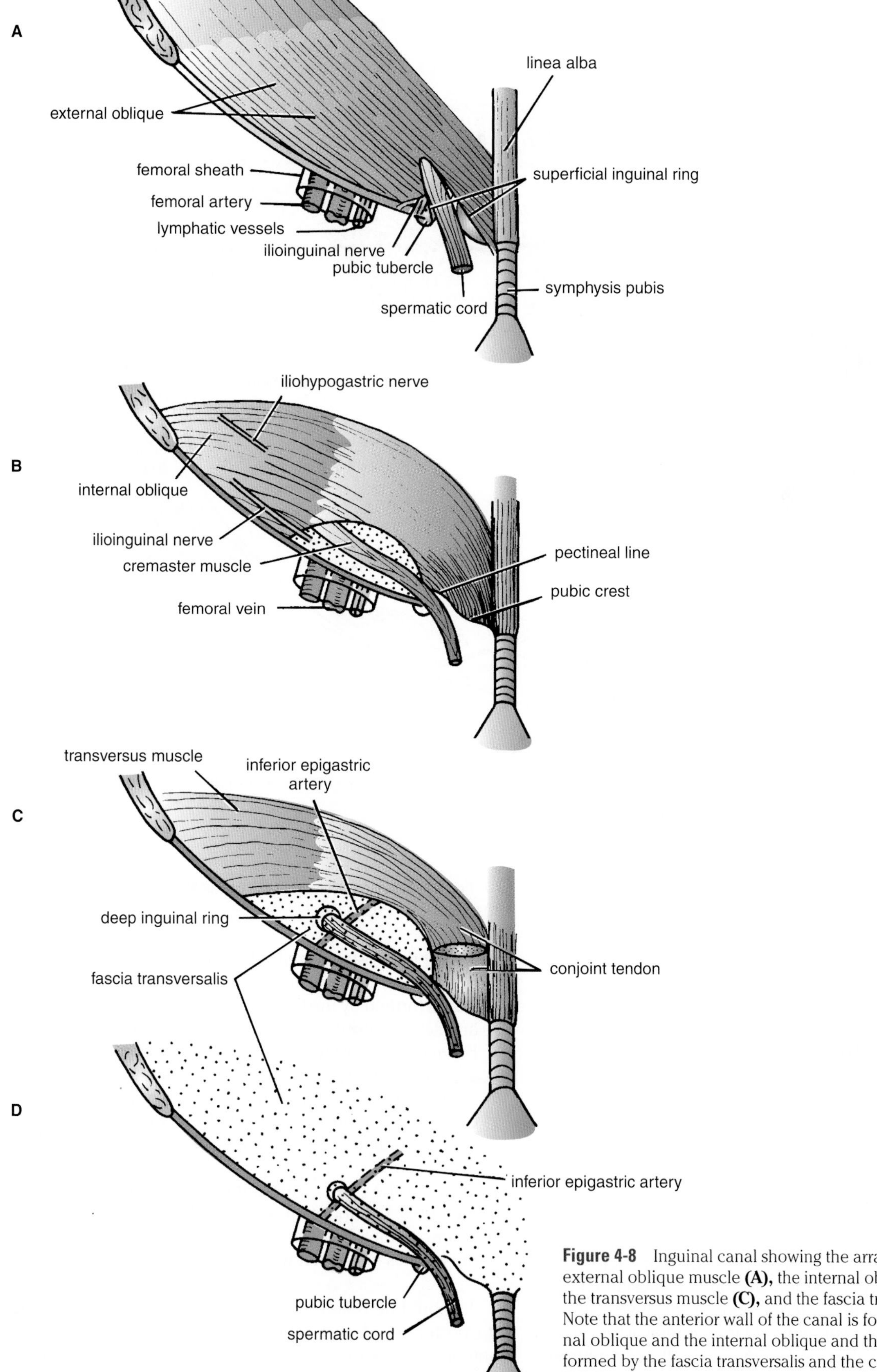

Figure 4-8 Inguinal canal showing the arrangement of the external oblique muscle **(A)**, the internal oblique muscle **(B)**, the transversus muscle **(C)**, and the fascia transversalis **(D)**. Note that the anterior wall of the canal is formed by the external oblique and the internal oblique and the posterior wall is formed by the fascia transversalis and the conjoint tendon. The deep inguinal ring lies lateral to the inferior epigastric artery.

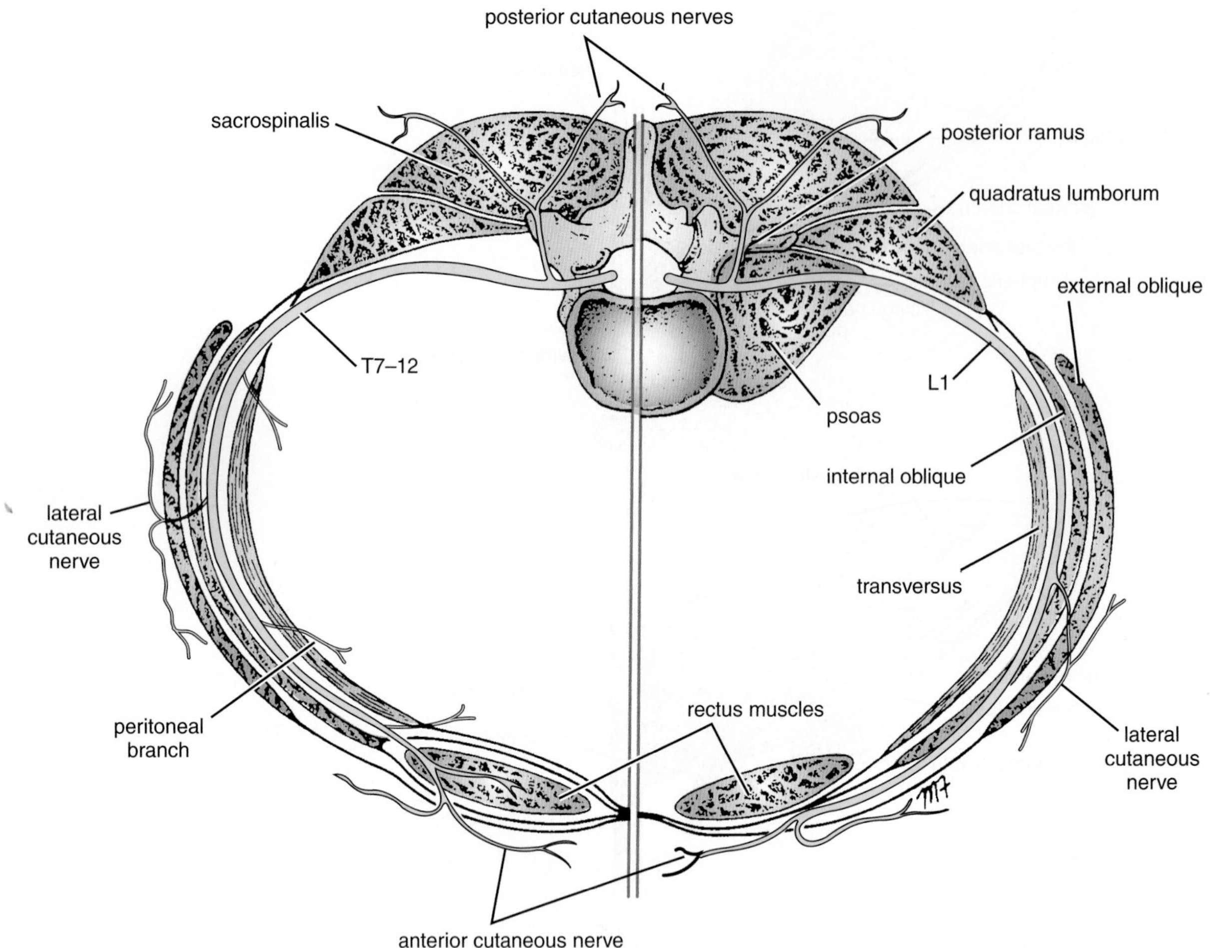

Figure 4-9 Cross section of the abdomen showing the courses of the lower thoracic and first lumbar nerves.

The rectus abdominis muscle is divided into distinct segments by three transverse **tendinous intersections:** one at the level of the xiphoid process, one at the level of the umbilicus, and one halfway between these two (Fig. 4-3). These intersections are strongly attached to the anterior wall of the **rectus sheath** (see below).

The rectus abdominis is enclosed between the aponeuroses of the external oblique, internal oblique, and transversus, which form the rectus sheath.

Pyramidalis

The pyramidalis muscle is often absent. It arises by its base from the anterior surface of the pubis and is inserted into the linea alba (Fig. 4-3). It lies in front of the lower part of the rectus abdominis.

Rectus Sheath

The rectus sheath is a long fibrous sheath that encloses the rectus abdominis muscle and pyramidalis muscle (if present) and contains the anterior rami of the lower six thoracic nerves and the superior and inferior epigastric vessels and lymph vessels. It is formed mainly by the aponeuroses of the three lateral abdominal muscles (Figs. 4-2, 4-3, and 4-10).

For ease of description the rectus sheath is considered at three levels (Fig. 4-13).

- Above the costal margin, the anterior wall is formed by the aponeurosis of the external oblique. The posterior wall is formed by the thoracic wall—that is, the fifth, sixth, and seventh costal cartilages and the intercostal spaces.
- Between the costal margin and the level of the anterior superior iliac spine, the aponeurosis of the internal oblique splits to enclose the rectus muscle; the external oblique aponeurosis is directed in front of the muscle, and the transversus aponeurosis is directed behind the muscle.
- Between the level of the anterosuperior iliac spine and the pubis, the aponeuroses of all three muscles form the anterior wall. The posterior wall is absent, and the rectus muscle lies in contact with the fascia transversalis.

It should be noted that where the aponeuroses forming the posterior wall pass in front of the rectus at the level of the anterior superior iliac spine, the posterior wall has a free, curved lower border called the **arcuate line** (Figs. 4-3 and 4-10). At this site, the inferior epigastric vessels enter the

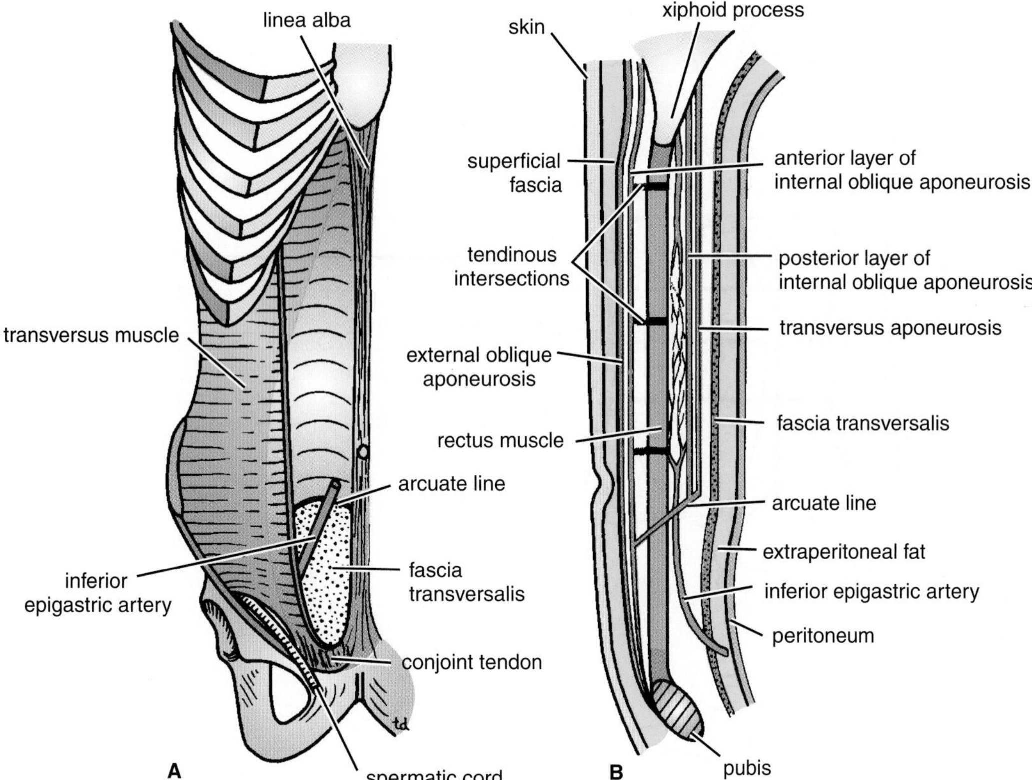

Figure 4-10 Rectus sheath in anterior view **(A)** and in sagittal section **(B).** Note the arrangement of the aponeuroses forming the rectus sheath.

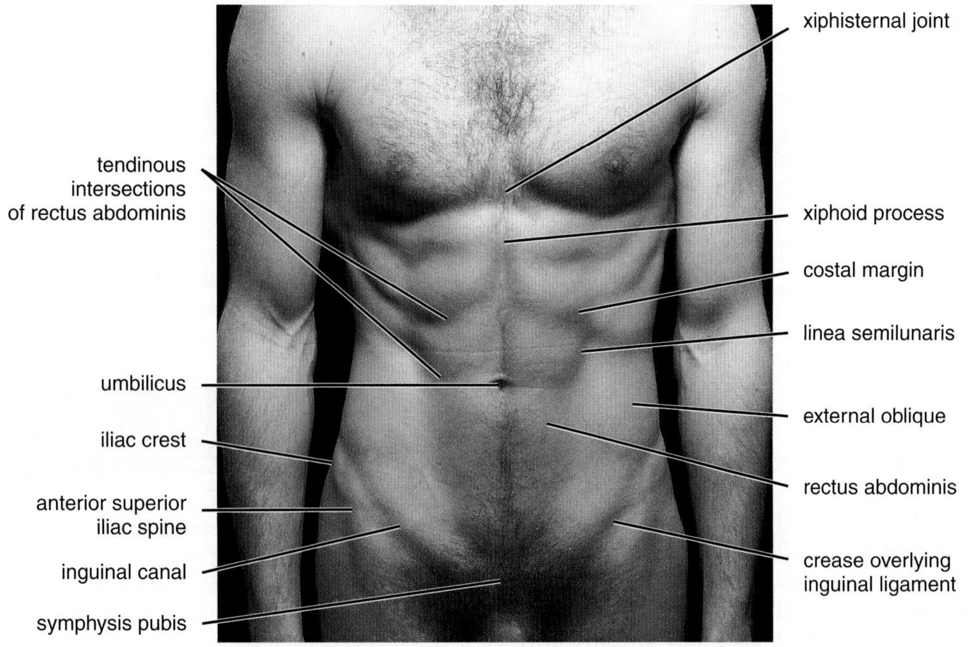

Figure 4-11 Anterior abdominal wall of a 27-year-old man.

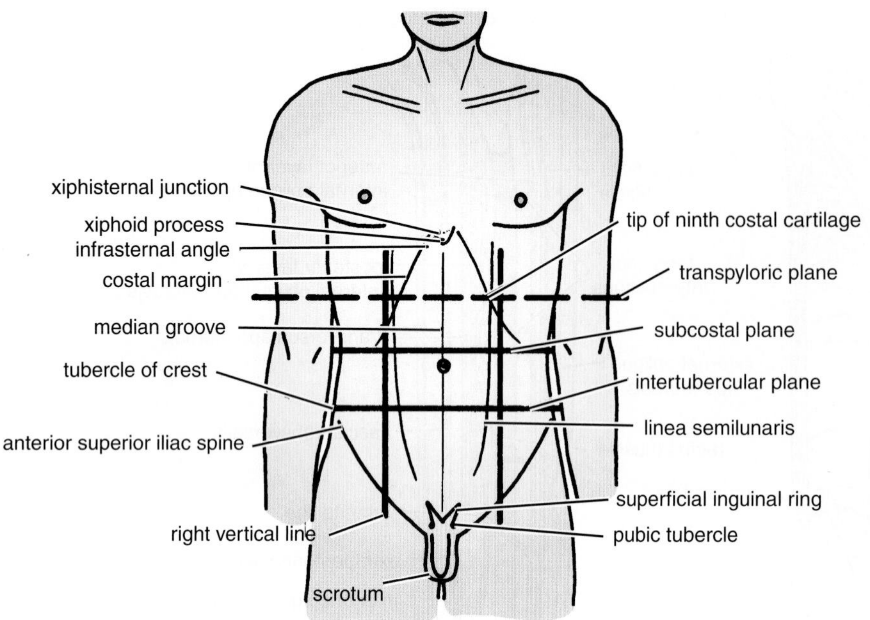

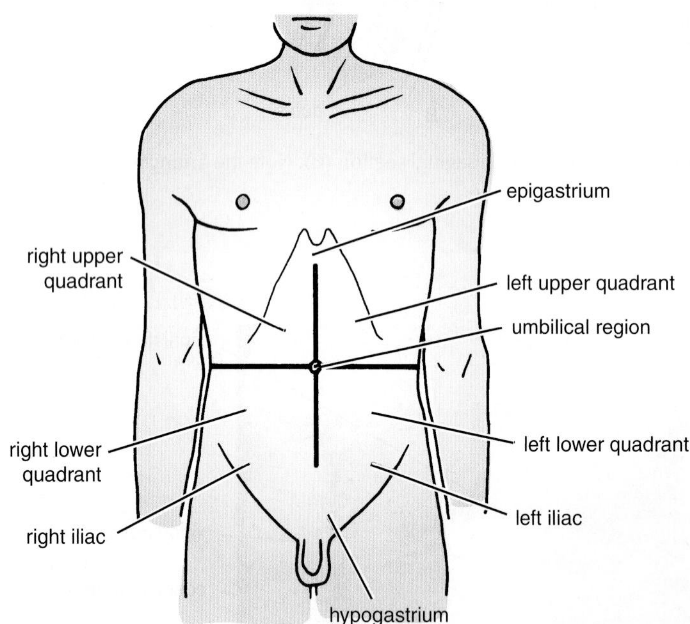

Figure 4-12 Surface landmarks and regions of the anterior abdominal wall.

rectus sheath and pass upward to anastomose with the superior epigastric vessels.

The rectus sheath is separated from its fellow on the opposite side by a fibrous band called the **linea alba** (Figs. 4-3, 4-7, and 4-13). This extends from the xiphoid process down to the symphysis pubis and is formed by the fusion of the aponeuroses of the lateral muscles of the two sides. Wider above the umbilicus, it narrows down below the umbilicus to be attached to the symphysis pubis.

The posterior wall of the rectus sheath is not attached to the rectus abdominis muscle. The anterior wall is firmly attached to it by the muscle's tendinous intersections (Figs. 4-3 and 4-10).

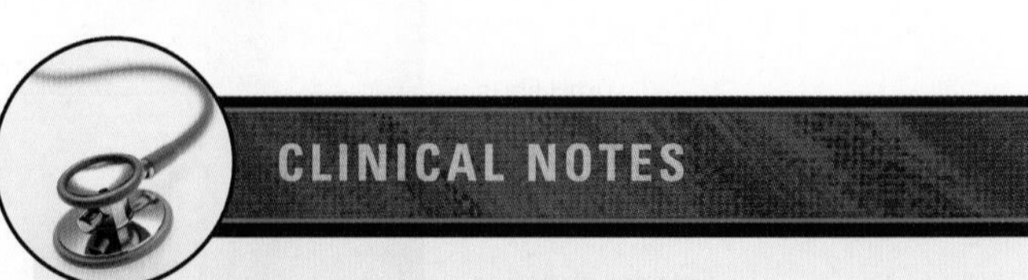

Hematoma of the Rectus Sheath

Hematoma of the rectus sheath is uncommon but important, since it is often overlooked. It occurs most often on the right side below the level of the umbilicus. The source of the bleeding is the inferior epigastric vein or, more rarely, the inferior epigastric artery. These vessels may be stretched during a severe bout of coughing or in the later months of pregnancy, which may predispose to the condition. The cause is usually blunt trauma to the abdominal wall, such as a fall or a kick. The symptoms that follow the trauma include midline abdominal pain. An acutely tender mass confined to one rectus sheath is diagnostic.

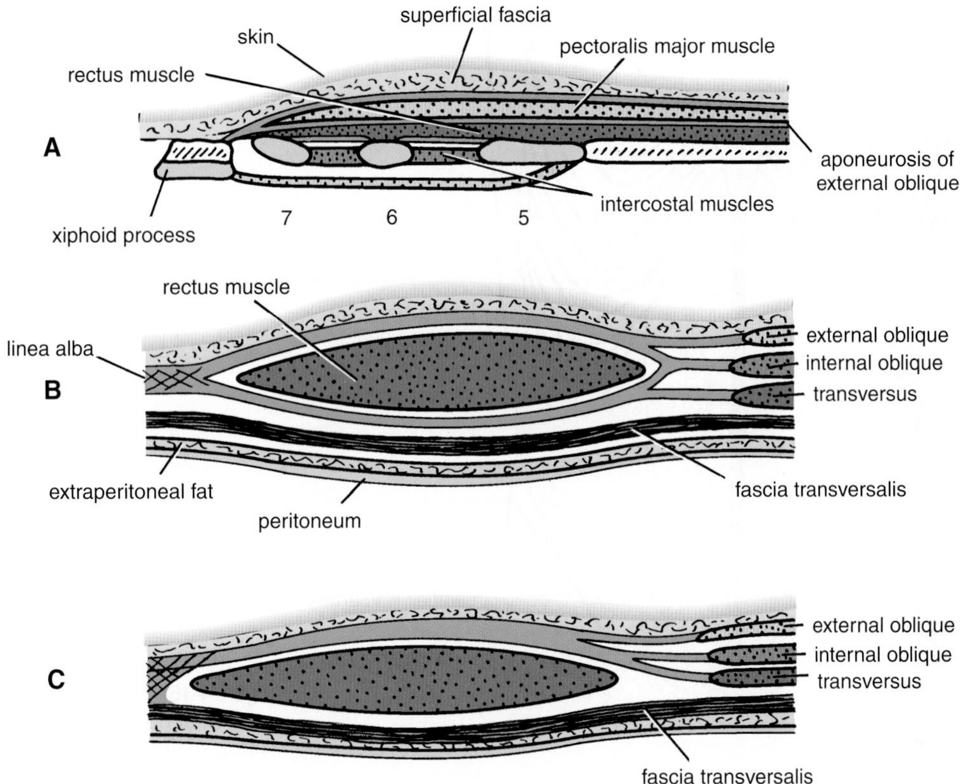

Figure 4-13 Transverse sections of the rectus sheath seen at three levels. **A.** Above the costal margin. **B.** Between the costal margin and the level of the anterior superior iliac spine. **C.** Below the level of the anterior superior iliac spine and above the pubis.

Function of the Anterior Abdominal Wall Muscles

The oblique muscles laterally flex and rotate the trunk (Fig. 4-14). The rectus abdominis flexes the trunk and stabilizes the pelvis, and the pyramidalis keeps the linea alba taut during the process.

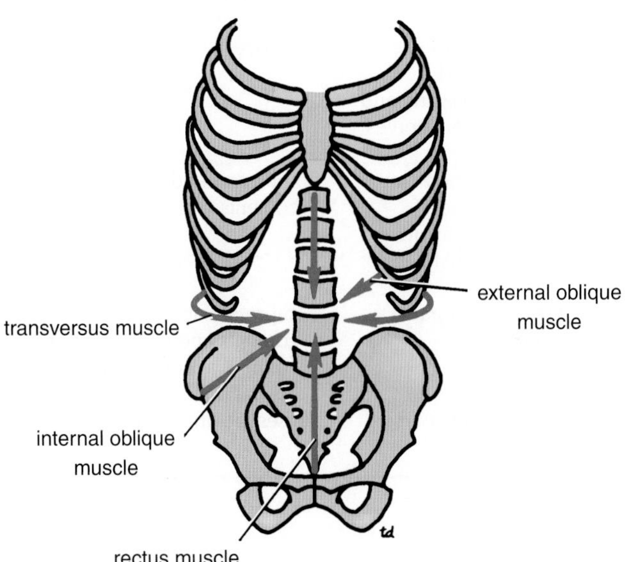

Figure 4-14 Action of the muscles of the anterior and lateral abdominal walls. Arrows indicate line of pull of different muscles.

The muscles of the anterior and lateral abdominal walls assist the diaphragm during inspiration by relaxing as the diaphragm descends so that the abdominal viscera can be accommodated.

The muscles assist in the act of forced expiration that occurs during coughing and sneezing by pulling down the ribs and sternum. Their tone plays an important part in supporting and protecting the abdominal viscera. By contracting simultaneously with the diaphragm, with the glottis of the larynx closed, they increase the intra-abdominal pressure and help in micturition, defecation, vomiting, and parturition.

Nerve Supply of Anterior Abdominal Wall Muscles

The oblique and transversus abdominis muscles are supplied by the lower six thoracic nerves and the iliohypogastric and ilioinguinal nerves (L1). The rectus muscle is supplied by the lower six thoracic nerves (Figs. 4-9 and 4-15). The pyramidalis is supplied by the 12th thoracic nerve.

A summary of the muscles of the anterior abdominal wall, their nerve supply, and their action is given in Table 4-1.

Fascia Transversalis

The fascia transversalis is a thin layer of fascia that lines the transversus abdominis muscle and is continuous with a similar layer lining the diaphragm and the iliacus muscle (Fig. 4-10).

The femoral sheath for the femoral vessels in the lower limbs is formed from the fascia transversalis and the fascia iliaca that covers the iliacus muscle (see page 579).

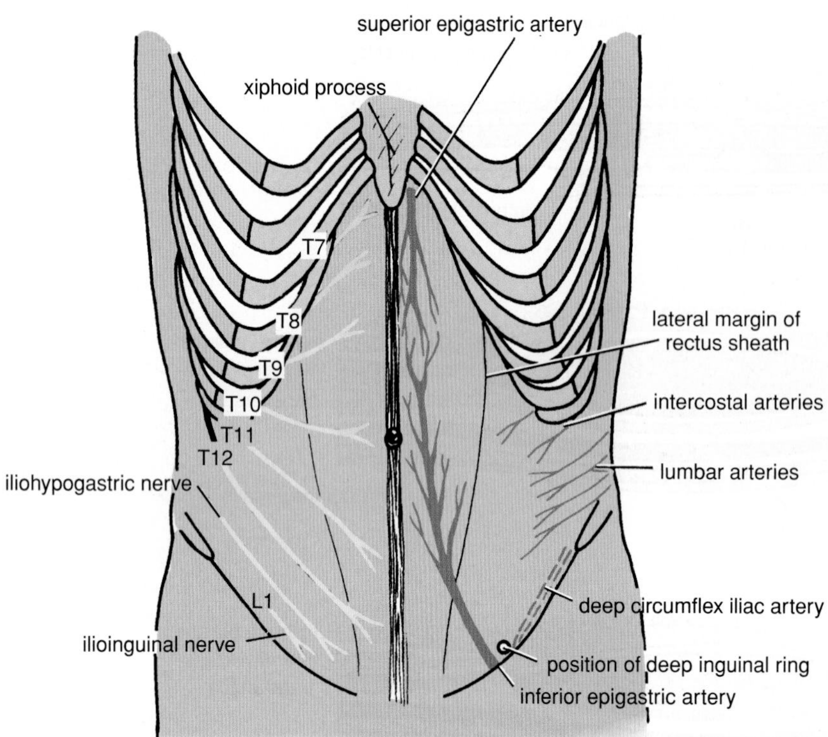

Figure 4-15 Segmental innervation of the anterior abdominal wall **(left)** and arterial supply to the anterior abdominal wall **(right).**

Table 4-1 Muscles of the Anterior Abdominal Wall

Name of Muscle	Origin	Insertion	Nerve Supply	Action
External oblique	Lower eight ribs	Xiphoid process, linea alba, pubic crest, pubic tubercle, iliac crest	Lower six thoracic nerves and iliohypogastric and ilioinguinal nerves (L1)	Supports abdominal contents; compresses abdominal contents; assists in flexing and rotation of trunk; assists in forced expiration, micturition, defecation, parturition, and vomiting
Internal oblique	Lumbar fascia, iliac crest, lateral two thirds of inguinal ligament	Lower three ribs and costal cartilages, xiphoid process, linea alba, symphysis pubis	Lower six thoracic nerves and iliohypogastric and ilioinguinal nerves (L1)	As above
Transversus	Lower six costal cartilages, lumbar fascia, iliac crest, lateral third of inguinal ligament	Xiphoid process linea alba, symphysis pubis	Lower six thoracic nerves and iliohypogastric and ilioinguinal nerves (L1)	Compresses abdominal contents
Rectus abdominis	Symphysis pubis and pubic crest	Fifth, sixth, and seventh costal cartilages and xiphoid process	Lower six thoracic nerves	Compresses abdominal contents and flexes vertebral column; accessory muscle of expiration
Pyramidalis (if present)	Anterior surface of pubis	Linea alba	12th thoracic nerve	Tenses the linea alba

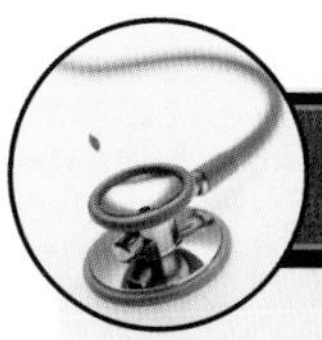

CLINICAL NOTES

Abdominal Muscles, Abdominothoracic Rhythm, and Visceroptosis

The abdominal muscles contract and relax with respiration, and the abdominal wall conforms to the volume of the abdominal viscera. There is an **abdominothoracic rhythm**. Normally, during inspiration, when the sternum moves forward and the chest expands, the anterior abdominal wall also moves forward. If, when the chest expands, the anterior abdominal wall remains stationary or contracts inward, it is highly probable that the parietal peritoneum is inflamed and has caused a reflex contraction of the abdominal muscles.

The shape of the anterior abdominal wall depends on the tone of its muscles. A middle-aged woman with poor abdominal muscles who has had multiple pregnancies is often incapable of supporting her abdominal viscera. The lower part of the anterior abdominal wall protrudes forward, a condition known as visceroptosis. This should not be confused with an abdominal tumor such as an ovarian cyst or with the excessive accumulation of fat in the fatty layer of the superficial fascia.

Extraperitoneal Fat

The extraperitoneal fat is a thin layer of connective tissue that contains a variable amount of fat and lies between the fascia transversalis and the parietal peritoneum (Fig. 4-10).

Parietal Peritoneum

The walls of the abdomen are lined with parietal peritoneum (Fig. 4-10). This is a thin serous membrane and is continuous below with the parietal peritoneum lining the pelvis (see pages 359 and 376).

Nerves of the Anterior Abdominal Wall

The nerves of the anterior abdominal wall are the anterior rami of the lower six thoracic and the first lumbar nerves (Figs. 4-9, 4-15, and 4-16). They pass forward in the interval between the internal oblique and the transversus muscles. The thoracic nerves are the lower five intercostal nerves and the subcostal nerves, and the first lumbar nerve is represented by the iliohypogastric and ilioinguinal nerves, branches of the lumbar plexus. They supply the skin of the anterior abdominal wall, the muscles, and the parietal peritoneum. (Compare with the intercostal nerves, which run forward in the intercostal spaces between the internal intercostal and the innermost intercostal muscles; see page 55). The lower six thoracic nerves pierce the posterior wall of the rectus sheath to supply the rectus muscle and the pyramidalis (T12 only). They terminate by piercing the anterior wall of the sheath and supplying the skin.

The first lumbar nerve has a similar course, but it does not enter the rectus sheath (Figs. 4-9, 4-15, and 4-16). It is represented by the iliohypogastric nerve, which pierces the external oblique aponeurosis above the superficial inguinal ring, and by the ilioinguinal nerve, which emerges through the ring. They end by supplying the skin just above the inguinal ligament and symphysis pubis.

The dermatome of T7 is located in the epigastrium over the xiphoid process, that of T10 includes the umbilicus, and that of L1 lies just above the inguinal ligament and the symphysis pubis. For the dermatomes of the anterior abdominal wall, see Figure 4-16.

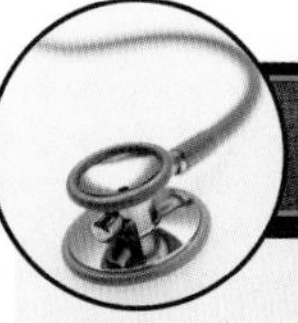

CLINICAL NOTES

Abdominal Pain

See also page 280.

Muscle Rigidity and Referred Pain

Sometimes it is difficult for a physician to decide whether the muscles of the anterior abdominal wall of a patient are rigid because of underlying inflammation of the parietal peritoneum or whether the patient is voluntarily contracting the muscles because he or she resents being examined or because the physician's hand is cold. This problem is usually easily solved by asking the patient, who is lying supine on the examination table, to rest the arms by the sides and draw up the knees to flex the hip joints. It is practically impossible for a patient to keep the abdominal musculature tensed when the thighs are flexed. Needless to say, the examiner's hand should be warm.

A pleurisy involving the lower costal parietal pleura causes pain in the overlying skin that may radiate down into the abdomen. Although it is unlikely to cause rigidity of the abdominal muscles, it may cause confusion in making a diagnosis unless these anatomic facts are remembered.

It is useful to remember the following:
Dermatomes over:

- The xiphoid process: T7
- The umbilicus: T10
- The pubis: L1

Anterior Abdominal Nerve Block

Area of Anesthesia

The area of anesthesia is the skin of the anterior abdominal wall. The nerves of the anterior and lateral abdominal walls are the anterior rami of the 7th through the 12th thoracic nerves and the first lumbar nerve (ilioinguinal and iliohypogastric nerves).

Indications

An anterior abdominal nerve block is performed to repair lacerations of the anterior abdominal wall.

(continues)

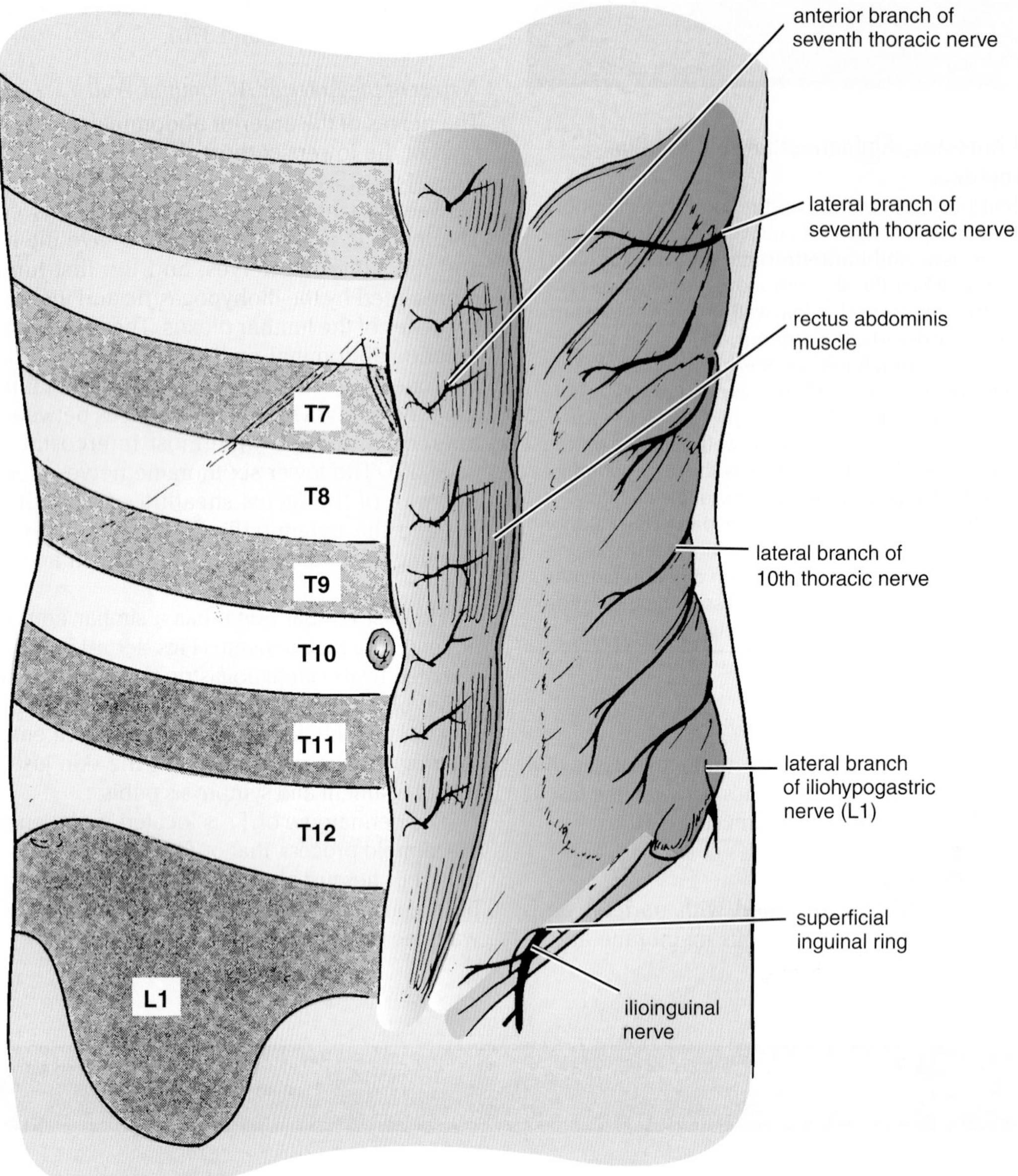

Figure 4-16 Dermatomes and distribution of cutaneous nerves on the anterior abdominal wall.

Clinical Notes, *continued*

Procedure

The anterior ends of intercostal nerves T7 through T11 enter the abdominal wall by passing posterior to the costal cartilages (Fig. 4-17). An abdominal field block is most easily carried out along the lower border of the costal margin and then infiltrating the nerves as they emerge between the xiphoid process and the 10th or 11th rib along the costal margin.

The ilioinguinal nerve passes forward in the inguinal canal and emerges through the superficial inguinal ring. The iliohypogastric nerve passes forward around the abdominal wall and pierces the external oblique aponeurosis above the superficial inguinal ring. The two nerves are easily blocked by inserting the anesthetic needle 1 in. (2.5 cm) above the anterior superior iliac spine on the spinoumbilical line (Fig. 4-17).

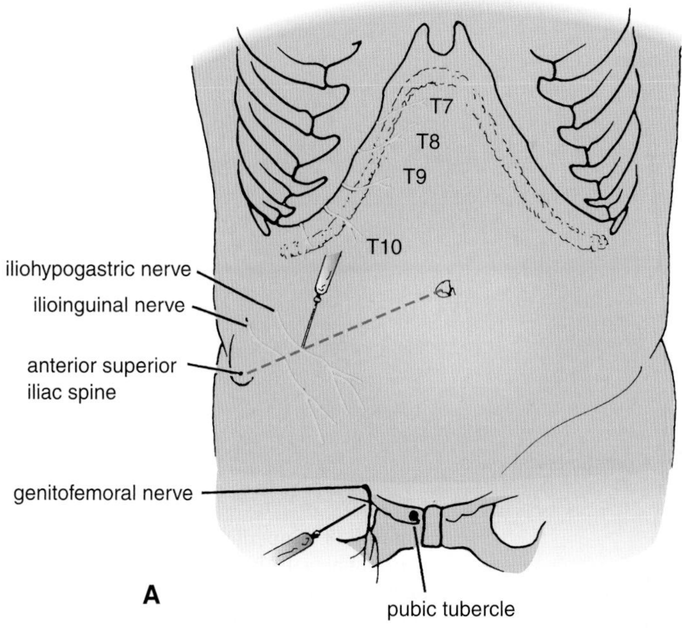

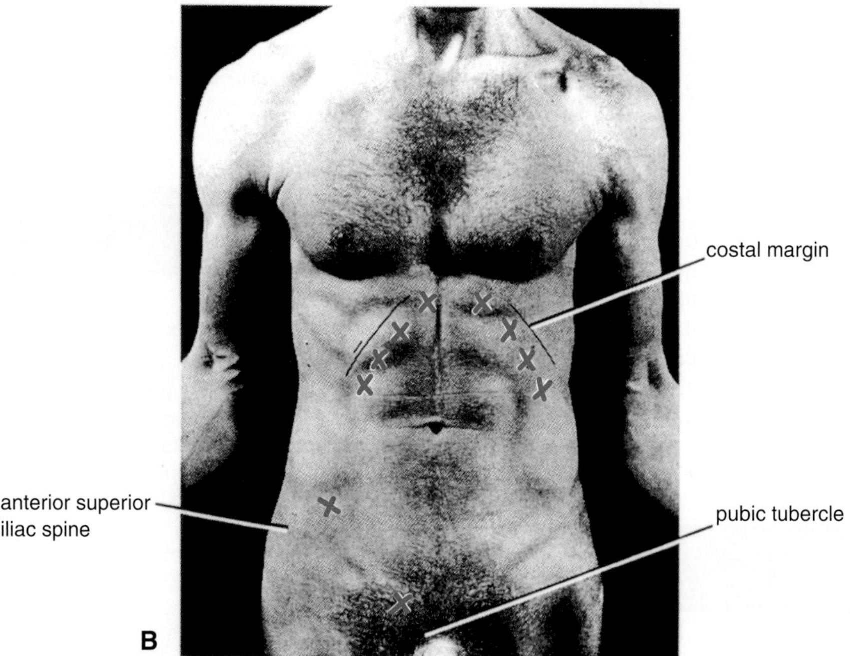

Figure 4-17 Anterior abdominal wall nerve blocks. T7 though T11 are blocked (*X*) as they emerge from beneath the costal margin. The iliohypogastric ilioinguinal nerves are blocked by inserting the needle about 1 in. (2.5 cm) above the anterior superior iliac spine on the spinoumbilical line (*X*). The terminal branches of the genitofemoral nerve are blocked by inserting the needle through the skin just lateral to the pubic tubercle and infiltrating the subcutaneous tissue with anesthetic solution (*X*).

Arteries of the Anterior Abdominal Wall

The **superior epigastric artery,** one of the terminal branches of the internal thoracic artery, enters the upper part of the rectus sheath between the sternal and costal origins of the diaphragm (Fig. 4-15). It descends behind the rectus muscle, supplying the upper central part of the anterior abdominal wall, and anastomoses with the inferior epigastric artery.

The inferior epigastric artery is a branch of the external iliac artery just above the inguinal ligament. It runs upward and medially along the medial side of the deep inguinal ring (Figs. 4-4, 4-8, and 4-15). It pierces the fascia transversalis to enter the rectus sheath anterior to the arcuate line (Fig. 4-10). It ascends behind the rectus muscle, supplying the lower central part of the anterior abdominal wall, and anastomoses with the superior epigastric artery.

The deep circumflex iliac artery is a branch of the external iliac artery just above the inguinal ligament (Fig. 4-15). It runs upward and laterally toward the anterosuperior iliac spine and then continues along the iliac crest. It supplies the lower lateral part of the abdominal wall.

The lower two posterior intercostal arteries, branches of the descending thoracic aorta, and the four lumbar arteries, branches of the abdominal aorta, pass forward between the muscle layers and supply the lateral part of the abdominal wall (Fig. 4-15).

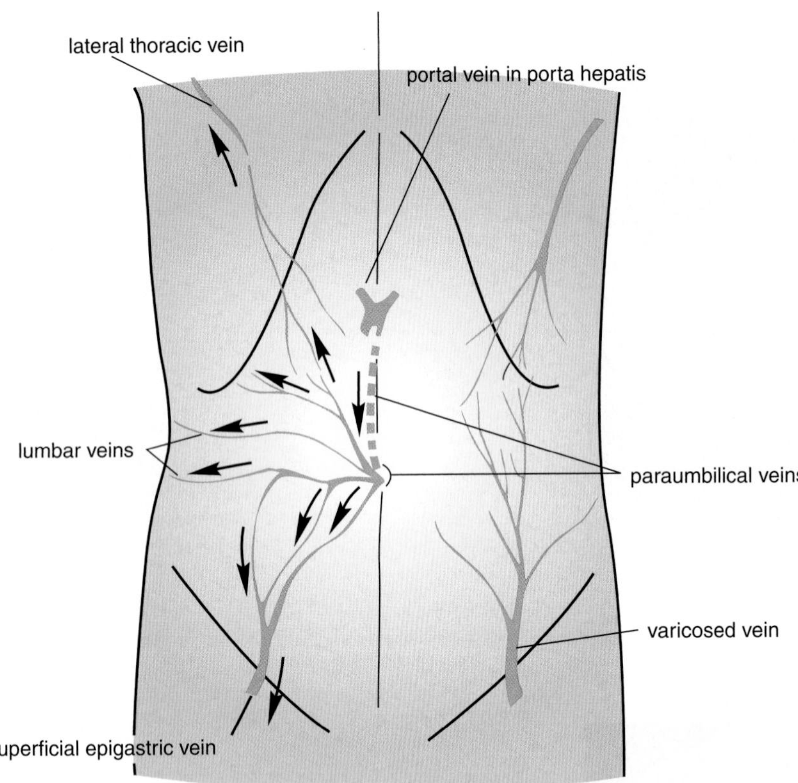

Figure 4-18 Superficial veins of the anterior abdominal wall. On the left are anastomoses between systemic veins and the portal vein via paraumbilical veins. Arrows indicate the direction taken by venous blood when the portal vein is obstructed. On the right is an enlarged anastomosis between the lateral thoracic vein and the superficial epigastric vein. This occurs if either the superior or the interior vena cava is obstructed.

Veins of the Anterior Abdominal Wall

Superficial Veins

The superficial veins form a network that radiates out from the umbilicus (Fig. 4-18). Above, the network is drained into the axillary vein via the lateral thoracic vein and, below, into the femoral vein via the superficial epigastric and great saphenous veins. A few small veins, the **paraumbilical veins,** connect the network through the umbilicus and along the ligamentum teres to the portal vein. This forms an important portal–systemic venous anastomosis.

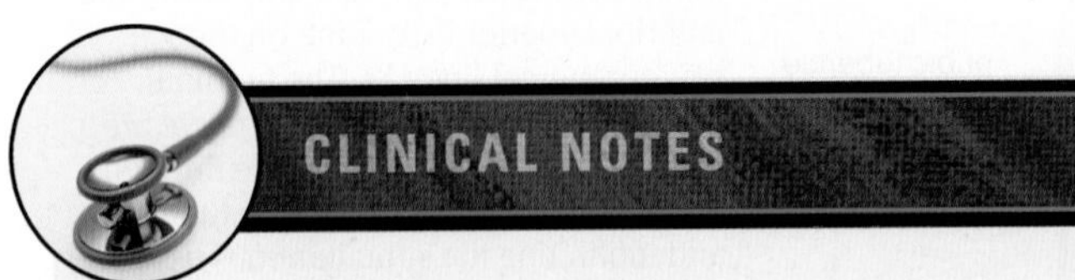

Portal Vein Obstruction

In cases of portal vein obstruction (Fig. 4-19), the superficial veins around the umbilicus and the paraumbilical veins become grossly distended. The distended subcutaneous veins radiate out from the umbilicus, producing in severe cases the clinical picture referred to as caput medusae.

Deep Veins

The deep veins of the abdominal wall, the superior epigastric, inferior epigastric, and deep circumflex iliac veins, follow the arteries of the same name and drain into the internal thoracic and external iliac veins. The posterior intercostal veins drain into the azygos veins, and the lumbar veins drain into the inferior vena cava.

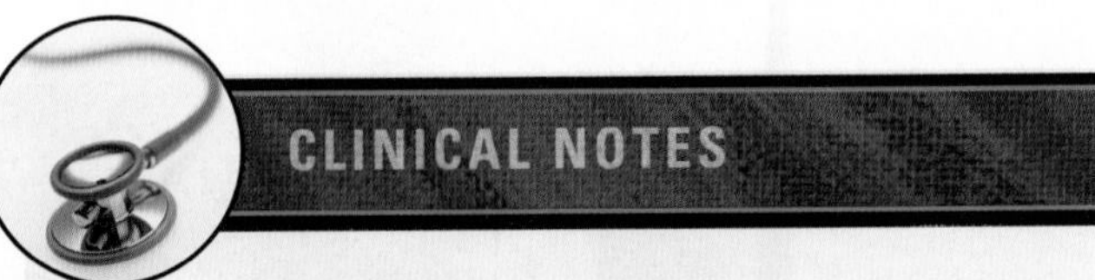

Caval Obstruction

If the superior or inferior vena cava is obstructed, the venous blood causes distention of the veins running from the anterior chest wall to the thigh. The lateral thoracic vein anastomoses with the superficial epigastric vein, a tributary of the great saphenous vein of the leg. In these circumstances, a tortuous varicose vein may extend from the axilla to the lower abdomen (Fig. 4-18).

Lymph Drainage of the Anterior Abdominal Wall

Superficial Lymph Vessels

The lymph drainage of the skin of the anterior abdominal wall above the level of the umbilicus is upward to the anterior axillary (pectoral) group of nodes, which can be palpated just beneath the lower border of the pectoralis major muscle. Below the level of the umbilicus, the lymph drains downward and laterally to the superficial inguinal nodes (Fig. 4-19). The lymph of the skin of the back above the level of the iliac crests is drained upward to the posterior axillary group of nodes, palpated on the posterior wall of the axilla; below the level of the iliac crests, it drains downward to the superficial inguinal nodes (Fig. 4-19).

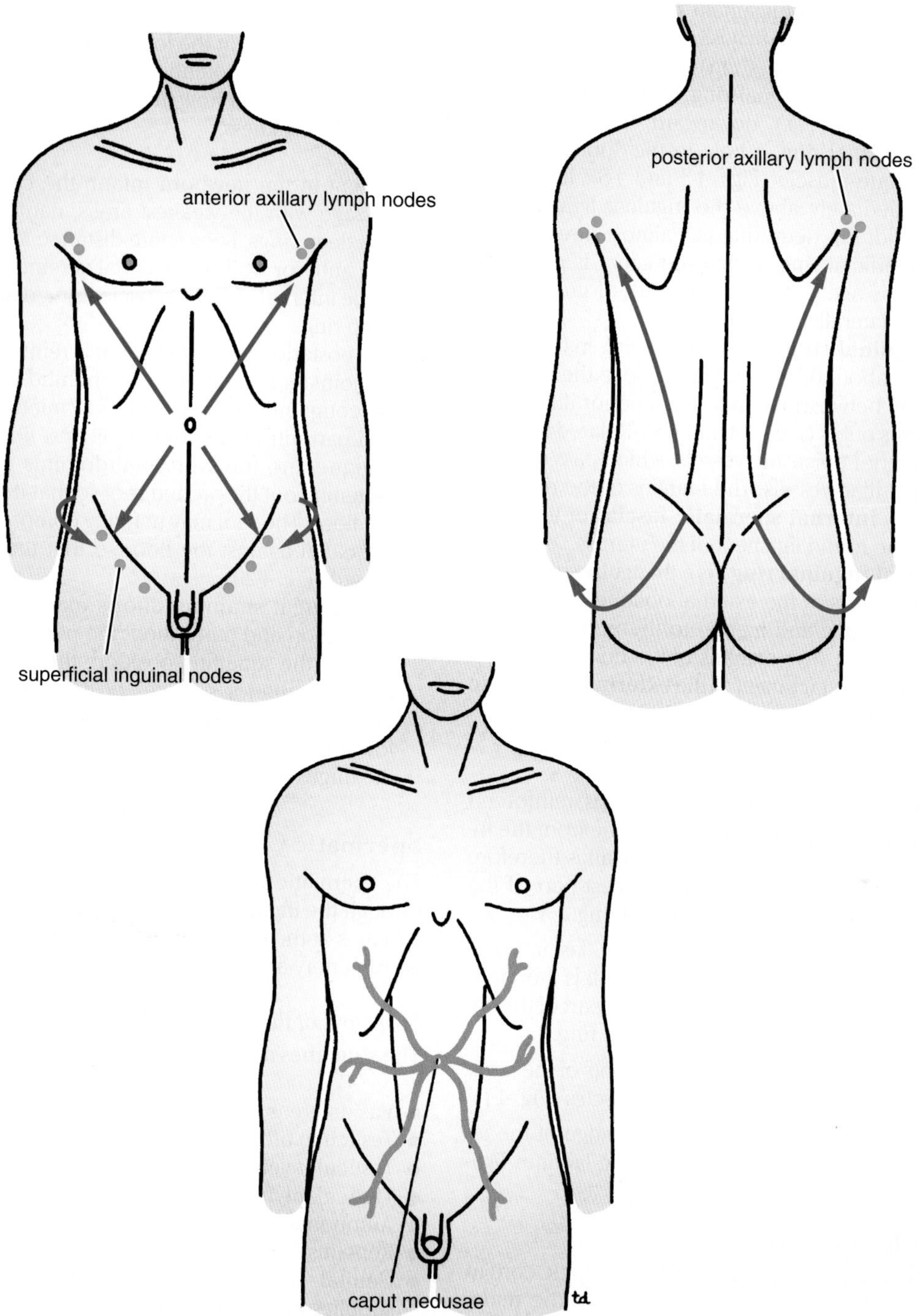

Figure 4-19 Lymph drainage of the skin of the anterior and posterior abdominal walls. Also shown is an example of caput medusae in a case of portal obstruction caused by cirrhosis of the liver.

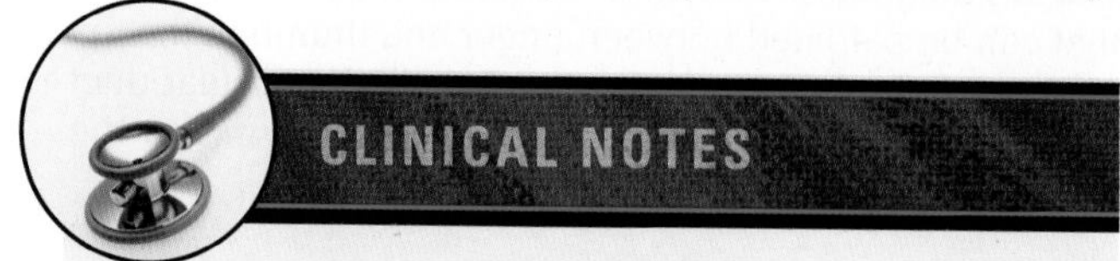

Skin and Its Regional Lymph Nodes

Knowledge of the areas of the skin that drain into a particular group of lymph nodes is clinically important. For example, it is possible to find a swelling in the groin (enlarged superficial inguinal node) caused by an infection or malignant tumor of the skin of the lower part of the anterior abdominal wall or that of the buttock.

Deep Lymph Vessels

The deep lymph vessels follow the arteries and drain into the internal thoracic, external iliac, posterior mediastinal, and para-aortic (lumbar) nodes.

Inguinal Canal

The inguinal canal is an oblique passage through the lower part of the anterior abdominal wall. In the males, it allows structures to pass to and from the testis to the abdomen. In females it allows the round ligament of the uterus to pass from the uterus to the labium majus.

The canal is about 1.5 in. (4 cm) long in the adult and extends from the deep inguinal ring, a hole in the fascia transversalis (see page 177), downward and medially to the superficial inguinal ring, a hole in the aponeurosis of the external oblique muscle (Figs. 4-3 and 4-8). It lies parallel to and immediately above the inguinal ligament. In the newborn child, the deep ring lies almost directly posterior to the superficial ring so that the canal is considerably shorter at this age. Later, as the result of growth, the deep ring moves laterally.

The **deep inguinal ring,*** an oval opening in the fascia transversalis, lies about 0.5 in. (1.3 cm) above the inguinal ligament midway between the anterior superior iliac spine and the symphysis pubis (Figs. 4-4 and 4-8). Related to it medially are the inferior epigastric vessels, which pass upward from the external iliac vessels. The margins of the ring give attachment to the **internal spermatic fascia** (or the internal covering of the round ligament of the uterus).

The **superficial inguinal ring*** is a triangular-shaped defect in the aponeurosis of the external oblique muscle and lies immediately above and medial to the pubic tubercle (Figs. 4-3, 4-5, and 4-8). The margins of the ring, sometimes called the **crura**, give attachment to the **external spermatic fascia.**

Walls of the Inguinal Canal

Anterior wall: External oblique aponeurosis, reinforced laterally by the origin of the internal oblique from the inguinal ligament (Figs. 4-3 and 4-8). This wall is therefore strongest where it lies opposite the weakest part of the posterior wall, namely, the deep inguinal ring.

Posterior wall: Conjoint tendon medially, fascia transversalis laterally (Figs. 4-4 and 4-8). This wall is therefore strongest where it lies opposite the weakest part of the anterior wall, namely, the superficial inguinal ring.

Roof or superior wall: Arching lowest fibers of the internal oblique and transversus abdominis muscles (Fig. 4-7)

Floor or inferior wall: Upturned lower edge of the inguinal ligament and, at its medial end, the lacunar ligament (Fig. 4-7).

Function of the Inguinal Canal

The inguinal canal allows structures of the spermatic cord to pass to and from the testis to the abdomen in the male. (Normal spermatogenesis takes place only if the testis leaves the abdominal cavity to enter a cooler environment in the scrotum.) In the female, the smaller canal permits the passage of the round ligament of the uterus from the uterus to the labium majus.

*A common frustration for medical students is the inability to observe these rings as openings. One must remember that the internal spermatic fascia is attached to the margins of the deep inguinal ring and the external spermatic fascia is attached to the margins of the superficial inguinal ring so that the edges of the rings cannot be observed externally. Compare this arrangement with the openings for the fingers seen inside a glove with the absence of openings for the fingers when the glove is viewed from the outside.

Mechanics of the Inguinal Canal

The inguinal canal in the lower part of the anterior abdominal wall is a site of potential weakness in both sexes. It is interesting to consider how the design of this canal attempts to lessen this weakness.

1. Except in the newborn infant, the canal is an oblique passage with the weakest areas, namely, the superficial and deep rings, lying some distance apart.
2. The anterior wall of the canal is reinforced by the fibers of the internal oblique muscle immediately in front of the deep ring.
3. The posterior wall of the canal is reinforced by the strong conjoint tendon immediately behind the superficial ring.
4. On coughing and straining, as in micturition, defecation, and parturition, the arching lowest fibers of the internal oblique and transversus abdominis muscles contract, flattening out the arched roof so that it is lowered toward the floor. The roof may actually compress the contents of the canal against the floor so that the canal is virtually closed (Fig. 4-20).
5. When great straining efforts may be necessary, as in defecation and parturition, the person naturally tends to assume the squatting position; the hip joints are flexed, and the anterior surfaces of the thighs are brought up against the anterior abdominal wall. By this means, the lower part of the anterior abdominal wall is protected by the thighs (Fig. 4-20).

Spermatic Cord

The spermatic cord is a collection of structures that pass through the inguinal canal to and from the testis (Fig. 4-21). It begins at the deep inguinal ring lateral to the inferior epigastric artery and ends at the testis.

Structures of the Spermatic Cord

The structures are as follows:

- Vas deferens
- Testicular artery
- Testicular veins (pampiniform plexus)
- Testicular lymph vessels
- Autonomic nerves
- Remains of the processus vaginalis
- Genital branch of the genitofemoral nerve, which supplies the cremaster muscle

Vas Deferens (Ductus Deferens)

The vas deferens is a cordlike structure (Figs. 4-5 and 4-21) that can be palpated between finger and thumb in the upper part of the scrotum. It is a thick-walled muscular duct that transports spermatozoa from the epididymis to the urethra.

Testicular Artery

A branch of the abdominal aorta (at the level of the second lumbar vertebra), the testicular artery is long and slender and descends on the posterior abdominal wall. It traverses the inguinal canal and supplies the testis and the epididymis (Fig. 4-21).

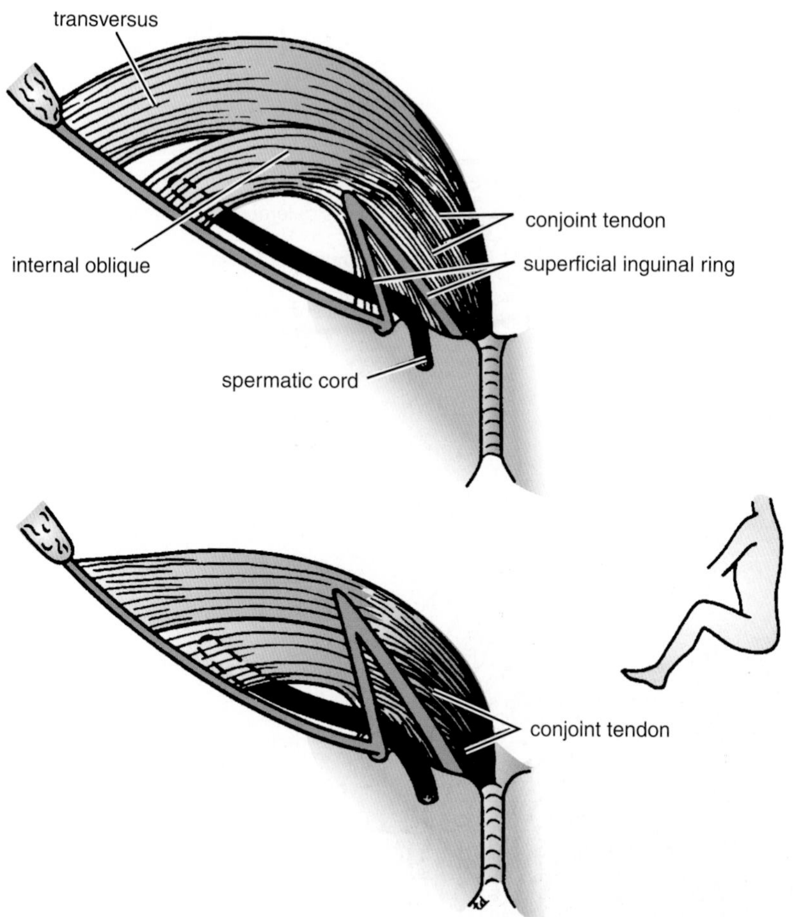

Figure 4-20 Action of the muscles on the inguinal canal. Note that the canal is "obliterated" when the muscles contract. Note also that the anterior surface of the thigh protects the inguinal region when one assumes the squatting position.

Testicular Veins

An extensive venous plexus, the **pampiniform plexus,** leaves the posterior border of the testis (Fig. 4-21). As the plexus ascends, it becomes reduced in size so that at about the level of the deep inguinal ring, a single testicular vein is formed. This runs up on the posterior abdominal wall and drains into the left renal vein on the left side and into the inferior vena cava on the right side.

Lymph Vessels

The testicular lymph vessels ascend through the inguinal canal and pass up over the posterior abdominal wall to reach the lumbar (para-aortic) lymph nodes on the side of the aorta at the level of the first lumbar vertebra (Fig. 4-22).

Autonomic Nerves

Sympathetic fibers run with the testicular artery from the renal or aortic sympathetic plexuses. Afferent sensory nerves accompany the efferent sympathetic fibers.

Processus Vaginalis

The remains of the processus vaginalis are present within the cord (see below).

Genital Branch of the Genitofemoral Nerve

This nerve supplies the cremaster muscle (Fig. 4-21) (see page 278).

Coverings of the Spermatic Cord (the Spermatic Fasciae)

The coverings of the spermatic cord are three concentric layers of fascia derived from the layers of the anterior abdominal wall. Each covering is acquired as the processus vaginalis descends into the scrotum through the layers of the abdominal wall (Fig. 4-23).

- **External spermatic fascia** derived from the external oblique aponeurosis and attached to the margins of the superficial inguinal ring
- **Cremasteric fascia** derived from the internal oblique muscle
- **Internal spermatic fascia** derived from the fascia transversalis and attached to the margins of the deep inguinal ring

To understand the coverings of the spermatic cord, one must first consider the development of the inguinal canal.

Development of the Inguinal Canal

Before the descent of the testis and the ovary from their site of origin high on the posterior abdominal wall (L1), a peritoneal diverticulum called the **processus vaginalis** is formed (Fig. 4-23). The processus vaginalis passes through the layers of the lower part of the anterior abdominal wall

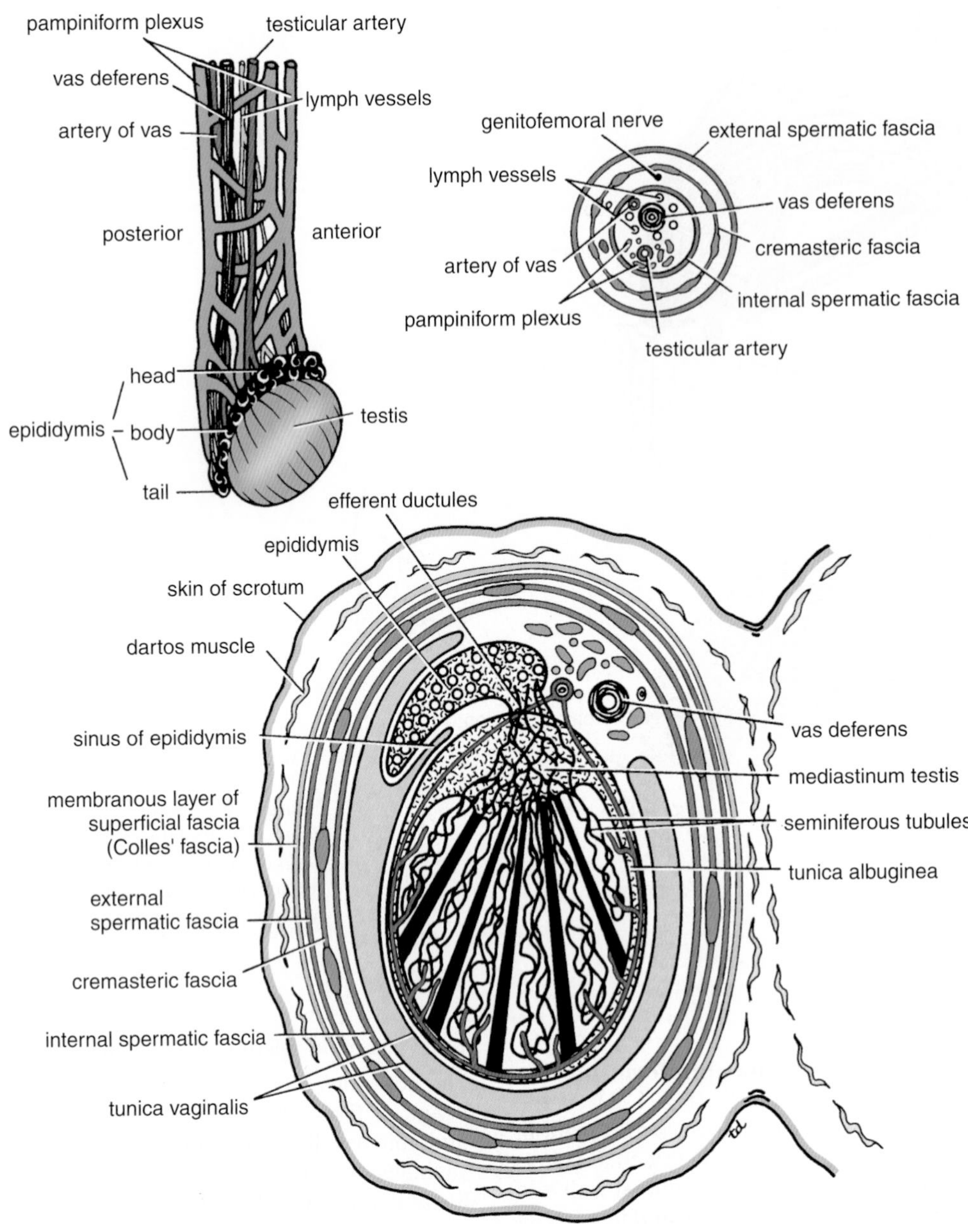

Figure 4-21 Testis and epididymis, spermatic cord, and scrotum. Also shown is the testis and epididymis cut across in horizontal section.

and, as it does so, acquires a tubular covering from each layer. It traverses the fascia transversalis at the deep inguinal ring and acquires a tubular covering, the **internal spermatic fascia** (Fig. 4-4). As it passes through the lower part of the internal oblique muscle, it takes with it some of its lowest fibers, which form the **cremaster muscle**. The muscle fibers are embedded in fascia, and thus the second tubular sheath is known as the **cremasteric fascia** (Fig. 4-4). The processus vaginalis passes under the arching fibers of the transversus abdominis muscle and therefore does not acquire a covering from this abdominal layer. On reaching the aponeurosis of the external oblique, it evaginates this to form the superficial inguinal ring and acquires a third tubular fascial coat, the **external spermatic fascia** (Figs. 4-4 and 4-5). It is in this manner that the inguinal canal is formed in both sexes. (In the female the term spermatic fascia should be replaced by the covering of the round ligament of the uterus.)

Meanwhile, a band of mesenchyme, extending from the lower pole of the developing gonad through the inguinal canal to the labioscrotal swelling, has condensed to form the **gubernaculum** (Fig. 4-23).

In the male, the testis descends through the pelvis and inguinal canal during the seventh and eighth months of fetal life. The normal stimulus for the descent of the testis is testosterone, which is secreted by the fetal testes. The testis follows the gubernaculum and descends behind the peritoneum on the posterior abdominal wall. The testis then passes behind the processus vaginalis and pulls down its duct, blood vessels, nerves, and lymph vessels. The testis

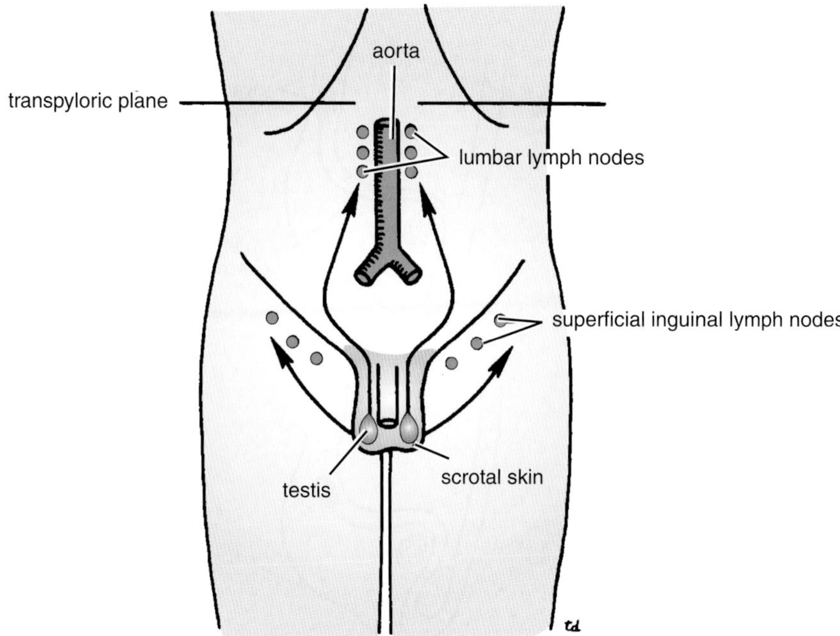

Figure 4-22 Lymph drainage of the testis and the skin of the scrotum.

takes up its final position in the developing scrotum by the end of the eighth month.

Because the testis and its accompanying vessels, ducts, and so on follow the course previously taken by the processus vaginalis, they acquire the same three coverings as they pass down the inguinal canal. Thus, the spermatic cord is covered by three concentric layers of fascia: the external spermatic fascia, the cremasteric fascia, and the internal spermatic fascia.

In the female, the ovary descends into the pelvis following the gubernaculum (Fig. 4-23). The gubernaculum becomes attached to the side of the developing uterus, and the gonad descends no farther. That part of the gubernaculum extending from the uterus into the developing labium majus persists as the **round ligament of the uterus**. Thus, in the female, the only structures that pass through the inguinal canal from the abdominal cavity are the round ligament of the uterus and a few lymph vessels. The lymph vessels convey a small amount of lymph from the body of the uterus to the superficial inguinal nodes.

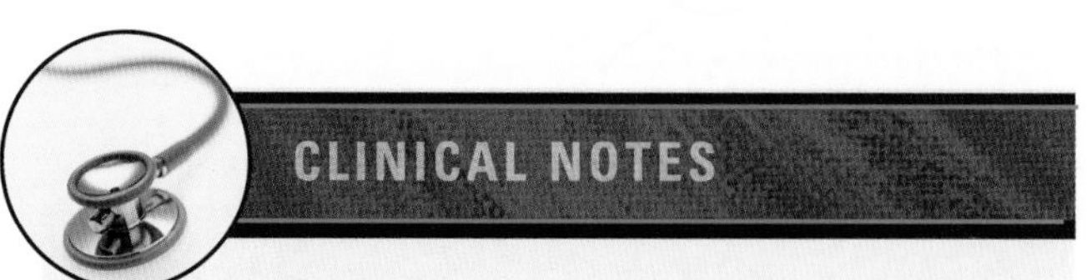

Vasectomy

Bilateral vasectomy is a simple operation performed to produce infertility. Under local anesthesia, a small incision is made in the upper part of the scrotal wall, and the vas deferens is divided between ligatures. Spermatozoa may be present in the first few postoperative ejaculations, but that is simply an emptying process. Now only the secretions of the seminal vesicles and prostate constitute the seminal fluid, which can be ejaculated as before.

Scrotum, Testis, and Epididymides

Scrotum

The scrotum is an outpouching of the lower part of the anterior abdominal wall. It contains the testes, the epididymides, and the lower ends of the spermatic cords (Figs. 4-4 and 4-21).

The wall of the scrotum has the following layers:

Skin: The skin of the scrotum is thin, wrinkled, and pigmented and forms a single pouch. A slightly raised ridge in the midline indicates the line of fusion of the two lateral labioscrotal swellings. (In the female, the swellings remain separate and form the labia majora.)

Superficial fascia: This is continuous with the fatty and membranous layers of the anterior abdominal wall; the fat is, however, replaced by smooth muscle called the dartos muscle. This is innervated by sympathetic nerve fibers and is responsible for the wrinkling of the overlying skin. The membranous layer of the superficial fascia (often referred to as Colles' fascia) is continuous in front with the membranous layer of the anterior abdominal wall (Scarpa's fascia), and behind it is attached to the perineal body and the posterior edge of the perineal membrane (Fig. 4-1). At the sides it is attached to the ischiopubic rami. Both layers of superficial fascia contribute to a median partition that crosses the scrotum and separates the testes from each other.

Spermatic fasciae: These three layers lie beneath the superficial fascia and are derived from the three layers of the anterior abdominal wall on each side, as previously explained. The external spermatic fascia is derived from the aponeurosis of the external oblique muscle; the cremasteric fascia is derived from the internal oblique muscle; and, finally, the internal spermatic fascia is derived from the fascia transversalis. The cremaster muscle is

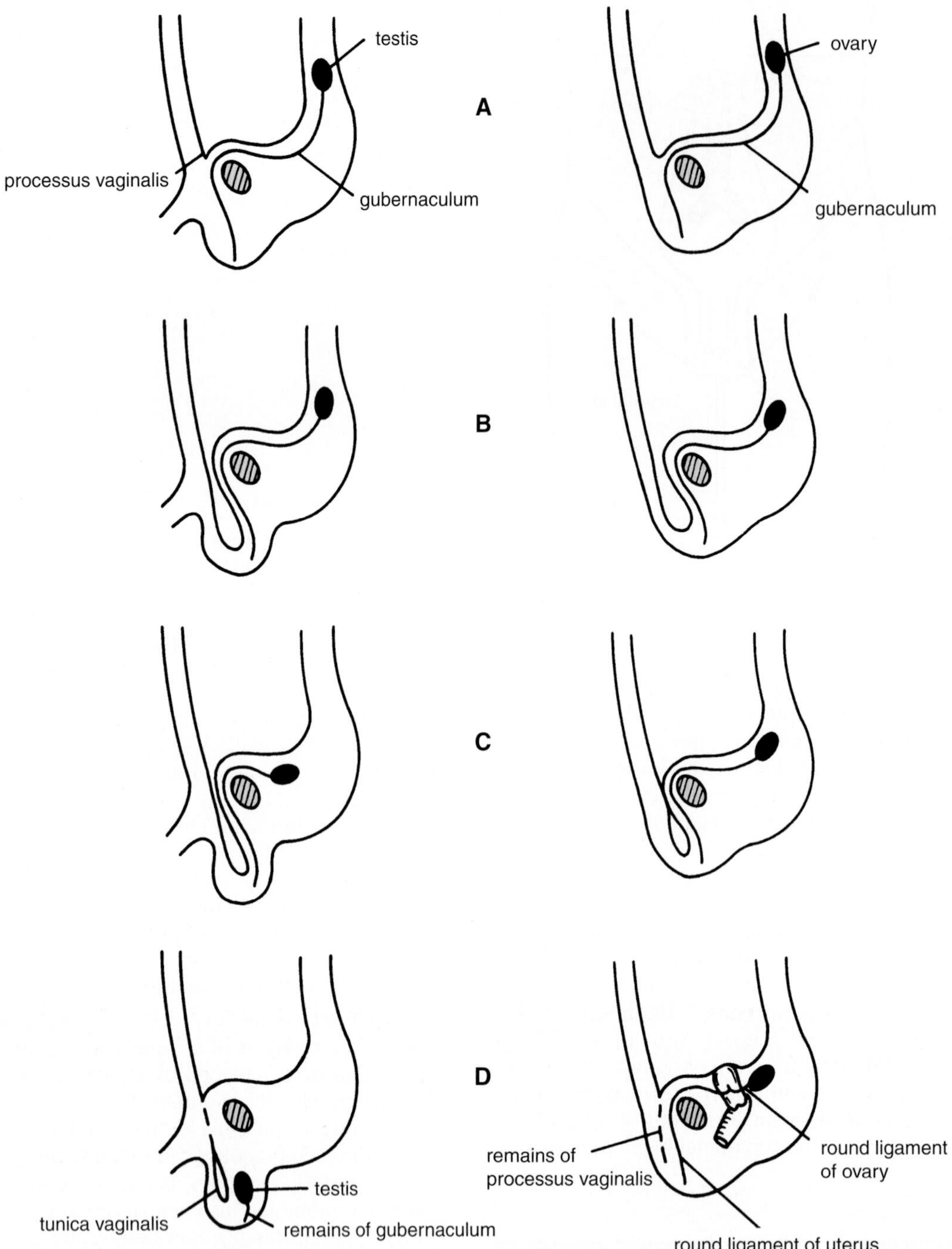

Figure 4-23 Origin, development, and fate of the processus vaginalis in the two sexes. Note the descent of the testis into the scrotum and the descent of the ovary into the pelvis.

supplied by the genital branch of the genitofemoral nerve (see page 279). The cremaster muscle can be made to contract by stroking the skin on the medial aspect of the thigh. This is called the **cremasteric reflex**. The afferent fibers of this reflex arc travel in the femoral branch of the genitofemoral nerve (L1 and 2), and the efferent motor nerve fibers travel in the genital branch of the genitofemoral nerve. The function of the cremaster muscle is to raise the testis and the scrotum upward for warmth and for protection against injury. For testicular temperature and fertility, see page 169.

Tunica vaginalis (Figs. 4-4, 4-5, and 4-21): This lies within the spermatic fasciae and covers the anterior, medial, and lateral surfaces of each testis. It is the lower expanded part of the processus vaginalis; normally, just before birth, it becomes shut off from the upper part of the processus and the peritoneal cavity. The tunica vaginalis is thus a closed sac, invaginated from behind by the testis.

Lymph Drainage of the Scrotum

Lymph from the skin and fascia, including the tunica vaginalis, drains into the superficial inguinal lymph nodes (Fig. 4-22).

Testis

The **testis** is a firm, mobile organ lying within the scrotum (Figs. 4-5 and 4-21). The left testis usually lies at a lower level than the right. Each testis is surrounded by a tough fibrous capsule, the **tunica albuginea.**

Extending from the inner surface of the capsule is a series of fibrous septa that divide the interior of the organ into **lobules**. Lying within each lobule are one to three coiled **seminiferous tubules**. The tubules open into a network of channels called the **rete testis**. Small **efferent ductules** connect the rete testis to the upper end of the epididymis (Fig. 4-21).

Normal spermatogenesis can occur only if the testes are at a temperature lower than that of the abdominal cavity. When they are located in the scrotum, they are at a temperature about 3°C lower than the abdominal temperature. The control of testicular temperature in the scrotum is not fully understood, but the surface area of the scrotal skin can be changed reflexly by the contraction of the dartos and cremaster muscles. It is now recognized that the testicular veins in the spermatic cord that form the pampiniform plexus—together with the branches of the testicular arteries, which lie close to the veins—probably assist in stabilizing the temperature of the testes by a countercurrent heat exchange mechanism. By this means, the hot blood arriving in the artery from the abdomen loses heat to the blood ascending to the abdomen within the veins.

Epididymis

The **epididymis** is a firm structure lying posterior to the testis, with the vas deferens lying on its medial side (Fig. 4-21). It has an expanded upper end, the **head,** a **body,** and a pointed **tail** inferiorly. Laterally, a distinct groove lies between the testis and the epididymis, which is lined with the inner visceral layer of the tunica vaginalis and is called the **sinus of the epididymis** (Fig. 4-21).

The epididymis is a much coiled tube nearly 20 ft (6 m) long, embedded in connective tissue. The tube emerges from the tail of the epididymis as the **vas deferens**, which enters the spermatic cord.

The long length of the duct of the epididymis provides storage space for the spermatozoa and allows them to mature. A main function of the epididymis is the absorption of fluid. Another function may be the addition of substances to the seminal fluid to nourish the maturing sperm.

Blood Supply of the Testis and Epididymis

The testicular artery is a branch of the abdominal aorta. The testicular veins emerge from the testis and the epididymis as a venous network, the **pampiniform plexus.** This becomes reduced to a single vein as it ascends through the inguinal canal. The right testicular vein drains into the inferior vena cava, and the left vein joins the left renal vein.

Lymph Drainage of the Testis and Epididymis

The lymph vessels (Fig. 4-22) ascend in the spermatic cord and end in the lymph nodes on the side of the aorta (lumbar or para-aortic) nodes at the level of the first lumbar vertebra (i.e., on the transpyloric plane). This is to be expected because during development the testis has migrated from high up on the posterior abdominal wall, down through the inguinal canal, and into the scrotum, dragging its blood supply and lymph vessels after it.

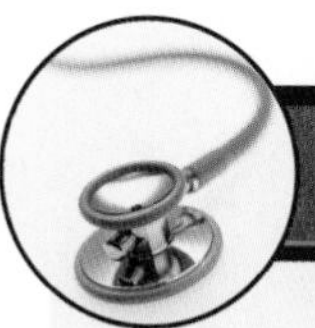

CLINICAL NOTES

Clinical Conditions Involving the Scrotum and Testis

Varicocele

A varicocele is a condition in which the veins of the pampiniform plexus are elongated and dilated. It is a common disorder in adolescents and young adults, with most occurring on the left side. This is thought to be because the right testicular vein joins the low-pressure inferior vena cava, whereas the left vein joins the left renal vein, in which the venous pressure is higher. Rarely, malignant disease of the left kidney extends along the renal vein and blocks the exit of the testicular vein. A rapidly developing left-sided variocele should therefore always lead one to examine the left kidney.

Malignant Tumor of the Testis

A malignant tumor of the testis spreads upward via the lymph vessels to the lumbar (para-aortic) lymph nodes at the level of the first lumbar vertebra. It is only later, when the tumor spreads locally to involve the tissues and skin of the scrotum, that the superficial inguinal lymph nodes are involved.

The process of the descent of the testis is shown in Figure 4-23. The testis may be subject to the following congenital anomalies:

Torsion of the Testis

Torsion of the testis is a rotation of the testis around the spermatic cord within the scrotum. It is often associated with an excessively large tunica vaginalis. Torsion commonly occurs in active young men and children and is accompanied by severe pain. If not treated quickly, the testicular artery may be occluded, followed by necrosis of the testis.

Processus Vaginalis

The formation of the processus vaginalis and its passage through the lower part of the anterior abdominal wall with the formation of the inguinal canal in both sexes were described elsewhere (see page 165). Normally, the upper part becomes obliterated just before birth and the lower part remains as the tunica vaginalis.

(continues)

Clinical Notes, *continued*

The processus is subject to the following common congenital anomalies:

- It may persist partially or in its entirety as a **preformed hernial sac** for an indirect inguinal hernia (Fig. 4-24).
- It may become very much narrowed, but its lumen remains in communication with the abdominal cavity. Peritoneal fluid accumulates in it, forming a **congenital hydrocele** (Fig. 4-24).
- The upper and lower ends of the processus may become obliterated, leaving a small intermediate cystic area referred to as an **encysted hydrocele of the cord** (Fig. 4-24).

The tunica vaginalis is closely related to the front and sides of the testis. It is therefore not surprising to find that inflammation of the testis can cause an accumulation of fluid within the tunica vaginalis. This is referred to simply as a **hydrocele** (Fig. 4-25). Most hydroceles are idiopathic.

To remove excess fluid from the tunica vaginalis, a procedure termed **tapping a hydrocele,** a fine trocar and cannula are inserted through the scrotal skin (Fig. 4-25). The following anatomic structures are traversed by the cannula: skin, dartos muscle and membranous layer of fascia (Colles' fascia), external spermatic fascia, cremasteric fascia, internal spermatic fascia, and parietal layer of the tunica vaginalis.

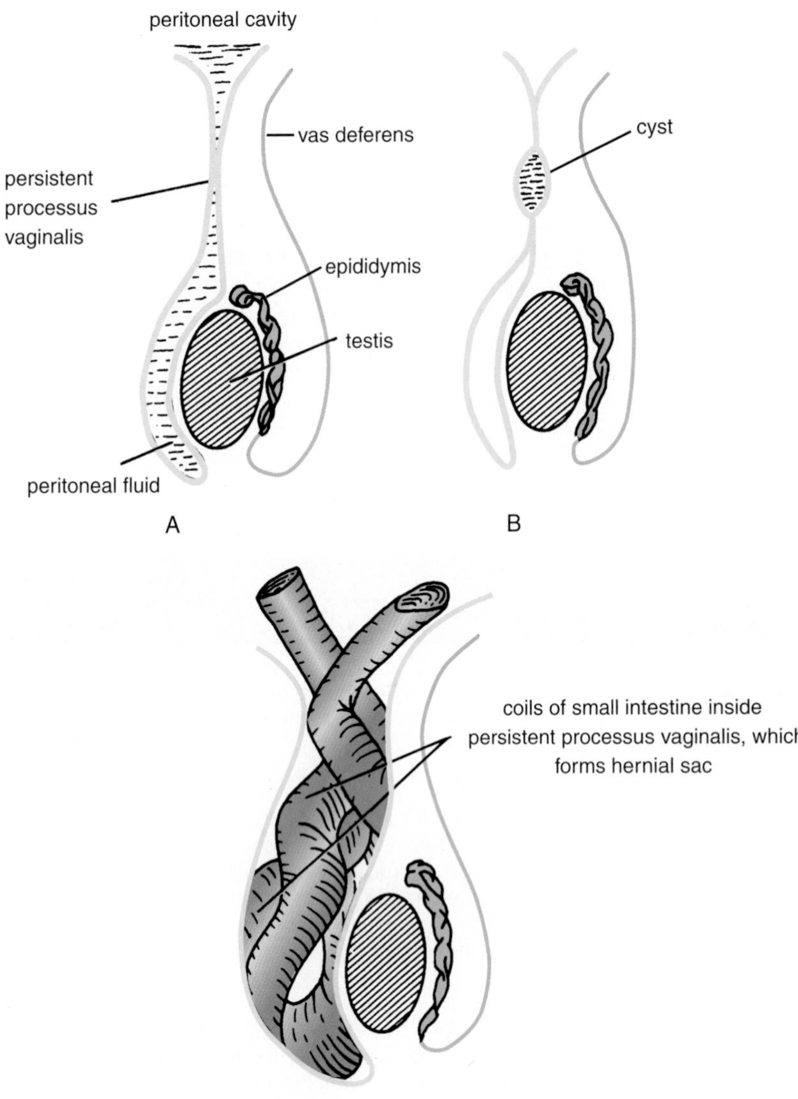

Figure 4-24 Common congenital anomalies of the processus vaginalis. **A.** Congenital hydrocele. **B.** Encysted hydrocele of the cord. **C.** Preformed hernial sac for indirect inguinal hernia.

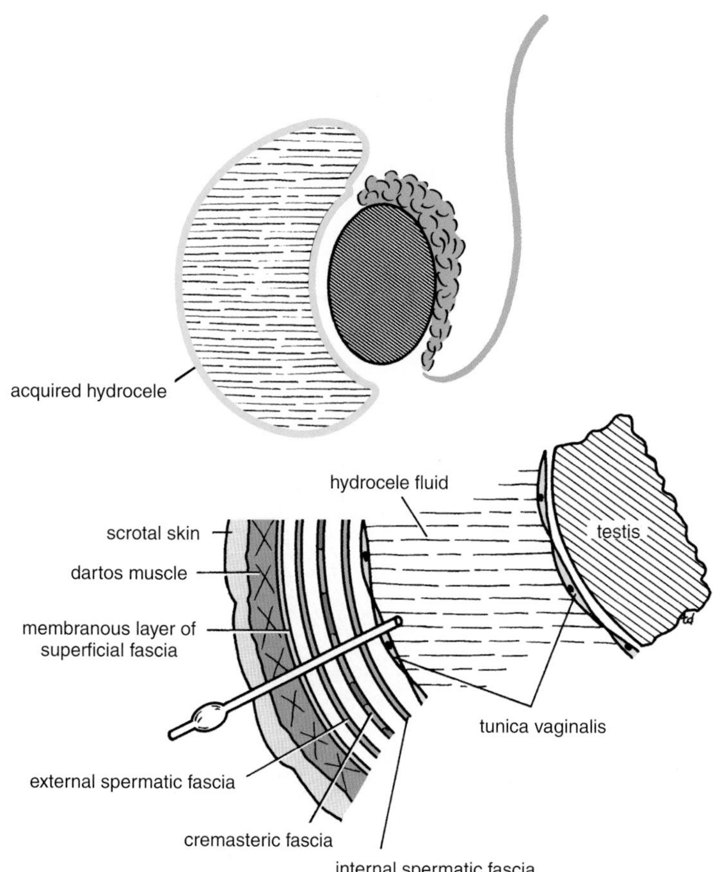

Figure 4-25 The tunica vaginalis distended with fluid (hydrocele). Also shown are the various anatomic layers traversed by a trocar and cannula when a hydrocele is tapped.

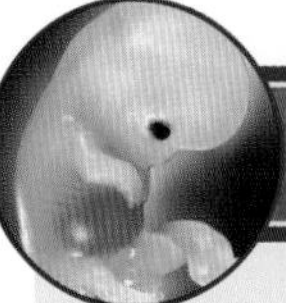

EMBRYOLOGIC NOTES

Development of the Testis

The male sex chromosome causes the genital ridge to secrete testosterone and induces the development of the testis and the other internal and external organs of reproduction.

The **sex cords** of the genital ridge become separated from the coelomic epithelium by the proliferation of the mesenchyme (Fig. 4-26). The outer part of the mesenchyme condenses to form a dense fibrous layer, the **tunica albuginea.** The sex cords become U-shaped and form the **seminiferous tubules.** The free ends of the tubules form the **straight tubules,** which join one another in the mediastinum testis to become the **rete testis.** The primordial sex cells in the seminiferous tubules form the **spermatogonia,** and the sex cord cells form the **Sertoli cells.** The mesenchyme in the developing gonad makes up the connective tissue and fibrous septa. The **interstitial cells,** which are already secreting testosterone, are also formed of mesenchyme. The rete testis becomes canalized, and the tubules extend into the mesonephric tissue, where they join the remnants of the mesonephric tubules; the latter tubules become the **efferent ductules** of the testis. The **duct of the epididymis,** the **vas deferens,** the **seminal vesicle,** and the **ejaculatory duct** are formed from the mesonephric duct (Fig. 4-26).

Descent of the Testis

The testis develops high up on the posterior abdominal wall, and in late fetal life it "descends" behind the peritoneum, dragging its blood supply, nerve supply, and lymphatic drainage after it (for details, see pages 166). The process of the descent of the testis is shown in Figure 4-23.

Congenital Anomalies of the Testis

The testis may be subject to the following congenital anomalies.

- **Anterior inversion,** in which the epididymis lies anteriorly and the testis and the tunica vaginalis lie posteriorly
- **Polar inversion,** in which the testis and epididymis are completely inverted
- **Imperfect descent (cryptorchidism): Incomplete descent** (Fig. 4-27), in which the testis, although traveling down its normal path, fails to reach the floor of the scrotum. It may be found within the abdomen, within the inguinal canal, at the superficial inguinal ring, or high up in the scrotum. **Maldescent** (Fig. 4-28), in which the testis travels down an abnormal path and fails to reach the scrotum. It may be found in the superficial fascia of the anterior abdominal wall above the inguinal ligament, in front of the pubis, in the perineum, or in the thigh.

It is necessary for the testes to leave the abdominal cavity because the temperature there retards the normal process of spermatogenesis. If an incompletely descended testis is brought down into the scrotum by surgery before puberty, it will develop

(continues)

Embryologic Notes, *continued*

and function normally. A maldescended testis, although often developing normally, is susceptible to traumatic injury and, for this reason, should be placed in the scrotum. Many authorities believe that the incidence of tumor formation is greater in testes that have not descended into the scrotum.

The **appendix of the testis** and the **appendix of the epididymis** are embryologic remnants found at the upper poles of these organs that may become cystic. The appendix of the testis is derived from the paramesonephric ducts, and the appendix of the epididymis is a remnant of the mesonephric tubules.

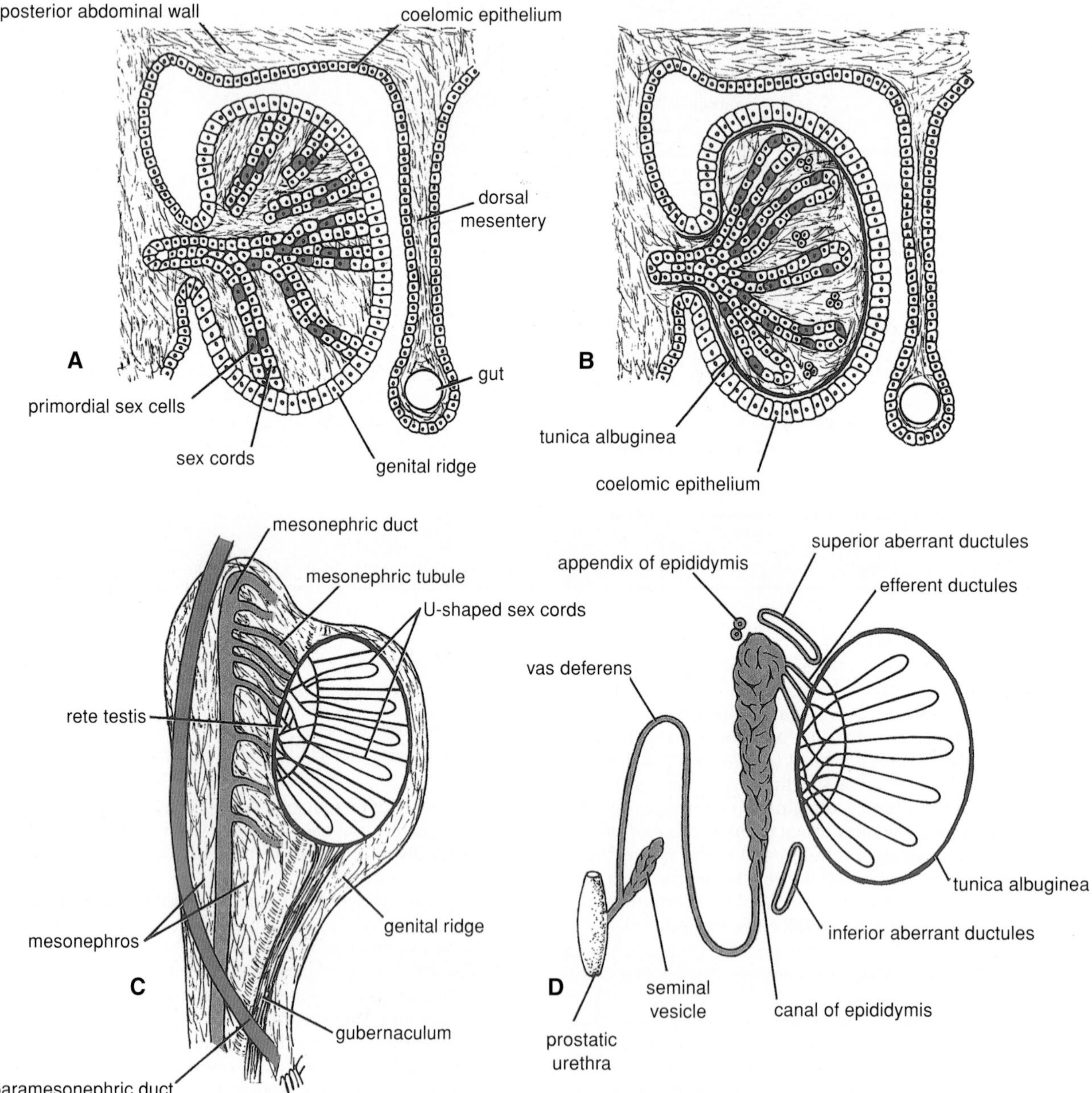

Figure 4-26 The formation of the testis and the ducts of the testis.

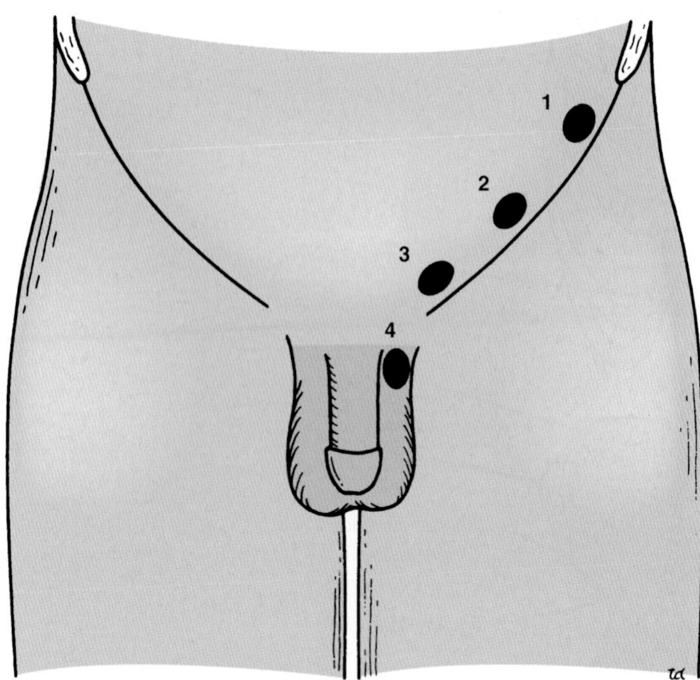

Figure 4-27 Four degrees of incomplete descent of the testis. **1.** In the abdominal cavity close to the deep inguinal ring. **2.** In the inguinal canal. **3.** At the superficial inguinal ring. **4.** In the upper part of scrotum.

Labia Majora

The labia majora are prominent, hair-bearing folds of skin formed by the enlargement of the genital swellings in the fetus. (In the male, the genital swellings fuse in the midline to form the scrotum.) Within the labia are a large amount of adipose tissue and the terminal strands of the round ligaments of the uterus. (For further details see page 367.)

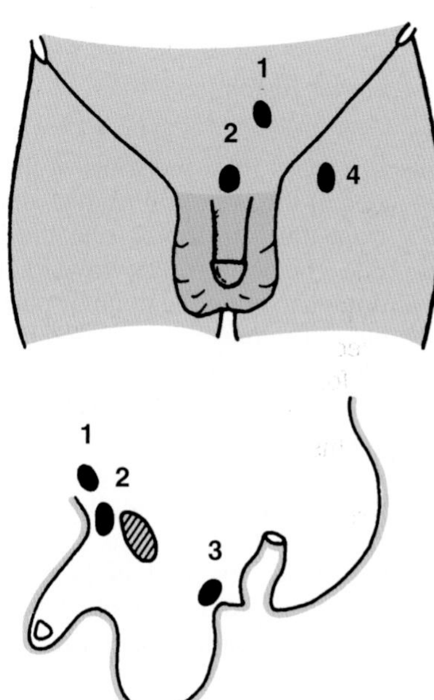

Figure 4-28 Four types of maldescent of the testis. **1.** In the superficial fascia of the anterior abdominal wall, above the superficial inguinal ring. **2.** At the root of the penis. **3.** In the perineum. **4.** In the thigh.

Structure of the Posterior Abdominal Wall

The posterior abdominal wall is formed in the midline by the five lumbar vertebrae and their intervertebral discs and laterally by the 12th ribs, the upper part of the bony pelvis (Fig. 4-29), the psoas muscles, the quadratus lumborum muscles, and the aponeuroses of origin of the transversus abdominis muscles. The iliacus muscles lie in the upper part of the bony pelvis.

Lumbar Vertebrae

The **body** of each vertebra (Fig. 4-30) is massive and kidney shaped, and it has to bear the greater part of the body weight. The fifth lumbar vertebra articulates with the base of the sacrum at the **lumbosacral joint.**

The **intervertebral discs** (Fig. 4-31) in the lumbar region are thicker than in other regions of the vertebral column. They are wedge shaped and are responsible for the normal posterior concavity in the curvature of the vertebral column in the lumbar region (lordosis). For a full description of the structure of the lumbar vertebrae and the intervertebral discs, see pages 855 and 858.

Twelfth Pair of Ribs

The ribs are described on page 47. It should be noted that the head of the 12th rib has a single facet for articulation with the body of the 12th thoracic vertebra. The anterior end is pointed and has a small costal cartilage, which is embedded in the musculature of the anterior abdominal wall. In many people it is so short that it fails to protrude beyond the lateral border of the erector spinae muscle on the back.

Ilium

The ilium, together with the ischium and pubis, forms the hip bone (Fig. 4-32); they meet one another at the acetabulum. The medial surface of the ilium is divided into two parts

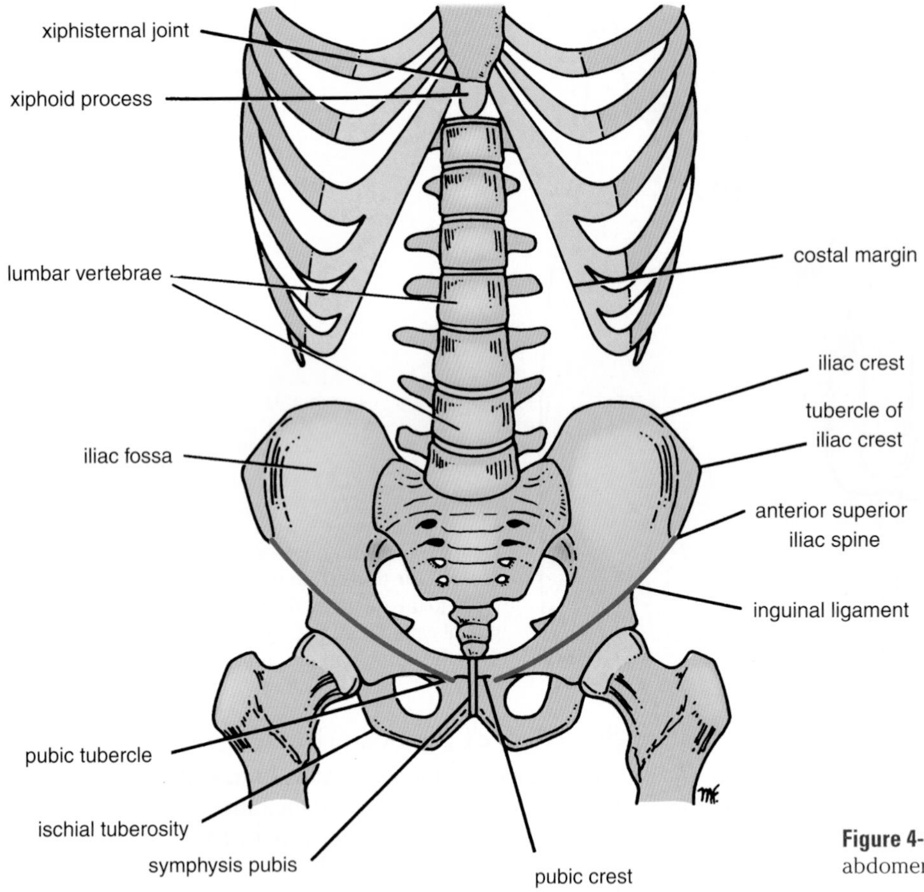

xiphisternal joint
xiphoid process
lumbar vertebrae
iliac fossa
pubic tubercle
ischial tuberosity
symphysis pubis
pubic crest
costal margin
iliac crest
tubercle of iliac crest
anterior superior iliac spine
inguinal ligament

Figure 4-29 Costal margin and bones of the abdomen.

by the **arcuate line.** Above this line is a concave surface called the iliac fossa; below this line is a flattened surface that is continuous with the medial surfaces of the pubis and ischium. It should be noted that the arcuate line of the ilium forms the posterior part of the **iliopectineal line,** and the **pectineal line** forms the anterior part of the iliopectineal line. The iliopectineal line runs forward and demarcates the false from the true pelvis. For further details on the structure of the hip bone, see page 316.

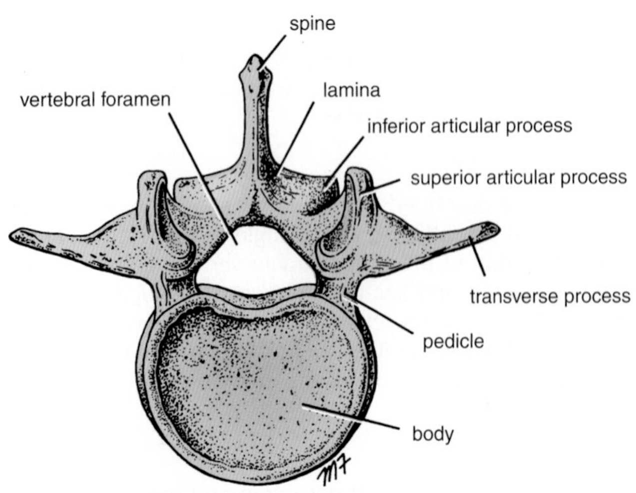

Figure 4-30 Fifth lumbar vertebra.

Muscles of the Posterior Abdominal Wall

Psoas Major

The psoas muscle* arises from the roots of the transverse processes, the sides of the vertebral bodies, and the intervertebral discs, from the 12th thoracic to the 5th lumbar vertebrae (Fig. 4-33). The fibers run downward and laterally and leave the abdomen to enter the thigh by passing behind the inguinal ligament. The muscle is inserted into the lesser trochanter of the femur. The psoas is enclosed in a fibrous sheath that is derived from the lumbar fascia. The sheath is thickened above to form the **medial arcuate ligament.**

- **Nerve supply:** This muscle is supplied by the lumbar plexus.
- **Action:** The psoas flexes the thigh at the hip joint on the trunk, or if the thigh is fixed, it flexes the trunk on the thigh, as in sitting up from a lying position.

*The psoas minor is a small muscle with a long tendon that lies anterior to the psoas major. It is unimportant and is absent in 40% of patients.

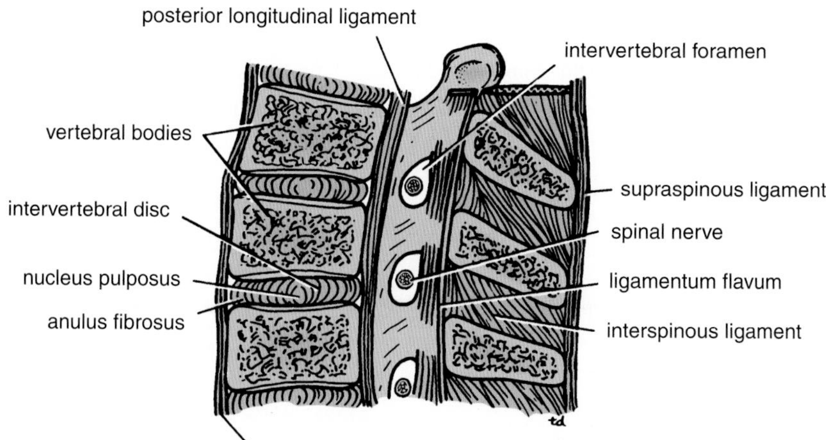

Figure 4-31 Sagittal section of the lumbar part of the vertebral column showing intervertebral discs and ligaments.

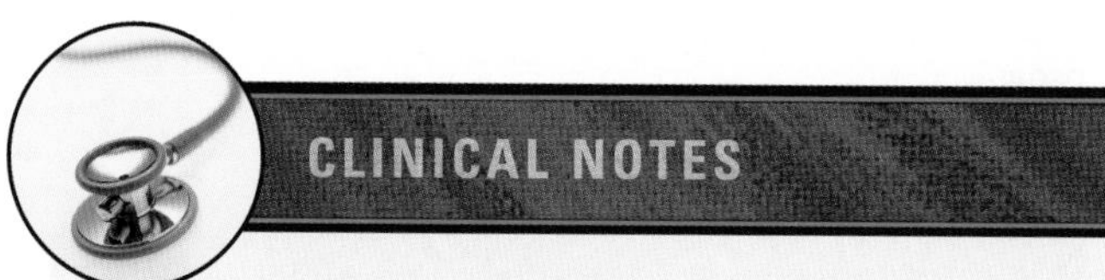

Psoas Fascia and Tuberculosis

The psoas fascia covers the anterior surface of the psoas muscle and can influence the direction taken by a tuberculous abscess. Tuberculous disease of the thoracolumbar region of the vertebral column results in the destruction of the vertebral bodies, with possible extension of pus laterally under the psoas fascia (Fig. 4-34). From there, the pus tracks downward, following the course of the psoas muscle, and appears as a swelling in the upper part of the thigh below the inguinal ligament. It may be mistaken for a femoral hernia.

Quadratus Lumborum

The quadratus lumborum is a flat, quadrilateral-shaped muscle that lies alongside the vertebral column. It arises below from the iliolumbar ligament, the adjoining part of the iliac crest, and the tips of the transverse processes of the lower lumbar vertebrae (Fig. 4-33). The fibers run upward and medially and are inserted into the lower border of the 12th rib and the transverse processes of the upper four lumbar vertebrae. The anterior surface of the muscle is covered by lumbar fascia, which is thickened above to form the **lateral arcuate ligament** and below to form the **iliolumbar ligament.**

- **Nerve supply:** This muscle is supplied by the lumbar plexus.

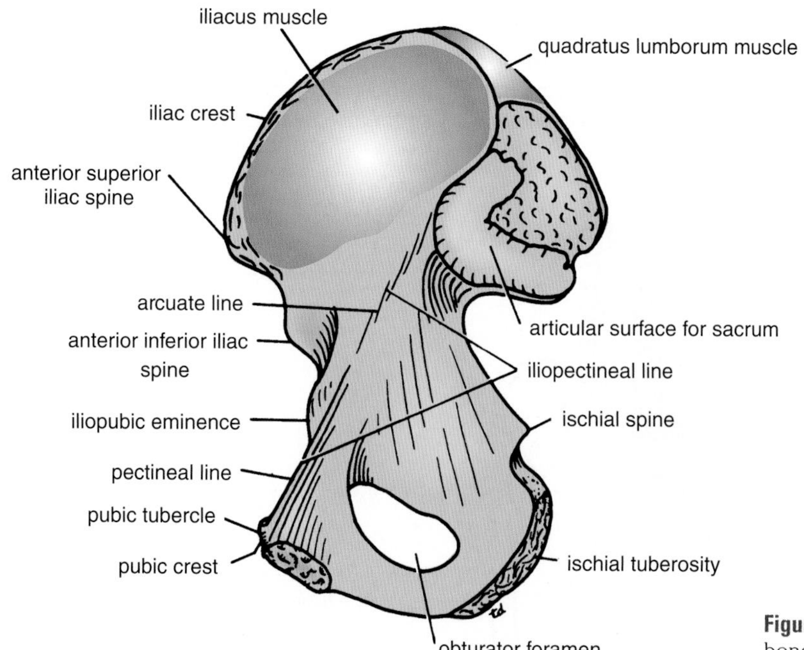

Figure 4-32 Internal aspect of the right hip bone.

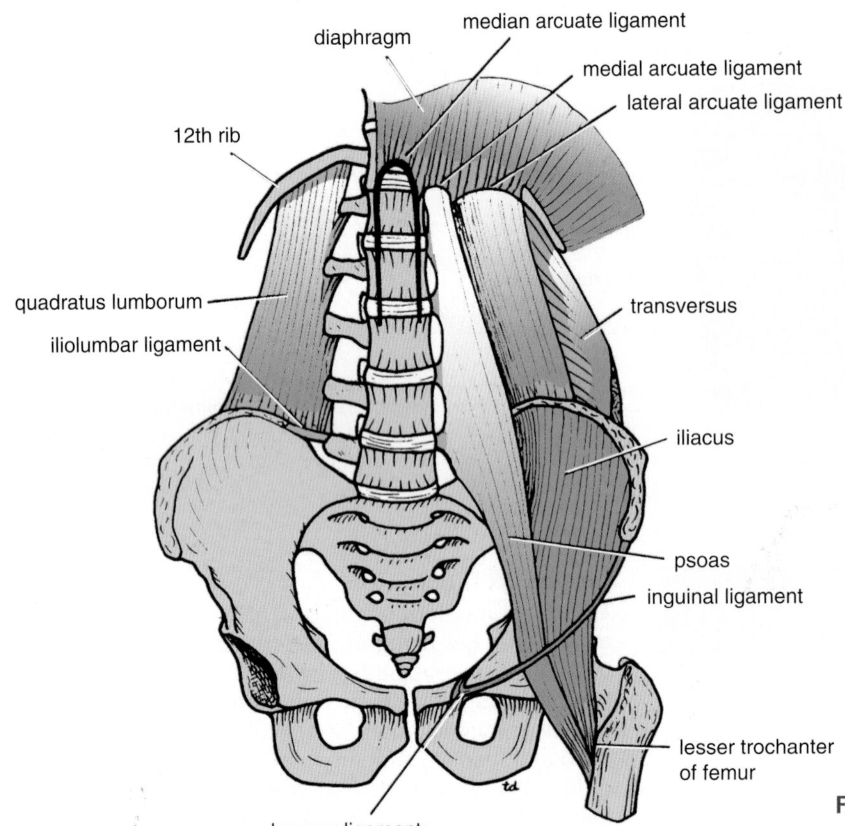

Figure 4-33 Muscles and bones forming the posterior abdominal wall.

- **Action:** It fixes or depresses the 12th rib during respiration (see page 102) and laterally flexes the vertebral column to the same side.

Transversus Abdominis

The transversus abdominis muscle is fully described on page 152.

Iliacus

The iliacus muscle is fan shaped and arises from the upper part of the iliac fossa (Figs. 4-32 and 4-33). Its fibers join the lateral side of the psoas tendon to be inserted into the lesser trochanter of the femur. The combined muscles are often referred to as the **iliopsoas.**

- **Nerve supply:** This muscle is supplied by the femoral nerve, a branch of the lumbar plexus.
- **Action:** The iliopsoas flexes the thigh on the trunk at the hip joint, or if the thigh is fixed, it flexes the trunk on the thigh.

The posterior part of the **diaphragm** (Fig. 4-33) also forms part of the posterior abdominal wall. It is described on page 57. A summary of the muscles of the posterior ab-

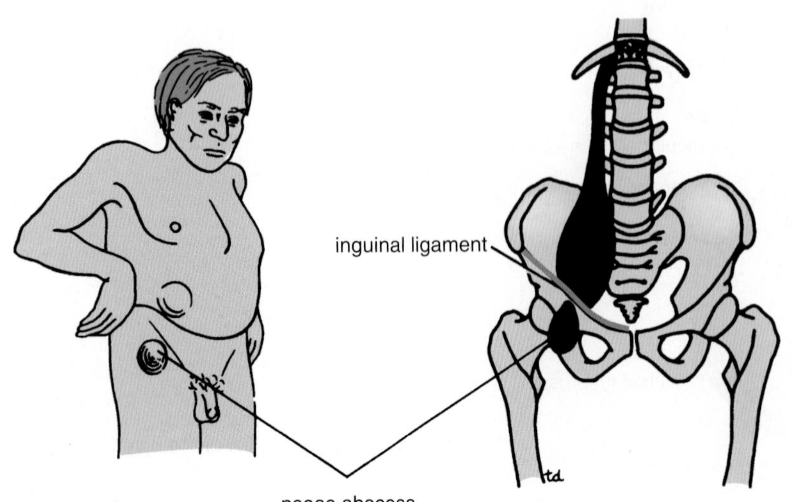

Figure 4-34 Case of advanced tuberculous disease of the thoracolumbar region of the vertebral column. A psoas abscess is present, and swellings occur in the right groin above and below the right inguinal ligament.

Table 4-2 **Muscles of the Posterior Abdominal Wall**

Name of Muscle	Origin	Insertion	Nerve Supply	Action
Psoas	Transverse processes, bodies, and intervertebral discs of 12th thoracic and five lumbar vertebrae	With iliacus into lesser trochanter of femur	Lumbar plexus	Flexes thigh on trunk; if thigh is fixed, it flexes trunk on thigh, as in sitting up from lying position
Quadratus lumborum	Iliolumbar ligament, iliac crest, tips of transverse processes of lower lumbar vertebrae	12th rib	Lumbar plexus	Fixes 12th rib during inspiration; depresses 12th rib during forced expiration; laterally flexes vertebral column same side
Iliacus	Iliac fossa	With psoas into lesser trochanter of femur	Femoral nerve	Flexes thigh on trunk; if thigh is fixed, it flexes the trunk on the thigh, as in sitting up from lying position

dominal wall, their nerve supply, and their action is given in Table 4-2.

Fascial Lining of the Abdominal Walls

As mentioned previously, the abdominal walls are lined by one continuous layer of connective tissue that lies between the parietal peritoneum and the muscles (Fig. 4-35). It is continuous below with a similar fascial layer lining the pelvic walls. It is customary to name the fascia according to the structure it overlies. For example, the **diaphragmatic fascia** covers the undersurface of the diaphragm, the **transversalis fascia** lines the transversus abdominis, the **psoas fascia** covers the psoas muscle, the **quadratus lumborum fascia** covers the quadratus lumborum, and the **iliaca fascia** covers the iliacus muscle.

The abdominal blood and lymph vessels lie within this fascial lining, whereas the principal nerves lie outside the fascia. This fact is important in the understanding of the femoral sheath (Fig. 4-35). This is simply a downward prolongation of the fascial lining around the femoral vessels and lymphatics, for about 1.5 in. (4 cm) into the thigh, behind the inguinal ligament. Because the femoral nerve lies outside the fascial envelope, it has no sheath (see page 582).

In certain areas of the abdominal wall, the fascial lining performs particularly important functions. Inferior to the level of the anterior superior iliac spines, the posterior wall of the rectus sheath is devoid of muscular aponeuroses (Figs. 4-10 and 4-13) and is formed by the fascia transversalis and peritoneum only (see page 154).

At the midpoint between the anterior superior iliac spine and the symphysis pubis, the spermatic cord pierces the fascia transversalis to form the deep inguinal ring (Fig. 4-8). From the margins of the ring, the fascia is continued over the cord as a tubular sheath, the internal spermatic fascia (Fig. 4-4).

Peritoneal Lining of the Abdominal Walls

The walls of the abdomen are lined with parietal peritoneum. This is a thin serous membrane consisting of a layer of mesothelium resting on connective tissue. It is continuous below with the parietal peritoneum lining the pelvis (Fig. 4-35). For further details, see pages 352 and 373.

Nerve Supply

The central part of the diaphragmatic peritoneum is supplied by the phrenic nerves, and the peripheral part is supplied by the lower intercostal nerves. The peritoneum lining the anterior and posterior abdominal walls is supplied segmentally by intercostal and lumbar nerves, which also supply the overlying muscles and skin.

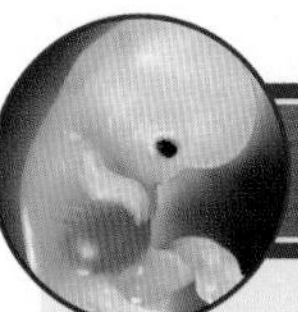

EMBRYOLOGIC NOTES

Development of the Abdominal Wall

Following segmentation of the mesoderm, the lateral mesoderm (see page 37) splits into a somatic and a splanchnic layer associated with ectoderm and entoderm, respectively (Fig. 4-36). The muscles of the anterior abdominal wall are derived from the somatopleuric mesoderm and retain their segmental innervation from the anterior rami of the spinal nerves. Unlike the thorax, the segmental arrangement becomes lost due to the absence of ribs, and the mesenchyme fuses to form large sheets of muscle. The rectus abdominis retains indications of its segmental origin, as seen by the presence of the tendinous intersections. The somatopleuric mesoderm becomes split tangentially into three layers, which form the external oblique, internal oblique, and transversus abdominis muscles. The anterior body

(continues)

Embryologic Notes, *continued*

wall finally closes in the midline at 3 months, when the right and left sides meet in the midline and fuse. The line of fusion of the mesenchyme forms the linea alba, and on either side of this, the rectus muscles come to lie within their rectus sheaths.

Development of the Umbilical Cord and the Umbilicus

As the tail fold of the embryo develops, the embryonic attachment of the body stalk to the caudal end of the embryonic disc comes to lie on the anterior surface of the embryo, close to the remains of the yolk sac (Fig. 4-37). The amnion and chorion now fuse, so that the amnion encloses the body stalk and the yolk sac with their blood vessels to form the tubular umbilical cord. The mesenchymal core of the cord forms the loose connective tissue called Wharton's jelly. Embedded in this are the remains of the yolk sac, the vitelline duct, the remains of the allantois, and the umbilical blood vessels.

The umbilical vessels consist of two arteries that carry deoxygenated blood from the fetus to the chorion (later the placenta). The two umbilical veins convey oxygenated blood from the placenta to the fetus. The right vein soon disappears (Fig. 4-37).

The umbilical cord is a twisted tortuous structure that measures about 0.75 in. (2 cm) in diameter. It increases in length until, at the end of pregnancy, it is about 20 in. (50 cm) long—that is, about the same length as the child.

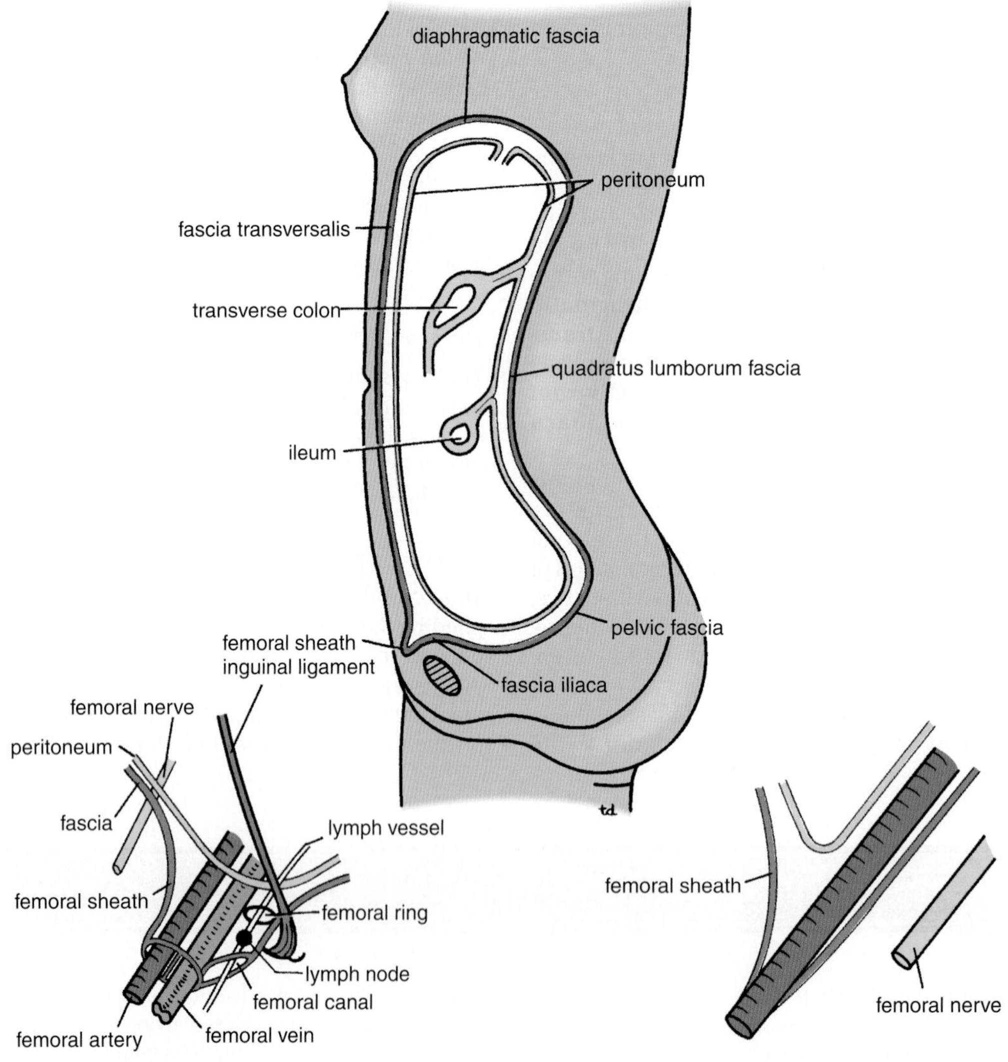

Figure 4-35 Sagittal section of the abdomen showing arrangement of the fascial and peritoneal linings of walls. The femoral sheath with its contained vessels is also shown. Note that the femoral nerve is devoid of a fascial sheath.

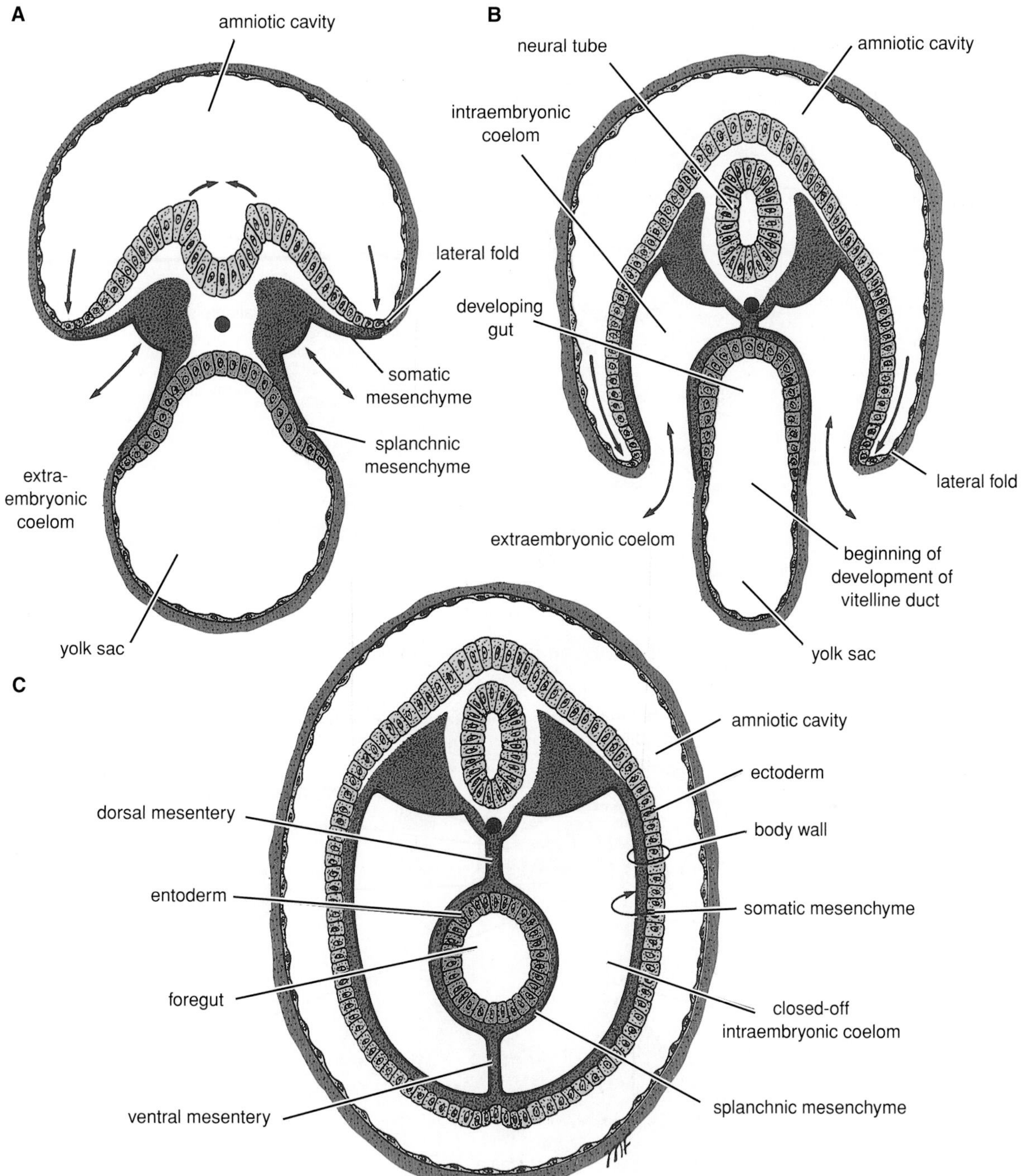

Figure 4-36 Transverse sections through the embryo at different stages of development showing the formation of the abdominal wall and peritoneal cavity. **A.** The intraembryonic coelom in free communication with the extraembryonic coelom (*double-headed arrows*). **B.** The development of the lateral folds of the embryo and the beginning of the closing off of the intraembryonic coelom. **C.** The lateral folds of the embryo finally fused in the midline and closing off the intraembryonic coelom or future peritoneal cavity. Most of the ventral mesentery will break down and disappear.

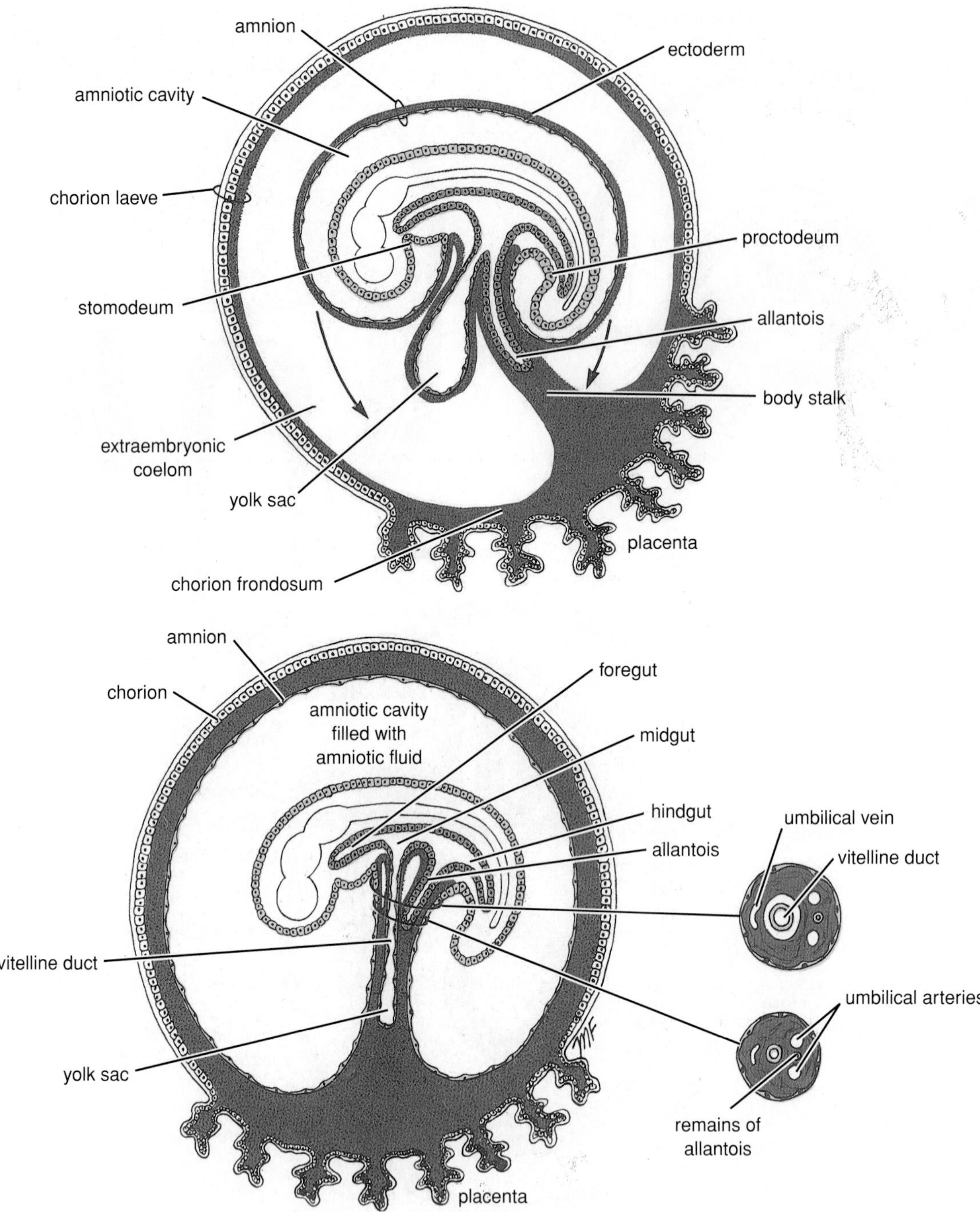

Figure 4-37 The formation of the umbilical cord. Note the expansion of the amniotic cavity (*arrows*) so that the cord becomes covered with amnion. Note also that the umbilical vessels have been reduced to one vein and two arteries.

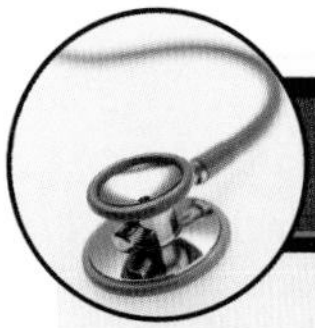

CLINICAL NOTES

Tying the Cord

At birth, the cord is tied off close to the umbilicus. About 2 in. (5 cm) of cord is left between the umbilicus and the ligature, since a piece of intestine may be present as an umbilical hernia in the remains of the extraembryonic coelom. After application of the ligature, the umbilical vessels constrict and thrombose. Later, the stump of the cord is shed and the umbilical scar tissue becomes retracted and assumes the shape of the umbilicus, or navel.

Patent Urachus

The urachus is the remains of the allantois of the fetus and normally persists as a fibrous cord that runs from the apex of the bladder to the umbilicus. Occasionally, the cavity of the allantois persists, and urine passes from the bladder through the umbilicus. In newborns, it usually reveals itself when a congenital urethral obstruction is present. More often, it remains undiscovered until old age, when enlargement of the prostate may obstruct the urethra (Fig. 4-38).

Vitellointestinal Duct

The vitelline duct in the early embryo connects the developing gut to the yolk sac. Normally, as development proceeds, the duct is obliterated, severs its connection with the small intestine, and disappears. Persistence of the vitellointestinal duct can result in

(continues)

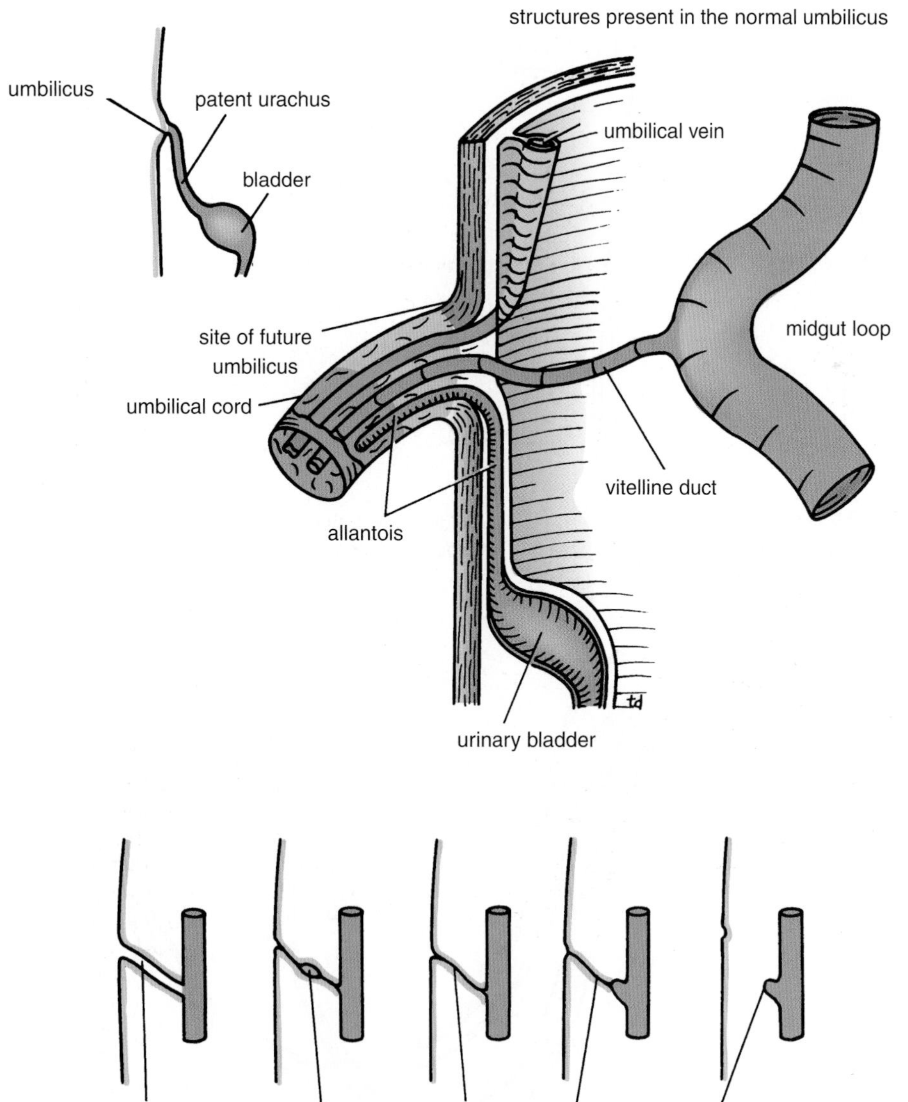

Figure 4-38 Umbilicus and some common congenital defects.

Clinical Notes, *continued*

an umbilical fecal fistula (Fig. 4-38). If the duct remains as a fibrous band, a loop of bowel can become wrapped around it, causing intestinal obstruction (Fig. 4-38).

Meckel's diverticulum is a congenital anomaly representing a persistent portion of the vitellointestinal duct. It occurs in 2% of patients (Fig. 4-38), is located about 2 ft (61 cm) from the ileocolic junction, and is about 2 in. (5 cm) long. It can become ulcerated or cause intestinal obstruction.

Umbilical Vessel Catheterization

The umbilical cord is surrounded by the fetal membrane, amnion, and contains Wharton's jelly. Embedded in this jelly are the remains of the vitellointestinal duct and the allantois, and the single umbilical vein and the two umbilical arteries (Fig. 4-39). The vein is a larger thin-walled vessel and is located at the 12 o'clock position when facing the umbilicus; the two arteries, which lie adjacent to one another and are located at the 4 and 8 o'clock positions when facing the umbilicus, are smaller and thick walled.

Indications for Umbilical Artery Catheterization

1. Administration of fluids or blood for resuscitation purposes
2. Arterial blood gas and blood pressure monitoring. The umbilical arteries may be cannulated most easily during the first few hours after birth, but they may be cannulated up to 6 days after delivery.

Anatomy of Procedure

One of the small, thick-walled arteries is identified in the Wharton's jelly in the umbilical stump. Because the umbilical arteries are branches of the internal iliac arteries in the pelvis, the

(continues)

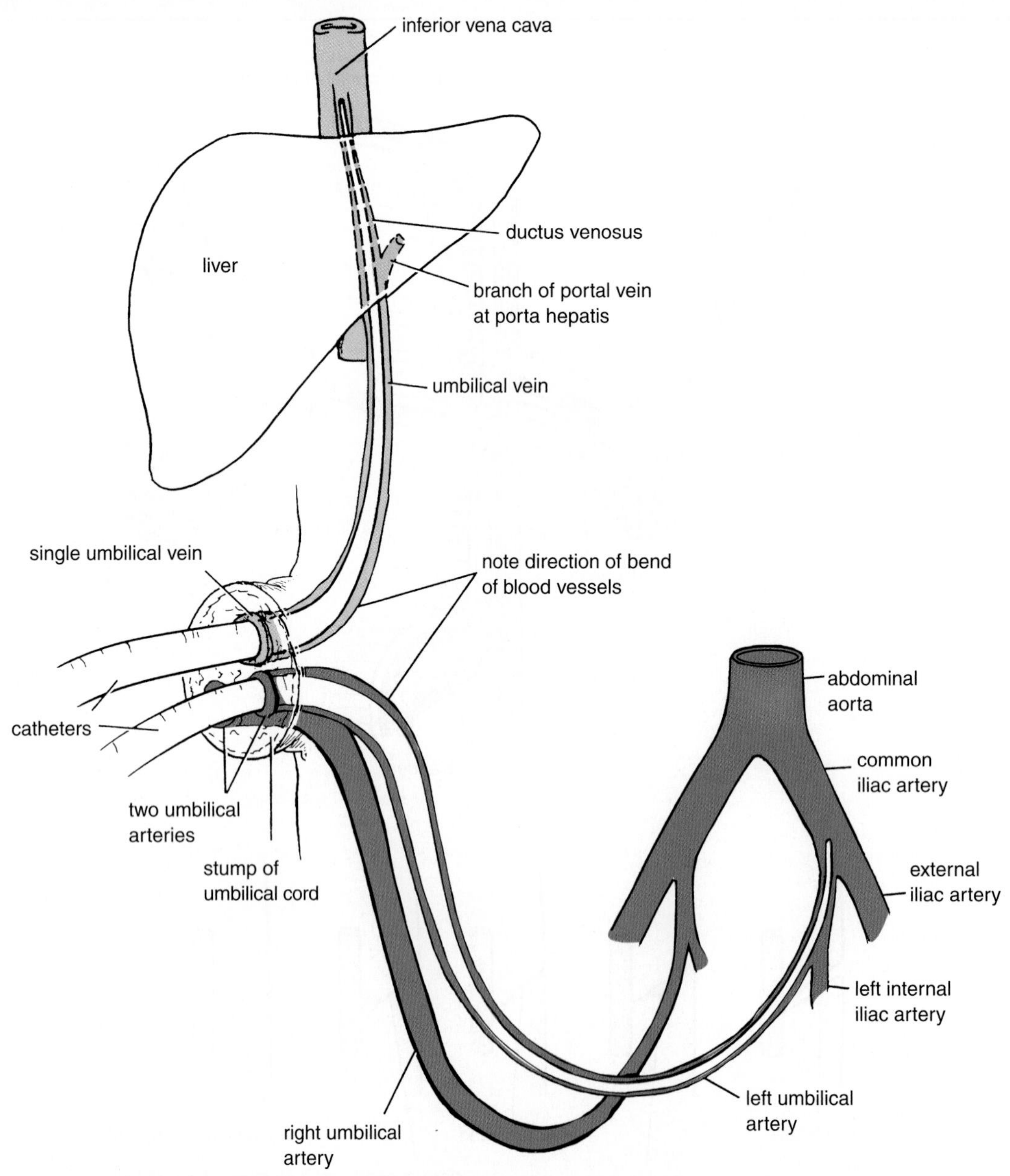

Figure 4-39 Catheterization of the umbilical blood vessels. Arrangement of the single umbilical vein and the two umbilical arteries in the umbilical cord and the paths taken by the catheter in the umbilical vein and the umbilical artery.

Clinical Notes, *continued*

catheter is introduced and advanced slowly in the direction of the feet. The catheter can be inserted for about 2.75 in. (7 cm) in a premature infant and 4.75 in. (12 cm) in a full-term infant. The course of the catheter can be confirmed on a radiograph and is as follows: (a) umbilical artery (directed downward into the pelvis), (b) internal iliac artery (acute turn into this artery), and (c) common iliac artery and the aorta.

Anatomy of Complications

- Catheter perforates arterial wall at a point where the artery turns downward toward the pelvis at the anterior abdominal wall.
- Catheter enters the thin-walled wider umbilical vein instead of the thick-walled smaller artery.
- Catheter enters the thin-walled persistent urachus (urine is returned into catheter).
- Vasospasm of the umbilical and the iliac arteries occurs, causing blanching of the leg.
- Perforation of arteries distal to the umbilical artery occurs, for example, the iliac arteries or even the aorta.
- Other complications include thrombosis, emboli, and infection of the umbilical stump.

Indications for Umbilical Vein Catheterization

1. Administration of fluids or blood for resuscitation purposes
2. Exchange transfusions. The umbilical vein may be cannulated up to 7 days after birth.

Anatomy of Procedure

The umbilical vein is located in the cord stump at the 12 o'clock position (Fig. 4-39), as described previously, and is easily recognized because of its thin wall and large lumen. The catheter is advanced gently and is directed toward the head, because the vein runs in the free margin of the falciform ligament to join the ductus venosus at the porta hepatis. The catheter may be advanced about 2 in. (5 cm) in a full-term infant. The course of the catheter may be confirmed by radiography and is as follows: (a) the umbilical vein, (b) the ductus venosus, and (c) the inferior vena cava (4 to 4.75 in. [10 to 12 cm]).

Anatomy of the Complications of Umbilical Vein Catheterization

- Catheter may perforate the venous wall. This is most likely to occur where the vein turns cranially at the abdominal wall.
- Other complications include liver necrosis, hemorrhage, and infection.

Abdominal Herniae

A hernia is the protrusion of part of the abdominal contents beyond the normal confines of the abdominal wall (Fig. 4-40). It consists of three parts: the sac, the contents of the sac, and the coverings of the sac. The hernial sac is a pouch (diverticulum) of peritoneum and has a neck and a body. The hernial contents may consist of any structure found within the abdominal cavity and may vary from a small piece of omentum to a large viscus such as the kidney. The hernial coverings are formed from the layers of the abdominal wall through which the hernial sac passes.

Abdominal herniae are of the following common types:

- Inguinal (indirect or direct)
- Femoral
- Umbilical (congenital or acquired)
- Epigastric

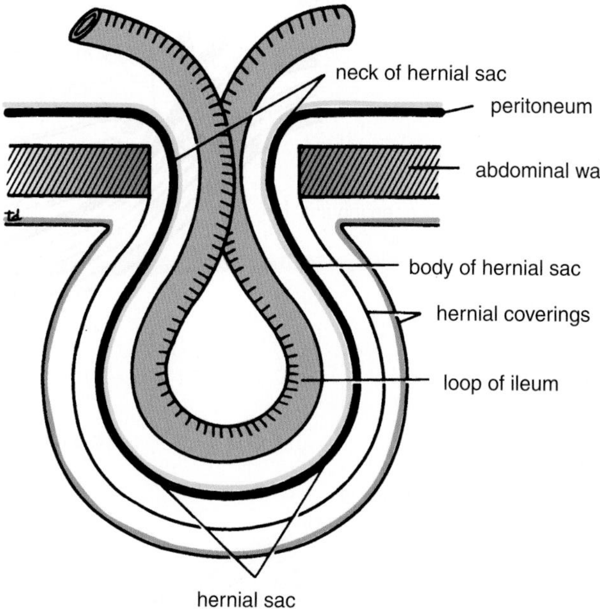

Figure 4-40 Different parts of a hernia.

- Separation of the recti abdominis
- Incisional
- Hernia of the linea semilunaris (Spigelian hernia)
- Lumbar (Petit's triangle hernia)
- Internal

Indirect Inguinal Hernia

The indirect inguinal hernia is the most common form of hernia and is believed to be congenital in origin (Fig. 4-41A). The hernial sac is the remains of the processus vaginalis (an outpouching of peritoneum that in the fetus is responsible for the formation of the inguinal canal [see page 165]). It follows that the sac enters the inguinal canal through the deep inguinal ring lateral to the inferior epigastric vessels (Fig. 4-41). It may extend part of the way along the canal or the full length, as far as the superficial inguinal ring. If the processus vaginalis has undergone no obliteration, then the hernia is complete and extends through the superficial inguinal ring down into the scrotum or labium majus. Under these circumstances the neck of the hernial sac lies at the deep inguinal ring lateral to the inferior epigastric vessels, and the body of the sac resides in the inguinal canal and scrotum (or base of labium majus).

An indirect inguinal hernia is about 20 times more common in males than in females, and nearly one third are bilateral. It is more common on the right (normally, the right processus vaginalis becomes obliterated after the left; the right testis descends later than the left). It is most common in children and young adults.

The indirect inguinal hernia can be summarized as follows:

- It is the remains of the processus vaginalis and therefore is congenital in origin.
- It is more common than a direct inguinal hernia.
- It is much more common in males than females.
- It is more common on the right side.
- It is most common in children and young adults.
- The hernial sac enters the inguinal canal through the deep inguinal ring and lateral to the inferior epigastric vessels. The neck of the sac is narrow.

(continues)

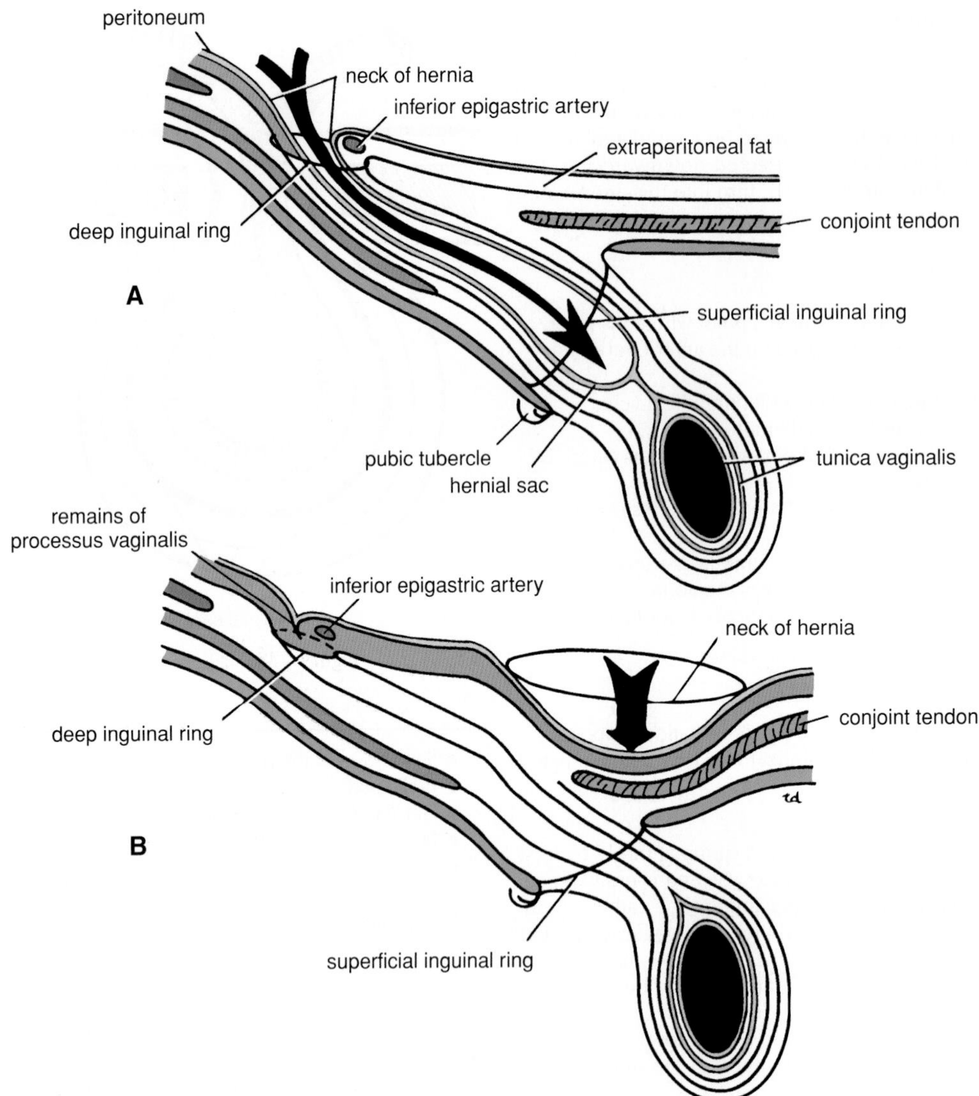

Figure 4-41 **A.** Indirect inguinal hernia. **B.** Direct inguinal hernia. Note that the neck of the indirect inguinal hernia lies lateral to the inferior epigastric artery, and the neck of the direct inguinal hernia lies medial to the inferior epigastric artery.

Clinical Notes, *continued*

- The hernial sac may extend through the superficial inguinal ring above and medial to the pubic tubercle. (Femoral hernia is located below and lateral to the pubic tubercle.)
- The hernial sac may extend down into the scrotum or labium majus.

Direct Inguinal Hernia

The direct inguinal hernia makes up about 15% of all inguinal hernias. The sac of a direct hernia bulges directly anteriorly through the posterior wall of the inguinal canal medial to the inferior epigastric vessels (Fig. 4-41B). Because of the presence of the strong conjoint tendon (combined tendons of insertion of the internal oblique and transversus muscles), this hernia is usually nothing more than a generalized bulge; therefore, the neck of the hernial sac is wide.

Direct inguinal hernias are rare in women and most are bilateral. It is a disease of old men with weak abdominal muscles.

A direct inguinal hernia can be summarized as follows:

- It is common in old men with weak abdominal muscles and is rare in women.
- The hernial sac bulges forward through the posterior wall of the inguinal canal medial to the inferior epigastric vessels.
- The neck of the hernial sac is wide.

An inguinal hernia can be distinguished from a femoral hernia by the fact that the sac, as it emerges through the superficial inguinal ring, lies above and medial to the pubic tubercle, whereas that of a femoral hernia lies below and lateral to the tubercle (Fig. 4-42).

Femoral Hernia

The hernial sac descends through the femoral canal within the femoral sheath, creating a femoral hernia. The femoral sheath, which is fully described on page 579, is a protrusion of the fascial

(continues)

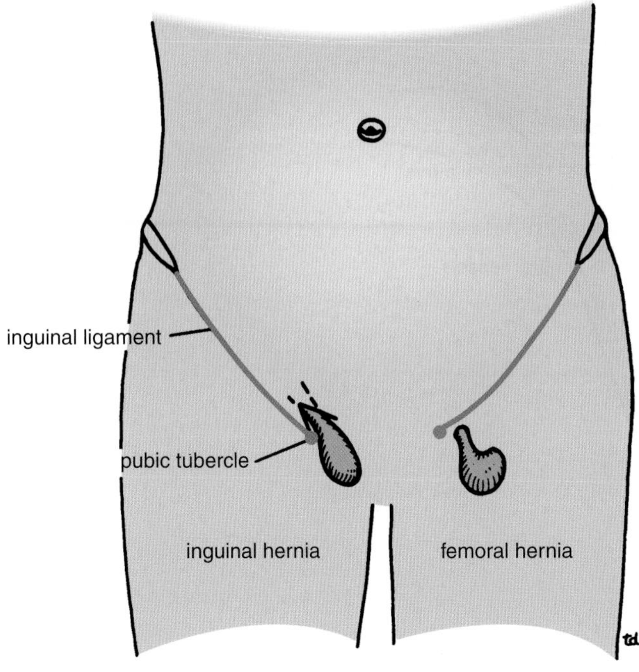

Figure 4-42 Relation of inguinal and femoral hernial sacs to the pubic tubercle.

Clinical Notes, *continued*

envelope lining the abdominal walls and surrounds the femoral vessels and lymphatics for about 1 in. (2.5 cm) below the inguinal ligament (Fig. 4-43). The **femoral artery,** as it enters the thigh below the inguinal ligament, occupies the lateral compartment of the sheath. The **femoral vein,** which lies on its medial side and is separated from it by a fibrous septum, occupies the intermediate compartment. The **lymph vessels,** which are separated from the vein by a fibrous septum, occupy the most medial compartment. The **femoral canal,** the compartment for the lymphatics, occupies the medial part of the sheath. It is about 0.5 in. (1.3 cm) long, and its upper opening is referred to as the **femoral ring.** The **femoral septum,** which is a condensation of extraperitoneal tissue, plugs the opening of the femoral ring.

A femoral hernia is more common in women than in men (possibly because of a wider pelvis and femoral canal). The hernial sac passes down the femoral canal, pushing the femoral septum before it. On escaping through the lower end, it expands to form a swelling in the upper part of the thigh deep to the deep fascia (Fig. 4-43). With further expansion, the hernial sac may turn upward to cross the anterior surface of the inguinal ligament.

The neck of the sac always lies below and lateral to the **pubic tubercle** (Fig. 4-42), which serves to distinguish it from an inguinal hernia. The neck of the sac is narrow and lies at the femoral ring. The ring is related anteriorly to the inguinal ligament, posteriorly to the pectineal ligament and the pubis, medially to the sharp free edge of the lacunar ligament, and laterally to the femoral vein. Because of the presence of these anatomic structures, the neck of the sac is unable to expand. Once an abdominal viscus has passed through the neck into the body of the sac, it may be difficult to push it up and return it to the abdominal cavity (**irreducible hernia**). Furthermore, after straining or coughing, a piece of bowel may be forced through the neck and its blood vessels may be compressed by the femoral ring, seriously impairing its blood supply (**strangulated hernia**). A femoral hernia is a dangerous disease and should always be treated surgically.

A femoral hernia can be summarized as follows:

- It is a protrusion of abdominal parietal peritoneum down through the femoral canal to form the hernial sac.
- It is more common in women than in men.
- The neck of the hernial sac lies below and lateral to the pubic tubercle.
- The neck of the hernial sac lies at the femoral ring and at that point is related anteriorly to the inguinal ligament, posteriorly to the pectineal ligament and the pubis, laterally to the femoral vein, and medially to the sharp free edge of the lacunar ligament.

Umbilical Herniae

Congenital umbilical hernia, or exomphalos (omphalocele), is caused by a failure of part of the midgut to return to the abdominal cavity from the extraembryonic coelom during fetal life. The hernial sac and its relationship to the umbilical cord are shown in Figure 4-44.

Acquired infantile umbilical hernia is a small hernia that sometimes occurs in children and is caused by a weakness in the scar of the umbilicus in the linea alba (Fig. 4-44). Most become smaller and disappear without treatment as the abdominal cavity enlarges.

Acquired umbilical hernia of adults is more correctly referred to as a **paraumbilical hernia.** The hernial sac does not protrude through the umbilical scar, but through the linea alba in the region of the umbilicus (Fig. 4-44). Paraumbilical herniae gradually increase in size and hang downward. The neck of the sac may be narrow, but the body of the sac often contains coils of small and large intestine and omentum. Paraumbilical herniae are much more common in women than in men.

Epigastric Hernia

Epigastric hernia occurs through the widest part of the linea alba, anywhere between the xiphoid process and the umbilicus. The

(continues)

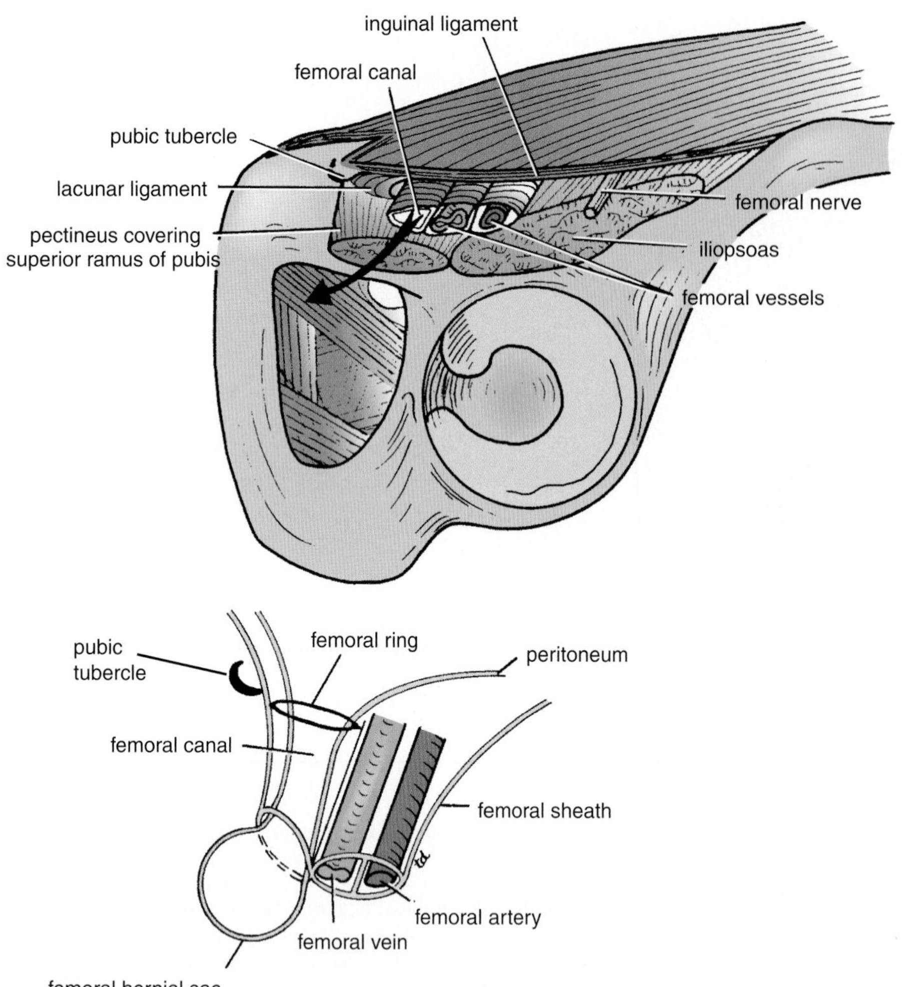

Figure 4-43 The femoral sheath as seen from below. Arrow emerging from the femoral canal indicates the path taken by the femoral hernial sac. Note relations of the femoral ring.

Clinical Notes, *continued*

hernia is usually small and starts off as a small protrusion of extraperitoneal fat between the fibers of the linea alba. During the following months or years the fat is forced farther through the linea alba and eventually drags behind it a small peritoneal sac. The body of the sac often contains a small piece of greater omentum. It is common in middle-aged manual workers.

Separation of the Recti Abdominis

Separation of the recti abdominis occurs in elderly multiparous women with weak abdominal muscles (Fig. 4-44). In this condition, the aponeuroses forming the rectus sheath become excessively stretched. When the patient coughs or strains, the recti separate widely, and a large hernial sac, containing abdominal viscera, bulges forward between the medial margins of the recti. This can be corrected by wearing a suitable abdominal belt.

Incisional Hernia

A postoperative incisional hernia is most likely to occur in patients in whom it was necessary to cut one of the segmental nerves supplying the muscles of the anterior abdominal wall; postoperative wound infection with death (necrosis) of the abdominal musculature is also a common cause. The neck of the sac is usually large, and adhesion and strangulation of its contents are rare complications. In very obese individuals the extent of the abdominal wall weakness is often difficult to assess.

Hernia of the Linea Semilunaris (Spigelian Hernia)

The uncommon hernia of the linea semilunaris occurs through the aponeurosis of the transversus abdominis just lateral to the lateral edge of the rectus sheath. It usually occurs just below the level of the umbilicus. The neck of the sac is narrow, so that adhesion and strangulation of its contents are common complications.

Lumbar Hernia

The lumbar hernia occurs through the lumbar triangle and is rare. The lumbar triangle (Petit's triangle) is a weak area in the posterior part of the abdominal wall. It is bounded anteriorly by the posterior margin of the external oblique muscle, posteriorly by the anterior border of the latissimus dorsi muscle, and inferiorly by the iliac crest. The floor of the triangle is formed by the internal oblique and the transversus abdominis muscles. The neck of the hernia is usually large, and the incidence of strangulation low.

Internal Hernia

Occasionally, a loop of intestine enters a peritoneal recess (e.g., the lesser sac or the duodenal recesses) and becomes strangulated at the edges of the recess (see page 214).

Abdominal Stab Wounds

Abdominal stab wounds may or may not penetrate the parietal peritoneum and violate the peritoneal cavity and consequently may or may not significantly damage the abdominal viscera. The

(continues)

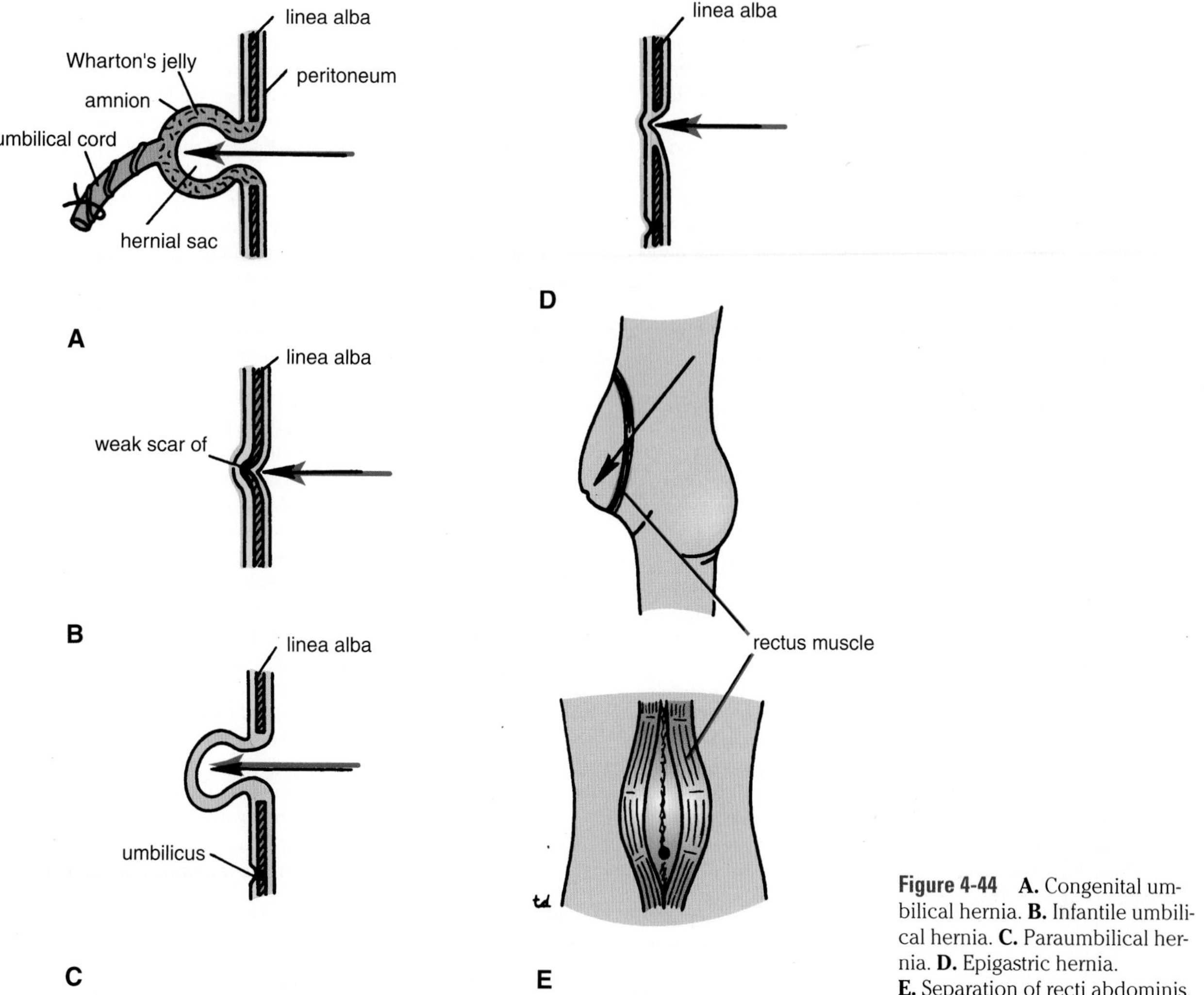

Figure 4-44 **A.** Congenital umbilical hernia. **B.** Infantile umbilical hernia. **C.** Paraumbilical hernia. **D.** Epigastric hernia. **E.** Separation of recti abdominis.

Clinical Notes, *continued*

structures in the various layers through which an abdominal stab wound penetrates depend on the anatomic location.

Lateral to the rectus sheath are the following: skin, fatty layer of superficial fascia, membranous layer of superficial fascia, thin layer of deep fascia, external oblique muscle or aponeurosis, internal oblique muscle or aponeurosis, transversus abdominis muscle or aponeurosis, fascia transversalis, extraperitoneal connective tissue (often fatty), and parietal peritoneum.

Anterior to the rectus sheath are the following: skin, fatty layer of superficial fascia, membranous layer of superficial fascia, thin layer of deep fascia, anterior wall of rectus sheath, rectus abdominis muscle with segmental nerves and epigastric vessels lying behind the muscle, posterior wall of rectus sheath, fascia transversalis, extraperitoneal connective tissue (often fatty), and parietal peritoneum.

In the midline are the following: skin, fatty layer of superficial fascia, membranous layer of superficial fascia, thin layer of deep fascia, fibrous linea alba, fascia transversalis, extraperitoneal connective tissue (often fatty), and parietal peritoneum.

In an abdominal stab wound, washing out the peritoneal cavity with saline solution (**peritoneal lavage**) can be used to determine whether any damage to viscera or blood vessels has occurred.

Abdominal Gunshot Wounds

Gunshot wounds are much more serious than stab wounds; in most patients, the peritoneal cavity has been entered, and significant visceral damage has ensued.

Surgical Incisions

The length and direction of surgical incisions through the anterior abdominal wall to expose the underlying viscera are largely governed by the position and direction of the nerves of the abdominal wall, the direction of the muscle fibers, and the arrangement of the aponeuroses forming the rectus sheath. Ideally, the incision should be made in the direction of the lines of cleavage in the skin so that a hairline scar is produced. The surgeon usually has to compromise, placing the safety of the patient first and the cosmetic result second.

Incisions that necessitate the division of one of the main segmental nerves lying within the abdominal wall result in paralysis of part of the anterior abdominal musculature and a segment of the rectus abdominis. The consequent weakness of the abdominal musculature causes an unsightly bulging forward of the abdominal wall and visceroptosis; extreme cases may require a surgical belt for support.

If the incision can be made in the line of the muscle fibers or aponeurotic fibers as each layer is traversed, on closing the incision the fibers fall back into position and function normally.

Incisions through the rectus sheath are widely used, provided that the rectus abdominis muscle and its nerve supply are kept intact. On closure of the incisions, the anterior and posterior walls of the sheath are sutured separately, and the rectus muscle springs back into position between the suture lines. The result is a very strong repair, with minimum interference with function.

(continues)

Clinical Notes, *continued*

The following incisions are commonly used.

- **Paramedian incision:** This may be supraumbilical, for exposure of the upper part of the abdominal cavity, or infraumbilical, for the lower abdomen and pelvis. In extensive operations in which a large exposure is required, the incision can run the full length of the rectus sheath. The anterior wall of the rectus sheath is exposed and incised about 1 in. (2.5 cm) from the midline. The medial edge of the incision is dissected medially, freeing the anterior wall of the sheath from the tendinous intersections of the rectus muscle. The rectus abdominis muscle is retracted laterally with its nerve supply intact, and the posterior wall of the sheath is exposed. The posterior wall is then incised, together with the fascia transversalis and the peritoneum. The wound is closed in layers.
- **Pararectus incision:** The anterior wall of the rectus sheath is incised medially and parallel to the lateral margin of the rectus muscle. The rectus is freed and retracted medially, exposing the segmental nerves entering its posterior surface. If the opening into the abdominal cavity is to be small, these nerves may be retracted upward and downward. The posterior wall of the sheath is then incised, as in the paramedian incision. The great disadvantage of this incision is that the opening is small, and any longitudinal extension requires that one or more segmental nerves to the rectus abdominis be divided, with resultant postoperative rectus muscle weakness.
- **Midline incision:** This incision is made through the linea alba. The fascia transversalis, the extraperitoneal connective tissue, and the peritoneum are then incised. It is easier to perform above the umbilicus because the linea alba is wider in that region. It is a rapid method of gaining entrance to the abdomen and has the obvious advantage that it does not damage muscles or their nerve and blood supplies. Midline incision has the additional advantage that it may be converted into a T-shaped incision for greater exposure. The anterior and posterior walls of the rectus sheath are then cut across transversely, and the rectus muscle is retracted laterally.
- **Transrectus incision:** The technique of making and closing of this incision is the same as that used in the paramedian incision, except that the rectus abdominis muscle is incised longitudinally and not retracted laterally from the midline. This incision has the great disadvantage of sectioning the nerve supply to that part of the muscle that lies medial to the muscle incision.
- **Transverse incision:** This can be made above or below the umbilicus and can be small or so large that it extends from flank to flank. It can be made through the rectus sheath and the rectus abdominis muscles and through the oblique and transversus abdominis muscles laterally. It is rare to damage more than one segmental nerve so that postoperative abdominal weakness is minimal. The incision gives good exposure and is well tolerated by the patient. Closure of the wound is made in layers. It is unnecessary to suture the cut ends of the rectus muscles, provided that the sheaths are carefully repaired.
- **Muscle splitting,** or McBurney's incision: This is chiefly used for cecostomy and appendectomy. It gives a limited exposure only, and should any doubt arise about the diagnosis, an infraumbilical right paramedian incision should be used instead.

An oblique skin incision is made in the right iliac region about 2 in. (5 cm) above and medial to the anterior superior iliac spine. The external and internal oblique and transversus muscles are incised or split in the line of their fibers and retracted to expose the fascia transversalis and the peritoneum. The latter are now incised and the abdominal cavity is opened. The incision is closed in layers, with no postoperative weakness.

- **Abdominothoracic incision:** This is used to expose the lower end of the esophagus, as, for example, in esophagogastric resection for carcinoma of this region. An upper oblique or paramedian abdominal incision is extended upward and laterally into the seventh, eighth, or ninth intercostal space, the costal arch is transected, and the diaphragm is incised. Wide exposure of the upper abdomen and thorax is then obtained by the use of a rib-spreading retractor.

On completion of the operation, the diaphragm is repaired with nonabsorbable sutures, the costal margin is reconstructed, and the abdominal and thoracic wounds are closed.

Paracentesis of the Abdomen

Paracentesis of the abdomen may be necessary to withdraw excessive collections of peritoneal fluid, as in ascites secondary to cirrhosis of the liver or malignant ascites secondary to advanced ovarian cancer. Under a local anesthetic, a needle or catheter is inserted through the anterior abdominal wall. The underlying coils of intestine are not damaged because they are mobile and are pushed away by the cannula.

(continues)

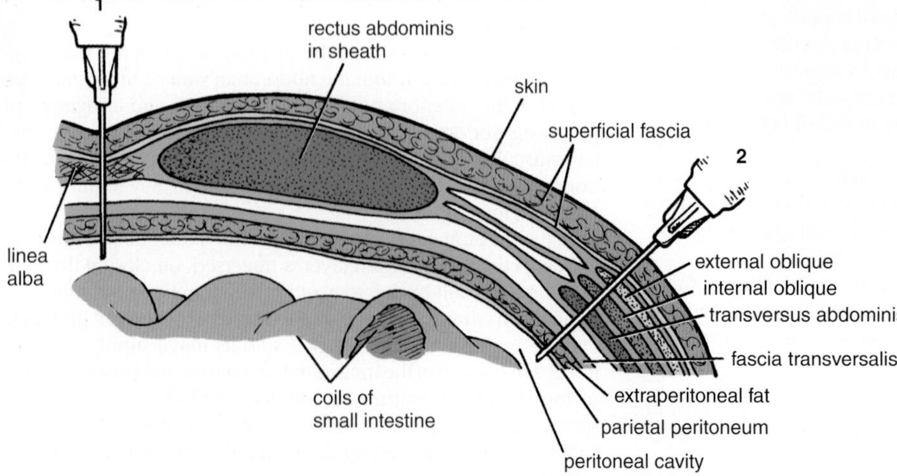

Figure 4-45 Paracentesis of the abdominal cavity in midline **(1)** and laterally **(2).**

Clinical Notes, *continued*

If the cannula is inserted in the midline (Fig. 4-45), it will pass through the following anatomic structures: skin, superficial fascia, deep fascia (very thin), linea alba (virtually bloodless), fascia transversalis, extraperitoneal connective tissue (fatty), and parietal peritoneum.

If the cannula is inserted in the flank (Fig. 4-45) lateral to the inferior epigastric artery and above the deep circumflex artery, it will pass through the following: skin, superficial fascia, deep fascia (very thin), aponeurosis or muscle of external oblique, internal oblique muscle, transversus abdominis muscle, fascia transversalis, extraperitoneal connective tissue (fatty), and parietal peritoneum.

Anatomy of Peritoneal Lavage

Peritoneal lavage is used to sample the intraperitoneal space for evidence of damage to viscera and blood vessels. It is generally employed as a diagnostic technique in certain cases of blunt abdominal trauma. In nontrauma situations, peritoneal lavage has been used to confirm the diagnosis of acute pancreatitis and primary peritonitis, to correct hypothermia, and to conduct dialysis.

The patient is placed in the supine position and the urinary bladder is emptied by catheterization. In small children the bladder is an abdominal organ (see page 348); in adults, the full bladder may rise out of the pelvis and reach as high as the umbilicus (see page 330). The stomach is emptied by a nasogastric tube because a distended stomach may extend to the anterior abdominal wall. The skin is anesthetized and a 2.25-in. (3-cm) vertical incision is made.

Midline Incision Technique

The following anatomic structures are penetrated, in order, to reach the parietal peritoneum (Fig. 4-46): skin, fatty layer of

(continues)

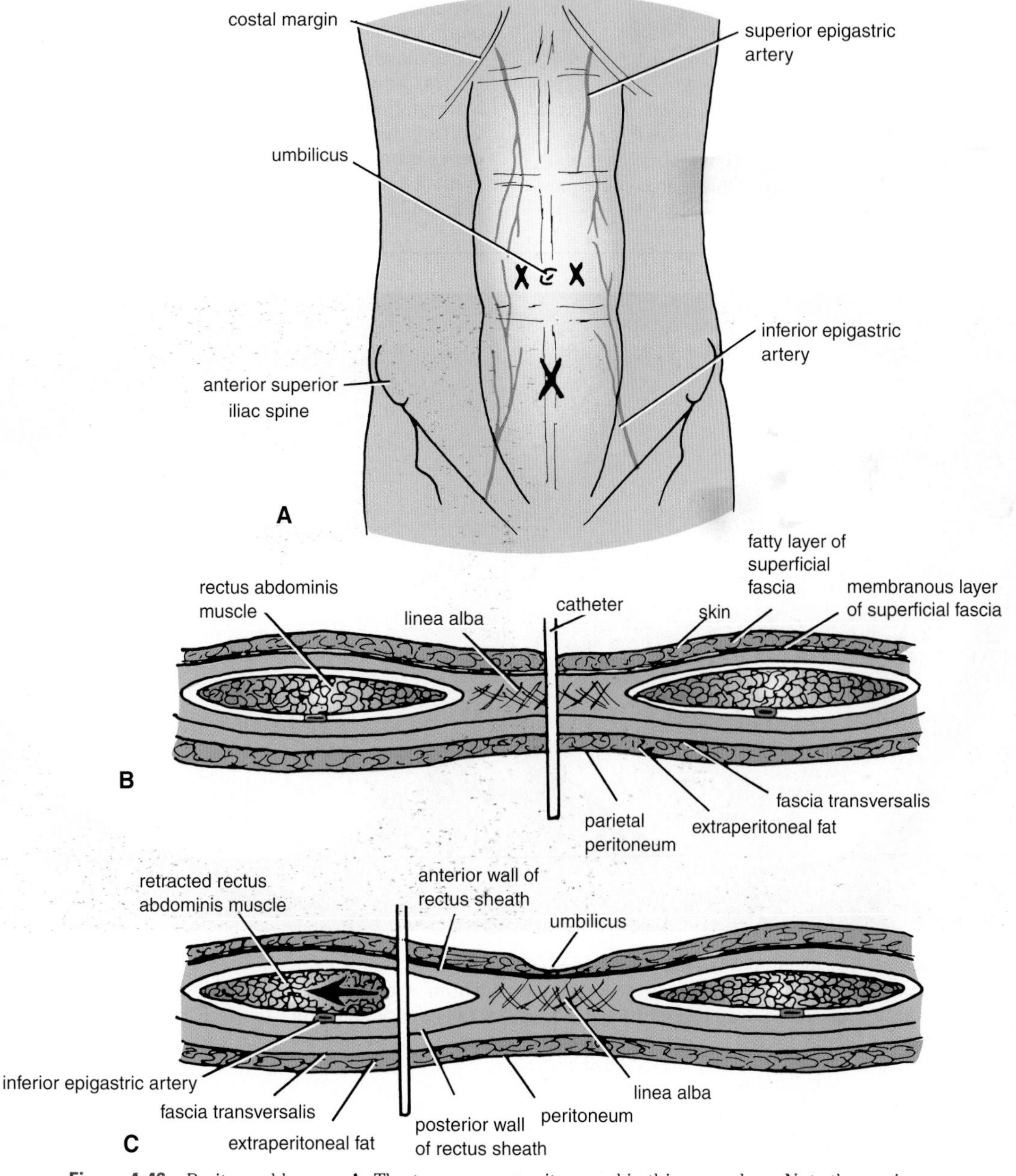

Figure 4-46 Peritoneal lavage. **A.** The two common sites used in this procedure. Note the positions of the superior and inferior epigastric arteries in the rectus sheath. **B.** Cross section of the anterior abdominal wall in the midline. Note the structures pierced by the catheter. **C.** Cross section of the anterior abdominal wall just lateral to the umbilicus. Note the structures pierced by the catheter. The rectus muscle has been retracted laterally.

Clinical Notes, *continued*

superficial fascia, membranous layer of superficial fascia, thin layer of deep fascia, linea alba, fascia transversalis, extraperitoneal fat, and parietal peritoneum.

Paraumbilical Incision Technique

The following anatomic structures are penetrated, in order, to reach the parietal peritoneum (Fig. 4-46): skin, fatty layer of superficial fascia, membranous layer of superficial fascia, thin layer of deep fascia, anterior wall of rectus sheath, the rectus abdominis muscle is retracted, posterior wall of the rectus sheath, fascia transversalis, extraperitoneal fat, and parietal peritoneum.

It is important that all the small blood vessels in the superficial fascia be secured, because bleeding into the peritoneal cavity might produce a false-positive result. These vessels are the terminal branches of the superficial and deep epigastric arteries and veins.

Anatomy of the Complications of Peritoneal Lavage

- In the midline technique, the incision or trocar may miss the linea alba, enter the rectus sheath, traverse the vascular rectus abdominis muscle and encounter branches of the epigastric vessels. Bleeding from this source could produce a false-positive result.
- Perforation of the gut by the scalpel or trocar
- Perforation of the mesenteric blood vessels or vessels on the posterior abdominal wall or pelvic walls
- Perforation of a full bladder
- Wound infection

Endoscopic Surgery

Endoscopic surgery on the gallbladder, bile ducts, and the appendix has become a common procedure. It involves the passage of the endoscope into the peritoneal cavity through small incisions in the anterior abdominal wall. The anatomic structures traversed by the instruments are similar to those enumerated for peritoneal lavage. Great care must be taken to preserve the integrity of the segmental nerves as they course down from the costal margin to supply the abdominal musculature.

The advantages of this surgical technique are that the anatomic and physiologic features of the anterior abdominal wall are disrupted only minimally and, consequently, convalescence is brief. The great disadvantages are that the surgical field is small and the surgeon is limited in the extent of the operation (Fig. 4-47).

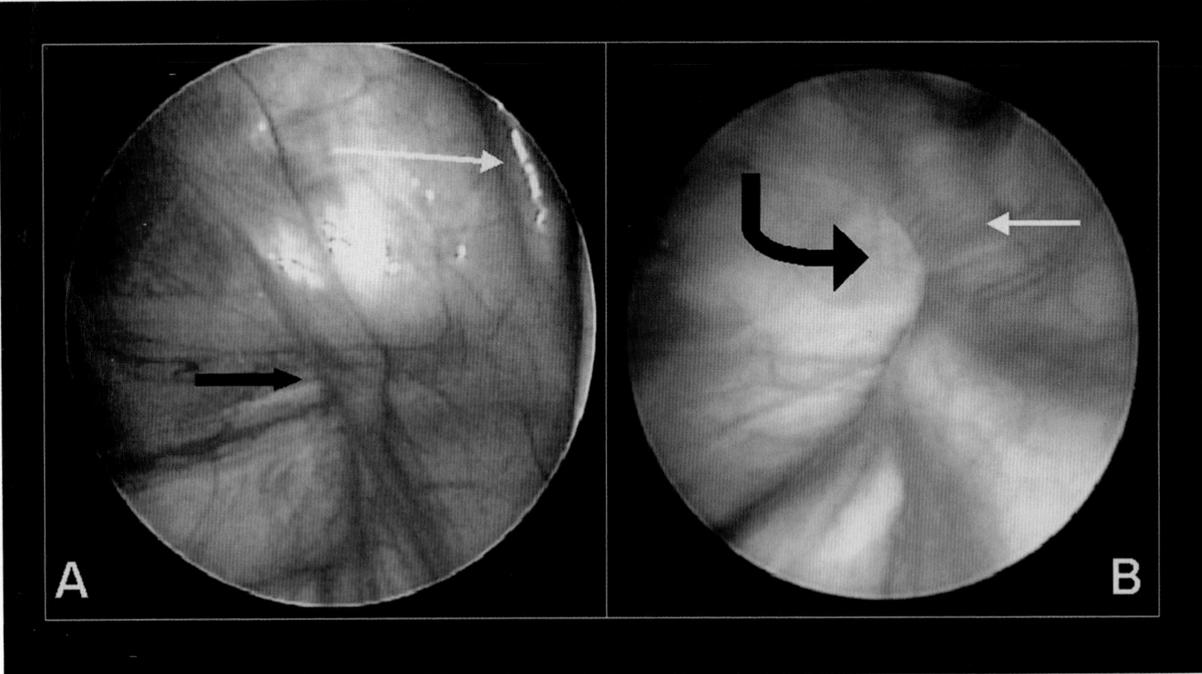

Figure 4-47 Inguinal canal anatomy as viewed during laparoscopic exploration of the peritoneal cavity. **A.** The normal anatomy of the inguinal region from within the peritoneal cavity. *Black arrow* indicates the closed deep inguinal ring; white arrow, the inferior epigastric vessels. **B.** An indirect inguinal hernia. *Curved black arrow* indicates the mouth of the hernial sac; *white arrow*, the inferior epigastric vessels. (Courtesy of N.S. Adzick.)

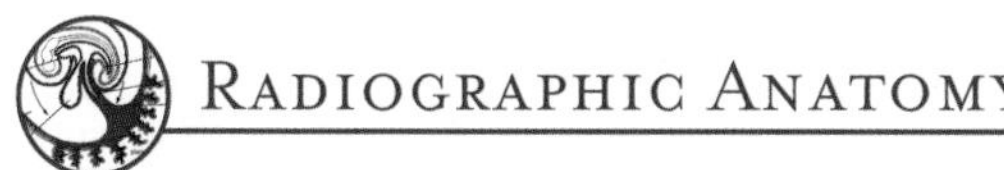

Radiographic Anatomy

For a detailed discussion, see page 282.

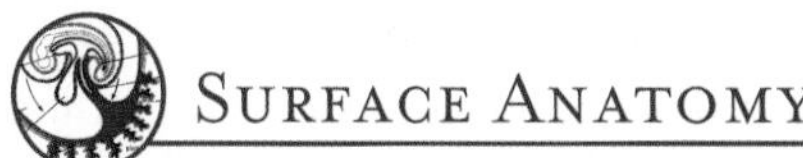

Surface Anatomy

Surface Landmarks of the Abdominal Wall

Xiphoid Process

The xiphoid process is the thin cartilaginous lower part of the sternum. It is easily palpated in the depression where the costal margins meet in the upper part of the anterior abdominal wall (Figs. 4-11 and 4-12). The **xiphisternal junction** is identified by feeling the lower edge of the body of the sternum, and it lies opposite the body of the ninth thoracic vertebra.

Costal Margin

The costal margin is the curved lower margin of the thoracic wall and is formed in front by the cartilages of the 7th, 8th, 9th, and 10th ribs (Figs. 4-11 and 4-12) and behind by the cartilages of the 11th and 12th ribs. The costal margin reaches its lowest level at the 10th costal cartilage, which lies opposite the body of the third lumbar vertebra. The 12th rib may be short and difficult to palpate.

Iliac Crest

The iliac crest can be felt along its entire length and ends in front at the **anterior superior iliac spine** (Figs. 4-11 and 4-12) and behind at the **posterior superior iliac spine** (Fig. 4-49). Its highest point lies opposite the body of the fourth lumbar vertebra.

About 2 in. (5 cm) posterior to the anterior superior iliac spine, the outer margin projects to form the tubercle of the crest (Fig. 4-12). The tubercle lies at the level of the body of the fifth lumbar vertebra.

Pubic Tubercle

The pubic tubercle is an important surface landmark. It may be identified as a small protuberance along the superior surface of the pubis (Figs. 4-3, 4-12, and 4-32).

Symphysis Pubis

The symphysis pubis is the cartilaginous joint that lies in the midline between the bodies of the pubic bones (Fig. 4-11). It is felt as a solid structure beneath the skin in the midline at the lower extremity of the anterior abdominal wall. The **pubic crest** is the name given to the ridge on the superior surface of the pubic bones medial to the pubic tubercle (Fig. 4-32).

Inguinal Ligament

The inguinal ligament lies beneath a skin crease in the groin. It is the rolled-under inferior margin of the aponeurosis of the external oblique muscle (Figs. 4-2, 4-6, and 4-11). It is attached laterally to the anterior superior iliac spine and curves downward and medially, to be attached to the pubic tubercle.

Superficial Inguinal Ring

The superficial inguinal ring is a triangular aperture in the aponeurosis of the external oblique muscle and is situated above and medial to the pubic tubercle (Figs. 4-2, 4-3, 4-8, and 4-12). In the adult male, the margins of the ring can be felt by invaginating the skin of the upper part of the scrotum with the tip of the little finger. The soft tubular **spermatic cord** can be felt emerging from the ring and descending over or medial to the pubic tubercle into the scrotum (Fig. 4-8). Palpate the spermatic cord in the upper part of the scrotum between the finger and thumb and note the presence of a firm cordlike structure in its posterior part called the **vas deferens** (Figs. 4-5 and 4-21).

In the female, the superficial inguinal ring is smaller and difficult to palpate; it transmits the round ligament of the uterus.

Scrotum

The scrotum is a pouch of skin and fascia containing the testes, the epididymides, and the lower ends of the spermatic cords. The skin of the scrotum is wrinkled and is covered with sparse hairs. The bilateral origin of the scrotum is indicated by the presence of a dark line in the midline, called the **scrotal raphe,** along the line of fusion. The **testis** on each side is a firm ovoid body surrounded on its lateral, anterior, and medial surfaces by the two layers of the **tunica vaginalis** (Fig. 4-21). The testis should therefore lie free and not tethered to the skin or subcutaneous tissue. Posterior to the testis is an elongated structure, the **epididymis** (Fig. 4-21). It has an enlarged upper end called the **head,** a **body,** and a narrow lower end, the **tail.** The vas deferens emerges from the tail and ascends medial to the epididymis to enter the spermatic cord at the upper end of the scrotum.

Linea Alba

The linea alba is a vertically running fibrous band that extends from the symphysis pubis to the xiphoid process and lies in the midline (Fig. 4-3). It is formed by the fusion of the aponeuroses of the muscles of the anterior abdominal wall and is represented on the surface by a slight median groove (Figs. 4-11 and 4-12).

Umbilicus

The umbilicus lies in the linea alba and is inconstant in position. It is a puckered scar and is the site of attachment of the umbilical cord in the fetus.

Rectus Abdominis

The rectus abdominis muscles lie on either side of the linea alba (Fig. 4-11) and run vertically in the abdominal wall; they can be made prominent by asking the patient to raise the shoulders while in the supine position without using the arms.

Tendinous Intersections of the Rectus Abdominis

The tendinous intersections are three in number and run across the rectus abdominis muscle. In muscular individuals they can be palpated as transverse depressions at the level of the tip of the xiphoid process, at the umbilicus, and halfway between the two (Fig. 4-11).

Linea Semilunaris

The linea semilunaris is the lateral edge of the rectus abdominis muscle and crosses the costal margin at the tip of the ninth costal cartilage (Figs. 4-11 and 4-12). To accentuate the semilunar lines, the patient is asked to lie on the back and raise the shoulders off the couch without using the arms. To accomplish this, the patient contracts the rectus abdominis muscles so that their lateral edges stand out.

Abdominal Lines and Planes

Vertical lines and horizontal planes (Fig. 4-12) are commonly used to facilitate the description of the location of diseased structures or the performing of abdominal procedures.

Vertical Lines

Each vertical line (right and left) passes through the midpoint between the anterior superior iliac spine and the symphysis pubis.

Transpyloric Plane

The horizontal transpyloric plane passes through the tips of the ninth costal cartilages on the two sides—that is, the point where the lateral margin of the rectus abdominis (linea semilunaris) crosses the costal margin (Fig. 4-12). It lies at the level of the body of the first lumbar vertebra. This plane passes through the pylorus of the stomach, the duodenojejunal junction, the neck of the pancreas, and the hila of the kidneys.

Subcostal Plane

The horizontal subcostal plane joins the lowest point of the costal margin on each side—that is, the 10th costal cartilage (Fig. 4-12). This plane lies at the level of the third lumbar vertebra.

Intercristal Plane

The intercristal plane passes across the highest points on the iliac crests and lies on the level of the body of the fourth lumbar vertebra. This is commonly used as a surface landmark when performing a lumbar spinal tap (see page 871).

Intertubercular Plane

The horizontal intertubercular plane joins the tubercles on the iliac crests (Fig. 4-12) and lies at the level of the fifth lumbar vertebra.

Abdominal Quadrants

It is common practice to divide the abdomen into quadrants by using a vertical and a horizontal line that intersect at the umbilicus (Fig. 4-12). The quadrants are the upper right, upper left, lower right, and lower left. The terms **epigastrium** and **periumbilical** are loosely used to indicate the area below the xiphoid process and above the umbilicus and the area around the umbilicus, respectively.

Surface Landmarks of the Abdominal Viscera

It must be emphasized that the positions of most of the abdominal viscera show individual variations as well as variations in the same person at different times. Posture and respiration have a profound influence on the position of viscera.

The following organs are more or less fixed, and their surface markings are of clinical value.

Liver

The liver lies under cover of the lower ribs, and most of its bulk lies on the right side (Fig. 4-48). In infants, until about the end of the third year, the lower margin of the liver extends one or two fingerbreadths below the costal margin (Fig. 4-48). In the adult who is obese or has a well-developed right rectus abdominis muscle, the liver is not palpable. In a thin adult, the lower edge of the liver may be felt a fingerbreadth below the costal margin. It is most easily felt when the patient inspires deeply and the diaphragm contracts and pushes down the liver.

Gallbladder

The fundus of the gallbladder lies opposite the tip of the right ninth costal cartilage—that is, where the lateral edge of the right rectus abdominis muscle crosses the costal margin (Fig. 4-48).

Spleen

The spleen is situated in the left upper quadrant and lies under cover of the 9th, 10th, and 11th ribs (Fig. 4-48). Its long axis corresponds to that of the 10th rib, and in the adult it does not normally project forward in front of the midaxillary line. In infants, the lower pole of the spleen may just be felt (Fig. 4-48).

Pancreas

The pancreas lies across the transpyloric plane. The head lies below and to the right, the neck lies on the plane, and the body and tail lie above and to the left.

Kidneys

The right kidney lies at a slightly lower level than the left kidney (because of the bulk of the right lobe of the liver), and the lower pole can be palpated in the right lumbar region at the end of deep inspiration in a person with poorly developed abdominal muscles. Each kidney moves about 1 in. (2.5 cm) in a vertical direction during full respiratory movement of the diaphragm. The normal left kidney, which is higher than the right kidney, is not palpable.

On the anterior abdominal wall the hilum of each kidney lies on the transpyloric plane, about three fingerbreadths from the midline (Fig. 4-49). On the back, the kidneys extend from the 12th thoracic spine to the third lumbar spine, and the hili are opposite the first lumbar vertebra (Fig. 4-49).

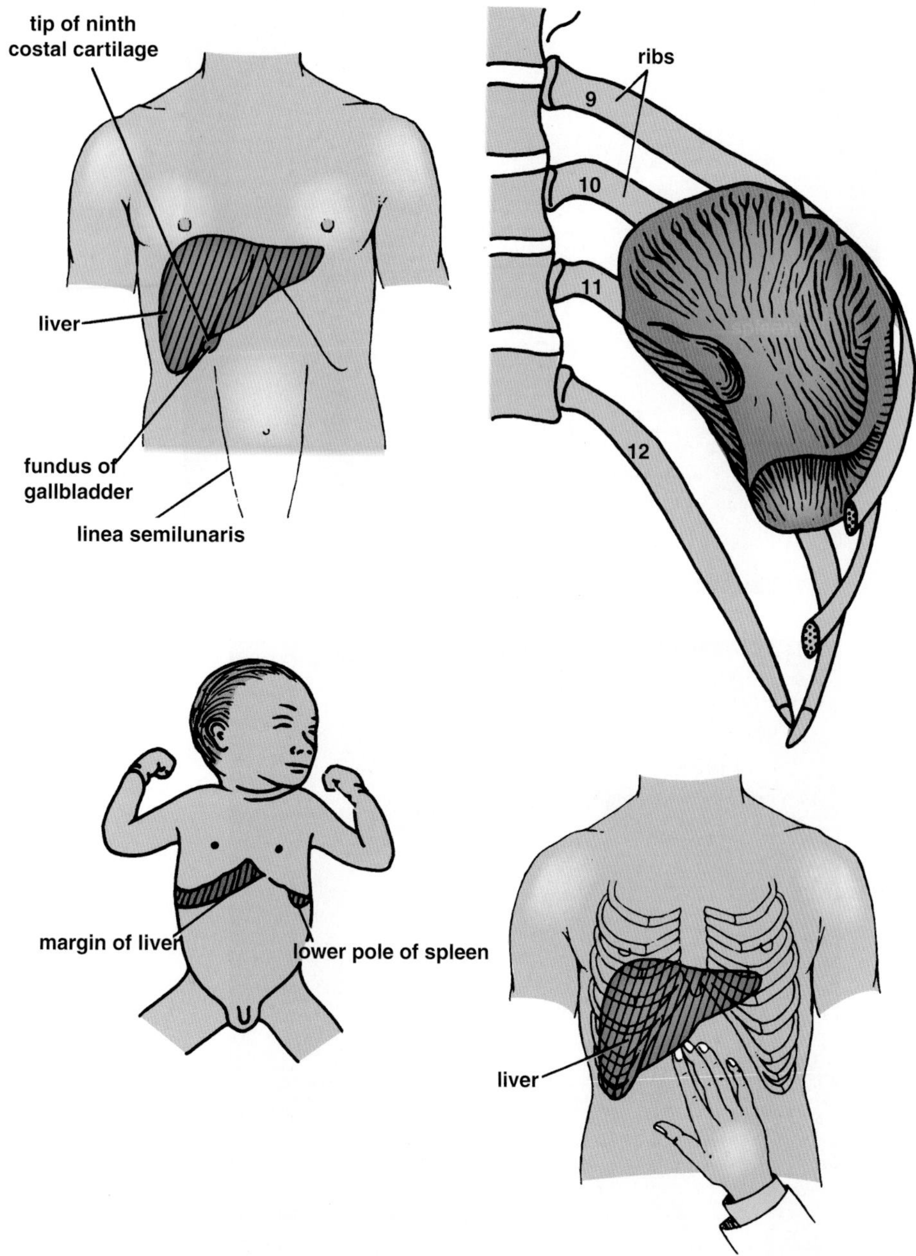

Figure 4-48 Surface markings of the fundus of the gallbladder, spleen, and liver. In a young child, the lower margin of the normal liver and the lower pole of the normal spleen can be palpated. In a thin adult, the lower margin of the normal liver may just be felt at the end of deep inspiration.

Stomach

The **cardioesophageal junction** lies about three fingerbreadths below and to the left of the xiphisternal junction (the esophagus pierces the diaphragm at the level of the 10th thoracic vertebra).

The **pylorus** lies on the transpyloric plane just to the right of the midline. The **lesser curvature** lies on a curved line joining the cardioesophageal junction and the pylorus. The **greater curvature** has an extremely variable position in the umbilical region or below.

Duodenum (First Part)

The duodenum lies on the transpyloric plane about four fingerbreadths to the right of the midline.

Cecum

The cecum is situated in the right lower quadrant. It is often distended with gas and gives a resonant sound when percussed. It can be palpated through the anterior abdominal wall.

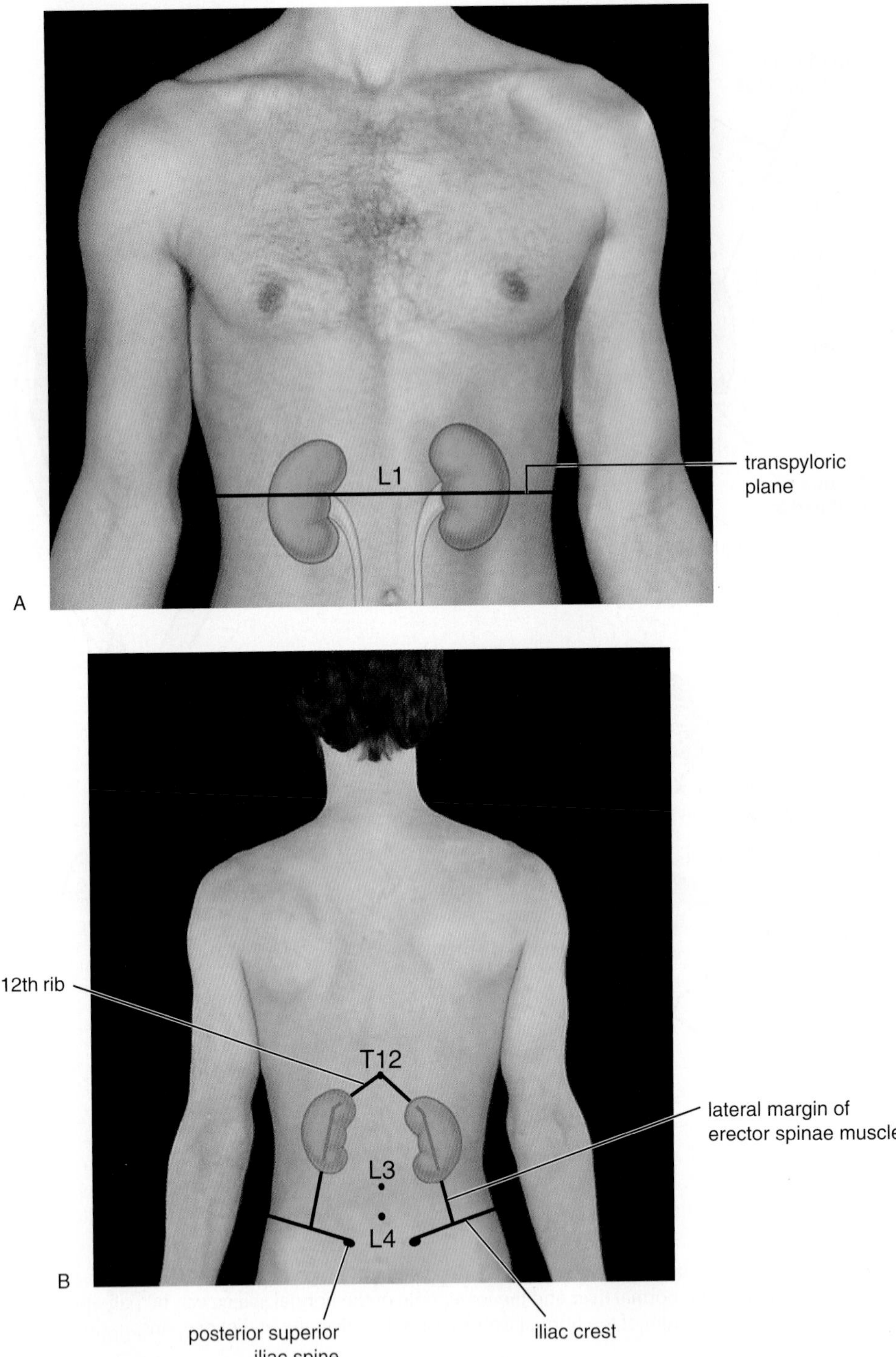

Figure 4-49 **A.** Surface anatomy of the kidneys and ureters on the anterior abdominal wall. Note the relationship of the hilum of each kidney to the transpyloric plane. **B.** Surface anatomy of the kidneys on the posterior abdominal wall.

Appendix

The appendix lies in the right lower quadrant. The base of the appendix is situated one third of the way up the line, joining the anterior superior iliac spine to the umbilicus (McBurney's point). The position of the free end of the appendix is variable.

Ascending Colon

The ascending colon extends upward from the cecum on the lateral side of the right vertical line and disappears under the right costal margin. It can be palpated through the anterior abdominal wall.

Transverse Colon

The transverse colon extends across the abdomen, occupying the umbilical region. It arches downward with its concavity directed upward. Because it has a mesentery, its position is variable.

Descending Colon

The descending colon extends downward from the left costal margin on the lateral side of the left vertical line. In the left lower quadrant it curves medially and downward to become continuous with the sigmoid colon. The descending colon has a smaller diameter than the ascending colon and can be palpated through the anterior abdominal wall.

Urinary Bladder and Pregnant Uterus

The full bladder and pregnant uterus can be palpated through the lower part of the anterior abdominal wall above the symphysis pubis (see page 330).

Aorta

The aorta lies in the midline of the abdomen and bifurcates below into the right and left common iliac arteries opposite the fourth lumbar vertebra—that is, on the intercristal plane. The pulsations of the aorta can be easily palpated through the upper part of the anterior abdominal wall just to the left of the midline.

External Iliac Artery

The pulsations of this artery can be felt as it passes under the inguinal ligament to become continuous with the femoral artery. It can be located at a point halfway between the anterior superior iliac spine and the symphysis pubis.

CLINICAL PROBLEM SOLVING

Study the following case histories and select the best answer to the questions following them.

An obese 40-year-old woman was seen in the emergency department complaining of a severe pain over the right shoulder and in her right side and back below the shoulder blade. She said that she had experienced the pain on several occasions before and that when she ate fatty foods it seemed to make the pain worse. Ultrasound demonstrated the presence of gallstones. Her condition was diagnosed as cholelithiasis, and the pain was attributed to gallstone colic.

1. The symptoms and signs displayed by this patient can be explained by the following statements except which?
   (a) The fundus of the gallbladder lies against the anterior abdominal wall next to the tip of the right ninth costal cartilage.
   (b) The parietal peritoneum in this area is innervated by the 10th and 11th intercostal nerves, which give rise to referred pain in the 10th and 11th dermatomes on the side and back.
   (c) The parietal peritoneum on the central part of the undersurface of the diaphragm is supplied by the phrenic nerve.
   (d) The spinal segmental nerves within the phrenic nerve are C3, C4, and C5.
   (e) The pain was referred to the shoulder along the supraclavicular nerves (C3 and C4).

An 8-year-old boy was admitted to the hospital with a temperature of 101°F, a furred tongue, and pain in the right lower quadrant. On examination, the skin on the right lower quadrant was tender to the touch, and the abdominal muscles were contracted and rigid. A diagnosis of acute appendicitis was made.

2. The symptoms and signs displayed by this patient can be explained by the following statements except which?
   (a) An acutely inflamed appendix produces an inflammation of the peritoneal coat covering it.
   (b) Should the inflammatory process spread, for example, if the appendix should rupture, the parietal peritoneum would become involved.
   (c) The parietal peritoneum, the abdominal muscles, and the overlying skin are supplied by the same segmental spinal nerves.
   (d) The segmental nerves supplying the right lower quadrant of the abdominal wall are T7, T8, and T9.
   (e) The pain in the right lower quadrant and the regional contraction of the abdominal muscles are an attempt by the body to keep the inflamed appendix immobile so that the inflammatory process remains localized.

A workman engaged in demolishing a building lost his balance and fell astride a girder on the floor below. On examination, he was found to have extensive swelling of his perineum, scrotum, and penis. He was unable to urinate normally, passing only a few drops of blood-stained urine. The lower part of the anterior abdominal wall was also swollen, but his thighs were normal.

3. The symptoms and signs displayed by this patient can be explained by the following statements except which?
   (a) The patient's fall ruptured the urethra in the perineum.
   (b) When the patient attempted to micturate, the urine extravasated beneath Colles' fascia.
   (c) The urine passed over the scrotum and penis under the membranous layer of superficial fascia.
   (d) The urine passed upward beneath the membranous layer of superficial fascia on the anterior abdominal wall.
   (e) The urine could not extend posteriorly because of the attachment of Colles' fascia to the tip of the coccyx.
   (f) The urine did not extend into the thigh because of the attachment of the membranous layer of superficial fascia to the fascia lata, just below the inguinal ligament.

A 45-year-old woman was shopping in a liquor store when an armed robbery took place. A shoot-out occurred and a bullet ricocheted off the wall and entered her left side. Fortunately, the bullet did not enter the peritoneal cavity. One year later, in addition to diminished skin sensation over the left lumbar region and umbilicus, she noticed a bulging forward of the left side of her anterior abdominal wall.

4. The symptoms and signs displayed by this patient can be explained by the following statements except which?
   (a) The bullet cut the 9th and 10th intercostal nerves just below the costal margin on the left side.
   (b) The diminished skin sensation was caused by the loss of the sensory nerve supply to the 9th and 10th thoracic dermatomes.
   (c) Portions of the oblique, transversus, and rectus abdominis muscles on the left side were paralyzed.
   (d) Atrophy of the pyramidalis muscle resulted in loss of support to the abdominal viscera, which then sagged forward.

A 9-week-old boy was admitted to the hospital with a swelling in the right groin that extended down into the upper part of the scrotum. When he cried, the swelling enlarged. On careful palpation it was possible to reduce the size of the swelling, and this procedure was accompanied by a gurgling noise.

5. The symptoms and signs displayed by this patient can be explained by the following statements except which?
   (a) The swelling was situated above and medial to the pubic tubercle on the right side.
   (b) The child had a right indirect inguinal hernia.
   (c) The processus vaginalis in its upper part had failed to become obliterated before birth.
   (d) The hernial sac in an indirect inguinal hernia emerges from the superficial inguinal ring.
   (e) The superficial inguinal ring lies above and medial to the pubic tubercle.
   (f) The contents of the hernial sac consisted only of the greater omentum.

A 75-year-old man with chronic bronchitis noticed that a bulge was developing in his left groin. On examination, an elongated swelling was seen above the medial end of the left inguinal ligament. When the patient coughed, the swelling enlarged but did not descend into the scrotum. The patient had weak abdominal muscles.

6. The symptoms and signs displayed by this patient can be explained by the following statements except which?
   (a) The inguinal swelling was a direct inguinal hernia.
   (b) The cause of the hernia was weak abdominal muscles.
   (c) The hernial sac was wide and in direct communication with the peritoneal cavity.
   (d) A rise in intra-abdominal pressure on coughing caused the hernial swelling to expand.
   (e) The swelling occurred lateral to the inferior epigastric artery.

A 40-year-old woman noticed a painful swelling in her right groin after helping her husband move some heavy furniture. On examination, a small tender swelling was noted in the right groin.

7. The symptoms and signs displayed by this patient can be explained by the following statements except which?
   (a) The excessive exertion caused a rise in intra-abdominal pressure.
   (b) A hernial sac formed of parietal peritoneum was forced downward.
   (c) The peritoneum was forced through the right femoral canal.
   (d) The patient had a right-sided femoral hernia.
   (e) The neck of a femoral hernial sac is situated below and medial to the pubic tubercle.

A 55-year-old man was admitted to the hospital with a large, hard, fixed, intra-abdominal mass. On examination of the abdomen the mass was situated on the transpyloric plane. The inguinal lymph nodes were normal.

8. The symptoms and signs displayed by this patient can be explained by the following statements except which?
   (a) Radiologic examination of the stomach showed nothing abnormal.
   (b) The right testicle was enlarged and was much harder than normal.
   (c) A diagnosis of malignant disease of the right testis was made.
   (d) The malignant tumor had metastasized to the lumbar lymph nodes lying on the transpyloric plane on the posterior abdominal wall, which is the normal lymphatic drainage of the testis.
   (e) In malignant disease of the testis the superficial inguinal lymph nodes only become involved if the tumor spreads to involve the scrotal skin.
   (f) The normal testis is tethered to the skin of the scrotum.

A 25-year-old man involved in purchasing drugs was knifed in the abdomen in the left upper quadrant. On examination in the emergency department, it was difficult to determine whether the knife had penetrated into the peritoneal cavity. It was decided to do a midline peritoneal lavage below the umbilicus to see if there was any free blood in the peritoneal cavity.

9. The following layers of tissue were penetrated by the trocar and cannula to enter the peritoneal cavity except which?
   (a) Skin
   (b) Fatty and membranous layers of superficial fascia
   (c) Rectus sheath and rectus abdominis muscle
   (d) Deep fascia
   (e) Fascia transversalis
   (f) Extraperitoneal tissue and parietal peritoneum

A 20-year-old soccer player was accidentally kicked on the left side of her chest. On returning to the locker room she said she felt faint and collapsed to the floor. On examination in the emergency department, she was found to be in hypovolemic shock. She had tenderness and muscle rigidity in the left upper quadrant of her abdomen. She also had extreme local tenderness over her left 10th rib in the midaxillary line.

10. The symptoms and signs displayed by this patient can be explained by the following statements except which?
   (a) Radiology revealed a fractured left 10th rib.
   (b) The spleen was severely bruised and the blood was initially confined to the spleen.
   (c) Later in the locker room the capsule of the spleen gave way and the blood escaped into the peritoneal cavity.
   (d) Blood does not irritate the parietal peritoneum.
   (e) Stimulation of the sensory nerves supplying the parietal peritoneum was responsible for the extreme tenderness of the left upper quadrant of the abdomen.
   (f) The muscles forming the anterior abdominal wall in that region were reflexly stimulated, producing muscle rigidity.

ANSWERS TO CLINICAL PROBLEMS

1. B. The parietal peritoneum in the region of the fundus of the gallbladder is innervated by the eighth and ninth intercostal nerves, which give rise to referred pain in the eighth and ninth thoracic dermatomes on the side and back.
2. D. The segmental nerves supplying the right lower quadrant of the abdominal wall are T11, T12, and L1.
3. E. The urine could not extend posteriorly because of the attachment of the Colles' fascia to the posterior edge of the perineal membrane.
4. D. The pyramidalis muscle (if present) is innervated by the 12th thoracic nerve.
5. F. The contents of this hernial sac included coils of small intestine, which were responsible for the gurgling noises that occurred as the hernia was reduced.
6. E. The swelling occurs medial to the inferior epigastric artery.
7. E. The neck of a femoral hernial sac is situated below and lateral to the pubic tubercle.
8. F. The normal testis is freely mobile within the scrotum and is not tethered to the subcutaneous tissue or skin.
9. C. The linea alba lies in the midline; the rectus sheath lies lateral to the linea alba.
10. D. Blood is very irritating to the parietal peritoneum.

REVIEW QUESTIONS

Multiple-Choice Questions

Select the best answer for each question.

1. The following structures form the walls of the inguinal canal except which?
   (a) The conjoint tendon
   (b) The aponeurosis of the external oblique muscle
   (c) The internal oblique muscle
   (d) The lacunar ligament
   (e) The fascia transversalis
2. The following statements concerning the walls of the inguinal canal are correct except which?
   (a) The inguinal ligament is made tense by flexing the hip joint.
   (b) The contracting internal oblique muscle reinforces the anterior wall of the canal in front of the weak deep inguinal ring.
   (c) The strong conjoint tendon reinforces the posterior wall of the canal behind the weak superficial inguinal ring.
   (d) Contraction of the arching fibers of the internal oblique and transversus abdominis muscles lowers the roof of the canal so that the canal is practically obliterated.
   (e) After birth, as the result of growth, the deep inguinal ring moves away from the superficial ring so that the canal becomes oblique and the two rings no longer lie opposite one another.
3. In the female, the inguinal canal contains the following structures except which?
   (a) Ilioinguinal nerve
   (b) Remnant of the processus vaginalis
   (c) Round ligament of the uterus
   (d) Inferior epigastric artery
   (e) Lymph vessels from the fundus of the uterus
4. The following statements concerning the spermatic cord are correct except which?
   (a) It extends from the deep inguinal ring to the scrotum.
   (b) It contains the testicular artery.
   (c) It is covered by five layers of spermatic fascia.

(d) It contains the pampiniform plexus.
(e) It contains lymph vessels that drain the testis.

5. The following structures are present in the inguinal canal in the male except which?
(a) Internal spermatic fascia
(b) Genital branch of the genitofemoral nerve
(c) Testicular vessels
(d) Deep circumflex iliac artery
(e) Ilioinguinal nerve
6. The following statements concerning the conjoint tendon are correct except which?
(a) It is attached to the pubic crest and the pectineal line.
(b) It is formed by the fusion of the aponeuroses of the transversus abdominis and internal oblique muscles.
(c) It is attached medially to the linea alba.
(d) It is continuous with the inguinal ligament.
(e) It may bulge forward in a direct inguinal hernia.
7. The following statements concerning an indirect inguinal hernia are correct except which?
(a) It is the most common form of abdominal hernia.
(b) The neck of the hernial sac lies medial to the inferior epigastric artery.
(c) The sac is the remains of the processus vaginalis.
(d) The hernial sac can extend into the scrotum.
(e) At the superficial inguinal ring, the hernial sac lies above and medial to the pubic tubercle.
8. To pass a needle into the cavity of the tunica vaginalis in the scrotum, the following structures have to be pierced except which?
(a) Skin
(b) Dartos muscle and Colles' fascia
(c) Tunica albuginea
(d) Internal spermatic fascia
(e) Cremasteric fascia
9. The following statements are correct concerning the muscles forming the posterior abdominal wall except which?
(a) The psoas major muscle has a fascial sheath that extends down into the thigh as far as the lesser trochanter of the femur.
(b) The quadratus lumborum is covered anteriorly by fascia that forms the lateral arcuate ligament.
(c) The iliacus muscle is innervated by the femoral nerve.
(d) The transversus abdominis muscle forms part of the posterior abdominal wall.
(e) The diaphragm does not contribute to the musculature on the posterior abdominal wall.

Matching Questions

Match each structure listed below with the region on the anterior abdominal wall in which it is located. Each lettered answer may be used more than once.

10. Appendix
11. Gallbladder
12. Cecum
13. Left colic flexure
(a) Right upper quadrant
(b) Left lower quadrant
(c) Right lower quadrant
(d) None of the above

Match each structure listed below with the structure with which it is most closely associated.

14. External spermatic fascia
15. Round ligament of the uterus
16. Cremasteric fascia
17. Internal spermatic fascia
18. Deep inguinal ring
(a) Internal oblique
(b) Fascia transversalis
(c) Gubernaculum
(d) External oblique
(e) None of the above

Match each structure listed below with the group of lymph nodes that drain it.

19. Testis
20. Skin of anterior abdominal wall below the level of the umbilicus
21. Epididymis
22. Skin of the scrotum
(a) Anterior axillary lymph nodes
(b) Para-aortic or lumbar lymph nodes
(c) Superficial inguinal lymph nodes
(d) External iliac nodes
(e) None of the above

Read the case histories and select the best answer to the question following them.

A 30-year-old man was seen in the emergency department with a stab wound in the right inguinal region.

23. Which of the following nerves supplies the skin of the inguinal region?
(a) The 11th thoracic nerve
(b) The 10th thoracic nerve
(c) The 12th thoracic nerve
(d) The first lumbar nerve
(e) The femoral nerve

Immediately after delivery, it was noted that a 7.5-lb male neonate had a large swelling on the anterior abdominal wall. The swelling consisted of a large sac, the walls of which were translucent and soft. The umbilical cord was attached to the apex of the sac, and the umbilical arteries and vein ran within its walls.

24. The following statements concerning this case are probably correct except which?
(a) On closer examination it was possible to see within the sac coils of small intestine and the lower margin of the liver.
(b) As the baby cried and started to swallow air, the sac became larger.
(c) Failure of the formation of adequate head and tail folds of the embryonic disc causes a defect in the anterior abdominal wall in the umbilical region.
(d) The defect in the anterior abdominal wall is filled with thin amnion, which forms the wall of the sac.
(e) The condition is known as exomphalos or omphalocele.

ANSWERS TO REVIEW QUESTIONS

1. D
2. A
3. D
4. C. The spermatic cord is covered by three layers of spermatic fascia, which are derived from the three layers of the anterior abdominal wall. The external spermatic fascia is from the aponeurosis of the external oblique muscle, the cremasteric fascia is derived from the internal oblique muscle, and the internal spermatic fascia is formed from the fascia transversalis.
5. D. The deep circumflex iliac artery is a branch of the external iliac artery and runs upward and laterally toward the anterior superior iliac spine away from the inguinal canal.
6. D
7. B
8. C
9. E
10. C
11. A
12. C
13. D
14. D
15. C
16. A
17. B
18. B
19. B
20. C
21. B
22. C
23. D. The first lumbar nerve, represented by the iliohypogastric and ilioinguinal nerves, supply the skin just above the inguinal ligament and the symphysis pubis.
24. C. The defect is caused by a failure of the formation of adequate lateral folds in the umbilical region, which is filled in by amnion only. During the first 24 hours after birth, the wall of the sac becomes dry and opaque and may rupture, causing evisceration. Bacteria at once gain entrance to the peritoneal cavity, producing peritonitis. The sac of amnion should be surgically excised as soon as possible after birth and the contained viscera returned to the abdominal cavity. The defect in the anterior abdominal wall should then be closed.

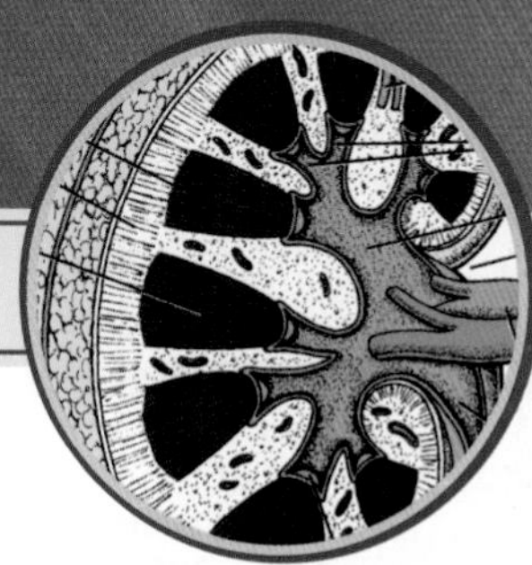

CHAPTER 5

THE ABDOMEN: PART II—THE ABDOMINAL CAVITY

A 15-year-old boy complaining of pain in the lower right part of the anterior abdominal wall was seen by a physician. On examination, he was found to have a temperature of 101°F (38.3°C). He had a furred tongue and was extremely tender in the lower right quadrant. The abdominal muscles in that area were found to be firm (rigid) on palpation and became more spastic when increased pressure was applied (guarding). A diagnosis of acute appendicitis was made.

Inflammation of the appendix initially is a localized disease giving rise to pain that is often referred to the umbilicus. Later, the inflammatory process spreads to involve the peritoneum covering the appendix, producing a localized peritonitis. If the appendix ruptures, further spread occurs and a more generalized peritonitis is produced. Inflammation of the peritoneum lining the anterior abdominal wall (parietal peritoneum) causes pain and reflex spasm of the anterior abdominal muscles. This can be explained by the fact that the parietal peritoneum, the abdominal muscles, and the overlying skin are supplied by the same segmental nerves. This is a protective mechanism to keep that area of the abdomen at rest so that the inflammatory process remains localized.

The understanding of the symptoms and signs of appendicitis depends on having a working knowledge of the anatomy of the appendix, including its nerve supply, blood supply, and relationships with other abdominal structures.

CHAPTER OUTLINE

Basic Anatomy 203
General Arrangement of the Abdominal Viscera 203
Liver 203
Gallbladder 203
Esophagus 203
Stomach 203
Small Intestine 204
Large Intestine 204
Pancreas 205
Spleen 205
Kidneys 205
Suprarenal Glands 205
Peritoneum 205
General Arrangement 205
Intraperitoneal and Retroperitoneal Relationships 206
Peritoneal Ligaments 206
Omenta 206
Mesenteries 207
Peritoneal Pouches, Recesses, Spaces, and Gutters 207
Nerve Supply of the Peritoneum 209
Functions of the Peritoneum 209
Gastrointestinal Tract 217
Esophagus (Abdominal Portion) 217
Gastroesophageal Sphincter 217
Stomach 219
Small Intestine 224
Duodenum 224
Jejunum and Ileum 227
Large Intestine 229
Cecum 229
Ileocecal Valve 230
Appendix 230
Ascending Colon 232
Transverse Colon 233
Descending Colon 234
Blood Supply of the Gastrointestinal Tract 240
Differences Between the Small and Large Intestine 246
Accessory Organs of the Gastrointestinal Tract 246
Liver 246
Bile Ducts of the Liver 250
Gallbladder 250
Pancreas 256
Spleen 259
Retroperitoneal Space 260
Urinary Tract 260
Kidneys 260
Ureter 266
Suprarenal Glands 269
Location and Description 269
Blood Supply 269
Lymph Drainage 269
Nerve Supply 269
Arteries on the Posterior Abdominal Wall 271
Aorta 271
Common Iliac Arteries 273
External Iliac Artery 274
Internal Iliac Artery 274
Veins on the Posterior Abdominal Wall 274
Inferior Vena Cava 274
Inferior Mesenteric Vein 276
Splenic Vein 276
Superior Mesenteric Vein 276
Portal Vein 276
Lymphatics on the Posterior Abdominal Wall 276
Lymph Nodes 276
Lymph Vessels 276
Nerves on the Posterior Abdominal Wall 278
Lumbar Plexus 278
Sympathetic Trunk (Abdominal Part) 279
Aortic Plexuses 280
Cross-Sectional Anatomy of the Abdomen 282
Radiographic Anatomy 282
Radiographic Appearances of the Abdomen 282
Radiographic Appearances of the Gastrointestinal Tract 282
Stomach 282
Duodenum 282
Jejunum and Ileum 289
Large Intestine 289
Radiographic Appearances of the Biliary Ducts 289
Radiographic Appearances of the Urinary Tract 295
Kidneys 295
Calyces, Renal Pelvis, and Ureter 295
Surface Anatomy of the Abdominal Viscera 298
Clinical Problem Solving 298
Answers to Clinical Problems 300
Review Questions 301
Answers to Review Questions 305

CHAPTER OBJECTIVES

- The abdominal cavity contains many vital organs, including the gastrointestinal tract, liver, biliary ducts, pancreas, spleen, and parts of the urinary system. These structures are closely packed within the abdominal cavity, and therefore disease of one can easily involve another. Gastrointestinal tract inflammation and bleeding, malignant disease, and penetrating trauma to the abdomen are just some of the problems facing the physician.
- Emergency problems involving the urinary system are common and may present diverse symptoms ranging from excruciating pain to failure to void urine.
- Within the abdomen also lie the aorta and its branches, the inferior vena cava and its tributaries, and the important portal vein.
- The purpose of this chapter is to give the student an understanding of the significant anatomy relative to clinical problems. Examiners can ask many good questions regarding this region.

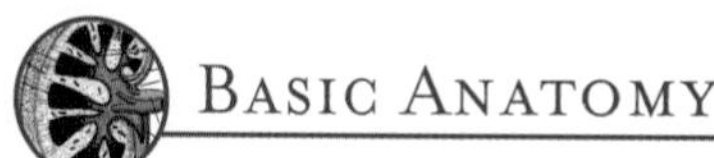

Basic Anatomy

General Arrangement of the Abdominal Viscera

Liver

The liver is a large organ that occupies the upper part of the abdominal cavity (Figs. 5-1 and 5-2). It lies almost entirely under cover of the ribs and costal cartilages and extends across the epigastric region.

Gallbladder

The gallbladder is a pear-shaped sac that is adherent to the undersurface of the right lobe of the liver; its blind end, or fundus, projects below the inferior border of the liver (Figs. 5-1 and 5-2).

Esophagus

The esophagus is a tubular structure that joins the pharynx to the stomach. The esophagus pierces the diaphragm slightly to the left of the midline and after a short course of about 0.5 in. (1.25 cm) enters the stomach on its right side. It is deeply placed, lying behind the left lobe of the liver (Fig. 5-1).

Stomach

The stomach is a dilated part of the alimentary canal between the esophagus and the small intestine (Figs. 5-1 and 5-2). It occupies the left upper quadrant, epigastric, and umbilical regions, and much of it lies under cover of the ribs. Its long axis passes downward and forward to the right and then backward and slightly upward.

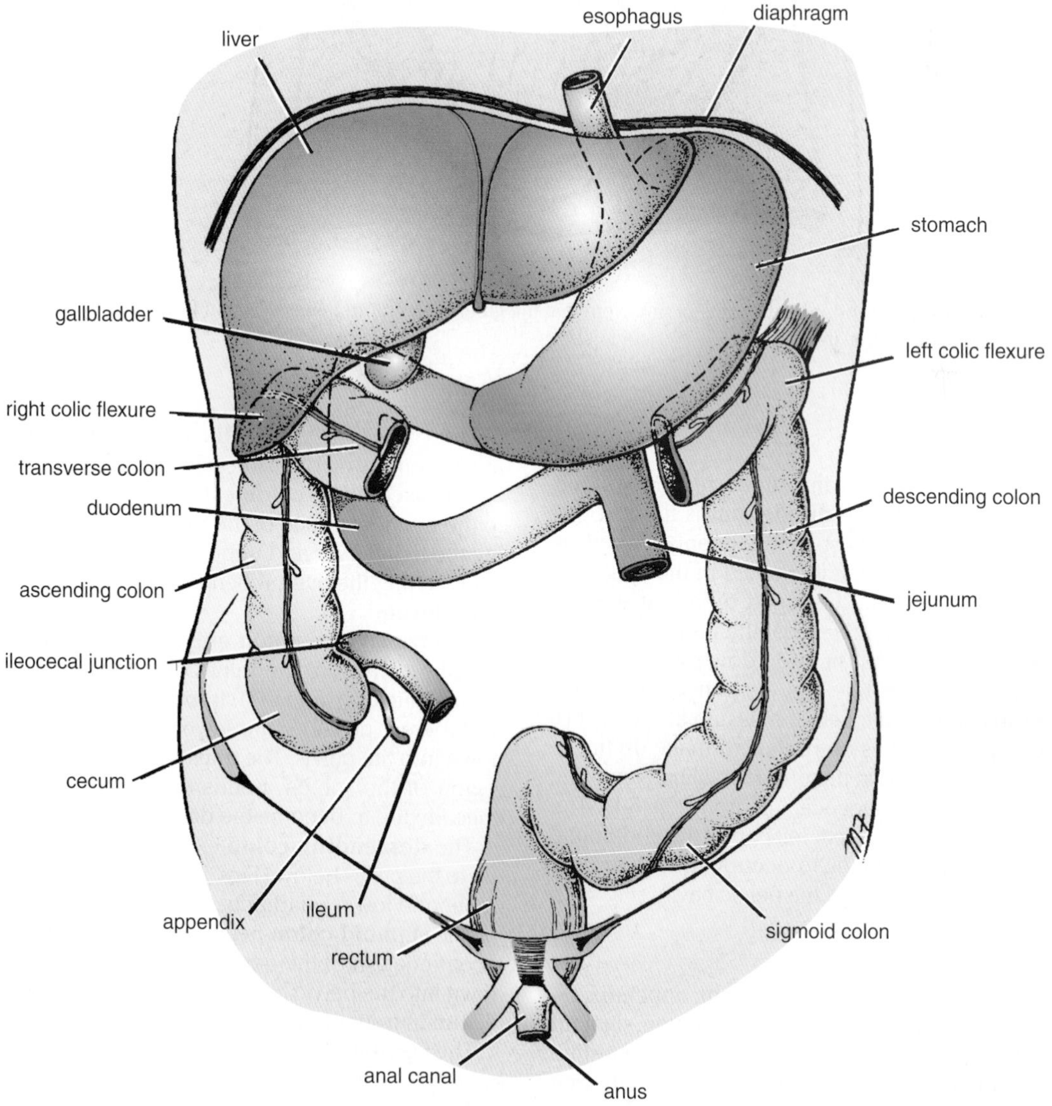

Figure 5-1 General arrangement of abdominal viscera.

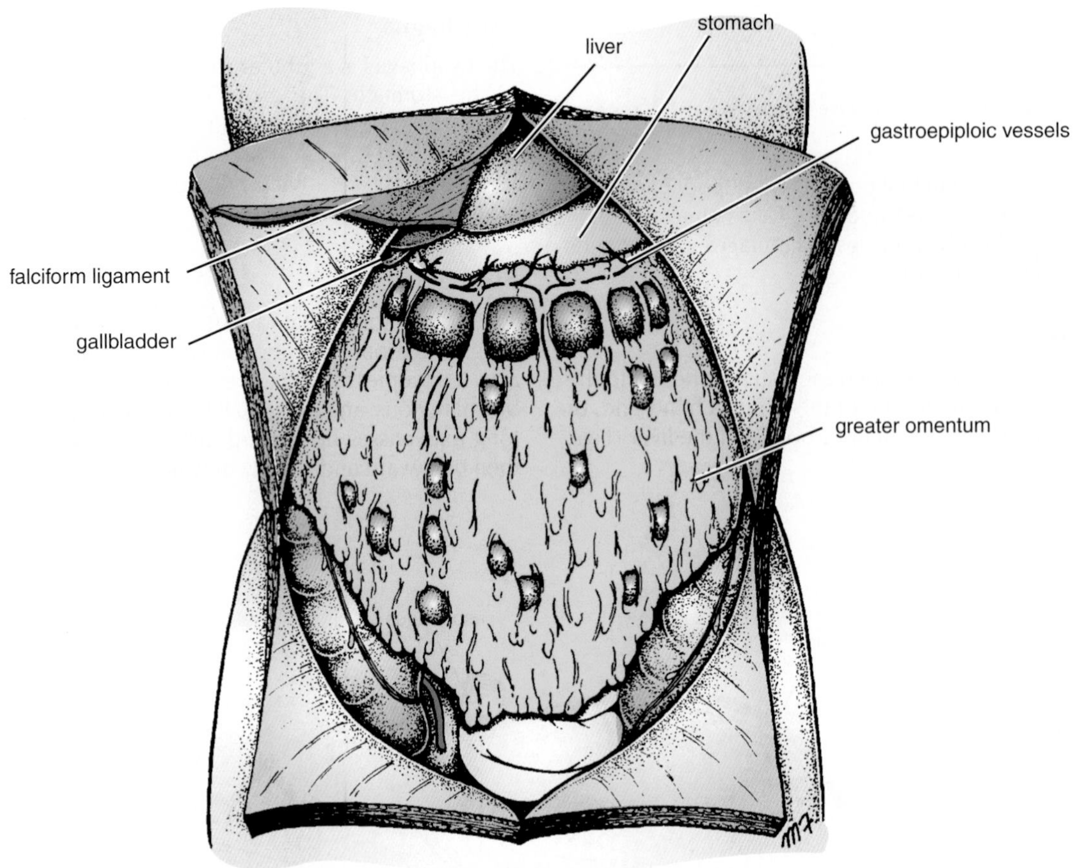

Figure 5-2 Abdominal organs in situ. Note that the greater omentum hangs down in front of the small and large intestines.

Small Intestine

The small intestine is divided into three regions: duodenum, jejunum, and ileum. The **duodenum** is the first part of the small intestine, and most of it is deeply placed on the posterior abdominal wall. It is situated in the epigastric and umbilical regions. It is a C-shaped tube that extends from the stomach around the head of the pancreas to join the jejunum (Fig. 5-1). About halfway down its length the small intestine receives the bile and the pancreatic ducts.

The **jejunum** and **ileum** together measure about 20 ft (6 m) long; the upper two fifths of this length make up the jejunum. The jejunum begins at the duodenojejunal junction, and the ileum ends at the ileocecal junction (Fig. 5-1). The coils of jejunum occupy the upper left part of the abdominal cavity, whereas the ileum tends to occupy the lower right part of the abdominal cavity and the pelvic cavity (Fig. 5-3).

Large Intestine

The large intestine is divided into the cecum, appendix, ascending colon, transverse colon, descending colon, sigmoid colon, rectum, and anal canal (Fig. 5-1). The large intestine arches around and encloses the coils of the small intestine (Fig. 5-3) and tends to be more fixed than the small intestine.

The **cecum** is a blind-ended sac that projects downward in the right iliac region below the ileocecal junction (Figs. 5-1 and 5-3). The **appendix** is a worm-shaped tube that arises from its medial side (Fig. 5-1).

The **ascending colon** extends upward from the cecum to the inferior surface of the right lobe of the liver, occupying the right lower and upper quadrants (Figs. 5-1 and 5-3). On reaching the liver, it bends to the left, forming the right colic flexure.

The **transverse colon** crosses the abdomen in the umbilical region from the right colic flexure to the left colic flexure (Figs. 5-1 and 5-3). It forms a wide U-shaped curve. In the erect position, the lower part of the U may extend down into the pelvis. The transverse colon, on reaching the region of the spleen, bends downward, forming the left colic flexure to become the descending colon.

The **descending colon** extends from the left colic flexure to the pelvis below (Figs. 5-1 and 5-3). It occupies the left upper and lower quadrants.

The **sigmoid colon** begins at the pelvic inlet, where it is a continuation of the descending colon (Fig. 5-1). It hangs down into the pelvic cavity in the form of a loop. It joins the rectum in front of the sacrum.

The **rectum** occupies the posterior part of the pelvic cavity (Fig. 5-1). It is continuous above with the sigmoid colon and descends in front of the sacrum to leave the pelvis by piercing the pelvic floor. Here, it becomes continuous with the anal canal in the perineum.

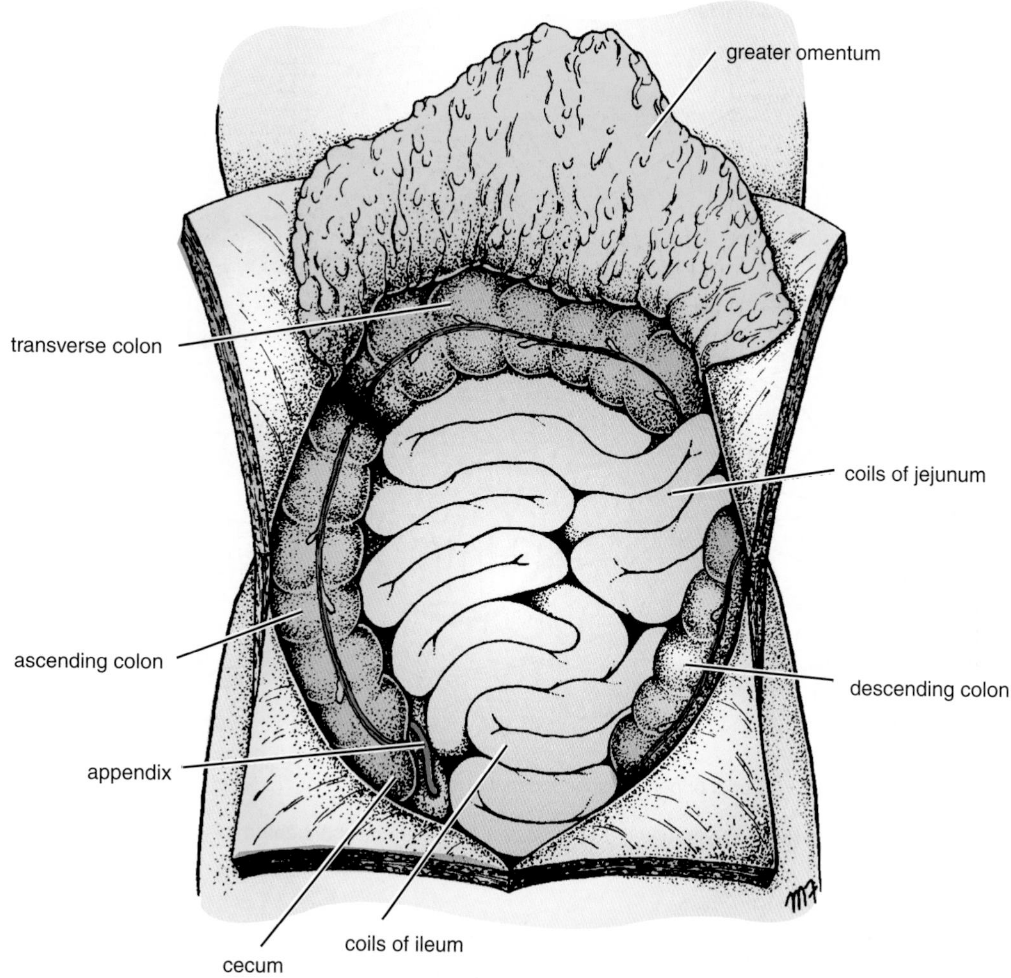

Figure 5-3 Abdominal contents after the greater omentum has been reflected upward. Coils of small intestine occupy the central part of the abdominal cavity, whereas ascending, transverse, and descending parts of the colon are located at the periphery.

Pancreas

The pancreas is a soft, lobulated organ that stretches obliquely across the posterior abdominal wall in the epigastric region (Fig. 5-4). It is situated behind the stomach and extends from the duodenum to the spleen.

Spleen

The spleen is a soft mass of lymphatic tissue that occupies the left upper part of the abdomen between the stomach and the diaphragm (Fig. 5-4). It lies along the long axis of the 10th left rib.

Kidneys

The kidneys are two reddish brown organs situated high up on the posterior abdominal wall, one on each side of the vertebral column (Fig. 5-4). The left kidney lies slightly higher than the right (because the left lobe of the liver is smaller than the right). Each kidney gives rise to a **ureter** that runs vertically downward on the psoas muscle.

Suprarenal Glands

The suprarenal glands are two yellowish organs that lie on the upper poles of the kidneys (Fig. 5-4) on the posterior abdominal wall.

Peritoneum

General Arrangement

The peritoneum is a thin serous membrane that lines the walls of the abdominal and pelvic cavities and clothes the viscera (Figs. 5-5 and 5-6). The peritoneum can be regarded as a balloon against which organs are pressed from outside. The **parietal peritoneum** lines the walls of the abdominal and pelvic cavities, and the **visceral peritoneum** covers the organs. The potential space between the parietal and visceral layers, which is in effect the inside space of the balloon, is called the **peritoneal cavity.** In males, this is a closed cavity, but in females, there is communication with the exterior through the uterine tubes, the uterus, and the vagina.

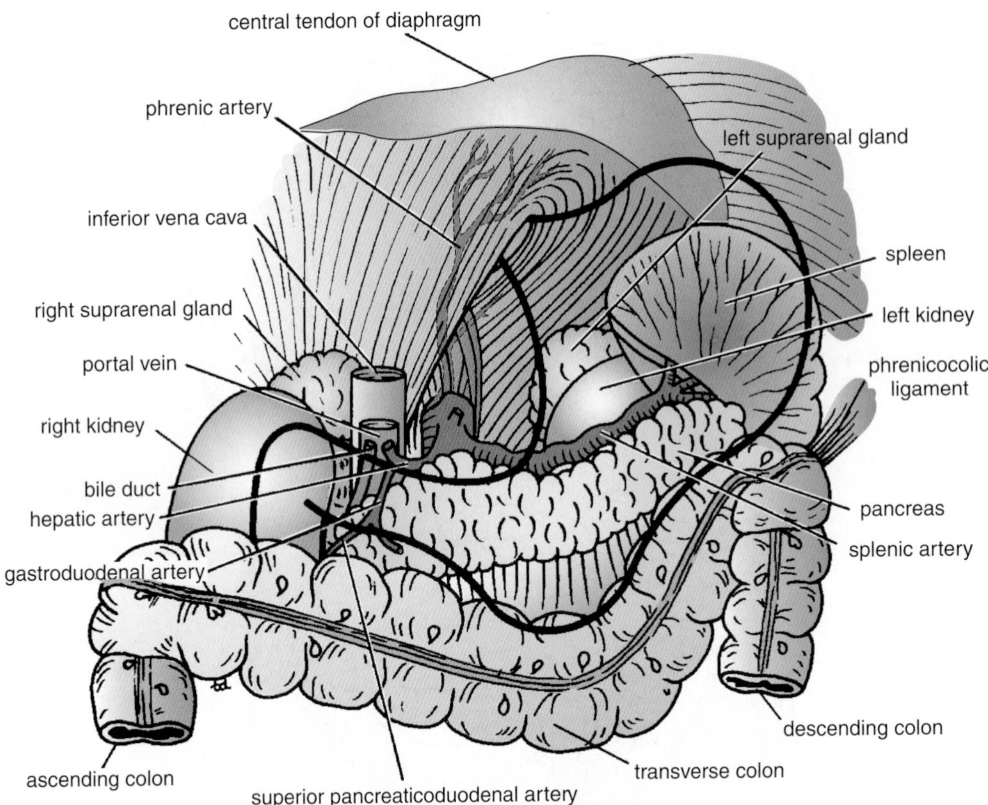

Figure 5-4 Structures situated on the posterior abdominal wall behind the stomach.

Between the parietal peritoneum and the fascial lining of the abdominal and pelvic walls is a layer of connective tissue called the **extraperitoneal tissue;** in the area of the kidneys this tissue contains a large amount of fat, which supports the kidneys.

The peritoneal cavity is the largest cavity in the body and is divided into two parts: the **greater sac** and the lesser sac (Fig. 5-5 and 5-6). The **greater sac** is the main compartment and extends from the diaphragm down into the pelvis. The **lesser sac** is smaller and lies behind the stomach. The greater and lesser sacs are in free communication with one another through an oval window called the **opening of the lesser sac,** or the **epiploic foramen** (Figs. 5-5 and 5-7). The peritoneum secretes a small amount of serous fluid, the **peritoneal fluid,** which lubricates the surfaces of the peritoneum and allows free movement between the viscera.

Intraperitoneal and Retroperitoneal Relationships

The terms **intraperitoneal** and **retroperitoneal** are used to describe the relationship of various organs to their peritoneal covering. An organ is said to be intraperitoneal when it is almost totally covered with visceral peritoneum. The stomach, jejunum, ileum, and spleen are good examples of intraperitoneal organs. Retroperitoneal organs lie behind the peritoneum and are only partially covered with visceral peritoneum. The pancreas and the ascending and descending parts of the colon are examples of retroperitoneal organs. No organ, however, is actually within the peritoneal cavity. An intraperitoneal organ, such as the stomach, appears to be surrounded by the peritoneal cavity, but it is covered with visceral peritoneum and is attached to other organs by omenta.

Peritoneal Ligaments

Peritoneal ligaments are two-layered folds of peritoneum that connect solid viscera to the abdominal walls. The liver, for example, is connected to the diaphragm by the **falciform ligament,** the **coronary ligament,** and the **right** and **left triangular ligaments** (Figs. 5-8 and 5-10).

Omenta

Omenta are two-layered folds of peritoneum that connect the stomach to another viscus. The **greater omentum** connects the greater curvature of the stomach to the transverse colon (Fig. 5-2). It hangs down like an apron in front of the coils of the small intestine and is folded back on itself to be attached to the transverse colon (Fig. 5-6). The **lesser omentum** suspends the lesser curvature of the stomach from the fissure of the ligamentum venosum and the porta hepatis on the undersurface of the liver (Fig. 5-6). The

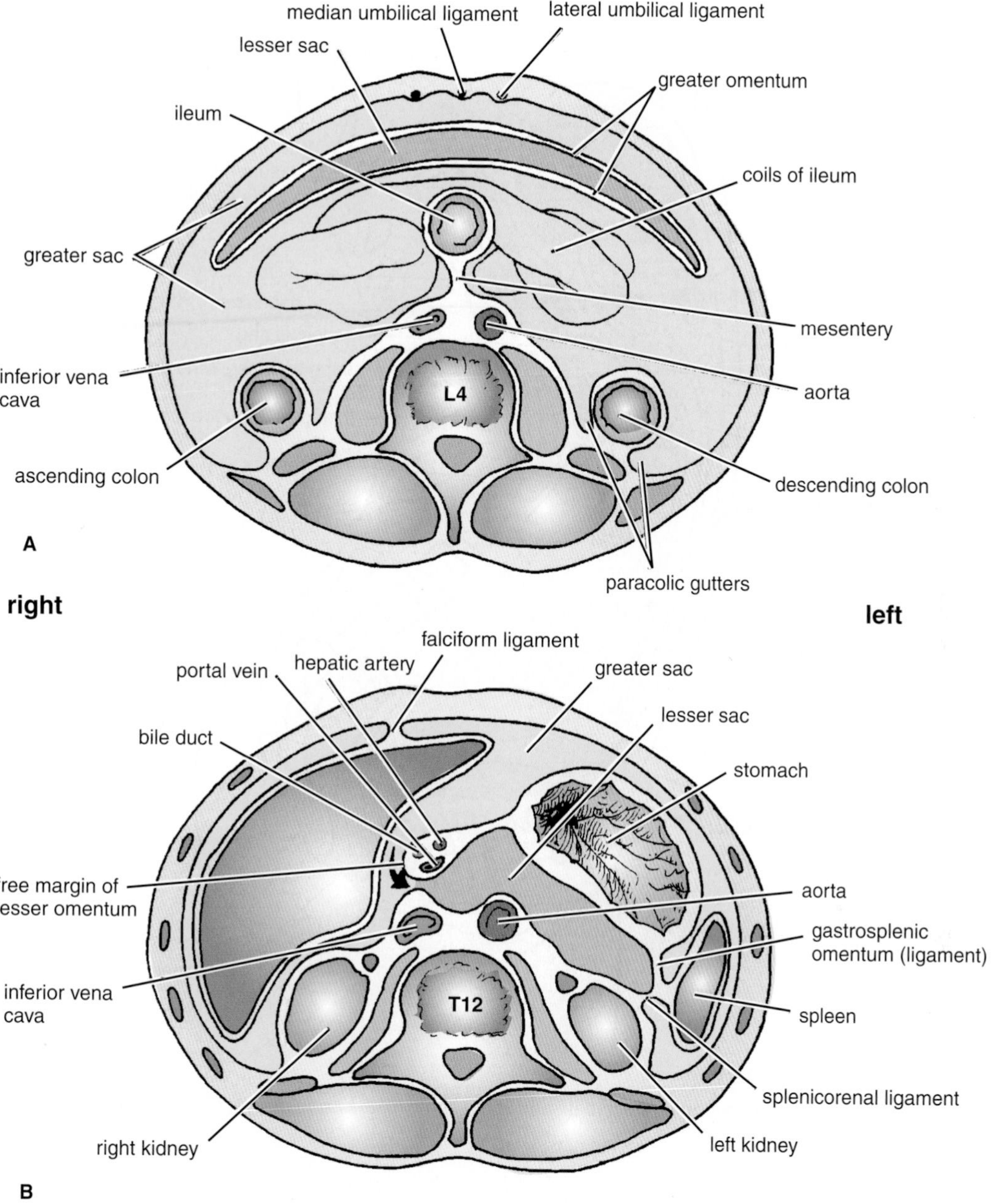

Figure 5-5 Transverse sections of the abdomen showing the arrangement of the peritoneum. The *arrow* in **B** indicates the position of the opening of the lesser sac. These sections are viewed from below.

gastrosplenic omentum (ligament) connects the stomach to the hilum of the spleen (Fig. 5-5).

Mesenteries

Mesenteries are two-layered folds of peritoneum connecting parts of the intestines to the posterior abdominal wall, for example, the **mesentery of the small intestine,** the **transverse mesocolon,** and the **sigmoid mesocolon** (Figs. 5-6 and 5-13).

The peritoneal ligaments, omenta, and mesenteries permit blood, lymph vessels, and nerves to reach the viscera.

The extent of the peritoneum and the peritoneal cavity should be studied in the transverse and sagittal sections of the abdomen seen in Figures 5-5 and 5-6.

Peritoneal Pouches, Recesses, Spaces, and Gutters

Lesser Sac

The lesser sac lies behind the stomach and the lesser omentum (Figs. 5-5, 5-6, and 5-11). It extends upward as far as the diaphragm and downward between the layers of the greater

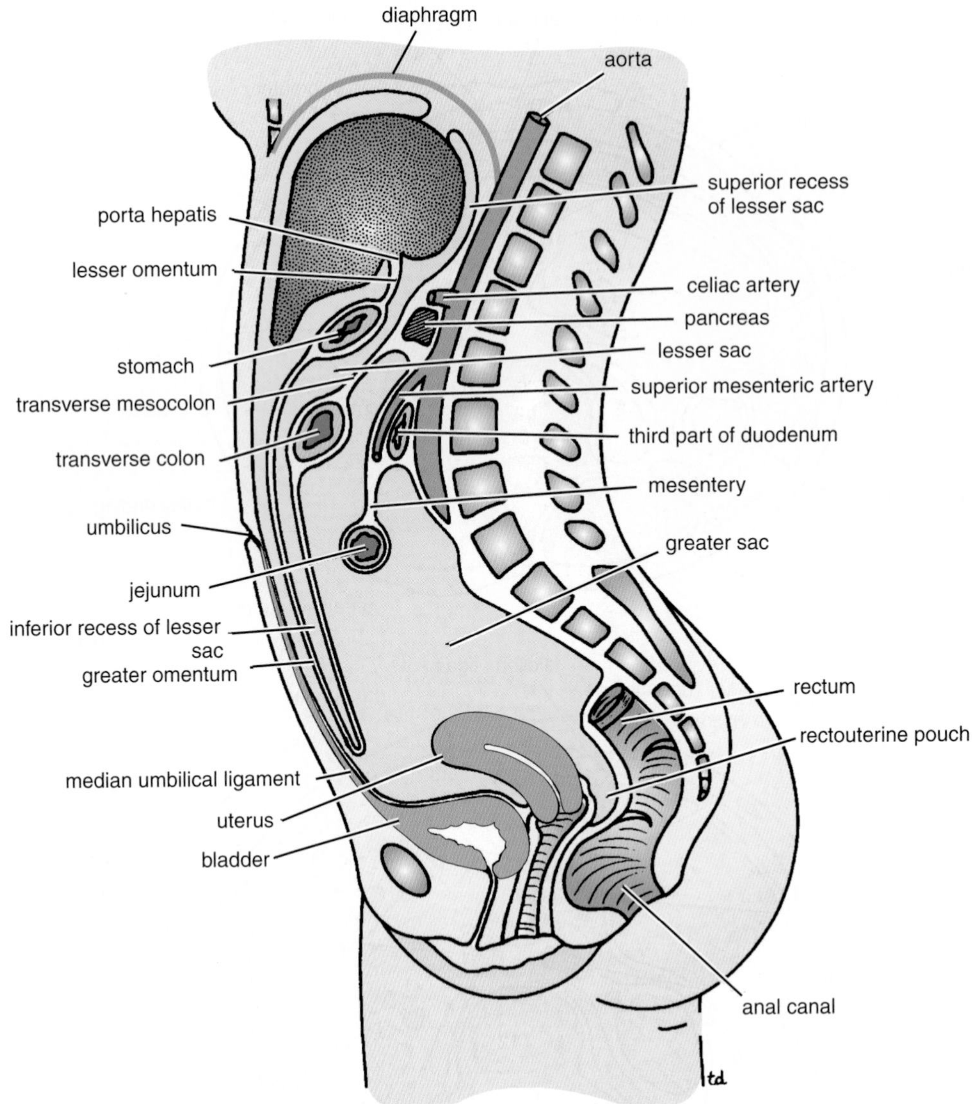

Figure 5-6 Sagittal section of the female abdomen showing the arrangement of the peritoneum.

omentum. The left margin of the sac is formed by the spleen (Fig. 5-11) and the gastrosplenic omentum and splenicorenal ligament. The right margin opens into the greater sac (the main part of the peritoneal cavity) through the **opening of the lesser sac,** or **epiploic foramen** (Fig. 5-7).

The opening into the lesser sac (epiploic foramen) has the following boundaries (Fig. 5-7):

- **Anteriorly:** Free border of the lesser omentum, the bile duct, the hepatic artery, and the portal vein (Fig. 5-11)
- **Posteriorly:** Inferior vena cava
- **Superiorly:** Caudate process of the caudate lobe of the liver
- **Inferiorly:** First part of the duodenum

Duodenal Recesses

Close to the duodenojejunal junction, there may be four small pocketlike pouches of peritoneum called the **superior duodenal, inferior duodenal, paraduodenal,** and **retroduodenal recesses** (Fig. 5-12).

Cecal Recesses

Folds of peritoneum close to the cecum produce three peritoneal recesses called the superior ileocecal, the inferior ileocecal, and the retrocecal recesses (Fig. 5-13).

Intersigmoid Recess

The intersigmoid recess is situated at the apex of the inverted, V-shaped root of the sigmoid mesocolon (Fig. 5-13); its mouth opens downward.

Subphrenic Spaces

The **right** and **left anterior subphrenic spaces** lie between the diaphragm and the liver, on each side of the falciform ligament (Fig. 5-14). The **right posterior subphrenic space** lies between the right lobe of the liver,

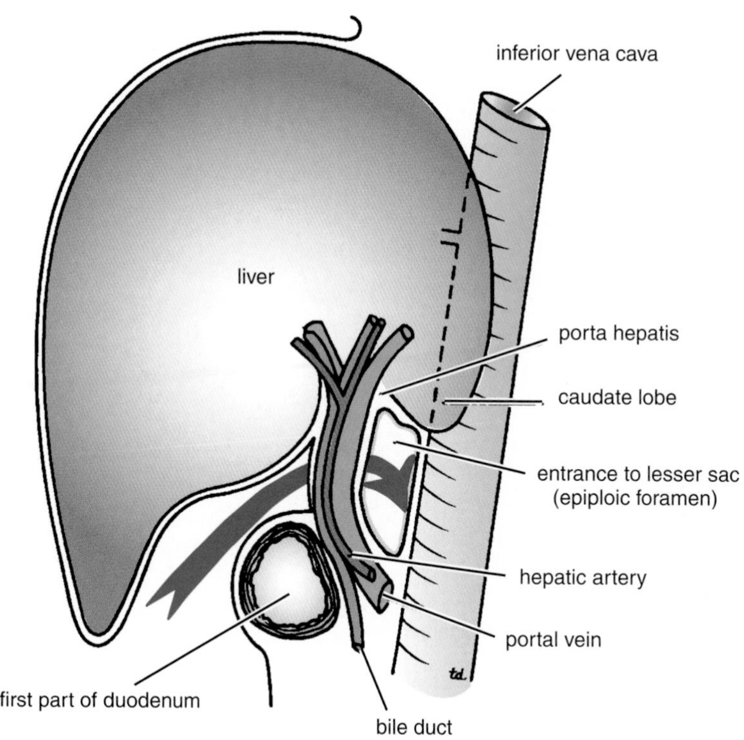

Figure 5-7 Sagittal section through the entrance into the lesser sac showing the important structures that form boundaries to the opening. (Note the arrow passing from the greater sac through the epiploic foramen into the lesser sac.)

the right kidney, and the right colic flexure (Fig. 5-15). The **right extraperitoneal space** lies between the layers of the coronary ligament and is therefore situated between the liver and the diaphragm (see page 247).

Paracolic Gutters

The paracolic gutters lie on the lateral and medial sides of the ascending and descending colons, respectively (Figs. 5-5 and 5-14).

The subphrenic spaces and the paracolic gutters are clinically important because they may be sites for the collection and movement of infected peritoneal fluid (see page 213).

Nerve Supply of the Peritoneum

The **parietal peritoneum** is sensitive to pain, temperature, touch, and pressure. The parietal peritoneum lining the anterior abdominal wall is supplied by the lower six thoracic and first lumbar nerves—that is, the same nerves that innervate the overlying muscles and skin. The central part of the diaphragmatic peritoneum is supplied by the phrenic nerves; peripherally, the diaphragmatic peritoneum is supplied by the lower six thoracic nerves. The parietal peritoneum in the pelvis is mainly supplied by the obturator nerve, a branch of the lumbar plexus.

The **visceral peritoneum** is sensitive only to stretch and tearing and is not sensitive to touch, pressure, or temperature. It is supplied by autonomic afferent nerves that supply the viscera or are traveling in the mesenteries. Overdistention of a viscus leads to the sensation of pain. The mesenteries of the small and large intestines are sensitive to mechanical stretching.

Functions of the Peritoneum

The peritoneal fluid, which is pale yellow and somewhat viscid, contains leukocytes. It is secreted by the peritoneum and ensures that the mobile viscera glide easily on one another. As a result of the movements of the diaphragm and the abdominal muscles, together with the peristaltic movements of the intestinal tract, the peritoneal fluid is not static. Experimental evidence has shown that particulate matter introduced into the lower part of the peritoneal cavity reaches the subphrenic peritoneal spaces rapidly, whatever the position of the body. It seems that intraperitoneal movement of fluid toward the diaphragm is continuous (Fig. 5-14), and there it is quickly absorbed into the subperitoneal lymphatic capillaries.

This can be explained on the basis that the area of peritoneum is extensive in the region of the diaphragm and the respiratory movements of the diaphragm aid lymph flow in the lymph vessels.

The peritoneal coverings of the intestine tend to stick together in the presence of infection. The greater omentum, which is kept constantly on the move by the peristalsis of the neighboring intestinal tract, may adhere to other peritoneal surfaces around a focus of infection. In this manner, many of the intraperitoneal infections are sealed off and remain localized.

The peritoneal folds play an important part in suspending the various organs within the peritoneal cavity and serve as a means of conveying the blood vessels, lymphatics, and nerves to these organs.

Large amounts of fat are stored in the peritoneal ligaments and mesenteries, and especially large amounts can be found in the greater omentum.

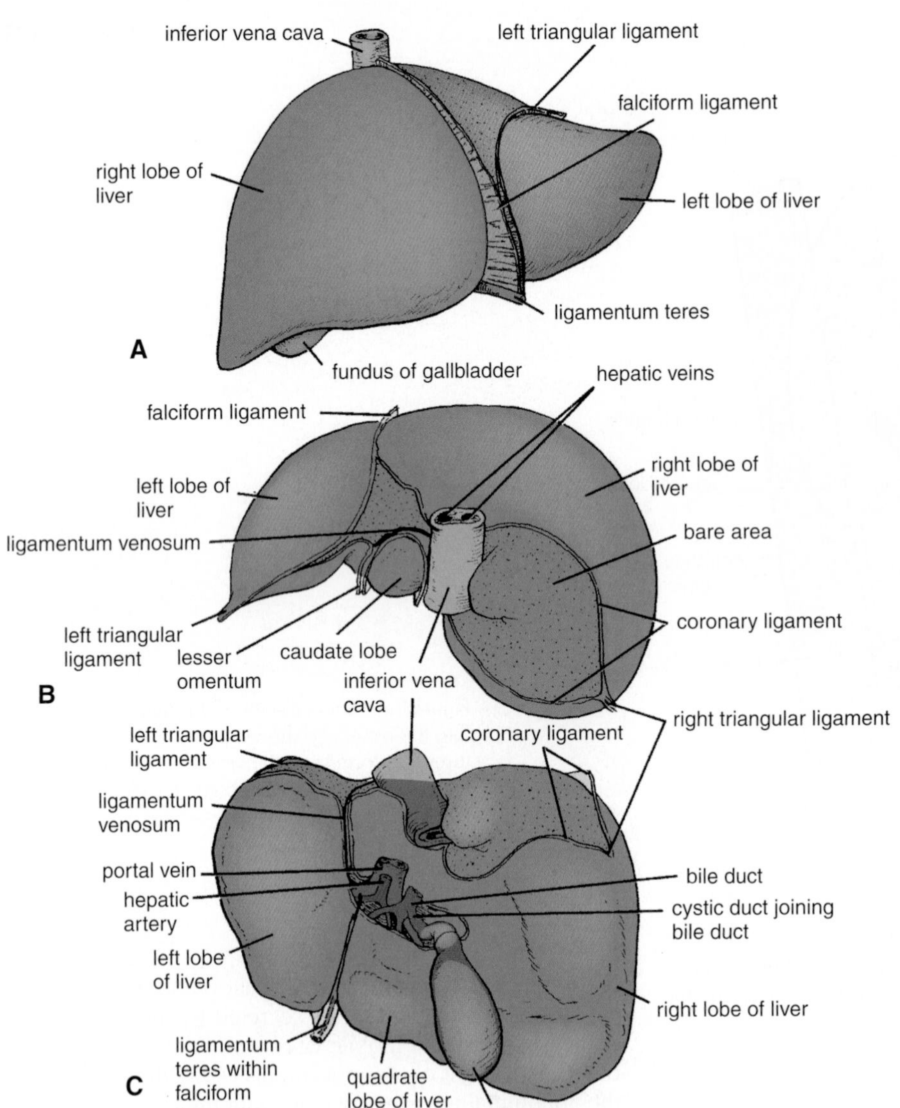

Figure 5-8 Liver as seen from in front **(A),** from above **(B),** and from behind **(C).** Note the position of the peritoneal reflections, the bare areas, and the peritoneal ligaments

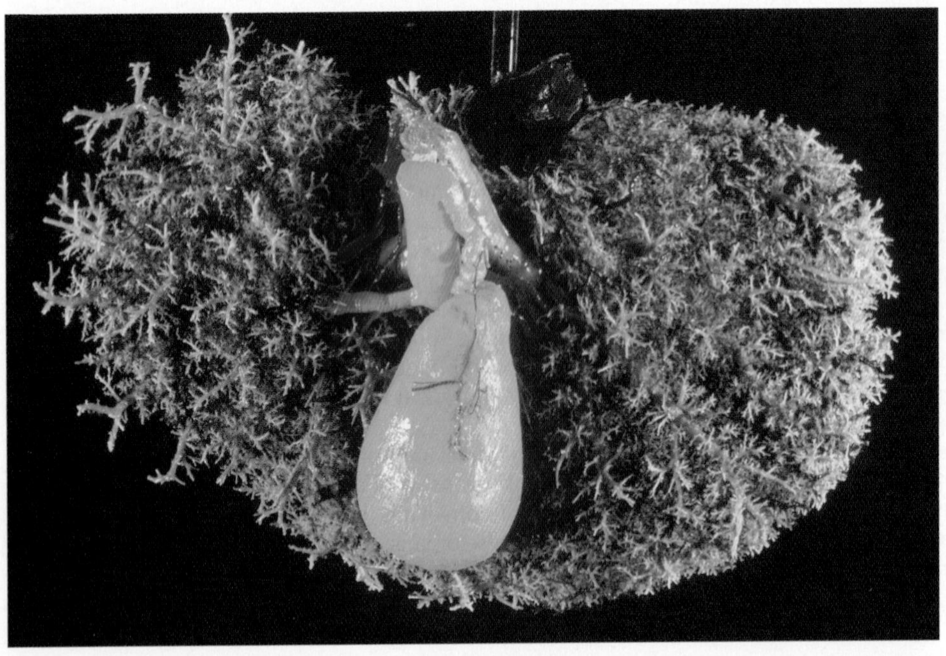

Figure 5-9 A plastinized specimen of the liver as seen on its posteroinferior (visceral) surface. The portal vein has been transfused with white plastic and the inferior vena cava with dark blue plastic. Outside the liver, the distended biliary ducts and gallbladder have been injected with yellow plastic and the hepatic artery with red plastic. The liver was then immersed in corrosive fluid to remove the liver tissue. Note the profuse branching of the portal vein as its white terminal branches enter the portal canals between the liver lobules; the dark blue tributaries of many of the hepatic veins can also be seen.

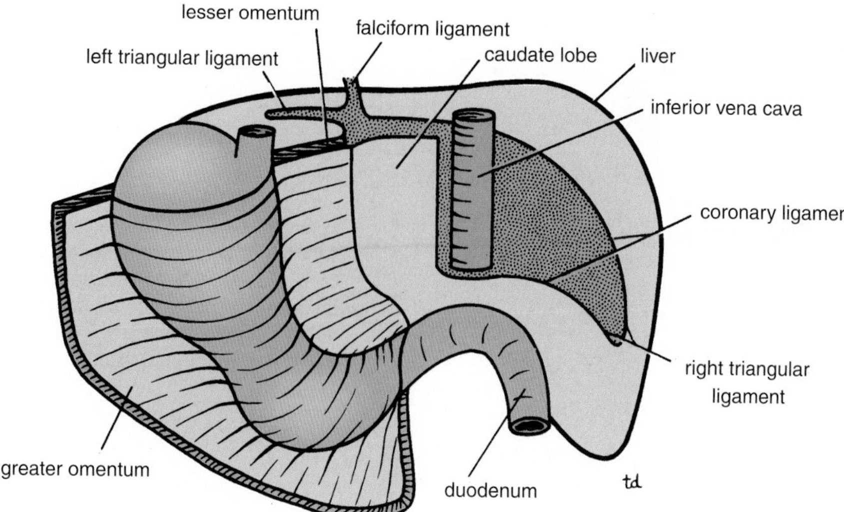

Figure 5-10 Attachment of the lesser omentum to the stomach and the posterior surface of the liver.

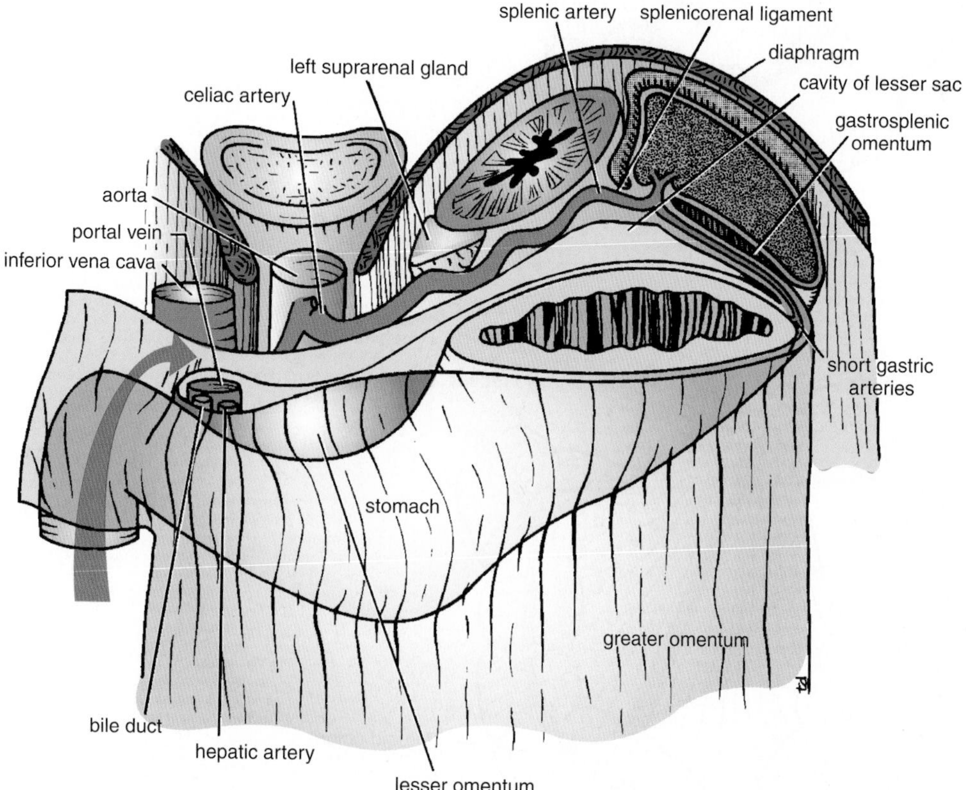

Figure 5-11 Transverse section of the lesser sac showing the arrangement of the peritoneum in the formation of the lesser omentum, the gastrosplenic omentum, and the splenicorenal ligament. Arrow indicates the position of the opening of the lesser sac.

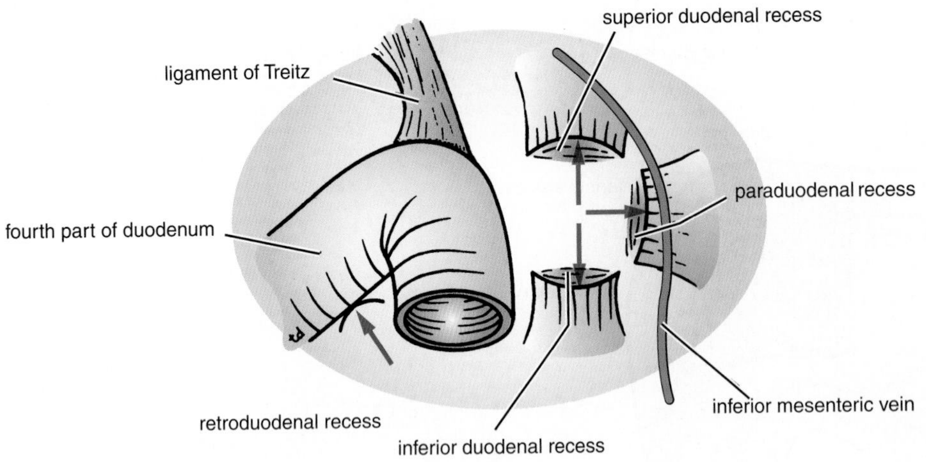

Figure 5-12 Peritoneal recesses, which may be present in the region of the duodenojejunal junction. Note the presence of the inferior mesenteric vein in the peritoneal fold, forming the paraduodenal recess.

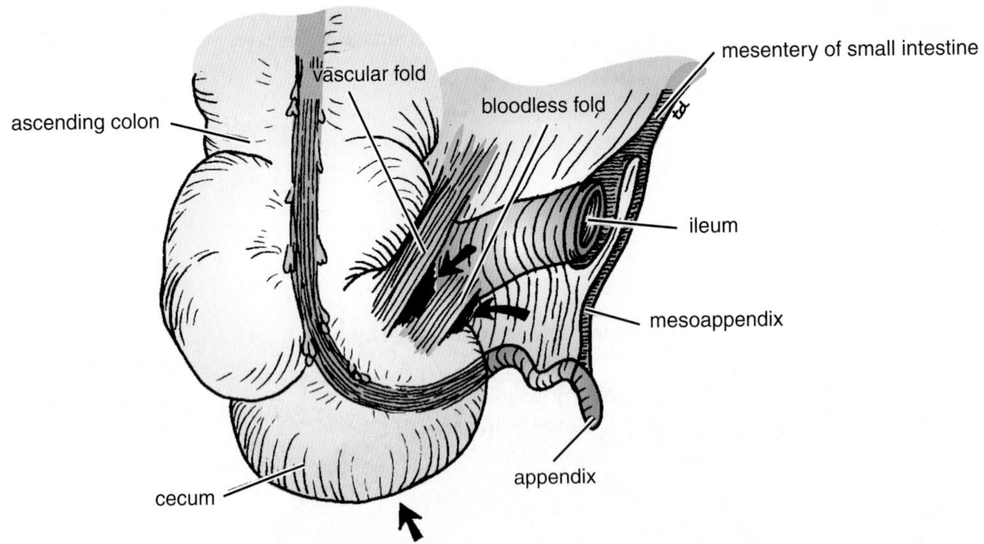

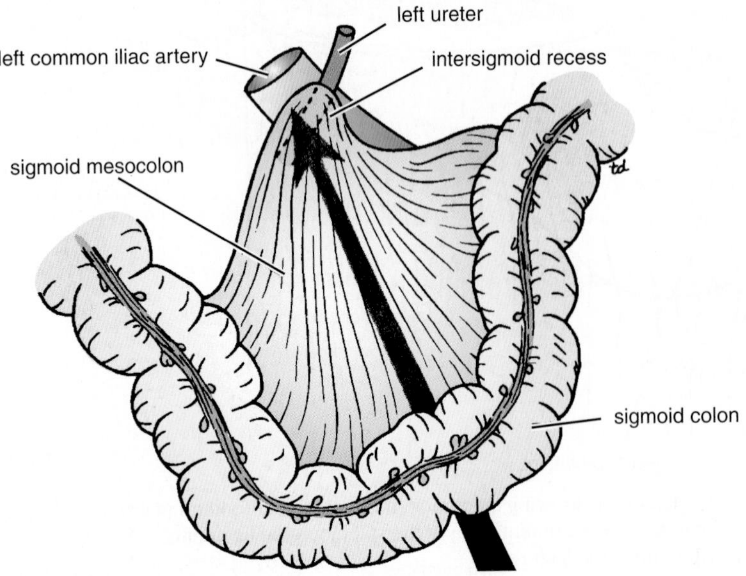

Figure 5-13 Peritoneal recesses (*arrows*) in the region of the cecum and the recess related to the sigmoid mesocolon.

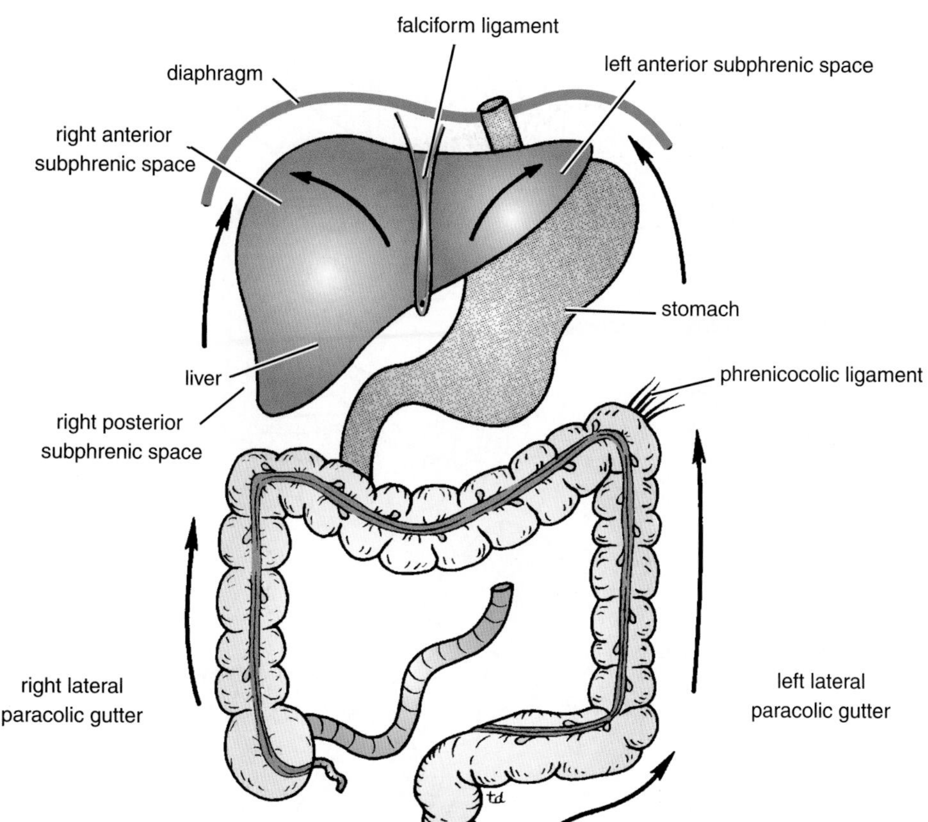

Figure 5-14 Normal direction of flow of the peritoneal fluid from different parts of the peritoneal cavity to the subphrenic spaces.

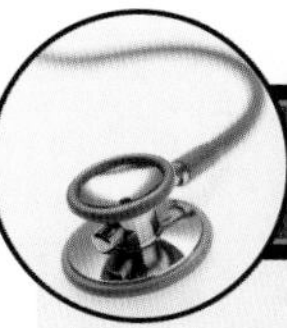

CLINICAL NOTES

The Peritoneum and Peritoneal Cavity

Movement of Peritoneal Fluid

The peritoneal cavity is divided into an upper part within the abdomen and a lower part in the pelvis. The abdominal part is further subdivided by the many peritoneal reflections into important recesses and spaces, which, in turn, are continued into the paracolic gutters (Fig. 5-15). The attachment of the transverse mesocolon and the mesentery of the small intestine to the posterior abdominal wall provides natural peritoneal barriers that may hinder the movement of infected peritoneal fluid from the upper part to the lower part of the peritoneal cavity.

It is interesting to note that when the patient is in the supine position the right subphrenic peritoneal space and the pelvic cavity are the lowest areas of the peritoneal cavity and the region of the pelvic brim is the highest area (Fig. 5-15).

Peritoneal Infection

Infection may gain entrance to the peritoneal cavity through several routes: from the interior of the gastrointestinal tract and gallbladder, through the anterior abdominal wall, via the uterine tubes in females (gonococcal peritonitis in adults and pneumococcal peritonitis in children occur through this route), and from the blood.

Collection of infected peritoneal fluid in one of the **subphrenic spaces** is often accompanied by infection of the pleural cavity. It is common to find a localized empyema in a patient with a subphrenic abscess. It is believed that the infection spreads from the peritoneum to the pleura via the diaphragmatic lymph vessels. A patient with a subphrenic abscess may complain of pain over the shoulder. (This also holds true for collections of blood under the diaphragm, which irritate the parietal diaphragmatic peritoneum.) The skin of the shoulder is supplied by the supraclavicular nerves (C3 and 4), which have the same segmental origin as the phrenic nerve, which supplies the peritoneum in the center of the undersurface of the diaphragm.

To avoid the accumulation of infected fluid in the subphrenic spaces and to delay the absorption of toxins from intraperitoneal infections, it is common nursing practice to sit a patient up in bed with the back at an angle of 45°. In this position, the infected peritoneal fluid tends to gravitate downward into the pelvic cavity, where the rate of toxin absorption is slow (Fig. 5-15).

Greater Omentum

Localization of Infection

The greater omentum is often referred to by the surgeons as the **abdominal policeman.** The lower and the right and left margins are free, and it moves about the peritoneal cavity in response to the peristaltic movements of the neighboring gut. In the first 2 years of life it is poorly developed and thus is less protective in a young child. Later, however, in an acutely inflamed appendix, for example, the inflammatory exudate causes the omentum to adhere to the appendix and wrap itself around the infected organ (Fig. 5-16).

(continues)

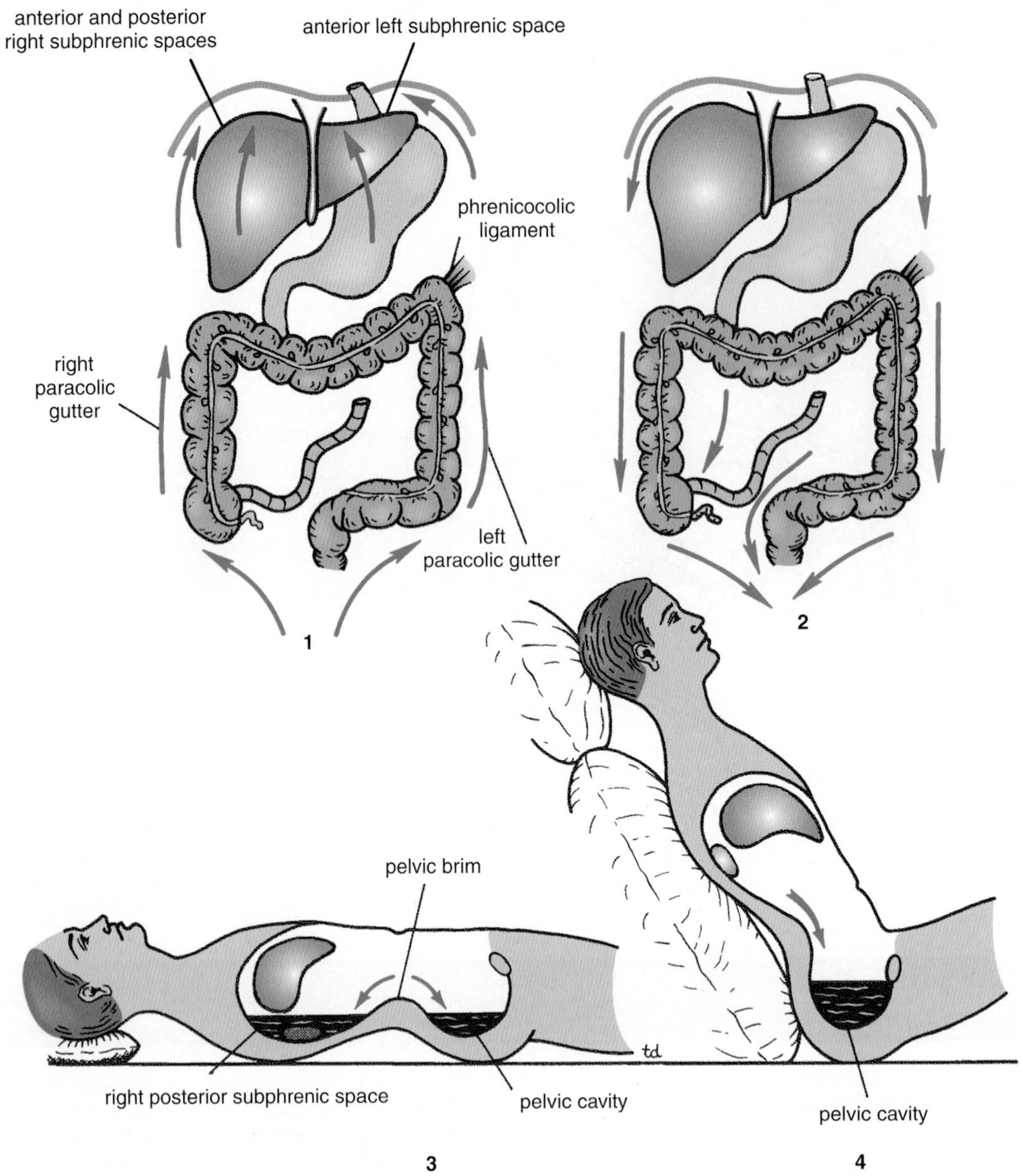

anterior and posterior right subphrenic spaces

anterior left subphrenic space

phrenicocolic ligament

right paracolic gutter

left paracolic gutter

1

2

pelvic brim

right posterior subphrenic space

pelvic cavity

pelvic cavity

3

4

Figure 5-15 Direction of flow of the peritoneal fluid. **1.** Normal flow upward to the subphrenic spaces. **2.** Flow of inflammatory exudate in peritonitis. **3.** The two sites where inflammatory exudate tends to collect when the patient is nursed in the supine position. **4.** Accumulation of inflammatory exudate in the pelvis when the patient is nursed in the inclined position.

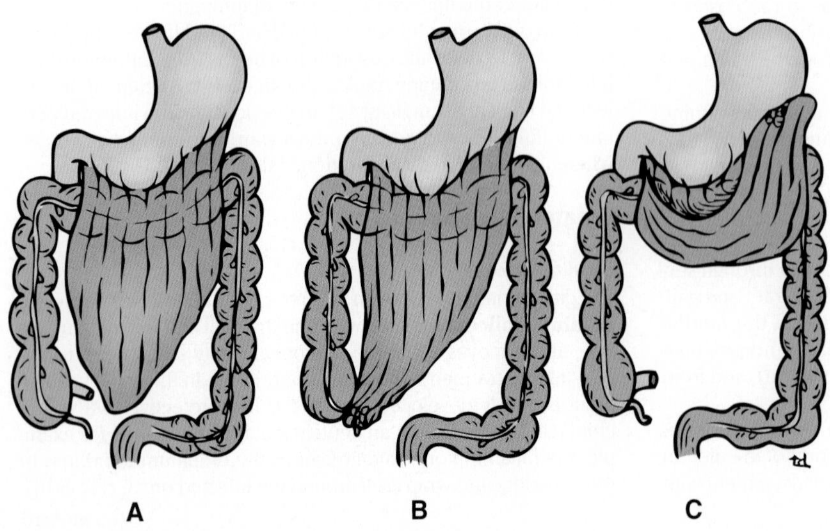

Figure 5-16 **A.** The normal greater omentum. **B.** The greater omentum wrapped around an inflamed appendix. **C.** The greater omentum adherent to the base of a gastric ulcer. One important function of the greater omentum is to attempt to limit the spread of intraperitoneal infections.

Clinical Notes, *continued*

By this means, the infection is often localized to a small area of the peritoneal cavity, thus saving the patient from a serious diffuse peritonitis.

Greater Omentum as a Hernial Plug

The greater omentum has been found to plug the neck of a hernial sac and prevent the entrance of coils of small intestine.

Greater Omentum in Surgery

Surgeons sometimes use the omentum to buttress an intestinal anastomosis or in the closure of a perforated gastric or duodenal ulcer.

Torsion of the Greater Omentum

The greater omentum may undergo torsion, and if extensive, the blood supply to a part of it may be cut off, causing necrosis.

Ascites

Ascites is essentially an excessive accumulation of peritoneal fluid within the peritoneal cavity. Ascites can occur secondary to hepatic cirrhosis (portal venous congestion), malignant disease (e.g., cancer of the ovary), or congestive heart failure (systemic venous congestion). In a thin patient, as much as 1500 mL has to accumulate before ascites can be recognized clinically. In obese individuals, a far greater amount has to collect before it can be detected. The withdrawal of peritoneal fluid from the peritoneal cavity is described on page 188.

Peritoneal Pain

From the Parietal Peritoneum

The parietal peritoneum lining the anterior abdominal wall is supplied by the lower six thoracic nerves and the first lumbar nerve. Abdominal pain originating from the parietal peritoneum is therefore of the somatic type and can be precisely localized; it is usually severe (see Abdominal Pain, page 281).

An inflamed parietal peritoneum is extremely sensitive to stretching. This fact is made use of clinically in diagnosing peritonitis. Pressure is applied to the abdominal wall with a single finger over the site of the inflammation. The pressure is then removed by suddenly withdrawing the finger. The abdominal wall rebounds, resulting in extreme local pain, which is known as **rebound tenderness.**

It should always be remembered that the parietal peritoneum in the pelvis is innervated by the obturator nerve and can be palpated by means of a rectal or vaginal examination. An inflamed appendix may hang down into the pelvis and irritate the parietal peritoneum. A pelvic examination can detect extreme tenderness of the parietal peritoneum on the right side (see page 345).

From the Visceral Peritoneum

The visceral peritoneum, including the mesenteries, is innervated by autonomic afferent nerves. Stretch caused by overdistension of a viscus or pulling on a mesentery gives rise to the sensation of pain. The sites of origin of visceral pain are shown in Figure 5-17.

Because the gastrointestinal tract arises embryologically as a midline structure and receives a bilateral nerve supply, pain is referred to the midline. Pain arising from an abdominal viscus is dull and poorly localized (see Abdominal Pain, page 281).

Peritoneal Dialysis

Because the peritoneum is a semipermeable membrane, it allows rapid bidirectional transfer of substances across itself. Because the surface area of the peritoneum is enormous, this transfer property has been made use of in patients with acute renal insufficiency. The efficiency of this method is only a fraction of that achieved by hemodialysis.

A watery solution, the dialysate, is introduced through a catheter through a small midline incision through the anterior abdominal wall below the umbilicus. The technique is the same as peritoneal lavage (see page 189). The products of metabolism, such as urea, diffuse through the peritoneal lining cells from the blood vessels into the dialysate and are removed from the patient.

Internal Abdominal Hernia

Occasionally, a loop of intestine enters a peritoneal pouch or recess (e.g., the lesser sac or the duodenal recesses) and becomes strangulated at the edges of the recess. Remember that important structures form the boundaries of the entrance into the lesser sac and that the inferior mesenteric vein often lies in the anterior wall of the paraduodenal recess.

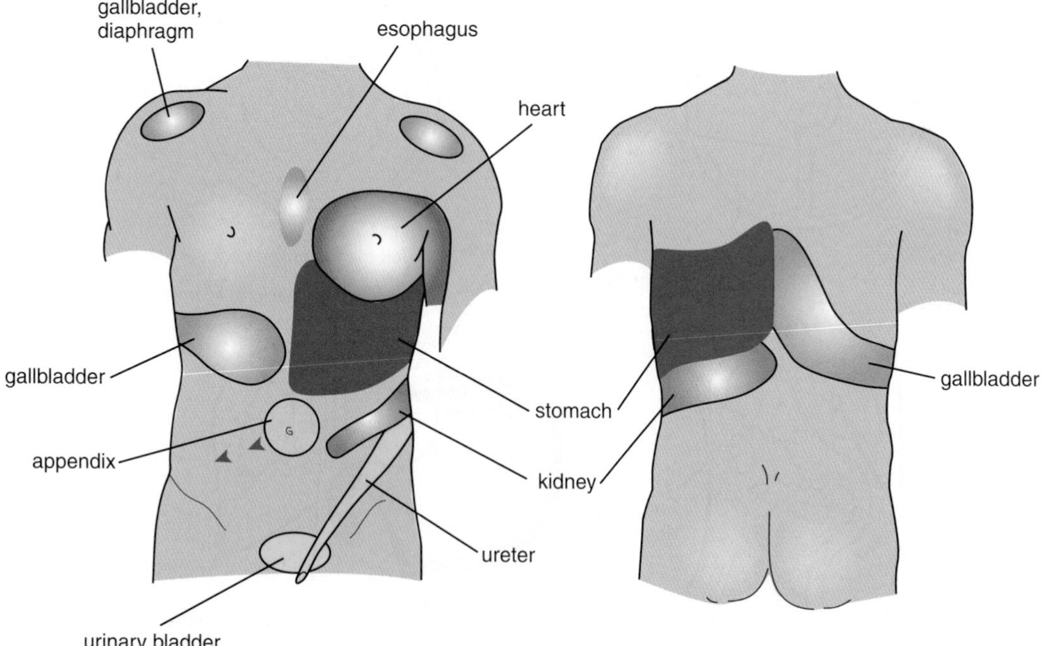

Figure 5-17 Some important skin areas involved in referred visceral pain.

EMBRYOLOGIC NOTES

Development of the Peritoneum and the Peritoneal Cavity

Once the lateral mesoderm has split into somatic and splanchnic layers, a cavity is formed between the two, called the **intraembryonic coelom.** The peritoneal cavity is derived from that part of the embryonic coelom situated caudal to the septum transversum. In the earliest stages, the peritoneal cavity is in free communication with the extraembryonic coelom on each side (see Fig. 4-36B). Later, with the development of the head, tail, and lateral folds of the embryo, this wide area of communication becomes restricted to the small area within the umbilical cord.

Early in development, the peritoneal cavity is divided into right and left halves by a central partition formed by the dorsal mesentery, the gut, and the small ventral mesentery (Fig. 5-18). However, the ventral mesentery extends only for a short distance along the gut (see below), so that below this level the right and left halves of the peritoneal cavity are in free communication (Fig. 5-18). As a result of the enormous growth of the liver and the enlargement of the developing kidneys, the capacity of the abdominal cavity becomes greatly reduced at about the sixth week of development. It is at this time that the small remaining communication between the peritoneal cavity and extraembryonic coelom becomes important. An intestinal loop is forced out of the abdominal cavity through the umbilicus into the umbilical cord. This physiologic herniation of the midgut takes place during the sixth week of development.

Formation of the Peritoneal Ligaments and Mesenteries

The peritoneal ligaments are developed from the ventral and dorsal mesenteries. The ventral mesentery is formed from the mesoderm of the septum transversum (derived from the cervical somites, which migrate downward). The ventral mesentery forms the **falciform ligament,** the **lesser omentum,** and the **coronary** and **triangular ligaments of the liver** (Fig. 5-18).

The dorsal mesentery is formed from the fusion of the splanchnopleuric mesoderm on the two sides of the embryo. It extends from the posterior abdominal wall to the posterior border of the abdominal part of the gut (Figs. 4-36 and 5-18). The dorsal mesentery forms the **gastrophrenic ligament,** the **gastrosplenic omentum,** the **splenicorenal ligament,** the **greater omentum,** and the **mesenteries of the small and large intestines.**

Formation of the Lesser and Greater Peritoneal Sacs

The extensive growth of the right lobe of the liver pulls the ventral mesentery to the right and causes rotation of the stomach and duodenum (Fig. 5-19). By this means, the upper right part of the peritoneal cavity becomes incorporated into the lesser sac. The right free border of the ventral mesentery becomes the right border of the lesser omentum and the anterior boundary of the entrance into the lesser sac.

The remaining part of the peritoneal cavity, which is not included in the lesser sac, is called the greater sac, and the two sacs are in communication through the **epiploic foramen.**

Formation of the Greater Omentum

The spleen is developed in the upper part of the dorsal mesentery, and the greater omentum is formed as a result of the rapid and extensive growth of the dorsal mesentery caudal to the spleen. To begin with, the greater omentum extends from the greater curvature of the stomach to the posterior abdominal wall superior to the transverse mesocolon. With continued growth, it reaches inferiorly as an apronlike double layer of peritoneum anterior to the transverse colon.

Later, the posterior layer of the omentum fuses with the transverse mesocolon; as a result, the greater omentum becomes attached to the anterior surface of the transverse colon (Fig. 5-19). As development proceeds, the omentum becomes laden with fat. The inferior recess of the lesser sac extends inferiorly between the anterior and the posterior layers of the fold of the greater omentum.

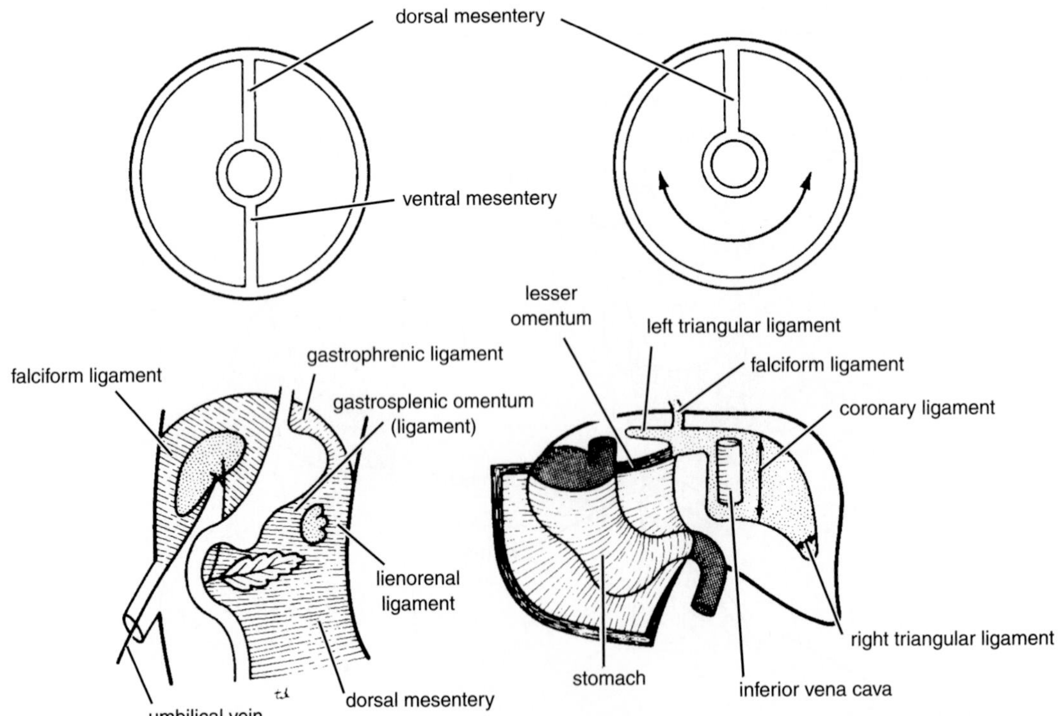

Figure 5-18 Ventral and dorsal mesenteries and the organs that develop within them.

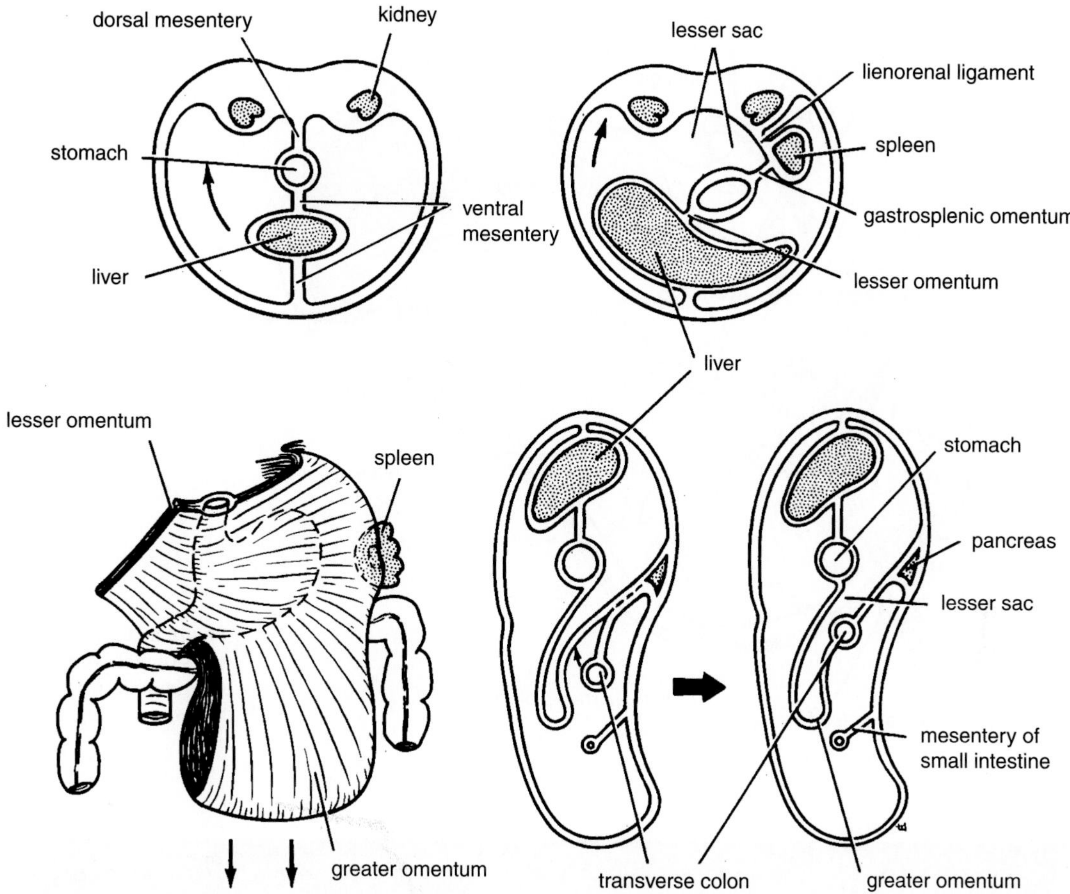

Figure 5-19 The rotation of the stomach and the formation of the greater omentum and lesser sac.

Gastrointestinal Tract

Esophagus (Abdominal Portion)

The esophagus is a muscular, collapsible tube about 10 in. (25 cm) long that joins the pharynx to the stomach. The greater part of the esophagus lies within the thorax (see page 127). The esophagus enters the abdomen through an opening in the right crus of the diaphragm (Fig. 5-4). After a course of about 0.5 in. (1.25 cm), it enters the stomach on its right side.

Relations

The esophagus is related anteriorly to the posterior surface of the left lobe of the liver and posteriorly to the left crus of the diaphragm. The left and right vagi lie on its anterior and posterior surfaces, respectively.

Blood Supply

Arteries

The arteries are branches from the left gastric artery (Fig. 5-20).

Veins

The veins drain into the left gastric vein, a tributary of the portal vein (see portal–systemic anastomosis, page 246).

Lymph Drainage

The lymph vessels follow the arteries into the left gastric nodes.

Nerve Supply

The nerve supply is the anterior and posterior gastric nerves (vagi) and sympathetic branches of the thoracic part of the sympathetic trunk.

Function

The esophagus conducts food from the pharynx into the stomach. Wavelike contractions of the muscular coat, called **peristalsis,** propel the food onward.

Gastroesophageal Sphincter

No anatomic sphincter exists at the lower end of the esophagus. However, the circular layer of smooth muscle in this region serves as a physiologic sphincter. As the food descends through the esophagus, relaxation of the muscle at the lower end occurs ahead of the peristaltic wave so that the food enters the stomach. The tonic contraction of this sphincter prevents the stomach contents from regurgitating into the esophagus.

The closure of the sphincter is under vagal control, and this can be augmented by the hormone gastrin and reduced in response to secretin, cholecystokinin, and glucagon.

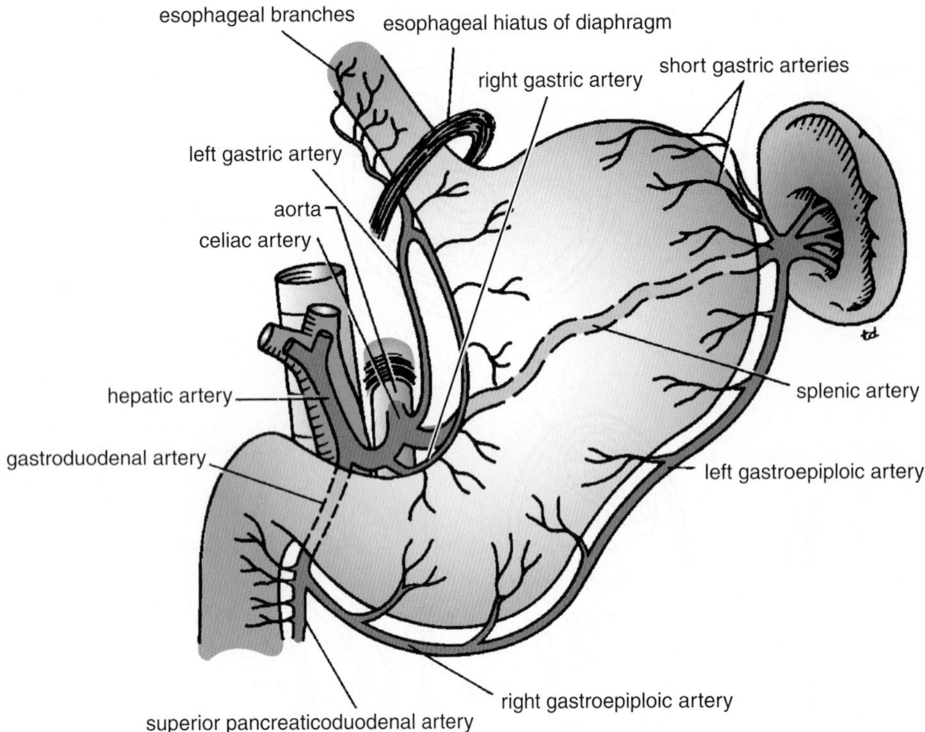

Figure 5-20 Arteries that supply the stomach. Note that all the arteries are derived from branches of the celiac artery.

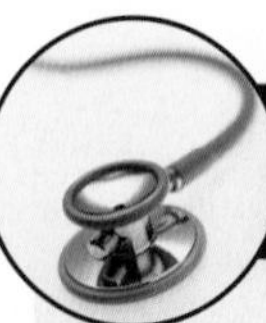

CLINICAL NOTES

The Esophagus

Narrow Areas of the Esophageal Lumen

The esophagus is narrowed at three sites: at the beginning, behind the cricoid cartilage of the larynx; where the left bronchus and the arch of the aorta cross the front of the esophagus; and where the esophagus enters the stomach. These three sites may offer resistance to the passage of a tube down the esophagus into the stomach (see Fig. 3-44).

Achalasia of the Cardia (Esophagogastric Junction)

The cause of achalasia is unknown, but it is associated with a degeneration of the parasympathetic plexus (Auerbach's plexus) in the wall of the esophagus. The primary site of the disorder may be in the innervation of the cardioesophageal sphincter by the vagus nerves. Dysphagia (difficulty in swallowing) and regurgitation are common symptoms that are later accompanied by proximal dilatation and distal narrowing of the esophagus.

Bleeding Esophageal Varices

At the lower third of the esophagus is an important **portal–systemic venous anastomosis** (see page 246). Here, the esophageal tributaries of the left gastric vein (which drains into the portal vein) anastomose with the esophageal tributaries of the azygos veins (systemic veins). Should the portal vein become obstructed, as, for example, in **cirrhosis of the liver,** portal hypertension develops, resulting in dilatation and varicosity of the portal–systemic anastomoses. Varicosed esophageal veins may rupture, causing severe vomiting of blood (hematemesis).

Anatomy of the Insertion of the Sengstaken-Blakemore Balloon for Esophageal Hemorrhage

The Sengstaken-Blakemore balloon is used for the control of massive esophageal hemorrhage from esophageal varices. A gastric balloon anchors the tube against the esophageal–gastric junction. An esophageal balloon occludes the esophageal varices by counterpressure. The tube is inserted through the nose or by using the oral route.

The lubricated tube is passed down into the stomach, and the gastric balloon is inflated. In the average adult the distance between the external orifices of the nose and the stomach is 17.2 in. (44 cm), and the distance between the incisor teeth and the stomach is 16 in. (41 cm).

Anatomy of the Complications

- Difficulty in passing the tube through the nose
- Damage to the esophagus from overinflation of the esophageal tube
- Pressure on neighboring mediastinal structures as the esophagus is expanded by the balloon within its lumen
- Persistent hiccups caused by irritation of the diaphragm by the distended esophagus and irritation of the stomach by the blood

Stomach

Location and Description

The stomach is the dilated portion of the alimentary canal and has three main functions: It stores food (in the adult it has a capacity of about 1500 mL), it mixes the food with gastric secretions to form a semifluid **chyme,** and it controls the rate of delivery of the chyme to the small intestine so that efficient digestion and absorption can take place.

The stomach is situated in the upper part of the abdomen, extending from beneath the left costal margin region into the epigastric and umbilical regions. Much of the stomach lies under cover of the lower ribs. It is roughly J-shaped and has two openings, the **cardiac** and **pyloric orifices;** two curvatures, the **greater** and **lesser curvatures;** and two surfaces, an **anterior** and a **posterior surface** (Fig. 5-21).

The stomach is relatively fixed at both ends but is very mobile in between. It tends to be high and transversely arranged in the short, obese person (steer-horn stomach) and elongated vertically in the tall, thin person (J-shaped stomach). Its shape undergoes considerable variation in the same person and depends on the volume of its contents, the position of the body, and the phase of respiration.

The stomach is divided into the following parts (Fig. 5-21):

- **Fundus:** This is dome-shaped and projects upward and to the left of the cardiac orifice. It is usually full of gas.
- **Body:** This extends from the level of the cardiac orifice to the level of the **incisura angularis,** a constant notch in the lower part of the lesser curvature (Fig. 5-21).
- **Pyloric antrum:** This extends from the incisura angularis to the pylorus (Fig. 5-21).

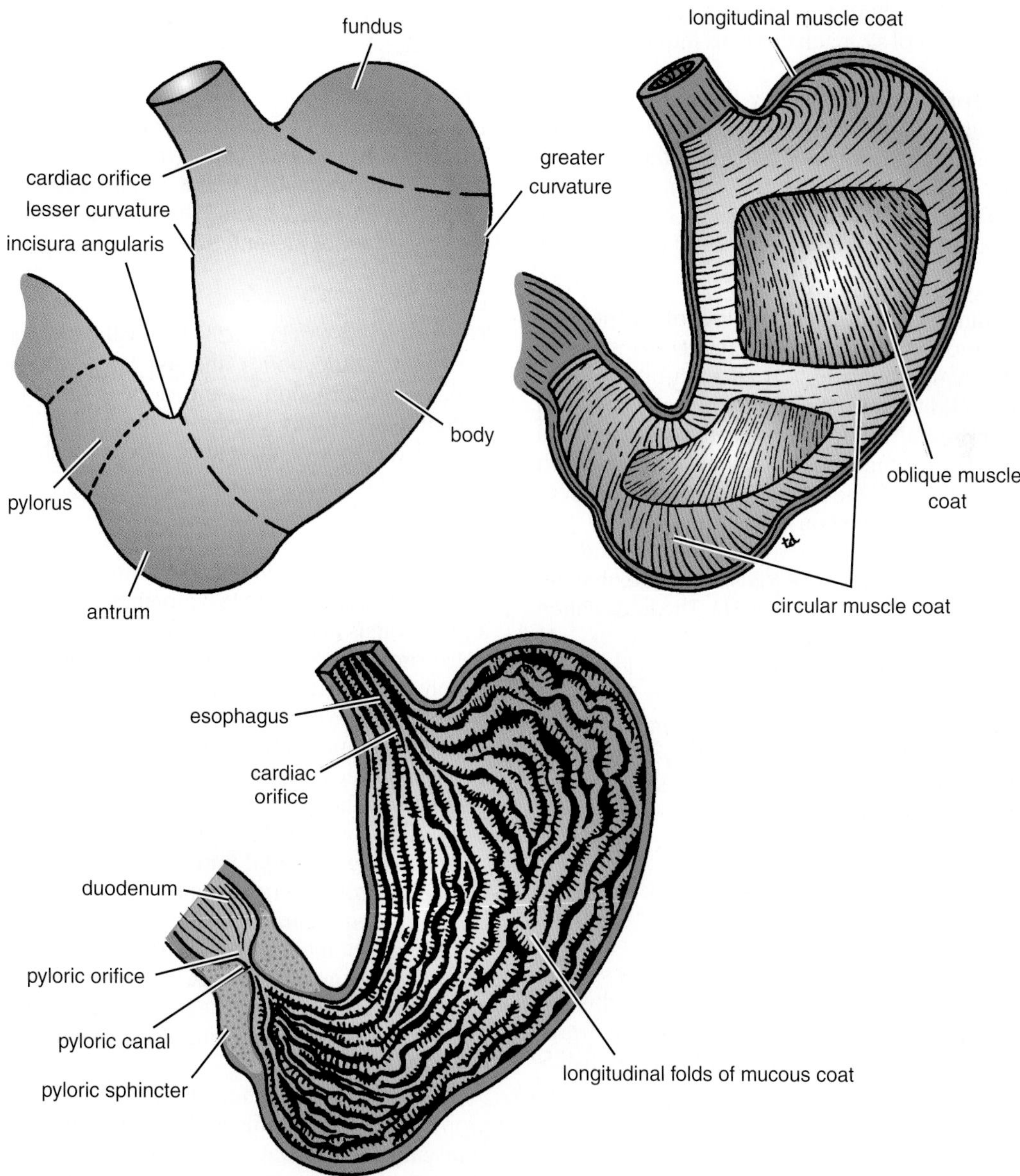

Figure 5-21 Stomach showing the parts, muscular coats, and mucosal lining. Note the increased thickness of the circular muscle forming the pyloric sphincter.

- **Pylorus:** This is the most tubular part of the stomach. The thick muscular wall is called the **pyloric sphincter,** and the cavity of the pylorus is the **pyloric canal** (Fig. 5-21).

The **lesser curvature** forms the right border of the stomach and extends from the cardiac orifice to the pylorus (Fig. 5-21). It is suspended from the liver by the lesser omentum. The **greater curvature** is much longer than the lesser curvature and extends from the left of the cardiac orifice, over the dome of the fundus, and along the left border of the stomach to the pylorus (Fig. 5-21). The gastrosplenic omentum (ligament) extends from the upper part of the greater curvature to the spleen, and the greater omentum extends from the lower part of the greater curvature to the transverse colon (Fig. 5-11).

The **cardiac orifice** is where the esophagus enters the stomach (Fig. 5-21). Although no anatomic sphincter can be demonstrated here, a physiologic mechanism exists that prevents regurgitation of stomach contents into the esophagus (see page 217).

The **pyloric orifice** is formed by the **pyloric canal,** which is about 1 in. (2.5 cm) long. The circular muscle coat of the stomach is much thicker here and forms the anatomic and physiologic **pyloric sphincter** (Fig. 5-21). The pylorus lies on the transpyloric plane, and its position can be recognized by a slight constriction on the surface of the stomach.

Function of the Pyloric Sphincter

The pyloric sphincter controls the outflow of gastric contents into the duodenum. The sphincter receives motor fibers from the sympathetic system and inhibitory fibers from the vagi. In addition, the pylorus is controlled by local nervous and hormonal influences from the stomach and duodenal walls. For example, the stretching of the stomach due to filling will stimulate the myenteric nerve plexus in its wall and reflexly cause relaxation of the sphincter.

The **mucous membrane** of the stomach is thick and vascular and is thrown into numerous folds, or **rugae,** that are mainly longitudinal in direction (Fig. 5-21). The folds flatten out when the stomach is distended.

The **muscular wall of the stomach** contains longitudinal fibers, circular fibers, and oblique fibers (Fig. 5-21).

The **peritoneum** (visceral peritoneum) completely surrounds the stomach. It leaves the lesser curvature as the lesser omentum and the greater curvature as the gastrosplenic omentum and the greater omentum.

Relations

- **Anteriorly:** The anterior abdominal wall, the left costal margin, the left pleura and lung, the diaphragm, and the left lobe of the liver (Figs. 5-2 and 5-6)
- **Posteriorly:** The lesser sac, the diaphragm, the spleen, the left suprarenal gland, the upper part of the left kidney, the splenic artery, the pancreas, the transverse mesocolon, and the transverse colon (Figs. 5-4, 5-6, and 5-11)

Blood Supply

Arteries

The arteries are derived from the branches of the celiac artery (Fig. 5-20).

The **left gastric artery** arises from the celiac artery. It passes upward and to the left to reach the esophagus and then descends along the lesser curvature of the stomach. It supplies the lower third of the esophagus and the upper right part of the stomach.

The **right gastric artery** arises from the hepatic artery at the upper border of the pylorus and runs to the left along the lesser curvature. It supplies the lower right part of the stomach.

The **short gastric arteries** arise from the splenic artery at the hilum of the spleen and pass forward in the gastrosplenic omentum (ligament) to supply the fundus.

The **left gastroepiploic artery** arises from the splenic artery at the hilum of the spleen and passes forward in the gastrosplenic omentum (ligament) to supply the stomach along the upper part of the greater curvature.

The **right gastroepiploic artery** arises from the gastroduodenal branch of the hepatic artery. It passes to the left and supplies the stomach along the lower part of the greater curvature.

Veins

The veins drain into the portal circulation (Fig. 5-22). The **left** and **right gastric veins** drain directly into the portal vein. The **short gastric veins** and the **left gastroepiploic veins** join the splenic vein. The **right gastroepiploic vein** joins the superior mesenteric vein.

Lymph Drainage

The lymph vessels (Fig. 5-23) follow the arteries into the left and right gastric nodes, the left and right gastroepiploic nodes, and the short gastric nodes. All lymph from the stomach eventually passes to the celiac nodes located around the root of the celiac artery on the posterior abdominal wall.

Nerve Supply

The nerve supply includes sympathetic fibers derived from the celiac plexus and parasympathetic fibers from the right and left vagus nerves (Fig. 5-24).

The **anterior vagal trunk,** which is formed in the thorax mainly from the left vagus nerve, enters the abdomen on the anterior surface of the esophagus. The trunk, which may be single or multiple, then divides into branches that supply the anterior surface of the stomach. A large hepatic branch passes up to the liver, and from this a pyloric branch passes down to the pylorus (Fig. 5-24).

The **posterior vagal trunk,** which is formed in the thorax mainly from the right vagus nerve, enters the abdomen on the posterior surface of the esophagus. The trunk then divides into branches that supply mainly the posterior surface of the stomach. A large branch passes to the celiac and superior mesenteric plexuses and is distributed to the intestine as far as the splenic flexure and to the pancreas (Fig. 5-24).

The sympathetic innervation of the stomach carries a proportion of pain-transmitting nerve fibers, whereas the parasympathetic vagal fibers are secretomotor to the gastric glands and motor to the muscular wall of the stomach. The pyloric sphincter receives motor fibers from the sympathetic system and inhibitory fibers from the vagi.

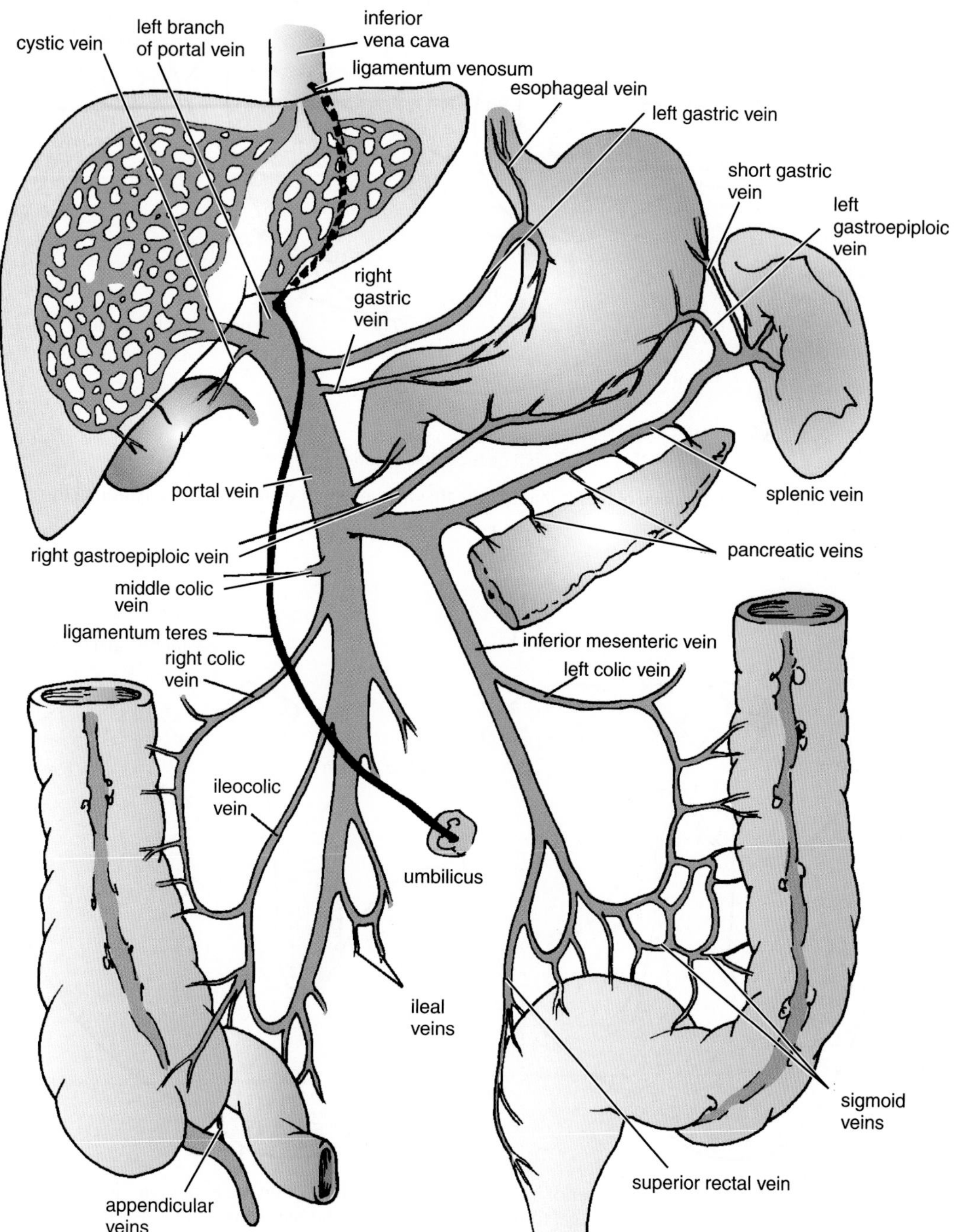

Figure 5-22 Tributaries of the portal vein.

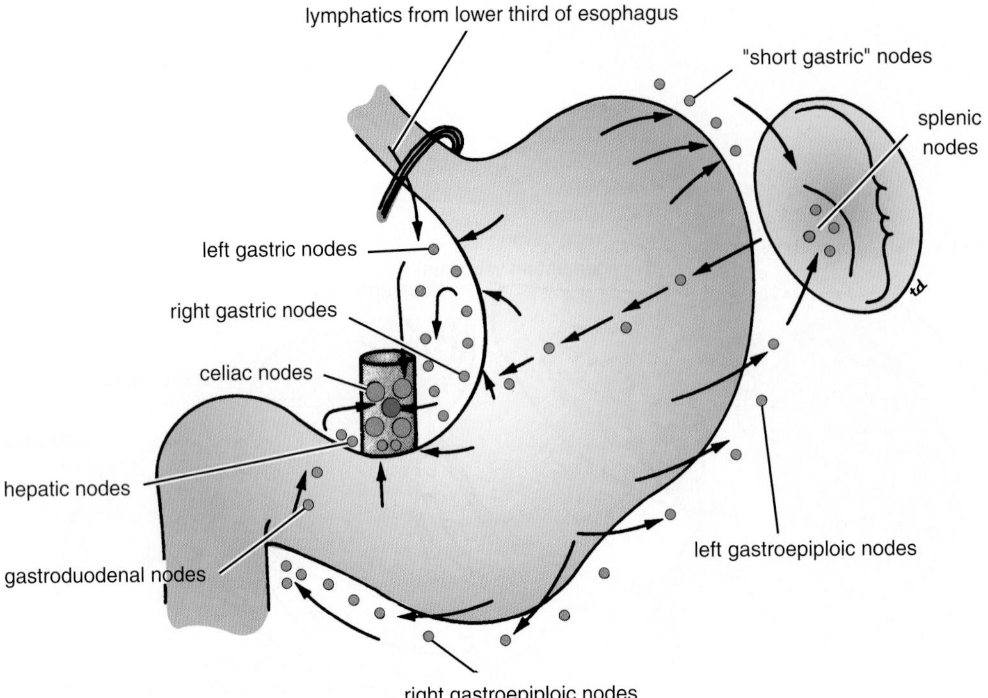

Figure 5-23 Lymph drainage of the stomach. Note that all the lymph eventually passes through the celiac lymph nodes.

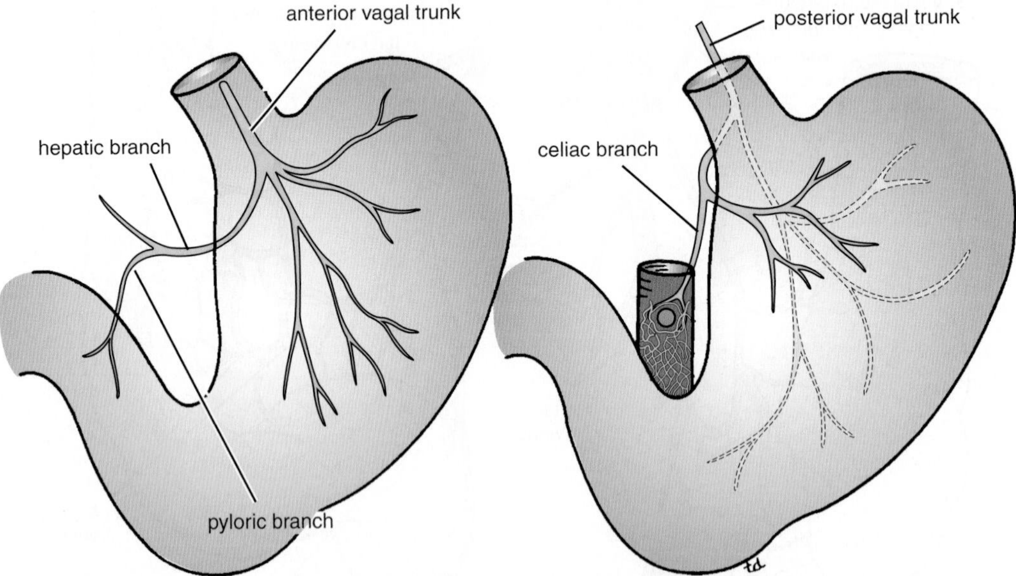

Figure 5-24 Distribution of the anterior and posterior vagal trunks within the abdomen. Note that the celiac branch of the posterior vagal trunk is distributed with the sympathetic nerves as far down the intestinal tract as the left colic flexure.

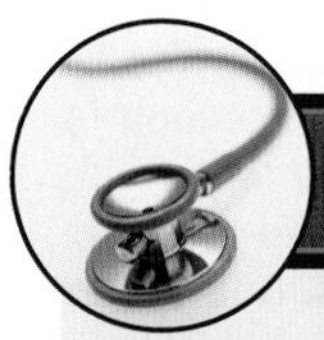

CLINICAL NOTES

Trauma to the Stomach

Apart from its attachment to the esophagus at the cardiac orifice and its continuity with the duodenum at the pylorus, the stomach is relatively mobile. It is protected on the left by the lower part of the rib cage. These factors greatly protect the stomach from blunt trauma to the abdomen. However, its large size makes it vulnerable to gunshot wounds.

Gastric Ulcer

The mucous membrane of the body of the stomach and, to a lesser extent, that of the fundus produce acid and pepsin. The secretion of the antrum and pyloric canal is mucous and weakly alkaline (Fig. 5-25). The secretion of acid and pepsin is controlled by two mechanisms: nervous and hormonal. The vagus nerves are responsible for the nervous control, and the hormone **gastrin,** produced by the antral mucosa, is responsible for the hormonal control. In the surgical treatment of chronic gastric and duodenal ulcers, attempts are made to reduce the amount of acid secretion by sectioning the vagus nerves (vagotomy) and by removing the gastrin-bearing area of mucosa, the antrum (partial gastrectomy).

Gastric ulcers occur in the alkaline-producing mucosa of the stomach, usually on or close to the lesser curvature. A chronic ulcer invades the muscular coats and, in time, involves the peritoneum so that the stomach adheres to neighboring structures. An ulcer situated on the posterior wall of the stomach may perforate into the lesser sac or become adherent to the pancreas. Erosion of the pancreas produces pain referred to the back. The splenic artery runs along the upper border of the pancreas, and erosion of this artery may produce fatal hemorrhage. A penetrating ulcer of the anterior stomach wall may result in the escape of stomach contents into the greater sac, producing diffuse peritonitis. The anterior stomach wall may, however, adhere to the liver, and the chronic ulcer may penetrate the liver substance.

Gastric Pain

The sensation of pain in the stomach is caused by the stretching or spasmodic contraction of the smooth muscle in its walls and is referred to the epigastrium. It is believed that the pain-transmitting fibers leave the stomach in company with the sympathetic nerves. They pass through the celiac ganglia and reach the spinal cord via the greater splanchnic nerves.

Cancer of the Stomach

Because the lymphatic vessels of the mucous membrane and submucosa of the stomach are in continuity, it is possible for cancer cells to travel to different parts of the stomach, some distance away from the primary site. Cancer cells also often pass through or bypass the local lymph nodes and are held up in the regional nodes. For these reasons, malignant disease of the stomach is treated by total gastrectomy, which includes the removal of the lower end of the esophagus and the first part of the duodenum; the spleen and the gastrosplenic and splenicorenal ligaments and their associated lymph nodes; the splenic vessels; the tail and body of the pancreas and their associated nodes; the nodes along the lesser curvature of the stomach; and the nodes along the greater curvature, along with the greater omentum. This radical operation is a desperate attempt to remove the stomach en bloc and, with it, its lymphatic field. The continuity of the gut is restored by anastomosing the esophagus with the jejunum.

Gastroscopy

Gastroscopy is the viewing of the mucous membrane of the stomach through an illuminated tube fitted with a lens system. The patient is anesthetized and the gastroscope is passed into the stomach, which is then inflated with air. With a flexible fiberoptic instrument, direct visualization of different parts of the gastric mucous membrane is possible. It is also possible to perform a mucosal biopsy through a gastroscope.

Nasogastric Intubation

Nasogastric intubation is a common procedure and is performed to empty the stomach, to decompress the stomach in cases of intestinal obstruction, or before operations on the gastrointestinal tract; it may also be performed to obtain a sample of gastric juice for biochemical analysis.

1. The patient is placed in the semiupright position or left lateral position to avoid aspiration.
2. The well-lubricated tube is inserted through the wider nostril and is directed backward along the nasal floor.
3. Once the tube has passed the soft palate and entered the oral pharynx, decreased resistance is felt, and the conscious patient will feel like gagging.
4. Some important distances in the adult may be useful. From the nostril (external nares) to the cardiac orifice of the stomach is about 17.2 in. (44 cm), and from the cardiac orifice to the pylorus of the stomach is 4.8 to 5.6 in. (12 to 14 cm). The curved course taken by the tube from the cardiac orifice to the pylorus is usually longer, 6.0 to 10.0 in. (15 to 25 cm) (see Fig. 3-51).

Anatomic Structures That May Impede the Passage of the Nasogastric Tube

- A deviated nasal septum makes the passage of the tube difficult on the narrower side.
- Three sites of esophageal narrowing may offer resistance to the nasogastric tube—at the beginning of the esophagus behind the cricoid cartilage (7.2 in. [18 cm]), where the left bronchus and the arch of the aorta cross the front of the esophagus (11.2 in. [28 cm]), and where the esophagus enters the stomach (17.2 in. [44 cm]). The upper esophageal narrowing may be overcome by gently grasping the wings of the thyroid cartilage and pulling the larynx forward. This maneuver opens the normally collapsed esophagus and permits the tube to pass down without further delay.

Anatomy of Complications

- The nasogastric tube enters the larynx instead of the esophagus.
- Rough insertion of the tube into the nose will cause nasal bleeding from the mucous membrane.
- Penetration of the wall of the esophagus or stomach. Always aspirate tube for gastric contents to confirm successful entrance into the stomach.

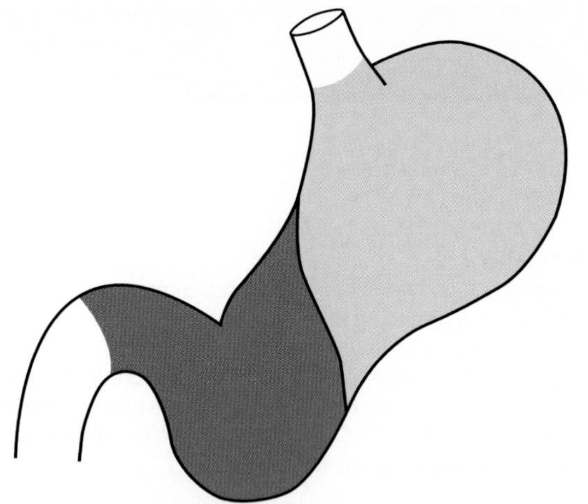

Figure 5-25 Areas of the stomach that produce acid and pepsin (*blue*) and alkali and gastrin (*red*).

Small Intestine

The small intestine is the longest part of the alimentary canal and extends from the pylorus of the stomach to the ileocecal junction (Fig. 5-1). The greater part of digestion and food absorption takes place in the small intestine. It is divided into three parts: the duodenum, the jejunum, and the ileum.

Duodenum

Location and Description

The duodenum is a C-shaped tube, about 10 in. (25 cm) long, which joins the stomach to the jejunum. It receives the openings of the bile and pancreatic ducts. The duodenum curves around the head of the pancreas (Fig. 5-26). The first inch (2.5 cm) of the duodenum resembles the stomach in that it is covered on its anterior and posterior surfaces with peritoneum and has the lesser omentum attached to its upper border and the greater omentum attached to its lower border; the lesser sac lies behind this short segment. The remainder of the duodenum is retroperitoneal, being only partially covered by peritoneum.

Parts of the Duodenum

The duodenum is situated in the epigastric and umbilical regions and, for purposes of description, is divided into four parts.

First Part of the Duodenum The first part of the duodenum begins at the pylorus and runs upward and backward on the transpyloric plane at the level of the first lumbar vertebra (Figs. 5-26 and 5-27).

The relations of this part are as follows:

- **Anteriorly:** The quadrate lobe of the liver and the gallbladder (Fig. 5-10)
- **Posteriorly:** The lesser sac (first inch only), the gastroduodenal artery, the bile duct and portal vein, and the inferior vena cava (Fig. 5-27)
- **Superiorly:** The entrance into the lesser sac (the epiploic foramen) (Figs. 5-7 and 5-11)
- **Inferiorly:** The head of the pancreas (Fig. 5-26)

Second Part of the Duodenum The second part of the duodenum runs vertically downward in front of the hilum of the right kidney on the right side of the second and third lumbar vertebrae (Figs. 5-26 and 5-27). About halfway down its medial border, the bile duct and the main pancreatic duct pierce the duodenal wall. They unite to form the ampulla that opens on the summit of the major duodenal

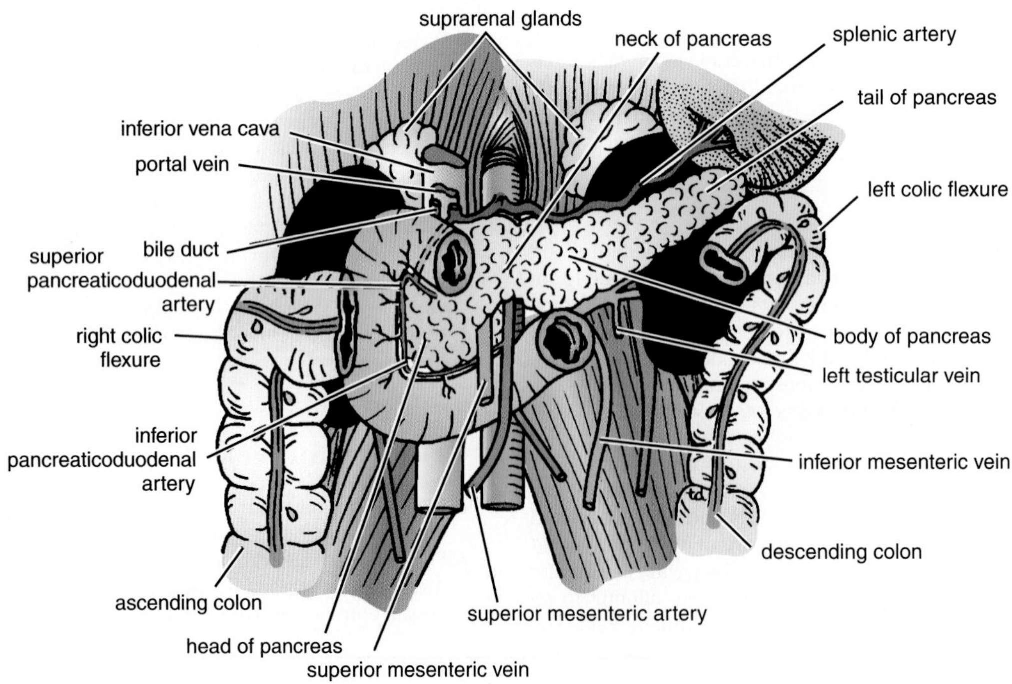

Figure 5-26 Pancreas and anterior relations of the kidneys.

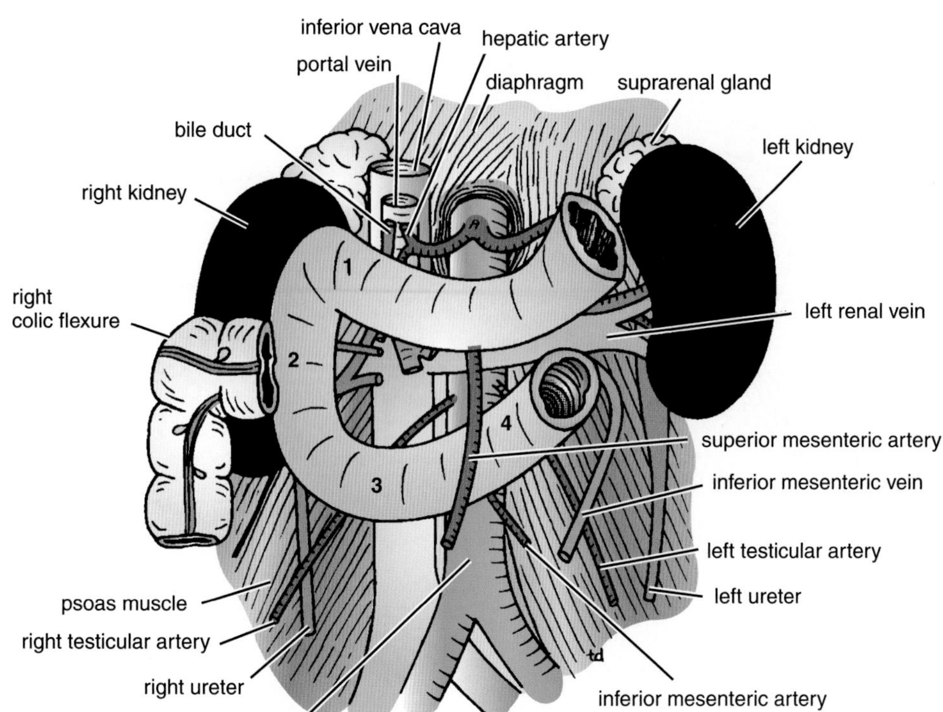

Figure 5-27 Posterior relations of the duodenum and the pancreas. The numbers represent the four parts of the duodenum.

papilla (Fig. 5-28). The accessory pancreatic duct, if present, opens into the duodenum a little higher up on the minor duodenal papilla (Figs. 5-27 and 5-28).

The relations of this part are as follows:

- **Anteriorly:** The fundus of the gallbladder and the right lobe of the liver, the transverse colon, and the coils of the small intestine (Fig. 5-29)
- **Posteriorly:** The hilum of the right kidney and the right ureter (Fig. 5-27)
- **Laterally:** The ascending colon, the right colic flexure, and the right lobe of the liver (Fig. 5-27)
- **Medially:** The head of the pancreas, the bile duct, and the main pancreatic duct (Figs. 5-27 and 5-28)

Third Part of the Duodenum The third part of the duodenum runs horizontally to the left on the subcostal plane, passing in front of the vertebral column and following the lower margin of the head of the pancreas (Figs. 5-26 and 5-27).

The relations of this part are as follows:

- **Anteriorly:** The root of the mesentery of the small intestine, the superior mesenteric vessels contained within it, and coils of jejunum (Figs. 5-26 and 5-27)
- **Posteriorly:** The right ureter, the right psoas muscle, the inferior vena cava, and the aorta (Fig. 5-27)
- **Superiorly:** The head of the pancreas (Fig. 5-26)
- **Inferiorly:** Coils of jejunum

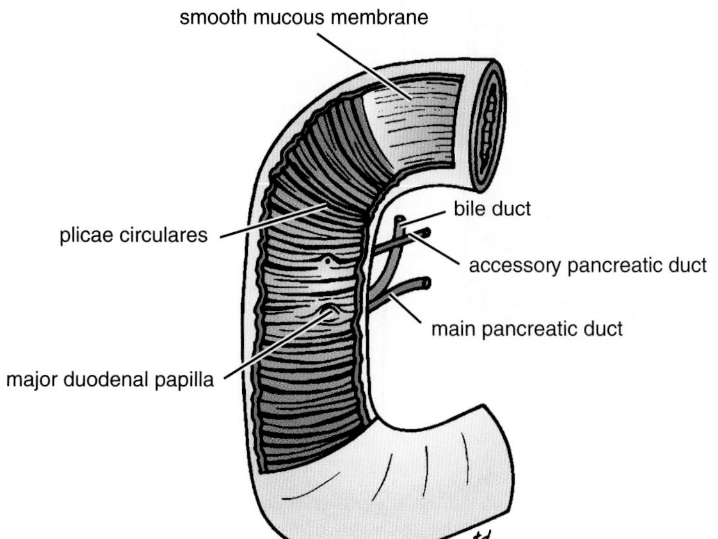

Figure 5-28 Entrance of the bile duct and the main and accessory pancreatic ducts into the second part of the duodenum. Note the smooth lining of the first part of the duodenum, the plicae circulares of the second part, and the major duodenal papilla.

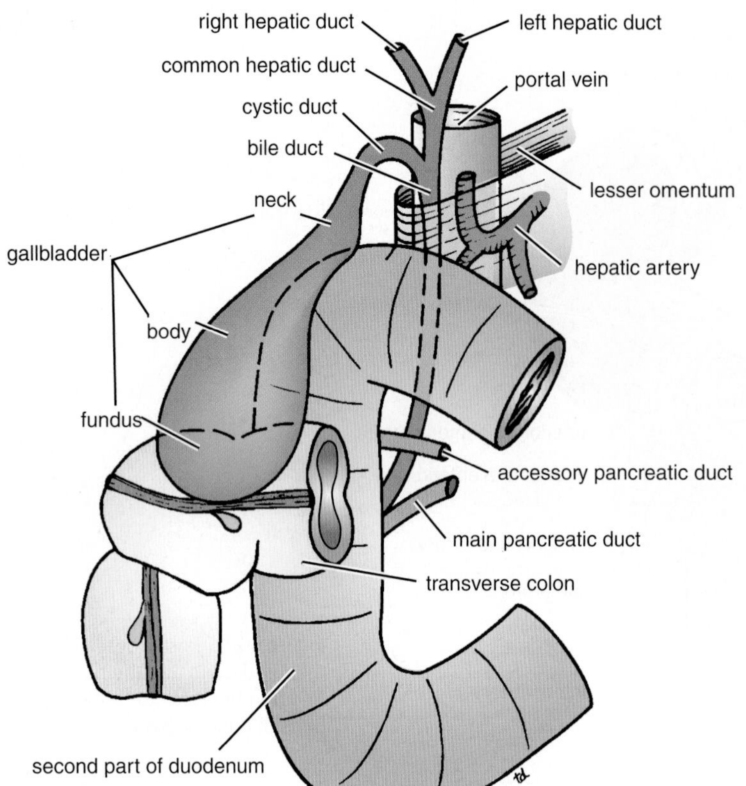

Figure 5-29 The bile ducts and the gallbladder. Note the relation of the gallbladder to the transverse colon and the duodenum.

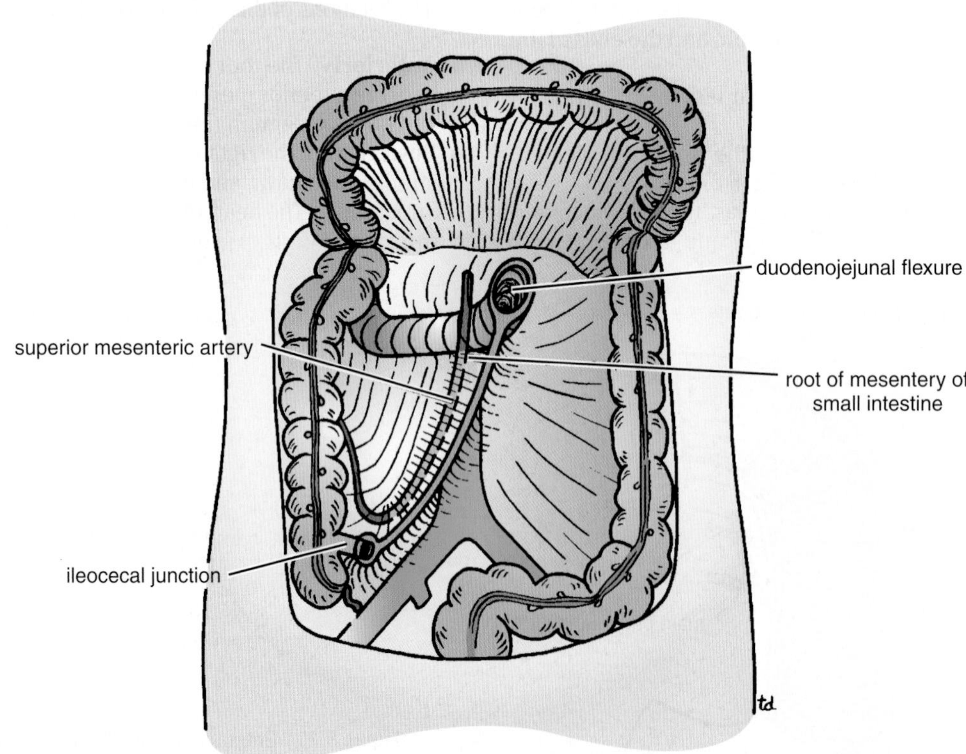

Figure 5-30 Attachment of the root of the mesentery of the small intestine to the posterior abdominal wall. Note that it extends from the duodenojejunal flexure on left of the aorta, downward and to the right to the ileocecal junction. The superior mesenteric artery lies in the root of the mesentery.

Fourth Part of the Duodenum The fourth part of the duodenum runs upward and to the left to the **duodenojejunal flexure** (Figs. 5-26 and 5-27). The flexure is held in position by a peritoneal fold, the **ligament of Treitz,** which is attached to the right crus of the diaphragm (Fig. 5-12).

The relations of this part are as follows:

- **Anteriorly:** The beginning of the root of the mesentery and coils of jejunum (Fig. 5-30)
- **Posteriorly:** The left margin of the aorta and the medial border of the left psoas muscle (Fig. 5-27)

Mucous Membrane and Duodenal Papillae

The **mucous membrane** of the duodenum is thick. In the first part of the duodenum it is smooth (Fig. 5-28). In the remainder of the duodenum it is thrown into numerous circular folds called the **plicae circulares.** At the site where the bile duct and the main pancreatic duct pierce the medial wall of the second part is a small, rounded elevation called the **major duodenal papilla** (Fig. 5-28). The accessory pancreatic duct, if present, opens into the duodenum on a smaller papilla about 0.75 in. (1.9 cm) above the major duodenal papilla.

Blood Supply

Arteries The upper half is supplied by the superior pancreaticoduodenal artery, a branch of the gastroduodenal artery (Figs. 5-20 and 5-26). The lower half is supplied by the inferior pancreaticoduodenal artery, a branch of the superior mesenteric artery.

Veins The superior pancreaticoduodenal vein drains into the portal vein; the inferior vein joins the superior mesenteric vein (Fig. 5-22).

Lymph Drainage

The lymph vessels follow the arteries and drain upward via pancreaticoduodenal nodes to the gastroduodenal nodes and then to the celiac nodes and downward via pancreaticoduodenal nodes to the superior mesenteric nodes around the origin of the superior mesenteric artery.

Nerve Supply

The nerves are derived from sympathetic and parasympathetic (vagus) nerves from the celiac and superior mesenteric plexuses.

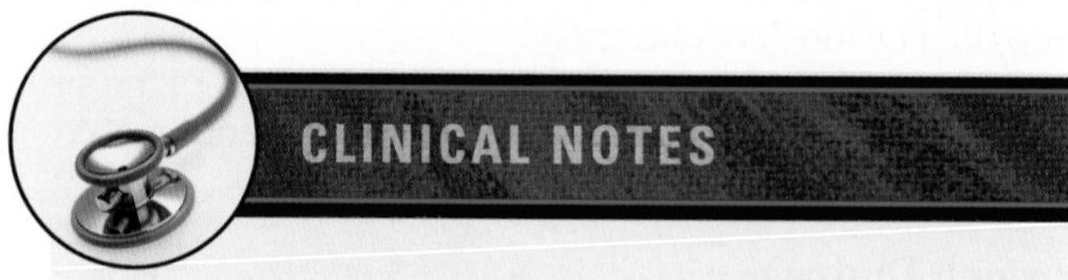

Trauma to the Duodenum

Apart from the first inch, the duodenum is rigidly fixed to the posterior abdominal wall by peritoneum and therefore cannot move away from crush injuries. In severe crush injuries to the anterior abdominal wall, the third part of the duodenum may be severely crushed or torn against the third lumbar vertebra.

Duodenal Ulcer

As the stomach empties its contents into the duodenum, the acid chyme is squirted against the anterolateral wall of the first

(continues)

Clinical Notes, *continued*

part of the duodenum. This is thought to be an important factor in the production of a duodenal ulcer at this site. An ulcer of the anterior wall of the first inch of the duodenum may perforate into the upper part of the greater sac, above the transverse colon. The transverse colon directs the escaping fluid into the right lateral paracolic gutter and thus down to the right iliac fossa. The differential diagnosis between a perforated duodenal ulcer and a perforated appendix may be difficult.

An ulcer of the posterior wall of the first part of the duodenum may penetrate the wall and erode the relatively large gastroduodenal artery, causing a severe hemorrhage.

The gastroduodenal artery is a branch of the hepatic artery, a branch of the celiac trunk (Fig. 5-4).

Duodenal Recesses

The importance of the duodenal recesses and the occurrence of herniae of the intestine were already alluded to on page 208.

Important Duodenal Relations

The relation to the duodenum of the gallbladder, the transverse colon, and the right kidney should be remembered. Cases have been reported in which a large gallstone ulcerated through the gallbladder wall into the duodenum. Operations on the colon and right kidney have resulted in damage to the duodenum.

Jejunum and Ileum

Location and Description

The jejunum and ileum measure about 20 ft (6 m) long; the upper two fifths of this length make up the jejunum. Each has distinctive features, but there is a gradual change from one to the other. The jejunum begins at the duodenojejunal flexure, and the ileum ends at the ileocecal junction.

The coils of jejunum and ileum re freely mobile and are attached to the posterior abdominal wall by a fan-shaped fold of peritoneum known as the **mesentery of the small intestine** (Fig. 5-30). The long free edge of the fold encloses the mobile intestine. The short root of the fold is continuous with the parietal peritoneum on the posterior abdominal wall along a line that extends downward and to the right from the left side of the second lumbar vertebra to the region of the right sacroiliac joint. The root of the mesentery permits the entrance and exit of the branches of the superior mesenteric artery and vein, lymph vessels, and nerves into the space between the two layers of peritoneum forming the mesentery.

In the living, the jejunum can be distinguished from the ileum by the following features:

- The jejunum lies coiled in the upper part of the peritoneal cavity below the left side of the transverse mesocolon; the ileum is in the lower part of the cavity and in the pelvis (Fig. 5-3).
- The jejunum is wider bored, thicker walled, and redder than the ileum. The jejunal wall feels thicker because the permanent infoldings of the mucous membrane, the plicae circulares, are larger, more numerous, and closely set in the jejunum, whereas in the upper part of the ileum

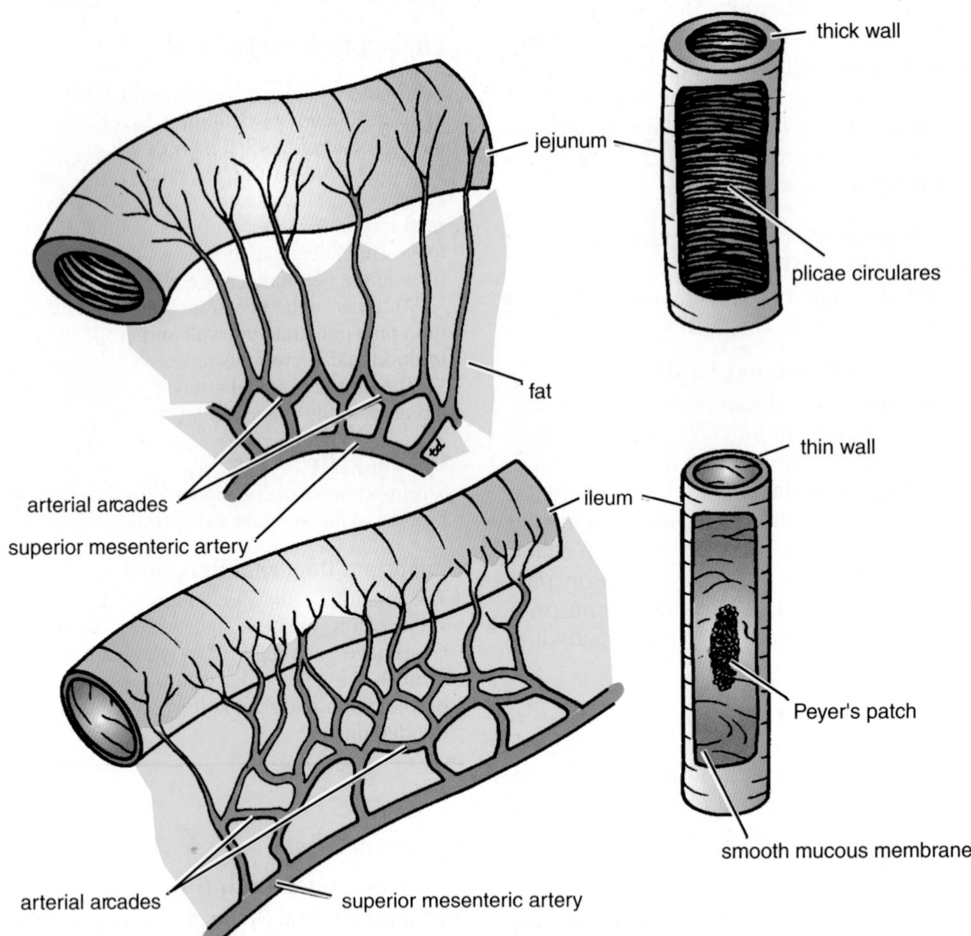

Figure 5-31 Some external and internal differences between the jejunum and the ileum.

they are smaller and more widely separated and in the lower part they are absent (Fig. 5-31).

- The jejunal mesentery is attached to the posterior abdominal wall above and to the left of the aorta, whereas the ileal mesentery is attached below and to the right of the aorta.
- The jejunal mesenteric vessels form only one or two arcades, with long and infrequent branches passing to the intestinal wall. The ileum receives numerous short terminal vessels that arise from a series of three or four or even more arcades (Fig. 5-31).
- At the jejunal end of the mesentery, the fat is deposited near the root and is scanty near the intestinal wall. At the ileal end of the mesentery the fat is deposited throughout so that it extends from the root to the intestinal wall (Fig. 5-31).
- Aggregations of lymphoid tissue (Peyer's patches) are present in the mucous membrane of the lower ileum along the antimesenteric border (Fig. 5-31). In the living these may be visible through the wall of the ileum from the outside.

Blood Supply

Arteries The arterial supply is from branches of the superior mesenteric artery (Fig. 5-32). The intestinal branches arise from the left side of the artery and run in the mesentery to reach the gut. They anastomose with one another to form a series of arcades. The lowest part of the ileum is also supplied by the ileocolic artery.

Veins The veins correspond to the branches of the superior mesenteric artery and drain into the superior mesenteric vein (Fig. 5-22).

Lymph Drainage

The lymph vessels pass through many intermediate mesenteric nodes and finally reach the superior mesenteric nodes, which are situated around the origin of the superior mesenteric artery.

Nerve Supply

The nerves are derived from the sympathetic and parasympathetic (vagus) nerves from the superior mesenteric plexus.

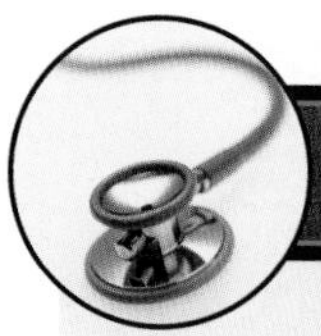

CLINICAL NOTES

Trauma to the Jejunum and Ileum

Because of its extent and position, the small intestine is commonly damaged by trauma. The extreme mobility and elasticity permit the coils to move freely over one another in instances of blunt trauma. Small, penetrating injuries may self-seal as a result of the mucosa plugging up the hole and the contraction of the smooth muscle wall. Material from large wounds leaks freely into the peritoneal cavity. The presence of the vertebral column and the prominent anterior margin of the first sacral vertebra may provide a firm background for intestinal crushing in cases of midline crush injuries.

Small-bowel contents have nearly a neutral pH and produce only slight chemical irritation to the peritoneum.

Recognition of the Jejunum and Ileum

A physician should be able to distinguish between the large and small intestine. He or she may be called on to examine a case of postoperative burst abdomen, where coils of gut are lying free in the bed. The macroscopic differences are described on page 227.

Tumors and Cysts of the Mesentery of the Small Intestine

The line of attachment of the small intestine to the posterior abdominal wall should be remembered. It extends from a point just to the left of the midline about 2 in. (5 cm) below the transpyloric plane (L1) downward to the right iliac fossa. A tumor or cyst of the mesentery, when palpated through the anterior abdominal wall, is more mobile in a direction at right angles to the line of attachment than along the line of attachment.

Pain Fibers from the Jejunum and Ileum

Pain fibers traverse the superior mesenteric sympathetic plexus and pass to the spinal cord via the splanchnic nerves. Referred pain from this segment of the gastrointestinal tract is felt in the dermatomes supplied by the 9th, 10th, and 11th thoracic nerves. Strangulation of a coil of small intestine in an inguinal hernia first gives rise to pain in the region of the umbilicus. Only later, when the parietal peritoneum of the hernial sac becomes inflamed, does the pain become more intense and localized to the inguinal region (see Abdominal Pain, page 281).

Mesenteric Arterial Occlusion

The superior mesenteric artery, a branch of the abdominal aorta, supplies an extensive territory of the gut, from halfway down the second part of the duodenum to the left colic flexure. Occlusion of the artery or one of its branches results in death of all or part of this segment of the gut. The occlusion may occur as the result of an embolus, a thrombus, an aortic dissection, or an abdominal aneurysm.

Mesenteric Vein Thrombosis

The superior mesenteric vein, which drains the same area of the gut supplied by the superior mesenteric artery, may undergo thrombosis after stasis of the venous bed. Cirrhosis of the liver with portal hypertension may predispose to this condition.

Meckel's Diverticulum

Meckel's diverticulum, a congenital anomaly of the ileum, is described on page 238.

Large Intestine

The large intestine extends from the ileum to the anus. It is divided into the cecum, appendix, ascending colon, transverse colon, descending colon, and sigmoid colon. The rectum and anal canal are considered in the sections on the pelvis and perineum. The primary function of the large intestine is the absorption of water and electrolytes and the storage of undigested material until it can be expelled from the body as feces.

Cecum

Location and Description

The cecum is that part of the large intestine that lies below the level of the junction of the ileum with the large intestine (Figs. 5-32 and 5-33). It is a blind-ended pouch that is situated in the right iliac fossa. It is about 2.5 in. (6 cm) long and is completely covered with peritoneum. It possesses a considerable amount of mobility, although it does not have a mesentery. Attached to its posteromedial surface is the appendix. The presence of peritoneal folds in the vicinity of the cecum (Fig. 5-33) creates the superior ileocecal, the inferior ileocecal, and the retrocecal recesses (see page 208).

As in the colon, the longitudinal muscle is restricted to three flat bands, the **teniae coli,** which converge on the base of the appendix and provide for it a complete longitudinal muscle coat (Fig. 5-33). The cecum is often distended with gas and can then be palpated through the anterior abdominal wall in the living patient.

The terminal part of the ileum enters the large intestine at the junction of the cecum with the ascending colon. The opening is provided with two folds, or lips, which form the so-called ileocecal valve (see below). The appendix communicates with the cavity of the cecum through an opening located below and behind the ileocecal opening.

Relations

- **Anteriorly:** Coils of small intestine, sometimes part of the greater omentum, and the anterior abdominal wall in the right iliac region
- **Posteriorly:** The psoas and the iliacus muscles, the femoral nerve, and the lateral cutaneous nerve of the thigh (Fig. 5-34). The appendix is commonly found behind the cecum.
- **Medially:** The appendix arises from the cecum on its medial side (Fig. 5-33).

Blood Supply

Arteries Anterior and posterior cecal arteries form the ileocolic artery, a branch of the superior mesenteric artery (Fig. 5-33).

Veins The veins correspond to the arteries and drain into the superior mesenteric vein.

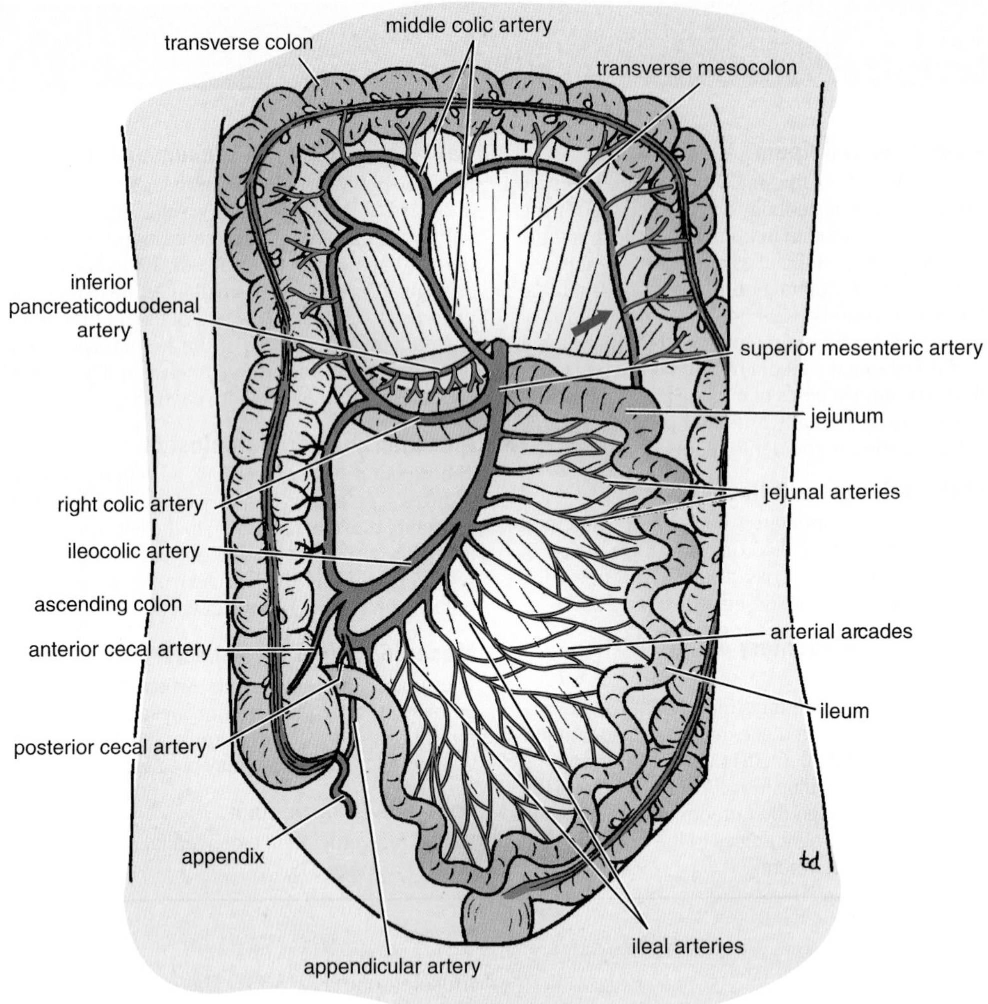

Figure 5-32 Superior mesenteric artery and its branches. Note that this artery supplies blood to the gut from halfway down the second part of the duodenum to the distal third of the transverse colon (*arrow*).

Lymph Drainage

The lymph vessels pass through several mesenteric nodes and finally reach the superior mesenteric nodes.

Nerve Supply

Branches from the sympathetic and parasympathetic (vagus) nerves form the superior mesenteric plexus.

Ileocecal Valve

A rudimentary structure, the ileocecal valve consists of two horizontal folds of mucous membrane that project around the orifice of the ileum. The valve plays little or no part in the prevention of reflux of cecal contents into the ileum. The circular muscle of the lower end of the ileum (called the **ileocecal sphincter** by physiologists) serves as a sphincter and controls the flow of contents from the ileum into the colon. The smooth muscle tone is reflexly increased when the cecum is distended; the hormone **gastrin,** which is produced by the stomach, causes relaxation of the muscle tone.

Appendix

Location and Description

The appendix (Fig. 5-1) is a narrow, muscular tube containing a large amount of lymphoid tissue. It varies in length from 3 to 5 in. (8 to 13 cm). The base is attached to the posteromedial surface of the cecum about 1 in. (2.5 cm) below the ileocecal junction (Fig. 5-33). The remainder of the appendix is free. It has a complete peritoneal covering, which is attached to the mesentery of the small intestine by a short mesentery of its own, the **mesoappendix.** The mesoappendix contains the appendicular vessels and nerves.

The appendix lies in the right iliac fossa, and in relation to the anterior abdominal wall its base is situated one third of the way up the line joining the right anterior superior iliac spine to the umbilicus (McBurney's point). Inside the abdomen, the base of the appendix is easily found by identifying the teniae coli of the cecum and tracing them to the base of the appendix, where they converge to form a continuous longitudinal muscle coat (Figs. 5-32 and 5-33).

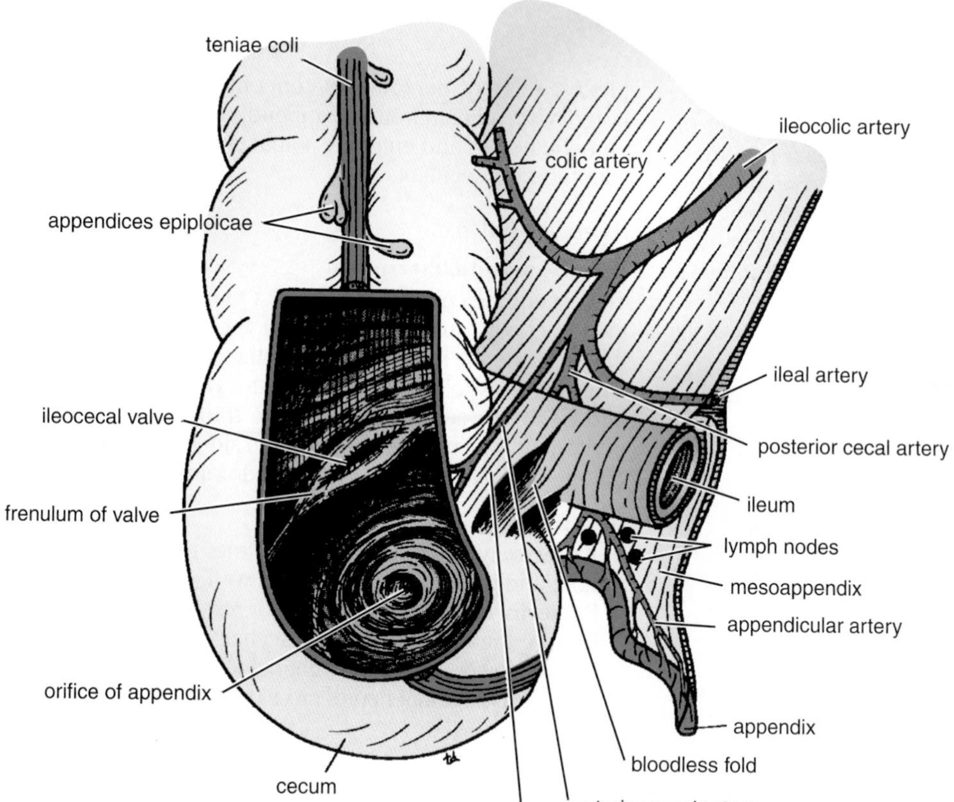

Figure 5-33 Cecum and appendix. Note that the appendicular artery is a branch of the posterior cecal artery. The edge of the mesoappendix has been cut to show the peritoneal layers.

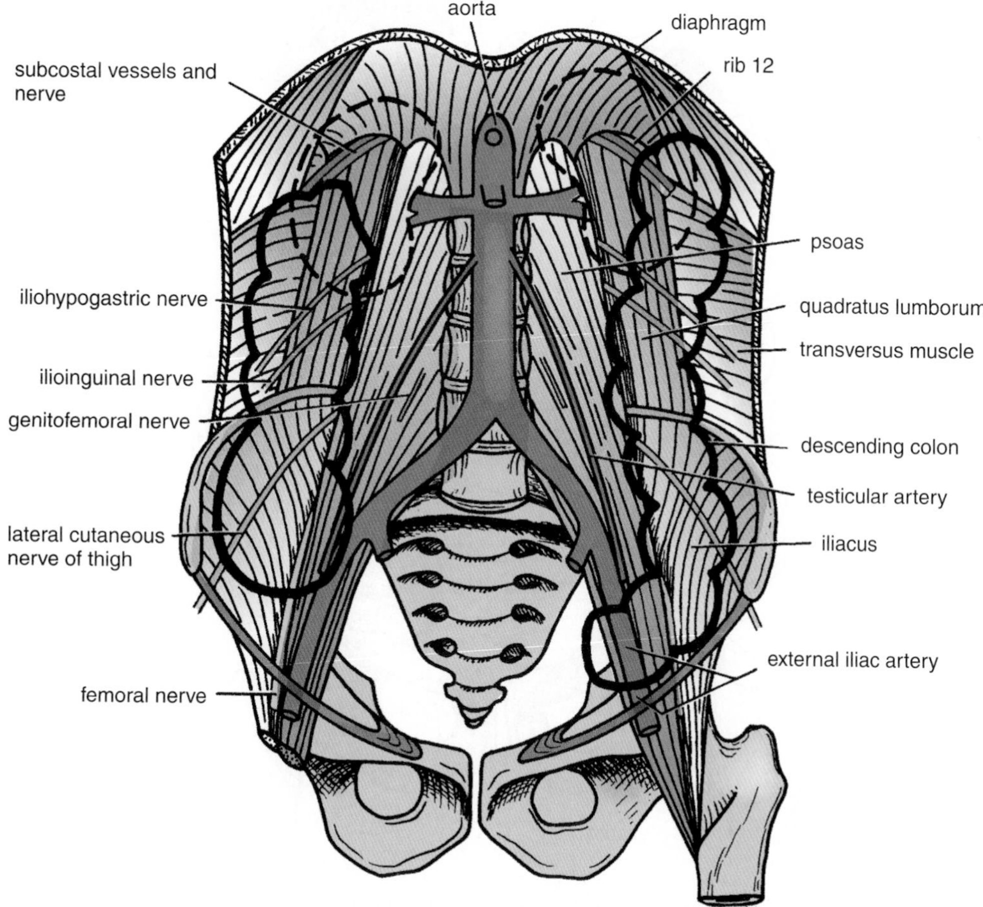

Figure 5-34 Posterior abdominal wall showing posterior relations of the kidneys and the colon.

Common Positions of the Tip of the Appendix

The tip of the appendix is subject to a considerable range of movement and may be found in the following positions: (a) hanging down into the pelvis against the right pelvic wall, (b) coiled up behind the cecum, (c) projecting upward along the lateral side of the cecum, and (d) in front of or behind the terminal part of the ileum. The first and second positions are the most common sites.

Blood Supply

Arteries The appendicular artery is a branch of the posterior cecal artery (Fig. 5-33).

Veins The appendicular vein drains into the posterior cecal vein.

Lymph Drainage

The lymph vessels drain into one or two nodes lying in the mesoappendix and then eventually into the superior mesenteric nodes.

Nerve Supply

The appendix is supplied by the sympathetic and parasympathetic (vagus) nerves from the superior mesenteric plexus. Afferent nerve fibers concerned with the conduction of visceral pain from the appendix accompany the sympathetic nerves and enter the spinal cord at the level of the 10th thoracic segment.

Ascending Colon

Location and Description

The ascending colon is about 5 in. (13 cm) long and lies in the right lower quadrant (Fig. 5-35). It extends upward from the cecum to the inferior surface of the right lobe of the liver, where it turns to the left, forming the **right colic flexure,** and becomes continuous with the transverse colon. The peritoneum covers the front and the sides of the ascending colon, binding it to the posterior abdominal wall.

Relations

- **Anteriorly:** Coils of small intestine, the greater omentum, and the anterior abdominal wall (Figs. 5-2 and 5-3)
- **Posteriorly:** The iliacus, the iliac crest, the quadratus lumborum, the origin of the transversus abdominis muscle, and the lower pole of the right kidney. The iliohypogastric and the ilioinguinal nerves cross behind it (Fig. 5-34).

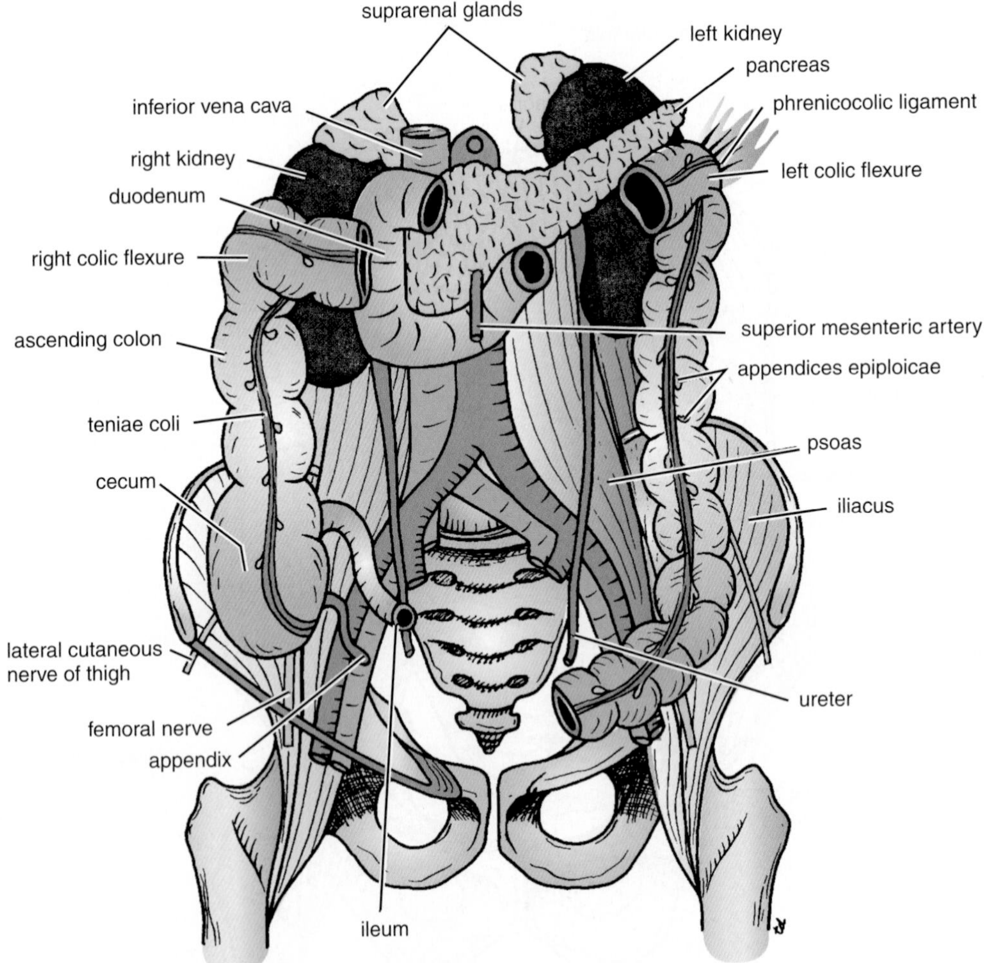

Figure 5-35 Abdominal cavity showing the terminal part of the ileum, the cecum, the appendix, the ascending colon, the right colic flexure, the left colic flexure, and the descending colon. Note the teniae coli and the appendices epiploicae.

Blood Supply

Arteries The ileocolic and right colic branches of the superior mesenteric artery (Fig. 5-32) supply this area.

Veins The veins correspond to the arteries and drain into the superior mesenteric vein.

Lymph Drainage

The lymph vessels drain into lymph nodes lying along the course of the colic blood vessels and ultimately reach the superior mesenteric nodes.

Nerve Supply

Sympathetic and parasympathetic (vagus) nerves from the superior mesenteric plexus supply this area of the colon.

Transverse Colon

Location and Description

The transverse colon is about 15 in. (38 cm) long and extends across the abdomen, occupying the umbilical region. It begins at the right colic flexure below the right lobe of the liver (Fig. 5-4) and hangs downward, suspended by the transverse mesocolon from the pancreas (Fig. 5-6). It then ascends to the **left colic flexure** below the spleen. The left colic flexure is higher than the right colic flexure and is suspended from the diaphragm by the **phrenicocolic ligament** (Fig. 5-35).

The **transverse mesocolon,** or mesentery of the transverse colon, suspends the transverse colon from the anterior border of the pancreas (Fig. 5-6). The mesentery is attached to the superior border of the transverse colon, and the posterior layers of the greater omentum are attached to the inferior border (Fig. 5-6). Because of the length of the transverse mesocolon, the position of the transverse colon is extremely variable and may sometimes reach down as far as the pelvis.

Relations

- **Anteriorly:** The greater omentum and the anterior abdominal wall (umbilical and hypogastric regions) (Fig. 5-6)
- **Posteriorly:** The second part of the duodenum, the head of the pancreas, and the coils of the jejunum and ileum (Fig. 5-35)

Blood Supply

Arteries The proximal two thirds are supplied by the middle colic artery, a branch of the superior mesenteric artery (Fig. 5-32). The distal third is supplied by the left colic artery, a branch of the inferior mesenteric artery (Fig. 5-36).

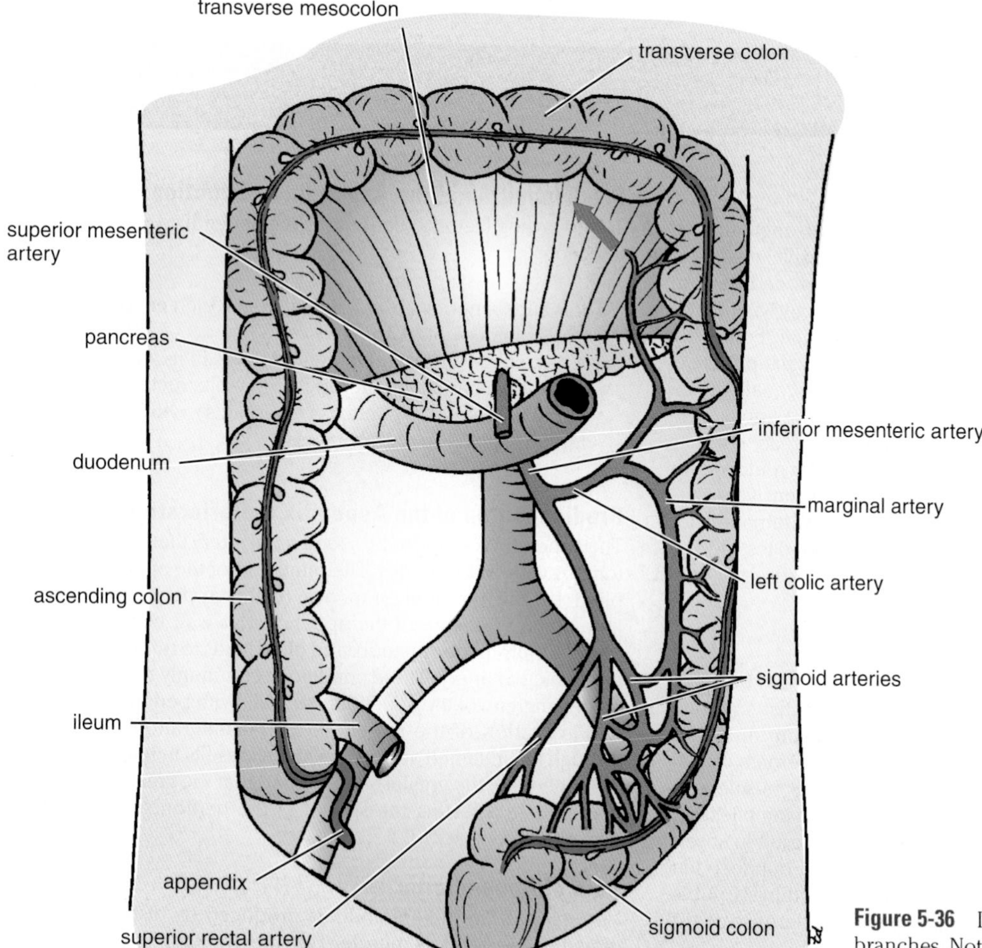

Figure 5-36 Inferior mesenteric artery and its branches. Note that this artery supplies the large bowel from the distal third of the transverse colon to halfway down the anal canal. It anastomoses with the middle colic branch of the superior mesenteric artery (*arrow*).

Veins The veins correspond to the arteries and drain into the superior and inferior mesenteric veins.

Lymph Drainage
The proximal two thirds drain into the colic nodes and then into the superior mesenteric nodes; the distal third drains into the colic nodes and then into the inferior mesenteric nodes.

Nerve Supply
The proximal two thirds are innervated by sympathetic and vagal nerves through the superior mesenteric plexus; the distal third is innervated by sympathetic and parasympathetic pelvic splanchnic nerves through the inferior mesenteric plexus.

Descending Colon

Location and Description
The descending colon is about 10 in. (25 cm) long and lies in the left upper and lower quadrants (Fig. 5-35). It extends downward from the left colic flexure, to the pelvic brim, where it becomes continuous with the sigmoid colon. (For the sigmoid colon, see page 338.) The peritoneum covers the front and the sides and binds it to the posterior abdominal wall.

Relations

- **Anteriorly:** Coils of small intestine, the greater omentum, and the anterior abdominal wall (Figs. 5-2 and 5-3)
- **Posteriorly:** The lateral border of the left kidney, the origin of the transversus abdominis muscle, the quadratus lumborum, the iliac crest, the iliacus, and the left psoas. The iliohypogastric and the ilioinguinal nerves, the lateral cutaneous nerve of the thigh, and the femoral nerve (Fig. 5-34) also lie posteriorly.

Blood Supply

Arteries The left colic and the sigmoid branches of the inferior mesenteric artery (Fig. 5-36) supply this area.

Veins The veins correspond to the arteries and drain into the inferior mesenteric vein.

Lymph Drainage
Lymph drains into the colic lymph nodes and the inferior mesenteric nodes around the origin of the inferior mesenteric artery.

Nerve Supply
The nerve supply is the sympathetic and parasympathetic pelvic splanchnic nerves through the inferior mesenteric plexus.

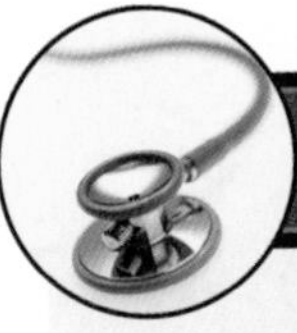

CLINICAL NOTES

Colonoscopy

Since colorectal cancer is a leading cause of death in the Western world, colonoscopy is now being extensively used for early detection of malignant tumors. In this procedure, the mucous membrane of the colon can be directly visualized through an elongated flexible tube, or endoscope. Following a thorough washing out of the large bowel, the patient is sedated, and the tube is gently inserted into the anal canal. The interior of the large bowel can be observed from the anus to the cecum (Fig. 5-37). Photographs of suspicious areas, such as polyps, can be taken and biopsy specimens can be removed for pathologic examination. Although a relatively expensive procedure, it provides a more complete screening examination for colorectal cancer than combined fecal occult blood testing and the examination of the distal colon with sigmoidoscopy (see page 339).

Variability of Position of the Appendix

The inconstancy of the position of the appendix should be borne in mind when attempting to diagnose an appendicitis. A retrocecal appendix, for example, may lie behind a cecum distended with gas, and thus it may be difficult to elicit tenderness on palpation in the right iliac region. Irritation of the psoas muscle, conversely, may cause the patient to keep the right hip joint flexed.

An appendix hanging down in the pelvis may result in absent abdominal tenderness in the right lower quadrant, but deep tenderness may be experienced just above the symphysis pubis. Rectal or vaginal examination may reveal tenderness of the peritoneum in the pelvis on the right side.

Predisposition of the Appendix to Infection

The following factors contribute to the appendix's predilection to infection:

- It is a long, narrow, blind-ended tube, which encourages stasis of large-bowel contents.
- It has a large amount of lymphoid tissue in its wall.
- The lumen has a tendency to become obstructed by hardened intestinal contents (enteroliths), which leads to further stagnation of its contents.

Predisposition of the Appendix to Perforation

The appendix is supplied by a long small artery that does not anastomose with other arteries. The blind end of the appendix is supplied by the terminal branches of the appendicular artery. Inflammatory edema of the appendicular wall compresses the blood supply to the appendix and often leads to thrombosis of the appendicular artery. These conditions commonly result in necrosis or gangrene of the appendicular wall, with perforation.

Perforation of the appendix or transmigration of bacteria through the inflamed appendicular wall results in infection of the peritoneum of the greater sac. The part that the greater omentum may play in arresting the spread of the peritoneal infection is described on page 213.

Pain of Appendicitis

Visceral pain in the appendix is produced by distention of its lumen or spasm of its muscle. The afferent pain fibers enter the

(continues)

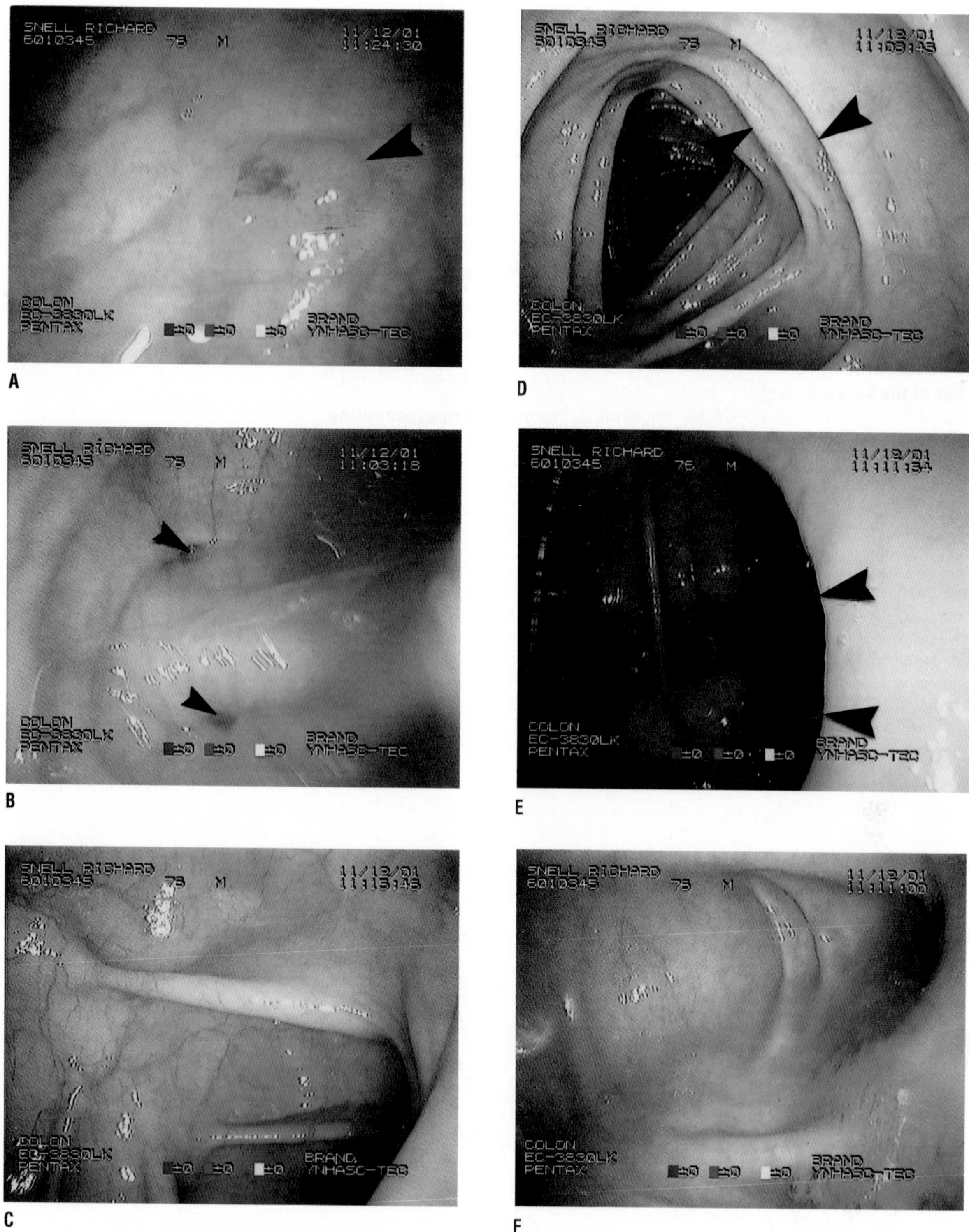

Figure 5-37 Series of the interior of the large bowel taken during a colonoscopy procedure. **A.** The rectal mucosa shows a small benign polyp (*arrowhead*). **B.** The sigmoid mucous membrane shows evidence of a mild diverticulosis. Arrowheads indicate the entrances into the mucosal pouches. **C.** The splenic flexure is normal. Note the light reflections from the drops of mucus on the mucous membrane. **D.** The transverse colon shows the characteristic normal folds or ridges (*arrowheads*) between the sacculations of the wall of the colon. **E.** The ileocecal valve shows the upper lip (*arrowheads*) of the valve, which has a normal appearance. **F.** Finally, the mucous membrane lining the inferior wall or floor of the cecum looks normal. (Courtesy of M.H. Brand.)

Clinical Notes, *continued*

spinal cord at the level of the 10th thoracic segment, and a **vague referred pain** is felt in the region of the umbilicus. Later, the pain shifts to where the inflamed appendix irritates the parietal peritoneum. Here the pain is **precise, severe,** and **localized** (see Abdominal Pain, page 281).

Trauma of the Cecum and Colon

Blunt or penetrating injuries to the colon occur. Blunt injuries most commonly occur where mobile parts of the colon (transverse and sigmoid) join the fixed parts (ascending and descending).

Penetrating injuries following stab wounds are common. The multiple anatomic relationships of the different parts of the colon explain why isolated colonic trauma is unusual.

Cancer of the Large Bowel

Cancer of the large bowel is relatively common in persons older than 50 years. The growth is restricted to the bowel wall for a considerable time before it spreads via the lymphatics. Bloodstream spread via the portal circulation to the liver occurs late. If a diagnosis is made early and a partial colectomy is performed, accompanied by removal of the lymph vessels and lymph nodes draining the area, then a cure can be anticipated.

Diverticulosis

Diverticulosis of the colon is a common clinical condition. It consists of a herniation of the lining mucosa through the circular muscle between the teniae coli and occurs at points where the circular muscle is weakest—that is, where the blood vessels pierce the muscle (Fig. 5-38). The common site for herniation is shown in Figure 5-38.

Cecostomy and Colostomy

Because of the anatomic mobility of the cecum, transverse colon, and sigmoid colon, they may be brought to the surface through a small opening in the anterior abdominal wall. If the cecum or transverse colon is then opened, the bowel contents may be allowed to drain by this route. These procedures are referred to as **cecostomy** or **colostomy,** respectively, and are used to relieve large-bowel obstructions.

Volvulus

Because of its extreme mobility, the sigmoid colon sometimes rotates around its mesentery. This may correct itself spontaneously or the rotation may continue until the blood supply of the gut is cut off completely.

Intussusception

Intussusception is the telescoping of a proximal segment of the bowel into the lumen of an adjoining distal segment. Needless to say, there is a grave risk of cutting off the blood supply to the gut and developing gangrene. It is common in children. Ileocolic, colocolic, and ileoileal forms do occur, but ileocolic is the most common.

The high incidence in children may be caused by the relatively large size of the large bowel compared with the small intestine at this time of life. Another factor may be the possible swelling of Peyer's patches secondary to infection. In the latter case, the swollen patch protrudes into the lumen and violent peristalsis of the ileal wall tries to pass it distally along the gut lumen.

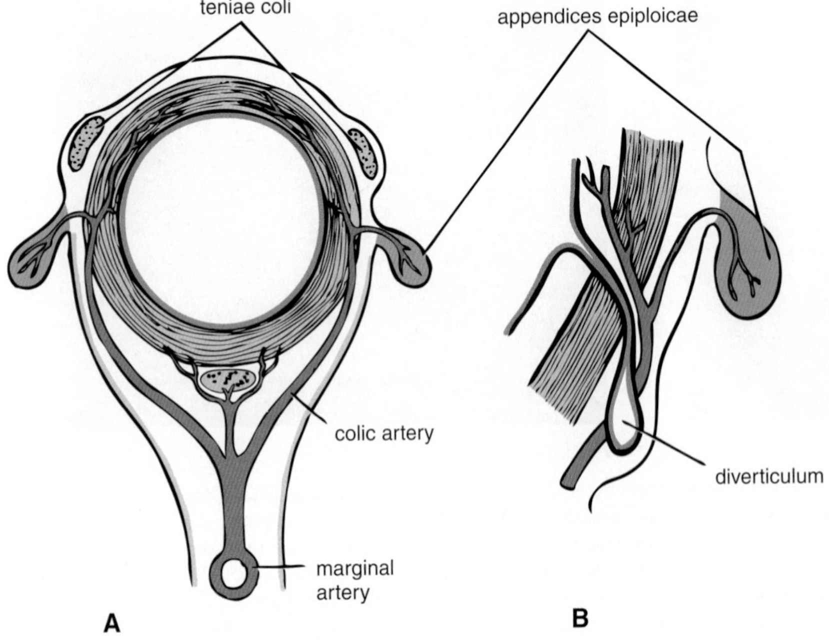

Figure 5-38 Blood supply to the colon **(A)** and formation of the diverticulum **(B).** Note the passage of the mucosal diverticulum through the muscle coat along the course of the artery.

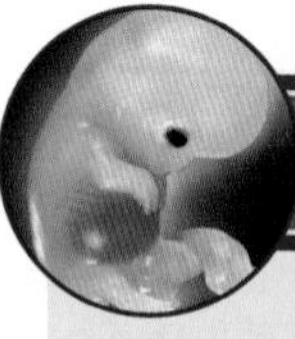

EMBRYOLOGIC NOTES

Development of the Digestive System

The digestive tube is formed from the yolk sac. The entoderm forms the epithelial lining, and the splanchnic mesenchyme forms the surrounding muscle and serous coats. The developing gut is divided into the **foregut, midgut,** and **hindgut** (Fig. 5-39).

Development of the Esophagus

The esophagus develops from the narrow part of the foregut that succeeds the pharynx (Fig. 5-39). At first, it is a short tube, but when the heart and diaphragm descend, it elongates rapidly.

Atresia of the Esophagus

Atresia of the esophagus, with and without fistula, with the trachea is considered in detail on page 99.

Esophageal Stenosis

Esophageal stenosis is a narrowing of the lumen of the esophagus, which commonly occurs in the lower part. It is treated by dilatation.

Congenital Short Esophagus

Abnormal shortness of the esophagus is caused by an esophageal hiatus hernia in the diaphragm. Stomach contents flow into the esophagus, resulting in **esophagitis.**

Development of the Stomach

The stomach develops as a dilatation of the foregut (Fig. 5-40). To begin with, it has a ventral and dorsal mesentery. Very active growth takes place along the dorsal border, which becomes convex and forms the **greater curvature.** The anterior border becomes concave and forms the lesser curvature. The fundus appears as a dilatation at the upper end of the stomach. At this stage, the stomach has a right and left surface to which the right and left vagus nerves are attached, respectively (Fig. 5-40). With the great growth of the right lobe of the liver, the stomach is gradually rotated to the right so that the left surface becomes anterior and the right surface, posterior. The ventral and dorsal mesenteries now change position as a result of rotation of the stomach, and they form the **omenta** and various peritoneal ligaments.

The pouch of peritoneum behind the stomach is known as the **lesser sac.**

Congenital Hypertrophic Pyloric Stenosis

Hypertrophic pyloric stenosis is a relatively common emergency in infants between the ages of 3 and 6 weeks. The child ejects the stomach contents with considerable force. The exact cause of the stenosis is unknown, although evidence suggests that the number of autonomic ganglion cells in the stomach wall is fewer than normal. This possibility leads to prenatal neuromuscular incoordination and localized muscular hypertrophy and hyperplasia of the pyloric sphincter. It is much more common in male children.

Development of the Duodenum

The duodenum is formed from the most caudal portion of the foregut and the most cephalic end of the midgut. This region rapidly grows to form a loop. At this time, the duodenum has a mesentery that extends to the posterior abdominal wall and is part of the dorsal mesentery. A small part of the ventral mesentery is also attached to the ventral border of the first part of the duodenum and the upper half of the second part of the duodenum. When the stomach rotates, the duodenal loop is forced to rotate to the right, where the second, third, and fourth parts adhere to the posterior abdominal wall. Now the peritoneum behind the duodenum disappears. However, some smooth muscle and fibrous tissue that belong to the dorsal mesentery remain as the **suspensory ligament of the duodenum (ligament of Treitz),** and this fixes the terminal part of the duodenum and prevents it from moving inferiorly (Fig. 5-41). The liver and pancreas arise as entodermal buds from the developing duodenum.

Atresia and Stenosis

During the development of the duodenum, the lining cells proliferate at such a rate that the lumen becomes completely obliterated. Later, as a result of degeneration of these cells, the gut becomes recanalized. Failure of recanalization could produce atresia or stenosis. Different forms of duodenal atresia and stenosis are shown in Figure 5-42. Vomiting is the most common presenting symptom, and the vomitus usually is bile stained. Surgical treatment during the first few days of life is essential.

Development of the Jejunum, Ileum, Cecum, Appendix, Ascending Colon, and Proximal Two Thirds of the Transverse Colon

Distal to the duodenum, the small intestine and the large intestine, as far as the distal third of the transverse colon, develop from the midgut. The midgut increases rapidly in length and forms a loop to the apex, on which is attached the **vitelline duct;** this duct passes through the widely open umbilicus (Fig. 5-39). At the same time, the dorsal mesentery elongates, and passing through it from the aorta to the yolk sac are the **vitelline arteries.** These arteries now fuse to form the **superior mesenteric artery,** which supplies the midgut and its derivatives. The rapidly growing liver and kidneys now encroach on the abdominal cavity, causing the midgut loop to herniate into the umbilical cord.

A diverticulum appears at the caudal end of the bowel loop, and this forms the **cecum.** At first the diverticulum is conical; later the upper part expands and forms the cecum, while the lower part remains rudimentary and forms the **appendix** (Fig. 5-43). After birth, the wall of the cecum grows unequally, and the appendix comes to lie on its medial side.

While the loop of gut is in the umbilical cord, its cephalic limb becomes greatly elongated and coiled and forms the future **jejunum** and greater part of the **ileum.** The caudal limb of the loop also increases in length, but it remains uncoiled and forms the future distal part of the ileum, the cecum, the appendix, the **ascending colon,** and the **proximal two thirds of the transverse colon.**

Rotation of the Midgut Loop in the Umbilical Cord and Its Return to the Abdominal Cavity

While in the umbilical cord, the midgut rotates around an axis formed by the superior mesenteric artery and the vitelline duct. As one views the embryo from the anterior aspect, a counterclockwise rotation of approximately 90° occurs (Fig. 5-44). Later, as the gut returns to the abdominal cavity, the midgut rotates counterclockwise an additional 180°. Thus, a total rotation of 270° counterclockwise has occurred (Fig. 5-45).

The rotation of the gut results in part of the large intestine (transverse colon) coming in front of the superior mesenteric artery and the second part of the duodenum; the third part of the

(continues)

Embryologic Notes, *continued*

duodenum comes to lie behind the artery. The cecum and appendix come into close contact with the right lobe of the liver. Later, the cecum and appendix descend into the right iliac fossa so that the ascending colon and right colic flexure are formed. Thus, the rotation of the gut has resulted in the large gut coming to lie laterally and encircle the centrally placed small gut.

The primitive mesenteries of the duodenum, ascending and descending colons now fuse with the parietal peritoneum on the posterior abdominal wall. This explains how these parts of the developing gut become retroperitoneal. The primitive mesenteries of the jejunum and ileum, the transverse colon, and the sigmoid colon persist as the mesentery of the small intestine, the transverse mesocolon, and the sigmoid mesocolon, respectively.

The rotation of the stomach and duodenum to the right is largely brought about by the great growth of the right lobe of the liver. The left surface of the stomach becomes anterior, and the right surface becomes posterior. A pouch of peritoneum becomes located behind the stomach and is called the lesser sac.

Fate of the Vitelline Duct

The midgut is at first connected with the yolk sac by the vitelline duct. By the time the gut returns to the abdominal cavity, the duct becomes obliterated and severs its connection with the gut.

Development of the Left Colic Flexure, Descending Colon, Sigmoid Colon, Rectum, and Upper Half of the Anal Canal

The left colic flexure, descending colon, sigmoid colon, rectum, and upper half of the anal canal are developed from the hindgut (see page 237).

Diverticula of the Intestine

All coats of the intestinal wall are found in the wall of a congenital diverticulum. In the duodenum, diverticula are found on the medial wall of the second and third parts (Fig. 5-42). Usually, these are symptomless. Jejunal diverticula occasionally occur and usually give rise to no symptoms. For Meckel's diverticulum of the ileum, see next column. A diverticulum of the cecum is commonly situated on the medial side of the cecum close to the ileocecal valve. It may be subject to acute inflammation and then is confused with appendicitis. Diverticula of the colon are acquired, not congenital (see page 236).

Atresia and Stenosis of the Intestine

The most common site of an atretic or stenotic obstruction is in the duodenum (see previous page). The next most common sites are the ileum and jejunum, respectively (Fig. 5-42). Frequently, the obstruction occurs at multiple sites. The cause is possibly the failure of the lumen to become recanalized after it has been blocked by epithelial proliferation of the cells of the mucous membrane. Other causes have been suggested, such as vascular damage associated with twisting or volvulus of the intestine. Persistent bile-stained vomiting occurs from birth. Surgical relief of the obstruction should be carried out as soon as possible.

Duplication of the Digestive System

In duplication of the digestive system, the normal degeneration of the mucous membrane cells, which have proliferated to temporarily block the lumen, occurs at two sites simultaneously instead of at one. In this way, two lumina are formed side by side. The additional segment of bowel should be removed as soon as possible, since it may cause obstruction or be the site of hemorrhage or perforation.

Arrested Rotation or Malrotation of the Midgut Loop

Complete Absence of Rotation or Incomplete Rotation

Complete absence of rotation is rare. In cases of incomplete rotation no further rotation occurs after the initial counterclockwise rotation of 90° in the umbilical cord. Thus, the duodenum, jejunum, and ileum remain on the right side of the abdomen, and the cecum and colon are on the left side of the abdomen (Fig. 5-42). In other cases, a counterclockwise rotation of 180° occurs, and although the duodenum may take up its correct position posterior to the superior mesenteric artery, the cecum comes to lie anterior and to the left of the duodenum. Abnormal adhesions form, which run across the anterior surface of the duodenum and cause obstruction to its second part.

Malrotation of the Midgut Loop

Counterclockwise rotation of 90° followed by clockwise rotation of 90° or 180° may occur. In these cases, the duodenum comes to lie anterior to the superior mesenteric artery, and the colon may come to lie anterior to the mesentery of the small intestine. Repeated vomiting is usually the presenting symptom and is caused by duodenal obstruction. Surgical correction of the incomplete rotation or malrotation of the gut is performed, and all adhesions are divided.

Persistence of the Vitellointestinal Duct

The vitelline duct in the early embryo connects the developing gut to the yolk sac (Fig. 5-46). Normally, as development proceeds, the duct is obliterated, severs its connection with the intestine, and disappears. Persistence of the vitellointestinal duct can result in an umbilical fistula (see Fig. 4-38). If the duct remains as a fibrous band, a loop of small intestine can become wrapped around it, causing intestinal obstruction (see Fig. 4-38).

Meckel's Diverticulum

Meckel's diverticulum, a congenital anomaly, represents a persistent portion of the vitellointestinal duct. The diverticulum is located on the antimesenteric border of the ileum about 2 ft (61 cm) from the ileocecal junction. It is about 2 in. (5 cm) long and occurs in about 2% of individuals. The diverticulum is important clinically, since it may possess a small area of gastric mucosa, and bleeding may occur from a "gastric" ulcer in its mucous membrane. Moreover, the pain from this ulcer may be confused with the pain from appendicitis. Should a fibrous band connect the diverticulum to the umbilicus, a loop of small bowel may become wrapped around it, causing intestinal obstruction.

Undescended Cecum and Appendix

In cases of undescended cecum and appendix, an inflammation of the appendix would give rise to tenderness in the right hypochondrium, which may lead to a mistaken diagnosis of inflammation of the gallbladder.

Anomalies of the Appendix

Agenesis of the appendix (failure to develop) is extremely rare; however, a few examples of double appendix have been reported (Fig. 5-42). The possibility of **left-sided appendix** in individuals with transposition of thoracic and abdominal viscera or in cases of arrested rotation of the midgut should always be remembered (Fig. 5-42).

Anomalies of the Colon

The congenital anomaly of undescended cecum or failure of rotation of the gut so that the cecum lies in the left iliac fossa may give rise to confusion in diagnosis. The pain of appendicitis, for example, although initially starting in the umbilical region, may shift not to the right iliac fossa, but to the right upper quadrant or to the left lower quadrant.

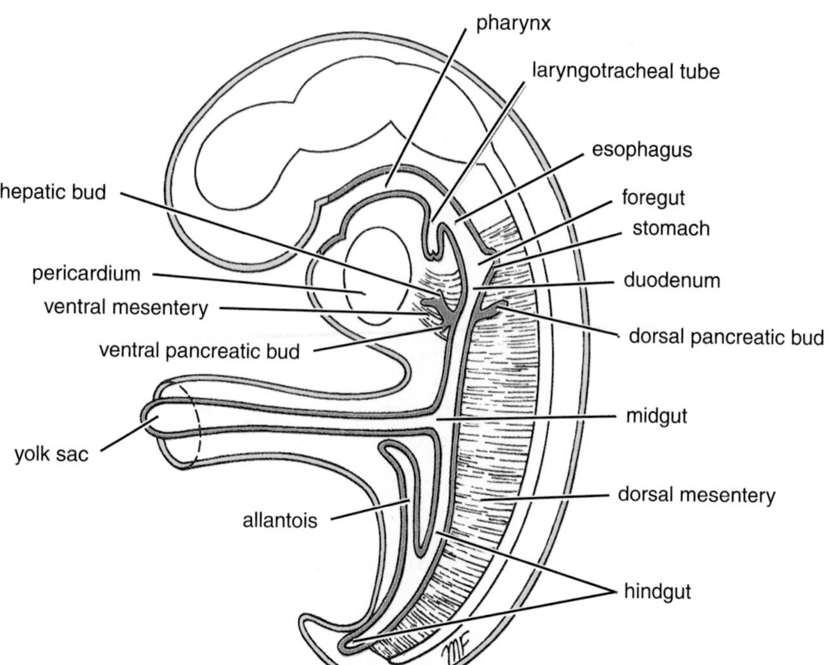

Figure 5-39 The foregut, midgut, and hindgut. The positions of the ventral and dorsal mesenteries, the hepatic bud, and the ventral and dorsal pancreatic buds are also shown.

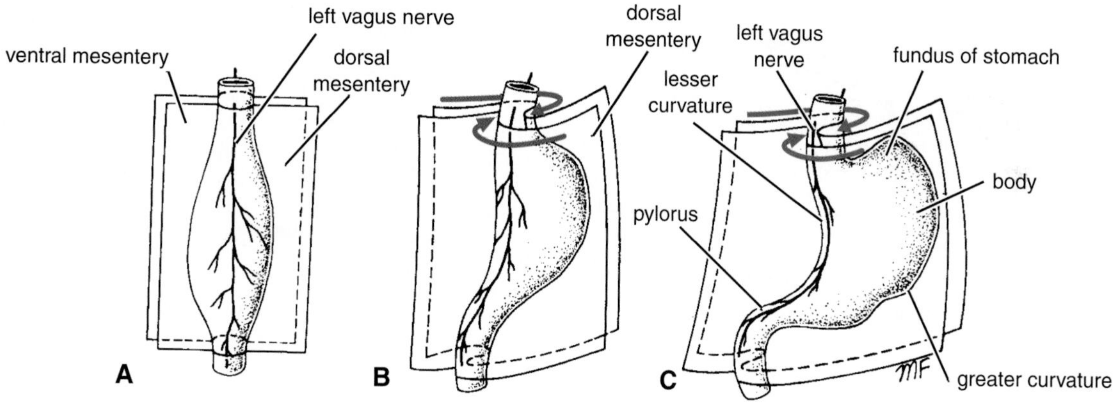

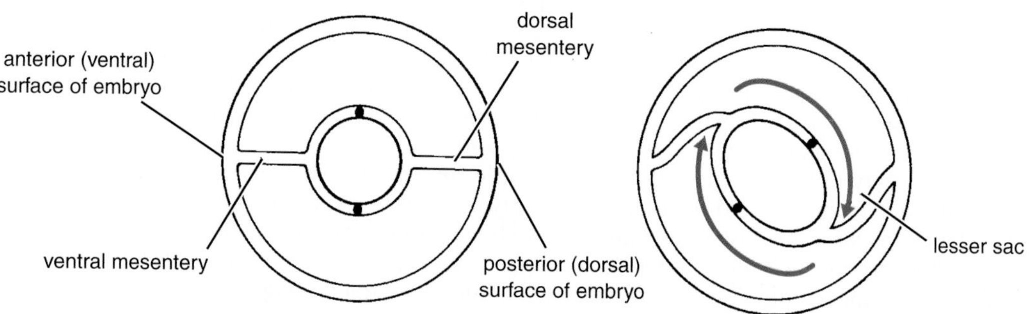

Figure 5-40 Development of the stomach in relation to the ventral and dorsal mesenteries. Note how the stomach rotates so that the left vagus nerve comes to lie on the anterior surface of the stomach. Note also the position of the lesser sac.

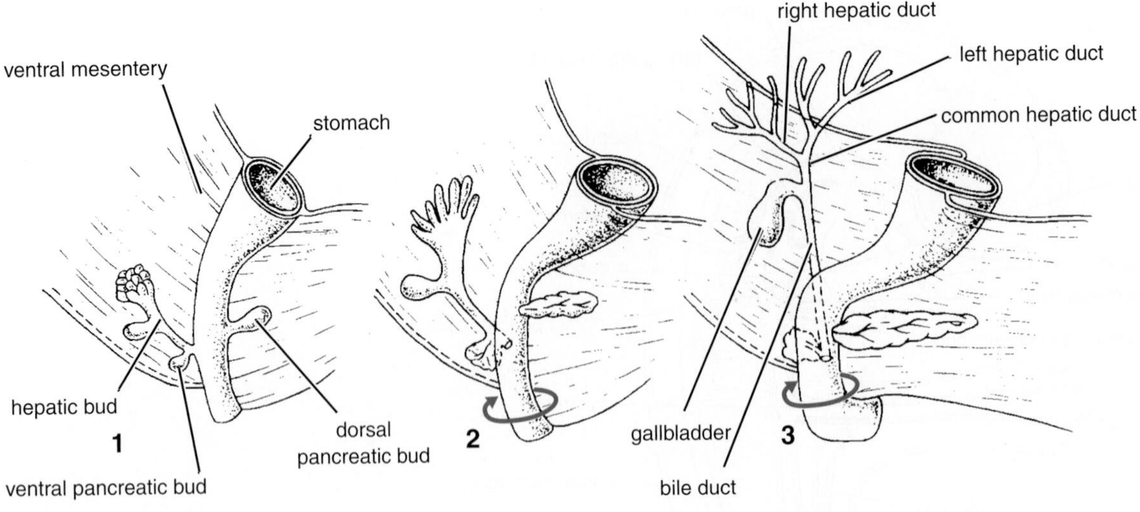

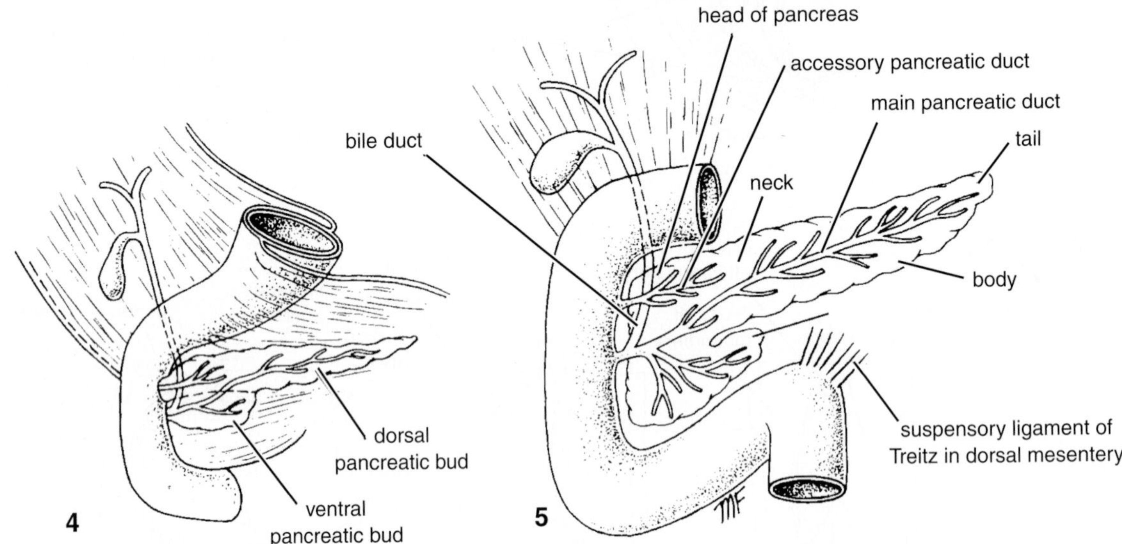

Figure 5-41 The development of the pancreas and the extrahepatic biliary apparatus.

Blood Supply of the Gastrointestinal Tract

Arterial Supply

The arterial supply to the gut and its relationship to the development of the different parts of the gut are illustrated diagrammatically in Figure 5-46. The celiac artery is the artery of the foregut and supplies the gastrointestinal tract from the lower one third of the esophagus down as far as the middle of the second part of the duodenum. The superior mesenteric artery is the artery of the midgut and supplies the gastrointestinal tract from the middle of the second part of the duodenum as far as the distal one third of the transverse colon. The inferior mesenteric artery is the artery of the hindgut and supplies the large intestine from the distal one third of the transverse colon to halfway down the anal canal.

Celiac Artery

The celiac artery or trunk is very short and arises from the commencement of the abdominal aorta at the level of the 12th thoracic vertebra (Fig. 5-20). It is surrounded by the celiac plexus and lies behind the lesser sac of peritoneum. It has three terminal branches: the left gastric, splenic, and hepatic arteries.

Left Gastric Artery The small left gastric artery runs to the cardiac end of the stomach, gives off a few esophageal branches, then turns to the right along the lesser curvature of the stomach. It anastomoses with the right gastric artery (Fig. 5-20).

Splenic Artery The large splenic artery runs to the left in a wavy course along the upper border of the pancreas and behind the stomach (Fig. 5-4). On reaching the left kidney the artery enters the splenicorenal ligament and runs to the hilum of the spleen (Fig. 5-11).

Branches

- **Pancreatic branches**
- The **left gastroepiploic artery** arises near the hilum of the spleen and reaches the greater curvature of the stomach in the gastrosplenic omentum. It passes to the right

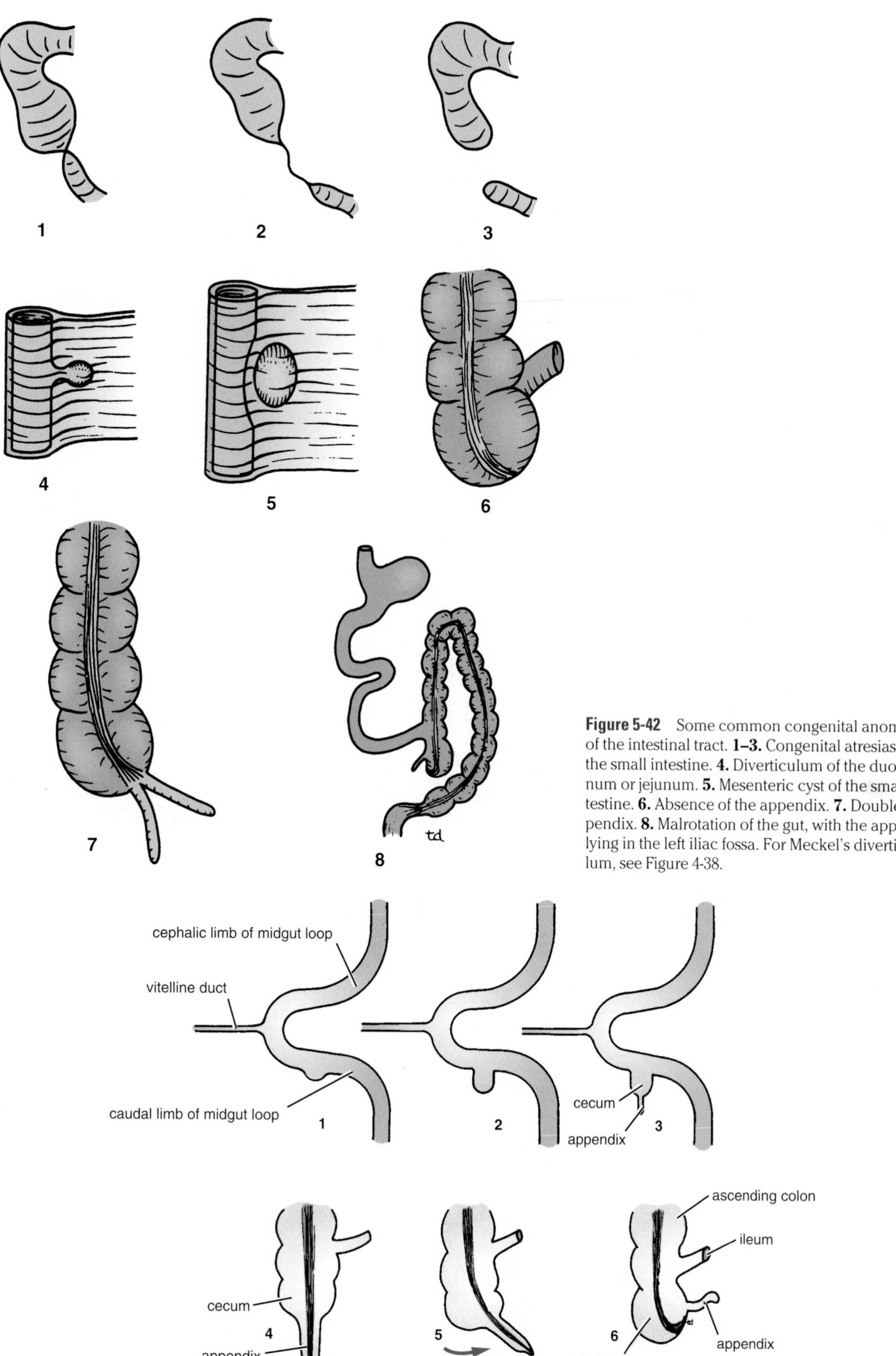

Figure 5-42 Some common congenital anomalies of the intestinal tract. **1–3.** Congenital atresias of the small intestine. **4.** Diverticulum of the duodenum or jejunum. **5.** Mesenteric cyst of the small intestine. **6.** Absence of the appendix. **7.** Double appendix. **8.** Malrotation of the gut, with the appendix lying in the left iliac fossa. For Meckel's diverticulum, see Figure 4-38.

Figure 5-43 Stages in the development of the cecum and appendix. The final stages of development (stages 4, 5, and 6) take place after birth.

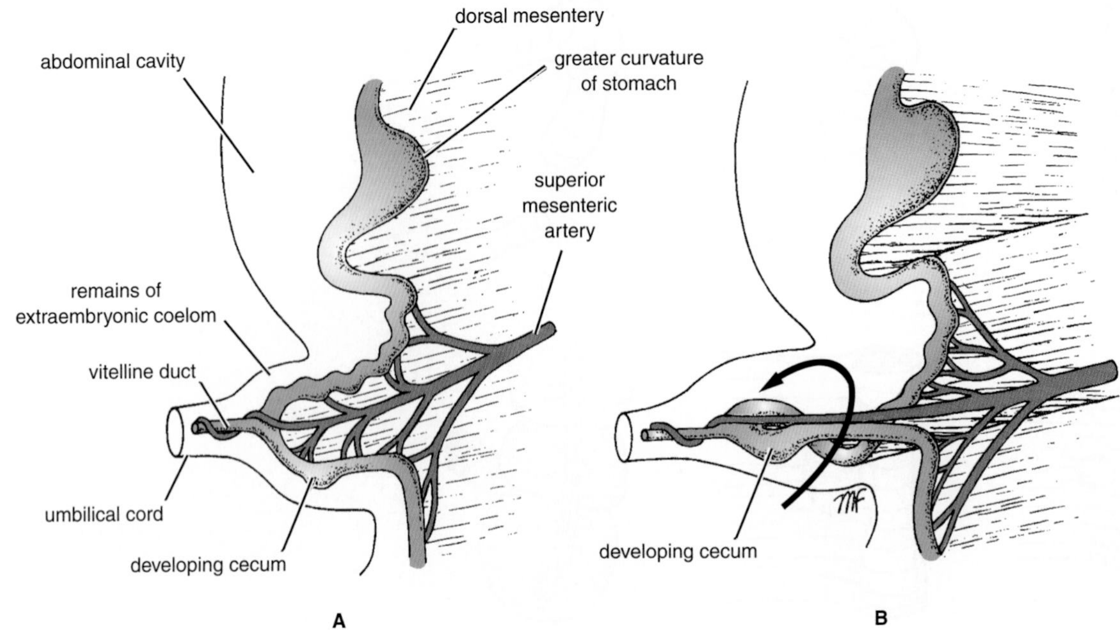

Figure 5-44 Left side views of the counterclockwise 90° rotation of the midgut loop while it is in the extraembryonic coelom in the umbilical cord.

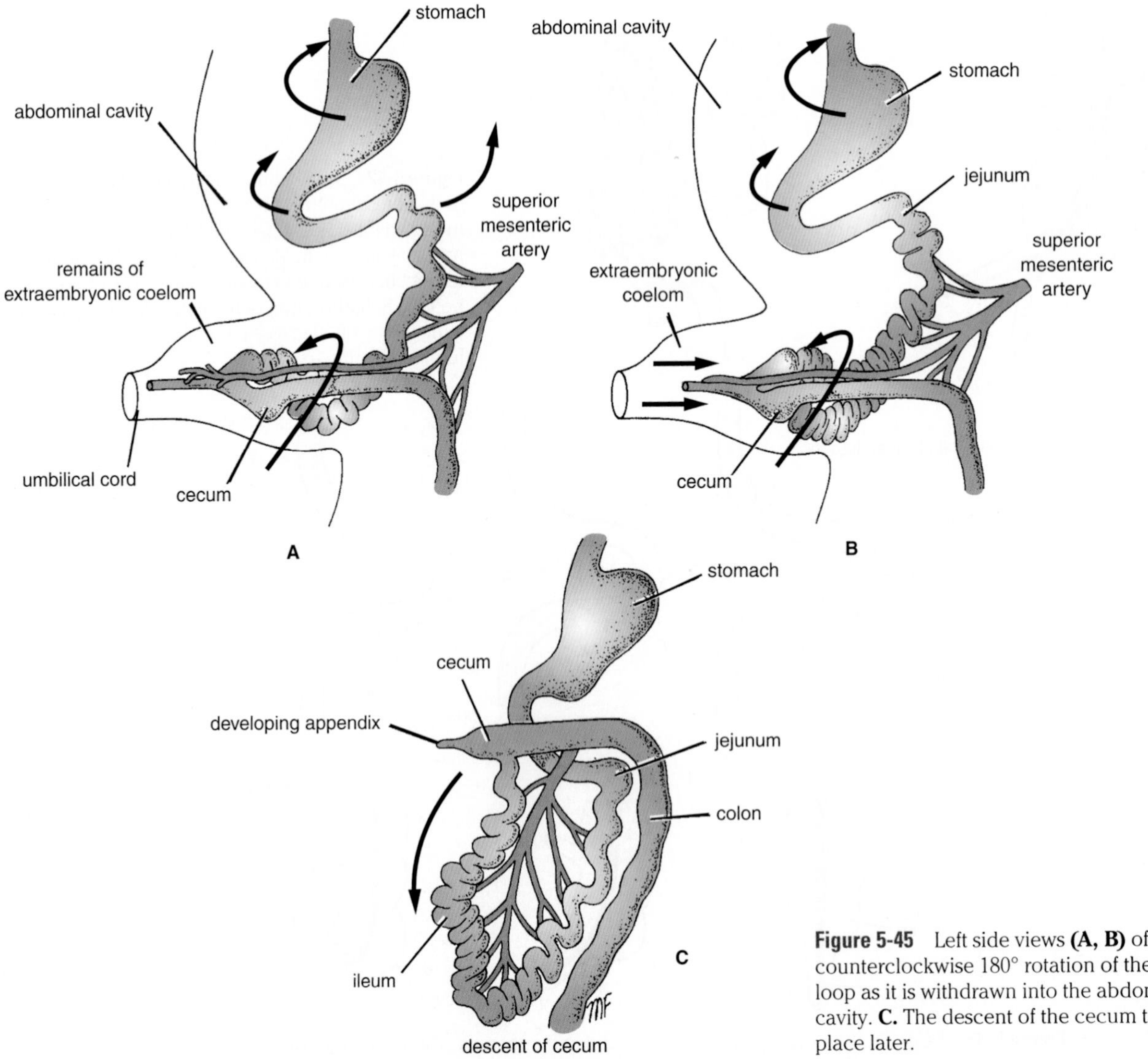

Figure 5-45 Left side views **(A, B)** of the counterclockwise 180° rotation of the midgut loop as it is withdrawn into the abdominal cavity. **C.** The descent of the cecum takes place later.

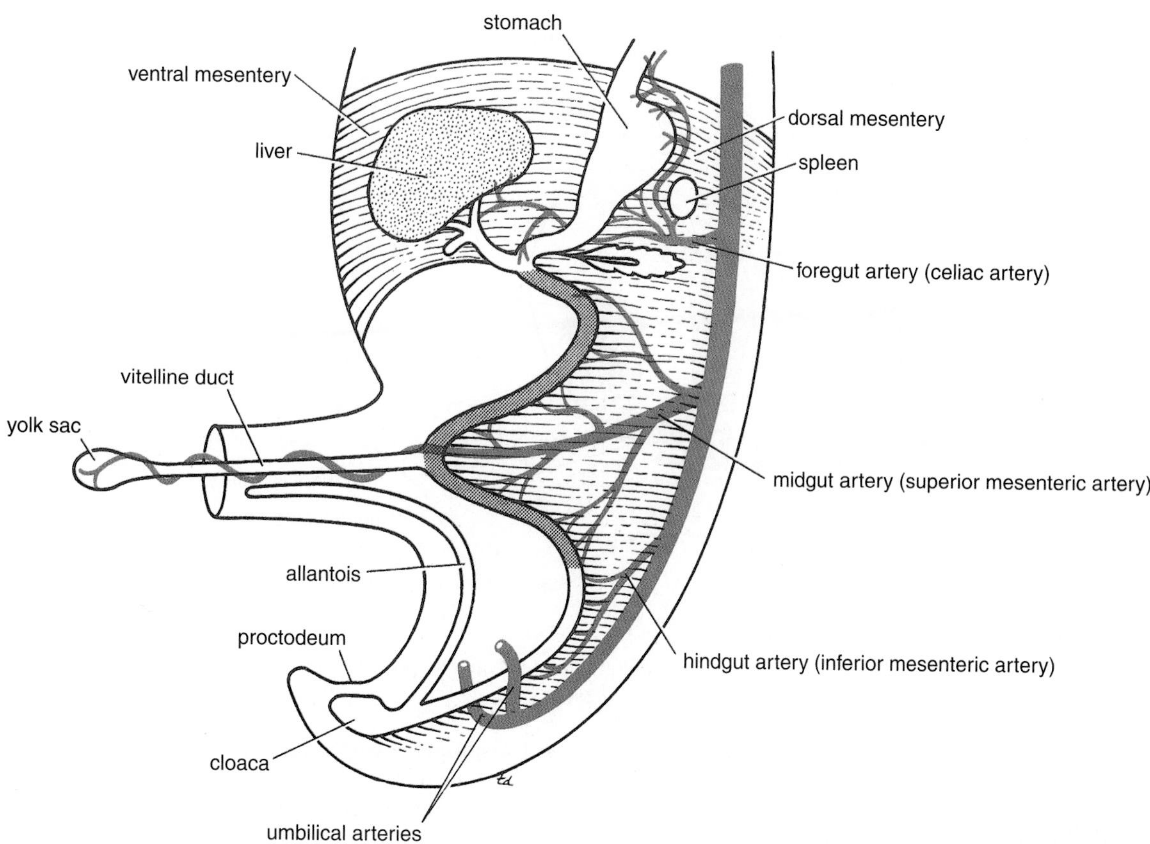

Figure 5-46 Formation of the midgut loop (*shaded*). Note how the superior mesenteric artery and vitelline duct form an axis for the future rotation of the midgut loop.

along the greater curvature of the stomach between the layers of the greater omentum. It anastomoses with the right gastroepiploic artery (Fig. 5-20).

- The **short gastric arteries,** five or six in number, arise from the end of the splenic artery and reach the fundus of the stomach in the gastrosplenic omentum. They anastomose with the left gastric artery and the left gastroepiploic artery (Fig. 5-20).

Hepatic Artery The medium-size hepatic artery* runs forward and to the right and then ascends between the layers of the lesser omentum (Figs. 5-7 and 5-11). It lies in front of the opening into the lesser sac and is placed to the left of the bile duct and in front of the portal vein. At the porta hepatis it divides into right and left branches to supply the corresponding lobes of the liver.

Branches

- The **right gastric artery** arises from the hepatic artery at the upper border of the pylorus and runs to the left in the lesser omentum along the lesser curvature of the stomach. It anastomoses with the left gastric artery (Fig. 5-20).
- The **gastroduodenal artery** is a large branch that descends behind the first part of the duodenum. It divides into the **right gastroepiploic artery** that runs along the greater curvature of the stomach between the layers of the greater omentum and the **superior pancreaticoduodenal artery** that descends between the second part of the duodenum and the head of the pancreas (Figs. 5-4 and 5-20).
- The **right** and **left hepatic arteries** enter the porta hepatis. The right hepatic artery usually gives off the **cystic artery,** which runs to the neck of the gallbladder (Fig. 5-47).

Superior Mesenteric Artery

The superior mesenteric artery supplies the distal part of the duodenum, the jejunum, the ileum, the cecum, the appendix, the ascending colon, and most of the transverse colon. It arises from the front of the abdominal aorta just below the celiac artery (Fig. 5-32) and runs downward and to the right behind the neck of the pancreas and in front of the third part of the duodenum. It continues downward to the right between the layers of the mesentery of the small intestine and ends by anastomosing with the ileal branch of its own ileocolic branch.

Branches

- The **inferior pancreaticoduodenal artery** passes to the right as a single or double branch along the upper border of the third part of the duodenum and the head of the pancreas. It supplies the pancreas and the adjoining part of the duodenum.

*For purposes of description, the hepatic artery is sometimes divided into the **common hepatic artery**, which extends from its origin to the gastroduodenal branch, and the **hepatic artery proper**, which is the remainder of the artery.

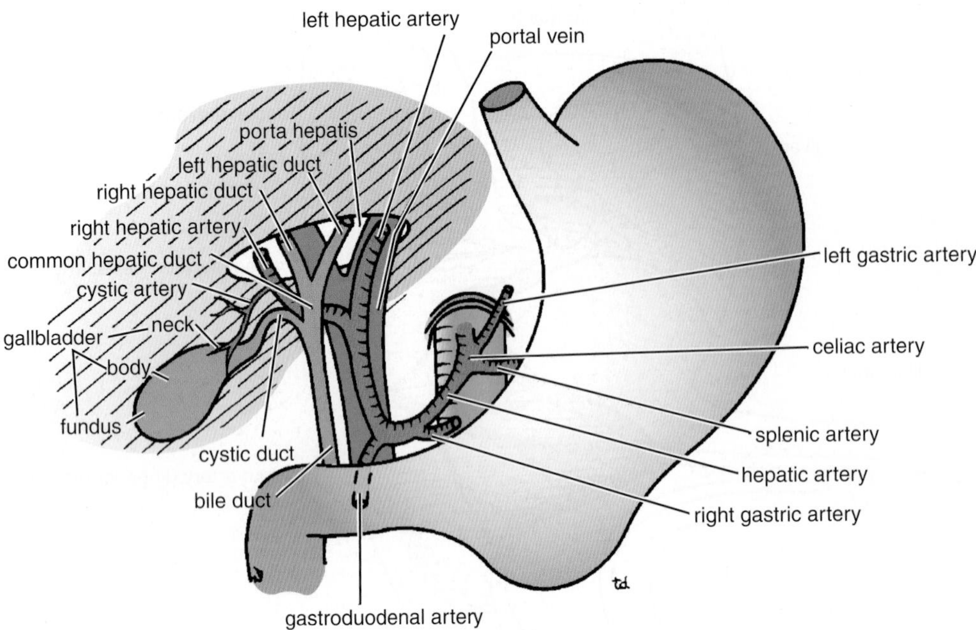

Figure 5-47 Structures entering and leaving the porta hepatis.

- The **middle colic artery** runs forward in the transverse mesocolon to supply the transverse colon and divides into right and left branches.
- The **right colic artery** is often a branch of the ileocolic artery. It passes to the right to supply the ascending colon and divides into ascending and descending branches.
- The **ileocolic artery** passes downward and to the right. It gives rise to a **superior branch** that anastomoses with the right colic artery and an **inferior branch** that anastomoses with the end of the superior mesenteric artery. The inferior branch gives rise to the **anterior** and **posterior cecal arteries;** the **appendicular artery** is a branch of the posterior cecal artery (Fig. 5-33).
- The **jejunal and ileal branches** are 12 to 15 in number and arise from the left side of the superior mesenteric artery (Fig. 5-32). Each artery divides into two vessels, which unite with adjacent branches to form a series of arcades. Branches from the arcades divide and unite to form a second, third, and fourth series of arcades. Fewer arcades supply the jejunum than supply the ileum. From the terminal arcades, small straight vessels supply the intestine.

Inferior Mesenteric Artery

The inferior mesenteric artery supplies the distal third of the transverse colon, the left colic flexure, the descending colon, the sigmoid colon, the rectum, and the upper half of the anal canal. It arises from the abdominal aorta about 1.5 in. (3.8 cm) above its bifurcation (Fig. 5-36). The artery runs downward and to the left and crosses the left common iliac artery. Here, it becomes the superior rectal artery.

Branches

- The **left colic artery** runs upward and to the left and supplies the distal third of the transverse colon, the left colic flexure, and the upper part of the descending colon. It divides into ascending and descending branches.
- The **sigmoid arteries** are two or three in number and supply the descending and sigmoid colon.
- The **superior rectal artery** is a continuation of the inferior mesenteric artery as it crosses the left common iliac artery. It descends into the pelvis behind the rectum. The artery supplies the rectum and upper half of the anal canal and anastomoses with the middle rectal and inferior rectal arteries.

Marginal Artery

The anastomosis of the colic arteries around the concave margin of the large intestine forms a single arterial trunk called the marginal artery. This begins at the ileocecal junction, where it anastomoses with the ileal branches of the superior mesenteric artery, and it ends where it anastomoses less freely with the superior rectal artery (Fig. 5-36).

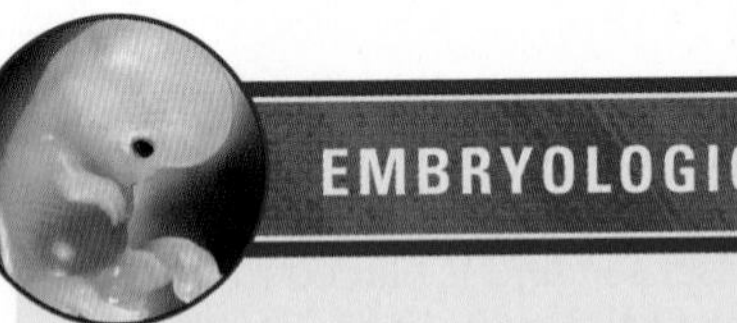

Explanation for the Blood Supply to the Gastrointestinal Tract

Foregut Arteries

The cephalic end of the foregut (which includes the pharynx) and the cervical and thoracic portions of the esophagus are supplied by the ascending pharyngeal arteries, palatine arteries, superior and inferior thyroid arteries, bronchial arteries, and esophageal branches from the aorta. The caudal end of the foregut (which includes the distal third of the esophagus, the stomach, and the proximal half of the duodenum) is supplied by a number of vessels that fuse to form a single trunk, the **celiac artery** (Fig. 5-46). It is interesting to note that this artery also supplies the liver and pancreas, which are glandular derivatives of this part of the gut. The spleen is also supplied by the

(continues)

Embryologic Notes, *continued*

same artery, which is not surprising, since this organ develops in the dorsal mesentery of the foregut; the artery to the spleen runs in the splenicorenal ligament.

Midgut Artery

The midgut, which extends from halfway along the second part of the duodenum to the left colic flexure, is supplied by the **superior mesenteric artery,** which represents the fused pair of vitelline arteries (Fig. 5-46).

Hindgut Artery

The hindgut, which extends from the left colic flexure to halfway down the anal canal, is supplied by the **inferior mesenteric artery** (Fig. 5-46). This represents a number of ventral branches of the aorta that fuse to form a single artery.

Venous Drainage

The venous blood from the greater part of the gastrointestinal tract and its accessory organs drains to the liver by the portal venous system.

The proximal tributaries drain directly into the portal vein, but the veins forming the distal tributaries correspond to the branches of the celiac artery and the superior and inferior mesenteric arteries.

Portal Vein (Hepatic Portal Vein)

The portal vein (Fig. 5-22) drains blood from the abdominal part of the gastrointestinal tract from the lower third of the esophagus to halfway down the anal canal; it also drains blood from the spleen, pancreas, and gallbladder. The portal vein enters the liver and breaks up into sinusoids, from which blood passes into the hepatic veins that join the inferior vena cava. The portal vein is about 2 in. (5 cm) long and is formed behind the neck of the pancreas by the union of the superior mesenteric and splenic veins (Fig. 5-48). It ascends to the right, behind the first part of the duodenum, and enters the lesser omentum (Figs. 5-7 and 5-11). It then runs upward in front of the opening into the lesser sac to the porta hepatis, where it divides into right and left terminal branches.

The portal circulation begins as a capillary plexus in the organs it drains and ends by emptying its blood into sinusoids within the liver.

For the relations of the portal vein in the lesser omentum, see Figures 5-7 and 5-11.

Tributaries of the Portal Vein The tributaries of the portal vein are the splenic vein, superior mesenteric vein, left gastric vein, right gastric vein, and cystic veins.

- **Splenic vein:** This vein leaves the hilum of the spleen and passes to the right in the splenicorenal ligament. It unites with the superior mesenteric vein behind the neck of the pancreas to form the portal vein (Fig. 5-48). It receives the short gastric, left gastroepiploic, inferior mesenteric, and pancreatic veins.
- **Inferior mesenteric vein:** This vein ascends on the posterior abdominal wall and joins the splenic vein behind the body of the pancreas (Fig. 5-48). It receives the superior rectal veins, the sigmoid veins, and the left colic vein.
- **Superior mesenteric vein:** This vein ascends in the root of the mesentery of the small intestine. It passes in front of the third part of the duodenum and joins the splenic vein behind the neck of the pancreas (Fig. 5-48). It receives the jejunal, ileal, ileocolic, right colic, middle colic, inferior pancreaticoduodenal, and right gastroepiploic veins.
- **Left gastric vein:** This vein drains the left portion of the lesser curvature of the stomach and the distal part of the esophagus. It opens directly into the portal vein (Fig. 5-22).
- **Right gastric vein:** This vein drains the right portion of the lesser curvature of the stomach and drains directly into the portal vein (Fig. 5-22).
- **Cystic veins:** These veins either drain the gallbladder directly into the liver or join the portal vein (Fig. 5-22).

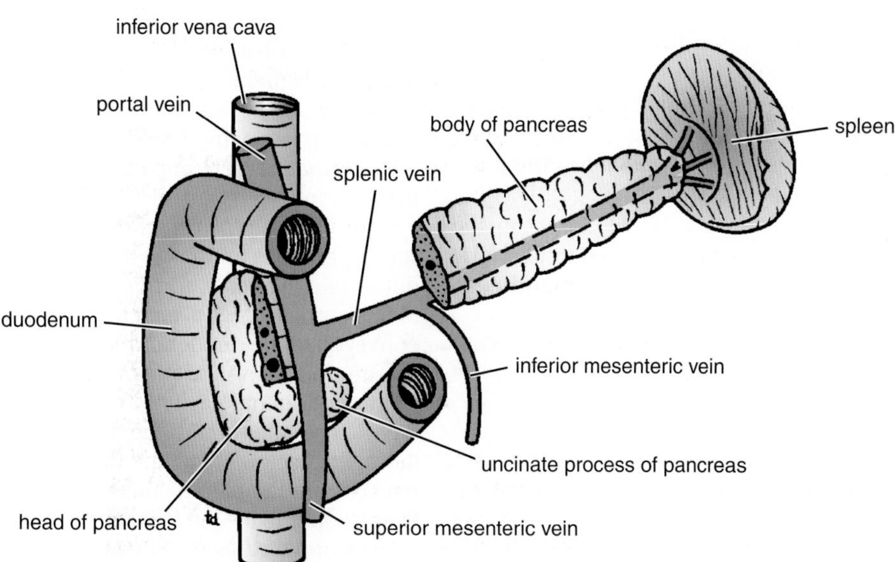

Figure 5-48 Formation of the portal vein behind the neck of the pancreas.

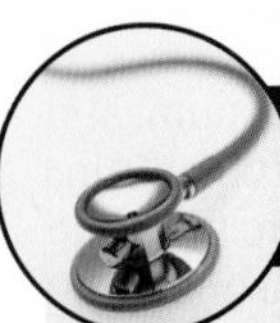

CLINICAL NOTES

Portal–Systemic Anastomoses

Under normal conditions, the portal venous blood traverses the liver and drains into the inferior vena cava of the systemic venous circulation by way of the hepatic veins. This is the direct route. However, other, smaller communications exist between the portal and systemic systems, and they become important when the direct route becomes blocked (Fig. 5-49).

These communications are as follows:

- At the lower third of the esophagus, the esophageal branches of the left gastric vein (portal tributary) anastomose with the esophageal veins draining the middle third of the esophagus into the azygos veins (systemic tributary).
- Halfway down the anal canal, the superior rectal veins (portal tributary) draining the upper half of the anal canal anastomose with the middle and inferior rectal veins (systemic tributaries), which are tributaries of the internal iliac and internal pudendal veins, respectively.
- The **paraumbilical veins** connect the left branch of the portal vein with the superficial veins of the anterior abdominal wall (systemic tributaries). The paraumbilical veins travel in the falciform ligament and accompany the ligamentum teres.
- The veins of the ascending colon, descending colon, duodenum, pancreas, and liver (portal tributary) anastomose with the renal, lumbar, and phrenic veins (systemic tributaries).

Portal Hypertension

Portal hypertension is a common clinical condition; thus, the list of portal–systemic anastomoses should be remembered. Enlargement of the portal–systemic connections is frequently accompanied by congestive enlargement of the spleen. **Portacaval shunts** for the treatment of portal hypertension may involve the anastomosis of the portal vein, because it lies within the lesser omentum, to the anterior wall of the inferior vena cava behind the entrance into the lesser sac. The splenic vein may be anastomosed to the left renal vein after removing the spleen.

Blood Flow in the Portal Vein and Malignant Disease

The portal vein conveys about 70% of the blood to the liver. The remaining 30% is oxygenated blood, which passes to the liver via the hepatic artery. The wide angle of union of the splenic vein with the superior mesenteric vein to form the portal vein leads to streaming of the blood flow in the portal vein. The right lobe of the liver receives blood mainly from the intestine, whereas the left lobe plus the quadrate and caudate lobes receive blood from the stomach and the spleen. This distribution of blood may explain the distribution of secondary malignant deposits in the liver.

Differences Between the Small and Large Intestine

External Differences (Fig. 5-50)

- The small intestine (with the exception of the duodenum) is mobile, whereas the ascending and descending parts of the colon are fixed.
- The caliber of the full small intestine is smaller than that of the filled large intestine.
- The small intestine (with the exception of the duodenum) has a mesentery that passes downward across the midline into the right iliac fossa.
- The longitudinal muscle of the small intestine forms a continuous layer around the gut. In the large intestine (with the exception of the appendix) the longitudinal muscle is collected into three bands, the teniae coli.
- The small intestine has no fatty tags attached to its wall. The large intestine has fatty tags, called the **appendices epiploicae.**
- The wall of the small intestine is smooth, whereas that of the large intestine is sacculated.

Internal Differences (Fig. 5-50)

- The mucous membrane of the small intestine has permanent folds, called **plicae circulares,** which are absent in the large intestine.
- The mucous membrane of the small intestine has villi, which are absent in the large intestine.
- Aggregations of lymphoid tissue called Peyer's patches are found in the mucous membrane of the small intestine; these are absent in the large intestine.

Accessory Organs of the Gastrointestinal Tract

Liver

Location and Description

The liver is the largest gland in the body and has a wide variety of functions. Three of its basic functions are production and secretion of bile, which is passed into the intestinal tract; involvement in many metabolic activities related to carbohydrate, fat, and protein metabolism; and filtration of the blood, removing bacteria and other foreign particles that have gained entrance to the blood from the lumen of the intestine.

The liver synthesizes heparin, an anticoagulant substance, and has an important detoxicating function. It produces bile pigments from the hemoglobin of worn-out red blood corpuscles and secretes bile salts; these together are conveyed to the duodenum by the biliary ducts.

The liver is soft and pliable and occupies the upper part of the abdominal cavity just beneath the diaphragm (Fig. 5-1). The greater part of the liver is situated under cover of the right costal margin, and the right hemidiaphragm separates it from the pleura, lungs, pericardium, and heart. The liver extends to the left to reach the left hemidiaphragm. The convex upper surface of the liver is molded to the undersurface of the domes of the diaphragm. The **posteroinferior,**

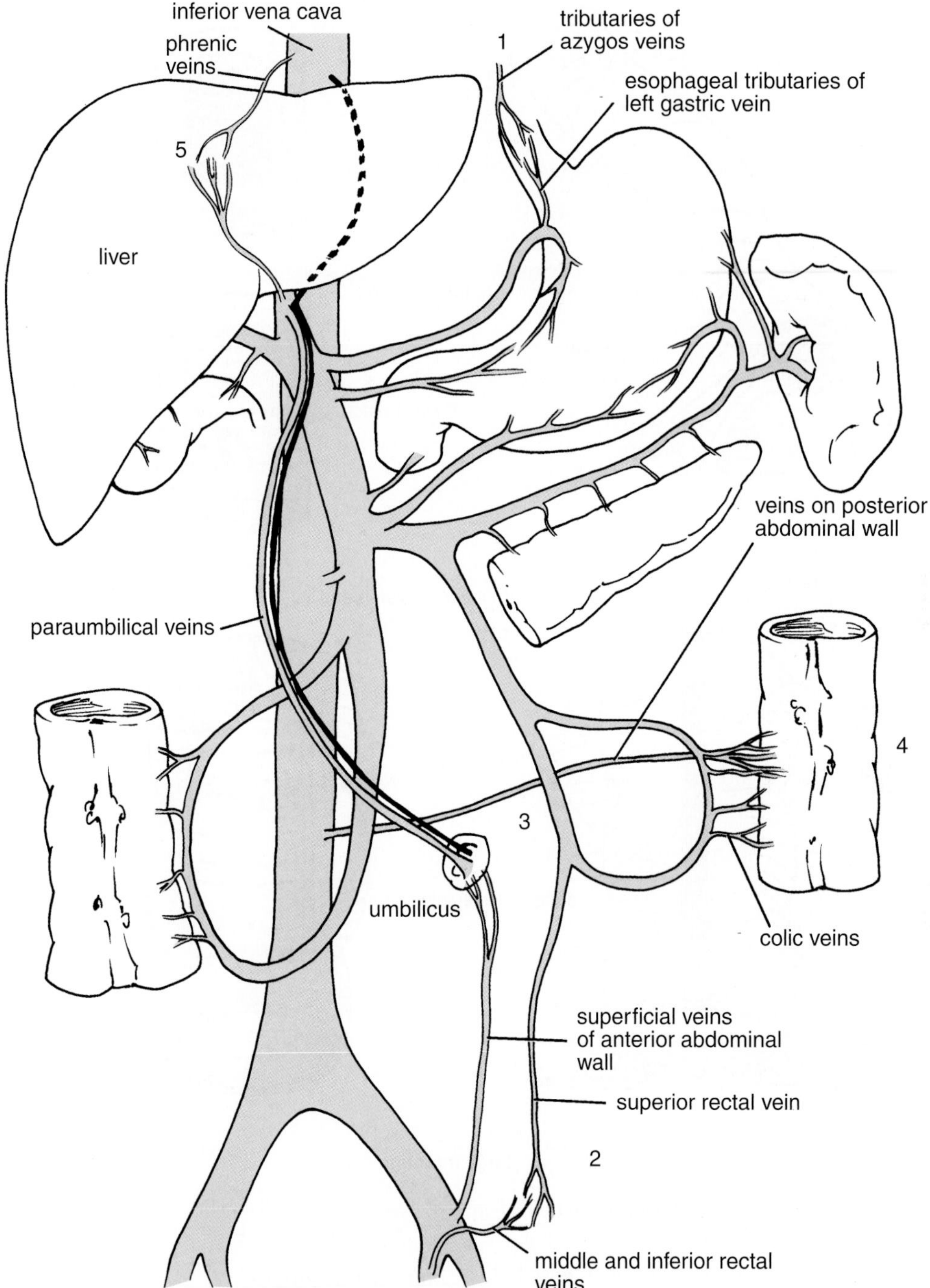

Figure 5-49 Important portal–systemic anastomoses.

or **visceral surface,** is molded to adjacent viscera and is therefore irregular in shape; it lies in contact with the abdominal part of the esophagus, the stomach, the duodenum, the right colic flexure, the right kidney and suprarenal gland, and the gallbladder.

The liver may be divided into a large **right lobe** and a small **left lobe** by the attachment of the peritoneum of the falciform ligament (Fig. 5-8). The right lobe is further divided into a **quadrate lobe** and a **caudate lobe** by the presence of the gallbladder, the fissure for the ligamentum teres, the inferior vena cava, and the fissure for the ligamentum venosum. Experiments have shown that, in fact, the quadrate and caudate lobes are a functional part of the left lobe of the liver. Thus, the right and left branches of the hepatic artery and portal vein, and the right and left hepatic ducts, are distributed to the right lobe and the left lobe (plus quadrate plus caudate lobes), respectively. Apparently, the two sides overlap very little.

The **porta hepatis,** or hilum of the liver, is found on the posteroinferior surface and lies between the caudate and quadrate lobes (Figs. 5-8 and 5-9). The upper part of the free edge of the lesser omentum is attached to its margins. In it

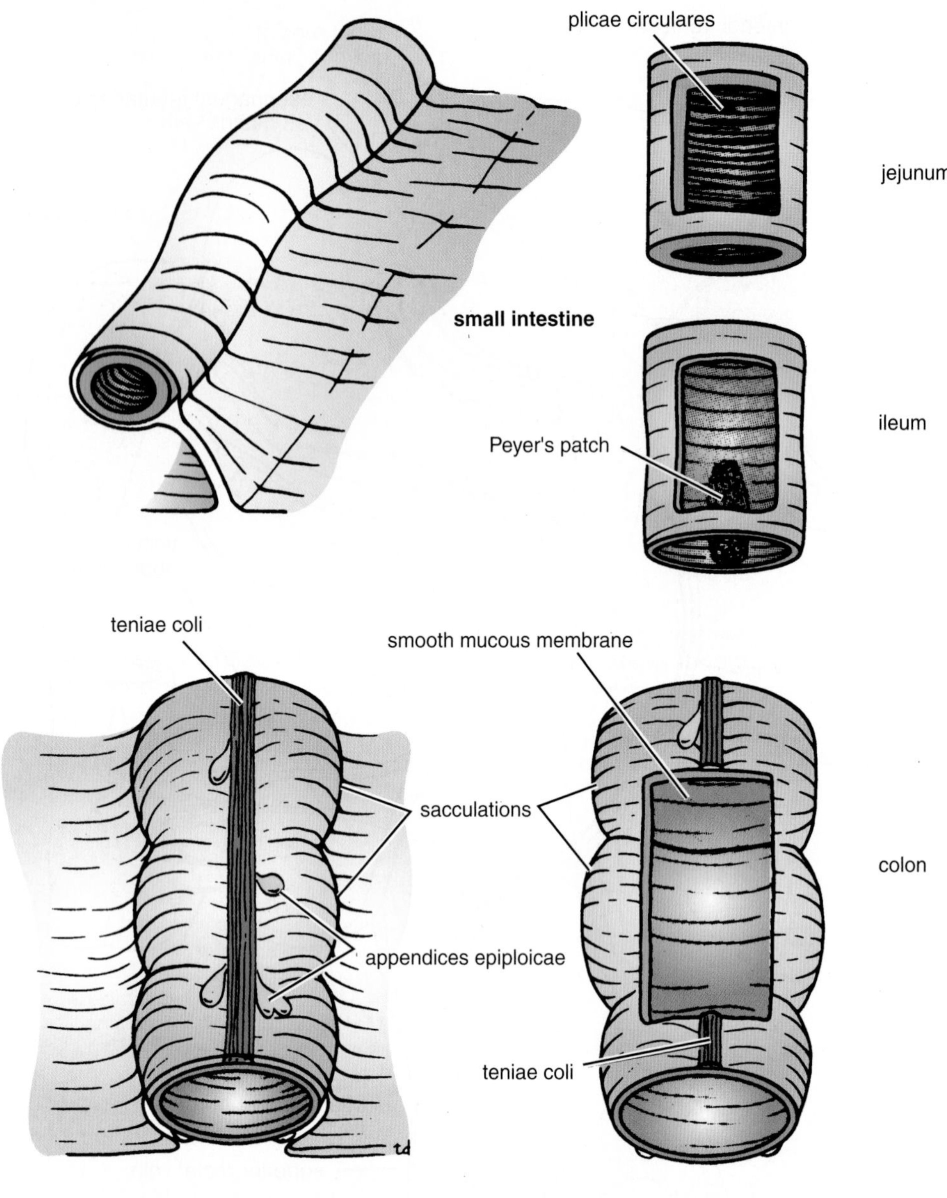

Figure 5-50 Some external and internal differences between the small and the large intestine.

lie the right and left hepatic ducts, the right and left branches of the hepatic artery, the portal vein, and sympathetic and parasympathetic nerve fibers (Fig. 5-47). A few hepatic lymph nodes lie here; they drain the liver and gallbladder and send their efferent vessels to the celiac lymph nodes.

The liver is completely surrounded by a fibrous capsule but only partially covered by peritoneum. The liver is made up of **liver lobules.** The **central vein** of each lobule is a tributary of the hepatic veins. In the spaces between the lobules are the **portal canals,** which contain branches of the hepatic artery, portal vein, and a tributary of a bile duct (portal triad). The arterial and venous blood passes between the liver cells by means of **sinusoids** and drains into the central vein.

Important Relations

- **Anteriorly:** Diaphragm, right and left costal margins, right and left pleura and lower margins of both lungs, xiphoid process, and anterior abdominal wall in the subcostal angle
- **Posteriorly:** Diaphragm, right kidney, hepatic flexure of the colon, duodenum, gallbladder, inferior vena cava, and esophagus and fundus of the stomach

Peritoneal Ligaments of the Liver

The **falciform ligament,** which is a two-layered fold of the peritoneum, ascends from the umbilicus to the liver (Fig. 5-8). It has a sickle-shaped free margin that contains the ligamentum teres, the remains of the umbilical vein. The falciform ligament passes on to the anterior and then the superior surfaces of the liver and then splits into two layers. The right layer forms the upper layer of the **coronary ligament;** the left layer forms the upper layer of the **left triangular ligament** (Fig. 5-8). The right extremity of the coronary ligament is known as the **right triangular ligament** of the liver. It should be noted that the peritoneal layers forming the coronary ligament are widely separated, leaving an area of liver devoid of peritoneum. Such an area is referred to as a **bare area of the liver** (Fig. 5-8).

The **ligamentum teres** passes into a fissure on the visceral surface of the liver and joins the left branch of the portal vein in the porta hepatis (Figs. 5-9 and 5-22). The **ligamentum venosum,** a fibrous band that is the remains of the **ductus venosus,** is attached to the left branch of the portal vein and ascends in a fissure on the visceral surface of the liver to be attached above to the inferior vena cava (Figs. 5-8 and 5-22). In the fetus, oxygenated blood is brought to the liver in the umbilical vein (ligamentum teres). The greater proportion of the blood bypasses the liver in the ductus venosus (ligamentum venosum) and joins the inferior vena cava. At birth, the umbilical vein and ductus venosus close and become fibrous cords.

The **lesser omentum** arises from the edges of the porta hepatis and the fissure for the ligamentum venosum and passes down to the lesser curvature of the stomach (Fig. 5-10).

Blood Supply

Arteries

The hepatic artery, a branch of the celiac artery, divides into right and left terminal branches that enter the porta hepatis.

Veins

The portal vein divides into right and left terminal branches that enter the porta hepatis behind the arteries. The **hepatic veins** (three or more) emerge from the posterior surface of the liver and drain into the inferior vena cava.

Blood Circulation through the Liver

The blood vessels (Fig. 5-47) conveying blood to the liver are the hepatic artery (30%) and portal vein (70%). The hepatic artery brings oxygenated blood to the liver, and the portal vein brings venous blood rich in the products of digestion, which have been absorbed from the gastrointestinal tract. The arterial and venous blood is conducted to the central vein of each liver lobule by the liver sinusoids. The central veins drain into the right and left hepatic veins, and these leave the posterior surface of the liver and open directly into the inferior vena cava.

Lymph Drainage

The liver produces a large amount of lymph—about one third to one half of all body lymph. The lymph vessels leave the liver and enter several lymph nodes in the porta hepatis. The efferent vessels pass to the celiac nodes. A few vessels pass from the bare area of the liver through the diaphragm to the posterior mediastinal lymph nodes.

Nerve Supply

Sympathetic and parasympathetic nerves form the celiac plexus. The anterior vagal trunk gives rise to a large hepatic branch, which passes directly to the liver.

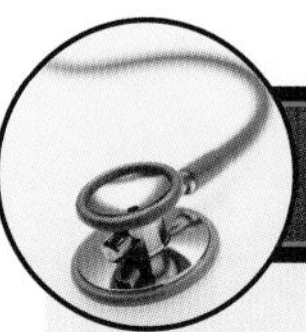

CLINICAL NOTES

Liver Supports and Surgery

The liver is held in position in the upper part of the abdominal cavity by the attachment of the hepatic veins to the inferior vena cava. The peritoneal ligaments and the tone of the abdominal muscles play a minor role in its support. This fact is important surgically because even if the peritoneal ligaments are cut, the liver can be only slightly rotated.

Liver Trauma

The liver is a soft, friable structure enclosed in a fibrous capsule. Its close relationship to the lower ribs must be emphasized. Fractures of the lower ribs or penetrating wounds of the thorax or upper abdomen are common causes of liver injury. Blunt traumatic injuries from automobile accidents are also common, and severe hemorrhage accompanies tears of this organ.

Because anatomic research has shown that the bile ducts, hepatic arteries, and portal vein are distributed in a segmental manner, appropriate ligation of these structures allows the surgeon to remove large portions of the liver in patients with severe traumatic lacerations of the liver or with a liver tumor. (Even large, localized carcinomatous metastatic tumors have been successfully removed.)

Liver Biopsy

Liver biopsy is a common diagnostic procedure. With the patient holding his or her breath in full expiration—to reduce the size of the costodiaphragmatic recess and the likelihood of damage to the lung—a needle is inserted through the right eighth or ninth intercostal space in the midaxillary line. The needle passes through the diaphragm into the liver, and a small specimen of liver tissue is removed for microscopic examination.

Subphrenic Spaces

The important subphrenic spaces and their relationship to the liver are described on page 208. Under normal conditions these are potential spaces only, and the peritoneal surfaces are in contact. An abnormal accumulation of gas or fluid is necessary for separation of the peritoneal surfaces. The anterior surface of the liver is normally dull on percussion. Perforation of a gastric ulcer is often accompanied by a loss of liver dullness caused by the accumulation of gas over the anterior surface of the liver and in the subphrenic spaces.

Bile Ducts of the Liver

Bile is secreted by the liver cells at a constant rate of about 40 mL per hour. When digestion is not taking place, the bile is stored and concentrated in the gallbladder; later, it is delivered to the duodenum. The bile ducts of the liver consist of the **right** and **left hepatic ducts,** the **common hepatic duct,** the **bile duct,** the **gallbladder,** and the **cystic duct.**

The smallest interlobular tributaries of the bile ducts are situated in the portal canals of the liver; they receive the bile canaliculi. The interlobular ducts join one another to form progressively larger ducts and, eventually, at the porta hepatis, form the right and left hepatic ducts. The right hepatic duct drains the right lobe of the liver and the left duct drains the left lobe, caudate lobe, and quadrate lobe.

Hepatic Ducts

The right and left hepatic ducts emerge from the right and left lobes of the liver in the porta hepatis (Fig. 5-47). After a short course, the hepatic ducts unite to form the common hepatic duct (Fig. 5-29).

The **common hepatic duct** is about 1.5 in. (4 cm) long and descends within the free margin of the lesser omentum. It is joined on the right side by the cystic duct from the gallbladder to form the bile duct (Fig. 5-29).

Bile Duct

The bile duct (common bile duct) is about 3 in. (8 cm) long. In the first part of its course, it lies in the right free margin of the lesser omentum in front of the opening into the lesser sac. Here, it lies in front of the right margin of the portal vein and on the right of the hepatic artery (Fig. 5-11). In the second part of its course, it is situated behind the first part of the duodenum (Fig. 5-7) to the right of the gastroduodenal artery (Fig. 5-4). In the third part of its course, it lies in a groove on the posterior surface of the head of the pancreas (Fig. 5-29). Here, the bile duct comes into contact with the main pancreatic duct.

The bile duct ends below by piercing the medial wall of the second part of the duodenum about halfway down its length (Fig. 5-51). It is usually joined by the main pancreatic duct, and together they open into a small ampulla in the duodenal wall, called the **hepatopancreatic ampulla (ampulla of Vater).** The ampulla opens into the lumen of the duodenum by means of a small papilla, the **major duodenal papilla** (Fig. 5-51). The terminal parts of both ducts and the ampulla are surrounded by circular muscle, known as the **sphincter of the hepatopancreatic ampulla (sphincter of Oddi)** (Fig. 5-51). Occasionally, the bile and pancreatic ducts open separately into the duodenum. The common variations of this arrangement are shown in Figure 5-52.

Gallbladder

Location and Description

The gallbladder is a pear-shaped sac lying on the undersurface of the liver (Figs. 5-8, 5-9, and 5-29). It has a capacity of 30 to 50 mL and stores bile, which it concentrates by absorbing water. The gallbladder is divided into the fundus, body, and neck. The **fundus** is rounded and projects below the inferior margin of the liver, where it comes in contact with the anterior abdominal wall at the level of the tip of the ninth right costal cartilage. The **body** lies in con-

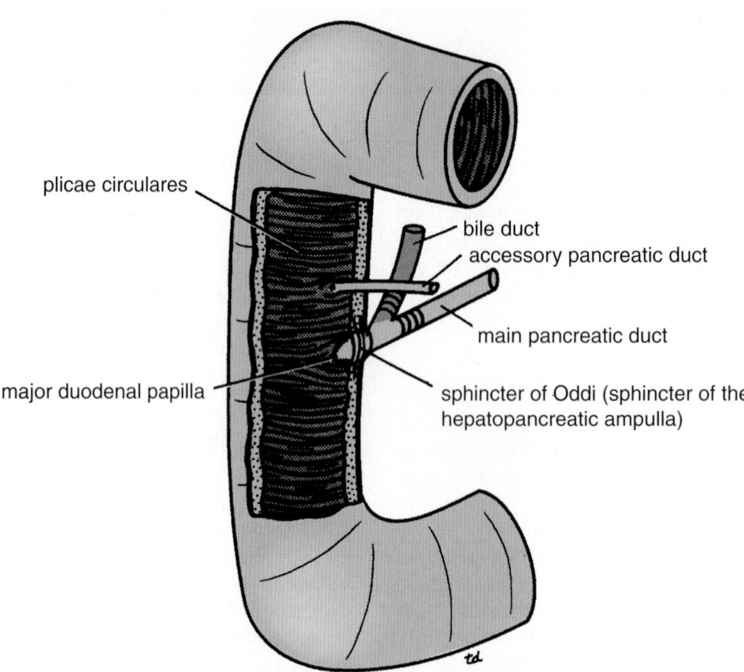

Figure 5-51 Terminal parts of the bile and pancreatic ducts as they enter the second part of the duodenum. Note the sphincter of Oddi and the smooth muscle around the ends of the bile duct and the main pancreatic duct.

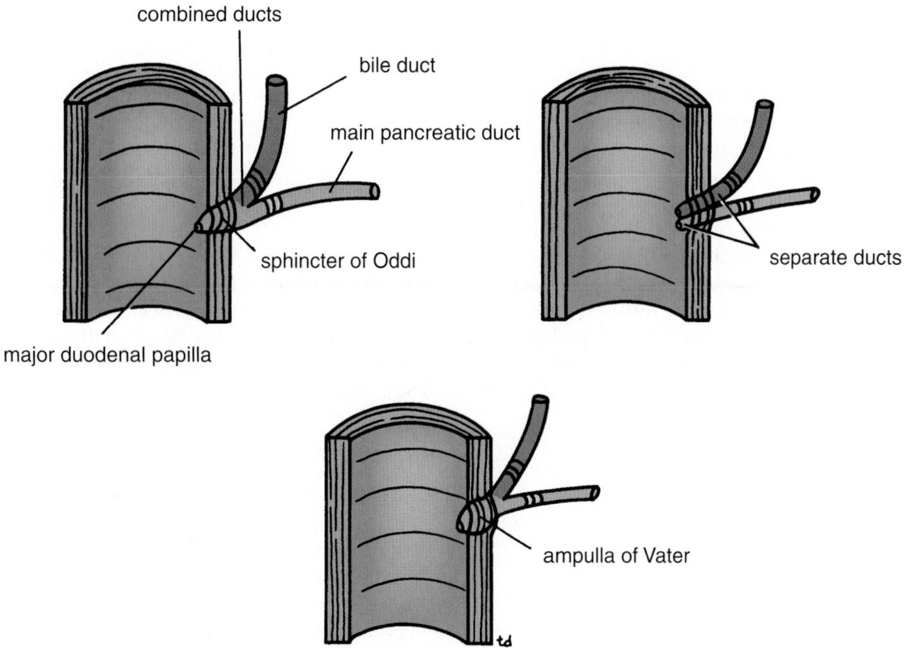

Figure 5-52 Three common variations of terminations of the bile and main pancreatic ducts as they enter the second part of the duodenum.

tact with the visceral surface of the liver and is directed upward, backward, and to the left. The **neck** becomes continuous with the cystic duct, which turns into the lesser omentum to join the common hepatic duct, to form the bile duct (Fig. 5-29).

The peritoneum completely surrounds the fundus of the gallbladder and binds the body and neck to the visceral surface of the liver.

Relations

- **Anteriorly:** The anterior abdominal wall and the inferior surface of the liver (Fig. 5-2)
- **Posteriorly:** The transverse colon and the first and second parts of the duodenum (Fig. 5-29)

Function of the Gallbladder

When digestion is not taking place, the sphincter of Oddi remains closed and bile accumulates in the gallbladder. The gallbladder concentrates bile; stores bile; selectively absorbs bile salts, keeping the bile acid; excretes cholesterol; and secretes mucus. To aid in these functions, the mucous membrane is thrown into permanent folds that unite with each other, giving the surface a honeycombed appearance. The columnar cells lining the surface have numerous microvilli on their free surface.

Bile is delivered to the duodenum as the result of contraction and partial emptying of the gallbladder. This mechanism is initiated by the entrance of fatty foods into the duodenum. The fat causes release of the hormone **cholecystokinin** from the mucous membrane of the duodenum; the hormone then enters the blood, causing the gallbladder to contract. At the same time, the smooth muscle around the distal end of the bile duct and the ampulla is relaxed, thus allowing the passage of concentrated bile into the duodenum. The bile salts in the bile are important in emulsifying the fat in the intestine and in assisting with its digestion and absorption.

Blood Supply

The **cystic artery,** a branch of the right hepatic artery (Fig. 5-47), supplies the gallbladder. The **cystic vein** drains directly into the portal vein. Several very small arteries and veins also run between the liver and gallbladder.

Lymph Drainage

The lymph drains into a **cystic lymph node** situated near the neck of the gallbladder. From here, the lymph vessels pass to the hepatic nodes along the course of the hepatic artery and then to the celiac nodes.

Nerve Supply

Sympathetic and parasympathetic vagal fibers form the celiac plexus. The gallbladder contracts in response to the hormone cholecystokinin, which is produced by the mucous membrane of the duodenum on the arrival of fatty food from the stomach.

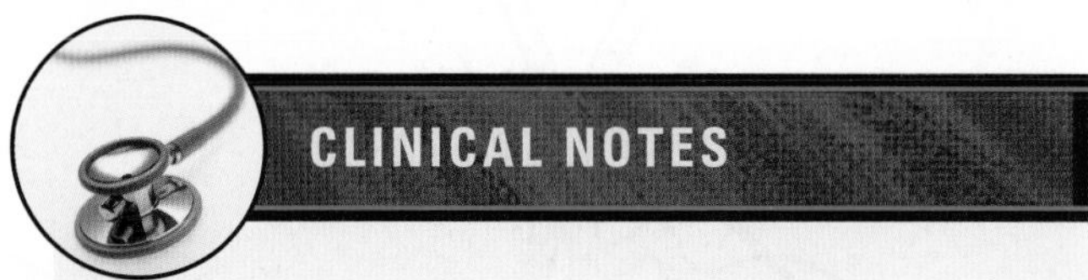

Gallstones

Gallstones are usually asymptomatic; however, they can give rise to gallstone colic or produce acute cholecystitis.

Biliary Colic

Biliary colic is usually caused by spasm of the smooth muscle of the wall of the gallbladder in an attempt to expel a gallstone.

(continues)

Clinical Notes, *continued*

Afferent nerve fibers ascend through the celiac plexus and the greater splanchnic nerves to the thoracic segments of the spinal cord. Referred pain is felt in the right upper quadrant or the epigastrium (T7, 8, and 9 dermatomes).

Obstruction of the biliary ducts with a gallstone or by compression by a tumor of the pancreas results in backup of bile in the ducts and development of **jaundice.** The impaction of a stone in the ampulla of Vater may result in the passage of infected bile into the pancreatic duct, producing **pancreatitis.** The anatomic arrangement of the terminal part of the bile duct and the main pancreatic duct is subject to considerable variation. The type of duct system present determines whether infected bile is likely to enter the pancreatic duct.

Gallstones have been known to ulcerate through the gallbladder wall into the transverse colon or the duodenum. In the former case, they are passed naturally per the rectum, but in the latter case, they may be held up at the ileocecal junction, producing intestinal obstruction.

Acute Cholecystitis

Acute cholecystitis produces discomfort in the right upper quadrant or epigastrium. Inflammation of the gallbladder may cause irritation of the subdiaphragmatic parietal peritoneum, which is supplied in part by the phrenic nerve (C3, 4, and 5). This may give rise to referred pain over the shoulder, because the skin in this area is supplied by the supraclavicular nerves (C3 and 4).

Cholecystectomy and the Arterial Supply to the Gallbladder

Before attempting a cholecystectomy operation, the surgeon must be aware of the many variations in the arterial supply to the gallbladder and the relationship of the vessels to the bile ducts (Fig. 5-53). Unfortunately, there have been several reported cases in which the common hepatic duct or the main bile duct have been included in the arterial ligature with disastrous consequences.

Gangrene of the Gallbladder

Unlike the appendix, which has a single arterial supply, the gallbladder rarely becomes gangrenous. In addition to the cystic artery, the gallbladder also receives small vessels from the visceral surface of the liver.

Sonograms can now be used to demonstrate the gallbladder (Fig. 5-54).

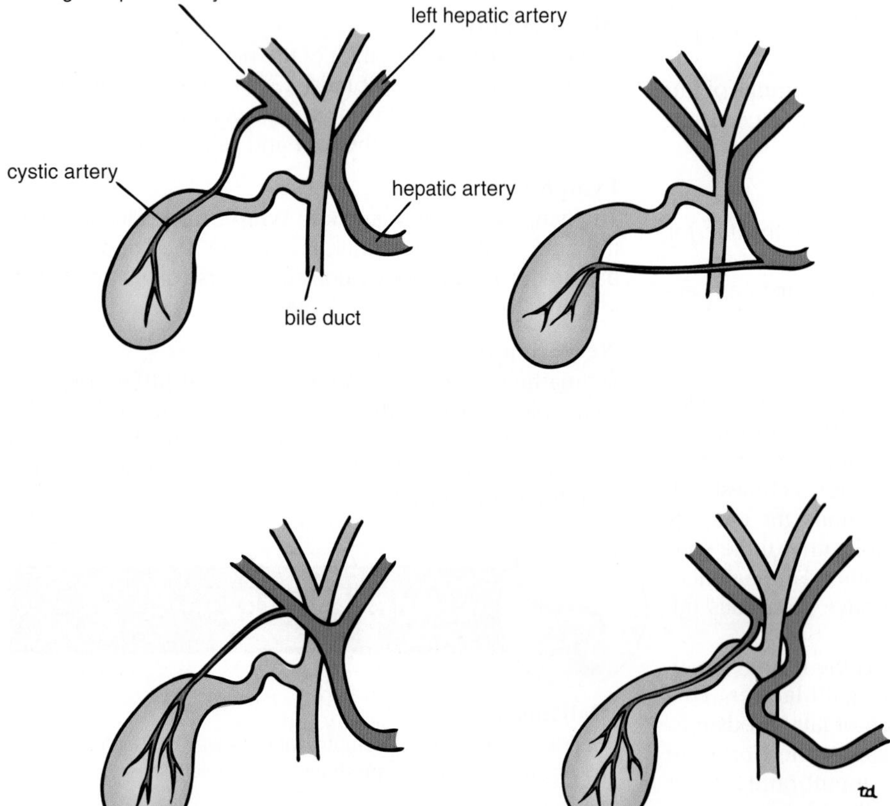

Figure 5-53 Some common variations of blood supply to the gallbladder.

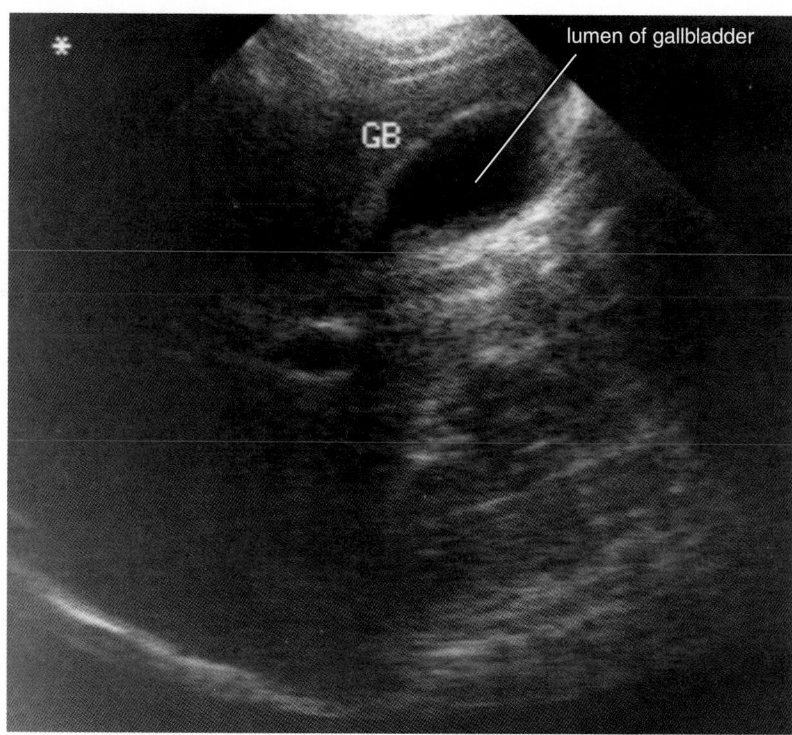

Figure 5-54 Longitudinal sonogram of the upper part of the abdomen showing the lumen of the gallbladder. (Courtesy of Dr. M.C. Hill.)

Cystic Duct

The **cystic duct** is about 1.5 in. (3.8 cm) long and connects the neck of the gallbladder to the common hepatic duct to form the bile duct (Fig. 5-29). It usually is somewhat S-shaped and descends for a variable distance in the right free margin of the lesser omentum.

The mucous membrane of the cystic duct is raised to form a spiral fold that is continuous with a similar fold in the neck of the gallbladder. The fold is commonly known as the "spiral valve." The function of the spiral valve is to keep the lumen constantly open.

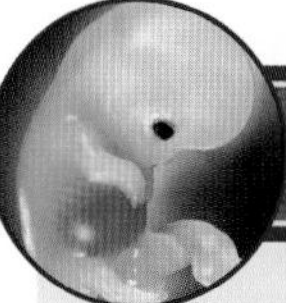

EMBRYOLOGIC NOTES

Development of the Liver and Bile Ducts

Liver

The liver arises from the distal end of the foregut as a solid bud of entodermal cells (Figs. 5-41 and 5-55). The site of origin lies at the apex of the loop of the developing duodenum and corresponds to a point halfway along the second part of the fully formed duodenum. The **hepatic bud** grows anteriorly into the mass of splanchnic mesoderm called the septum transversum. The end of the bud now divides into right and left branches, from which columns of entodermal cells grow into the vascular mesoderm. The paired vitelline veins and umbilical veins that course through the septum transversum become broken up by the invading columns of liver cells and form the **liver sinusoids.** The columns of entodermal cells form the liver cords. The connective tissue of the liver is formed from the mesenchyme of the septum transversum.

The main hepatic bud and its right and left terminal branches now become canalized to form the **common hepatic duct** and the **right** and **left hepatic ducts.** The liver grows rapidly in size and comes to occupy the greater part of the abdominal cavity; the right lobe becomes much larger than the left lobe.

Gallbladder and Cystic Duct

The gallbladder develops from the hepatic bud as a solid outgrowth of cells (Fig. 5-41). The end of the outgrowth expands to form the gallbladder, while the narrow stem remains as the cystic duct. Later, the gallbladder and cystic duct become canalized. The cystic duct now opens into the **common hepatic duct** to form the **bile duct.**

Biliary Atresia

Failure of the bile ducts to canalize during development causes atresia. The various forms of atresia are shown in Figure 5-56. Jaundice appears soon after birth; clay-colored stools and very dark colored urine are also present. Surgical correction of the atresia should be attempted when possible. If the atresia cannot be corrected, the child will die of liver failure.

Absence of the Gallbladder

Occasionally, the outgrowth of cells from the hepatic bud fails to develop. In these cases, there is no gallbladder and no cystic duct (Fig. 5-57).

(continues)

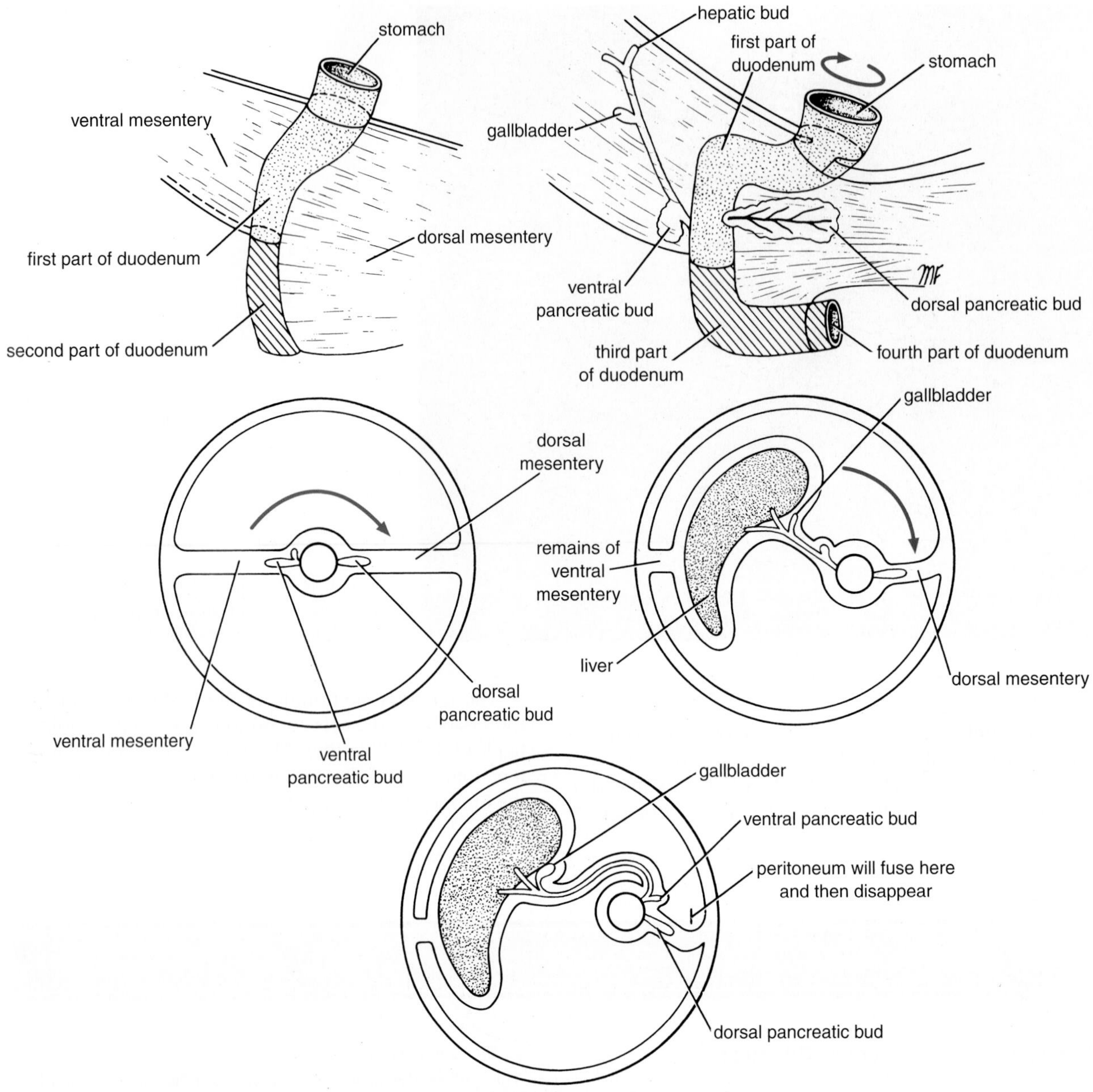

Figure 5-55 Development of the duodenum in relation to the ventral and dorsal mesenteries. Stippled area, foregut; crosshatched area, midgut.

Embryologic Notes, *continued*

Double Gallbladder

Rarely, the outgrowth of cells from the hepatic bud bifurcates so that two gallbladders are formed (Fig. 5-57).

Absence of the Cystic Duct

In absence of the cystic duct, the entire outgrowth of cells from the hepatic bud develops into the gallbladder and fails to leave the narrow stem that would normally form the cystic duct. The gallbladder drains directly into the bile duct. The condition may not be recognized when performing a cholecystectomy, and the bile duct may be seriously damaged by the surgeon (Fig. 5-57).

Accessory Bile Duct

A small accessory bile duct may open directly from the liver into the gallbladder, which may cause leakage of bile into the peritoneal cavity after cholecystectomy if it is not recognized at the time of surgery (Fig. 5-57).

Congenital Choledochal Cyst

Rarely, a choledochal cyst develops because of an area of weakness in the wall of the bile duct. A cyst can contain 1 to 2 L of bile. The anomaly is important in that it may press on the bile duct and cause obstructive jaundice (Fig. 5-57).

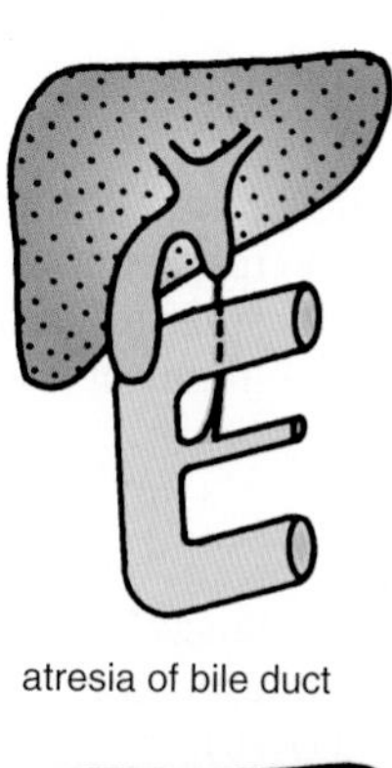
atresia of bile duct

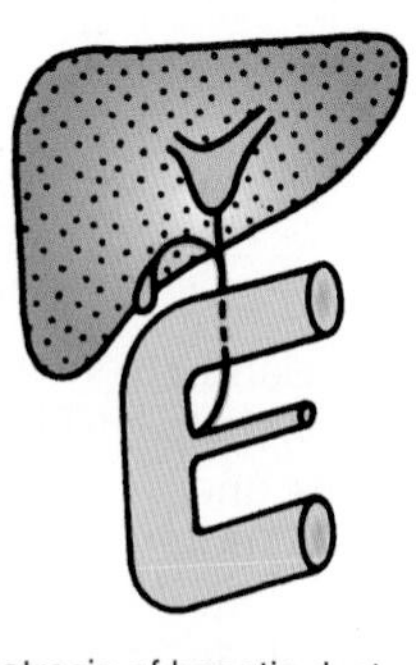
atresia of hepatic duct

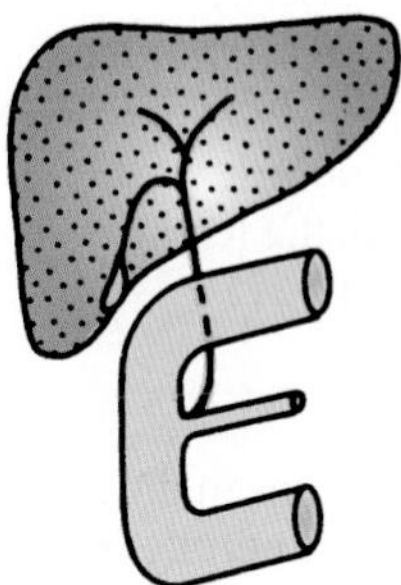
atresia of entire extrahepatic apparatus

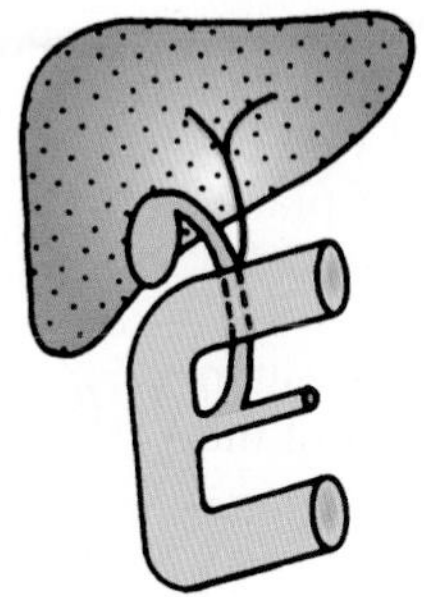
atresia of hepatic ducts

Figure 5-56 Some common congenital anomalies of the biliary ducts.

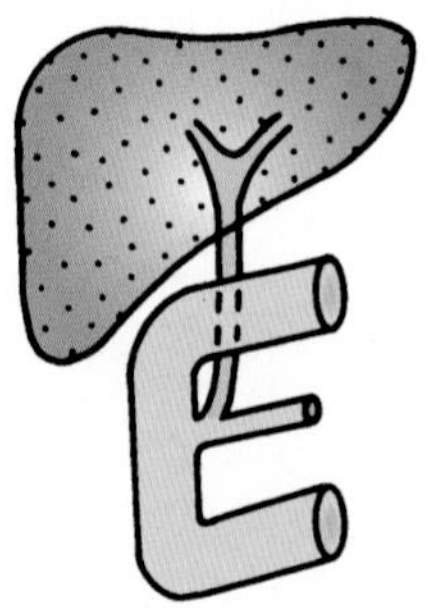
congenital absence of gallbladder

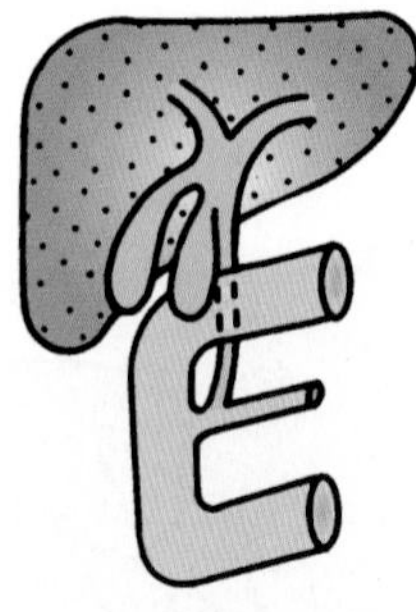
double gallbladder

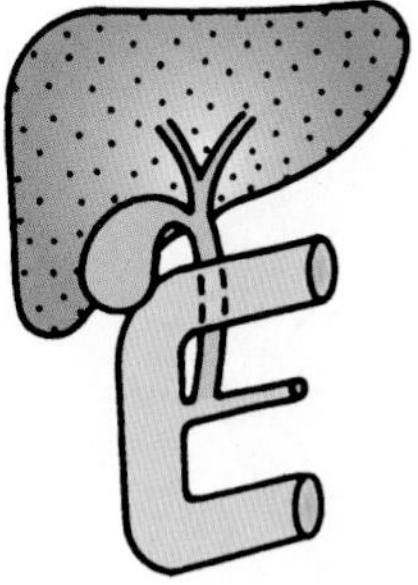
absence of cystic duct

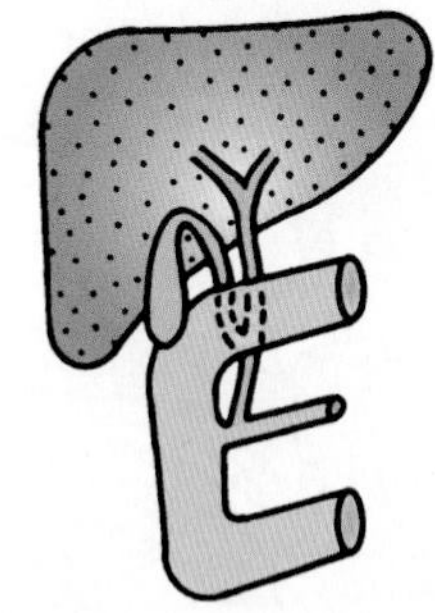
abnormally long cystic duct

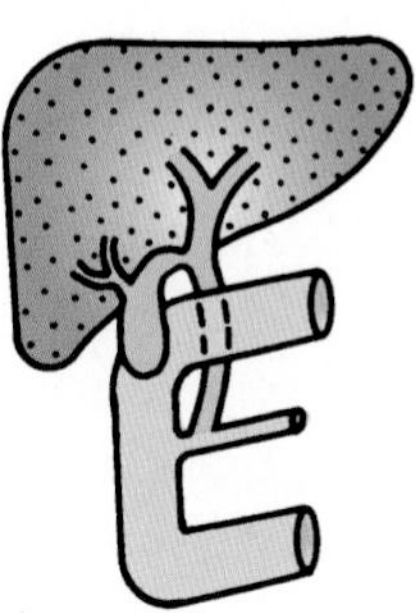
accessory bile duct

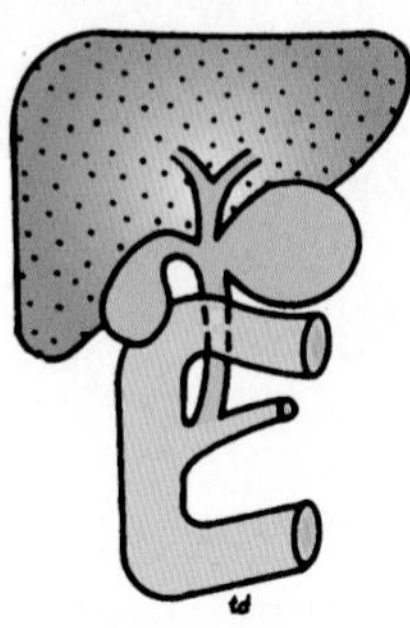
choledochal cyst

Figure 5-57 Some common congenital anomalies of the gallbladder.

Pancreas

Location and Description

The pancreas is both an exocrine and an endocrine gland. The exocrine portion of the gland produces a secretion that contains enzymes capable of hydrolyzing proteins, fats, and carbohydrates. The endocrine portion of the gland, the **pancreatic islets (islets of Langerhans),** produces the hormones **insulin** and **glucagon,** which play a key role in carbohydrate metabolism.

The pancreas is an elongated structure that lies in the epigastrium and the left upper quadrant. It is soft and lobulated and situated on the posterior abdominal wall behind the peritoneum. It crosses the transpyloric plane. The pancreas is divided into a head, neck, body, and tail (Fig. 5-58).

The **head** of the pancreas is disc shaped and lies within the concavity of the duodenum (Fig. 5-58). A part of the head extends to the left behind the superior mesenteric vessels and is called the **uncinate process.**

The **neck** is the constricted portion of the pancreas and connects the head to the body. It lies in front of the beginning of the portal vein and the origin of the superior mesenteric artery from the aorta (Fig. 5-26).

The **body** runs upward and to the left across the midline (Fig. 5-4). It is somewhat triangular in cross section.

The **tail** passes forward in the splenicorenal ligament and comes in contact with the hilum of the spleen (Fig. 5-4).

Relations

- **Anteriorly:** From right to left: the transverse colon and the attachment of the transverse mesocolon, the lesser sac, and the stomach (Figs. 5-4 and 5-6)
- **Posteriorly:** From right to left: the bile duct, the portal and splenic veins, the inferior vena cava, the aorta, the origin of the superior mesenteric artery, the left psoas muscle, the left suprarenal gland, the left kidney, and the hilum of the spleen (Figs. 5-4 and 5-27)

Pancreatic Ducts

The **main duct of the pancreas** begins in the tail and runs the length of the gland, receiving numerous tributaries on the way (Fig. 5-58). It opens into the second part of the duodenum at about its middle with the bile duct on the **major duodenal papilla** (Fig. 5-51). Sometimes the main duct drains separately into the duodenum.

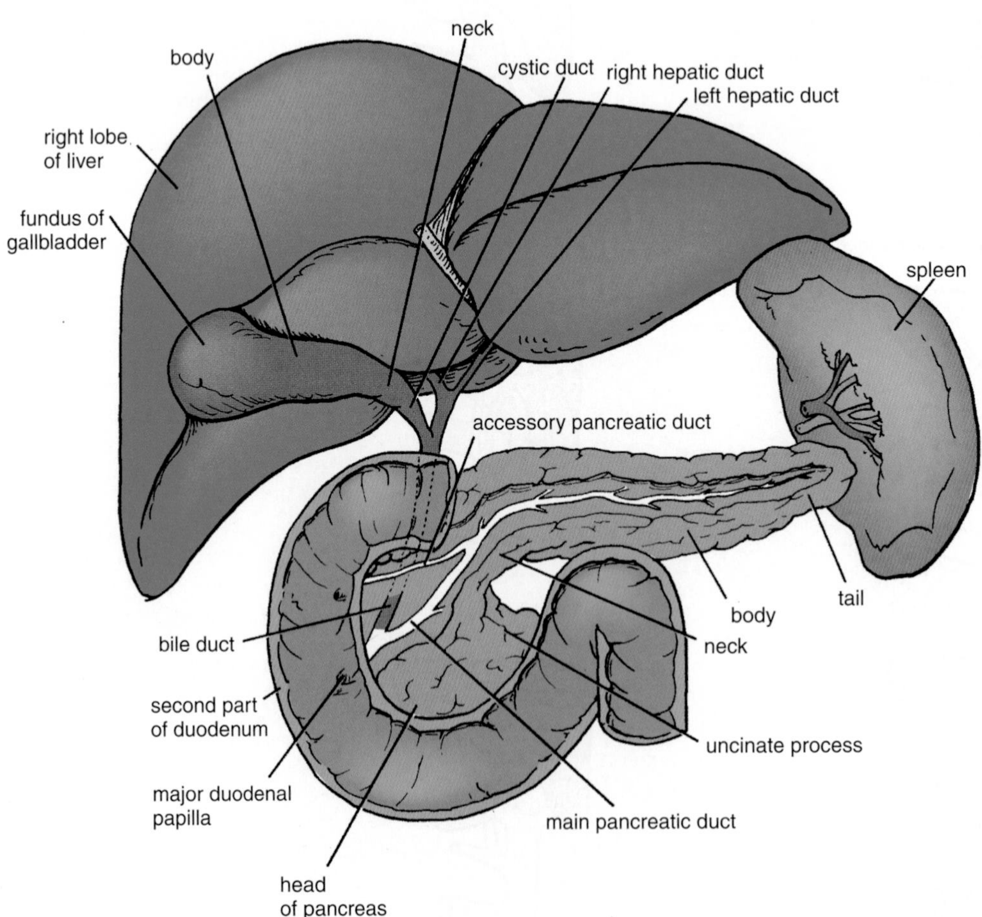

Figure 5-58 Different parts of the pancreas dissected to reveal the duct system.

The **accessory duct** of the pancreas, when present, drains the upper part of the head and then opens into the duodenum a short distance above the main duct on the **minor duodenal papilla** (Figs. 5-51 and 5-58). The accessory duct frequently communicates with the main duct.

Blood Supply

Arteries

The splenic and the superior and inferior pancreaticoduodenal arteries (Fig. 5-26) supply the pancreas.

Veins

The corresponding veins drain into the portal system.

Lymph Drainage

Lymph nodes are situated along the arteries that supply the gland. The efferent vessels ultimately drain into the celiac and superior mesenteric lymph nodes.

Nerve Supply

Sympathetic and parasympathetic (vagal) nerve fibers supply the area.

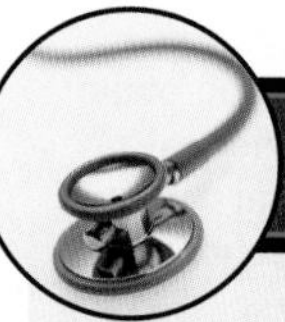

CLINICAL NOTES

Diagnosis of Pancreatic Disease

The deep location of the pancreas sometimes gives rise to problems of diagnosis for the following reasons:

- Pain from the pancreas is commonly referred to the back.
- Because the pancreas lies behind the stomach and transverse colon, disease of the gland can be confused with that of the stomach or transverse colon.
- Inflammation of the pancreas can spread to the peritoneum forming the posterior wall of the lesser sac. This in turn can lead to adhesions and the closing off of the lesser sac to form a pseudocyst.

Trauma of the Pancreas

The pancreas is deeply placed within the abdomen and is well protected by the costal margin and the anterior abdominal wall. However, blunt trauma, such as in a sports injury when a sudden blow to the abdomen occurs, can compress and tear the pancreas against the vertebral column. The pancreas is most commonly damaged by gunshot or stab wounds.

Damaged pancreatic tissue releases activated pancreatic enzymes that produce the signs and symptoms of acute peritonitis.

Cancer of the Head of the Pancreas and the Bile Duct

Because of the close relation of the head of the pancreas to the bile duct, cancer of the head of the pancreas often causes obstructive jaundice.

The Pancreatic Tail and Splenectomy

The presence of the tail of the pancreas in the splenicorenal ligament sometimes results in its damage during splenectomy. The damaged pancreas releases enzymes that start to digest surrounding tissues, with serious consequences.

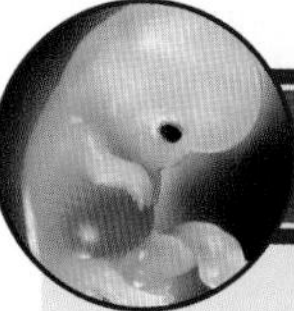

EMBRYOLOGIC NOTES

Development of the Pancreas

The pancreas develops from a **dorsal** and **ventral bud** of entodermal cells that arise from the foregut. The dorsal bud originates a short distance above the ventral bud and grows into the dorsal mesentery. The ventral bud arises in common with the hepatic bud, close to the junction of the foregut with the midgut (Fig. 5-41). A canalized duct system now develops in each bud. The rotation of the stomach and duodenum, together with the rapid growth of the left side of the duodenum, results in the ventral bud's coming into contact with the dorsal bud, and fusion occurs (Fig. 5-59).

Fusion also occurs between the ducts, so that the **main pancreatic duct** is derived from the entire ventral pancreatic duct and the distal part of the dorsal pancreatic duct. The main pancreatic duct joins the bile duct and enters the second part of the duodenum. The proximal part of the dorsal pancreatic duct may persist as an **accessory duct,** which may or may not open into the duodenum about 0.75 in. (2 cm) above the opening of the main duct.

Continued growth of the entodermal cells of the now-fused ventral and dorsal pancreatic buds extends into the surrounding mesenchyme as columns of cells. These columns give off side branches, which later become canalized to form collecting ducts. Secretory acini appear at the ends of the ducts.

The **pancreatic islets** arise as small buds from the developing ducts. Later, these cells sever their connection with the duct system and form isolated groups of cells that start to secrete **insulin** and **glucagon** at about the fifth month.

The inferior part of the head and the uncinate process of the pancreas are formed from the ventral pancreatic bud; the superior part of the head, the neck, the body, and the tail of the pancreas are formed from the dorsal pancreatic bud (Fig. 5-59).

(continues)

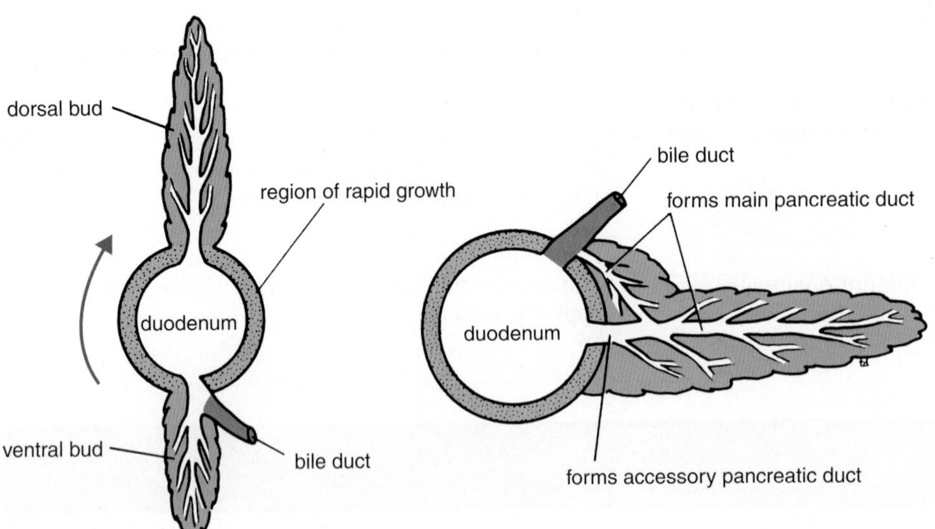

Figure 5-59 The rotation of the duodenum and the unequal growth of the duodenal wall lead to the fusing of the ventral and dorsal pancreatic buds.

Embryologic Notes, *continued*

Entrance of the Bile Duct and Pancreatic Duct into the Duodenum

As seen from development, the bile duct and the main pancreatic duct are joined to one another. They pass obliquely through the wall of the second part of the duodenum to open on the summit of the **major duodenal papilla,** which is surrounded by the **sphincter of Oddi** (Fig. 5-52). In some individuals, they pass separately through the duodenal wall, although in close contact, and open separately on the summit of the duodenal papilla. In other individuals, the two ducts join and form a common dilatation, the **hepatopancreatic ampulla (ampulla of Vater).** This opens on the summit of the duodenal papilla.

Anular Pancreas

In anular pancreas, the ventral pancreatic bud becomes fixed so that, when the stomach and duodenum rotate, the ventral bud is pulled around the right side of the duodenum to fuse with the dorsal bud of the pancreas, thus encircling the duodenum (Fig. 5-60). This may cause obstruction of the duodenum, and vomiting may start a few hours after birth. Early surgical relief of the obstruction is necessary.

Ectopic Pancreas

Ectopic pancreatic tissue may be found in the submucosa of the stomach, duodenum, small intestine (including Meckel's diverticulum), and gallbladder, and in the spleen. It is important in that it may protrude into the lumen of the gut and be responsible for causing intussusception.

Congenital Fibrocystic Disease

Basically, congenital fibrocystic disease in the pancreas is caused by an abnormality in the secretion of mucus. The mucus produced is excessively viscid and obstructs the pancreatic duct, which leads to pancreatitis with subsequent fibrosis. The condition also involves the lungs, kidneys, and liver.

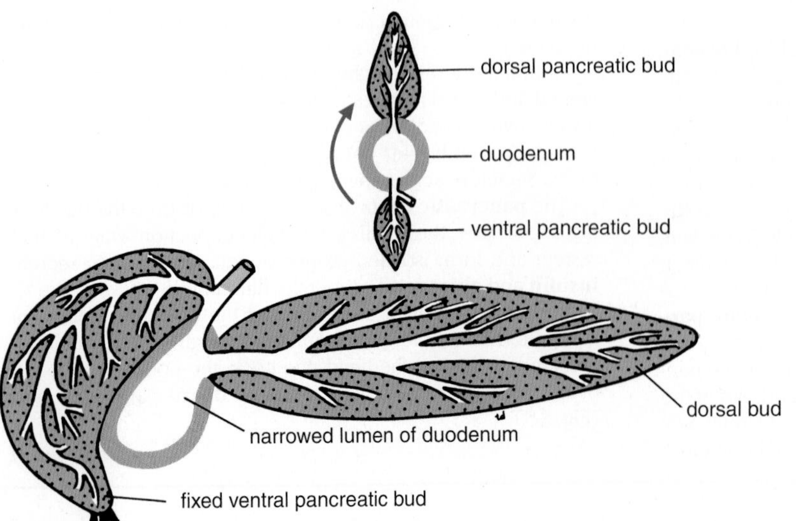

Figure 5-60 Formation of the anular pancreas, producing duodenal obstruction. Note the narrowing of the duodenum.

Spleen

Location and Description

The spleen is reddish and is the largest single mass of lymphoid tissue in the body. It is oval shaped and has a notched anterior border. It lies just beneath the left half of the diaphragm close to the 9th, 10th, and 11th ribs. The long axis lies along the shaft of the 10th rib, and its lower pole extends forward only as far as the midaxillary line and cannot be palpated on clinical examination (Fig. 5-61).

The spleen is surrounded by peritoneum (Figs. 5-5 and 5-61), which passes from it at the hilum as the gastrosplenic omentum (ligament) to the greater curvature of the stomach (carrying the short gastric and left gastroepiploic vessels). The peritoneum also passes to the left kidney as the splenicorenal ligament (carrying the splenic vessels and the tail of the pancreas).

Relations

- **Anteriorly:** The stomach, tail of the pancreas, and left colic flexure. The left kidney lies along its medial border (Figs. 5-4 and 5-11).
- **Posteriorly:** The diaphragm; left pleura (left costodiaphragmatic recess); left lung; and 9th, 10th, and 11th ribs (Figs. 5-11 and 5-61)

Blood Supply

Arteries

The large splenic artery is the largest branch of the celiac artery. It has a tortuous course as it runs along the upper border of the pancreas. The splenic artery then divides into about six branches, which enter the spleen at the hilum.

Veins

The splenic vein leaves the hilum and runs behind the tail and the body of the pancreas. Behind the neck of the pancreas, the splenic vein joins the superior mesenteric vein to form the portal vein.

Lymph Drainage

The lymph vessels emerge from the hilum and pass through a few lymph nodes along the course of the splenic artery and then drain into the celiac nodes.

Nerve Supply

The nerves accompany the splenic artery and are derived from the celiac plexus.

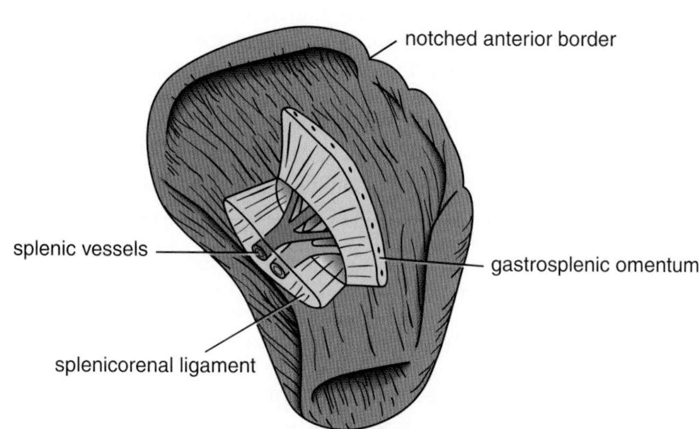

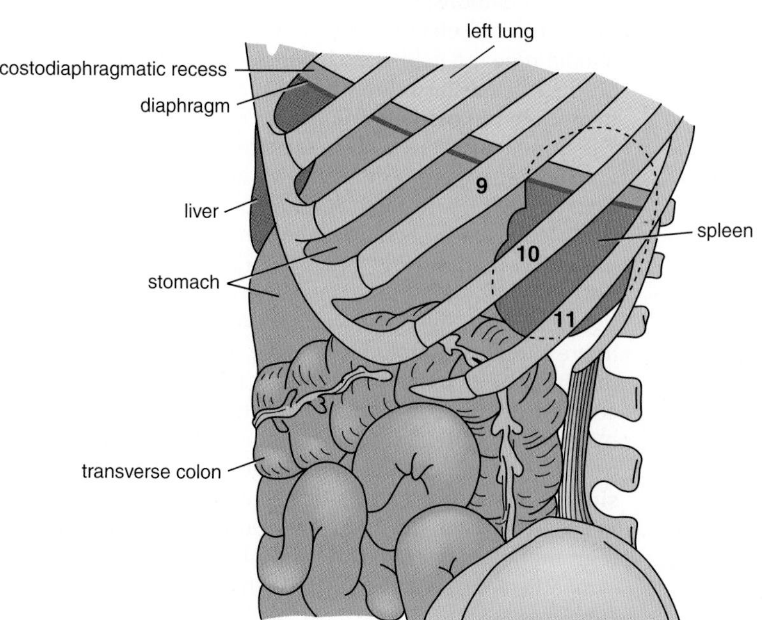

Figure 5-61 Spleen, with its notched anterior border, and its relation to adjacent structures.

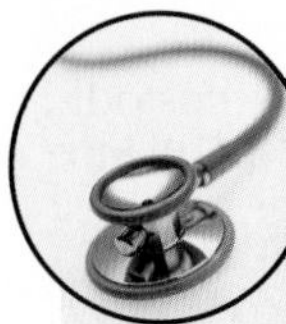

CLINICAL NOTES

Splenic Enlargement

A pathologically enlarged spleen extends downward and medially. The left colic flexure and the phrenicocolic ligament prevent a direct downward enlargement of the organ. As the enlarged spleen projects below the left costal margin, its notched anterior border can be recognized by palpation through the anterior abdominal wall.

The spleen is situated at the beginning of the splenic vein, and in cases of portal hypertension it often enlarges from venous congestion.

Trauma to the Spleen

Although anatomically the spleen gives the appearance of being well protected, automobile accidents of the crushing or run-over type commonly produce laceration of the spleen. Penetrating wounds of the lower left thorax can also damage the spleen.

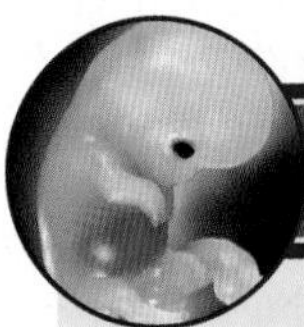

EMBRYOLOGIC NOTES

Development of the Spleen

The spleen develops as a thickening of the mesenchyme in the dorsal mesentery (Fig. 5-46). In the earliest stages, the spleen consists of a number of mesenchymal masses that later fuse. The notches along its anterior border are permanent and indicate that the mesenchymal masses never completely fuse.

The part of the dorsal mesentery that extends between the hilum of the spleen and the greater curvature of the stomach is called the **gastrosplenic omentum;** the part that extends between the spleen and the left kidney on the posterior abdominal wall is called the **splenicorenal ligament.** The spleen is supplied by a branch of the foregut artery (celiac artery), the **splenic artery.**

Supernumerary Spleen

In 10% of people, one or more supernumerary spleens may be present, either in the gastrosplenic omentum or in the splenicorenal ligament. Their clinical importance is that they may hypertrophy after removal of the major spleen and be responsible for a recurrence of symptoms of the disease for which splenectomy was initially performed.

Retroperitoneal Space

The retroperitoneal space lies on the posterior abdominal wall behind the parietal peritoneum. It extends from the 12th thoracic vertebra and the 12th rib to the sacrum and the iliac crests below (Fig. 5-62).

The floor or posterior wall of the space is formed from medial to lateral by the psoas and quadratus lumborum muscles and the origin of the transversus abdominis muscle. Each of these muscles is covered on the anterior surface by a definite layer of fascia. In front of the fascial layers is a variable amount of fatty connective tissue that forms a bed for the suprarenal glands, the kidneys, the ascending and descending parts of the colon, and the duodenum. The retroperitoneal space also contains the ureters and the renal and gonadal blood vessels.

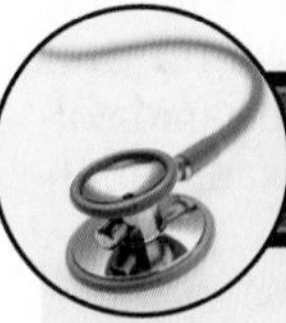

CLINICAL NOTES

Trauma to Organs in the Retroperitoneal Space

Palpation of the anterior abdominal wall in the lumbar and iliac regions may give rise to signs indicative of peritoneal irritation (the peritoneum forms the anterior boundary of the space; Fig. 5-62). In other words, tenderness and muscle spasm (rigidity) may be present. Palpation of the back in the interval between the 12th rib and the vertebral column may reveal tenderness suggestive of kidney disease.

Abdominal radiographs may reveal air in the extraperitoneal tissues, indicating perforation of a viscus (e.g., ascending or descending colon). Computed tomography scans can often accurately define the extent of the injury to the extraperitoneal organs.

Abscess Formation

Infection originating in retroperitoneal organs, such as the kidneys, lymph nodes, and retrocecal appendix, may extend widely into the retroperitoneal space.

Leaking Aortic Aneurysm

The blood may first be confined to the retroperitoneal space before rupturing into the peritoneal cavity.

Urinary Tract

Kidneys

Location and Description

The two kidneys function to excrete most of the waste products of metabolism. They play a major role in controlling the water and electrolyte balance within the body and in maintaining the acid–base balance of the blood. The waste products leave the kidneys as **urine,** which passes down the **ureters** to the **urinary bladder,** located within the pelvis. The urine leaves the body in the **urethra.**

The kidneys are reddish brown and lie behind the peritoneum high up on the posterior abdominal wall on either side of the vertebral column; they are largely under cover of the costal margin (Fig. 5-63). The right kidney lies slightly lower than the left kidney because of the large size of the right lobe of the liver. With contraction of the diaphragm during respiration, both kidneys move downward in a vertical direction by as much as 1 in. (2.5 cm). On the medial concave border of each kidney is a vertical slit that is bounded by thick lips of renal substance and is called the **hilum** (Fig. 5-64). The hilum extends into a large cavity called the **renal sinus.** The hilum transmits, from the front backward, the renal vein, two branches of the renal artery, the ureter, and the third branch of the renal artery (VAUA). Lymph vessels and sympathetic fibers also pass through the hilum.

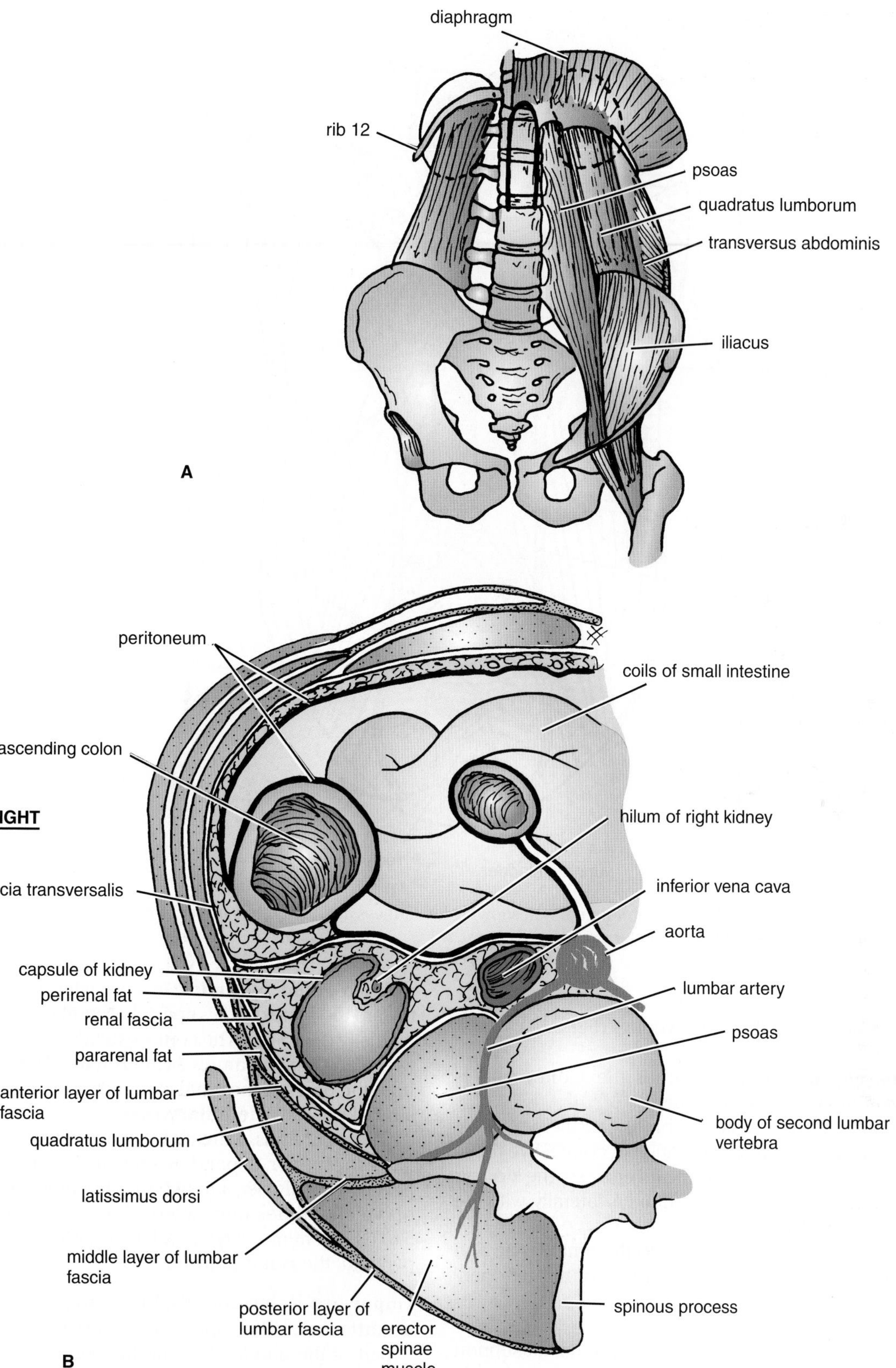

Figure 5-62 Retroperitoneal space. **A.** Structures present on the posterior abdominal wall behind the peritoneum. **B.** Transverse section of the posterior abdominal wall showing structures in the retroperitoneal space as seen from below.

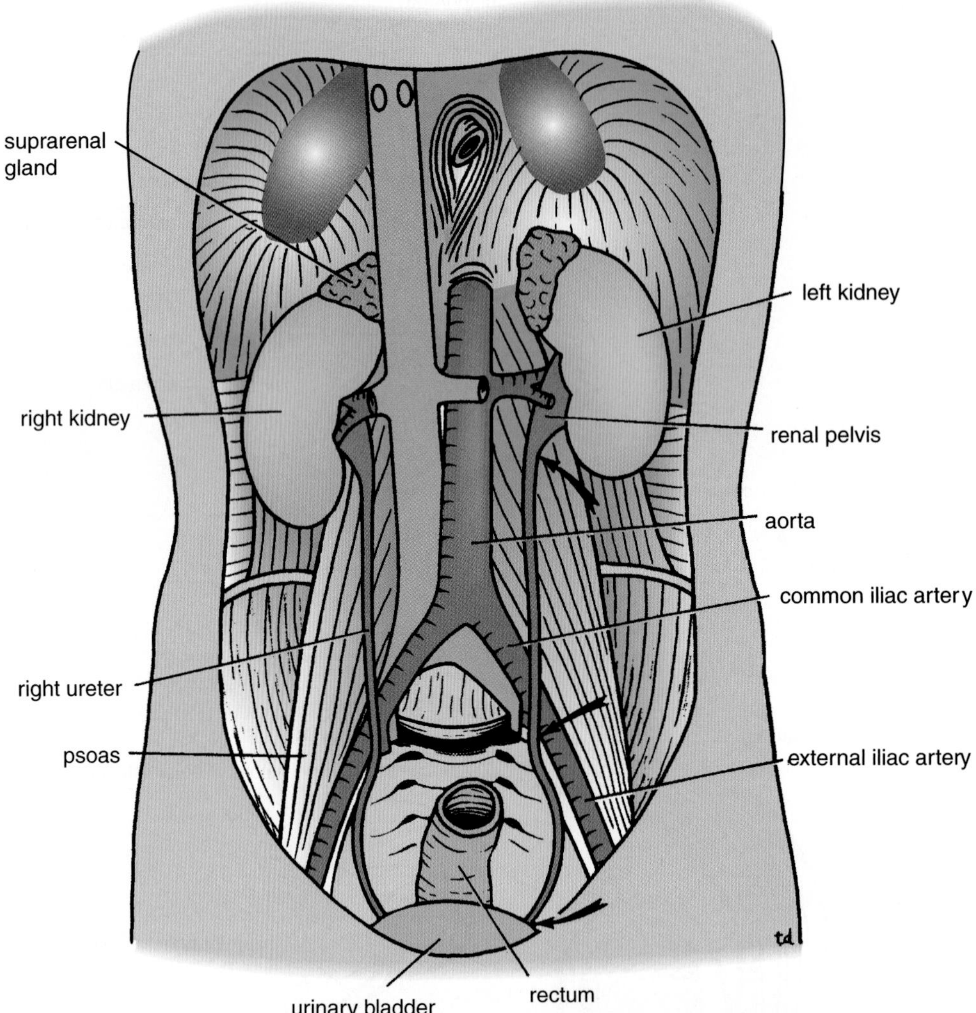

Figure 5-63 Posterior abdominal wall showing the kidneys and the ureters in situ. *Arrows* indicate three sites where the ureter is narrowed.

Coverings

The kidneys have the following coverings (Fig. 5-64):

- **Fibrous capsule:** This surrounds the kidney and is closely applied to its outer surface.
- **Perirenal fat:** This covers the fibrous capsule.
- **Renal fascia:** This is a condensation of connective tissue that lies outside the perirenal fat and encloses the kidneys and suprarenal glands; it is continuous laterally with the fascia transversalis.
- **Pararenal fat:** This lies external to the renal fascia and is often in large quantity. It forms part of the retroperitoneal fat.

The perirenal fat, renal fascia, and pararenal fat support the kidneys and hold them in position on the posterior abdominal wall.

Renal Structure

Each kidney has a dark brown outer **cortex** and a light brown inner **medulla.** The medulla is composed of about a dozen **renal pyramids,** each having its base oriented toward the cortex and its apex, the **renal papilla,** projecting medially (Fig. 5-64). The cortex extends into the medulla between adjacent pyramids as the **renal columns.** Extending from the bases of the renal pyramids into the cortex are striations known as **medullary rays.**

The renal sinus, which is the space within the hilum, contains the upper expanded end of the ureter, the **renal pelvis.** This divides into two or three **major calyces,** each of which divides into two or three **minor calyces** (Fig. 5-64). Each minor calyx is indented by the apex of the renal pyramid, the **renal papilla.**

Important Relations, Right Kidney

- **Anteriorly:** The suprarenal gland, the liver, the second part of the duodenum, and the right colic flexure (Figs. 5-4 and 5-65)
- **Posteriorly:** The diaphragm; the costodiaphragmatic recess of the pleura; the 12th rib; and the psoas, quadratus lumborum, and transversus abdominis muscles. The subcostal (T12), iliohypogastric, and ilioinguinal nerves (L1) run downward and laterally (Fig. 5-34).

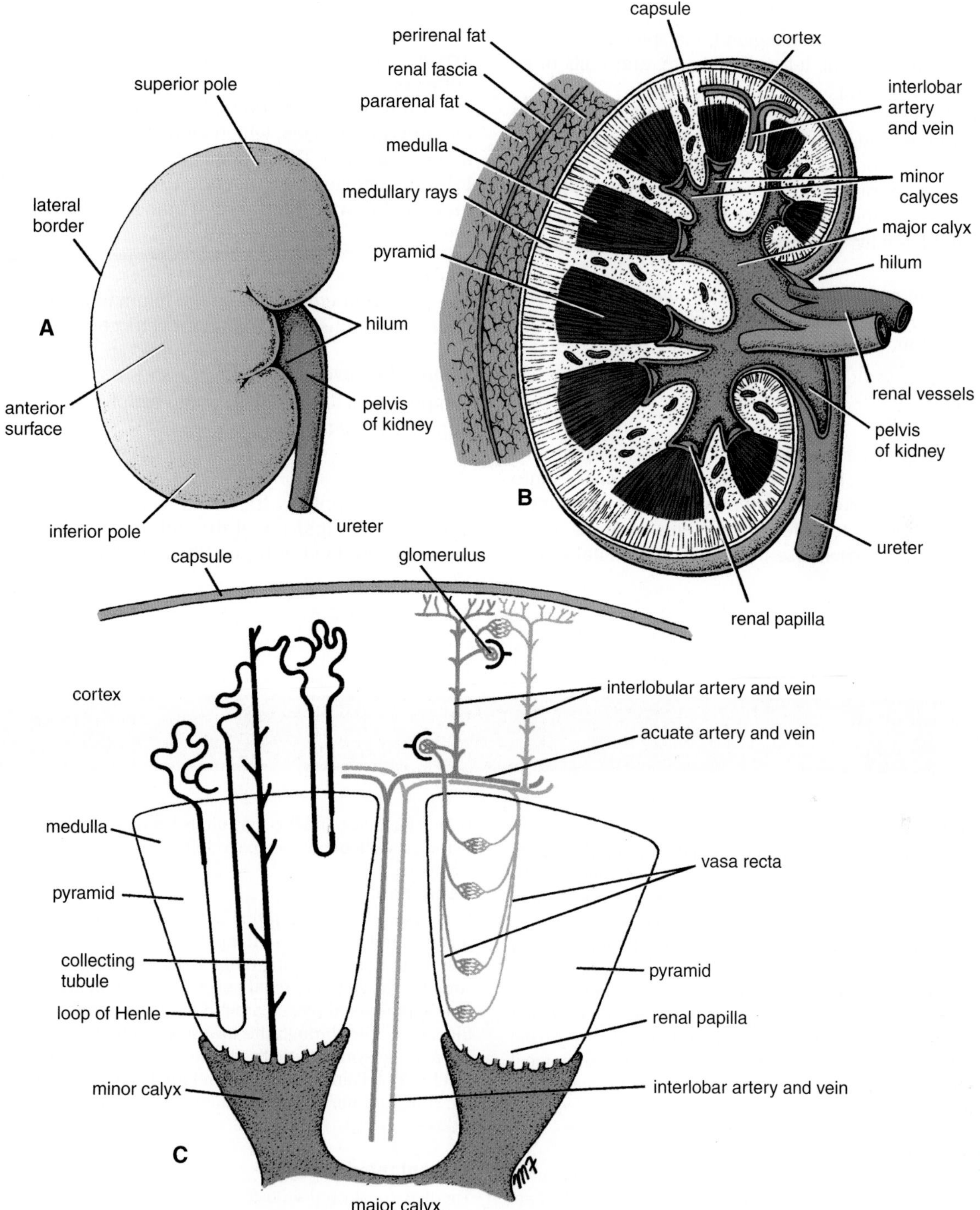

Figure 5-64 **A.** Right kidney, anterior surface. **B.** Right kidney, coronal section showing the cortex, medulla, pyramids, renal papillae, and calyces. **C.** Section of the kidney showing the position of the nephrons and the arrangement of the blood vessels within the kidney.

Important Relations, Left Kidney

- **Anteriorly:** The suprarenal gland, the spleen, the stomach, the pancreas, the left colic flexure, and coils of jejunum (Figs. 5-4 and 5-65)
- **Posteriorly:** The diaphragm; the costodiaphragmatic recess of the pleura; the 11th (the left kidney is higher) and 12th ribs; and the psoas, quadratus lumborum, and transversus abdominis muscles. The subcostal (T12), iliohypogastric, and ilioinguinal nerves (L1) run downward and laterally (Fig. 5-34).

Note that many of the structures are directly in contact with the kidneys, whereas others are separated by visceral layers of peritoneum. For details, see Figure 5-65.

Blood Supply

Arteries

The renal artery arises from the aorta at the level of the second lumbar vertebra. Each renal artery usually divides into five **segmental arteries** that enter the hilum of the kidney. They are distributed to different segments or areas of the kidney. **Lobar arteries** arise from each segmental artery, one for each renal pyramid. Before entering the renal substance, each lobar artery gives off two or three **interlobar arteries** (Fig. 5-64). The interlobar arteries run toward the cortex on each side of the renal pyramid. At the junction of the cortex and the medulla, the interlobar arteries give off the **arcuate arteries,** which arch over the bases of the pyramids (Fig. 5-65). The arcuate arteries give off several **interlobular arteries** that ascend in the cortex. The **afferent glomerular arterioles** arise as branches of the interlobular arteries.

Veins

The renal vein emerges from the hilum in front of the renal artery and drains into the inferior vena cava.

Lymph Drainage

Lymph drains to the lateral aortic lymph nodes around the origin of the renal artery.

Nerve Supply

The nerve supply is the renal sympathetic plexus. The afferent fibers that travel through the renal plexus enter the spinal cord in the 10th, 11th, and 12th thoracic nerves.

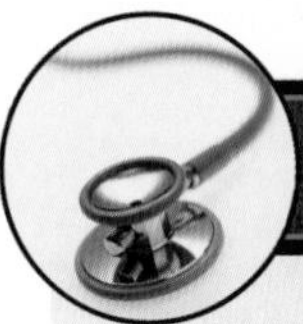

CLINICAL NOTES

Renal Mobility

The kidneys are maintained in their normal position by intra-abdominal pressure and by their connections with the perirenal fat and renal fascia. Each kidney moves slightly with respiration. The right kidney lies at a slightly lower level than the left kidney, and the lower pole may be palpated in the right lumbar region at the end of deep inspiration in a person with poorly developed abdominal musculature. Should the amount of perirenal fat be reduced, the mobility of the kidney may become excessive and produce symptoms of renal colic caused by kinking of the ureter. Excessive mobility of the kidney leaves the suprarenal gland undisturbed because the latter occupies a separate compartment in the renal fascia.

Kidney Trauma

The kidneys are well protected by the lower ribs, the lumbar muscles, and the vertebral column. However, a severe blunt injury applied to the abdomen may crush the kidney against the last rib and the vertebral column. Depending on the severity of the blow, the injury varies from a mild bruising to a complete laceration of the organ. Penetrating injuries are usually caused by stab wounds or gunshot wounds and often involve other viscera. Because 25% of the cardiac outflow passes through the kidneys, renal injury can result in rapid blood loss. A summary of the injuries to the kidneys is shown in Figure 5-66.

Kidney Tumors

Malignant tumors of the kidney have a strong tendency to spread along the renal vein. The left renal vein receives the left testicular vein in the male, and this may rarely become blocked, producing left-sided **varicocele** (see page 169).

Renal Pain

Renal pain varies from a dull ache to a severe pain in the flank that may radiate downward into the lower abdomen. Renal pain can result from stretching of the kidney capsule or spasm of the smooth muscle in the renal pelvis. The afferent nerve fibers pass through the renal plexus around the renal artery and ascend to the spinal cord through the lowest splanchnic nerve in the thorax and the sympathetic trunk. They enter the spinal cord at the level of T12. Pain is commonly referred along the distribution of the subcostal nerve (T12) to the flank and the anterior abdominal wall.

Transplanted Kidneys

The iliac fossa on the posterior abdominal wall is the usual site chosen for transplantation of the kidney. The fossa is exposed through an incision in the anterior abdominal wall just above the inguinal ligament. The iliac fossa in front of the iliacus muscle is approached retroperitoneally. The kidney is positioned and the vascular anastomosis constructed. The renal artery is anastomosed end-to-end to the internal iliac artery and the renal vein is anastomosed end-to-side to the external iliac vein (Fig. 5-67). Anastomosis of the branches of the internal iliac arteries on the two sides is sufficient so that the pelvic viscera on the side of the renal arterial anastomosis are not at risk. Ureterocystostomy is then performed by opening the bladder and providing a wide entrance of the ureter through the bladder wall.

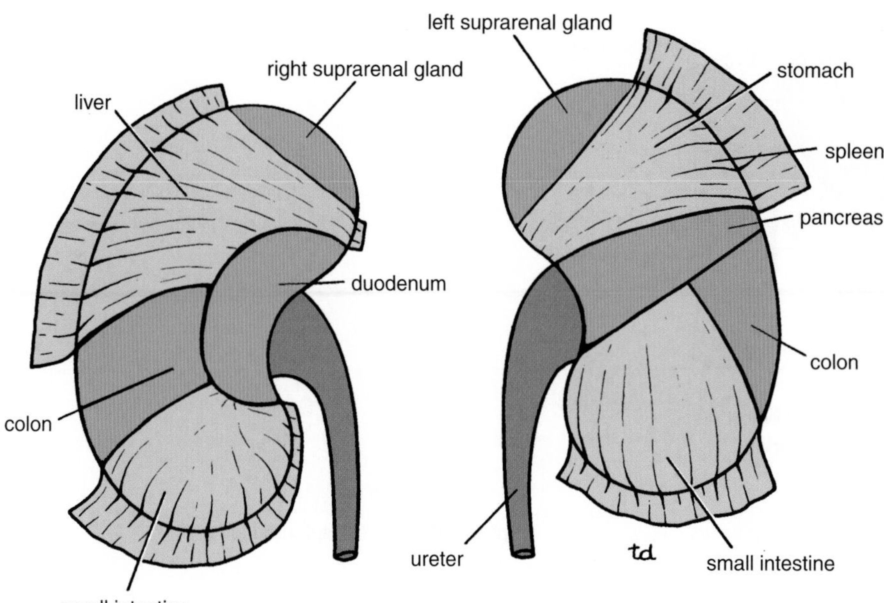

Figure 5-65 Anterior relations of both kidneys. Visceral peritoneum covering the kidneys has been left in position. Brown areas indicate where the kidney is in direct contact with the adjacent viscera.

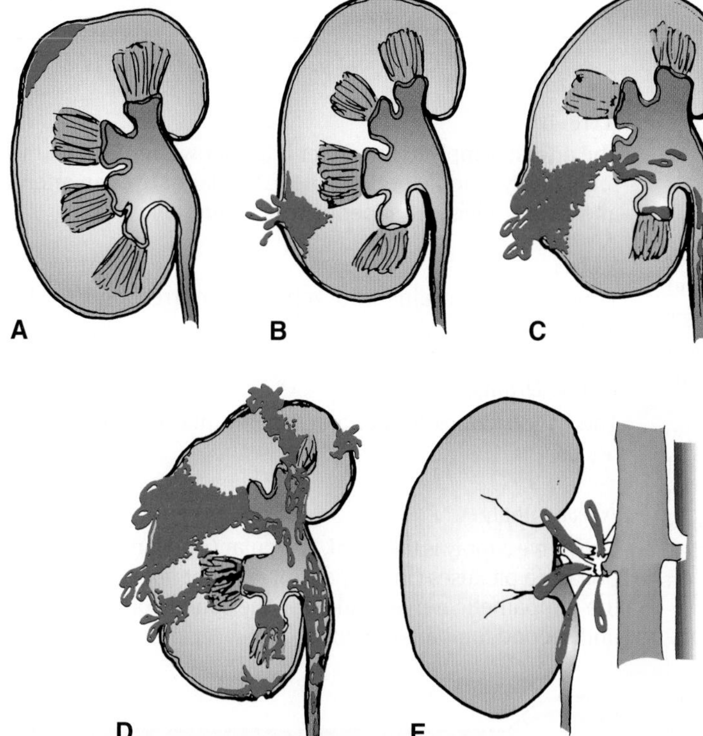

Figure 5-66 Injuries to the kidney. **A.** Contusion, with hemorrhage confined to the cortex beneath the intact fibrous capsule. **B.** Tearing of the capsule and cortex with bleeding occurring into the perirenal fat. **C.** Tearing of the capsule, the cortex, and the medulla. Note the escape of blood into the calyces and therefore the urine. Urine as well as blood may extravasate into the perirenal and pararenal fat and into the peritoneal cavity. **D.** Shattered kidney with extensive hemorrhage and extravasation of blood and urine into the perirenal and pararenal fat; blood also enters the calyces and appears in the urine. **E.** Injury to the renal pedicle involving the renal vessels and possibly the renal pelvis.

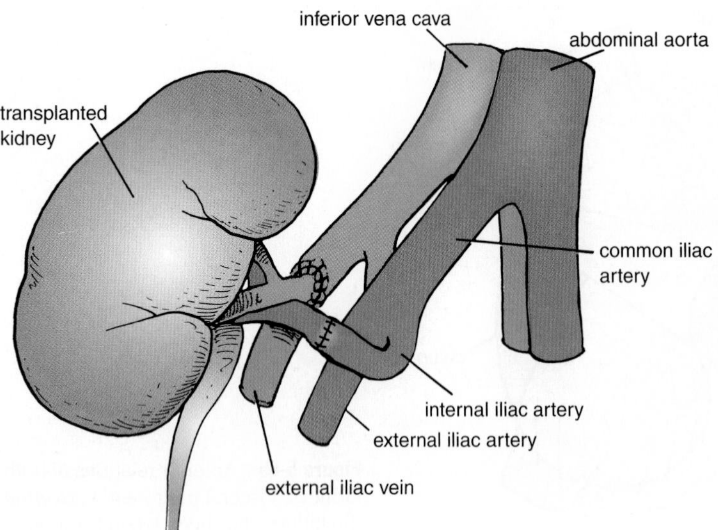

Figure 5-67 The transplanted kidney.

Ureter

Location and Description

The two ureters are muscular tubes that extend from the kidneys to the posterior surface of the urinary bladder (Fig. 5-63). The urine is propelled along the ureter by peristaltic contractions of the muscle coat, assisted by the filtration pressure of the glomeruli.

Each ureter measures about 10 in. (25 cm) long and resembles the esophagus (also 10 in. long) in having three constrictions along its course: where the renal pelvis joins the ureter, where it is kinked as it crosses the pelvic brim, and where it pierces the bladder wall (Fig. 5-63).

The renal pelvis is the funnel-shaped expanded upper end of the ureter. It lies within the hilum of the kidney and receives the major calyces (Fig. 5-64). The ureter emerges from the hilum of the kidney and runs vertically downward behind the parietal peritoneum (adherent to it) on the psoas muscle, which separates it from the tips of the transverse processes of the lumbar vertebrae. It enters the pelvis by crossing the bifurcation of the common iliac artery in front of the sacroiliac joint (Fig. 5-63). The ureter then runs down the lateral wall of the pelvis to the region of the ischial spine and turns forward to enter the lateral angle of the bladder. The pelvic course of the ureter is described in detail on pages 347 and 355.

Relations, Right Ureter

- **Anteriorly:** The duodenum, the terminal part of the ileum, the right colic and ileocolic vessels, the right testicular or ovarian vessels, and the root of the mesentery of the small intestine (Fig. 5-27)
- **Posteriorly:** The right psoas muscle, which separates it from the lumbar transverse processes, and the bifurcation of the right common iliac artery (Fig. 5-63)

Relations, Left Ureter

- **Anteriorly:** The sigmoid colon and sigmoid mesocolon, the left colic vessels, and the left testicular or ovarian vessels (Figs. 5-13 and 5-27)
- **Posteriorly:** The left psoas muscle, which separates it from the lumbar transverse processes, and the bifurcation of the left common iliac artery (Fig. 5-63)

The inferior mesenteric vein lies along the medial side of the left ureter (Fig. 5-27).

Blood Supply

Arteries

The arterial supply to the ureter is as follows: upper end, the renal artery; middle portion, the testicular or ovarian artery; and in the pelvis, the superior vesical artery.

Veins

Venous blood drains into veins that correspond to the arteries.

Lymph Drainage

The lymph drains to the lateral aortic nodes and the iliac nodes.

Nerve Supply

The nerve supply is the renal, testicular (or ovarian), and hypogastric plexuses (in the pelvis). Afferent fibers travel with the sympathetic nerves and enter the spinal cord in the first and second lumbar segments.

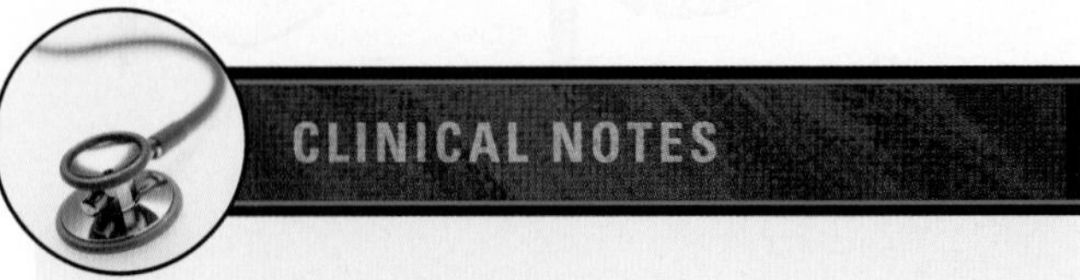

Traumatic Ureteral Injuries

Because of its protected position and small size, injuries to the ureter are rare. Most injuries are caused by gunshot wounds and, in a few individuals, penetrating stab wounds. Because

(continues)

Clinical Notes, *continued*

the ureters are retroperitoneal in position, urine may escape into the retroperitoneal tissues on the posterior abdominal wall.

Ureteric Stones

There are three sites of anatomic narrowing of the ureter where stones may be arrested, namely, the pelviureteral junction, the pelvic brim, and where the ureter enters the bladder. Most stones, although radiopaque, are small enough to be impossible to see definitely along the course of the ureter on plain radiographic examination. An intravenous pyelogram is usually necessary. The ureter runs down in front of the tips of the transverse processes of the lumbar vertebrae, crosses the region of the sacroiliac joint, swings out to the ischial spine, and then turns medially to the bladder.

Renal Colic

The renal pelvis and the ureter send their afferent nerves into the spinal cord at segments T11 and 12 and L1 and 2. In renal colic, strong peristaltic waves of contraction pass down the ureter in an attempt to pass the stone onward. The spasm of the smooth muscle causes an agonizing colicky pain, which is referred to the skin areas that are supplied by these segments of the spinal cord, namely, the flank, loin, and groin.

When a stone enters the low part of the ureter, the pain is felt at a lower level and is often referred to the testis or the tip of the penis in the male and the labium majus in the female. Sometimes ureteral pain is referred along the femoral branch of the genitofemoral nerve (L1 and 2) so that pain is experienced in the front of the thigh. The pain is often so severe that afferent pain impulses spread within the central nervous system, giving rise to nausea

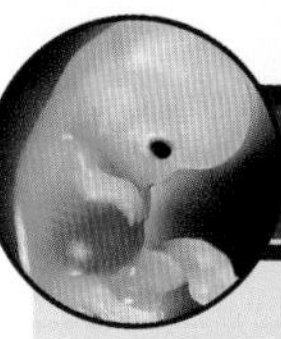

EMBRYOLOGIC NOTES

Development of the Kidneys and Ureters

Three sets of structures in the urinary system appear, called the **pronephros, mesonephros,** and **metanephros.** In the human, the metanephros is responsible for the permanent kidney. The metanephros develops from two sources: the ureteric bud from the mesonephric duct and the metanephrogenic cap from the intermediate cell mass of mesenchyme of the lower lumbar and sacral regions.

Ureteric Bud

The ureteric bud arises as an outgrowth of the mesonephric duct (Figs. 5-68 and 5-69). It forms the **ureter,** which dilates at its upper end to form the **pelvis of the ureter.** The pelvis later gives off branches that form the **major calyces,** and these in turn divide and branch to form the **minor calyces** and the **collecting tubules.**

Metanephrogenic Cap

The metanephrogenic cap condenses around the ureteric bud (Fig. 5-69) and forms the **glomerular capsules,** the **proximal** and **distal convoluted tubules,** and the **loops of Henle.** The glomerular capsule becomes invaginated by a cluster of capillaries that form the **glomerulus.** Each distal convoluted tubule formed from the metanephrogenic cap tissue becomes joined to a collecting tubule derived from the ureteric bud. The surface of the kidney is lobulated at first, but after birth, this lobulation usually soon disappears.

The developing kidney is initially a pelvic organ and receives its blood supply from the pelvic continuation of the aorta, the middle sacral artery. Later, the kidneys "ascend" up the posterior abdominal wall. This so-called ascent is caused mainly by the growth of the body in the lumbar and sacral regions and by the straightening of its curvature. The ureter elongates as the ascent continues.

The kidney is vascularized at successively higher levels by successively higher lateral splanchnic arteries, branches of the aorta. The kidneys reach their final position opposite the second lumbar vertebra. Because of the large size of the right lobe of the liver, the right kidney lies at a slightly lower level than the left kidney.

Polycystic Kidney

A hereditary disease, polycystic kidneys can be transmitted by either parent. It may be associated with congenital cysts of the liver, pancreas, and lung. Both kidneys are enormously enlarged and riddled with cysts. Polycystic kidney is thought to be caused by a failure of union between the developing convoluted tubules and collecting tubules. The accumulation of urine in the proximal tubules results in the formation of retention cysts.

Pelvic Kidney

In pelvic kidney, the kidney is arrested in some part of its normal ascent; it usually is found at the brim of the pelvis (Fig. 5-70). Such a kidney may present with no signs or symptoms and may function normally. However, should an ectopic kidney become inflamed, it may—because of its unusual position—give rise to a mistaken diagnosis.

Horseshoe Kidney

When the caudal ends of both kidneys fuse as they develop, the result is horseshoe kidney (Fig. 5-70). Both kidneys commence to ascend from the pelvis, but the interconnecting bridge becomes trapped behind the inferior mesenteric artery so that the kidneys come to rest in the low lumbar region. Both ureters are kinked as they pass inferiorly over the bridge of renal tissue, producing urinary stasis, which may result in infection and stone formation. Surgical division of the bridge corrects the condition.

Unilateral Double Kidney

The kidney on one side may be double, with separate ureters and blood vessels. In unilateral double kidney, the ureteric bud on one side crosses the midline as it ascends, and its upper pole fuses with the lower pole of the normally placed kidney (Fig.

(continues)

Embryologic Notes, *continued*

5-70). Here again, angulation of the ureter may result in stasis of the urine and may require surgical treatment.

Rosette Kidney
Both kidneys may fuse together at their hila, and they usually remain in the pelvis. The two kidneys together form a rosette (Fig. 5-70). This is the result of the early fusion of the two ureteric buds in the pelvis.

Supernumerary Renal Arteries
Supernumerary renal arteries are relatively common. They represent persistent fetal renal arteries, which grow in sequence from the aorta to supply the kidney as it ascends from the pelvis. Their occurrence is clinically important because a supernumerary artery may cross the pelviureteral junction and obstruct the outflow of urine, producing dilatation of the calyces and pelvis, a condition known as **hydronephrosis** (Fig. 5-70).

Double Pelvis
Double pelvis of the ureter is usually unilateral (Fig. 5-71). The upper pelvis is small and drains the upper group of calyces; the larger lower pelvis drains the middle and lower groups of calyces. The cause is a premature division of the ureteric bud near its termination.

Bifid Ureter
In bifid ureter, the ureters may join in the lower third of their course, may open through a common orifice into the bladder, or may open independently into the bladder (Fig. 5-71). In the latter case, one ureter crosses its fellow and may produce urinary obstruction. The cause of bifid ureter is a premature division of the ureteric bud.

Cases of double pelvis and double ureters may be found by chance on radiologic investigation of the urinary tract. They are more liable to become infected or to be the seat of calculus formation than a normal ureter.

Megaloureter
Megaloureter may be unilateral or bilateral and shows complete absence of motility (Fig. 5-71). The cause is unknown. Because of the urinary stasis, the ureter is prone to infection. Plastic surgery is required to improve the rate of drainage.

Postcaval Ureter
The right ureter may ascend posterior to the inferior vena cava and may be obstructed by it (Fig. 5-71). Surgical rerouting of the ureter with reimplantation of the distal end into the bladder is the treatment of choice.

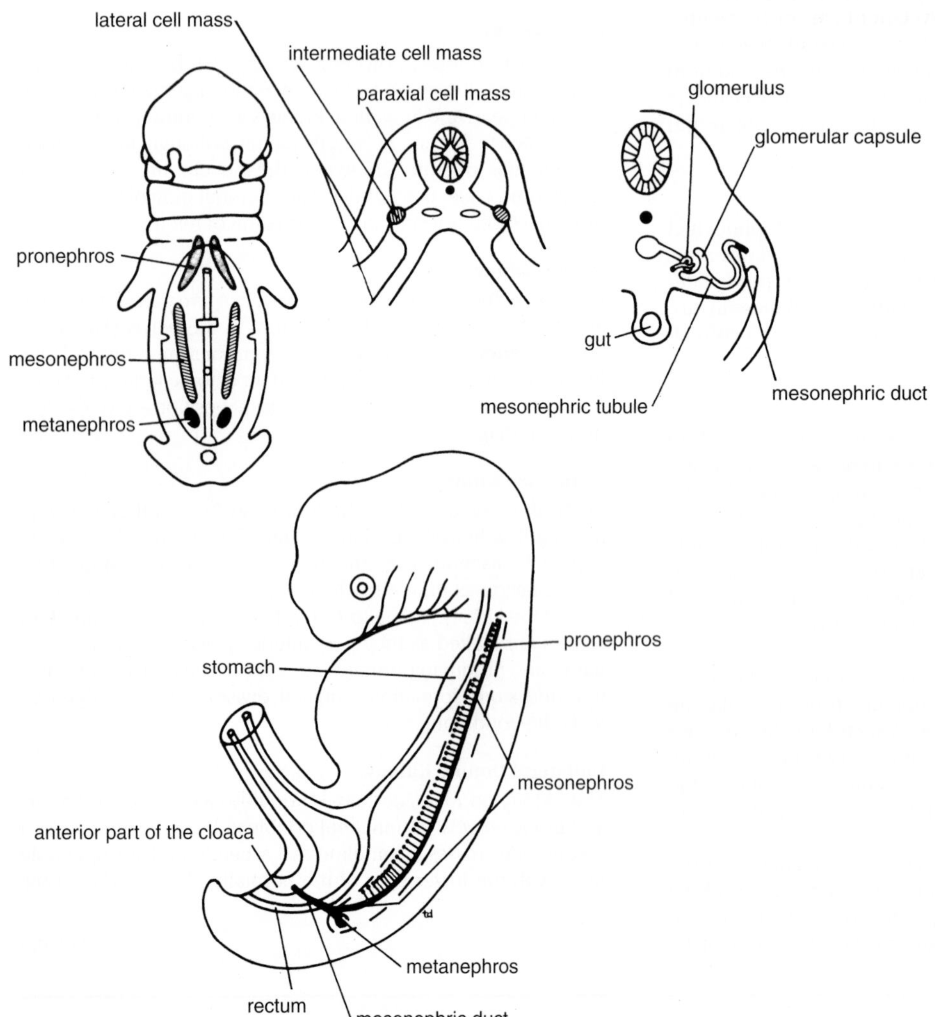

Figure 5-68 The origins and positions of the pronephros, mesonephros, and metanephros.

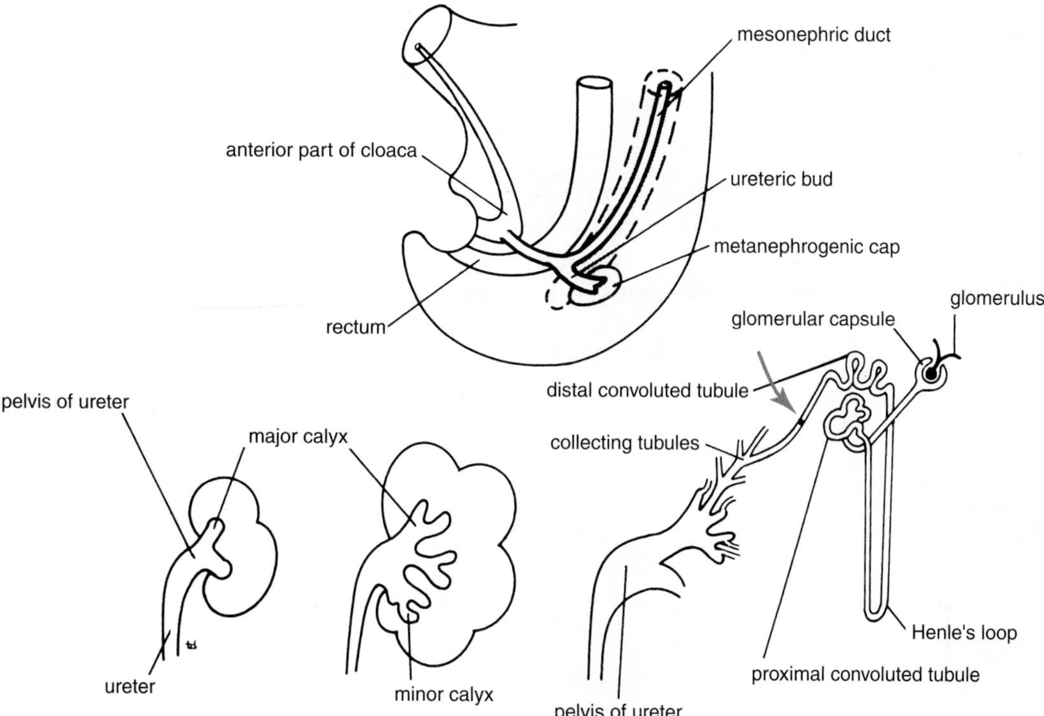

Figure 5-69 The origin of the ureteric bud from the mesonephric duct and the formation of the major and minor calyces and the collecting tubules. *Arrow* indicates the point of union between the collecting tubules and the convoluted tubules.

Suprarenal Glands

Location and Description

The two suprarenal glands are yellowish retroperitoneal organs that lie on the upper poles of the kidneys. They are surrounded by renal fascia (but are separated from the kidneys by the perirenal fat). Each gland has a yellow **cortex** and a dark brown **medulla.**

The cortex of the suprarenal glands secretes hormones that include **mineral corticoids,** which are concerned with the control of fluid and electrolyte balance; **glucocorticoids,** which are concerned with the control of the metabolism of carbohydrates, fats, and proteins; and small amounts of **sex hormones,** which probably play a role in the prepubertal development of the sex organs. The medulla of the suprarenal glands secretes the catecholamines **epinephrine** and **norepinephrine.**

The **right suprarenal gland** is pyramid shaped and caps the upper pole of the right kidney (Fig. 5-4). It lies behind the right lobe of the liver and extends medially behind the inferior vena cava. It rests posteriorly on the diaphragm.

The **left suprarenal gland** is crescentic in shape and extends along the medial border of the left kidney from the upper pole to the hilus (Fig. 5-4). It lies behind the pancreas, the lesser sac, and the stomach and rests posteriorly on the diaphragm.

Blood Supply

Arteries

The arteries supplying each gland are three in number: inferior phrenic artery, aorta, and renal artery.

Veins

A single vein emerges from the hilum of each gland and drains into the inferior vena cava on the right and into the renal vein on the left.

Lymph Drainage

The lymph drains into the lateral aortic nodes.

Nerve Supply

Preganglionic sympathetic fibers derived from the splanchnic nerves supply the glands. Most of the nerves end in the medulla of the gland.

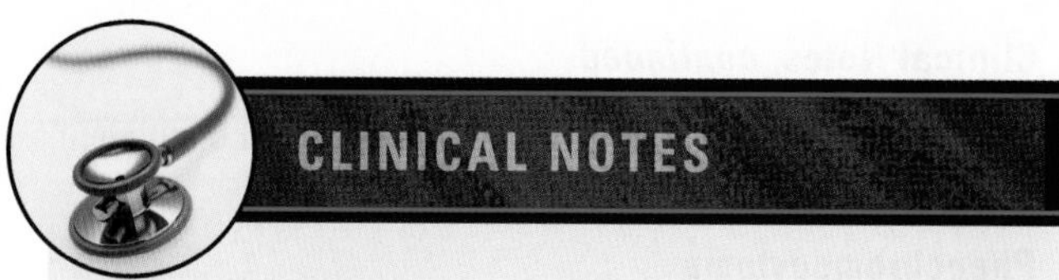

Cushing's Syndrome

Suprarenal cortical hyperplasia is the most common cause of Cushing's syndrome, the clinical manifestations of which include moon-shaped face, truncal obesity, abnormal hairiness (hirsutism), and hypertension; if the syndrome occurs later in life, it may result from an adenoma or carcinoma of the cortex.

Addison's Disease

Adrenocortical insufficiency (Addison's disease), which is characterized clinically by increased pigmentation, muscular weak-

(continues)

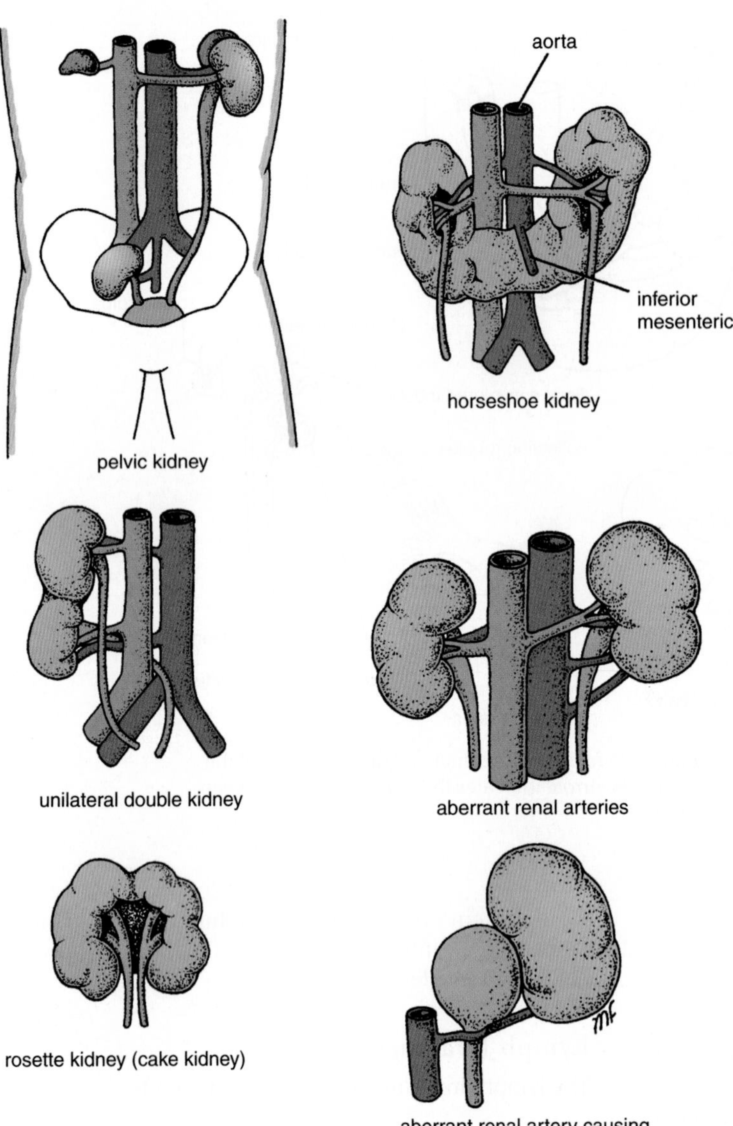

Figure 5-70 Some common congenital anomalies of the kidney.

Clinical Notes, *continued*

ness, weight loss, and hypotension, may be caused by tuberculous destruction or bilateral atrophy of both cortices.

Pheochromocytoma

Pheochromocytoma, a tumor of the medulla, produces a paroxysmal or sustained hypertension. The symptoms and signs result from the production of a large amount of catecholamines, which are then poured into the bloodstream.

Because of their position on the posterior abdominal wall, few tumors of the suprarenal glands can be palpated. Computed tomography (CT) scans can be used to visualize the glandular enlargement; however, when interpreting CT scans, remember the close relationship of the suprarenal glands to the crura of the diaphragm.

Surgical Significance of the Renal Fascia

The suprarenal glands, together with the kidneys, are enclosed within the renal fascia; the suprarenal glands, however, lie in a separate compartment, which allows the two organs to be separated easily at operation.

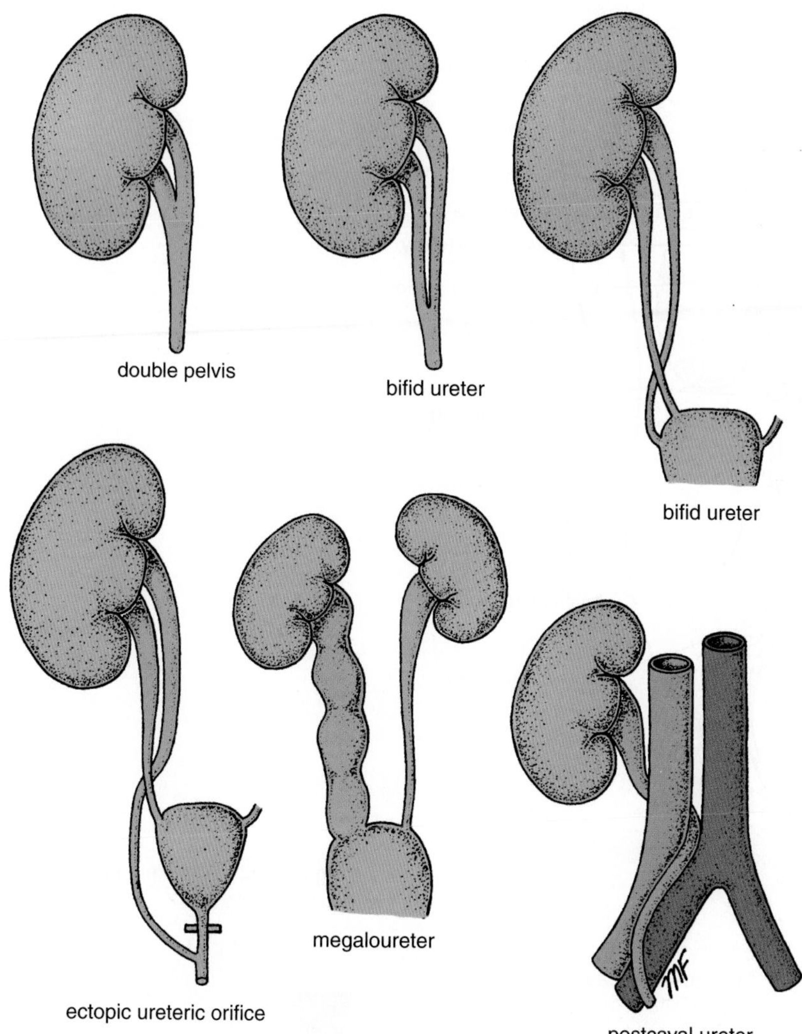

Figure 5-71 Some common congenital anomalies of the ureter.

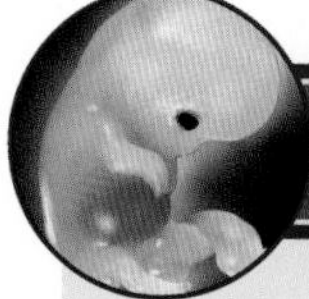

EMBRYOLOGIC NOTES

Development of the Suprarenal Glands

The cortex develops from the coelomic mesothelium covering the posterior abdominal wall. At first, a **fetal cortex** is formed; later, it becomes covered by a second final cortex. After birth, the fetal cortex retrogresses, and its involution is largely completed in the first few weeks of life.

The **medulla** is formed from the sympathochromaffin cells of the neural crest. These invade the cortex on its medial side. By this means, the medulla comes to occupy a central position and is arranged in cords and clusters. Preganglionic sympathetic nerve fibers grow into the medulla and influence the activity of the medullary cells.

Susceptibility to Trauma at Birth

At birth, the suprarenal glands are relatively large because of the presence of the fetal cortex; later, when this part of the cortex involutes, the gland becomes reduced in size. During the process of involution, the cortex is friable and susceptible to damage and severe hemorrhage.

Arteries on the Posterior Abdominal Wall

Aorta

Location and Description

The aorta enters the abdomen through the aortic opening of the diaphragm in front of the 12th thoracic vertebra (Fig. 5-72). It descends behind the peritoneum on the anterior surface of the bodies of the lumbar vertebrae. At the level of the fourth lumbar vertebra, it divides into the two common iliac arteries (Fig. 5-72). On its right side lie the inferior vena cava, the cisterna chyli, and the beginning of the azygos vein. On its left side lies the left sympathetic trunk.

The surface markings of the aorta are shown in Figure 5-73.

Branches (Fig. 5-72)

- Three anterior visceral branches: the celiac artery, superior mesenteric artery, and inferior mesenteric artery
- Three lateral visceral branches: the suprarenal artery, renal artery, and testicular or ovarian artery

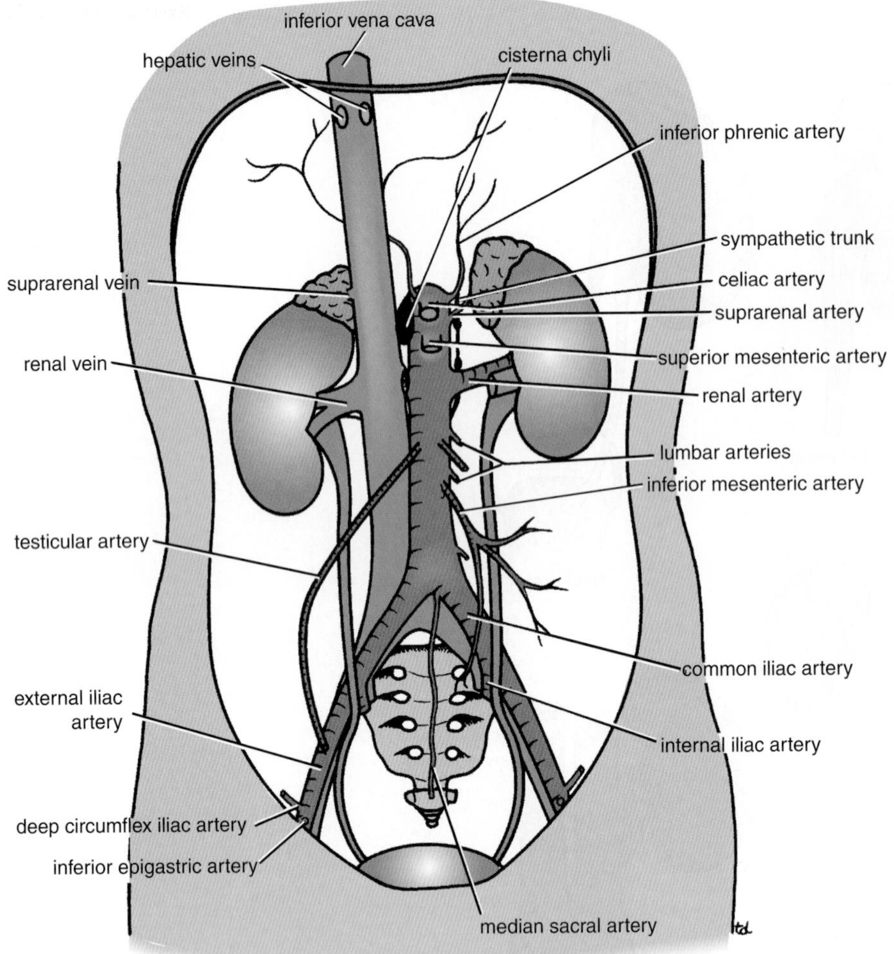

Figure 5-72 Aorta and inferior vena cava.

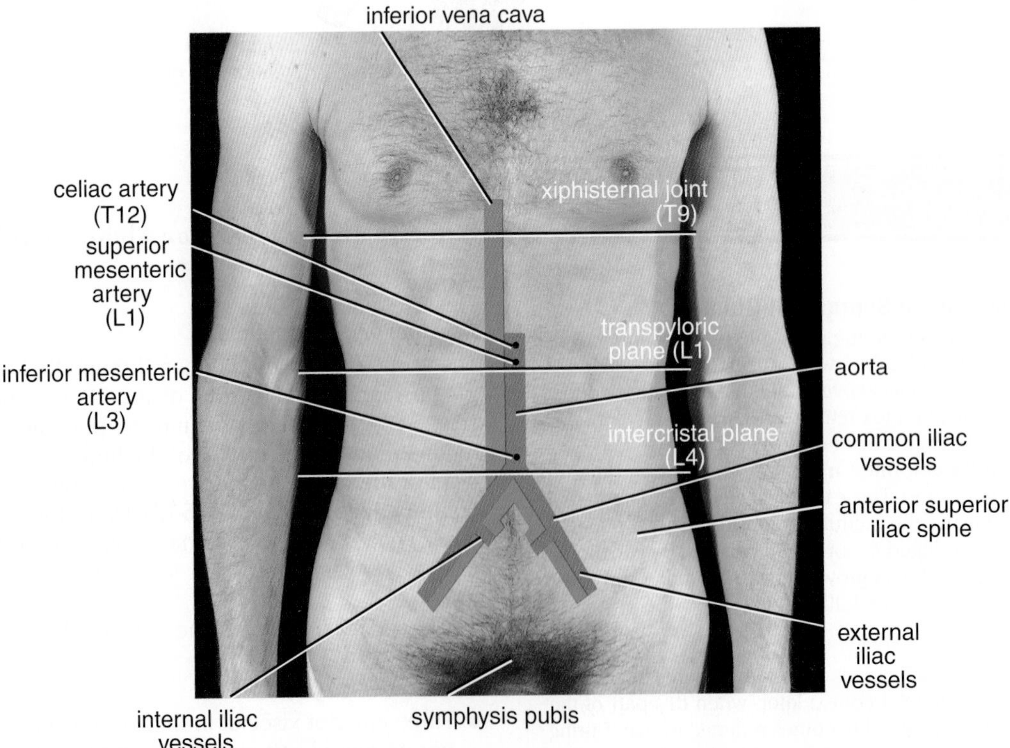

Figure 5-73 Surface markings of the aorta and its branches and the inferior vena cava on the anterior abdominal wall.

Diagram 5-1 Branches of Abdominal Aorta

- 1. Three anterior visceral branches
  - a. Celiac artery
    - left gastric artery
    - splenic artery
      - short gastric arteries (six)
      - splenic arteries (six)
      - left gastroepiploic artery
    - hepatic artery
      - cystic artery
      - right gastric artery
      - gastroduodenal artery
        - right gastroepiploic artery
        - superior pancreatico-duodenal artery
      - right hepatic artery
      - left hepatic artery
  - b. Superior mesenteric artery
    - jejunal and ileal arteries
    - inferior pancreaticoduodenal artery
    - middle colic artery
    - right colic artery
    - ileocolic artery
      - anterior cecal artery
      - posterior cecal artery—appendicular artery
      - ileal artery
      - colic artery
  - c. Inferior mesenteric artery
    - left colic artery
    - sigmoid arteries (two or three)
    - superior rectal artery
- 2. Three lateral visceral branches
  - a. Suprarenal artery
  - b. Renal artery
  - c. Testicular or ovarian artery
- 3. Five lateral abdominal wall branches
  - a. Inferior phrenic artery
  - b. Four lumbar arteries
- 4. Three terminal branches
  - a. Two common iliac arteries
    - external iliac artery
    - internal iliac artery
  - b. Median sacral artery

- Five lateral abdominal wall branches: the inferior phrenic artery and four lumbar arteries
- Three terminal branches: the two common iliac arteries and the median sacral artery

These branches are summarized in Diagram 5-1.

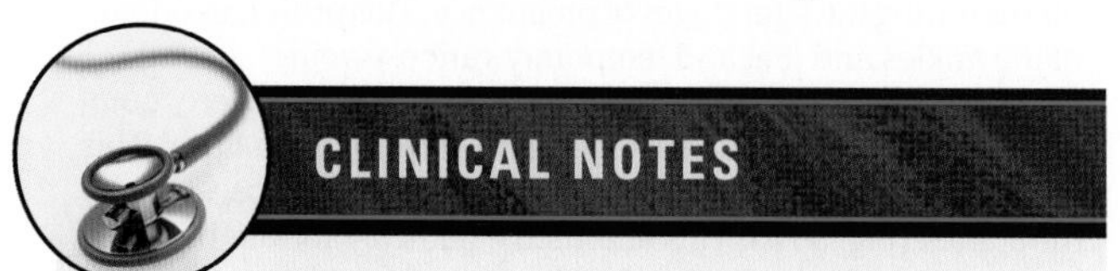

CLINICAL NOTES

Aortic Aneurysms

Localized or diffuse dilatations of the abdominal part of the aorta (aneurysms) usually occur below the origin of the renal arteries. Most result from atherosclerosis, which causes weakening of the arterial wall, and occur most commonly in elderly men. Large aneurysms should be surgically excised and replaced with a prosthetic graft.

(continues)

Clinical Notes, *continued*

Embolic Blockage of the Abdominal Aorta

The bifurcation of the abdominal aorta where the lumen suddenly narrows may be a lodging site for an embolus discharged from the heart. Severe ischemia of the lower limbs results.

Common Iliac Arteries

The right and left common iliac arteries are the terminal branches of the aorta. They arise at the level of the fourth lumbar vertebra and run downward and laterally along the medial border of the psoas muscle (Figs. 5-63 and 5-72). Each artery ends in front of the sacroiliac joint by dividing into the external and internal iliac arteries. At the bifurcation, the common iliac artery on each side is crossed anteriorly by the ureter (Fig. 5-72).

External Iliac Artery

The external iliac artery runs along the medial border of the psoas, following the pelvic brim (Fig. 5-63). It gives off the **inferior epigastric** and **deep circumflex iliac** branches (Fig. 5-72).

The artery enters the thigh by passing under the inguinal ligament to become the femoral artery. The inferior epigastric artery arises just above the inguinal ligament. It passes upward and medially along the medial margin of the deep inguinal ring (Fig. 4-4) and enters the rectus sheath behind the rectus abdominis muscle. The deep circumflex iliac artery arises close to the inferior epigastric artery (Fig. 5-72). It ascends laterally to the anterior superior iliac spine and the iliac crest, supplying the muscles of the anterior abdominal wall.

Internal Iliac Artery

The internal iliac artery passes down into the pelvis in front of the sacroiliac joint (Fig. 5-72). Its further course is described on page 328.

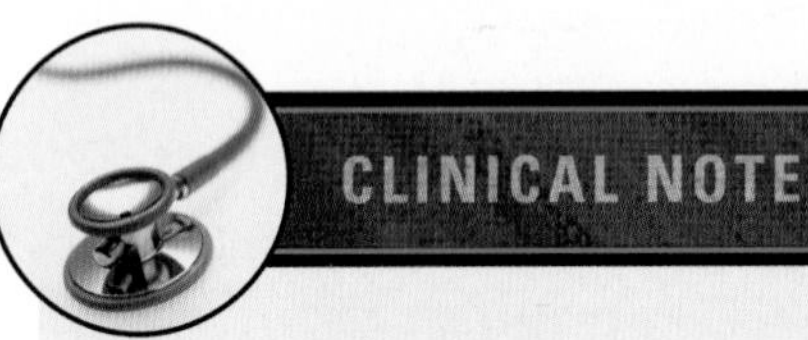

Obliteration of the Abdominal Aorta and Iliac Arteries

Gradual occlusion of the bifurcation of the abdominal aorta, produced by atherosclerosis, results in the characteristic clinical symptoms of pain in the legs on walking (claudication) and impotence, the latter caused by lack of blood in the internal iliac arteries. In otherwise healthy individuals, surgical treatment by thromboendarterectomy or a bypass graft should be considered. Because the progress of the disease is slow, some collateral circulation is established, but it is physiologically inadequate. However, the collateral blood flow does prevent tissue death in both lower limbs, although skin ulcers may occur.

The collateral circulation of the abdominal aorta is shown in Figure 5-74.

Veins on the Posterior Abdominal Wall

Inferior Vena Cava

Location and Description

The inferior vena cava conveys most of the blood from the body below the diaphragm to the right atrium of the heart. It is formed by the union of the common iliac veins behind the right common iliac artery at the level of the fifth lumbar vertebra (Fig. 5-72). It ascends on the right side of the aorta, pierces the central tendon of the diaphragm at the level of the eighth thoracic vertebra, and drains into the right atrium of the heart.

The right sympathetic trunk lies behind its right margin and the right ureter lies close to its right border. The entrance into the lesser sac separates the inferior vena cava from the portal vein (Fig. 5-7).

The surface markings of the inferior vena cava are shown in Figure 5-73.

Tributaries

The inferior vena cava has the following tributaries (Fig. 5-72):

- Two anterior visceral tributaries: the hepatic veins
- Three lateral visceral tributaries: the right suprarenal vein (the left vein drains into the left renal vein), renal veins, and right testicular or ovarian vein (the left vein drains into the left renal vein)
- Five lateral abdominal wall tributaries: the inferior phrenic vein and four lumbar veins
- Three veins of origin: two common iliac veins and the median sacral vein

The tributaries of the inferior vena cava are summarized in Diagram 5-2.

If one remembers that the venous blood from the abdominal portion of the gastrointestinal tract drains to the liver by means of the tributaries of the portal vein, and that the left suprarenal and testicular or ovarian veins drain first into the left renal vein, then it is apparent that the tributaries of the inferior vena cava correspond rather closely to the branches of the abdominal portion of the aorta.

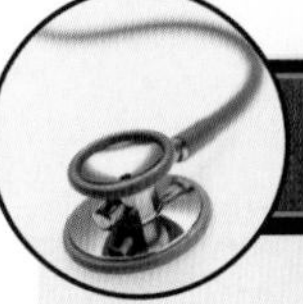

CLINICAL NOTES

Trauma to the Inferior Vena Cava

Injuries to the inferior vena cava are commonly lethal, despite the fact that the contained blood is under low pressure. The anatomic inaccessibility of the vessel behind the liver, duodenum, and mesentery of the small intestine and the blocking presence of the right costal margin make a surgical approach difficult. Moreover, the thin wall of the vena cava makes it prone to extensive tears.

Because of the multiple anastomoses of the tributaries of the inferior vena cava (Fig. 5-75), it is impossible in an emergency to ligate the vessel. Most patients have venous congestion of the lower limbs.

Compression of the Inferior Vena Cava

The inferior vena cava is commonly compressed by the enlarged uterus during the later stages of pregnancy. This produces edema of the ankles and feet and temporary varicose veins.

Malignant retroperitoneal tumors can cause severe compression and eventual blockage of the inferior vena cava. This results in the dilatation of the extensive anastomoses of the tributaries (Fig. 5-75). This alternative pathway for the blood to return to the right atrium of the heart is commonly referred to as the **caval–caval shunt.** The same pathway comes into effect in patients with a superior mediastinal tumor compressing the superior vena cava. Clinically, the enlarged subcutaneous anastomosis between the lateral thoracic vein, a tributary of the axillary vein, and the superficial epigastric vein, a tributary of the femoral vein, may be seen on the thoracoabdominal wall (Fig. 5-75).

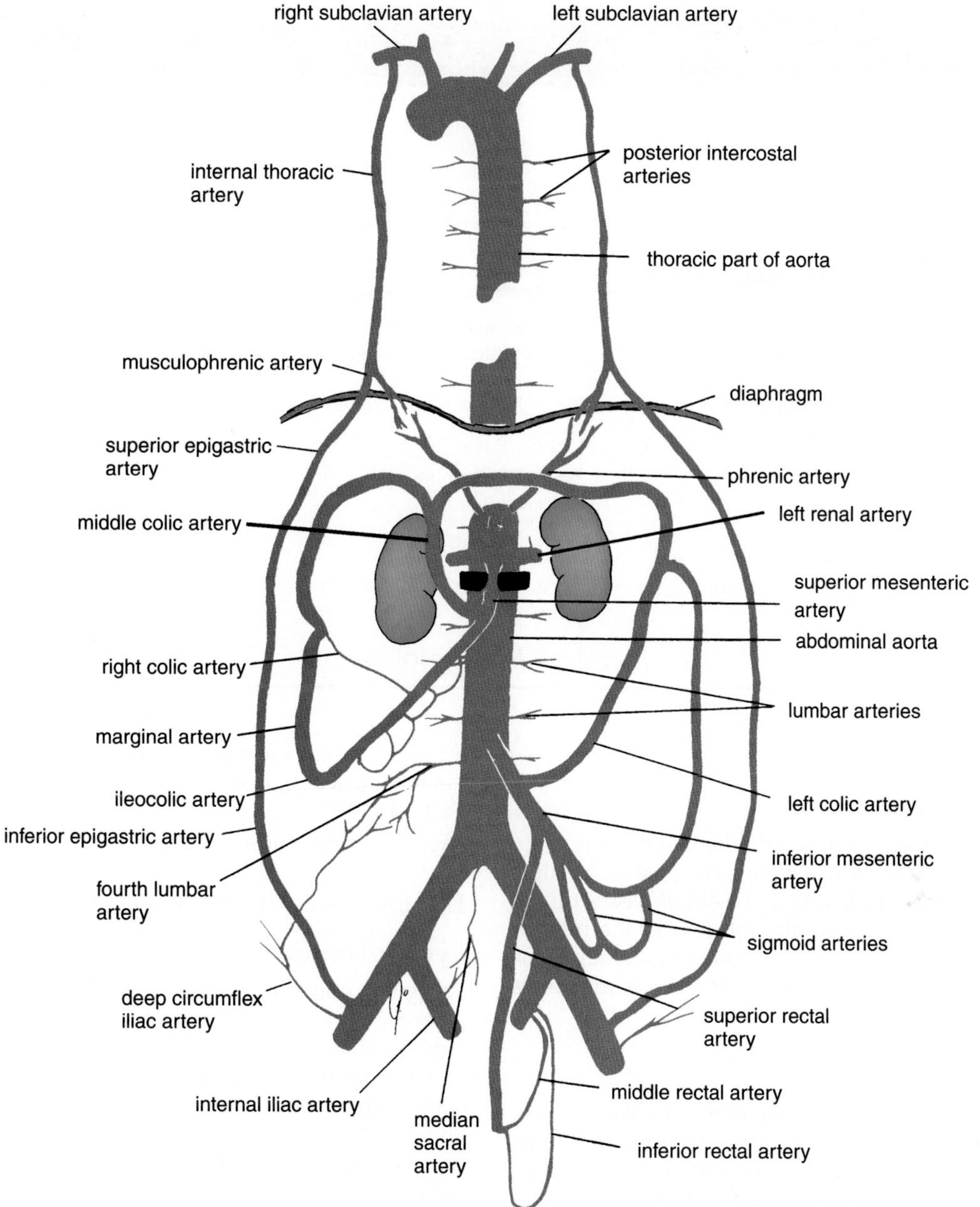

Figure 5-74 The possible collateral circulations of the abdominal aorta. Note the great dilatation of the mesenteric arteries and their branches, which occurs if the aorta is slowly blocked just below the level of the renal arteries (*black bar*).

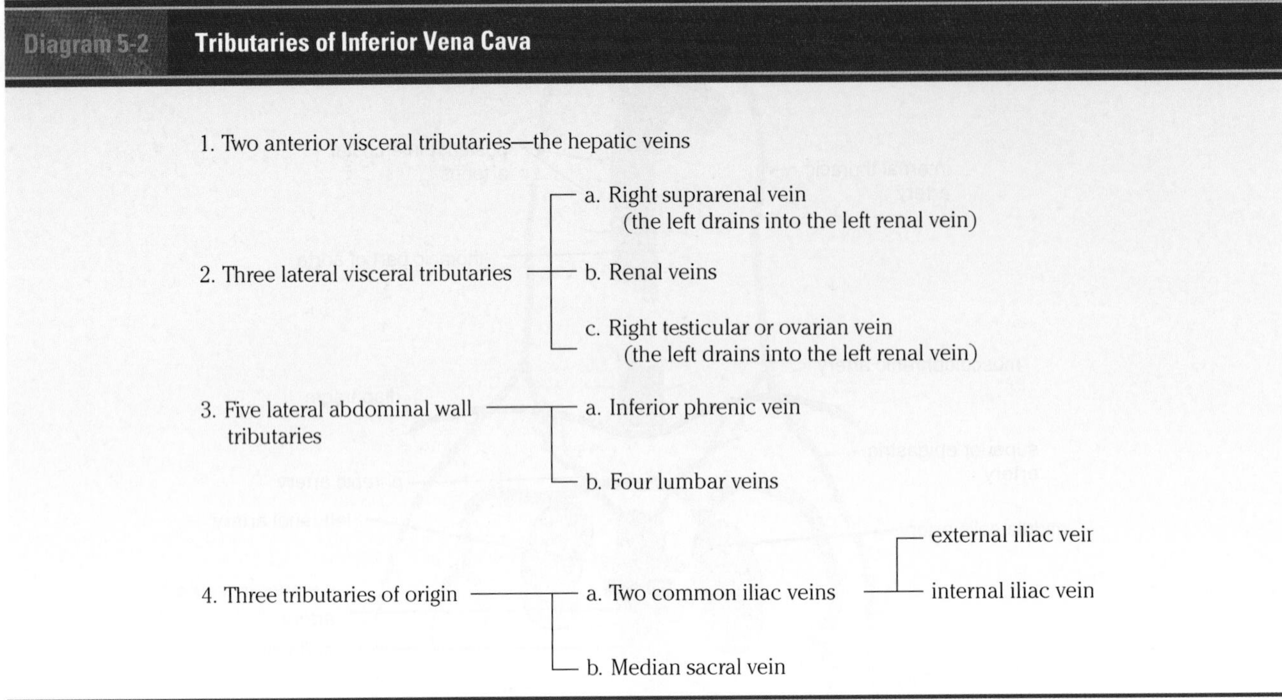

Inferior Mesenteric Vein

The inferior mesenteric vein is a tributary of the portal circulation. It begins halfway down the anal canal as the superior rectal vein (Figs. 5-22, 5-26, and 5-48). It passes up the posterior abdominal wall on the left side of the inferior mesenteric artery and the duodenojejunal flexure and joins the splenic vein behind the pancreas. It receives tributaries that correspond to the branches of the artery.

Splenic Vein

The splenic vein is a tributary of the portal circulation. It begins at the hilum of the spleen by the union of several veins and is then joined by the short gastric and the left gastroepiploic veins (Figs. 5-22 and 5-48). It passes to the right within the splenicorenal ligament and runs behind the pancreas. It joins the superior mesenteric vein behind the neck of the pancreas to form the portal vein. It is joined by veins from the pancreas and the inferior mesenteric vein.

Superior Mesenteric Vein

The superior mesenteric vein is a tributary of the portal circulation (Figs. 5-22, 5-26, and 5-48). It begins at the ileocecal junction and runs upward on the posterior abdominal wall within the root of the mesentery of the small intestine and on the right side of the superior mesenteric artery. It passes in front of the third part of the duodenum and behind the neck of the pancreas, where it joins the splenic vein to form the portal vein. It receives tributaries that correspond to the branches of the superior mesenteric artery and also receives the inferior pancreaticoduodenal vein and the right gastroepiploic vein (Fig. 5-22).

Portal Vein

The portal vein is described on page 245.

Lymphatics on the Posterior Abdominal Wall

Lymph Nodes

The lymph nodes are closely related to the aorta and form a preaortic and a right and left lateral aortic (para-aortic or lumbar) chain (Fig. 5-76).

The **preaortic lymph nodes** lie around the origins of the celiac, superior mesenteric, and inferior mesenteric arteries and are referred to as the **celiac, superior mesenteric,** and **inferior mesenteric lymph nodes,** respectively. They drain the lymph from the gastrointestinal tract, extending from the lower one third of the esophagus to halfway down the anal canal, and from the spleen, pancreas, gallbladder, and greater part of the liver. The efferent lymph vessels form the large intestinal trunk (see Fig. 1-18 and below).

The **lateral aortic (para-aortic or lumbar) lymph nodes** drain lymph from the kidneys and suprarenals; from the testes in the male and from the ovaries, uterine tubes, and fundus of the uterus in the female; from the deep lymph vessels of the abdominal walls; and from the common iliac nodes. The efferent lymph vessels form the **right** and **left lumbar trunks** (see Fig. 1-18 and below).

Lymph Vessels

The **thoracic duct** commences in the abdomen as an elongated lymph sac, the **cisterna chyli.** This lies just below the diaphragm in front of the first two lumbar vertebrae and on the right side of the aorta (Fig. 5-76).

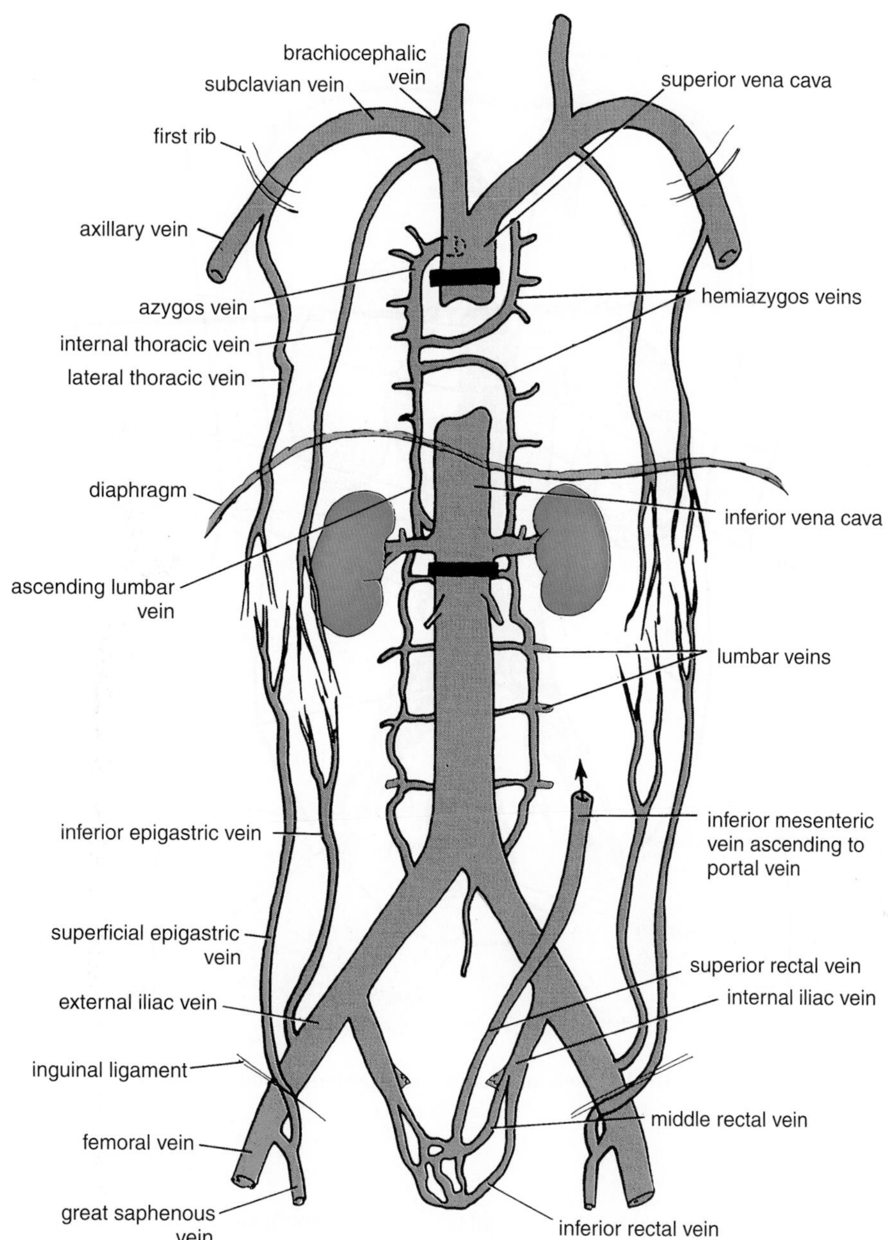

Figure 5-75 The possible collateral circulations of the superior and inferior venae cavae. Note the alternative pathways that exist for blood to return to the right atrium of the heart if the superior vena cava becomes blocked below the entrance of the azygos vein (*upper black bar*). Similar pathways exist if the inferior vena cava becomes blocked below the renal veins (*lower black bar*). Note also the connections that exist between the portal circulation and the systemic veins in the anal canal.

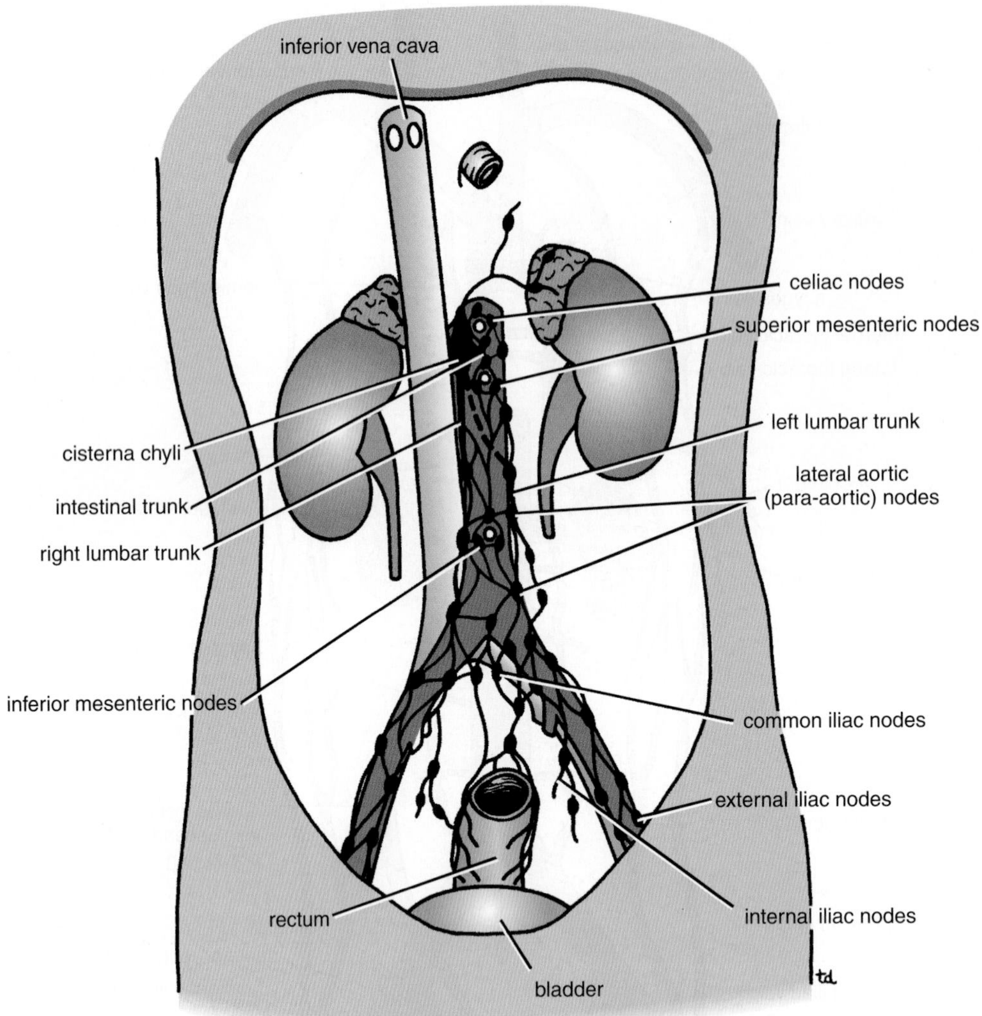

Figure 5-76 Lymph vessels and nodes on the posterior abdominal wall.

The cisterna chyli receives the intestinal trunk, the right and left lumbar trunks, and some small lymph vessels that descend from the lower part of the thorax.

Lymphatic Drainage of the Gonads

The importance of the lymph drainage of the testis was emphasized on page 169.

Nerves on the Posterior Abdominal Wall

Lumbar Plexus

The lumbar plexus, which is one of the main nervous pathways supplying the lower limb, is formed in the psoas muscle from the anterior rami of the upper four lumbar nerves (Fig. 5-77). The anterior rami receive gray rami communicantes from the sympathetic trunk, and the upper two give off white rami communicantes to the sympathetic trunk. The branches of the plexus emerge from the lateral and medial borders of the muscle and from its anterior surface.

The iliohypogastric nerve, ilioinguinal nerve, lateral cutaneous nerve of the thigh, and femoral nerve emerge from the lateral border of the psoas, in that order from above downward (Fig. 5-34). The **iliohypogastric** and **ilioinguinal nerves** (L1) enter the lateral and anterior abdominal walls (see page 157). The iliohypogastric nerve supplies the skin of the lower part of the anterior abdominal wall, and the ilioinguinal nerve passes through the inguinal canal to supply the skin of the groin and the scrotum or labium majus. The **lateral cutaneous nerve of the thigh** crosses the iliac fossa in front of the iliacus muscle and enters the thigh behind the lateral end of the inguinal ligament (see page 568). It supplies the skin over the lateral surface of the thigh. The **femoral nerve** (L2, 3, and 4) is the largest branch of the lumbar plexus. It runs downward and laterally between the psoas and the iliacus muscles and enters the thigh behind the inguinal ligament and lateral to the femoral vessels and the femoral sheath. In the abdomen it supplies the iliacus muscle.

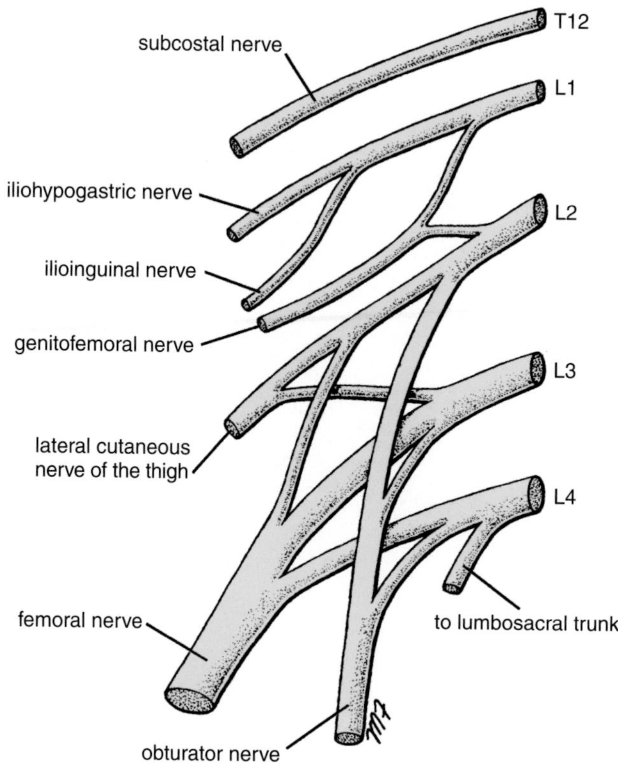

Figure 5-77 Lumbar plexus of nerves.

The obturator nerve and the fourth lumbar root of the lumbosacral trunk emerge from the medial border of the psoas at the brim of the pelvis. The **obturator nerve** (L2, 3, and 4) crosses the pelvic brim in front of the sacroiliac joint and behind the common iliac vessels. It leaves the pelvis by passing through the obturator foramen into the thigh. (For a description of its course in the pelvis see page 326 and in the thigh see page 586). The **fourth lumbar root of the lumbosacral trunk** takes part in the formation of the sacral plexus (see page 325). It descends anterior to the ala of the sacrum and joins the first sacral nerve.

The **genitofemoral nerve** (L1 and 2) emerges on the anterior surface of the psoas. It runs downward in front of the muscle and divides into a **genital branch,** which enters the spermatic cord and supplies the cremaster muscle, and a **femoral branch,** which supplies a small area of the skin of the thigh (see page 568). It is the nervous pathway involved in the **cremasteric reflex,** in which stimulation of the skin of the thigh in the male results in reflex contraction of the cremaster muscle and the drawing upward of the testis within the scrotum.

The branches of the lumbar plexus and their distribution are summarized in Table 5-1.

Sympathetic Trunk (Abdominal Part)

The abdominal part of the sympathetic trunk is continuous above with the thoracic and below with the pelvic parts of the sympathetic trunk. It runs downward along the medial border of the psoas muscle on the bodies of the lumbar vertebrae (Fig. 5-78). It enters the abdomen from behind the medial arcuate ligament and gains entrance to the pelvis below by passing behind the common iliac vessels. The **right sympathetic trunk** lies behind the right border of the inferior vena cava; the **left sympathetic trunk** lies close to the left border of the aorta.

The sympathetic trunk possesses four or five segmentally arranged ganglia, the first and second often being fused together.

Branches

- **White rami communicantes** join the first two ganglia to the first two lumbar spinal nerves. A white ramus contains preganglionic nerve fibers and afferent sensory nerve fibers.
- **Gray rami communicantes** join each ganglion to a corresponding lumbar spinal nerve. A gray ramus contains postganglionic nerve fibers. The postganglionic fibers are

Table 5-1 Branches of the Lumbar Plexus and Their Distribution

Branches	Distribution
Iliohypogastric nerve	External oblique, internal oblique, transversus abdominis muscles of anterior abdominal wall; skin over lower anterior abdominal wall and buttock
Ilioinguinal nerve	External oblique, internal oblique, transversus abdominis muscles of anterior abdominal wall; skin of upper medial aspect of thigh; root of penis and scrotum in the male; mons pubis and labia majora in the female
Lateral cutaneous nerve of the thigh	Skin of anterior and lateral surfaces of the thigh
Genitofemoral nerve (L1, 2)	Cremaster muscle in scrotum in male; skin over anterior surface of thigh; nervous pathway for cremasteric reflex
Femoral nerve (L2, 3, 4)	Iliacus, pectineus, sartorius, quadriceps femoris muscles, and intermediate cutaneous branches to the skin of the anterior surface of the thigh and by saphenous branch to the skin of the medial side of the leg and foot; articular branches to hip and knee joints
Obturator nerve (L2, 3, 4)	Gracilis, adductor brevis, adductor longus, obturator externus, pectineus, adductor magnus (adductor portion), and skin on medial surface of thigh; articular branches to hip and knee joints
Segmental branches	Quadratus lumborum and psoas muscles

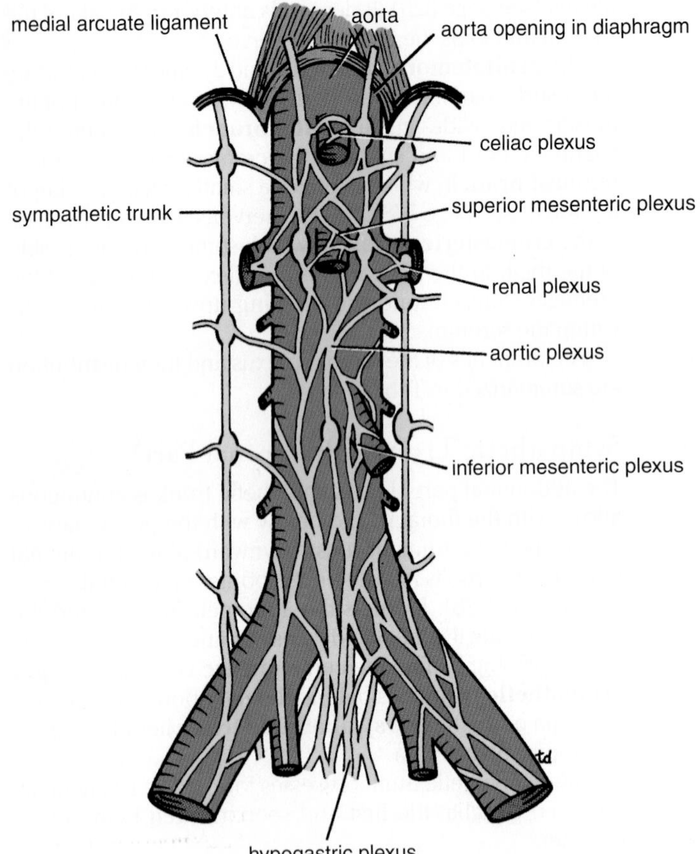

Figure 5-78 Aorta and related sympathetic plexuses.

distributed through the branches of the spinal nerves to the blood vessels, sweat glands, and arrector pili muscles of the skin (see Fig. 1-4).

- Fibers pass medially to the sympathetic plexuses on the abdominal aorta and its branches. (These plexuses also receive fibers from splanchnic nerves and the vagus.)
- Fibers pass downward and medially in front of the common iliac vessels into the pelvis, where, together with branches from sympathetic nerves in front of the aorta, they form a large bundle of fibers called the **superior hypogastric plexus** (Fig. 5-78).

Aortic Plexuses

Preganglionic and postganglionic sympathetic fibers, preganglionic parasympathetic fibers, and visceral afferent fibers form a plexus of nerves, the **aortic plexus,** around the abdominal part of the aorta (Fig. 5-78). Regional concentrations of this plexus around the origins of the celiac, renal, superior mesenteric, and inferior mesenteric arteries form the **celiac plexus, renal plexus, superior mesenteric plexus,** and **inferior mesenteric plexus,** respectively.

The celiac plexus consists mainly of two **celiac ganglia** connected together by a large network of fibers that surrounds the origin of the celiac artery. The ganglia receive the greater and lesser splanchnic nerves (preganglionic sympathetic fibers). Postganglionic branches accompany the branches of the celiac artery and follow them to their distribution. Parasympathetic vagal fibers also accompany the branches of the artery.

The renal and superior mesenteric plexuses are smaller than the celiac plexus. They are distributed along the branches of the corresponding arteries. The inferior mesenteric plexus is similar but receives parasympathetic fibers from the sacral parasympathetic.

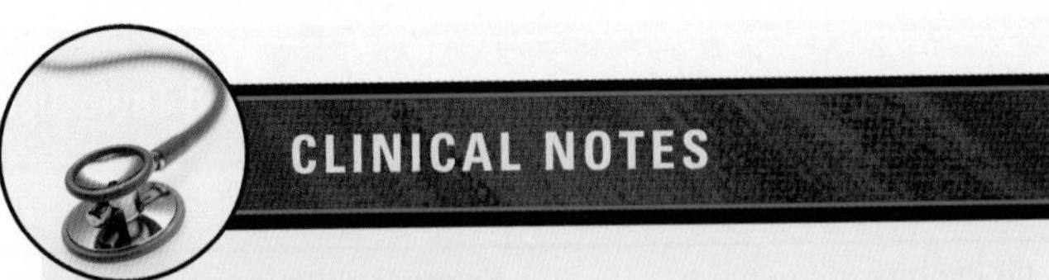

Lumbar Sympathectomy

Lumbar sympathectomy is performed mainly to produce a vasodilatation of the arteries of the lower limb in patients with vasospastic disorders. The preganglionic sympathetic fibers that supply the vessels of the lower limb leave the spinal cord from segments T11 to L2. They synapse in the lumbar and sacral ganglia of the sympathetic trunks. The postganglionic fibers join the lumbar and sacral nerves and are distributed to the vessels of the limb as branches of these nerves. Additional postganglionic fibers pass directly from the lumbar ganglia to the common and external iliac arteries, but they follow the latter artery only down as far as the inguinal ligament. In the male a bilateral lumbar sympathectomy may be followed by loss of ejaculatory power, but erection is not impaired.

(continues)

Clinical Notes, *continued*

Abdominal Pain

Abdominal pain is one of the most important problems facing the physician. This section provides an anatomic basis for the different forms of abdominal pain found in clinical practice.

Three distinct forms of pain exist: somatic, visceral, and referred pain.

Somatic Abdominal Pain

Somatic abdominal pain in the abdominal wall can arise from the skin, fascia, muscles, and parietal peritoneum. It can be severe and precisely localized. When the origin is on one side of the midline, the pain is also lateralized. The somatic pain impulses from the abdomen reach the central nervous system in the following segmental spinal nerves:

- **Central part of the diaphragm:** Phrenic nerve (C3, 4, and 5)
- **Peripheral part of the diaphragm:** Intercostal nerves (T7 to 11)
- **Anterior abdominal wall:** Thoracic nerves (T7 to 12) and the first lumbar nerve
- **Pelvic wall:** Obturator nerve (L2, 3, and 4)

The inflamed parietal peritoneum is extremely sensitive, and because the full thickness of the abdominal wall is innervated by the same nerves, it is not surprising to find cutaneous hypersensitivity (hyperesthesia) and tenderness. Local reflexes involving the same nerves bring about a protective phenomenon in which the abdominal muscles increase in tone. This increased tone or rigidity, sometimes called **guarding,** is an attempt to rest and localize the inflammatory process.

Rebound tenderness occurs when the parietal peritoneum is inflamed. Any movement of that inflamed peritoneum, even when that movement is elicited by removing the examining hand from a site distant from the inflamed peritoneum, brings about tenderness.

Examples of acute, severe, localized pain originating in the parietal peritoneum are seen in the later stages of appendicitis. Cutaneous hyperesthesia, tenderness, and muscular spasm or rigidity occur in the lower right quadrant of the anterior abdominal wall. A perforated peptic ulcer, in which the parietal peritoneum is chemically irritated, produces the same symptoms and signs but involves the right upper and lower quadrants.

Visceral Abdominal Pain

Visceral abdominal pain arises in abdominal organs, visceral peritoneum, and the mesenteries. The causes of visceral pain include stretching of a viscus or mesentery, distention of a hollow viscus, impaired blood supply (ischemia) to a viscus, and chemical damage (e.g., acid gastric juice) to a viscus or its covering peritoneum. Pain arising from an abdominal viscus is dull and poorly localized. Visceral pain is referred to the midline, probably because the viscera develop embryologically as midline structures and receive a bilateral nerve supply; many viscera later move laterally as development proceeds, taking their nerve supply with them.

Colic is a form of visceral pain produced by the violent contraction of smooth muscle; it is commonly caused by luminal obstruction as in intestinal obstruction, in the passage of a gallstone in the biliary ducts, or in the passage of a stone in the ureters.

Many visceral afferent fibers that enter the spinal cord participate in reflex activity. Reflex sweating, salivation, nausea, vomiting, and increased heart rate may accompany visceral pain.

The sensations that arise in viscera reach the central nervous system in afferent nerves that accompany the sympathetic nerves and enter the spinal cord through the posterior roots. The significance of this pathway is better understood in the following discussion on referred visceral pain.

Referred Abdominal Pain

Referred abdominal pain is the feeling of pain at a location other than the site of origin of the stimulus but in an area supplied by the same or adjacent segments of the spinal cord. Both somatic and visceral structures can produce referred pain.

In the case of referred somatic pain, the possible explanation is that the nerve fibers from the diseased structure and the area where the pain is felt ascend in the central nervous system along a common pathway, and the cerebral cortex is incapable of distinguishing between the sites. Examples of referred somatic pain follow. Pleurisy involving the lower part of the costal parietal pleura can give rise to referred pain in the abdomen because the lower parietal pleura receives its sensory innervation from the lower five intercostal nerves, which also innervate the skin and muscles of the anterior abdominal wall.

Visceral pain from the stomach is commonly referred to the epigastrium (Fig. 5-79). The afferent pain fibers from the stomach ascend in company with the sympathetic nerves and pass through the celiac plexus and the greater splanchnic nerves. The sensory fibers enter the spinal cord at segments T5 to 9 and give rise to referred pain in dermatomes T5 to 9 on the lower chest and abdominal walls.

Visceral pain from the appendix (Fig. 5-79), which is produced by distension of its lumen or spasm of its smooth muscle coat, travels in nerve fibers that accompany sympathetic nerves through the superior mesenteric plexus and the lesser splanchnic nerve to the spinal cord (T10 segment). The vague referred pain is felt in the region of the umbilicus (T10 dermatome). Later, if the inflammatory process involves the parietal peritoneum, the severe somatic pain dominates the clinical picture and is localized precisely in the right lower quadrant.

Visceral pain from the gallbladder, as occurs in patients with cholecystitis or gallstone colic, travels in nerve fibers that accompany sympathetic nerves. They pass through the celiac plexus and greater splanchnic nerves to the spinal cord (segments T5 to 9). The vague referred pain is felt in the dermatomes (T5 to 9) on the lower chest and upper abdominal walls (Fig. 5-79). If the inflammatory process spreads to involve the parietal peritoneum of the anterior abdominal wall or peripheral diaphragm, the severe somatic pain is felt in the right upper quadrant and through to the back below the inferior angle of the scapula. Involvement of the central diaphragmatic parietal peritoneum, which is innervated by the phrenic nerve (C3, 4, and 5), can give rise to referred pain over the shoulder because the skin in this area is innervated by the supraclavicular nerves (C3 and 4).

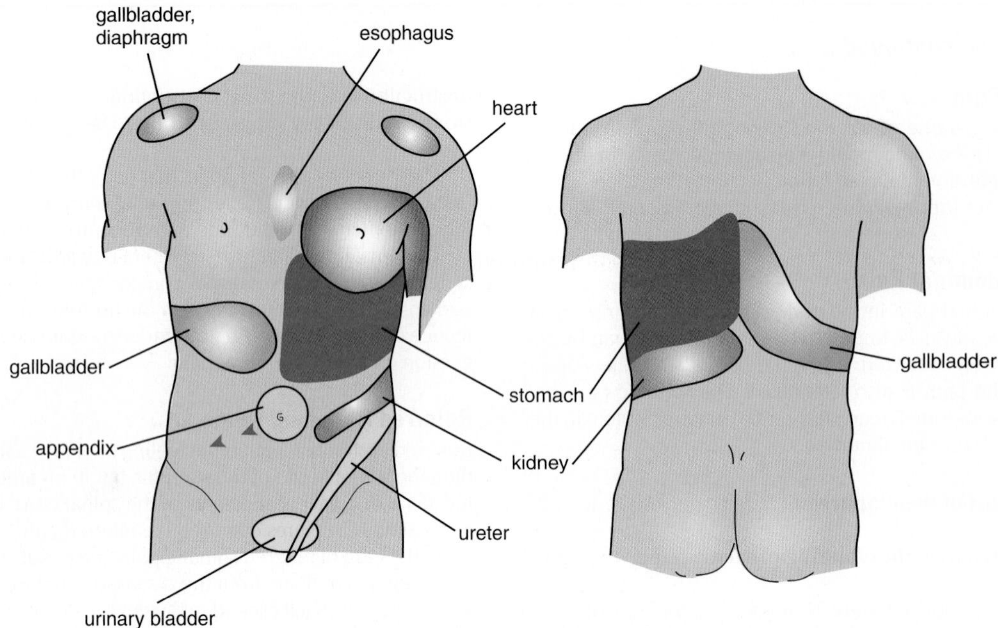

Figure 5-79 Some important skin areas involved in referred visceral pain.

Cross-Sectional Anatomy of the Abdomen

To assist in interpretation of computed tomography (CT) scans of the abdomen, study the labeled cross sections of the abdomen shown in Figures 5-80 and 5-81. The sections have been photographed on their **inferior surfaces.** Also see Figure 5-82 for an example of a CT scan.

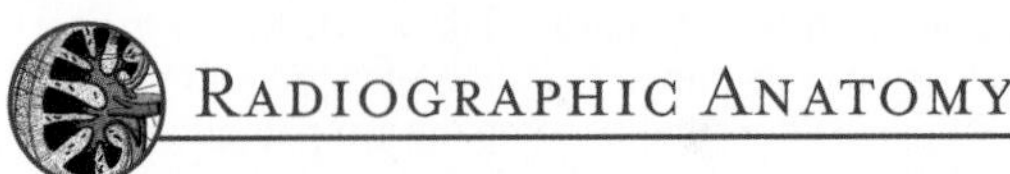

RADIOGRAPHIC ANATOMY

Radiographic Appearances of the Abdomen

Only the more important features seen in a standard anteroposterior radiograph of the abdomen, with the patient in the supine position, are described (Figs. 5-83 and 5-84).

Examine the following in a systematic order.

1. **Bones.** In the upper part of the radiograph the lower ribs are seen. Running down the middle of the radiograph are the lower thoracic and lumbar vertebrae and the sacrum and coccyx. On either side are the sacroiliac joints, the pelvic bones, and the hip joints.
2. **Diaphragm.** This casts dome-shaped shadows on each side; the one on the right is slightly higher than the one on the left (not shown in Fig. 5-83).
3. **Psoas muscle.** On either side of the vertebral column, the lateral borders of the psoas muscle cast a shadow that passes downward and laterally from the 12th thoracic vertebra.
4. **Liver.** This forms a homogeneous opacity in the upper part of the abdomen.
5. **Spleen.** This may cast a soft shadow, which can be seen in the left 9th and 10th intercostal spaces (not shown in Fig. 5-83).
6. **Kidneys.** These are usually visible because the perirenal fat surrounding the kidneys produces a transradiant line.
7. **Stomach and intestines.** Gas may be seen in the fundus of the stomach and in the intestines. Fecal material may also be seen in the colon.
8. **Urinary bladder.** If this contains sufficient urine, it will cast a shadow in the pelvis.

Radiographic Appearances of the Gastrointestinal Tract

Stomach

The stomach can be demonstrated radiologically (Figs. 5-85 and 5-86) by the administration of a watery suspension of barium sulfate (barium meal). With the patient in the erect position, the first few mouthfuls pass into the stomach and form a triangular shadow with the apex downward. The gas bubble in the fundus shows above the fluid level at the top of the barium shadow. As the stomach is filled, the greater and lesser curvatures are outlined and the body and pyloric portions are recognized. The pylorus is seen to move downward and come to lie at the level of the third lumbar vertebra.

Fluoroscopic examination of the stomach as it is filled with the barium emulsion reveals peristaltic waves of contraction of the stomach wall, which commence near the middle of the body and pass to the pylorus. The respiratory movements of the diaphragm cause displacement of the fundus.

Duodenum

A barium meal passes into the first part of the duodenum and forms a triangular homogeneous shadow, the **duodenal cap,** which has its base toward the pylorus (Fig. 5-87).

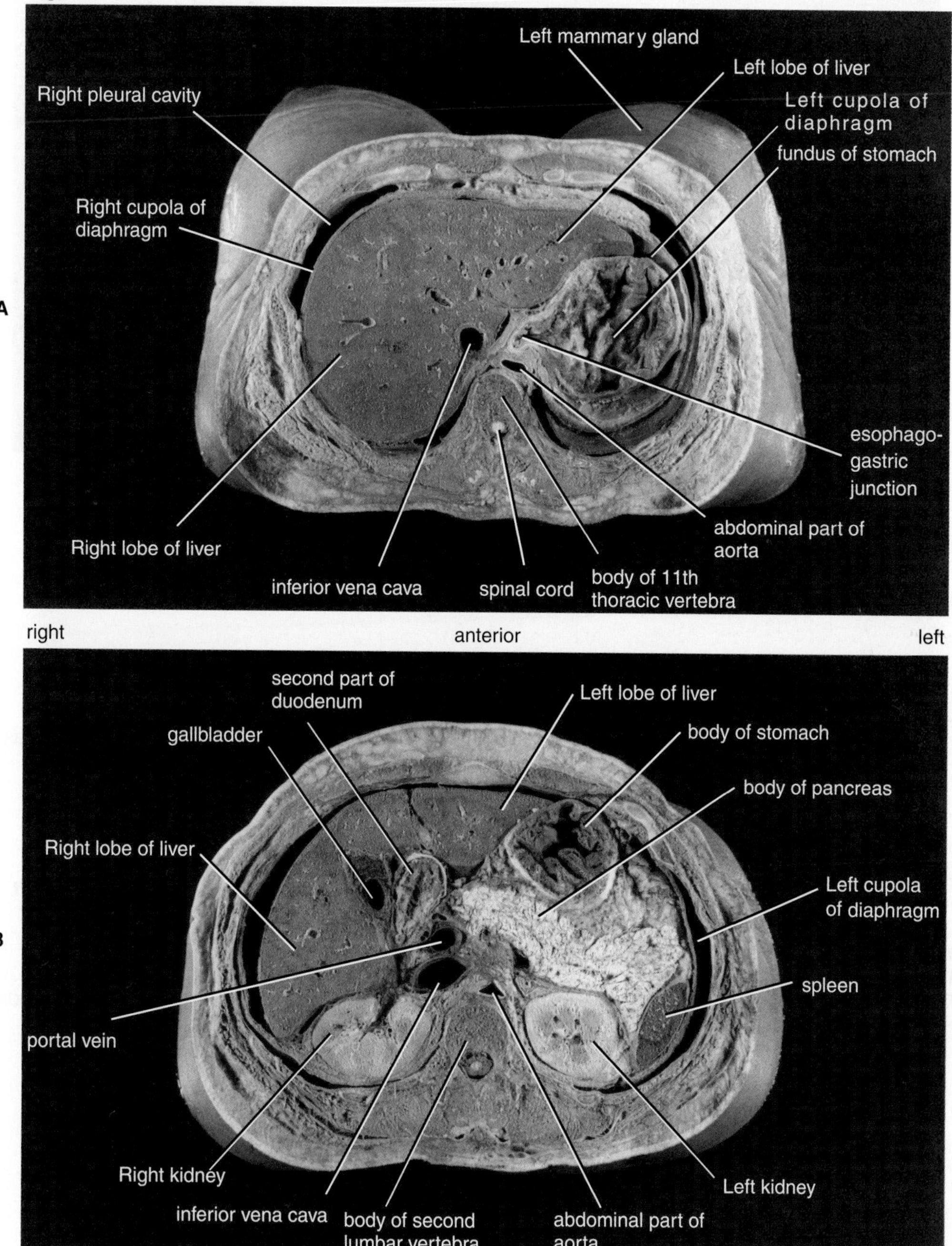

Figure 5-80 **A.** Cross section of the abdomen at the level of the body of the 11th thoracic vertebra, viewed from below. Note that the large size of the pleural cavity is an artifact caused by the embalming process. **B.** Cross section of the abdomen at the level of the body of the second lumbar vertebra, viewed from below.

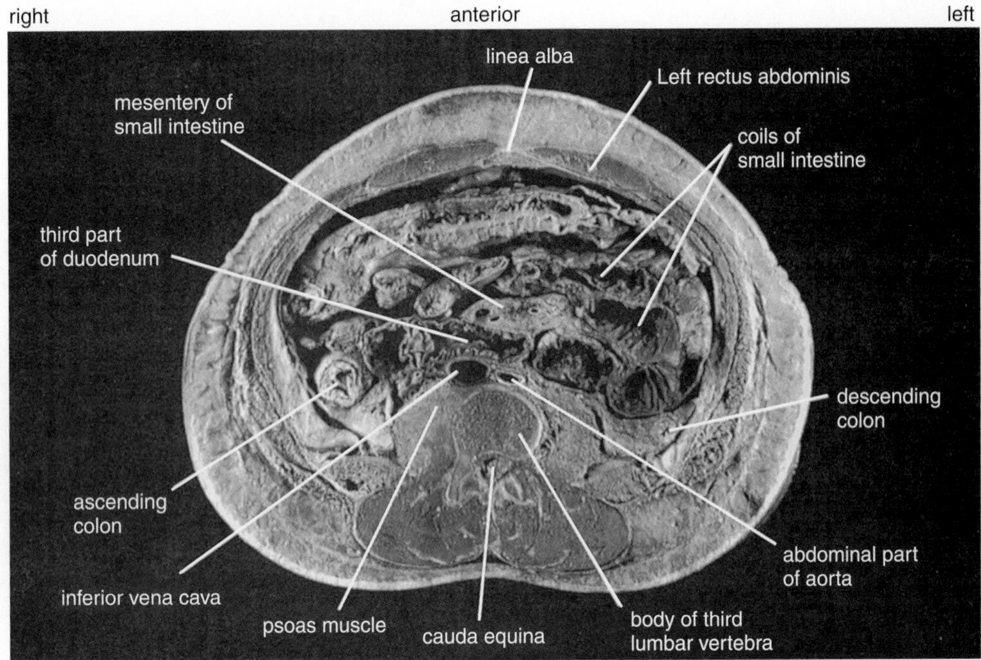

Figure 5-81 Cross section of the abdomen at the level of the body of the third lumbar vertebra, viewed from below.

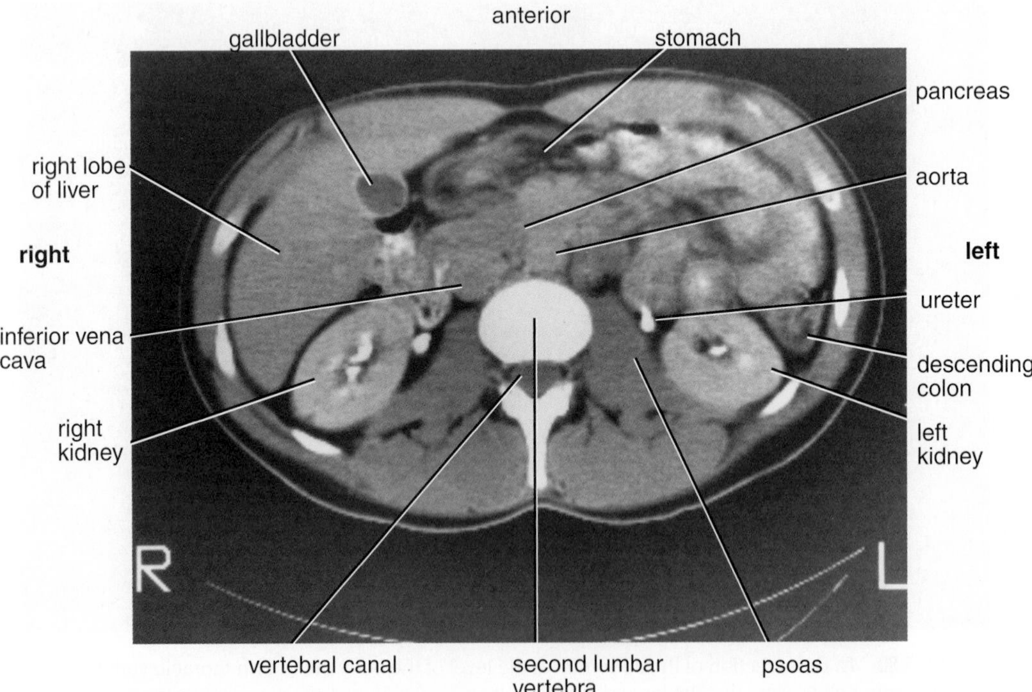

Figure 5-82 Computed tomography scan of the abdomen at the level of the second lumbar vertebra after intravenous pyelography. The radiopaque material can be seen in the renal pelvis and the ureters. The section is viewed from below.

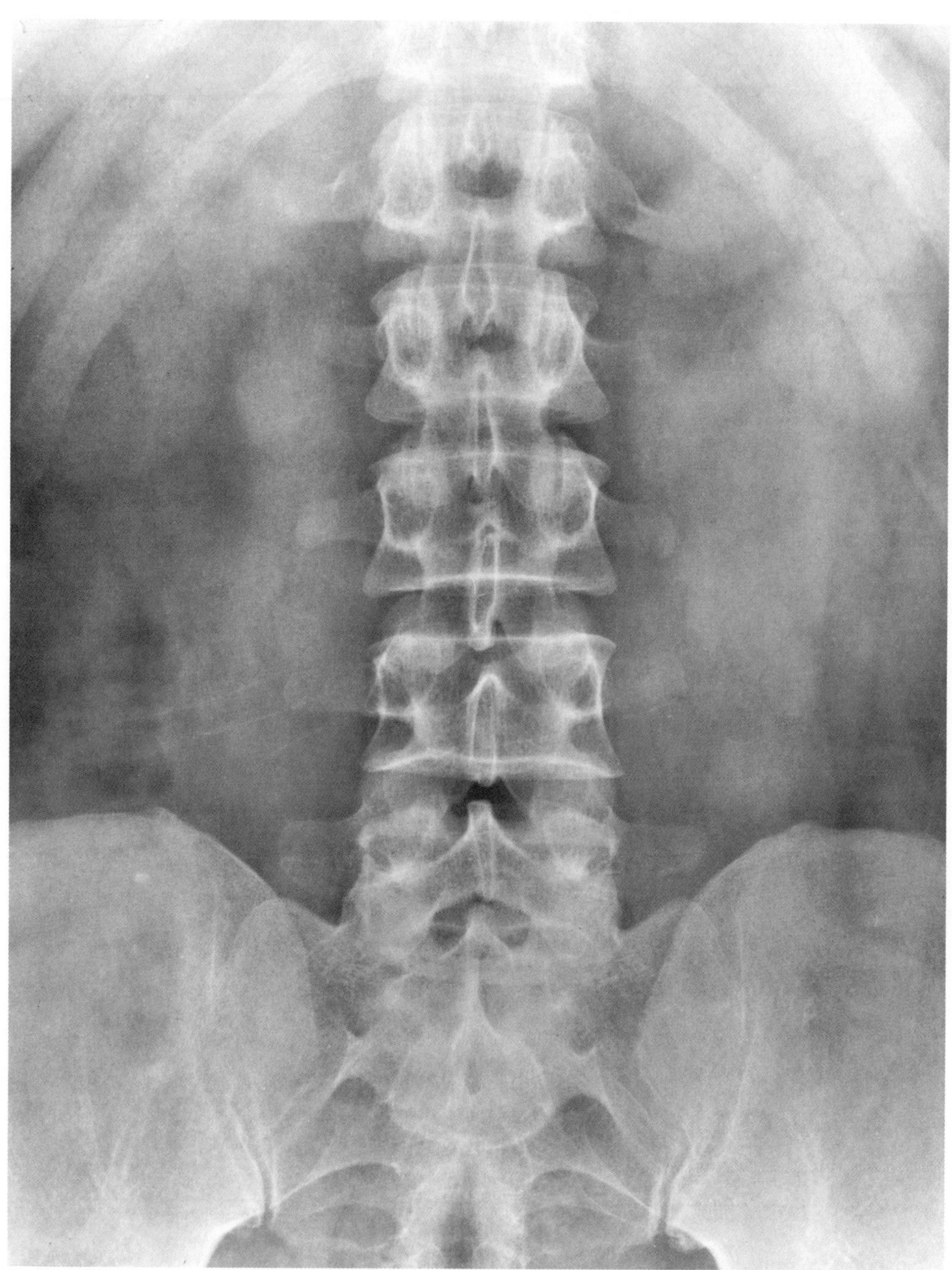

Figure 5-83 Anteroposterior radiograph of the abdomen.

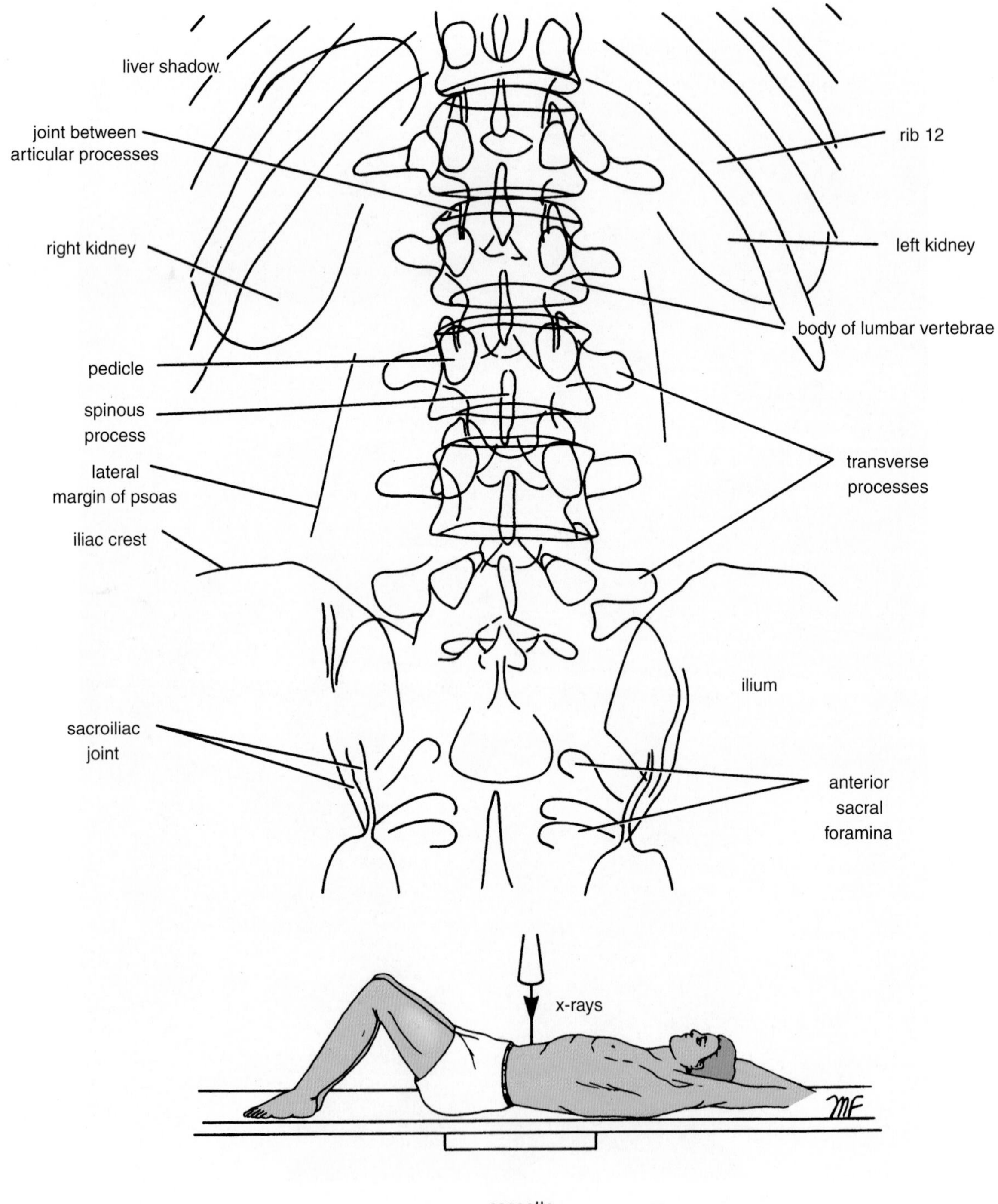

Figure 5-84 Representation of the main features seen in the anteroposterior radiograph in Figure 5-83.

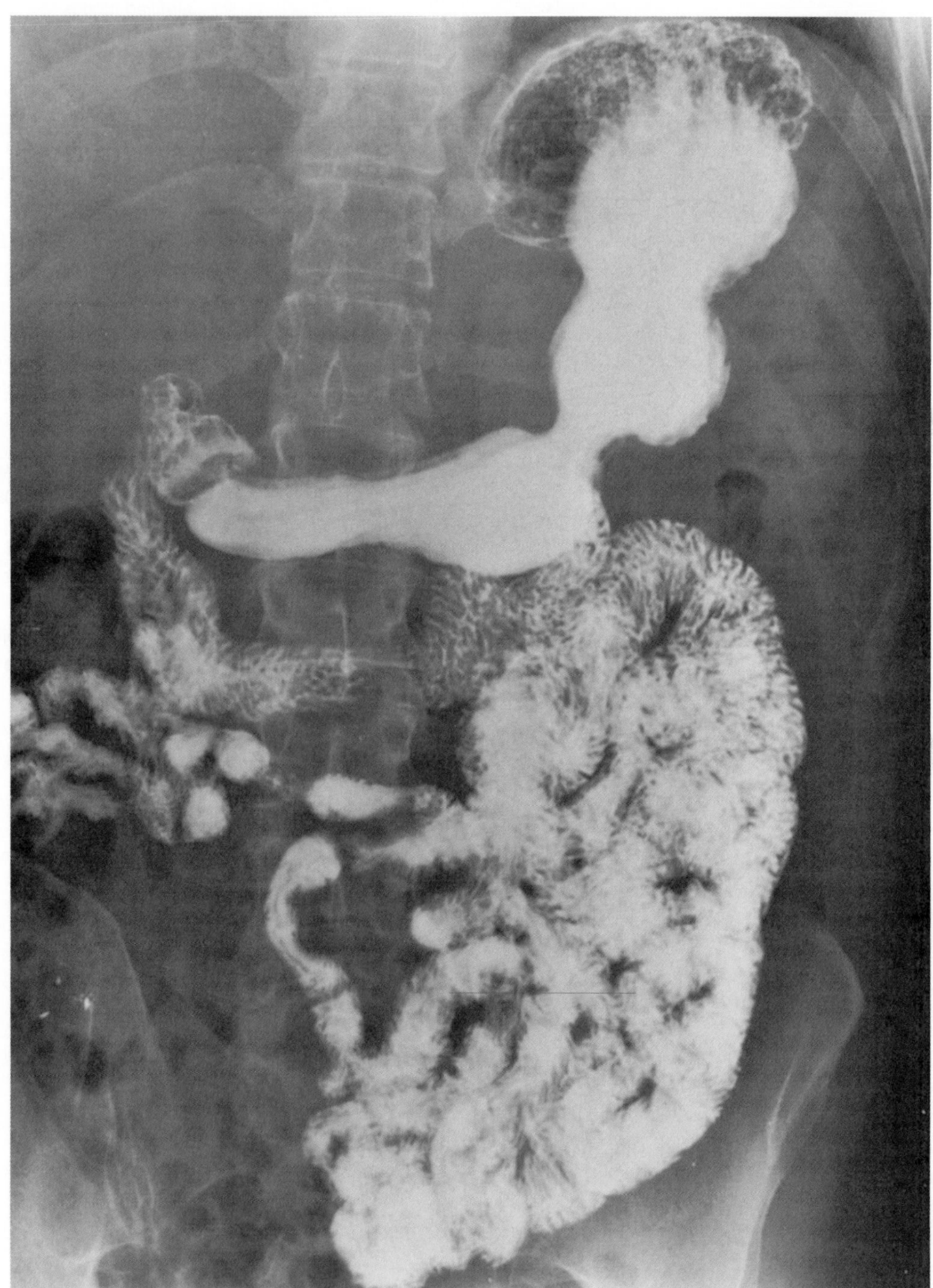

Figure 5-85 Anteroposterior radiograph of the stomach and the small intestine after ingestion of barium meal.

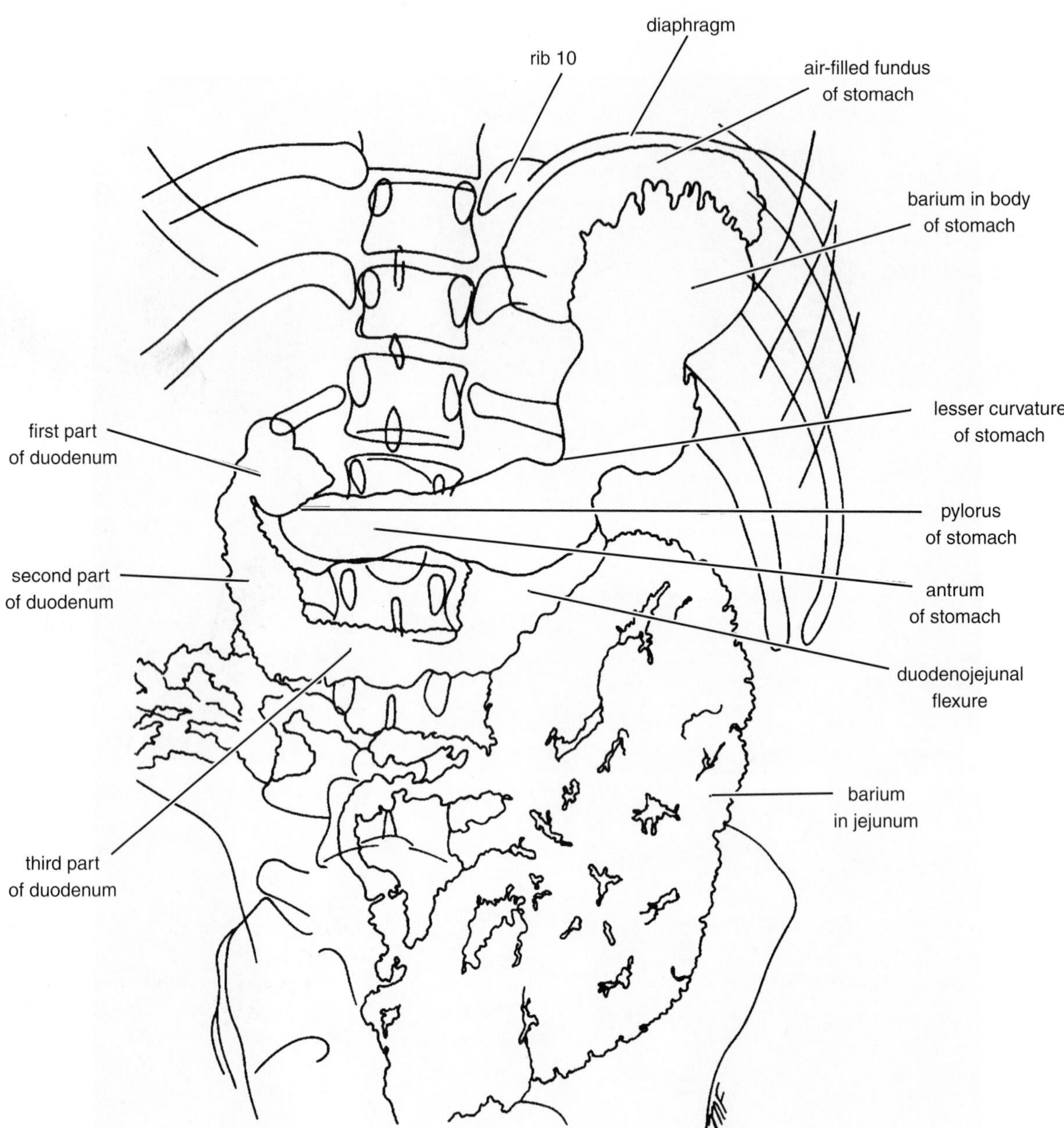

Figure 5-86 Representation of the main features seen in the radiograph in Figure 5-85.

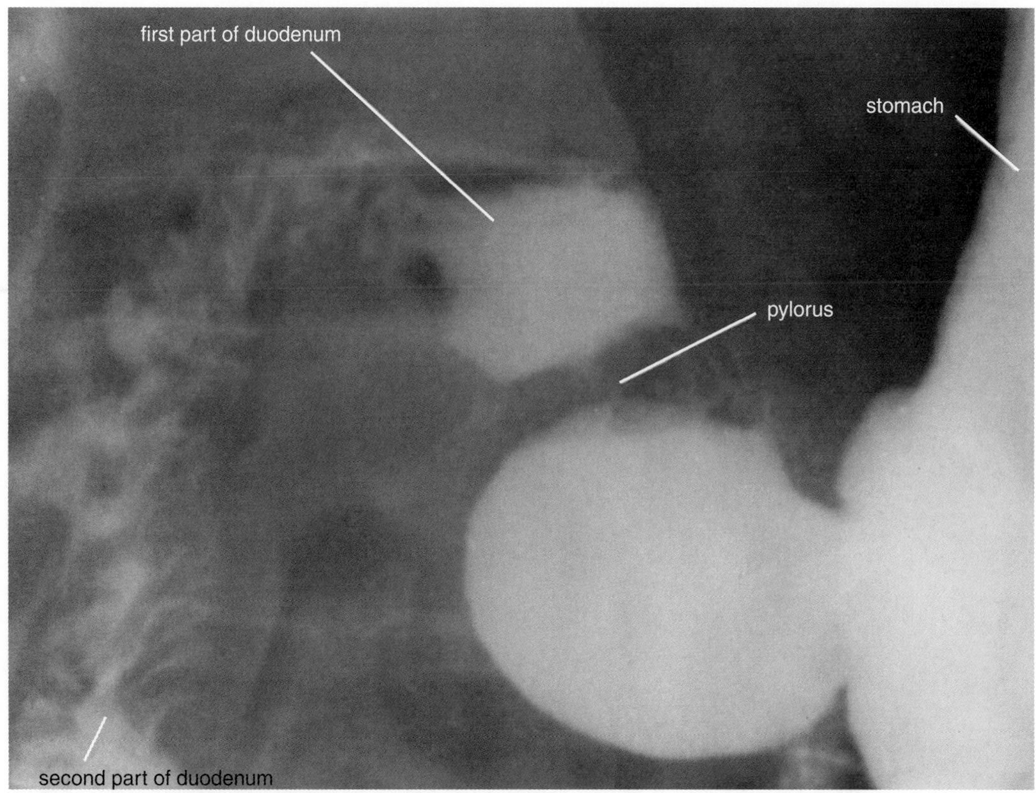

Figure 5-87 Anteroposterior radiograph of the duodenum after ingestion of barium meal.

Under the influence of peristalsis, the barium quickly leaves the duodenal cap and passes rapidly through the remaining portions of the duodenum. The outline of the barium shadow in the first part of the duodenum is smooth because of the absence of mucosal folds. In the remainder of the duodenum, the presence of plicae circulares breaks up the barium emulsion, giving it a floccular appearance.

Jejunum and Ileum

A barium meal enters the jejunum in a few minutes and reaches the ileocecal junction in 30 minutes to 2 hours, and the greater part has left the small intestine in 6 hours. In the jejunum and upper part of the ileum, the mucosal folds and the peristaltic activity scatter the barium shadow (Figs. 5-85 and 5-88). In the last part of the ileum, the barium meal tends to form a continuous mass of barium.

Large Intestine

The large intestine can be demonstrated by the administration of a barium enema or a barium meal. The former is more satisfactory.

The bowel may be outlined by the administration of 2 to 3 pints (1 L) of barium sulfate emulsion through the anal canal. When the large intestine is filled, the entire outline can be seen in an anteroposterior projection (Figs. 5-89 and 5-90). Oblique and lateral views of the colic flexures may be necessary. The characteristic sacculations are well seen when the bowel is filled, and, after the enema has been evacuated, the mucosal pattern is clearly demonstrated.

The appendix frequently fills with barium after an enema. The radiographic appearances of the sigmoid colon and rectum are described on page 377.

The arterial supply to the gastrointestinal tract can be demonstrated by arteriography. A catheter is inserted into the femoral artery and threaded upward under direct vision on a screen into the abdominal aorta. The end of the catheter is then manipulated into the opening of the appropriate artery. Radiopaque material is injected through the catheter and an arteriogram is obtained (Fig. 5-91).

Radiographic Appearances of the Biliary Ducts

The bile passages normally are not visible on a radiograph. Their lumina can be outlined by the administration of various iodine-containing compounds orally or by injection. When taken orally, the compound is absorbed from the small intestine, carried to the liver, and excreted with the bile. On reaching the gallbladder, it is concentrated with the bile. The concentrated iodine compound, mixed with the bile, is now radiopaque and reveals the gallbladder as a pear-shaped opacity in the angle between the right 12th rib and the vertebral column (Figs. 5-92 and 5-93). If the patient is given a fatty meal, the gallbladder contracts, and the cystic and bile ducts become visible as the opaque medium passes down to the second part of the duodenum.

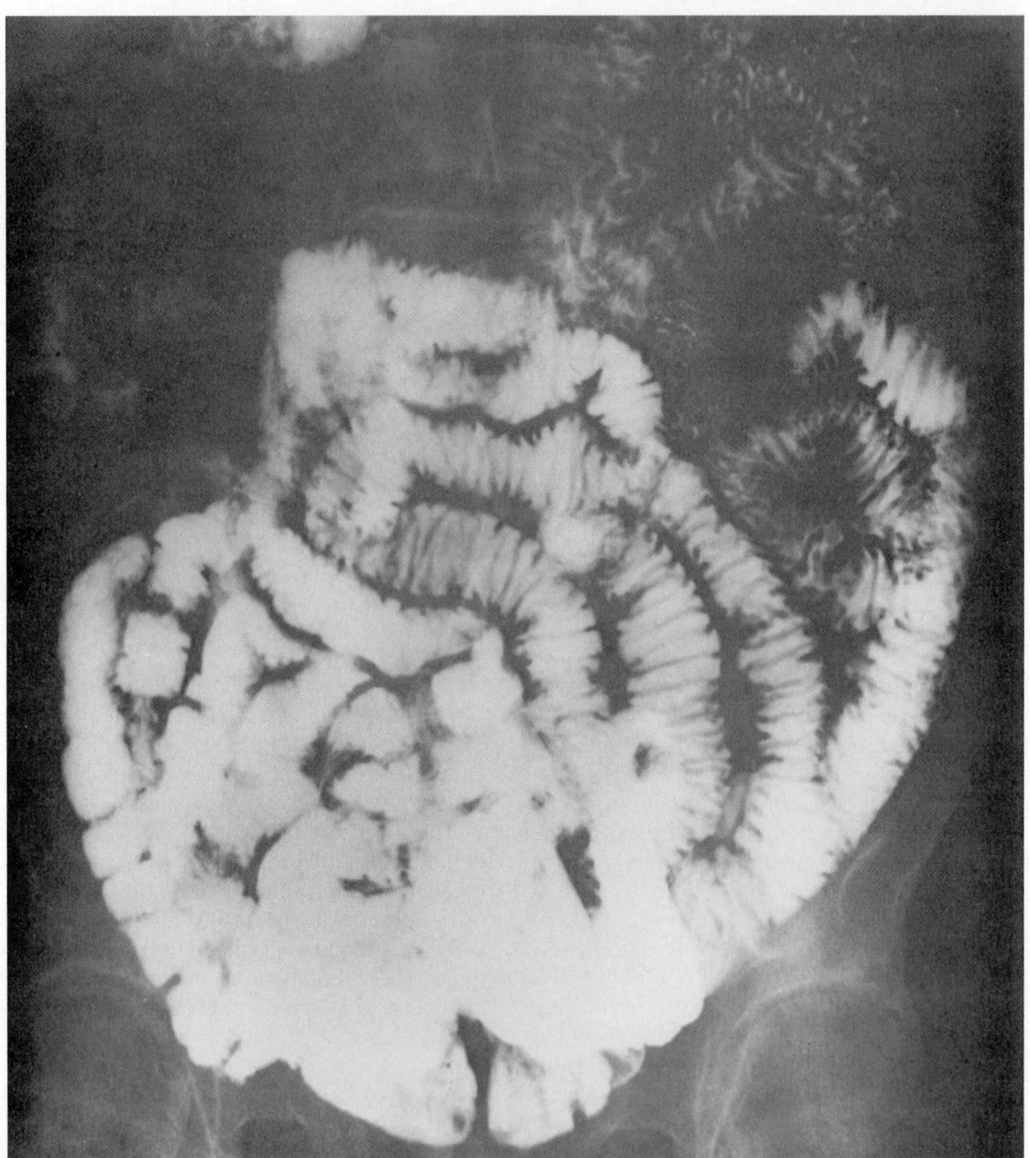

Figure 5-88 Anteroposterior radiograph of the small intestine after ingestion of barium meal.

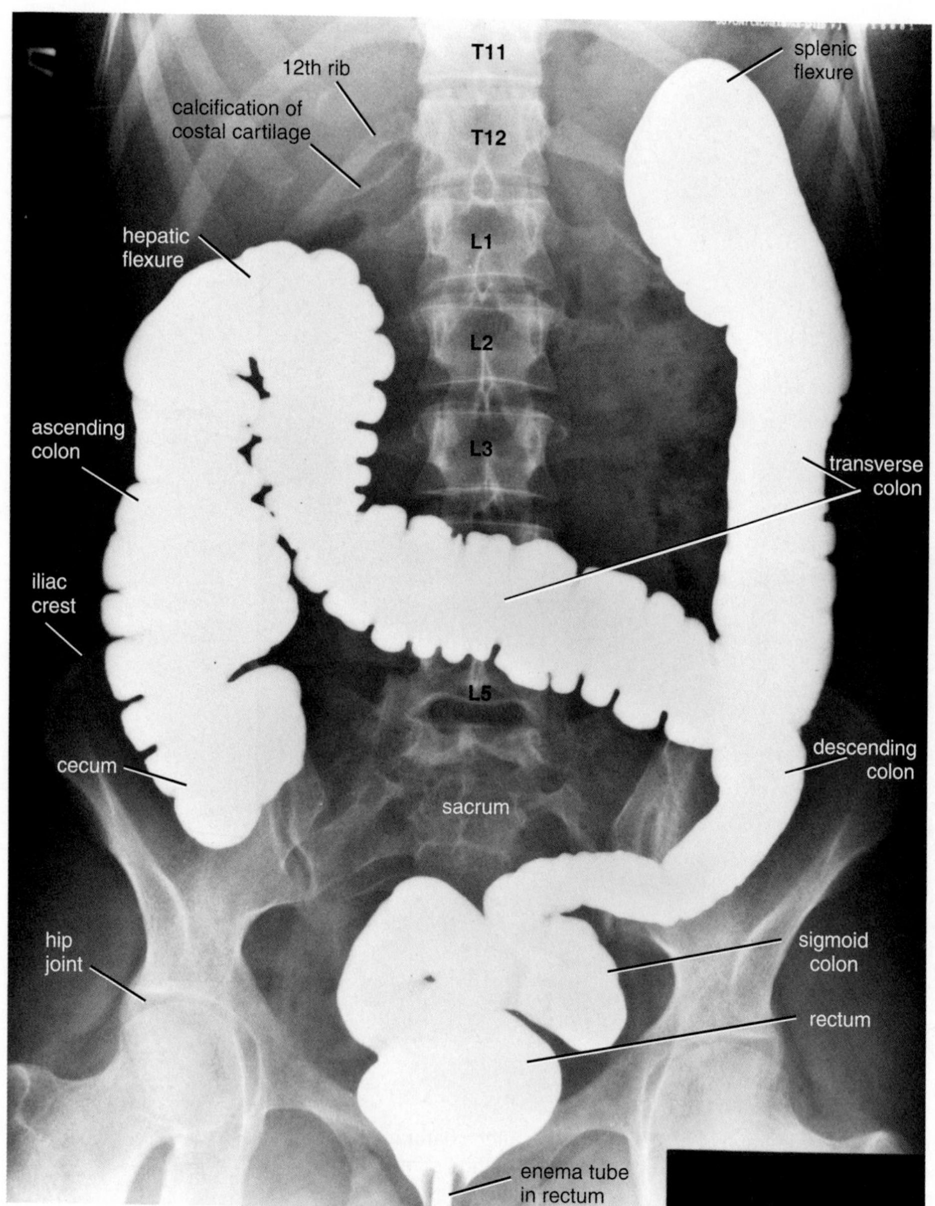

Figure 5-89 Anteroposterior radiograph of the large intestine after a barium enema.

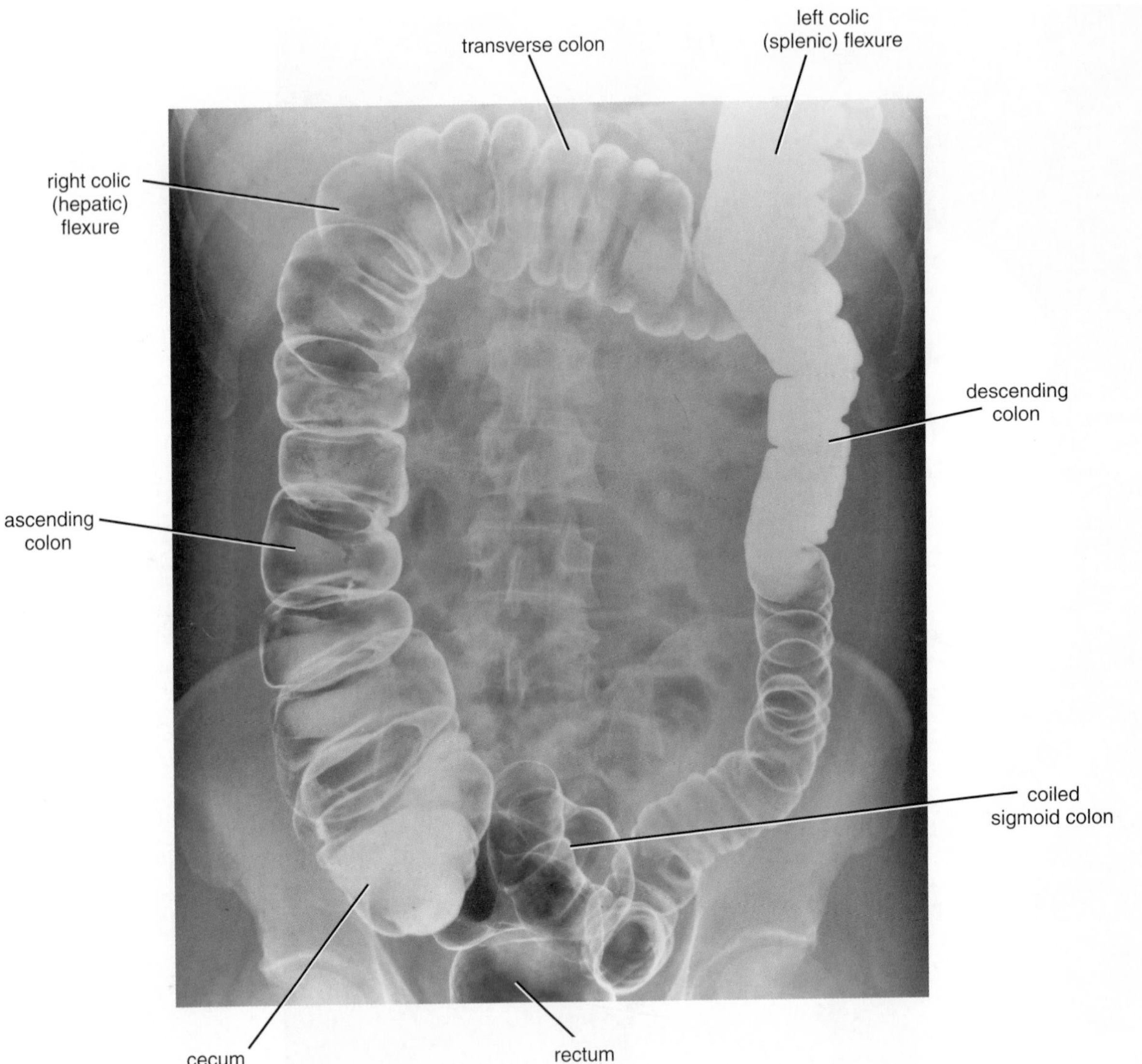

Figure 5-90 Anteroposterior radiograph of the large intestine after a barium enema. Air has been introduced into the intestine through the enema tube after evacuation of most of the barium. This procedure is referred to as a contrast enema.

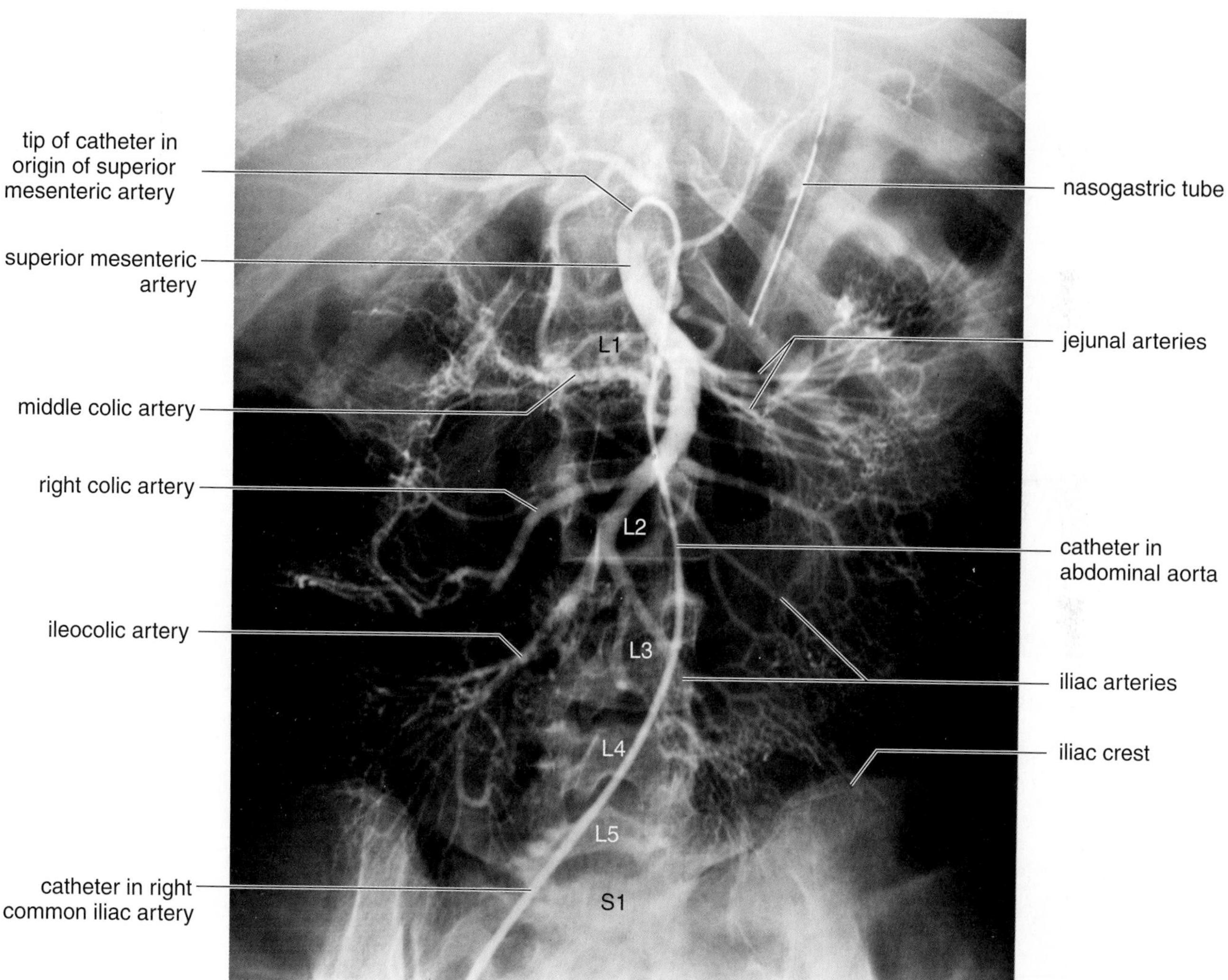

Figure 5-91 An arteriogram of the superior mesenteric artery. The catheter has been inserted into the right femoral artery and has passed up the external and common iliac arteries to ascend the aorta to the origin of the superior mesenteric artery. A nasogastric tube is also in position.

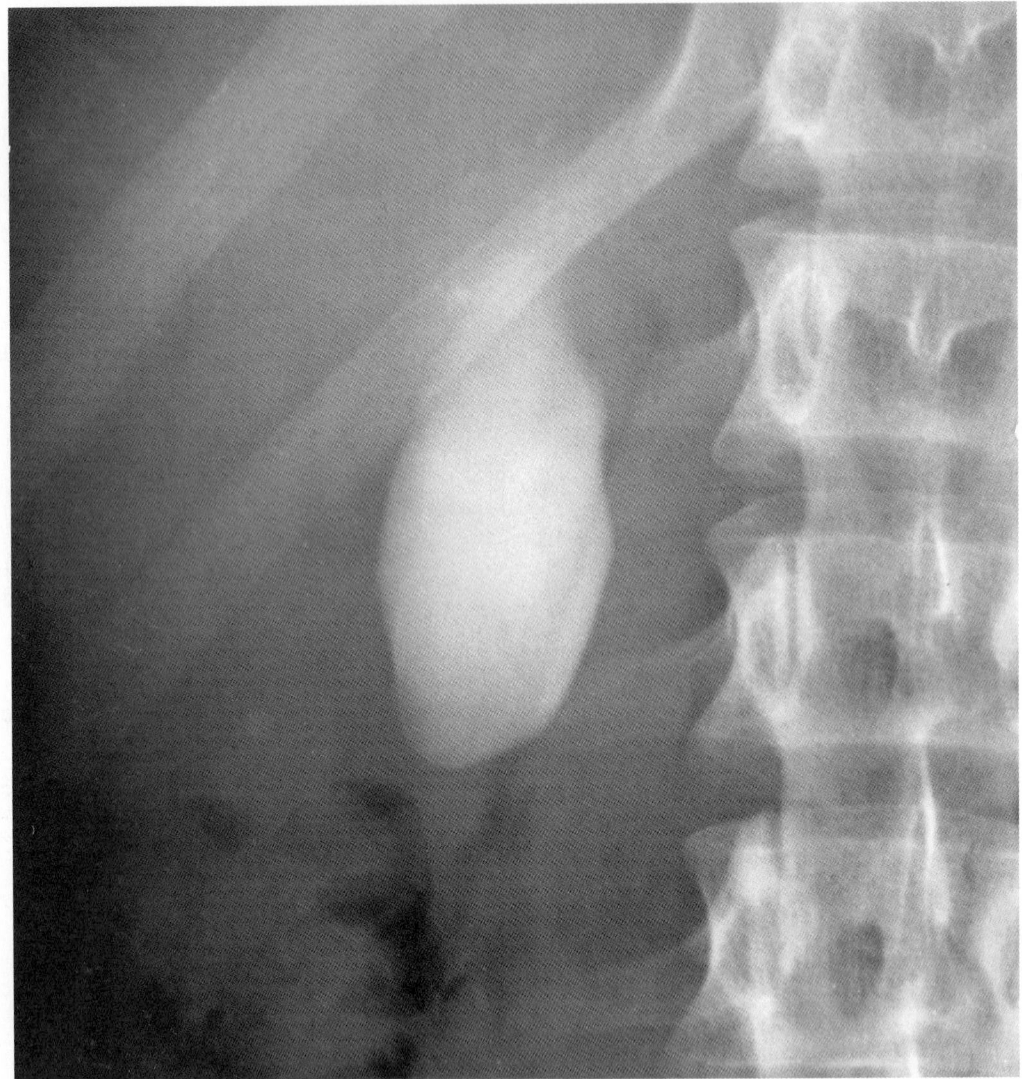

Figure 5-92 Anteroposterior radiograph of the gallbladder after administration of an iodine-containing compound.

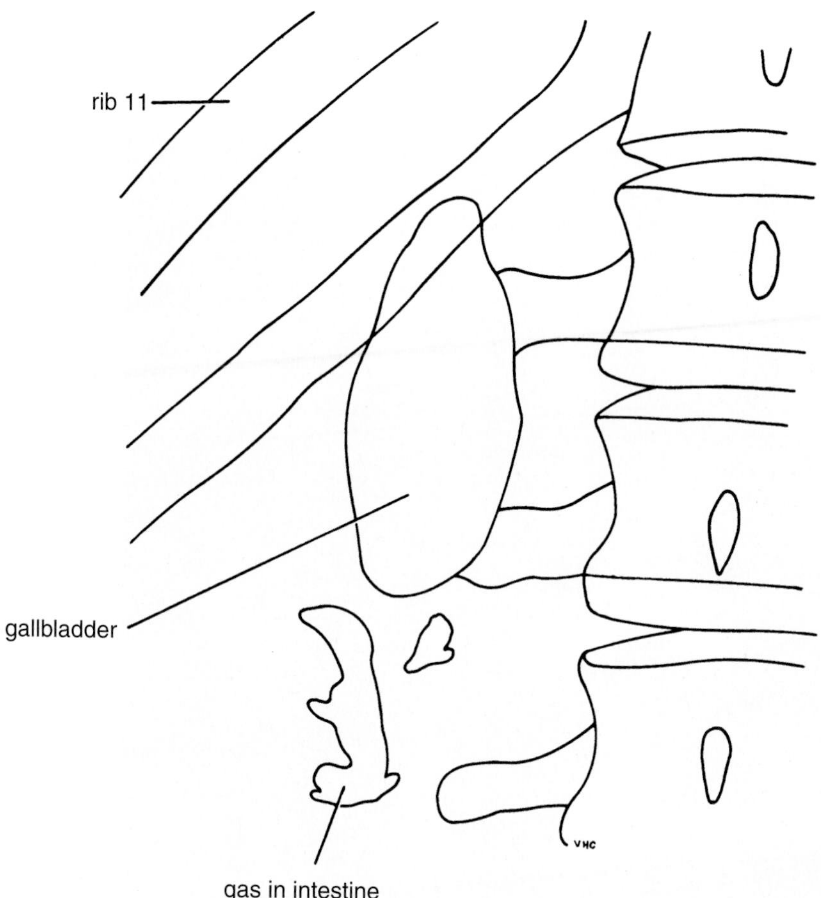

Figure 5-93 Representation of the main features seen in the radiograph in Figure 5-92.

A sonogram of the upper part of the abdomen can be used to show the lumen of the gallbladder (Fig. 5-54).

Radiographic Appearances of the Urinary Tract

Kidneys

The kidneys are usually visible on a standard anteroposterior radiograph of the abdomen because the perirenal fat surrounding the kidneys produces a transradiant line.

Calyces, Renal Pelvis, and Ureter

Calyces, the renal pelvis, and the ureter are not normally visible on a standard radiograph. The lumen can be demonstrated by the use of radiopaque compounds in intravenous pyelography or retrograde pyelography.

With **intravenous pyelography,** an iodine-containing compound is injected into a subcutaneous arm vein. It is excreted and concentrated by the kidneys, thus rendering the calyces and ureter opaque to x-rays (Figs. 5-94, 5-95, and 5-96). When enough of the opaque medium has been excreted, the bladder is also revealed. The ureters are seen superimposed on the transverse processes of the lumbar vertebrae. They cross the sacroiliac joints and enter the pelvis. In the vicinity of the ischial spines, they turn medially to enter the bladder. The three normal constrictions of the ureters (at the junction of the renal pelvis with the ureter, at the pelvic brim, and where the ureter enters the bladder) can be recognized.

With **retrograde pyelography,** a cystoscope is passed through the urethra into the bladder, and a ureteric catheter is inserted into the ureter. A solution of sodium iodide is then injected along the catheter into the ureter. When the minor calyces become filled with the radiopaque medium, the detailed anatomic features of the minor and major calyces and the pelvis of the ureter can be clearly seen. Each minor calyx has a cup-shaped appearance caused by the renal papilla projecting into it.

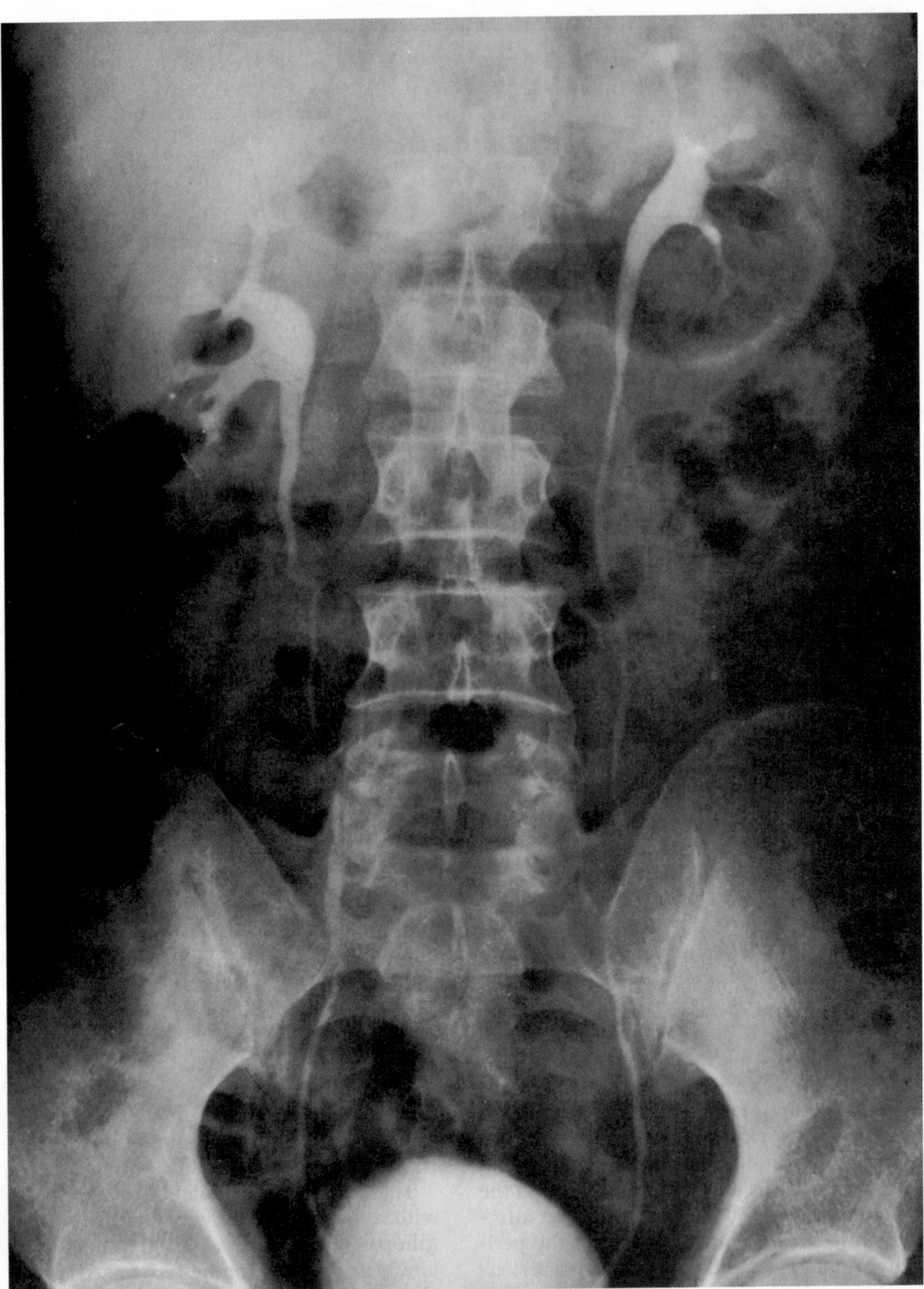

Figure 5-94 Anteroposterior radiograph of the ureter and renal pelvis after intravenous injection of an iodine-containing compound, which is excreted by the kidney. Major and minor calyces are also shown.

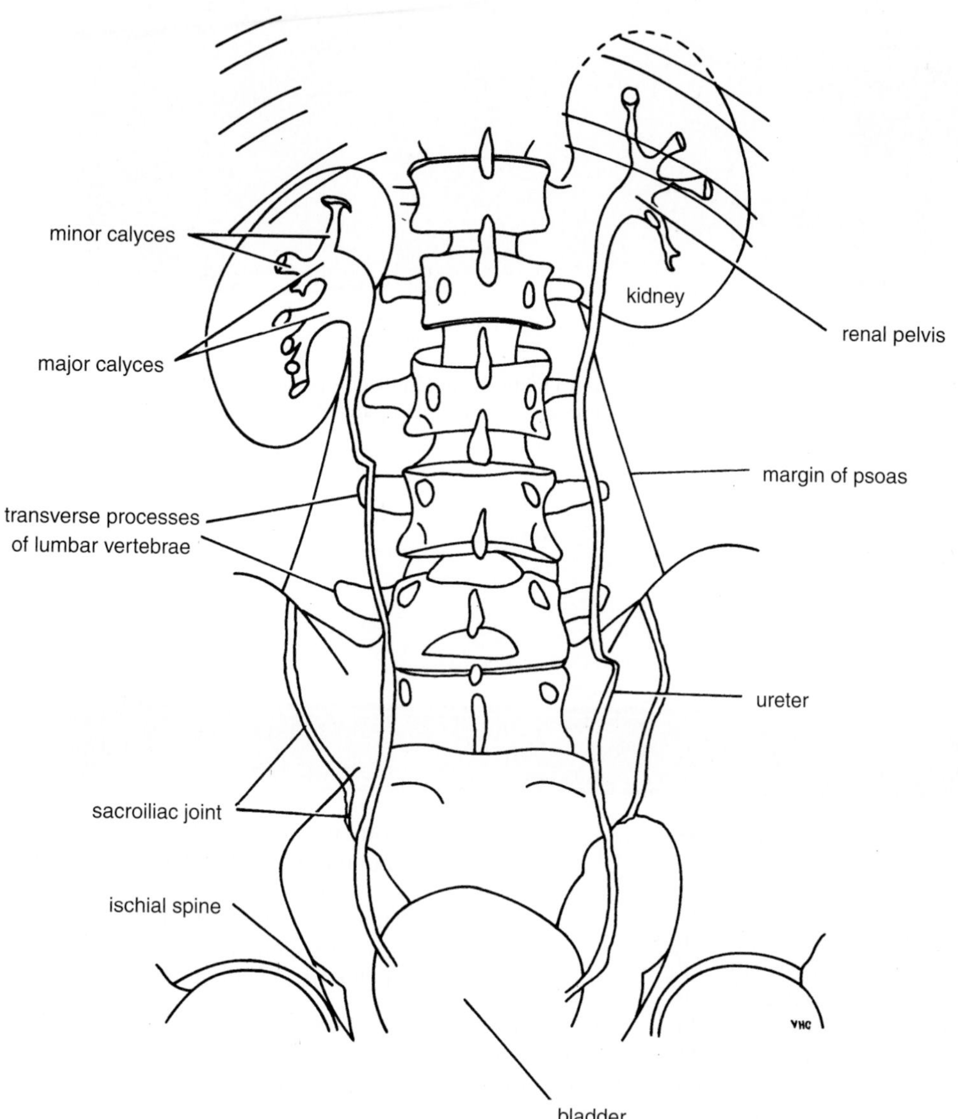

Figure 5-95 Representation of the main features seen in the radiograph in Figure 5-94.

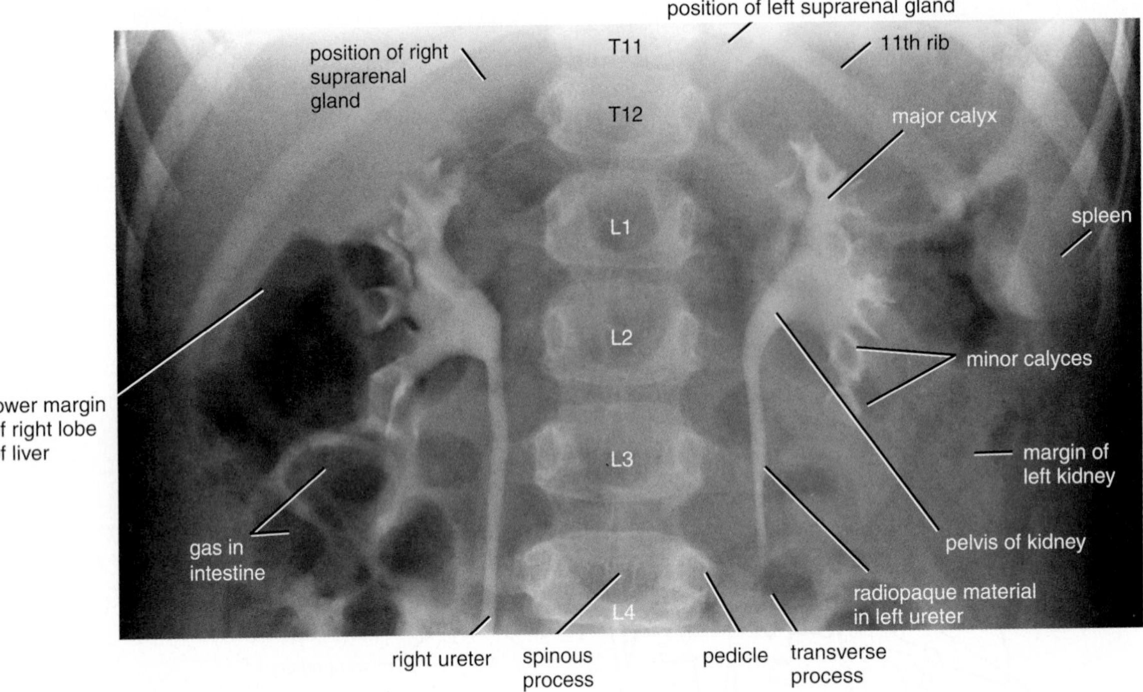

Figure 5-96 Anteroposterior radiograph of both kidneys 15 minutes after intravenous injection of an iodine-containing compound. The calyces, the renal pelvis, and the upper parts of the ureters are clearly seen (5-year-old girl).

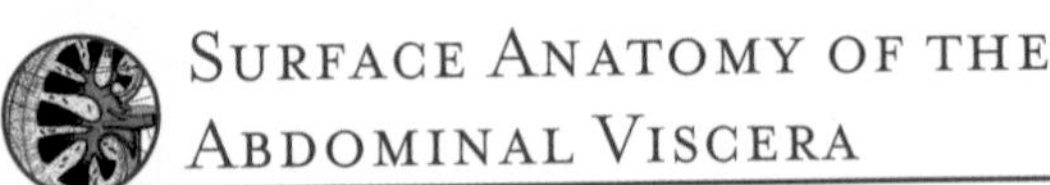

Surface Anatomy of the Abdominal Viscera

The surface anatomy of the abdominal viscera is fully described on page 192.

CLINICAL PROBLEM SOLVING

Study the following case histories and select the best answers to the question following them.

A 45-year-old man was admitted to the emergency department complaining of severe pain in the right lower quadrant of the anterior abdominal wall. He had repeatedly vomited, and his temperature and pulse rate were elevated. His history indicated that he had acute appendicitis and that the pain had suddenly increased. On examination, the muscles of the lower part of the anterior abdominal wall in the right lower quadrant showed rigidity. The diagnosis of peritonitis after perforation of the appendix was made.

1. The symptoms and signs displayed by this patient can be explained by the following statements except which?
   (a) The perforation of the appendix had resulted in the spread of the infection from the appendix to involve the parietal peritoneum.
   (b) The parietal peritoneum in the right iliac region, the muscles of the anterior abdominal wall, and the overlying skin are all supplied by the segmental nerves T12 and L1.
   (c) Irritation of the parietal peritoneum reflexly increases the tone of the abdominal muscles, causing rigidity.
   (d) The greater omentum tends to become stuck down to the appendix and restricts the spread of infection.
   (e) The pain was intensified after perforation of the appendix because of stimulation of the autonomic pain endings in the parietal peritoneum.

A 63-year-old man with a long history of a duodenal ulcer was seen in the emergency department after vomiting blood-stained fluid and exhibiting all the signs and symptoms of severe hypovolemic shock.

2. The following statements concerning duodenal ulcers could apply to the patient's condition except which?
   (a) Hemorrhage from a duodenal ulcer often reveals itself by the passage of black stools on defecation.
   (b) The pyloric sphincter prevents most of the blood from the duodenal lumen from passing up into the stomach.
   (c) The gastroduodenal artery lies behind the first part of the duodenum and was probably eroded by the ulcer.
   (d) The gastroduodenal artery is a small branch of the hepatic artery.

(e) The duodenal ulcer was most likely to be situated on the posterior wall of the first part of the duodenum.

A 47-year-old woman was operated on for the treatment of a chronic gastric ulcer that had not responded to medical treatment. At operation for partial gastrectomy, it was found that the posterior wall of the stomach was stuck down to the posterior abdominal wall. The surgeon had to proceed with great care to avoid damaging important structures lying on the posterior abdominal wall.

3. The following structures located on the posterior abdominal wall were possibly involved in the disease process except which?
   (a) The right kidney
   (b) The pancreas
   (c) The left suprarenal gland
   (d) The left kidney
   (e) The lesser sac of peritoneum
   (f) The splenic artery

A 58-year-old man was in a restaurant when he suddenly started to vomit blood. He was taken unconscious to the emergency department of a local hospital. On examination, he had all the signs of severe hypovolemic shock. On palpation of the anterior abdominal wall, the right lobe of the liver was felt three fingerbreadths below the costal margin. Several enlarged superficial veins could be seen around the umbilicus. His wife said that he had vomited blood 3 months previously and had nearly died. She admitted that he was a chronic alcoholic. The diagnosis was cirrhosis of the liver secondary to chronic alcoholism.

4. The symptoms and signs displayed by this patient can be explained by the following statements except which?
   (a) The normal flow of portal blood through the liver is impaired by cirrhosis of the liver.
   (b) The portal–systemic anastomoses become enlarged in this condition.
   (c) At the lower end of the esophagus, a branch from the right gastric vein anastomoses with an esophageal tributary of the azygos vein.
   (d) Rupture of a varicosed esophageal vein could produce a severe hemorrhage so that the patient would vomit up blood.
   (e) With portal hypertension the paraumbilical veins linking the superficial veins of the skin (systemic veins) to the portal vein become congested and visible.

A 55-year-old woman with a history of flatulent dyspepsia suddenly experienced an excruciating colicky pain across the upper part of the abdomen. On examination in the emergency department, she was found to have some rigidity and tenderness in the right upper quadrant. A diagnosis of biliary colic was made.

5. The following statements would explain this patient's symptoms except which?
   (a) The pain of gallstone colic is caused by spasm of the smooth muscle in the wall of the gallbladder and distention of the bile ducts by the stones.
   (b) The pain fibers from the gallbladder and bile ducts ascend through the superior mesenteric plexus and the greater splanchnic nerves to enter the thoracic segments of the spinal cord.
   (c) Referred pain is felt in the right upper quadrant or the epigastrium.
   (d) T7 through T9 dermatomes are involved.
   (e) The violent contractions of the gallbladder wall are attempts to expel the gallstones.

On examination of the abdomen of a 31-year-old woman, a large swelling was found to extend downward and medially below the left costal margin. On percussion, a continuous band of dullness was noted to extend upward from the left of the umbilicus to the left axillary region. On palpation, a notch was felt along the anterior border of the swelling. A diagnosis of splenic enlargement was made.

6. The signs displayed by this patient can be explained by the following statements except which?
   (a) The spleen has a notched anterior border caused by incomplete fusion of its parts during development.
   (b) Because of the presence of the left colic flexure and the phrenicocolic ligament, the spleen is unable to expand vertically downward.
   (c) A pathologically enlarged spleen extends downward and forward, toward the umbilicus.
   (d) The spleen is situated in the upper left quadrant of the abdomen beneath the diaphragm.
   (e) The long axis of the spleen lies along the 12th rib.

A 48-year-old woman with a history of repeated vomiting was admitted to the hospital with a diagnosis of large bowel obstruction. To decompress the stomach a nasogastric tube was passed.

7. When passing a nasogastric tube some important anatomic statements should be considered except which?
   (a) The well-lubricated tube is inserted through the wider nostril.
   (b) The tube is directed backward along the nasal floor and not upward because it may become caught on the nasal choanae.
   (c) The distance between the nostril and the cardiac orifice of the stomach is about 23 in. (57.5 cm).
   (d) The distance between the cardiac orifice and the pylorus is 4.8 to 5.6 in. (12 to 14 cm).
   (e) Esophageal narrowing may offer resistance to the tube behind the cricoid cartilage, 7.21 in. (18 cm) from the nostril.
   (f) The left bronchus and the arch of the aorta cross in front of the esophagus and may impede the descent of the tube, 11.2 in. (28 cm) from the nostril.
   (g) Where the esophagus enters the stomach is a slight resistance to the descent of the tube.

A 16-year-old boy received a severe kick in the right flank while playing football at school. On examination in the emergency department, his right flank was severely bruised, and his right costovertebral angle was extremely tender on palpation. A specimen of urine showed microscopic hematuria. A diagnosis of damage to the right kidney was made.

8. The following statements concerning blunt trauma to the kidney are correct except which?
   (a) The kidney tends to be crushed between the 12th rib and the vertebral column.
   (b) The kidney can be injured by fractures of the 12th rib (right kidney) or 11th and 12th ribs (left kidney).

(c) In most patients the kidney damage is mild and results in nothing more than microscopic hematuria, as in this patient.
(d) In severe kidney lacerations, extensive hemorrhage and extravasation of blood and urine into the pararenal fat occurs.
(e) In severe kidney lacerations, a mass caused by extravasated blood and urine behind the peritoneum may be palpated, especially on the right side.
(f) Both kidneys lie on the posterior abdominal wall and are at the same vertebral level.

A 17-year-old boy was involved in a gang fight. It started as an argument but quickly worsened into a street brawl with the use of knives. He was examined in the emergency department and found to have a bleeding stab wound in his left flank. A urine specimen revealed frank blood.

9. Stab wounds of the kidneys involve other abdominal organs in a high percentage of cases. Of the organs listed, which one is least likely to be damaged in this patient?
   (a) Stomach
   (b) Spleen
   (c) Inferior vena cava
   (d) Left colic flexure
   (e) Left suprarenal gland
   (f) Coils of jejunum
   (g) Body of the pancreas

A 56-year-old man visited his physician complaining that he experiences severe pain in both legs when taking long walks. He noticed recently that the cramplike pain occurs after walking only a hundred yards. On questioning, he said that the pain quickly disappears on rest only to return after he walks the same distance. When the physician asked about his sex life the patient admitted that he was experiencing difficulty with erection.

10. The symptoms and signs displayed by this patient can be explained by the following statements except which?
   (a) Arteriography of the abdominal aorta revealed blockage in the region of the bifurcation.
   (b) Only the right common iliac artery was involved by disease.
   (c) The gradual blockage of the aorta was caused by advanced arteriosclerosis.
   (d) An insufficient amount of blood was reaching both legs, causing pain (claudication) on walking.
   (e) The lack of blood entering both internal iliac arteries was responsible for the difficulty with erection.

A 23-year-old woman, who was 8 months pregnant, told her obstetrician that she had recently noticed that her feet and ankles were swollen at the end of the day. She said that the swelling was worse if she had been standing for long periods. She also noticed that the veins around her ankles were becoming prominent.

11. The symptoms and signs displayed by this patient can be explained by the following statements except which?
   (a) The enlarged uterus is an abdominal organ and often compresses the inferior vena cava.
   (b) Venous back pressure causes the tissue fluid to accumulate in the subcutaneous tissues of the feet and ankles.
   (c) Venous back pressure impairs the venous return in the superficial veins in both the legs, leading to varicose veins.
   (d) High levels of progesterone in the blood during pregnancy cause the smooth muscle in the wall of the veins to relax, thus permitting the veins to dilate.
   (e) The pregnant uterus presses on the sympathetic trunks, causing vasodilatation of the blood vessels of the legs.

A 27-year-old woman was involved in a head-on automobile accident. When examined in a neighboring hospital, she was in a state of severe shock, with a rapid pulse and low blood pressure. Extensive bruising was seen on the lower part of the anterior abdominal wall. Further examination showed that the abdomen was becoming rapidly distended. Exploratory surgery revealed a ruptured abdominal aorta.

12. The following statements concerning this case would explain her clinical condition except which?
   (a) The patient was wearing a seat belt, which explained the bruising on the anterior abdominal wall.
   (b) The aorta is located on the posterior abdominal wall lateral to the left side of the vertebral column.
   (c) The aorta lies behind the peritoneum in the retroperitoneal space.
   (d) The blood did not immediately escape into the peritoneal cavity because it is retroperitoneal in position and the tear was small in size.
   (e) A seat belt may hold the patient securely in the seat, but in some individuals the kidneys continue forward after impact and the renal artery may be torn from the side of the aorta.

ANSWERS TO CLINICAL PROBLEMS

1. E. In the parietal peritoneum lining the anterior abdominal wall in the right iliac fossa, the sensation of pain originates in the nerve endings of somatic spinal nerves (T12 and L1).
2. D. The gastroduodenal artery is a large branch of the hepatic artery.
3. A
4. C. At the lower end of the esophagus, a branch from the left gastric vein anastomoses with an esophageal tributary of the azygos vein.
5. B. The pain fibers from the gallbladder and bile ducts ascend through the celiac plexus.
6. E. The long axis of the spleen lies along the 10th rib.
7. C. The distance between the nostril and the cardiac orifice of the stomach is about 17.2 in. (44 cm).
8. F. Because of the large size of the right lobe of the liver, the right kidney lies at a lower level than the left kidney.
9. C

10. B. The blockage of the aorta in the region of the bifurcation had effectively blocked the entrances into both common iliac arteries.
11. E. The sympathetic trunks are not pressed on by the pregnant uterus.
12. B. The aorta descends through the abdomen behind the peritoneum on the anterior surface of the bodies of the lumbar vertebrae.

REVIEW QUESTIONS

Multiple-Choice Questions

Select the best answer for each question.

1. The following statements concerning the liver are correct except which?
   (a) The quadrate lobe drains into the right hepatic duct.
   (b) The lesser omentum suspends the stomach from the visceral surface of the liver.
   (c) The left triangular ligament of the liver lies anterior to the abdominal part of the esophagus.
   (d) The attachment of the hepatic veins to the inferior vena cava is one of the most important supports of the liver.
   (e) The ligamentum venosum is attached to the left branch of the portal vein in the porta hepatis.
2. The following statements concerning the pancreas are correct except which?
   (a) The pancreas receives part of the arterial supply from the splenic artery.
   (b) The main pancreatic duct opens into the third part of the duodenum.
   (c) The uncinate process of the pancreas projects from the head of the pancreas.
   (d) The bile duct (common bile duct) lies posterior to the head of the pancreas.
   (e) The transverse mesocolon is attached to the anterior border of the pancreas.
3. The following statements concerning the ileum are correct except which?
   (a) The circular smooth muscle of the lower end of the ileum serves as a sphincter at the junction of the ileum and the cecum.
   (b) The branches of the superior mesenteric artery serving the ileum form more arcades than those serving the jejunum.
   (c) Peyer's patches are present in the mucous membrane of the lower ileum along the antimesenteric border.
   (d) The plicae circulares are more prominent at the distal end of the ileum than in the jejunum.
   (e) The parasympathetic innervation of the ileum is from the vagus nerves.
4. The hilum of the right kidney contains the following important structures except which?
   (a) The renal pelvis
   (b) Tributaries of the renal vein
   (c) Sympathetic nerve fibers
   (d) Part of the right suprarenal gland
   (e) Branches of the renal artery
5. The following statements concerning the left suprarenal gland are correct except which?
   (a) The gland extends along the medial border of the left kidney from the upper pole to the hilus.
   (b) The gland's vein drains into the left renal vein.
   (c) The gland is separated from the left kidney by perirenal fat.
   (d) The gland lies behind the lesser sac of peritoneum.
   (e) The medulla is innervated by postganglionic sympathetic nerve fibers.
6. The following statements concerning the abdominal aorta are correct except which?
   (a) The aorta bifurcates into the two common iliac arteries in front of the fourth lumbar vertebra.
   (b) The aorta lies on the right side of the inferior vena cava.
   (c) From the aorta's anterior surface arise the celiac, superior mesenteric, and inferior mesenteric arteries.
   (d) The aorta enters the abdomen in front of the 12th thoracic vertebra.
   (e) The thoracic duct leaves the abdomen through the aortic opening of the diaphragm on the right side of the aorta.
7. The following statements concerning the abdominal part of the sympathetic trunk are correct except which?
   (a) The trunk enters the abdomen from behind the medial arcuate ligament.
   (b) The trunk possesses four or five segmentally arranged ganglia.
   (c) All the ganglia receive white rami communicantes.
   (d) Gray rami communicantes are given off to the lumbar spinal nerves.
   (e) Nerve fibers pass medially to the sympathetic plexuses on the abdominal aorta and its branches.
8. The following statements concerning the lumbar plexus are correct except which?
   (a) The plexus lies within the psoas muscle.
   (b) The plexus is formed from the posterior rami of the upper four lumbar nerves.
   (c) The femoral nerve emerges from the lateral border of the psoas muscle.
   (d) The obturator nerve emerges from the medial border of the psoas muscle.
   (e) The iliohypogastric nerve emerges from the lateral border of the psoas muscle.
9. The following veins form important portal–systemic anastomoses except which?
   (a) Esophageal branches of the left gastric vein and tributaries of the azygos veins
   (b) Superior rectal vein and inferior vena cava

(c) Paraumbilical veins and superficial veins of the anterior abdominal wall
(d) Veins of the ascending and descending parts of the colon with the lumbar veins
(e) Veins from the bare areas of the liver with the phrenic veins

10. The following statements concerning the ureters are correct except which?
(a) Both ureters have three anatomic sites that are constricted.
(b) Both ureters receive their blood supply from the testicular or ovarian arteries.
(c) Both ureters are separated from the transverse processes of the lumbar vertebrae by the psoas muscles.
(d) Both ureters pass anterior to the testicular or ovarian vessels.
(e) Both ureters lie anterior to the sacroiliac joints.

11. The following statements concerning the inferior mesenteric artery are correct except which?
(a) The mesenteric artery's colic branch supplies the descending colon.
(b) The mesenteric artery gives off the inferior pancreaticoduodenal artery.
(c) The mesenteric artery supplies the sigmoid colon.
(d) The mesenteric artery's branches contribute to the marginal artery.
(e) The mesenteric artery arises from the aorta immediately below the third part of the duodenum.

12. The following structures are present within the lesser omentum except which?
(a) The portal vein
(b) The bile duct
(c) The inferior vena cava
(d) The hepatic artery
(e) The lymph nodes

Matching Questions

Match the numbered structures shown on the posteroanterior radiograph of the stomach and small intestine—after ingestion of a barium meal—with the appropriate lettered structures (38-year-old male).

13. Structure 1

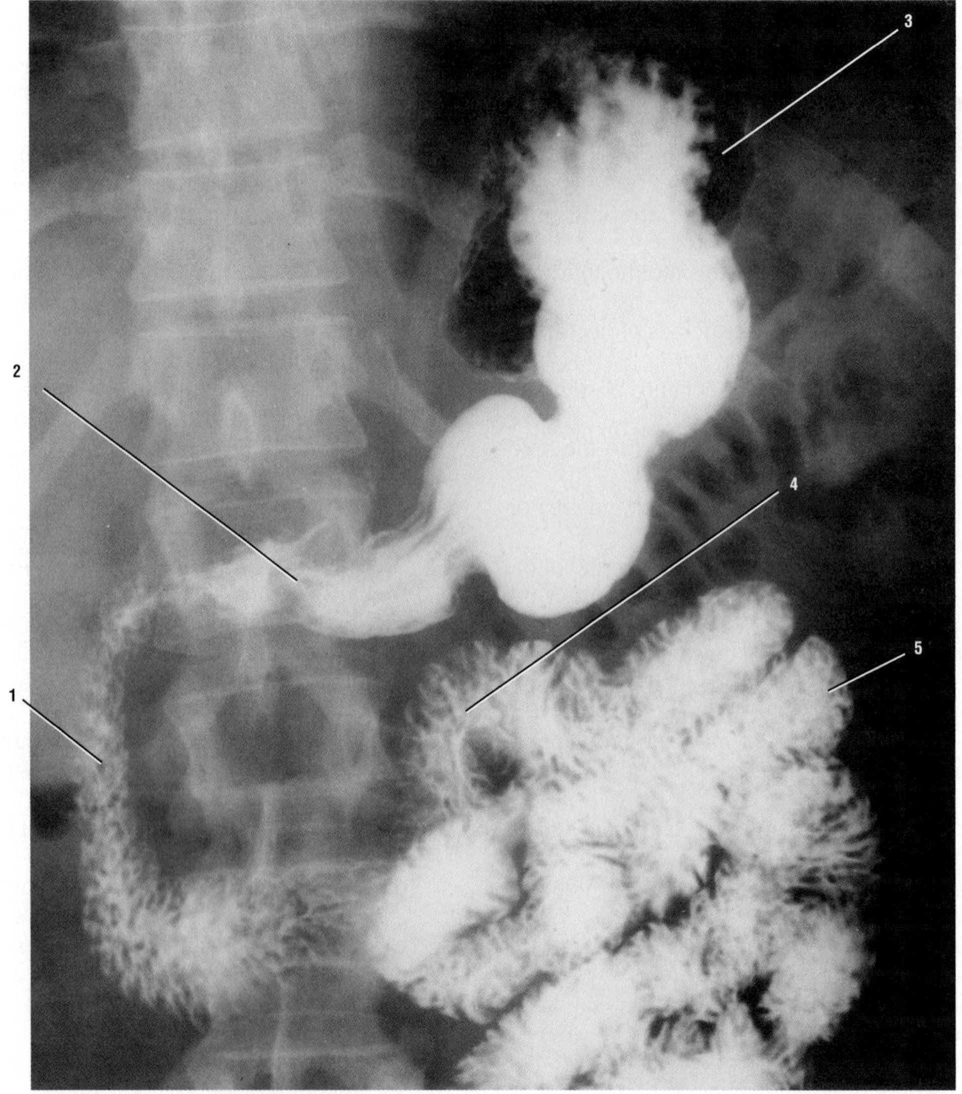

14. Structure 2
15. Structure 3
16. Structure 4
17. Structure 5
    (a) First part of duodenum
    (b) Second part of duodenum
    (c) Third part of duodenum
    (d) Air-filled fundus of stomach
    (e) Jejunum
    (f) Pylorus of stomach
    (g) None of the above

Match the numbered structures shown on the posteroanterior radiograph of the large intestine—after evacuation of a barium enema—with the appropriate lettered lymphatic drainage (20-year-old female).

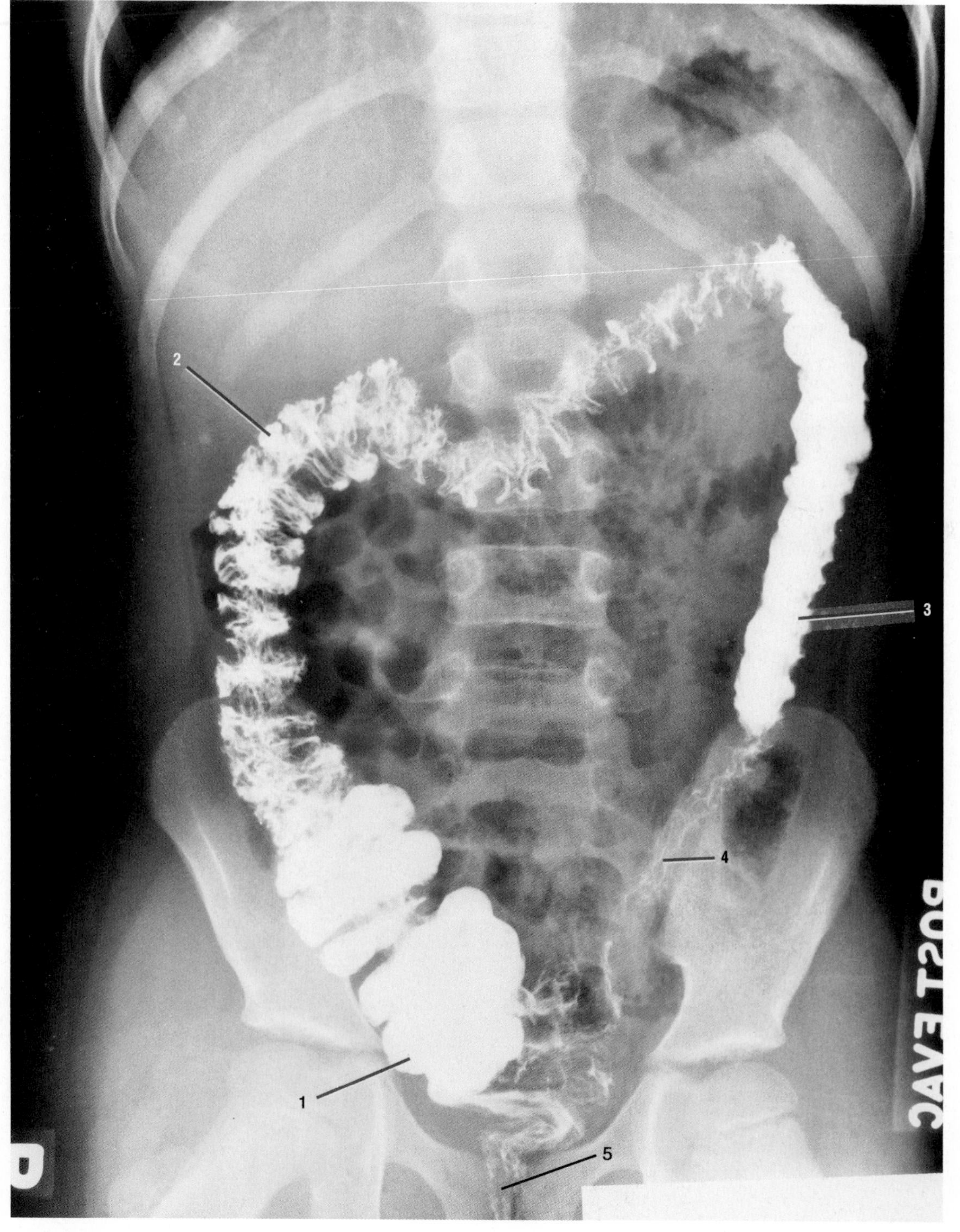

18. Structure 1
19. Structure 2
20. Structure 3
21. Structure 4
22. Structure 5
    (a) Appendix
    (b) Splenic flexure
    (c) Transverse colon
    (d) Cecum
    (e) Rectum
    (f) Sigmoid colon
    (g) Descending colon
    (h) None of the above

Match the numbered structures shown on the intravenous pyelogram—obtained 20 minutes after injection of a suitable contrast medium—with the appropriate lettered structure (5-year-old female).

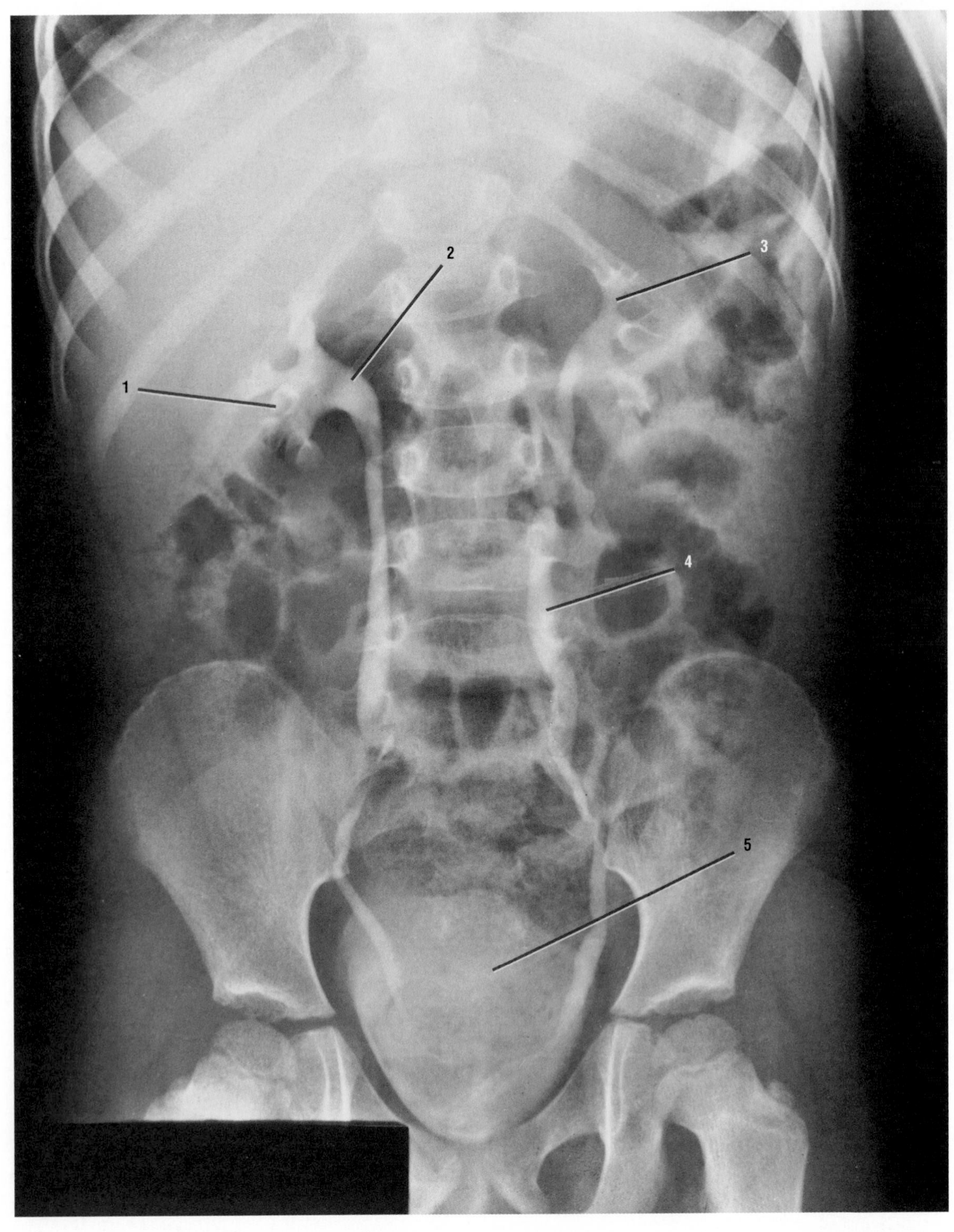

23. Structure 1
24. Structure 2
25. Structure 3
26. Structure 4
27. Structure 5
    (a) Rectum
    (b) Pelvis of ureter
    (c) Sacrum
    (d) Ureter
    (e) Urinary bladder
    (f) Major calyx
    (g) None of the above

Multiple-Choice Questions

Read the case histories and select the best answer to the question following them.

A mother took her 20-day-old baby boy to a pediatrician because he had started to vomit after his feeds. The baby was breast-fed. For the first 15 days after birth, the baby had taken his feeds very well and had slept contentedly in his crib following the normal after-feed burp. However, in the previous 5 days, the baby had begun to vomit toward the end of each feed, shooting the milk out of his mouth for a distance of 1 to 2 ft. After carefully questioning the mother and after a physical examination of the boy, the pediatrician made the diagnosis of congenital hypertrophic pyloric stenosis.

28. He was able to ascertain the following additional signs and symptoms except which?
    (a) Once the milk had been vomited, the child immediately would feed again, only to repeat the same performance.
    (b) On gentle palpation of the anterior abdominal wall, a small firm swelling was felt just below and medial to the tip of the left eighth costal cartilage.
    (c) On observing the anterior abdominal wall, an occasional wave of gastric peristalsis was seen traveling across the epigastrium from left to right.
    (d) The stools were small in quantity and infrequent.
    (e) The child showed signs of dehydration as evidenced by a depressed anterior fontanelle of the skull.

A 6-year-old girl was examined by a pediatrician because she had a history of recurrent pain in the region of the umbilicus. The pain was dull and aching in nature and lasted for about 1 week. It had recurred on four occasions in the previous 2 years. Then, 2 days before the examination, the child had severe rectal bleeding and had fainted.

29. On examination of the child, the pediatrician found the following signs and symptoms consistent with the diagnosis of Meckel's diverticulum except which?
    (a) Tenderness of the anterior abdominal wall in the right iliac region
    (b) Anemia
    (c) Stools streaked with dark red blood
    (d) Pyrexia of 102°F

ANSWERS TO REVIEW QUESTIONS

1. A. The quadrate lobe and the caudate lobe are in fact parts of the left lobe. Thus, the right and left branches of the hepatic artery and portal vein and the right and left hepatic ducts are distributed to the right lobe and the left lobe plus the quadrate and caudate lobes.

2. B. The main pancreatic duct opens into the second part of the duodenum, at about its middle, with the bile duct on the major duodenal papilla. Sometimes, the main duct drains separately into the duodenum.

3. D. The plicae circulares are absent from the distal end of the ileum.

4. D. The right suprarenal gland caps the upper pole of the right kidney and does not extend downward to the hilum of the kidney.

5. E. The medulla of the suprarenal gland is innervated by preganglionic sympathetic nerve fibers.

6. B. The abdominal aorta lies on the left side of the inferior vena cava.

7. C. The white rami communicantes join the first two ganglia to the first two lumbar spinal nerves.

8. B. The lumbar plexus is formed from the anterior rami of the upper four lumbar spinal nerves.

9. B. The superior rectal veins (tributaries of the portal vein) anastomose with the middle and inferior rectal veins (systemic tributaries).

10. D. The ureters are crossed on their anterior surfaces by the testicular and ovarian vessels.

11. B. The inferior pancreaticoduodenal artery is a branch of the superior mesenteric artery.

12. C. The inferior vena cava lies on the posterior abdominal wall behind the parietal peritoneum. It is separated from the lesser omentum by the epiploic foramen.

13. B

14. F

15. D

16. G. The duodenojejunal junction

17. E

18. D

19. H. Right colic flexure

20. G

21. F

22. E

23. G. Minor calyx
24. B
25. F
26. D
27. E
28. B. In congenital hypertrophic pyloric stenosis, there is a localized muscular hypertrophy and hyperplasia of the pyloric sphincter, which is larger than normal and can usually be palpated just below and medial to the tip of the right ninth costal cartilage.
29. D. In many cases of Meckel's diverticulum, a small area of ectopic gastric mucosa is present, which is capable of producing hydrochloric acid and pepsin. In the adjoining mucous membrane, this child had a chronic ulcer that was responsible for the umbilical pain. Sudden severe hemorrhage from an artery in the floor of the ulcer was the cause of the rectal bleeding and fainting attack. The condition is not associated with a pyrexia. After restoration of the blood volume and hemoglobin to a normal level, a child with this condition should be operated on and the diverticulum should be widely excised. The cut ends of the ileum then are joined by an end-to-end anastomosis.

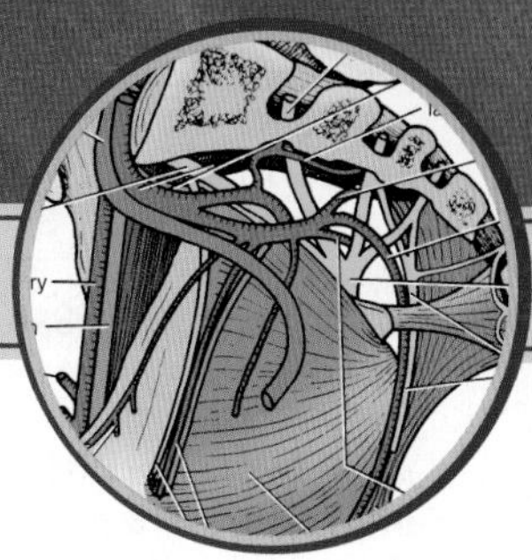

CHAPTER 6

THE PELVIS: PART I—THE PELVIC WALLS

A 51-year-old man was involved in a light-plane accident. He was flying home from a business trip when, because of fog, he had to make a forced landing in a plowed field. On landing, the plane came abruptly to rest on its nose. His companion was killed on impact, and he was thrown from the cockpit. On admission to the emergency department, he was unconscious and showed signs of severe hypovolemic (loss of circulating blood) shock. He had extensive bruising of the lower part of the anterior abdominal wall, and the front of his pelvis was prominent on the right side. During examination of the penis, it was possible to express a drop of blood-stained fluid from the external orifice. No evidence of external hemorrhage was present.

Radiographic examination of the pelvis showed a dislocation of the symphysis pubis and a linear fracture through the lateral part of the sacrum on the right side. The urethra was damaged by the shearing forces applied to the pelvic area, which explained the blood-stained fluid from the external orifice of the penis. The pelvic radiograph (later confirmed on computed tomography scan) also revealed the presence of a large collection of blood in the loose connective tissue outside the peritoneum, which was caused by the tearing of the large, thin-walled pelvic veins by the fractured bone and accounted for the hypovolemic shock.

This patient illustrates the fact that in-depth knowledge of the anatomy of the pelvic region is necessary before a physician can even contemplate making an initial examination and start treatment in cases of pelvic injury.

CHAPTER OUTLINE

Basic Anatomy 308
The Pelvis 308
Orientation of the Pelvis 308
False Pelvis 309
True Pelvis 309
Structure of the Pelvic Walls 310
Anterior Pelvic Wall 310
Posterior Pelvic Wall 310
Lateral Pelvic Wall 316
Inferior Pelvic Wall, or Pelvic Floor 318
Pelvic Diaphragm 318
Pelvic Fascia 319
Parietal Pelvic Fascia 319
Visceral Layer of Pelvic Fascia 321
Pelvic Peritoneum 321
Nerves of the Pelvis 325
Sacral Plexus 325
Branches of the Lumbar Plexus 326
Autonomic Nerves 327
Arteries of the Pelvis 327
Common Iliac Artery 327
External Iliac Artery 328
Arteries of the True Pelvis 328
Internal Iliac Artery 328
Veins of the Pelvis 329
External Iliac Vein 329
Internal Iliac Vein 329
Median Sacral Veins 329
Lymphatics of the Pelvis 329
Joints of the Pelvis 329
Sacroiliac Joints 329
Symphysis Pubis 329
Sacrococcygeal Joint 329
Sex Differences of the Pelvis 330
Radiographic Anatomy 330
Surface Anatomy 330
Surface Landmarks 330
Iliac Crest 330
Anterior Superior Iliac Spine 330
Posterior Superior Iliac Spine 330
Pubic Tubercle 330
Pubic Crest 330
Symphysis Pubis 330
Spinous Processes of Sacrum 330
Sacral Hiatus 330
Coccyx 330
Viscera 330
Urinary Bladder 330
Uterus 332
Rectal and Vaginal Examinations as a Means of Palpating the Pelvic Viscera 332
Clinical Problem Solving 334
Answers to Clinical Problems 335
Review Questions 335
Answers to Review Questions 336

CHAPTER OBJECTIVES

- The pelvis is a bowl-shaped bony structure that protects the terminal parts of the gastrointestinal tract and the urinary system and the male and female internal organs of reproduction.
- It also contains important nerves, blood vessels, and lymphatic tissues.
- The purpose of this chapter is to review the significant anatomy of the pelvic walls relative to clinical problems. Particular attention is paid to age and sexual differences and to the anatomic features associated with pelvic examinations.

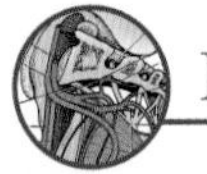

Basic Anatomy

The pelvis* is the region of the trunk that lies below the abdomen. Although the abdominal and pelvic cavities are continuous, the two regions are described separately.

The Pelvis

The bony pelvis's main function is to transmit the weight of the body from the vertebral column to the femurs. In addition, it contains, supports, and protects the pelvic viscera and provides attachment for trunk and lower limb muscles. The bony pelvis is composed of four bones: the two **hip bones,** which form the lateral and anterior walls, and the **sacrum** and the **coccyx,** which are part of the vertebral column and form the back wall (Fig. 6-1).

The two hip bones articulate with each other anteriorly at the **symphysis pubis** and posteriorly with the sacrum at the **sacroiliac joints.** The bony pelvis thus forms a strong basin-shaped structure that contains and protects the lower parts of the intestinal and urinary tracts and the internal organs of reproduction.

The pelvis is divided into two parts by the **pelvic brim,** which is formed by the **sacral promontory** (anterior and upper margin of the first sacral vertebra) behind, the **iliopectineal lines** (a line that runs downward and forward around the inner surface of the ileum) laterally, and the **symphysis pubis** (joint between bodies of pubic bones) anteriorly. Above the brim is the **false pelvis,** which forms part of the abdominal cavity. Below the brim is the **true pelvis.**

Orientation of the Pelvis

It is important for the student, at the outset, to understand the correct orientation of the bony pelvis relative to the trunk, with the individual standing in the anatomic position. The front of the symphysis pubis and the anterior superior iliac spines should lie in the same vertical plane. This means

*The term **pelvis** is loosely used to describe the region where the trunk and lower limbs meet. The word **pelvis** means "a basin" and is more correctly applied to the skeleton of the region—that is, the pelvic girdle or bony pelvis.

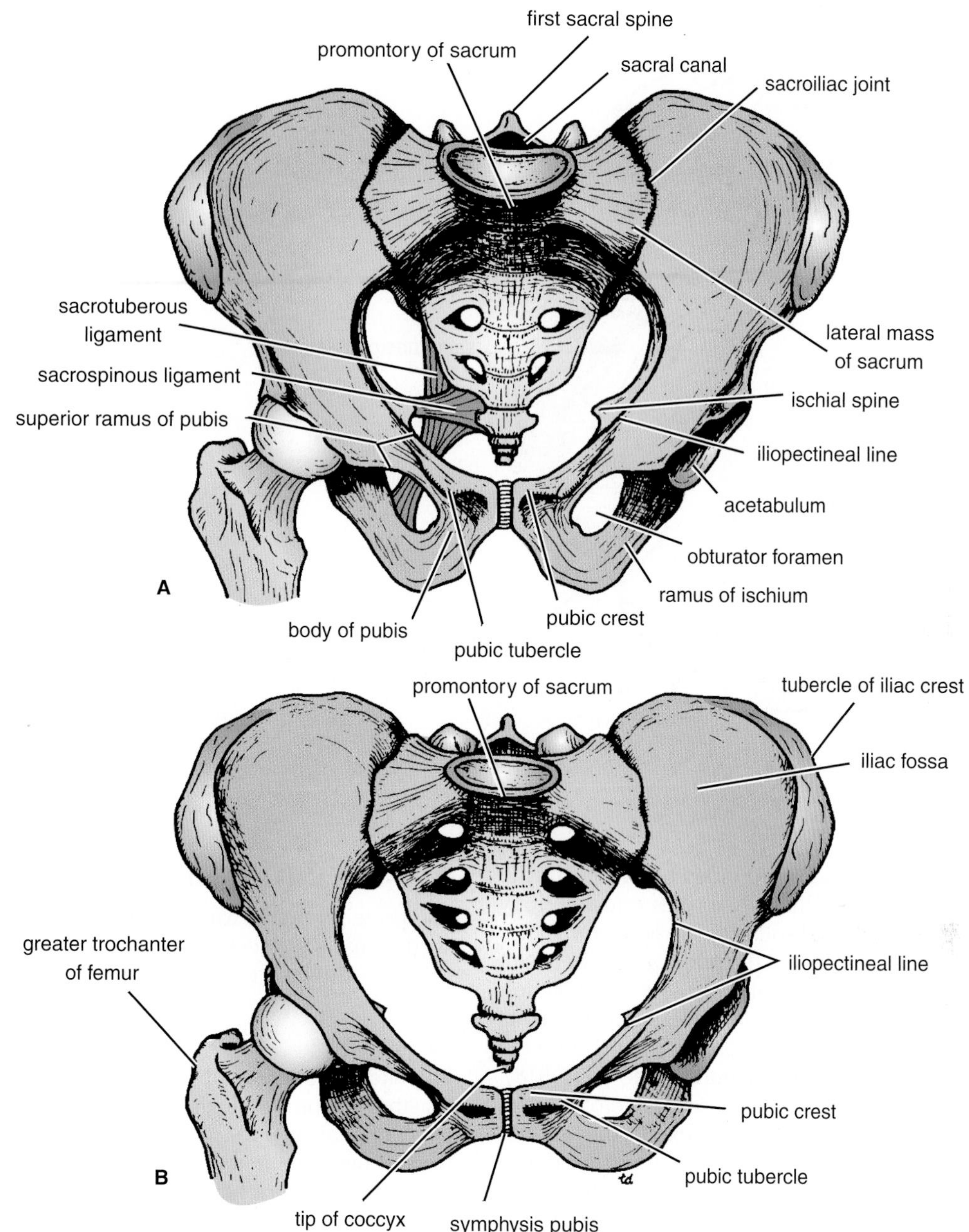

Figure 6-1 Anterior view of the male pelvis **(A)** and female pelvis **(B).**

that the pelvic surface of the symphysis pubis faces upward and backward and the anterior surface of the sacrum is directed forward and downward.

False Pelvis

The false pelvis is of little clinical importance. It is bounded behind by the lumbar vertebrae, laterally by the iliac fossae and the iliacus muscles, and in front by the lower part of the anterior abdominal wall. The false pelvis flares out at its upper end and should be considered as part of the abdominal cavity. It supports the abdominal contents and after the third month of pregnancy helps support the gravid uterus. During the early stages of labor, it helps guide the fetus into the true pelvis.

True Pelvis

Knowledge of the shape and dimensions of the female pelvis is of great importance for obstetrics, because it is the bony canal through which the child passes during birth.

The true pelvis has an inlet, an outlet, and a cavity.

- The **pelvic inlet,** or **pelvic brim** (Fig. 6-2), is bounded posteriorly by the sacral promontory, laterally by the iliopectineal lines, and anteriorly by the symphysis pubis (Fig. 6-1).

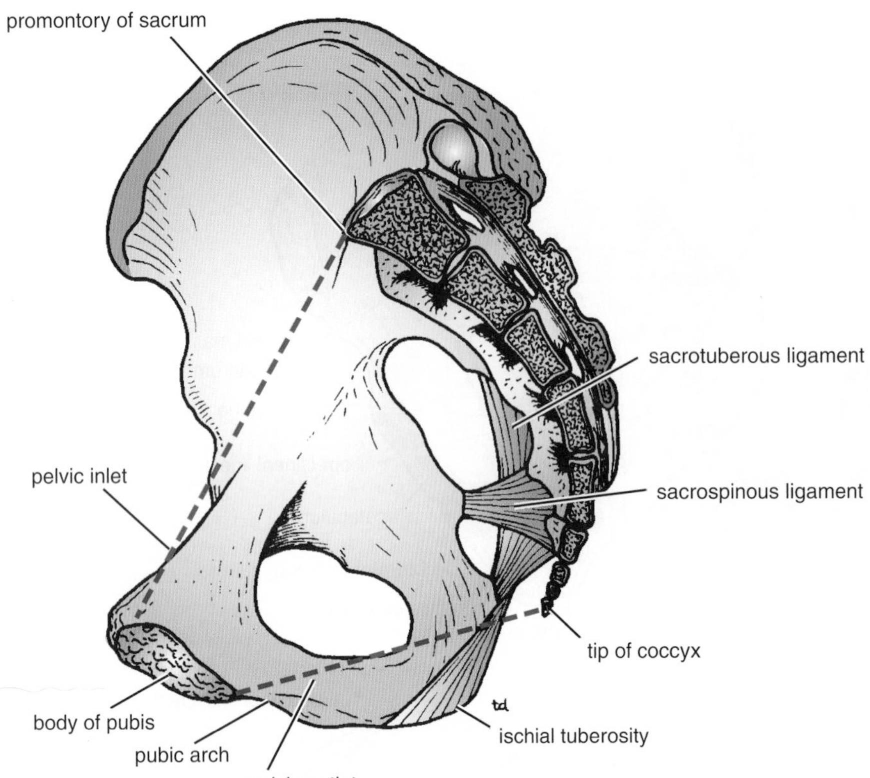

Figure 6-2 Right half of the pelvis showing the pelvic inlet, pelvic outlet, and sacrotuberous and sacrospinous ligaments.

- The **pelvic outlet** (Fig. 6-2) is bounded posteriorly by the coccyx, laterally by the ischial tuberosities, and anteriorly by the **pubic arch** (Figs. 6-2 and 6-3). The pelvic outlet has three wide notches. Anteriorly, the pubic arch is between the ischiopubic rami, and laterally are the sciatic notches. The sciatic notches are divided by the **sacrotuberous** and **sacrospinous ligaments** (Figs. 6-1 and 6-2) into the **greater** and **lesser sciatic foramina** (see page 318). From an obstetric standpoint, because the sacrotuberous ligaments are strong and relatively inflexible, they should be considered to form part of the perimeter of the pelvic outlet. Thus, the outlet is diamond shaped, with the ischiopubic rami and the symphysis pubis forming the boundaries in front and the sacrotuberous ligaments and the coccyx forming the boundaries behind.
- The **pelvic cavity** lies between the inlet and the outlet. It is a short, curved canal, with a shallow anterior wall and a much deeper posterior wall (Fig. 6-2).

Structure of the Pelvic Walls

The walls of the pelvis are formed by bones and ligaments that are partly lined with muscles covered with fascia and parietal peritoneum. The pelvis has anterior, posterior, and lateral walls and an inferior wall or floor (Fig. 6-6).

Anterior Pelvic Wall

The anterior pelvic wall is the shallowest wall and is formed by the bodies of the pubic bones, the pubic rami, and the symphysis pubis (Fig. 6-7).

Posterior Pelvic Wall

The posterior pelvic wall is extensive and is formed by the sacrum and coccyx (Fig. 6-8) and by the piriformis muscles (Fig. 6-9) and their covering of parietal pelvic fascia.

Sacrum

The sacrum consists of five rudimentary vertebrae fused together to form a single wedge-shaped bone with a forward concavity (Figs. 6-2 and 6-8). The upper border or base of the bone articulates with the fifth lumbar vertebra. The narrow inferior border articulates with the coccyx. Laterally, the sacrum articulates with the two iliac bones to form the **sacroiliac joints** (Fig. 6-1). The anterior and upper margins of the first sacral vertebra bulge forward as the posterior margin of the pelvic inlet—the **sacral promontory** (Fig. 6-2)—which is an important obstetric landmark used when measuring the size of the pelvis.

The vertebral foramina together form the **sacral canal.** The laminae of the fifth sacral vertebra, and sometimes those of the fourth, fail to meet in the midline, forming the sacral hiatus (Fig. 6-8). The sacral canal contains the anterior and posterior roots of the lumbar, sacral, and coccygeal spinal nerves; the filum terminale; and fibrofatty material. It also contains the lower part of the subarachnoid space down as far as the lower border of the second sacral vertebra (Fig. 6-10).

The anterior and posterior surfaces of the sacrum possess on each side four foramina for the passage of the anterior and posterior rami of the upper four sacral nerves (Fig. 6-8).

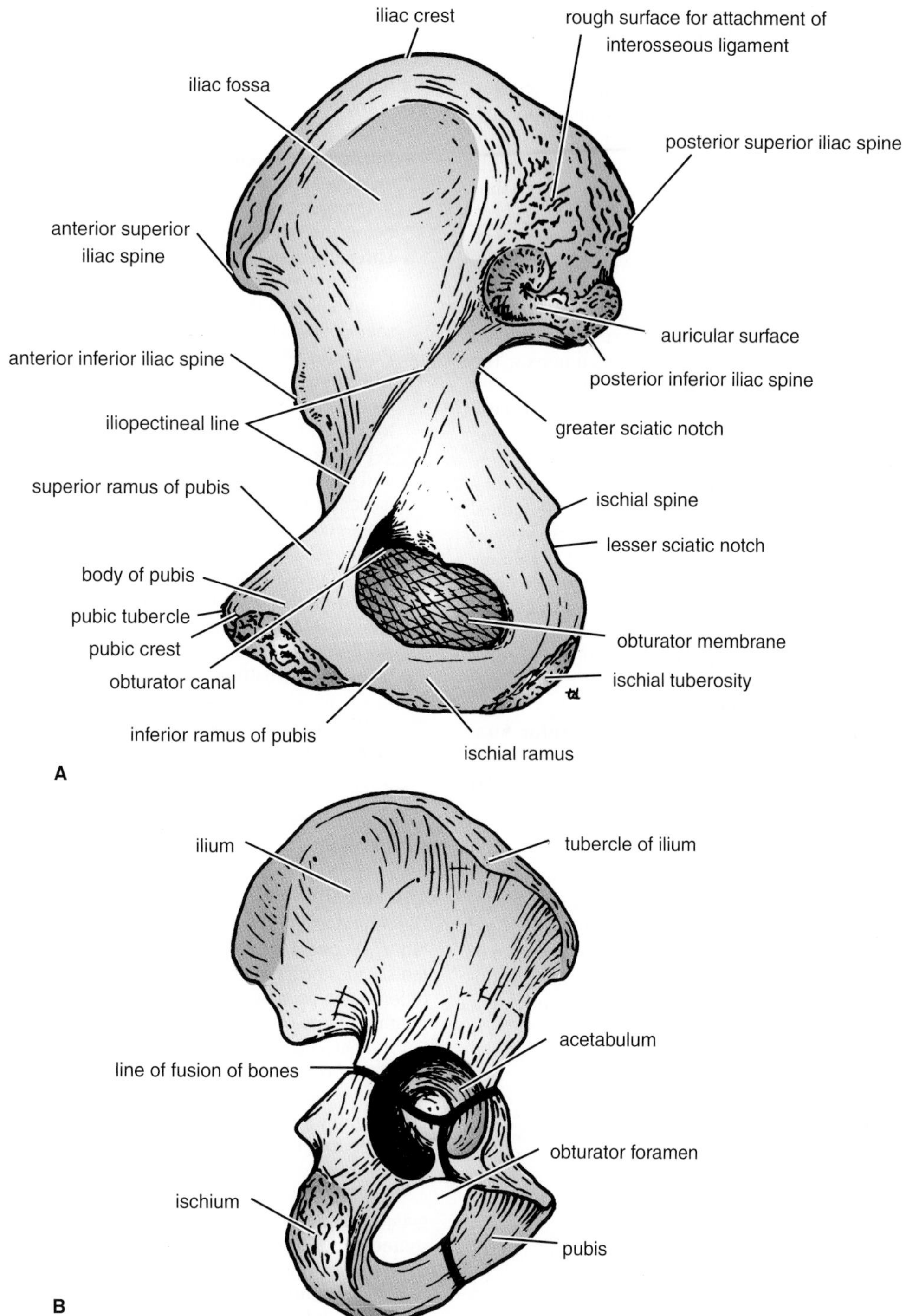

Figure 6-3 Right hip bone. **A.** Medial surface. **B.** Lateral surface. Note the lines of fusion between the three bones—the ilium, the ischium, and the pubis.

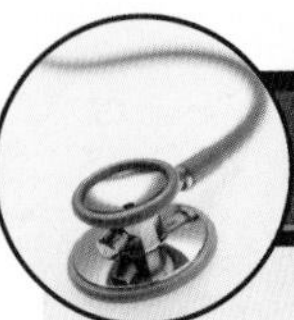

CLINICAL NOTES

Clinical Concept: The Pelvis Is a Basin with Holes in Its Walls

The walls of the pelvis are formed by bones and ligaments; these are partly lined with muscles (obturator internus and piriformis) covered with fascia and parietal peritoneum. On the outside of the pelvis are the attachments of the gluteal muscles and the obturator externus muscle. The greater part of the bony pelvis is thus sandwiched between inner and outer muscles.

The basin has anterior, posterior, and lateral walls and an inferior wall or floor formed by the important levator ani and coccygeus muscles and their covering fascia.

The basin has many holes: The posterior wall has holes on the anterior surface of the sacrum, the **anterior sacral foramina,** for the passage of the anterior rami of the sacral spinal nerves. The **sacrotuberous** and **sacrospinous ligaments** convert the greater and lesser sciatic notches into the **greater** and **lesser sciatic foramina.** The greater sciatic foramen provides an exit from the true pelvis into the gluteal region for the sciatic nerve, the pudendal nerve, and the gluteal nerves and vessels; the lesser sciatic foramen provides an entrance into the perineum from the gluteal region for the pudendal nerve and the internal pudendal vessels. (One can make a further analogy here: For the wires to gain entrance to the apartment below, without going through the floor, they have to pierce the wall [greater sciatic foramen] to get outside the building and then return through a second hole [lesser sciatic foramen]. In the case of the human body, the pudendal nerve and internal pudendal vessels are the wires and the levator ani and the coccygeus muscles are the floor.)

The lateral pelvic wall has a large hole, the **obturator foramen,** which is closed by the **obturator membrane,** except for a small opening that permits the obturator nerve to leave the pelvis and enter the thigh.

Pelvic Measurements in Obstetrics

The capacity and shape of the female pelvis are of fundamental importance in obstetrics. The female pelvis is well adapted for the process of childbirth. The pelvis is shallower and the bones are smoother than in the male. The size of the pelvic inlet is similar in the two sexes, but in the female, the cavity is larger and cylindrical and the pelvic outlet is wider in both the anteroposterior and the transverse diameters.

Four terms relating to areas of the pelvis are commonly used in clinical practice:

- The **pelvic inlet** or **brim** of the true pelvis (Fig. 6-4) is bounded anteriorly by the symphysis pubis, laterally by the iliopectineal lines, and posteriorly by the sacral promontory.
- The **pelvic outlet** of the true pelvis (Fig. 6-4) is bounded in front by the pubic arch, laterally by the ischial tuberosities, and posteriorly by the coccyx. The sacrotuberous ligaments also form part of the margin of the outlet.
- The **pelvic cavity** is the space between the inlet and the outlet (Fig. 6-4).
- The **axis of the pelvis** is an imaginary line joining the central points of the anteroposterior diameters from the inlet to the outlet and is the curved course taken by the baby's head as it descends through the pelvis during childbirth (Figs. 6-4 and 6-5A).

Internal Pelvic Assessments

Internal pelvic assessments are made by vaginal examination during the later weeks of pregnancy, when the pelvic tissues are softer and more yielding than in the newly pregnant condition.

- **Pubic arch:** Spread the fingers under the pubic arch and examine its shape. Is it broad or angular? The examiner's four fingers should be able to rest comfortably in the angle below the symphysis.
- **Lateral walls:** Palpate the lateral walls and determine whether they are concave, straight, or converging. The prominence of the ischial spines and the position of the sacrospinous ligaments are noted.
- **Posterior wall:** The sacrum is palpated to determine whether it is straight or well curved. Finally, if the patient has relaxed the perineum sufficiently, an attempt is made to palpate the promontory of the sacrum. The second finger of the examining hand is placed on the promontory, and the index finger of the free hand, outside the vagina, is placed at the point on the examining hand where it makes contact with the lower border of the symphysis. The fingers are then withdrawn and the distance measured (Fig. 6-5B), providing the measurement of the **diagonal conjugate,** which is normally about 5 in. (13 cm). The anteroposterior diameter from the sacrococcygeal joint to the lower border of the symphysis is then estimated.
- **Ischial tuberosities:** The distance between the ischial tuberosities may be estimated by using the closed fist (Fig. 6-5D). It measures about 4 in. (10 cm), but it is difficult to measure exactly.

Needless to say, considerable clinical experience is required to be able to assess the shape and size of the pelvis by vaginal examination.

The Female Pelvis

Deformities of the pelvis may be responsible for **dystocia** (difficult labor). A contracted pelvis may obstruct the normal passage of the fetus. It may be indirectly responsible for dystocia by causing conditions such as malpresentation or malposition of the fetus, premature rupture of the fetal membranes, and uterine inertia.

The cause of pelvic deformities may be congenital (rare) or acquired from disease, poor posture, or fractures caused by injury. Pelvic deformities are more common in women who have grown up in a poor environment and are undernourished. It is probable that these women suffered in their youth from minor degrees of rickets.

In 1933, Caldwell and Moloy classified pelves into four groups: gynecoid, android, anthropoid, and platypelloid (Fig. 6-5C). The **gynecoid** type, present in about 41% of women, is the typical female pelvis, which was previously described.

The **android** type, present in about 33% of white females and 16% of black females, is the male or funnel-shaped pelvis with a contracted outlet.

The **anthropoid** type, present in about 24% of white females and 41% of black females, is long, narrow, and oval shaped.

The **platypelloid** type, present in only about 2% of women, is a wide pelvis flattened at the brim, with the promontory of the sacrum pushed forward.

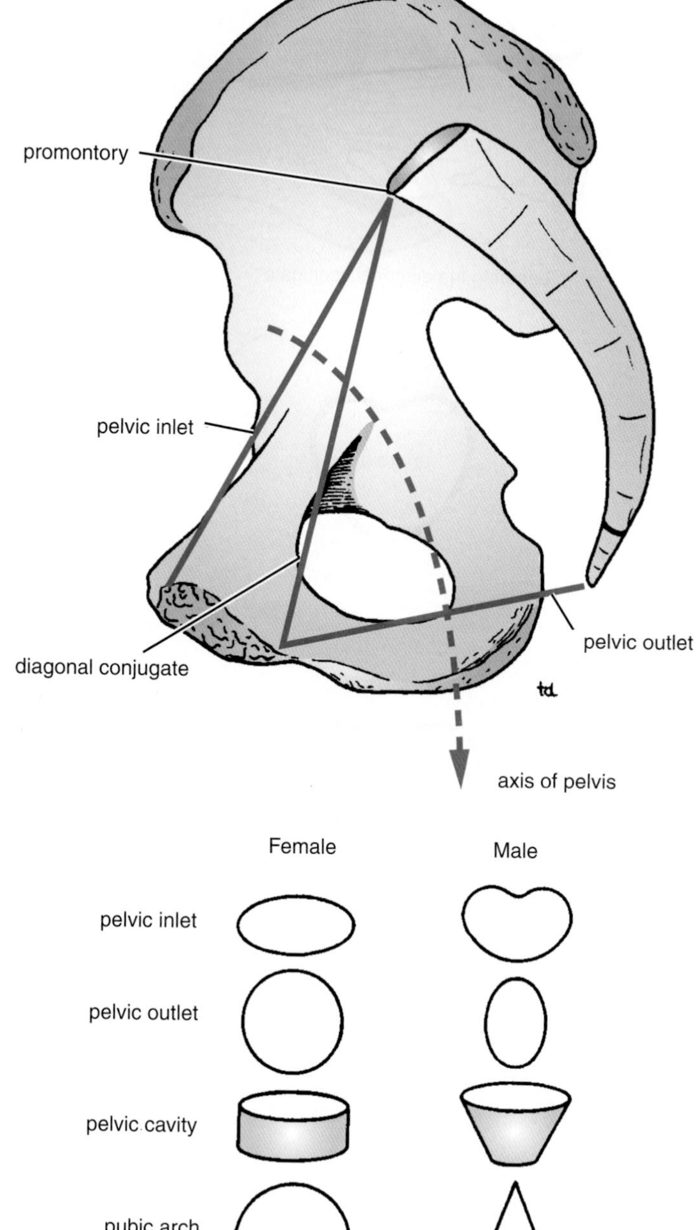

Figure 6-4 Pelvic inlet, pelvic outlet, diagonal conjugate, and axis of the pelvis. Some of the main differences between the female and the male pelvis are also shown.

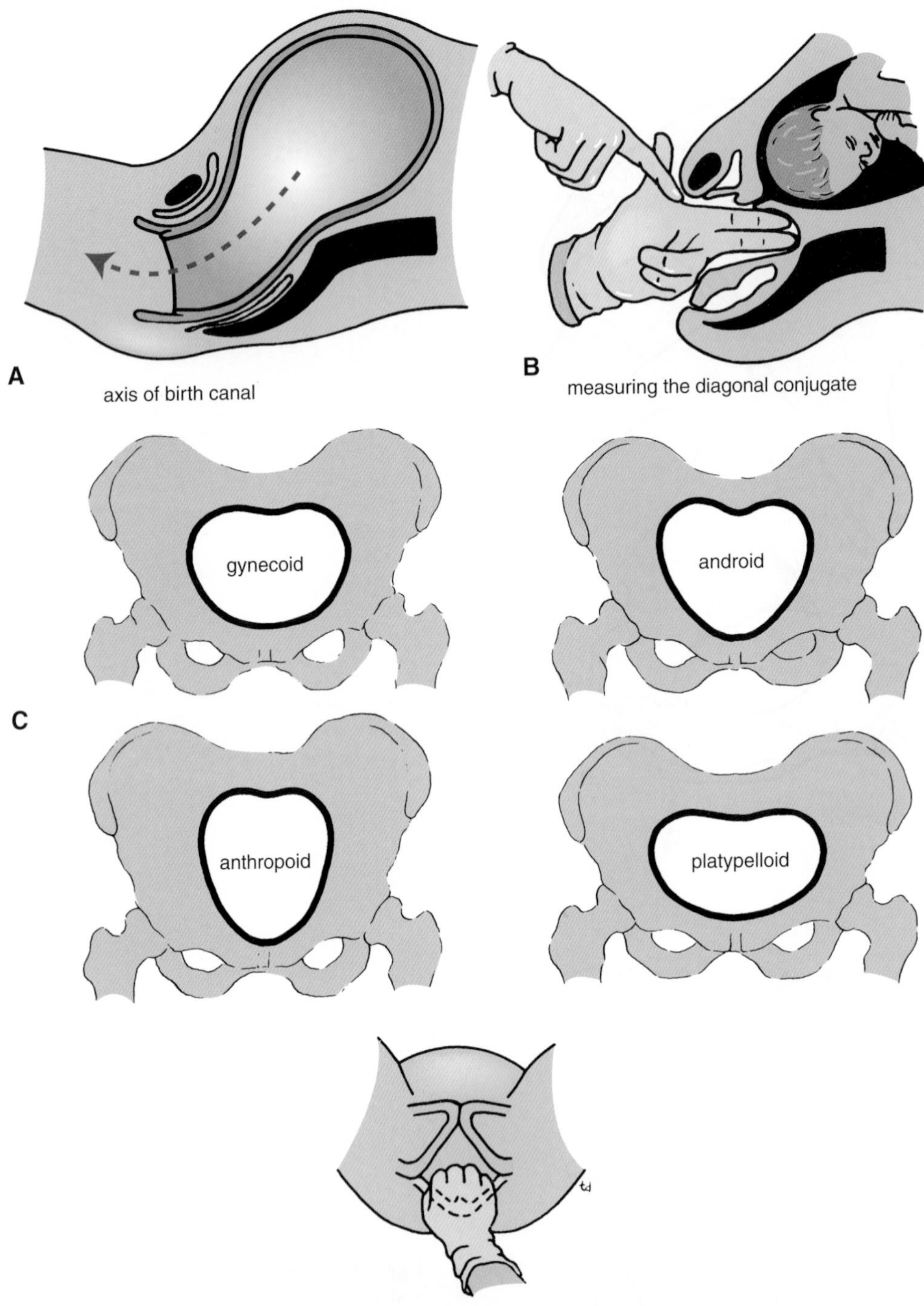

Figure 6-5 **A.** Birth canal. Interrupted line indicates the axis of the canal. **B.** Procedure used in measuring the diagonal conjugate. **C.** Different types of pelvic inlets, according to Caldwell and Moloy. **D.** Estimation of the width of the pelvic outlet by means of a closed fist.

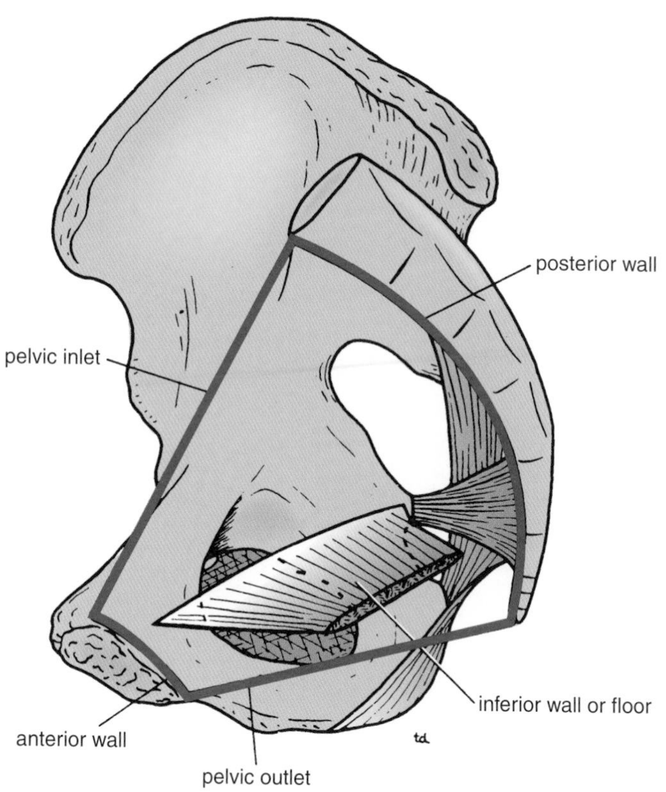

Figure 6-6 Right half of the pelvis showing the pelvic walls.

The sacrum is usually wider in proportion to its length in the female than in the male. The sacrum is tilted forward so that it forms an angle with the fifth lumbar vertebra, called the **lumbosacral angle.**

Coccyx

The coccyx consists of four vertebrae fused together to form a small triangular bone, which articulates at its base with the lower end of the sacrum (Fig. 6-8).

The coccygeal vertebrae consist of bodies only, but the first vertebra possesses a rudimentary **transverse process** and **cornua.** The cornua are the remains of the pedicles and superior articular processes and project upward to articulate with the sacral cornua (Fig. 6-8).

Piriformis Muscle

The piriformis muscle arises from the front of the lateral mass of the sacrum and leaves the pelvis to enter the gluteal

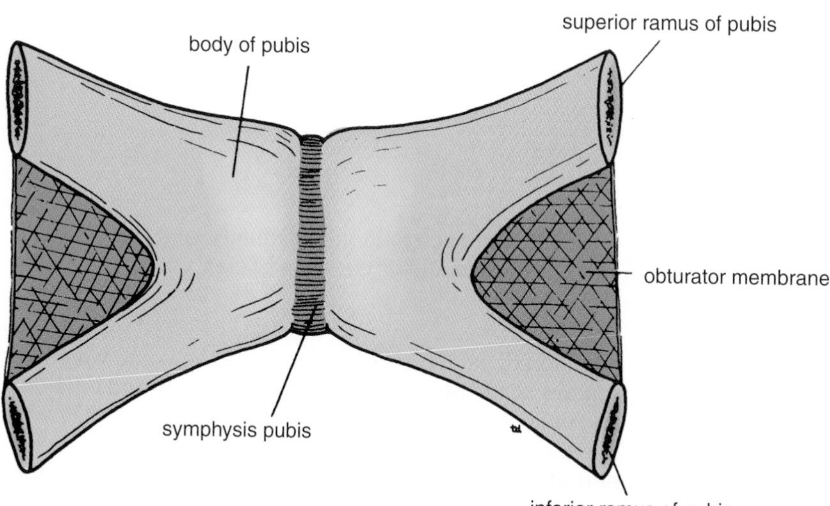

Figure 6-7 Anterior wall of the pelvis (posterior view).

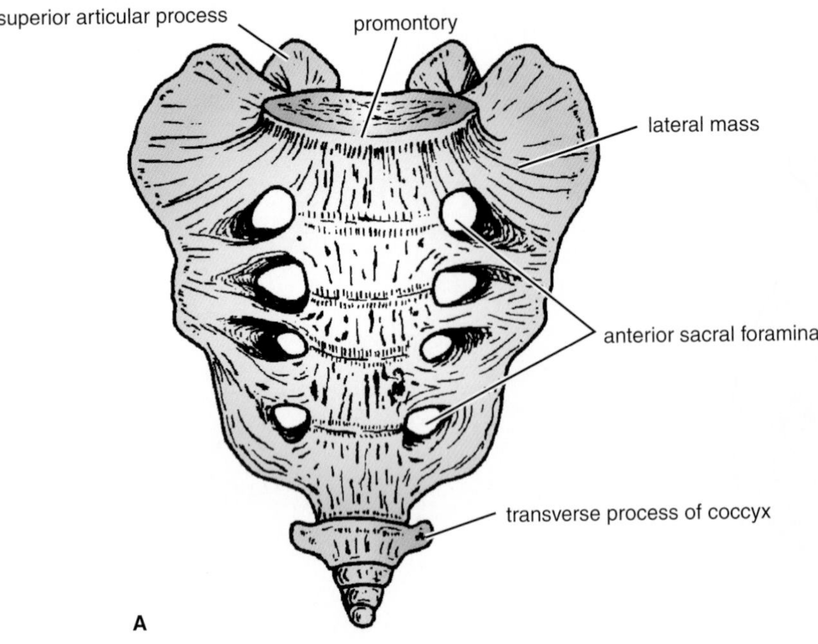

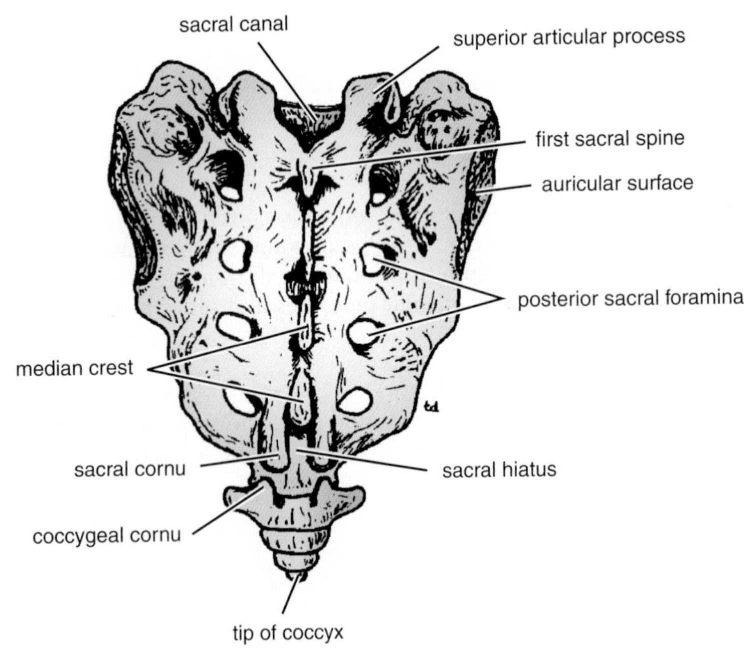

Figure 6-8 Sacrum. **A.** Anterior view. **B.** Posterior view.

region by passing laterally through the greater sciatic foramen (Fig. 6-9). It is inserted into the upper border of the greater trochanter of the femur.

- **Action:** It is a lateral rotator of the femur at the hip joint.
- **Nerve supply:** It receives branches from the sacral plexus.

Lateral Pelvic Wall

The lateral pelvic wall is formed by part of the hip bone below the pelvic inlet, the obturator membrane, the sacrotuberous and sacrospinous ligaments, and the obturator internus muscle and its covering fascia.

Hip Bone

In children, each hip bone consists of the ilium, which lies superiorly; the ischium, which lies posteriorly and inferiorly; and the pubis, which lies anteriorly and inferiorly (Fig. 6-3). The three separate bones are joined by cartilage at the **acetabulum.** At puberty, these three bones fuse together to form one large, irregular bone. The hip bones articulate with the sacrum at the sacroiliac joints and form the anterolateral

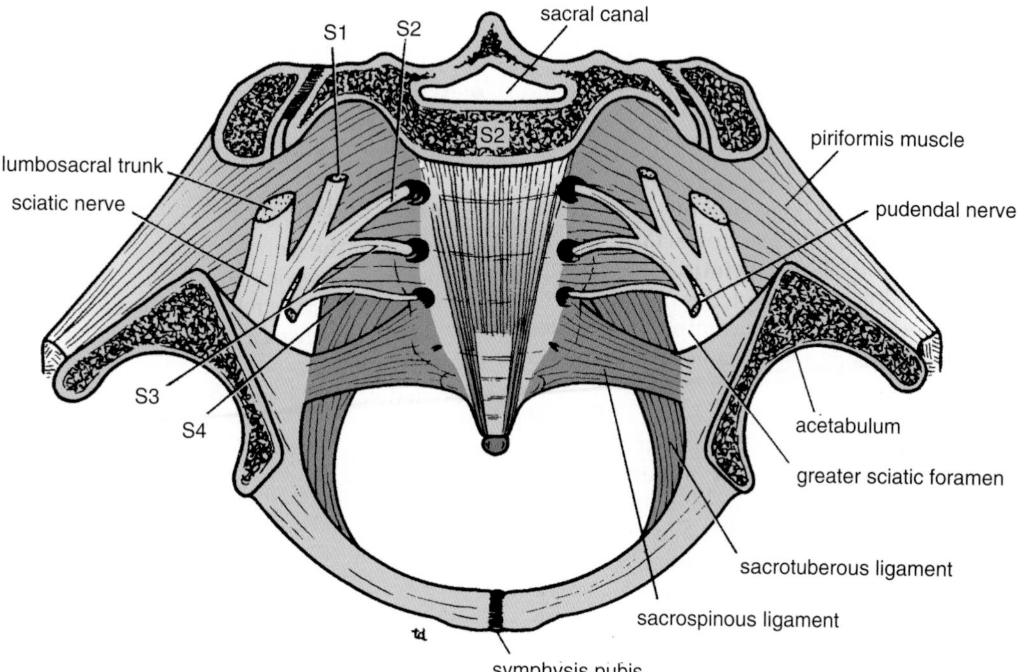

Figure 6-9 Posterior wall of the pelvis.

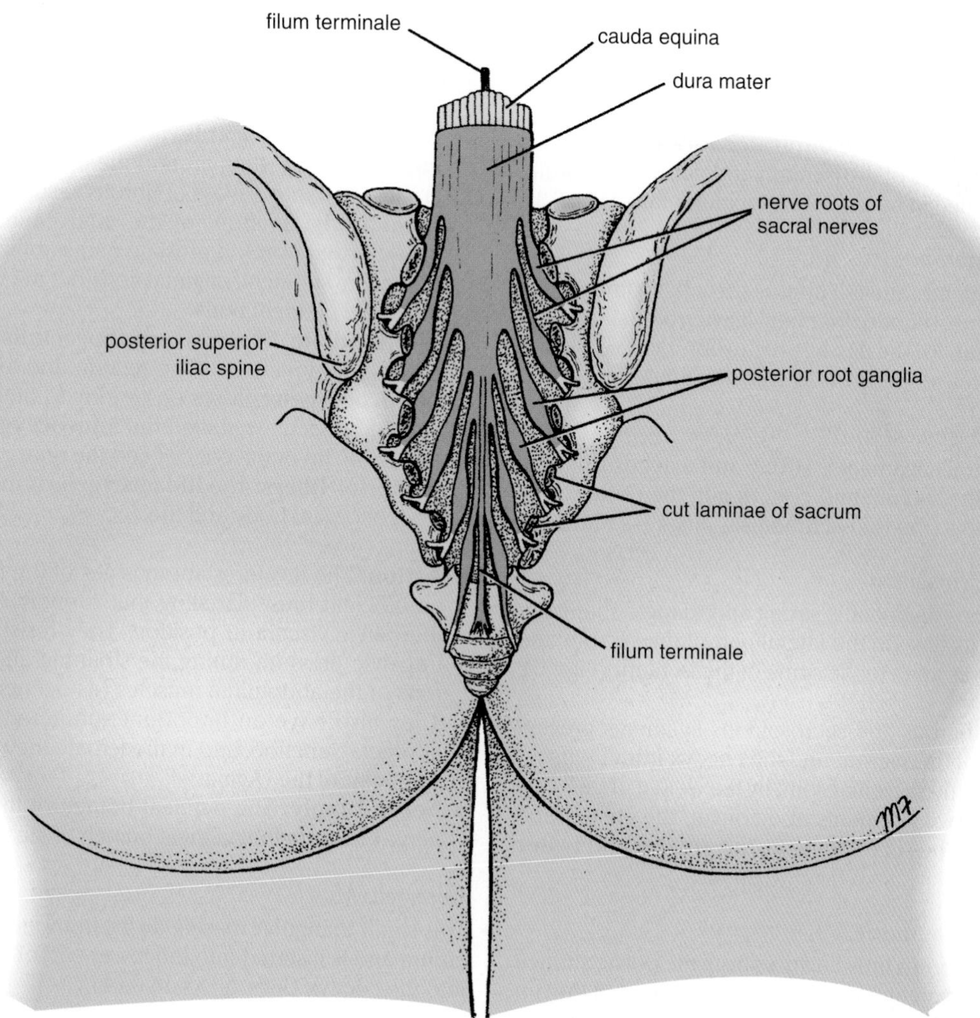

Figure 6-10 Sacrum from behind. Laminae have been removed to show the sacral nerve roots lying within the sacral canal. Note that in the adult the spinal cord ends below, at the level of the lower border of the first lumbar vertebra.

walls of the pelvis; they also articulate with one another anteriorly at the symphysis pubis.

On the outer surface of the hip bone is a deep depression, the **acetabulum,** which articulates with the hemispherical head of the femur (Figs. 6-1 and 6-3). Behind the acetabulum is a large notch, the **greater sciatic notch,** which is separated from the **lesser sciatic notch** by the **spine of the ischium.** The sciatic notches are converted into the **greater** and **lesser sciatic foramina** by the presence of the **sacrotuberous** and **sacrospinous ligaments** (Fig. 6-2).

The **ilium,** which is the upper flattened part of the hip bone, possesses the **iliac crest** (Fig. 6-3). The iliac crest runs between the **anterior** and **posterior superior iliac spines.** Below these spines are the corresponding anterior and posterior inferior iliac spines. On the inner surface of the ilium is the large **auricular surface** for articulation with the sacrum. The **iliopectineal line** runs downward and forward around the inner surface of the ilium and serves to divide the false from the true pelvis.

The **ischium** is the inferior and posterior part of the hip bone and possesses an **ischial spine** and an **ischial tuberosity** (Fig. 6-3).

The **pubis** is the anterior part of the hip bone and has a **body** and **superior** and **inferior pubic rami.** The body of the pubis bears the **pubic crest** and the **pubic tubercle** and articulates with the pubic bone of the opposite side at the **symphysis pubis** (Fig. 6-1). In the lower part of the hip bone is a large opening, the **obturator foramen,** which is bounded by the parts of the ischium and pubis. The obturator foramen is filled in by the obturator membrane (Fig. 6-3).

Obturator Membrane

The obturator membrane is a fibrous sheet that almost completely closes the obturator foramen, leaving a small gap, the **obturator canal,** for the passage of the obturator nerve and vessels as they leave the pelvis to enter the thigh (Fig. 6-3).

Sacrotuberous Ligament

The sacrotuberous ligament is strong and extends from the lateral part of the sacrum and coccyx and the posterior inferior iliac spine to the ischial tuberosity (Figs. 6-2 and 6-9).

Sacrospinous Ligament

The sacrospinous ligament is strong and triangle shaped. It is attached by its base to the lateral part of the sacrum and coccyx and by its apex to the spine of the ischium (Figs. 6-2 and 6-9).

The sacrotuberous and sacrospinous ligaments prevent the lower end of the sacrum and the coccyx from being rotated upward at the sacroiliac joint by the weight of the body (Fig. 6-11). The two ligaments also convert the greater and lesser sciatic notches into foramina, the **greater** and **lesser sciatic foramina.**

Obturator Internus Muscle

The obturator internus muscle arises from the pelvic surface of the obturator membrane and the adjoining part of the hip bone (Fig. 6-12). The muscle fibers converge to a tendon, which leaves the pelvis through the lesser sciatic foramen and is inserted into the greater trochanter of the femur.

- **Action:** It laterally rotates the femur at the hip joint.
- **Nerve supply:** The nerve to the obturator internus, a branch from the sacral plexus

Inferior Pelvic Wall, or Pelvic Floor

The floor of the pelvis supports the pelvic viscera and is formed by the pelvic diaphragm.

The pelvic floor stretches across the pelvis and divides it into the main pelvic cavity above, which contains the pelvic viscera, and the perineum below. The perineum is considered in detail in Chapter 8.

Pelvic Diaphragm

The pelvic diaphragm is formed by the important levatores ani muscles and the small coccygeus muscles and their covering fasciae (Fig. 6-13). It is incomplete anteriorly to allow passage of the urethra in males and the urethra and the vagina in females.

Levator Ani Muscle

The levator ani muscle is a wide thin sheet that has a linear origin from the back of the body of the pubis, a tendinous arch formed by a thickening of the fascia covering the obturator internus, and the spine of the ischium (Fig. 6-13). From this extensive origin, groups of fibers sweep downward and medially to their insertion (Fig. 6-14), as follows:

1. **Anterior fibers:** The **levator prostatae** or **sphincter vaginae** form a sling around the prostate or vagina and are inserted into a mass of fibrous tissue, called the **perineal body,** in front of the anal canal. The levator prostatae support the prostate and stabilize the perineal body. The sphincter vaginae constrict the vagina and stabilize the perineal body.
2. **Intermediate fibers:** The **puborectalis** forms a sling around the junction of the rectum and anal canal. The **pubococcygeus** passes posteriorly to be inserted into a small fibrous mass, called the **anococcygeal body,** between the tip of the coccyx and the anal canal.
3. **Posterior fibers:** The **iliococcygeus** is inserted into the anococcygeal body and the coccyx.

- **Action:** The levatores ani muscles of the two sides form an efficient muscular sling that supports and maintains the pelvic viscera in position. They resist the rise in intrapelvic pressure during the straining and expulsive efforts of the abdominal muscles (as occurs in coughing). They also have an important sphincter action on the anorectal junction, and in the female they serve also as a sphincter of the vagina.
- **Nerve supply:** The perineal branch of the fourth sacral nerve and from the perineal branch of the pudendal nerve

Coccygeus Muscle

This small triangular muscle arises from the spine of the ischium and is inserted into the lower end of the sacrum and into the coccyx (Figs. 6-13 and 6-14).

- **Action:** The two muscles assist the levatores ani in supporting the pelvic viscera.

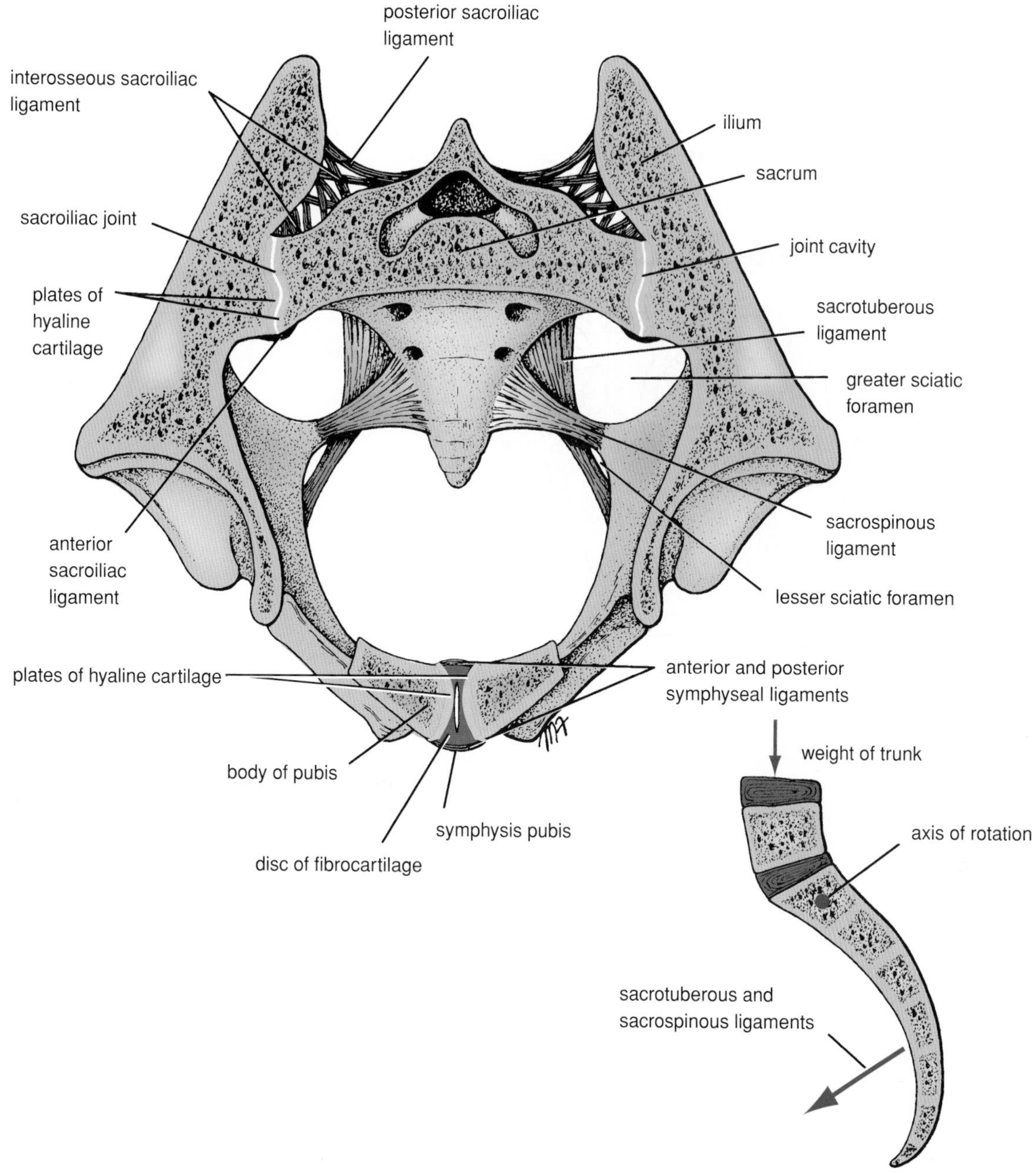

Figure 6-11 Horizontal section through the pelvis showing the sacroiliac joints and the symphysis pubis. The lower diagram shows the function of the sacrotuberous and sacrospinous ligaments in resisting the rotation force exerted on the sacrum by the weight of the trunk.

- **Nerve supply:** A branch of the fourth and fifth sacral nerves

A summary of the attachments of the muscles of the pelvic walls and floor, their nerve supply, and their action is given in Table 6-1.

Pelvic Fascia

The pelvic fascia is formed of connective tissue and is continuous above with the fascia lining the abdominal walls. Below, the fascia is continuous with the fascia of the perineum. The pelvic fascia can be divided into parietal and visceral layers.

Parietal Pelvic Fascia

The parietal pelvic fascia lines the walls of the pelvis and is named according to the muscle it overlies (Fig. 6-17). Where the pelvic diaphragm is deficient anteriorly, the parietal pelvic fascia becomes continuous through the opening with the fascia covering the inferior surface of the pelvic diaphragm, in the perineum. It covers the sphincter urethrae muscle and the perineal membrane (see page

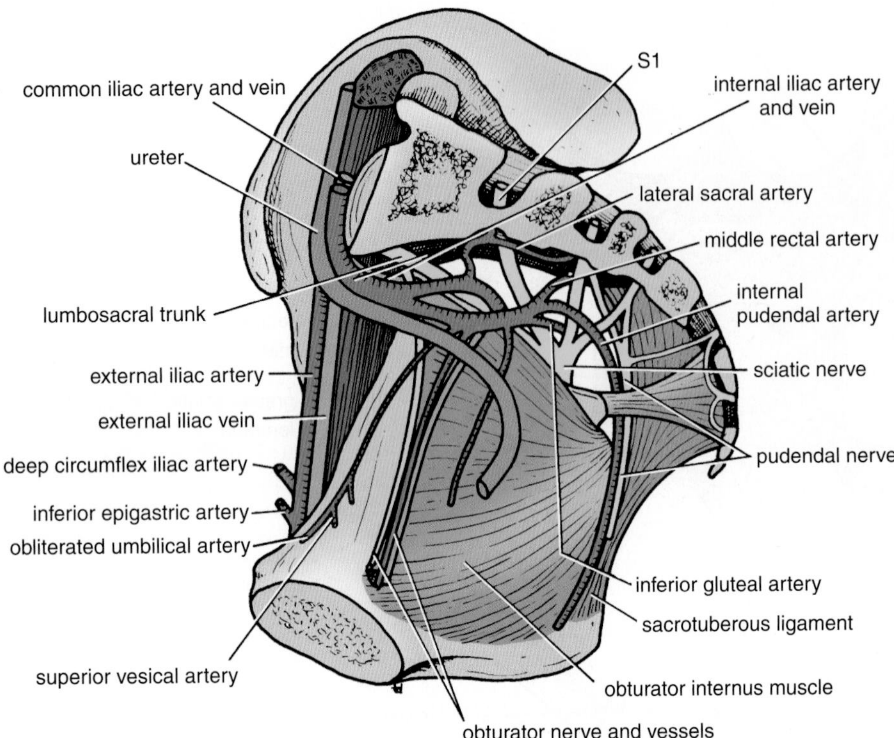

Figure 6-12 Lateral wall of the pelvis.

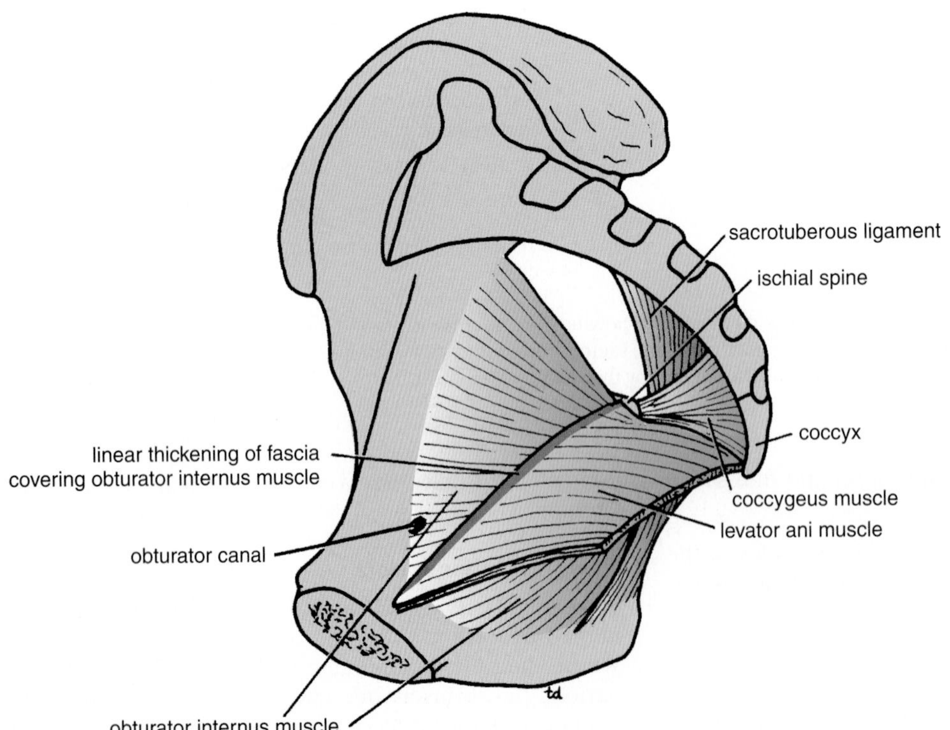

Figure 6-13 Inferior wall or floor of the pelvis.

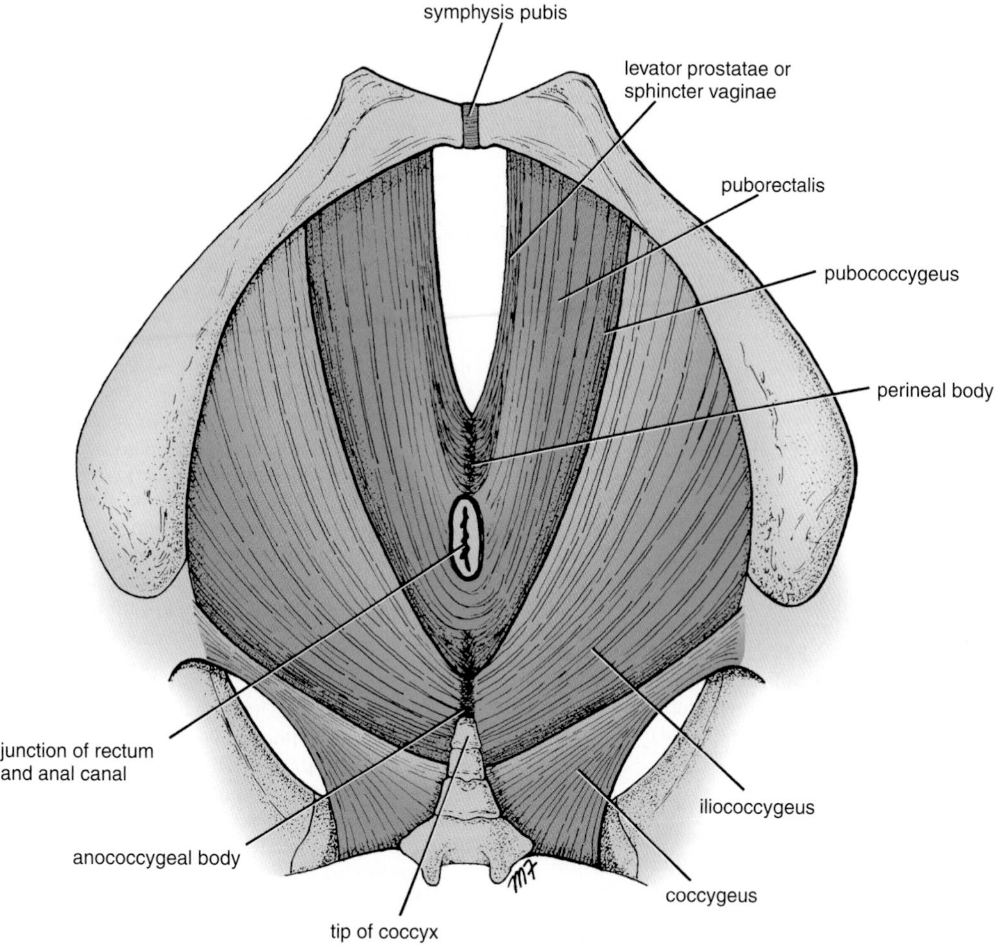

Figure 6-14 Levator ani muscle and coccygeus muscle seen on their inferior aspects. Note that the levator ani is made up of several different muscle groups. The levator ani and coccygeus muscles with their fascial coverings form a continuous muscular floor to the pelvis, known as the pelvic diaphragm.

401) and forms the superior fascial layer of the urogenital diaphragm.

Visceral Layer of Pelvic Fascia

The visceral layer of pelvic fascia covers and supports all the pelvic viscera. In certain locations the fascia thickens and extends from the viscus to the pelvic walls and provides support. These fascial ligaments are named according to their attachments, for example, the pubovesical and the sacrocervical ligaments.

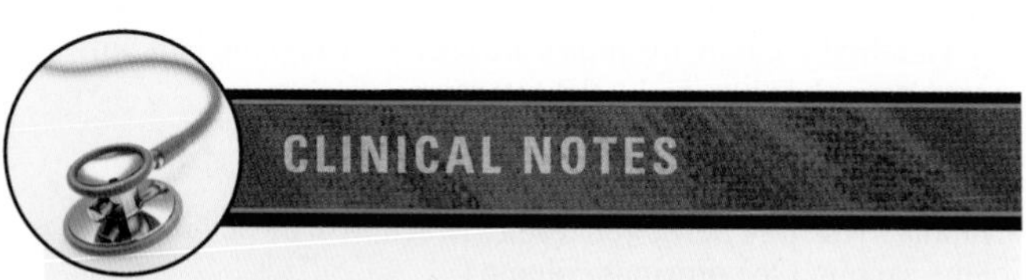

Fascial Ligaments of the Uterine Cervix

In the female the fascial ligaments attached to the uterine cervix are of particular clinical importance because they assist with the support of the uterus and thus prevent uterine prolapse (see page 366). The visceral pelvic fascia around the uterine cervix and vagina is commonly referred to as the **parametrium.**

Pelvic Peritoneum

The parietal peritoneum lines the pelvic walls and is reflected onto the pelvic viscera and becomes continuous with the visceral peritoneum (Fig. 6-17). For further details, see pages 356 to 376.

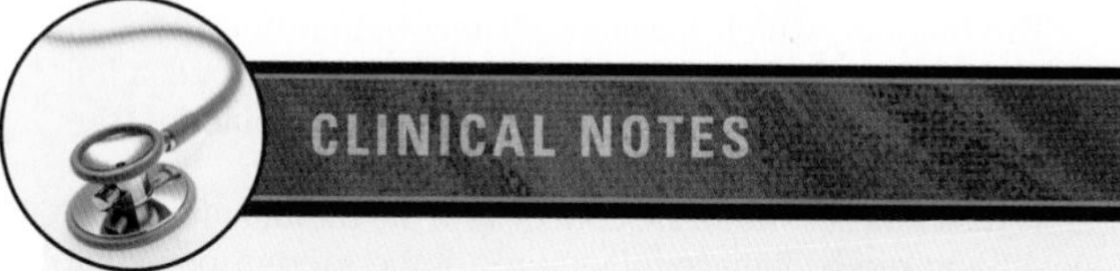

Fractures of the Pelvis

Fractures of the False Pelvis

Fractures of the false pelvis caused by direct trauma occasionally occur. The upper part of the ilium is seldom displaced because of the attachment of the iliacus muscle on the inside and the gluteal muscles on the outside.

Fractures of the True Pelvis

The mechanism of fractures of the true pelvis can be better understood if the pelvis is regarded not only as a basin but also as

(continues)

Clinical Notes, *continued*

a rigid ring (Fig. 6-15). The ring is made up of the pubic rami, the ischium, the acetabulum, the ilium, and the sacrum, joined by strong ligaments at the sacroiliac and symphyseal joints. If the ring breaks at any one point, the fracture will be stable and no displacement will occur. However, if two breaks occur in the ring, the fracture will be unstable and displacement will occur, because the postvertebral and abdominal muscles will shorten and elevate the lateral part of the pelvis (Fig. 6-15). The break in the ring may occur not as the result of a fracture but as the result of disruption of the sacroiliac or symphyseal joints. Fracture of bone on either side of the joint is more common than disruption of the joint.

The forces responsible for the disruption of the bony ring may be anteroposterior compression, lateral compression, or shearing.

A heavy fall on the greater trochanter of the femur may drive the head of the femur through the floor of the acetabulum into the pelvic cavity.

Fractures of the Sacrum and Coccyx

Fractures of the lateral mass of the sacrum may occur as part of a pelvic fracture. Fractures of the coccyx are rare. However, **coccydynia** is common and is usually caused by direct trauma to the coccyx, as in falling down a flight of concrete steps. The anterior surface of the coccyx can be palpated with a rectal examination.

Minor Fractures of the Pelvis

The anterior superior iliac spine may be pulled off by the forcible contraction of the sartorius muscle in athletes (Fig. 6-15). In a similar manner the anterior inferior iliac spine may be avulsed by the contraction of the rectus femoris muscle (origin of the straight head). The ischial tuberosity can be avulsed by the contraction of the hamstring muscles. Healing may occur by fibrous union, possibly resulting in elongation of the muscle unit and some reduction in muscular efficiency.

Anatomy of Complications of Pelvic Fractures

Fractures of the true pelvis are commonly associated with injuries to the soft pelvic tissues.

If damaged, the thin pelvic veins—namely, the internal iliac veins and their tributaries—that lie in the parietal pelvic fascia beneath the parietal peritoneum can be the source of a massive hemorrhage, which may be life threatening.

The male urethra is often damaged, especially in vertical shear fractures that may disrupt the urogenital diaphragm (see page 407).

The bladder, which lies immediately behind the pubis in both sexes, is occasionally damaged by spicules of bone; a full bladder is more likely to be injured than an empty bladder (see page 353).

The rectum lies within the concavity of the sacrum and is protected and rarely damaged. Fractures of the sacrum or ischial spine may be thrust into the pelvic cavity, tearing the rectum.

Nerve injuries can follow sacral fractures; the laying down of fibrous tissue around the anterior or posterior nerve roots or the branches of the sacral spinal nerves can result in persistent pain.

Damage to the sciatic nerve may occur in fractures involving the boundaries of the greater sciatic notch. The peroneal part of the sciatic nerve is most often involved, resulting in the inability of a conscious patient to dorsiflex the ankle joint or failure of an unconscious patient to reflexly plantar-flex (ankle jerk) the foot (see page 659).

Pelvic Floor

The pelvic diaphragm is a gutter-shaped sheet of muscle formed by the levatores ani and coccygeus muscles and their covering fasciae. From their origin, the muscle fibers on the two sides slope downward and backward to the midline, producing a gutter that slopes downward and forward.

A rise in the intra-abdominal pressure, caused by the contraction of the diaphragm and the muscles of the anterior and lateral abdominal walls, is counteracted by the contraction of the muscles forming the pelvic floor. By this means, the pelvic viscera are supported and do not "drop out" through the pelvic outlet. Contraction of the puborectalis fibers greatly assists the anal sphincters in maintaining continence under these conditions by pulling the anorectal junction upward and forward. During the act of defecation, however, the levator ani continues to support the pelvic viscera but the puborectalis fibers relax with the anal sphincters.

Functional Significance of the Pelvic Floor in the Female

The female pelvic floor serves an important function during the second stage of labor (Fig. 6-16). At the pelvic inlet, the widest diameter is transverse so that the longest axis of the baby's head (anteroposterior) takes up the transverse position. When the head reaches the pelvic floor, the gutter shape of the floor tends to cause the baby's head to rotate so that its long axis comes to lie in the anteroposterior position. The occipital part of the head now moves downward and forward along the gutter until it lies under the pubic arch. As the baby's head passes through the lower part of the birth canal, the small gap that exists in the anterior part of the pelvic diaphragm becomes enormously enlarged so that the head may slip through into the perineum. Once the baby has passed through the perineum, the levatores ani muscles recoil and take up their previous position.

Injury to the Pelvic Floor

Injury to the pelvic floor during a difficult childbirth can result in the loss of support for the pelvic viscera leading to **uterine** and **vaginal prolapse,** herniation of the bladder **(cystocele),** and alteration in the position of the bladder neck and urethra, leading to **stress incontinence.** In the latter condition, the patient dribbles urine whenever the intra-abdominal pressure is raised, as in coughing. **Prolapse of the rectum** may also occur.

Partial Fusion of the Sacral Vertebrae

The first sacral vertebra can be partly or completely separated from the second sacral vertebra. Occasionally, on radiographs of the vertebral column, examples are seen in which the fifth lumbar vertebra has fused with the first sacral vertebra.

Trauma to the True Pelvis

Trauma to the true pelvis can result in fracture of the lateral mass of the sacrum (see previous column).

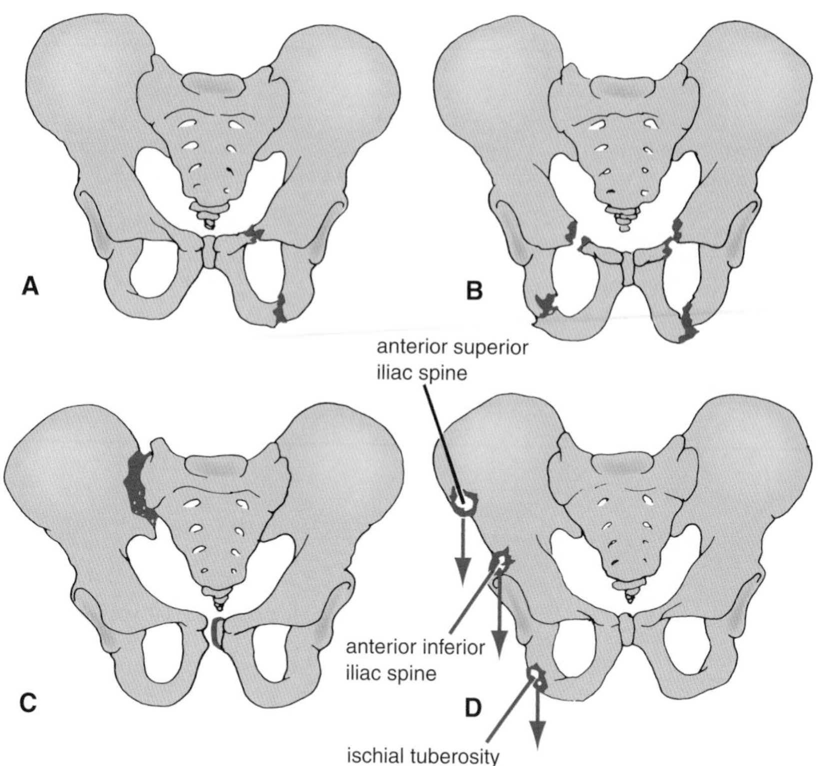

Figure 6-15 **A–C.** Different types of fractures of the pelvic basin. **D.** Avulsion fractures of the pelvis. The sartorius muscle is responsible for the avulsion of the anterior superior iliac spine; the straight head of the rectus femoris muscle, for the avulsion of the anterior inferior iliac spine; and the hamstring muscles, for the avulsion of the ischial tuberosity.

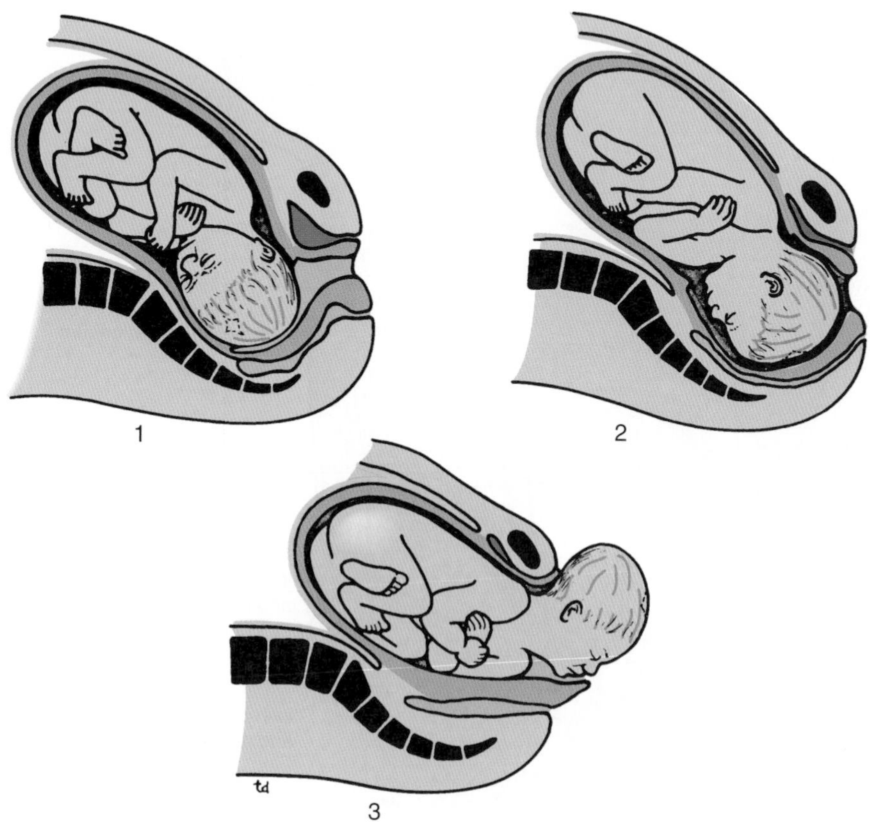

Figure 6-16 Stages in rotation of the baby's head during the second stage of labor. The shape of the pelvic floor plays an important part in this process.

Table 6-1 Muscles of the Pelvic Walls and Floor

Name of Muscle	Origin	Insertion	Nerve Supply	Action
Piriformis	Front of sacrum	Greater trochanter of femur	Sacral plexus	Lateral rotator of femur at hip joint
Obturator internus	Obturator membrane and adjoining part of hip bone	Greater trochanter of femur	Nerve to obturator internus from sacral plexus	Lateral rotator of femur at hip joint
Levator ani	Body of pubis, fascia of obturator internus, spine of ischium	Perineal body; anococcygeal body; walls of prostate, vagina, rectum, and anal canal	Fourth sacral nerve, pudendal nerve	Supports pelvic viscera; sphincter to anorectal junction and vagina
Coccygeus	Spine of ischium	Lower end of sacrum; coccyx	Fourth and fifth sacral nerve	Assists levator ani to support pelvic viscera; flexes coccyx

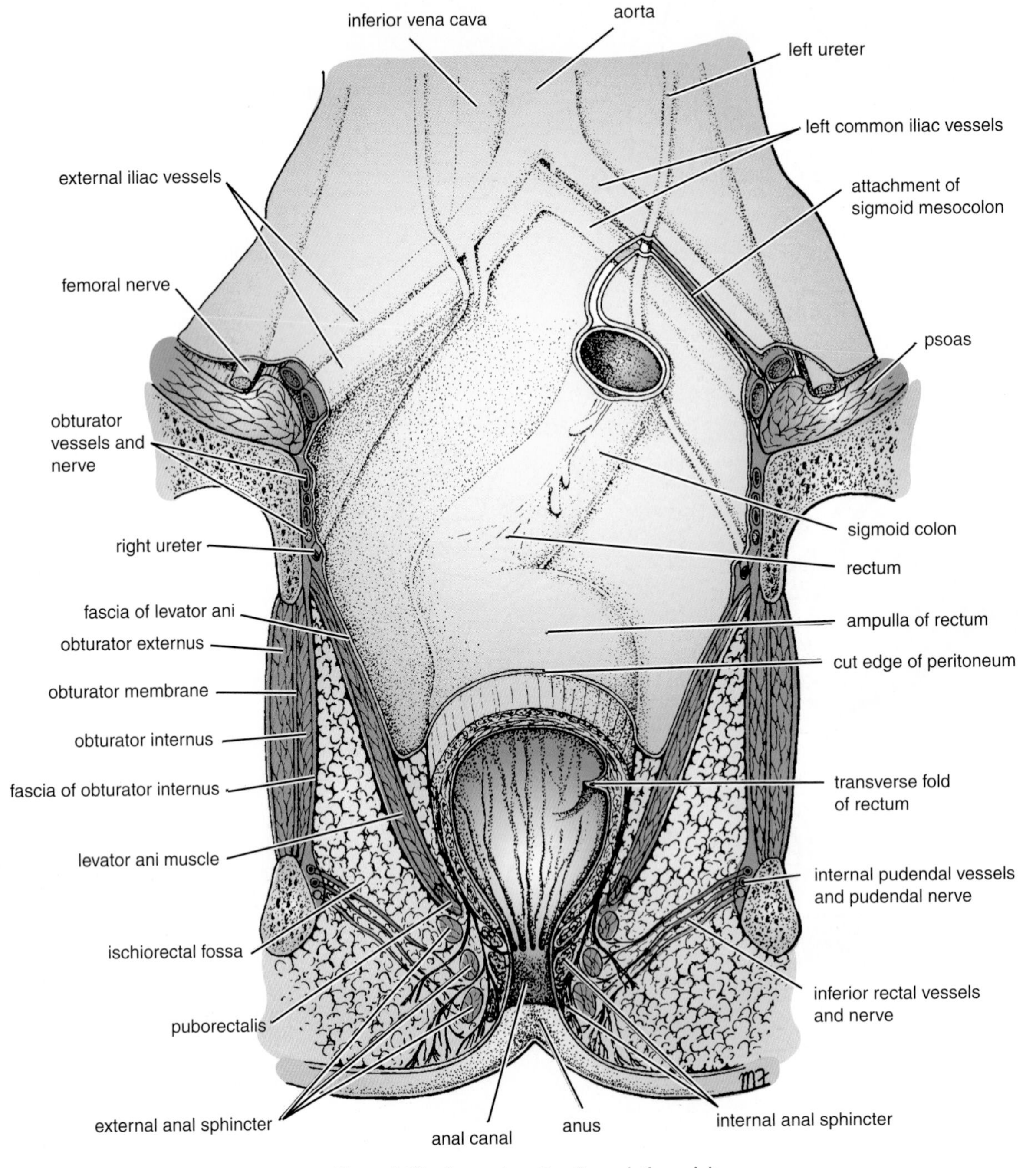

Figure 6-17 Coronal section through the pelvis.

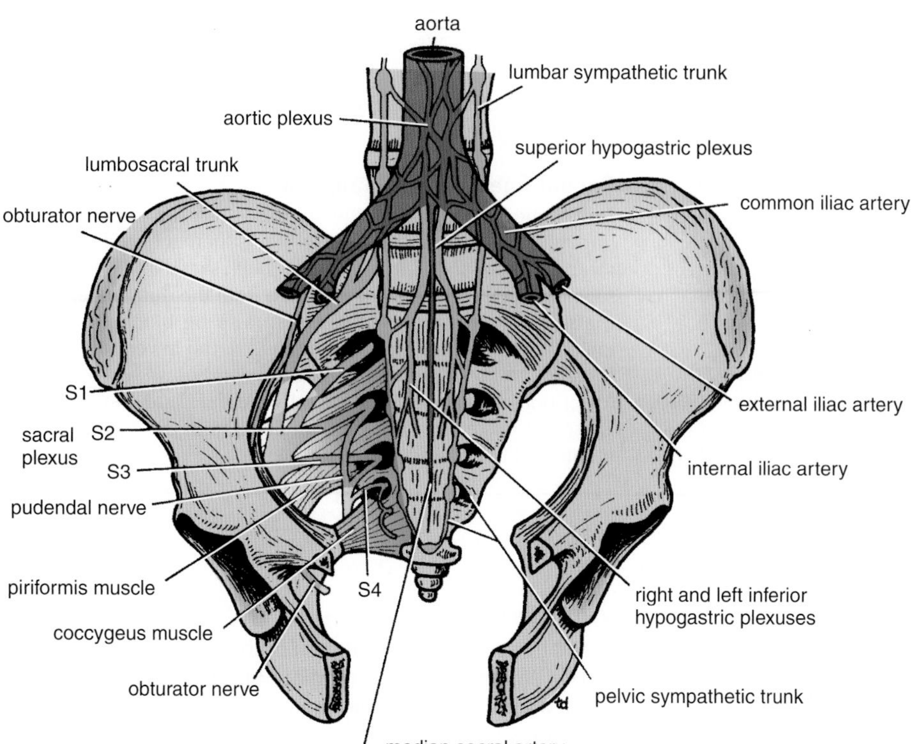

Figure 6-18 Posterior pelvic wall showing the sacral plexus, superior hypogastric plexus, and right and left inferior hypogastric plexuses. Pelvic parts of the sympathetic trunks are also shown.

Nerves of the Pelvis

Sacral Plexus

The sacral plexus lies on the posterior pelvic wall in front of the piriformis muscle (Fig. 6-18). It is formed from the anterior rami of the fourth and fifth lumbar nerves and the anterior rami of the first, second, third, and fourth sacral nerves (Fig. 6-19). The fourth lumbar nerve joins the fifth lumbar nerve to form the **lumbosacral trunk.** The lumbosacral trunk passes down into the pelvis and joins the sacral nerves as they emerge from the anterior sacral foramina.

Relations

- **Anteriorly:** The internal iliac vessels and their branches, and the rectum (Fig. 6-12)
- **Posteriorly:** The piriformis muscle (Fig. 6-18)

Branches

- Branches to the lower limb that leave the pelvis through the greater sciatic foramen (Fig. 6-12):

1. The **sciatic nerve** (L4 and 5; S1, 2, and 3), the largest branch of the plexus and the largest nerve in the body (Fig. 6-9)
2. The **superior gluteal nerve,** which supplies the gluteus medius and minimus and the tensor fasciae latae muscles
3. The **inferior gluteal nerve,** which supplies the gluteus maximus muscle
4. The **nerve to the quadratus femoris muscle,** which also supplies the inferior gemellus muscle
5. The **nerve to the obturator internus muscle,** which also supplies the superior gemellus muscle
6. The **posterior cutaneous nerve of the thigh,** which supplies the skin of the buttock and the back of the thigh

- Branches to the pelvic muscles, pelvic viscera, and perineum:

1. The **pudendal nerve** (S2, 3, and 4), which leaves the pelvis through the greater sciatic foramen and enters the perineum through the lesser sciatic foramen (Fig. 6-12)
2. The **nerves to the piriformis muscle**
3. The **pelvic splanchnic nerves,** which constitute the sacral part of the parasympathetic system and arise from the second, third, and fourth sacral nerves. They are distributed to the pelvic viscera.

- The **perforating cutaneous nerve,** which supplies the skin of the lower medial part of the buttock

The branches of the sacral plexus and their distribution are summarized in Table 6-2.

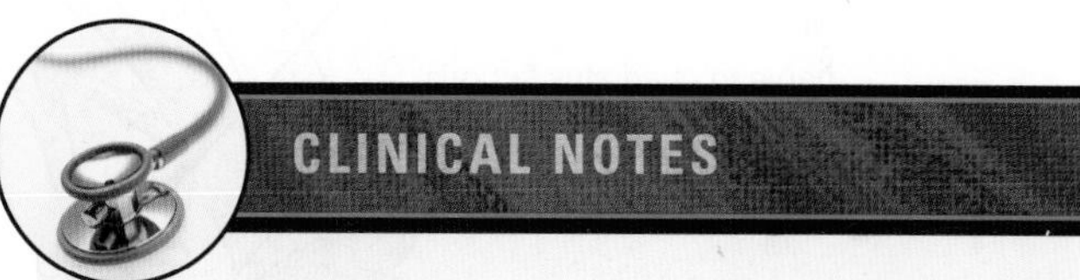

Sacral Plexus

Pressure from the Fetal Head

During the later stages of pregnancy, when the fetal head has descended into the pelvis, the mother often complains of discomfort or aching pain extending down one of the lower

(continues)

Clinical Notes, *continued*

limbs. The discomfort, caused by pressure from the fetal head, is often relieved by changing position, such as lying on the side in bed.

Invasion by Malignant Tumors

The nerves of the sacral plexus can become invaded by malignant tumors extending from neighboring viscera. A carcinoma of the rectum, for example, can cause severe intractable pain down the lower limbs.

Referred Pain from the Obturator Nerve

The obturator nerve lies on the lateral wall of the pelvis and supplies the parietal peritoneum. An inflamed appendix hanging down into the pelvic cavity could cause irritation of the obturator nerve endings, leading to referred pain down the inner side of the right thigh. Inflammation of the ovaries can produce similar symptoms.

Caudal Anesthesia (Analgesia)

Anesthetic solutions can be injected into the sacral canal through the sacral hiatus. The solutions then act on the spinal roots of the second, third, fourth, and fifth sacral and coccygeal segments of the cord as they emerge from the dura mater. The roots of higher spinal segments can also be blocked by this method. The needle must be confined to the lower part of the sacral canal, because the meninges extend down as far as the lower border of the second sacral vertebra. Caudal anesthesia is used in obstetrics to block pain fibers from the cervix of the uterus and to anesthetize the perineum.

Branches of the Lumbar Plexus

Lumbosacral Trunk

Part of the anterior ramus of the fourth lumbar nerve emerges from the medial border of the psoas muscle and joins the anterior ramus of the fifth lumbar nerve to form the lumbosacral trunk (Figs. 6-18 and 6-19). This trunk now enters the pelvis by passing down in front of the sacroiliac joint and joins the sacral plexus.

Obturator Nerve

The obturator nerve is a branch of the lumbar plexus (L2, 3, and 4), emerges from the medial border of the psoas muscle in the abdomen, and accompanies the lumbosacral trunk down into the pelvis. It crosses the front of the sacroiliac joint and runs forward on the lateral pelvic wall in the angle between the internal and external iliac vessels (Fig. 6-12). On reaching the obturator canal (that is, the upper part of the obturator foramen, which is devoid of the obturator

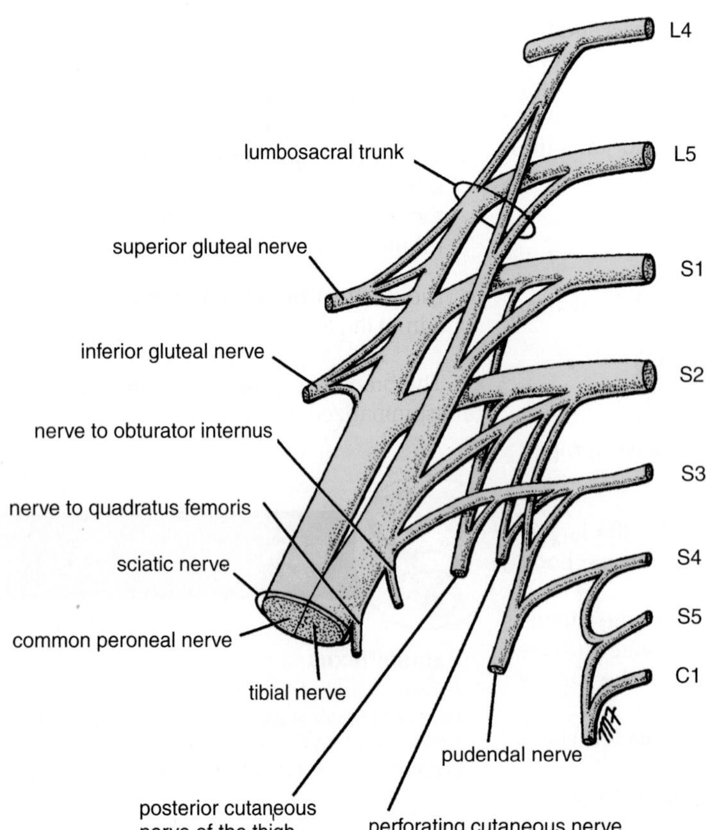

Figure 6-19 Sacral plexus.

Table 6-2 Branches of the Sacral Plexus and Their Distribution

Branches	Distribution
Superior gluteal nerve	Gluteus medius, gluteus minimus, and tensor fasciae latae muscles
Inferior gluteal nerve	Gluteus maximus muscle
Nerve to piriformis	Piriformis muscle
Nerve to obturator internus	Obturator internus and superior gemellus muscles
Nerve to quadratus femoris	Quadratus femoris and inferior gemellus muscles
Perforating cutaneous nerve	Skin over medial aspect of buttock
Posterior cutaneous nerve of thigh	Skin over posterior surface of thigh and popliteal fossa, also over lower part of buttock, scrotum, or labium majus
Sciatic nerve (L4, 5; S1, 2, 3) Tibial portion	Hamstring muscles (semitendinosus, biceps femoris [long head], adductor magnus [hamstring part]), gastrocnemius, soleus, plantaris, popliteus, tibialis posterior, flexor digitorum longus, flexor hallucis longus, and via medial and lateral plantar branches to muscles of sole of foot; sural branch supplies skin on lateral side of leg and foot
Common peroneal portion	Biceps femoris muscle (short head) and via deep peroneal branch: tibialis anterior, extensor hallucis longus, extensor digitorum longus, peroneus tertius, and extensor digitorum brevis muscles; skin over cleft between first and second toes. The superficial peroneal branch supplies the peroneus longus and brevis muscles and skin over lower third of anterior surface of leg and dorsum of foot
Pudendal nerve	Muscles of perineum including the external anal sphincter, mucous membrane of lower half of anal canal, perianal skin, skin of penis, scrotum, clitoris, and labia majora and minora

membrane), it splits into anterior and posterior divisions that pass through the canal to enter the adductor region of the thigh. The distribution of the obturator nerve in the thigh is considered on page 586.

Branches

Sensory branches supply the parietal peritoneum on the lateral wall of the pelvis.

Autonomic Nerves

Pelvic Part of the Sympathetic Trunk

The pelvic part of the sympathetic trunk is continuous above, behind the common iliac vessels, with the abdominal part (Fig. 6-18). It runs down behind the rectum on the front of the sacrum, medial to the anterior sacral foramina. The sympathetic trunk has four or five segmentally arranged ganglia. Below, the two trunks converge and finally unite in front of the coccyx.

Branches

- Gray rami communicantes to the sacral and coccygeal nerves
- Fibers that join the hypogastric plexuses

Pelvic Splanchnic Nerves

The pelvic splanchnic nerves form the parasympathetic part of the autonomic nervous system in the pelvis. The preganglionic fibers arise from the second, third, and fourth sacral nerves and synapse in ganglia in the inferior hypogastric plexus or in the walls of the viscera.

Some of the parasympathetic fibers ascend through the hypogastric plexuses and thence via the aortic plexus to the inferior mesenteric plexus. The fibers are then distributed along branches of the inferior mesenteric artery to supply the large bowel from the left colic flexure to the upper half of the anal canal.

Superior Hypogastric Plexus

The superior hypogastric plexus is situated in front of the promontory of the sacrum (Fig. 6-18). It is formed as a continuation of the aortic plexus and from branches of the third and fourth lumbar sympathetic ganglia. It contains sympathetic and sacral parasympathetic nerve fibers and visceral afferent nerve fibers. The superior hypogastric plexus divides inferiorly to form the **right** and **left hypogastric nerves.**

Inferior Hypogastric Plexuses

The inferior hypogastric plexuses lie on each side of the rectum, the base of the bladder, and the vagina (Fig. 6-18). Each plexus is formed from a hypogastric nerve (from the superior hypogastric plexus) and from the pelvic splanchnic nerve. It contains postganglionic sympathetic fibers, preganglionic and postganglionic parasympathetic fibers, and visceral afferent fibers. Branches pass to the pelvic viscera via small subsidiary plexuses.

Arteries of the Pelvis

Common Iliac Artery

Each common iliac artery ends at the pelvic inlet in front of the sacroiliac joint by dividing into the external and internal iliac arteries (Figs. 6-12 and 6-18).

External Iliac Artery

The external iliac artery runs along the medial border of the psoas muscle, following the pelvic brim (Fig. 6-12), and gives off the **inferior epigastric** and **deep circumflex iliac** branches. It leaves the false pelvis by passing under the inguinal ligament to become the **femoral artery.**

Arteries of the True Pelvis

The following arteries enter the pelvic cavity:

- Internal iliac artery
- Superior rectal artery
- Ovarian artery
- Median sacral artery

Internal Iliac Artery

The internal iliac artery passes down into the pelvis to the upper margin of the greater sciatic foramen, where it divides into anterior and posterior divisions (Fig. 6-12). The branches of these divisions supply the pelvic viscera, the perineum, the pelvic walls, and the buttocks. The origin of the terminal branches is subject to variation, but the usual arrangement is shown in Diagram 6-1.

Branches of the Anterior Division

- **Umbilical artery:** From the proximal patent part of the umbilical artery arises the **superior vesical artery,** which supplies the upper portion of the bladder (Fig. 6-12).
- **Obturator artery:** This artery runs forward along the lateral wall of the pelvis with the obturator nerve and leaves the pelvis through the obturator canal.
- **Inferior vesical artery:** This artery supplies the base of the bladder and the prostate and seminal vesicles in the male; it also gives off the **artery to the vas deferens.**
- **Middle rectal artery:** Commonly, this artery arises with the inferior vesical artery (Fig. 6-12). It supplies the muscle of the lower rectum and anastomoses with the superior rectal and inferior rectal arteries.
- **Internal pudendal artery:** This artery leaves the pelvis through the greater sciatic foramen and enters the gluteal region below the piriformis muscle (Fig. 6-12). It then enters the perineum by passing through the lesser sciatic foramen and passes forward in the pudendal canal with the pudendal nerve. Its branches supply the musculature of the anal canal and the skin and muscles of the perineum.
- **Inferior gluteal artery:** This artery leaves the pelvis through the greater sciatic foramen below the piriformis muscle (Fig. 6-12). It passes between the first and second or second and third sacral nerves.
- **Uterine artery:** This artery runs medially on the floor of the pelvis and **crosses the ureter superiorly** (see Fig. 7-28). It passes above the lateral fornix of the vagina to reach the uterus. Here, it ascends between the layers of the broad ligament along the lateral margin of the uterus. It ends by following the uterine tube laterally, where it anastomoses with the ovarian artery. The uterine artery gives off a vaginal branch.
- **Vaginal artery:** This artery usually takes the place of the inferior vesical artery present in the male. It supplies the vagina and the base of the bladder.

Branches of the Posterior Division

- **Iliolumbar artery:** This artery ascends across the pelvic inlet posterior to the external iliac vessels, psoas, and iliacus muscles.
- **Lateral sacral arteries:** These arteries descend in front of the sacral plexus, giving off branches to neighboring structures (Fig. 6-12).
- **Superior gluteal artery:** This artery leaves the pelvis through the greater sciatic foramen above the piriformis muscle. It supplies the gluteal region.

Superior Rectal Artery

The superior rectal artery is a direct continuation of the inferior mesenteric artery. The name changes as the latter artery crosses the common iliac artery. It supplies the mucous membrane of the rectum and the upper half of the anal canal.

Ovarian Artery

(The testicular artery enters the inguinal canal and does not enter the pelvis.) The ovarian artery arises from the

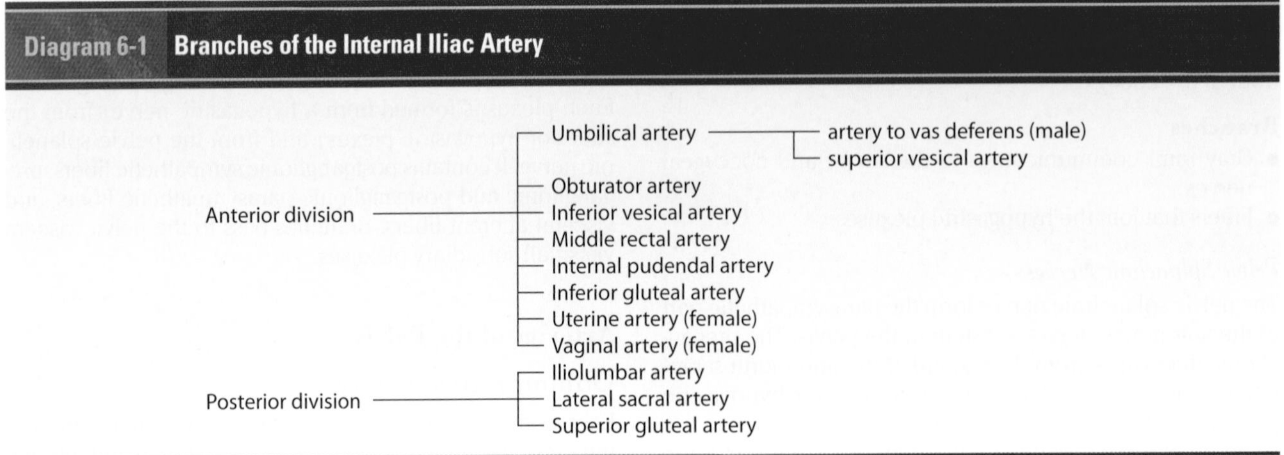

abdominal part of the aorta at the level of the first lumbar vertebra. The artery is long and slender and passes downward and laterally behind the peritoneum. It crosses the external iliac artery at the pelvic inlet and enters the suspensory ligament of the ovary. It then passes into the broad ligament and enters the ovary by way of the mesovarium.

Median Sacral Artery

The median sacral artery is a small artery that arises at the bifurcation of the aorta (Fig. 6-18). It descends over the anterior surface of the sacrum and coccyx.

The distribution of the visceral branches of the pelvic arteries is discussed in detail with the individual viscera in Chapter 7.

Veins of the Pelvis

External Iliac Vein

The external iliac vein begins behind the inguinal ligament as a continuation of the femoral vein. It runs along the medial side of the corresponding artery and joins the internal iliac vein to form the **common iliac vein** (Fig. 6-12). It receives the **inferior epigastric** and **deep circumflex iliac veins.**

Internal Iliac Vein

The internal iliac vein begins by the joining together of tributaries that correspond to the branches of the internal iliac artery. It passes upward in front of the sacroiliac joint and joins the external iliac vein to form the common iliac vein (Fig. 6-12).

Median Sacral Veins

The median sacral veins accompany the corresponding artery and end by joining the left common iliac vein.

Lymphatics of the Pelvis

The lymph nodes and vessels are arranged in a chain along the main blood vessels. The nodes are named after the blood vessels with which they are associated. Thus, there are **external iliac nodes, internal iliac nodes,** and **common iliac nodes.**

Joints of the Pelvis

Sacroiliac Joints

The sacroiliac joints are strong synovial joints and are formed between the auricular surfaces of the sacrum and the iliac bones (Fig. 6-11). The sacrum carries the weight of the trunk, and, apart from the interlocking of the irregular articular surfaces, the shape of the bones contributes little to the stability of the joints. The strong **posterior** and **interosseous sacroiliac ligaments** suspend the sacrum between the two iliac bones. The **anterior sacroiliac ligament** is thin and lies in front of the joint.

The weight of the trunk tends to thrust the upper end of the sacrum downward and rotate the lower end of the bone upward (Fig. 6-11). This rotatory movement is prevented by the strong **sacrotuberous** and **sacrospinous ligaments** described previously. The **iliolumbar ligament** connects the tip of the fifth lumbar transverse process to the iliac crest.

Movements

A small but limited amount of movement is possible at these joints. In older people, the synovial cavity disappears and the joint becomes fibrosed. Their primary function is to transmit the weight of the body from the vertebral column to the bony pelvis.

Nerve Supply

The nerve supply is from branches of the sacral spinal nerves.

Symphysis Pubis

The symphysis pubis is a cartilaginous joint between the two pubic bones (Fig. 6-11). The articular surfaces are covered by a layer of hyaline cartilage and are connected together by a fibrocartilaginous disc. The joint is surrounded by ligaments that extend from one pubic bone to the other.

Movements

Almost no movement is possible at this joint.

Sacrococcygeal Joint

The sacrococcygeal joint is a cartilaginous joint between the bodies of the last sacral vertebra and the first coccygeal vertebra. The cornua of the sacrum and coccyx are joined by ligaments.

Movements

Extensive flexion and extension are possible at this joint.

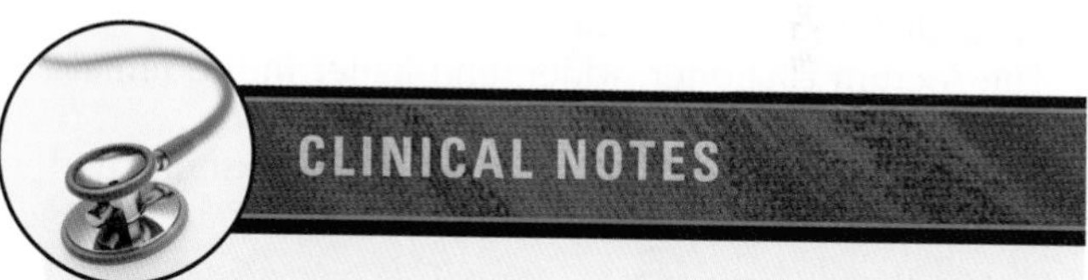

Pelvic Joints

Changes with Pregnancy

During pregnancy, the symphysis pubis and the ligaments of the sacroiliac and sacrococcygeal joints undergo softening in response to hormones, thus increasing the mobility and increasing the potential size of the pelvis during childbirth. The hormones responsible are estrogen and progesterone produced by the ovary and the placenta. An additional hormone, called relaxin, produced by these organs can also have a relaxing effect on the pelvic ligaments.

Changes with Age

Obliteration of the cavity in the sacroiliac joint occurs in both sexes after middle age.

Sacroiliac Joint Disease

The sacroiliac joint is innervated by the lower lumbar and sacral nerves so that disease in the joint can produce low back pain and pain referred along the sciatic nerve (sciatica).

The sacroiliac joint is inaccessible to clinical examination. However, a small area located just medial to and below the

(continues)

Clinical Notes, *continued*

posterior superior iliac spine is where the joint comes closest to the surface. In disease of the lumbosacral region, movements of the vertebral column in any direction cause pain in the lumbosacral part of the column. In sacroiliac disease, pain is extreme on rotation of the vertebral column and is worst at the end of forward flexion. The latter movement causes pain because the hamstring muscles (see page 587) hold the hip bones in position while the sacrum is rotating forward as the vertebral column is flexed.

Sex Differences of the Pelvis

The sex differences of the bony pelvis are easily recognized. The more obvious differences result from the adaptation of the female pelvis for childbearing. The stronger muscles in the male are responsible for the thicker bones and more prominent bony markings (Figs. 6-1 and 6-4).

- The false pelvis is shallow in the female and deep in the male.
- The pelvic inlet is transversely oval in the female but heart shaped in the male because of the indentation produced by the promontory of the sacrum in the male.
- The pelvic cavity is roomier in the female than in the male, and the distance between the inlet and the outlet is much shorter.
- The pelvic outlet is larger in the female than in the male. In the female the ischial tuberosities are everted and in the male they are turned in.
- The sacrum is shorter, wider, and flatter in the female than in the male.
- The subpubic angle, or pubic arch, is more rounded and wider in the female than in the male.

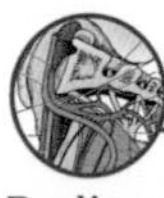

Radiographic Anatomy

Radiographic anatomy of the pelvis is fully described on page 377.

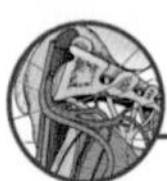

Surface Anatomy

Surface Landmarks

Iliac Crest

The iliac crest can be felt through the skin along its entire length (Figs. 6-20, 6-21, and 6-22).

Anterior Superior Iliac Spine

The anterior superior iliac spine is situated at the anterior end of the iliac crest and lies at the upper lateral end of the fold of the groin (Figs. 6-20, 6-21, and 6-22).

Posterior Superior Iliac Spine

The posterior superior iliac spine is situated at the posterior end of the iliac crest (Fig. 6-22). It lies at the bottom of a small skin dimple and on a level with the second sacral spine, which coincides with the lower limit of the subarachnoid space; it also coincides with the level of the middle of the sacroiliac joint.

Pubic Tubercle

The pubic tubercle can be felt on the upper border of the pubis (Figs. 6-20, 6-21, and 6-22). Attached to it is the medial end of the inguinal ligament. The tubercle can be palpated easily in the male by invaginating the scrotum from below with the examining finger. In the female, the pubic tubercle can be palpated through the lateral margin of the labium majus.

Pubic Crest

The pubic crest is the ridge of bone on the superior surface of the pubic bone, medial to the pubic tubercle (Figs. 6-1 and 6-22).

Symphysis Pubis

The symphysis pubis (Figs. 6-1 and 6-22) lies in the midline between the bodies of the pubic bones and can be palpated as a solid structure through the fat that is present in this region.

Spinous Processes of Sacrum

The spinous processes of the sacrum (Fig. 6-22) are fused with each other in the midline to form the median sacral crest. The crest can be felt beneath the skin in the uppermost part of the cleft between the buttocks.

Sacral Hiatus

The sacral hiatus is situated on the posterior aspect of the lower end of the sacrum, where the extradural space terminates (Fig. 6-22). The hiatus lies about 2 in. (5 cm) above the tip of the coccyx and beneath the skin of the cleft between the buttocks.

Coccyx

The inferior surface and tip of the coccyx (Fig. 6-22) can be palpated in the cleft between the buttocks about 1 in. (2.5 cm) behind the anus. The anterior surface of the coccyx can be palpated with the gloved finger in the anal canal.

Viscera

Urinary Bladder

In adults, the empty bladder is a pelvic organ and lies posterior to the symphysis pubis. As the bladder fills, it rises up out of the pelvis into the abdomen, where it can be palpated through the anterior abdominal wall above the symphysis pubis (Fig. 6-23). The peritoneum covering the distended bladder becomes peeled off from the anterior abdominal wall so that the front of the bladder is in direct contact with the abdominal wall (see page 349).

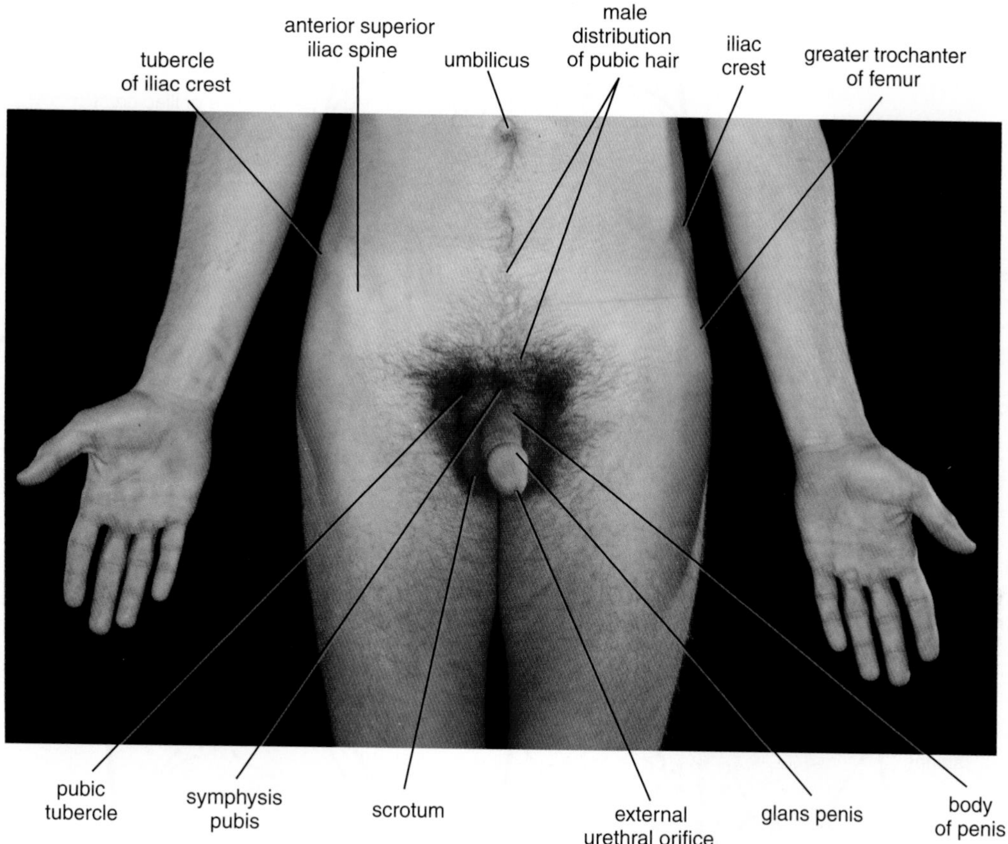

Figure 6-20 Anterior view of the pelvis of a 27-year-old man.

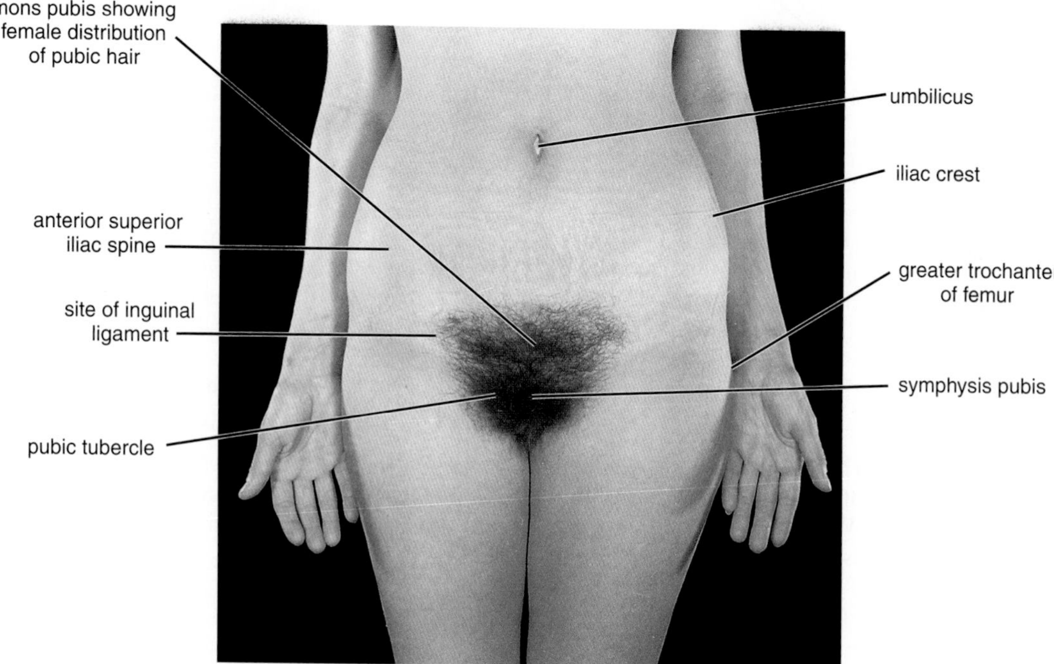

Figure 6-21 Anterior view of the pelvis of a 29-year-old woman.

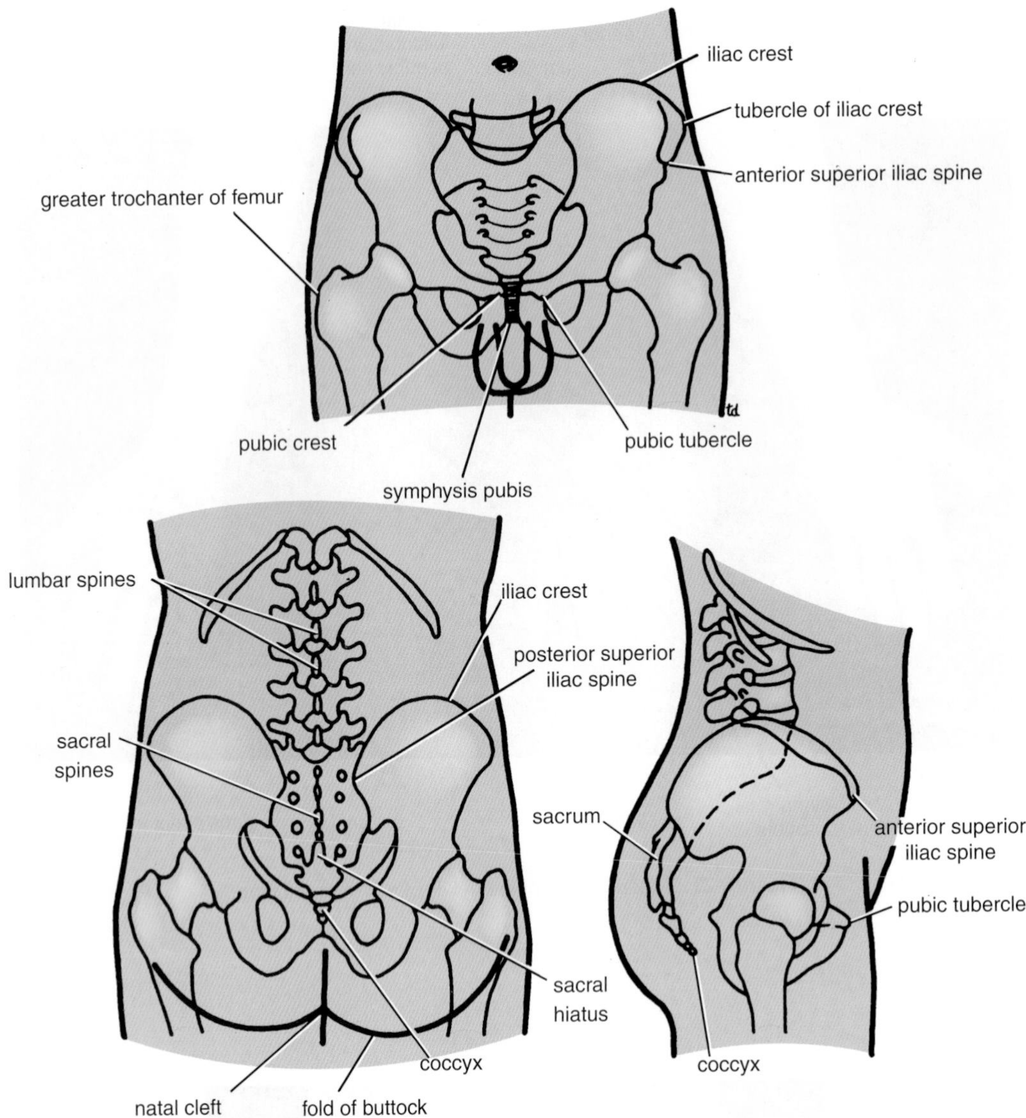

Figure 6-22 Relationship between different parts of the pelvis and the body surface.

In children, until the age of 6 years, the bladder is an abdominal organ even when empty because the capacity of the pelvic cavity is not great enough to contain it. The neck of the bladder lies just below the level of the upper border of the symphysis pubis.

Uterus

Toward the end of the second month of pregnancy, the fundus of the uterus can be palpated through the lower part of the anterior abdominal wall. With the progressive enlargement of the uterus, the fundus rises above the level of the umbilicus and reaches the region of the xiphoid process by the ninth month of pregnancy (Fig. 6-23). Later, when the presenting part of the fetus, usually the head, descends into the pelvis, the fundus of the uterus descends also.

Rectal and Vaginal Examinations as a Means of Palpating the Pelvic Viscera

Bimanual rectoabdominal and vaginal–abdominal examinations are extremely valuable methods of palpating the pelvic viscera; they are described in detail on pages 397 and 412.

A

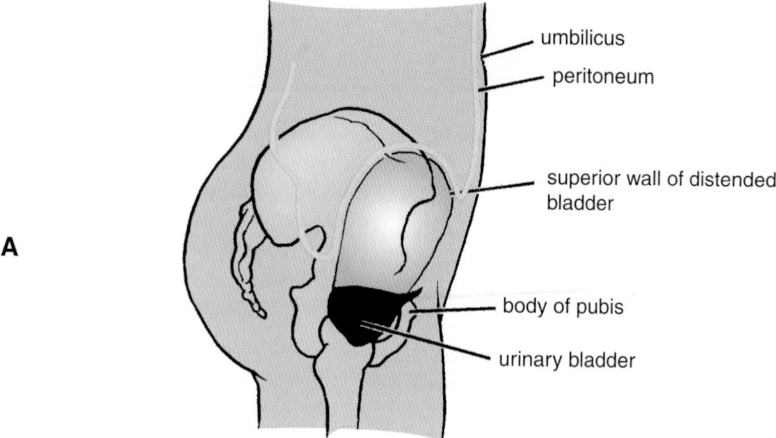

B

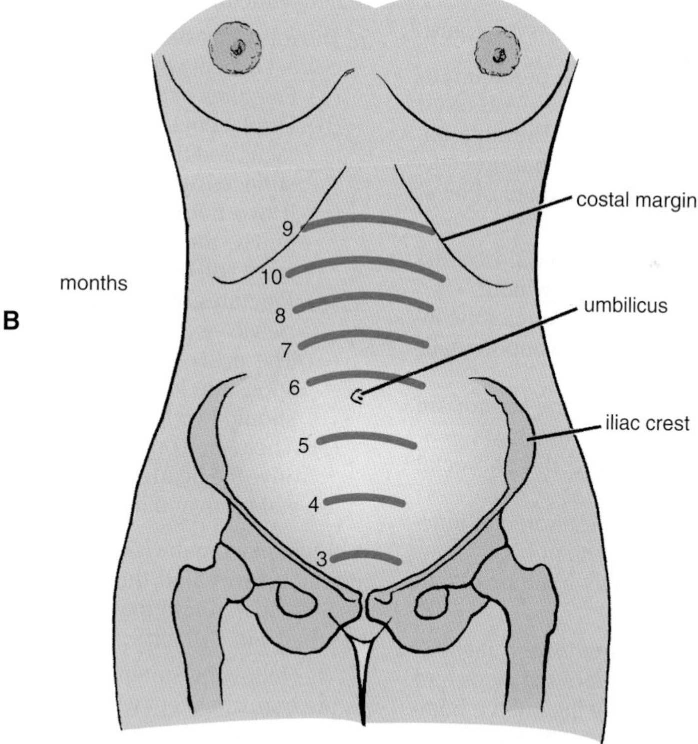

Figure 6-23 **A.** Surface anatomy of the empty bladder and the full bladder **B.** Height of the fundus of the uterus at various months of pregnancy. Note that the peritoneum covering the distended bladder becomes peeled off from the anterior abdominal wall so that the front of the bladder comes to lie in direct contact with the abdominal wall.

CLINICAL PROBLEM SOLVING

Study the following case histories and select the best answer to the questions following them.

A 65-year-old man with a history of prostatic enlargement complained that he could not micturate. The last time that he passed urine had been 6 hours previously. He was found lying on his bed in great distress, clutching his anterior abdominal wall with both hands and pleading for something to be done quickly. On examination, a large ovoid swelling could be palpated through the abdominal wall above the symphysis pubis.

1. In this patient the following statements are correct except which?
   (a) In the adult, the urinary bladder is a pelvic structure.
   (b) When the bladder fills the superior wall of the bladder rises out of the pelvis.
   (c) When the bladder becomes filled it never reaches a level above the umbilicus.
   (d) The swelling is dull on percussion.
   (e) Pressure on the swelling exacerbates the symptoms.

A 43-year-old woman was operated on in the perineum to drain an ischial rectal abscess. The abscess extended deeply to the region of the anorectal junction. The surgeon, to obtain better drainage, decided to cut the puborectalis muscle. Then, 3 days later, the patient complained of fecal incontinence.

2. The symptoms displayed by this patient could be explained by the following statements except which?
   (a) Anal continence is maintained by the tone of the internal and external sphincters and the puborectalis muscle.
   (b) The puborectalis fibers are a part of the levator ani muscle.
   (c) The puborectalis fibers pass around the anorectal junction.
   (d) The puborectalis muscle slings the anorectal junction up to the back of the body of the pubis.
   (e) The puborectalis muscle plays only a minor role in preserving anal continence.

A heavily built, middle-aged man running down a flight of stone steps misjudged the position of one of the steps and fell suddenly onto his buttocks. Following the fall, he complained of severe bruising of the area of the cleft between the buttocks and persistent pain in this area.

3. The following statements concerning this patient are correct except which?
   (a) The lower end of the vertebral column was traumatized by the stone step.
   (b) The coccyx can be palpated beneath the skin in the natal cleft.
   (c) The anterior surface of the coccyx cannot be felt clinically.
   (d) The coccyx is usually severely bruised or fractured.
   (e) The pain is felt in the distribution of dermatomes S4 and S5.

A 28-year-old pregnant woman was very frightened by the thought of going through the pain of childbirth. She asked her obstetrician if it was possible to relieve the pain without having a general anesthetic. She was told that she could have a relatively simple procedure called caudal anesthesia.

4. When performing caudal anesthesia, the syringe needle is inserted into the sacral canal by piercing the following anatomic structures except which?
   (a) Skin
   (b) Fascia
   (c) Ligaments
   (d) Sacral hiatus
   (e) Dura mater

An elderly woman was run over by an automobile as she was crossing the road. Radiographic examination of the pelvis in the emergency department of the local hospital revealed a fracture of the ilium and iliac crest on the left side.

5. The following statements about fractures of the pelvis are correct except which?
   (a) Fractures of the ilium have little displacement.
   (b) Displacement is prevented by the presence of the iliacus and the gluteal muscles on the inner and outer surfaces of this bone, respectively.
   (c) If two fractures occur in the ring forming the true pelvis, the fracture will be unstable and displacement will occur.
   (d) Fractures of the true pelvis do not cause injury to the pelvic viscera.
   (e) The postvertebral and abdominal muscles are responsible for elevating the lateral part of the pelvis should two fractures occur.
   (f) A heavy fall on the greater trochanter of the femur may drive the head of the femur through the floor of the acetabulum and into the pelvic cavity.

A pregnant woman visited an antenatal clinic. A vaginal examination revealed that the sacral promontory could be easily palpated and that the diagonal conjugate measured less than 4 in. (10 cm).

6. The following statements concerning this examination are correct except which?
   (a) Normally it is difficult or impossible to feel the sacral promontory by means of a vaginal examination.
   (b) The normal diagonal conjugate measures about 10 in. (25 cm).
   (c) This patient's pelvis was flattened anteroposteriorly, and the sacral promontory projected too far forward.
   (d) It is likely that this patient would have an obstructed labor.
   (e) This patient was advised to have a cesarean section.

ANSWERS TO CLINICAL PROBLEMS

1. C. In extreme cases of urethral obstruction in the male, the superior wall of the bladder has been known to reach the costal margin.
2. E. The puborectalis muscle is one of the most important sphincters of the anal canal.
3. C. The anterior surface of the coccyx can be palpated with a gloved finger placed in the anal canal.
4. E. The dura mater extends down in the sacral canal only as far as the lower border of the second sacral vertebra. It lies about 2 in. (50 mm) above the sacral hiatus in the adult.
5. D. Fractures of the true pelvis are commonly associated with injuries to the soft pelvic viscera, especially the bladder and the urethra.
6. B. The normal diagonal conjugate measures about 5 in. (11.5 cm).

REVIEW QUESTIONS

Multiple-Choice Questions

Select the best answer for each question.

1. The following statements concerning the pelvis are correct except which?
   (a) The ilium, ischium, and pubis are three separate bones that fuse together to form the hip bone in the 25th year of life.
   (b) The platypelloid type of pelvis occurs in about 2% of women.
   (c) External pelvic measurements have little practical importance in determining whether a disproportion between the size of the fetal head and the size of the pelvic inlet is likely.
   (d) The pelvic outlet is formed by the symphysis pubis anteriorly, the ischial tuberosities laterally, the sacrotuberous ligaments laterally, and the coccyx posteriorly.
   (e) The sacrum is shorter, wider, and flatter in the female than in the male.
2. The following statements concerning structures that leave the pelvis are correct except which?
   (a) The sciatic nerve leaves the pelvis through the greater sciatic foramen.
   (b) The piriformis muscle leaves the pelvis through the greater sciatic foramen.
   (c) The external iliac artery passes beneath the inguinal ligament to become the femoral artery.
   (d) The obturator nerve leaves the pelvis through the lesser sciatic foramen.
   (e) The inferior gluteal artery leaves the pelvis through the greater sciatic foramen.
3. The following statements concerning the muscles and fascia in the pelvis are correct except which?
   (a) The levator ani muscle is innervated by the perineal branch of the fourth sacral nerve and from the perineal branch of the pudendal nerve.
   (b) In the pelvis, the fascia is divided into parietal and visceral layers.
   (c) The iliococcygeus muscle arises from a thickening of the obturator internus fascia.
   (d) The pelvic diaphragm is strong and has no openings.
   (e) The visceral layer of pelvic fascia forms important ligaments that help support the uterus.
4. The following statements concerning the nerves of the pelvic cavity are correct except which?
   (a) The inferior hypogastric plexus contains both sympathetic and parasympathetic nerves.
   (b) The sacral plexus lies behind the rectum.
   (c) The pelvic part of the sympathetic trunk possesses both white and gray rami communicantes.
   (d) The superior hypogastric plexus is formed from the aortic sympathetic plexus and branches of the lumbar sympathetic ganglia.
   (e) The anterior rami of the upper four sacral nerves emerge into the pelvis through the anterior sacral foramina.
5. The following statements concerning the bony pelvis are correct except which?
   (a) When the patient is in the standing position, the anterior superior iliac spines lie vertically above the anterior surface of the symphysis pubis.
   (b) Very little movement is possible at the sacrococcygeal joint.
   (c) The false pelvis helps guide the fetus into the true pelvis during labor.
   (d) The female sex hormones cause a relaxation of the ligaments of the pelvis during pregnancy.
   (e) Obliteration of the cavity of the sacroiliac joint often occurs in both sexes after middle age.
6. The statements concerning the segmental origin of the following nerves are correct except which?
   (a) The sciatic nerve is derived from the segments L4 and 5 and S1, 2, and 3.
   (b) The pudendal nerve is derived from the segments L3, 4, and 5.
   (c) The pelvic splanchnic nerve is derived from the segments S2, 3, and 4.
   (d) The obturator nerve is derived from the segments L2, 3, and 4.
   (e) The lumbosacral trunk is derived from the segments L4 and 5.

7. The statements concerning the origin of the following arteries are correct except which?
   (a) The superior rectal artery is derived from the inferior mesenteric artery.
   (b) The ovarian artery is derived from the renal artery.
   (c) The uterine artery is derived from the internal iliac artery.
   (d) The middle rectal artery is derived from the internal iliac artery.
   (e) The superior gluteal artery is derived from the internal iliac artery.
8. The statements concerning the motor nerve supply of the muscles of the pelvic walls are correct except which?
   (a) The sacral nerves or plexus supply the obturator internus muscle.
   (b) The obturator nerve supplies the piriformis muscle.
   (c) The sacral nerves, or plexus, supply the iliococcygeus muscle.
   (d) The sacral nerves, or plexus, supply the coccygeus muscle.
   (e) The perineal branch of the fourth sacral nerve and the perineal branch of the pudendal nerve supply the levator ani muscle.

Read the case history and select the best answer to the question following it.

A 37-year-old woman was involved in a severe automobile accident in which the car, traveling at high speed, swerved off the road and hit a tree. She was evaluated in the emergency department and found to have multiple injuries. Radiographic examination of her pelvis showed a fracture of her right ilium and iliac crest.

9. From your knowledge of anatomy, determine which of the following treatments was correct.
   (a) An attempt was made to immobilize the bony fragments by encasing the patient in a plaster cast extending from the subcostal region down both thighs to just above the knee.
   (b) The right gluteal region was strapped with a strong Elastoplast bandage.
   (c) The patient was operated on and the bony fragments were replaced in their correct anatomic position and secured with screws.
   (d) Splinting of the fractured bone was unnecessary.
   (e) Because of the fear of avascular necrosis, the smaller bony fragments were surgically removed.

ANSWERS TO REVIEW QUESTIONS

1. A. At puberty the three separate bones—the ilium, ischium, and pubis—fuse together to form one large irregular bone, the hip bone.

2. D. The obturator nerve leaves the pelvis through the obturator canal, which is the upper part of the obturator foramen, devoid of the obturator membrane.

3. D. The pelvic diaphragm is a gutter-shaped sheet of muscle formed by the levatores ani and coccygeus muscles and their covering fasciae. Its function is to support the pelvic viscera. The pelvic diaphragm is incomplete anteriorly, forming an opening to allow passage of the urethra in males and the urethra and the vagina in females.

4. C. The pelvic part of the sympathetic trunk gives rise to only gray postganglionic nerve fibers, which are distributed to the pelvic viscera and blood vessels.

5. B. The sacrococcygeal joint is a cartilaginous joint and can perform a great deal of movement.

6. B. The pudendal nerve is a branch of the sacral plexus and is derived from S2, 3, and 4.

7. B. Both the right and the left ovarian arteries are branches of the abdominal aorta.

8. B. The piriformis muscle receives its motor nerve supply from the sacral plexus.

9. D. Most fractures of the upper part of the ilium have little displacement of the bone fragments. This is because the iliacus muscle is attached to the inner surface and the gluteal muscles are attached to the outer surface. Splinting the bones is unnecessary because of the attachment of these muscles. The muscular attachments also provide an adequate blood supply to the bone fragments.

CHAPTER 7

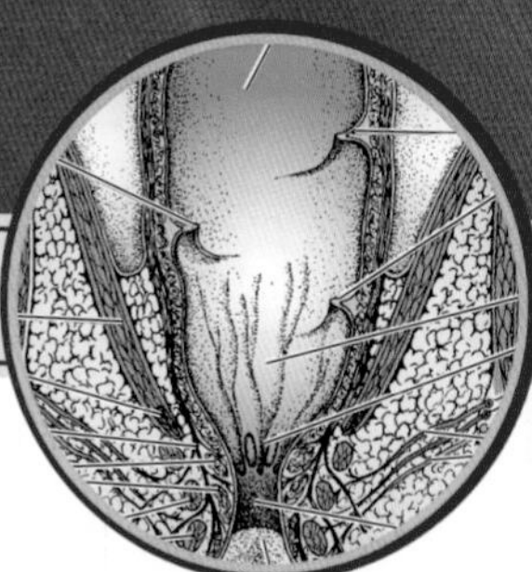

THE PELVIS: PART II—THE PELVIC CAVITY

A 62-year-old man visited his physician for an annual physical examination. He appeared to be in very good health and had no complaints. A general examination revealed nothing abnormal. The physician then told the patient that he was about to perform a rectal examination. At first the patient objected, saying that he did not feel it was necessary because nothing abnormal was found a year ago. The physician persisted and finally the patient agreed to the examination.

A small hard nodule was found projecting from the posterior surface of the prostate. No other abnormalities were discovered. The patient was informed of the findings, and the possibility that the nodule was malignant was explained. The patient was very upset, especially because he had no abnormal urinary symptoms.

Additional laboratory and radiologic tests were performed, and the prostate-specific antigen (PSA) level in the blood was found to be well above the normal range. No evidence of pelvic lymphatic enlargement was seen on pelvic computed tomography (CT) scans and no evidence of bone metastases was seen on bone scans. A diagnosis of early cancer of the prostate was made and was later confirmed by a needle biopsy of prostatic tissue through the anterior wall of the rectum.

This case illustrates how a physician in general practice who has good knowledge of the relevant anatomic features of the pelvis can recognize an abnormal prostate when it is palpated through the anterior rectal wall. This patient later had the prostate removed, and the prognosis was excellent.

CHAPTER OUTLINE

Basic Anatomy 338
Contents of the Pelvic Cavity 338
Sigmoid Colon 338
Rectum 341
Pelvic Viscera in the Male 347
Ureters 347
Urinary Bladder 348
Male Genital Organs 352
Vas Deferens 352
Seminal Vesicles 352
Ejaculatory Ducts 353
Prostate 353
Prostatic Urethra 356
Visceral Pelvic Fascia 356
Peritoneum 356
Pelvic Viscera in the Female 356
Ureters 356
Urinary Bladder 356
Female Genital Organs 361
Ovary 361
Uterine Tube 363
Uterus 364
Vagina 372
Visceral Pelvic Fascia 376
Peritoneum 376
Cross-Sectional Anatomy of the Pelvis 377
Radiographic Anatomy 377
Radiographic Appearances of the Bony Pelvis 377
Radiographic Appearances of the Sigmoid Colon and Rectum 377
Barium Enema 377
Radiographic Appearances of the Female Genital Tract 381
Surface Anatomy 381
Clinical Problem Solving 382
Answers to Clinical Problems 383
Review Questions 384
Answers to Review Questions 385

CHAPTER OBJECTIVES

- The pelvic cavity contains the lower ends of the intestinal and urinary tracts and the internal organs of reproduction as well as their nerve supply, blood supply, and lymphatic drainage.
- The organs project up into the peritoneal cavity, causing the peritoneum to be draped over them in folds, producing important fossae that are the sites for the accumulation of blood and pus in different types of pelvic disease.
- The physician is often confronted with problems involving infections, injuries, and prolapses of the rectum, uterus, and vagina.
- Emergency situations involving the bladder, the pregnant uterus, ectopic pregnancy, spontaneous abortion, and acute pelvic inflammatory disease are examples of problems found in the female.
- The urinary bladder and the prostate in the male are frequent sites of disease.
- The purpose of this chapter is to consider the important anatomy relative to common clinical conditions involving the pelvic organs.

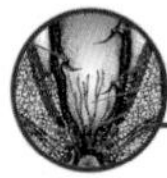

BASIC ANATOMY

The pelvic cavity, or cavity of the true pelvis, can be defined as the area between the pelvic inlet and the pelvic outlet. It is customary to subdivide it by the pelvic diaphragm into the main pelvic cavity above and the perineum below (Fig. 7-1). This chapter is concerned with the contents of the main pelvic cavity. A detailed description of the perineum is given in Chapter 8.

Contents of the Pelvic Cavity

Sigmoid Colon

Location and Description

The sigmoid colon is 10 to 15 in. (25 to 38 cm) long and begins as a continuation of the descending colon in front of the pelvic brim. Below, it becomes continuous with the rectum in front of the third sacral vertebra. The sigmoid colon is mobile and hangs down into the pelvic cavity in the form of a loop.

The sigmoid colon is attached to the posterior pelvic wall by the fan-shaped **sigmoid mesocolon.**

Relations

- **Anteriorly:** In the male, the urinary bladder; in the female, the posterior surface of the uterus and the upper part of the vagina
- **Posteriorly:** The rectum and the sacrum. The sigmoid colon is also related to the lower coils of the terminal part of the ileum.

Blood Supply

Arteries

Sigmoid branches of the inferior mesenteric artery.

Veins

The veins drain into the inferior mesenteric vein, which joins the portal venous system.

Lymph Drainage

The lymph drains into nodes along the course of the sigmoid arteries; from these nodes, the lymph travels to the inferior mesenteric nodes.

Nerve Supply

The sympathetic and parasympathetic nerves from the inferior hypogastric plexuses.

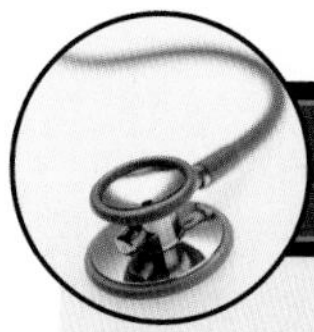

CLINICAL NOTES

Variation in Length and Location of the Sigmoid Colon

The sigmoid colon shows great variation in length and may measure as much as 36 in. (91 cm). In the young child, because the pelvis is small, this segment of the colon may lie mainly in the abdomen.

Cancer of the Sigmoid Colon

The sigmoid colon is a common site for cancer of the large bowel. Because the lymphatic vessels of this segment of the colon drain ultimately into the inferior mesenteric nodes, it follows that an extensive resection of the gut and its associated lymphatic field is necessary to extirpate the growth and its local lymphatic metastases. The colon is removed from the left colic flexure to the distal end of the sigmoid colon, and the transverse colon is anastomosed to the rectum.

Volvulus

Because of its extreme mobility, the sigmoid colon sometimes rotates around its mesentery. This may correct itself spontaneously, or the rotation may continue until the blood supply of the gut is cut off completely. The rotation commonly occurs in a counterclockwise direction and is referred to as volvulus.

Diverticula

Diverticula of the mucous membrane along the course of the arteries supplying the sigmoid colon is a common clinical condition and is described on page 236. In patients with diverticulitis or ulcerative colitis, the sigmoid colon may become adherent to the bladder, rectum, ileum, or ureter and produce an internal fistula.

Sigmoidoscopy

Because the sigmoid colon lies only a short distance from the anus (6.5 in. [17 cm]), it is possible to examine the mucous membrane under direct vision for pathologic conditions. A flexible tube fitted with lenses and illuminated internally is introduced through the anus and carefully passed up through the anal canal, rectum, sigmoid colon, and descending colon. This examination, called sigmoidoscopy, can be carried out without an anesthetic in an outpatient clinic. Biopsy specimens of the mucous membrane can be obtained through this instrument.

Anatomic Facts Relevant to Sigmoidoscopy

- The patient is placed in the left lateral position with the left knee flexed and the right knee extended (Fig. 7-2). Alternatively, the patient is placed kneeling in the knee–chest position.
- The sigmoidoscope is gently inserted into the anus and anal canal in the direction of the umbilicus to ensure that the instrument passes along the long axis of the canal. Gentle but firm pressure is applied to overcome the resistance of the anal sphincters (Fig. 7-3).
- After a distance of about 1.5 in. (4 cm), the instrument enters the ampulla of the rectum. At this point, the tip of the sigmoidoscope should be directed posteriorly in the midline to follow the sacral curve of the rectum (Fig. 7-2).
- Slow advancement is made under direct vision. Some slight side-to-side movement may be necessary to bypass the **transverse rectal folds.**
- At approximately 6.5 in. (16.25 cm) from the anal margin, the rectosigmoid junction will be reached. The sigmoid colon here bends forward and to the left, and the lumen appears to end in a blind cul-de-sac. To negotiate this angulation, the tip of the sigmoidoscope must be directed anteriorly and to the patient's left side. This maneuver can cause some discomfort in the anal canal from distortion of the anal sphincters by the shaft of the sigmoidoscope. Another possibility is that the point of the instrument may stretch the wall of the colon, giving rise to colicky pain in the lower abdomen.
- Once the instrument has entered the sigmoid colon, it should be possible to pass it smoothly along its full extent and, using the full length of the sigmoidoscope, enter the descending colon.
- The sigmoidoscope may now be slowly withdrawn, carefully inspecting the mucous membrane. The normal rectal and colonic mucous membrane is smooth and glistening and pale pink with an orange tinge, and blood vessels in the submucosa can be clearly seen. The mucous membrane is supple and moves easily over the end of the sigmoidoscope.

Anatomy of Complications of Sigmoidoscopy

Perforation of the bowel at the rectosigmoid junction can occur. This is almost invariably caused by the operator failing to negotiate carefully the curve between the rectum and the sigmoid colon. In some patients, the curve is in the form of an acute angulation, which may frustrate the overzealous advancement of the sigmoidoscope. Perforation of the sigmoid colon results in the escape of colonic contents into the peritoneal cavity.

Colonoscopy

Direct inspection of the lining of the entire colon including the cecum has become an important weapon in the early diagnosis of mucosal polyps and large bowel cancer in recent years. Not only can the colon be observed and suspicious areas photographed for future reference, but also biopsy specimens can be removed for pathologic examination.

For the diagnosis of early cancer, physicians previously relied almost entirely on rectal examination, sigmoidoscopy, and the detection of occult blood in the feces. The disadvantage of colonoscopy is the high cost (see Fig. 5-37).

Following a regime in which the large bowel is thoroughly washed out, the patient is relaxed under a light anesthetic. The flexible endoscopic tube is introduced through the anus into the anal canal, rectum, and colon. Colonoscopy can also be used in the diagnosis and treatment of ulcerative colitis and Crohn's disease.

Colostomy

The sigmoid colon is often selected as a site for performing a colostomy in patients with carcinoma of the rectum. Its mobility allows the surgeon to bring out a loop of colon, with its blood supply intact, through a small incision in the left iliac region of the anterior abdominal wall. Its mobility also makes it suitable for implantation of the ureters after surgical removal of the bladder.

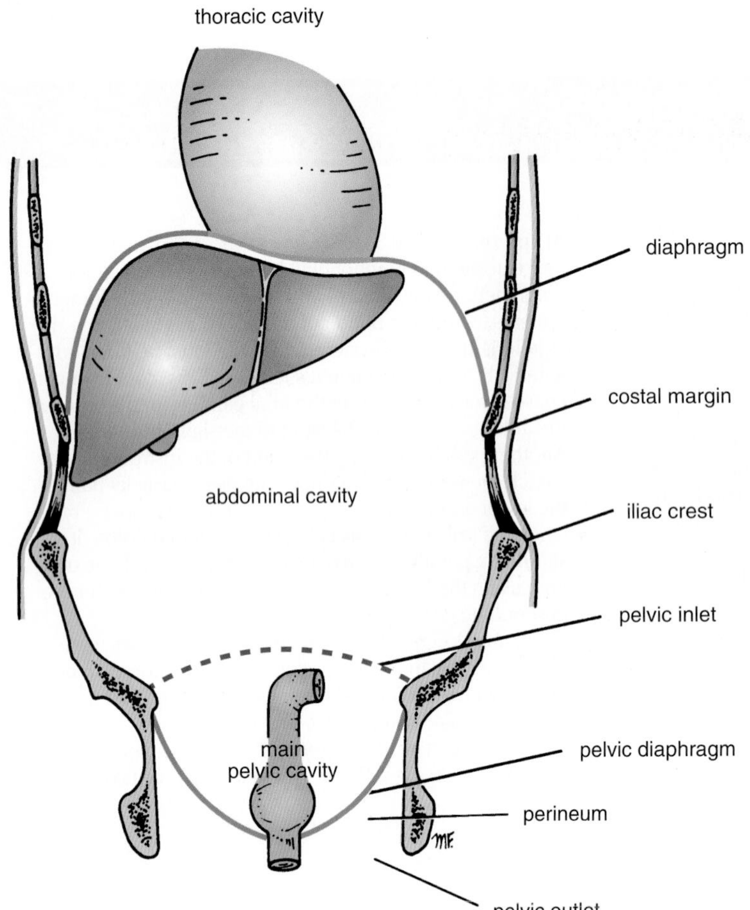

Figure 7-1 Coronal section through the thorax, abdomen, and pelvis showing the thoracic, abdominal, and pelvic cavities and the perineum.

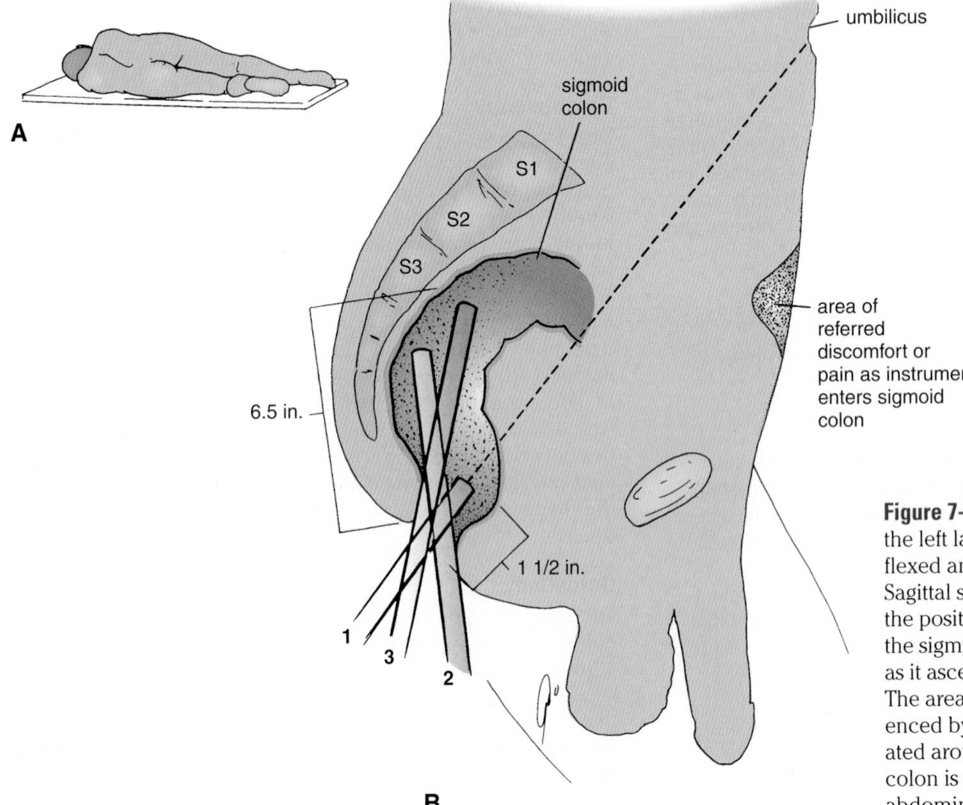

Figure 7-2 Sigmoidoscopy. **A.** Patient in the left lateral position with the left knee flexed and the right knee extended. **B.** Sagittal section of the male pelvis showing the positions (*1*, *2*, and *3*) of the tube of the sigmoidoscope relative to the patient as it ascends the anal canal and rectum. The area of discomfort or pain experienced by the patient as the tube is negotiated around the bend into the sigmoid colon is referred to the skin of the anterior abdominal wall below the umbilicus.

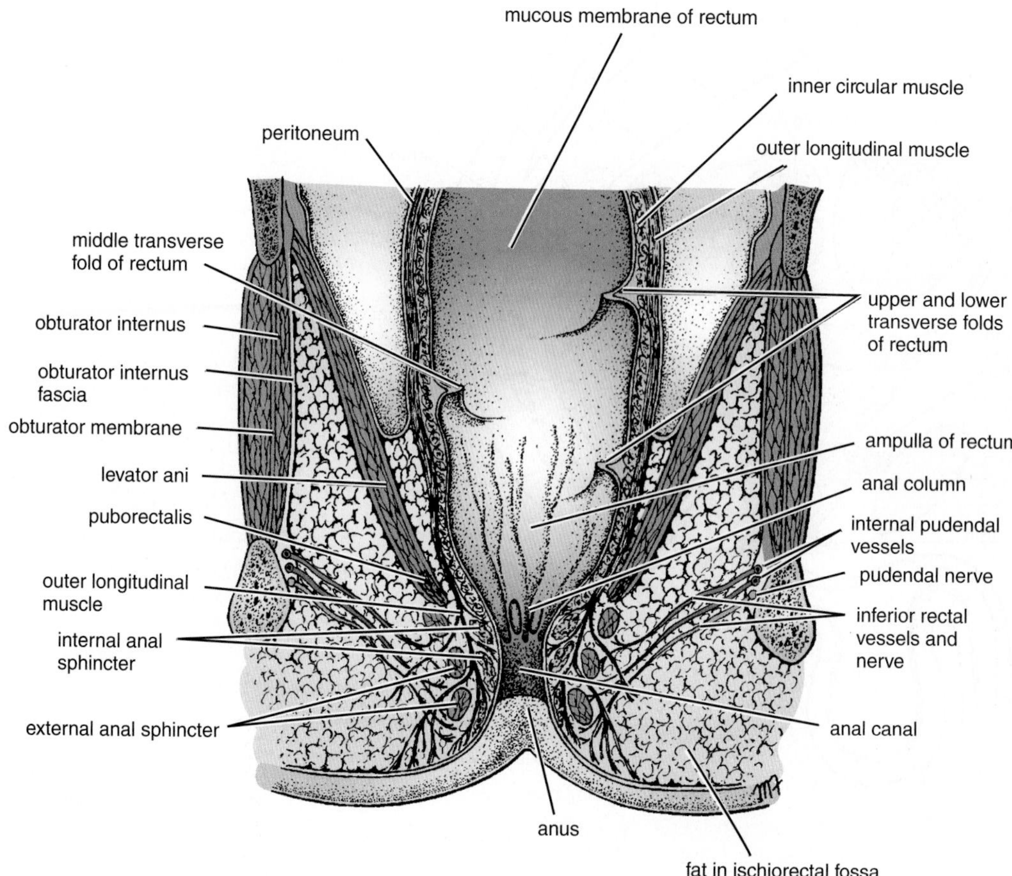

Figure 7-3 Coronal section through the pelvis showing the rectum and the pelvic floor.

Rectum

Location and Description

The rectum is about 5 in. (13 cm) long and begins in front of the third sacral vertebra as a continuation of the sigmoid colon. It passes downward, following the curve of the sacrum and coccyx, and ends in front of the tip of the coccyx by piercing the pelvic diaphragm and becoming continuous with the anal canal. The lower part of the rectum is dilated to form the **rectal ampulla.**

The rectum deviates to the left, but it quickly returns to the median plane (Fig. 7-3). On lateral view, the rectum follows the anterior concavity of the sacrum before bending downward and backward at its junction with the anal canal (Fig. 7-4).

The puborectalis portion of the levator ani muscles forms a sling (see page 318) at the junction of the rectum with the anal canal and pulls this part of the bowel forward, producing the anorectal angle.

The **peritoneum** covers the anterior and lateral surfaces of the first third of the rectum and only the anterior surface of the middle third, leaving the lower third devoid of peritoneum (Figs. 7-4 and 7-5).

The **muscular coat** of the rectum is arranged in the usual outer longitudinal and inner circular layers of smooth muscle. The three teniae coli of the sigmoid colon, however, come together so that the longitudinal fibers form a broad band on the anterior and posterior surfaces of the rectum.

The **mucous membrane** of the rectum, together with the circular muscle layer, forms two or three semicircular permanent folds called the **transverse folds of the rectum** (Fig. 7-3); they vary in position.

Relations

- **Posteriorly:** The rectum is in contact with the sacrum and coccyx; the piriformis, coccygeus, and levatores ani muscles; the sacral plexus; and the sympathetic trunks (see Fig. 6-18).
- **Anteriorly: In the male,** the upper two thirds of the rectum, which is covered by peritoneum, is related to the sigmoid colon and coils of ileum that occupy the rectovesical pouch. The lower third of the rectum, which is devoid of peritoneum, is related to the posterior surface of the bladder, to the termination of the vas deferens and the seminal vesicles on each side, and to the prostate (Fig. 7-4).

In the female, the upper two thirds of the rectum, which is covered by peritoneum, is related to the sigmoid colon and coils of ileum that occupy the rectouterine pouch (pouch of Douglas). The lower third of the rectum, which is devoid of peritoneum, is related to the posterior surface of the vagina (Fig. 7-5).

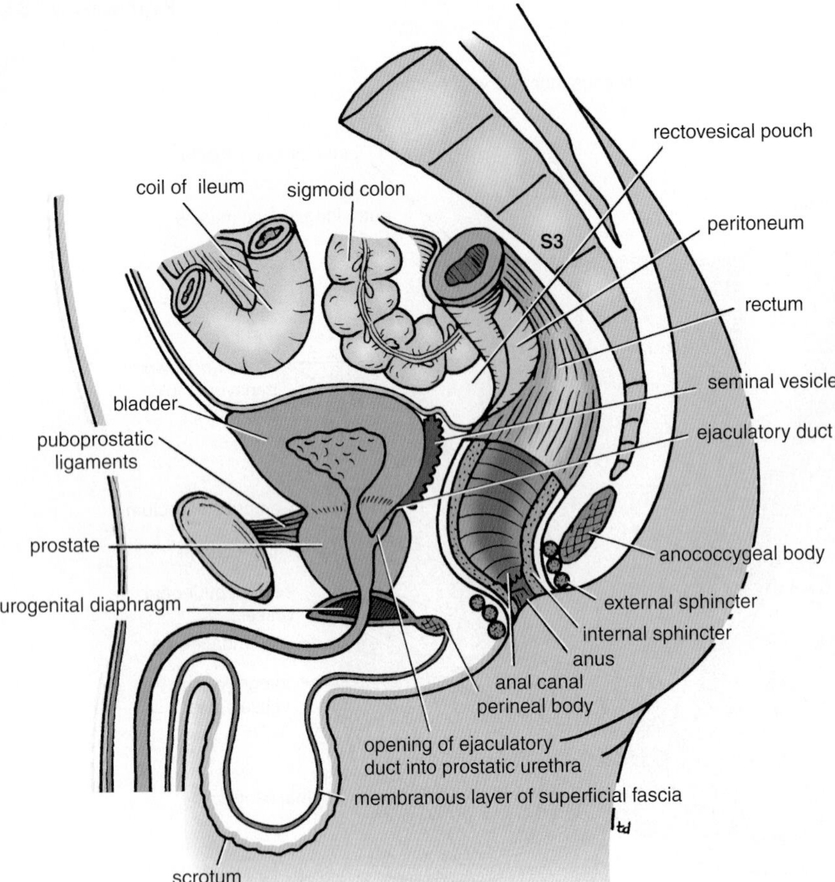

Figure 7-4 Sagittal section of the male pelvis.

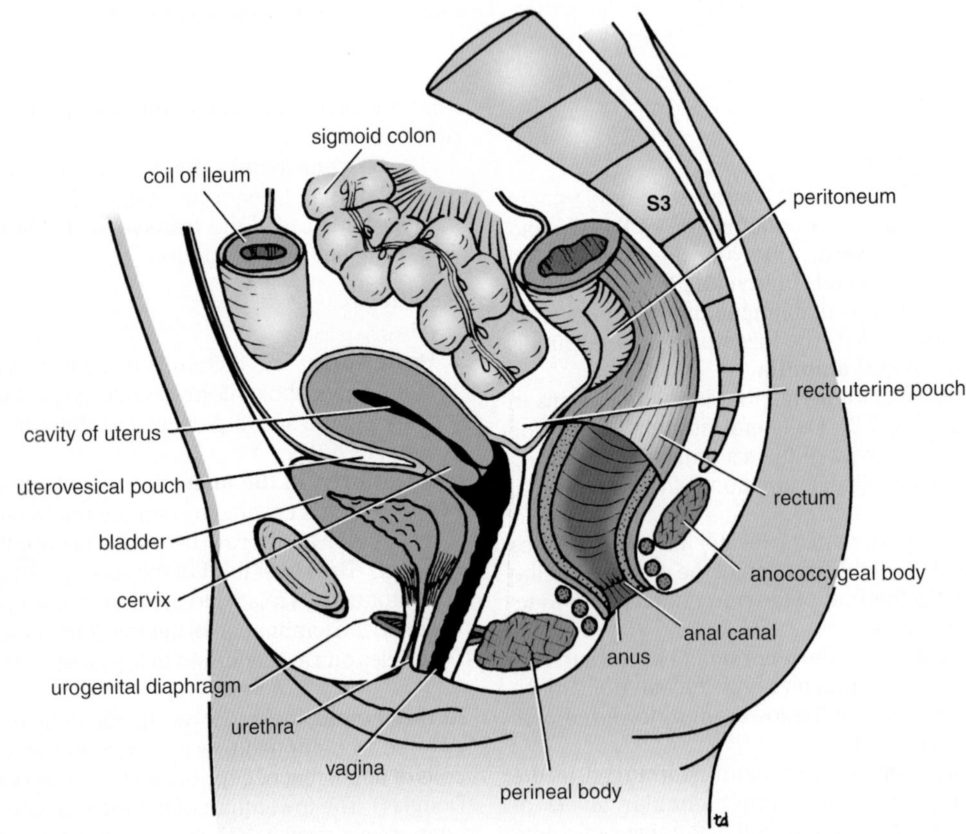

Figure 7-5 Sagittal section of the female pelvis.

Blood Supply

Arteries

The superior, middle, and inferior rectal arteries (Fig. 7-6) supply the rectum.

The **superior rectal artery** is a direct continuation of the inferior mesenteric artery and is the chief artery supplying the mucous membrane. It enters the pelvis by descending in the root of the sigmoid mesocolon and divides into right and left branches, which pierce the muscular coat and supply the mucous membrane. They anastomose with one another and with the middle and inferior rectal arteries.

The **middle rectal artery** is a small branch of the internal iliac artery and is distributed mainly to the muscular coat.

The **inferior rectal artery** is a branch of the internal pudendal artery in the perineum. It anastomoses with the middle rectal artery at the anorectal junction.

Veins

The veins of the rectum correspond to the arteries. The **superior rectal vein** is a tributary of the portal circulation and drains into the inferior mesenteric vein. The **middle** and **inferior rectal veins** drain into the internal iliac and internal pudendal veins, respectively. The union between

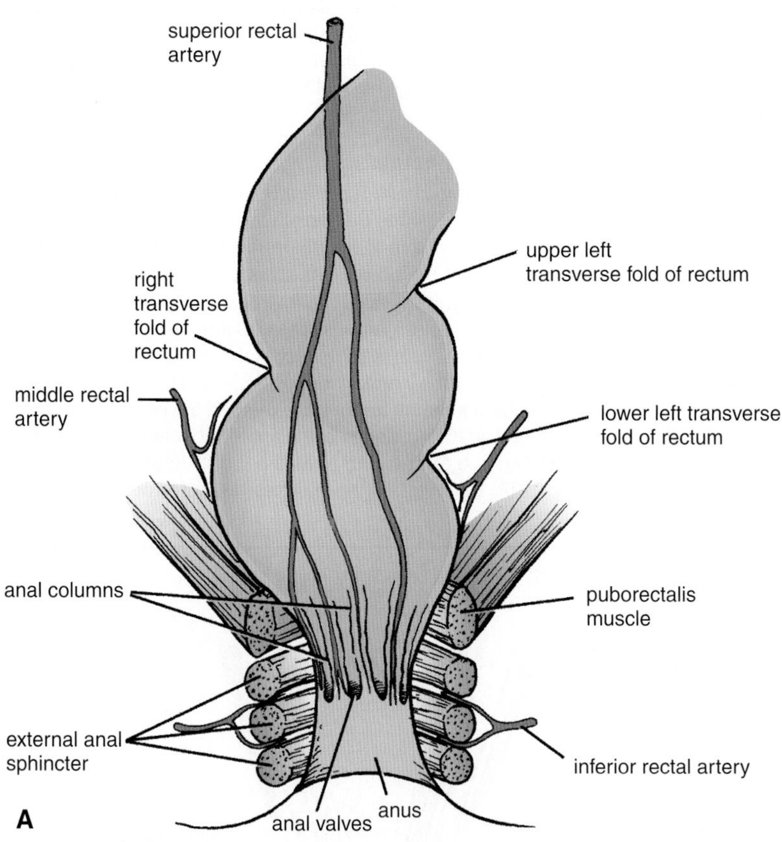

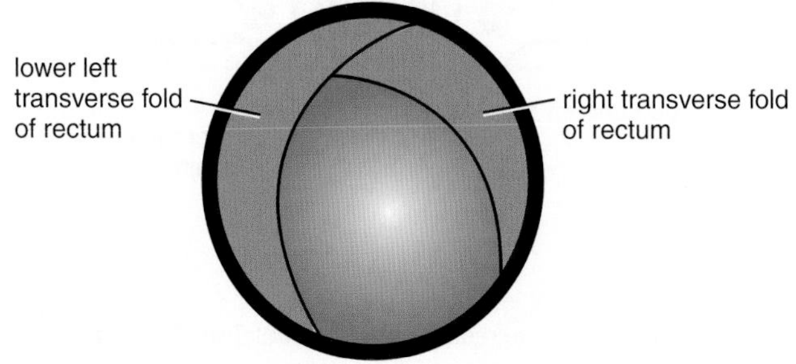

Figure 7-6 **A.** Blood supply to the rectum. **B.** The transverse folds of the rectum as seen through a sigmoidoscope.

the rectal veins forms an important portal–systemic anastomosis (see Chapter 5).

Lymph Drainage

The lymph vessels of the rectum drain first into the **pararectal nodes** and then into inferior mesenteric nodes. Lymph vessels from the lower part of the rectum follow the middle rectal artery to the internal iliac nodes.

Nerve Supply

The nerve supply is from the sympathetic and parasympathetic nerves from the inferior hypogastric plexuses. The rectum is sensitive **only** to stretch.

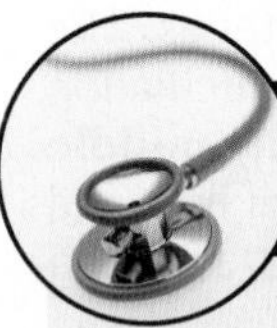

CLINICAL NOTES

Rectal Curves and Mucosal Folds

The anteroposterior flexure of the rectum, as it follows the curvature of the sacrum and coccyx, and the lateral flexures must be remembered when one is passing a sigmoidoscope to avoid causing the patient unnecessary discomfort.

The crescentic transverse mucosal folds of the rectum must also be borne in mind when passing an instrument into the rectum. It is thought that these folds serve to support the weight of the feces and to prevent excessive distention of the rectal ampulla.

Blood Supply and Internal Hemorrhoids

The chief arterial supply to the rectum is from the superior rectal artery, a continuation of the inferior mesenteric artery. In front of the third sacral vertebra, the artery divides into right and left branches. Halfway down the rectum, the right branch divides into an anterior and a posterior branch. The tributaries of the superior rectal vein are arranged in a similar manner, so that it is not surprising to find that **internal hemorrhoids** are arranged in three groups (see Chapter 8): two on the right side of the lower rectum and anal canal and one on the left.

Partial and Complete Prolapse of the Rectum

Partial and complete prolapses of the rectum through the anus are relatively common clinical conditions. In partial prolapse, the rectal mucous membrane and submucous coat protrude for a short distance outside the anus (Fig. 7-7). In complete prolapse, the whole thickness of the rectal wall protrudes through the anus. In both conditions, many causative factors may be involved. However, damage to the levatores ani muscles as the result of childbirth and poor muscle tone in the aged are important contributing factors. A complete rectal prolapse may be regarded as a sliding hernia through the pelvic diaphragm.

Cancer of the Rectum

Cancer (carcinoma) of the rectum is a common clinical finding that remains localized to the rectal wall for a considerable time. At first, it tends to spread locally in the lymphatics around the circumference of the bowel. Later, it spreads upward and laterally along the lymph vessels, following the superior rectal and middle rectal arteries. Venous spread occurs late, and because the superior rectal vein is a tributary of the portal vein, the liver is a common site for secondary deposits.

Once the malignant tumor has extended beyond the confines of the rectal wall, knowledge of the anatomic relations of the rectum will enable a physician to assess the structures and organs likely to be involved. In both sexes, a posterior penetration

(continues)

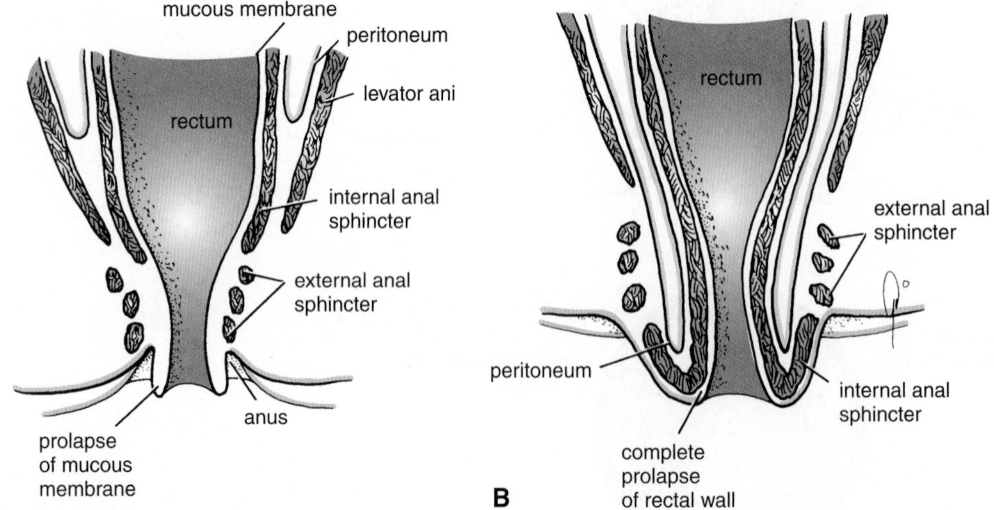

Figure 7-7 Coronal section of the rectum and anal canal. **A.** Incomplete rectal (mucosal) prolapse. **B.** Complete rectal prolapse.

Clinical Notes, *continued*

involves the sacral plexus and can cause severe intractable pain down the leg in the distribution of the sciatic nerve. A lateral penetration may involve the ureter. An anterior penetration in the male may involve the prostate, seminal vesicles, or bladder; in the female, the vagina and uterus may be invaded.

It is clear from the anatomic features of the rectum and its lymph drainage that a wide resection of the rectum with its lymphatic field offers the best chance of cure. When the tumor has spread to contiguous organs and is of a low grade of malignancy, some form of pelvic evisceration may be justifiable.

It is most important for a medical student to remember that the interior of the lower part of the rectum can be examined by a gloved index finger introduced through the anal canal. The anal canal is about 1.5 in. (4 cm) long so that the pulp of the index finger can easily feel the mucous membrane lining the lower end of the rectum. Most cancers of the rectum can be diagnosed by this means. This examination can be extended in both sexes by placing the other hand on the lower part of the anterior abdominal wall. With the bladder empty, the anterior rectal wall can be examined bimanually. In the female, the placing of one finger in the vagina and another in the rectum may enable the physician to make a thorough examination of the lower part of the anterior rectal wall.

Rectal Injuries

The management of penetrating rectal injuries will be determined by the site of penetration relative to the peritoneal covering. The upper third of the rectum is covered on the anterior and lateral surfaces by peritoneum, the middle third is covered only on its anterior surface, and the lower third is devoid of a peritoneal covering (Figs. 7-3, 7-4, and 7-5). The treatment of penetration of the intraperitoneal portion of the rectum is identical to that of the colon, because the peritoneal cavity has been violated. In the case of penetration of the extraperitoneal portion, the rectum is treated by diverting the feces through a temporary abdominal colostomy, administering antibiotics, and repairing and draining the tissue in front of the sacrum.

Pelvic Appendix

If an inflamed appendix is hanging down into the pelvis, abdominal tenderness in the right iliac region may not be felt, but deep tenderness may be experienced above the symphysis pubis. Rectal examination (or vaginal examination in the female) may reveal tenderness of the peritoneum in the pelvis on the right side. If such an inflamed appendix perforates, a localized pelvic peritonitis may result.

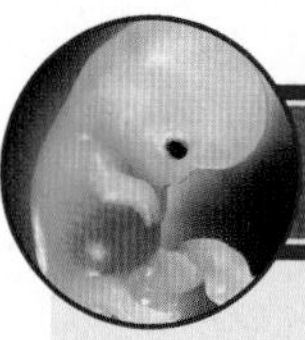

EMBRYOLOGIC NOTES

Development of the Distal Part of the Large Bowel

The left colic flexure, descending colon, sigmoid colon, rectum, and upper half of the anal canal are developed from the hindgut. Distally, this terminates as a blind sac of entoderm, which is in contact with a shallow ectodermal depression called the **proctodeum.** The apposed layers of ectoderm and entoderm form the **cloacal membrane,** which separates the cavity of the hindgut from the surface (Fig. 7-8). The hindgut sends off a diverticulum, the **allantois,** that passes into the umbilical cord. Distal to the allantois, the hindgut dilates to form the **entodermal cloaca** (Fig. 7-8). In the interval between the allantois and the hindgut, a wedge of mesenchyme invaginates the entoderm. With continued proliferation of the mesenchyme, a septum is formed that grows inferiorly and divides the cloaca into anterior and posterior parts. The septum is called the **urorectal septum,** the anterior part of the cloaca becomes the **primitive bladder** and the **urogenital sinus,** and the posterior part of the cloaca forms the **anorectal canal.** On reaching the cloacal membrane, the urorectal septum fuses with it and forms the future **perineal body** (Fig. 7-8). The fates of the primitive bladder and the urogenital sinus in both sexes are considered in detail on page 357.

The anorectal canal forms the **rectum** and the superior half of the **anal canal.** The lining of the inferior half of the anal canal is formed from the ectoderm of the proctodeum (Fig. 7-9). The posterior part of the cloacal membrane breaks down so that the gut opens onto the surface of the embryo.

Hindgut Artery

The hindgut, which extends from the left colic flexure to halfway down the anal canal, is supplied by the **inferior mesenteric artery** (see Fig. 5-46). Here, a number of ventral branches of the aorta fuse to form a single artery.

Meconium

At full term, the large intestine is filled with a mixture of intestinal gland secretions, bile, and amniotic fluid. This substance is dark green in color and is called meconium. It starts to accumulate at 4 months and reaches the rectum at the fifth month.

Primary Megacolon (Hirschsprung Disease)

Hirschsprung disease shows a familial tendency and is more common in males than in females. Symptoms usually appear during the first few days after birth. The child fails to pass meconium, and the abdomen becomes enormously distended. The sigmoid colon is greatly distended and hypertrophied, while the rectum and anal canal are constricted (Fig. 7-10). It is the constricted segment of the bowel that causes the obstruction, and histologic examination reveals a complete failure of development of the parasympathetic ganglion cells in this region. The treatment is operative excision of the aganglionic segment of the bowel.

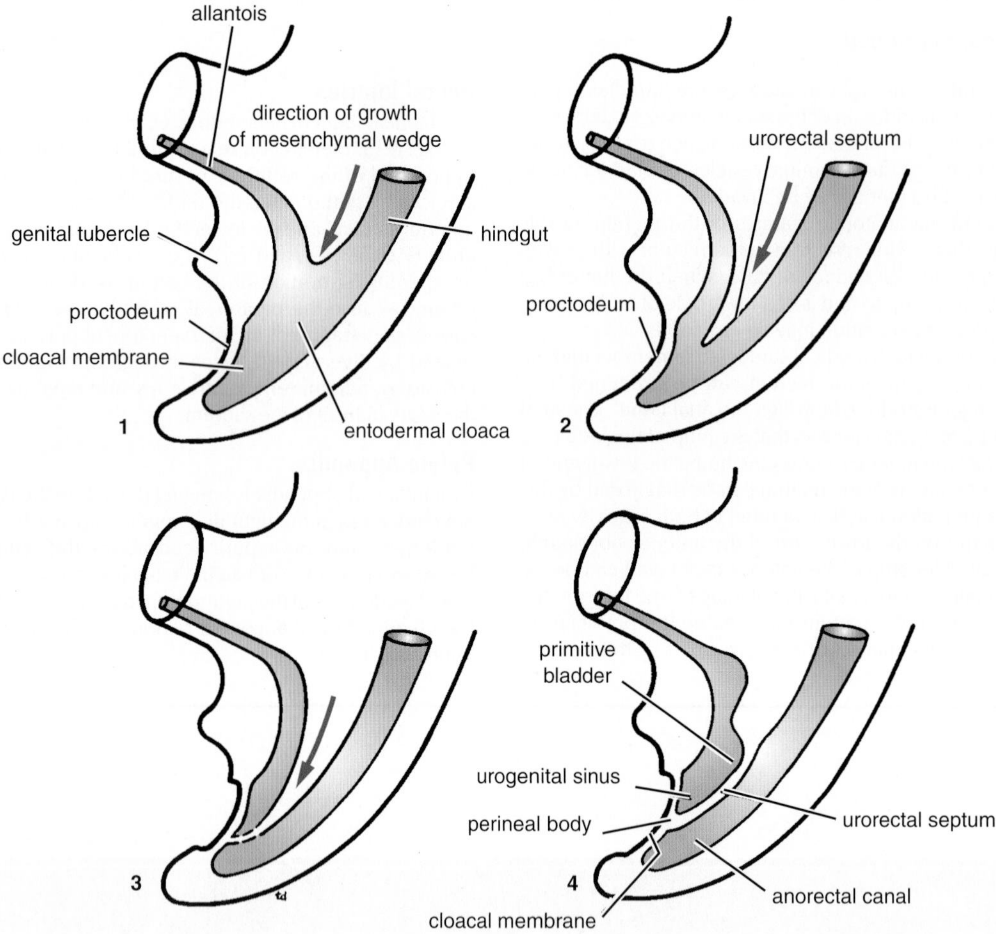

Figure 7-8 Progressive stages (*1–4*) in the formation of the urorectal septum, which divides the cloaca into an anterior part (the primitive bladder and the urogenital sinus) and a posterior part (the anorectal canal).

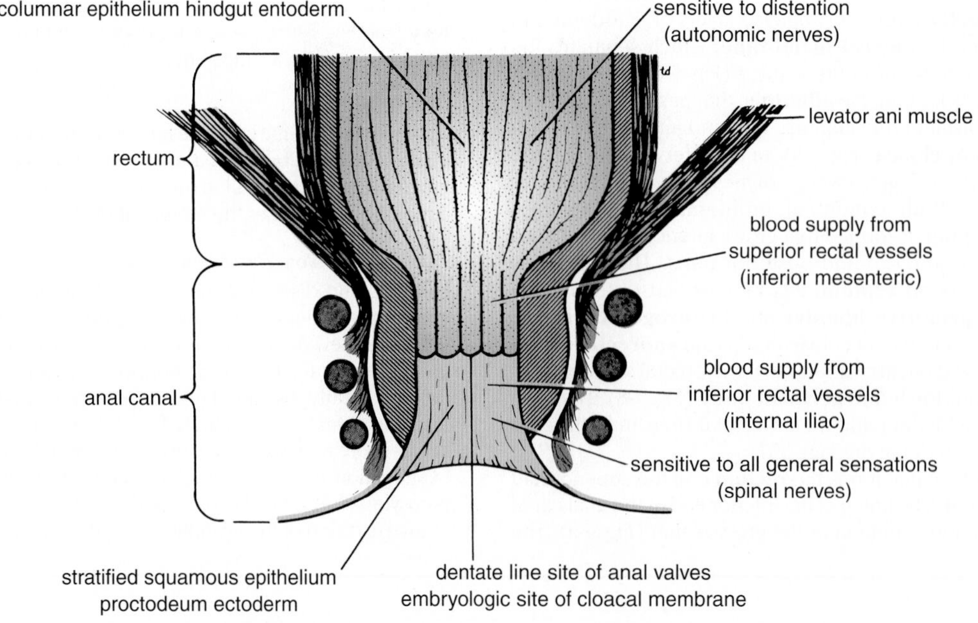

Figure 7-9 Structure of the anal canal and its embryologic origin.

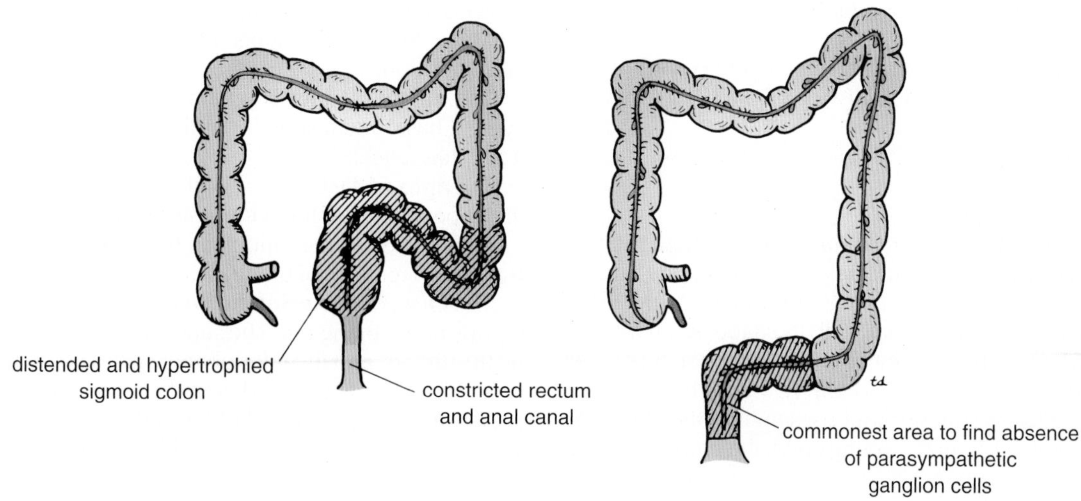

Figure 7-10 Main characteristics of primary megacolon (Hirschsprung disease).

Pelvic Viscera in the Male

The rectum, sigmoid colon, and terminal coils of ileum occupy the posterior part of the pelvic cavity in both sexes, as described above. The contents of the anterior part of the pelvic cavity in the male are described in the following sections.

Ureters

Each ureter is a muscular tube that extends from the kidney to the posterior surface of the bladder. Its abdominal course is described on page 266.

The ureter enters the pelvis by crossing the bifurcation of the common iliac artery in front of the sacroiliac joint. Each ureter then runs down the lateral wall of the pelvis in front of the internal iliac artery to the region of the ischial spine and turns forward to enter the lateral angle of the bladder (Fig. 7-11). Near its termination, it is crossed by the vas deferens. The ureter passes obliquely through the wall of the bladder for about 0.75 in. (1.9 cm) before opening into the bladder.

Constrictions

The ureter possesses three constrictions: where the renal pelvis joins the ureter in the abdomen, where it is kinked as

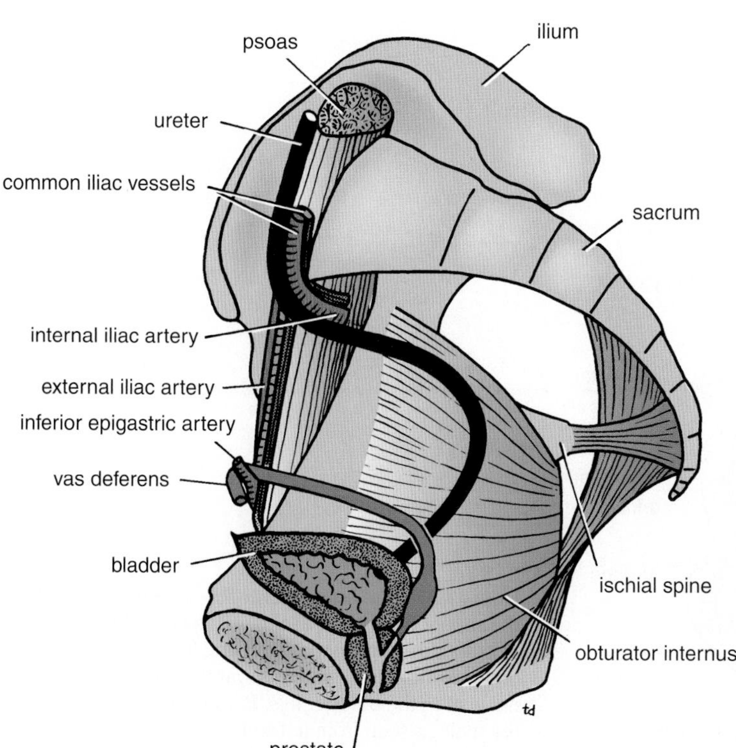

Figure 7-11 Right half of the pelvis showing relations of the ureter and vas deferens.

it crosses the pelvic brim to enter the pelvis, and where it pierces the bladder wall.

The blood supply, lymph drainage, and nerve supply of the ureter are described on page 266.

Urinary Bladder

Location and Description

The urinary bladder is situated immediately behind the pubic bones (Fig. 7-4) within the pelvis. It stores urine and in the adult has a maximum capacity of about 500 mL. The bladder has a strong muscular wall. Its shape and relations vary according to the amount of urine that it contains. The empty bladder in the adult lies entirely within the pelvis; as the bladder fills, its superior wall rises up into the hypogastric region (Fig. 7-12). In the young child, the empty bladder projects above the pelvic inlet; later, when the pelvic cavity enlarges, the bladder sinks into the pelvis to take up the adult position.

The empty bladder is pyramidal (Fig. 7-13), having an apex, a base, and a superior and two inferolateral surfaces; it also has a neck.

The **apex** of the bladder points anteriorly and lies behind the upper margin of the symphysis pubis (Figs. 7-4 and 7-12). It is connected to the umbilicus by the **median umbilical ligament** (remains of urachus).

The **base,** or **posterior surface** of the bladder, faces posteriorly and is triangular. The superolateral angles are joined by the ureters, and the inferior angle gives rise to the urethra (Fig. 7-13). The two vasa deferentia lie side by side on the posterior surface of the bladder and separate the seminal vesicles from each other (Fig. 7-13). The upper part of the

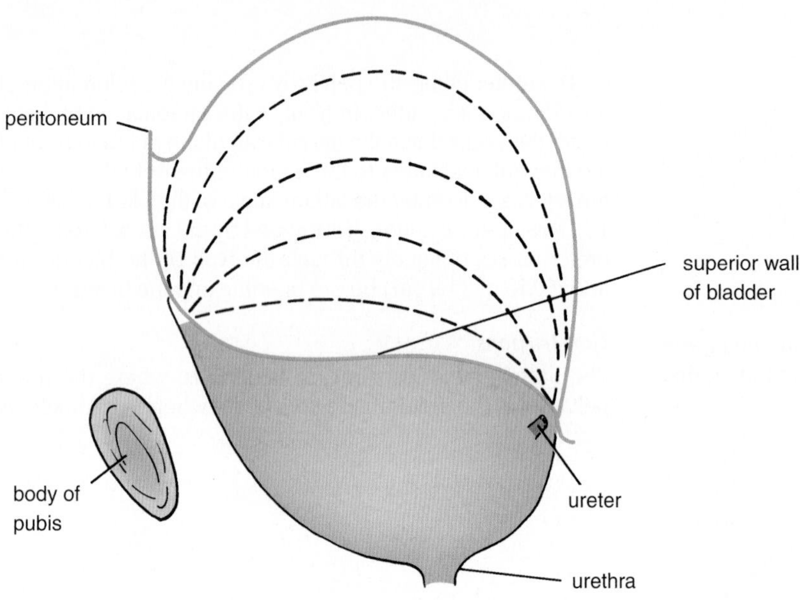

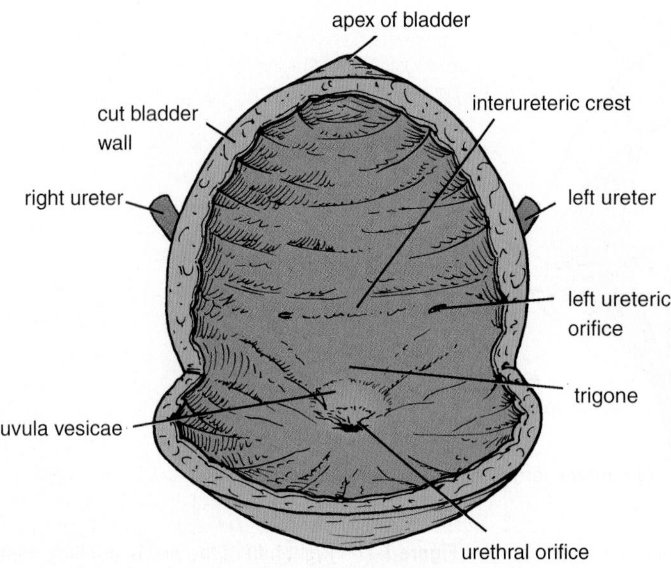

Figure 7-12 **A.** Lateral view of the bladder. Note that the superior wall rises as the viscus fills with urine. Note also that the peritoneum covering the superior surface of the bladder is peeled off from the anterior abdominal wall as the bladder fills. **B.** Interior of the bladder in the male as seen from in front.

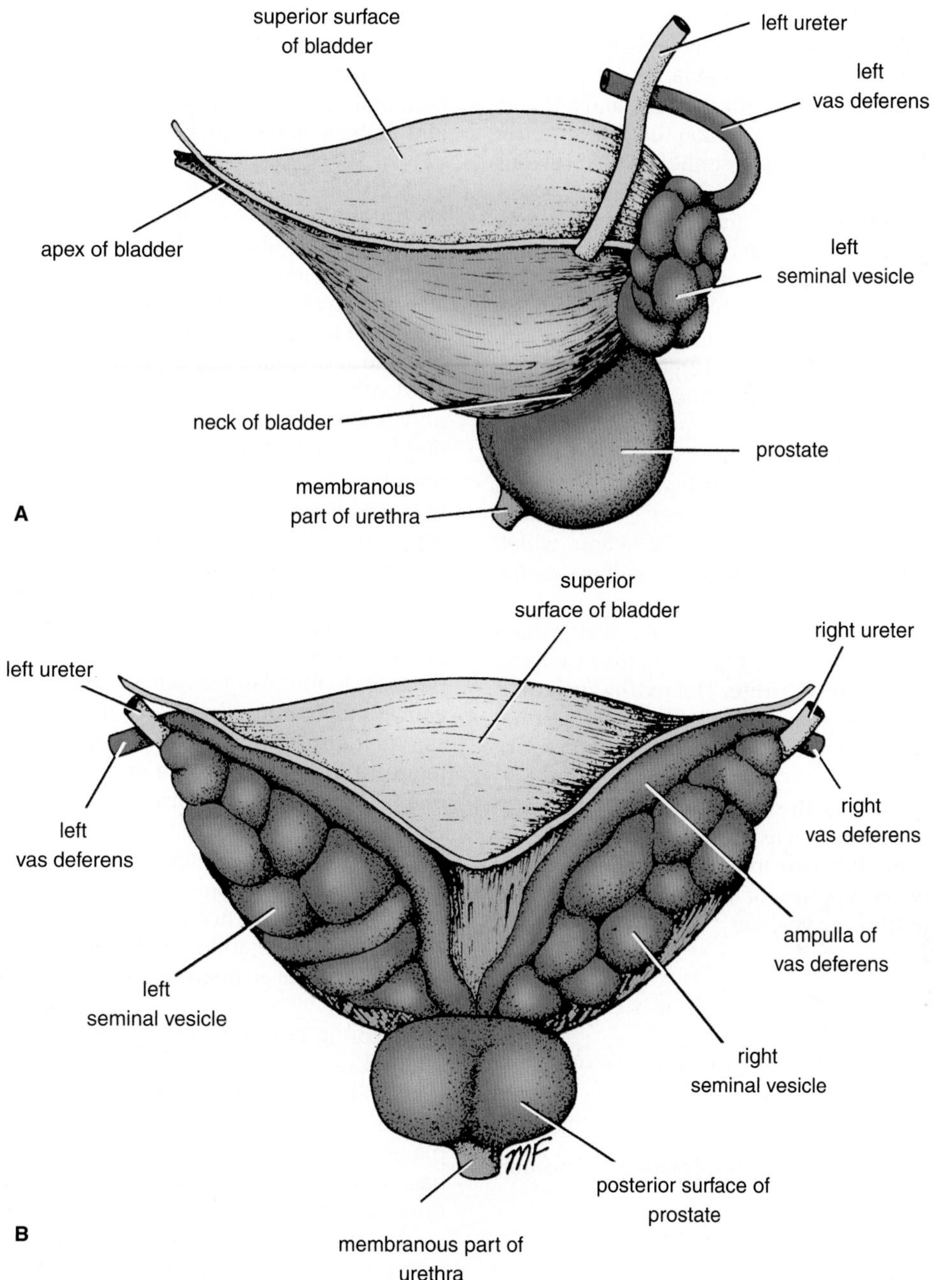

Figure 7-13 **A.** Lateral view of the bladder, prostate, and left seminal vesicle. **B.** Posterior view of the bladder, prostate, vasa deferentia, and seminal vesicles.

posterior surface of the bladder is covered by peritoneum, which forms the anterior wall of the rectovesical pouch. The lower part of the posterior surface is separated from the rectum by the vasa deferentia, the seminal vesicles, and the rectovesical fascia (Fig. 7-4).

The **superior surface** of the bladder is covered with peritoneum and is related to coils of ileum or sigmoid colon (Fig. 7-4). Along the lateral margins of this surface, the peritoneum passes to the lateral pelvic walls.

As the bladder fills, it becomes ovoid, and the superior surface bulges upward into the abdominal cavity. The peritoneal covering is peeled off the lower part of the anterior abdominal wall so that the bladder comes into direct contact with the anterior abdominal wall.

The **inferolateral surfaces** are related in front to the **retropubic pad of fat** and the pubic bones. More posteriorly, they lie in contact with the obturator internus muscle above and the levator ani muscle below.

The **neck** of the bladder lies inferiorly and rests on the upper surface of the prostate (Fig. 7-13). Here, the smooth muscle fibers of the bladder wall are continuous with those of the prostate. The neck of the bladder is held in position by the **puboprostatic ligaments** in the male; these are called the **pubovesical ligaments** in the female. These ligaments are thickenings of the pelvic fascia.

When the bladder fills, the posterior surface and neck remain more or less unchanged in position, but the superior surface rises into the abdomen, as described in the previous paragraphs.

The **mucous membrane** of the greater part of the empty bladder is thrown into folds that disappear when the bladder is full. The area of mucous membrane covering the internal surface of the base of the bladder is called the **trigone.** Here, the mucous membrane is always smooth, even when the viscus is empty (Fig. 7-12), because the mucous membrane is firmly adherent to the underlying muscular coat.

The superior angles of the trigone correspond to the openings of the ureters, and the inferior angle to the internal urethral orifice (Fig. 7-12). The ureters pierce the bladder wall obliquely, and this provides a valvelike action, which prevents a reverse flow of urine toward the kidneys as the bladder fills.

The trigone is limited above by a muscular ridge, which runs from the opening of one ureter to that of the other and is known as the **interureteric ridge.** The **uvula vesicae** is a small elevation situated immediately behind the urethral orifice, which is produced by the underlying median lobe of the prostate.

The **muscular coat of the bladder** is composed of smooth muscle and is arranged as three layers of interlacing bundles known as the **detrusor muscle.** At the neck of the bladder, the circular component of the muscle coat is thickened to form the **sphincter vesicae.**

Blood Supply

Arteries

The superior and inferior vesical arteries, branches of the internal iliac arteries.

Veins

The veins form the **vesical venous plexus** which drains into the internal iliac vein.

Lymph Drainage

Internal and external iliac nodes.

Nerve Supply

The inferior hypogastric plexuses. The sympathetic postganglionic fibers originate in the first and second lumbar ganglia and descend to the bladder via the hypogastric plexuses. The parasympathetic preganglionic fibers arise as the pelvic splanchnic nerves from the second, third, and fourth sacral nerves; they pass through the inferior hypogastric plexuses to reach the bladder wall, where they synapse with postganglionic neurons. Most afferent sensory fibers arising in the bladder reach the central nervous system via the pelvic splanchnic nerves. Some afferent fibers travel with the sympathetic nerves via the hypogastric plexuses and enter the first and second lumbar segments of the spinal cord.

The sympathetic nerves* inhibit contraction of the detrusor muscle of the bladder wall and stimulate closure of the sphincter vesicae. The parasympathetic nerves stimulate contraction of the detrusor muscle of the bladder wall and inhibit the action of the sphincter vesicae.

Micturition

Micturition is a reflex action that, in the toilet-trained individual, is controlled by higher centers in the brain. The reflex is initiated when the volume of urine reaches about 300 mL; stretch receptors in the bladder wall are stimulated and transmit impulses to the central nervous system, and the individual has a conscious desire to micturate. Most afferent impulses pass up the pelvic splanchnic nerves and enter the second, third, and fourth sacral segments of the spinal cord (Fig. 7-14). Some afferent impulses travel with the sympathetic nerves via the hypogastric plexuses and enter the first and second lumbar segments of the spinal cord.

Efferent parasympathetic impulses leave the cord from the second, third, and fourth sacral segments and pass via the parasympathetic preganglionic nerve fibers through the pelvic splanchnic nerves and the inferior hypogastric plexuses to the bladder wall, where they synapse with postganglionic neurons. By means of this nervous pathway, the smooth muscle of the bladder wall (the detrusor muscle) is made to contract, and the sphincter vesicae is made to relax. Efferent impulses also pass to the urethral sphincter via the pudendal nerve (S2, 3, and 4), and this undergoes relaxation. Once urine enters the urethra, additional afferent impulses pass to the spinal cord from the urethra and reinforce the reflex action. Micturition can be assisted by contraction of the abdominal muscles to raise the intra-abdominal and pelvic pressures and exert external pressure on the bladder.

In young children, micturition is a simple reflex act and takes place whenever the bladder becomes distended. In the adult, this simple stretch reflex is inhibited by the activity of the cerebral cortex until the time and place for micturition are favorable. The inhibitory fibers pass downward with the corticospinal tracts to the second, third, and fourth sacral segments of the cord. Voluntary control of micturition is accomplished by contracting the sphincter urethrae, which closes the urethra; this is assisted by the sphincter vesicae, which compresses the bladder neck.

Voluntary control of micturition is normally developed during the second or third year of life.

*The sympathetic nerves to the detrusor muscle are now thought to have little or no action on the smooth muscle of the bladder wall and are distributed mainly to the blood vessels. The sympathetic nerves to the sphincter vesicae are thought to play only a minor role in causing contraction of the sphincter in maintaining urinary continence. However, in males, the sympathetic innervation of the sphincter causes active contraction of the bladder neck during ejaculation (brought about by sympathetic action), thus preventing seminal fluid from entering the bladder.

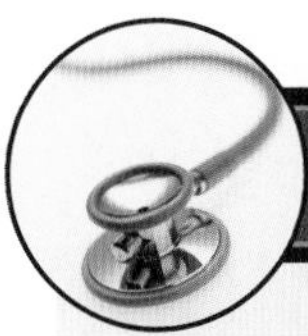

CLINICAL NOTES

Ureteric Calculi

Ureteric calculi are discussed on page 266. The ureter is narrowed anatomically where it bends down into the pelvis at the pelvic brim and where it passes through the bladder wall. It is at these sites that urinary stones may be arrested.

When a calculus enters the lower pelvic part of the ureter, the pain is often referred to the testis and the tip of the penis in the male and the labium majus in the female.

Palpation of the Urinary Bladder

The full bladder in the adult projects up into the abdomen and may be palpated through the anterior abdominal wall above the symphysis pubis.

Bimanual palpation of the empty bladder with or without a general anesthetic is an important method of examining the bladder. In the male, one hand is placed on the anterior abdominal wall above the symphysis pubis, and the gloved index finger of the other hand is inserted into the rectum. From their knowledge of anatomy, students can see that the bladder wall can be palpated between the examining fingers. In the female, an abdominovaginal examination can be similarly made. In the child, the bladder is in a higher position than in the adult because of the relatively smaller size of the pelvis.

Bladder Distention

The normal adult bladder has a capacity of about 500 mL. In the presence of urinary obstruction in males, the bladder may become greatly distended without permanent damage to the bladder wall; in such cases, it is routinely possible to drain 1000 to 1200 mL of urine through a catheter.

Urinary Retention

In adult males, urinary retention is commonly caused by obstruction to the urethra by a benign or malignant enlargement of the prostate. An acute urethritis or prostatitis can also be responsible. Acute retention occurs much less frequently in females. The only anatomic cause of urinary retention in females is acute inflammation around the urethra (e.g., from herpes).

Suprapubic Aspiration

As the bladder fills, the superior wall rises out of the pelvis and peels the peritoneum off the posterior surface of the anterior abdominal wall. In cases of acute retention of urine, when catheterization has failed, it is possible to pass a needle into the bladder through the anterior abdominal wall above the symphysis pubis, without entering the peritoneal cavity. This is a simple method of draining off the urine in an emergency.

Cystoscopy

The mucous membrane of the bladder, the two ureteric orifices, and the urethral meatus can easily be observed by means of a cystoscope. With the bladder distended with fluid, an illuminated tube fitted with lenses is introduced into the bladder through the urethra. Over the trigone, the mucous membrane is pink and smooth. If the bladder is partially emptied, the mucous membrane over the trigone remains smooth, but it is thrown into folds elsewhere. The ureteric orifices are slitlike and eject a drop of urine at intervals of about 1 minute. The interureteric ridge and the uvula vesicae can easily be recognized.

Bladder Injuries

The bladder may rupture intraperitoneally or extraperitoneally. Intraperitoneal rupture usually involves the superior wall of the bladder and occurs most commonly when the bladder is full and has extended up into the abdomen. Urine and blood escape freely into the peritoneal cavity. Extraperitoneal rupture involves the anterior part of the bladder wall below the level of the peritoneal reflection; it most commonly occurs in fractures of the pelvis when bony fragments pierce the bladder wall. Lower abdominal pain and blood in the urine (hematuria) are found in most patients.

In young children, the bladder is an abdominal organ, so abdominal trauma can injure the empty bladder.

Difficulty with Micturition After Spinal Cord Injury

After injuries to the spinal cord, the nervous control of micturition is disrupted.

The **normal bladder** is innervated as follows:

- **Sympathetic outflow** is from the first and second lumbar segments of the spinal cord. The sympathetic nerves (see the footnote on page 350) inhibit contraction of the detrusor muscle of the bladder wall and stimulate closure of the sphincter vesicae.
- **Parasympathetic outflow** is from the second, third, and fourth sacral segments of the spinal cord. The parasympathetic nerves stimulate the contraction of the detrusor muscle of the bladder wall and inhibit the action of the sphincter vesicae.
- **Sensory nerve fibers** enter the spinal cord at the above segments. The normal process of micturition is described on page 350.

Disruption of the process of micturition by spinal cord injuries may produce the following types of bladder.

The **atonic bladder** occurs during the phase of spinal shock, immediately after the injury, and may last for a few days to several weeks. The bladder wall muscle is relaxed, the sphincter vesicae tightly contracted, and the sphincter urethrae relaxed. The bladder becomes greatly distended and finally overflows. Depending on the level of the cord injury, the patient either is or is not aware that the bladder is full.

The **automatic reflex bladder** (Fig. 7-15) occurs after the patient has recovered from spinal shock, provided that the cord lesion lies above the level of the parasympathetic outflow (S2, 3, and 4). It is the type of bladder normally found in infancy. The bladder fills and empties reflexly. Stretch receptors in the bladder wall are stimulated as the bladder fills, and the afferent impulses pass to the spinal cord (segments S2, 3, and 4). Efferent impulses pass down to the bladder muscle, which contracts; the sphincter vesicae and the urethral sphincter both relax. This simple reflex occurs every 1 to 4 hours.

The **autonomous bladder** (Fig. 7-15) is the condition that occurs if the sacral segments of the spinal cord are destroyed. The sacral segments of the spinal cord are situated in the upper part of the lumbar region of the vertebral column (see page 871). The bladder is without any external reflex control. The bladder wall is flaccid, and the capacity of the bladder is greatly increased. It merely fills to capacity and overflows; continual dribbling is the result. The bladder may be partially emptied by manual compression of the lower part of the anterior abdominal wall, but infection of the urine and back-pressure effects on the ureters and kidneys are inevitable.

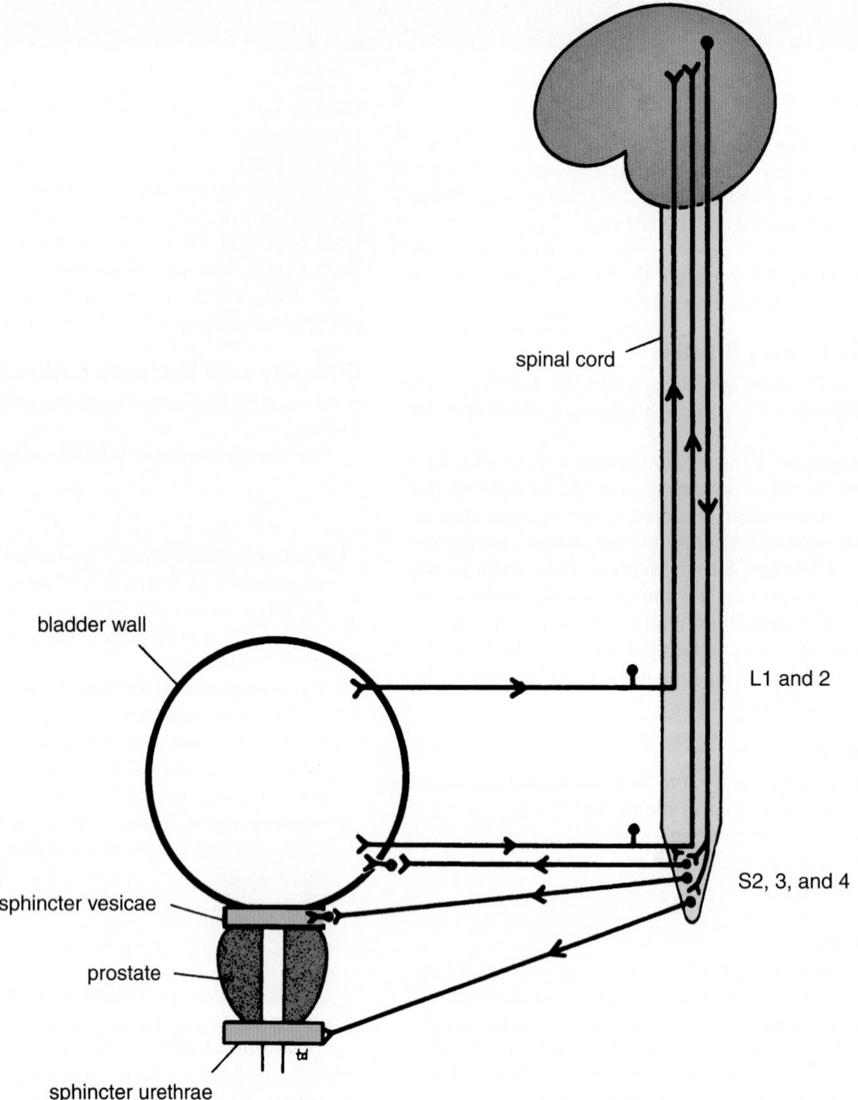

Figure 7-14 Nervous control of the bladder. Sympathetic fibers have been omitted for simplification.

Male Genital Organs

The **testes** and **epididymides** are described on page 169.

Vas Deferens

The vas deferens is a thick-walled tube about 18 in. (45 cm) long that conveys mature sperm from the epididymis to the ejaculatory duct and the urethra. It arises from the lower end or tail of the epididymis and passes through the inguinal canal. It emerges from the deep inguinal ring and passes around the lateral margin of the inferior epigastric artery (Fig. 7-11). It then passes downward and backward on the lateral wall of the pelvis and crosses the ureter in the region of the ischial spine. The vas deferens then runs medially and downward on the posterior surface of the bladder (Fig. 7-11). The terminal part of the vas deferens is dilated to form the **ampulla of the vas deferens.** The inferior end of the ampulla narrows down and joins the duct of the seminal vesicle to form the **ejaculatory duct.**

Seminal Vesicles

The seminal vesicles are two lobulated organs about 2 in. (5 cm) long lying on the posterior surface of the bladder (Fig. 7-13). On the medial side of each vesicle lies the terminal part of the vas deferens. Posteriorly, the seminal vesicles are related to the rectum (Fig. 7-4). Inferiorly, each seminal vesicle narrows and joins the vas deferens of the same side to form the **ejaculatory duct.**

Each seminal vesicle consists of a much-coiled tube embedded in connective tissue.

Blood Supply

Arteries

The inferior vesicle and middle rectal arteries.

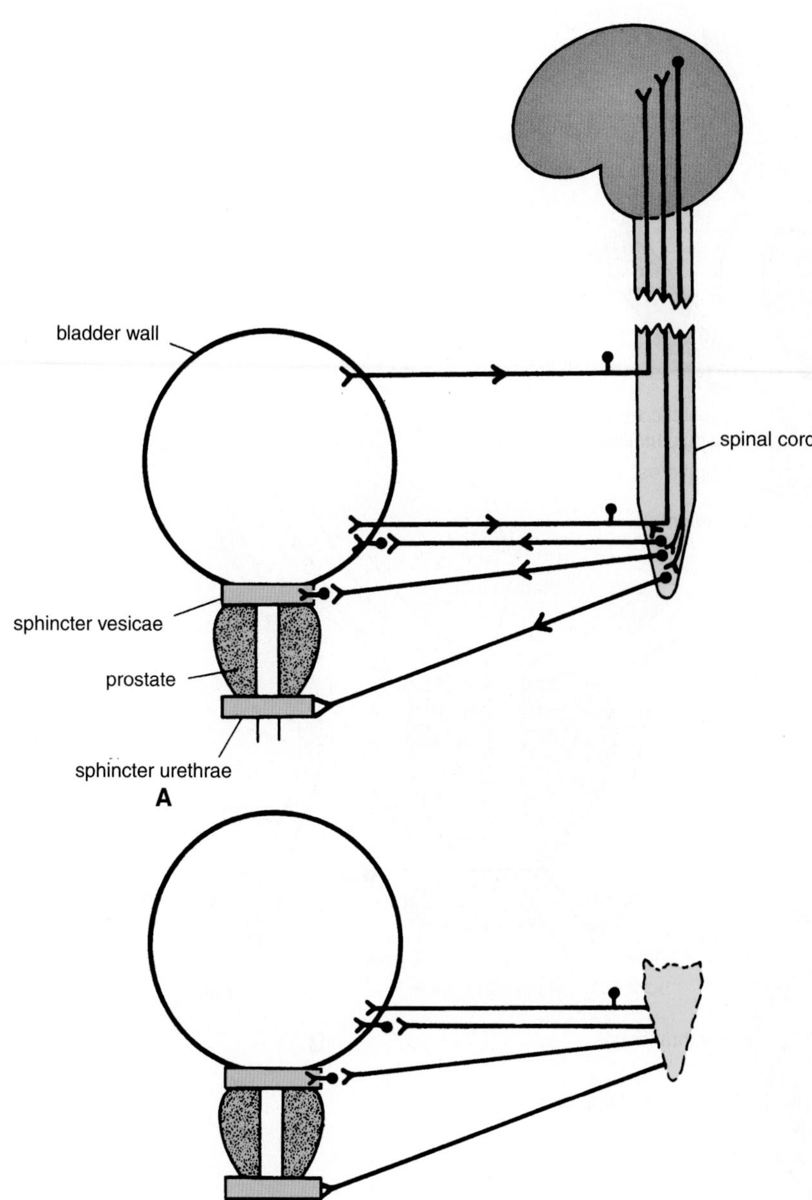

Figure 7-15 **A.** Nervous control of the bladder after section of the spinal cord in the upper thoracic region. Destruction of the sacral segments of the spinal cord. **B.** The afferent sensory fibers from the bladder entering the central nervous system and the parasympathetic efferent fibers passing to the bladder are shown; the sympathetic fibers have been omitted for clarity.

Veins

The veins drain into the internal iliac veins.

Lymph Drainage

The internal iliac nodes.

Function

The function of the seminal vesicles is to produce a secretion that is added to the seminal fluid. The secretions nourish the spermatozoa. During ejaculation the seminal vesicles contract and expel their contents into the ejaculatory ducts, thus washing the spermatozoa out of the urethra.

Ejaculatory Ducts

The two ejaculatory ducts are each less than 1 in. (2.5 cm) long and are formed by the union of the vas deferens and the duct of the seminal vesicle (Fig. 7-16). The ejaculatory ducts pierce the posterior surface of the prostate and open into the prostatic part of the urethra, close to the margins of the prostatic utricle; their function is to drain the seminal fluid into the prostatic urethra.

Prostate

Location and Description

The prostate is a fibromuscular glandular organ that surrounds the prostatic urethra (Figs. 7-4 and 7-16). It is about 1.25 in. (3 cm) long and lies between the neck of the bladder above and the urogenital diaphragm below (Fig. 7-16).

The prostate is surrounded by a fibrous capsule (Fig. 7-16). The somewhat conical prostate has a **base,** which lies against the bladder neck above, and an **apex,** which lies

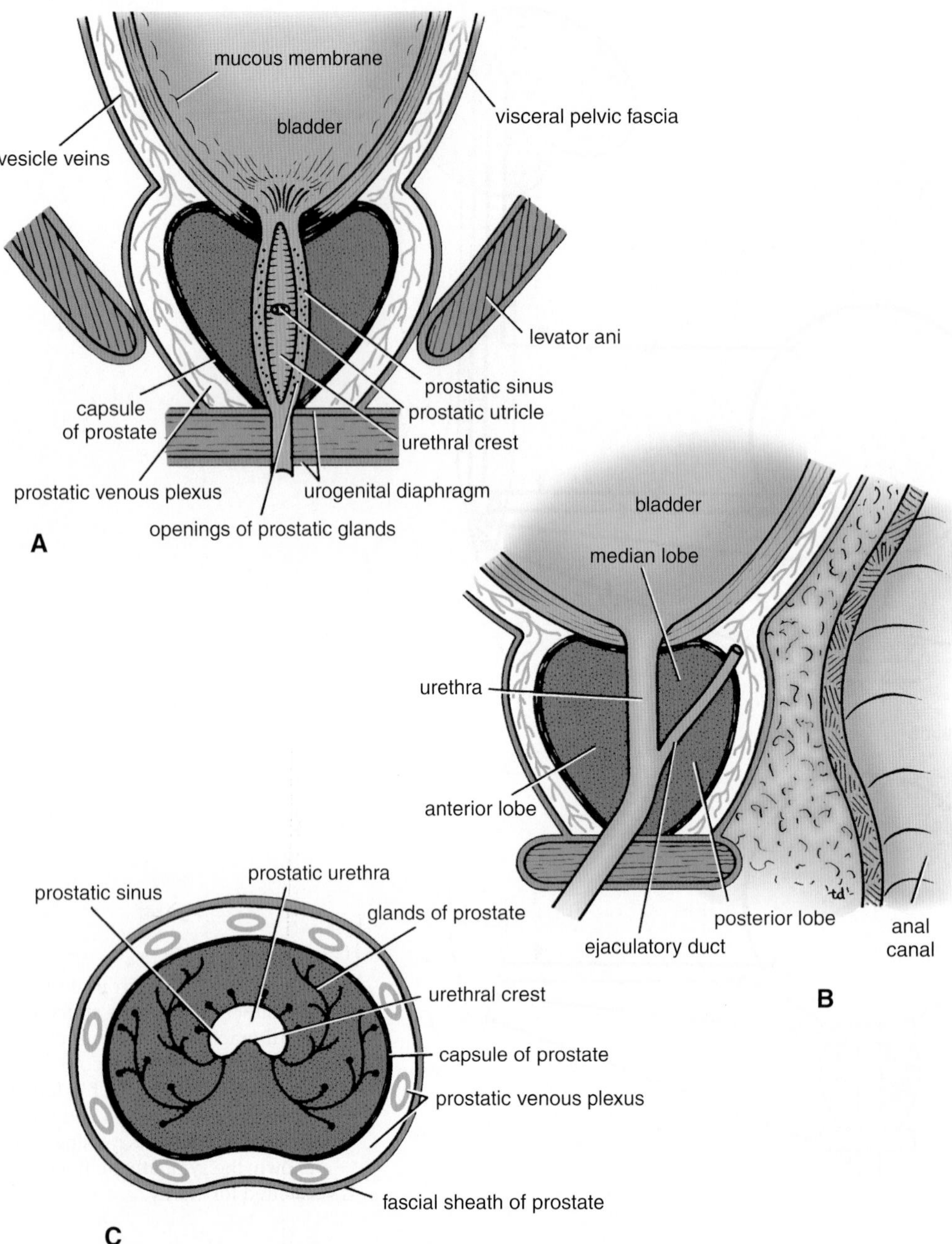

Figure 7-16 Prostate in coronal section **(A),** sagittal section **(B),** and horizontal section **(C).** In the coronal section, note the openings of the ejaculatory ducts on the margin of the prostatic utricle.

against the urogenital diaphragm below. The two ejaculatory ducts pierce the upper part of the posterior surface of the prostate to open into the prostatic urethra at the lateral margins of the prostatic utricle (Fig. 7-16).

Relations

- **Superiorly:** The base of the prostate is continuous with the neck of the bladder, the smooth muscle passing without interruption from one organ to the other. The urethra enters the center of the base of the prostate (Fig. 7-4).
- **Inferiorly:** The apex of the prostate lies on the upper surface of the urogenital diaphragm. The urethra leaves the prostate just above the apex on the anterior surface (Fig. 7-16).
- **Anteriorly:** The prostate is related to the symphysis pubis, separated from it by the **extraperitoneal fat** in the retropubic space **(cave of Retzius).** The prostate is connected to the posterior aspect of the pubic bones by the fascial **puboprostatic ligaments** (Fig. 7-4).
- **Posteriorly:** The prostate (Figs. 7-4 and 7-16) is closely related to the anterior surface of the rectal ampulla and is

separated from it by the **rectovesical septum (fascia of Denonvilliers).** This septum is formed in fetal life by the fusion of the walls of the lower end of the rectovesical pouch of peritoneum, which originally extended down to the perineal body.

- **Laterally:** The prostate is embraced by the anterior fibers of the levator ani as they run posteriorly from the pubis (Fig. 7-16).

Structure of the Prostate

The numerous glands of the prostate are embedded in a mixture of smooth muscle and connective tissue, and their ducts open into the prostatic urethra.

The prostate is incompletely divided into five lobes (Fig. 7-16). The **anterior lobe** lies in front of the urethra and is devoid of glandular tissue. The **median,** or **middle, lobe** is the wedge of gland situated between the urethra and the ejaculatory ducts. Its upper surface is related to the trigone of the bladder; it is rich in glands. The **posterior lobe** is situated behind the urethra and below the ejaculatory ducts and also contains glandular tissue. The **right** and **left lateral lobes** lie on either side of the urethra and are separated from one another by a shallow vertical groove on the posterior surface of the prostate. The lateral lobes contain many glands.

Function of the Prostate

The prostate produces a thin, milky fluid containing citric acid and acid phosphatase that is added to the seminal fluid at the time of ejaculation. The smooth muscle, which surrounds the glands, squeezes the secretion into the prostatic urethra. The prostatic secretion is alkaline and helps neutralize the acidity in the vagina.

Blood Supply

Arteries

Branches of the inferior vesical and middle rectal arteries.

Veins

The veins form the **prostatic venous plexus,** which lies outside the capsule of the prostate (Fig. 7-16). The prostatic plexus receives the deep dorsal vein of the penis and numerous vesical veins and drains into the internal iliac veins.

Lymph Drainage

Internal iliac nodes.

Nerve Supply

Inferior hypogastric plexuses. The sympathetic nerves stimulate the smooth muscle of the prostate during ejaculation.

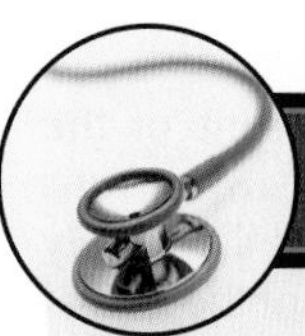

CLINICAL NOTES

Prostate Examination

The prostate can be examined clinically by palpation by performing a rectal examination (see page 397). The examiner's gloved finger can feel the posterior surface of the prostate through the anterior rectal wall.

Prostate Activity and Disease

It is now generally believed that the normal glandular activity of the prostate is controlled by the androgens and estrogens circulating in the bloodstream. The secretions of the prostate are poured into the urethra during ejaculation and are added to the seminal fluid. Acid phosphatase is an important enzyme present in the secretion in large amounts. When the glandular cells producing this enzyme cannot discharge their secretion into the ducts, as in carcinoma of the prostate, the serum acid phosphatase level of the blood rises.

It has been shown that trace amounts of proteins produced specifically by prostatic epithelial cells are found in peripheral blood. In certain prostatic diseases, notably cancer of the prostate, this protein appears in the blood in increased amounts. The specific protein level can be measured by a simple laboratory test called the **PSA** (prostate-specific antigen) test.

Benign Enlargement of the Prostate

Benign enlargement of the prostate is common in men older than 50 years. The cause is possibly an imbalance in the hormonal control of the gland. The median lobe of the gland enlarges upward and encroaches within the sphincter vesicae, located at the neck of the bladder. The leakage of urine into the prostatic urethra causes an intense reflex desire to micturate. The enlargement of the median and lateral lobes of the gland produces elongation and lateral compression and distortion of the urethra so that the patient experiences difficulty in passing urine and the stream is weak. Back-pressure effects on the ureters and both kidneys are a common complication. The enlargement of the uvula vesicae (owing to the enlarged median lobe) results in the formation of a pouch of stagnant urine behind the urethral orifice within the bladder (Fig. 7-17). The stagnant urine frequently becomes infected, and the inflamed bladder **(cystitis)** adds to the patient's symptoms.

In all operations on the prostate, the surgeon regards the prostatic venous plexus with respect. The veins have thin walls, are valveless, and are drained by several large trunks directly into the internal iliac veins. Damage to these veins can result in a severe hemorrhage.

Prostate Cancer and the Prostatic Venous Plexus

Many connections between the prostatic venous plexus and the vertebral veins exist. During coughing and sneezing or abdominal straining, it is possible for prostatic venous blood to flow in a reverse direction and enter the vertebral veins. This explains the frequent occurrence of skeletal metastases in the lower vertebral column and pelvic bones of patients with carcinoma of the prostate. Cancer cells enter the skull via this route by floating up the valveless prostatic and vertebral veins.

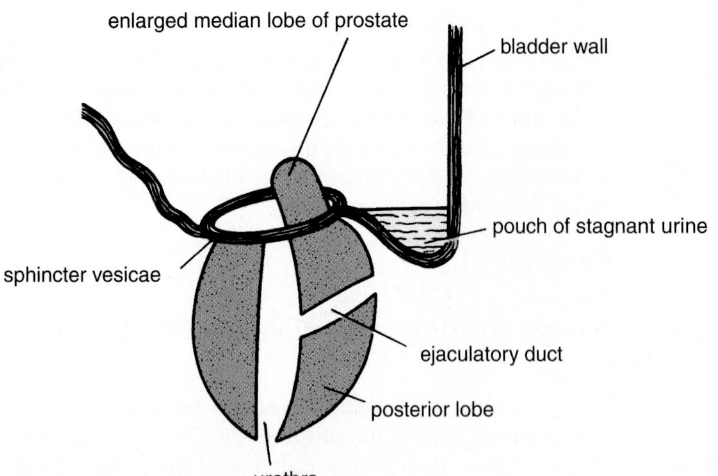

Figure 7-17 Sagittal section of a prostate that had undergone benign enlargement of the median lobe. Note the bladder pouch filled with stagnant urine behind the prostate.

Prostatic Urethra

The prostatic urethra is about 1.25 in. (3 cm) long and begins at the neck of the bladder. It passes through the prostate from the base to the apex, where it becomes continuous with the membranous part of the urethra (Fig. 7-16).

The **prostatic urethra is the widest and most dilatable portion of the entire urethra.** On the posterior wall is a longitudinal ridge called the **urethral crest** (Fig. 7-16). On each side of this ridge is a groove called the **prostatic sinus;** the prostatic glands open into these grooves. On the summit of the urethral crest is a depression, the **prostatic utricle,** which is an analog of the uterus and vagina in females. On the edge of the mouth of the utricle are the openings of the two ejaculatory ducts (Fig. 7-16).

Visceral Pelvic Fascia

The visceral pelvic fascia is a layer of connective tissue that covers and supports the pelvic viscera (Fig.7-16).

Peritoneum

The peritoneum is best understood by tracing it around the pelvis in a sagittal plane (Fig. 7-4).

The peritoneum passes down from the anterior abdominal wall onto the upper surface of the urinary bladder. It then runs down on the posterior surface of the bladder for a short distance until it reaches the upper ends of the seminal vesicles. Here it sweeps backward to reach the anterior aspect of the rectum, forming the shallow **rectovesical pouch.** The peritoneum then passes up on the front of the middle third of the rectum and the front and lateral surfaces of the upper third of the rectum. It then becomes continuous with the parietal peritoneum on the posterior abdominal wall. It is thus seen that the lowest part of the abdominopelvic peritoneal cavity, when the patient is in the erect position, is the rectovesical pouch (Fig. 7-4).

The peritoneum covering the superior surface of the bladder passes laterally to the lateral pelvic walls and does not cover the lateral surfaces of the bladder. It is important to remember that as the bladder fills, the superior wall rises up into the abdomen and peels off the peritoneum from the anterior abdominal wall so that the bladder becomes directly in contact with the abdominal wall.

Pelvic Viscera in the Female

The rectum, sigmoid colon, and terminal coils of ileum occupy the posterior part of the pelvic cavity (Fig. 7-5), as described previously. The contents of the anterior part of the pelvic cavity in the female are described in the following sections.

Ureters

The ureter crosses over the pelvic inlet in front of the bifurcation of the common iliac artery (Fig. 7-18). It runs downward and backward in front of the internal iliac artery and behind the ovary until it reaches the region of the ischial spine. It then turns forward and medially beneath the base of the broad ligament, where it is crossed by the uterine artery (Figs. 7-18 and 7-19). The ureter then runs forward, lateral to the lateral fornix of the vagina, to enter the bladder.

Urinary Bladder

As in the male, the urinary bladder is situated immediately behind the pubic bones (Fig. 7-5). Because of the absence of the prostate, the bladder lies at a lower level than in the male pelvis, and the neck rests directly on the upper surface of the urogenital diaphragm. The close relation of the bladder to the uterus and the vagina is of considerable clinical importance (Fig. 7-5).

The **apex** of the bladder lies behind the symphysis pubis (Fig. 7-5). The **base,** or **posterior surface,** is separated by the vagina from the rectum. The **superior surface** is related to the uterovesical pouch of peritoneum and to the body of the uterus. The **inferolateral surfaces** are related in front to the **retropubic pad of fat** and the pubic bones. More posteriorly, they lie in contact with the obturator internus muscle above and the levator ani muscle below. The **neck** of the bladder rests on the upper surface of the urogenital diaphragm.

The general shape and structure of the bladder; its blood supply, lymph drainage, and nerve supply; and the process of micturition are identical to those in the male.

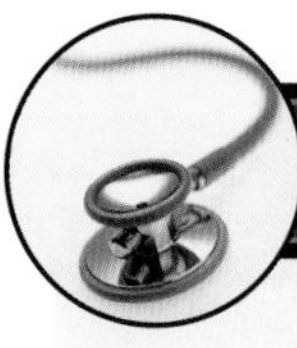

CLINICAL NOTES

Stress Incontinence

The bladder is normally supported by the visceral pelvic fascia, which in certain areas is condensed to form ligaments. However, the most important support for the bladder is the tone of the levatores ani muscles. In the female, a difficult labor, especially one in which forceps is used, excessively stretches the supports of the bladder neck, and the normal angle between the urethra and the posterior wall of the bladder is lost. This injury causes stress incontinence, a condition of partial urinary incontinence occurring when the patient coughs or strains or laughs excessively.

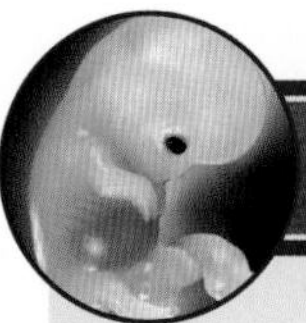

EMBRYOLOGIC NOTES

Development of the Bladder in Both Sexes

The division of the cloaca into anterior and posterior parts by the development of the **urorectal septum** is described on page 345. The posterior portion forms the **anorectal canal** (Fig. 7-20). The entrance of the distal ends of the mesonephric ducts into the anterior part of the cloaca on each side permits one, for purposes of description, to divide the anterior part of the cloaca into an area above the duct entrances called the **primitive bladder** and another area below called the **urogenital sinus.**

The caudal ends of the mesonephric ducts now become absorbed into the lower part of the bladder so that the ureters and ducts have individual openings in the dorsal wall (Fig. 7-20). With differential growth of the dorsal bladder wall, the ureters come to open through the lateral angles of the bladder, and the mesonephric ducts open close together in what will be the urethra. That part of the dorsal bladder wall marked off by the openings of these four ducts forms the **trigone** of the bladder (Fig. 7-21). Thus, it is seen that in the earliest stages the lining of the bladder over the trigone is mesodermal in origin; later, this mesodermal tissue is thought to be replaced by epithelium of entodermal origin. The smooth muscle of the bladder wall is derived from the splanchnopleuric mesoderm.

The primitive bladder may now be divided into an upper dilated portion, the **bladder,** and a lower narrow portion, the **urethra** (Fig. 7-20). The apex of the bladder is continuous with the **allantois,** which now becomes obliterated and forms a fibrous core, the **urachus.** The urachus persists throughout life as a ligament that runs from the apex of the bladder to the umbilicus and is called the **median umbilical ligament.**

Congenital Anomalies of the Bladder

Exstrophy of the Bladder (Ectopia Vesicae)

Exstrophy of the bladder occurs three times more commonly in males than in females. The posterior bladder wall protrudes through a defect in the anterior abdominal wall below the umbilicus (Fig. 7-22). The condition is caused by a failure of the embryonic mesenchyme to invade the embryonic disc caudal to the cloacal membrane (Fig. 7-22). The absence of intervening mesenchyme between the ectoderm and entoderm produces an unstable state, which is followed by breakdown of this area.

Because of the urinary incontinence and almost certain occurrence of ascending urinary infection, surgical reconstruction of the bladder is attempted.

Fate of the Mesonephric Duct in Both Sexes

In both sexes, the mesonephric (or Wolffian) duct gives origin on each side to the **ureteric bud,** which forms the **ureter,** the **pelvis of the ureter,** the **major** and **minor calyces,** and the **collecting tubules of the kidney** (see page 267). Its inferior end is absorbed into the developing bladder and forms the trigone and part of the urethra.

In the male, its upper or cranial end is joined to the developing testis by the efferent ductules of the testis, and so it becomes the **duct of the epididymis,** the **vas deferens,** and the **ejaculatory duct.** From the latter, a small diverticulum arises that forms the **seminal vesicle** (see Fig. 4-26).

In the female, the mesonephric duct largely disappears. Only small remnants persist—as the **duct of the epoophoron** and the **duct of the paroophoron.** The caudal end may persist and extend from the epoophoron to the hymen as **Gartner's duct.**

Development of the Urethra

In the male, the **prostatic urethra** is formed from two sources. The proximal part, as far as the openings of the ejaculatory ducts, is derived from the mesonephric ducts. The distal part of the prostatic urethra is formed from the urogenital sinus (Fig. 7-21). The **membranous urethra** and the greater part of the **penile urethra** also are formed from the urogenital sinus. The distal end of the penile urethra is derived from an ingrowth of ectodermal cells on the glans penis.

In the female, the upper two thirds of the urethra are derived from the mesonephric ducts. The lower end of the urethra is formed from the urogenital sinus (Fig. 7-21).

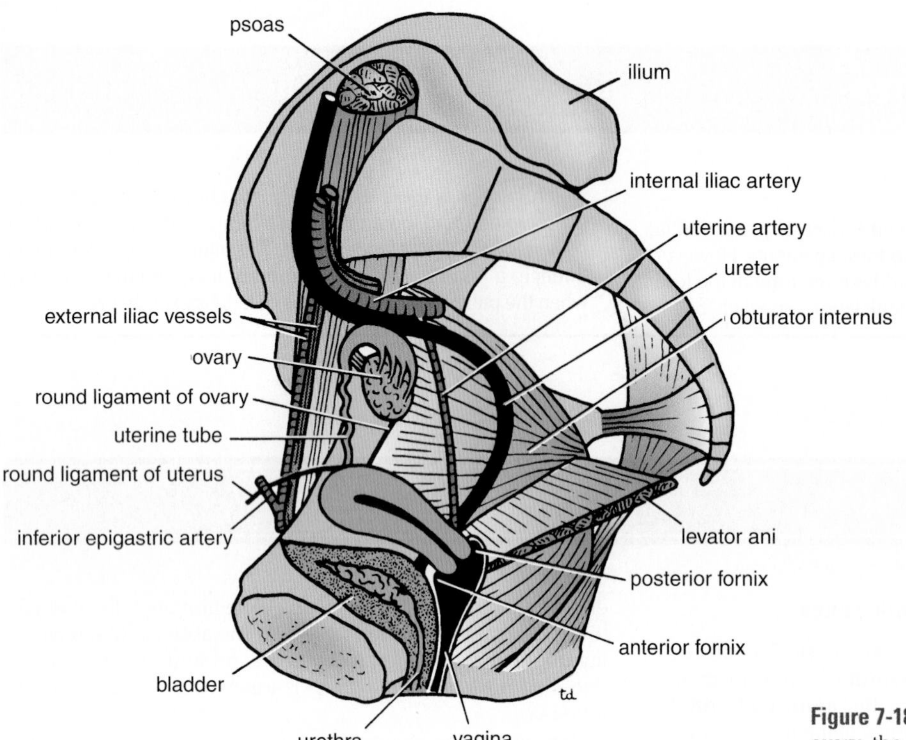

Figure 7-18 Right half of the pelvis showing the ovary, the uterine tube, and the vagina.

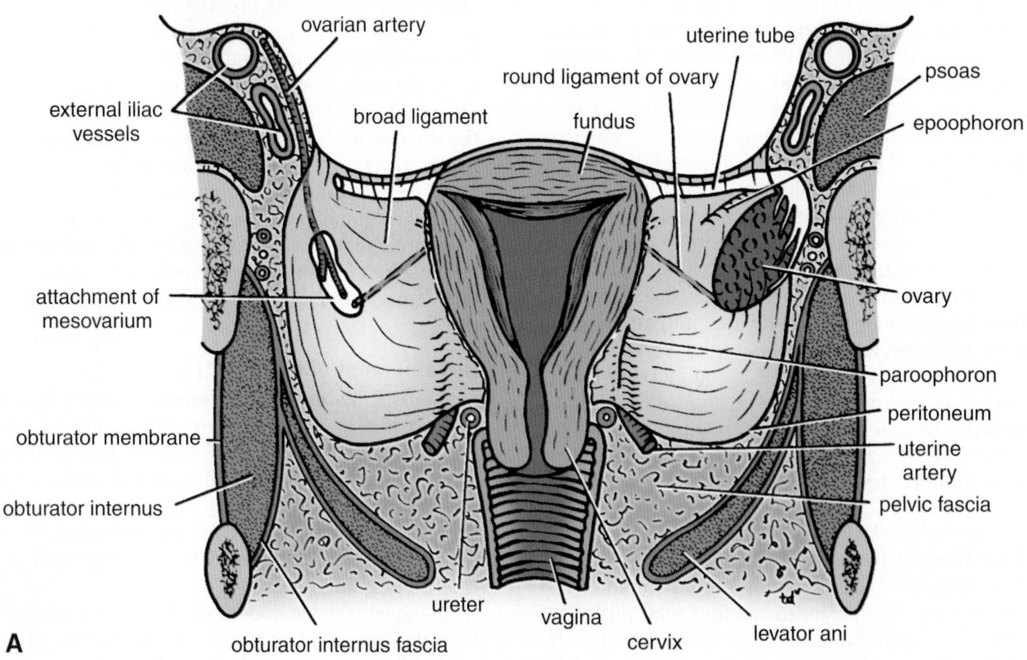

Figure 7-19 **A.** Coronal section of the pelvis showing the uterus, broad ligaments, and right ovary on posterior view. The left ovary and part of the left uterine tube have been removed for clarity.

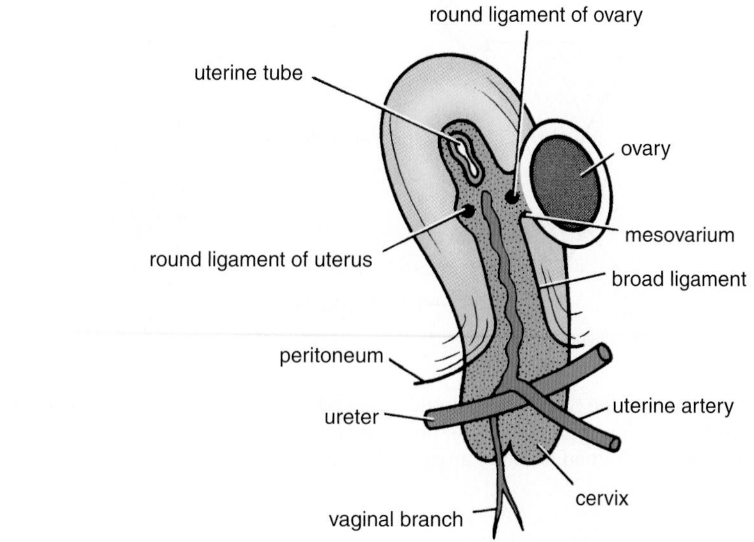

Figure 7-19 *(continued)* **B.** Uterus on lateral view. Note the structures that lie within the broad ligament. Note that the uterus has been retroverted into the plane of the vaginal lumen in both diagrams.

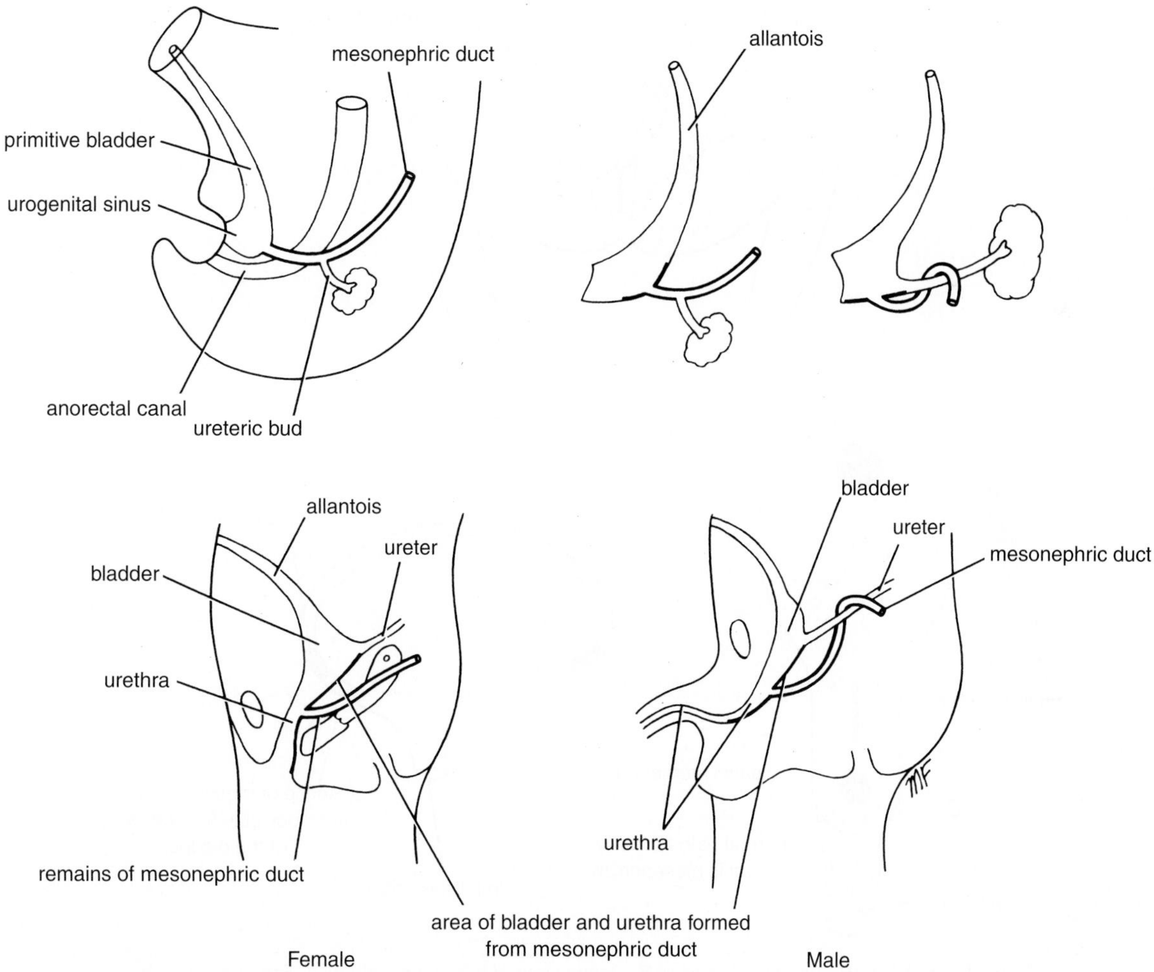

mesonephric duct
allantois
primitive bladder
urogenital sinus
anorectal canal
ureteric bud
allantois
bladder
ureter
urethra
remains of mesonephric duct
bladder
ureter
mesonephric duct
urethra
area of bladder and urethra formed from mesonephric duct
Female
Male

Figure 7-20 Formation of the urinary bladder from the anterior part of the cloaca and the terminal parts of the mesonephric ducts in both sexes. The mesonephric ducts and the ureteric buds are drawn into the developing bladder.

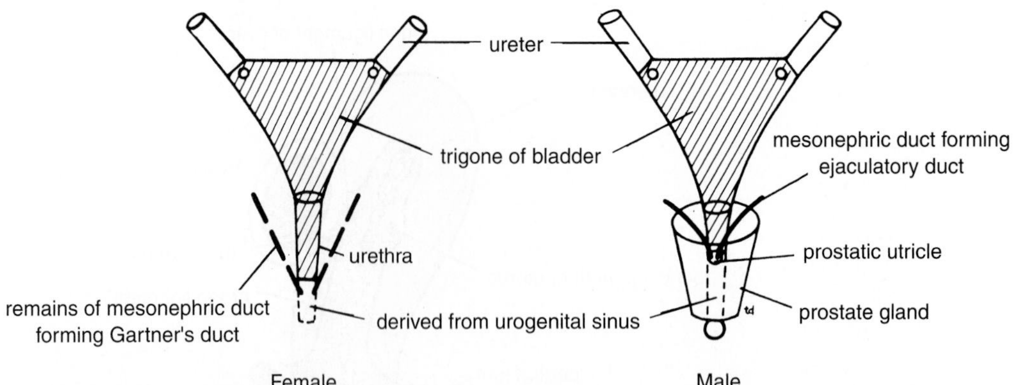

Figure 7-21 Parts of the bladder and urethra derived from the mesonephric ducts in both sexes (*hatch marks*). The lower end of the urethra in the female and the lower part of the prostatic urethra in the male are formed from the urogenital sinus.

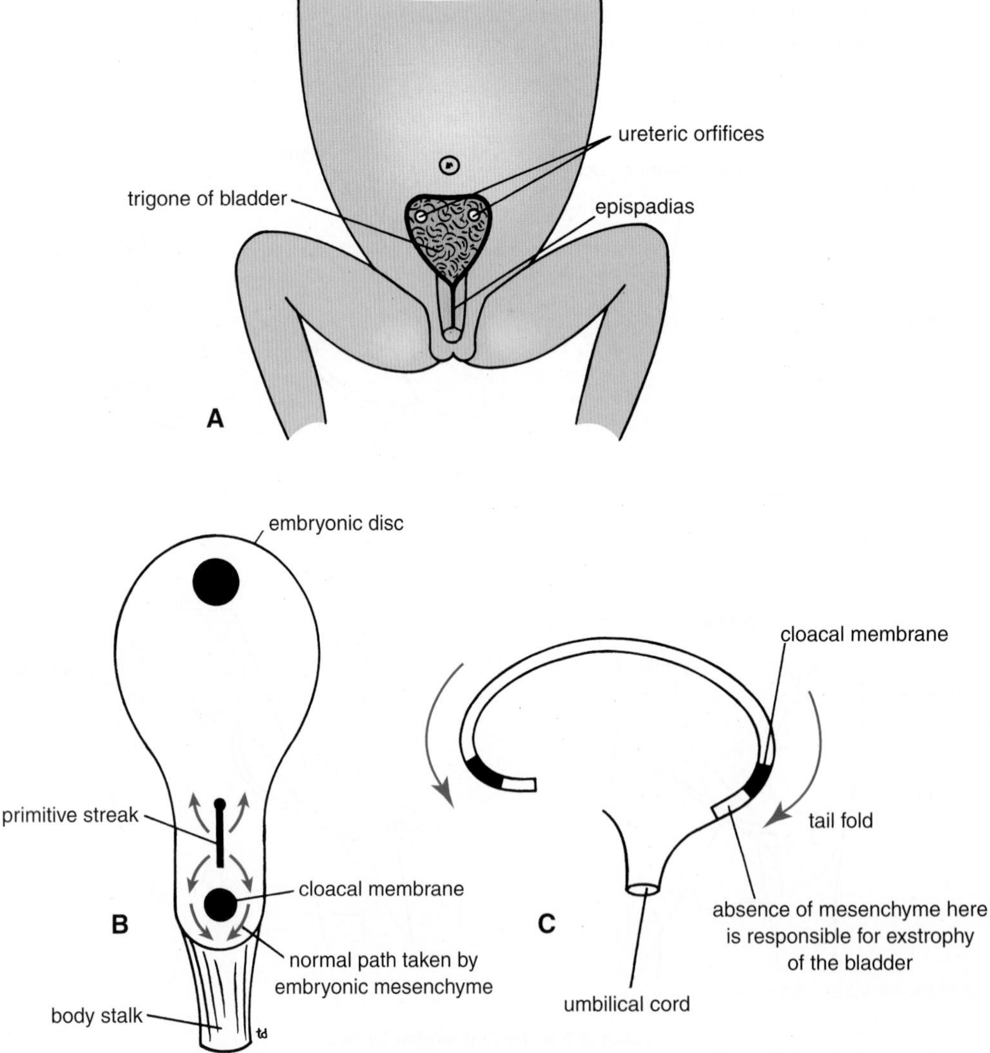

Figure 7-22 **A.** Exstrophy of the bladder. **B.** Dorsal view of the embryonic disc. The normal path taken by the growing embryonic mesenchyme in the region of the cloaca is shown. **C.** Fetus as seen from the side. The head and tail folds have developed, but the mesenchyme has failed to enter the ventral body wall between the cloaca and the umbilical cord.

Female Genital Organs

Ovary

Location and Description

Each ovary is oval shaped, measuring 1.5 by 0.75 in. (4 by 2 cm), and is attached to the back of the broad ligament by the **mesovarium** (Fig. 7-19).

That part of the broad ligament extending between the attachment of the mesovarium and the lateral wall of the pelvis is called the **suspensory ligament of the ovary** (Fig. 7-19).

The **round ligament of the ovary,** which represents the remains of the upper part of the gubernaculum, connects the lateral margin of the uterus to the ovary (Figs. 7-18 and 7-19).

The ovary usually lies against the lateral wall of the pelvis in a depression called the **ovarian fossa,** bounded by the external iliac vessels above and by the internal iliac vessels behind (Fig. 7-18). The position of the ovary is, however, extremely variable, and it is often found hanging down in the rectouterine pouch (pouch of Douglas). During pregnancy, the enlarging uterus pulls the ovary up into the abdominal cavity. After childbirth, when the broad ligament is lax, the ovary takes up a variable position in the pelvis.

The ovaries are surrounded by a thin fibrous capsule, the **tunica albuginea.** This capsule is covered externally by a modified area of peritoneum called the **germinal epithelium.** The term **germinal epithelium** is a misnomer because the layer does not give rise to ova. Oogonia develop before birth from primordial germ cells.

Before puberty, the ovary is smooth, but after puberty, the ovary becomes progressively scarred as successive corpora lutea degenerate. After menopause, the ovary becomes shrunken and its surface is pitted with scars.

Function

The ovaries are the organs responsible for the production of the female germ cells, the **ova,** and the female sex hormones, **estrogen** and **progesterone,** in the sexually mature female.

Blood Supply

Arteries

The **ovarian artery** arises from the abdominal aorta at the level of the first lumbar vertebra.

Veins

The ovarian vein drains into the inferior vena cava on the right side and into the left renal vein on the left side.

Lymph Drainage

The lymph vessels of the ovary follow the ovarian artery and drain into the para-aortic nodes at the level of the first lumbar vertebra.

Nerve Supply

The nerve supply to the ovary is derived from the aortic plexus and accompanies the ovarian artery.

The blood supply, lymph drainage, and nerve supply of the ovary pass over the pelvic inlet and cross the external iliac vessels (Fig. 7-19). They reach the ovary by passing through the lateral end of the broad ligament, the part known as the suspensory ligament of the ovary. The vessels and nerves finally enter the hilum of the ovary via the mesovarium. (Compare the blood supply and the lymph drainage of the ovary with those of the testis.)

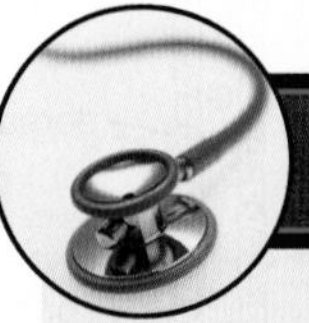

CLINICAL NOTES

Position of the Ovary

The ovary is kept in position by the broad ligament and the mesovarium. After pregnancy, the broad ligament is lax, and the ovaries may prolapse into the rectouterine pouch (pouch of Douglas). In these circumstances, the ovary may be tender and cause discomfort on sexual intercourse **(dyspareunia).** An ovary situated in the rectouterine pouch may be palpated through the posterior fornix of the vagina.

Cysts of the Ovary

Follicular cysts are common and originate in unruptured graafian follicles; they rarely exceed 0.6 in. (1.5 cm) in diameter. **Luteal cysts** are formed in the corpus luteum. Fluid is retained, and the corpus luteum cannot become fibrosed. Luteal cysts rarely exceed 1.2 in. (3 cm) in diameter.

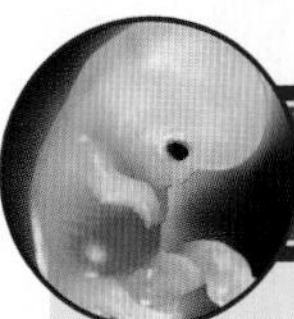

EMBRYOLOGIC NOTES

Development of the Ovary

The female sex chromosome causes the **genital ridge** on the posterior abdominal wall to secrete estrogens. The presence of estrogen and the absence of testosterone induce the development of the ovary and the other female genital organs.

The **sex cords** contained within the genital ridges contain groups of primordial germ cells. These become broken up into irregular cell clusters by the proliferating mesenchyme (Fig. 7-23). The germ cells differentiate into **oogonia,** and by the third month, they start to undergo a number of mitotic divisions within the cortex of the ovary to form **primary oocytes.** These primary oocytes become surrounded by a single layer of cells derived from the sex cords, called the **granulosa cells.** Thus, **primordial follicles** have been formed, but later, many degenerate. The mesenchyme that surrounds the follicles provides the ovarian stroma. The relationship of the ovary to the developing uterine tube is shown in Figure 7-24.

Ovarian Dysgenesis

Complete failure of both ovaries to develop is found in Turner's syndrome. The classic features of this syndrome are webbed neck, short stocky build, increased carrying angle of the elbows, lack of secondary sex characteristics, and amenorrhea.

Imperfect Descent of the Ovary

The ovary may fail to descend into the pelvis or very rarely may be drawn downward with the round ligament of the uterus into the inguinal canal or even into the labium majus.

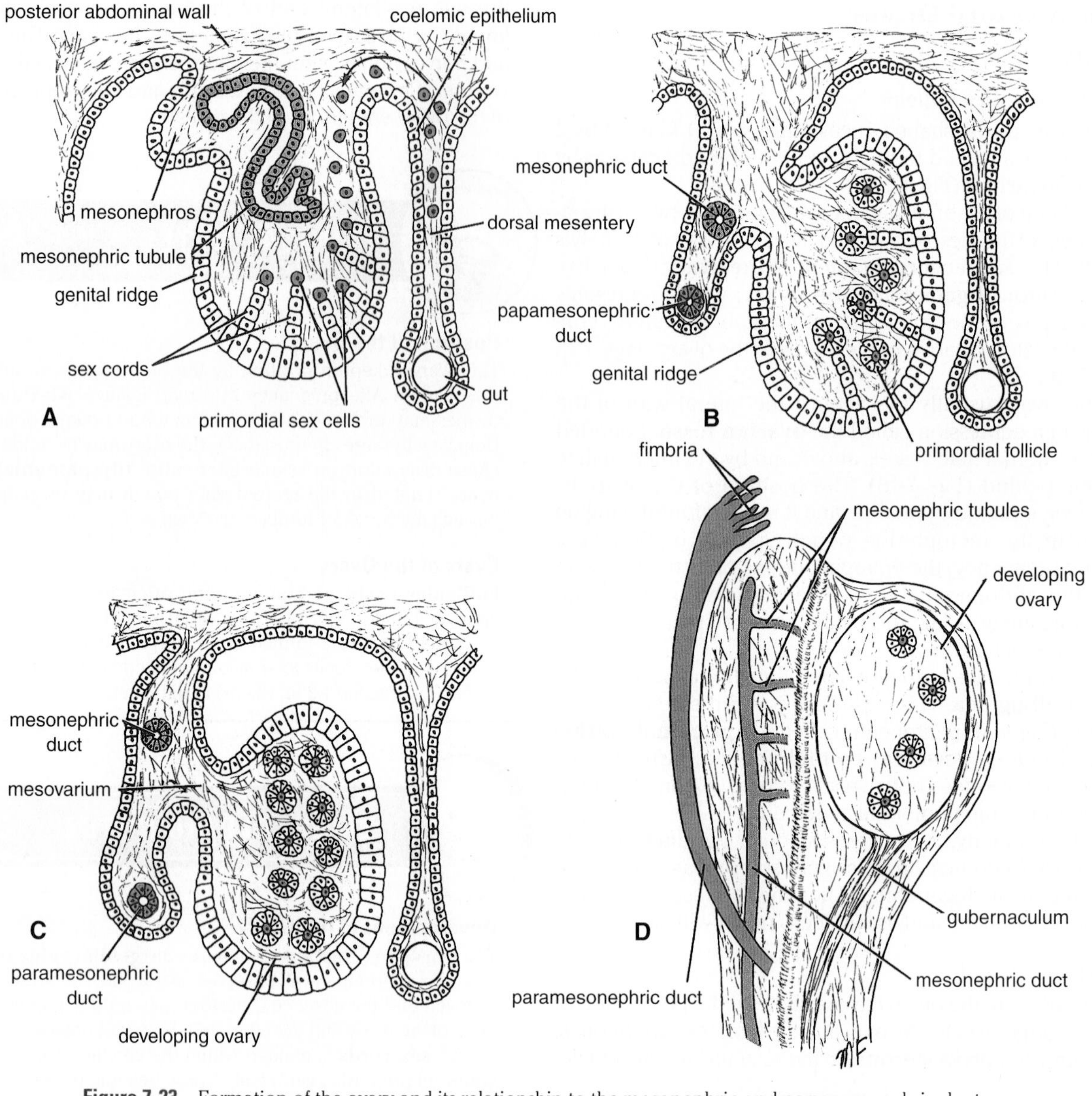

Figure 7-23 Formation of the ovary and its relationship to the mesonephric and paramesonephric ducts.

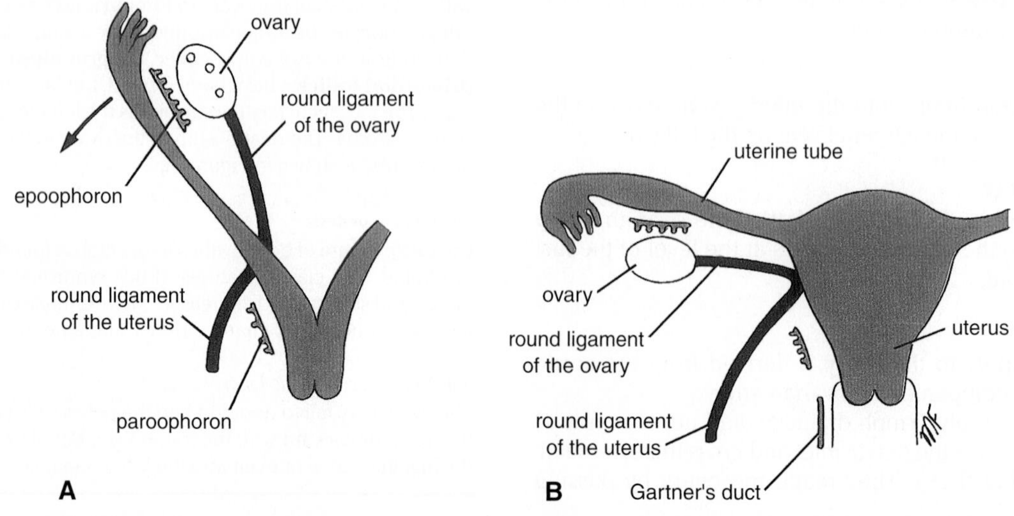

Figure 7-24 The descent of the ovary and its relationship to the developing uterine tube and uterus.

Uterine Tube

Location and Description

The two uterine tubes are each about 4 in. (10 cm) long and lie in the upper border of the broad ligament (Figs. 7-18 and 7-19). Each connects the peritoneal cavity in the region of the ovary with the cavity of the uterus. The uterine tube is divided into four parts:

1. The **infundibulum** is the funnel-shaped lateral end that projects beyond the broad ligament and overlies the ovary. The free edge of the funnel has several fingerlike processes, known as **fimbriae,** which are draped over the ovary (Figs. 7-19 and 7-25).
2. The **ampulla** is the widest part of the tube (Fig. 7-25).
3. The **isthmus** is the narrowest part of the tube and lies just lateral to the uterus (Fig. 7-25).
4. The **intramural part** is the segment that pierces the uterine wall (Fig. 7-25).

Function

The uterine tube receives the ovum from the ovary and provides a site where fertilization of the ovum can take place (usually in the ampulla). It provides nourishment for the fertilized ovum and transports it to the cavity of the uterus. The tube serves as a conduit along which the spermatozoa travel to reach the ovum.

Blood Supply

Arteries

The uterine artery from the internal iliac artery and the ovarian artery from the abdominal aorta (Fig. 7-25).

Veins

The veins correspond to the arteries.

Lymph Drainage

The internal iliac and para-aortic nodes.

Nerve Supply

Sympathetic and parasympathetic nerves from the inferior hypogastric plexuses.

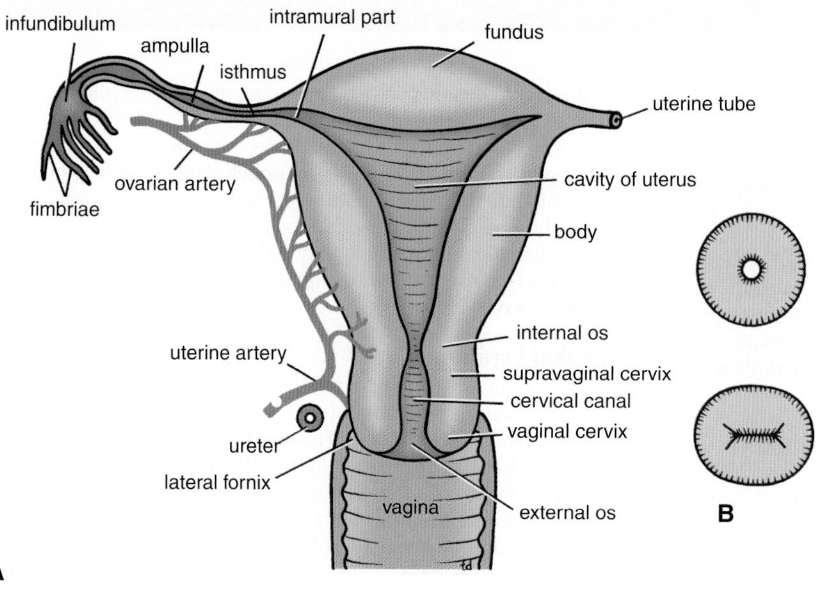

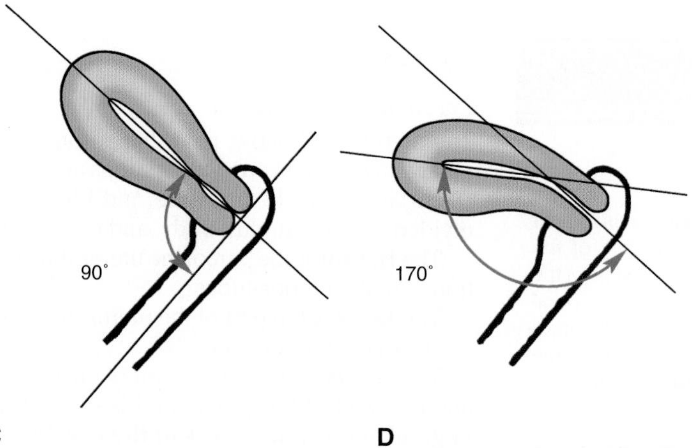

Figure 7-25 **A.** Different parts of the uterine tube and the uterus. **B.** External os of the cervix: **(above)** nulliparous; **(below)** parous. **C.** Anteverted position of the uterus. **D.** Anteverted and anteflexed position of the uterus.

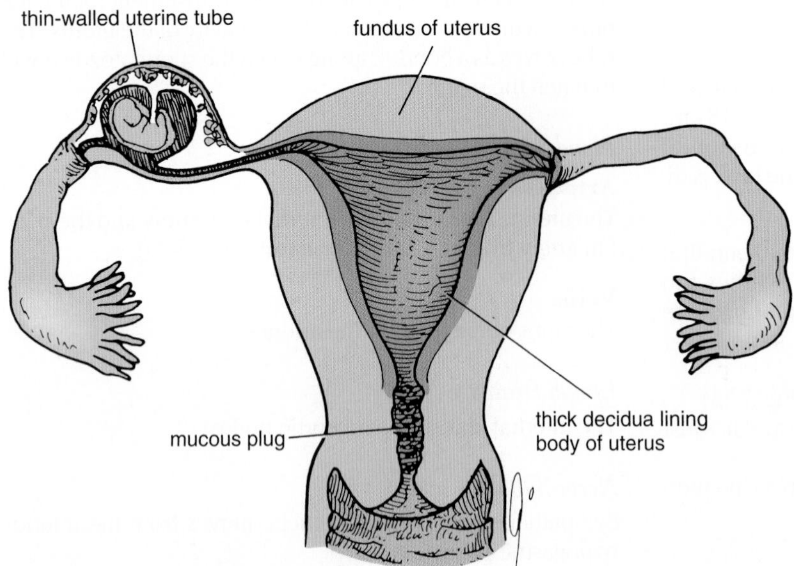

Figure 7-26 An ectopic pregnancy located where the ampulla of the uterine tube narrows down to join the isthmus. Note the thin tubal wall compared to the thick decidua that lines the body of the uterus.

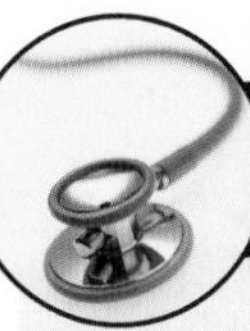

CLINICAL NOTES

The Uterine Tube as a Conduit for Infection

The uterine tube lies in the upper free border of the broad ligament and is a direct route of communication from the vulva through the vagina and uterine cavity to the peritoneal cavity.

Pelvic Inflammatory Disease

The pathogenic organism(s) enter the body through sexual contact and ascend through the uterus and enter the uterine tubes. **Salpingitis** may follow, with leakage of pus into the peritoneal cavity, causing pelvic peritonitis. A pelvic abscess usually follows, or the infection spreads farther, causing general peritonitis.

Ectopic Pregnancy

Implantation and growth of a fertilized ovum may occur outside the uterine cavity in the wall of the uterine tube (Fig. 7-26). This is a variety of **ectopic pregnancy.** There being no decidua formation in the tube, the eroding action of the trophoblast quickly destroys the wall of the tube. Tubal abortion or rupture of the tube, with the effusion of a large quantity of blood into the peritoneal cavity, is the common result.

The blood pours down into the rectouterine pouch (pouch of Douglas) or into the uterovesical pouch. The blood may quickly ascend into the general peritoneal cavity, giving rise to severe abdominal pain, tenderness, and guarding. Irritation of the subdiaphragmatic peritoneum (supplied by phrenic nerves C3, 4, and 5) may give rise to referred pain to the shoulder skin (supraclavicular nerves C3 and 4).

Tubal Ligation

Ligation and division of the uterine tubes is a method of obtaining permanent birth control and is usually restricted to women who already have children. The ova that are discharged from the ovarian follicles degenerate in the tube proximal to the obstruction. If, later, the woman wishes to have an additional child, restoration of the continuity of the uterine tubes can be attempted, and, in about 20% of women, fertilization occurs.

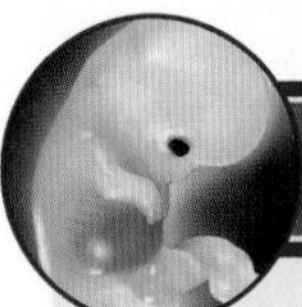

EMBRYOLOGIC NOTES

Development of the Uterine Tube

Early on in development, the **paramesonephric ducts** appear on the posterior abdominal wall on the lateral side of the mesonephros. The uterine tube on each side is formed from the cranial vertical and middle horizontal parts of the paramesonephric duct (Fig. 7-27). The tube elongates and becomes coiled; differentiation of the muscle and mucous membrane takes place; the **fimbriae** develop; and the **infundibulum, ampulla,** and **isthmus** are identifiable.

Uterus

Location and Description

The uterus is a hollow, pear-shaped organ with thick muscular walls. In the young nulliparous adult, it measures 3 in. (8 cm) long, 2 in. (5 cm) wide, and 1 in. (2.5 cm) thick. It is divided into the fundus, body, and cervix (Fig. 7-25).

The **fundus** is the part of the uterus that lies above the entrance of the uterine tubes.

The **body** is the part of the uterus that lies below the entrance of the uterine tubes.

The **cervix** is the narrow part of the uterus. It pierces the anterior wall of the vagina and is divided into the **supravaginal** and **vaginal parts of the cervix.**

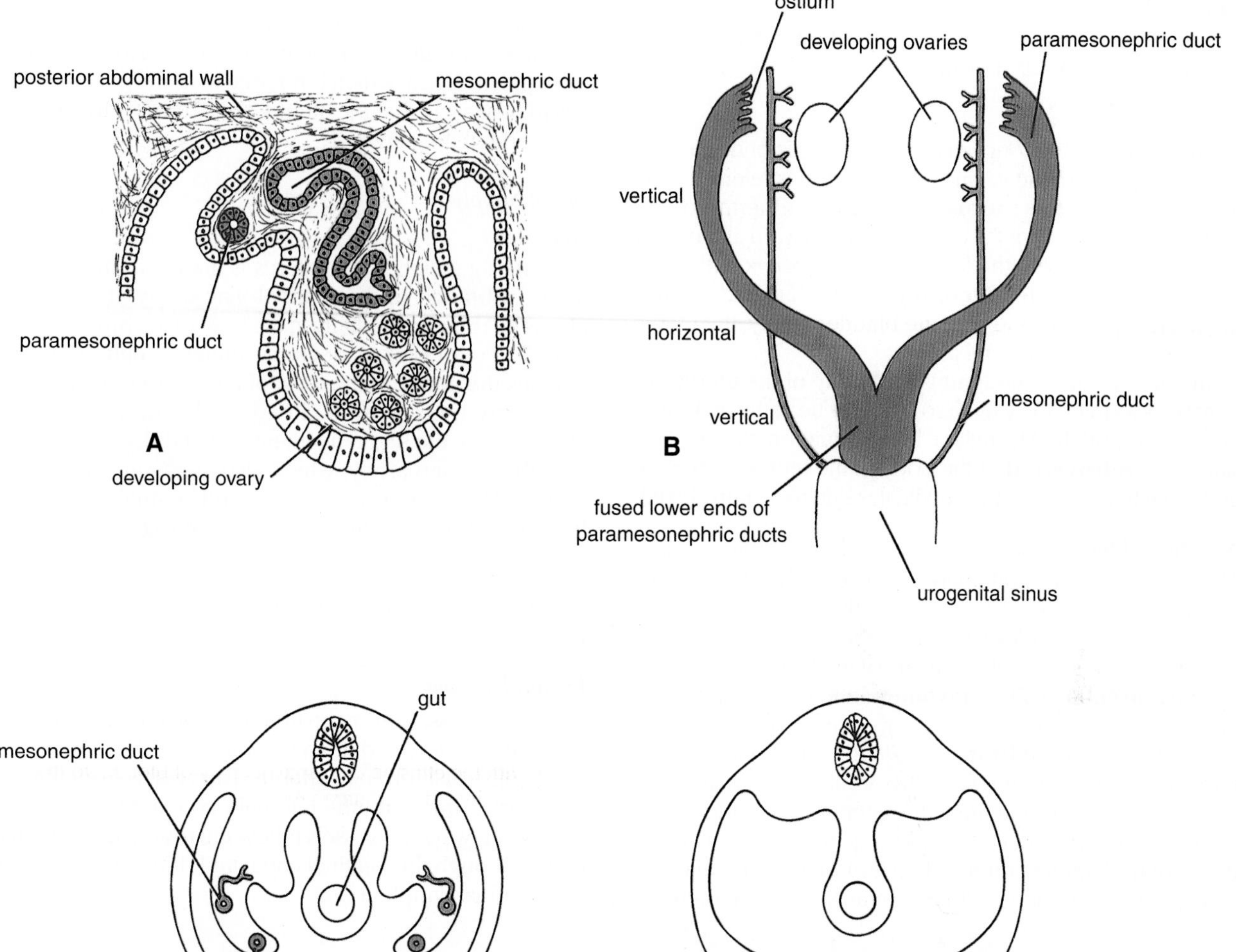

Figure 7-27 The relationship of the mesonephric and paramesonephric ducts to the developing ovary. **A.** Cross section of a developing ovary. **B.** Anterior view of ovaries and ducts. **C and D.** Mesonephric and paramesonephric ducts in a cross section of the pelvis. Note the developing broad ligament.

The **cavity** of the uterine body is triangular in coronal section, but it is merely a cleft in the sagittal plane (Fig. 7-25). The cavity of the cervix, the **cervical canal,** communicates with the cavity of the body through the **internal os** and with that of the vagina through the **external os.** Before the birth of the first child, the external os is circular. In a parous woman, the vaginal part of the cervix is larger, and the external os becomes a transverse slit so that it possesses an anterior lip and a posterior lip (Fig. 7-25).

Relations

- **Anteriorly:** The body of the uterus is related anteriorly to the uterovesical pouch and the superior surface of the bladder (Fig. 7-5). The supravaginal cervix is related to the superior surface of the bladder. The vaginal cervix is related to the anterior fornix of the vagina.
- **Posteriorly:** The body of the uterus is related posteriorly to the rectouterine pouch (pouch of Douglas) with coils of ileum or sigmoid colon within it (Fig. 7-5).
- **Laterally:** The body of the uterus is related laterally to the broad ligament and the uterine artery and vein (Fig. 7-19). The supravaginal cervix is related to the ureter as it passes forward to enter the bladder. The vaginal cervix is related to the lateral fornix of the vagina. The uterine tubes enter the superolateral angles of the uterus, and the round ligaments of the ovary and of the uterus are attached to the uterine wall just below this level.

Function

The uterus serves as a site for the reception, retention, and nutrition of the fertilized ovum.

Positions of the Uterus

In most women, the long axis of the uterus is bent forward on the long axis of the vagina. This position is referred to as **anteversion of the uterus** (Fig. 7-25). Furthermore, the long axis of the body of the uterus is bent forward at the level of the internal os with the long axis of the cervix. This position is termed **anteflexion of the uterus** (Fig. 7-25). Thus, in the erect position and with the bladder empty, the uterus lies in an almost horizontal plane.

In some women, the fundus and body of the uterus are bent backward on the vagina so that they lie in the rectouterine pouch (pouch of Douglas). In this situation, the uterus is said to be **retroverted.** If the body of the uterus is, in addition, bent backward on the cervix, it is said to be retroflexed.

Structure of the Uterus

The uterus is covered with peritoneum except anteriorly, below the level of the internal os, where the peritoneum passes forward onto the bladder. Laterally, there is also a space between the attachment of the layers of the broad ligament.

The **muscular wall,** or **myometrium,** is thick and made up of smooth muscle supported by connective tissue.

The **mucous membrane** lining the body of the uterus is known as the **endometrium.** It is continuous above with the mucous membrane lining the uterine tubes and below with the mucous membrane lining the cervix. The endometrium is applied directly to the muscle, there being no submucosa. From puberty to menopause, the endometrium undergoes extensive changes during the menstrual cycle in response to the ovarian hormones.

The supravaginal part of the cervix is surrounded by visceral pelvic fascia, which is referred to as the **parametrium.** It is in this fascia that the uterine artery crosses the ureter on each side of the cervix.

Blood Supply

Arteries

The arterial supply to the uterus is mainly from the uterine artery, a branch of the internal iliac artery. It reaches the uterus by running medially in the base of the broad ligament (Fig. 7-19). It crosses above the ureter at right angles and reaches the cervix at the level of the internal os (Fig. 7-25). The artery then ascends along the lateral margin of the uterus within the broad ligament and ends by anastomosing with the ovarian artery, which also assists in supplying the uterus. The uterine artery gives off a small descending branch that supplies the cervix and the vagina.

Veins

The uterine vein follows the artery and drains into the internal iliac vein.

Lymph Drainage

The lymph vessels from the fundus of the uterus accompany the ovarian artery and drain into the para-aortic nodes at the level of the first lumbar vertebra. The vessels from the body and cervix drain into the internal and external iliac lymph nodes. A few lymph vessels follow the round ligament of the uterus through the inguinal canal and drain into the superficial inguinal lymph nodes.

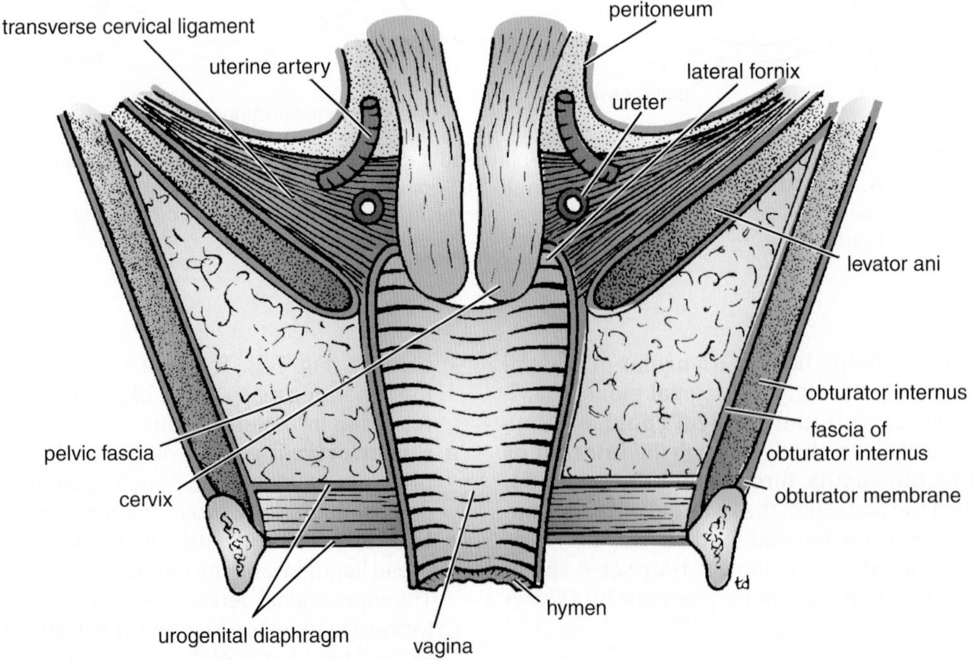

Figure 7-28 Coronal section of the pelvis showing relation of the levatores ani muscles and transverse cervical ligaments to the uterus and vagina. Note that the transverse cervical ligaments are formed from a condensation of visceral pelvic fascia.

Nerve Supply

Sympathetic and parasympathetic nerves from branches of the inferior hypogastric plexuses

Supports of the Uterus

The uterus is supported mainly by the tone of the levatores ani muscles and the condensations of pelvic fascia, which form three important ligaments.

The Levatores Ani Muscles and the Perineal Body

The origin and the insertion of the levatores ani muscles are described in Chapter 6. They form a broad muscular sheet stretching across the pelvic cavity, and, together with the pelvic fascia on their upper surface, they effectively support the pelvic viscera and resist the intra-abdominal pressure transmitted downward through the pelvis. The medial edges of the anterior parts of the levatores ani muscles are attached to the cervix of the uterus by the pelvic fascia (Fig. 7-28).

Some of the fibers of levator ani are inserted into a fibromuscular structure called the **perineal body** (Fig. 7-5). This structure is important in maintaining the integrity of the pelvic floor; if the perineal body is damaged during childbirth, prolapse of the pelvic viscera may occur. The perineal body lies in the perineum between the vagina and the anal canal. It is slung up to the pelvic walls by the levatores ani and thus supports the vagina and, indirectly, the uterus.

The Transverse Cervical, Pubocervical, and Sacrocervical Ligaments

These three ligaments are subperitoneal condensations of pelvic fascia on the upper surface of the levatores ani muscles. They are attached to the cervix and the vault of the vagina and play an important part in supporting the uterus and keeping the cervix in its correct position (Figs. 7-28 and 7-29).

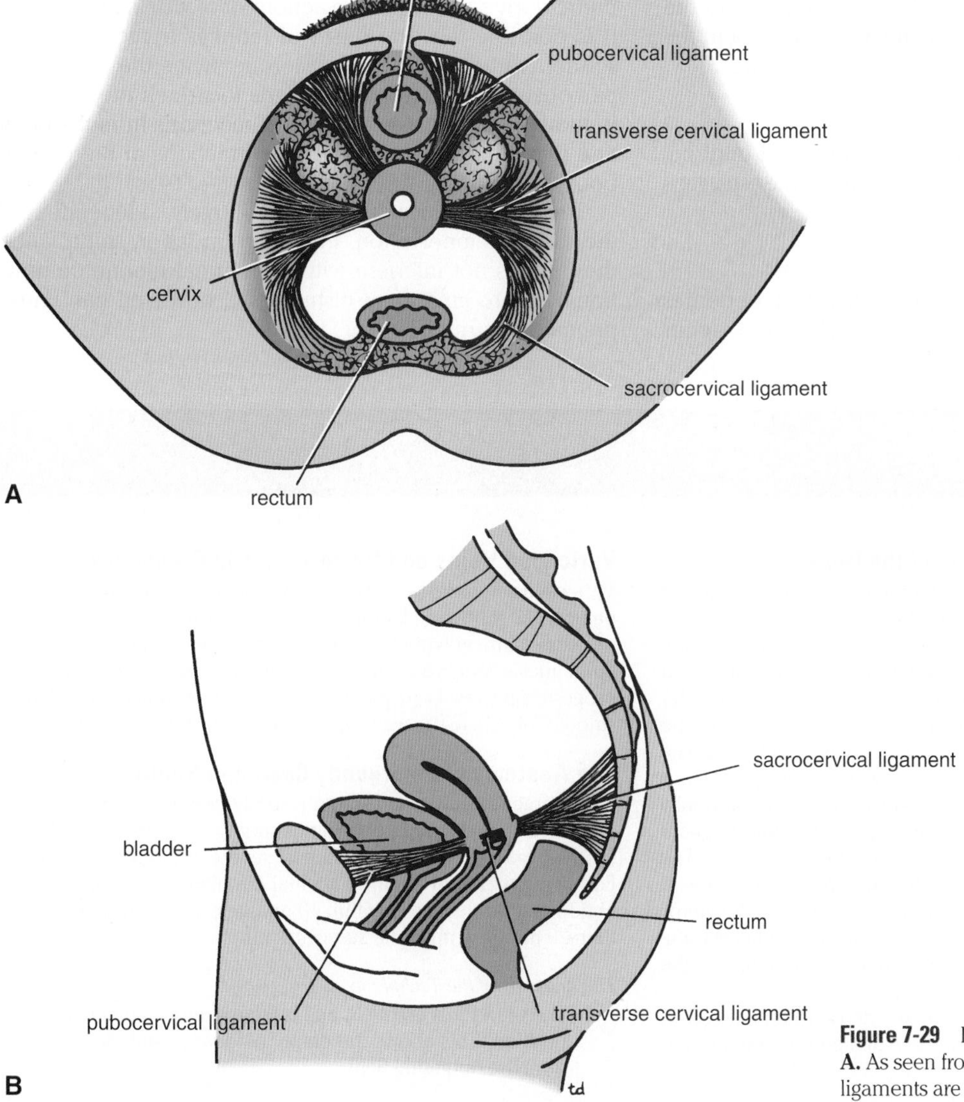

Figure 7-29 Ligamentous supports of uterus. **A.** As seen from below. **B.** Lateral view. These ligaments are formed from visceral pelvic fascia.

Transverse Cervical (Cardinal) Ligaments Transverse cervical ligaments are fibromuscular condensations of pelvic fascia that pass to the cervix and the upper end of the vagina from the lateral walls of the pelvis.

Pubocervical Ligaments The pubocervical ligaments consist of two firm bands of connective tissue that pass to the cervix from the posterior surface of the pubis. They are positioned on either side of the neck of the bladder, to which they give some support **(pubovesical ligaments).**

Sacrocervical Ligaments The sacrocervical ligaments consist of two firm fibromuscular bands of pelvic fascia that pass to the cervix and the upper end of the vagina from the lower end of the sacrum. They form two ridges, one on either side of the rectouterine pouch (pouch of Douglas).

The broad ligaments and the round ligaments of the uterus are lax structures, and the uterus can be pulled up or pushed down for a considerable distance before they become taut. Clinically, they are considered to play a minor role in supporting the uterus.

The **round ligament of the uterus,** which represents the remains of the lower half of the gubernaculum, extends between the superolateral angle of the uterus, through the deep inguinal ring and inguinal canal, to the subcutaneous tissue of the labium majus (Fig. 7-18). It helps keep the uterus anteverted (tilted forward) and anteflexed (bent forward) but is considerably stretched during pregnancy.

Uterus in the Child

The fundus and body of the uterus remain small until puberty, when they enlarge greatly in response to the estrogens secreted by the ovaries.

Uterus After Menopause

After menopause, the uterus atrophies and becomes smaller and less vascular. These changes occur because the ovaries no longer produce estrogens and progesterone.

Uterus in Pregnancy

During pregnancy, the uterus becomes greatly enlarged as a result of the increasing production of estrogens and progesterone, first by the corpus luteum of the ovary and later by the placenta. At first it remains as a pelvic organ, but by the third month the fundus rises out of the pelvis, and by the ninth month it has reached the xiphoid process. The increase in size is largely a result of hypertrophy of the smooth muscle fibers of the myometrium, although some hyperplasia takes place.

Role of the Uterus in Labor

Labor, or parturition, is the series of processes by which the baby, the fetal membranes, and the placenta are expelled from the genital tract of the mother. Normally this process takes place at the end of the 10th lunar month, at which time the pregnancy is said to be at **term.**

The cause of the onset of labor is not definitely known. By the end of pregnancy, the contractility of the uterus has been fully developed in response to estrogen, and it is particularly sensitive to the actions of oxytocin at this time. It is possible that the onset of labor is triggered by the sudden withdrawal of progesterone. Once the presenting part (usually the fetal head) starts to stretch the cervix, it is thought that a nervous reflex mechanism is initiated and increases the force of the contractions of the uterine body.

The uterine muscular activity is largely independent of the extrinsic innervation. In women in labor, spinal anesthesia does not interfere with the normal uterine contractions. Severe emotional disturbance, however, can cause premature parturition.

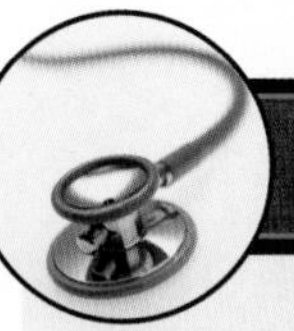

CLINICAL NOTES

Bimanual Pelvic Examination of the Uterus

A great deal of useful clinical information can be obtained about the state of the uterus, uterine tubes, and ovaries from a bimanual examination. The examination is easiest in parous women who are able to relax while the examination is in progress. In patients in whom it causes distress, the examination may be performed under an anesthetic. With the bladder empty, the vaginal portion of the cervix is first palpated with the index finger of the right hand. The external os is circular in the nulliparous woman but has anterior and posterior lips in the multiparous woman. The cervix normally has the consistency of the end of the nose, but in the pregnant uterus it is soft and vascular and has the consistency of the lips. The left hand is then placed gently on the anterior abdominal wall above the symphysis pubis, and the fundus and body of the uterus may be palpated between the abdominal and vaginal fingers situated in the anterior fornix. The size, shape, and mobility of the uterus can then be ascertained.

In most women, the uterus is anteverted and anteflexed. A retroverted, retroflexed uterus can be palpated through the posterior vaginal fornix.

Varicosed Veins and Hemorrhoids in Pregnancy

Varicosed veins and hemorrhoids are common conditions in pregnancy. The following factors probably contribute to their cause: pressure of the gravid uterus on the inferior vena cava and the inferior mesenteric vein, impairing venous return, and increased progesterone levels in the blood, leading to relaxation of the smooth muscle in the walls of the veins and venous dilatation.

The Anatomy of Emergency Cesarean Section

An emergency cesarean section is rarely performed. However, a physician may need to perform this surgery in cases in which the mother may die after suffering a severe traumatic incident. Following maternal death, placental circulation ceases, and the child must be delivered within 10 minutes; after a delay of more than 20 minutes, neonatal survival is rare.

The Anatomy of the Technique

1. The bladder is emptied, and an indwelling catheter is left in position. This allows the empty bladder to sink down away from the operating field.

(continues)

Clinical Notes, *continued*

2. A midline skin incision is made that extends from just below the umbilicus to just above the symphysis pubis. The following structures are then incised: superficial fascia, fatty layer, and the membranous layer; deep fascia (thin layer); linear alba; fascia transversalis; extraperitoneal fatty layer; and parietal peritoneum. To avoid damaging loops of the small intestine or the greater omentum, which might be lying beneath the parietal peritoneum, a fold of peritoneum is raised between two hemostats; an incision is then made between the hemostats.
3. The bladder is identified, and a cut is made in the floor of the uterovesical pouch. The bladder is then separated from the lower part of the body of the uterus and depressed downward into the pelvis.
4. The uterus is palpated to identify the presenting part of the fetus.
5. A transverse incision about 1 in. (2.5 cm) long is made into the exposed lower segment of the body of the uterus. Care is taken that the uterine wall is not immediately penetrated and the fetus injured.
6. When the uterine cavity is entered, the amniotic cavity is opened, and amniotic fluid spurts. The uterine incision is then enlarged sufficiently to deliver the head and trunk of the fetus. When possible, the large tributaries and branches of the uterine vessels in the myometrial wall are avoided. Great care has to be taken to avoid the large uterine arteries that course along the lateral margin of the uterus.
7. Once the fetus is delivered, the umbilical cord is clamped and divided.
8. The contracting uterus will cause the placenta to bulge through the uterine incision. The placenta and fetal membranes are then delivered.
9. The uterine incision is closed with a full-thickness continuous suture. The peritoneum over the bladder and lower part of the uterine body is then repaired to restore the integrity of the uterovesical pouch. Finally, the abdominal wall incision is closed in layers.

Prolapse of the Uterus

The great importance of the tone of the levatores ani muscles in supporting the uterus has already been emphasized. The importance of the transverse cervical, pubocervical, and sacrocervical ligaments in positioning the cervix within the pelvic cavity has been considered. Damage to these structures during childbirth or general poor body muscular tone may result in downward displacement of the uterus called **uterine prolapse.** It most commonly reveals itself after menopause, when the visceral pelvic fascia tends to atrophy along with the pelvic organs. In advanced cases, the cervix descends the length of the vagina and may protrude through the orifice.

Because of the attachment of the cervix to the vaginal vault, it follows that prolapse of the uterus is always accompanied by some prolapse of the vagina.

Hysterectomy and Damage to the Ureter

During the surgical procedure of hysterectomy, great care must be exercised to not damage the ureters. When the surgeon is looking for the uterine artery on each side at the base of the broad ligament, it is essential that he or she first identifies the ureter before clamping and tying off the artery. The uterine artery passes forward from the internal iliac artery and crosses the ureter at right angles to reach the cervix at the level of the internal os.

Sonography of the Female Pelvis

A sonogram of the female pelvis can be used to visualize the uterus and the developing fetus and the vagina (Figs. 7-30, 7-31, and 7-32).

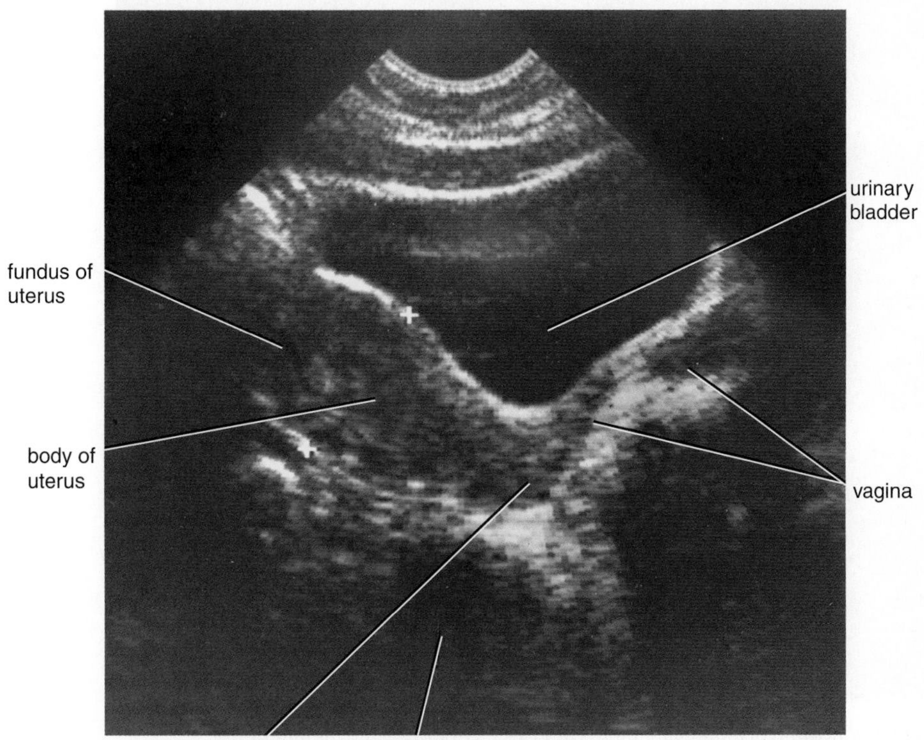

Figure 7-30 Longitudinal sonogram of the female pelvis showing the uterus, the vagina, and the bladder. (Courtesy of M.C. Hill.)

anterior

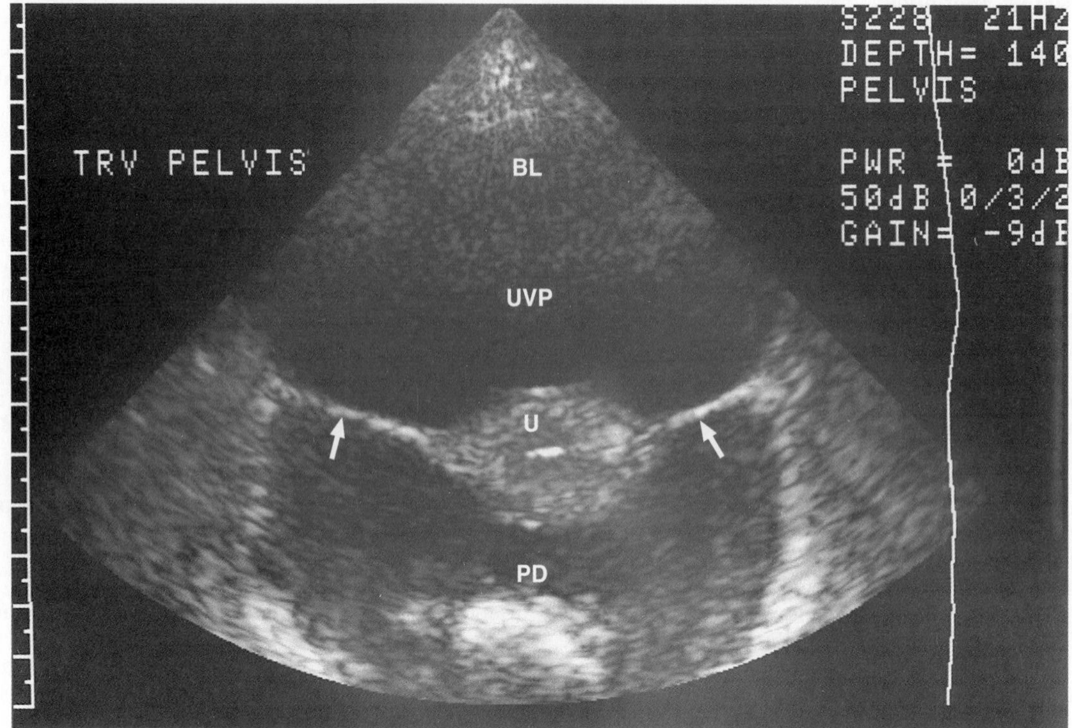

posterior

Figure 7-31 Transverse sonogram of the pelvis in a woman after an automobile accident, in which the liver was lacerated and blood escaped into the peritoneal cavity. The bladder (*BL*), the body of the uterus (*U*), and the broad ligaments (*white arrows*) are identified. Note the presence of blood (*dark areas*) in the uterovesical pouch (*UVP*) and the pouch of Douglas (*PD*). (Courtesy of L. Scoutt.)

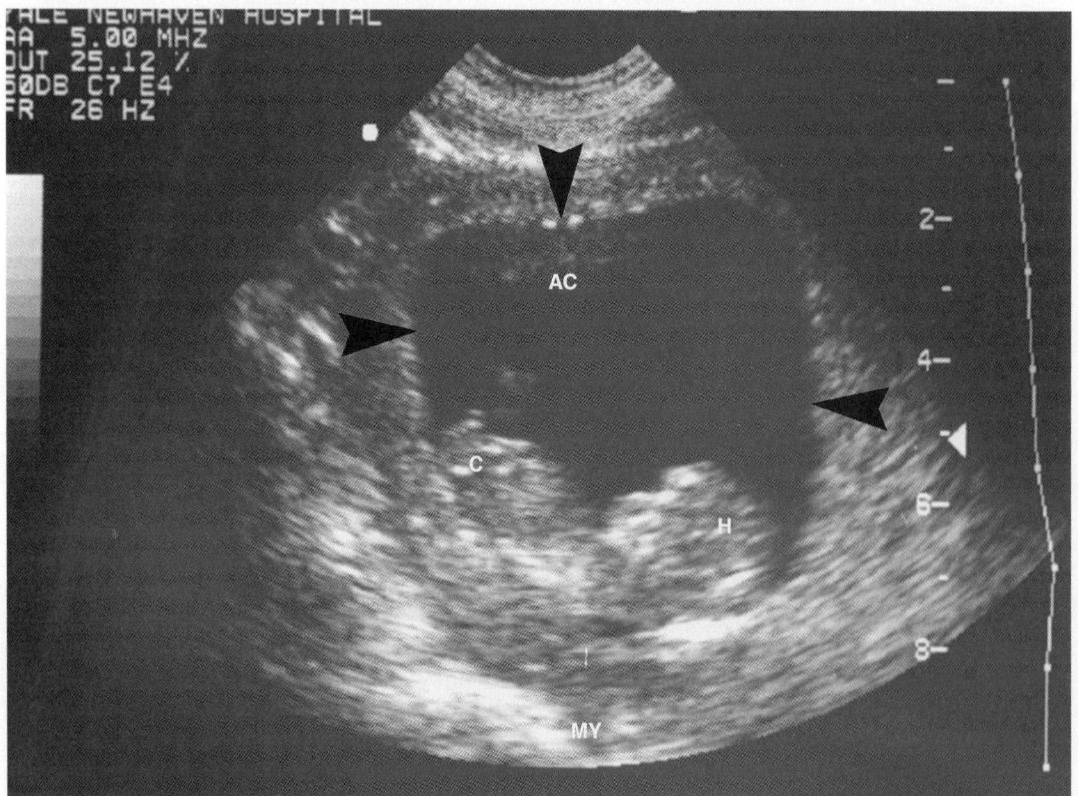

Figure 7-32 Longitudinal sonogram of a pregnant uterus at 11 weeks showing the intrauterine gestational sac (*black arrowheads*) and the amniotic cavity (*AC*) filled with amniotic fluid; the fetus is seen in longitudinal section with the head (*H*) and coccyx (*C*) well displayed. The myometrium (*MY*) of the uterus can be identified. (Courtesy of L. Scoutt.)

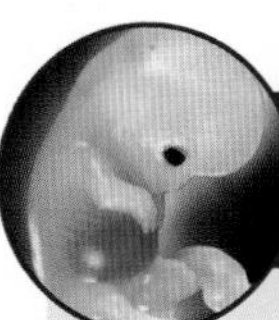

EMBRYOLOGIC NOTES

Development of the Uterus

The uterus is derived from the fused caudal vertical parts of the paramesonephric ducts (Fig. 7-33), and the site of their angular junction becomes a convex dome and forms the **fundus** of the uterus. The fusion between the ducts is incomplete at first, a septum persisting between the lumina. Later, the septum disappears so that a single cavity remains. The upper part of the cavity forms the lumen of the **body** and **cervix** of the uterus. The myometrium is formed from the surrounding mesenchyme.

Agenesis of the Uterus

Rarely the uterus will be absent as the result of a failure of the paramesonephric ducts to develop.

Infantile Uterus

Some adults may have an infantile uterus, a condition in which the uterus is much smaller than normal and resembles that present before puberty. Amenorrhea is present, but the vagina and ovaries may be normal.

Failure of Fusion of the Paramesonephric Ducts

Failure of the paramesonephric ducts to fuse may cause a variety of uterine defects: (a) The uterus may be duplicated with two bodies and two cervices. (b) There may be a complete septum through the uterus, making two uterine cavities and two cervices. (c) There may be two separate uterine bodies with one cervix. (d) One paramesonephric duct may fail to develop, leaving one uterine tube and half of the body of the uterus. Clinically, the main problems with a double uterus may be seen when pregnancy occurs. Abortion is frequent, and the nonpregnant half of the uterus may cause obstruction at labor.

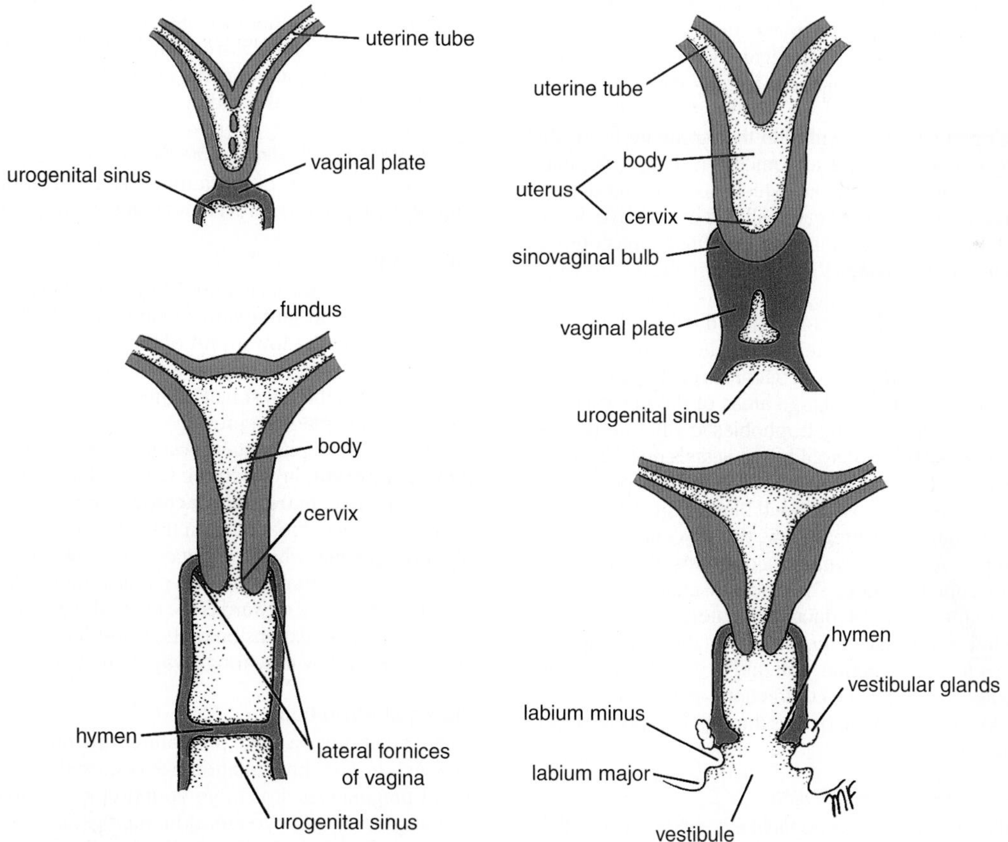

Figure 7-33 Formation of the uterine tubes, the uterus, and the vagina.

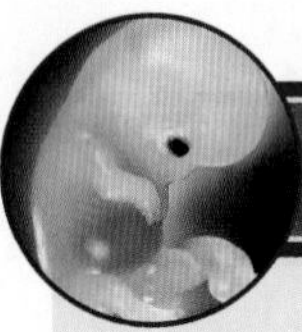

Brief Summary of the Implantation of the Fertilized Ovum in the Uterus

The blastocyst enters the uterine cavity between the fourth and ninth days after ovulation. Normal implantation takes place in the endometrium of the body of the uterus, most frequently on the upper part of the posterior wall near the midline (Fig. 7-34). As the result of the enzymatic digestion of the uterine epithelium by the trophoblast of the embryo, the blastocyst sinks beneath the surface epithelium and becomes embedded in the stroma by the 11th or 12th day.

Vagina

Location and Description

The vagina is a muscular tube that extends upward and backward from the vulva to the uterus (Fig. 7-5). It measures about 3 in. (8 cm) long and has anterior and posterior walls, which are normally in apposition. At its upper end, the anterior wall is pierced by the cervix, which projects downward and backward into the vagina. It is important to remember that the upper half of the vagina lies above the pelvic floor and the lower half lies within the perineum (Figs. 7-5 and 7-28). The area of the vaginal lumen, which surrounds the cervix, is divided into four regions, or **fornices:** anterior, posterior, right lateral, and left lateral. The vaginal orifice in a virgin possesses a thin mucosal fold called the **hymen,** which is perforated at its center. After childbirth the hymen usually consists only of tags.

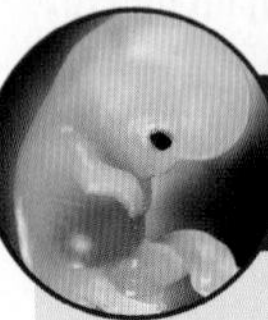

A Summary of the Formation of the Placenta

The placenta is the organ that carries out respiration, excretion, and nutrition for the embryo, and it is fully formed during the fourth month. The formation of the placenta is complicated and is essentially the development of an organ by mother and child in symbiosis and consists of fetal and maternal parts.

The fetal part develops as follows. The trophoblast becomes a highly developed structure, with villi that continue to erode and penetrate deeper into the endometrium. Large irregular spaces known as **lacunae** appear, which become filled with maternal blood. At the center of each villus is connective tissue containing fetal blood vessels that will eventually anastomose with one another and converge to form the umbilical cord (Fig. 7-35).

The maternal part develops as follows. Under the influence of progesterone, secreted first by the corpus luteum and later by the placenta itself, the endometrium becomes greatly thickened and is known as the **decidua.** Large areas of the decidua become excavated by the invading trophoblastic villi to form the **intervillous spaces.** The maternal blood vessels open into the spaces so that the outer surfaces of the villi of the fetal part of the placenta become bathed in oxygenated blood (Fig. 7-35).

By the fourth month of pregnancy, the placenta is a well-developed organ. As the pregnancy continues, the placenta increases in area and thickness. The placental attachment occupies one third of the internal surface of the uterus.

At birth, a few minutes after the delivery of the child, the placenta separates from the uterine wall and is expelled from the uterine cavity as the result of the contractions of the uterine musculature. The line of separation occurs through the spongy layer of the decidua (Fig. 7-35).

Gross Appearance of the Placenta at Birth

At full term, the placenta has a spongelike consistency. It is flattened and circular, with a diameter of about 8 in. (20 cm) and a thickness of about 1 in. (2.5 cm), and weighs about 1 lb (500 g). It thins out at the edges, where it is continuous with the fetal membranes (Fig. 7-36).

The outer, or maternal, surface of a freshly shed placenta is rough on palpation, is dark red, and oozes blood from the torn maternal blood vessels.

The inner, or fetal, surface is smooth and shiny and is raised in ridges by the umbilical blood vessels, which radiate from the attachment of the umbilical cord near its center.

The fetal membranes (see Fig. 4-36), which surround and enclose the amniotic fluid, are continuous with the edge of the placenta. They are the amnion, the chorion, and a small amount of the adherent maternal decidua.

The Placenta and Bleeding in Late Pregnancy

The common causes of substantial vaginal bleeding in the third trimester are placenta previa and placental abruption.

Placenta Previa

Placenta previa occurs in about 1 of every 200 pregnancies. It is more common in multiparous women and in those who have had surgery on the lower part of the uterus. Normally, the placenta is situated in the upper half of the uterus. Should implantation occur in the lower half of the body of the uterus, the condition is called placenta previa.

Three types of placenta previa may be recognized: a **central placenta previa,** in which the entire internal os is covered by placental tissue; **marginal placenta previa,** when the edge of the placenta is encroaching on the internal os; and a **low-lying placenta previa,** when the placenta lies low down in the uterus, lateral to the internal os. Severe, painless hemorrhage occurring from the 28th week onward is the clinical sign of placenta previa and is caused by expansion of the lower half of the uterine wall at this time and by its tearing away from the placenta.

Placental Abruption

Placental abruption is the premature separation of the placenta in which normal implantation has occurred. It occurs in about 1% of pregnancies. It is more common in multiparous women and in women with hypertension in pregnancy. As the placenta separates, hemorrhage occurs; the blood clot dissects the fetal membranes away from the uterine wall. The blood usually escapes through the cervix or ruptures into the amniotic cavity. The blood irritates the myometrium, and uterine muscle tone is increased, which results in contractions. The placental circulation is compromised by the placental separation and the increased pressure on the placenta by the increased uterine tone.

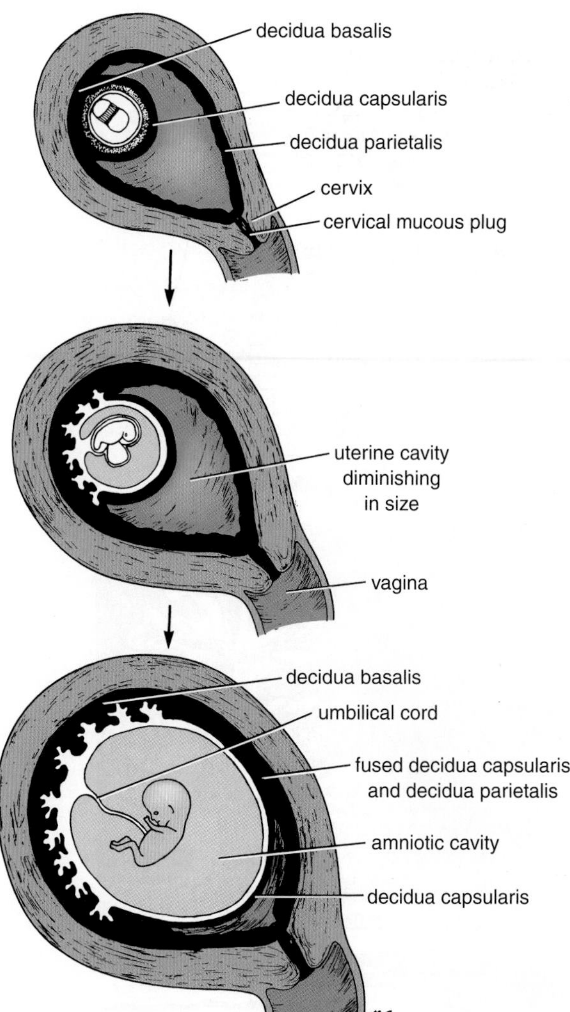

Figure 7-34 Sagittal section of the uterus showing the developing conceptus expanding into the uterine cavity. The three different regions of the decidua can be recognized. By the 16th week, the uterine cavity is obliterated by the fusion of the decidua capsularis with the decidua parietalis.

Relations

- **Anteriorly:** The vagina is closely related to the bladder above and to the urethra below (Fig. 7-5).
- **Posteriorly:** The upper third of the vagina is related to the rectouterine pouch (pouch of Douglas) and its middle third to the ampulla of the rectum. The lower third is related to the perineal body, which separates it from the anal canal (Fig. 7-5).
- **Laterally:** In its upper part, the vagina is related to the ureter; its middle part is related to the anterior fibers of the levator ani, as they run backward to reach the perineal body and hook around the anorectal junction (Figs. 7-19 and 7-28). Contraction of the fibers of levator ani compresses the walls of the vagina together. In its lower part, the vagina is related to the urogenital diaphragm (see Chapter 8) and the bulb of the vestibule.

Function

The vagina not only is the female genital canal, but it also serves as the excretory duct for the menstrual flow and forms part of the birth canal.

Blood Supply

Arteries

The vaginal artery, a branch of the internal iliac artery, and the vaginal branch of the uterine artery supply the vagina.

Veins

The vaginal veins form a plexus around the vagina that drains into the internal iliac vein.

Lymph Drainage

The upper third of the vagina drains to the external and internal iliac nodes, the middle third drains to the internal iliac nodes, and the lower third drains to the superficial inguinal nodes.

Nerve Supply

The inferior hypogastric plexuses.

Supports of the Vagina

The upper part of the vagina is supported by the levatores ani muscles and the transverse cervical, pubocervical, and sacrocervical ligaments. These structures are attached to the vaginal wall by pelvic fascia (Figs. 7-28 and 7-29).

The middle part of the vagina is supported by the urogenital diaphragm (see Chapter 8).

The lower part of the vagina, especially the posterior wall, is supported by the perineal body (Fig. 7-5).

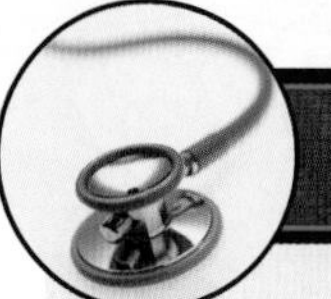

CLINICAL NOTES

Vaginal Examination

The anatomic relations of the vagina are of great clinical importance. Many pathologic conditions occurring in the female pelvis may be diagnosed using a simple vaginal examination.

The following structures can be palpated through the vaginal walls from above downward:

- **Anteriorly:** The bladder and the urethra
- **Posteriorly:** Loops of ileum and the sigmoid colon in the rectouterine peritoneal pouch (pouch of Douglas), the rectal ampulla, and the perineal body
- **Laterally:** The ureters, the pelvic fascia and the anterior fibers of the levatores ani muscles, and the urogenital diaphragm

Prolapse of the Vagina

The vaginal vault is supported by the same structures that support the uterine cervix. Prolapse of the uterus is necessarily associated with some degree of sagging of the vaginal walls. However, if the supports of the bladder, urethra, or anterior rectal wall are damaged in childbirth, prolapse of the vaginal walls occurs, with the uterus remaining in its correct position.

(continues)

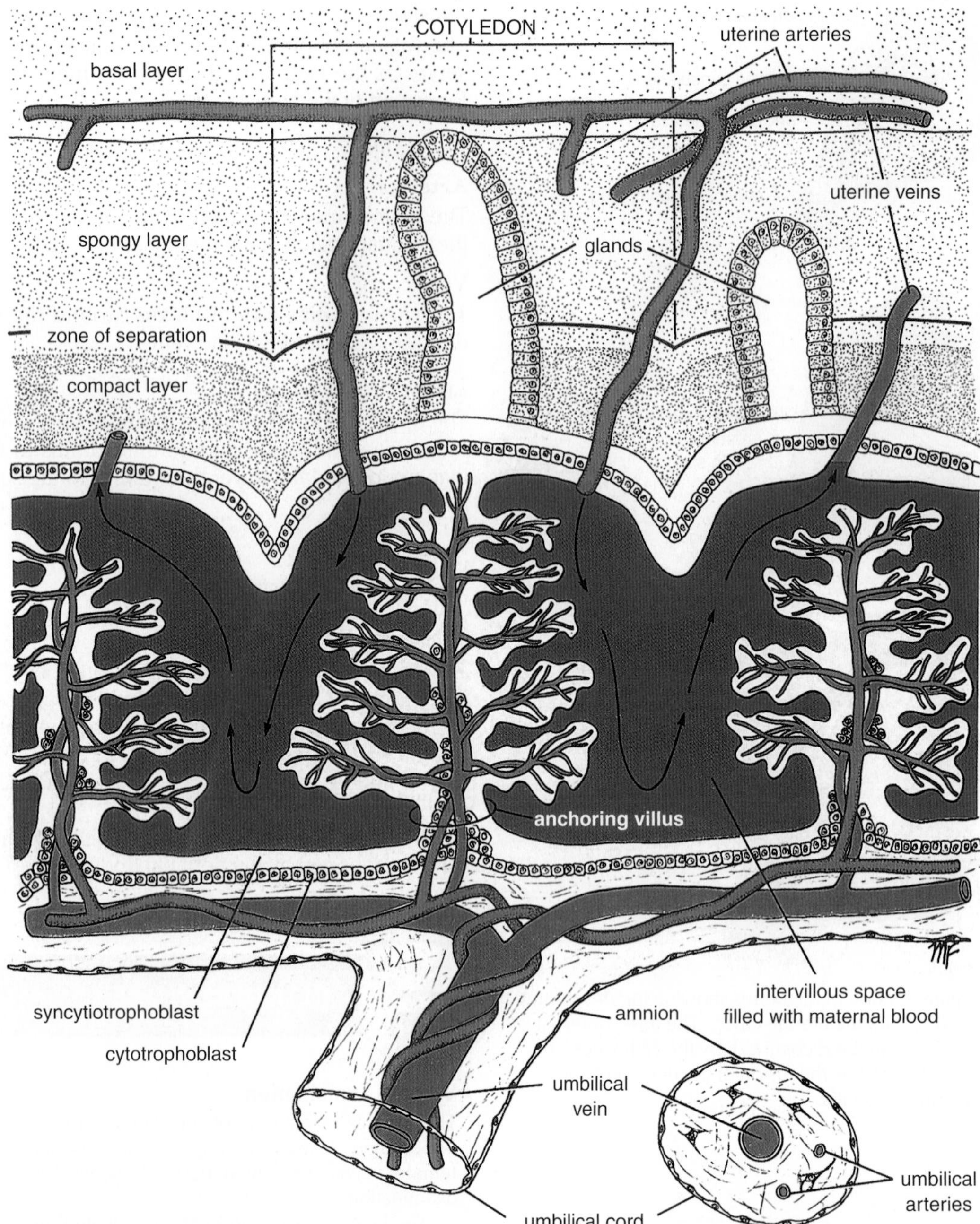

Figure 7-35 A section through the placenta showing the maternal **(top)** and fetal **(bottom)** parts. Note that the maternal part is divided into the basal layer, the spongy layer, and the compact layer. The heavy solid line in the spongy layer indicates where separation occurs between the maternal and fetal parts of the placenta during the third stage of labor.

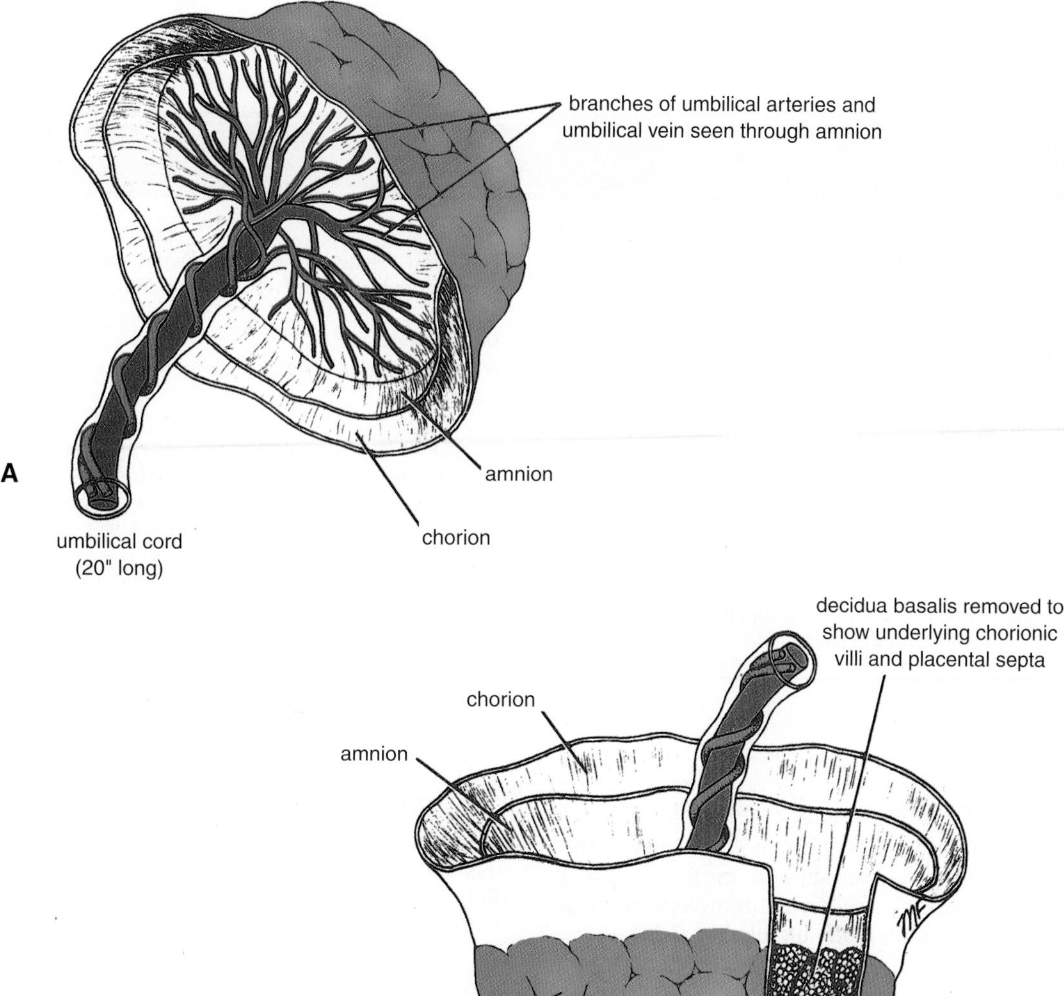

Figure 7-36 The mature placenta as seen from the fetal surface **(A)** and from the maternal surface **(B).**

Clinical Notes, *continued*

Sagging of the bladder results in the bulging of the anterior wall of the vagina, a condition known as a **cystocele.** When the ampulla of the rectum sags against the posterior vaginal wall, the bulge is called a **rectocele.**

Culdocentesis

The closeness of the peritoneal cavity to the posterior vaginal fornix enables the physician to drain a pelvic abscess through the vagina without performing a major operation. It is also possible to identify blood or pus in the peritoneal cavity by the passage of a needle through the posterior fornix.

Anatomic Structures Through Which the Needle Passes

The needle passes through the mucous membrane of the vagina, muscular coat of the vagina, connective tissue coat of the vagina, visceral layer of pelvic fascia, and visceral layer of peritoneum.

Anatomic Features of the Complications of Culdocentesis

Complications are as follows: (a) The loops of ileum and the sigmoid colon, structures that are normally present within the pouch of Douglas, could be impaled by the needle. However, the presence of blood or pus within the pouch tends to deflect the viscera superiorly. (b) Occasionally, when the uterus is somewhat retroflexed, the needle may enter the posterior wall of the body of the uterus.

Vaginal Trauma

Coital injury, picket fence–type of impalement injury, and vaginal perforation caused by water under pressure, as occurs in water skiing, are common injuries. Lacerations of the vaginal wall involving the posterior fornix may violate the pouch of Douglas of the peritoneal cavity and cause prolapse of the small intestine into the vagina.

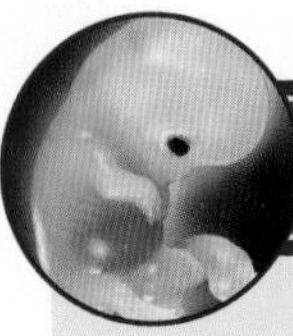

EMBRYOLOGIC NOTES

Development of the Vagina

The vagina is developed from the wall of the **urogenital sinus** (Fig. 7-33). The fused lower ends of the paramesonephric ducts form the body and cervix of the uterus, and once the solid end of the fused ducts reaches the posterior wall of the urogenital sinus, two outgrowths occur from the sinus, called the **sinovaginal bulbs.** The cells of the sinovaginal bulbs proliferate rapidly and form the **vaginal plate.** The vaginal plate thickens and elongates and extends around the solid end of the fused paramesonephric ducts. Later, the plate is completely canalized and the vaginal fornices are formed.

Vaginal Agenesis

If the paramesonephric ducts fail to develop, the wall of the urogenital sinus will fail to form the vaginal plate. In these patients, there is an absence of the vagina, uterus, and uterine tubes. Plastic surgical construction of a vagina should be attempted.

Double Vagina

A double vagina is caused by incomplete canalization of the vaginal plate.

Imperforate Vagina and Imperforate Hymen

Imperforate vagina is caused by a failure of the cells to degenerate in the center of the vaginal plates. Imperforate hymen is caused by a failure of the cells of the lower part of the vaginal plate and wall of the urogenital sinus to degenerate. These conditions lead to retention of the menstrual flow, a clinical condition called **hematocolpos.** Surgical incision of the obstruction, followed by dilatation, relieves the condition.

Visceral Pelvic Fascia

The visceral pelvic fascia is a layer of connective tissue, which, as in the male, covers and supports the pelvic viscera. It is condensed to form the pubocervical, transverse cervical, and sacrocervical ligaments of the uterus. (Fig. 7-29).

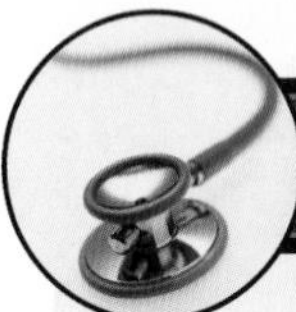

CLINICAL NOTES

Visceral Pelvic Fascia and Infection

Clinically, the pelvic fascia in the region of the uterine cervix is often referred to as the **parametrium.** It is a common site for the spread of acute infections from the uterus and vagina, and here the infection often becomes chronic (pelvic inflammatory disease).

Peritoneum

The peritoneum in the female, as in the male, is best understood by tracing it around the pelvis in a sagittal plane (Fig. 7-5).

The peritoneum passes down from the anterior abdominal wall onto the upper surface of the urinary bladder. It then runs directly onto the anterior surface of the uterus, at the level of the internal os. The peritoneum now passes upward over the anterior surface of the body and fundus of the uterus and then downward over the posterior surface. It continues downward and covers the upper part of the posterior surface of the vagina, where it forms the anterior wall of the rectouterine pouch (pouch of Douglas). The peritoneum then passes onto the front of the rectum, as in the male.

In the female, the lowest part of the abdominopelvic peritoneal cavity in the erect position is the rectouterine pouch.

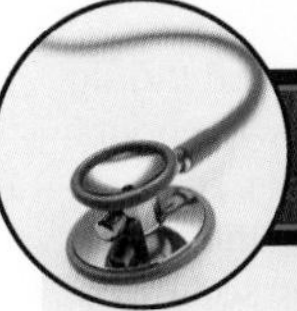

CLINICAL NOTES

The Rectouterine Pouch and Disease

Since the rectouterine pouch (pouch of Douglas) is the most dependent part of the entire peritoneal cavity (when the patient is in the standing position), it frequently becomes the site for the accumulation of blood (from a ruptured ectopic pregnancy) or pus (from a ruptured pelvic appendicitis or in gonococcal peritonitis).

Because the pouch lies directly behind the posterior fornix of the vagina, it is commonly violated by misguided nonsterile instruments, which pierce the wall of the posterior fornix in a failed attempt at an illegal abortion. Pelvic peritonitis, often with fatal consequences, is the almost certain result.

A needle may be passed into the pouch through the posterior fornix in the procedure known as **culdocentesis** (see page 375). Surgically, the pouch may be entered in **posterior colpotomy.**

The interior of the female pelvic peritoneal cavity may be viewed for evidence of disease through an endoscope; the instrument is introduced through a small colpotomy incision.

Broad Ligaments

The broad ligaments are two-layered folds of peritoneum that extend across the pelvic cavity from the lateral margins of the uterus to the lateral pelvic walls (Fig. 7-19). Superiorly, the two layers are continuous and form the upper free edge. Inferiorly, at the base of the ligament, the layers separate to cover the pelvic floor. The ovary is attached to the posterior layer by the **mesovarium.** The part of the broad ligament that lies lateral to the attachment of the mesovarium forms the **suspensory ligament of the ovary.** The part of the broad ligament between the uterine tube and the mesovarium is called the **mesosalpinx.**

At the base of the broad ligament, the uterine artery crosses the ureter (Figs. 7-19 and 7-28).

Each broad ligament contains the following:

- The uterine tube in its upper free border
- The round ligament of the ovary and the round ligament of the uterus. They represent the remains of the gubernaculum.
- The uterine and ovarian blood vessels, lymph vessels, and nerves
- The epoophoron, a vestigial structure that lies in the broad ligament above the attachment of the mesovarium. It represents the remains of the mesonephros (Fig. 7-19).
- The paroophoron, also a vestigial structure that lies in the broad ligament just lateral to the uterus. It is a mesonephric remnant (Fig. 7-19).

Cross-Sectional Anatomy of the Pelvis

To assist in the interpretation of CT scans of the pelvis, students should study the labeled cross sections of the pelvis shown in Figures 7-37 and 7-38.

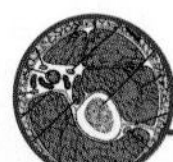

Radiographic Anatomy

Radiographic Appearances of the Bony Pelvis

A routine anteroposterior view of the pelvis is taken with the patient in the supine position and with the cassette underneath the tabletop. A somewhat distorted view of the lower part of the sacrum and coccyx is obtained, and these bones may be partially obscured by the symphysis pubis. A better view of the sacrum and coccyx can be obtained by slightly tilting the x-ray tube.

An anteroposterior radiograph should be systematically examined (Figs. 7-39 through 7-42). The lower lumbar vertebrae, sacrum, and coccyx may be looked at first, followed by the sacroiliac joints, the different parts of the hip bones, and finally the hip joints and the upper ends of the femurs. Gas and fecal material may be seen in the large bowel, and soft tissue shadows of the skin and subcutaneous tissues may also be visualized.

To demonstrate the sacrum and sacroiliac joints more clearly, lateral and oblique views of the pelvis are often taken.

Radiographic Appearances of the Sigmoid Colon and Rectum

Barium Enema

The pelvic colon and rectum can be demonstrated by the administration of 2 to 3 pints (1 L) of barium sulfate emulsion slowly through the anus. The appearances of the pelvic colon are similar to those seen in the more proximal parts of the colon, but a distended sigmoid colon usually shows no sacculations. The rectum is seen to have a wider caliber than the colon.

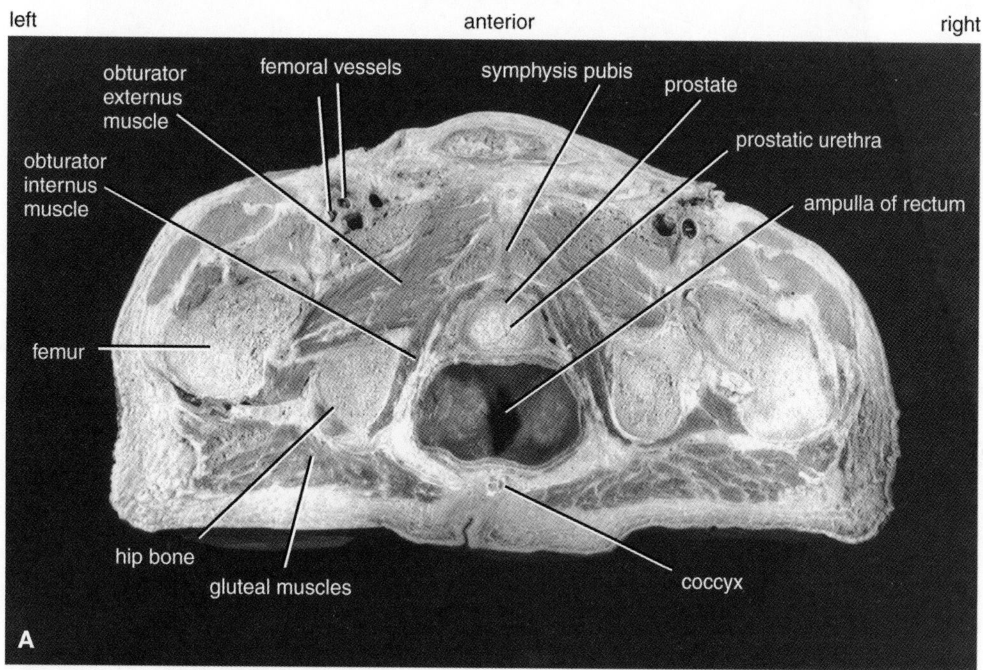

Figure 7-37 **A.** Cross section of the male pelvis as seen from above.

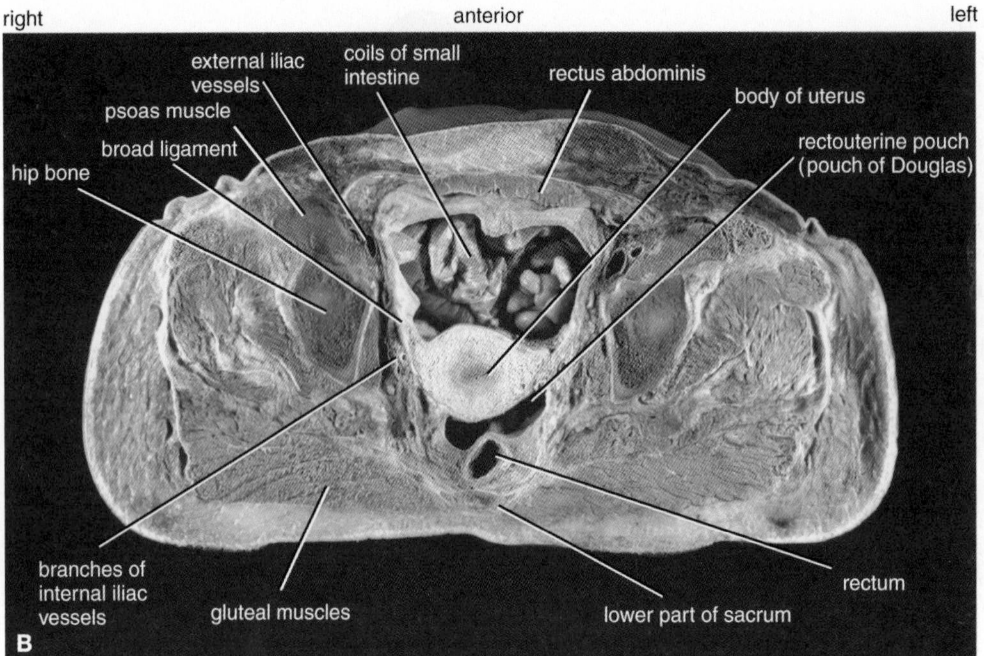

Figure 7-37 *(continued)* **B.** Cross section of the female pelvis as seen from below.

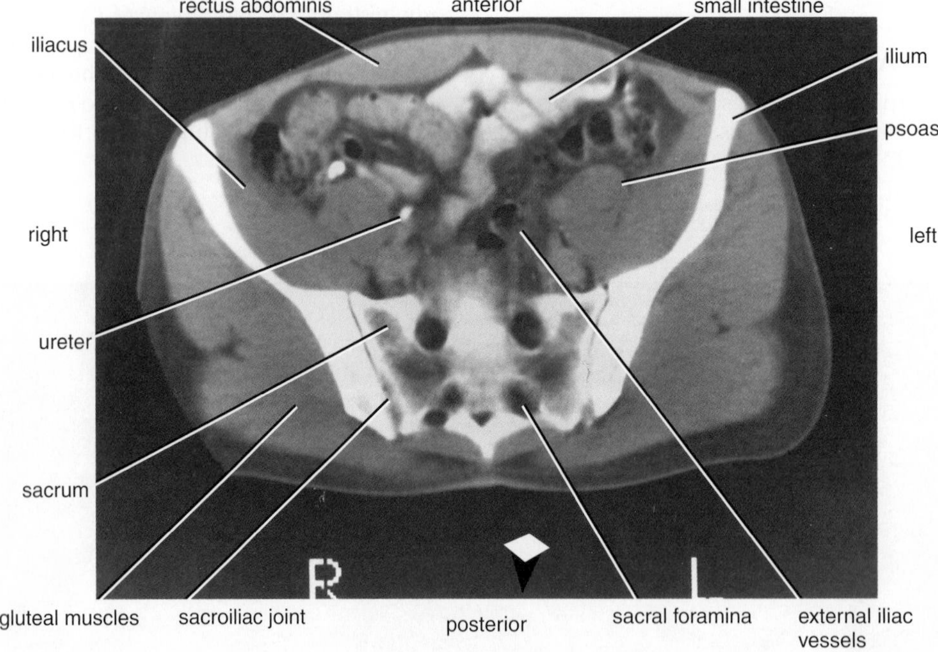

Figure 7-38 Computed tomography scan of the pelvis after a barium meal and intravenous pyelography. Note the presence of the radiopaque material in the small intestine and the right ureter. The section is viewed from below.

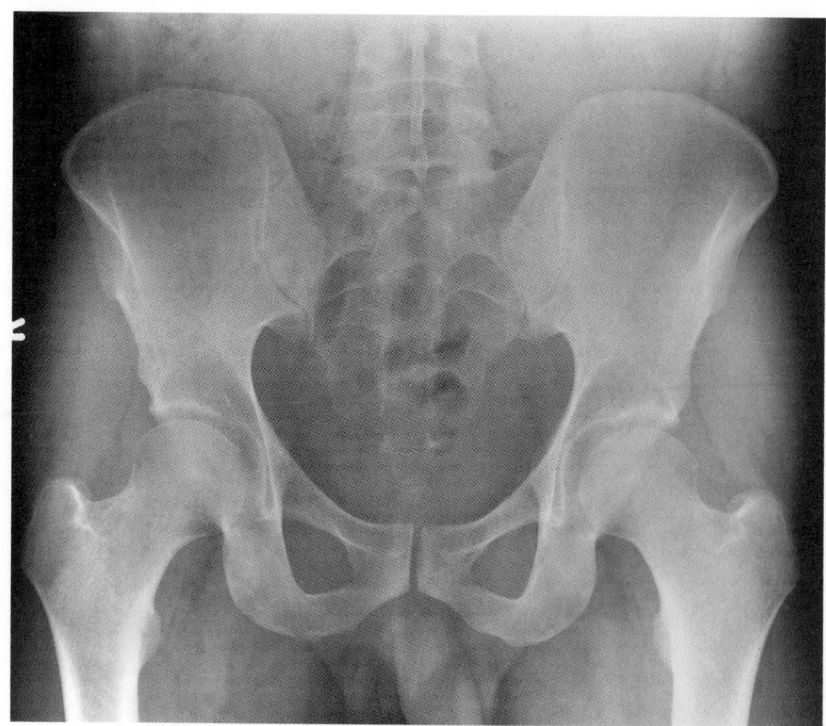

Figure 7-39 Anteroposterior radiograph of the male pelvis.

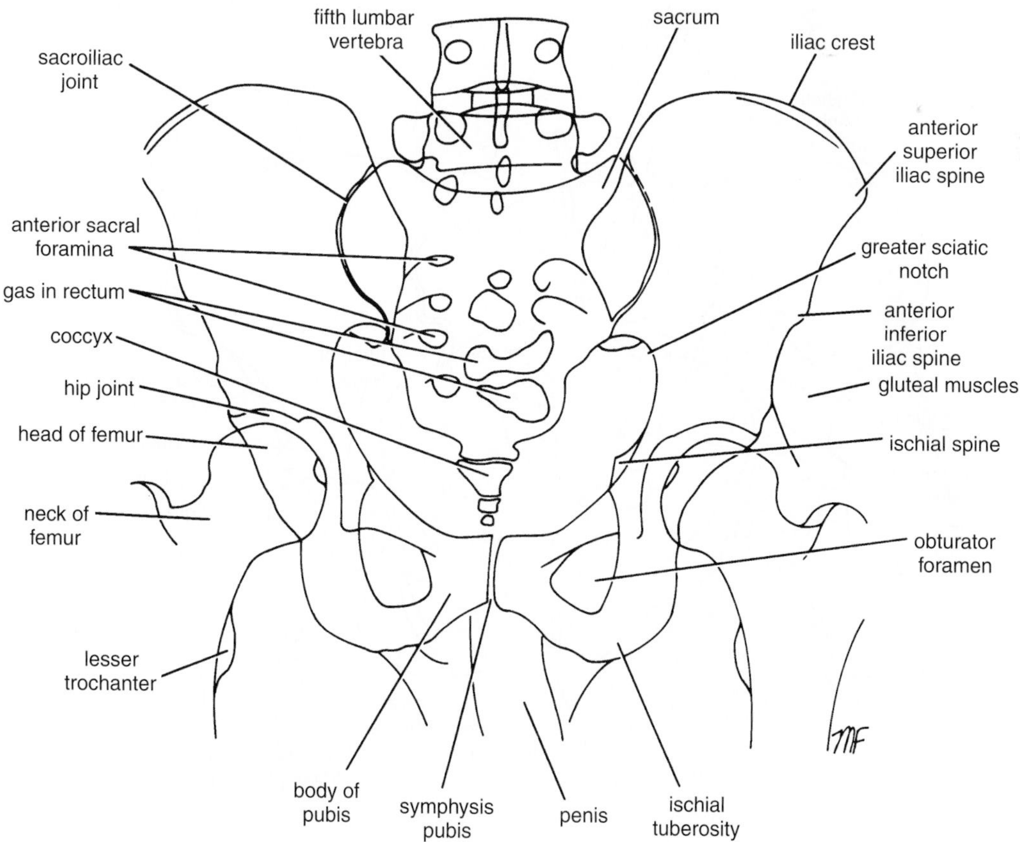

Figure 7-40 Representation of the radiograph of the pelvis seen in Figure 7-39.

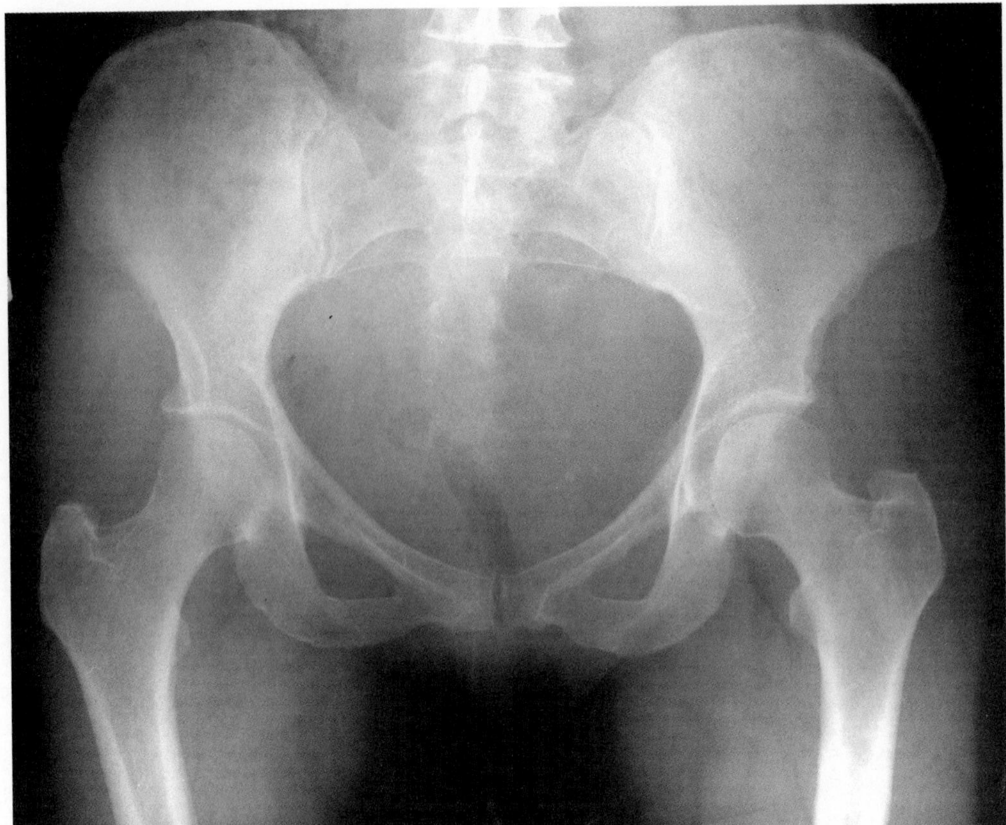

Figure 7-41 Anteroposterior radiograph of the adult female pelvis.

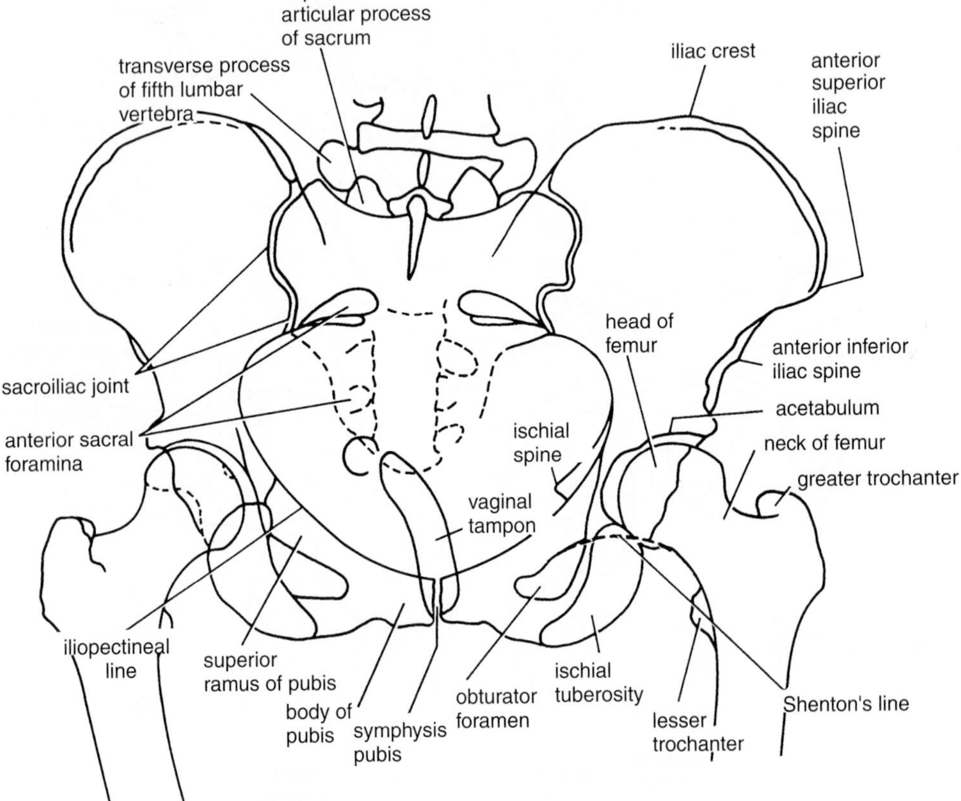

Figure 7-42 Representation of the radiograph of the pelvis seen in Figure 7-41.

A **contrast enema** is sometimes useful for examining the mucous membrane of the sigmoid colon. The barium enema is partly evacuated and air is injected into the colon. By this means the walls of the colon become outlined (see Fig. 5-90).

Radiographic Appearances of the Female Genital Tract

The instillation of viscous iodine preparations through the external os of the uterus allows the lumen of the cervical canal, the uterine cavity, and the different parts of the uterine tubes to be visualized (Fig. 7-43). This procedure is known as **hysterosalpingography.** The patency of these structures is demonstrated by the entrance into the peritoneal cavity of some of the opaque medium.

A sonogram of the female pelvis shows the uterus and the vagina (Figs. 7-30, 7-31, and 7-32).

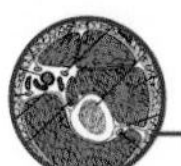

Surface Anatomy

The surface anatomy of the pelvic viscera is considered on page 330.

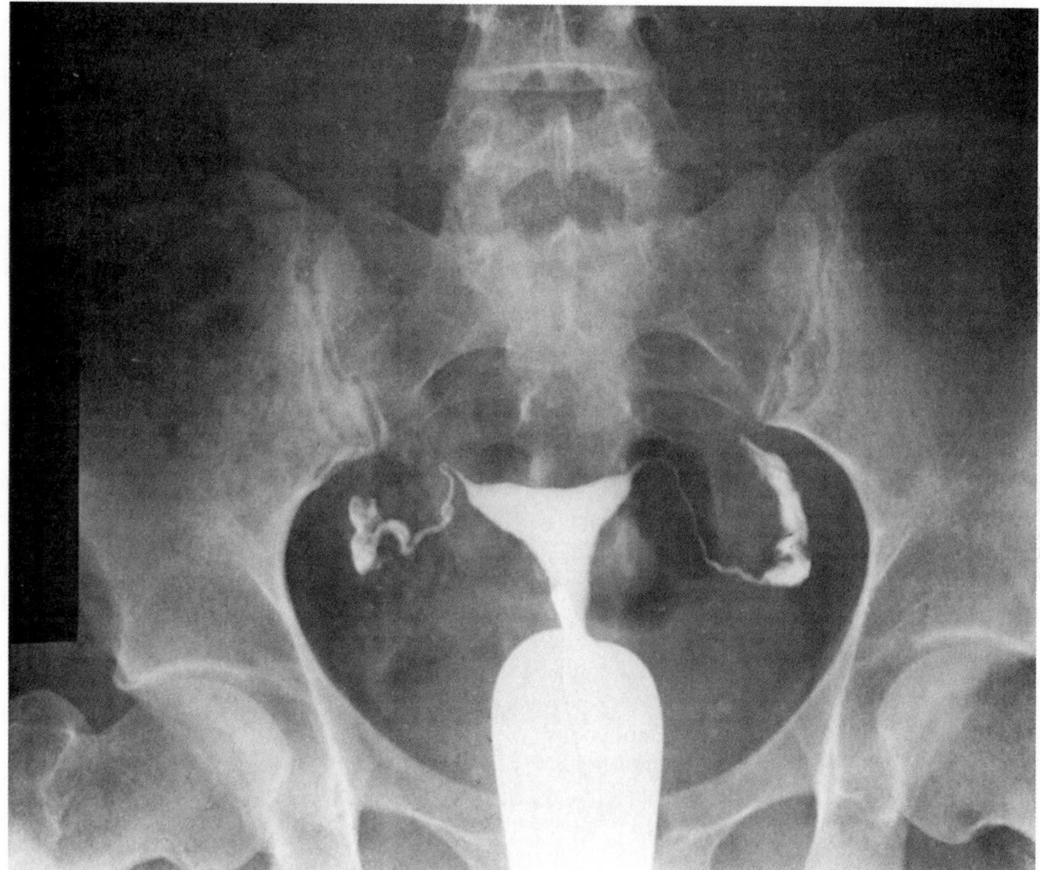

Figure 7-43 Anteroposterior radiograph of the female pelvis after injection of radiopaque compound into the uterine cavity (hysterosalpingogram).

CLINICAL PROBLEM SOLVING

Study the following case histories and select the best answers to the questions following them.

A 30-year-old man involved in a barroom brawl was seen in the emergency department. He was found to have a blood-stained tear on the seat of his trousers and lacerations of the anal margin. During the fight he was knocked down and fell in the sitting position on the leg of an upturned bar stool. While under observation he developed the signs and symptoms of peritonitis.

1. The signs and symptoms displayed by this patient could be explained by the following anatomic statements except which?
   (a) The patient had impaled his rectum on the leg of the upturned bar stool.
   (b) At operation, a laceration of the anterior wall of the middle of the rectum was found.
   (c) The leg of the bar stool had entered the rectovesical pouch.
   (d) The rectal contents had contaminated the peritoneal cavity and were responsible for the development of peritonitis.
   (e) The anterior surface of the middle third of the rectum has no peritoneal covering.

A 46-year-old man had been treating himself for hemorrhoids for the past 3 years. He had noticed that his feces was often slightly blood stained. For the past 12 months, he had noticed that when he had his bowels open, he always felt that more was to come. Sometimes he went to the toilet several times a day but was only able to pass flatus and blood-stained mucus. Recently, pain had developed down the outside of his right leg. Digital examination of the rectum revealed a large, hard-based ulcer on the posterior wall of the rectum with extensive induration of the pararectal tissues. A diagnosis of advanced carcinoma of the rectum was made.

2. The following statements about this patient are probably correct except which?
   (a) Some of the bleeding was from the carcinomatous ulcer of the rectum as well as from the hemorrhoids.
   (b) The lymphatic drainage of the rectum takes place first into the pararectal lymph nodes.
   (c) Carcinoma of the rectum never metastasizes to the liver.
   (d) Examination of the right leg revealed some weakness of the muscles supplied by the sciatic nerve.
   (e) The carcinoma had extended posteriorly to involve the sacral plexus.
   (f) The patient indicated that the leg pain was felt in skin areas supplied by branches of the sciatic nerve.

An inebriated 40-year-old man was involved in a fight over a woman. The woman's husband gave the man a severe blow on the lower part of the anterior abdominal wall, whereupon he doubled up with pain and collapsed on the floor. On admission to the emergency department of the local hospital the man was in a state of shock and complaining of severe pain in the lower abdominal region. He was unable to pass urine since the fight. A diagnosis of ruptured urinary bladder was made.

3. The following statements concerning this patient are correct except which?
   (a) Rectal examination revealed a bulging backward of the rectovesical fossa.
   (b) Although the patient had consumed a considerable volume of liquor, dullness was not present on percussion of the anterior abdominal wall above the symphysis pubis.
   (c) The urine accumulated in the rectovesical pouch.
   (d) A full bladder is more likely to be ruptured by a blow on the anterior abdominal wall than an empty bladder.
   (e) In the adult as the normal bladder fills, its superior wall extends upward into the abdomen, leaving the covering of parietal peritoneum behind.

A 56-year-old woman was seen by her obstetrician and gynecologist complaining of a "bearing-down" feeling in the pelvis and of a low backache. On vaginal examination, the external os of the cervix was found to be located just within the vaginal orifice. A diagnosis of uterine prolapse was made.

4. The following anatomic statements concerning uterine prolapse are correct except which?
   (a) The most important support to the uterus is the tone of the levator ani muscles.
   (b) The transverse cervical, pubocervical, and sacrocervical ligaments play an important role in supporting the uterus.
   (c) Damage to the levator ani and the cervical ligaments during childbirth can be responsible for prolapse of the uterus.
   (d) Prolapse most commonly reveals itself before menopause.
   (e) Prolapse of the uterus is always accompanied by some prolapse of the vagina.

A 25-year-old woman was seen in the emergency department complaining of severe pain in the right iliac region. Just before admission she had fainted. On physical examination, her abdominal wall was extremely tender on palpation in the lower right quadrant, and some rigidity and guarding of the lower abdominal muscles were noticed. A vaginal examination revealed a rather soft cervix with a circular external os. A tender "doughlike mass" could be felt through the posterior fornix. The patient had missed her last period.

5. The following statements concerning this patient are correct except which?
   (a) A diagnosis of ruptured ectopic pregnancy was made.
   (b) Tubal pregnancies commonly occur where the ampulla narrows to join the isthmus.
   (c) Each uterine tube is situated in the base of the broad ligament.

(d) An ectopic tubal pregnancy almost invariably results in rupture of the tube with severe intraperitoneal hemorrhage.
(e) Tubal rupture occurs as a result of the eroding action of the trophoblast.
(f) Once a tubal pregnancy dies, the decidual lining of the uterus begins to be shed because of lack of hormonal support, and this causes vaginal bleeding.
(g) The doughlike mass is produced by the accumulation of blood in the pouch of Douglas.

A 39-year-old woman was admitted to the local hospital after experiencing a gunshot wound to the lower part of her back. Radiographic examination revealed that the bullet was lodged in the vertebral canal at the level of the third lumbar vertebra. A comprehensive neurologic examination indicated that a complete lesion of the cauda equina had occurred.

6. The following statements concerning this patient are likely to be true except which?
   (a) The cauda equina, which consists of anterior and posterior nerve roots below the level of the first lumbar segment, was sectioned at the level of the third lumbar vertebra.
   (b) The preganglionic sympathetic nerve fibers to the vesical sphincter that descend in the anterior roots of the fourth and fifth lumbar nerves were sectioned.
   (c) The preganglionic parasympathetic fibers to the detrusor muscle that descend in the anterior roots of the second, third, and fourth sacral nerves were sectioned.
   (d) The patient would have an autonomous bladder.
   (e) The bladder would fill to capacity and then overflow.
   (f) Micturition could be activated by powerful contraction of the abdominal muscles and manual pressure on the anterior abdominal wall in the suprapubic region.

A 65-year-old man with a history of prostatic disease was found on radiologic examination of his skeleton to have extensive carcinomatous metastases in the skull and lumbar vertebrae. The PSA level in his blood was found to be excessively high.

7. The following statements concerning this patient are correct except which?
   (a) The patient has advanced carcinoma of the prostate that has spread some distance from the primary site.
   (b) The prostate is surrounded by the prostatic venous plexus, which drains into the internal iliac veins.
   (c) Large veins with valves connect the prostatic venous plexus to the vertebral veins.
   (d) Coughing, sneezing, or straining at stool can force the blood from the prostatic plexus into the vertebral veins.
   (e) Dislodged cancer cells can be carried with the blood to the vertebral column and skull.

A 72-year-old woman was suspected of having a tumor of the sigmoid colon. The physician decided to confirm the diagnosis by performing a sigmoidoscopy.

8. The following anatomic statements are correct concerning the procedure of sigmoidoscopy except which?
   (a) After inserting the instrument into the anus, the lighted end enters the ampulla of the rectum after a distance of about 1.5 in. (4 cm).
   (b) Some side-to-side movement may be necessary to avoid the transverse rectal folds.
   (c) The rectosigmoid junction will be reached approximately 6.5 in. (16.25 cm) from the anal margin.
   (d) To negotiate the rectosigmoid junction, the tip of the sigmoidoscope should be directed anteriorly and to the patient's left.
   (e) Stretching of the colonic wall may give rise to colicky pain in the upper part of the abdomen in the region of the xiphoid process.

ANSWERS TO CLINICAL PROBLEMS

1. E. The upper third of the rectum has peritoneum on its anterior and lateral surfaces; the middle third has peritoneum on its anterior surface; and the lower third has no peritoneal covering.
2. C. Advanced carcinoma of the rectum not only extends to the pararectal and inferior mesenteric nodes, but may also spread via the superior rectal, inferior mesenteric, splenic, and portal veins to the liver.
3. E. In the adult as the normal bladder fills, its superior wall bulges upward into the abdomen, peeling off the peritoneum from the posterior surface of the anterior abdominal wall.
4. D. Prolapse of the uterus most often reveals itself after menopause, when the pelvic fascia tends to atrophy.
5. C. Each uterine tube is situated in the upper free margin of the broad ligament.
6. B. The preganglionic sympathetic nerve fibers to the vesical sphincter descend in the anterior roots of the first and second lumbar nerves and were left intact.
7. C. The large veins that connect the prostatic venous plexus to the valveless vertebral veins are also devoid of valves.
8. E. Colicky pain from the colon is referred to the lower part of the anterior abdominal wall above the symphysis pubis.

REVIEW QUESTIONS

Multiple-Choice Questions

Select the best answer for each question.

1. The following statements concerning the uterus are correct except which?
   (a) The fundus is part of the uterus above the openings of the uterine tubes.
   (b) The long axis of the uterus is usually bent anteriorly on the long axis of the vagina (anteversion).
   (c) The nerve supply of the uterus is from the inferior hypogastric plexuses.
   (d) The anterior surface of the cervix is completely covered with peritoneum.
   (e) The uterine veins drain into the internal iliac veins.
2. The following statements concerning the ductus (vas) deferens are correct except which?
   (a) It emerges from the deep inguinal ring and passes around the lateral margin of the inferior epigastric artery.
   (b) It crosses the ureter in the region of the ischial spine.
   (c) The terminal part is dilated to form the ampulla.
   (d) It lies on the posterior surface of the prostate but is separated from it by the peritoneum.
   (e) It joins the duct of the seminal vesicle to form the ejaculatory duct.
3. The following statements concerning the pelvic part of the ureter are correct except which?
   (a) It enters the pelvis in front of the bifurcation of the common iliac artery.
   (b) The ureter enters the bladder by passing directly through its wall, there being no valvular mechanism at its entrance.
   (c) It has a close relationship to the ischial spine before it turns medially toward the bladder.
   (d) The blood supply of the distal part of the ureter is from the superior vesical artery.
   (e) It enters the bladder at the upper lateral angle of the trigone.
4. The following statements concerning the seminal vesicle are correct except which?
   (a) The seminal vesicles are related posteriorly to the rectum and can be palpated through the rectal wall.
   (b) The seminal vesicles are two lobulated organs that store spermatozoa.
   (c) The upper ends of the seminal vesicles are covered by peritoneum.
   (d) The function of the seminal vesicles is to produce a secretion that is added to the seminal fluid.
   (e) The seminal vesicles are related anteriorly to the bladder, and no peritoneum separates these structures.
5. The following statements concerning the ovary are correct except which?
   (a) The lymph drainage is into the para-aortic (lumbar) lymph nodes at the level of the first lumbar vertebra.
   (b) The round ligament of the ovary extends from the ovary to the upper end of the lateral wall of the body of the uterus.
   (c) The ovarian fossa is bounded above by the external iliac vessels and behind by the internal iliac vessels.
   (d) The left ovarian artery is a branch of the left internal iliac artery.
   (e) The obturator nerve lies lateral to the ovary.
6. The following statements concerning the nerve supply to the urinary bladder are correct except which?
   (a) The sympathetic postganglionic fibers originate in the first and second lumbar ganglia.
   (b) The parasympathetic postganglionic fibers originate in the inferior hypogastric plexuses.
   (c) The afferent sensory fibers arising in the bladder wall reach the spinal cord via the pelvic splanchnic nerves and also travel with the sympathetic nerves.
   (d) The parasympathetic preganglionic fibers arise from the second, third, and fourth sacral segments of the spinal cord.
   (e) The parasympathetic postganglionic fibers are responsible for closing the vesical sphincter during ejaculation.
7. The following statements concerning the vagina are correct except which?
   (a) The area of the vaginal lumen around the cervix is divided into four fornices.
   (b) The upper part of the vagina is supported by the levator ani muscles and the transverse cervical ligaments.
   (c) The perineal body lies posterior to and supports the lower part of the vagina.
   (d) The upper part of the vagina is not covered with peritoneum.
   (e) The vaginal wall receives a branch of the uterine artery.
8. The following statements concerning the visceral layer of pelvic fascia in the female are correct except which?
   (a) In the region of the cervix of the uterus, it is called the parametrium.
   (b) It is considered to form the pubocervical, transverse cervical, and sacrocervical ligaments of the uterus.
   (c) It covers the obturator internus muscle.
   (d) It does not become continuous above with the fascia transversalis.
   (e) On the lateral wall of the pelvis, it fuses with the parietal layer of pelvic fascia.
9. The following statements concerning the lymphatic drainage of pelvic structures are correct except which?
   (a) Lymph from the cervix of the uterus drains into the internal and external iliac lymph nodes.
   (b) Lymph from the prostate drains into the external iliac lymph nodes.
   (c) Lymph from the posterior fornix of the vagina drains into the internal and external iliac lymph nodes.
   (d) Lymph from the trigone of the bladder drains into the internal and external iliac lymph nodes.
   (e) Lymph from the fundus of the uterus drains into the para-aortic lymph nodes at the level of the first lumbar vertebra.

10. The following statements concerning the main venous drainage of pelvic structures are correct except which?
    (a) The venous blood from the left ovary drains into the inferior vena cava.
    (b) The venous blood from the prostate drains into the internal iliac veins.
    (c) The venous blood from the urinary bladder drains into the internal iliac veins.
    (d) The venous blood from the mucous membrane of the rectum drains into the superior rectal vein.
    (e) The venous drainage of the seminal vesicles drains into the internal iliac veins.

Read the case histories and select the best answer to the question following them.

A 3-week-old boy was taken to a pediatrician because of repeated vomiting and reluctance to feed. On questioning, the mother said the child had started to vomit on the first day of life and had vomited at least once a day since then. Early on, the mother had been reassured and told that the baby was taking his feedings too quickly and that the vomiting eventually would cease. While initially accepting this reassurance, the mother now noticed that the child did not seem hungry at feeding time; moreover, she could see that the abdomen was becoming distended. She added that the child definitely was constipated; very occasionally, hard meconium was passed. After a thorough physical examination of the child, the pediatrician made the diagnosis of primary megacolon (Hirschsprung disease).

11. The examination of the child revealed the following possible signs except which?
    (a) The abdomen was found to be distended.
    (b) A rectal examination with the gloved little finger resulted in the passage of a large amount of flatus and the abdominal distention became visibly less.
    (c) A low barium enema followed by a radiographic examination showed a normal rectum.
    (d) On the radiograph, above the rectum, a narrowed part of the colon led to a funnel-shaped expansion, which in turn led to a greatly dilated descending colon and transverse colon.
    (e) On placing a stethoscope on the abdominal wall, the physician could not hear sounds of peristalsis.

After the birth of a baby boy, a moist, red, protruding area was noted on the lower part of his anterior abdominal wall above the symphysis pubis. The pediatrician made the diagnosis of exstrophy of the bladder.

12. On further clinical examination, the following physical signs might have been noted except which?
    (a) The abdominal skin was seen to be continuous with the margin of the red area.
    (b) The child had epispadias and bilateral undescended testes.
    (c) Radiographic examination of the lower abdominal area showed a normal symphysis pubis.
    (d) On closer examination, jets of urine could be seen discharging through the upper lateral corners of the red protruding area.
    (e) The scrotum was wide and shallow.

ANSWERS TO REVIEW QUESTIONS

1. D. The anterior surface of the cervix lies in direct contact with the posterior surface of the urinary bladder and there is no peritoneum separating the two structures.

2. D. The ductus (vas) deferens lies in direct contact with the posterior surface of the bladder. The inferior end of the ampulla narrows down and joins the duct of the seminal vesicle to form the ejaculator duct.

3. B. The ureters pierce the bladder wall obliquely, and this provides a valvelike mechanism that prevents urine from reentering the ureter from the bladder cavity.

4. B. The seminal vesicles do not store spermatozoa; they produce a secretion that nourishes the spermatozoa.

5. D. The right and the left ovarian arteries are branches of the abdominal aorta at the level of the first lumbar vertebra.

6. E. The sympathetic nerves are responsible for the contraction of the sphincter vesicae during ejaculation.

7. D. The upper third of the posterior wall of the vagina is covered with peritoneum and is related to the rectouterine pouch (pouch of Douglas).

8. C. The obturator internus muscle is covered with the parietal layer of pelvic fascia and is called the obturator internus fascia.

9. B. The lymph from the prostate drains into the internal iliac nodes.

10. A. The venous blood from the left ovary drains into the left renal vein.

11. E. In patients with primary megacolon, the muscle of the colon immediately proximal to the obstruction is hypertrophied as the result of attempting to force the meconium and feces onward. Usually very active peristalsis is heard on listening to the abdomen with a stethoscope.

12. C. Exstrophy of the bladder is believed to result from a failure of the embryonic mesenchyme to invade the embryonic disc caudal to the cloacal membrane. This produces an unstable state, which is followed by a breakdown of this area of the abdominal wall with exposure of the red mucous membrane of the trigone of the bladder. This results in the separation of the pubes and anomalies in the development of the external genitalia.

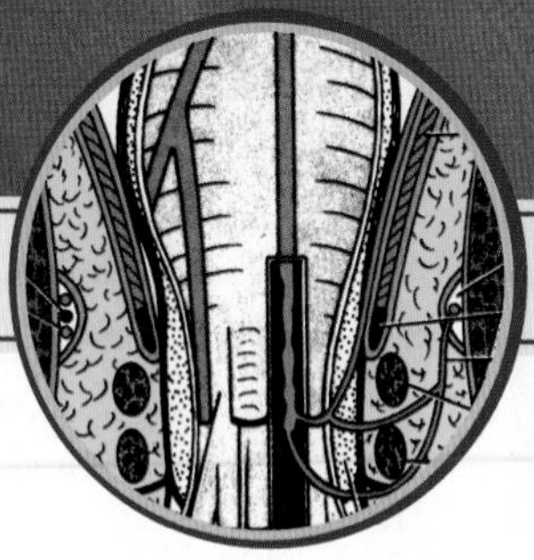

CHAPTER 8

THE PERINEUM

A 51-year-old woman was seen by her physician for complaints of breathlessness, which she noticed was worse on climbing stairs. On questioning, she said that the problem started about 3 years ago and was getting worse. On examination, the patient was found to have a healthy appearance, although the conjunctivae and lips were paler than normal, suggesting anemia. The cardiovascular and respiratory systems were normal. On further questioning, the patient said that she frequently passed blood-stained stools and was often constipated.

Digital examination of the anal canal revealed nothing abnormal apart from the presence of some blood-stained mucus on the glove. Proctoscopic examination revealed that the mucous membrane of the anal canal had three congested swellings that bulged into the lumen at the 3-, 7-, and 11-o'clock positions (the patient was in the lithotomy position). Laboratory examination of the blood showed the red blood cells to be smaller than normal, and the red blood cell count was very low; the hemoglobin level was also low. The diagnosis was microcytic hypochromic anemia, secondary to prolonged bleeding from internal hemorrhoids.

The severe anemia explained the patient's breathlessness. The hemorrhoids were dilatations of the tributaries of the superior rectal vein in the wall of the anal canal. Repeated abrasion of the hemorrhoids by hard stools caused the bleeding and loss of blood. Without knowledge of the anatomic position of the veins in the anal canal, the physician would not have been able to make a diagnosis.

CHAPTER OUTLINE

Basic Anatomy 388
Definition of Perineum 388
Pelvic Diaphragm 388
Contents of Anal Triangle 388
Anal Canal 388
Defecation 394
Ischiorectal Fossa 394
Urogenital Triangle 400
Superficial Fascia 400
Superficial Perineal Pouch 401
Urogenital Diaphragm 401
Contents of the Male Urogenital Triangle 402
Penis 402
Scrotum 405
Contents of the Superficial Perineal Pouch in the Male 405
Contents of the Deep Perineal Pouch in the Male 406
Erection of the Penis 406
Ejaculation 406
Male Urethra 407
Contents of the Female Urogenital Triangle 408
Clitoris 408
Contents of the Superficial Perineal Pouch in the Female 408
Contents of the Deep Perineal Pouch in the Female 409
Erection of the Clitoris 409
Orgasm in the Female 409
Female Urethra 409
Greater Vestibular Glands 409
Vagina 409
Vulva 411
Radiographic Anatomy 417
Surface Anatomy 417
Symphysis Pubis 417
Coccyx 417
Ischial Tuberosity 419
Anal Triangle 419
Anus 419
Male Urogenital Triangle 419
Penis 419
Scrotum 419
Testes 419
Epididymides 419
Female Urogenital Triangle 419
Vulva 419
Orifices of the Ducts of the Greater Vestibular Glands 419
Clinical Problem Solving 421
Answers to Clinical Problems 422
Review Questions 422
Answers to Review Questions 424

CHAPTER OBJECTIVES

- Infections, injuries, and prolapses involving the anal canal, the urethra, and the female external genitalia are common problems facing the physician.
- Urethral obstruction, traumatic rupture of the penile urethra, and infections of the epididymis and testis are frequently seen in the male.
- The purpose of this chapter is to cover the significant anatomy relative to these clinical problems. Because the descent of the testes and the structure of the scrotum are intimately related to the development of the inguinal canal, they are dealt with in detail in Chapter 4.

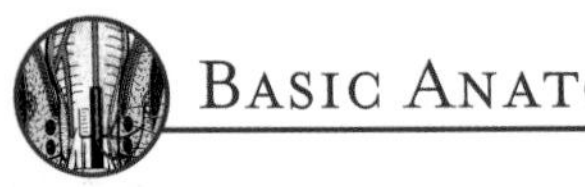

BASIC ANATOMY

Definition of Perineum

The cavity of the pelvis is divided by the pelvic diaphragm into the main pelvic cavity above and the perineum below (Fig. 8-1). When seen from below with the thighs abducted, the perineum is diamond shaped and is bounded anteriorly by the symphysis pubis, posteriorly by the tip of the coccyx, and laterally by the ischial tuberosities (Fig. 8-2).

Pelvic Diaphragm

The pelvic diaphragm is formed by the important levatores ani muscles and the small coccygeus muscles and their covering fasciae (Fig. 8-1). It is incomplete anteriorly to allow passage of the urethra in males and the urethra and the vagina in females (for details see page 318).

Contents of Anal Triangle

The anal triangle is bounded behind by the tip of the coccyx and on each side by the ischial tuberosity and the sacrotuberous ligament, overlapped by the border of the gluteus maximus muscle (Fig. 8-3). The **anus,** or lower opening of the anal canal, lies in the midline, and on each side is the ischiorectal fossa. The skin around the anus is supplied by the inferior rectal (hemorrhoidal) nerve. The lymph vessels of the skin drain into the medial group of the superficial inguinal nodes.

Anal Canal

Location and Description

The anal canal is about 1.5 in. (4 cm) long and passes downward and backward from the rectal ampulla to the anus (Fig. 8-4). Except during defecation, its lateral walls are kept in apposition by the levatores ani muscles and the anal sphincters.

Relations

- **Posteriorly:** The **anococcygeal body,** which is a mass of fibrous tissue lying between the anal canal and the coccyx (Fig. 8-4)
- **Laterally:** The fat-filled ischiorectal fossae (Fig. 8-5)
- **Anteriorly:** In the male, the perineal body, the urogenital diaphragm, the membranous part of the urethra, and

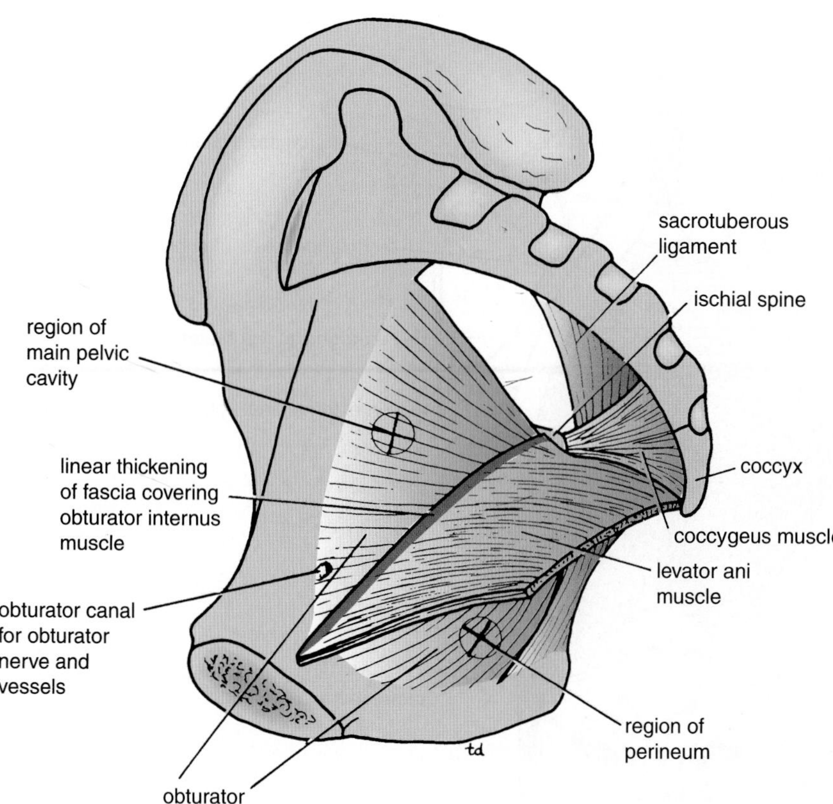

Figure 8-1 Right half of the pelvis showing the muscles forming the pelvic floor. Note that the levator ani and coccygeus muscles and their covering fascia form the pelvic diaphragm. Note also that the region of the main pelvic cavity lies above the pelvic diaphragm and the region of the perineum lies below the diaphragm.

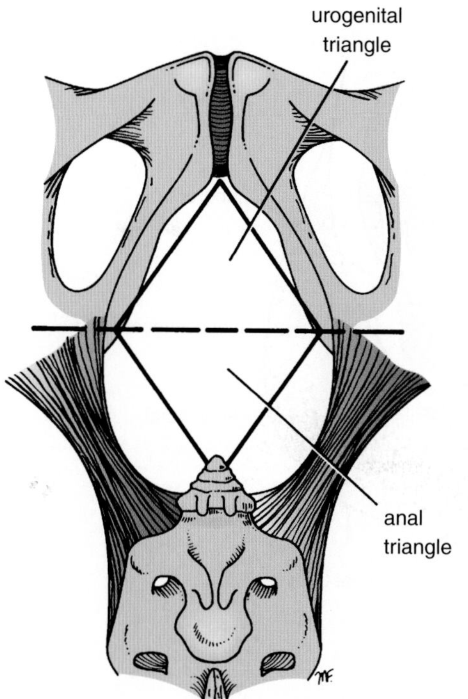

Figure 8-2 Diamond-shaped perineum divided by a broken line into the urogenital triangle and the anal triangle.

the bulb of the penis (Fig. 8-4). In the female, the perineal body, the urogenital diaphragm, and the lower part of the vagina (Fig. 8-4).

Structure

The **mucous membrane of the upper half of the anal canal** is derived from hindgut entoderm (Fig. 8-6). It has the following important anatomic features:

- It is lined by columnar epithelium.
- It is thrown into vertical folds called **anal columns,** which are joined together at their lower ends by small semilunar folds called **anal valves** (remains of proctodeal membrane) (Figs. 8-5 and 8-7).
- The nerve supply is the same as that for the rectal mucosa and is derived from the autonomic hypogastric plexuses. It is sensitive only to stretch (Fig. 8-6).
- The arterial supply is that of the hindgut—namely, the superior rectal artery, a branch of the inferior mesenteric artery (Fig. 8-6). The venous drainage is mainly by the superior rectal vein, a tributary of the inferior mesenteric vein, and the portal vein (Fig. 8-5).
- The lymphatic drainage is mainly upward along the superior rectal artery to the pararectal nodes and then eventually to the inferior mesenteric nodes (Fig. 8-6).

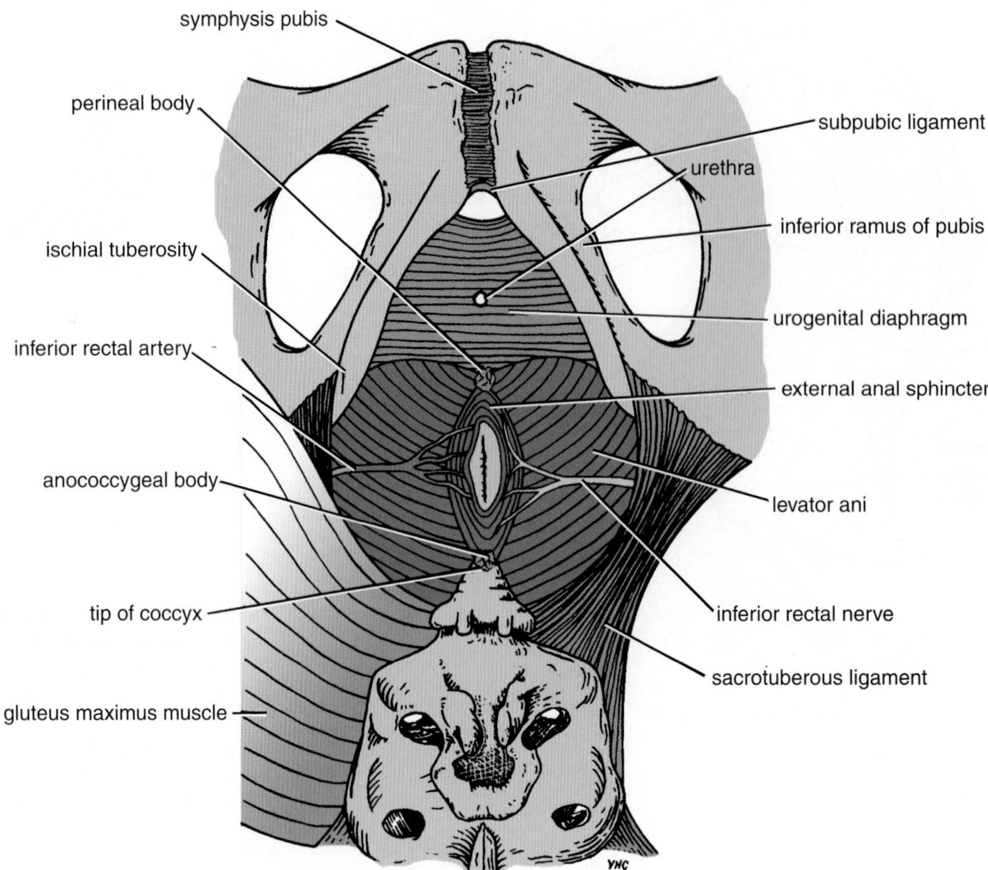

Figure 8-3 Anal triangle and urogenital triangle in the male as seen from below.

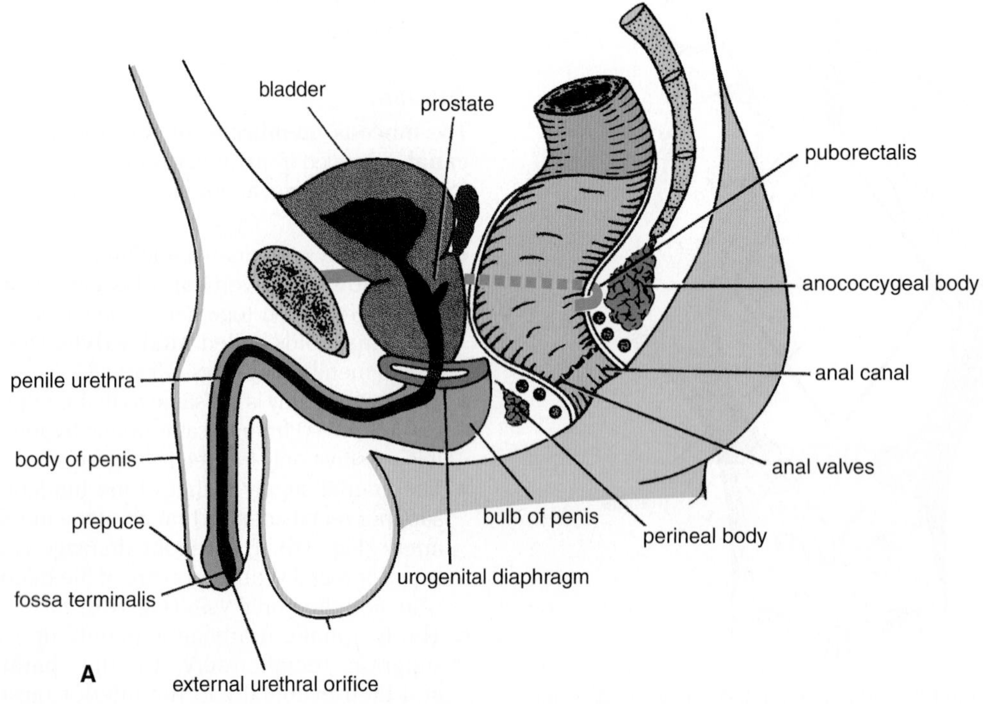

Figure 8-4 Sagittal sections of the male (**A**) pelvis.

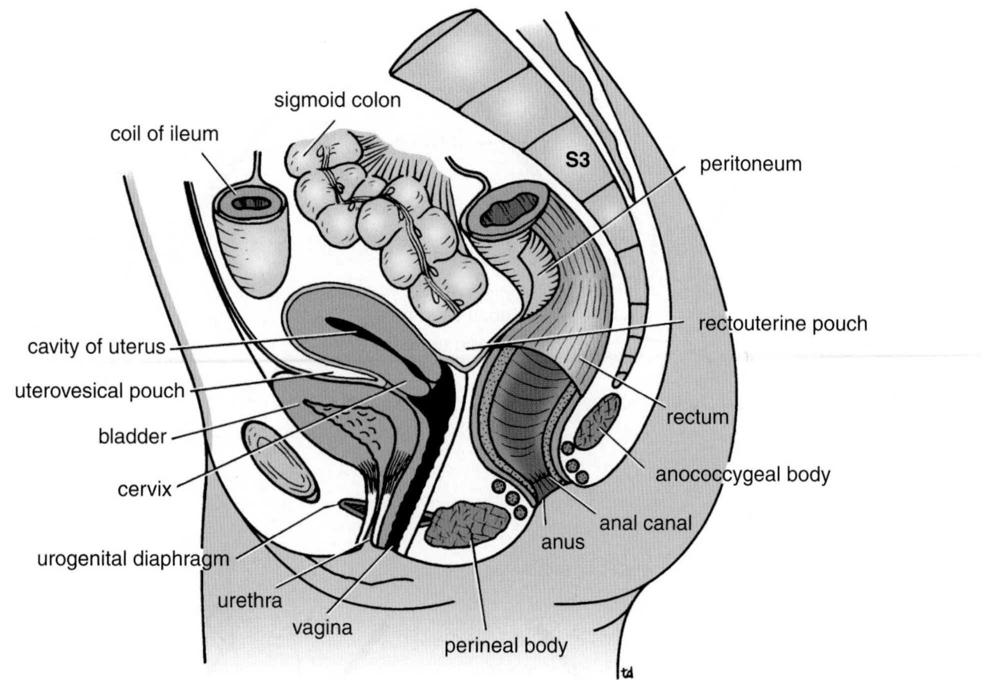

Figure 8-4 *(continued)* Sagittal sections of the female (**B**) pelvis.

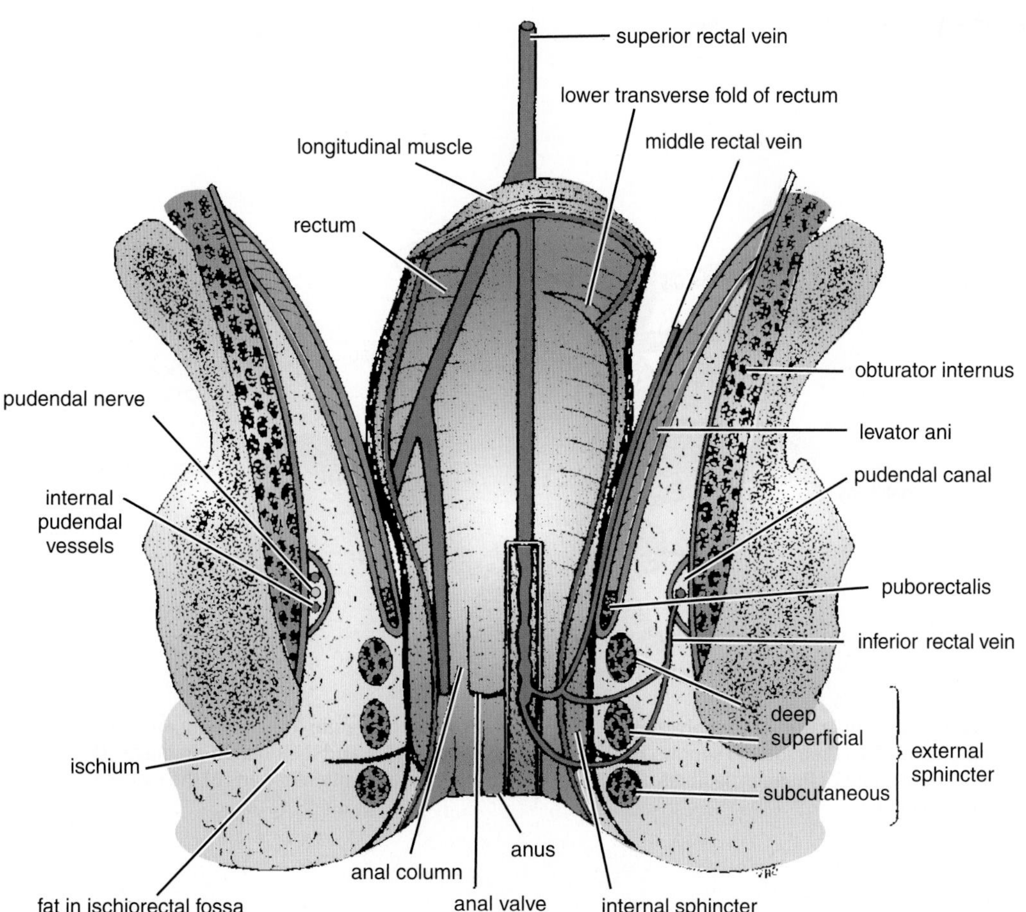

Figure 8-5 Coronal section of the pelvis and the perineum showing venous drainage of the anal canal.

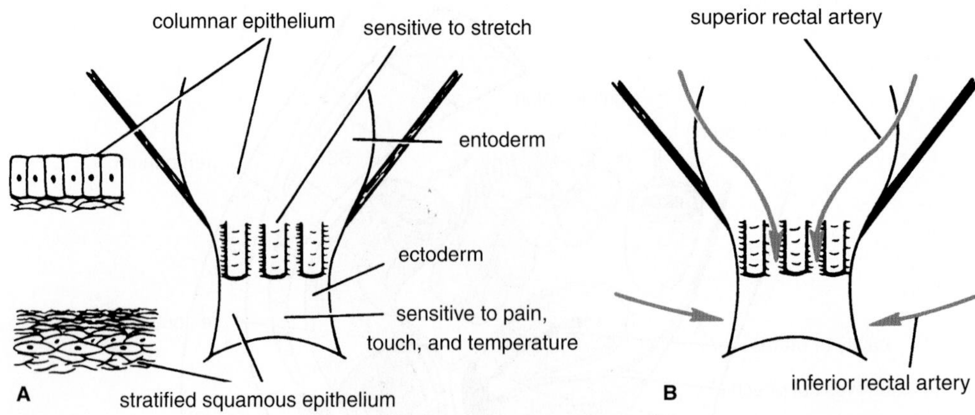

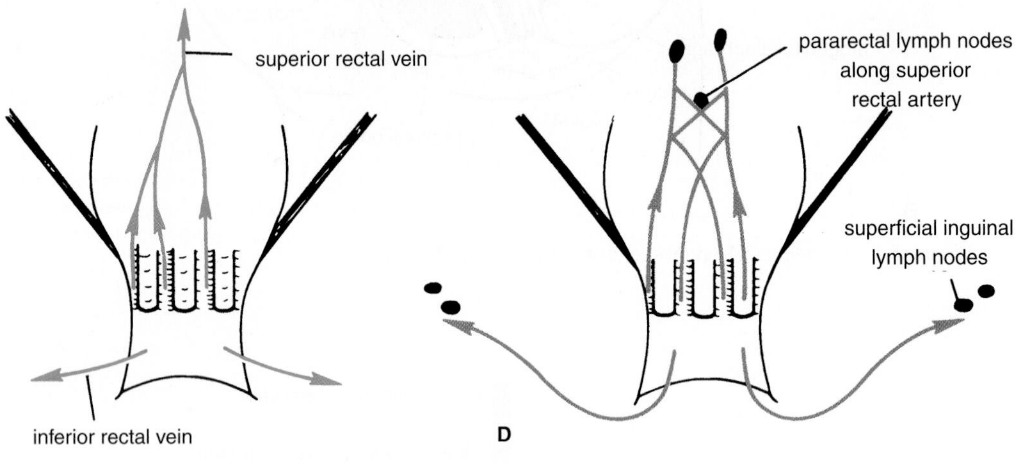

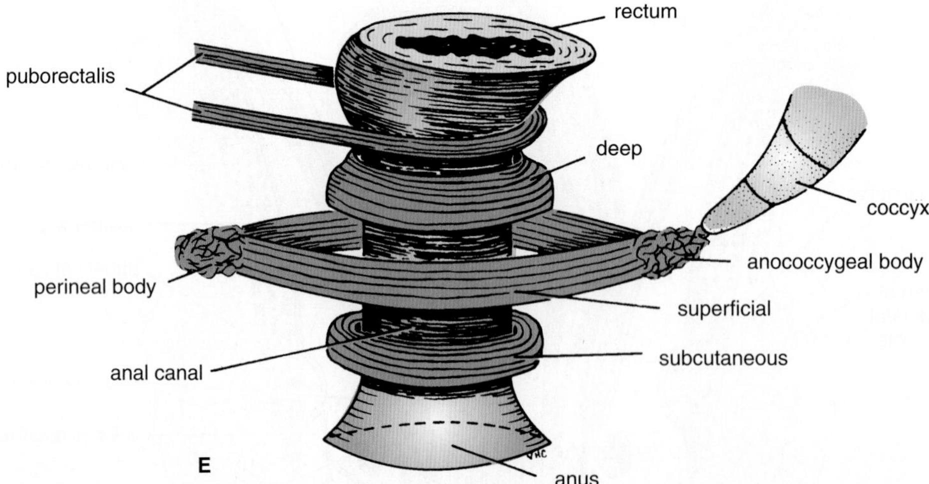

Figure 8-6 Upper and lower halves of the anal canal showing their embryologic origin and lining epithelium (**A**), their arterial supply (**B**), their venous drainage (**C**), and their lymph drainage (**D**). **E.** Arrangement of the muscle fibers of the puborectalis muscle and different parts of the external anal sphincter.

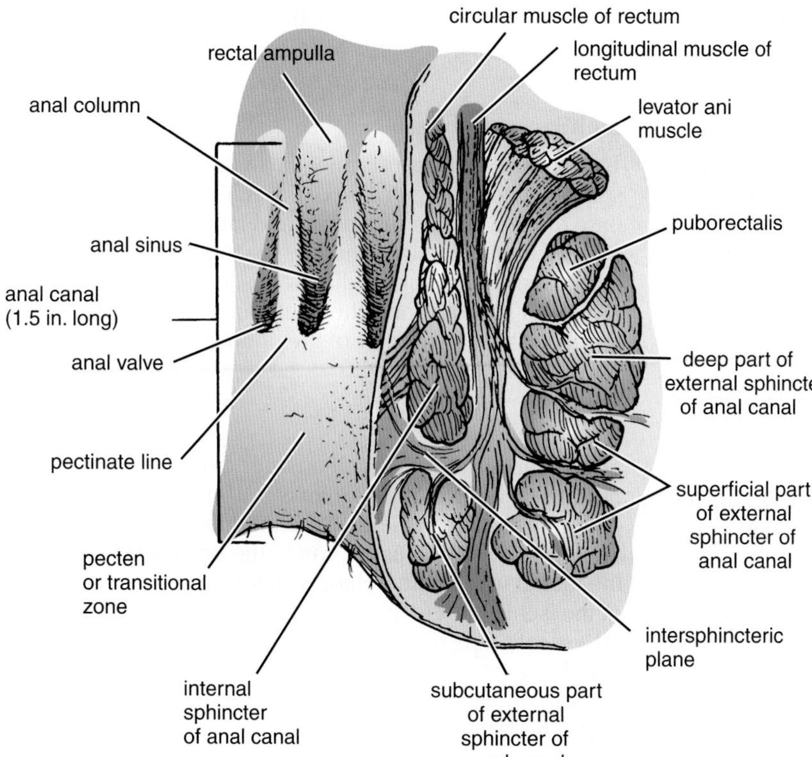

Figure 8-7 Coronal section of the anal canal showing the detailed anatomy of the mucous membrane and the arrangement of the internal and external anal sphincters. Note that the terms pectinate line (the line at the level of the anal valves) and pecten (the transitional zone between the skin and the mucous membrane) are sometimes used by clinicians.

The **mucous membrane of the lower half of the anal canal** is derived from ectoderm of the proctodeum. It has the following important features:

- It is lined by stratified squamous epithelium, which gradually merges at the anus with the perianal epidermis (Fig. 8-6).
- There are *no* anal columns (Fig. 8-7).
- The nerve supply is from the somatic inferior rectal nerve; it is thus sensitive to pain, temperature, touch, and pressure (Figs. 8-3 and 8-6).
- The arterial supply is the inferior rectal artery, a branch of the internal pudendal artery (Fig. 8-3). The venous drainage is by the inferior rectal vein, a tributary of the internal pudendal vein, which drains into the internal iliac vein (Figs. 8-5 and 8-6).
- The lymph drainage is downward to the medial group of superficial inguinal nodes (Fig. 8-6).

The **pectinate line** indicates the level where the upper half of the anal canal joins the lower half (Fig. 8-7).

Muscle Coat

As in the upper parts of the intestinal tract, it is divided into an outer longitudinal and an inner circular layer of smooth muscle (Fig. 8-5).

Anal Sphincters

The anal canal has an involuntary internal sphincter and a voluntary external sphincter.

The **internal sphincter** is formed from a thickening of the smooth muscle of the circular coat at the upper end of the anal canal. The internal sphincter is enclosed by a sheath of striped muscle that forms the voluntary external sphincter (Figs. 8-5, 8-6, and 8-7).

The **external sphincter** can be divided into three parts:

- A **subcutaneous part,** which encircles the lower end of the anal canal and has no bony attachments
- A **superficial part,** which is attached to the coccyx behind and the perineal body in front
- A **deep part,** which encircles the upper end of the anal canal and has no bony attachments

The **puborectalis** fibers of the two levatores ani muscles blend with the deep part of the external sphincter (Figs. 8-5, 8-6, and 8-7). The puborectalis fibers of the two sides form a sling, which is attached in front to the pubic bones and passes around the junction of the rectum and the anal canal, pulling the two forward at an acute angle (Fig. 8-6).

The longitudinal smooth muscle of the anal canal is continuous above with that of the rectum. It forms a continuous coat around the anal canal and descends in the interval between the internal and external anal sphincters. Some of the longitudinal fibers are attached to the mucous membrane of the anal canal, whereas others pass laterally into the ischiorectal fossa or are attached to the perianal skin (Fig. 8-5).

At the junction of the rectum and anal canal (Fig. 8-6), the internal sphincter, the deep part of the external sphincter, and the puborectalis muscles form a distinct ring, called the **anorectal ring,** which can be felt on rectal examination.

Blood Supply

Arteries

The superior artery supplies the upper half and the inferior artery supplies the lower half (Fig. 8-6).

Veins

The upper half is drained by the superior rectal vein into the inferior mesenteric vein and the lower half is drained by the inferior rectal vein into the internal pudendal vein.

Lymph Drainage

The upper half of the anal canal drains into the pararectal nodes and then the inferior mesenteric nodes. The lower half drains into the medial group of superficial inguinal nodes (Fig. 8-6).

Nerve Supply

The mucous membrane of the upper half is sensitive to stretch and is innervated by sensory fibers that ascend through the hypogastric plexuses. The lower half is sensitive to pain, temperature, touch, and pressure and is innervated by the inferior rectal nerves. The involuntary internal sphincter is supplied by sympathetic fibers from the inferior hypogastric plexuses. The voluntary external sphincter is supplied by the inferior rectal nerve, a branch of the pudendal nerve (Fig. 8-3), and the perineal branch of the fourth sacral nerve.

Defecation

The time, place, and frequency of defecation are a matter of habit. Some adults defecate once a day, some defecate several times a day, and some perfectly normal people defecate once in several days.

The desire to defecate is initiated by stimulation of the stretch receptors in the wall of the rectum by the presence of feces in the lumen. The act of defecation involves a coordinated reflex that results in the emptying of the descending colon, sigmoid colon, rectum, and anal canal. It is assisted by a rise in intra-abdominal pressure brought about by contraction of the muscles of the anterior abdominal wall. The tonic contraction of the internal and external anal sphincters, including the puborectalis muscles, is now voluntarily inhibited, and the feces are evacuated through the anal canal. Depending on the laxity of the submucous coat, the mucous membrane of the lower part of the anal canal is extruded through the anus ahead of the fecal mass. At the end of the act, the mucosa is returned to the anal canal by the tone of the longitudinal fibers of the anal walls and the contraction and upward pull of the puborectalis muscle. The empty lumen of the anal canal is now closed by the tonic contraction of the anal sphincters.

Ischiorectal Fossa

The ischiorectal fossa (ischioanal fossa) is a wedge-shaped space located on each side of the anal canal (Fig. 8-5). The base of the wedge is superficial and formed by the skin. The edge of the wedge is formed by the junction of the medial and lateral walls. The medial wall is formed by the sloping levator ani muscle and the anal canal. The lateral wall is formed by the lower part of the obturator internus muscle, covered with pelvic fascia.

Contents of Fossa

The ischiorectal fossa is filled with dense fat, which supports the anal canal and allows it to distend during defecation. The pudendal nerve and internal pudendal vessels are embedded in a fascial canal, the **pudendal canal,** on the lateral wall of the ischiorectal fossa, on the medial side of the ischial tuberosity (Figs. 8-5 and 8-8). The inferior rectal vessels and nerve cross the fossa to reach the anal canal.

Pudendal Nerve

The pudendal nerve is a branch of the sacral plexus and leaves the main pelvic cavity through the greater sciatic foramen (Fig. 8-8). After a brief course in the gluteal region of the lower limb, it enters the perineum through the lesser sciatic foramen. The nerve then passes forward in the pudendal canal and, by means of its branches, supplies the external anal sphincter and the muscles and skin of the perineum.

Branches

- **Inferior rectal nerve:** This runs medially across the ischiorectal fossa and supplies the external anal sphincter, the mucous membrane of the lower half of the anal canal, and the perianal skin (Fig. 8-3).
- **Dorsal nerve of the penis (or clitoris):** This is distributed to the penis (or clitoris) (Fig. 8-8).
- **Perineal nerve:** This supplies the muscles in the urogenital triangle (Fig. 8-8) and the skin on the posterior surface of the scrotum (or labia majora).

Internal Pudendal Artery

The internal pudendal artery is a branch of the internal iliac artery and passes from the pelvis through the greater sciatic foramen and enters the perineum through the lesser sciatic foramen.

Branches

- **Inferior rectal artery:** This supplies the lower half of the anal canal (Fig. 8-3).
- **Branches to the penis** in the male and **to the labia and clitoris** in the female

Internal Pudendal Vein

The internal pudendal vein receives tributaries that correspond to the branches of the internal pudendal artery.

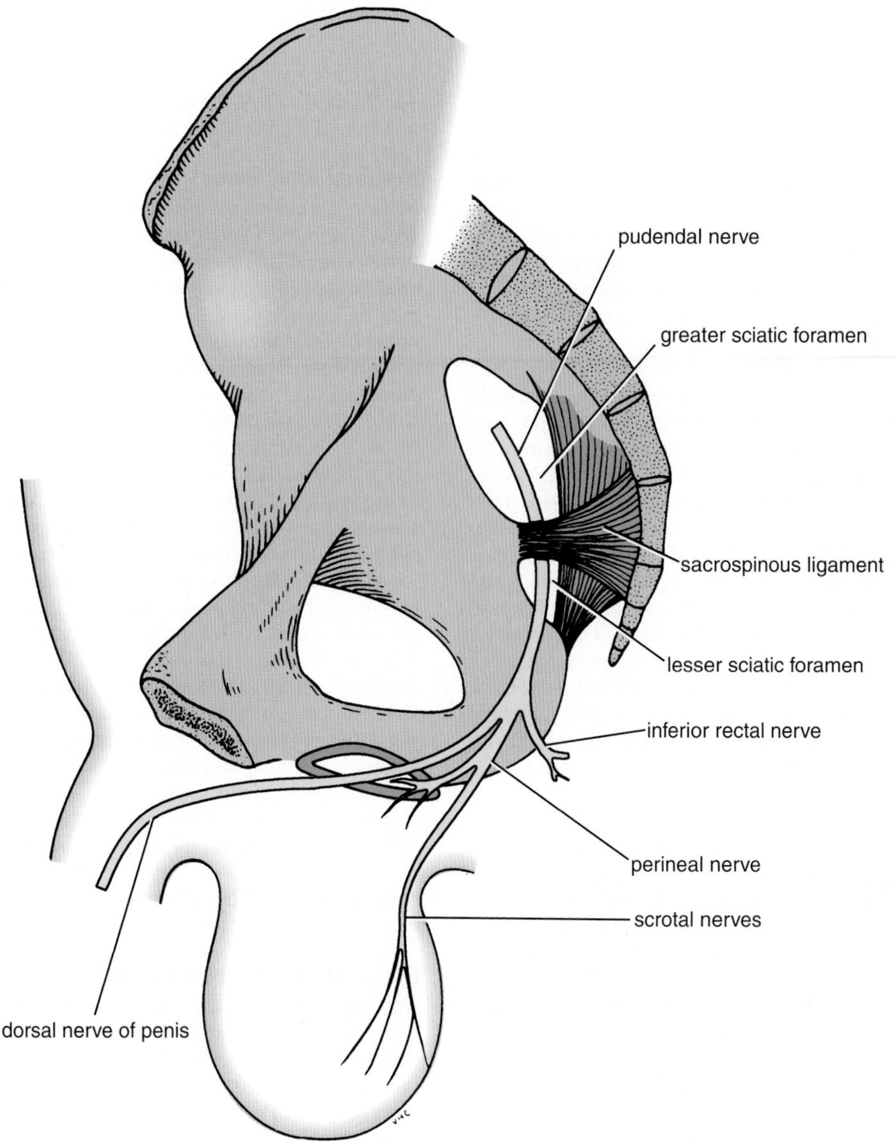

Figure 8-8 Course and branches of the pudendal nerve in the male.

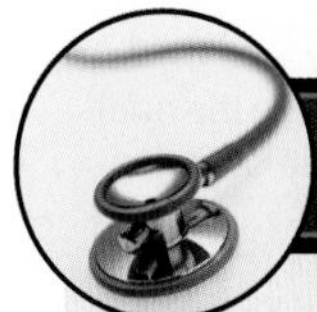

CLINICAL NOTES

Portal–Systemic Anastomosis

The rectal veins form an important portal–systemic anastomosis because the superior rectal vein drains ultimately into the portal vein and the inferior rectal vein drains into the systemic system.

Internal Hemorrhoids (Piles)

Internal hemorrhoids are varicosities of the tributaries of the superior rectal (hemorrhoidal) vein and are covered by mucous membrane (Fig. 8-9). The tributaries of the vein, which lie in the anal columns at the 3-, 7-, and 11-o'clock positions when the patient is viewed in the lithotomy position,* are particularly liable to become varicosed. Anatomically, a hemorrhoid is therefore a fold of mucous membrane and submucosa containing a varicosed tributary of the superior rectal vein and a terminal branch of the

* The patient is in the supine position with both hip joints flexed and abducted; the feet are held in position by stirrups. The position is commonly used for pelvic examinations of the female.

(continues)

Clinical Notes, *continued*

superior rectal artery. Internal hemorrhoids are initially contained within the anal canal (first degree). As they enlarge, they extrude from the canal on defecation but return at the end of the act (second degree). With further elongation, they prolapse on defecation and remain outside the anus (third degree).

Because internal hemorrhoids occur in the upper half of the anal canal, where the mucous membrane is innervated by autonomic afferent nerves, they are painless and are sensitive only to stretch. This may explain why large internal hemorrhoids give rise to an aching sensation rather than acute pain.

The causes of internal hemorrhoids are many. They frequently occur in members of the same family, which suggests a congenital weakness of the vein walls. Varicose veins of the legs and hemorrhoids often go together. The superior rectal vein is the most dependent part of the portal circulation and is valveless. The weight of the column of venous blood is thus greatest in the veins in the upper half of the anal canal. Here, the loose connective tissue of the submucosa gives little support to the walls of the veins. Moreover, the venous return is interrupted by the contraction of the muscular coat of the rectal wall during defecation. Chronic constipation, associated with prolonged straining at stool, is a common predisposing factor. Pregnancy hemorrhoids are common owing to pressure on the superior rectal veins by the gravid uterus. Portal hypertension as a result of cirrhosis of the liver can also cause hemorrhoids. The possibility that cancerous tumors of the rectum are blocking the superior rectal vein must never be overlooked.

External Hemorrhoids

External hemorrhoids are varicosities of the tributaries of the inferior rectal (hemorrhoidal) vein as they run laterally from the anal margin. They are covered by skin (Fig. 8-9) and are commonly associated with well-established internal hemorrhoids.

External hemorrhoids are covered by the mucous membrane of the lower half of the anal canal or the skin, and they are innervated by the inferior rectal nerves. They are sensitive to pain, temperature, touch, and pressure, which explains why external hemorrhoids tend to be painful. Thrombosis of an external hemorrhoid is common. Its cause is unknown, although coughing or straining may produce distention of the hemorrhoid followed by stasis. The presence of a small, acutely tender swelling at the anal margin is immediately recognized by the patient.

Perianal Hematoma

A perianal hematoma is a small collection of blood beneath the perianal skin (Fig. 8-9). It is caused by a rupture of a small subcutaneous vein, possibly an external hemorrhoid, and is extremely painful.

Anal Fissure

The lower ends of the anal columns are connected by small folds called **anal valves** (Fig. 8-10). In people suffering from chronic constipation, the anal valves may be torn down to the anus as the result of the edge of the fecal mass catching on the fold of mucous membrane. The elongated ulcer so formed, known as an **anal fissure** (Fig. 8-10), is extremely painful. The fissure occurs most commonly in the midline posteriorly or, less commonly, anteriorly, and this may be caused by the lack of support provided by the superficial part of the external sphincter in these areas. (The superficial part of the external sphincter does not encircle the anal canal, but sweeps past its lateral sides.)

The site of the anal fissure in the sensitive lower half of the anal canal, which is innervated by the inferior rectal nerve, results in reflex spasm of the external anal sphincter, aggravating the condition. Because of the intense pain, anal fissures may have to be examined under local anesthesia.

Perianal Abscesses

Perianal abscesses are produced by fecal trauma to the anal mucosa (Fig. 8-10). Infection may gain entrance to the submucosa through a small mucosal lesion, or the abscess may complicate an anal fissure or the infection of an anal mucosal gland. The abscess may be localized to the submucosa (submucous abscess), may occur beneath the perianal skin (subcutaneous abscess), or may occupy the ischiorectal fossa (ischiorectal abscess). Large ischiorectal abscesses sometimes extend posteriorly around the side of the anal canal to invade the ischiorectal fossa of the opposite side (horseshoe abscess). An abscess may be found in the space between the ampulla of the rectum and the upper surface of the levator ani (pelvirectal abscess). Anatomically, these abscesses are closely related to the different parts of the external sphincter and levator ani muscles, as seen in Figure 8-10.

Anal fistulae develop as the result of spread or inadequate treatment of anal abscesses. The fistula opens at one end at the lumen of the anal canal or lower rectum and at the other end on the skin surface close to the anus (Fig. 8-10). If the abscess opens onto only one surface, it is known as a **sinus,** not a fistula. The high-level fistulae are rare and run from the rectum to the perianal skin. They are located above the anorectal ring; as a result, fecal material constantly soils the clothes. The low-level fistulae occur below the level of the anorectal ring, as shown in Figure 8-10.

The most important part of the sphincteric mechanism of the anal canal is the **anorectal ring.** It consists of the deep part of the external sphincter, the internal sphincter, and the puborectalis part of the levator ani. Surgical operations on the anal canal that result in damage to the anorectal ring will produce fecal incontinence.

Removal of Anorectal Foreign Bodies

Normally, the anal canal is kept closed by the tone of the internal and external anal sphincters and the tone of the puborectalis part of the levator ani muscles. The rectal contents are supported by the levator ani muscles, possibly assisted by the transverse rectal mucosal folds. For these reasons, the removal of a large foreign body, such as a vase or electric light bulb, from the rectum may be a formidable problem.

The following procedure is usually successful:

1. The foreign body must first be fixed so that the sphincteric tone, together with external attempts to grab the object, do not displace the object farther up the rectum.
2. Large, irregular, or fragile foreign bodies may not be removed so easily, and it may be necessary to paralyze the anal sphincter by giving the patient a general anesthetic or by performing an anal sphincter nerve block.

Anal Sphincter Nerve Block and Anesthetizing the Perianal Skin

By blocking the branches of the inferior rectal nerve and the perineal branch of the fourth sacral nerve, the anal sphincters will be relaxed and the perianal skin anesthetized.

The procedure is as follows:

1. An intradermal wheal is produced by injecting a small amount of anesthetic solution behind the anus in the midline.
2. A gloved index finger is inserted into the anal canal to serve as a guide.
3. A long needle attached to a syringe filled with anesthetic solution is inserted through the cutaneous wheal into the sphincter muscles along the posterior and lateral surfaces of the anal canal. The procedure is repeated on the oppo-

(continues)

Clinical Notes, *continued*

site side. The purpose of the finger in the anal canal is to guide the needle and to prevent penetration of the anal mucous membrane.

Incontinence Associated with Rectal Prolapse

Fecal incontinence can accompany severe rectal prolapse of long duration. It is thought that the prolonged and excessive stretching of the anal sphincters is the cause of the condition. The condition can be treated by restoring the anorectal angle by tightening the puborectalis part of the levator ani muscles and the external anal sphincters behind the anorectal junction.

Incontinence After Trauma

Trauma, such as childbirth, or damage to the sphincters during surgery or perianal abscesses or fistulae can be responsible for incontinence after trauma.

Incontinence After Spinal Cord Injury

After severe spinal cord injuries, the patient is not aware of rectal distention. Moreover, the parasympathetic influence on the peristaltic activity of the descending colon, sigmoid colon, and rectum is lost. In addition, control over the abdominal musculature and sphincters of the anal canal may be severely impaired. The rectum, now an isolated structure, responds by contracting when the pressure within its lumen rises. This local reflex response is much more efficient if the sacral segments of the spinal cord are spared. At best, however, the force of the contractions of the rectal wall is small, and constipation and impaction of feces are the usual outcome.

Rectal Examination

The following structures can be palpated by the gloved index finger inserted into the anal canal and rectum in the normal patient.

Anteriorly

In the male:

- **Opposite the terminal phalanx** are the contents of the rectovesical pouch, the posterior surface of the bladder, the seminal vesicles, and the vasa deferentia (Fig. 8-11).
- **Opposite the middle phalanx** are the rectoprostatic fascia and the prostate.
- **Opposite the proximal phalanx** are the perineal body, the urogenital diaphragm, and the bulb of the penis.

In the female:

- **Opposite the terminal phalanx** are the rectouterine pouch, the vagina, and the cervix.
- **Opposite the middle phalanx** are the urogenital diaphragm and the vagina.
- **Opposite the proximal phalanx** are the perineal body and the lower part of the vagina.

Posteriorly

The sacrum, coccyx, and anococcygeal body can be felt.

Laterally

The ischiorectal fossae and ischial spines can be palpated.

Cancer and the Lymph Drainage of the Anal Canal

The upper half of the mucous membrane of the anal canal is drained upward to lymph nodes along the course of the superior rectal artery. The lower half of the mucous membrane is drained downward to the medial group of superficial inguinal nodes. Many patients have thought they had an inguinal hernia, and the physician has found a cancer of the lower half of the anal canal, with secondary deposits in the inguinal lymph nodes.

The Ischiorectal Fossa and Infection

The ischiorectal fossae (ischioanal fossae) are filled with fat that is poorly vascularized. The close proximity to the anal canal makes them particularly vulnerable to infection. Infection commonly tracks laterally from the anal mucosa through the external anal sphincter. Infection of the perianal hair follicles or sweat glands may also be the cause of infection in the fossae. Rarely, a perirectal abscess bursts downward through the levator ani muscle. An ischiorectal abscess may involve the opposite fossa by the spread of infection across the midline behind the anal canal.

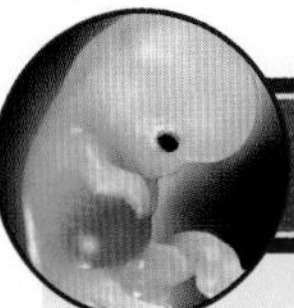

EMBRYOLOGIC NOTES

Development of the Anal Canal

The distal end of the hindgut terminates as a blind sac of entoderm called the **cloaca** (see Fig. 7-8). The cloaca lies in contact with a shallow ectodermal depression called the **proctodeum.** The apposed layers of ectoderm and entoderm form the **cloacal membrane,** which separates the cavity of the hindgut from the surface (see Fig. 7-8). The cloaca becomes divided into anterior and posterior parts by the **urorectal septum;** the posterior part of the cloaca is called the **anorectal canal.** The anorectal canal forms the rectum and the upper half of the anal canal. The lining of the superior half of the anal canal is formed from entoderm, and that of the inferior half of the anal canal is formed from the ectoderm of the proctodeum (see Fig. 7-8). The sphincters of the anal canal are formed from the surrounding mesenchyme. The posterior part of the cloacal membrane breaks down so that the gut opens onto the surface of the embryo.

Imperforate Anus

About 1 child in 4000 is born with imperforate anus caused by an imperfect fusion of the entodermal cloaca with the proctodeum.

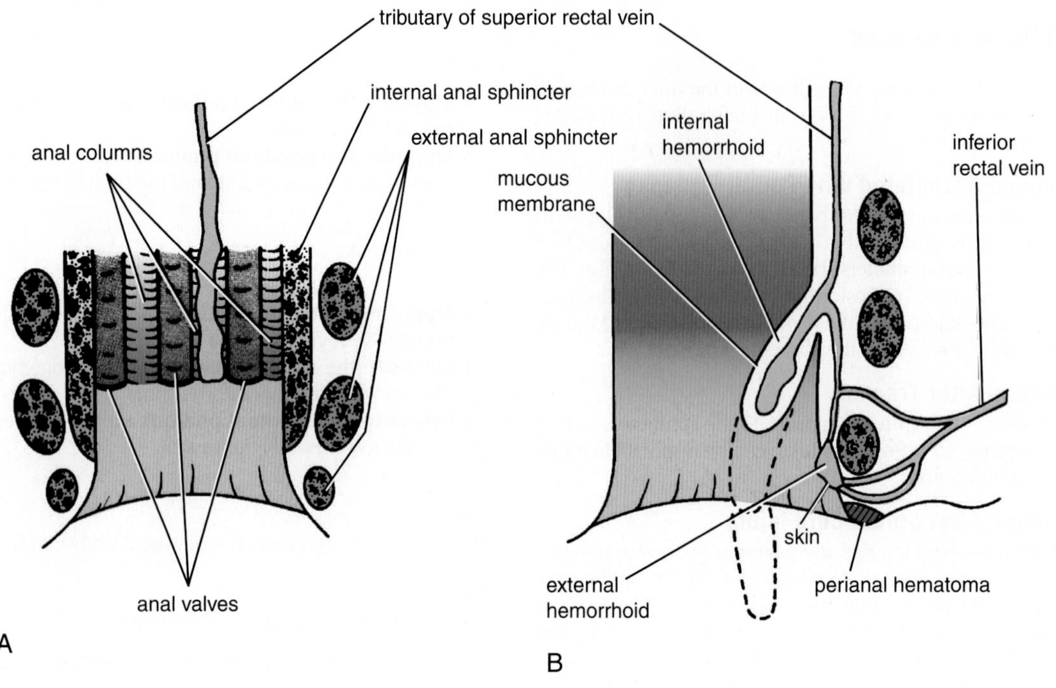

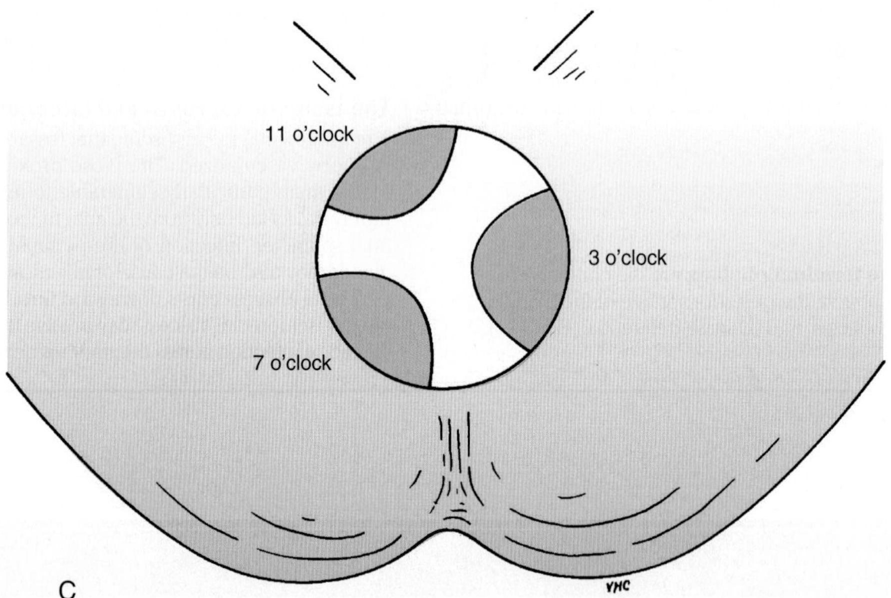

Figure 8-9 **A.** Normal tributary of the superior rectal vein within the anal column. **B.** Varicosed tributary of the superior rectal vein forming the internal hemorrhoid. Dotted lines indicate degrees of severity of condition. **C.** Positions of three internal hemorrhoids as seen through a proctoscope with the patient in the lithotomy position.

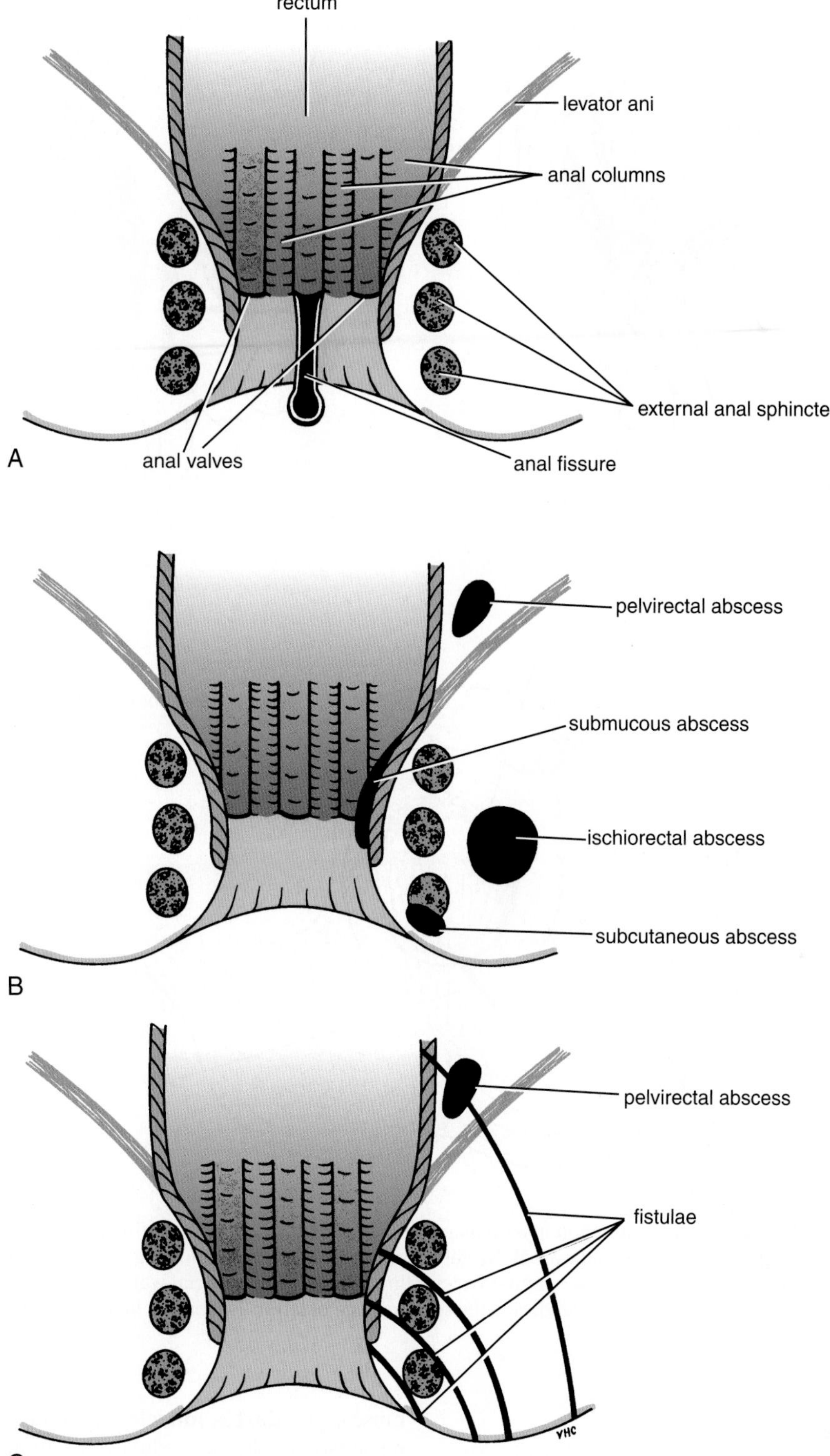

Figure 8-10 **A.** Tearing downward of the anal valve to form an anal fissure. **B.** Common locations of perianal abscesses. **C.** Common positions of perianal fistulae.

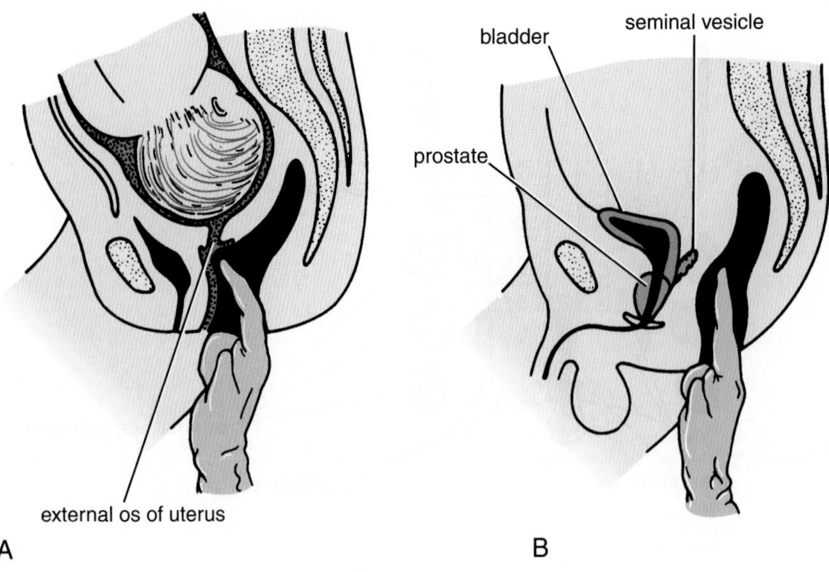

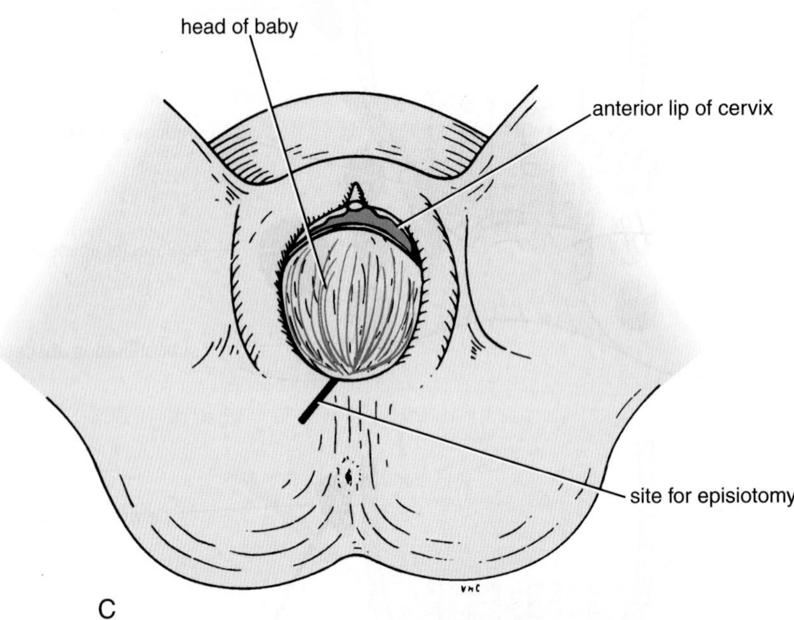

Figure 8-11 **A.** Rectal examination in a pregnant woman showing how it is possible to palpate the cervix through the anterior rectal wall. **B.** Rectal examination in the male showing how it is possible to palpate the prostate and the seminal vesicles through the anterior rectal wall. **C.** Position of the episiotomy incision in a woman during the second stage of labor. The baby's head is presenting at the vaginal orifice.

Urogenital Triangle

The urogenital triangle is bounded in front by the pubic arch and laterally by the ischial tuberosities (Fig. 8-3).

Superficial Fascia

The superficial fascia of the urogenital triangle can be divided into a fatty layer and a membranous layer.

The **fatty layer** (fascia of Camper) is continuous with the fat of the ischiorectal fossa (Fig. 8-12) and the superficial fascia of the thighs. In the scrotum, the fat is replaced by smooth muscle, the **dartos muscle.** The dartos muscle contracts in response to cold and reduces the surface area of the scrotal skin (see testicular temperature and fertility, page 169).

The **membranous layer** (Colles' fascia) is attached posteriorly to the posterior border of the urogenital diaphragm (Fig. 8-12) and laterally to the margins of the pubic arch; anteriorly it is continuous with the membranous layer of superficial fascia of the anterior abdominal wall (Scarpa's fascia). The fascia is continued over the penis (or clitoris) as a tubular sheath (Fig. 8-13). In the scrotum (or labia majora) it forms a distinct layer (Fig. 8-12).

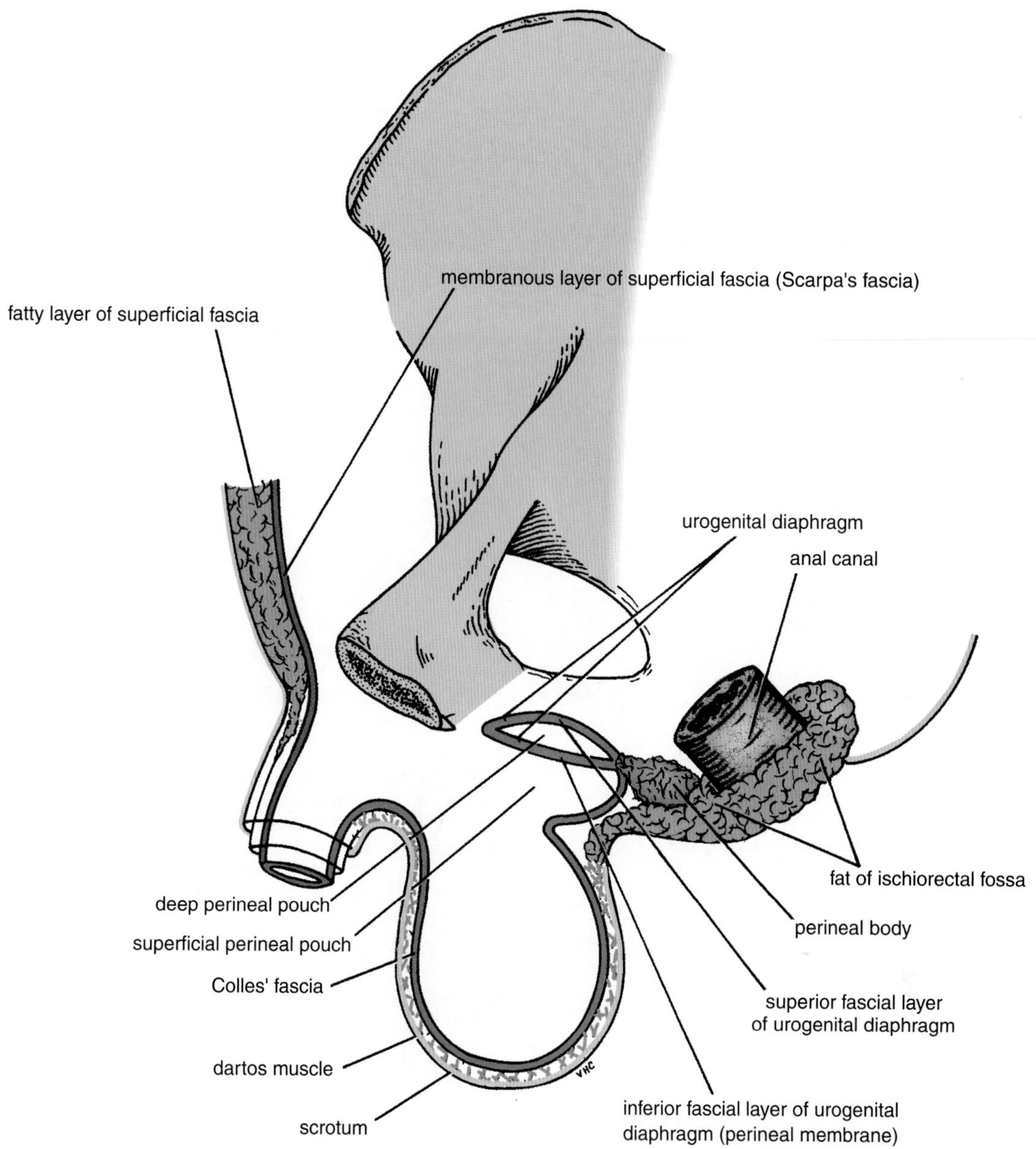

Figure 8-12 Arrangement of the superficial fascia in the urogenital triangle. Note the superficial and deep perineal pouches.

Superficial Perineal Pouch

The superficial perineal pouch is bounded below by the membranous layer of superficial fascia and above by the urogenital diaphragm (Fig. 8-12). It is closed behind by the fusion of its upper and lower walls. Laterally, it is closed by the attachment of the membranous layer of superficial fascia and the urogenital diaphragm to the margins of the pubic arch (Figs. 8-14 and 8-15). Anteriorly, the space communicates freely with the potential space lying between the superficial fascia of the anterior abdominal wall and the anterior abdominal muscles.

The contents of the superficial perineal pouch in both sexes are described on pages 405 and 408.

Urogenital Diaphragm

The urogenital diaphragm is a triangular musculofascial diaphragm situated in the anterior part of the perineum, filling in the gap of the pubic arch (Figs. 8-12, 8-14, and 8-15). It is formed by the sphincter urethrae and the deep transverse perineal muscles, which are enclosed between a superior and an inferior layer of fascia of the urogenital diaphragm. The inferior layer of fascia is often referred to as the **perineal membrane.**

Anteriorly, the two layers of fascia fuse, leaving a small gap beneath the symphysis pubis. Posteriorly, the two layers of fascia fuse with each other and with the membranous layer of the superficial fascia and the perineal body (Fig. 8-

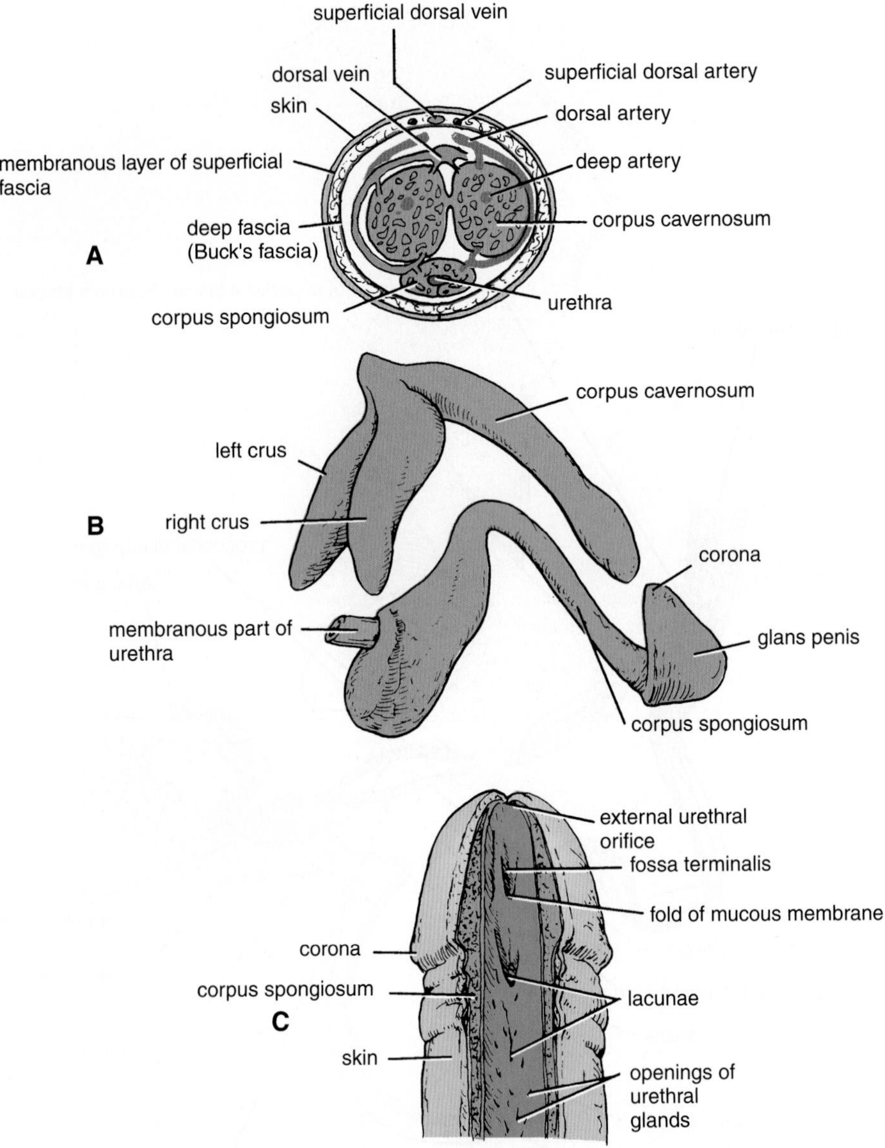

Figure 8-13 The penis. **A and B.** The three bodies of erectile tissue, the two corpora cavernosa, and the corpus spongiosum with the glans. **C.** The penile urethra slit open to show the folds of mucous membrane and glandular orifices in the roof of the urethra.

12). Laterally, the layers of fascia are attached to the pubic arch. The closed space that is contained between the superficial and deep layers of fascia is known as the **deep perineal pouch** (Figs. 8-12, 8-14, and 8-15).

The contents of the deep perineal pouch in both sexes are described in subsequent sections.

Contents of the Male Urogenital Triangle

In the male, the triangle contains the penis and scrotum.

Penis

Location and Description

The penis has a fixed root and a body that hangs free (Figs. 8-4 and 8-16).

Root of the Penis

The root of the penis is made up of three masses of erectile tissue called the **bulb of the penis** and the **right** and **left crura of the penis** (Figs. 8-13, 8-16, and 8-17). The bulb is situated in the midline and is attached to the undersurface of the urogenital diaphragm. It is traversed by the urethra and is covered on its outer surface by the **bulbospongiosus muscles.** Each crus is attached to the side of the pubic arch and is covered on its outer surface by the **ischiocavernosus muscle.** The bulb is continued forward into the body of the penis and forms the **corpus spongiosum** (Fig. 8-17). The two crura converge anteriorly and come to lie side by side in the dorsal part of the body of the penis, forming the **corpora cavernosa** (Figs. 8-13 and 8-16).

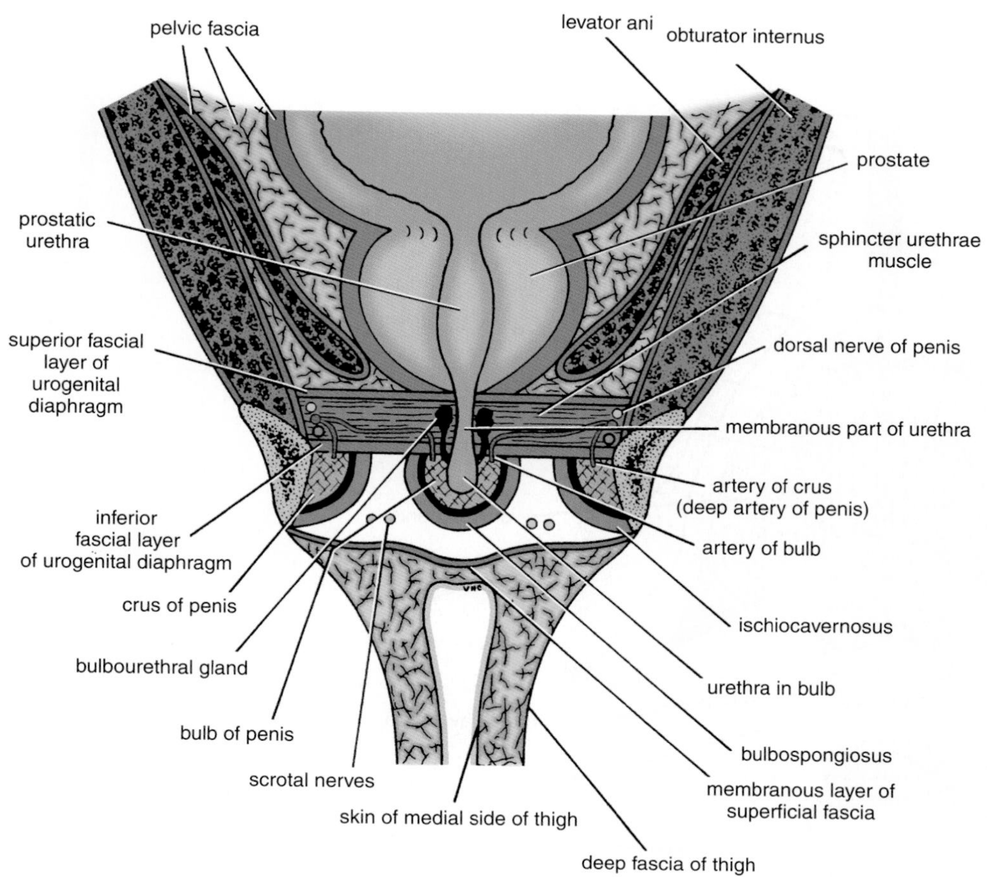

Figure 8-14 Coronal section of the male pelvis showing the prostate, the urogenital diaphragm, and the contents of the superficial perineal pouch.

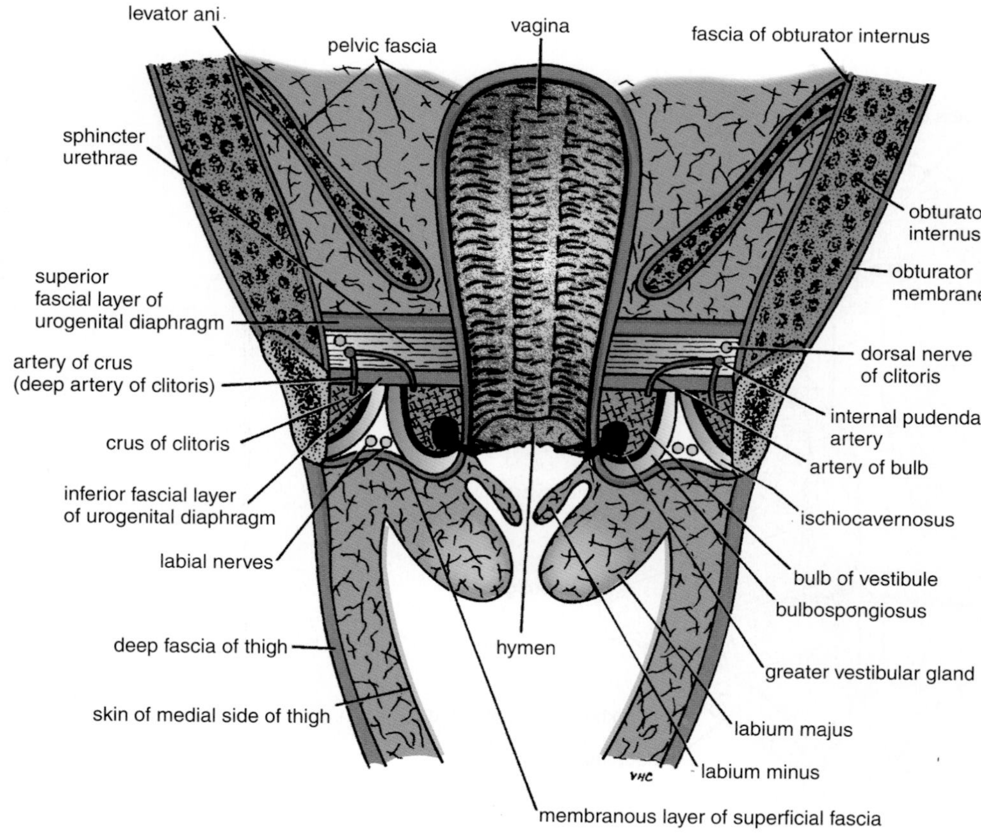

Figure 8-15 Coronal section of the female pelvis showing the vagina, the urogenital diaphragm, and the contents of the superficial perineal pouch.

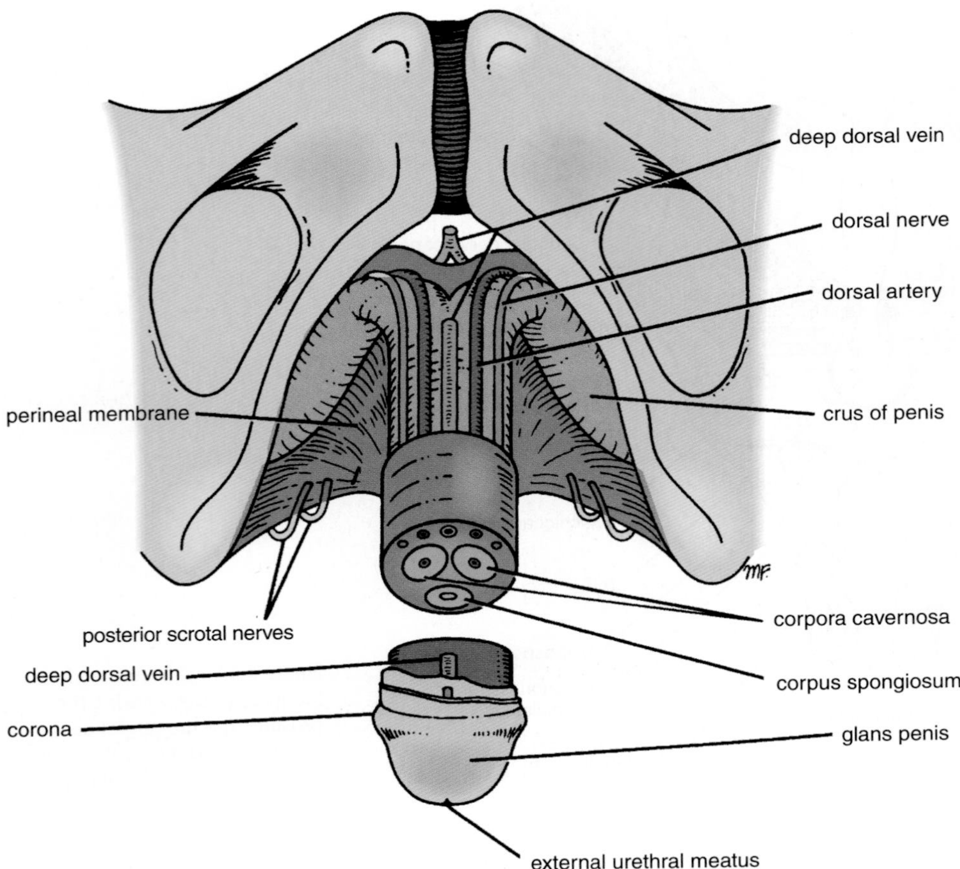

Figure 8-16 Root and body of the penis.

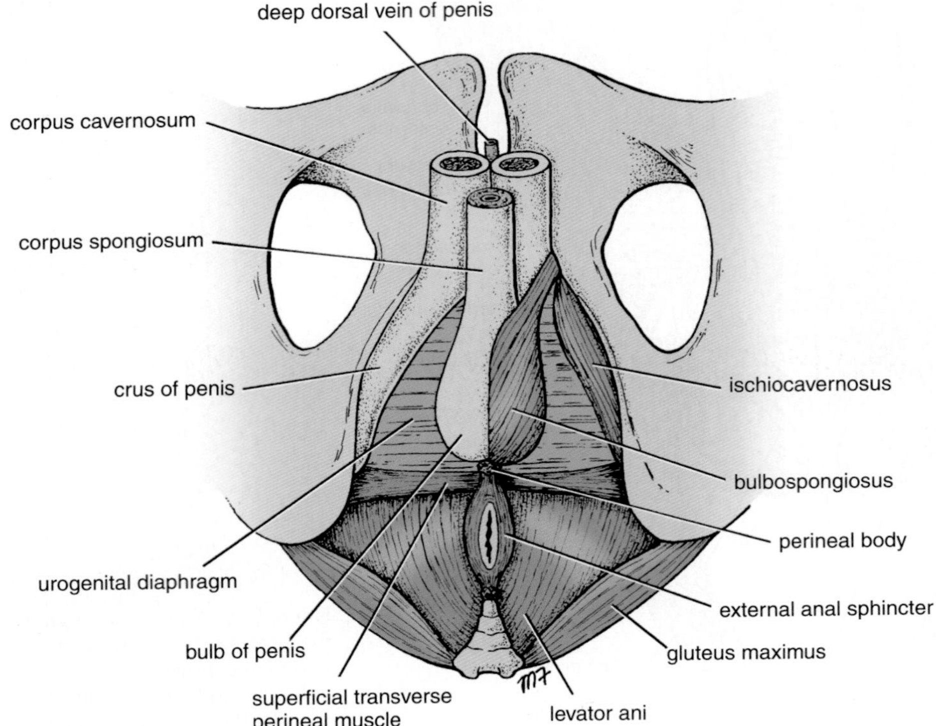

Figure 8-17 Root of penis and perineal muscles.

Body of the Penis

The body of the penis is essentially composed of three cylinders of erectile tissue enclosed in a tubular sheath of fascia **(Buck's fascia).** The erectile tissue is made up of two dorsally placed corpora cavernosa and a single corpus spongiosum applied to their ventral surface (Figs. 8-13 and 8-16). At its distal extremity, the corpus spongiosum expands to form the **glans penis,** which covers the distal ends of the corpora cavernosa. On the tip of the glans penis is the slitlike orifice of the urethra, called the **external urethral meatus.**

The **prepuce** or **foreskin** is a hoodlike fold of skin that covers the glans. It is connected to the glans just below the urethral orifice by a fold called the **frenulum.**

The body of the penis is supported by two condensations of deep fascia that extend downward from the linea alba and symphysis pubis to be attached to the fascia of the penis.

Blood Supply

Arteries

The corpora cavernosa are supplied by the **deep arteries of the penis** (Fig. 8-13); the corpus spongiosum is supplied by the **artery of the bulb.** In addition, there is the **dorsal artery of the penis.** All the above arteries are branches of the internal pudendal artery.

Veins

The veins drain into the internal pudendal veins.

Lymph Drainage

The skin of the penis is drained into the medial group of superficial inguinal nodes. The deep structures of the penis are drained into the internal iliac nodes.

Nerve Supply

The nerve supply is from the pudendal nerve and the pelvic plexuses.

Scrotum

Location and Description

The scrotum is an outpouching of the lower part of the anterior abdominal wall and contains the testes, the epididymides, and the lower ends of the spermatic cords (see Fig. 4-21).

The wall of the scrotum has the following layers:

- Skin
- Superficial fascia; the dartos muscle, which is smooth muscle, replaces the fatty layer of the anterior abdominal wall, and Scarpa's fascia (membranous layer) is now called Colles' fascia.
- External spermatic fascia derived from the external oblique
- Cremasteric fascia derived from the internal oblique
- Internal spermatic fascia derived from the fascia transversalis
- Tunica vaginalis, which is a closed sac that covers the anterior, medial, and lateral surfaces of each testis

Because the structure of the scrotum, the descent of the testes, and the formation of the inguinal canal are interrelated, they are fully described in Chapter 4.

Blood Supply

Subcutaneous plexuses and arteriovenous anastomoses promote heat loss and thus assist in the environmental control of the temperature of the testes.

Arteries

The external pudendal branches of the femoral and scrotal branches of the internal pudendal arteries supply the scrotum.

Veins

The veins accompany the corresponding arteries.

Lymph Drainage

The wall of the scrotum is drained into the medial group of superficial inguinal lymph nodes. The lymph drainage of the testis and epididymis ascends in the spermatic cord and ends in the lumbar (para-aortic) lymph nodes at the level of the first lumbar vertebra. This is to be expected, because the testis during development has migrated from high up on the posterior abdominal wall, down through the inguinal canal, and into the scrotum, dragging its blood supply and lymph vessels after it.

Nerve Supply

The anterior surface of the scrotum is supplied by the ilioinguinal nerves and the genital branch of the genitofemoral nerves, and the posterior surface is supplied by branches of the perineal nerves and the posterior cutaneous nerves of the thigh.

Contents of the Superficial Perineal Pouch in the Male

The superficial perineal pouch contains structures forming the root of the penis, together with the muscles that cover them—namely, the bulbospongiosus muscles and the ischiocavernosus muscles (Fig. 8-17). The **bulbospongiosus muscles,** situated one on each side of the midline (Fig. 8-17), cover the bulb of the penis and the posterior portion of the corpus spongiosum. Their function is to compress the penile part of the urethra and empty it of residual urine or semen. The anterior fibers also compress the deep dorsal vein of the penis, thus impeding the venous drainage of the erectile tissue and thereby assisting in the process of erection of the penis.

Ischiocavernosus Muscles

The ischiocavernosus muscles cover the crus penis on each side (Fig. 8-17). The action of each muscle is to compress the crus penis and assist in the process of erection of the penis.

Superficial Transverse Perineal Muscles

The superficial transverse perineal muscles lie in the posterior part of the superficial perineal pouch (Fig. 8-17). Each muscle arises from the ischial ramus and is inserted into the perineal body. The function of these muscles is to fix the perineal body in the center of the perineum.

Nerve Supply

All the muscles of the superficial perineal pouch are supplied by the perineal branch of the pudendal nerve.

Perineal Body

This small mass of fibrous tissue is attached to the center of the posterior margin of the urogenital diaphragm (Figs. 8-12 and 8-17). It serves as a point of attachment for the following muscles: external anal sphincter, bulbospongiosus muscle, and superficial transverse perineal muscles.

Perineal Branch of the Pudendal Nerve

The perineal branch of the pudendal nerve on each side terminates in the superficial perineal pouch by supplying the muscles and skin (Fig. 8-8).

Contents of the Deep Perineal Pouch in the Male

The deep perineal pouch contains the membranous part of the urethra, the sphincter urethrae, the bulbourethral glands, the deep transverse perineal muscles, the internal pudendal vessels and their branches, and the dorsal nerves of the penis.

Membranous Part of the Urethra

The membranous part of the urethra is about 0.5 in. (1.3 cm) long and lies within the urogenital diaphragm, surrounded by the sphincter urethrae muscle; it is continuous above with the prostatic urethra and below with the penile urethra. It is the shortest and least dilatable part of the urethra (Fig. 8-14).

Sphincter Urethrae Muscle

The sphincter urethrae muscle surrounds the urethra in the deep perineal pouch. It arises from the pubic arch on the two sides and passes medially to encircle the urethra (Fig. 8-14).

Nerve Supply

The perineal branch of the pudendal nerve supplies the sphincter.

Action

The muscle compresses the membranous part of the urethra and relaxes during micturition. It is the means by which micturition can be voluntarily stopped.

Bulbourethral Glands

The bulbourethral glands are two small glands that lie beneath the sphincter urethrae muscle (Fig. 8-14). Their ducts pierce the perineal membrane (inferior fascial layer of the urogenital diaphragm) and enter the penile portion of the urethra. The secretion is poured into the urethra as a result of erotic stimulation.

Deep Transverse Perineal Muscles

The deep transverse perineal muscles lie posterior to the sphincter urethrae muscle. Each muscle arises from the ischial ramus and passes medially to be inserted into the perineal body. These muscles are clinically unimportant.

Internal Pudendal Artery

The internal pudenal artery (Fig. 8-14) on each side enters the deep perineal pouch and passes forward, giving rise to the **artery to the bulb of the penis;** the **arteries to the crura of the penis** (deep artery of penis); and the **dorsal artery of the penis,** which supplies the skin and fascia of the penis.

Dorsal Nerve of the Penis

The dorsal nerve of the penis on each side passes forward through the deep perineal pouch and supplies the skin of the penis (Fig. 8-14).

Erection of the Penis

Erection in the male is gradually built up as a consequence of various sexual stimuli. Pleasurable sight, sound, smell, and other psychic stimuli, fortified later by direct touch sensory stimuli from the general body skin and genital skin, result in a bombardment of the central nervous system by afferent stimuli. Efferent nervous impulses pass down the spinal cord to the parasympathetic outflow in the second, third, and fourth sacral segments. The parasympathetic preganglionic fibers enter the inferior hypogastric plexuses and synapse on the postganglionic neurons. The postganglionic fibers join the internal pudendal arteries and are distributed along their branches, which enter the erectile tissue at the root of the penis. Vasodilatation of the arteries now occurs, producing a great increase in blood flow through the blood spaces of the erectile tissue. The corpora cavernosa and the corpus spongiosum become engorged with blood and expand, compressing their draining veins against the surrounding fascia. By this means, the outflow of blood from the erectile tissue is retarded so that the internal pressure is further accentuated and maintained. The penis thus increases in length and diameter and assumes the erect position.

Once the climax of sexual excitement is reached and ejaculation takes place, or the excitement passes off or is inhibited, the arteries supplying the erectile tissue undergo vasoconstriction. The penis then returns to its flaccid state.

Ejaculation

During the increasing sexual excitement that occurs during sex play, the external urinary meatus of the glans penis becomes moist as a result of the secretions of the bulbourethral glands.

Friction on the glans penis, reinforced by other afferent nervous impulses, results in a discharge along the sympathetic nerve fibers to the smooth muscle of the duct of the epididymis and the vas deferens on each side, the seminal vesicles, and the prostate. The smooth muscle contracts, and the spermatozoa, together with the secretions of the seminal vesicles and prostate, are discharged into the prostatic urethra. The fluid now joins the secretions of the bulbourethral glands and penile urethral glands and is then ejected from the penile urethra as a result of the rhythmic contractions of the bulbospongiosus muscles, which compress the urethra. Meanwhile, the sphincter of the bladder contracts and prevents a reflux of the spermatozoa into the bladder. The spermatozoa and the secretions of the several accessory glands constitute the **seminal fluid,** or **semen.**

At the climax of male sexual excitement, a mass discharge of nervous impulses takes place in the central nervous system. Impulses pass down the spinal cord to the sympathetic outflow (T1 to L2). The nervous impulses that pass to the genital organs are thought to leave the cord at the first and second lumbar segments in the preganglionic sympathetic fibers. Many of these fibers synapse with postganglionic neurons in the first and second lumbar ganglia. Other fibers may synapse in ganglia in the lower lumbar or pelvic parts of the sympathetic trunks. The postganglionic fibers are then distributed to the vas deferens, the seminal vesicles, and the prostate via the inferior hypogastric plexuses.

Male Urethra

The male urethra is about 8 in. (20 cm) long and extends from the neck of the bladder to the external meatus on the glans penis (Fig. 8-4). It is divided into three parts: prostatic, membranous, and penile.

The **prostatic urethra** is described on page 356. It is about 1.25 in. (3 cm) long and passes through the prostate from the base to the apex (Fig. 8-14). It is the widest and most dilatable portion of the urethra.

The **membranous urethra** is about 0.5 in. (1.25 cm) long and lies within the urogenital diaphragm, surrounded by the sphincter urethrae muscle. It is the least dilatable portion of the urethra (Fig. 8-14).

The **penile urethra** is about 6 in. (15.75 cm) long and is enclosed in the bulb and the corpus spongiosum of the penis (Figs. 8-4, 8-14, 8-16, and 8-17). The external meatus is the narrowest part of the entire urethra. The part of the urethra that lies within the glans penis is dilated to form the

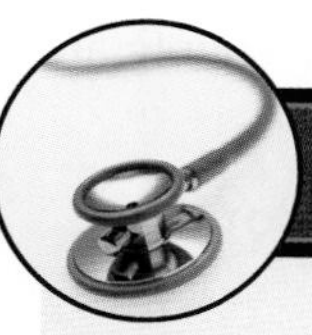

CLINICAL NOTES

Circumcision

Circumcision is the operation of removing the greater part of the prepuce, or foreskin. In many newborn males, the prepuce cannot be retracted over the glans. This can result in infection of the secretions beneath the prepuce, leading to inflammation, swelling, and fibrosis of the prepuce. Repeated inflammation leads to constriction of the orifice of the prepuce **(phimosis)** with obstruction to urination. It is now generally believed that chronic inflammation of the prepuce predisposes to carcinoma of the glans penis. For these reasons prophylactic circumcision is commonly practiced. For Jews, it is a religious rite.

Catheterization of the Male

The following anatomic facts should be remembered before passing a catheter or other instrument along the male urethra:

- The external orifice at the glans penis is the narrowest part of the entire urethra.
- Within the glans, the urethra dilates to form the **fossa terminalis** (navicular fossa).
- Near the posterior end of the fossa, a fold of mucous membrane projects into the lumen from the roof (Fig. 8-13).
- The membranous part of the urethra is narrow and fixed.
- The prostatic part of the urethra is the widest and most dilatable part of the urethra.
- By holding the penis upward, the S-shaped curve to the urethra is converted into a J-shaped curve.

If the point of the catheter passes through the external orifice and is then directed toward the urethral floor until it has passed the mucosal fold, it should easily pass along a normal urethra into the bladder.

Anatomy of the Procedure of Catheterization

The procedure is as follows:

1. The patient lies in a supine position.
2. With gentle traction, the penis is held erect at right angles to the anterior abdominal wall. The lubricated catheter is passed through the narrow external urethral meatus. The catheter should pass easily along the penile urethra. On reaching the membranous part of the urethra, a slight resistance is felt because of the tone of the urethral sphincter and the surrounding rigid perineal membrane.
3. The penis is then lowered toward the thighs, and the catheter is gently pushed through the sphincter.
4. Passage of the catheter through the prostatic urethra and bladder neck should not present any difficulty.

Urethral Infection

The most dependent part of the male urethra is that which lies within the bulb. Here, it is subject to chronic inflammation and stricture formation.

The many glands that open into the urethra—including those of the prostate, the bulbourethral glands, and many small penile urethral glands—are commonly the site of chronic gonococcal infection.

Injuries to the penis may occur as the result of blunt trauma, penetrating trauma, or strangulation. Amputation of the entire penis should be repaired by anastomosis using microsurgical techniques to restore continuity of the main blood vessels.

Rupture of the Urethra

Rupture of the urethra may complicate a severe blow on the perineum. The common site of rupture is within the bulb of the penis, just below the perineal membrane. The urine extravasates into the superficial perineal pouch and then passes forward over the scrotum beneath the membranous layer of the superficial fascia, as described in Chapter 4. If the membranous part of the urethra is ruptured, urine escapes into the deep perineal pouch and can extravasate upward around the prostate and bladder or downward into the superficial perineal pouch.

Erection and Ejaculation After Spinal Cord Injuries

Erection of the penis is controlled by the parasympathetic nerves that originate from the second, third, and fourth sacral segments of the spinal cord. Bilateral damage to the reticulospinal nerve tracts in the spinal cord will result in loss of erection. Later, when the effects of spinal shock have disappeared, spontaneous or reflex erection may occur if the sacral segments of the spinal cord are intact.

Ejaculation is controlled by sympathetic nerves that originate in the first and second lumbar segments of the spinal cord. As in the case of erection, severe bilateral damage to the spinal cord results in loss of ejaculation. Later, reflex ejaculation may be possible in patients with spinal cord transections in the thoracic or cervical regions.

Scrotum

See page 167.

fossa terminalis (navicular fossa) (Fig. 8-4). The bulbourethral glands open into the penile urethra below the urogenital diaphragm.

Contents of the Female Urogenital Triangle

In the female, the triangle contains the external genitalia and the orifices of the urethra and the vagina.

Clitoris

Location and Description

The clitoris, which corresponds to the penis in the male, is situated at the apex of the vestibule anteriorly. It has a structure similar to the penis. The glans of the clitoris is partly hidden by the prepuce.

Root of the Clitoris

The root of the clitoris is made up of three masses of erectile tissue called the bulb of the vestibule and the right and left crura of the clitoris (Figs. 8-15 and 8-18).

The **bulb of the vestibule** corresponds to the bulb of the penis, but because of the presence of the vagina, it is divided into two halves (Fig. 8-18). It is attached to the undersurface of the urogenital diaphragm and is covered by the **bulbospongiosus muscles.**

The **crura of the clitoris** correspond to the crura of the penis and become the corpora cavernosa anteriorly. Each remains separate and is covered by an **ischiocavernosus muscle** (Fig. 8-18).

Body of the Clitoris

The body of the clitoris consists of the two **corpora cavernosa** covered by their **ischiocavernosus muscles.** The corpus spongiosum of the male is represented by a small amount of erectile tissue leading from the vestibular bulbs to the glans.

Glans of the Clitoris

The glans of the clitoris is a small mass of erectile tissue that caps the body of the clitoris. It is provided with numerous sensory endings. The glans is partly hidden by the **prepuce.**

Blood Supply, Lymph Drainage, and Nerve Supply

The blood supply, lymph drainage, and nerve supply are similar to those of the penis.

Contents of the Superficial Perineal Pouch in the Female

The superficial perineal pouch contains structures forming the root of the clitoris and the muscles that cover them, namely, the bulbospongiosus muscles and the ischiocavernosus muscles (Figs. 8-15 and 8-18).

Bulbospongiosus Muscle

The bulbospongiosus muscle surrounds the orifice of the vagina and covers the vestibular bulbs. Its fibers extend forward to gain attachment to the corpora cavernosa of the clitoris. The bulbospongiosus muscle reduces the size of the vaginal orifice and compresses the deep dorsal vein of the

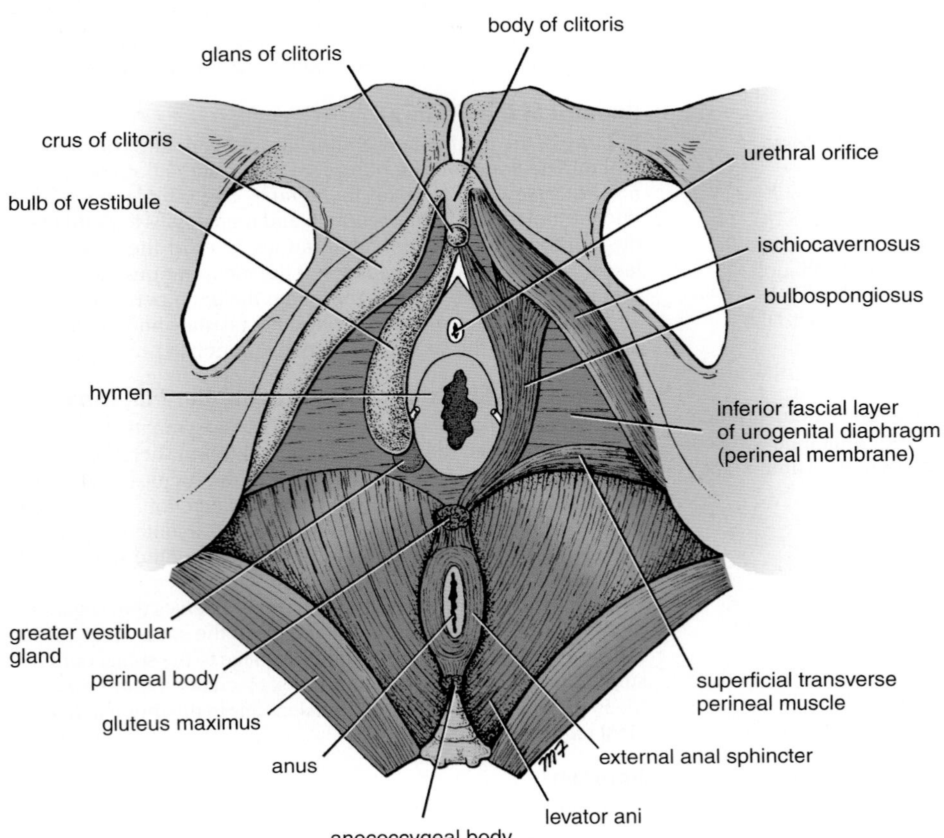

Figure 8-18 Root and body of the clitoris and the perineal muscles.

clitoris, thereby assisting in the mechanism of erection in the clitoris.

Ischiocavernosus Muscle

The ischiocavernosus muscle on each side covers the crus of the clitoris. Contraction of this muscle assists in causing the erection of the clitoris.

Superficial Transverse Perineal Muscles

The superficial transverse perineal muscles are identical in structure and function to those of the male.

Nerve Supply

All the muscles of the superficial perineal pouch are supplied by the perineal branch of the pudendal nerve.

Perineal Body

The perineal body is larger than that of the male and is clinically important. It is a wedge-shaped mass of fibrous tissue situated between the lower end of the vagina and the anal canal (Figs. 8-4 and 8-18). It is the point of attachment of many perineal muscles (as in the male), including the levatores ani muscles; the latter assist the perineal body in supporting the posterior wall of the vagina.

Perineal Branch of Pudendal Nerve

The perineal branch of the pudendal nerve on each side terminates in the superficial perineal pouch by supplying the muscles and skin (Fig. 8-8).

Contents of the Deep Perineal Pouch in the Female

The deep perineal pouch (Fig. 8-15) contains part of the urethra; part of the vagina; the sphincter urethrae, which is pierced by the urethra and the vagina; the deep transverse perineal muscles; the internal pudendal vessels and their branches; and the dorsal nerves of the clitoris.

The urethra and the vagina are described in the next column.

The **sphincter urethrae** and the **deep transverse perineal muscles** are described on page 406. The **internal pudendal vessels** and the **dorsal nerves of the clitoris** have an arrangement similar to the corresponding structures found in the male.

A summary of the muscles of the perineum, their nerve supply, and their action is given in Table 8-1.

Erection of the Clitoris

Sexual excitement produces engorgement of the erectile tissue within the clitoris in exactly the same manner as in the male.

Orgasm in the Female

As in the male, vision, hearing, smell, touch, and other psychic stimuli gradually build up the intensity of sexual excitement. During this process the vaginal walls become moist because of transudation of fluid through the congested mucous membrane. In addition, the greater vestibular glands at the vaginal orifice secrete a lubricating mucus.

The upper part of the vagina, which resides in the pelvic cavity, is supplied by the hypogastric plexuses and is sensitive only to stretch. The region of the vaginal orifice, the labia minora, and the clitoris are extremely sensitive to touch and are supplied by the ilioinguinal nerves and the dorsal nerves of the clitoris.

Appropriate sexual stimulation of these sensitive areas, reinforced by afferent nervous impulses from the breasts and other regions, results in a climax of pleasurable sensory impulses reaching the central nervous system. Impulses then pass down the spinal cord to the sympathetic outflow (T1 to L2).

The nervous impulses that pass to the genital organs are thought to leave the cord at the first and second lumbar segments in preganglionic sympathetic fibers. Many of these fibers synapse with postganglionic neurons in the first and second lumbar ganglia; other fibers may synapse in ganglia in the lower lumbar or pelvic parts of the sympathetic trunks. The postganglionic fibers are then distributed to the smooth muscle of the vaginal wall, which rhythmically contracts. In addition, nervous impulses travel in the pudendal nerve (S2, 3, and 4) to reach the bulbospongiosus and ischiocavernosus muscles, which also undergo rhythmic contraction. In many women, a single orgasm brings about sexual contentment, but other women require a series of orgasms to feel replete.

Female Urethra

The female urethra is about 1.5 in. (3.8 cm) long. It extends from the neck of the bladder to the **external meatus,** where it opens into the vestibule about 1 in. (2.5 cm) below the clitoris (Figs. 8-4 and 8-18). It traverses the sphincter urethrae and lies immediately in front of the vagina. At the sides of the external urethral meatus are the small openings of the ducts of the paraurethral glands. The urethra can be dilated relatively easily.

Paraurethral Glands

The paraurethral glands, which correspond to the prostate in the male, open into the vestibule by small ducts on either side of the urethral orifice (Fig. 8-19).

Greater Vestibular Glands

The greater vestibular glands are a pair of small mucus-secreting glands that lie under cover of the posterior parts of the bulb of the vestibule and the labia majora (Figs. 8-15 and 8-18). Each drains its secretion into the vestibule by a small duct, which opens into the groove between the hymen and the posterior part of the labium minus (Fig. 8-19). These glands secrete a lubricating mucus during sexual intercourse.

Vagina

Location and Description

The vagina not only is the female genital canal but also serves as the excretory duct for the menstrual flow from the uterus and forms part of the birth canal. This muscular tube extends upward and backward between the vulva and the uterus (Fig. 8-4). It measures about 3 in. (8 cm) long. The cervix of the uterus pierces its anterior wall. The vaginal orifice in a virgin possesses a thin mucosal fold,

Table 8-1 Muscles of Perineum

Muscle	Origin	Insertion	Nerve Supply	Action
External anal sphincter				
Subcutaneous part	Encircles anal canal, no bony attachments		Inferior rectal nerve and perineal branch of fourth sacral nerve	Together with puborectalis muscle forms voluntary sphincter of anal canal
Superficial part	Perineal body	Coccyx		
Deep part	Encircles anal canal, no bony attachments			
Puborectalis (part of levator ani)	Pubic bones	Sling around junction of rectum and anal canal	Perineal branch of fourth sacral nerve and from perineal branch of pudendal nerve	Together with external anal sphincter forms voluntary sphincter for anal canal
Male Urogenital Muscles				
Bulbospongiosus	Perineal body	Fascia of bulb of penis and corpus spongiosum and cavernosum	Perineal branch of pudendal nerve	Compresses urethra and assists in erection of penis
Ischiocavernosus	Ischial tuberosity	Fascia covering corpus cavernosum	Perineal branch of pudendal nerve	Assists in erection of penis
Sphincter urethrae	Pubic arch	Surrounds urethra	Perineal branch of pudendal nerve	Voluntary sphincter of urethra
Superficial transverse perineal muscle	Ischial tuberosity	Perineal body	Perineal branch of pudendal nerve	Fixes perineal body
Deep transverse perineal muscle	Ischial ramus	Perineal body	Perineal branch of pudendal nerve	Fixes perineal body
Female Urogenital Muscles				
Bulbospongiosus	Perineal body	Fascia of corpus cavernosum	Perineal branch of pudendal nerve	Sphincter of vagina and assists in erection of clitoris
Ischiocavernosus	Ischial tuberosity	Fascia covering corpus cavernosum	Perineal branch of pudendal nerve	Causes erection of clitoris
Sphincter urethrae	Same as in male			
Superficial transverse perineal muscle	Same as in male			
Deep transverse perineal muscle	Same as in male			

called the **hymen,** which is perforated at its center. The upper half of the vagina lies above the pelvic floor within the pelvis between the bladder anteriorly and the rectum posteriorly; the lower half lies within the perineum between the urethra anteriorly and the anal canal posteriorly (Fig. 8-18).

Supports of the Vagina

- **Upper third:** Levatores ani muscles and transverse cervical, pubocervical, and sacrocervical ligaments
- **Middle third:** Urogenital diaphragm
- **Lower third:** Perineal body

Blood Supply

Arteries

The vaginal artery, a branch of the internal iliac artery, and the vaginal branch of the uterine artery supply the vagina.

Veins

Vaginal veins drain into the internal iliac veins.

Lymph Drainage

- **Upper third:** Internal and external iliac nodes
- **Middle third:** Internal iliac nodes
- **Lower third:** Superficial inguinal nodes

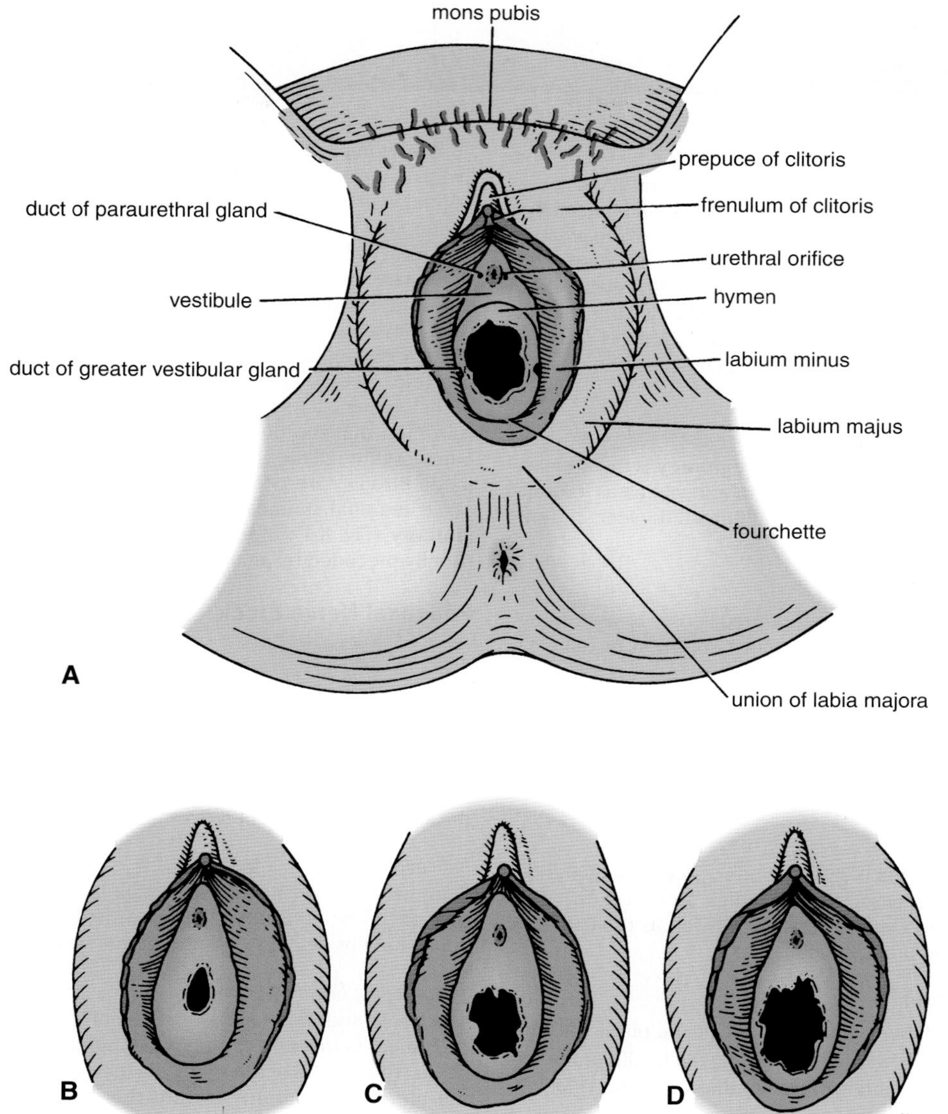

Figure 8-19 **A.** Vulva. Note the different appearances of the hymen in a virgin (**B**), a woman who has had sexual intercourse (**C**), and a multiparous woman (**D**).

Nerve Supply

The vagina is supplied by nerves from the inferior hypogastric plexuses.

Vulva

The term **vulva** is the collective name for the female external genitalia and includes the mons pubis, labia majora and minora, the clitoris, the vestibule of the vagina, the vestibular bulb, and the greater vestibular glands.

Blood Supply

Branches of the external and internal pudendal arteries on each side

The skin of the vulva is drained into the medial group of superficial inguinal nodes.

Lymph Drainage

Medial group of superficial inguinal nodes

Nerve Supply

The anterior parts of the vulva are supplied by the ilioinguinal nerves and the genital branch of the genitofemoral nerves. The posterior parts of the vulva are supplied by the branches of the perineal nerves and the posterior cutaneous nerves of the thigh.

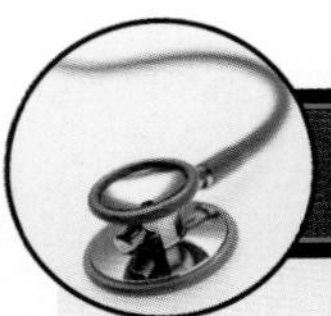

CLINICAL NOTES

Vulval Infection

In the region of the vulva, the presence of numerous glands and ducts opening onto the surface makes this area prone to infection. The sebaceous glands of the labia majora, the ducts of the greater vestibular glands, the vagina (with its indirect communication with the peritoneal cavity), the urethra, and the paraurethral glands can all become infected. The vagina itself has no glands and is lined with stratified squamous epithelium. Provided that the pH of its interior is kept low, it is capable of resisting infection to a remarkable degree.

The Vulva and Pregnancy

An important sign in the **diagnosis of pregnancy** is the appearance of a bluish discoloration of the vulva and vagina as a result of venous congestion. It appears at the 8th to 12th week and increases as the pregnancy progresses.

Urethral Infection

The short length of the female urethra predisposes to ascending infection; consequently, **cystitis** is more common in females than in males.

Urethral Injuries

Because of the short length of the urethra, injuries are rare. In fractures of the pelvis the urethra may be damaged by shearing forces as it emerges from the fixed urogenital diaphragm.

Catheterization

Because the female urethra is shorter, wider, and more dilatable, catheterization is much easier than in males. Moreover, the urethra is straight, and only minor resistance is felt as the catheter passes through the urethral sphincter.

Vaginal Examination

Digital examination of the vagina may provide the physician with much valuable information concerning the health of the vaginal walls, the uterus, and the surrounding structures (Fig. 8-4). Thus, the anatomic relations of the vagina must be known; they are considered in detail in Chapter 7.

Injury to the Perineum During Childbirth

The **perineal body** is a wedge of fibromuscular tissue that lies between the lower part of the vagina and the anal canal. It is held in position by the insertion of the perineal muscles and by the attachment of the levator ani muscles. In the female, it is a much larger structure than in the male, and it serves to support the posterior wall of the vagina. Damage by laceration during childbirth can be followed by permanent weakness of the pelvic floor.

Few women escape some injury to the birth canal during delivery. In most, this is little more than an abrasion of the posterior vaginal wall. Spontaneous delivery of the child with the patient unattended can result in a severe tear of the lower third of the posterior wall of the vagina, the perineal body, and overlying skin. In severe tears, the lacerations may extend backward into the anal canal and damage the external sphincter. In these cases, it is imperative that an accurate repair of the walls of the anal canal, vagina, and perineal body be undertaken as soon as possible.

In the management of childbirth, when it is obvious to the obstetrician that the perineum will tear before the baby's head emerges through the vaginal orifice, a planned surgical incision is made through the perineal skin in a posterolateral direction to avoid the anal sphincters. This procedure is known as an **episiotomy** (Fig. 8-4). Breech deliveries and forceps deliveries are usually preceded by an episiotomy.

Pudendal Nerve Block

Area of Anesthesia

The area anesthetized is the skin of the perineum; this nerve block does not, however, abolish sensation from the anterior part of the perineum, which is innervated by the ilioinguinal nerve and the genitofemoral nerve. Needless to say, it does not abolish pain from uterine contractions that ascend to the spinal cord via the sympathetic afferent nerves.

Indications

During the second stage of a difficult labor, when the presenting part of the fetus, usually the head, is descending through the vulva, forceps delivery and episiotomy may be necessary.

Transvaginal Procedure

The bony landmark used is the ischial spine (Fig. 8-20). The index finger is inserted through the vagina to palpate the ischial spine. The needle of the syringe is then passed through the vaginal mucous membrane toward the ischial spine. On passing through the sacrospinous ligament, the anesthetic solution is injected around the pudendal nerve (Fig. 8-20).

Perineal Procedure

The bony landmark is the ischial tuberosity (Fig. 8-20). The tuberosity is palpated subcutaneously through the buttock, and the needle is introduced into the pudendal canal along the medial side of the tuberosity. The canal lies about 1 in. (2.5 cm) deep to the free surface of the ischial tuberosity. The local anesthetic is then infiltrated around the pudendal nerve.

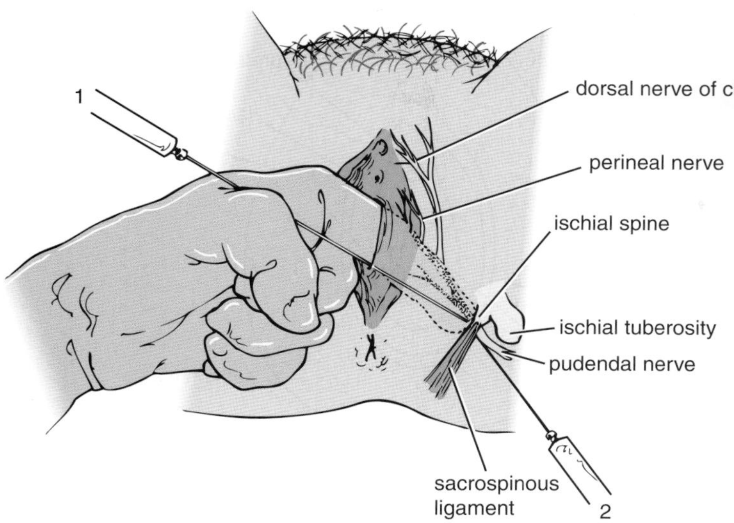

Figure 8-20 Pudendal nerve block. *1,* Transvaginal method. The needle is passed through the vaginal mucous membrane toward the ischial spine. After the needle is passed through the sacrospinous ligament, the anesthetic solution is injected around the pudendal nerve. *2,* Perineal method. The ischial tuberosity is palpated subcutaneously through the buttock. The needle is inserted on the medial side of the ischial tuberosity to a depth of about 1 in. (2.5 cm) from the free surface of the tuberosity. The anesthetic is injected around the pudendal nerve.

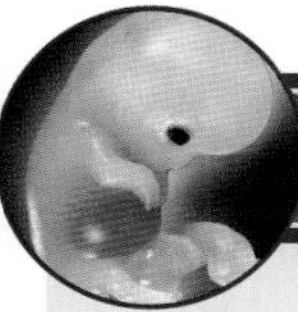

EMBRYOLOGIC NOTES

Development of the External Genitalia

Early in development, the embryonic mesenchyme grows around the cloacal membrane and causes the overlying ectoderm to be raised up to form three swellings. One swelling occurs between the cloacal membrane and the umbilical cord in the midline and is called the **genital tubercle** (Fig. 8-21). On each side of the membrane, another swelling, called the **genital fold,** appears. At the seventh week, the genital tubercle elongates to form the glans. The anterior part of the cloacal membrane, the **urogenital membrane,** now ruptures so that the urogenital sinus opens onto the surface. The entodermal cells of the urogenital sinus proliferate and grow into the root of the phallus, forming a **urethral plate.** Meanwhile, a second pair of lateral swellings, called the **genital swellings,** appears lateral to the genital folds. At this stage of development, the genitalia of the two sexes are identical.

Male Genitalia

In the male, the phallus now rapidly elongates and pulls the genital folds anteriorly onto its ventral surface so that they form the lateral edges of a groove, the **urethral groove** (Fig. 8-22). The floor of the groove is formed by the entodermal **urethral plate.** The penile urethra develops as the result of the two genital folds fusing together progressively along the shaft of the phallus to the root of the glans penis. During the fourth month, the remainder of the urethra in the glans is developed from a bud of ectodermal cells from the tip of the glans. This cord of cells later becomes canalized so that the penile urethra opens at the tip of the glans.

The **prepuce** or **foreskin** is formed from a fold of skin at the base of the glans (Figs. 8-21 and 8-22). The fold of skin remains tethered to the ventral aspect of the root of the glans to form the **frenulum.** The **erectile tissue**—the corpus spongiosum and the corpora cavernosa—develops within the mesenchymal core of the penis.

Female Genitalia

The changes in the female are less extensive than those in the male. The phallus becomes bent and forms the **clitoris** (Fig. 8-21). The genital folds do not fuse to form the urethra, as in the male, but develop into the **labia minora.** The **labia majora** are formed by the enlargement of the genital swellings.

Meatal Stenosis

The external urinary meatus normally is the narrowest part of the male urethra, but occasionally the opening is excessively small and may cause back pressure effect on the entire urinary system. In severe cases, dilatation of the orifice by incision is necessary.

Hypospadias

Hypospadias is the most common congenital anomaly affecting the male urethra. The external meatus is situated on the ventral or undersurface of the penis anywhere between the glans and the perineum. Five degrees of severity may occur, the first of which is the most common: (1) glandular, (2) coronal, (3) penile, (4) penoscrotal, and (5) perineal (Fig. 8-23). In all except the first type, the penis is curved in a downward or ventral direction, a condition referred to as **chordee.**

Types 1 and 2 are caused by a failure of the bud of ectodermal cells from the tip of the glans to grow into the substance of the glans and join the entodermal cells lining the penile urethra. Types 3, 4, and 5 are caused by a failure of the genital folds to unite on the undersurface of the developing penis and so convert the urethral groove into the penile urethra. In the penoscrotal variety, the genital swellings fail to fuse completely, so that the meatal orifice occurs in the midline of the scrotum. Type 1 requires no treatment; for the remainder, plastic surgery is necessary.

Epispadias

Epispadias is a relatively rare condition and is more commonly found in the male. In the male, the external meatus is situated on the dorsal or upper surface of the penis between the glans and the anterior abdominal wall (Fig. 8-24). The most severe type is associated with exstrophy of the bladder (see page 361). In the female, the urethra is split dorsally and is associated with a double clitoris. It is thought that epispadias is caused by failure of the embryonic mesenchyme to develop in the lower part of the anterior abdominal wall, so that when the cloacal membrane breaks down the urogenital sinus opens onto the surface of the cranial aspect of the penis. Plastic surgery is the required treatment

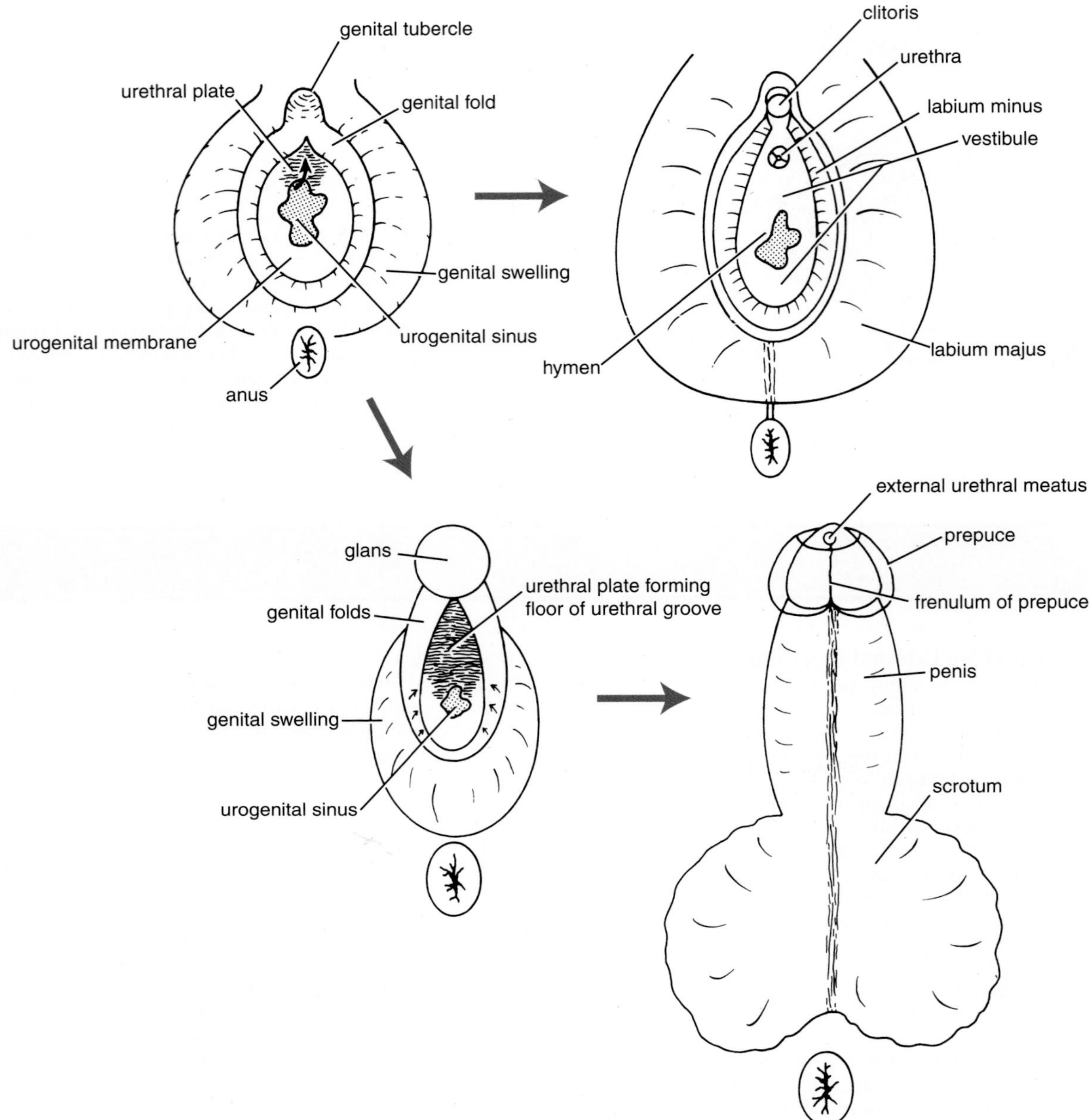

Figure 8-21 The development of the external genitalia in the female and male.

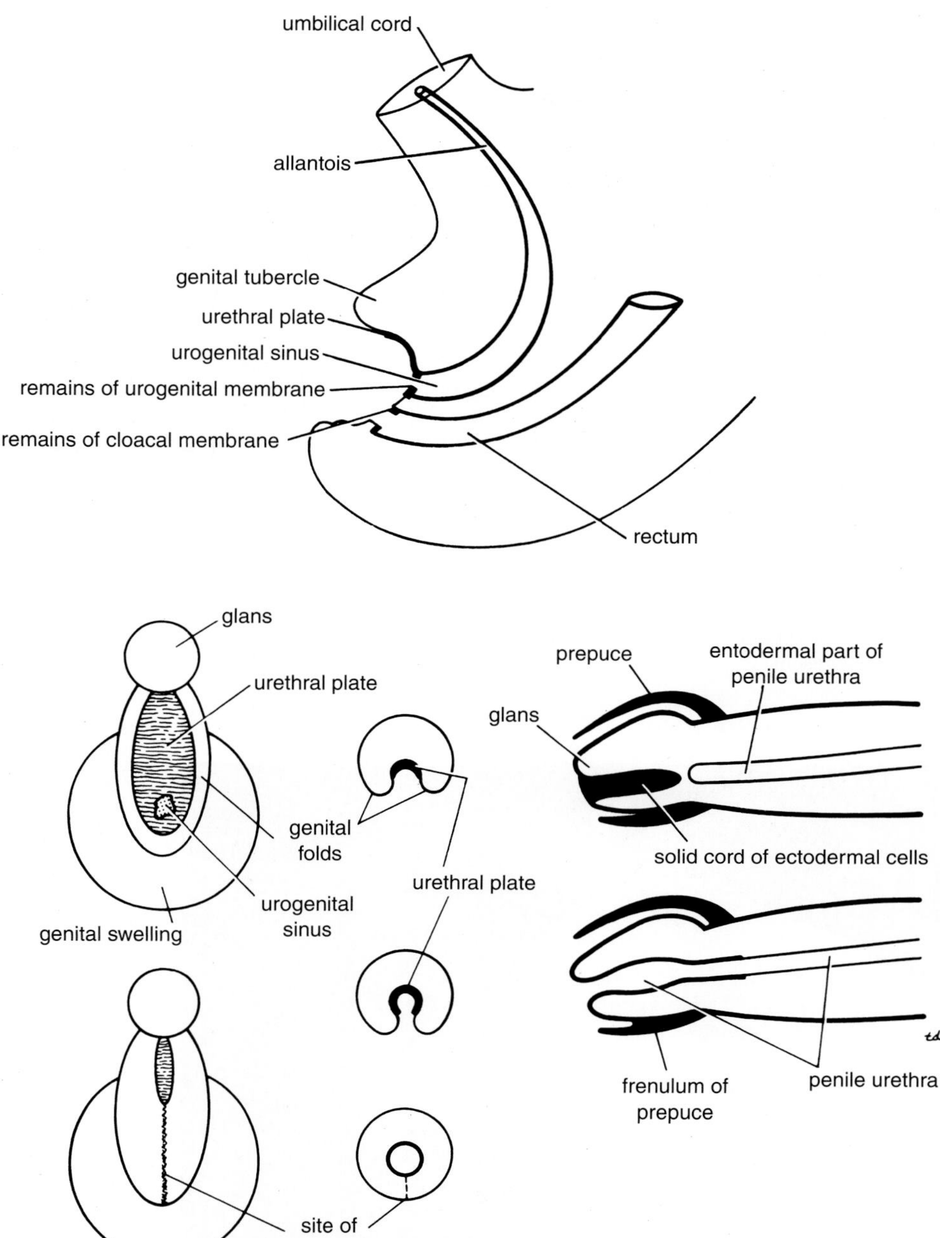

Figure 8-22 The development of the penile portion of the male urethra.

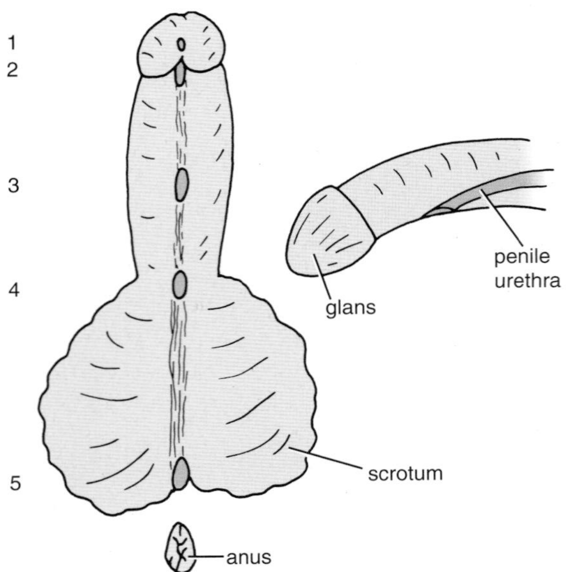

Figure 8-23 Types of hypospadias: (*1*) glandular, (*2*) coronal, (*3*) penile, (*4*) penoscrotal, and (*5*) perineal. Ventral flexion (chordee) of the penis also is present.

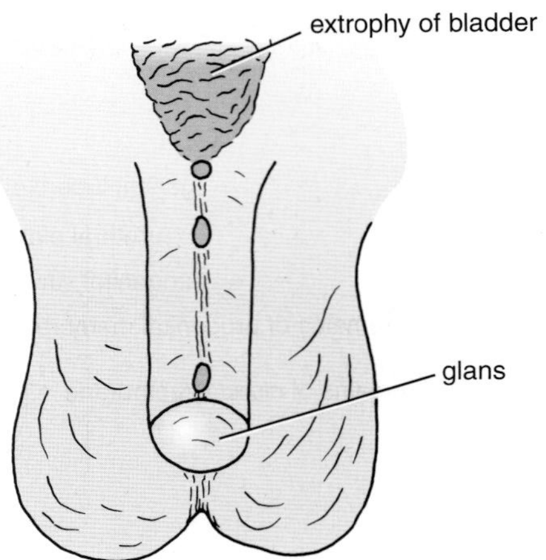

Figure 8-24 Types of epispadias.

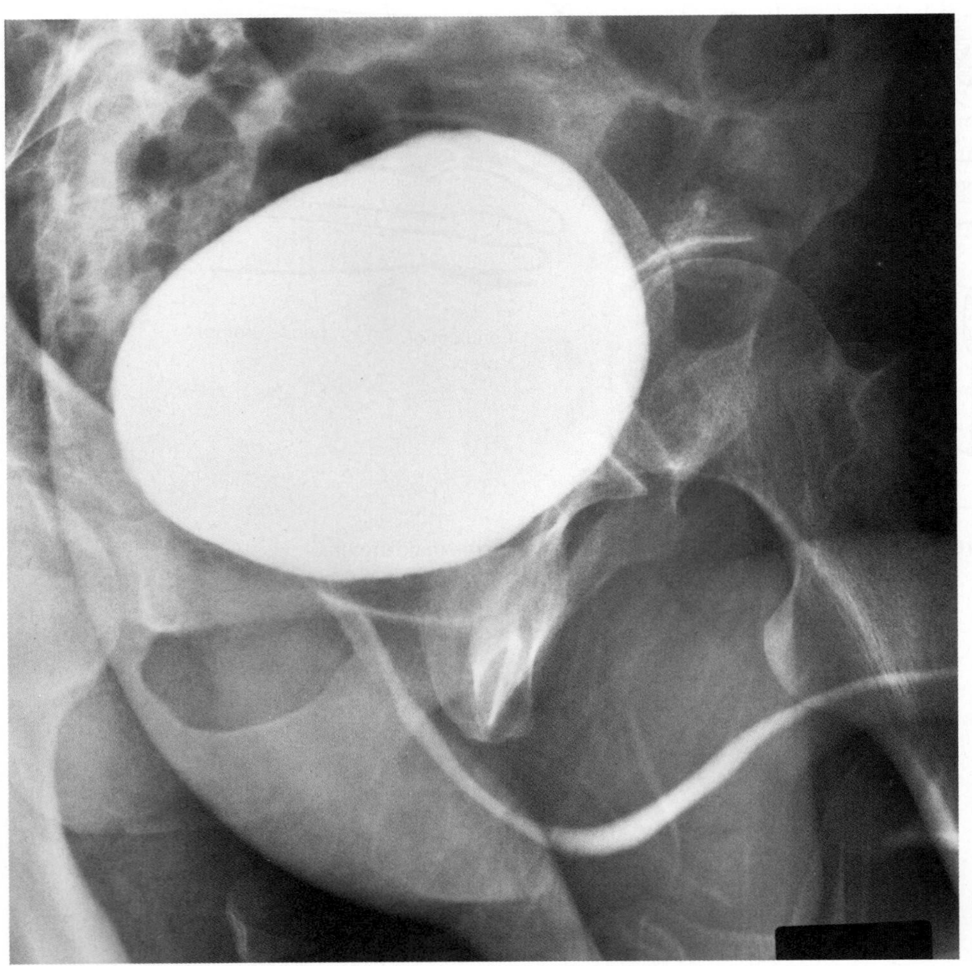

Figure 8-25 Cystourethrogram after intravenous injection of contrast medium (28-year-old man).

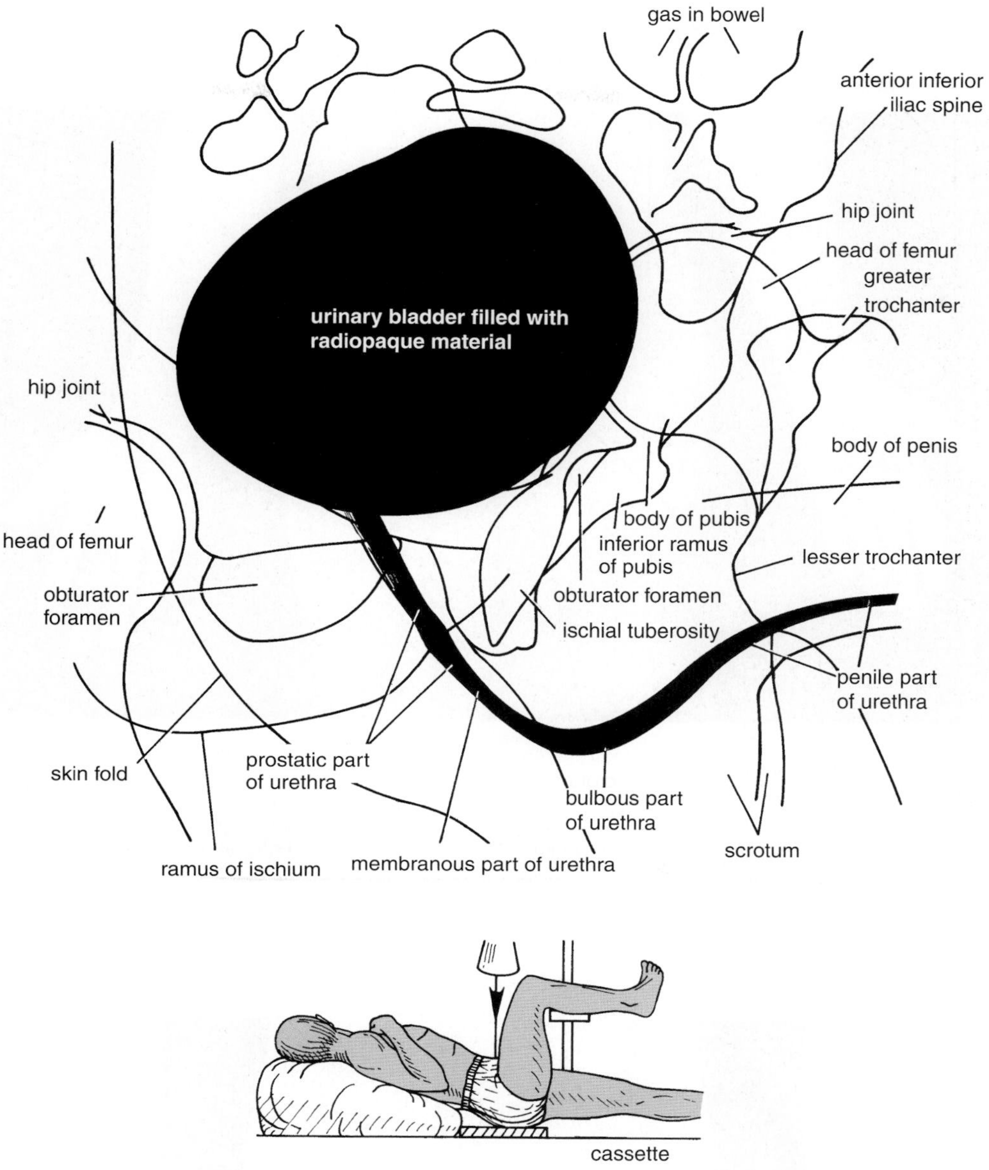

Figure 8-26 The main features seen in the cystourethrogram shown in Figure 8-25.

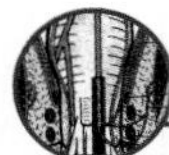

Radiographic Anatomy

The radiographic anatomy of the bones forming the boundaries of the perineum is shown in Figures 7-39, 7-41, and 7-43. A cystourethrogram of the male urethra is shown in Figures 8-25 and 8-26.

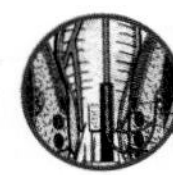

Surface Anatomy

The perineum when seen from below with the thighs abducted (Fig. 8-2) is diamond shaped and is bounded anteriorly by the **symphysis pubis,** posteriorly by the tip of the **coccyx,** and laterally by the **ischial tuberosities.**

Symphysis Pubis

The symphysis pubis is the cartilaginous joint that lies in the midline between the bodies of the pubic bones (Figs. 8-3, 8-27, and 8-28). It is felt as a solid structure beneath the skin in the midline at the lower extremity of the anterior abdominal wall.

Coccyx

The inferior surface and tip of the coccyx can be palpated in the cleft between the buttocks about 1 in. (2.5 cm) behind the anus (Fig. 8-3).

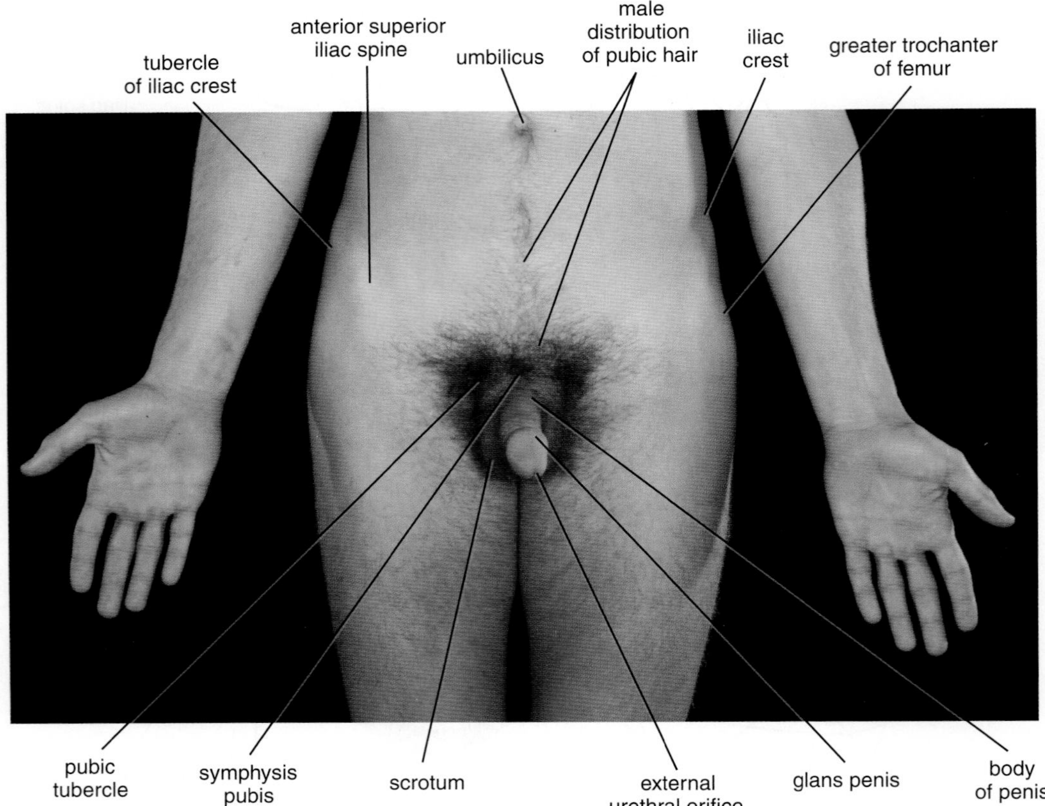

Figure 8-27 Anterior view of the pelvis of a 27-year-old man.

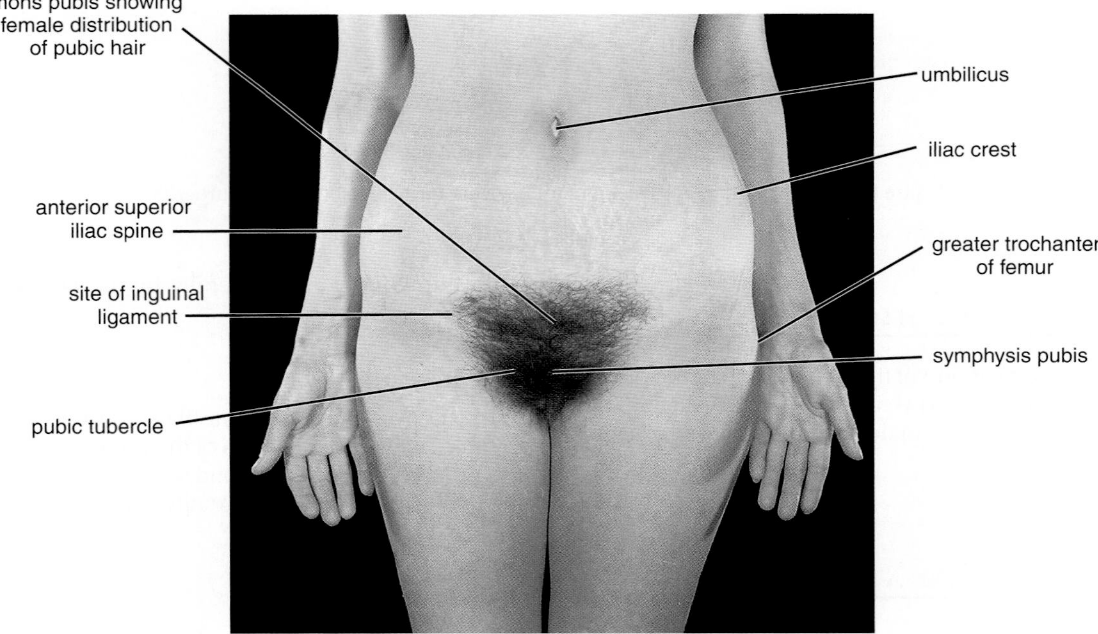

Figure 8-28 Anterior view of the pelvis of a 29-year-old woman.

Ischial Tuberosity

The ischial tuberosity can be palpated in the lower part of the buttock (Fig. 8-3). In the standing position, the tuberosity is covered by the gluteus maximus. In the sitting position, the ischial tuberosity emerges from beneath the lower border of the gluteus maximus and supports the weight of the body.

It is customary to divide the perineum into two triangles by joining the ischial tuberosities with an imaginary line (Fig. 8-2). The posterior triangle, which contains the anus, is called the **anal triangle;** the anterior triangle, which contains the urogenital orifices, is called the **urogenital triangle.**

Anal Triangle

Anus

The anus is the lower opening of the anal canal and lies in the midline. In the living the anal margin is reddish brown and is puckered by the contraction of the **external anal sphincter.** Around the anal margin are coarse hairs (Fig. 8-29).

Male Urogenital Triangle

The male urogenital triangle contains the penis and the scrotum.

Penis

The penis consists of a root, a body, and a glans (Figs. 8-13, 8-16, and 8-27). The **root of the penis** consists of three masses of erectile tissue called the **bulb of the penis** and the **right** and **left crura of the penis.** The bulb can be felt on deep palpation in the midline of the perineum, posterior to the scrotum.

The **body of the penis** is the free portion of the penis, which is suspended from the symphysis pubis. Note that the dorsal surface (anterior surface of the flaccid organ) usually possesses a **superficial dorsal vein** in the midline (Figs. 8-13).

The **glans penis** forms the extremity of the body of the penis (Figs. 8-13, 8-16, and 8-27). At the summit of the glans is the **external urethral meatus.** Extending from the lower margin of the external meatus is a fold connecting the glans to the prepuce called the **frenulum.** The edge of the base of the glans is called the **corona** (Fig. 8-16). The **prepuce** or **foreskin** is formed by a fold of skin attached to the neck of the penis. The prepuce covers the glans for a variable extent, and it should be possible to retract it over the glans.

Scrotum

The scrotum is a sac of skin and fascia (Figs. 8-12 and 8-27) containing the testes and the epididymides. The skin of the scrotum is rugose and is covered with sparse hairs. The bilateral origin of the scrotum is indicated by the presence of a dark line in the midline, called the **scrotal raphe,** along the line of fusion.

Testes

The testes should be palpated. They are oval shaped and have a firm consistency. They lie free within the tunica vaginalis (see Fig. 4-21) and are not tethered to the subcutaneous tissue or skin.

Epididymides

Each epididymis can be palpated on the posterolateral surface of the testis. The epididymis is a long, narrow, firm structure having an expanded upper end or **head,** a **body,** and a pointed **tail** inferiorly (see Fig. 4-21). The cordlike **vas deferens** emerges from the tail and ascends medial to the epididymis to enter the spermatic cord at the upper end of the scrotum.

Female Urogenital Triangle

Vulva

Vulva is the term applied to the female external genitalia (Figs. 8-19, 8-28, and 8-29).

Mons Pubis

The mons pubis is the rounded, hair-bearing elevation of skin found anterior to the pubis (Figs. 8-19 and 8-28). The pubic hair in the female has an abrupt horizontal superior margin, whereas in the male it extends upward to the umbilicus.

Labia Majora

The labia majora are prominent, hair-bearing folds of skin extending posteriorly from the mons pubis to unite posteriorly in the midline (Figs. 8-19 and 8-29).

Labia Minora

The labia minora are two smaller, hairless folds of soft skin that lie between the labia majora (Fig. 8-19). Their posterior ends are united to form a sharp fold, the **fourchette.** Anteriorly, they split to enclose the clitoris, forming an anterior **prepuce** and a posterior **frenulum** (Figs. 8-19 and 8-29).

Vestibule

The vestibule is a smooth triangular area bounded laterally by the labia minora, with the clitoris at its apex and the fourchette at its base (Figs. 8-19 and 8-29).

Vaginal Orifice

The vaginal orifice is protected in virgins by a thin mucosal fold called the **hymen,** which is perforated at its center (Fig. 8-19). At the first coitus, the hymen tears, usually posteriorly or posterolaterally, and after childbirth only a few tags of the hymen remain (Fig. 8-19).

Orifices of the Ducts of the Greater Vestibular Glands

Small orifices, one on each side, are found in the groove between the hymen and the posterior part of the labium minus (Fig. 8-19).

Clitoris

This is situated at the apex of the vestibule anteriorly (Fig. 8-19). The **glans of the clitoris** is partly hidden by the **prepuce** (Fig. 8-29).

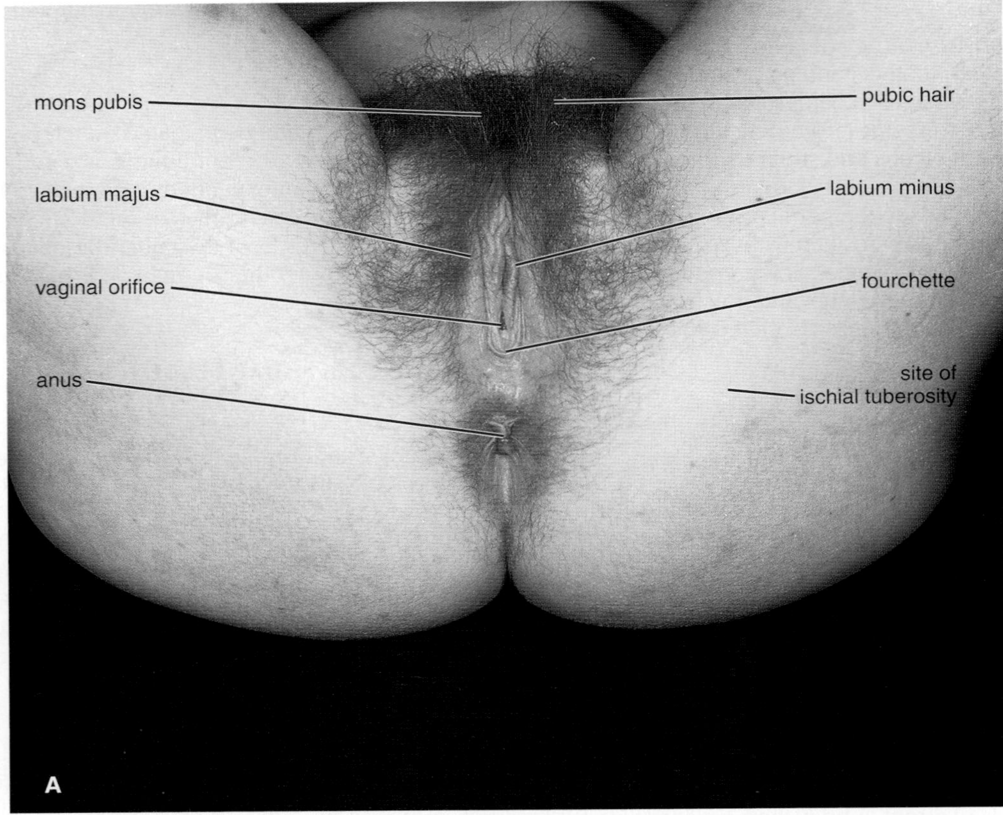

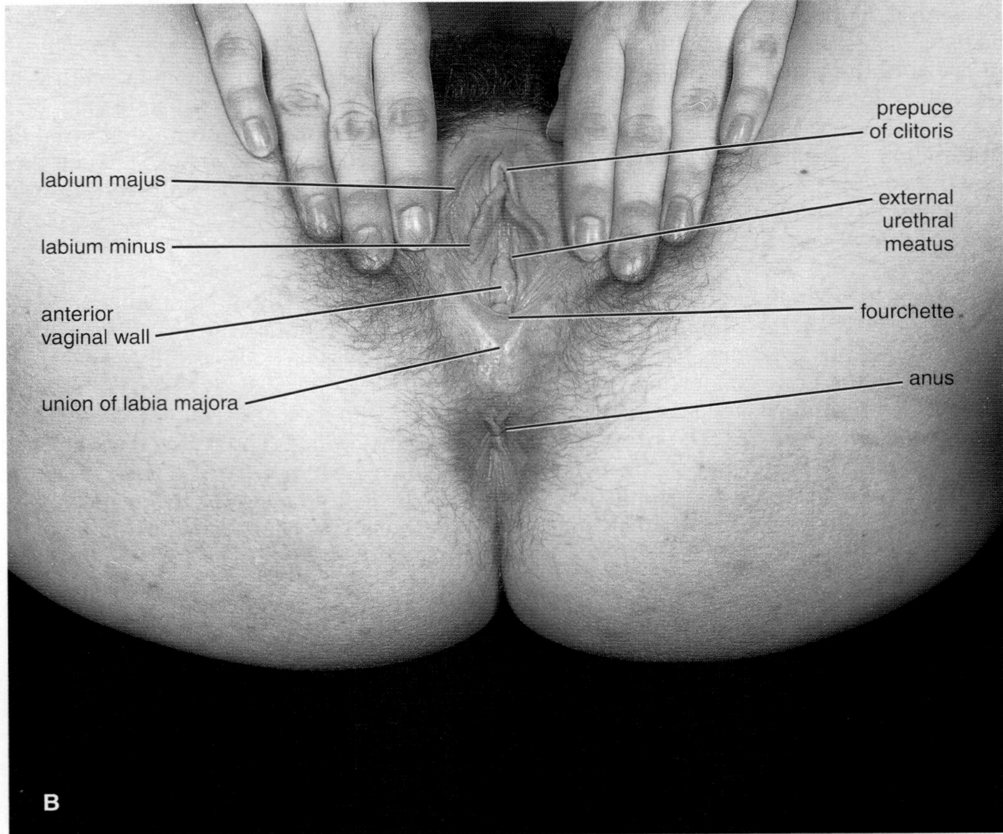

Figure 8-29 The perineum in a 25-year-old woman, inferior view. **A.** With labia together. **B.** With labia separated.

CLINICAL PROBLEM SOLVING

Read the following case histories and select the best answer to the question following them.

A 53-year-old man complained that for the past 4 years he had frequently passed blood-stained stools. Recently, he had noticed that his "bowel" protruded from his anus after defecation, and this caused him considerable discomfort.

1. The following symptoms and signs in this patient were consistent with a diagnosis of third-degree internal hemorrhoids except which?
   (a) The patient suffered from intense perianal irritation caused by the mucous secretions from the prolapsed mucous membrane.
   (b) Proctoscopic examination revealed three pink swellings of mucous membrane at the level of the anal valves.
   (c) The swellings were situated at 1, 4, and 9 o'clock with the patient in the lithotomy position.
   (d) The swellings bulged downward when the patient was asked to strain.
   (e) Large, congested veins were seen in the swellings.
   (f) The swellings remained outside the anus after defecation.
   (g) Abrasion of the mucous membrane was responsible for the bleeding.

A 42-year-old woman visited her physician because she experienced an agonizing pain in the rectum, which occurred on defecation. She had first noticed the pain a week before when she tried to defecate. The pain lasted for about an hour, then passed off, only to return with the next bowel movement. She said that she suffered from constipation and admitted that sometimes her stools were streaked with blood. After a careful examination, a diagnosis of anal fissure was made.

2. The following statements concerning this case are correct except which?
   (a) Examination of the anal canal was difficult because any attempt to insert a gloved finger into the canal caused severe pain.
   (b) The anus was kept tightly closed by the spasm of the external anal sphincter.
   (c) Gentle eversion of the anal margin under local anesthesia revealed the lower edge of a linear tear in the posterior wall of the anal canal; a small tag of skin projected from the lower end of the tear.
   (d) The forward edge of a hard fecal mass may have caught one of the anal valves and torn it downward as it descended.
   (e) Anal fissures tend to occur on the anterior and posterior walls of the anal canal because the mucous membrane is poorly supported in this region by the superficial external sphincter muscle.
   (f) The mucous membrane of the lower half of the anal canal is innervated by autonomic afferent nerves and is sensitive only to stretch.

A 16-year-old boy was taking part in a bicycle race when, on approaching a steep hill, he stood up on the pedals to increase the speed. His right foot slipped off the pedal and he fell violently, his perineum hitting the bar of the bicycle. Several hours later he was admitted to the hospital unable to micturate. On examination, he was found to have extensive swelling of the penis and scrotum. A diagnosis of ruptured urethra was made.

3. The following statements concerning this case are correct except which?
   (a) Rupture of the bulbous part of the urethra had taken place.
   (b) The urine had escaped from the urethra and extravasated into the superficial perineal pouch.
   (c) The urine had passed forward over the scrotum and penis to enter the anterior abdominal wall.
   (d) The urine had extended posteriorly into the ischiorectal fossae.
   (e) The urine was located beneath the membranous layer of superficial fascia.

A 34-year-old man was suffering from postoperative retention of urine after an appendectomy. The patient's urinary tract was otherwise normal. Because the patient was in considerable discomfort, the resident decided to pass a catheter.

4. The following statements concerning the catheterization of a male patient are correct except which?
   (a) Because the external urethral orifice is the narrowest part of the urethra, once the tip of the catheter has passed this point, the further passage should be easy.
   (b) Near the posterior end of the fossa terminalis, a fold of mucous membrane projects from the roof and may catch the end of the catheter.
   (c) The membranous part of the urethra is narrow and fixed and may produce some resistance to the passage of the catheter.
   (d) The prostatic part of the urethra is the widest and most easily dilated part of the urethra and should cause no difficulty to the passage of the catheter.
   (e) The bladder neck is surrounded by the sphincter vesicae and always strongly resists the passage of the tip of the catheter.

A 41-year-old woman was seen in the emergency department complaining of a painful swelling in the region of the anus. On examination, a hot, red, tender swelling was found on the right side of the anal margin. A diagnosis of ischiorectal abscess was made.

5. The following statements concerning this case are probably correct except which?
   (a) An ischiorectal abscess is a common complication of anal fissure.
   (b) The fat in the ischiorectal fossa is prone to infection that might extend laterally through the base of the anal fissure.

(c) The fat in the ischiorectal fossa has a profuse blood supply.
(d) A surgical incision of the abscess should provide adequate drainage of the pus.
(e) The surgeon should avoid the inferior rectal nerve and vessels that cross the ischiorectal fossa from the lateral to the medial side.

A 35-year-old woman was seen by her obstetrician and gynecologist complaining of a swelling in the genital region. On examination, a tense cystic swelling was found beneath the posterior two thirds of the right labium majus and minus. A diagnosis of a cyst of the right greater vestibular gland (Bartholin's cyst) was made.

6. The following statements concerning this case are probably correct except which?
   (a) The cyst of the greater vestibular gland is produced by the retention of secretion caused by the blockage of the duct.
   (b) Infection of the duct by the gonococcus is a common cause of the blockage.
   (c) Infection of the cyst may occur, forming a painful abscess.
   (d) The lymphatic drainage of this area is into the lateral group of superficial inguinal nodes.
   (e) A small tender swelling was detected below and medial to the inguinal ligament.

ANSWERS TO CLINICAL PROBLEMS

1. C. The swellings of internal hemorrhoids are situated at 3, 7, and 11 o'clock with the patient in the lithotomy position. These swellings are caused by a dilatation of the three main tributaries of the superior rectal vein.
2. F. The mucous membrane of the lower half of the anal canal is innervated by the inferior rectal nerve and is very sensitive to pain, temperature, touch, and pressure.
3. D. The superficial perineal pouch is closed off posteriorly by the attachment of the membranous layer of superficial fascia to the posterior margin of the urogenital diaphragm. Because of this attachment the extravasated urine cannot enter the ischiorectal fossae.
4. E. The bladder neck does not cause obstruction to the passage of the catheter. In this patient, the sphincter may provide some minor resistance that is easily overcome.
5. C. The fat in the ischiorectal fossa has a poor blood supply.
6. D. The lymphatic drainage of this area is into the medial group of superficial inguinal nodes situated below the inguinal ligament. The spread of infection can result in an enlargement of one of the nodes, as in this case, which becomes tender to palpation.

REVIEW QUESTIONS

Multiple-Choice Questions

Select the best answer for each question.

1. The following statements concerning the female urethra are correct except which?
   (a) It lies immediately anterior to the vagina.
   (b) Its external orifice lies about 2 in. (5 cm) from the clitoris.
   (c) It is about 1.5 in. (3.75 cm) long.
   (d) It pierces the urogenital diaphragm.
   (e) It is straight, and only minor resistance is felt as a catheter is passed through the urethral sphincter.
2. The following structures can be palpated by a vaginal examination except which?
   (a) Sigmoid colon
   (b) Ureters
   (c) Perineal body
   (d) Ischial spines
   (e) Iliopectineal line
3. The following statements concerning the ischiorectal fossa are correct except which?
   (a) The pudendal nerve lies in its lateral wall.
   (b) The floor is formed by the superficial fascia and skin.
   (c) The lateral wall is formed by the obturator internus muscle and its fascia.
   (d) The medial wall is formed in part by the levator ani muscles.
   (e) The roof is formed by the urogenital diaphragm.
4. The following statements concerning the penis are correct except which?
   (a) Its root is formed in the midline by the bulb of the penis, which continues anteriorly as the corpus spongiosum.
   (b) Its roots laterally are formed by the crura, which continue anteriorly as the corpora cavernosa.
   (c) The penile urethra lies within the corpus spongiosum.

(d) The glans penis is a distal expansion of the fused corpora cavernosa.
(e) The penis is suspended from the lower part of the anterior abdominal wall by two condensations of deep fascia.

5. The following statements concerning perineal structures are correct except which?
   (a) The anorectal ring is formed by the subcutaneous, superficial, and deep fibers of the external anal sphincter.
   (b) The urogenital diaphragm is attached laterally to the inferior ramus of the pubis and the ischial ramus.
   (c) The bulbourethral glands are situated in the deep perineal pouch.
   (d) The anococcygeal body is rarely damaged in childbirth.
   (e) The lymph drainage of the skin around the anus is into the medial group of superficial inguinal nodes.
6. The urogenital diaphragm is formed by the following structures except which?
   (a) Deep transverse perineal muscle
   (b) Perineal membrane
   (c) Sphincter urethrae
   (d) Colles' fascia (membranous layer of superficial fascia)
   (e) Parietal pelvic fascia covering the upper surface of the sphincter urethrae muscle
7. In the male, the following structures can be palpated on rectal examination except which?
   (a) Bulb of the penis
   (b) Urogenital diaphragm
   (c). Anorectal ring
   (d) The anterior surface of the sacrum
   (e) Ureter
8. The following statements concerning the anal canal are correct except which?
   (a) It is about 1.5 in. (3.8 cm) long.
   (b) It pierces the urogenital diaphragm.
   (c) It is related laterally to the external anal sphincter.
   (d) It is the site of an important portal–systemic anastomosis.
   (e) The mucous membrane of the lower half receives its arterial supply from the inferior rectal artery.
9. The following statements concerning the subcutaneous part of the external anal sphincter are correct except which?
   (a) It encircles the anal canal.
   (b) It is not attached to the anococcygeal body.
   (c) It is composed of striated muscle fibers.
   (d) It is not responsible for causing the anal canal and rectum to join at an acute angle.
   (e) It is innervated by the middle rectal nerve.
10. The following statements concerning defecation are correct except which?
    (a) The act is often preceded by the entrance of feces into the rectum, which gives rise to the desire to defecate.
    (b) The muscles of the anterior abdominal wall contract.
    (c) The external anal sphincters and the puborectalis relax.
    (d) The internal sphincter contracts and causes the evacuation of the feces.
    (e) The mucous membrane of the lower part of the anal canal is extruded through the anus ahead of the fecal mass.
11. The process of ejaculation depends on the following processes except which?
    (a) The sphincter of the bladder contracts.
    (b) The sympathetic preganglionic nerve fibers arising from the first and second lumbar segments of the spinal cord must be intact.
    (c) The smooth muscle of the epididymis, ductus (vas) deferens, seminal vesicles, and prostate contracts.
    (d) The bulbourethral glands and the urethral glands are active.
    (e) The bulbospongiosus muscles relax.
12. The following structures receive innervation from branches of the pudendal nerve except which?
    (a) Labia minora
    (b) Urethral sphincter
    (c) The posterior fornix of the vagina
    (d) Ischiocavernosus muscles
    (e) Skin of the penis or clitoris

Read the case history and select the best answer to the questions following it.

While bathing her 5-month-old boy, a mother noticed that his penis tended to curve downward. She decided to seek advice from a pediatrician.

13. The pediatrician examined the child and made the following possible correct observations and statements except which?
    (a) The penis had a definite downward curvature (chordee).
    (b) Both testes were in the scrotum.
    (c) The external urethral meatus opened halfway along the undersurface of the penis.
    (d) The fusion of the genital folds on the ventral or undersurface of the shaft of the penis was incomplete so that the urethra opened on the ventral surface.
    (e) The condition is a rare congenital anomaly.
14. The pediatrician made the following possible correct statements to the mother regarding the diagnosis and treatment except which?
    (a) The child has hypospadias associated with chordee.
    (b) The proximal portion of the penile urethra had developed normally but was incomplete.
    (c) The bud of cells (ectodermal) on the tip of the glans penis had failed to grow into the substance of the glans and join up with the cells (entodermal cells) of the penile urethra.
    (d) The treatment is the surgical correction of the chordee, which is followed by the plastic reconstruction of the penile urethra.
    (e) In view of the delicate tissues involved, the treatment should be delayed until the child is at least 10 years old.

ANSWERS TO REVIEW QUESTIONS

1. B. The female urethra opens into the vestibule at the external meatus about 1 in. (2.5 cm) below the clitoris.
2. E. The iliopectineal line lies at the brim of the bony pelvis and is far beyond the reach of a vaginal examination.
3. E. The roof of the ischiorectal fossa is formed by the junction of the medial and lateral walls. The medial wall is formed by the sloping levator ani muscle, and the anal canal and the lateral wall are formed by the lower part of the obturator internus muscle, covered with pelvic fascia.
4. D. The glans penis is a distal expansion of the corpus spongiosum.
5. A. At the junction of the rectum and anal canal, the internal sphincter, the deep part of the external sphincter, and the puborectalis muscles form a distinct ring, called the anorectal ring.
6. D. Colles' fascia (membranous layer of superficial fascia) takes no part in the formation of the urogenital diaphragm; it is too superficial and lies just beneath the skin.
7. E. The ureters cannot be felt on rectal examination in both sexes. An abnormal ureter, thickened by disease, can be felt on vaginal examination.
8. B. The anal canal lies posterior to the urogenital diaphragm and, therefore, does not pierce it.
9. E. The subcutaneous part of the external anal sphincter is innervated by the inferior rectal nerve, which is a branch of the pudendal nerve.
10. D. The internal anal sphincter is relaxed during defecation.
11. E. During ejaculation, the bulbospongiosus muscles rhythmically contract and compress the urethra, forcing the seminal fluid out of the external meatus.
12. C. The posterior fornix of the vagina is innervated by the inferior hypogastric plexuses.
13. E. The clinical condition is one of the commonest congenital anomalies affecting the male urethra.
14. E. The surgical treatment should start at about the age of 2 years and be complete before the child goes to school. Little boys like to look the same as other little boys.

CHAPTER 9

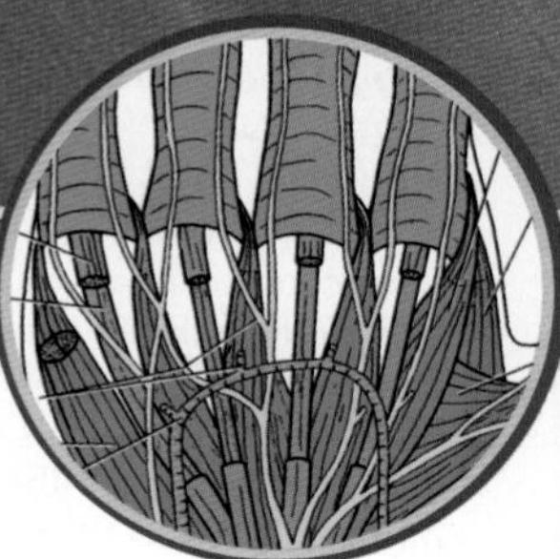

THE UPPER LIMB

A 64-year-old woman fell down the stairs and was admitted to the emergency department with severe left shoulder pain. While she was sitting up her left arm was by her side and her left elbow was flexed and supported by her right hand. Inspection of the left shoulder showed loss of the normal rounded curvature and evidence of a slight swelling below the left clavicle. The physician then systematically tested the cutaneous sensibility of the left upper limb and found severe sensory deficits involving the skin of the back of the arm down as far as the elbow, the lower lateral surface of the arm down to the elbow, the middle of the posterior surface of the forearm as far as the wrist, the lateral half of the dorsal surface of the hand, and the dorsal surface of the lateral three and a half fingers proximal to the nail beds.

A diagnosis of subcoracoid dislocation of the left shoulder joint was made, complicated by damage to the axillary and radial nerves. The head of the humerus was displaced downward to below the coracoid process of the scapula by the initial trauma and was displaced further by the pull of the muscles (subscapularis, pectoralis major). The loss of shoulder curvature was caused by the displacement of the humerus (greater tuberosity) medially so that it no longer pushed the overlying muscle (deltoid) laterally. The extensive loss of skin sensation to the left upper limb was the result of damage to the axillary and radial nerves.

For a physician to be able to make a diagnosis in this case and to be able to interpret the clinical findings, he or she must have considerable knowledge of the anatomy of the shoulder joint. Furthermore, the physician must know the relationship of the axillary and radial nerves to the joint and the distribution of these nerves to the parts of the upper limb.

CHAPTER OUTLINE

Basic Anatomy 427
The Pectoral Region and the Axilla 427
The Breasts 427
Bones of the Shoulder Girdle and Arm 432
The Axilla 437
Walls of the Axilla 437
Contents of the Axilla 444
The Superficial Part of the Back and the Scapular Region 454
Skin 454
Bones of the Back 454
Muscles 454
Rotator Cuff 454
Nerves 458
Arterial Anastomosis Around the Shoulder Joint 458
Sternoclavicular Joint 459
Acromioclavicular Joint 460
Shoulder Joint 462
The Scapular–Humeral Mechanism 465
The Upper Arm 465
Skin 465
Fascial Compartments of the Upper Arm 469
Contents of the Anterior Fascial Compartment of the Upper Arm 469
Contents of the Posterior Fascial Compartment of the Upper Arm 474
The Cubital Fossa 476
Bones of the Forearm 477
Bones of the Hand 480
The Forearm 482
Skin 482
Fascial Compartments of the Forearm 483
Interosseous Membrane 484
Flexor and Extensor Retinacula 484
Contents of the Anterior Fascial Compartment of the Forearm 485
Contents of the Lateral Fascial Compartment of the Forearm 495
Contents of the Posterior Fascial Compartment of the Forearm 495
The Region of the Wrist 499
Structures on the Anterior Aspect of the Wrist 499
Structures on the Posterior Aspect of the Wrist 499
The Palm of the Hand 499
Skin 499
Deep Fascia 500
The Palmar Aponeurosis 500
The Carpal Tunnel 500
Fibrous Flexor Sheaths 500
Synovial Flexor Sheaths 501
Insertion of the Long Flexor Tendons 502
Small Muscles of the Hand 502
Short Muscles of the Thumb 502
Short Muscles of the Little Finger 502
Arteries of the Palm 503
Veins of the Palm 504
Lymph Drainage of the Palm 504
Nerves of the Palm 505
Fascial Spaces of the Palm 508
Pulp Space of the Fingers 508
The Dorsum of the Hand 508
Skin 508
Dorsal Venous Arch 509
Insertion of the Long Extensor Tendons 509
The Radial Artery on the Dorsum of the Hand 509
Joints of the Upper Limb 509
Elbow Joint 509
Proximal Radioulnar Joint 512
Distal Radioulnar Joint 513
Wrist Joint (Radiocarpal Joint) 513
Joints of the Hand and Fingers 516
The Hand as a Functional Unit 517
Radiographic Anatomy 523
Radiographic Appearances of the Upper Limb 523
Surface Anatomy 523
Anterior Surface of the Chest 523
Suprasternal Notch 523
Sternal Angle (Angle of Louis) 523
Xiphisternal Joint 523
Costal Margin 523
Clavicle 523
Ribs 530
Deltopectoral Triangle 530
Axillary Folds 530
Axilla 530
Posterior Surface of the Chest 530
Spinous Processes of Cervical and Thoracic Vertebrae 530
Scapula 531
The Breast 531
The Elbow Region 533
The Wrist and Hand 533
Important Structures Lying in Front of the Wrist 533
Important Structures Lying on the Lateral Side of the Wrist 533
Important Structures Lying on the Back of the Wrist 535
Important Structures Lying in the Palm 535
Important Structures Lying on the Dorsum of the Hand 535
Clinical Notes on the Arteries of the Upper Limb 535
Clinical Notes on the Nerves of the Upper Limb 536
Clinical Problem Solving 542
Answers to Clinical Problems 544
Review Questions 545
Answers to Review Questions 547

CHAPTER OBJECTIVES

- Pain, fractures, dislocations, and nerve injuries of the upper limb are commonly seen by the physician. Wrist and hand injuries deserve particular attention because the goal is to preserve as much function as possible. The pincer action of the thumb and index finger and the unique ability of the thumb to be drawn across the palm to the other fingers must be preserved at all costs.
- A physician must be familiar with the nerves, bones, joints, tendons, and blood and lymphatic vessels and their anatomic relationships.
- The basic anatomy of the breast is of considerable clinical importance because of the frequent development of cancer in the glands and the subsequent dissemination of the malignant cells along the lymph vessels to the lymph nodes in the armpit.
- The primary concern of this chapter is to present to the student the basic anatomy of the upper limb so that as a practicing medical professional he or she will be able to make an accurate diagnosis and initiate prompt treatment.

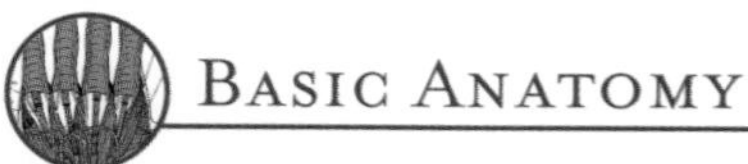

Basic Anatomy

The upper limb is a multijointed lever that is freely movable on the trunk at the shoulder joint. At the distal end of the upper limb is the prehensile organ, the hand. Much of the importance of the hand depends on the pincerlike action of the thumb, which enables one to grasp objects between the thumb and index finger.

The upper limb is divided into the shoulder (junction of the trunk with the arm), arm, elbow, forearm, wrist, and hand.

The Pectoral Region and the Axilla

The Breasts

Location and Description

The breasts are specialized accessory glands of the skin that secrete milk (Fig. 9-1). They are present in both sexes. In males and immature females, they are similar in structure. The **nipples** are small and surrounded by a colored area of skin called the **areola.** The breast tissue consists of a system of ducts embedded in connective tissue that does not extend beyond the margin of the areola.

Puberty

At puberty in females, the breasts gradually enlarge and assume their hemispherical shape under the influence of the ovarian hormones (Fig. 9-1). The ducts elongate, but the increased size of the glands is mainly from the deposition of fat. The base of the breast extends from the second to the sixth rib and from the lateral margin of the sternum to the midaxillary line. The greater part of the gland lies in the superficial fascia. A small part, called the **axillary tail** (Fig. 9-1), extends upward and laterally, pierces the deep fascia at the lower border of the pectoralis major muscle, and enters the axilla.

Each breast consists of 15 to 20 **lobes,** which radiate out from the nipple. The main duct from each lobe opens separately on the summit of the nipple and possesses a dilated **ampulla** just before its termination. The base of the nipple is surrounded by the **areola** (Fig. 9-1). Tiny tubercles on the areola are produced by the underlying **areolar glands.**

The lobes of the gland are separated by fibrous septa that serve as **suspensory ligaments** (Fig. 9-1). Behind the breasts is a space filled by loose connective tissue called the **retromammary space** (Fig. 9-1).

Young Women

In young women the breasts tend to protrude forward from a circular base.

Pregnancy

Early In the early months of pregnancy, there is a rapid increase in length and branching in the duct system (Fig. 9-2). The secretory alveoli develop at the ends of the smaller ducts and the connective tissue becomes filled with expanding and budding secretory alveoli. The vascularity of the connective tissue also increases to provide adequate nourishment for the developing gland. The nipple enlarges, and the areola becomes darker and more extensive as a result of increased deposits of melanin pigment in the epidermis. The areolar glands enlarge and become more active.

Late During the second half of pregnancy, the growth process slows. The breasts, however, continue to enlarge, mostly because of the distention of the secretory alveoli with the fluid secretion called **colostrum.**

Postweaning Once the baby has been weaned, the breasts return to their inactive state. The remaining milk is absorbed, the secretory alveoli shrink, and most of them disappear. The interlobular connective tissue thickens. The breasts and the nipples shrink and return nearly to their original size. The pigmentation of the areola fades, but the area never lightens to its original color.

Postmenopause

After the menopause, the breast atrophies (Fig. 9-2). Most of the secretory alveoli disappear, leaving behind the ducts. The amount of adipose tissue may increase or decrease. The breasts tend to shrink in size and become more pendulous. The atrophy after menopause is caused by an absence of ovarian estrogens and progesterone.

Blood Supply

Arteries

The branches to the breasts include the perforating branches of the internal thoracic artery and the intercostal arteries. The axillary artery also supplies the gland via its lateral thoracic and thoracoacromial branches.

Veins

The veins correspond to the arteries.

Lymph Drainage

The lymph drainage of the mammary gland is of great clinical importance because of the frequent development of cancer in the gland and the subsequent dissemination of the malignant cells along the lymph vessels to the lymph nodes.

The lateral quadrants of the breast drain into the anterior axillary or pectoral group of nodes (Fig. 9-3) (situated just posterior to the lower border of the pectoralis major muscle). The medial quadrants drain by means of vessels that pierce the intercostal spaces and enter the internal thoracic group of nodes (situated within the thoracic cavity along the course of the internal thoracic artery). A few lymph vessels follow the posterior intercostal arteries and drain posteriorly into the posterior intercostal nodes (situated along the course of the posterior intercostal arteries); some vessels communicate with the lymph vessels of the opposite breast and with those of the anterior abdominal wall.

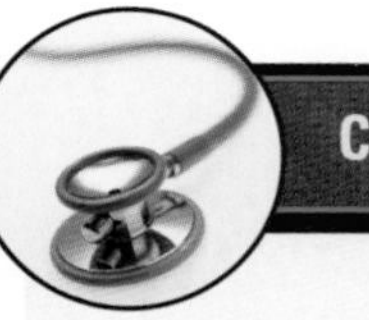

CLINICAL NOTES

Witch's Milk in the Newborn

While the fetus is in the uterus, the maternal and placental hormones cross the placental barrier and cause proliferation of the duct epithelium and the surrounding connective tissue. This proliferation may cause swelling of the mammary glands in both sexes during the first week of life; in some cases a milky fluid, called witch's milk, may be expressed from the nipples. The condition is resolved spontaneously as the maternal hormone levels in the child fall.

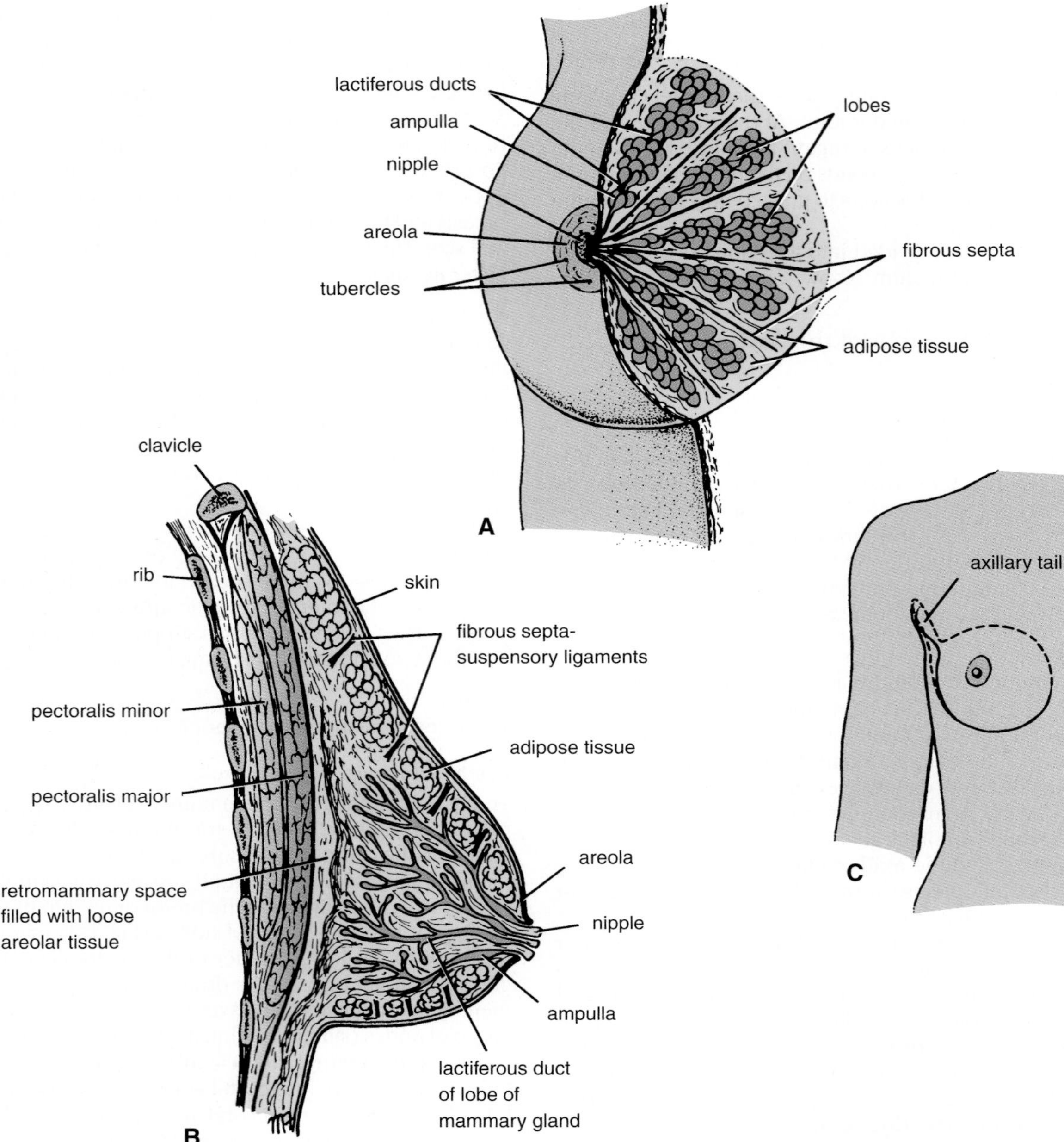

Figure 9-1 Mature breast in the female. **A.** Anterior view with skin partially removed to show internal structure. **B.** Sagittal section. **C.** The axillary tail, which pierces the deep fascia and extends into the axilla.

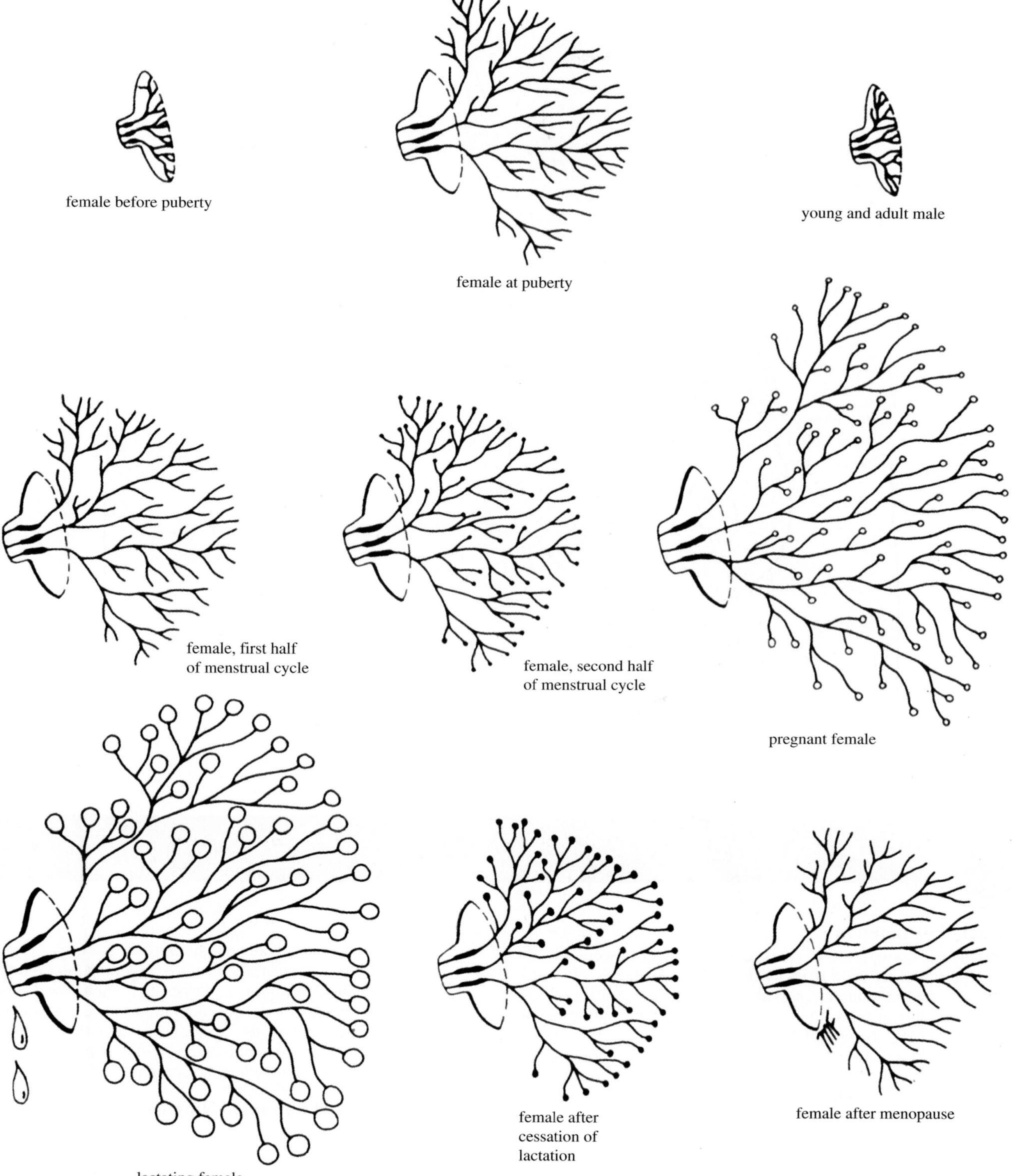

Figure 9-2 Extent of the development of the ducts and secretory alveoli in the breasts in both sexes at different stages of activity.

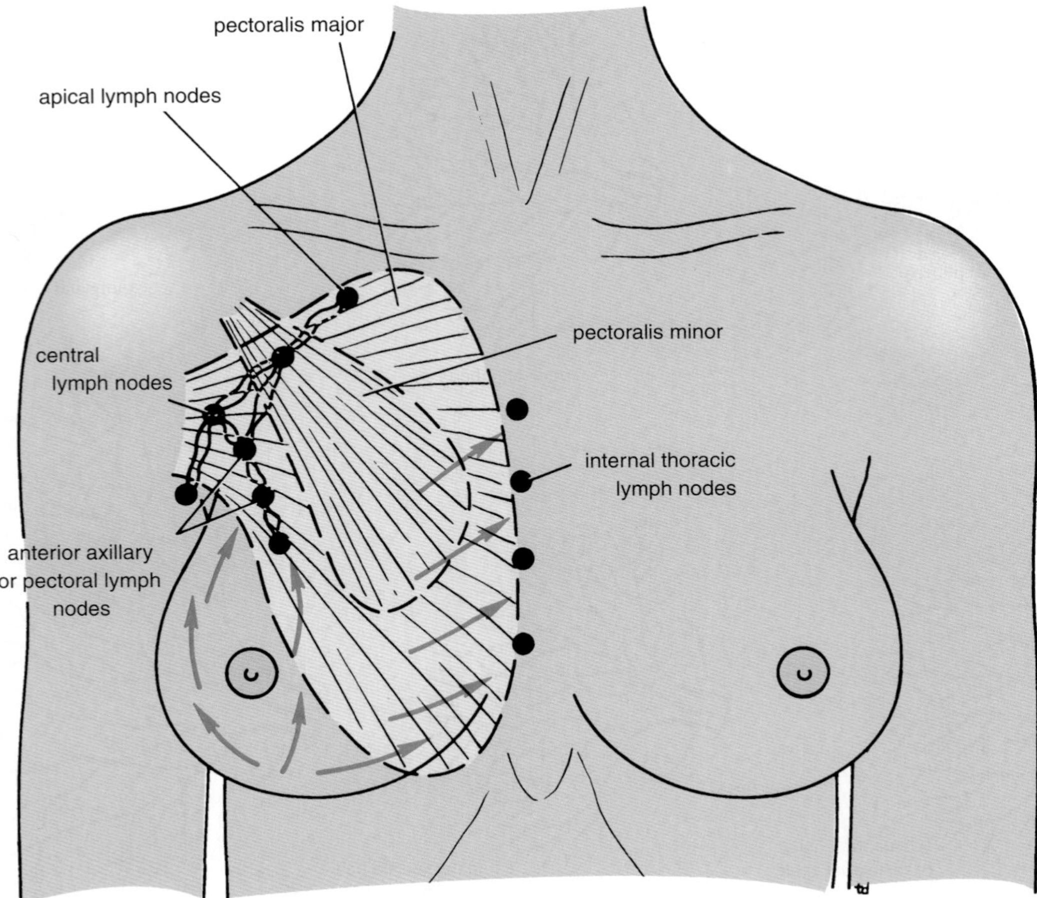

Figure 9-3 Lymph drainage of the breast.

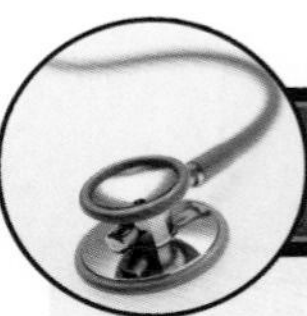

CLINICAL NOTES

Breast Examination

The breast is one of the common sites of cancer in women. It is also the site of different types of benign tumors and may be subject to acute inflammation and abscess formation. For these reasons, the clinical personnel must be familiar with the development, structure, and lymph drainage of this organ.

With the patient undressed to the waist and sitting upright, the breasts are first inspected for symmetry. Some degree of asymmetry is common and is the result of unequal breast development. Any swelling should be noted. A swelling can be caused by an underlying tumor, a cyst, or abscess formation. The nipples should be carefully examined for evidence of retraction. A carcinoma within the breast substance can cause retraction of the nipple by pulling on the lactiferous ducts. The patient is then asked to lie down so that the breasts can be palpated against the underlying thoracic wall. Finally, the patient is asked to sit up again and raise both arms above her head. With this maneuver, a carcinoma tethered to the skin, the suspensory ligaments, or the lactiferous ducts produces dimpling of the skin or retraction of the nipple.

Mammography

Mammography is a radiographic examination of the breast (Fig. 9-4). This technique is extensively used for screening the breasts for benign and malignant tumors and cysts. Extremely low doses of x-rays are used so that the dangers are minimal and the examination can be repeated often. Its success is based on the fact that a lesion measuring only a few millimeters in diameter can be detected long before it is felt by clinical examination.

Supernumerary and Retracted Nipples

Supernumerary nipples occasionally occur along a line extending from the axilla to the groin; they may or may not be associated with breast tissue (see page 432). This minor congenital anomaly may result in a mistaken diagnosis of warts or moles. A long-standing retracted nipple is a congenital deformity caused by a failure in the complete development of the nipple. A retracted nipple of recent occurrence is usually caused by an underlying carcinoma pulling on the lactiferous ducts.

(continues)

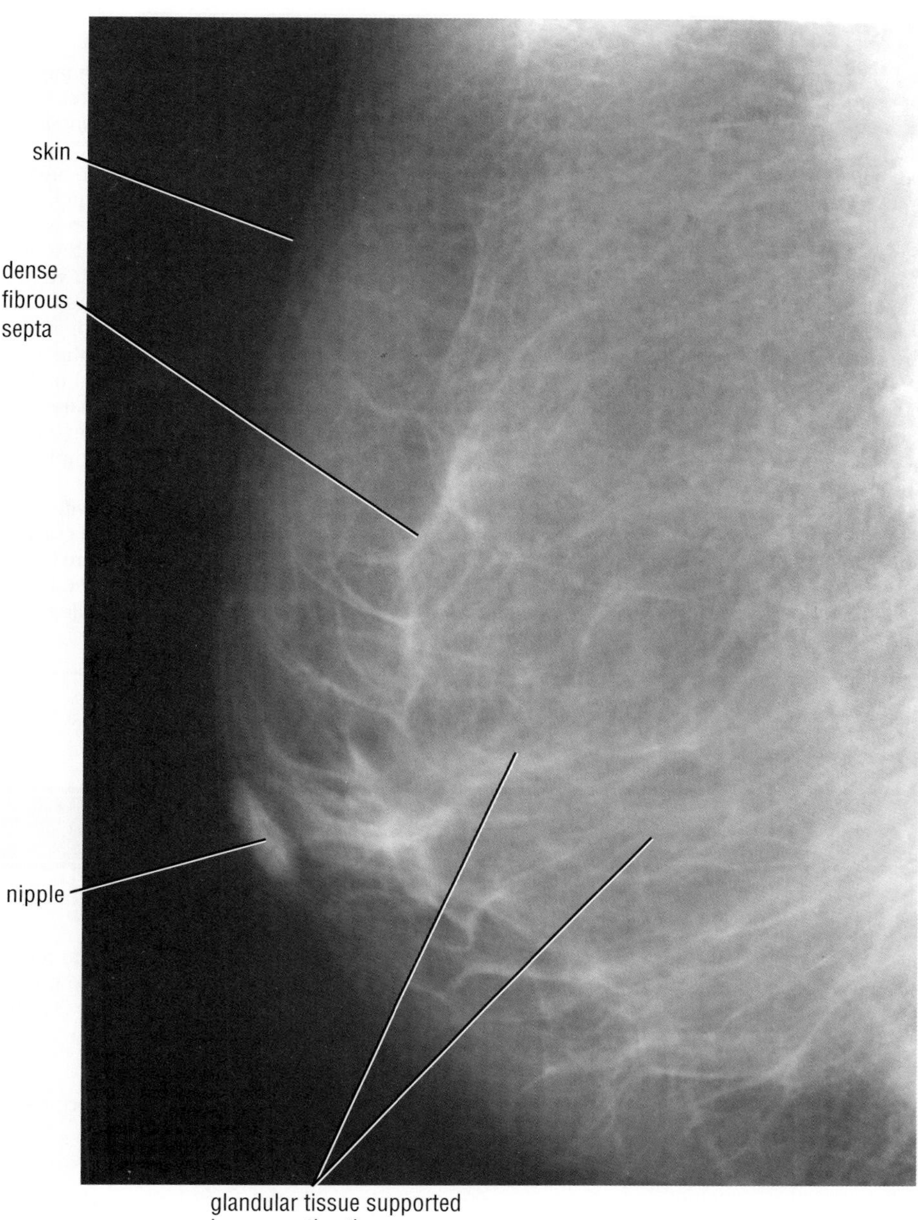

Figure 9-4 Mediolateral mammogram showing the glandular tissue supported by the connective tissue septa.

Clinical Notes, *continued*

The Importance of Fibrous Septa

The interior of the breast is divided into 15 to 20 compartments that radiate from the nipple by fibrous septa that extend from the deep surface of the skin. Each compartment contains a lobe of the gland. Normally, the skin feels completely mobile over the breast substance. However, should the fibrous septa become involved in a scirrhous carcinoma or in a disease such as a breast abscess, which results in the production of contracting fibrous tissue, the septa will be pulled on, causing dimpling of the skin. The fibrous septa are sometimes referred to as the suspensory ligaments of the mammary gland.

An acute infection of the mammary gland may occur during lactation. Pathogenic bacteria gain entrance to the breast tissue through a crack in the nipple. Because of the presence of the fibrous septa, the infection remains localized to one compartment or lobe to begin with. Abscesses should be drained through a radial incision to avoid spreading of the infection into neighboring compartments; a radial incision also minimizes the damage to the radially arranged ducts.

Lymph Drainage and Carcinoma of the Breast

The importance of knowing the lymph drainage of the breast in relation to the spread of cancer from that organ cannot be overemphasized. The lymph vessels from the medial quadrants of the breast pierce the second, third, and fourth intercostal spaces and enter the thorax to drain into the lymph nodes alongside the

(continues)

Clinical Notes, *continued*

internal thoracic artery. The lymph vessels from the lateral quadrants of the breast drain into the anterior or pectoral group of axillary nodes. It follows, therefore, that a cancer occurring in the lateral quadrants of the breast tends to spread to the axillary nodes. Thoracic metastases are difficult or impossible to treat, but the lymph nodes of the axilla can be removed surgically.

Approximately 60% of carcinomas of the breast occur in the upper lateral quadrant. The lymphatic spread of cancer to the opposite breast, to the abdominal cavity, or into lymph nodes in the root of the neck is caused by obstruction of the normal lymphatic pathways by malignant cells or destruction of lymph vessels by surgery or radiotherapy. The cancer cells are swept along the lymph vessels and follow the lymph stream. The entrance of cancer cells into the blood vessels accounts for the metastases in distant bones.

In patients with localized cancer of the breast, most surgeons do a simple mastectomy or a lumpectomy, followed by radiotherapy to the axillary lymph nodes and/or hormone therapy. In patients with localized cancer of the breast with early metastases in the axillary lymph nodes, most authorities agree that radical mastectomy offers the best chance of cure. In patients in whom the disease has already spread beyond these areas (e.g., into the thorax), simple mastectomy, followed by radiotherapy or hormone therapy, is the treatment of choice.

Radical mastectomy is designed to remove the primary tumor and the lymph vessels and nodes that drain the area. This means that the breast and the associated structures containing the lymph vessels and nodes must be removed en bloc. The excised mass is therefore made up of the following: a large area of skin overlying the tumor and including the nipple; all the breast tissue; the pectoralis major and associated fascia through which the lymph vessels pass to the internal thoracic nodes; the pectoralis minor and associated fascia related to the lymph vessels passing to the axilla; all the fat, fascia, and lymph nodes in the axilla; and the fascia covering the upper part of the rectus sheath, the serratus anterior, the subscapularis, and the latissimus dorsi muscles. The axillary blood vessels, the brachial plexus, and the nerves to the serratus anterior and the latissimus dorsi are preserved. Some degree of postoperative edema of the arm is likely to follow such a radical removal of the lymph vessels draining the upper limb.

A modified form of radical mastectomy for patients with clinically localized cancer is also a common procedure and consists of a simple mastectomy in which the pectoral muscles are left intact. The axillary lymph nodes, fat, and fascia are removed. This procedure removes the primary tumor and permits pathologic examination of the lymph nodes for possible metastases.

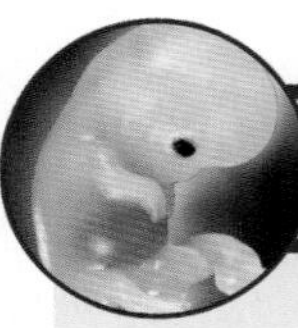

EMBRYOLOGIC NOTES

Development of the Breasts

In the young embryo a linear thickening of ectoderm appears called the **milk ridge,** which extends from the axilla obliquely to the inguinal region. In animals, several mammary glands are formed along this ridge. In the human, the ridge disappears except for a small part in the pectoral region. This localized area thickens, becomes slightly depressed, and sends off 15 to 20 solid cords, which grow into the underlying mesenchyme. Meanwhile, the underlying mesenchyme proliferates, and the depressed ectodermal thickening becomes raised to form the **nipple.** At the fifth month, the **areola** is recognized as a circular pigmented area of skin around the future nipple.

Polythelia

Supernumerary nipples occasionally occur along a line corresponding to the position of the milk ridge. They are liable to be mistaken for moles.

Retracted Nipple or Inverted Nipple

Retracted nipple is a failure in the development of the nipple during its later stages. It is important clinically, because normal suckling of an infant cannot take place, and the nipple is prone to infection (see also page 430).

Micromastia

An excessively small breast on one side occasionally occurs, resulting from lack of development.

Macromastia

Diffuse hypertrophy of one or both breasts occasionally occurs at puberty in otherwise normal girls.

Gynecomastia

Unilateral or bilateral enlargement of the male breast occasionally occurs, usually at puberty. The cause is unknown, but the condition is probably related to some form of hormonal imbalance.

Bones of the Shoulder Girdle and Arm

The shoulder girdle consists of the clavicle and the scapula, which articulate with one another at the acromioclavicular joint.

Clavicle

The clavicle is a long, slender bone that lies horizontally across the root of the neck just beneath the skin. It articulates with the sternum and first costal cartilage medially and with the acromion process of the scapula laterally (Fig. 9-5). The clavicle acts as a strut that holds the arm away from the trunk. It also transmits forces from the upper limb to the axial skeleton and provides attachment for muscles.

The medial two thirds of the clavicle is convex forward and its lateral third is concave forward. The important muscles and ligaments attached to the clavicle are shown in Figure 9-6.

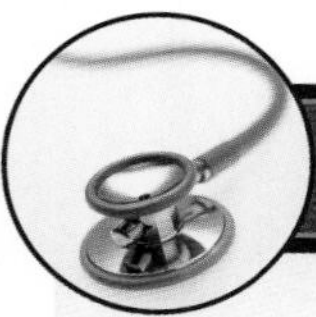

CLINICAL NOTES

Fractures of the Clavicle

The clavicle is a strut that holds the arm laterally so that it can move freely on the trunk. Unfortunately, because of its position, it is exposed to trauma and transmits forces from the upper limb to the trunk. *It is the most commonly fractured bone in the body.* The fracture usually occurs as a result of a fall on the shoulder or outstretched hand. The force is transmitted along the clavicle, which breaks at its weakest point, the junction of the middle and outer thirds. After the fracture, the lateral fragment is depressed by the weight of the arm, and it is pulled medially and forward by the strong adductor muscles of the shoulder joint, especially the pectoralis major. The medial end is tilted upward by the sternocleidomastoid muscle.

The close relationship of the supraclavicular nerves to the clavicle may result in their involvement in callus formation after fracture of the bone. This may be the cause of persistent pain over the side of the neck.

Compression of the Brachial Plexus, Subclavian Artery, and Subclavian Vein by the Clavicle

The interval between the clavicle and the first rib in some patients may become narrowed and thus is responsible for compression of nerves and blood vessels. (See discussion of thoracic outlet syndrome on page 52.)

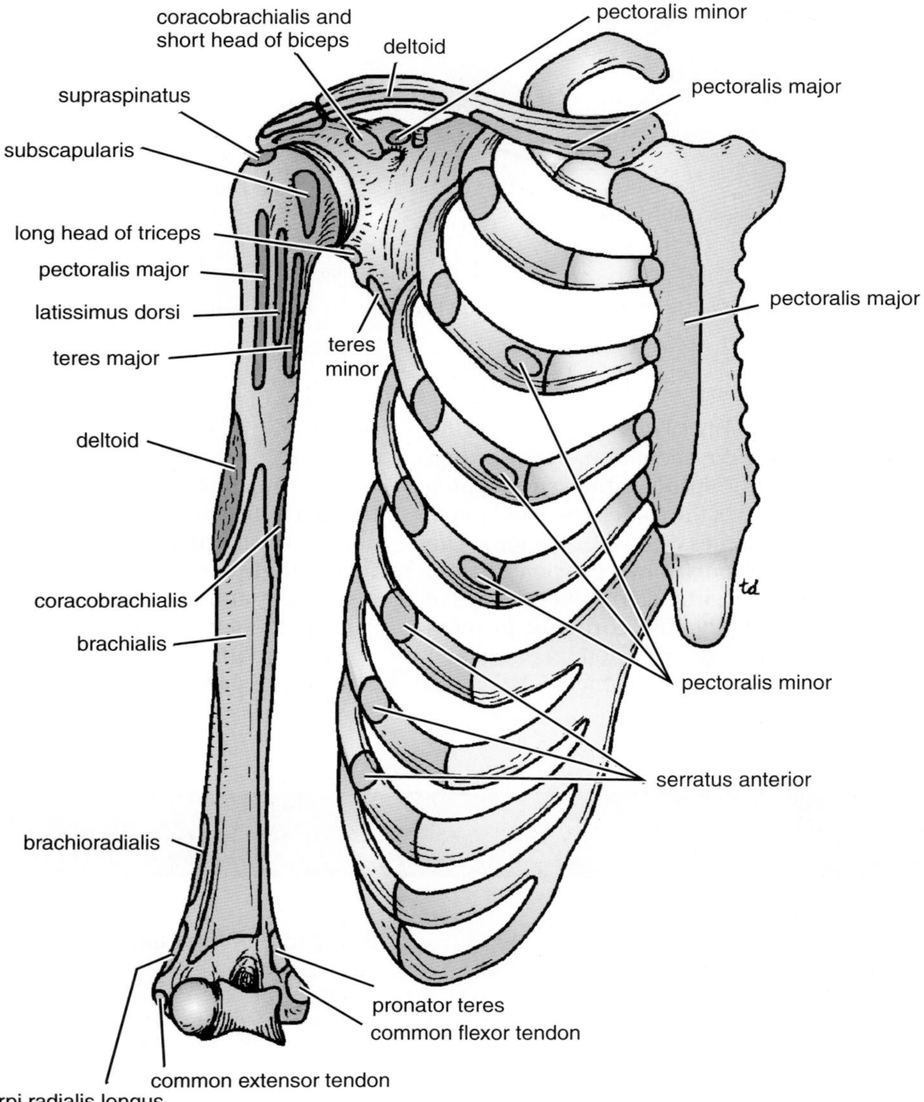

Figure 9-5 Muscle attachments to the bones of the thorax, clavicle, scapula, and humerus.

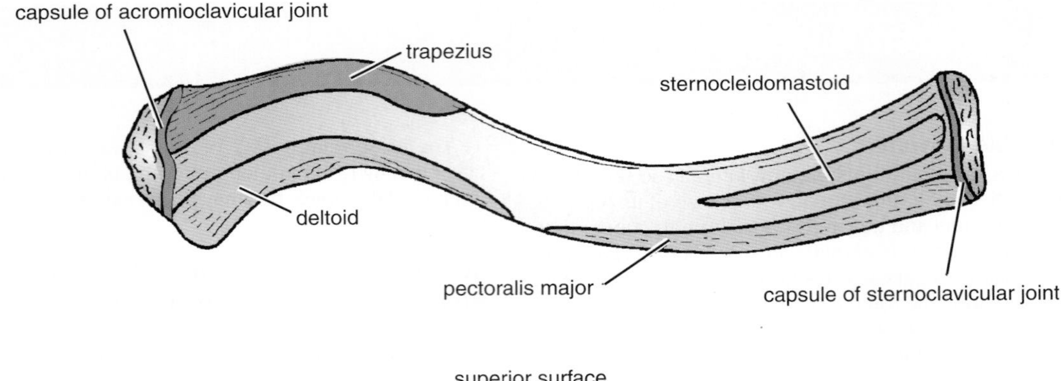

superior surface

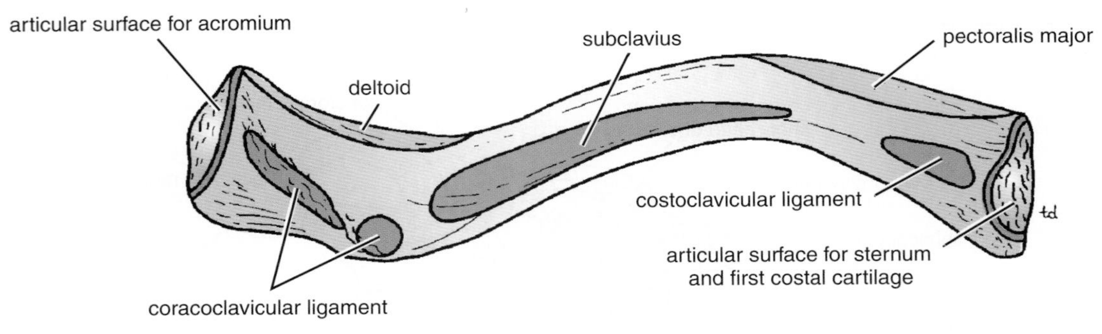

inferior surface

Figure 9-6 Important muscular and ligamentous attachments to the right clavicle.

Scapula

The scapula is a flat triangular bone (Fig. 9-7) that lies on the posterior chest wall between the second and the seventh ribs. On its posterior surface, the **spine of the scapula** projects backward. The lateral end of the spine is free and forms the **acromion,** which articulates with the clavicle. The superolateral angle of the scapula forms the pear-shaped **glenoid cavity,** or **fossa,** which articulates with the head of the humerus at the shoulder joint. The **coracoid process** projects upward and forward above the glenoid cavity and provides attachment for muscles and ligaments. Medial to the base of the coracoid process is the **suprascapular notch** (Fig. 9-7).

The anterior surface of the scapula is concave and forms the shallow **subscapular fossa.** The posterior surface of the scapula is divided by the spine into the **supraspinous fossa** above and an **infraspinous fossa** below (Fig. 9-5). The **inferior angle** of the scapula can be palpated easily in the living subject and marks the level of the seventh rib and the spine of the seventh thoracic vertebra.

The important muscles and ligaments attached to the scapula are shown in Figure 9-7.

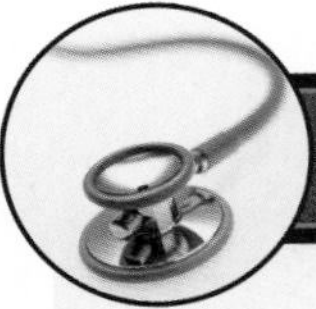

CLINICAL NOTES

Fractures of the Scapula

Fractures of the scapula are usually the result of severe trauma, such as occurs in run-over accident victims or in occupants of automobiles involved in crashes. Injuries are usually associated with fractured ribs. Most fractures of the scapula require little treatment because the muscles on the anterior and posterior surfaces adequately splint the fragments.

Dropped Shoulder and Winged Scapula

The position of the scapula on the posterior wall of the thorax is maintained by the tone and balance of the muscles attached to it. If one of these muscles is paralyzed, the balance is upset, as in dropped shoulder, which occurs with paralysis of the trapezius, or winged scapula (Fig. 9-8), caused by paralysis of the serratus anterior. Such imbalance can be detected by careful physical examination.

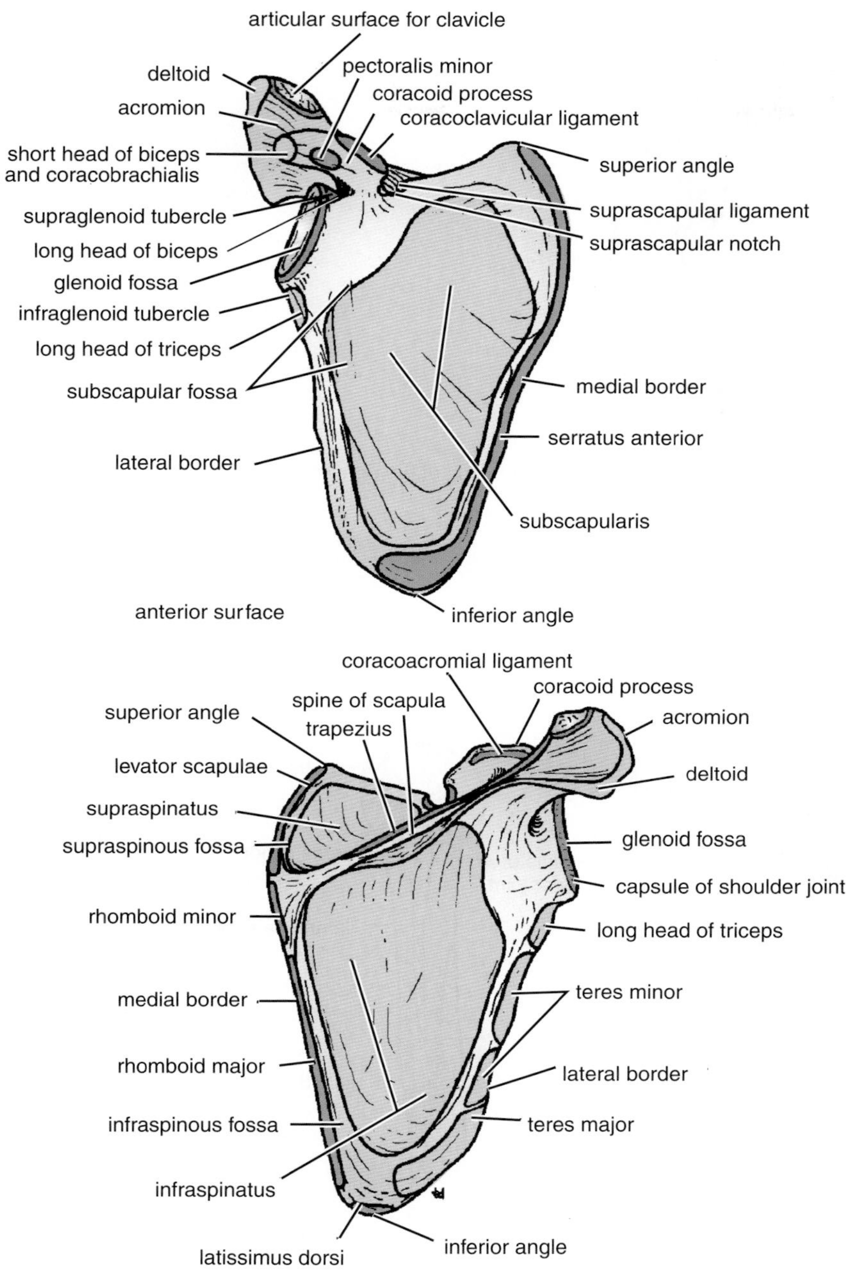

Figure 9-7 Important muscular and ligamentous attachments to the right scapula.

Humerus

The humerus articulates with the scapula at the shoulder joint and with the radius and ulna at the elbow joint. The upper end of the humerus has a **head** (Fig. 9-9), which forms about one third of a sphere and articulates with the glenoid cavity of the scapula. Immediately below the head is the **anatomic neck.** Below the neck are the **greater** and **lesser tuberosities,** separated from each other by the **bicipital groove.** Where the upper end of the humerus joins the shaft is a narrow **surgical neck.** About halfway down the lateral aspect of the shaft is a roughened elevation called the **deltoid tuberosity.** Behind and below the tuberosity is a **spiral groove,** which accommodates the radial nerve (Fig. 9-9).

The lower end of the humerus possesses the **medial** and **lateral epicondyles** for the attachment of muscles and ligaments, the rounded **capitulum** for articulation with the head of the radius, and the pulley-shaped **trochlea** for articulation with the trochlear notch of the ulna (Fig. 9-9). Above the capitulum is the **radial fossa,** which receives the head of the radius when the elbow is flexed. Above the trochlea anteriorly is the **coronoid fossa,** which during the same movement receives the coronoid process of the ulna. Above the trochlea pos-

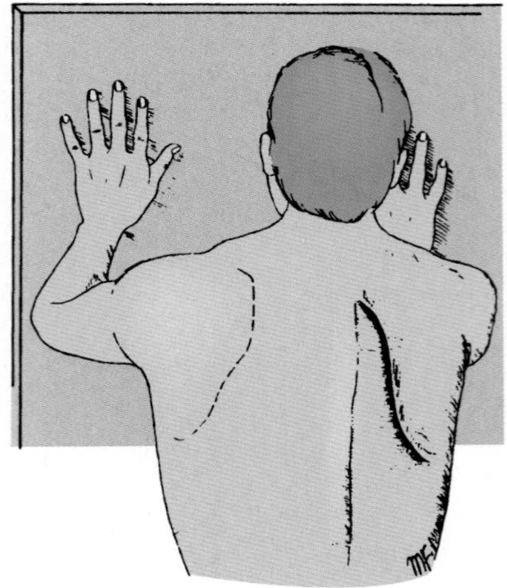

Figure 9-8 Winging of the right scapula.

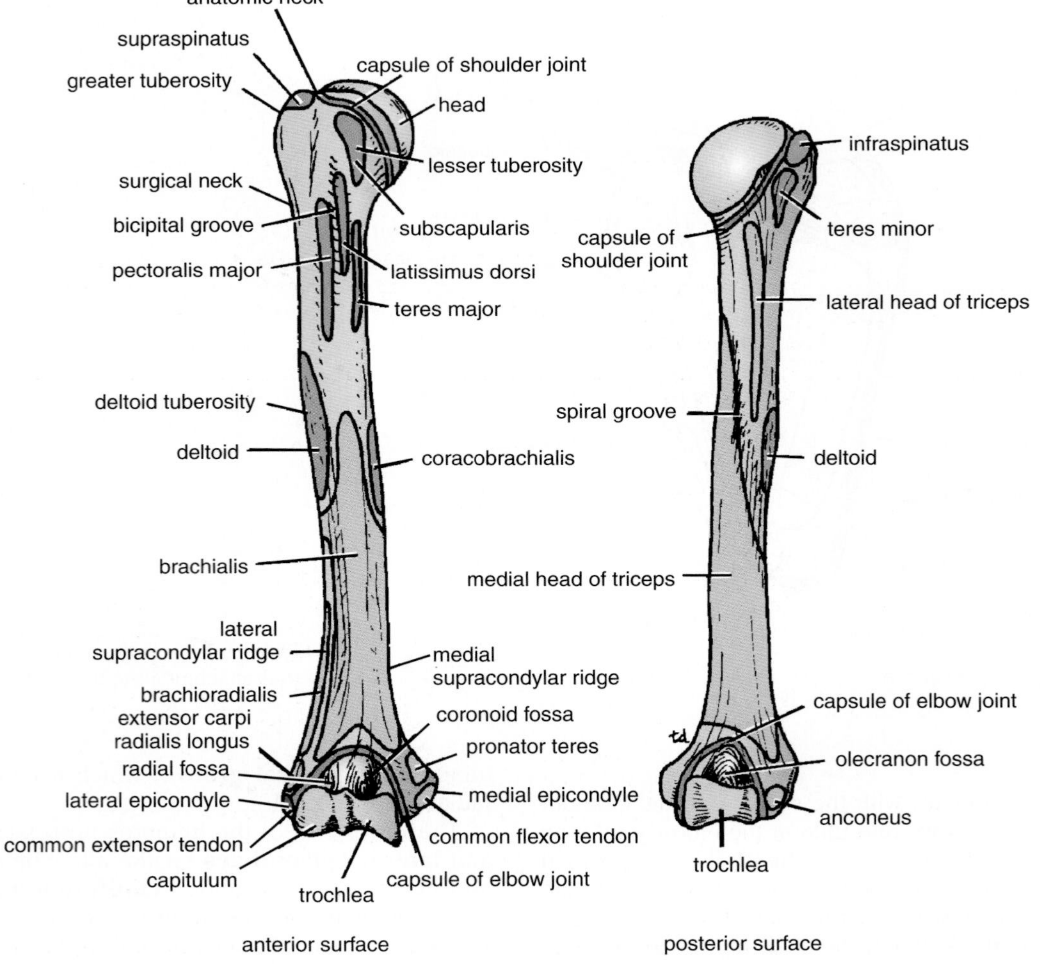

Figure 9-9 Important muscular and ligamentous attachments to the right humerus.

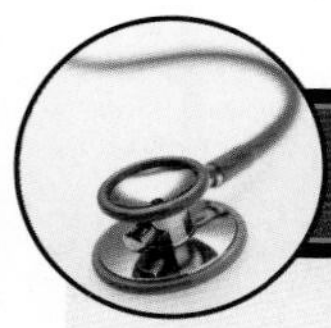

CLINICAL NOTES

Fractures of the Proximal End of the Humerus

Humeral Head Fractures

Fractures of the humeral head (Fig. 9-10) can occur during the process of anterior and posterior dislocations of the shoulder joint. The fibrocartilaginous glenoid labrum of the scapula produces the fracture, and the labrum can become jammed in the defect, making reduction of the shoulder joint difficult.

Greater Tuberosity Fractures

The greater tuberosity of the humerus can be fractured by direct trauma, displaced by the glenoid labrum during dislocation of the shoulder joint, or avulsed by violent contractions of the supraspinatus muscle. The bone fragment will have the attachments of the supraspinatus, teres minor, and infraspinatus muscles, whose tendons form part of the rotator cuff. When associated with a shoulder dislocation, severe tearing of the cuff with the fracture can result in the greater tuberosity remaining displaced posteriorly after the shoulder joint has been reduced. In this situation, open reduction of the fracture is necessary to attach the rotator cuff back into place.

Lesser Tuberosity Fractures

Occasionally, a lesser tuberosity fracture accompanies posterior dislocation of the shoulder joint. The bone fragment receives the insertion of the subscapularis tendon (Fig. 9-10), a part of the rotator cuff.

Surgical Neck Fractures

The surgical neck of the humerus (Fig. 9-10), which lies immediately distal to the lesser tuberosity, can be fractured by a direct blow on the lateral aspect of the shoulder or in an indirect manner by falling on the outstretched hand.

Fractures of the Shaft of the Humerus

Fractures of the humeral shaft are common; displacement of the fragments depends on the relation of the site of fracture to the insertion of the deltoid muscle (Fig. 9-10). When the fracture line is proximal to the deltoid insertion, the proximal fragment is adducted by the pectoralis major, latissimus dorsi, and teres major muscles; the distal fragment is pulled proximally by the deltoid, biceps, and triceps. When the fracture is distal to the deltoid insertion, the proximal fragment is abducted by the deltoid, and the distal fragment is pulled proximally by the biceps and triceps. The radial nerve can be damaged where it lies in the spiral groove on the posterior surface of the humerus under cover of the triceps muscle.

Fractures of the Distal End of the Humerus

Supracondylar fractures (Fig. 9-10) are common in children and occur when the child falls on the outstretched hand with the elbow partially flexed. Injuries to the median, radial, and ulnar nerves are not uncommon, although function usually quickly returns after reduction of the fracture. Damage to or pressure on the brachial artery can occur at the time of the fracture or from swelling of the surrounding tissues; the circulation to the forearm may be interfered with, leading to Volkmann's ischemic contracture (see page 483).

The medial epicondyle (Fig. 9-10) can be avulsed by the medial collateral ligament of the elbow joint if the forearm is forcibly abducted. The ulnar nerve can be injured at the time of the fracture, can become involved later in the repair process of the fracture (in the callus), or can undergo irritation on the irregular bony surface after the bone fragments are reunited.

---

teriorly is the **olecranon fossa,** which receives the olecranon process of the ulna when the elbow joint is extended (Fig. 9-9).

The important muscles and ligaments attached to the humerus are shown in Figure 9-9.

The Axilla

The axilla, or armpit, is a pyramid-shaped space between the upper part of the arm and the side of the chest (Fig. 9-11). It forms an important passage for nerves, blood, and lymph vessels as they travel from the root of the neck to the upper limb. The upper end of the axilla, or **apex,** is directed into the root of the neck and is bounded in front by the clavicle, behind by the upper border of the scapula, and medially by the outer border of the first rib (Fig. 9-11). The lower end, or **base,** is bounded in front by the anterior axillary fold (formed by the lower border of the pectoralis major muscle), behind by the posterior axillary fold (formed by the tendon of latissimus dorsi and the teres major muscle), and medially by the chest wall (Fig. 9-11).

Walls of the Axilla

The walls of the axilla are made up as follows:

- **Anterior wall:** By the pectoralis major, subclavius, and pectoralis minor muscles (Figs. 9-12, 9-13, and 9-14)
- **Posterior wall:** By the subscapularis, latissimus dorsi, and teres major muscles from above down (Figs. 9-13, 9-14, 9-15, and 9-16)
- **Medial wall:** By the upper four or five ribs and the intercostal spaces covered by the serratus anterior muscle (Figs. 9-14, 9-15, and 9-16)
- **Lateral wall:** By the coracobrachialis and biceps muscles in the bicipital groove of the humerus (Figs. 9-14, 9-15, and 9-16)

The **base** is formed by the skin stretching between the anterior and posterior walls (Fig. 9-14).

The axilla contains the principal vessels and nerves to the upper limb and many lymph nodes.

The origins, insertions, nerve supply, and actions of the muscles forming the walls of the axilla are described in Tables 9-1, 9-2, and 9-3.

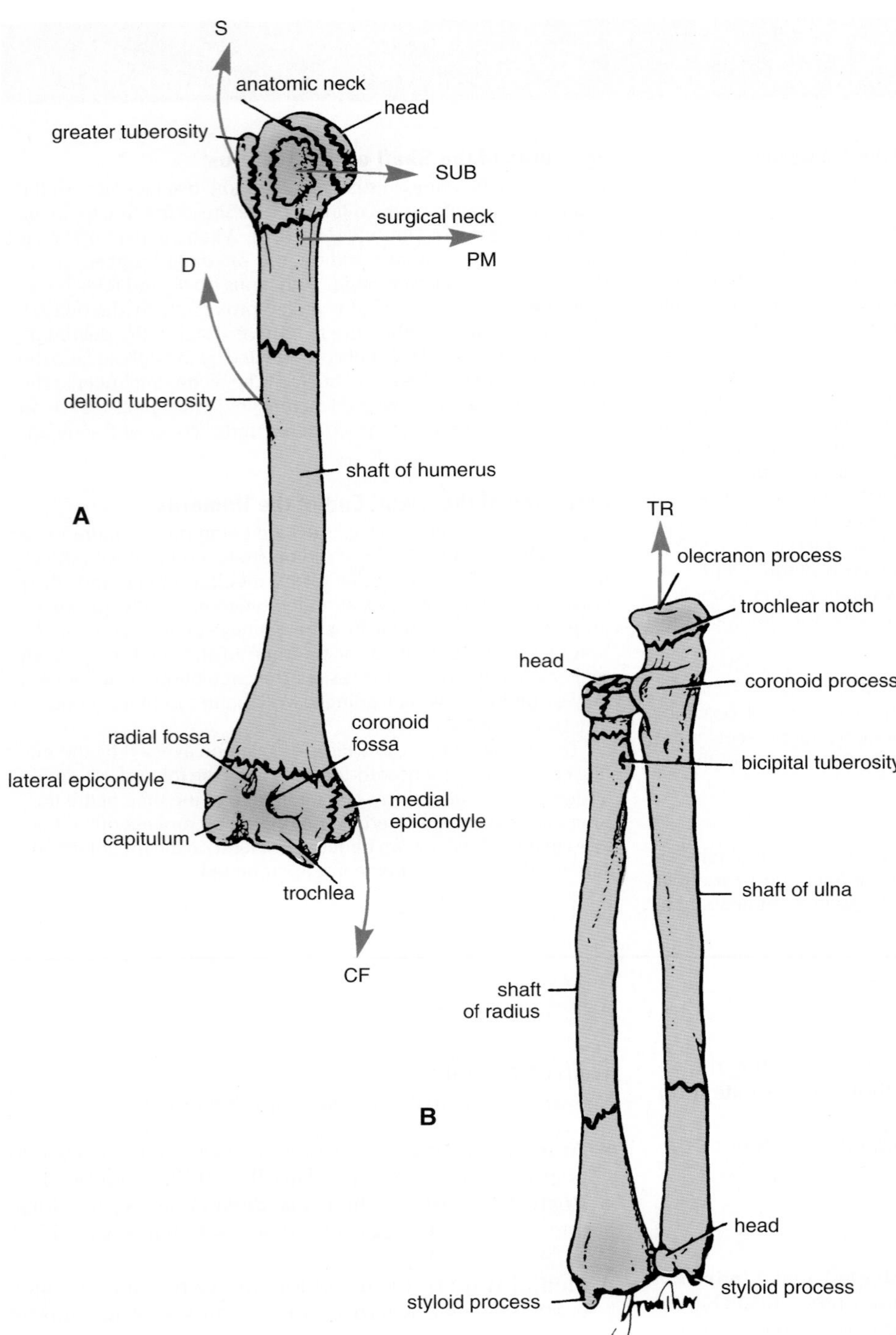

Figure 9-10 **A.** Common fractures of the humerus. **B.** Common fractures of the radius and ulna. The displacement of the bony fragments on the site of the fracture line and the pull of the muscles. S, supraspinatus; D, deltoid; PM, pectoralis major; CF, pull of common flexure muscles; TR, triceps; SUB, subscapularis.

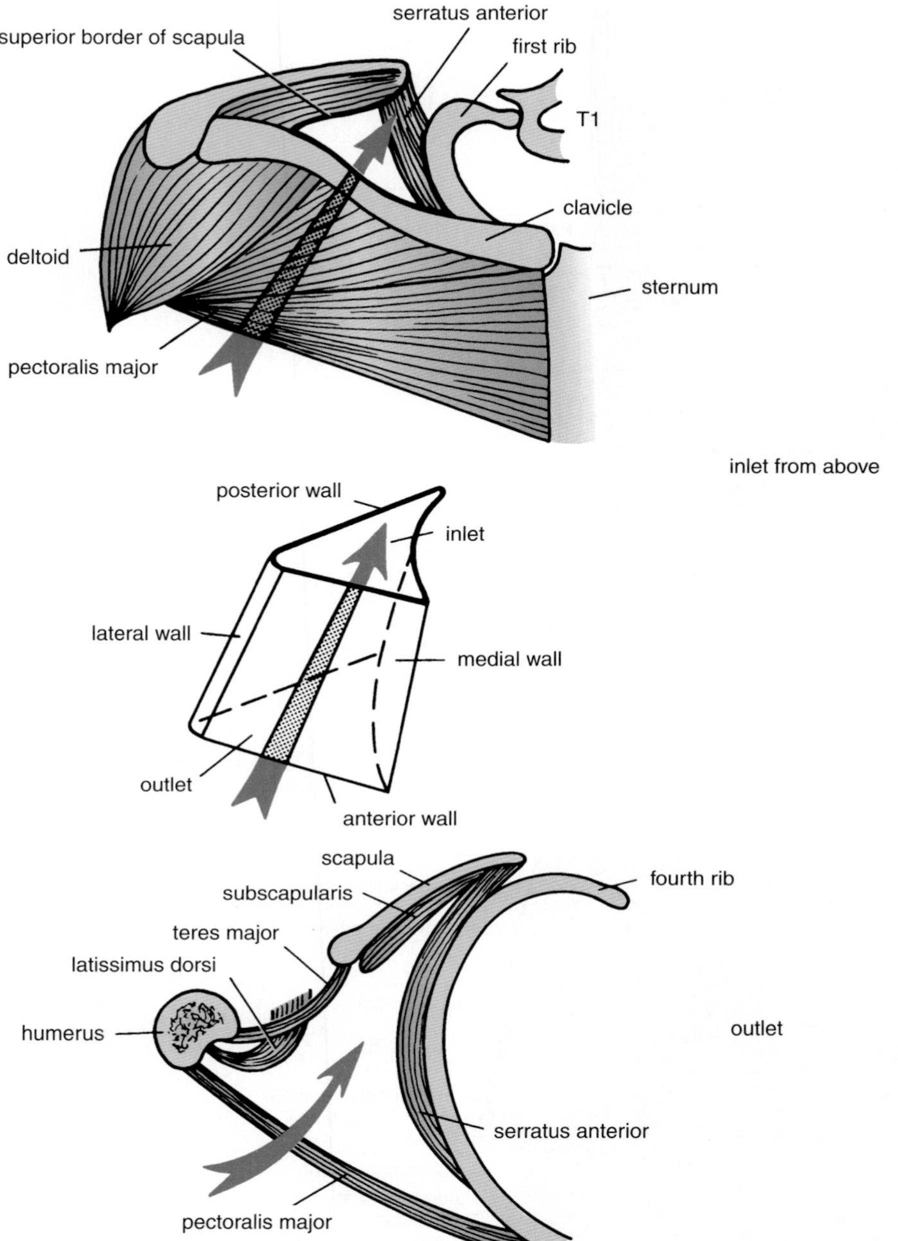

Figure 9-11 Inlet, walls, and outlet of the right axilla.

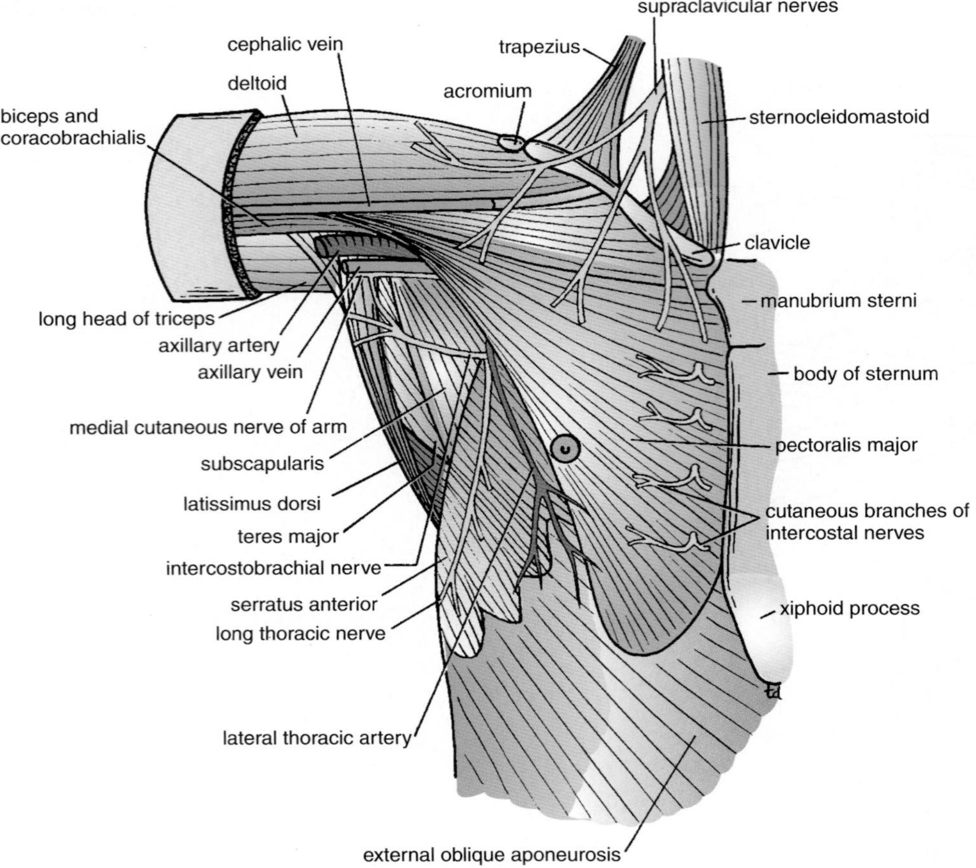

Figure 9-12 Pectoral region and axilla.

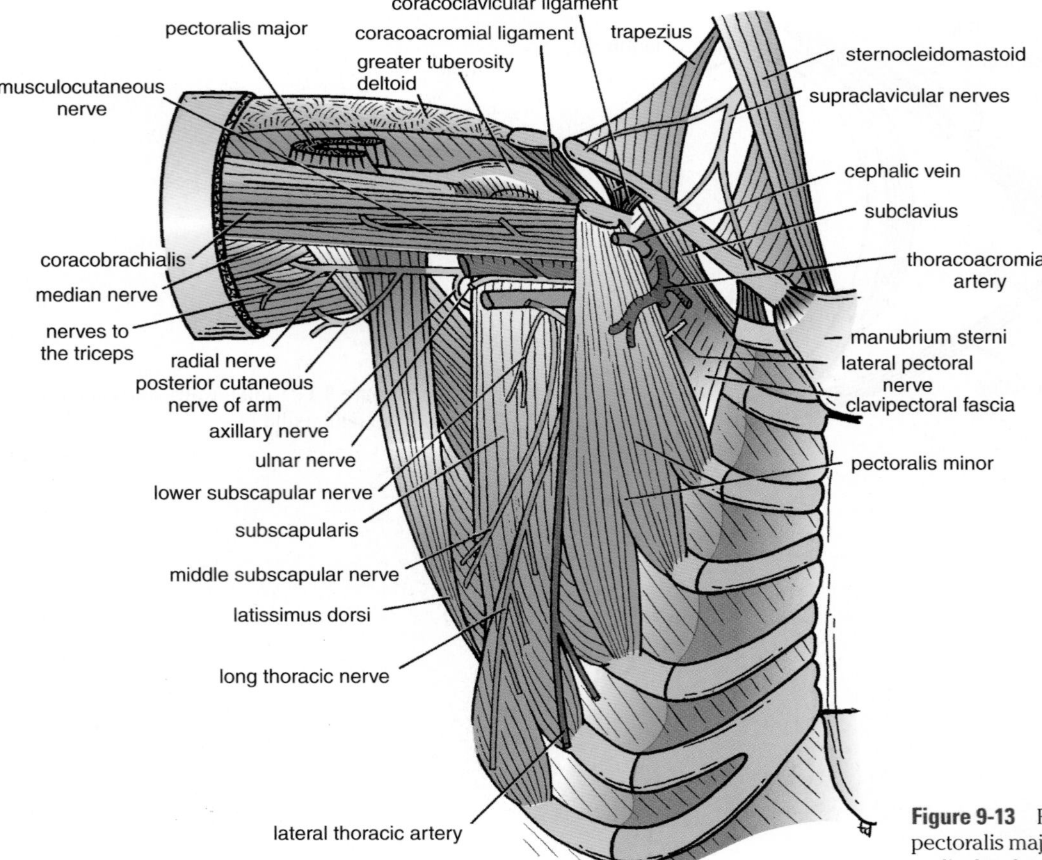

Figure 9-13 Pectoral region and axilla; the pectoralis major muscle has been removed to display the underlying structures.

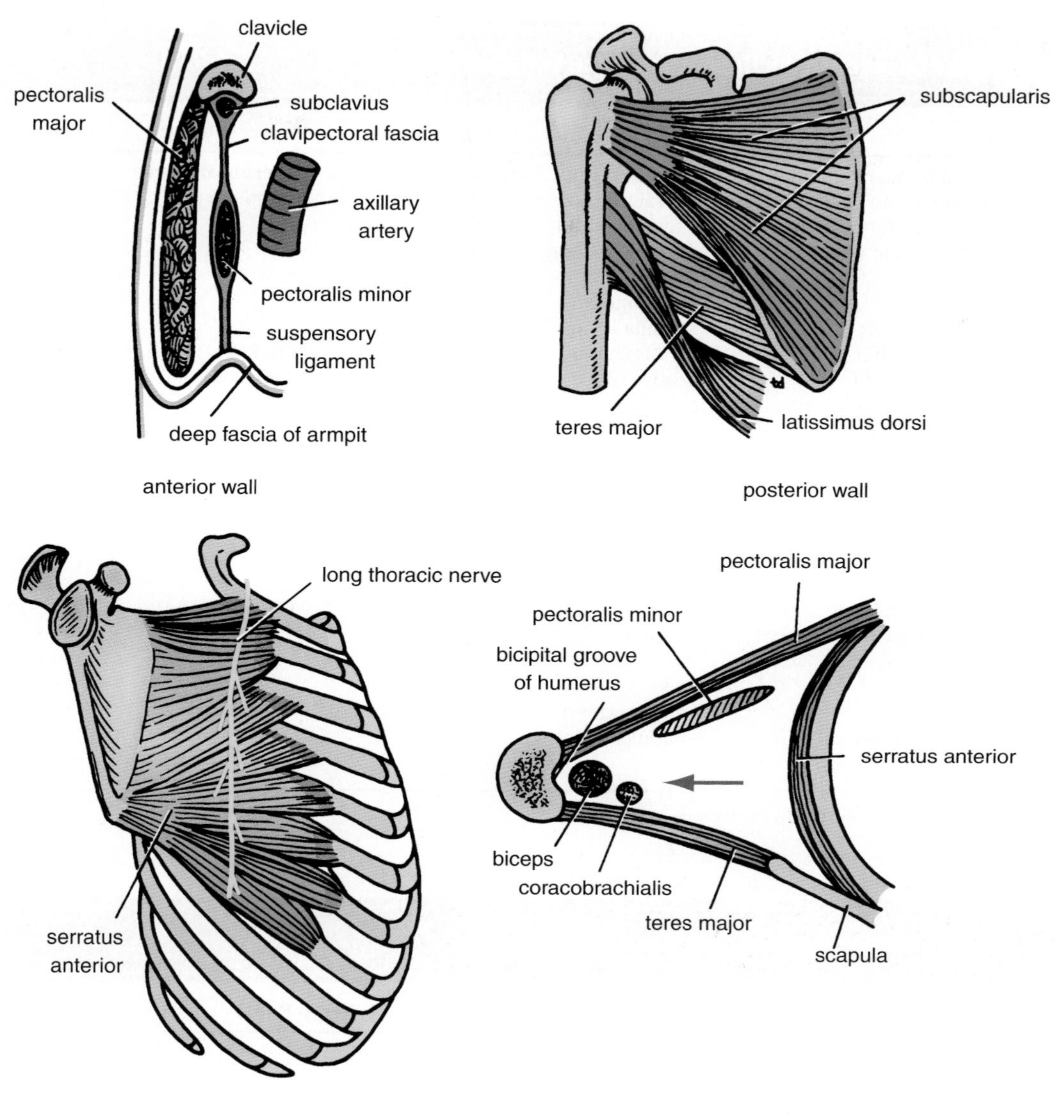

Figure 9-14 Structures that form the walls of the axilla. The lateral wall is indicated by the arrow.

Table 9-1 Muscles Connecting the Upper Limb to the Thoracic Wall

Muscle	Origin	Insertion	Nerve Supply	Nerve Roots[a]	Action
Pectoralis major	Clavicle, sternum, and upper six costal cartilages	Lateral lip of bicipital groove of humerus	Medial and lateral pectoral nerves from brachial plexus	C5, **6, 7, 8;** T1	Adducts arm and rotates it medially; clavicular fibers also flex arm
Pectoralis minor	Third, fourth, and fifth ribs	Coracoid process of scapula	Medial pectoral nerve from brachial plexus	C6, **7,** 8	Depresses point of shoulder; if the scapula is fixed, it elevates the ribs of origin
Subclavius	First costal cartilage	Clavicle	Nerve to subclavius from upper trunk of brachial plexus	**C5,** 6	Depresses the clavicle and steadies this bone during movements of the shoulder girdle
Serratus anterior	Upper eight ribs	Medial border and inferior angle of scapula	Long thoracic nerve	C5, **6, 7**	Draws the scapula forward around the thoracic wall; rotates scapula

[a] The predominant nerve root supply is indicated by boldface type.

Table 9-2 Muscles Connecting the Upper Limb to the Vertebral Column

Muscle	Origin	Insertion	Nerve Supply	Nerve Roots[a]	Action
Trapezius	Occipital bone, ligamentum nuchae, spine of seventh cervical vertebra, spines of all thoracic vertebrae	Upper fibers into lateral third of clavicle; middle and lower fibers into acromion and spine of scapula	Spinal part of accessory nerve (motor) and C3 and 4 (sensory)	XI **cranial nerve** (spinal part)	Upper fibers elevate the scapula; middle fibers pull scapula medially; lower fibers pull medial border of scapula downward
Latissimus dorsi	Iliac crest, lumbar fascia, spines of lower six thoracic vertebrae, lower three or four ribs, and inferior angle of scapula	Floor of bicipital groove of humerus	Thoracodorsal nerve	C6, **7,** 8,	Extends, adducts, and medially rotates the arm
Levator scapulae	Transverse processes of first four cervical vertebrae	Medial border of scapula	C3 and 4 and dorsal scapular nerve	C3, 4, 5	Raises medial border of scapula
Rhomboid minor	Ligamentum nuchae and spines of seventh cervical and first thoracic vertebrae	Medial border of scapula	Dorsal scapular nerve	**C4,** 5	Raises medial border of scapula upward and medially
Rhomboid major	Second to fifth thoracic spines	Medial border of scapula	Dorsal scapular nerve	**C4,** 5	Raises medial border of scapula upward and medially

[a] The predominant nerve root supply is indicated by boldface type.

Table 9-3 Muscles Connecting the Scapula to the Humerus

Muscle	Origin	Insertion	Nerve Supply	Nerve Roots[a]	Action
Deltoid	Lateral third of clavicle, acromion, spine of scapula	Middle of lateral surface of shaft of humerus	Axillary nerve	**C5,** 6	Abducts arm; anterior fibers flex and medially rotate arm; posterior fibers extend and laterally rotate arm
Supraspinatus	Supraspinous fossa of scapula	Greater tuberosity of humerus; capsule of shoulder joint	Suprascapular nerve	C4, **5,** 6	Abducts arm and stabilizes shoulder joint
Infraspinatus	Infraspinous fossa of scapula	Greater tuberosity of humerus; capsule of shoulder joint	Suprascapular nerve	(C4), **5, 6**	Laterally rotates arm and stabilizes shoulder joint
Teres major	Lower third of lateral border of scapula	Medial lip of bicipital groove of humerus	Lower subscapular nerve	**C6,** 7	Medially rotates and adducts arm and stabilizes shoulder joint
Teres minor	Upper two thirds of lateral border of scapula	Greater tuberosity of humerus; capsule of shoulder joint	Axillary nerve	(C4), **C5,** 6	Laterally rotates arm and stabilizes shoulder joint
Subscapularis	Subscapular fossa	Lesser tuberosity of humerus	Upper and lower subscapular nerves	C5, **6,** 7	Medially rotates arm and stabilizes shoulder joint

[a] The predominant nerve root supply is indicated by boldface type.

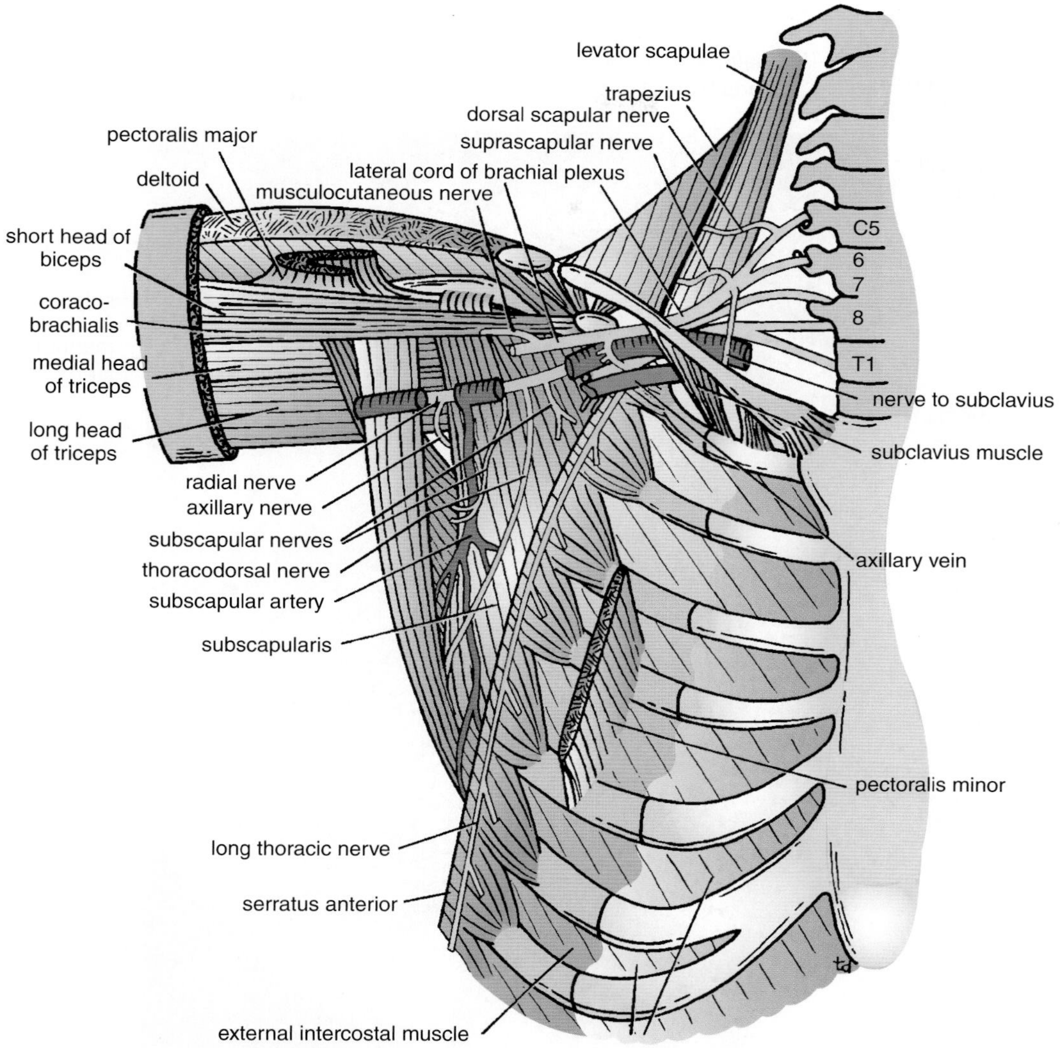

Figure 9-15 Pectoral region and axilla; the pectoralis major and minor muscles and the clavipectoral fascia have been removed to display the underlying structures.

Key Muscles in the Axilla

Pectoralis Minor

The pectoralis minor is a thin triangular muscle that lies beneath the pectoralis major (Fig. 9-13). It arises from the third, fourth, and fifth ribs and runs upwards and laterally to be inserted by its apex into the coracoid process of the scapula. It crosses the axillary artery and the brachial plexus of nerves. It is used when describing the axillary artery to divide it into three parts (see page 445).

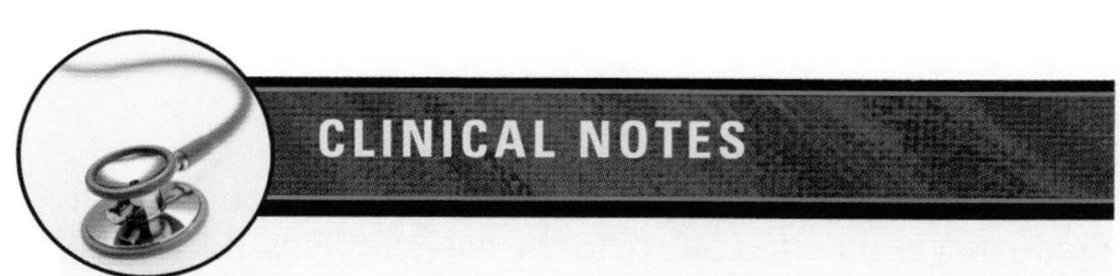

Absent Pectoralis Major

Occasionally, parts of the pectoralis major muscle may be absent. The sternocostal origin is the most commonly missing part, and this causes weakness in adduction and medial rotation of the shoulder joint.

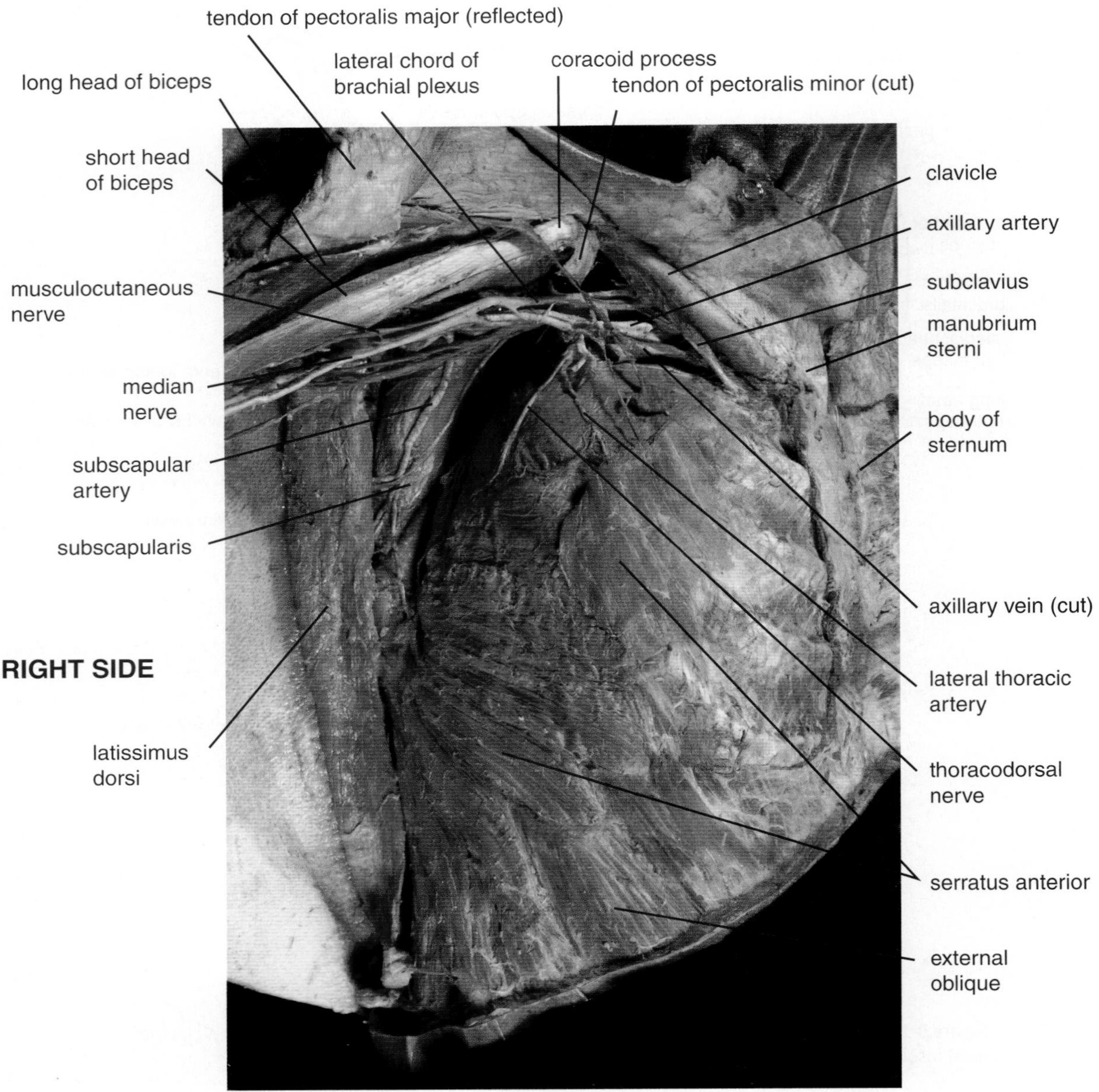

Figure 9-16 Dissection of the right axilla. The pectoralis major and minor muscles and the clavipectoral fascia have been removed to display the underlying structures.

Clavipectoral Fascia

The clavipectoral fascia is a strong sheet of connective tissue that is attached above to the clavicle (Figs. 9-13 and 9-14). Below, it splits to enclose the pectoralis minor muscle and then continues downward as the **suspensory ligament of the axilla** and joins the fascial floor of the armpit.

Contents of the Axilla

The axilla contains the axillary artery and its branches, which supply blood to the upper limb; the axillary vein and its tributaries, which drain blood from the upper limb; and lymph vessels and lymph nodes, which drain lymph from the upper limb and the breast and from the skin of the trunk, down as far as the level of the umbilicus. Lying among these structures in the axilla is an important nerve plexus, the brachial plexus, which innervates the upper limb. These structures are embedded in fat.

Axillary Artery

The axillary artery (Figs. 9-12, 9-13, 9-15, and 9-16) begins at the lateral border of the first rib as a continuation of the subclavian (Fig. 9-17) and ends at the lower border of the teres major muscle, where it continues as the brachial artery. Throughout its course, the artery is closely related to the cords of the brachial plexus and their branches and is enclosed with them in a connective tissue sheath called the **axillary sheath.** If this sheath is traced upward into the root

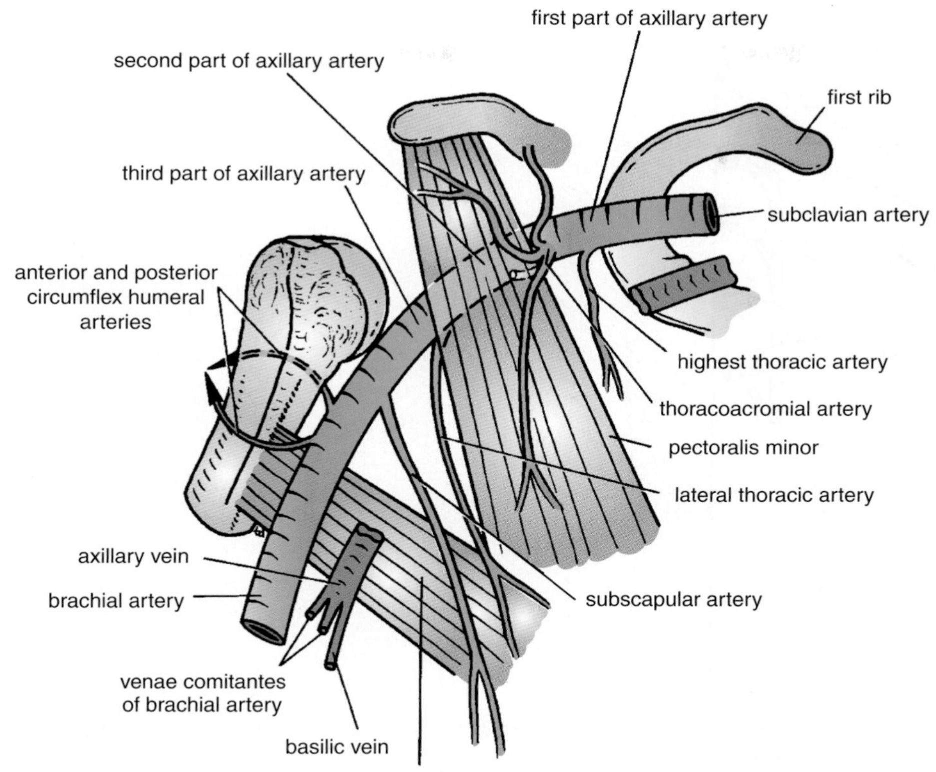

Figure 9-17 Parts of the axillary artery and its branches. Note formation of the axillary vein at the lower border of the teres major muscle.

of the neck, it is seen to be continuous with the prevertebral fascia.

The pectoralis minor muscle crosses in front of the axillary artery and divides it into three parts (Figs. 9-13, 9-15, and 9-17).

First Part of the Axillary Artery This extends from the lateral border of the first rib to the upper border of the pectoralis minor (Fig. 9-17).

Relations

- **Anteriorly:** The pectoralis major and the skin. The cephalic vein crosses the artery (Figs. 9-13 and 9-15).
- **Posteriorly:** The long thoracic nerve (nerve to the serratus anterior) (Fig. 9-15)
- **Laterally:** The three cords of the brachial plexus (Fig. 9-15)
- **Medially:** The axillary vein (Fig. 9-15 and 9-16)

Second Part of the Axillary Artery This lies behind the pectoralis minor muscle (Fig. 9-17).

Relations

- **Anteriorly:** The pectoralis minor, the pectoralis major, and the skin (Figs. 9-13 and 9-17)
- **Posteriorly:** The posterior cord of the brachial plexus, the subscapularis muscle, and the shoulder joint (Fig. 9-15)
- **Laterally:** The lateral cord of the brachial plexus (Figs. 9-13, 9-15, and 9-16)
- **Medially:** The medial cord of the brachial plexus and the axillary vein (Figs. 9-15, 9-16, and 9-20)

Third Part of the Axillary Artery This extends from the lower border of the pectoralis minor to the lower border of the teres major (Fig. 9-17).

Relations

- **Anteriorly:** The pectoralis major for a short distance; lower down the artery it is crossed by the medial root of the median nerve (Fig. 9-13).
- **Posteriorly:** The subscapularis, the latissimus dorsi, and the teres major. The axillary and radial nerves also lie behind the artery (Figs. 9-15 and 9-16).
- **Laterally:** The coracobrachialis, the biceps, and the humerus. The lateral root of the median and the musculocutaneous nerves also lie on the lateral side (Figs. 9-13 and 9-16).
- **Medially:** The ulnar nerve, the axillary vein, and the medial cutaneous nerve of the arm (Fig. 9-13)

Branches of the Axillary Artery

From the first part:

The **highest thoracic artery** is small and runs along the upper border of the pectoralis minor.

From the second part:

The **thoracoacromial artery** immediately divides into terminal branches.

The **lateral thoracic artery** runs along the lower border of the pectoralis minor (Fig. 9-17).

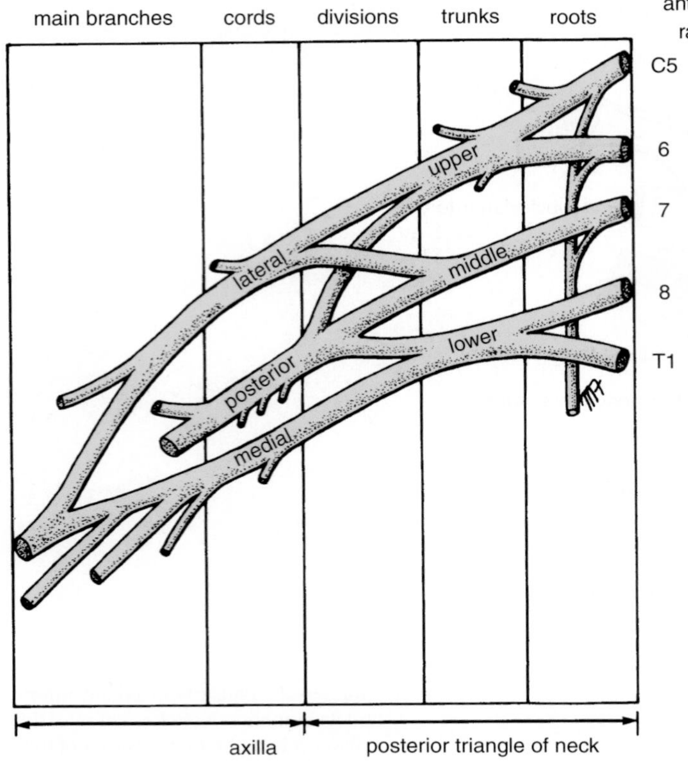

Figure 9-18 The formation of the main parts of the brachial plexus. Note the locations of the different parts.

From the third part:

The **subscapular artery** runs along the lower border of the subscapularis muscle.

The **anterior** and **posterior circumflex humeral arteries** wind around the front and the back of the surgical neck of the humerus, respectively (Fig. 9-17).

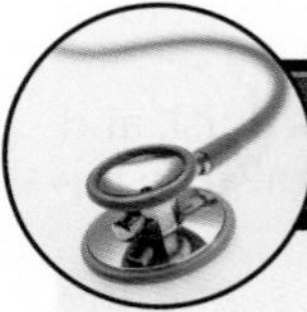

CLINICAL NOTES

The Axillary Sheath and a Brachial Plexus Nerve Block

Because the axillary sheath encloses the axillary vessels and the brachial plexus, a brachial plexus nerve block can easily be obtained. The distal part of the sheath is closed with finger pressure, and a syringe needle is inserted into the proximal part of the sheath. The anesthetic solution is then injected into the sheath, and the solution is massaged along the sheath to produce the nerve block. The position of the sheath can be verified by feeling the pulsations of the third part of the axillary artery.

Axillary Vein

The axillary vein (Fig. 9-12) is formed at the lower border of the teres major muscle by the union of the venae comitantes of the brachial artery and the basilic vein (Fig. 9-17). It runs upward on the medial side of the axillary artery and ends at the lateral border of the first rib by becoming the subclavian vein.

The vein receives tributaries, which correspond to the branches of the axillary artery, and the cephalic vein.

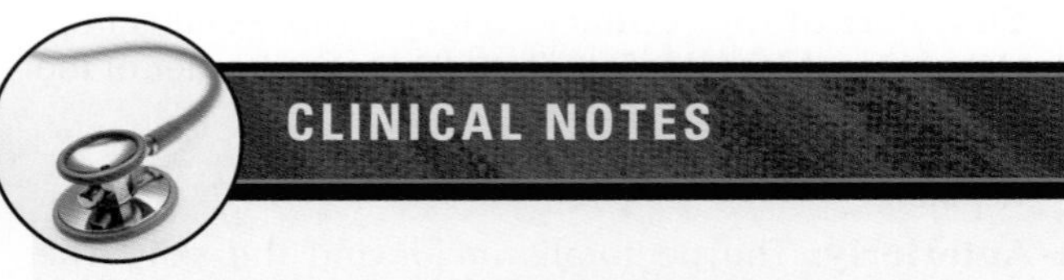

Spontaneous Thrombosis of the Axillary Vein

Spontaneous thrombosis of the axillary vein occasionally occurs after excessive and unaccustomed movements of the arm at the shoulder joint.

Brachial Plexus

The nerves entering the upper limb provide the following important functions: sensory innervation to the skin and deep structures, such as the joints; motor innervation to the muscles; influence over the diameters of the blood vessels by the sympathetic vasomotor nerves; and sympathetic secretomotor supply to the sweat glands.

At the root of the neck, the nerves form a complicated plexus called the **brachial plexus.** This allows the nerve fibers derived from different segments of the spinal cord to be arranged and distributed efficiently in different nerve trunks to the various parts of the upper limb. The brachial plexus is formed in the posterior triangle of the neck by the union of the anterior rami of the fifth, sixth, seventh, and eighth cervical and the first thoracic spinal nerves (Figs. 9-18 and 9-19).

The plexus can be divided into **roots, trunks, divisions,** and **cords** (Fig. 9-18). The roots of C5 and 6 unite to form the **upper trunk,** the root of C7 continues as the **middle trunk,** and the roots of C8 and T1 unite to form the **lower trunk.** Each trunk then divides into anterior and posterior divisions. The anterior divisions of the upper and middle trunks unite to form the **lateral cord,** the anterior division of the lower trunk continues as the **medial cord,** and the posterior divisions of all three trunks join to form the **posterior cord.**

The roots, trunks, and divisions of the brachial plexus reside in the lower part of the posterior triangle of the neck and are fully described on page 771. The cords become arranged around the axillary artery in the axilla (Fig. 9-15). Here, the brachial plexus and the axillary artery and vein are enclosed in the axillary sheath.

Cords of the Brachial Plexus All three cords of the brachial plexus lie above and lateral to the first part of the axillary artery (Figs. 9-15 and 9-20). The medial cord crosses behind the artery to reach the medial side of the second part of the artery (Fig. 9-20). The posterior cord lies behind the second part of the artery, and the lateral cord lies on the lateral side of the second part of the artery (Fig. 9-20). Thus, the cords of the plexus have the relationship to the second part of the axillary artery that is indicated by their names.

Most branches of the cords that form the main nerve trunks of the upper limb continue this relationship to the artery in its third part (Fig. 9-20).

The **branches** of the different parts of the brachial plexus (Figs. 9-19 and 9-21) are as follows:

- **Roots**
  Dorsal scapular nerve (C5)
  Long thoracic nerve (C5, 6, and 7)
- **Upper trunk**
  Nerve to subclavius (C5 and 6)
  Suprascapular nerve (supplies the supraspinatus and infraspinatus muscles)
- **Lateral cord**
  Lateral pectoral nerve
  Musculocutaneous nerve
  Lateral root of median nerve

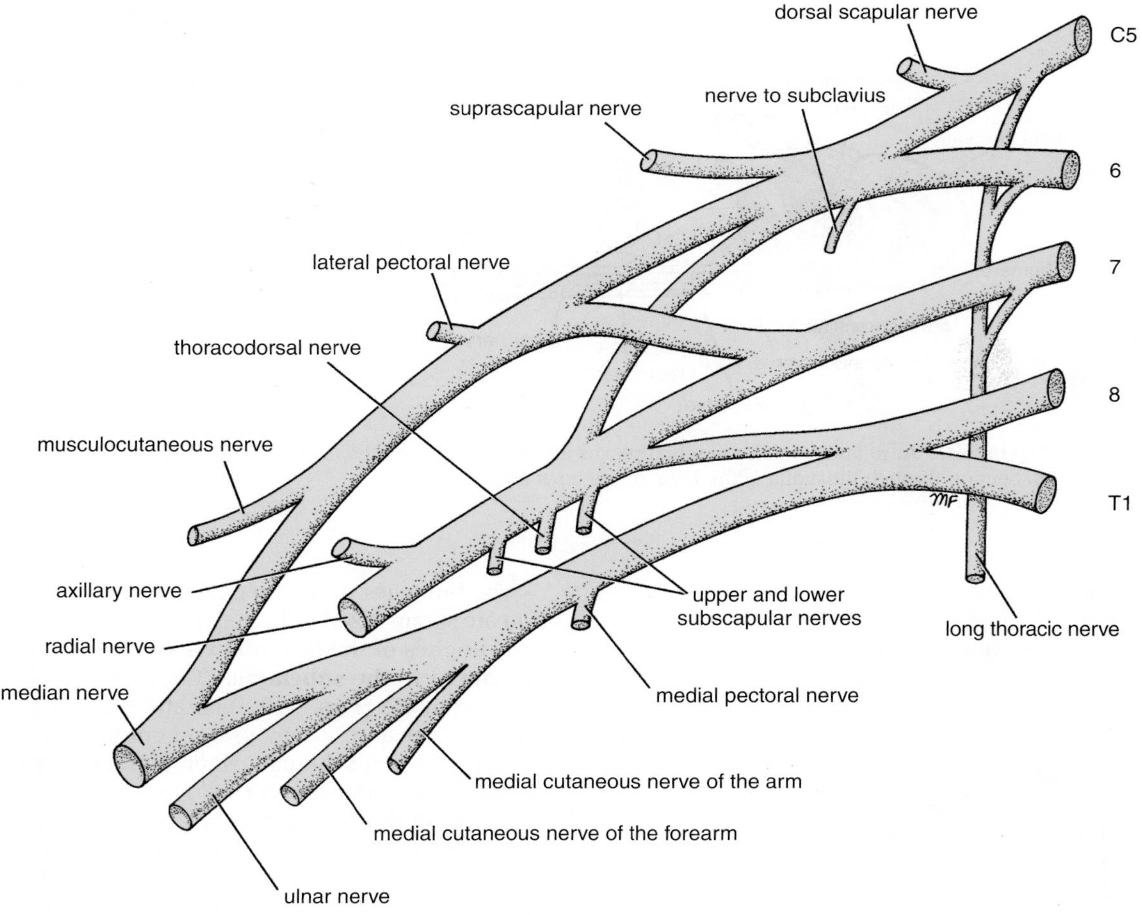

Figure 9-19 Roots, trunks, divisions, cords, and terminal branches of the brachial plexus.

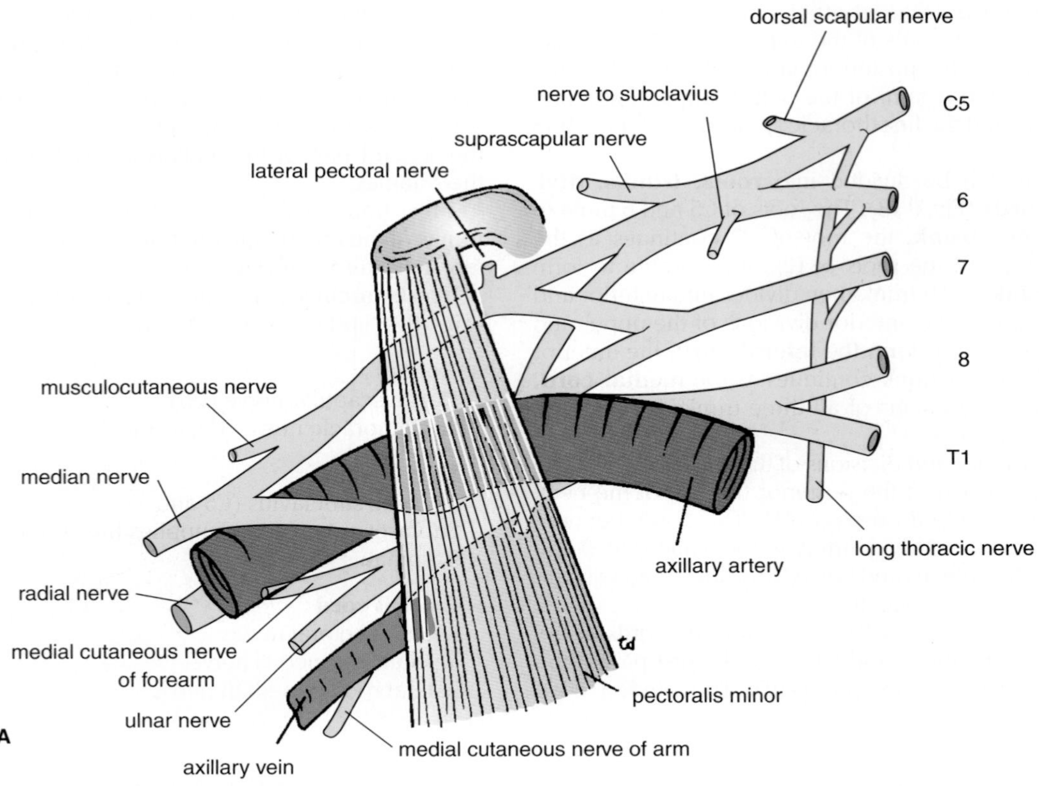

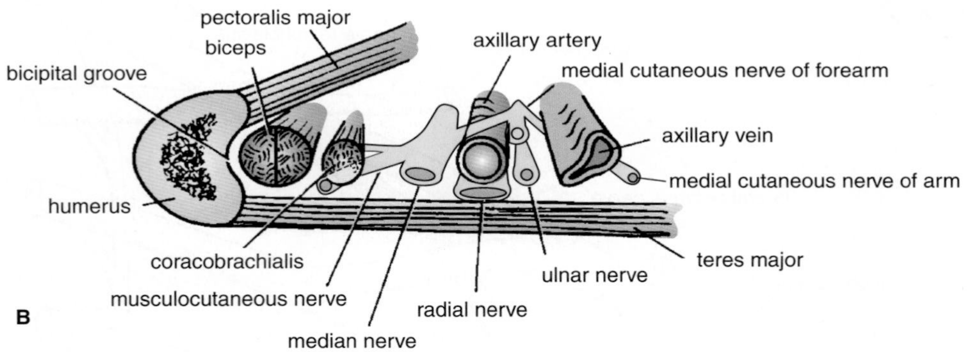

Figure 9-20 **A.** Relations of the brachial plexus and its branches to the axillary artery and vein. **B.** Section through the axilla at the level of the teres major muscle.

- **Medial cord**
  Medial pectoral nerve
  Medial cutaneous nerve of arm and medial cutaneous nerve of forearm
  Ulnar nerve
  Medial root of median nerve
- **Posterior cord**
  Upper and lower subscapular nerves
  Thoracodorsal nerve
  Axillary nerve
  Radial nerve

The branches of the brachial plexus and their distribution are summarized in Table 9-4.

Branches of the Brachial Plexus Found in the Axilla The **nerve to the subclavius** (C5 and 6) supplies the subclavius muscle (Figs. 9-15, 9-19, and 9-20). It is important clinically because it may give a contribution (C5) to the phrenic nerve; this branch, when present, is referred to as the **accessory phrenic nerve.**

The **long thoracic nerve** (C5, 6, and 7) arises from the roots of the brachial plexus in the neck and enters the axilla by passing down over the lateral border of the first rib behind the axillary vessels and brachial plexus (Figs. 9-15 and

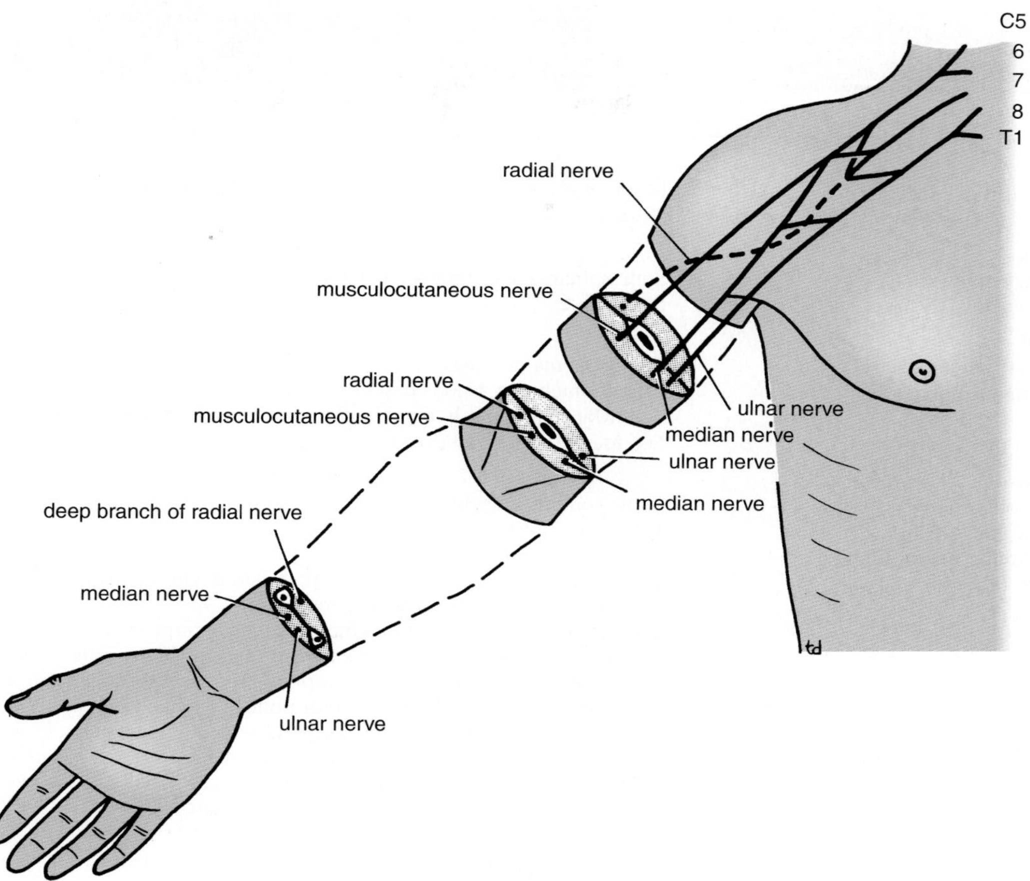

Figure 9-21 Distribution of the main branches of the brachial plexus to different fascial compartments of the arm and forearm.

9-19). It descends over the lateral surface of the serratus anterior muscle, which it supplies.

The **lateral pectoral nerve** arises from the lateral cord of the brachial plexus and supplies the pectoralis major muscle (Figs. 9-13 and 9-20).

The **musculocutaneous nerve** arises from the lateral cord of the brachial plexus, supplies the coracobrachialis muscle, and leaves the axilla by piercing that muscle (Figs. 9-13 and 9-20). A summary of the complete distribution of the musculocutaneous nerve is given in Figure 9-22.

The **lateral root of the median nerve** is the direct continuation of the lateral cord of the brachial plexus (Figs. 9-13 and 9-19). It is joined by the medial root to form the median nerve trunk, and this passes downward on the lateral side of the axillary artery. The median nerve gives off no branches in the axilla.

The **medial pectoral nerve** arises from the medial cord of the brachial plexus, supplies and pierces the pectoralis minor muscle, and supplies the pectoralis major muscle (Fig. 9-19).

The **medial cutaneous nerve of the arm** (T1) arises from the medial cord of the brachial plexus (Figs. 9-12 and 9-20) and is joined by the intercostobrachial nerve (lateral cutaneous branch of the second intercostal nerve). It supplies the skin on the medial side of the arm.

The **medial cutaneous nerve of the forearm** arises from the medial cord of the brachial plexus and descends in front of the axillary artery (Fig. 9-20).

The **ulnar nerve** (C8 and T1) arises from the medial cord of the brachial plexus and descends in the interval between the axillary artery and vein (Figs. 9-13 and 9-20). The ulnar nerve gives off no branches in the axilla. A summary of the complete distribution of the ulnar nerve is given in Figure 9-23.

The **medial root of the median nerve** arises from the medial cord of the brachial plexus and crosses in front of the third part of the axillary artery to join the lateral root of the median nerve (Figs. 9-13 and 9-20). A summary diagram of the complete distribution of the median nerve is given in Figure 9-22.

The **upper and lower subscapular nerves** arise from the posterior cord of the brachial plexus and supply the upper and lower parts of the subscapularis muscle. In addition, the lower subscapular nerve supplies the teres muscle (Figs. 9-15 and 9-19).

Table 9-4 Summary of the Branches of the Brachial Plexus and Their Distribution

Branches	Distribution
Roots	
Dorsal scapular nerve (C5)	Rhomboid minor, rhomboid major, levator scapulae muscles
Long thoracic nerve (C5, 6, 7)	Serratus anterior muscle
Upper Trunk	
Suprascapular nerve (C5, 6)	Supraspinatus and infraspinatus muscles
Nerve to subclavius (C5, 6)	Subclavius
Lateral Cord	
Lateral pectoral nerve (C5, 6, 7)	Pectoralis major muscle
Musculocutaneous nerve (C5, 6, 7)	Coracobrachialis, biceps brachii, brachialis muscles; supplies skin along lateral border of forearm when it becomes the lateral cutaneous nerve of forearm
Lateral root of median nerve (C5, 6, 7)	See medial root of median nerve
Posterior Cord	
Upper subscapular nerve (C5, 6)	Subscapularis muscle
Thoracodorsal nerve (C6, 7, 8)	Latissimus dorsi muscle
Lower subscapular nerve (C5, 6)	Subscapularis and teres major muscles
Axillary nerve (C5, 6)	Deltoid and teres minor muscles; upper lateral cutaneous nerve of arm supplies skin over lower half of deltoid muscle
Radial nerve (C5, 6, 7, 8; T1)	Triceps, anconeus, part of brachialis, extensor carpi radialis longus; via deep radial nerve branch supplies extensor muscles of forearm: supinator, extensor carpi radialis brevis, extensor carpi ulnaris, extensor digitorum, extensor digiti minimi, extensor indicis, abductor pollicis longus, extensor pollicis longus, extensor pollicis brevis; skin, lower lateral cutaneous nerve of arm, posterior cutaneous nerve of arm, and posterior cutaneous nerve of forearm; skin on lateral side of dorsum of hand and dorsal surface of lateral three and a half fingers; articular branches to elbow, wrist, and hand
Medial Cord	
Medial pectoral nerve (C8; T1)	Pectoralis major and minor muscles
Medial cutaneous nerve of arm joined by intercostal brachial nerve from second intercostal nerve (C8; T1, 2)	Skin of medial side of arm
Medial cutaneous nerve of forearm (C8; T1)	Skin of medial side of forearm
Ulnar nerve (C8; T1)	Flexor carpi ulnaris and medial half of flexor digitorum profundus, flexor digiti minimi, opponens digiti minimi, abductor digiti minimi, adductor pollicis, third and fourth lumbricals, interossei, palmaris brevis, skin of medial half of dorsum of hand and palm, skin of palmar and dorsal surfaces of medial one and a half fingers
Medial root of median nerve (with lateral root) forms median nerve (C5, 6, 7, 8; T1)	Pronator teres, flexor carpi radialis, palmaris longus, flexor digitorum superficialis, abductor pollicis brevis, flexor pollicis brevis, opponens pollicis, first two lumbricals (by way of anterior interosseous branch), flexor pollicis longus, flexor digitorum profundus (lateral half), pronator quadratus; palmar cutaneous branch to lateral half of palm and digital branches to palmar surface of lateral three and a half fingers; articular branches to elbow, wrist, and carpal joints

The **thoracodorsal nerve** arises from the posterior cord of the brachial plexus and runs downward to supply the latissimus dorsi muscle (Figs. 9-15 and 9-19).

The **axillary nerve** is one of the terminal branches of the posterior cord of the brachial plexus (Figs. 9-15 and 9-19). It turns backward and passes through the quadrangular space (see page 458). Having given off a branch to the shoulder joint, it divides into anterior and posterior branches (see page 458). A summary of the complete distribution of the axillary nerve is given in Figure 9-24.

The **radial nerve** is the largest branch of the brachial plexus and lies behind the axillary artery (Figs. 9-15, 9-19, and 9-20). It gives off branches to the long and medial heads of the triceps muscle and the posterior cutaneous nerve of the arm (Fig. 9-13). The latter branch is distributed to the skin on the middle of the back of the arm. A summary of the complete distribution of the radial nerve is given in Figure 9-25.

Lesions of the brachial plexus and its branches are described on page 536.

Lymph Nodes of the Axilla

The axillary lymph nodes (20 to 30 in number) drain lymph vessels from the lateral quadrants of the breast, the superficial

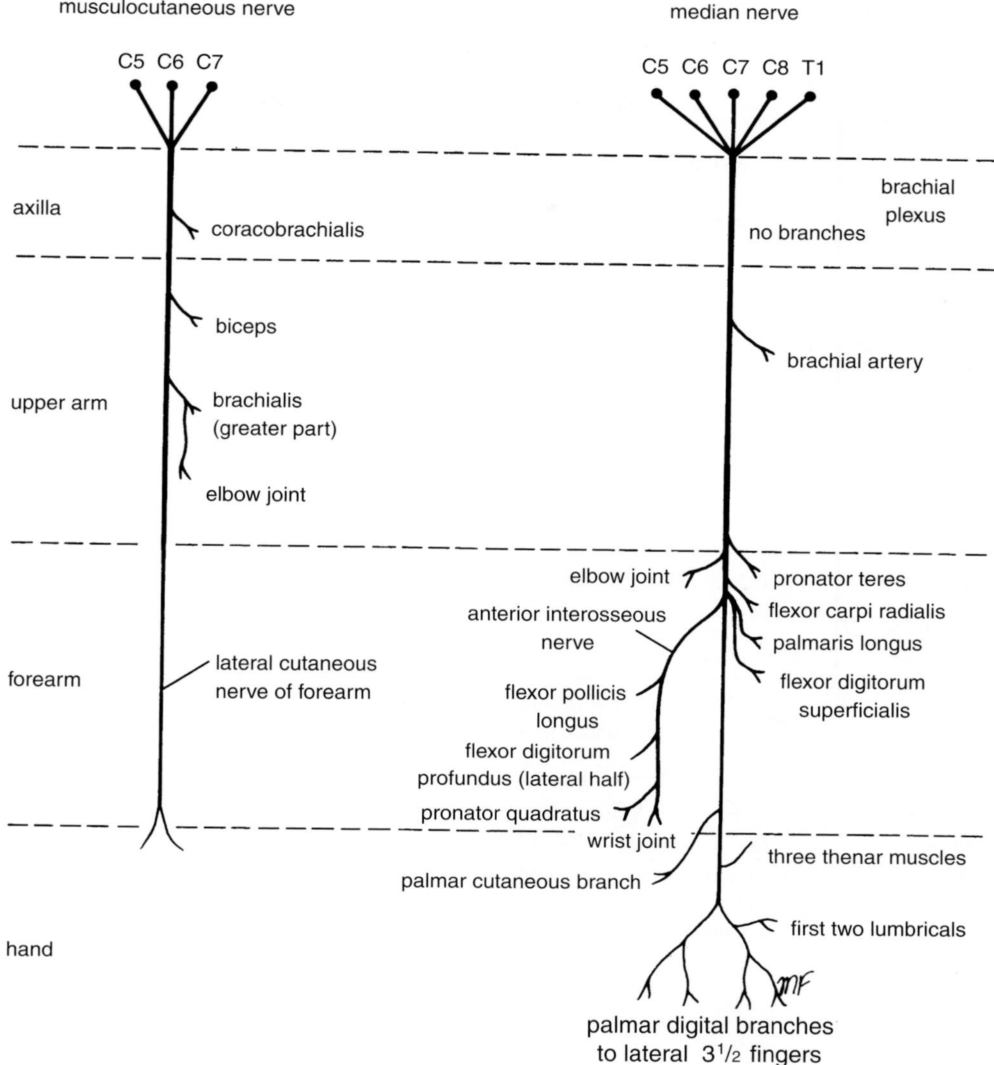

Figure 9-22 Summary of the main branches of the musculocutaneous and median nerves.

lymph vessels from the thoracoabdominal walls above the level of the umbilicus, and the vessels from the upper limb.

The lymph nodes are arranged in six groups (Fig. 9-26).

- **Anterior (pectoral) group:** Lying along the lower border of the pectoralis minor behind the pectoralis major, these nodes receive lymph vessels from the lateral quadrants of the breast and superficial vessels from the anterolateral abdominal wall above the level of the umbilicus.
- **Posterior (subscapular) group:** Lying in front of the subscapularis muscle, these nodes receive superficial lymph vessels from the back, down as far as the level of the iliac crests.
- **Lateral group:** Lying along the medial side of the axillary vein, these nodes receive most of the lymph vessels of the upper limb (except those superficial vessels draining the lateral side—see infraclavicular nodes, below).
- **Central group:** Lying in the center of the axilla in the axillary fat, these nodes receive lymph from the above three groups.
- **Infraclavicular (deltopectoral) group:** These nodes are not strictly axillary nodes because they are located outside the axilla. They lie in the groove between the deltoid and pectoralis major muscles and receive superficial lymph vessels from the lateral side of the hand, forearm, and arm.
- **Apical group:** Lying at the apex of the axilla at the lateral border of the first rib, these nodes receive the efferent lymph vessels from all the other axillary nodes.

The apical nodes drain into the **subclavian lymph trunk.** On the left side, this trunk drains into the thoracic duct; on the right side, it drains into the right lymph trunk. Alternatively, the lymph trunks may drain directly into one of the large veins at the root of the neck.

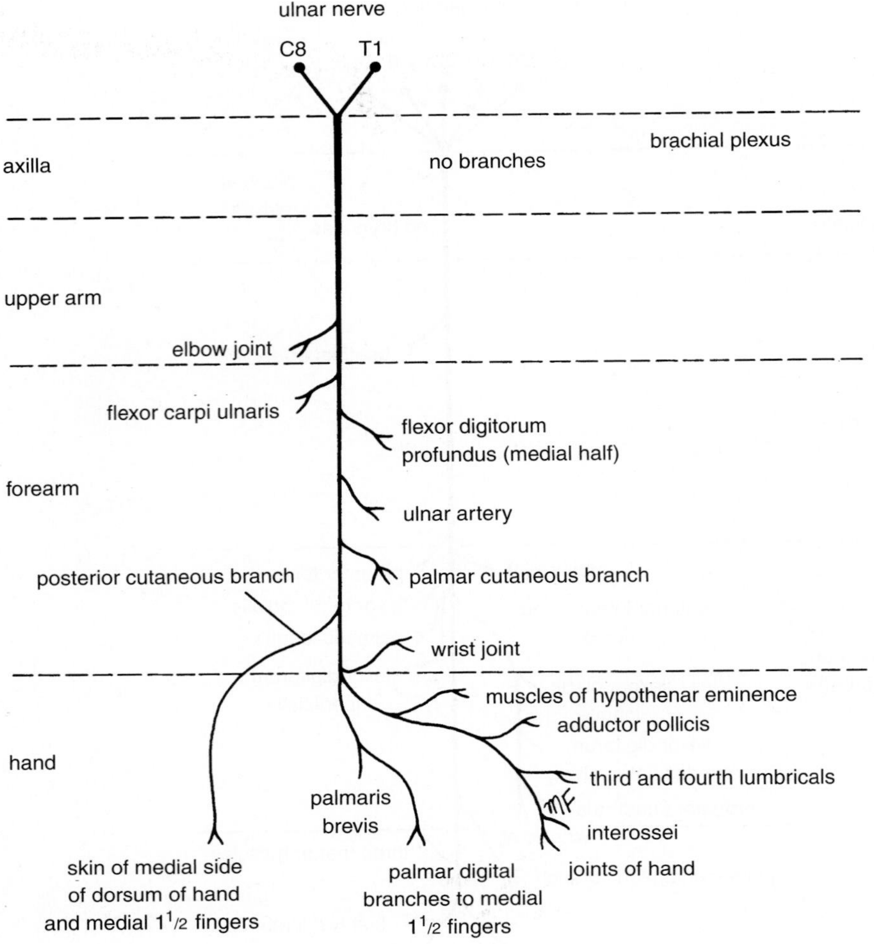

Figure 9-23 Summary of the main branches of the ulnar nerve.

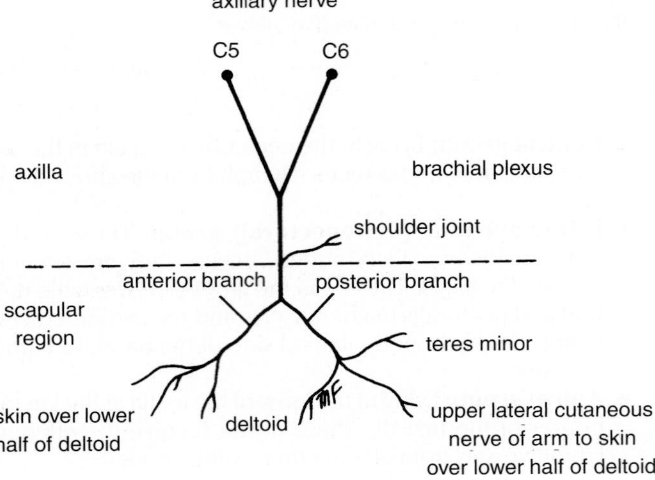

Figure 9-24 Summary of the main branches of the axillary nerve.

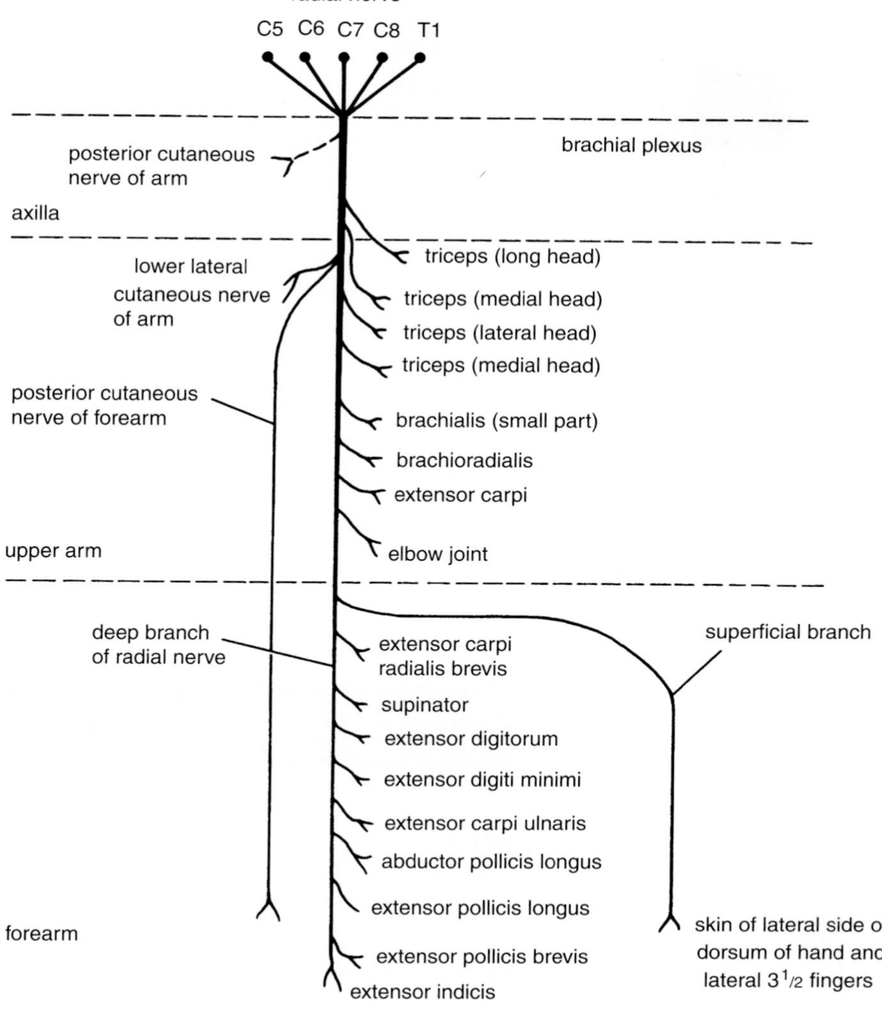

Figure 9-25 Summary of the main branches of the radial nerve.

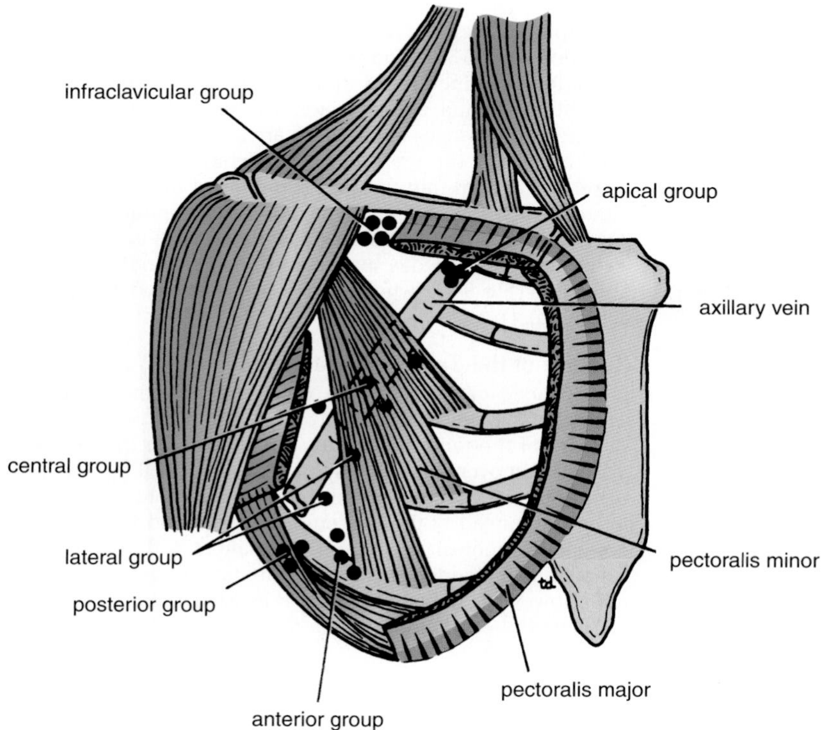

Figure 9-26 Different groups of lymph nodes in the axilla.

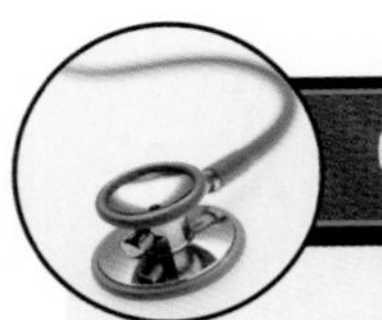

CLINICAL NOTES

Examination of the Axillary Lymph Nodes

With the patient standing or sitting, he or she is asked to place the hand of the side to be examined on the hip and push hard medially. This action of adduction of the shoulder joint causes the pectoralis major muscle to contract maximally so that it becomes hard like a board. The examiner then palpates the axillary nodes (Fig. 9-26) as follows:

- The **anterior (pectoral) nodes** may be palpated by pressing forward against the posterior surface of the pectoralis major muscle on the anterior wall of the axilla.
- The **posterior (subscapular) nodes** may be palpated by pressing backward against the anterior surface of the subscapularis muscle on the posterior wall of the axilla.
- The **lateral nodes** may be palpated against the medial side of the axillary vein. The examiner's fingers are pressed laterally against the subclavian vein and the pulsating axillary artery.
- The **central nodes** may be palpated in the center of the axilla between the pectoralis major (anterior wall) and the subscapularis (posterior wall).
- For the **apical nodes,** the patient is asked to relax the shoulder muscles and let the upper limb hang down at the side. The examiner then gently places the tips of the fingers of the examining hand high up in the axilla to the outer border of the first rib. If the nodes are enlarged they can be felt.

The examination of the axillary lymph nodes always forms part of the clinical examination of the breast.

The Superficial Part of the Back and the Scapular Region

Skin

The **sensory nerve supply** to the skin of the back is from the posterior rami of the spinal nerves (see Fig. 1-24). The first and eighth cervical nerves do not supply the skin, and the posterior rami of the upper three lumbar nerves run downward to supply the skin over the buttock.

The **blood supply** to the skin is from the posterior branches of the posterior intercostal arteries and the lumbar arteries. The veins correspond to the arteries and drain into the azygos veins and the inferior vena cava.

The **lymph drainage** of the skin of the back above the level of the iliac crests is upward into the posterior group of axillary lymph nodes.

Bones of the Back

The underlying bones of the back are shown in Figure 9-27 and are described in detail in Chapter 12.

Muscles

The muscles on the back connecting the upper limb to the thoracic wall and the vertebral column are shown in Figure 9-28 and are described in Tables 9-1 and 9-2, and the muscles connecting the scapula to the humerus are shown in Figure 9-29 and are described in Table 9-3.

Rotator Cuff

The rotator cuff is the name given to the tendons of the subscapularis, supraspinatus, infraspinatus, and teres minor muscles, which are fused to the underlying capsule of the shoulder joint (Fig. 9-34). The cuff plays a very important role in stabilizing the shoulder joint. The tone of these muscles assists in holding the head of the humerus in the glenoid cavity of the scapula during movements at the shoulder joint. The cuff lies on the anterior, superior, and posterior aspects of the joint. The cuff is deficient inferiorly, and this is a site of potential weakness.

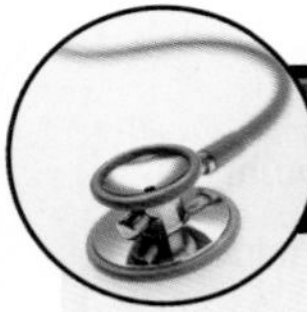

CLINICAL NOTES

Rotator Cuff Tendinitis

The rotator cuff, consisting of the tendons of the subscapularis, supraspinatus, infraspinatus, and teres minor muscles, which are fused to the underlying capsule of the shoulder joint, plays an important role in stabilizing the shoulder joint. Lesions of the cuff are a common cause of pain in the shoulder region. Excessive overhead activity of the upper limb may be the cause of tendinitis, although many cases appear spontaneously. During abduction of the shoulder joint, the supraspinatus tendon is exposed to friction against the acromion (Fig. 9-30). Under normal conditions, the amount of friction is reduced to a minimum by the large subacromial bursa, which extends laterally beneath the deltoid. Degenerative changes in the bursa are followed by degenerative changes in the underlying supraspinatus tendon, and these may extend into the other tendons of the rotator cuff. Clinically, the condition is known as **subacromial bursitis, supraspinatus tendinitis,** or **pericapsulitis.** It is characterized by the presence of a spasm of pain in the middle range of abduction (Fig. 9-30), when the diseased area impinges on the acromion.

Rupture of the Supraspinatus Tendon

In advanced cases of rotator cuff tendinitis, the necrotic supraspinatus tendon can become calcified or rupture. Rupture of the tendon seriously interferes with the normal abduction movement of the shoulder joint. It will be remembered that the main function of the supraspinatus muscle is to hold the head of the humerus in the glenoid fossa at the commencement of abduction. The patient with a ruptured supraspinatus tendon is unable to initiate abduction of the arm. However, if the arm is passively assisted for the first 15° of abduction, the deltoid can then take over and complete the movement to a right angle.

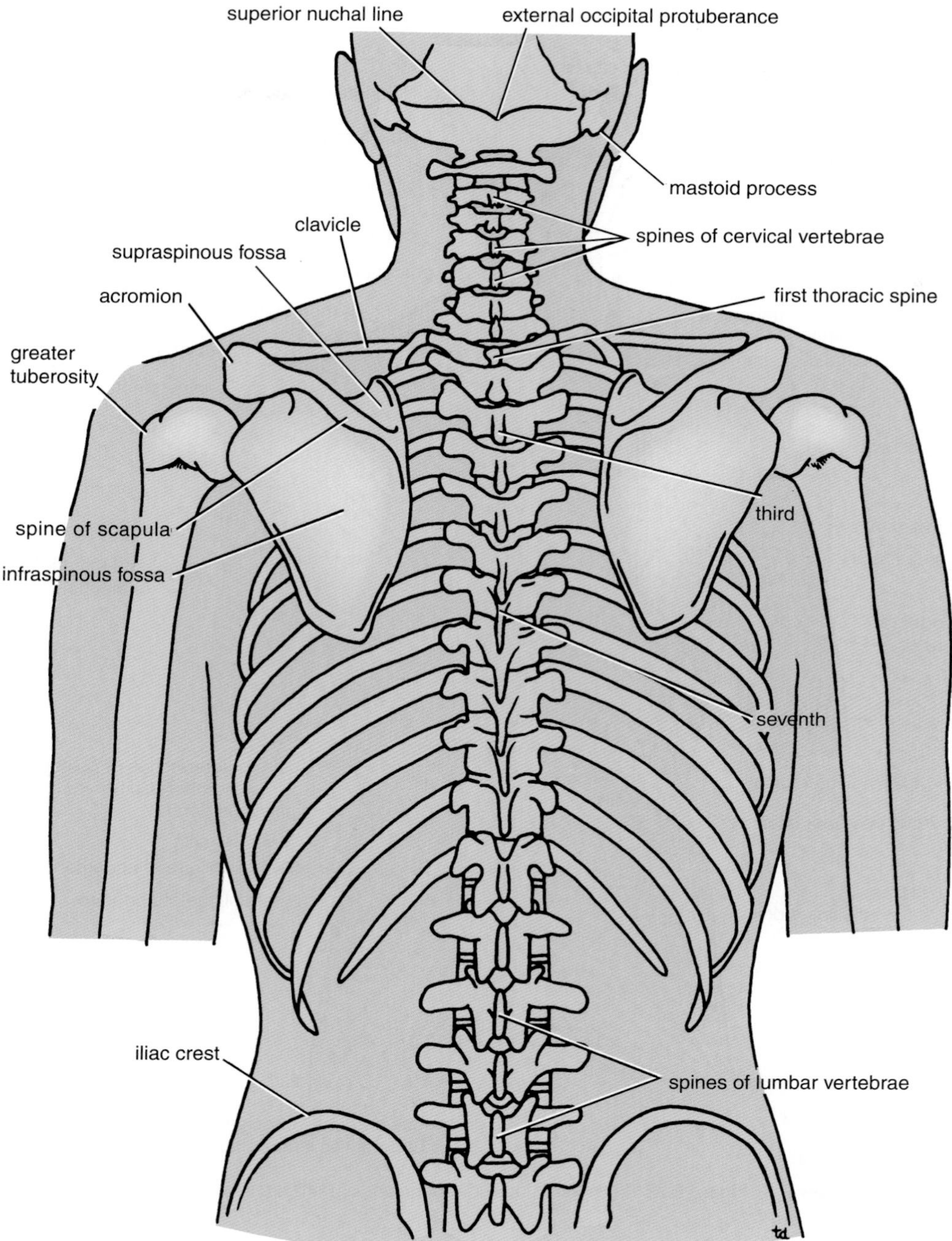

Figure 9-27 Bones of the back.

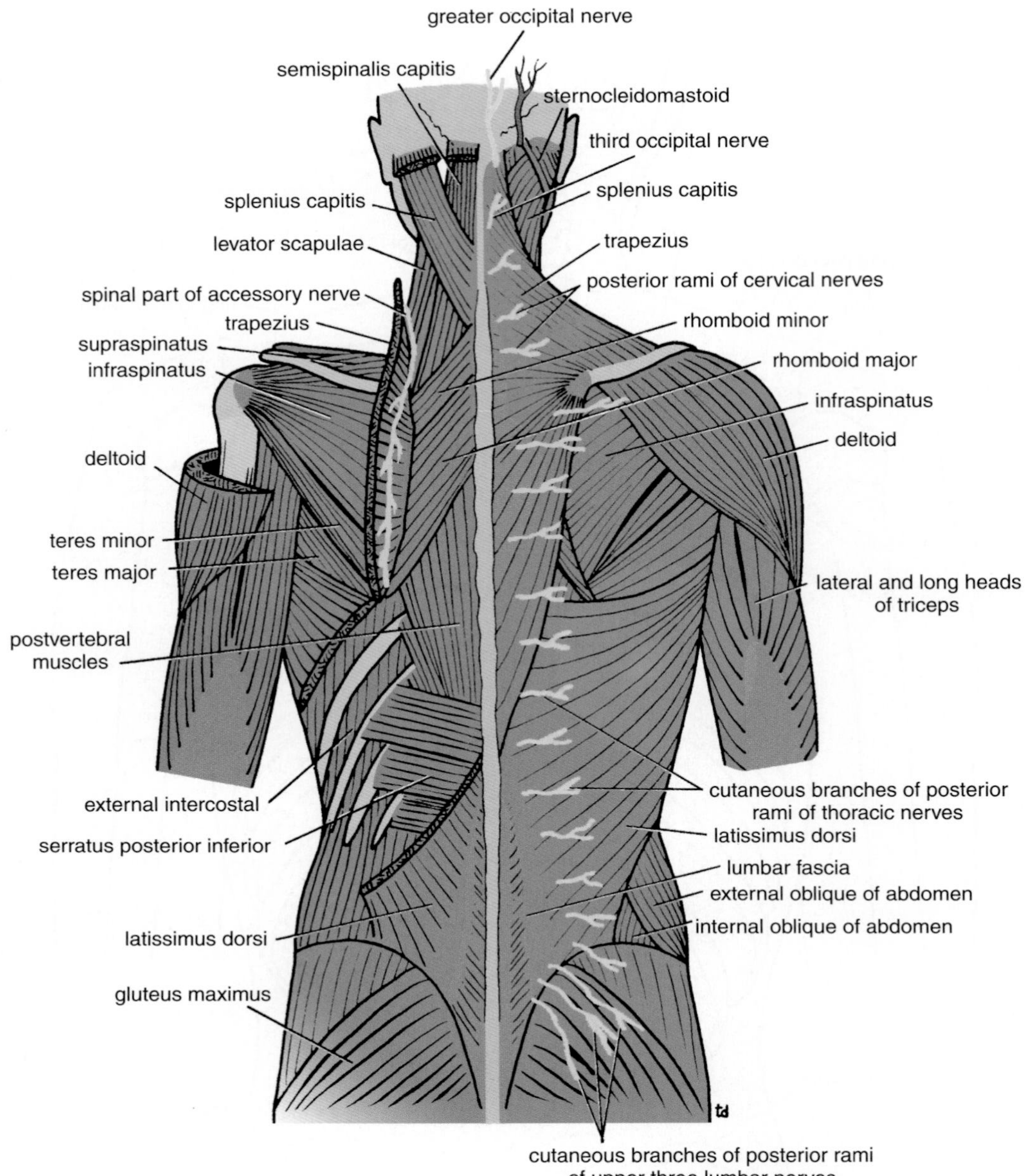

Figure 9-28 Superficial and deep muscles of the back.

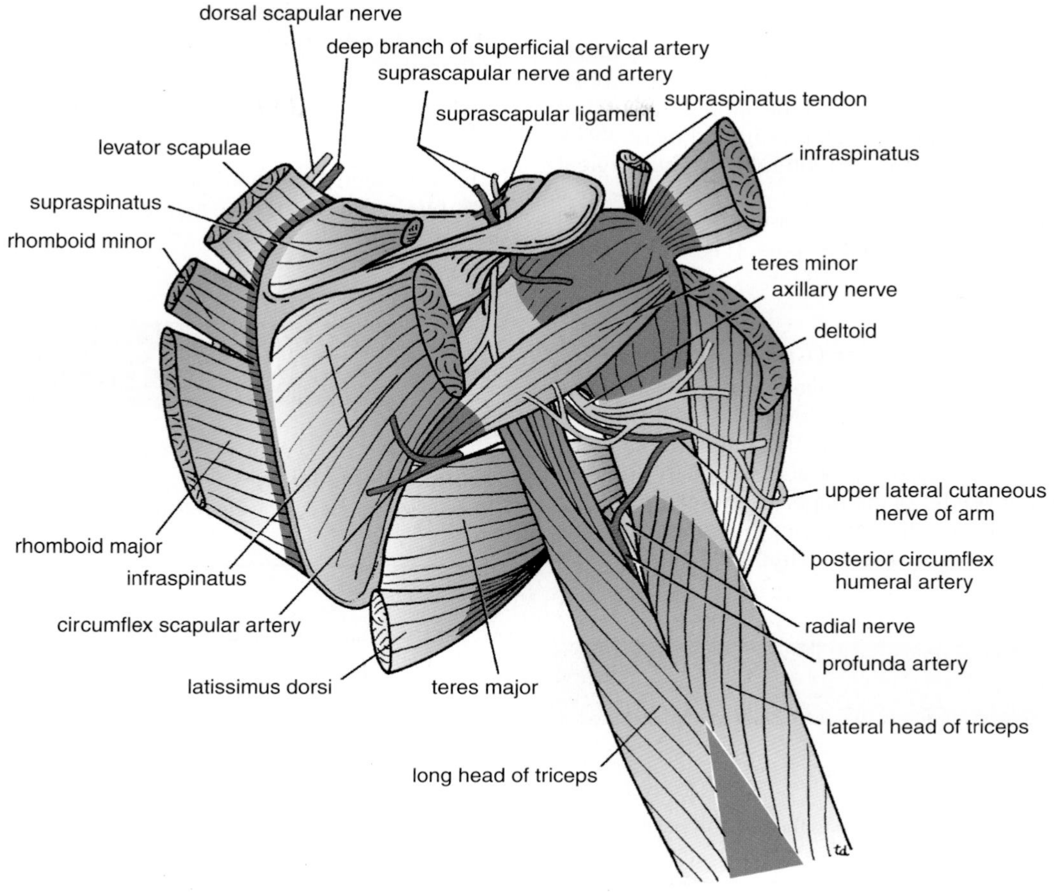

Figure 9-29 Muscles, nerves, and blood vessels of the scapular region. Note the close relation of the axillary nerve to the shoulder joint.

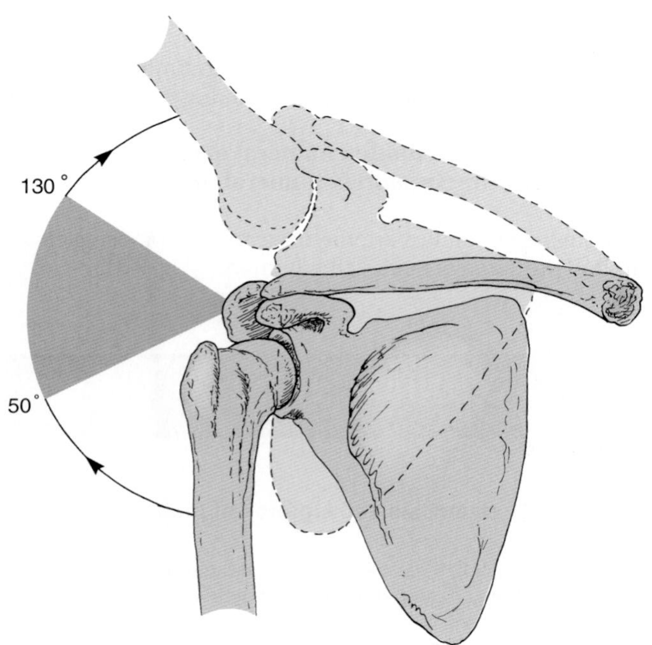

Figure 9-30 Subacromial bursitis, supraspinatus tendinitis, or pericapsulitis showing the painful arc in the middle range of abduction, when the diseased area impinges on the lateral edge of the acromion.

Quadrangular Space

The quadrangular space is an intermuscular space, located immediately below the shoulder joint. It is bounded above by the subscapularis and capsule of the shoulder joint and below by the teres major muscle. It is bounded medially by the long head of the triceps and laterally by the surgical neck of the humerus.

The axillary nerve and the posterior circumflex humeral vessels pass backward through this space (Fig. 9-29).

Nerves

Spinal Part of the Accessory Nerve (Cranial Nerve XI)

The spinal part of the accessory nerve runs downward in the posterior triangle of the neck on the levator scapulae muscle. It is accompanied by branches from the anterior rami of the third and fourth cervical nerves. The accessory nerve runs beneath the anterior border of the trapezius muscle (Fig. 9-28) at the junction of its middle and lower thirds and, together with the cervical nerves, supplies the trapezius muscle.

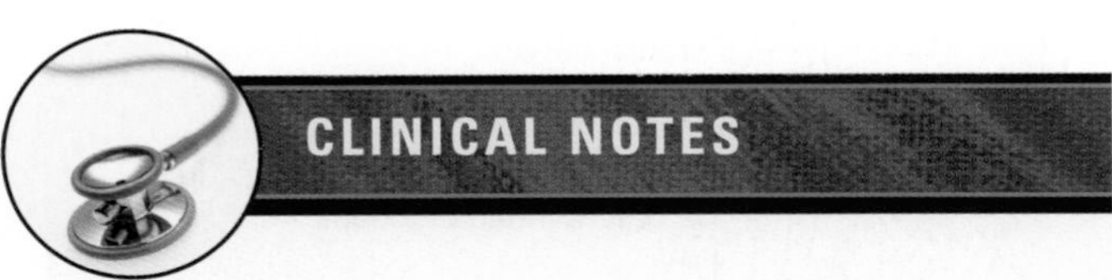

Accessory Nerve Injury

The accessory nerve can be injured as the result of stab wounds to the neck.

Suprascapular Nerve

The suprascapular nerve arises from the upper trunk of the brachial plexus (C5 and 6) in the posterior triangle in the neck. It runs downward and laterally and passes beneath the **suprascapular ligament,** which bridges the suprascapular notch, to reach the supraspinous fossa (Fig. 9-29). It supplies the supraspinatus and infraspinatus muscles and the shoulder joint.

Axillary Nerve

The axillary nerve arises from the posterior cord of the brachial plexus (C5 and 6) in the axilla (see page 450). It passes backward and enters the quadrangular space with the posterior circumflex humeral artery (Fig. 9-29). As the nerve passes through the space, it comes into close relationship with the inferior aspect of the capsule of the shoulder joint and with the medial side of the surgical neck of the humerus. It terminates by dividing into anterior and posterior branches (Fig. 9-29).

Branches

The axillary nerve has the following branches:

- An **articular branch** to the shoulder joint
- An **anterior terminal branch,** which winds around the surgical neck of the humerus beneath the deltoid muscle; it supplies the deltoid and the skin that covers its lower part.
- A **posterior terminal branch,** which gives off a **branch to the teres minor muscle** and a few branches to the deltoid, then emerges from the posterior border of the deltoid as the **upper lateral cutaneous nerve of the arm** (Fig. 9-29)

It is thus seen that the axillary nerve supplies the shoulder joint, two muscles, and the skin covering the lower half of the deltoid muscle.

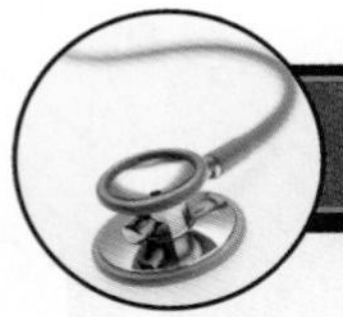
CLINICAL NOTES

Axillary Nerve Injury

The axillary nerve can be injured in dislocations of the shoulder joint.

Arterial Anastomosis Around the Shoulder Joint

The extreme mobility of the shoulder joint may result in kinking of the axillary artery and a temporary occlusion of its lumen. To compensate for this, an important arterial anastomosis exists between the branches of the subclavian artery and the axillary artery, thus ensuring that an adequate blood flow takes place into the upper limb irrespective of the position of the arm (Fig. 9-31).

Branches from the Subclavian Artery

- The **suprascapular artery,** which is distributed to the supraspinous and infraspinous fossae of the scapula
- The **superficial cervical artery,** which gives off a deep branch that runs down the medial border of the scapula

Branches from the Axillary Artery

- The **subscapular artery** and its circumflex scapular branch supply the subscapular and infraspinous fossae of the scapula, respectively.
- The **anterior circumflex humeral artery**
- The **posterior circumflex humeral artery**

Both the circumflex arteries form an anastomosing circle around the surgical neck of the humerus (Fig. 9-31).

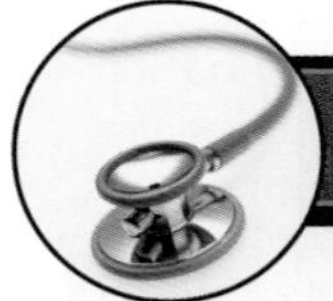
CLINICAL NOTES

Arterial Anastomosis and Ligation of the Axillary Artery

The existence of the anastomosis around the shoulder joint is vital to preserving the upper limb should it be necessary to ligate the axillary artery.

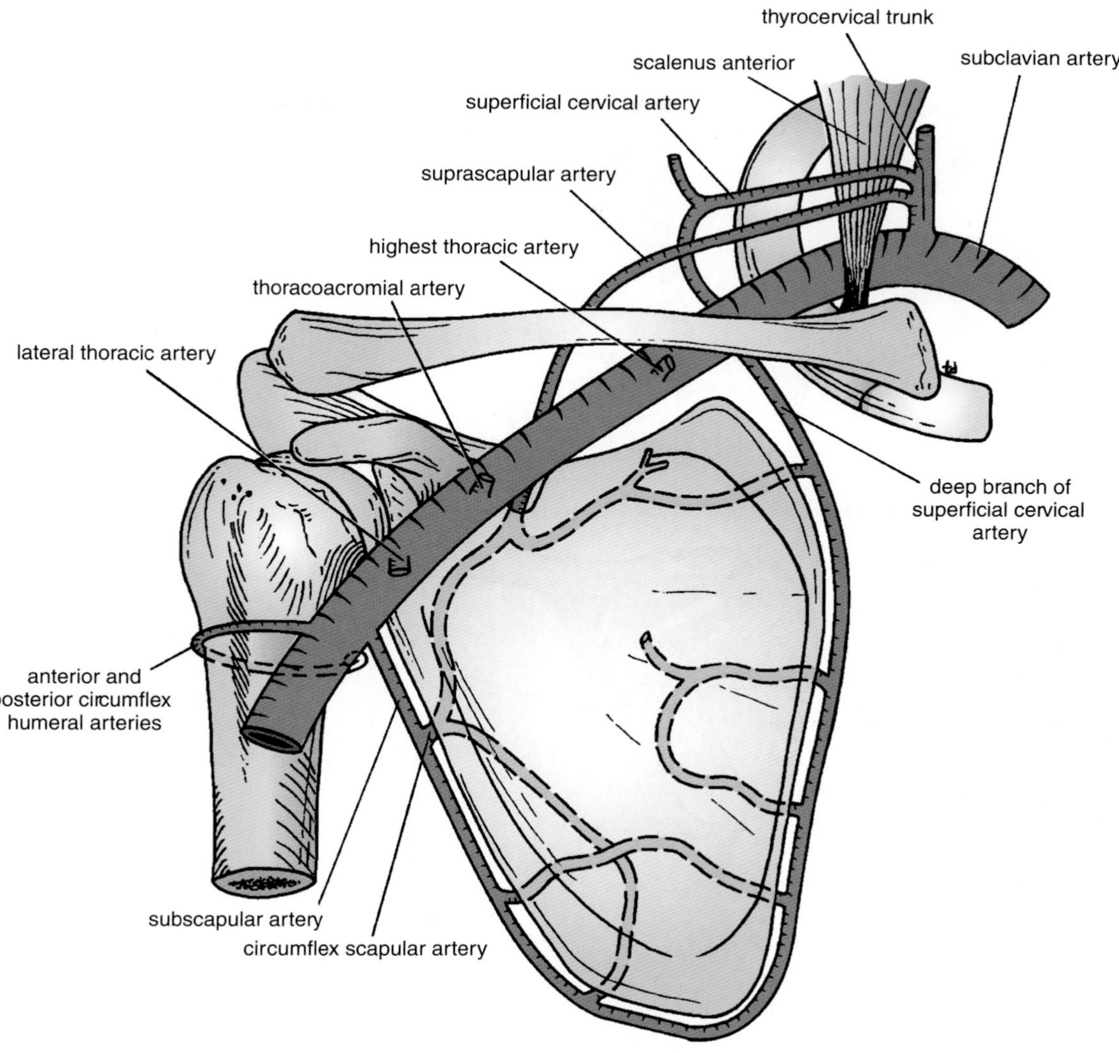

Figure 9-31 Arteries that take part in anastomosis around the shoulder joint.

Sternoclavicular Joint

- **Articulation:** This occurs between the sternal end of the clavicle, the manubrium sterni, and the first costal cartilage (Fig. 9-32).
- **Type:** Synovial double-plane joint
- **Capsule:** This surrounds the joint and is attached to the margins of the articular surfaces.
- **Ligaments:** The capsule is reinforced in front of and behind the joint by the strong **sternoclavicular ligaments.**
- **Articular disc:** This flat fibrocartilaginous disc lies within the joint and divides the joint's interior into two compartments (Fig. 9-32). Its circumference is attached to the interior of the capsule, but it is also strongly attached to the superior margin of the articular surface of the clavicle above and to the first costal cartilage below.
- **Accessory ligament:** The **costoclavicular ligament** is a strong ligament that runs from the junction of the first rib with the first costal cartilage to the inferior surface of the sternal end of the clavicle (Fig. 9-32).
- **Synovial membrane:** This lines the capsule and is attached to the margins of the cartilage covering the articular surfaces.
- **Nerve supply:** The supraclavicular nerve and the nerve to the subclavius muscle

Movements

Forward and backward movement of the clavicle takes place in the medial compartment. Elevation and depression of the clavicle take place in the lateral compartment.

Muscles Producing Movement

The forward movement of the clavicle is produced by the serratus anterior muscle. The backward movement is produced by the trapezius and rhomboid muscles. Elevation of the clavicle is produced by the trapezius, sternocleidomastoid, levator scapulae, and rhomboid muscles. Depression of the clavicle is produced by the pectoralis minor and the subclavius muscles (Fig. 9-33).

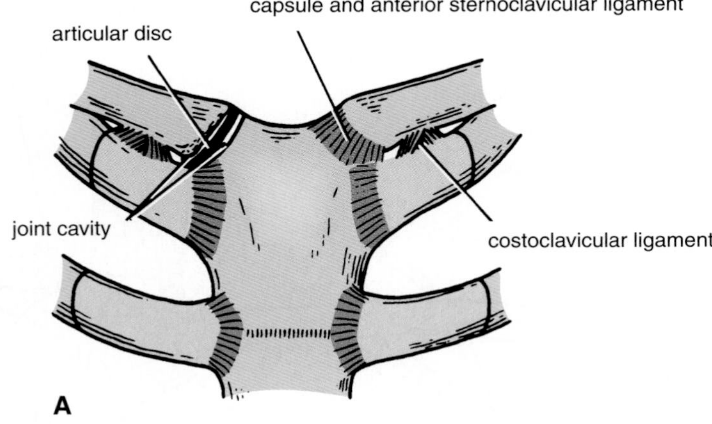

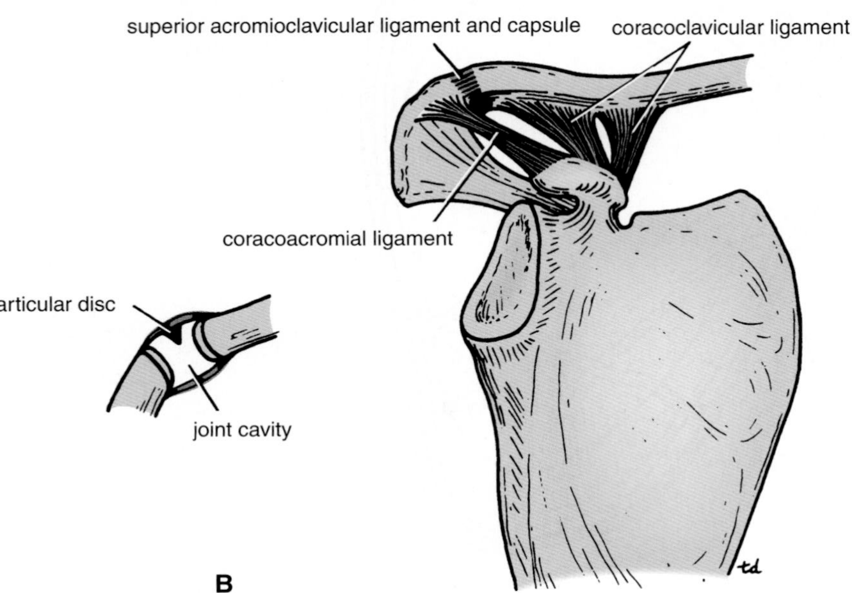

Figure 9-32 **A.** Sternoclavicular joint. **B.** Acromioclavicular joint.

Important Relations

- **Anteriorly:** The skin and some fibers of the sternocleidomastoid and pectoralis major muscles
- **Posteriorly:** The sternohyoid muscle; on the right, the brachiocephalic artery; on the left, the left brachiocephalic vein and the left common carotid artery

Acromioclavicular Joint

- **Articulation:** This occurs between the acromion of the scapula and the lateral end of the clavicle (Fig. 9-32).
- **Type:** Synovial plane joint
- **Capsule:** This surrounds the joint and is attached to the margins of the articular surfaces.

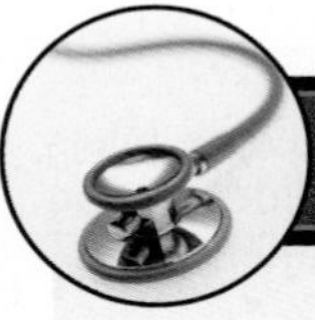

CLINICAL NOTES

Sternoclavicular Joint Injuries

The strong costoclavicular ligament firmly holds the medial end of the clavicle to the first costal cartilage. Violent forces directed along the long axis of the clavicle usually result in fracture of that bone, but dislocation of the sternoclavicular joint takes place occasionally.

Anterior dislocation results in the medial end of the clavicle projecting forward beneath the skin; it may also be pulled upward by the sternocleidomastoid muscle.

Posterior dislocation usually follows direct trauma applied to the front of the joint that drives the clavicle backward. This type is the more serious because the displaced clavicle may press on the trachea, the esophagus, and major blood vessels in the root of the neck.

If the costoclavicular ligament ruptures completely, it is difficult to maintain the normal position of the clavicle once reduction has been accomplished.

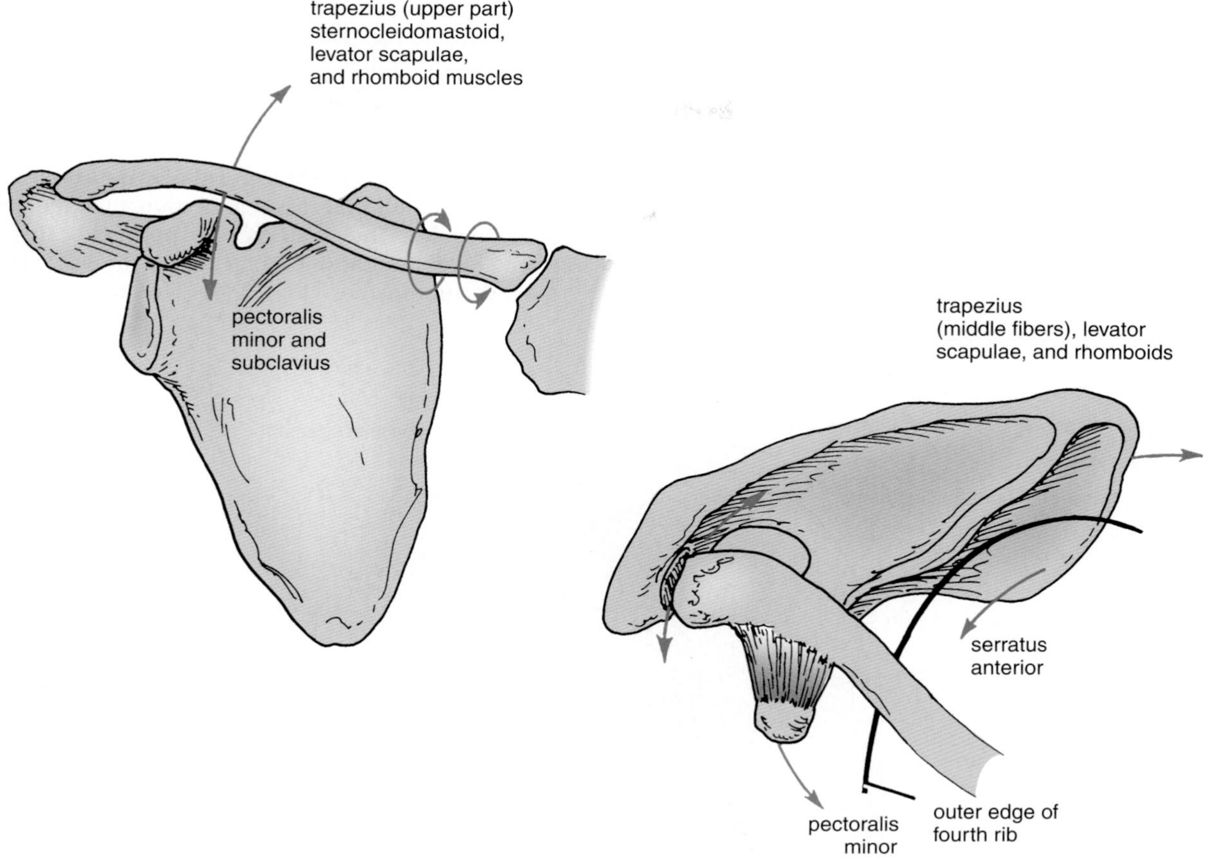

Figure 9-33 The wide range of movements possible at the sternoclavicular and acromioclavicular joints gives great mobility to the clavicle and the upper limb.

- **Ligaments: Superior** and **inferior acromioclavicular ligaments** reinforce the capsule; from the capsule, a wedge-shaped **fibrocartilaginous disc** projects into the joint cavity from above (Fig. 9-32).
- **Accessory ligament:** The very strong **coracoclavicular ligament** extends from the coracoid process to the undersurface of the clavicle (Fig. 9-32). It is largely responsible for suspending the weight of the scapula and the upper limb from the clavicle.
- **Synovial membrane:** This lines the capsule and is attached to the margins of the cartilage covering the articular surfaces.
- **Nerve supply:** The suprascapular nerve

Movements

A gliding movement takes place when the scapula rotates or when the clavicle is elevated or depressed (Fig. 9-33).

Important Relations

- **Anteriorly:** The deltoid muscle
- **Posteriorly:** The trapezius muscle
- **Superiorly:** The skin

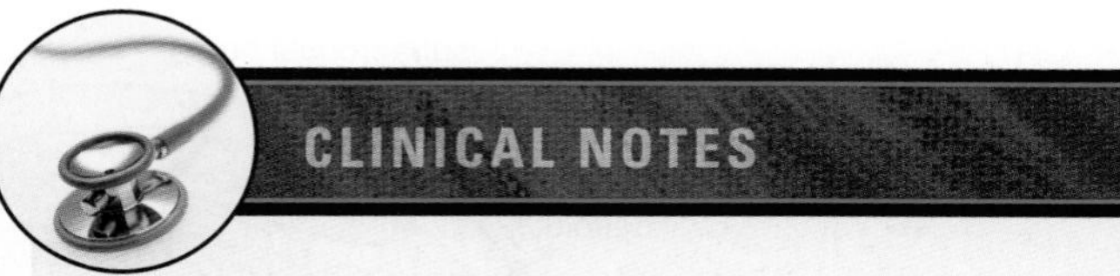

Acromioclavicular Joint Injuries

The plane of the articular surfaces of the acromioclavicular joint passes downward and medially so that there is a tendency for the lateral end of the clavicle to ride up over the upper surface of the acromion. The strength of the joint depends on the strong coracoclavicular ligament, which binds the coracoid process to the undersurface of the lateral part of the clavicle. The greater part of the weight of the upper limb is transmitted to the clavicle through this ligament, and rotary movements of the scapula occur at this important ligament.

Acromioclavicular Dislocation

A severe blow on the point of the shoulder, as is incurred during blocking or tackling in football or any severe fall, can result in the acromion being thrust beneath the lateral end of the clavicle, tearing the coracoclavicular ligament. This condition is known as **shoulder separation.** The displaced outer end of the clavicle is easily palpable. As in the case of the sternoclavicular joint, the dislocation is easily reduced, but withdrawal of support results in immediate redislocation.

Shoulder Joint

- **Articulation:** This occurs between the rounded head of the humerus and the shallow, pear-shaped glenoid cavity of the scapula. The articular surfaces are covered by hyaline articular cartilage, and the glenoid cavity is deepened by the presence of a fibrocartilaginous rim called the **glenoid labrum** (Figs. 9-34 and 9-35).
- **Type:** Synovial ball-and-socket joint
- **Capsule:** This surrounds the joint and is attached medially to the margin of the glenoid cavity outside the labrum; laterally it is attached to the anatomic neck of the humerus (Fig. 9-35). The capsule is thin and lax, allowing a wide range of movement. It is strengthened by fibrous slips from the tendons of the subscapularis, supraspinatus, infraspinatus, and teres minor muscles (the rotator cuff muscles).
- **Ligaments:** The **glenohumeral ligaments** are three weak bands of fibrous tissue that strengthen the front of the capsule. The **transverse humeral ligament** strengthens the capsule and bridges the gap between the two tuberosities (Fig. 9-34). The **coracohumeral**

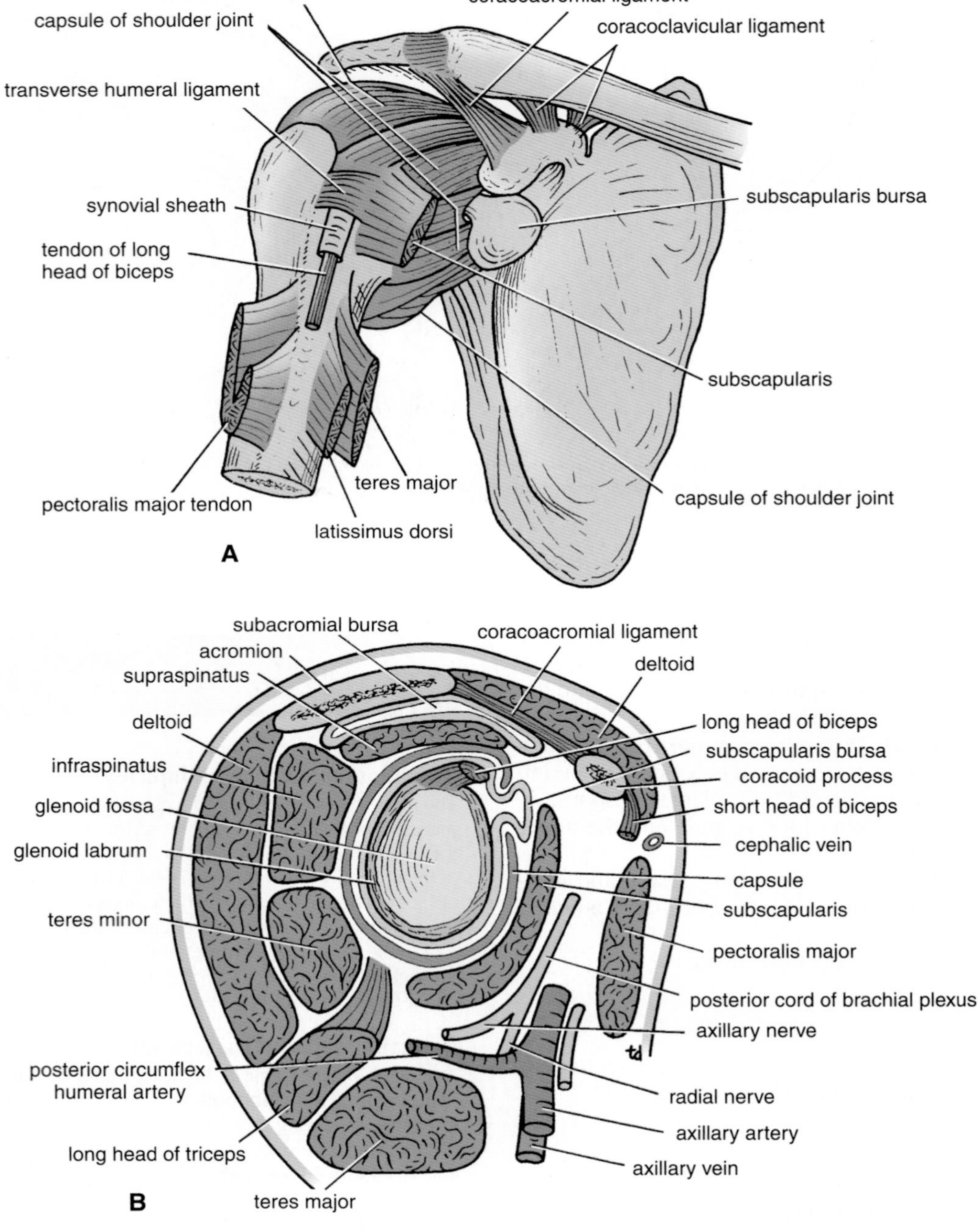

Figure 9-34 Shoulder joint and its relations. **A.** Anterior view. **B.** Sagittal section.

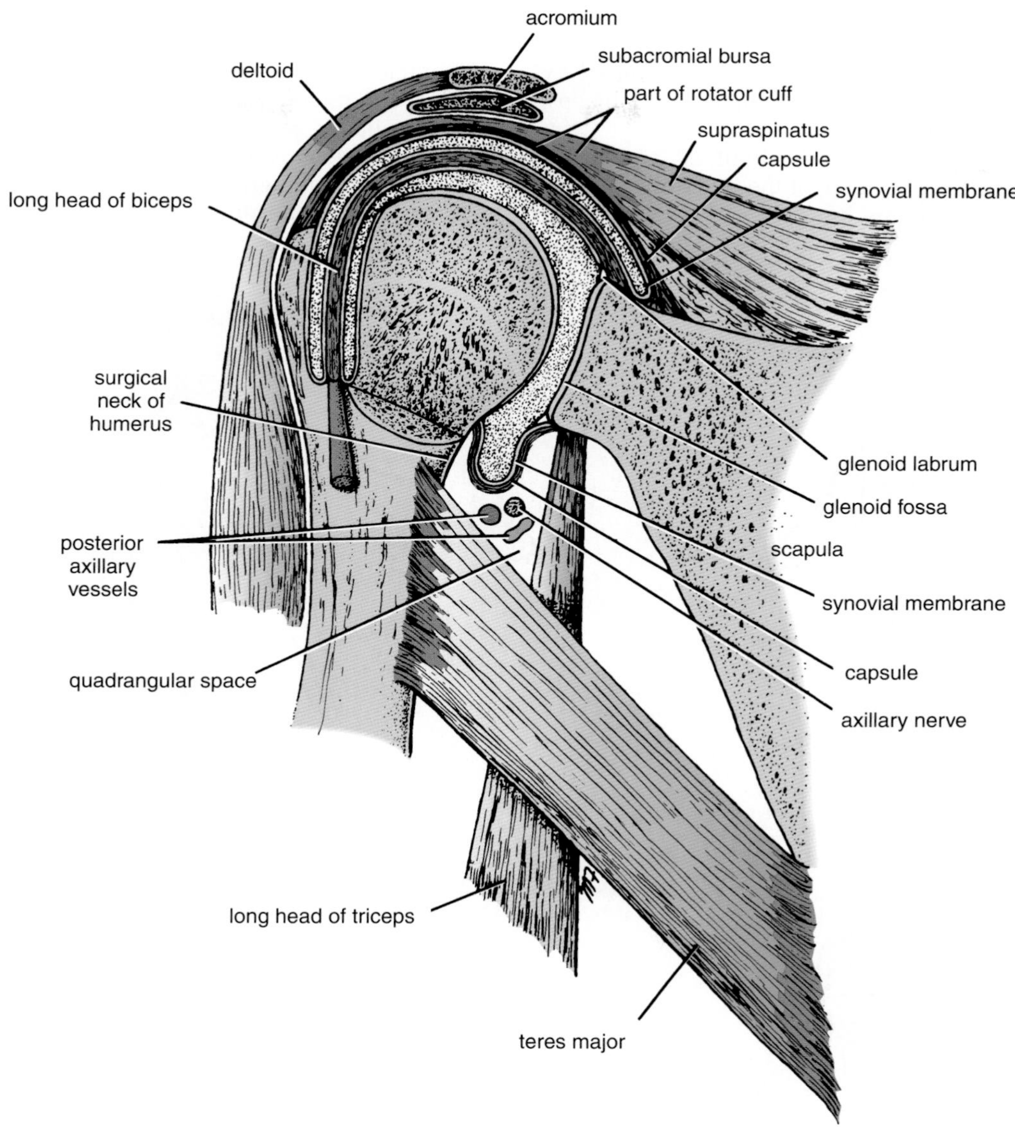

Figure 9-35 Interior of the shoulder joint.

ligament strengthens the capsule above and stretches from the root of the coracoid process to the greater tuberosity of the humerus (Fig. 9-34).

- **Accessory ligaments:** The **coracoacromial ligament** extends between the coracoid process and the acromion. Its function is to protect the superior aspect of the joint (Fig. 9-34).
- **Synovial membrane:** This lines the capsule and is attached to the margins of the cartilage covering the articular surfaces (Figs. 9-34 and 9-35). It forms a tubular sheath around the tendon of the long head of the biceps brachii. It extends through the anterior wall of the capsule to form the **subscapularis bursa** beneath the subscapularis muscle (Fig. 9-34).
- **Nerve supply:** The axillary and suprascapular nerves

Movements

The shoulder joint has a wide range of movement, and the stability of the joint has been sacrificed to permit this. (Compare with the hip joint, which is stable but limited in its movements.) The strength of the joint depends on the tone of the short rotator cuff muscles that cross in front, above, and behind the joint—namely, the subscapularis, supraspinatus, infraspinatus, and teres minor. When the joint is abducted, the lower surface of the head of the humerus is supported by the long head of the triceps, which bows downward because of its length and gives little actual support to the humerus. In addition, the inferior part of the capsule is the weakest area.

The following movements are possible (Fig. 9-36):

- **Flexion:** Normal flexion is about 90° and is performed by the anterior fibers of the deltoid, pectoralis major, biceps, and coracobrachialis muscles.
- **Extension:** Normal extension is about 45° and is performed by the posterior fibers of the deltoid, latissimus dorsi, and teres major muscles.
- **Abduction:** Abduction of the upper limb occurs both at the shoulder joint and between the scapula and the thoracic wall (see scapular–humeral mechanism, page 465). The middle fibers of the deltoid, assisted by the supraspinatus, are involved. The supraspinatus muscle initiates the movement of abduction and holds the head of the humerus against the glenoid fossa of the scapula; this latter function allows the deltoid muscle

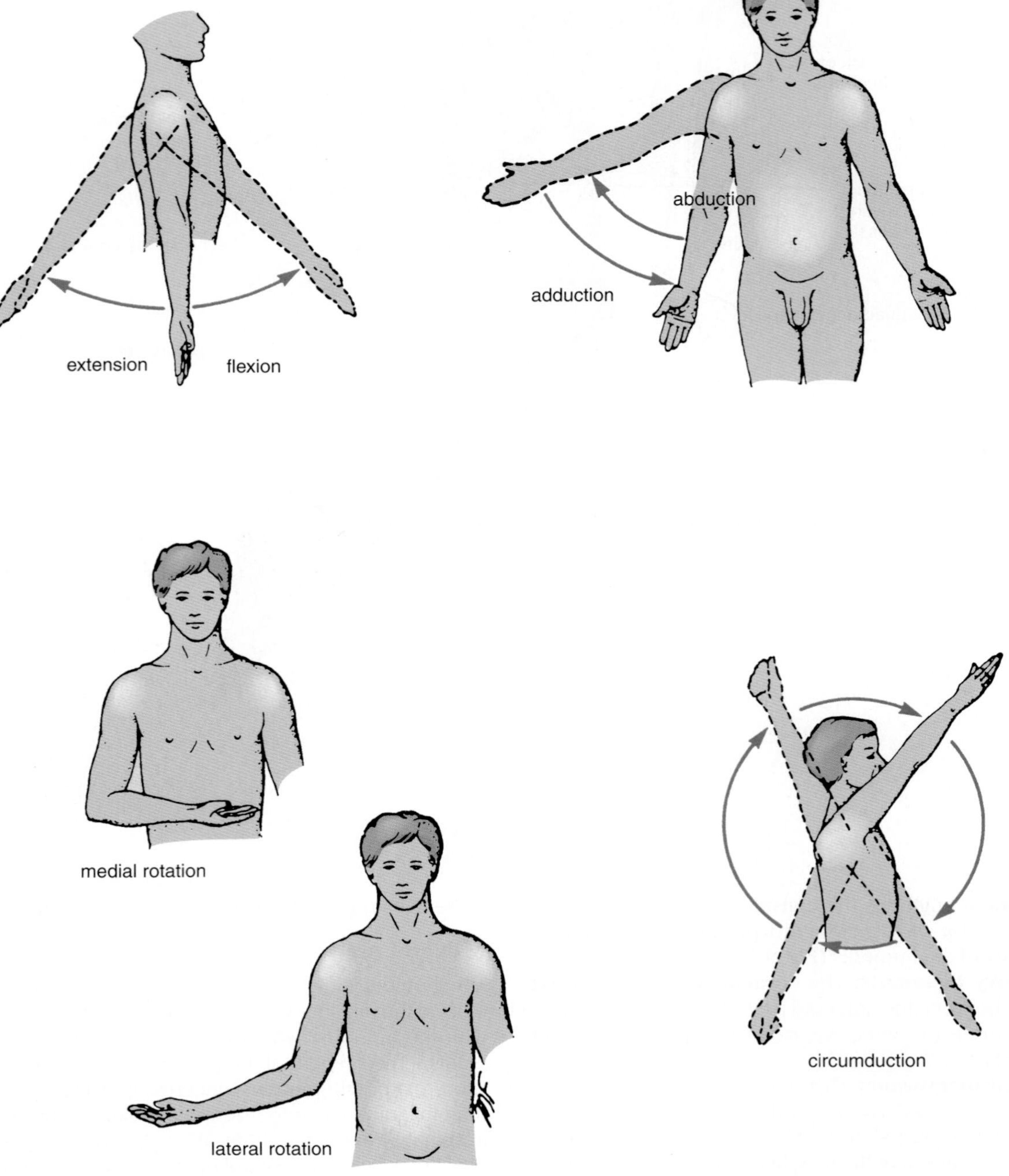

Figure 9-36 The movements possible at the shoulder joint. Pure glenohumeral abduction is possible only as much as about 120°; further movement of the upper limb above the level of the shoulder requires rotation of the scapula (see text).

to contract and abduct the humerus at the shoulder joint.

- **Adduction:** Normally, the upper limb can be swung 45° across the front of the chest. This is performed by the pectoralis major, latissimus dorsi, teres major, and teres minor muscles.
- **Lateral rotation:** Normal lateral rotation is 40° to 45°. This is performed by the infraspinatus, the teres minor, and the posterior fibers of the deltoid muscle.
- **Medial rotation:** Normal medial rotation is about 55°. This is performed by the subscapularis, the latissimus dorsi, the teres major, and the anterior fibers of the deltoid muscle.
- **Circumduction:** This is a combination of the above movements.

Important Relations

- **Anteriorly:** The subscapularis muscle and the axillary vessels and brachial plexus
- **Posteriorly:** The infraspinatus and teres minor muscles
- **Superiorly:** The supraspinatus muscle, subacromial bursa, coracoacromial ligament, and deltoid muscle
- **Inferiorly:** The long head of the triceps muscle, the axillary nerve, and the posterior circumflex humeral vessels

The tendon of the long head of the biceps muscle passes through the joint and emerges beneath the transverse ligament.

The Scapular–Humeral Mechanism

The scapula and upper limb are suspended from the clavicle by the strong coracoclavicular ligament assisted by the tone of muscles. When the scapula rotates on the chest wall so that the position of the glenoid fossa is altered, the axis of rotation may be considered to pass through the coracoclavicular ligament.

Abduction of the arm involves rotation of the scapula as well as movement at the shoulder joint. For every 3° of abduction of the arm, a 2° abduction occurs in the shoulder joint and a 1° abduction occurs by rotation of the scapula. At about 120° of abduction of the arm, the greater tuberosity of the humerus comes into contact with the lateral edge of the acromion. Further elevation of the arm above the head is accomplished by rotating the scapula. Figure 9-37 summarizes the movements of abduction of the arm and shows the direction of pull of the muscles responsible for these movements.

The Upper Arm

Skin

Superficial Sensory Nerves

The sensory nerve supply (Fig. 9-38) to the skin over the point of the shoulder to halfway down the deltoid muscle is from the **supraclavicular nerves** (C3 and 4). The skin over

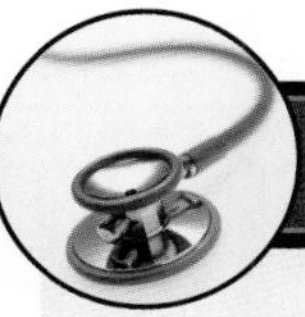

CLINICAL NOTES

Stability of the Shoulder Joint

The shallowness of the glenoid fossa of the scapula and the lack of support provided by weak ligaments make this joint an unstable structure. Its strength almost entirely depends on the tone of the short muscles that bind the upper end of the humerus to the scapula—namely, the subscapularis in front, the supraspinatus above, and the infraspinatus and teres minor behind. The tendons of these muscles are fused to the underlying capsule of the shoulder joint. Together, these tendons form the rotator cuff.

The least supported part of the joint lies in the inferior location, where it is unprotected by muscles.

Dislocations of the Shoulder Joint

The shoulder joint is the most commonly dislocated large joint.

Anterior Inferior Dislocation

Sudden violence applied to the humerus with the joint fully abducted tilts the humeral head downward onto the inferior weak part of the capsule, which tears, and the humeral head comes to lie inferior to the glenoid fossa. During this movement, the acromion has acted as a fulcrum. The strong flexors and adductors of the shoulder joint now usually pull the humeral head forward and upward into the subcoracoid position.

Posterior Dislocations

Posterior dislocations are rare and are usually caused by direct violence to the front of the joint. On inspection of the patient with shoulder dislocation, the rounded appearance of the shoulder is seen to be lost because the greater tuberosity of the humerus is no longer bulging laterally beneath the deltoid muscle. A subglenoid displacement of the head of the humerus into the quadrangular space can cause damage to the axillary nerve, as indicated by paralysis of the deltoid muscle and loss of skin sensation over the lower half of the deltoid. Downward displacement of the humerus can also stretch and damage the radial nerve.

Shoulder Pain

The synovial membrane, capsule, and ligaments of the shoulder joint are innervated by the axillary nerve and the suprascapular nerve. The joint is sensitive to pain, pressure, excessive traction, and distention. The muscles surrounding the joint undergo reflex spasm in response to pain originating in the joint, which in turn serves to immobilize the joint and thus reduce the pain.

Injury to the shoulder joint is followed by pain, limitation of movement, and muscle atrophy owing to disuse. It is important to appreciate that pain in the shoulder region can be caused by disease elsewhere and that the shoulder joint may be normal; for example, diseases of the spinal cord and vertebral column and the pressure of a cervical rib (see page 50) can cause shoulder pain. Irritation of the diaphragmatic pleura or peritoneum can produce referred pain via the phrenic and supraclavicular nerves.

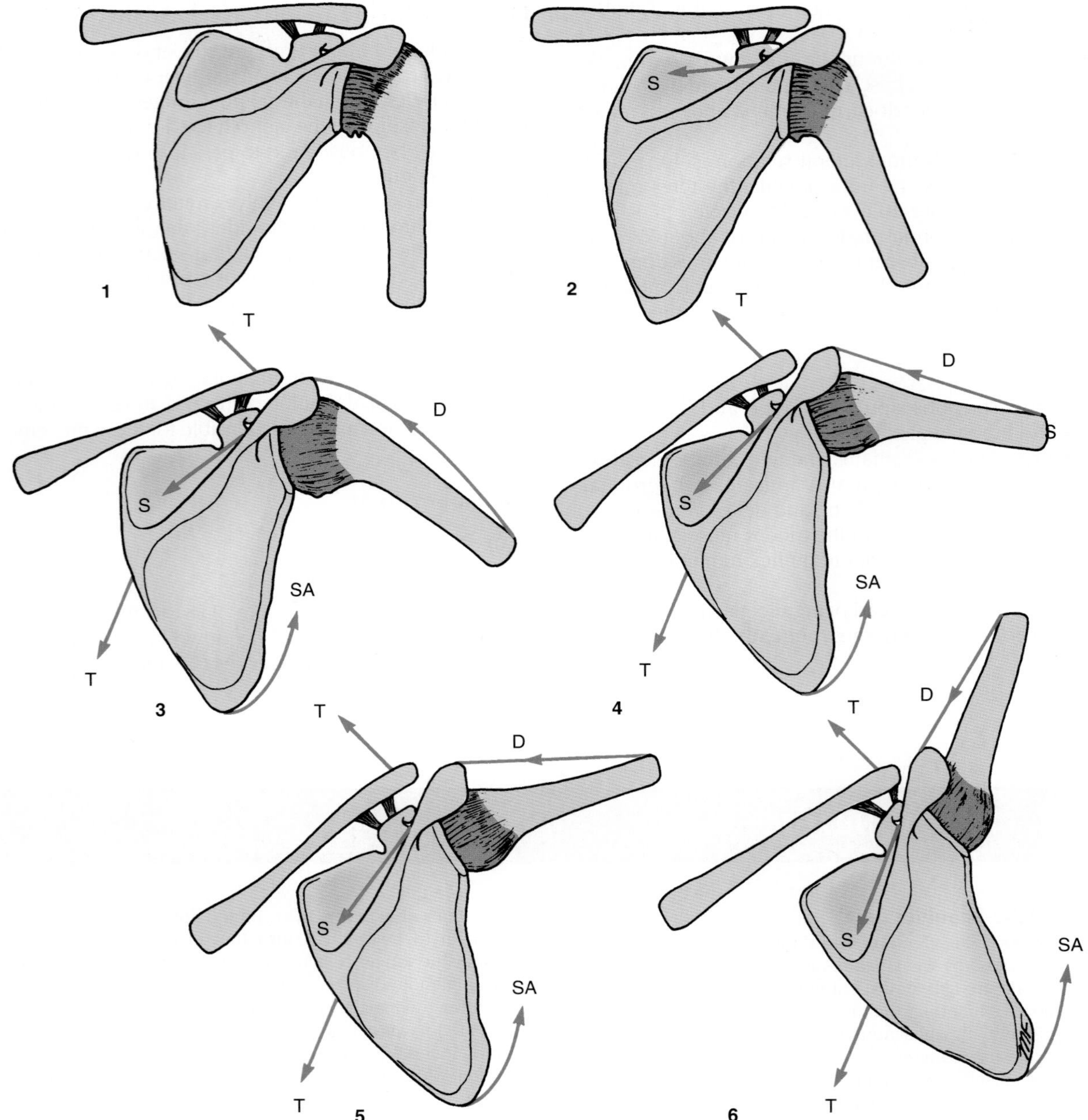

Figure 9-37 Movements of abduction of the shoulder joint and rotation of the scapula and the muscles producing these movements. Note that for every 3° of abduction of the arm, a 2° abduction occurs in the shoulder joint, and 1° occurs by rotation of the scapula. At about 120° of abduction, the greater tuberosity of the humerus hits the lateral edge of the acromion. Elevation of the arm above the head is accomplished by rotating the scapula. S, supraspinatus; D, deltoid; T, trapezius; SA, serratus anterior.

the lower half of the deltoid is supplied by the **upper lateral cutaneous nerve of the arm,** a branch of the axillary nerve (C5 and 6). The skin over the lateral surface of the arm below the deltoid is supplied by the **lower lateral cutaneous nerve of the arm,** a branch of the radial nerve (C5 and 6). The skin of the armpit and the medial side of the arm is supplied by the **medial cutaneous nerve of the arm** (T1) and the **intercostobrachial nerves** (T2). The skin of the back of the arm (Fig. 9-38) is supplied by the **posterior cutaneous nerve of the arm,** a branch of the radial nerve (C8).

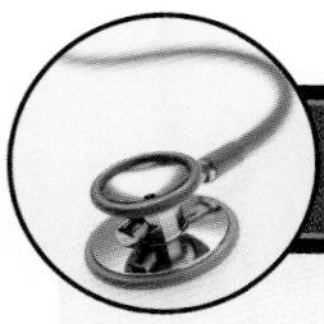

CLINICAL NOTES

Dermatomes and Cutaneous Nerves

It may be necessary for a physician to test the integrity of the spinal cord segments of C3 through T1. The diagrams in Figures 1-23 and 1-24 show the arrangement of the dermatomes of the upper limb. It is seen that the dermatomes for the upper cervical segments C3 to 6 are located along the lateral margin of the upper limb; the C7 dermatome is situated on the middle finger; and the dermatomes for C8, T1, and T2 are along the medial margin of the limb. The nerve fibers from a particular segment of the spinal cord, although they exit from the cord in a spinal nerve of the same segment, pass to the skin in two or more different cutaneous nerves.

The skin over the point of the shoulder and halfway down the lateral surface of the deltoid muscle is supplied by the supraclavicular nerves (C3 and 4). Pain may be referred to this region as a result of inflammatory lesions involving the diaphragmatic pleura or peritoneum. The afferent stimuli reach the spinal cord via the phrenic nerves (C3, 4, and 5). Pleurisy, peritonitis, subphrenic abscess, or gallbladder disease may therefore be responsible for shoulder pain.

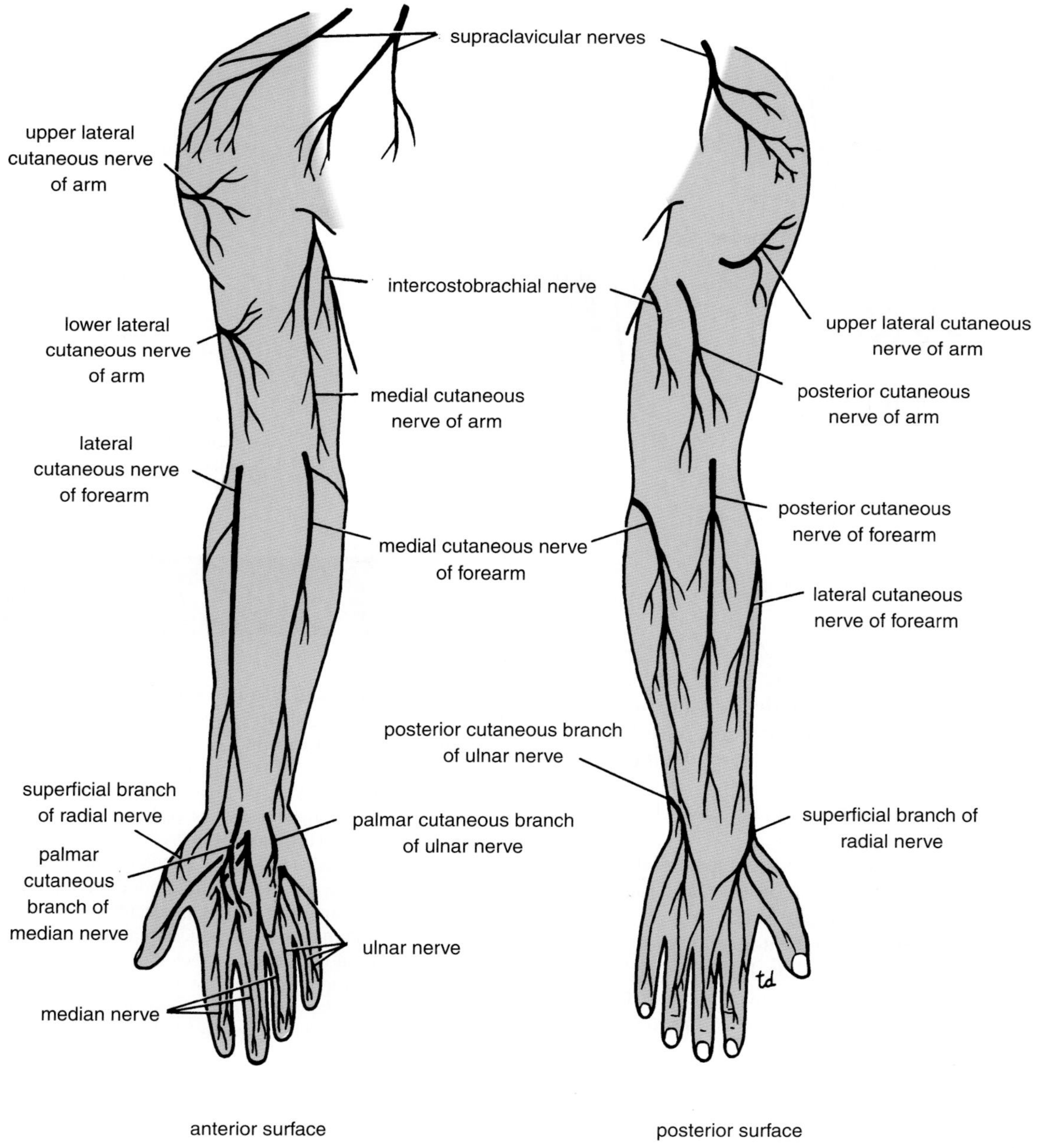

Figure 9-38 Cutaneous innervation of the upper limb.

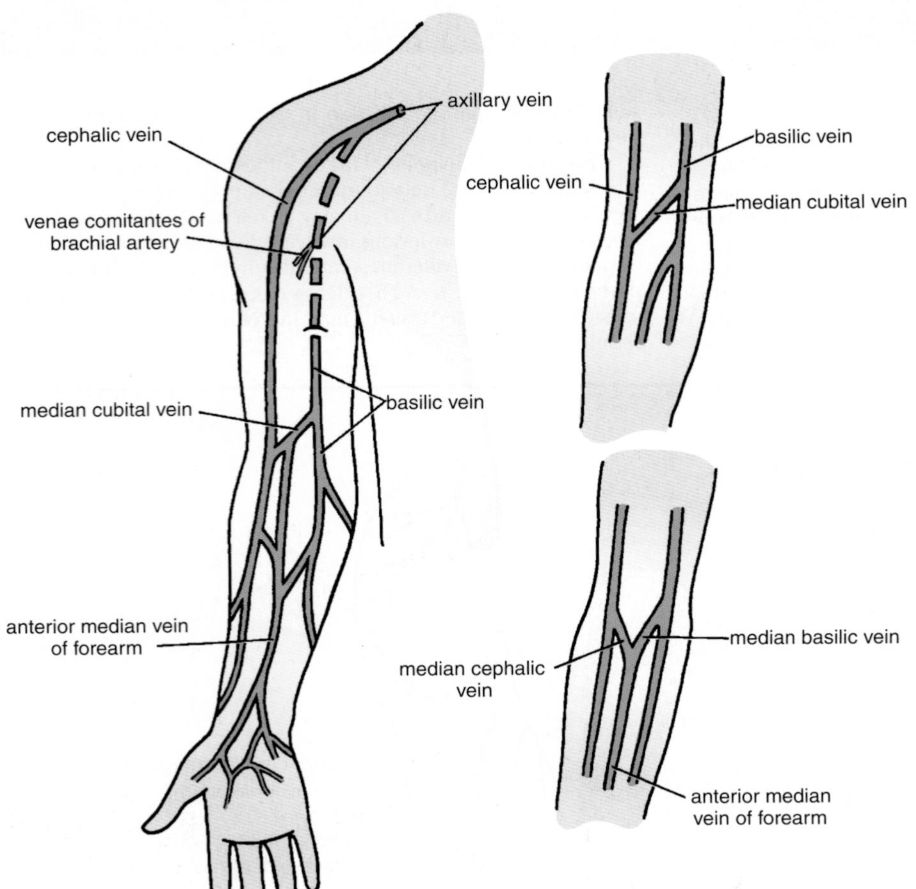

Figure 9-39 Superficial veins of the upper limb. Note the common variations seen in the region of the elbow.

Superficial Veins

The veins of the upper limb can be divided into two groups: superficial and deep. The deep veins comprise the venae comitantes, which accompany all the large arteries, usually in pairs, and the axillary vein.

The superficial veins of the arm (Fig. 9-39) lie in the superficial fascia.

The **cephalic vein** ascends in the superficial fascia on the lateral side of the biceps and, on reaching the infraclavicular fossa, drains into the axillary vein.

The **basilic vein** ascends in the superficial fascia on the medial side of the biceps (Fig. 9-39). Halfway up the arm, it pierces the deep fascia and at the lower border of the teres major joins the venae comitantes of the brachial artery to form the axillary vein.

Nerve Supply of the Veins

Like the arteries, the smooth muscle in the wall of the veins is innervated by sympathetic postganglionic nerve fibers that provide vasomotor tone. The origin of these fibers is similar to those of the arteries.

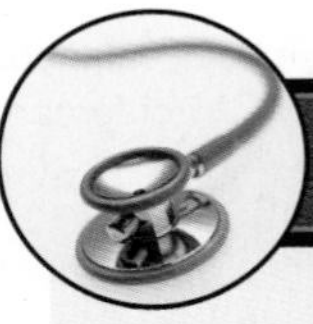

CLINICAL NOTES

Venipuncture and Blood Transfusion

The superficial veins are clinically important and are used for venipuncture, transfusion, and cardiac catheterization. Every clinical professional, in an emergency, should know where to obtain blood from the arm. When a patient is in a state of shock, the superficial veins are not always visible. The cephalic vein lies fairly constantly in the superficial fascia, immediately posterior to the styloid process of the radius. In the cubital fossa, the median cubital vein is separated from the underlying brachial artery by the bicipital aponeurosis. This is important because it protects the artery from the mistaken introduction into its lumen of irritating drugs that should have been injected into the vein. The cephalic vein, in the deltopectoral triangle, frequently communicates with the external jugular vein by a small vein that crosses in front of the clavicle. Fracture of the clavicle can result in rupture of this communicating vein, with the formation of a large hematoma.

Intravenous Transfusion and Hypovolemic Shock

In extreme hypovolemic shock, excessive venous tone may inhibit venous blood flow and thus delay the introduction of intravenous blood into the vascular system.

(continues)

Clinical Notes, *continued*

Anatomy of Basilic and Cephalic Vein Catheterization

The median basilic or basilic veins are the veins of choice for central venous catheterization, because from the cubital fossa until the basilic vein reaches the axillary vein, the basilic vein increases in diameter and is in direct line with the axillary vein (Fig. 9-39). The valves in the axillary vein may be troublesome, but abduction of the shoulder joint may permit the catheter to move past the obstruction.

The cephalic vein does not increase in size as it ascends the arm, and it frequently divides into small branches as it lies within the deltopectoral triangle. One or more of these branches may ascend over the clavicle and join the external jugular vein. In its usual method of termination, the cephalic vein joins the axillary vein at a right angle. It may be difficult to maneuver the catheter around this angle.

Superficial Lymph Vessels

The superficial lymph vessels draining the superficial tissues of the upper arm pass upward to the axilla (Fig. 9-40). Those from the lateral side of the arm follow the cephalic vein to the infraclavicular group of nodes; those from the medial side follow the basilic vein to the lateral group of axillary nodes.

The **deep lymphatic vessels** draining the muscles and deep structures of the arm drain into the lateral group of axillary nodes.

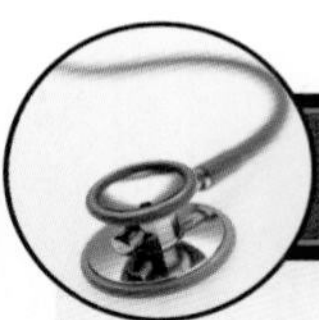

CLINICAL NOTES

Lymphangitis

Infection of the lymph vessels (lymphangitis) of the arm is common. Red streaks along the course of the lymph vessels are characteristic of the condition. The lymph vessels from the thumb and index finger and the lateral part of the hand follow the cephalic vein to the infraclavicular group of axillary nodes; those from the middle, ring, and little fingers and from the medial part of the hand follow the basilic vein to the supratrochlear node, which lies in the superficial fascia just above the medial epicondyle of the humerus, and thence to the lateral group of axillary nodes.

Lymphadenitis

Once the infection reaches the lymph nodes, they become enlarged and tender, a condition known as lymphadenitis. Most of the lymph vessels from the fingers and palm pass to the dorsum of the hand before passing up into the forearm. This explains the frequency of inflammatory edema, or even abscess formation, which may occur on the dorsum of the hand after infection of the fingers or palm.

Fascial Compartments of the Upper Arm

The upper arm is enclosed in a sheath of deep fascia (Fig. 9-41). Two fascial septa, one on the medial side and one on the lateral side, extend from this sheath and are attached to the medial and lateral supracondylar ridges of the humerus, respectively. By this means, the upper arm is divided into an anterior and a posterior fascial compartment, each having its muscles, nerves, and arteries.

Contents of the Anterior Fascial Compartment of the Upper Arm

- **Muscles:** Biceps brachii, coracobrachialis, and brachialis
- **Blood supply:** Brachial artery (Fig. 9-42)
- **Nerve supply to the muscles:** Musculocutaneous nerve
- **Structures passing through the compartment:** Musculocutaneous, median, and ulnar nerves; brachial artery and basilic vein. The radial nerve is present in the lower part of the compartment.

Muscles of the Anterior Fascial Compartment

The muscles of the anterior fascial compartment are shown in Figures 9-43 and 9-44 and are described in Table 9-5. Note that the biceps brachii is a powerful supinator and this action is made use of in twisting the corkscrew into the cork or driving the screw into wood with a screwdriver. The biceps also is a powerful flexor of the elbow joint and a weak flexor of the shoulder joint.

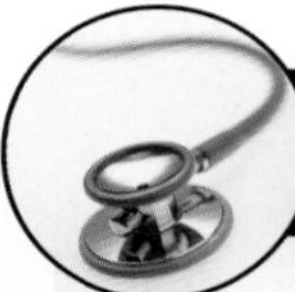

CLINICAL NOTES

Biceps Brachii and Osteoarthritis of the Shoulder Joint

The tendon of the long head of biceps is attached to the supraglenoid tubercle within the shoulder joint. Advanced osteoarthritic changes in the joint can lead to erosion and fraying of the tendon by osteophytic outgrowths, and rupture of the tendon can occur.

Structures Passing Through the Anterior Fascial Compartment

Brachial Artery The brachial artery (Figs. 9-42 and 9-43) begins at the lower border of the teres major muscle as a continuation of the axillary artery. It provides the main arterial supply to the arm (Fig. 9-42). It terminates opposite the neck of the radius by dividing into the radial and ulnar arteries.

Relations

- **Anteriorly:** The vessel is superficial and is overlapped from the lateral side by the coracobrachialis and biceps. The medial cutaneous nerve of the forearm lies in front of the upper part; the median nerve crosses its middle part; and the bicipital aponeurosis crosses its lower part (Fig. 9-43).
- **Posteriorly:** The artery lies on the triceps, the coracobrachialis insertion, and the brachialis (Fig. 9-43).

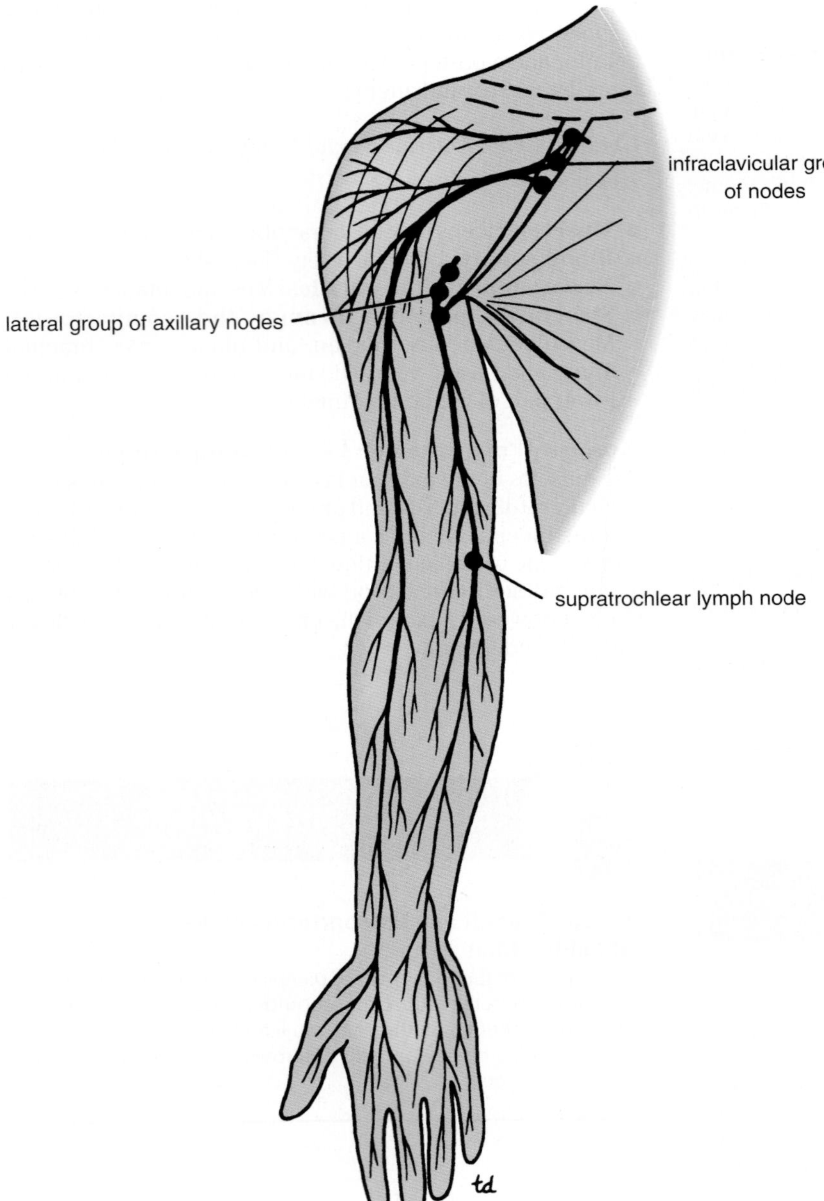

Figure 9-40 Superficial lymphatics of the upper limb. Note the positions of the lymph nodes.

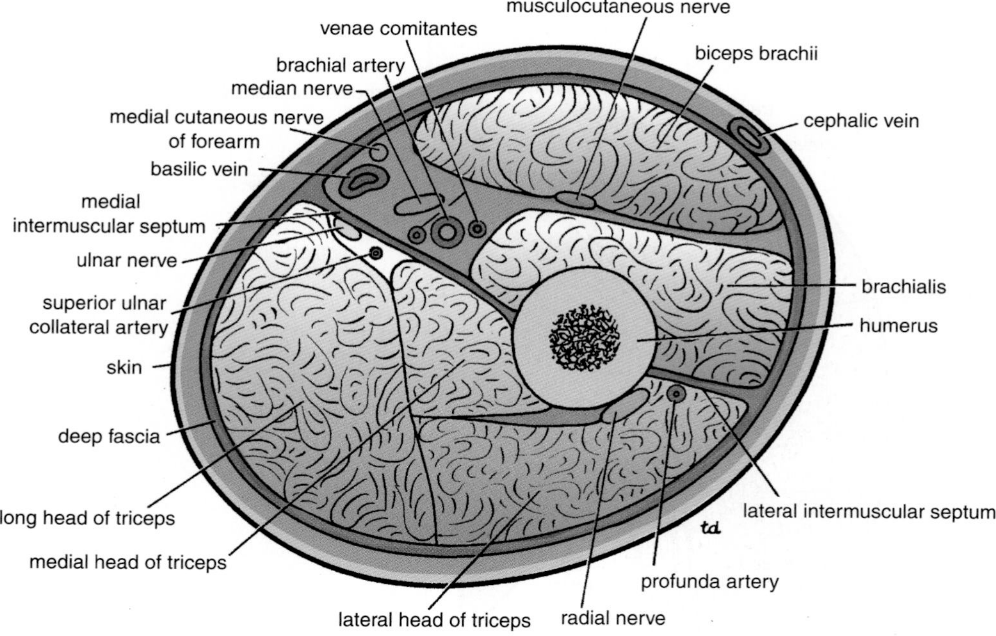

Figure 9-41 Cross section of the upper arm just below the level of insertion of the deltoid muscle. Note the division of the arm by the humerus and the medial and lateral intermuscular septa into anterior and posterior compartments.

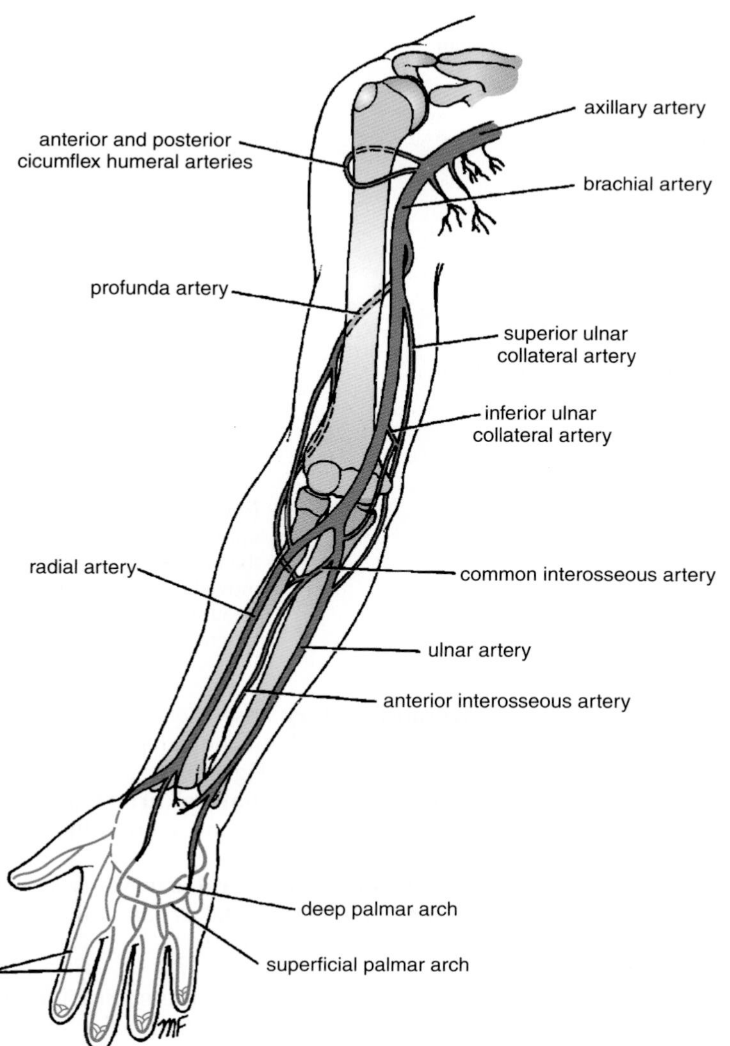

Figure 9-42 The main arteries of the upper limb.

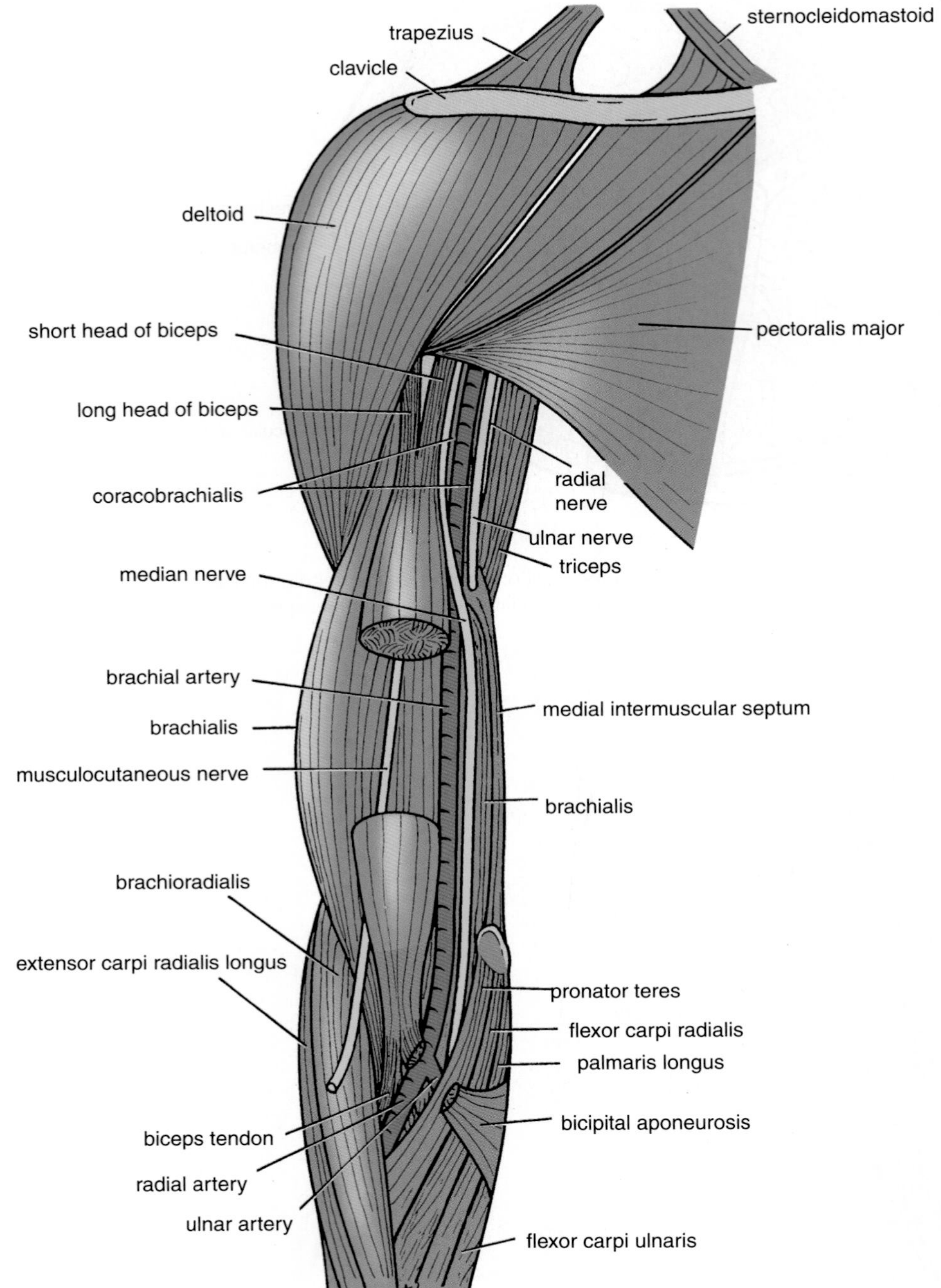

Figure 9-43 Anterior view of the upper arm. The middle portion of the biceps brachii has been removed to show the musculocutaneous nerve lying in front of the brachialis.

- **Medially:** The ulnar nerve and the basilic vein in the upper part of the arm; in the lower part of the arm, the median nerve lies on its medial side (Fig. 9-43).
- **Laterally:** The median nerve and the coracobrachialis and biceps muscles above; the tendon of the biceps lies lateral to the artery in the lower part of its course (Fig. 9-43).

Branches

- **Muscular branches** to the anterior compartment of the upper arm
- The **nutrient artery** to the humerus
- The **profunda artery** arises near the beginning of the brachial artery and follows the radial nerve into the spiral groove of the humerus (Fig. 9-45).
- The **superior ulnar collateral artery** arises near the middle of the upper arm and follows the ulnar nerve (Fig. 9-45).
- The **inferior ulnar collateral artery** arises near the termination of the artery and takes part in the anastomosis around the elbow joint (Fig. 9-45).

Musculocutaneous Nerve The origin of the musculocutaneous nerve from the lateral cord of the brachial plexus

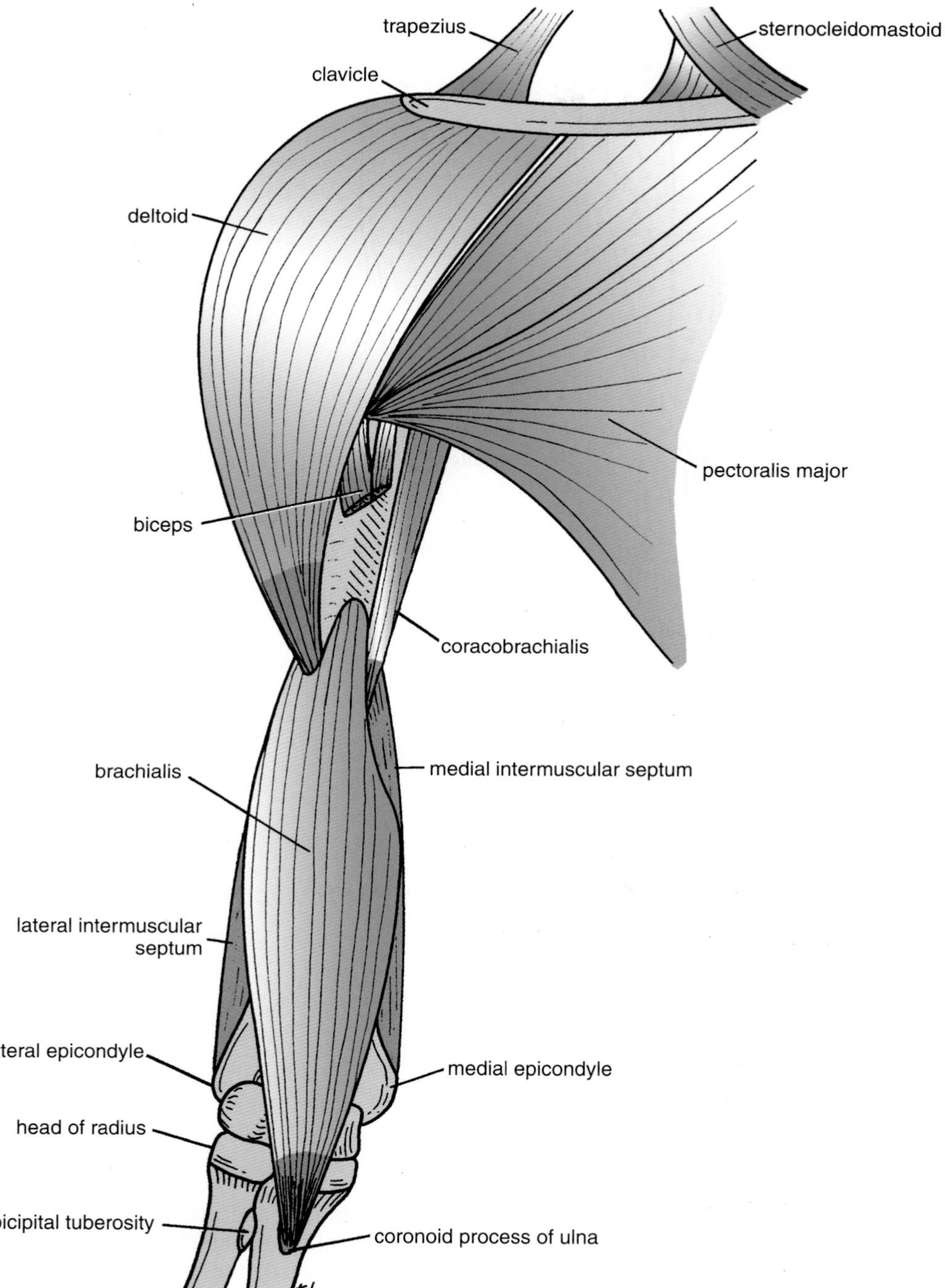

Figure 9-44 Anterior view of the upper arm showing the insertion of the deltoid and the origin and insertion of the brachialis.

(C5, 6, and 7) in the axilla is described on page 449. It runs downward and laterally, pierces the coracobrachialis muscle (Fig. 9-15), and then passes downward between the biceps and brachialis muscles (Fig. 9-43). It appears at the lateral margin of the biceps tendon and pierces the deep fascia just above the elbow. It runs down the lateral aspect of the forearm as the lateral cutaneous nerve of the forearm (Fig. 9-38).

Branches

- **Muscular branches** to the biceps, coracobrachialis, and brachialis (Fig. 9-22)
- **Cutaneous branches;** the **lateral cutaneous nerve of the forearm** supplies the skin of the front and lateral aspects of the forearm down as far as the root of the thumb.
- **Articular branches** to the elbow joint

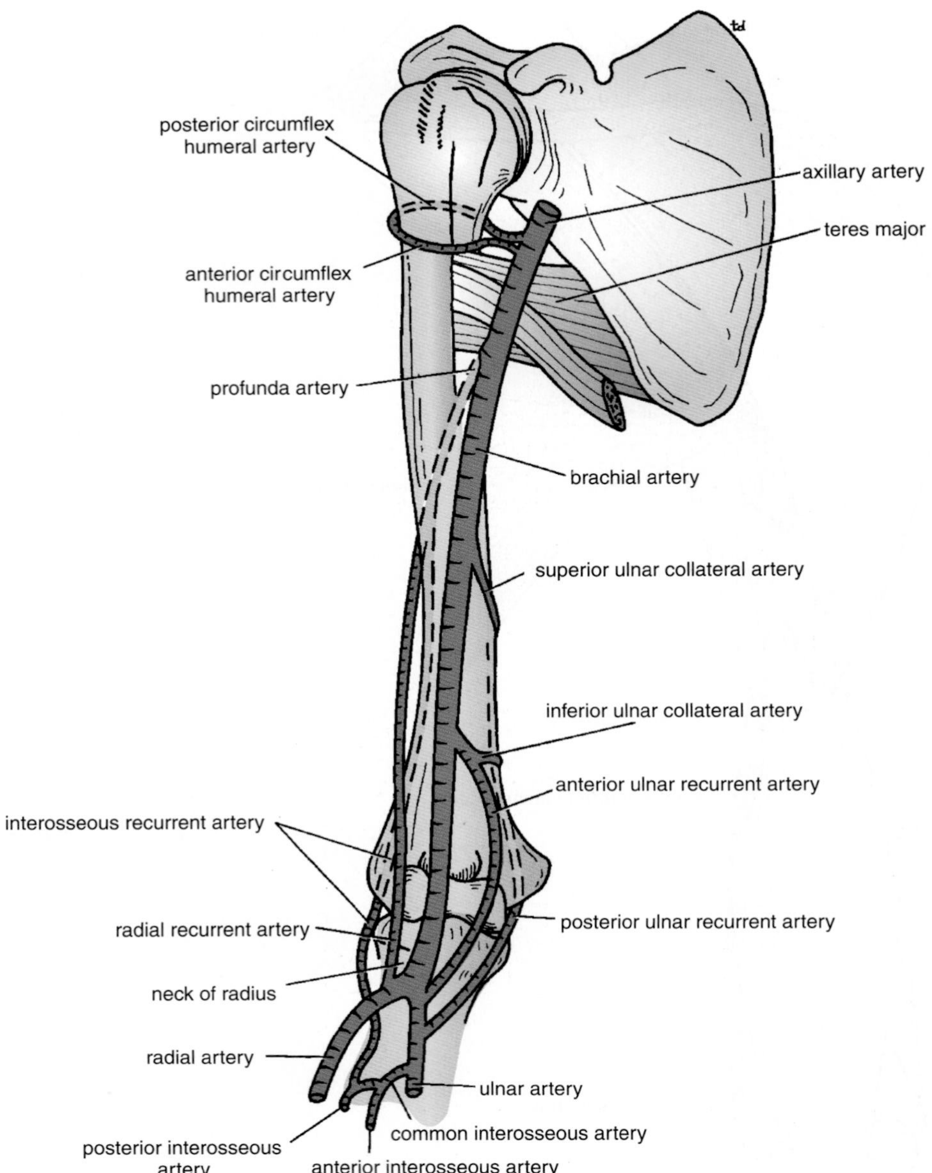

Figure 9-45 Main arteries of the upper arm. Note the arterial anastomosis around the elbow joint.

Median Nerve The origin of the median nerve from the medial and lateral cords of the brachial plexus in the axilla is described on page 449. It runs downward on the lateral side of the brachial artery (Fig. 9-43). Halfway down the upper arm, it crosses the brachial artery and continues downward on its medial side.

The nerve, like the artery, is therefore superficial, but at the elbow, it is crossed by the bicipital aponeurosis. The further course of this nerve is described on page 489.

The median nerve has no branches in the upper arm (Fig. 9-22), except for a small vasomotor nerve to the brachial artery.

Ulnar Nerve The origin of the ulnar nerve from the medial cord of the brachial plexus in the axilla is described on page 449. It runs downward on the medial side of the brachial artery as far as the middle of the arm (Fig. 9-43). Here, at the insertion of the coracobrachialis, the nerve pierces the medial fascial septum, accompanied by the superior ulnar collateral artery, and enters the posterior compartment of the arm; the nerve passes behind the medial epicondyle of the humerus.

The ulnar nerve has no branches in the anterior compartment of the upper arm (Fig. 9-23).

Radial Nerve On leaving the axilla, the radial nerve immediately enters the posterior compartment of the arm and enters the anterior compartment just above the lateral epicondyle.

Contents of the Posterior Fascial Compartment of the Upper Arm

- **Muscle:** The three heads of the triceps muscle
- **Nerve supply to the muscle:** Radial nerve

Table 9-5 Muscles of the Arm

Muscle	Origin	Insertion	Nerve Supply	Nerve Roots[a]	Action
Anterior Compartment					
Biceps brachii					
Long head	Supraglenoid tubercle of scapula	Tuberosity of radius and bicipital aponeurosis into deep fascia of forearm	Musculocutaneous nerve	C5, **6**	Supinator of forearm and flexor of elbow joint; weak flexor of shoulder joint
Short head	Coracoid process of scapula				
Coracobrachialis	Coracoid process of scapula	Medial aspect of shaft of humerus	Musculocutaneous nerve	C5, **6,** 7	Flexes arm and also weak adductor
Brachialis	Front of lower half of humerus	Coronoid process of ulna	Musculocutaneous nerve	C5, **6**	Flexor of elbow joint
Posterior Compartment					
Triceps					
Long head	Infraglenoid tubercle of scapula				
Lateral head	Upper half of posterior surface of shaft of humerus	Olecranon process of ulna	Radial nerve	C6, 7, **8**	Extensor of elbow joint
Medial head	Lower half of posterior surface of shaft of humerus				

[a] The predominant nerve root supply is indicated by boldface type.

- **Blood supply:** Profunda brachii and ulnar collateral arteries
- **Structures passing through the compartment:** Radial nerve and ulnar nerve

Muscle of the Posterior Fascial Compartment

The triceps muscle is seen in Figure 9-46 and is described in Table 9-5.

Structures Passing Through the Posterior Fascial Compartment

Radial Nerve The origin of the radial nerve from the posterior cord of the brachial plexus in the axilla is described on page 450. The nerve winds around the back of the arm in the spiral groove on the back of the humerus between the heads of the triceps (Fig. 9-46). It pierces the lateral fascial septum above the elbow and continues downward into the cubital fossa in front of the elbow, between the brachialis and the brachioradialis muscles (Fig. 9-47). In the spiral groove, the nerve is accompanied by the profunda vessels, and it lies directly in contact with the shaft of the humerus (Fig. 9-46).

Branches

- In the **axilla,** branches (Fig. 9-25) are given to the long and medial heads of the triceps, and the **posterior cutaneous nerve of the arm** is given off.
- In the **spiral groove** (Fig. 9-46), branches are given to the lateral and medial heads of the triceps and to the anconeus. The **lower lateral cutaneous nerve of the arm** supplies the skin over the lateral and anterior aspects of the lower part of the arm. The **posterior cutaneous nerve of the forearm** runs down the middle of the back of the forearm as far as the wrist.
- In the **anterior compartment of the arm,** after the nerve has pierced the lateral fascial septum, it gives branches to the brachialis, the brachioradialis, and the extensor carpi radialis longus muscles (Fig. 9-47). It also gives **articular branches** to the elbow joint.

Ulnar Nerve Having pierced the medial fascial septum halfway down the upper arm, the ulnar nerve descends behind the septum, covered posteriorly by the medial head of

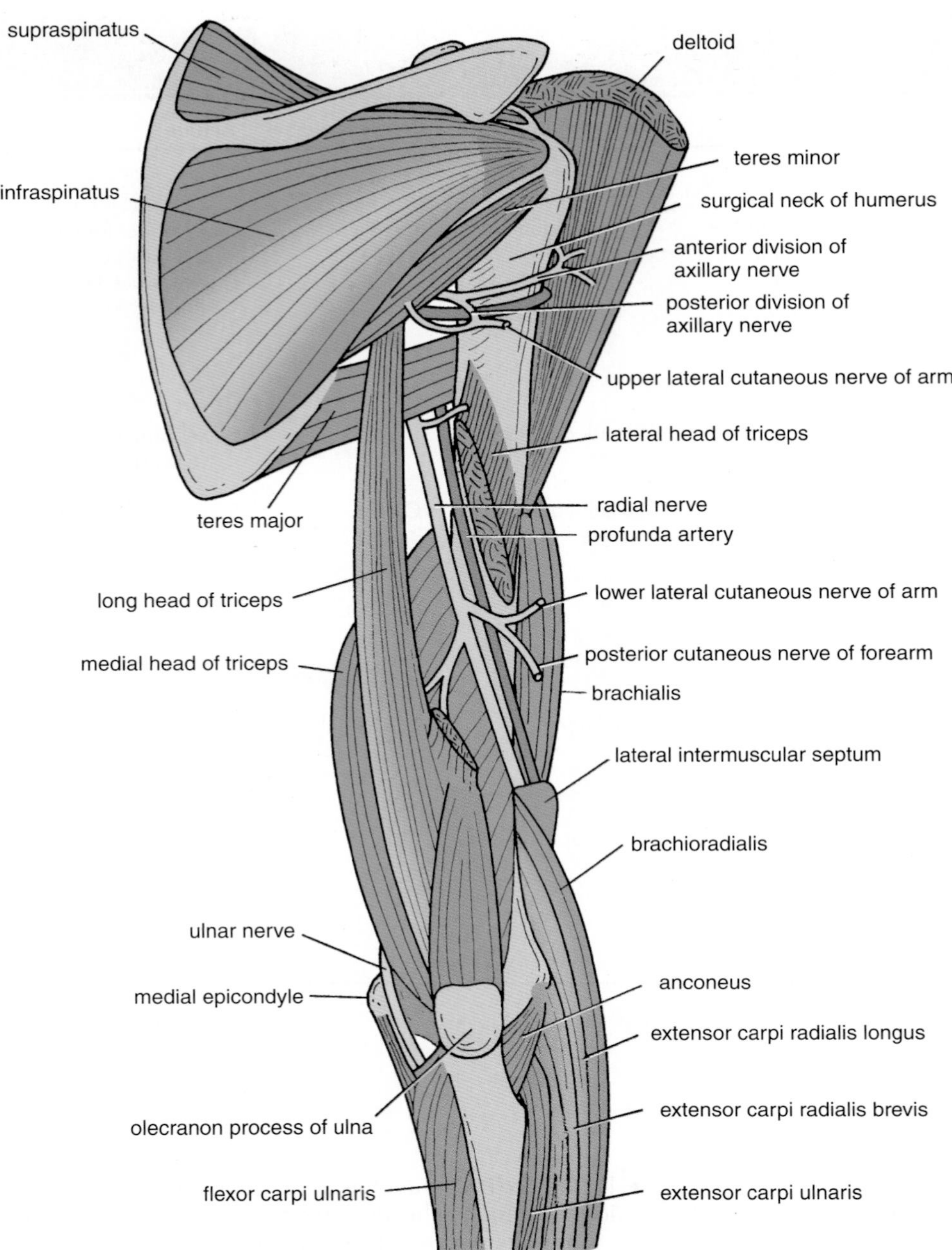

Figure 9-46 Posterior view of the upper arm. The lateral head of the triceps has been divided to display the radial nerve and the profunda artery in the spiral groove of the humerus.

the triceps. The nerve is accompanied by the superior ulnar collateral vessels. At the elbow, it lies behind the medial epicondyle of the humerus (Fig. 9-46) on the medial ligament of the elbow joint. It continues downward to enter the forearm between the two heads of origin of the flexor carpi ulnaris (see page 493).

Branches The ulnar nerve has an articular branch to the elbow joint (Fig. 9-23).

Profunda Brachii Artery The profunda brachii artery arises from the brachial artery near its origin (Fig. 9-45). It accompanies the radial nerve through the spiral groove, supplies the triceps muscle, and takes part in the anastomosis around the elbow joint.

Superior and Inferior Ulnar Collateral Arteries The superior and inferior ulnar collateral arteries arise from the brachial artery and take part in the anastomosis around the elbow joint.

The Cubital Fossa

The cubital fossa is a triangular depression that lies in front of the elbow (Figs. 9-47 and 9-48).

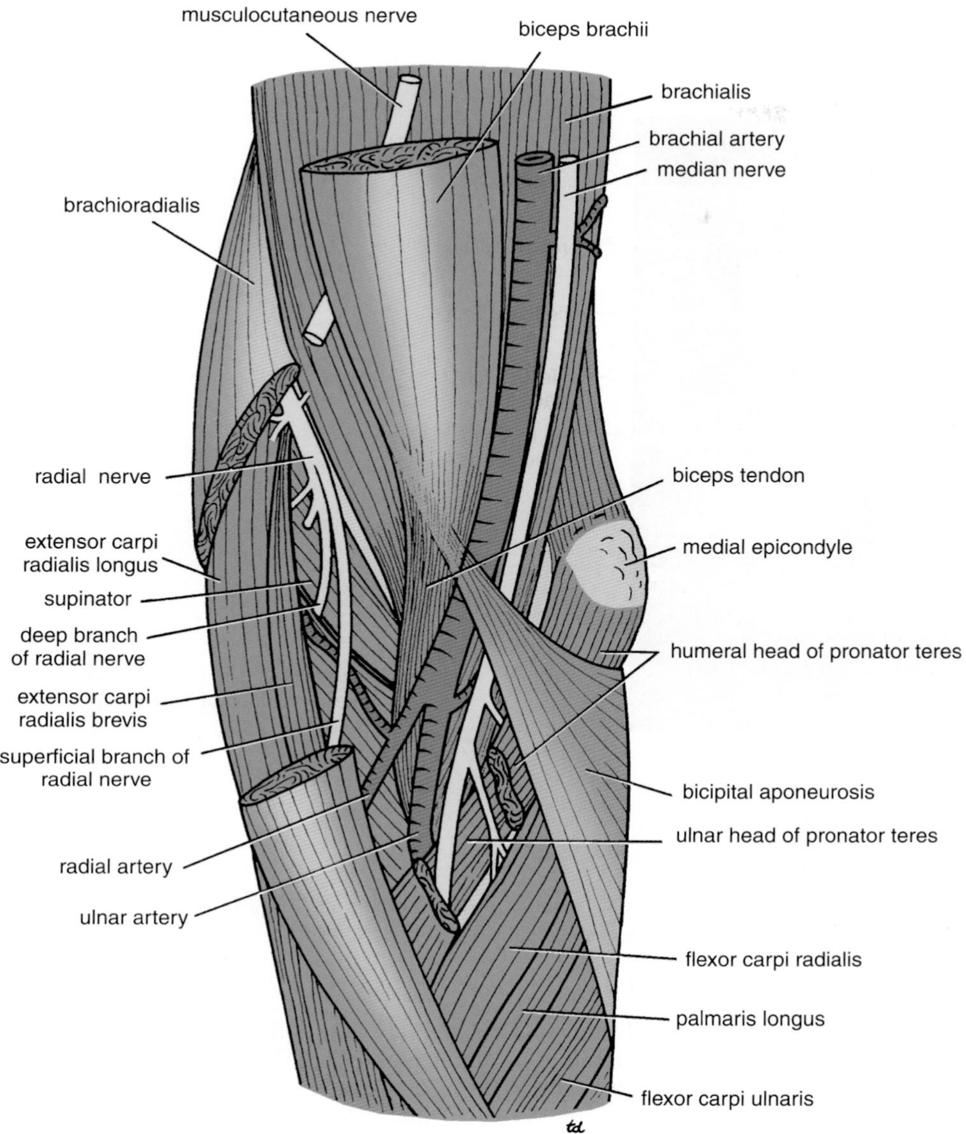

Figure 9-47 Right cubital fossa.

Boundaries

- **Laterally:** The brachioradialis muscle
- **Medially:** The pronator teres muscle

The **base** of the triangle is formed by an imaginary line drawn between the two epicondyles of the humerus. The **floor** of the fossa is formed by the supinator muscle laterally and the brachialis muscle medially. The **roof** is formed by skin and fascia and is reinforced by the bicipital aponeurosis.

Contents

The cubital fossa (Fig. 9-47) contains the following structures, enumerated from the medial to the lateral side: the median nerve, the bifurcation of the brachial artery into the ulnar and radial arteries, the tendon of the biceps muscle, and the radial nerve and its deep branch.

The **supratrochlear lymph node** lies in the superficial fascia over the upper part of the fossa, above the trochlea (Fig. 9-40). It receives afferent lymph vessels from the third, fourth, and fifth fingers; the medial part of the hand; and the medial side of the forearm. The efferent lymph vessels pass up to the axilla and enter the lateral axillary group of nodes (Fig. 9-40).

Bones of the Forearm

The forearm contains two bones: the radius and the ulna.

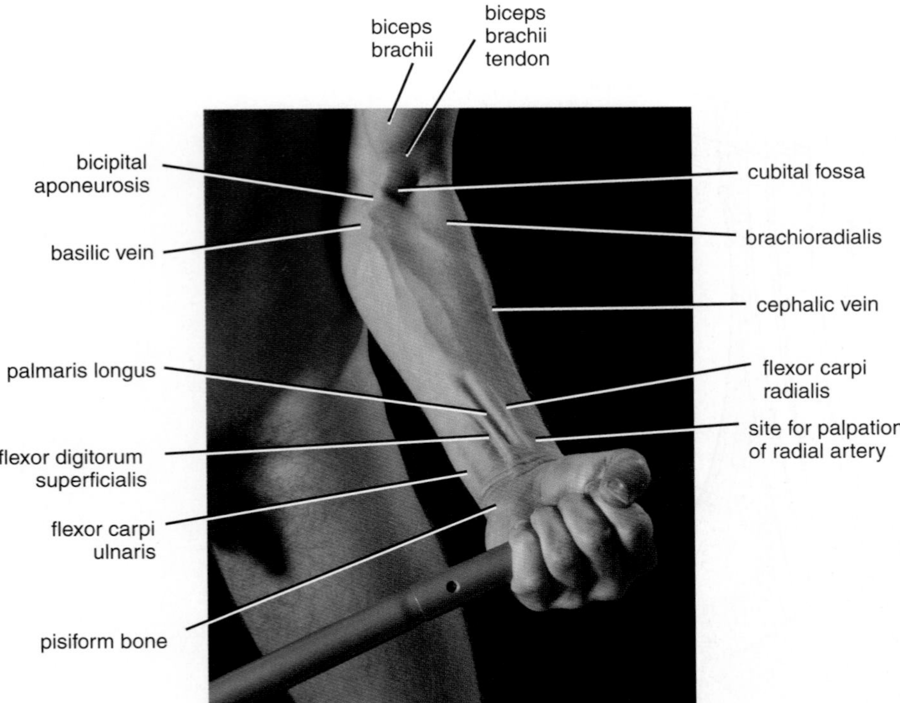

Figure 9-48 The cubital fossa and anterior surface of the forearm in a 27-year-old man.

Radius

The radius is the lateral bone of the forearm (Fig. 9-49). Its proximal end articulates with the humerus at the elbow joint and with the ulna at the proximal radioulnar joint. Its distal end articulates with the scaphoid and lunate bones of the hand at the wrist joint and with the ulna at the distal radioulnar joint.

At the proximal end of the radius is the small circular **head** (Fig. 9-49). The upper surface of the head is concave and articulates with the convex capitulum of the humerus. The circumference of the head articulates with the radial notch of the ulna. Below the head the bone is constricted to form the **neck.** Below the neck is the **bicipital tuberosity** for the insertion of the biceps muscle.

The shaft of the radius, in contradistinction to that of the ulna, is wider below than above (Fig. 9-49). It has a sharp **interosseous border** medially for the attachment of the interosseous membrane that binds the radius and ulna together. The **pronator tubercle,** for the insertion of the pronator teres muscle, lies halfway down on its lateral side.

At the distal end of the radius is the **styloid process;** this projects distally from its lateral margin (Fig. 9-49). On the medial surface is the **ulnar notch,** which articulates with the round head of the ulna. The inferior articular surface articulates with the scaphoid and lunate bones. On the posterior aspect of the distal end is a small tubercle, the **dorsal tubercle,** which is grooved on its medial side by the tendon of the extensor pollicis longus (Fig. 9-49).

The important muscles and ligaments attached to the radius are shown in Figure 9-49.

Ulna

The ulna is the medial bone of the forearm (Fig. 9-49). Its proximal end articulates with the humerus at the elbow joint and with the head of the radius at the proximal radioulnar joint. Its distal end articulates with the radius at the distal radioulnar joint, but it is excluded from the wrist joint by the articular disc.

The proximal end of the ulna is large and is known as the **olecranon process** (Fig. 9-49); this forms the prominence of the elbow. It has a notch on its anterior surface, the **trochlear notch,** which articulates with the trochlea of the humerus. Below the trochlear notch is the triangular **coronoid process,** which has on its lateral surface the **radial notch** for articulation with the head of the radius.

The **shaft** of the ulna tapers from above down (Fig. 9-49). It has a sharp **interosseous border** laterally for the attachment of the interosseous membrane. The posterior border is rounded and subcutaneous and can be easily palpated throughout its length. Below the radial notch is the **supinator crest** that gives origin to the supinator muscle.

At the distal end of the ulna is the small rounded **head,** which has projecting from its medial aspect the styloid process (Fig. 9-49).

The important muscles and ligaments attached to the ulna are shown in Figure 9-49.

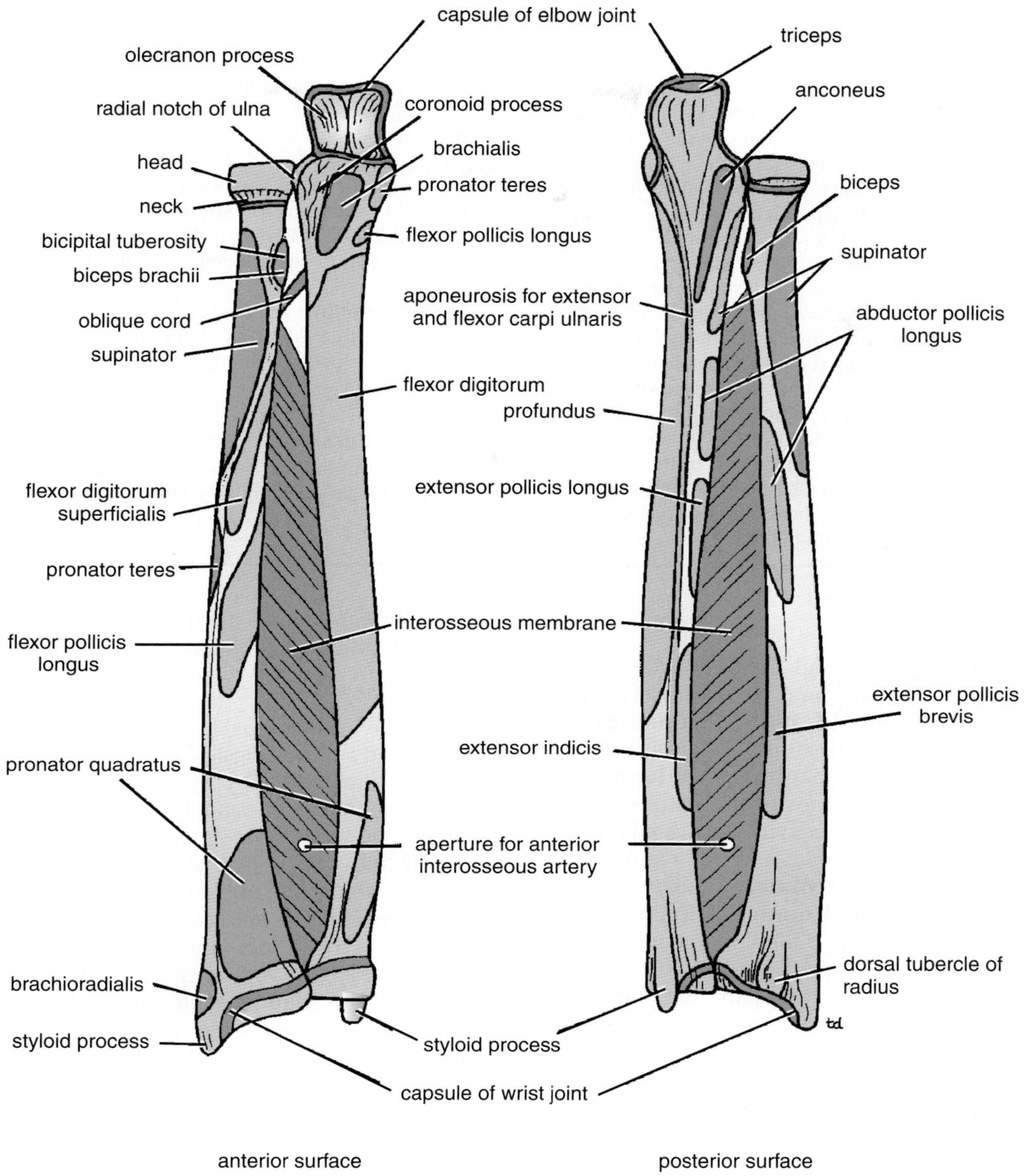

Figure 9-49 Important muscular and ligamentous attachments to the radius and the ulna.

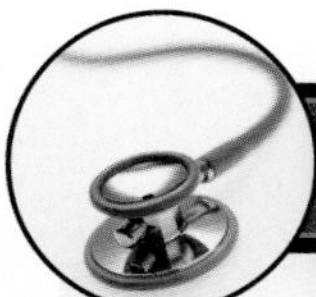

CLINICAL NOTES

Fractures of the Radius and Ulna

Fractures of the head of the radius can occur from falls on the outstretched hand. As the force is transmitted along the radius, the head of the radius is driven sharply against the capitulum, splitting or splintering the head (Fig. 9-10).

Fractures of the neck of the radius occur in young children from falls on the outstretched hand (Fig. 9-10).

Fractures of the shafts of the radius and ulna may or may not occur together (Fig. 9-10). Displacement of the fragments is usually considerable and depends on the pull of the attached muscles. The proximal fragment of the radius is supinated by the supinator and the biceps brachii muscles (Fig. 9-10). The distal fragment of the radius is pronated and pulled medially by the pronator quadratus muscle. The strength of the brachioradialis

(continues)

Clinical Notes, *continued*

and extensor carpi radialis longus and brevis shortens and angulates the forearm. In fractures of the ulna, the ulna angulates posteriorly. To restore the normal movements of pronation and supination, the normal anatomic relationship of the radius, ulna, and interosseous membrane must be regained.

A fracture of one forearm bone may be associated with a dislocation of the other bone. In **Monteggia's fracture,** for example, the shaft of the ulna is fractured by a force applied from behind. There is a bowing forward of the ulnar shaft and an anterior dislocation of the radial head with rupture of the anular ligament. In **Galeazzi's fracture,** the proximal third of the radius is fractured and the distal end of the ulna is dislocated at the distal radioulnar joint.

Fractures of the olecranon process can result from a fall on the flexed elbow or from a direct blow. Depending on the location of the fracture line, the bony fragment may be displaced by the pull of the triceps muscle, which is inserted on the olecranon process (Fig. 9-10). Avulsion fractures of part of the olecranon process can be produced by the pull of the triceps muscle. Good functional return after any of these fractures depends on the accurate anatomic reduction of the fragment.

Colles' fracture is a fracture of the distal end of the radius resulting from a fall on the outstretched hand. It commonly occurs in patients older than 50 years. The force drives the distal fragment posteriorly and superiorly, and the distal articular surface is inclined posteriorly (Fig. 9-50). This posterior displacement produces a posterior bump, sometimes referred to as the "dinner-fork deformity" because the forearm and wrist resemble the shape of that eating utensil. Failure to restore the distal articular surface to its normal position will severely limit the range of flexion of the wrist joint.

Smith's fracture is a fracture of the distal end of the radius and occurs from a fall on the back of the hand. It is a reversed Colles' fracture because the distal fragment is displaced anteriorly (Fig. 9-50).

Olecranon Bursitis

A small subcutaneous bursa is present over the olecranon process of the ulna, and repeated trauma often produces chronic bursitis.

Bones of the Hand

There are eight carpal bones, made up of two rows of four (Figs. 9-51 and 9-52). The **proximal row** consists of (from lateral to medial) the **scaphoid, lunate, triquetral,** and **pisiform** bones. The **distal row** consists of (from lateral to medial) the **trapezium, trapezoid, capitate,** and **hamate** bones. Together, the bones of the carpus present on their anterior surface a concavity, to the lateral and medial edges of which is attached a strong membranous band called the **flexor retinaculum.** In this manner, an osteofascial tunnel, the **carpal tunnel,** is formed for the passage of the median nerve and the flexor tendons of the fingers.

The bones of the hand are cartilaginous at birth. The capitate begins to ossify during the first year, and the others begin to ossify at intervals thereafter until the 12th year, when all the bones are ossified.

A detailed knowledge of the bones of the hand is unnecessary. The position, shape, and size of the scaphoid bone, however, should be studied, because it is commonly fractured. The ridge of the trapezium and the hook of the hamate should be examined.

The Metacarpals and Phalanges

There are five metacarpal bones, each of which has a **base,** a **shaft,** and a **head** (Figs. 9-51 and 9-52).

The first metacarpal bone of the thumb is the shortest and most mobile. It does not lie in the same plane as the others but occupies a more anterior position. It is also rotated medially through a right angle so that its extensor surface is directed laterally and not backward.

The bases of the metacarpal bones articulate with the distal row of the carpal bones; the heads, which form the knuckles, articulate with the proximal phalanges (Figs. 9-51 and 9-52). The shaft of each metacarpal bone is slightly concave forward and is triangular in transverse section. Its surfaces are posterior, lateral, and medial.

There are three phalanges for each of the fingers but only two for the thumb.

The important muscles attached to the bones of the hand and fingers are shown in Figures 9-51 and 9-52.

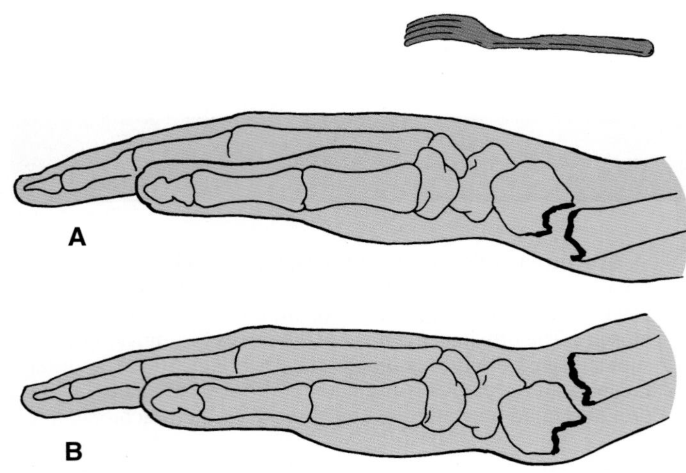

Figure 9-50 Fractures of the distal end of the radius. **A.** Colles' fracture. **B.** Smith's fracture.

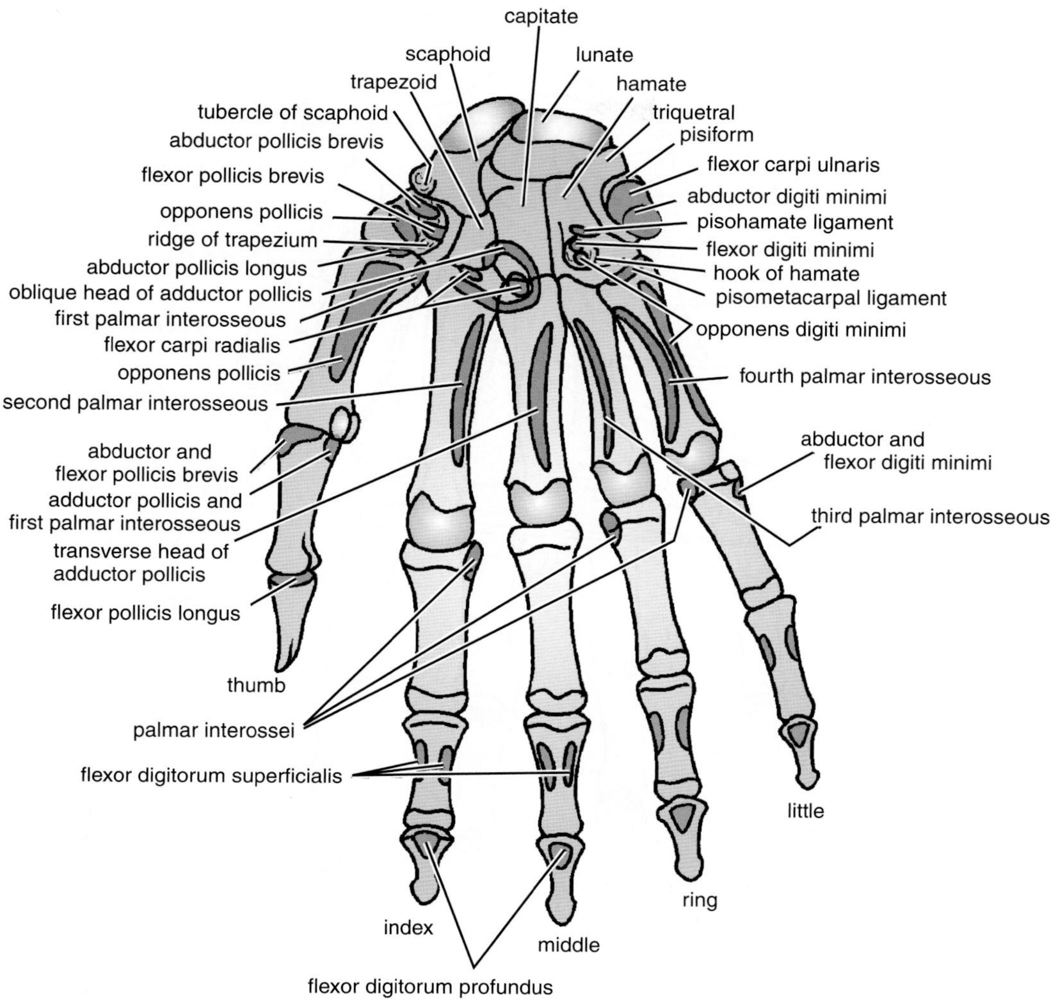

Figure 9-51 Important muscular attachments to the anterior surfaces of the bones of the hand.

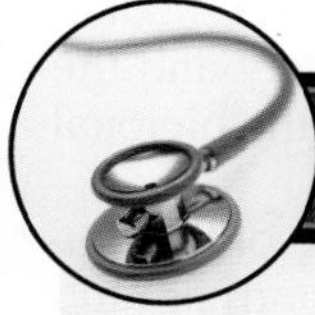

CLINICAL NOTES

Injuries to the Bones of the Hand

Fracture of the scaphoid bone is common in young adults; unless treated effectively, the fragments will not unite, and permanent weakness and pain of the wrist will result, with the subsequent development of osteoarthritis. The fracture line usually goes through the narrowest part of the bone, which, because of its location, is bathed in synovial fluid. The blood vessels to the scaphoid enter its proximal and distal ends, although the blood supply is occasionally confined to its distal end. If the latter occurs, a fracture deprives the proximal fragment of its arterial supply, and this fragment undergoes avascular necrosis. Deep tenderness in the anatomic snuffbox after a fall on the outstretched hand in a young adult makes one suspicious of a fractured scaphoid.

Dislocation of the lunate bone occasionally occurs in young adults who fall on the outstretched hand in a way that causes hyperextension of the wrist joint. Involvement of the median nerve is common.

Fractures of the metacarpal bones can occur as a result of direct violence, such as the clenched fist striking a hard object. The fracture always angulates dorsally. The "boxer's fracture" commonly produces an oblique fracture of the neck of the fifth and sometimes the fourth metacarpal bones. The distal fragment is commonly displaced proximally, thus shortening the finger posteriorly.

Bennett's fracture is a fracture of the base of the metacarpal of the thumb caused when violence is applied along the long axis of the thumb or the thumb is forcefully abducted. The fracture is oblique and enters the carpometacarpal joint of the thumb, causing joint instability.

Fractures of the phalanges are common and usually follow direct injury.

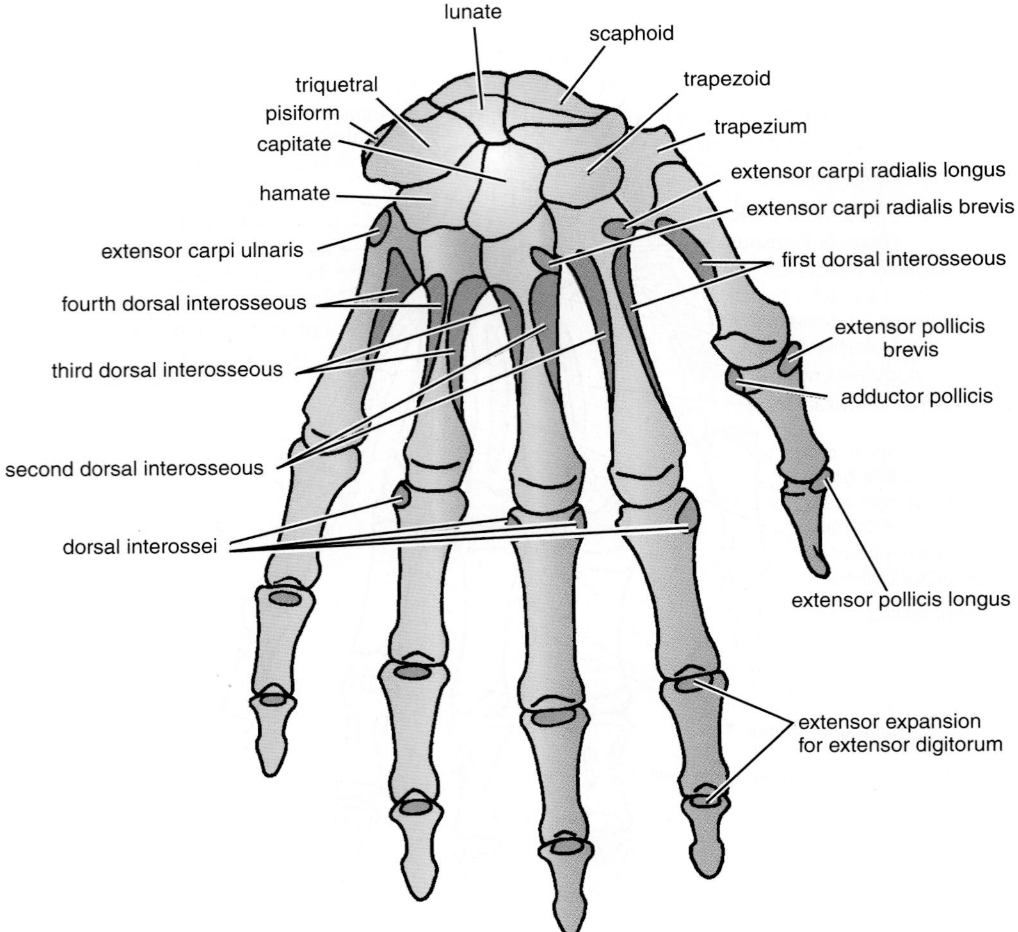

Figure 9-52 Important muscular attachments to the posterior surfaces of the bones of the hand.

The Forearm

Skin

The **sensory nerve supply** to the skin of the forearm is from the anterior and posterior branches of the lateral cutaneous nerve of the forearm, a continuation of the musculocutaneous nerve, and from the anterior and posterior branches of the medial cutaneous nerve of the forearm (Fig. 9-38). A narrow strip of skin down the middle of the posterior surface of the forearm is supplied by the posterior cutaneous nerve of the forearm.

The **superficial veins** of the forearm lie in the superficial fascia (Fig. 9-39). The **cephalic vein** arises from the lateral side of the dorsal venous arch on the back of the hand and winds around the lateral border of the forearm; it then ascends into the cubital fossa and up the front of the arm on the lateral side of the biceps. It terminates in the axillary vein in the deltopectoral triangle (see page 530). As the cephalic vein passes up the upper limb, it receives a variable number of tributaries from the lateral and posterior surfaces of the limb (Fig. 9-39). The **median cubital vein,** a branch of the cephalic vein in the cubital fossa, runs upward and medially and joins the basilic vein. In the cubital fossa, the median cubital vein crosses in front of the brachial artery and the median nerve, but it is separated from them by the bicipital aponeurosis.

The **basilic vein** arises from the medial side of the dorsal venous arch on the back of the hand and winds around the medial border of the forearm; it then ascends into the cubital fossa and up the front of the arm on the medial side of the biceps (Fig. 9-39). Its termination, by joining the venae comitantes of the brachial artery to form the axillary vein, is described on page 446. It receives the median cubital vein and a variable number of tributaries from the medial and posterior surfaces of the upper limb.

The **superficial lymph vessels** from the thumb and lateral fingers and the lateral areas of the hand and forearm follow the cephalic vein to the infraclavicular group of nodes (Fig. 9-40). Those from the medial fingers and the medial areas of the hand and forearm follow the basilic vein to the cubital fossa. Here, some of the vessels drain into the **supratrochlear lymph node,** whereas others bypass the node and accompany the basilic vein to the axilla, where they drain into the lateral group of axillary nodes. The effer-

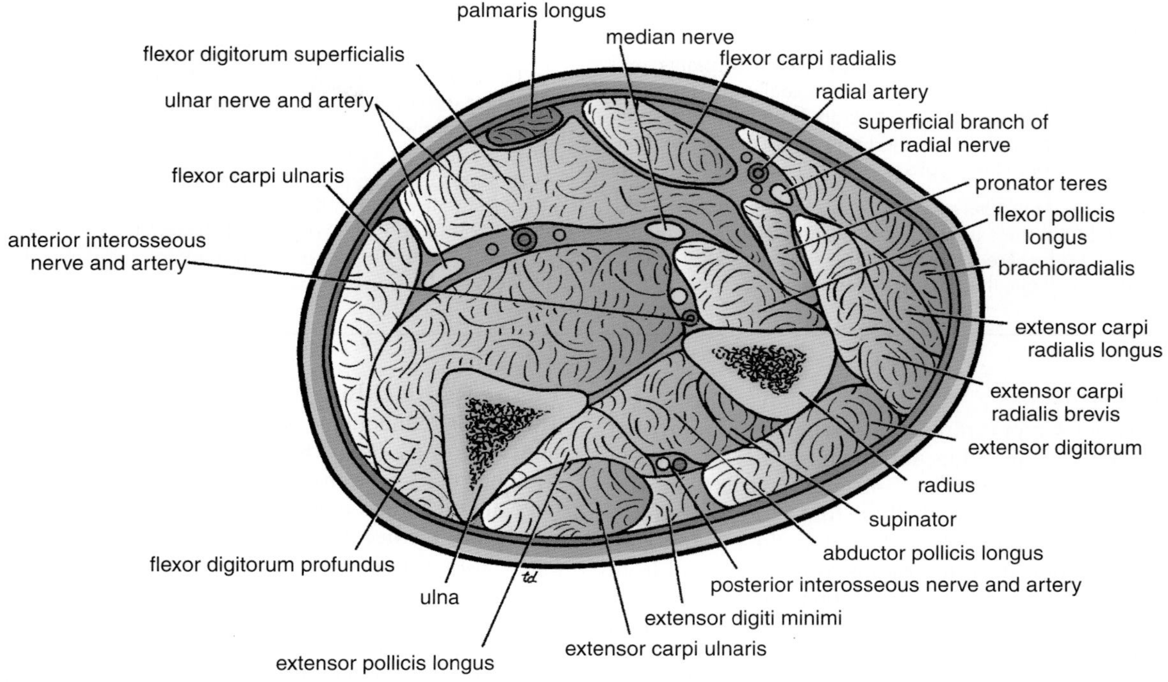

Figure 9-53 Cross section of the forearm at the level of insertion of the pronator teres muscle.

ent vessels from the supratrochlear node also drain into the lateral axillary nodes (Fig. 9-40).

Fascial Compartments of the Forearm

The forearm is enclosed in a sheath of deep fascia, which is attached to the periosteum of the posterior subcutaneous border of the ulna (Fig. 9-53). This fascial sheath, together with the interosseous membrane and fibrous intermuscular septa, divides the forearm into several compartments, each having its own muscles, nerves, and blood supply.

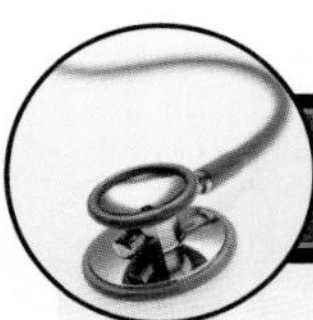

CLINICAL NOTES

Compartment Syndrome of the Forearm

The forearm is enclosed in a sheath of deep fascia, which is attached to the periosteum of the posterior subcutaneous border of the ulna (Fig. 9-53). This fascial sheath, together with the interosseous membrane and fibrous intermuscular septa, divides the forearm into several compartments, each having its own muscles, nerves, and blood supply. There is very little room within each compartment, and any edema can cause secondary vascular compression of the blood vessels; the veins are first affected, and later the arteries.

Soft tissue injury is a common cause, and early diagnosis is critical. Early signs include altered skin sensation (caused by ischemia of the sensory nerves passing through the compartment), pain disproportionate to any injury (caused by pressure on nerves within the compartment), pain on passive stretching of muscles that pass through the compartment (caused by muscle ischemia), tenderness of the skin over the compartment (a late sign caused by edema), and absence of capillary refill in the nail beds (caused by pressure on the arteries within the compartment). Once the diagnosis is made, the deep fascia must be incised surgically to decompress the affected compartment. A delay of as little as 4 hours can cause irreversible damage to the muscles.

Volkmann's Ischemic Contracture

Volkmann's ischemic contracture is a contracture of the muscles of the forearm that commonly follows fractures of the distal end of the humerus or fractures of the radius and ulna. In this syndrome a localized segment of the brachial artery goes into spasm, reducing the arterial flow to the flexor and the extensor muscles so that they undergo ischemic necrosis. The flexor muscles are larger than the extensor muscles, and they are therefore the ones mainly affected.

(continues)

Clinical Notes, *continued*

The muscles are replaced by fibrous tissue, which contracts, producing the deformity. The arterial spasm is usually caused by an overtight cast, but in some cases the fracture itself may be responsible. The deformity can be explained only by understanding the anatomy of the region. Three types of deformity exist:

- The long flexor muscles of the carpus and fingers are more contracted than the extensor muscles, and the wrist joint is flexed; the fingers are extended. If the wrist joint is extended passively, the fingers become flexed.
- The long extensor muscles to the fingers, which are inserted into the extensor expansion that is attached to the proximal phalanx, are greatly contracted; the metacarpophalangeal joints and the wrist joint are extended, and the interphalangeal joints of the fingers are flexed.
- Both the flexor and the extensor muscles of the forearm are contracted. The wrist joint is flexed, the metacarpophalangeal joints are extended, and the interphalangeal joints are flexed.

Interosseous Membrane

The interosseous membrane is a strong membrane that unites the shafts of the radius and the ulna; it is attached to their interosseous borders (Figs. 9-49 and 9-53). Its fibers run obliquely downward and medially so that a force applied to the lower end of the radius (e.g., falling on the outstretched hand) is transmitted from the radius to the ulna and from there to the humerus and scapula. Its fibers are taut when the forearm is in the midprone position—that is, the position of function. The interosseous membrane provides attachment for neighboring muscles.

Flexor and Extensor Retinacula

The flexor and extensor retinacula are strong bands of deep fascia that hold the long flexor and extensor tendons in position at the wrist.

Flexor Retinaculum

The flexor retinaculum is a thickening of deep fascia that holds the long flexor tendons in position at the wrist. It stretches across the front of the wrist and converts the concave anterior surface of the hand into an osteofascial tunnel, the **carpal tunnel,** for the passage of the median nerve and the flexor tendons of the thumb and fingers (Fig. 9-54). It is attached medially to the pisiform bone and the hook of the hamate and laterally to the tubercle of the scaphoid and the trapezium bones. The attachment to the trapezium consists of superficial and deep parts and forms a synovial-lined tunnel for passage of the tendon of the flexor carpi radialis.

The upper border of the retinaculum corresponds to the distal transverse skin crease in front of the wrist and is continuous with the deep fascia of the forearm. The lower border is attached to the palmar aponeurosis (Fig. 9-55).

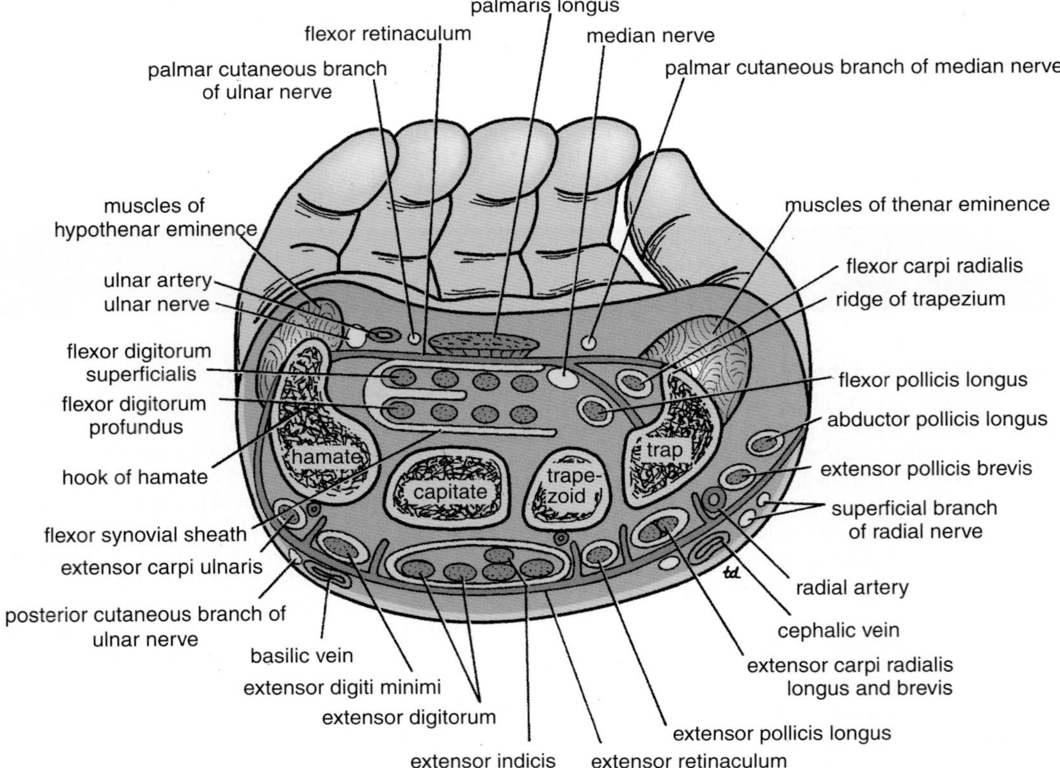

Figure 9-54 Cross section of the hand showing the relation of the tendons, nerves, and arteries to the flexor and extensor retinacula.

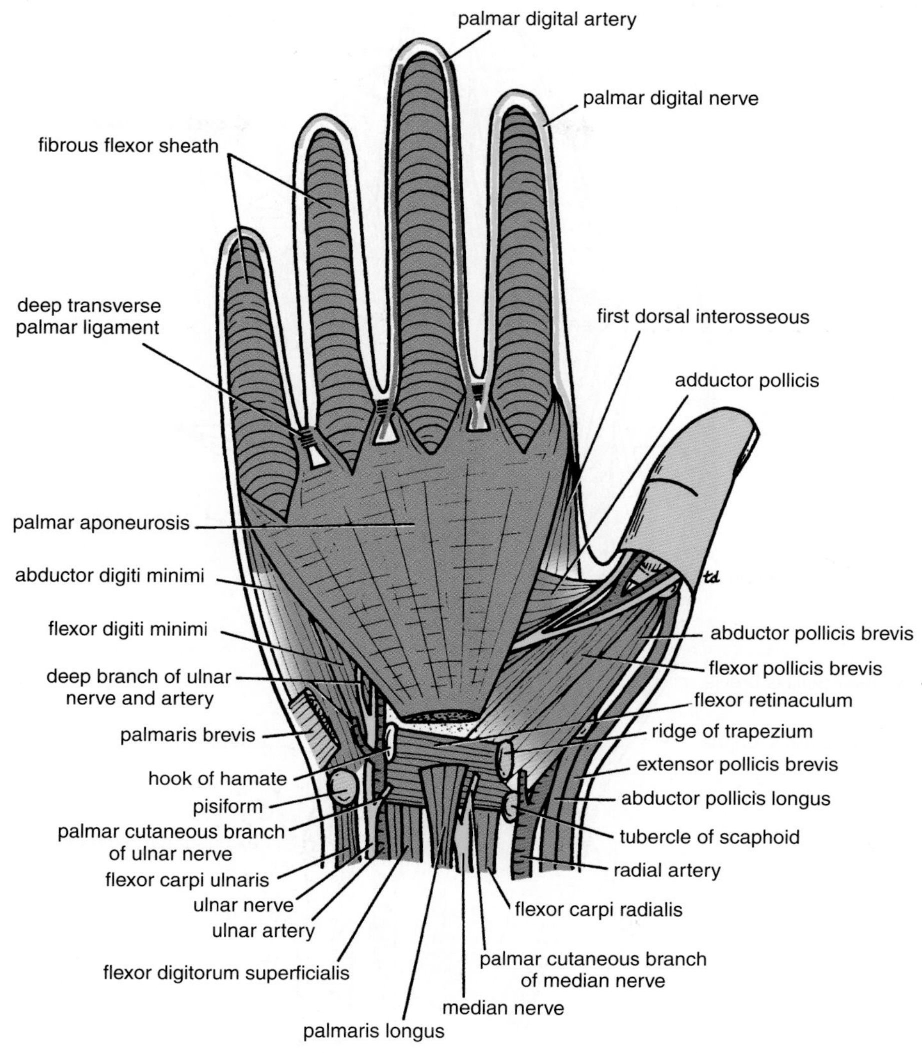

Figure 9-55 Anterior view of the palm of the hand. The palmar aponeurosis has been left in position.

Extensor Retinaculum

The extensor retinaculum is a thickening of deep fascia that stretches across the back of the wrist and holds the long extensor tendons in position (Figs. 9-56 and 9-57). It converts the grooves on the posterior surface of the distal ends of the radius and ulna into six separate tunnels for the passage of the long extensor tendons. Each tunnel is lined with a synovial sheath, which extends above and below the retinaculum on the tendons. The tunnels are separated from one another by fibrous septa that pass from the deep surface of the retinaculum to the bones.

The retinaculum is attached medially to the pisiform bone and the hook of the hamate and laterally to the distal end of the radius. The upper and lower borders of the retinaculum are continuous with the deep fascia of the forearm and hand, respectively.

The contents of the tunnels beneath the extensor retinaculum are described on page 499.

Carpal Tunnel

The bones of the hand and the flexor retinaculum form the carpal tunnel (Fig. 9-54). The median nerve lies in a **restricted space** between the tendons of the flexor digitorum superficialis and the flexor carpi radialis muscles. For further details, see page 500.

Contents of the Anterior Fascial Compartment of the Forearm

- **Muscles:** A **superficial group,** consisting of the pronator teres, the flexor carpi radialis, the palmaris longus, and the flexor carpi ulnaris; an **intermediate group** consisting of the flexor digitorum superficialis; and a **deep group** consisting of the flexor pollicis longus, the flexor digitorum profundus, and the pronator quadratus
- **Blood supply to the muscles:** Ulnar and radial arteries

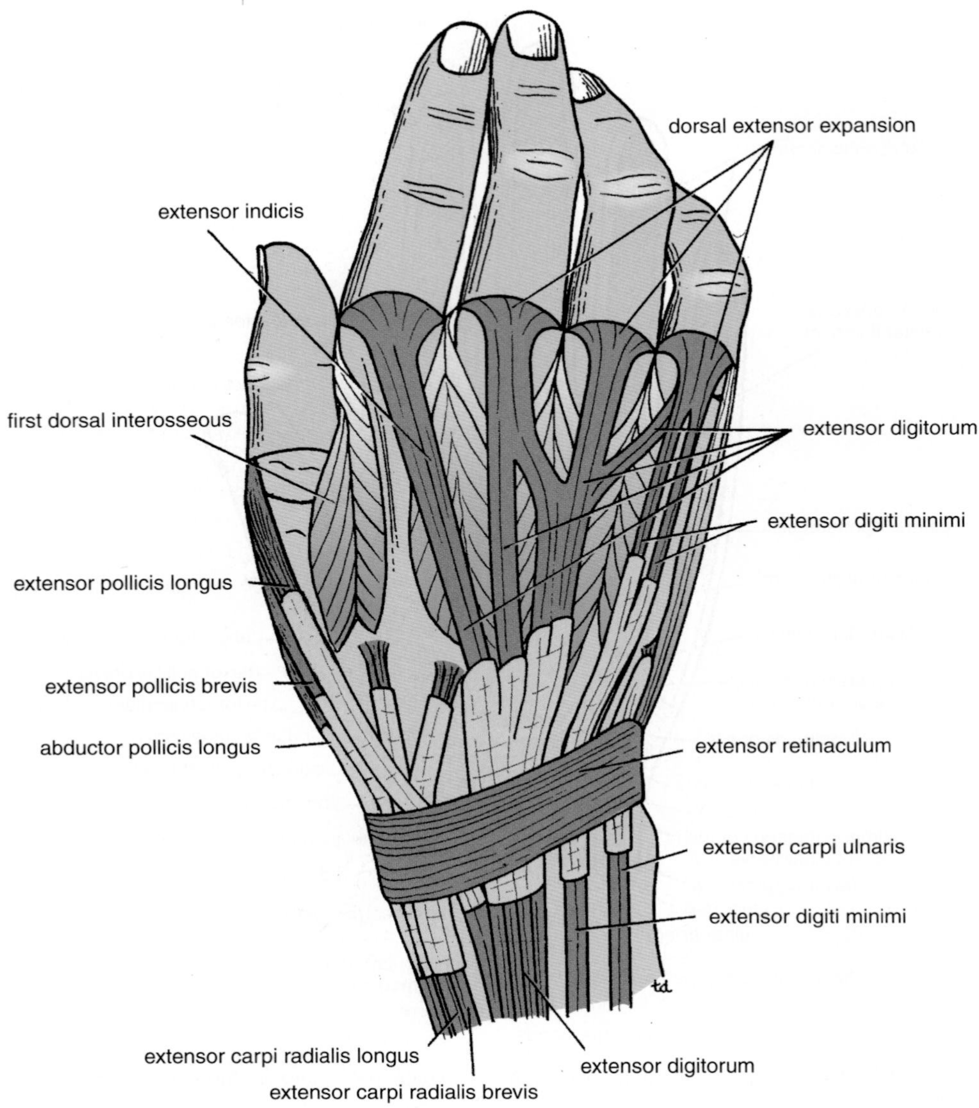

Figure 9-56 Dorsal surface of the hand showing the long extensor tendons and their synovial sheaths.

- **Nerve supply to the muscles:** All the muscles are supplied by the median nerve and its branches, except the flexor carpi ulnaris and the medial part of the flexor digitorum profundus, which are supplied by the ulnar nerve.

CLINICAL NOTES

Absent Palmaris Longus

The palmaris longus muscle may be absent on one or both sides of the forearm in about 10% of persons. Others show variation in form, such as centrally or distally placed muscle belly in the place of a proximal one. Because the muscle is relatively weak, its absence produces no disability.

Muscles of the Anterior Fascial Compartment of the Forearm

The muscles of the anterior fascial compartment are seen in Figures 9-58, 9-59, 9-60, and 9-61 and are described in Table 9-6. Note that the superficial group of muscles possesses a common tendon of origin, which is attached to the medial epicondyle of the humerus.

Arteries of the Anterior Fascial Compartment of the Forearm

Ulnar Artery The ulnar artery is the larger of the two terminal branches of the brachial artery (Figs. 9-42 and 9-60). It begins in the cubital fossa at the level of the neck of the radius. It descends through the anterior compartment of the forearm and enters the palm **in front of** the flexor retinaculum in company with the ulnar nerve (Fig. 9-62). It ends by forming the **superficial palmar arch,** often anastomosing with the superficial palmar branch of the radial artery (Fig. 9-62).

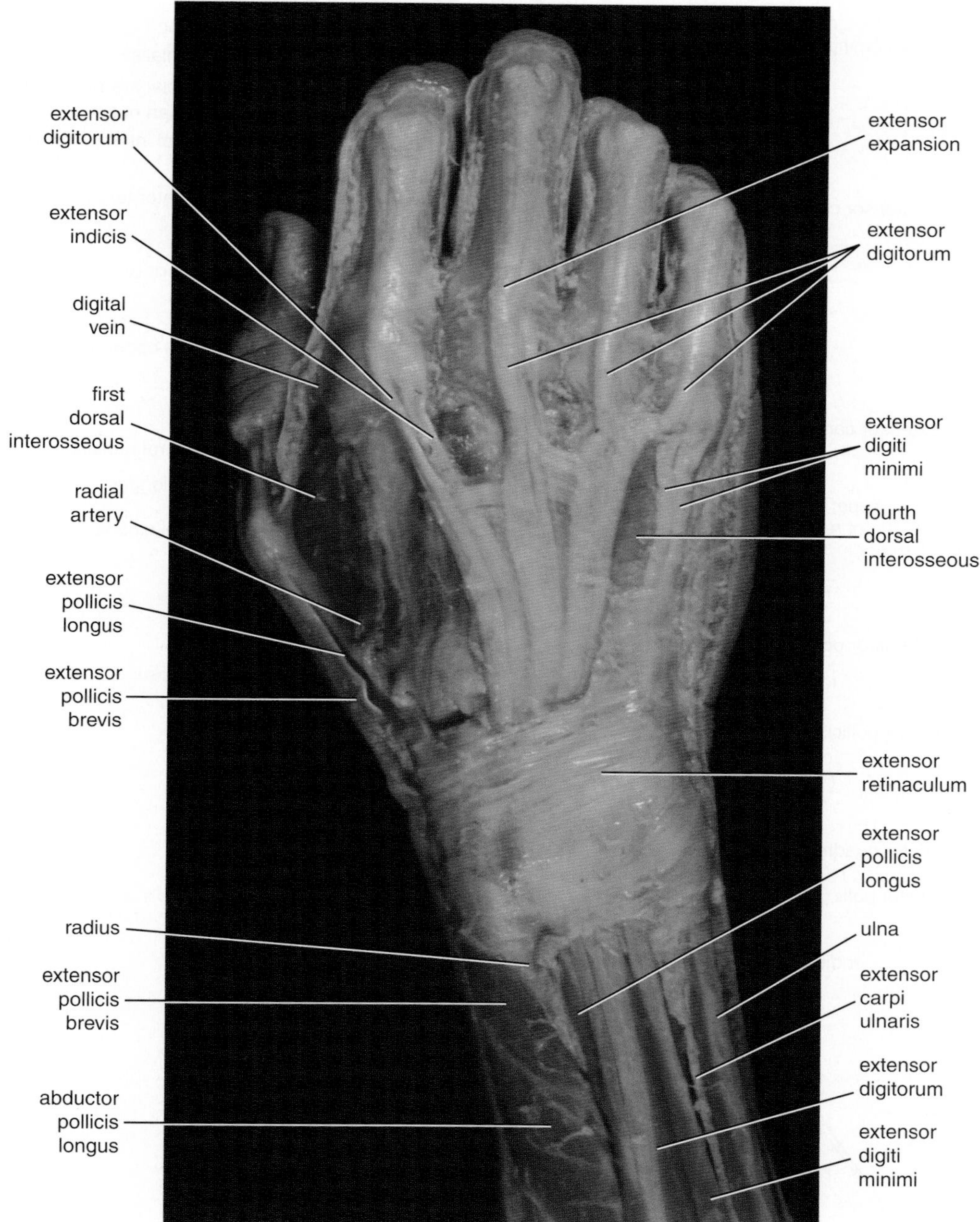

Figure 9-57 Dissection of the dorsal surface of the right hand showing the long extensor tendons and the extensor retinaculum.

In the upper part of its course, the ulnar artery lies deep to most of the flexor muscles. Below, it becomes superficial and lies between the tendons of the flexor carpi ulnaris and the tendons of the flexor digitorum superficialis. In front of the flexor retinaculum, it lies just lateral to the pisiform bone and is covered only by skin and fascia (site for taking ulnar pulse).

Branches

- **Muscular branches** to neighboring muscles
- **Recurrent branches** that take part in the arterial anastomosis around the elbow joint (Fig. 9-61)
- **Branches that take part in the arterial anastomosis around the wrist joint**
- The **common interosseous artery,** which arises from the upper part of the ulnar artery and after a brief course divides into the **anterior** and **posterior interosseous arteries** (Fig. 9-61). The interosseous arteries are distributed to the muscles lying in front of and behind the interosseous membrane; they provide nutrient arteries to the radius and ulna bone.

Radial Artery The radial artery is the smaller of the terminal branches of the brachial artery. It begins in the cubital fossa at the level of the neck of the radius (Figs. 9-58, 9-59, and 9-60). It passes downward and laterally, be-

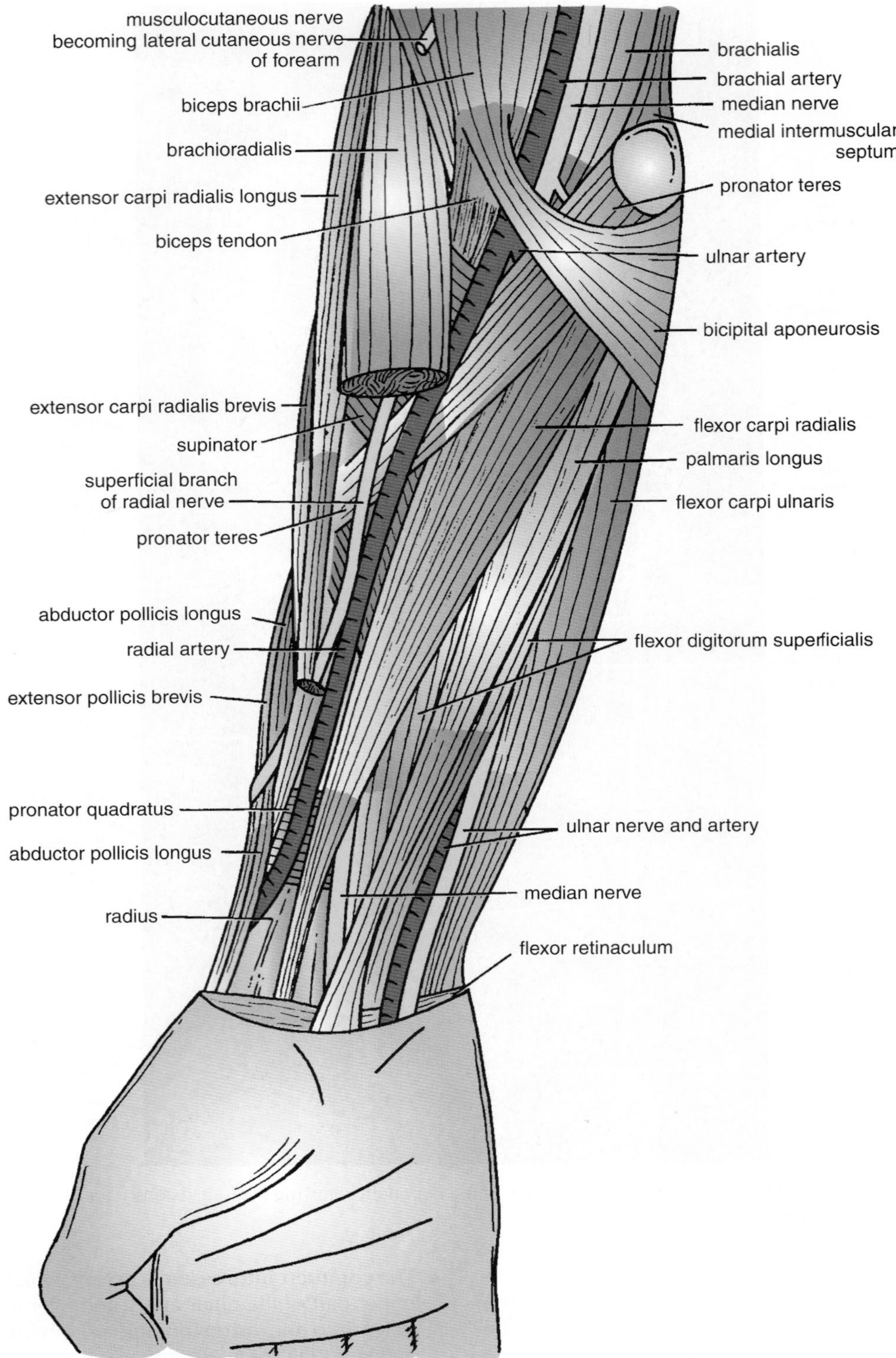

Figure 9-58 Anterior view of the forearm. The middle portion of the brachioradialis muscle has been removed to display the superficial branch of the radial nerve and the radial artery.

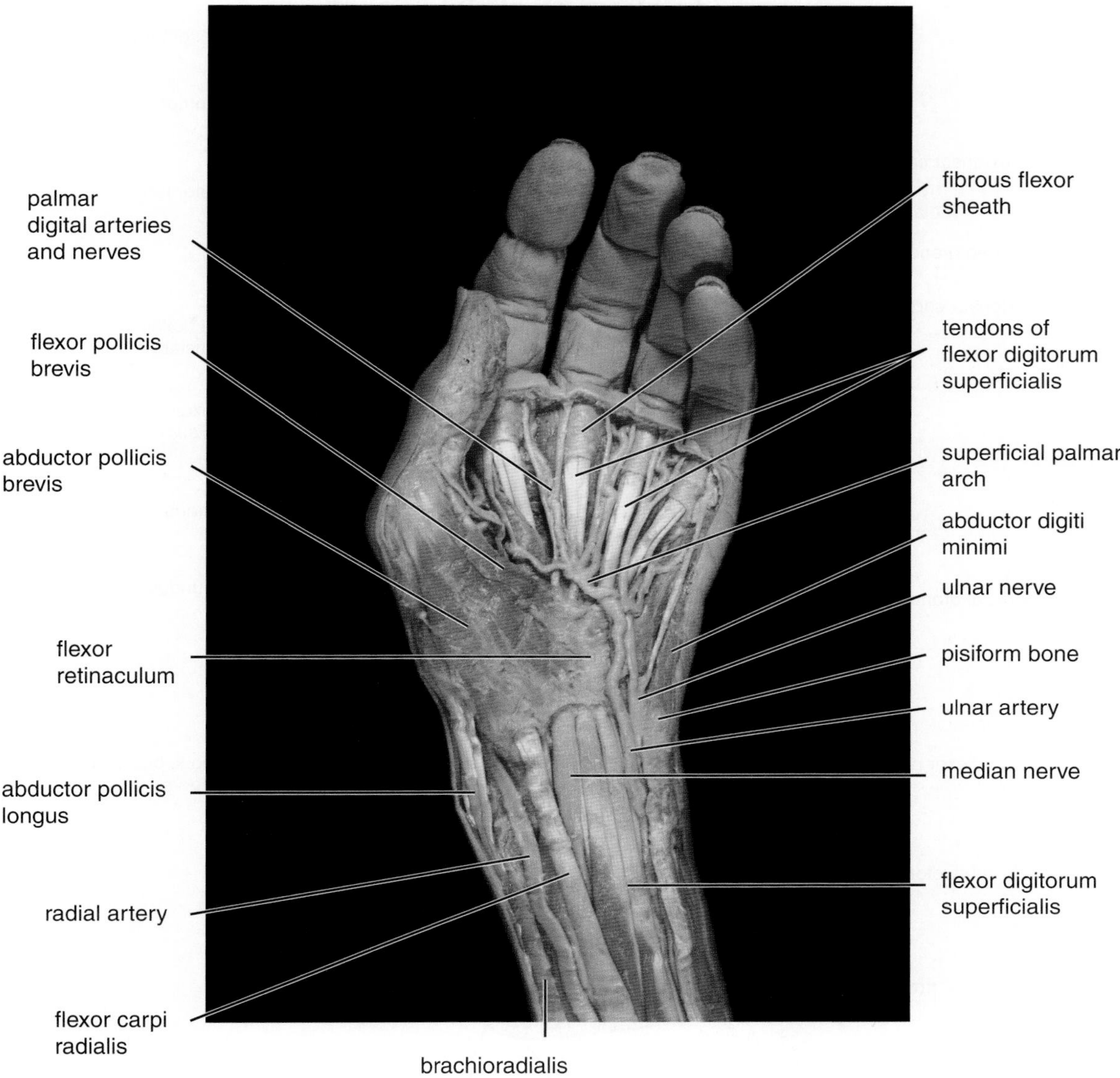

Figure 9-59 Dissection of the front of the left forearm and hand showing the superficial structures.

neath the brachioradialis muscle and resting on the deep muscles of the forearm. In the middle third of its course, the superficial branch of the radial nerve lies on its lateral side.

In the distal part of the forearm, the radial artery lies on the anterior surface of the radius and is covered only by skin and fascia. Here, the artery has the tendon of brachioradialis on its lateral side and the tendon of flexor carpi radialis on its medial side (site for taking the radial pulse).

The radial artery leaves the forearm by winding around the lateral aspect of the wrist to reach the posterior surface of the hand (see page 509).

Branches in the Forearm

- **Muscular branches** to neighboring muscles
- **Recurrent branch,** which takes part in the arterial anastomosis around the elbow joint (Fig. 9-60)
- **Superficial palmar branch,** which arises just above the wrist (Fig. 9-60), enters the palm of the hand, and frequently joins the ulnar artery to form the **superficial palmar arch**

Nerves of the Anterior Fascial Compartment of the Forearm

Median Nerve The median nerve leaves the cubital fossa by passing between the two heads of the pronator teres (Fig. 9-60). It continues downward behind the flexor digitorum superficialis and rests posteriorly on the flexor digitorum profundus. At the wrist, the median nerve emerges from the lateral border of the flexor digitorum superficialis muscle and lies behind the tendon of the palmaris longus (Figs. 9-58, 9-59, and 9-60). It enters the palm by passing **behind** the flexor retinaculum (see pages 499 and 500).

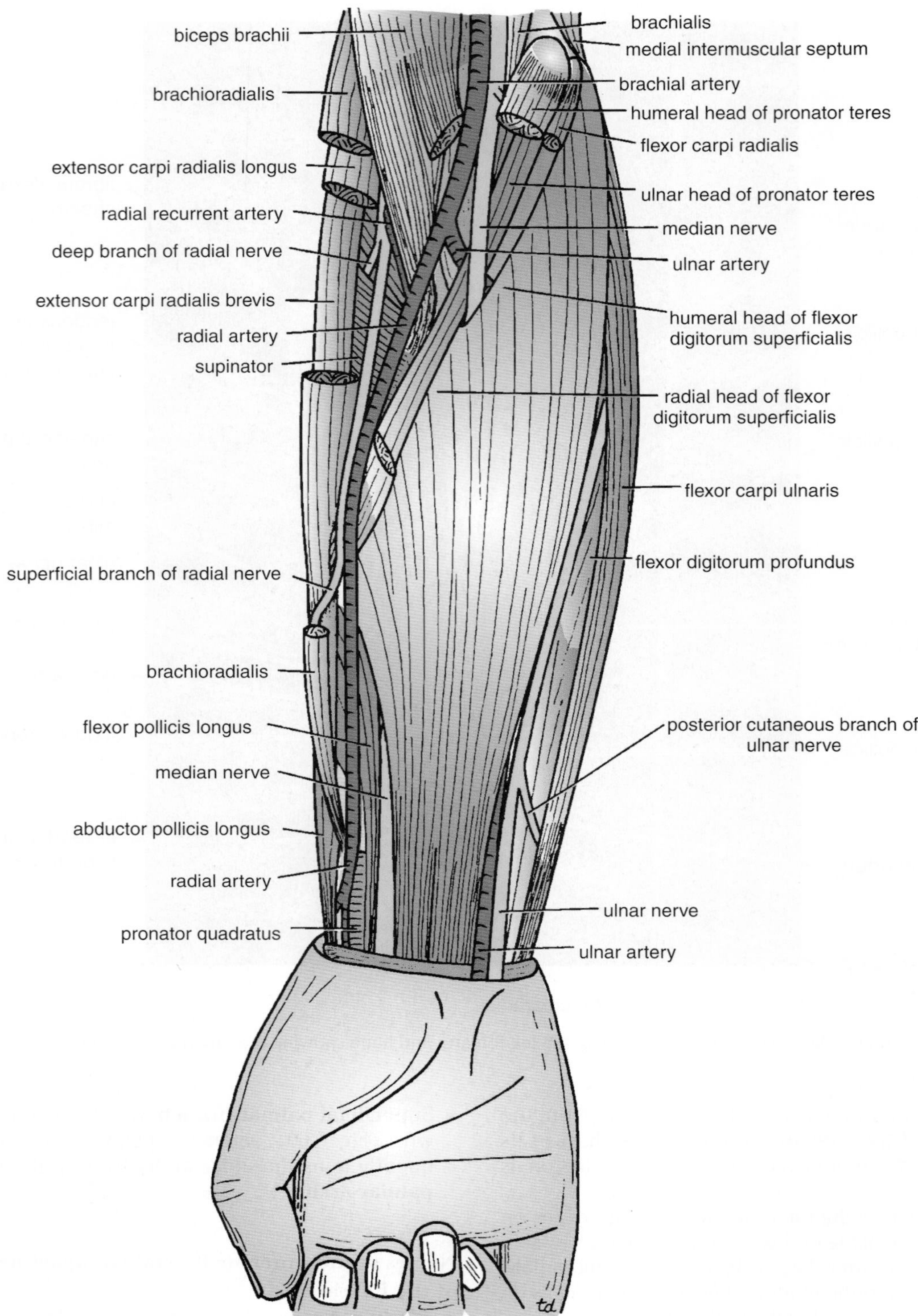

Figure 9-60 Anterior view of the forearm. Most of the superficial muscles have been removed to display the flexor digitorum superficialis, median nerve, superficial branch of the radial nerve, and radial artery. Note that the ulnar head of the pronator teres separates the median nerve from the ulnar artery.

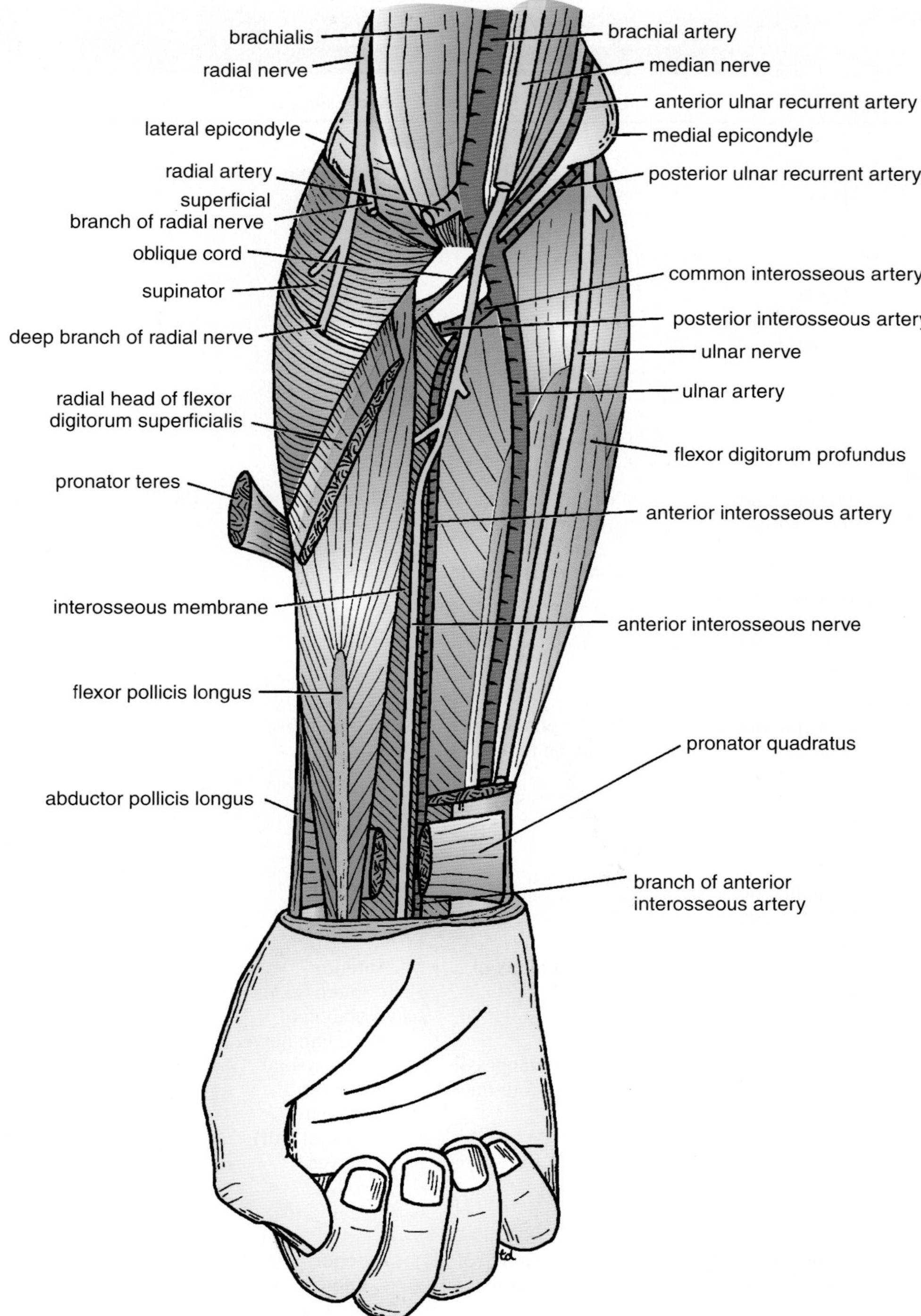

Figure 9-61 Anterior view of the forearm showing the deep structures.

Table 9-6 Muscles of the Anterior Fascial Compartment of the Forearm

Muscle	Origin	Insertion	Nerve Supply	Nerve Roots[a]	Action
Pronator Teres					
Humeral head	Medial epicondyle of humerus	Lateral aspect of shaft of radius	Median nerve	C6, **7**	Pronation and flexion of forearm
Ulnar head	Medial border of coronoid process of ulna				
Flexor carpi radialis	Medial epicondyle of humerus	Bases of second and third metacarpal bones	Median nerve	C6, **7**	Flexes and abducts hand at wrist joint
Palmaris longus	Medial epicondyle of humerus	Flexor retinaculum and palmar aponeurosis	Median nerve	C7, 8	Flexes hand
Flexor Carpi Ulnaris					
Humeral head	Medial epicondyle of humerus	Pisiform bone, hook of the hamate, base at fifth metacarpal bone	Ulnar nerve	C8; T1	Flexes and adducts hand at wrist joint
Ulnar head	Medial aspect of olecranon process and posterior border of ulna				
Flexor Digitorum Superficialis					
Humeroulnar head	Medial epicondyle of humerus; medial border of coronoid process of ulna	Middle phalanx of medial four fingers	Median nerve	C7, **8**; T1	Flexes middle phalanx of fingers and assists in flexing proximal phalanx and hand
Radial head	Oblique line on anterior surface of shaft of radius				
Flexor pollicis longus	Anterior surface of shaft of radius	Distal phalanx of thumb	Anterior interosseous branch of median nerve	**C8**; T1	Flexes distal phalanx of thumb
Flexor digitorum profundus	Anteromedial surface of shaft of ulna	Distal phalanges of medial four fingers	Ulnar (medial half) and median (lateral half) nerves	**C8**; T1	Flexes distal phalanx of fingers; then assists in flexion of middle and proximal phalanges and wrist
Pronator quadratus	Anterior surface of shaft of ulna	Anterior surface of shaft of radius	Anterior interosseous branch of median nerve	**C8**; T1	Pronates forearm

[a] The predominant nerve root supply is indicated by boldface type.

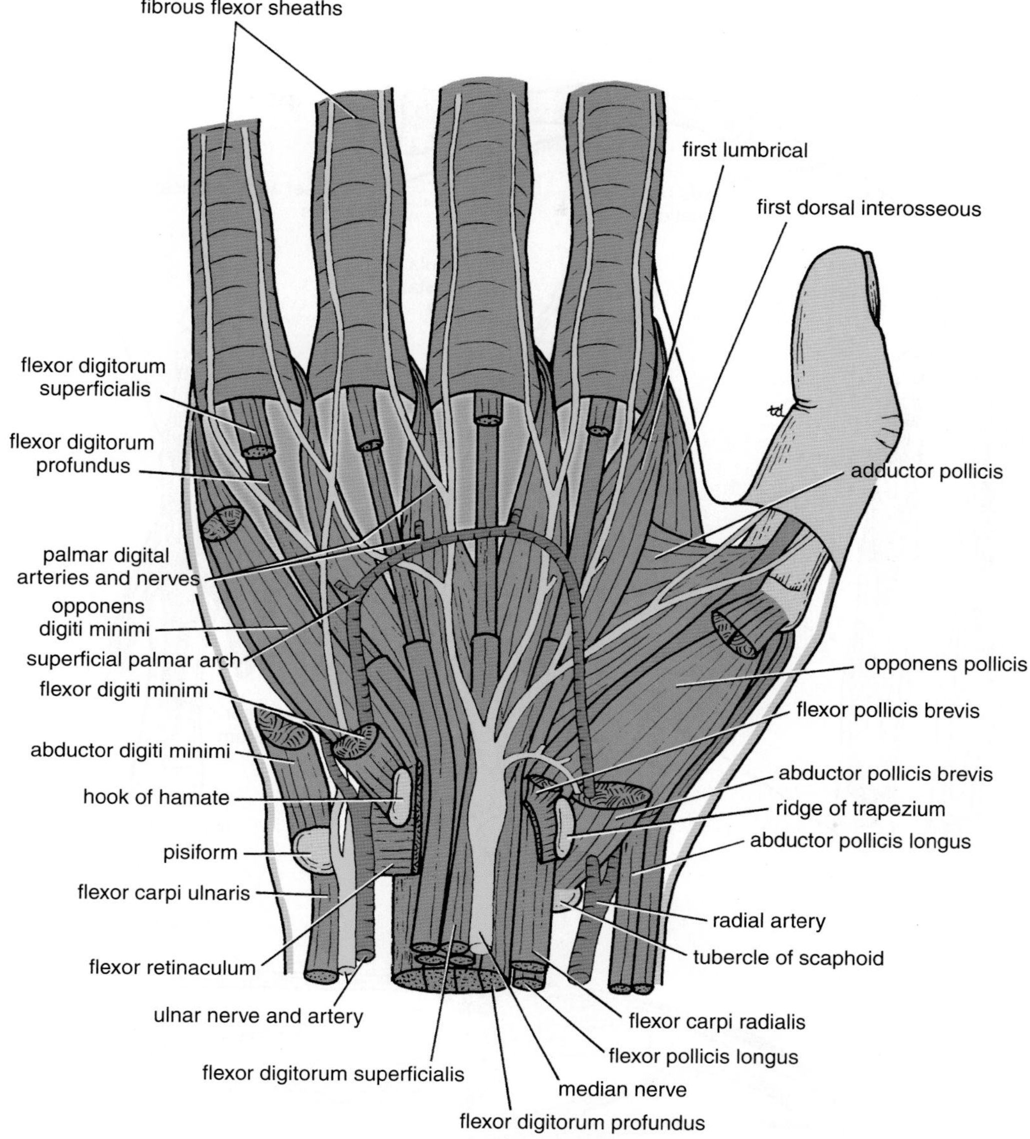

Figure 9-62 . Anterior view of the palm of the hand. The palmar aponeurosis and the greater part of the flexor retinaculum have been removed to display the superficial palmar arch, the median nerve, and the long flexor tendons. Segments of the tendons of the flexor digitorum superficialis have been removed to show the underlying tendons of the flexor digitorum profundus.

Branches

- **Muscular branches** in the cubital fossa to the pronator teres, the flexor carpi radialis, the palmaris longus, and the flexor digitorum superficialis (Fig. 9-22)
- **Articular branches** to the elbow joint
- **Anterior interosseous nerve**
- **Palmar cutaneous branch.** This arises in the lower part of the forearm and is distributed to the skin over the lateral part of the palm (Fig. 9-38).

Anterior Interosseous Nerve The anterior interosseous nerve arises from the median nerve as it emerges from between the two heads of the pronator teres. It passes downward on the anterior surface of the interosseous membrane, between the flexor pollicis longus and the flexor digitorum profundus (Fig. 9-61). It ends on the anterior surface of the carpus.

Branches

- **Muscular branches** to the flexor pollicis longus, the pronator quadratus, and the lateral half of the flexor digitorum profundus
- **Articular branches** to the wrist and distal radioulnar joints. It also supplies the joints of the hand.

Ulnar Nerve The ulnar nerve (Fig. 9-61) passes from behind the medial epicondyle of the humerus, crosses the medial ligament of the elbow joint, and enters the front of the forearm by passing between the two heads of the flexor carpi ulnaris. It then runs down the forearm between the

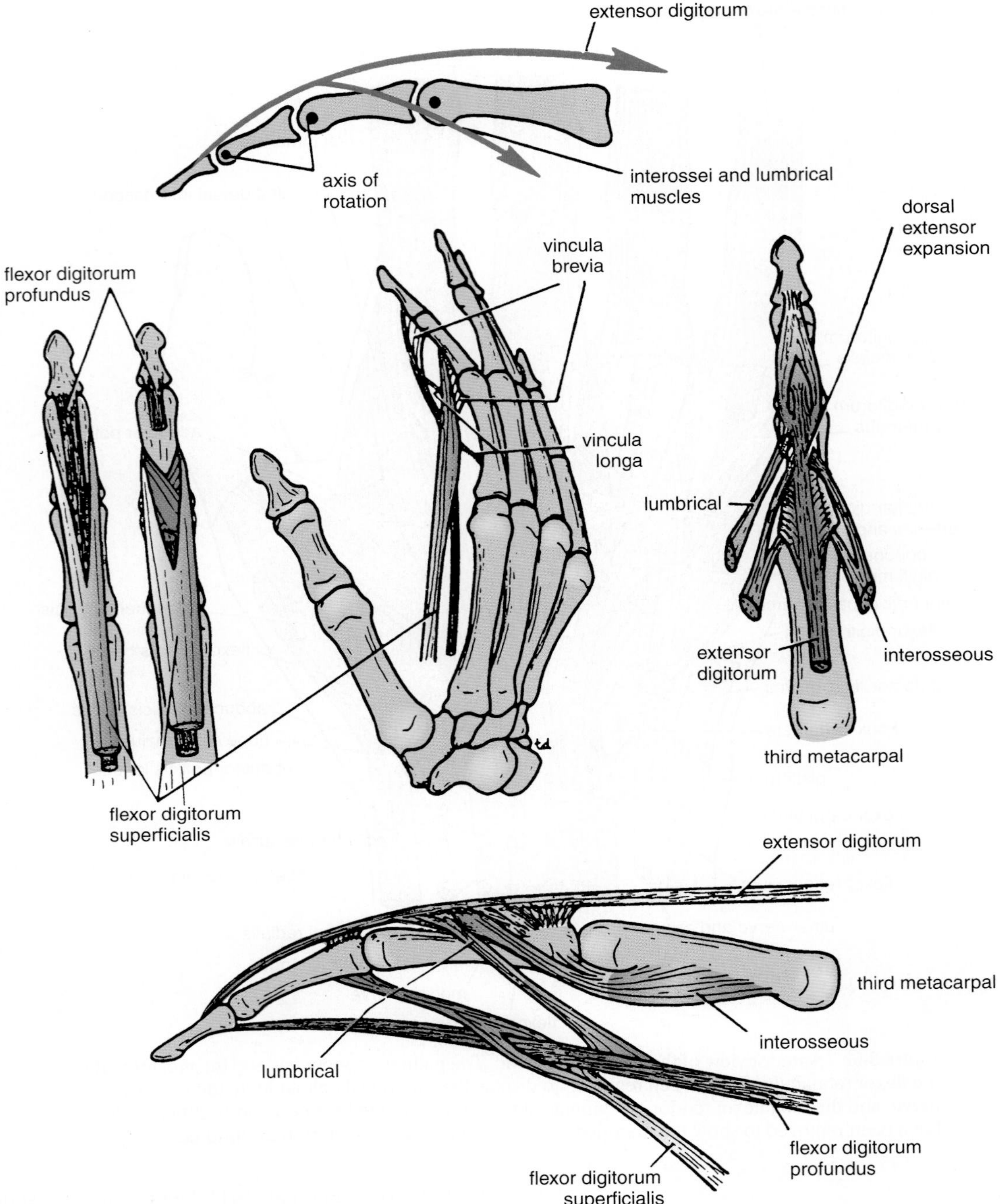

Figure 9-63 Insertions of long flexor and extensor tendons in the fingers. Insertions of the lumbrical and interossei muscles are also shown. The uppermost figure illustrates the action of the lumbrical and interossei muscles in flexing the metacarpophalangeal joints and extending the interphalangeal joints.

flexor carpi ulnaris and the flexor digitorum profundus muscles. In the distal two thirds of the forearm, the ulnar artery lies on the lateral side of the ulnar nerve (Fig. 9-61). At the wrist, the ulnar nerve becomes superficial and lies between the tendons of the flexor carpi ulnaris and flexor digitorum superficialis muscles (Figs. 9-58 and 9-59). The ulnar nerve enters the palm of the hand by passing **in front of** the flexor retinaculum and lateral to the pisiform bone; here it has the ulnar artery lateral to it (see page 499).

Branches

- **Muscular branches** to the flexor carpi ulnaris and to the medial half of the flexor digitorum profundus (Fig. 9-23)
- **Articular branches** to the elbow joint
- The **palmar cutaneous branch** is a small branch that arises in the middle of the forearm (Fig. 9-38) and supplies the skin over the hypothenar eminence.
- The **dorsal posterior cutaneous branch** is a large branch that arises in the distal third of the forearm. It passes medially between the tendon of the flexor carpi ulnaris and the ulna and is distributed on the posterior surface of the hand and fingers.

Contents of the Lateral Fascial Compartment of the Forearm

The lateral fascial compartment may be regarded as part of the posterior fascial compartment.

- **Muscles:** Brachioradialis and extensor carpi radialis longus
- **Blood supply:** Radial and brachial arteries
- **Nerve supply to the muscles:** Radial nerve

Muscles of the Lateral Fascial Compartment of the Forearm

The muscles of the lateral fascial compartment of the forearm are seen in Figures 9-58 and 9-60 and are described in Table 9-7.

Arteries of the Lateral Compartment of the Forearm

The arterial supply is derived from branches of the radial and brachial arteries.

Nerve of the Lateral Compartment of the Forearm

Radial Nerve The radial nerve pierces the lateral intermuscular septum in the lower part of the arm and passes forward into the cubital fossa (Fig. 9-47). It then passes downward in front of the lateral epicondyle of the humerus, lying between the brachialis on the medial side and the brachioradialis and extensor carpi radialis longus on the lateral side (Fig. 9-60). At the level of the lateral epicondyle, it divides into superficial and deep branches (Figs. 9-60 and 9-61).

Branches

- **Muscular branches** to the brachioradialis, to the extensor carpi radialis longus, and a small branch to the lateral part of the brachialis muscle (Fig. 9-25)
- **Articular branches** to the elbow joint
- **Deep branch of the radial nerve.** This winds around the neck of the radius, within the supinator muscle (Fig. 9-61), and enters the posterior compartment of the forearm (Fig. 9-61).
- **Superficial branch of the radial nerve**

Superficial Branch of the Radial Nerve The superficial branch of the radial nerve is the direct continuation of the nerve after its main stem has given off its deep branch in front of the lateral epicondyle of the humerus (Fig. 9-60). It runs down under cover of the brachioradialis muscle on the lateral side of the radial artery. In the distal part of the forearm, it leaves the artery and passes backward under the tendon of the brachioradialis (Fig. 9-60). It reaches the posterior surface of the wrist, where it divides into terminal branches that supply the skin on the lateral two thirds of the posterior surface of the hand (Fig. 9-38) and the posterior surface over the proximal phalanges of the lateral three and a half fingers. The area of skin supplied by the nerve on the dorsum of the hand is variable.

Contents of the Posterior Fascial Compartment of the Forearm

- **Muscles:** The **superficial group** includes the extensor carpi radialis brevis, extensor digitorum, extensor digiti minimi, extensor carpi ulnaris, and anconeus. These muscles possess a common tendon of origin, which is attached to the lateral epicondyle of the humerus. The **deep group** includes the supinator, abductor pollicis longus, extensor pollicis brevis, extensor pollicis longus, and extensor indicis.
- **Blood supply:** Posterior and anterior interosseous arteries
- **Nerve supply to the muscles:** Deep branch of the radial nerve

Muscles of the Posterior Fascial Compartment of the Forearm

The muscles of the posterior fascial compartment are seen in Figures 9-64 and 9-65 and are described in Table 9-8.

Table 9-7 Muscles of the Lateral Fascial Compartment of the Forearm

Muscle	Origin	Insertion	Nerve Supply	Nerve Roots[a]	Action
Brachioradialis	Lateral supracondylar ridge of humerus	Base of styloid process of radius	Radial nerve	C5, **6,** 7	Flexes forearm at elbow joint; rotates forearm to the midprone position
Extensor carpi radialis longus	Lateral supracondylar ridge of humerus	Posterior surface of base of second metacarpal bone	Radial nerve	C6, 7	Extends and abducts hand at wrist joint

[a] The predominant nerve root supply is indicated by boldface type.

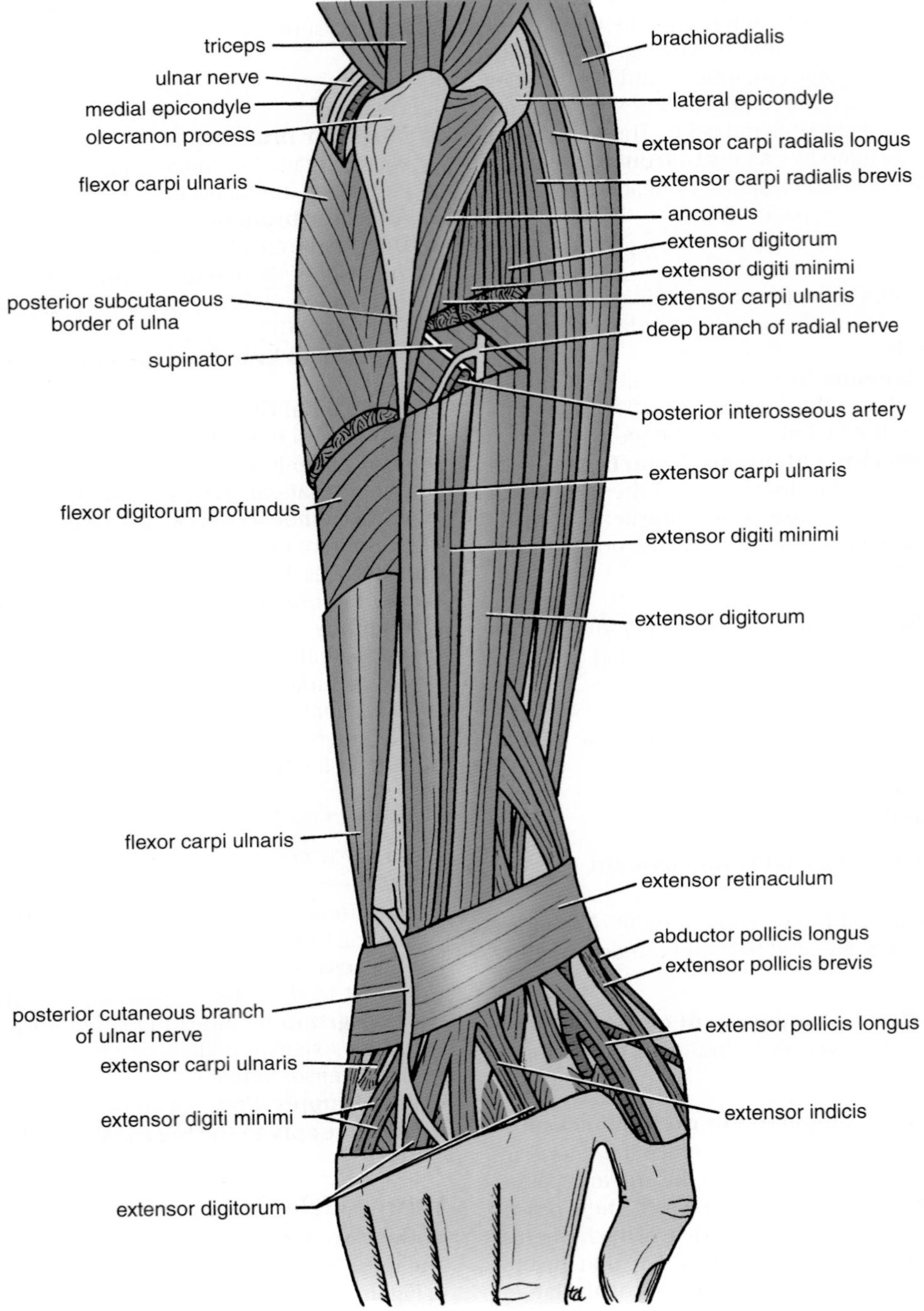

Figure 9-64 Posterior view of the forearm. Parts of the extensor digitorum, extensor digiti minimi, and extensor carpi ulnaris have been removed to show the deep branch of the radial nerve and the posterior interosseous artery.

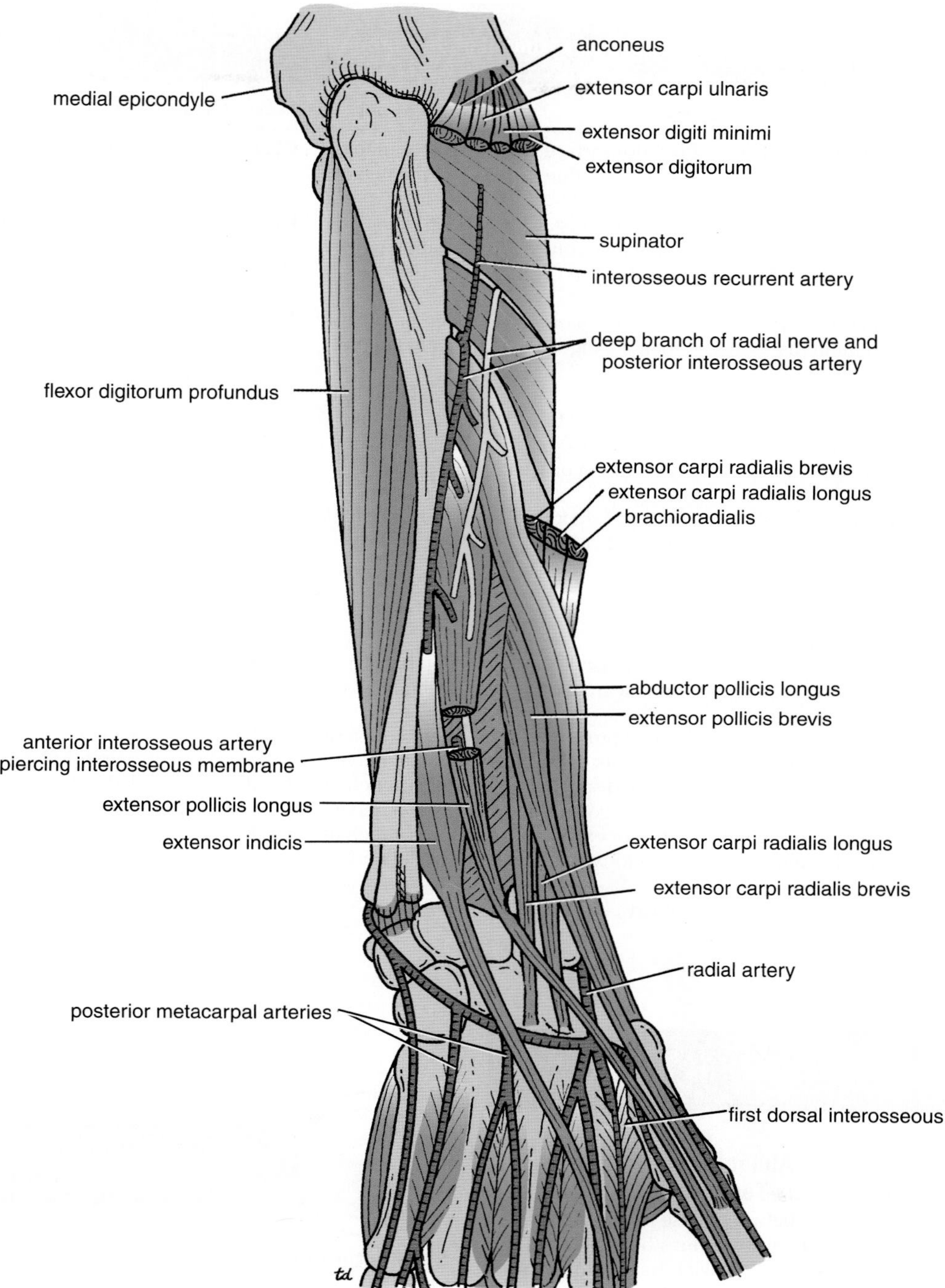

Figure 9-65 Posterior view of the forearm. The superficial muscles have been removed to display the deep structures.

Table 9-8 Muscles of the Posterior Fascial Compartment of the Forearm

Muscle	Origin	Insertion	Nerve Supply	Nerve Roots[a]	Action
Extensor carpi radialis brevis	Lateral epicondyle of humerus	Posterior surface of base of third metacarpal bone	Deep branch of radial nerve	**C7,** 8	Extends and abducts hand at wrist joint
Extensor digitorum	Lateral epicondyle of humerus	Middle and distal phalanges of medial four fingers	Deep branch of radial nerve	**C7,** 8	Extends fingers and hand (see text for details)
Extensor digiti minimi	Lateral epicondyle of humerus	Extensor expansion of little finger	Deep branch of radial nerve	**C7,** 8	Extends metacarpal phalangeal joint of little finger
Extensor carpi ulnaris	Lateral epicondyle of humerus	Base of fifth metacarpal bone	Deep branch of radial nerve	C7, **8**	Extends and adducts hand at wrist joint
Anconeus	Lateral epicondyle of humerus	Lateral surface of olecranon process of ulna	Radial nerve	C7, 8; T1	Extends elbow joint
Supinator	Lateral epicondyle of humerus, anular ligament of proximal radioulnar joint, and ulna	Neck and shaft of radius	Deep branch of radial nerve	C5, 6	Supination of forearm
Abductor pollicis longus	Posterior surface of shafts of radius and ulna	Base of first metacarpal bone	Deep branch of radial nerve	C7, **8**	Abducts and extends thumb
Extensor pollicis brevis	Posterior surface of shaft of radius	Base of proximal phalanx of thumb	Deep branch of radial nerve	C7, **8**	Extends metacarpophalangeal joints of thumb
Extensor pollicis longus	Posterior surface of shaft of ulna	Base of distal phalanx of thumb	Deep branch of radial nerve	C7, **8**	Extends distal phalanx of thumb
Extensor indicis	Posterior surface of shaft of ulna	Extensor expansion of index finger	Deep branch of radial nerve	C7, **8**	Extends metacarpophalangeal joint of index finger

[a] The predominant nerve root supply is indicated by boldface type.

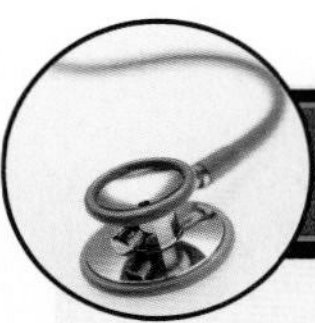

CLINICAL NOTES

Stenosing Synovitis of the Abductor Pollicis Longus and Extensor Pollicis Brevis Tendons

As a result of repeated friction between these tendons and the styloid process of the radius, they sometimes become edematous and swell. Later, fibrosis of the synovial sheath produces a condition known as **stenosing tenosynovitis** in which movement of the tendons becomes restricted. Advanced cases require surgical incision along the constricting sheath.

Arteries of the Posterior Fascial Compartment of the Forearm

The **anterior** and **posterior interosseous arteries** arise from the common interosseous artery, a branch of the ulnar artery (Figs. 9-61 and 9-65). They pass downward on the anterior and posterior surfaces of the interosseous membrane, respectively, and supply the adjoining muscles and bones. They end by taking part in the anastomosis around the wrist joint.

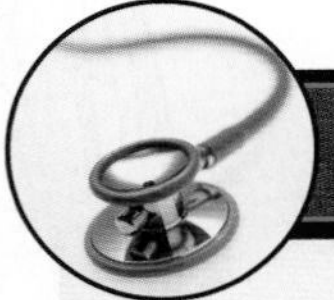

CLINICAL NOTES

Rupture of the Extensor Pollicis Longus Tendon

Rupture of this tendon can occur after fracture of the distal third of the radius. Roughening of the dorsal tubercle of the radius by the fracture line can cause excessive friction on the tendon, which can then rupture. Rheumatoid arthritis can also cause rupture of this tendon.

"Anatomic Snuffbox"

The anatomic snuffbox is a term commonly used to describe a triangular skin depression on the lateral side of the wrist that is bounded medially by the tendon of the extensor pollicis longus and laterally by the tendons of the abductor pollicis longus and extensor pollicis brevis (Fig. 9-64). Its clinical importance lies in the fact that the scaphoid bone is most easily palpated here and that the pulsations of the radial artery can be felt here (Fig. 9-100).

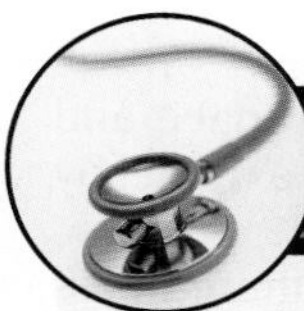

CLINICAL NOTES

Tennis Elbow

Tennis elbow is caused by a partial tearing or degeneration of the origin of the superficial extensor muscles from the lateral epicondyle of the humerus. It is characterized by pain and tenderness over the lateral epicondyle of the humerus, with pain radiating down the lateral side of the forearm; it is common in tennis players, violinists, and housewives.

Nerve of the Posterior Fascial Compartment of the Forearm

Deep Branch of the Radial Nerve The deep branch arises from the radial nerve in front of the lateral epicondyle of the humerus in the cubital fossa (Fig. 9-61). It pierces the supinator and winds around the lateral aspect of the neck of the radius in the substance of the muscle to reach the posterior compartment of the forearm. The nerve descends in the interval between the superficial and deep groups of muscles (Fig. 9-65). It eventually reaches the posterior surface of the wrist joint.

Branches

- **Muscular branches** to the extensor carpi radialis brevis and the supinator, the extensor digitorum, the extensor digiti minimi, the extensor carpi ulnaris, the abductor pollicis longus, the extensor pollicis brevis, the extensor pollicis longus, and the extensor indicis
- **Articular branches** to the wrist and carpal joints

The Region of the Wrist

Before learning the anatomy of the hand, it is essential that a student have a sound knowledge of the arrangement of the tendons, arteries, and nerves in the region of the wrist joint. From a clinical standpoint, the wrist is a common site for injury.

In a transverse section through the wrist (Fig. 9-54), identify the structures from medial to lateral. At the same time, examine your own wrist and identify as many of the structures as possible.

Structures on the Anterior Aspect of the Wrist

The following structures pass superficial to the flexor retinaculum from medial to lateral (Fig. 9-54):

- **Flexor carpi ulnaris tendon,** ending on the pisiform bone. (This tendon does not actually cross the flexor retinaculum but is included for the sake of completeness.)
- **Ulnar nerve** lies lateral to the pisiform bone.
- **Ulnar artery** lies lateral to the ulnar nerve.
- **Palmar cutaneous branch of the ulnar nerve**
- **Palmaris longus tendon** (if present), passing to its insertion into the flexor retinaculum and the palmar aponeurosis
- **Palmar cutaneous branch of the median nerve**

The following structures pass beneath the flexor retinaculum from medial to lateral (Fig. 9-54):

- **Flexor digitorum superficialis tendons** and, posterior to these, the tendons of the flexor digitorum profundus; both groups of tendons share a common synovial sheath.
- **Median nerve**
- **Flexor pollicis longus tendon** surrounded by a synovial sheath
- **Flexor carpi radialis tendon** going through a split in the flexor retinaculum. The tendon is surrounded by a synovial sheath.

Structures on the Posterior Aspect of the Wrist

The following structures pass superficial to the extensor retinaculum from medial to lateral (Fig. 9-54):

- **Dorsal (posterior) cutaneous branch of the ulnar nerve**
- **Basilic vein**
- **Cephalic vein**
- **Superficial branch of the radial nerve**

The following structures pass beneath the extensor retinaculum from medial to lateral (Fig. 9-54):

- **Extensor carpi ulnaris tendon,** which grooves the posterior aspect of the head of the ulna
- **Extensor digiti minimi tendon** is situated posterior to the distal radioulnar joint.
- **Extensor digitorum** and **extensor indicis tendons** share a common synovial sheath and are situated on the lateral part of the posterior surface of the radius.
- **Extensor pollicis longus tendon** winds around the medial side of the dorsal tubercle of the radius.
- **Extensor carpi radialis longus** and **brevis tendons** share a common synovial sheath and are situated on the lateral part of the posterior surface of the radius.
- **Abductor pollicis longus** and the **extensor pollicis brevis tendons** have separate synovial sheaths but share a common compartment.

Beneath the extensor retinaculum, fibrous septa pass to the underlying radius and ulna and form six compartments that contain the tendons of the extensor muscles. Each compartment is provided with a synovial sheath, which extends above and below the retinaculum.

The radial artery reaches the back of the hand by passing between the lateral collateral ligament of the wrist joint and the tendons of the abductor pollicis longus and extensor pollicis brevis (Fig. 9-65).

The Palm of the Hand

Skin

The skin of the palm of the hand is thick and hairless. It is bound down to the underlying deep fascia by numerous fibrous bands. The skin shows many flexure creases at the sites of skin movement, which are not necessarily placed at the site of joints. Sweat glands are present in large numbers.

The **palmaris brevis** (Fig. 9-55) is a small muscle that arises from the flexor retinaculum and palmar aponeurosis and is inserted into the skin of the palm. It is supplied by the superficial branch of the ulnar nerve. Its function is to corrugate the skin at the base of the hypothenar eminence and so improve the grip of the palm in holding a rounded object.

The **sensory nerve** supply to the skin of the palm (Figs. 9-38 and 9-55) is derived from the **palmar cutaneous branch of the median nerve,** which crosses in front of the flexor retinaculum and supplies the lateral part of the palm, and the **palmar cutaneous branch of the ulnar nerve;** the latter nerve also crosses in front of the flexor retinaculum (Fig. 9-54) and supplies the medial part of the palm.

The skin over the base of the thenar eminence is supplied by the **lateral cutaneous nerve of the forearm** or the **superficial branch of the radial nerve** (Fig. 9-38).

Deep Fascia

The deep fascia of the wrist and palm is thickened to form the **flexor retinaculum** (described on page 484) and the **palmar aponeurosis.**

The Palmar Aponeurosis

The palmar aponeurosis is triangular and occupies the central area of the palm (Fig. 9-55). The apex of the palmar aponeurosis is attached to the distal border of the flexor retinaculum and receives the insertion of the palmaris longus tendon (Fig. 9-55). The base of the aponeurosis divides at the bases of the fingers into four slips. Each slip divides into two bands, one passing superficially to the skin and the other passing deeply to the root of the finger; here each deep band divides into two, which diverge around the flexor tendons and finally fuse with the fibrous flexor sheath and the deep transverse ligaments.

The medial and lateral borders of the palmar aponeurosis are continuous with the thinner deep fascia covering the hypothenar and thenar muscles. From each of these borders, fibrous septa pass posteriorly into the palm and take part in the formation of the palmar fascial spaces (see page 508).

The function of the palmar aponeurosis is to give firm attachment to the overlying skin and so improve the grip and to protect the underlying tendons.

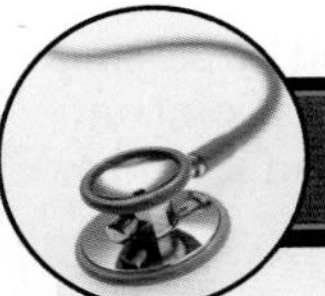

CLINICAL NOTES

Dupuytren's Contracture

Dupuytren's contracture is a localized thickening and contracture of the palmar aponeurosis. It commonly starts near the root of the ring finger and draws that finger into the palm, flexing it at the metacarpophalangeal joint. Later, the condition involves the little finger in the same manner. In long-standing cases, the pull on the fibrous sheaths of these fingers results in flexion of the proximal interphalangeal joints. The distal interphalangeal joints are not involved and are actually extended by the pressure of the fingers against the palm.

The Carpal Tunnel

The carpus is deeply concave on its anterior surface and forms a bony gutter. The gutter is converted into a tunnel by the flexor retinaculum (Fig. 9-54).

The long flexor tendons to the fingers and thumb pass through the tunnel and are accompanied by the median nerve. The four separate tendons of the flexor digitorum superficialis muscle are arranged in anterior and posterior rows, those to the middle and ring fingers lying in front of those to the index and little fingers. At the lower border of the flexor retinaculum, the four tendons diverge and become arranged on the same plane (Fig. 9-62).

The tendons of the flexor digitorum profundus muscle are on the same plane and lie behind the superficialis tendons.

All eight tendons of the flexor digitorum superficialis and profundus invaginate a common synovial sheath from the lateral side (Fig. 9-54). This allows the arterial supply to the tendons to enter them from the lateral side.

The tendon of the flexor pollicis longus muscle runs through the lateral part of the tunnel in its own synovial sheath.

The median nerve passes beneath the flexor retinaculum in a **restricted** space between the flexor digitorum superficialis and the flexor carpi radialis muscles (Fig. 9-54).

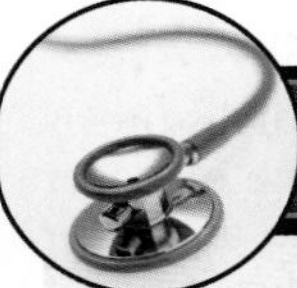

CLINICAL NOTES

Carpal Tunnel Syndrome

The carpal tunnel, formed by the concave anterior surface of the carpal bones and closed by the flexor retinaculum, is tightly packed with the long flexor tendons of the fingers, with their surrounding synovial sheaths, and the median nerve (Fig. 9-54). Clinically, the syndrome consists of a burning pain or "pins and needles" along the distribution of the median nerve to the lateral three and a half fingers and weakness of the thenar muscles. It is produced by compression of the median nerve within the tunnel. The exact cause of the compression is difficult to determine, but thickening of the synovial sheaths of the flexor tendons or arthritic changes in the carpal bones are thought to be responsible in many cases. As you would expect, no paresthesia occurs over the thenar eminence because this area of skin is supplied by the palmar cutaneous branch of the median nerve, which passes superficially to the flexor retinaculum. The condition is dramatically relieved by decompressing the tunnel by making a longitudinal incision through the flexor retinaculum.

Fibrous Flexor Sheaths

The anterior surface of each finger, from the head of the metacarpal to the base of the distal phalanx, is provided with a strong fibrous sheath that is attached to the sides of the phalanges (Fig. 9-66). The proximal end of the fibrous sheath is open, whereas the distal end of the sheath is closed and is attached to the base of the distal phalanx. The sheath and the bones form a blind tunnel in which the flexor tendons of the finger lie.

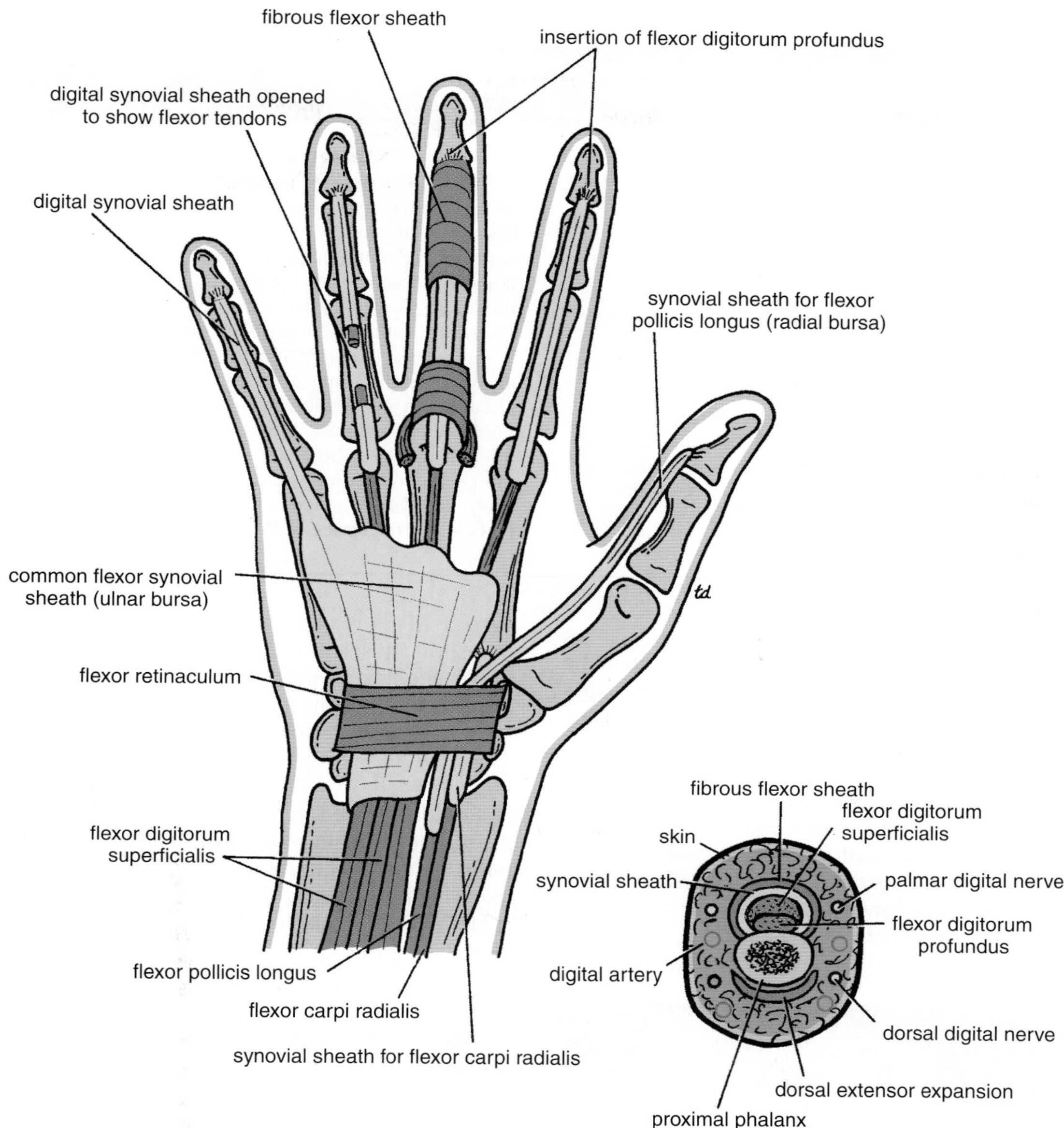

Figure 9-66 Anterior view of the palm of the hand showing the flexor synovial sheaths. Cross section of a finger is also shown.

In the thumb, the osteofibrous tunnel contains the tendon of the flexor pollicis longus. In the case of the four medial fingers, the tunnel is occupied by the tendons of the flexor digitorum superficialis and profundus (Fig. 9-66). The fibrous sheath is thick over the phalanges but thin and lax over the joints.

Synovial Flexor Sheaths

In the hand, the tendons of the flexor digitorum superficialis and profundus muscles invaginate a common synovial sheath from the lateral side (Fig. 9-54). The medial part of this common sheath extends distally without interruption on the tendons of the little finger. The lateral part of the sheath stops abruptly on the middle of the palm, and the distal ends of the long flexor tendons of the index, the middle, and the ring fingers acquire **digital synovial sheaths** as they enter the fingers. The flexor pollicis longus tendon has its own synovial sheath that passes into the thumb. These sheaths allow the long tendons to move smoothly, with a minimum of friction, beneath the flexor retinaculum and the fibrous flexor sheaths.

The synovial sheath of the flexor pollicis longus (sometimes referred to as the **radial bursa)** communicates with the common synovial sheath of the superficialis and profundus tendons (sometimes referred to as the **ulnar bursa)** at the level of the wrist in about 50% of subjects.

The **vincula longa** and **brevia** are small vascular folds of synovial membrane that connect the tendons to the anterior surface of the phalanges (Fig. 9-63). They resemble a mesentery and convey blood vessels to the tendons.

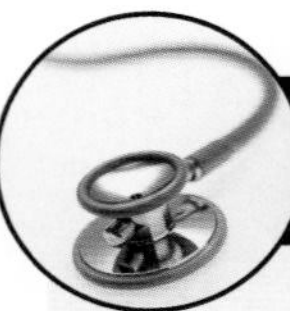

CLINICAL NOTES

Tenosynovitis of the Synovial Sheaths of the Flexor Tendons

Tenosynovitis is an infection of a synovial sheath. It most commonly results from the introduction of bacteria into a sheath through a small penetrating wound, such as that made by the point of a needle or thorn. Rarely, the sheath may become infected by extension of a pulp-space infection.

Infection of a digital sheath results in distention of the sheath with pus; the finger is held semiflexed and is swollen. Any attempt to extend the finger is accompanied by extreme pain because the distended sheath is stretched. As the inflammatory process continues, the pressure within the sheath rises and may compress the blood supply to the tendons that travel in the vincula longa and brevia (Fig. 9-63). Rupture or later severe scarring of the tendons may follow.

A further increase in pressure can cause the sheath to rupture at its proximal end. Anatomically, the digital sheath of the index finger is related to the thenar space, whereas that of the ring finger is related to the midpalmar space. The sheath for the middle finger is related to both the thenar and midpalmar spaces. These relationships explain how infection can extend from the digital synovial sheaths and involve the palmar fascial spaces.

In the case of infection of the digital sheaths of the little finger and thumb, the ulnar and radial bursae are quickly involved. Should such an infection be neglected, pus may burst through the proximal ends of these bursae and enter the fascial space of the forearm between the flexor digitorum profundus anteriorly and the pronator quadratus and the interosseous membrane posteriorly. This fascial space in the forearm is commonly referred to clinically as the **space of Parona.**

Insertion of the Long Flexor Tendons

Each tendon of the flexor digitorum superficialis enters the fibrous flexor sheath; opposite the proximal phalanx it divides into two halves, which pass around the profundus tendon and meet on its deep or posterior surface, where partial decussation of the fibers takes place (Fig. 9-63). The superficialis tendon, having united again, divides almost at once into two further slips, which are attached to the borders of the middle phalanx. Each tendon of the flexor digitorum profundus, having passed through the division of the superficialis tendon, continues downward, to be inserted into the anterior surface of the base of the distal phalanx (Fig. 9-63).

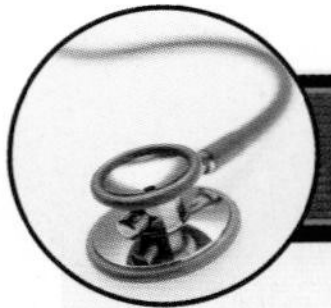

CLINICAL NOTES

Trigger Finger

In trigger finger, there is a palpable and even audible snapping when a patient is asked to flex and extend the fingers. It is caused by the presence of a localized swelling of one of the long flexor tendons that catches on a narrowing of the fibrous flexor sheath anterior to the metacarpophalangeal joint. It may take place either in flexion or in extension. A similar condition occurring in the thumb is called trigger thumb. The situation can be relieved surgically by incising the fibrous flexor sheath.

Small Muscles of the Hand

The small muscles of the hand include the four lumbrical muscles, the eight* interossei muscles, the short muscles of the thumb, and the short muscles of the little finger. The muscles are seen in Figures 9-55, 9-67, 9-68, and 9-69 and are described in Table 9-9.

* There are eight interossei, consisting of four dorsal and four palmar muscles. Some authors describe only three palmar interossei and state that the first palmar interosseous is in reality a second head to the flexor pollicis brevis: others believe that it is part of the adductor pollicis muscle.

Short Muscles of the Thumb

The short muscles of the thumb are the abductor pollicis brevis, the flexor pollicis brevis, the opponens pollicis, and the adductor pollicis (Figs. 9-59, 9-62, and 9-67). The first three of these muscles form the **thenar eminence.**

Opposition of the Thumb

It should be noted that the opponens pollicis muscle pulls the thumb medially and forward across the palm so that the palmar surface of the tip of the thumb may come into contact with the palmar surface of the tips of the other fingers. It is an important muscle and enables the thumb to form one claw in the pincerlike action used for picking up objects. This complex movement involves a flexion of the carpometacarpal and metacarpophalangeal joints and a small amount of abduction and medial rotation of the metacarpal bone at the carpometacarpal joint.

Abduction of the Thumb

Abduction of the thumb may be defined as a movement forward of the thumb in the anteroposterior plane. It takes place at the carpometacarpal joint and the metacarpophalangeal joint.

Adduction of the Thumb

This movement can be defined as a movement backward of the abducted thumb in the anteroposterior plane. It restores the thumb to its anatomic position, which is flush with the palm. The adductor pollicis is the muscle that, in association with the flexor pollicis longus and the opponens pollicis muscles, is largely responsible for the power of the pincers grip of the thumb. Adduction of the thumb occurs at the carpometacarpal and at the metacarpophalangeal joint.

Short Muscles of the Little Finger

The short muscles of the little finger are the abductor digiti minimi, the flexor digiti minimi brevis, and the opponens digiti minimi, which together form the **hypothenar eminence** (Figs 9-59, 9-62, and 9-67).

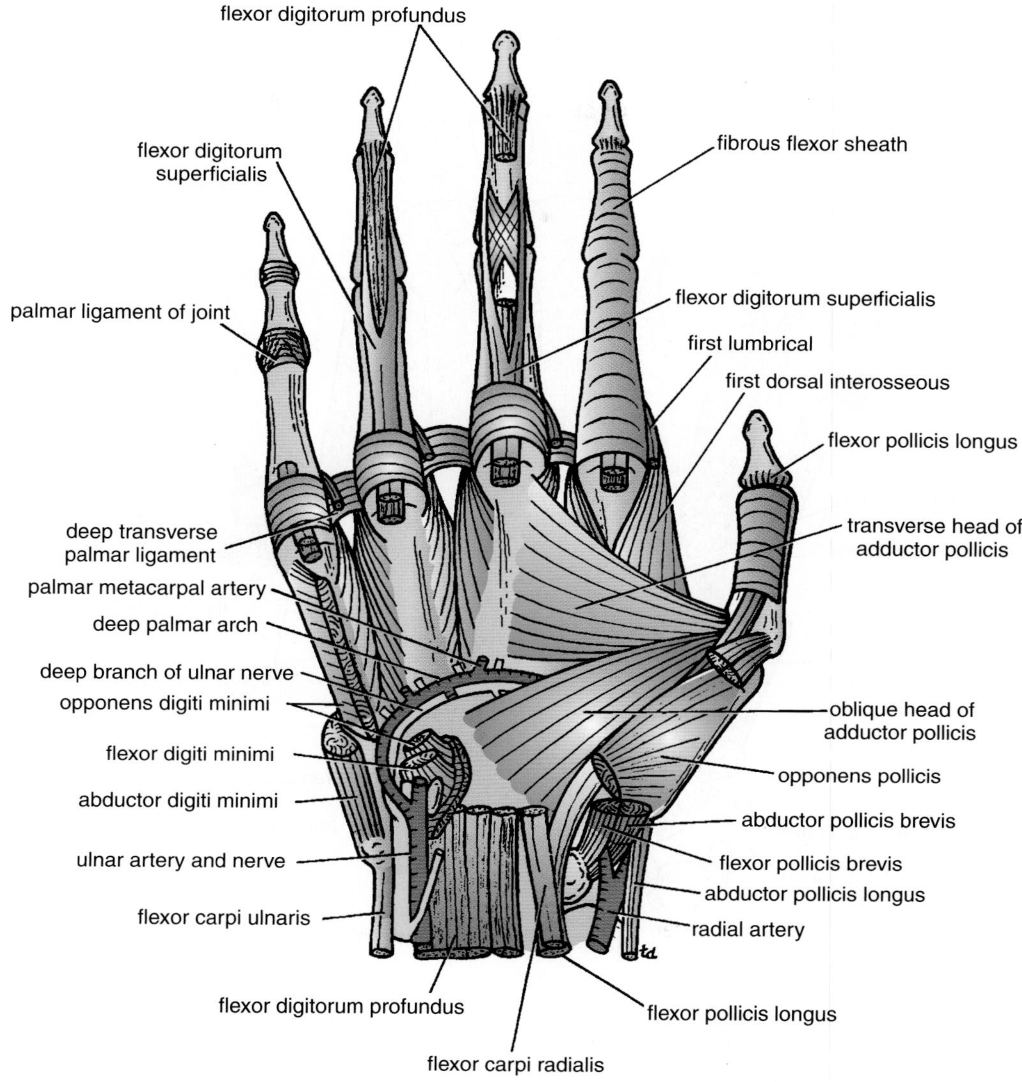

Figure 9-67 Anterior view of the palm of the hand. The long flexor tendons have been removed from the palm, but their method of insertion into the fingers is shown.

Opposition of the Little Finger

The opponens digiti minimi muscle is only capable of rotating the fifth metacarpal bone to a slight degree. However, it assists the flexor digiti minimi in flexing the carpometacarpal joint of the little finger, thereby pulling the fifth metacarpal bone forward and cupping the palm.

Arteries of the Palm

Ulnar Artery

The ulnar artery enters the hand anterior to the flexor retinaculum on the lateral side of the ulnar nerve and the pisiform bone (Fig. 9-62). The artery gives off a deep branchand then continues into the palm as the superficial palmar arch.

The **superficial palmar arch** is a direct continuation of the ulnar artery (Fig. 9-62). On entering the palm, it curves laterally behind the palmar aponeurosis and in front of the long flexor tendons. The arch is completed on the lateral side by one of the branches of the radial artery. The curve of the arch lies across the palm, level with the distal border of the fully extended thumb.

Four **digital arteries** arise from the convexity of the arch and pass to the fingers (Fig. 9-62).

The **deep branch of the ulnar artery** arises in front of the flexor retinaculum, passes between the abductor digiti minimi and the flexor digiti minimi, and joins the radial artery to complete the deep palmar arch (Figs. 9-67 and 9-68).

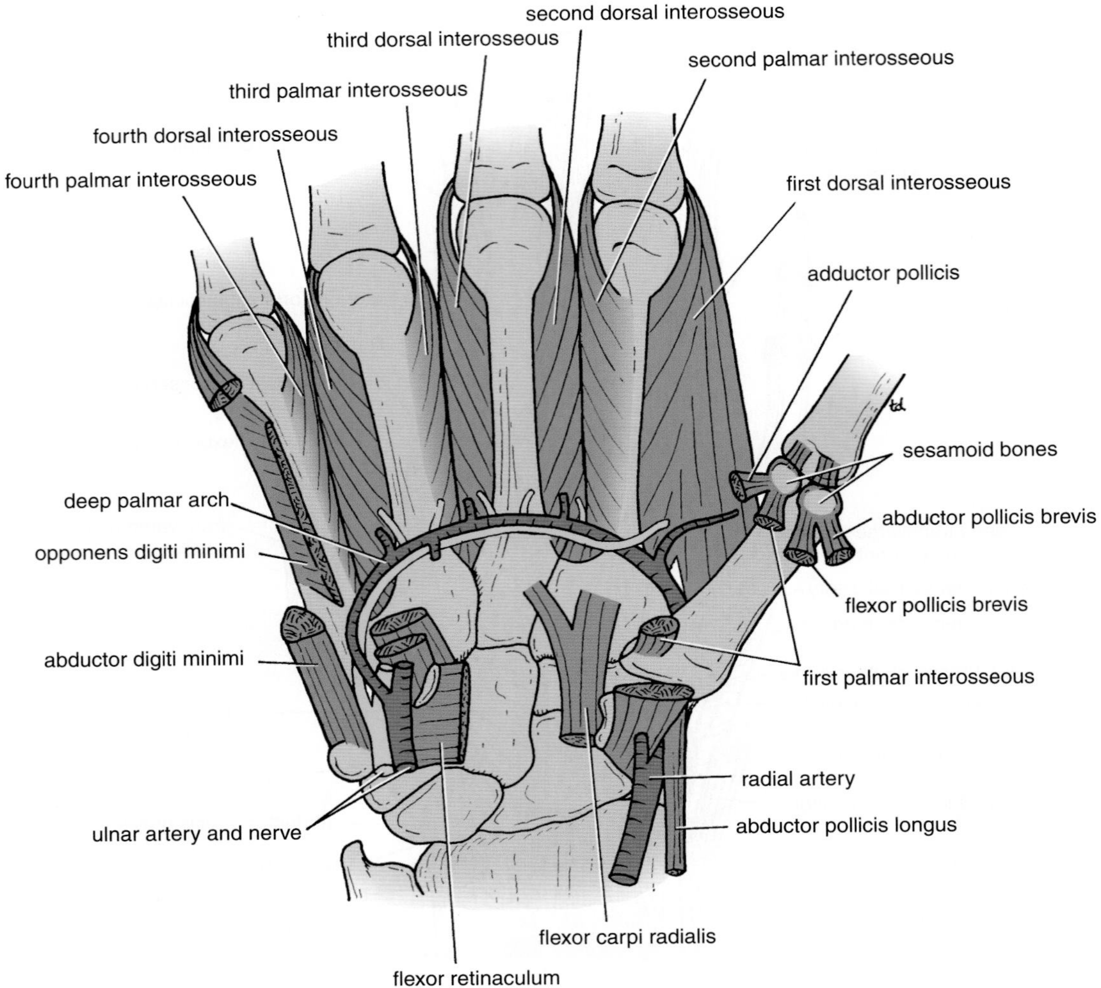

Figure 9-68 Anterior view of the palm of the hand showing the deep palmar arch and the deep terminal branch of the ulnar nerve. The interossei are also shown.

Radial Artery

The radial artery leaves the dorsum of the hand by turning forward between the proximal ends of the first and second metacarpal bones and the two heads of the first dorsal interosseous muscle (see page 509). On entering the palm, it curves medially between the oblique and transverse heads of the adductor pollicis and continues as the deep palmar arch (Figs. 9-67 and 9-68).

The **deep palmar arch** is a direct continuation of the radial artery (Fig. 9-68). It curves medially beneath the long flexor tendons and in front of the metacarpal bones and the interosseous muscles. The arch is completed on the medial side by the deep branch of the ulnar artery. The curve of the arch lies at a level with the proximal border of the extended thumb.

The deep palmar arch sends branches superiorly, which take part in the anastomosis around the wrist joint, and inferiorly, to join the digital branches of the superficial palmar arch.

Branches of the Radial Artery in the Palm

Immediately on entering the palm, the radial artery gives off the **arteria radialis indicis,** which supplies the lateral side of the index finger, and the **arteria princeps pollicis,** which divides into two and supplies the lateral and medial sides of the thumb.

Veins of the Palm

Superficial and deep palmar arterial arches are accompanied by superficial and deep palmar venous arches, receiving corresponding tributaries.

Lymph Drainage of the Palm

The lymph vessels of the fingers pass along their borders to reach the webs. From here the vessels ascend onto the dorsum of the hand. Lymph vessels on the palm form a plexus that is drained by vessels that ascend in front of the forearm or pass around the medial and lateral borders to join vessels on the dorsum of the hand.

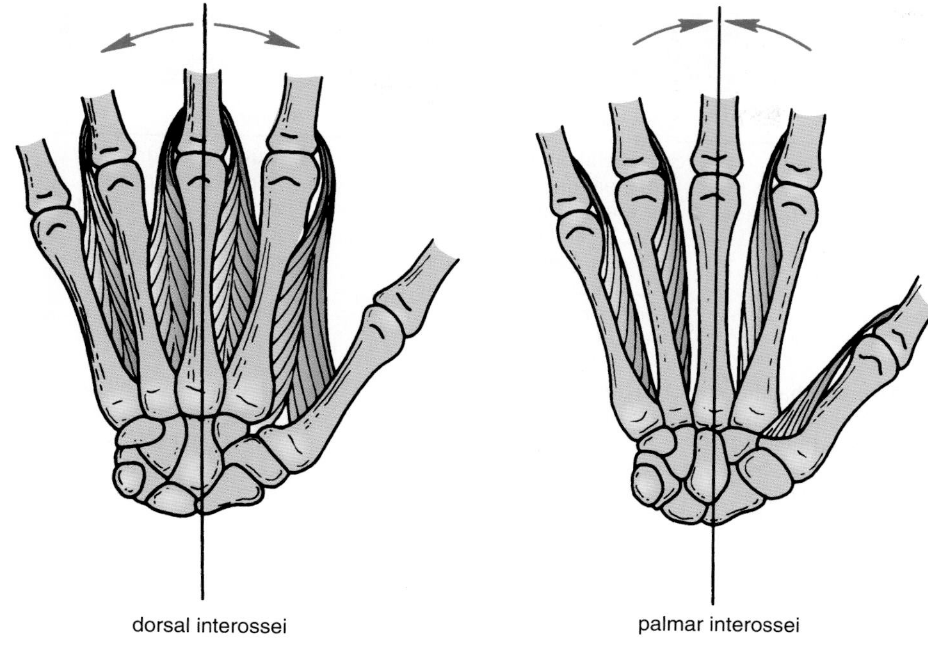

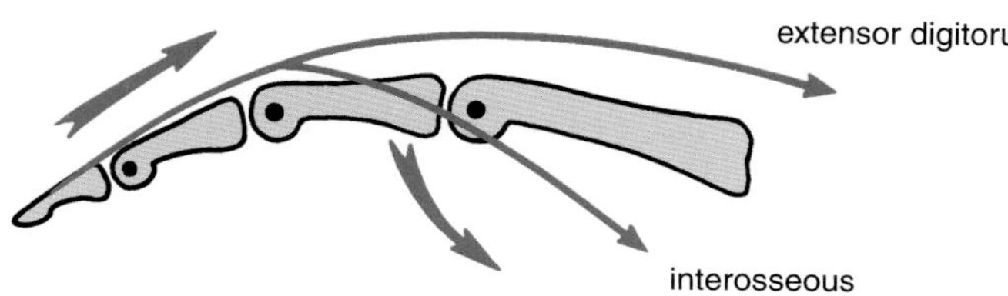

Figure 9-69 Origins and insertion of the palmar and the dorsal interossei muscles. The actions of these muscles are also shown.

The lymph from the medial side of the hand ascends in vessels that accompany the basilic vein; they drain into the **supratrochlear nodes** and then ascend to drain into the **lateral axillary nodes.** The lymph from the lateral side of the hand ascends in vessels that accompany the cephalic vein; they drain into the **infraclavicular nodes,** and some drain into the **lateral axillary nodes.**

Nerves of the Palm

Median Nerve

The median nerve enters the palm by passing **behind** the flexor retinaculum and through the **carpal tunnel.** It immediately divides into lateral and medial branches.

The **muscular branch** takes a recurrent course around the lower border of the flexor retinaculum and lies about one fingerbreadth distal to the tubercle of the scaphoid; it supplies the muscles of the thenar eminence (the abductor pollicis brevis, the flexor pollicis brevis, and the opponens pollicis) and the first lumbrical muscle.

The **cutaneous branches** supply the palmar aspect of the lateral three and a half fingers and the distal half of the dorsal aspect of each finger. One of these branches also supplies the second lumbrical muscle.

Note also that the **palmar cutaneous branch** of the median nerve given off in the front of the forearm (Fig. 9-55) crosses **anterior** to the flexor retinaculum and supplies the skin over the lateral part of the palm (Fig. 9-38).

Ulnar Nerve

The ulnar nerve enters the palm **anterior** to the flexor retinaculum alongside the lateral border of the pisiform bone (Figs. 9-55 and 9-62). As it crosses the retinaculum it divides into a superficial and a deep terminal branch.

Superficial Branch of the Ulnar Nerve

The superficial branch of the ulnar nerve descends into the palm, lying in the subcutaneous tissue between the pisiform bone and the hook of the hamate (Figs. 9-55 and 9-62). The ulnar artery is on its lateral side. Here, the nerve and artery may lie in a fibro-osseous tunnel, the **tunnel of Guyon,** created by fibrous tissue derived from the superficial part of the flexor retinaculum. The nerve may be compressed at this site, giving rise to clinical signs and symptoms.

The nerve gives off the following branches: a **muscular branch** to the palmaris brevis and **cutaneous branches** to the palmar aspect of the medial side of the little finger and the adjacent sides of the little and ring fingers (Fig. 9-62). It also supplies the distal half of the dorsal aspect of each finger.

Deep Branch of thIe Ulnar Nerve

The deep branch of the ulnar nerve runs backward between the abductor digiti minimi and the flexor digiti minimi (Fig. 9-67). It pierces the opponens digiti minimi, winds around the lower border of the hook of the hamate, and passes laterally within the concavity of the deep palmar arch. The nerve lies

Table 9-9 Small Muscles of the Hand

Muscle	Origin	Insertion	Nerve Supply	Nerve Roots[a]	Action
Palmaris brevis	Flexor retinaculum, palmar aponeurosis	Skin of palm	Superficial branch of ulnar nerve	C8; **T1**	Corrugates skin to improve grip of palm
Lumbricals (4)	Tendons of flexor digitorum profundus	Extensor expansion of medial four fingers	First and second, (i.e., lateral two) median nerve; third and fourth deep branch of ulnar nerve	C8; **T1**	Flex metacarpophalangeal joints and extend interphalangeal joints of fingers except thumb
Interossei (8)					
Palmar (4)	First arises from base of first metacarpal; remaining three from anterior surface of shafts of second, fourth, and fifth metacarpals	Proximal phalanges of thumb and index, ring, and little fingers and dorsal extensor expansion of each finger (Fig. 9-69)	Deep branch of ulnar nerve	C8; **T1**	Palmar interossei adduct fingers toward center of third finger
Dorsal (4)	Contiguous sides of shafts of metacarpal bones	Proximal phalanges of index, middle, and ring fingers and dorsal extensor expansion (Fig. 9-69)	Deep branch of ulnar nerve	C8; **T1**	Dorsal interossei abduct fingers from center of third finger; both palmar and dorsal flex metacarpophalangeal joints and extend interphalangeal joints
Short Muscles of Thumb					
Abductor pollicis brevis	Scaphoid, trapezium, flexor retinaculum	Base of proximal phalanx of thumb	Median nerve	**C8**; T1	Abduction of thumb
Flexor pollicis brevis	Flexor retinaculum	Base of proximal phalanx of thumb	Median nerve	C8; T1	Flexes metacarpophalangeal joint of thumb
Opponens pollicis	Flexor retinaculum	Shaft of metacarpal bone of thumb	Median nerve	**C8**; T1	Pulls thumb medially and forward across palm
Adductor pollicis	Oblique head; second and third metacarpal bones; transverse head; third metacarpal bone	Base of proximal phalanx of thumb	Deep branch of ulnar nerve	C8; **T1**	Adduction of thumb
Short Muscles of Little Finger					
Abductor digiti minimi	Pisiform bone	Base of proximal phalanx of little finger	Deep branch of ulnar nerve	C8; **T1**	Abducts little finger
Flexor digiti minimi	Flexor retinaculum	Base of proximal phalanx of little finger	Deep branch of ulnar nerve	C8; **T1**	Flexes little finger
Opponens digiti minimi	Flexor retinaculum	Medial border fifth metacarpal bone	Deep branch of ulnar nerve	C8; **T1**	Pulls fifth metacarpal forward as in cupping the palm

[a] The predominant nerve root supply is indicated by boldface type.

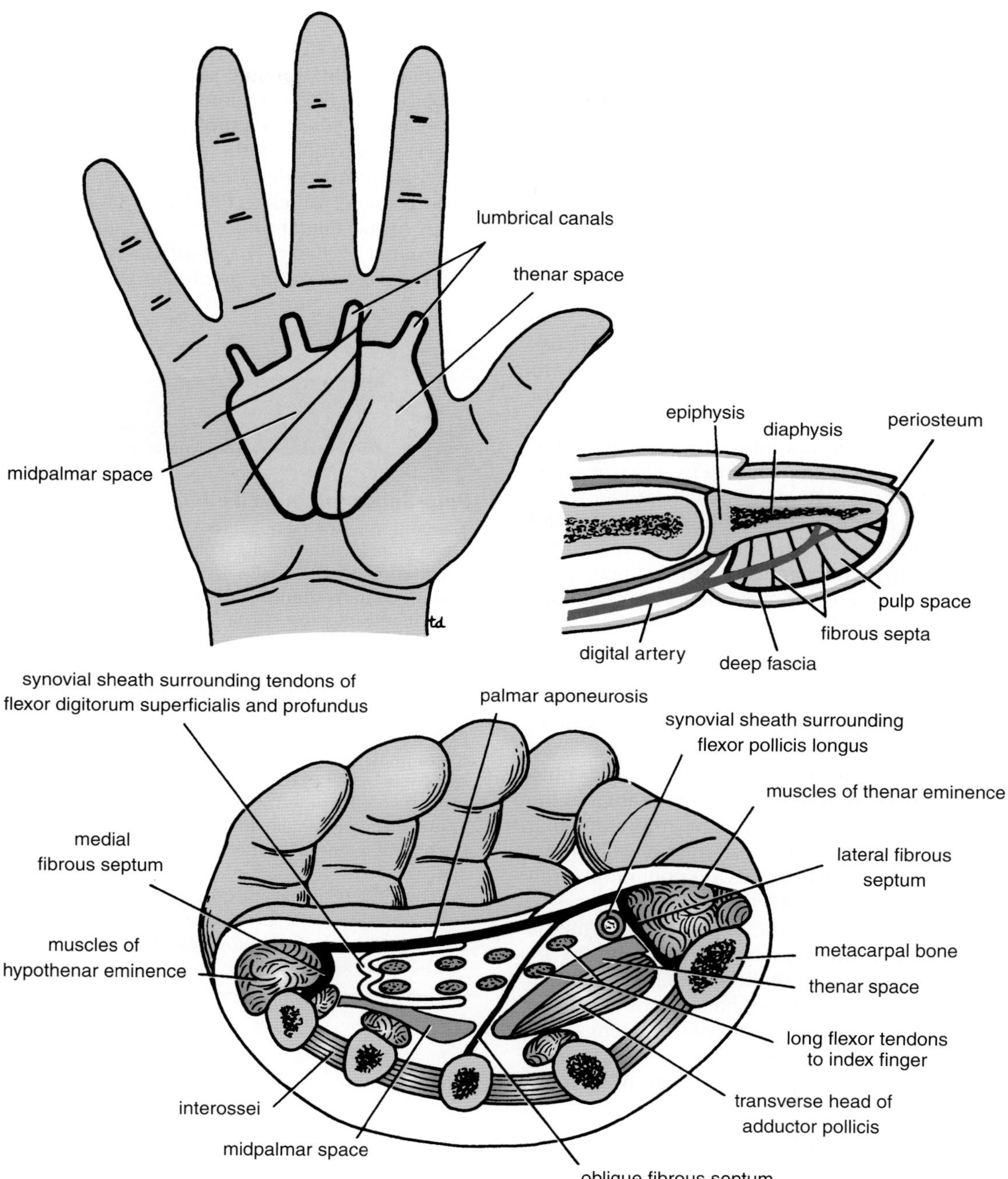

Figure 9-70 Palmar and pulp fascial spaces.

behind the long flexor tendons and in front of the metacarpal bones and interosseous muscles. It gives off **muscular branches** to the three muscles of the hypothenar eminence, namely, the abductor digiti minimi, the flexor digiti minimi, and the opponens digiti minimi. It supplies all the palmar and dorsal interossei, the third and fourth lumbrical muscles, and both heads of the adductor pollicis muscle.

The **palmar cutaneous branch** of the ulnar nerve given off in the front of the forearm crosses **anterior** to the flexor retinaculum (Fig. 9-54) and supplies the skin over the medial part of the palm (Fig. 9-38).

Fascial Spaces of the Palm

Normally, the fascial spaces of the palm are potential spaces filled with loose connective tissue. Their boundaries are important clinically because they may limit the spread of infection in the palm.

The triangular palmar aponeurosis fans out from the lower border of the flexor retinaculum (Fig. 9-55). From its medial border a fibrous septum passes backward and is attached to the anterior border of the fifth metacarpal bone (Fig. 9-70). Medial to this septum is a fascial compartment containing the three hypothenar muscles; this compartment is unimportant clinically. From the lateral border of the palmar aponeurosis, a second fibrous septum passes obliquely backward to the anterior border of the third metacarpal bone (Fig. 9-70). Usually, the septum passes between the long flexor tendons of the index and middle fingers. This second septum divides the palm into the **thenar space,** which lies lateral to the septum (and must not be confused with the fascial compartment containing the thenar muscles), and the **midpalmar space,** which lies medial to the septum (Fig. 9-70). Proximally, the thenar and midpalmar spaces are closed off from the forearm by the walls of the carpal tunnel. Distally, the two spaces are continuous with the appropriate lumbrical canals (Fig. 9-70).

The **thenar space** contains the first lumbrical muscle and lies posterior to the long flexor tendons to the index finger and in front of the adductor pollicis muscle (Fig. 9-70).

The **midpalmar space** contains the second, third, and fourth lumbrical muscles and lies posterior to the long flexor tendons to the middle, ring, and little fingers. It lies in front of the interossei and the third, fourth, and fifth metacarpal bones (Fig. 9-70).

The **lumbrical canal** is a potential space surrounding the tendon of each lumbrical muscle and is normally filled with connective tissue. Proximally, it is continuous with one of the palmar spaces.

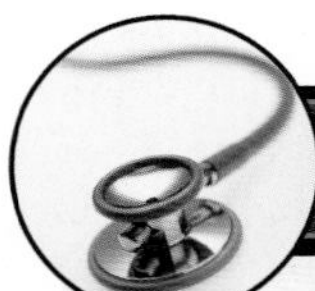

CLINICAL NOTES

Fascial Spaces of the Palm and Infection

The fascial spaces of the palm (Fig. 9-70) are clinically important because they can become infected and distended with pus as a result of the spread of infection in acute suppurative tenosynovitis; rarely, they can become infected after penetrating wounds such as falling on a dirty nail.

Pulp Space of the Fingers

The deep fascia of the pulp of each finger fuses with the periosteum of the terminal phalanx just distal to the insertion of the long flexor tendons and closes off a fascial compartment known as the pulp space (Fig. 9-70). Each pulp space is subdivided by the presence of numerous septa, which pass from the deep fascia to the periosteum. Through the pulp space, which is filled with fat, runs the terminal branch of the digital artery that supplies the diaphysis of the terminal phalanx. The epiphysis of the distal phalanx receives its blood supply proximal to the pulp space.

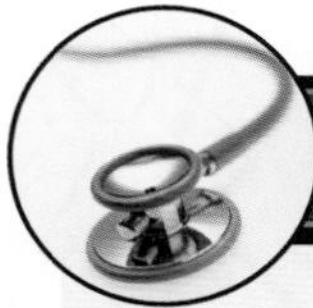

CLINICAL NOTES

Pulp-Space Infection (Felon)

The pulp space of the fingers is a closed fascial compartment situated in front of the terminal phalanx of each finger (Fig. 9-70). Infection of such a space is common and serious, occurring most often in the thumb and index finger. Bacteria are usually introduced into the space by pinpricks or sewing needles. Because each space is subdivided into numerous smaller compartments by fibrous septa, it is easily understood that the accumulation of inflammatory exudate within these compartments causes the pressure in the pulp space to quickly rise. If the infection is left without decompression, infection of the terminal phalanx can occur. In children, the blood supply to the diaphysis of the phalanx passes through the pulp space, and pressure on the blood vessels could result in necrosis of the diaphysis. The proximally located epiphysis of this bone is saved because it receives its arterial supply just proximal to the pulp space.

The close relationship of the proximal end of the pulp space to the digital synovial sheath accounts for the involvement of the sheath in the infectious process when the pulp-space infection has been neglected.

The Dorsum of the Hand

Skin

The skin on the dorsum of the hand is thin, hairy, and freely mobile on the underlying tendons and bones.

The **sensory nerve supply** to the skin on the dorsum of the hand is derived from the superficial branch of the radial nerve and the posterior cutaneous branch of the ulnar nerve.

The **superficial branch of the radial nerve** winds around the radius deep to the brachioradialis tendon, descends over the extensor retinaculum, and supplies the lateral two thirds of the dorsum of the hand (Fig. 9-38). It divides into several dorsal digital nerves that supply the thumb, the index and middle fingers, and the lateral side of the ring finger. The area of skin on the back of the hand and fingers supplied by the radial nerve is subject to variation. Frequently, a dorsal digital nerve, a branch of the ulnar nerve, also supplies the lateral side of the ring finger.

The **posterior cutaneous branch of the ulnar nerve** winds around the ulna deep to the flexor carpi ulnaris tendon, descends over the extensor retinaculum, and supplies the medial third of the dorsum of the hand (Fig. 9-38). It divides into several dorsal digital nerves that supply the medial side of the ring and the sides of the little fingers.

The dorsal digital branches of the radial and ulnar nerves do not extend far beyond the proximal phalanx. The remainder of the dorsum of each finger receives its nerve supply from palmar digital nerves.

Dorsal Venous Arch (or Network)

The dorsal venous arch lies in the subcutaneous tissue proximal to the metacarpophalangeal joints and drains on the lateral side into the cephalic vein and, on the medial side, into the basilic vein (Fig. 9-100). The greater part of the blood from the whole hand drains into the arch, which receives digital veins and freely communicates with the deep veins of the palm through the interosseous spaces.

Insertion of the Long Extensor Tendons

The four tendons of the extensor digitorum emerge from under the extensor retinaculum and fan out over the dorsum of the hand (Figs. 9-56 and 9-57). The tendons are embedded in the deep fascia, and together they form the roof of a **subfascial space,** which occupies the whole width of the dorsum of the hand. Strong oblique fibrous bands connect the tendons to the little, ring, and middle fingers, proximal to the heads of the metacarpal bones. The tendon to the index finger is joined on its medial side by the tendon of the extensor indicis, and the tendon to the little finger is joined on its medial side by the two tendons of the extensor digiti minimi (Fig. 9-55).

On the posterior surface of each finger, the extensor tendon joins the fascial expansion called the **extensor expansion** (Figs. 9-56 and 9-57). Near the proximal interphalangeal joint, the extensor expansion splits into three parts: a **central part,** which is inserted into the base of the middle phalanx, and **two lateral parts,** which converge to be inserted into the base of the distal phalanx (Fig. 9-63).

The dorsal extensor expansion receives the tendon of insertion of the corresponding interosseous muscle on each side and farther distally receives the tendon of the lumbrical muscle on the lateral side (Fig. 9-63).

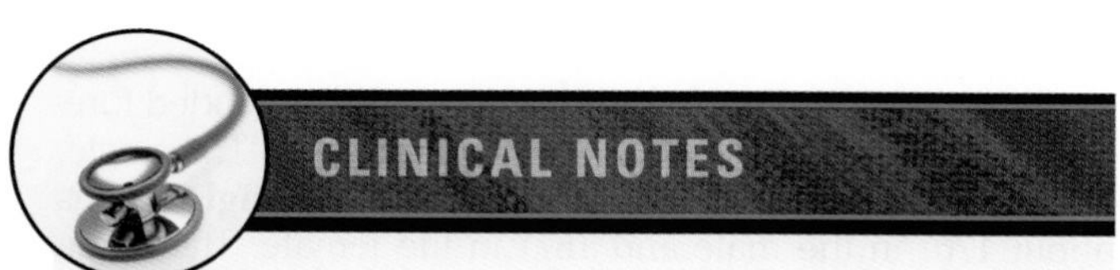

Mallet Finger

Avulsion of the insertion of one of the extensor tendons into the distal phalanges can occur if the distal phalanx is forcibly flexed when the extensor tendon is taut. The last 20° of active extension is lost, resulting in a condition known as mallet finger (Fig. 9-71).

(continues)

Clinical Notes, *continued*

Boutonnière Deformity

Avulsion of the central slip of the extensor tendon proximal to its insertion into the base of the middle phalanx results in a characteristic deformity (Fig. 9-71C). The deformity results from flexing of the proximal interphalangeal joint and hyperextension of the distal interphalangeal joint. This injury can result from direct end-on trauma to the finger, direct trauma over the back of the proximal interphalangeal joint, or laceration of the dorsum of the finger.

The Radial Artery on the Dorsum of the Hand

The radial artery winds around the lateral margin of the wrist joint, beneath the tendons of the abductor pollicis longus and extensor pollicis brevis, and lies on the lateral ligament of the joint (Fig. 9-65). On reaching the dorsum of the hand, the artery descends beneath the tendon of the extensor pollicis longus to reach the interval between the two heads of the first dorsal interosseous muscle; here the artery turns forward to enter the palm of the hand (see page 504).

Branches of the radial artery on the dorsum of the hand take part in the anastomosis around the wrist joint. Dorsal digital arteries pass to the thumb and index finger (Fig. 9-65).

Joints of the Upper Limb

The sternoclavicular joint, the acromioclavicular joint, and the shoulder joint are fully described on pages 459 and 460.

Elbow Joint

- **Articulation:** This occurs between the trochlea and capitulum of the humerus and the trochlear notch of the ulna and the head of the radius (Fig. 9-72). The articular surfaces are covered with hyaline cartilage.
- **Type:** Synovial hinge joint
- **Capsule: Anteriorly** it is attached above to the humerus along the upper margins of the coronoid and radial fossae and to the front of the medial and lateral epicondyles and below to the margin of the coronoid process of the ulna and to the anular ligament, which surrounds the head of the radius. **Posteriorly** it is attached above to the margins of the olecranon fossa of the humerus and below to the upper margin and sides of the olecranon process of the ulna and to the anular ligament.
- **Ligaments:** The **lateral ligament** (Fig. 9-72) is triangular and is attached by its apex to the lateral epicondyle of the humerus and by its base to the upper margin of the anular ligament. The **medial ligament** is also triangular and consists principally of three strong bands: the anterior band, which passes from the medial epicondyle of the humerus to the medial margin of the coronoid process; the posterior band, which passes from the medial epicondyle of the humerus to the medial side of the olecranon; and the transverse band, which passes between the ulnar attachments of the two preceding bands.
- **Synovial membrane:** This lines the capsule and covers fatty pads in the floors of the coronoid, radial, and ole-

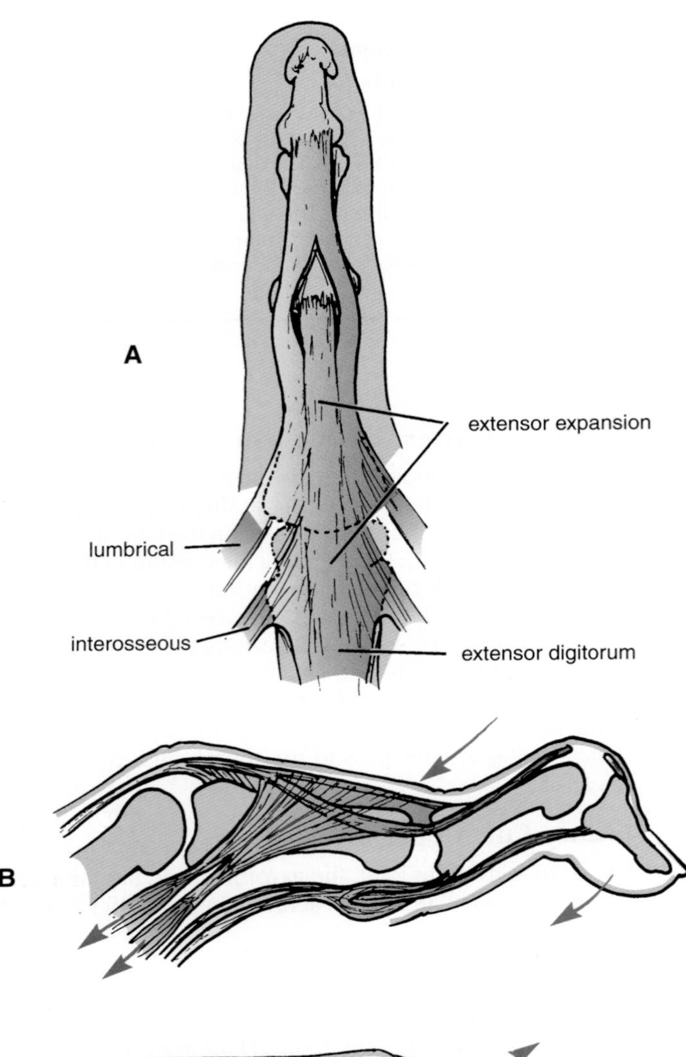

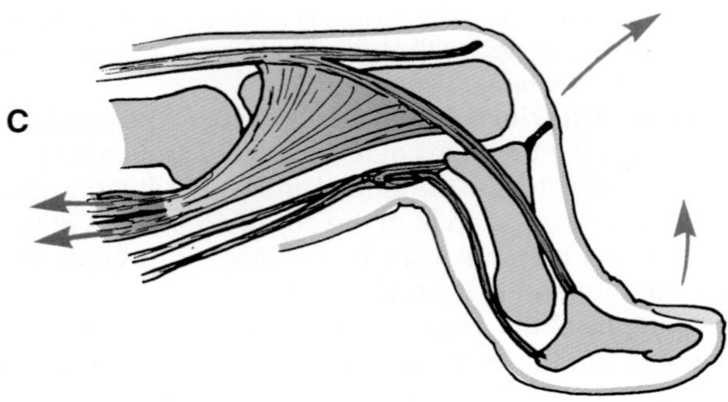

Figure 9-71 **A.** Posterior view of normal dorsal extensor expansion. The extensor expansion near the proximal interphalangeal joint splits into three parts: a central part, which is inserted into the base of the middle phalanx, and two lateral parts, which converge to be inserted into the base of the distal phalanx. **B.** Mallet or baseball finger. The insertion of the extensor expansion into the base of the distal phalanx ruptured; sometimes a flake of bone on the base of the phalanx is pulled off. **C.** Boutonnière deformity. The insertion of the extensor expansion into the base of the middle phalanx is ruptured. The arrows indicate the direction of the pull of the muscles and the deformity.

cranon fossae; it is continuous below with the synovial membrane of the proximal radioulnar joint.

- **Nerve supply:** Branches from the median, ulnar, musculocutaneous, and radial nerves

Movements

The elbow joint is capable of flexion and extension. **Flexion** is limited by the anterior surfaces of the forearm and arm coming into contact. **Extension** is checked by the tension of the anterior ligament and the brachialis muscle. Flexion is performed by the brachialis, biceps brachii, brachioradialis, and pronator teres muscles. Extension is performed by the triceps and anconeus muscles.

It should be noted that the long axis of the extended forearm lies at an angle to the long axis of the arm. This angle, which opens laterally, is called the **carrying angle** and is about 170° in the male and 167° in the female. The angle disappears when the elbow joint is fully flexed.

Important Relations

- **Anteriorly:** The brachialis, the tendon of the biceps, the median nerve, and the brachial artery
- **Posteriorly:** The triceps muscle, a small bursa intervening
- **Medially:** The **ulnar nerve passes behind the medial epicondyle and crosses the medial ligament of the joint.**
- **Laterally:** The common extensor tendon and the supinator.

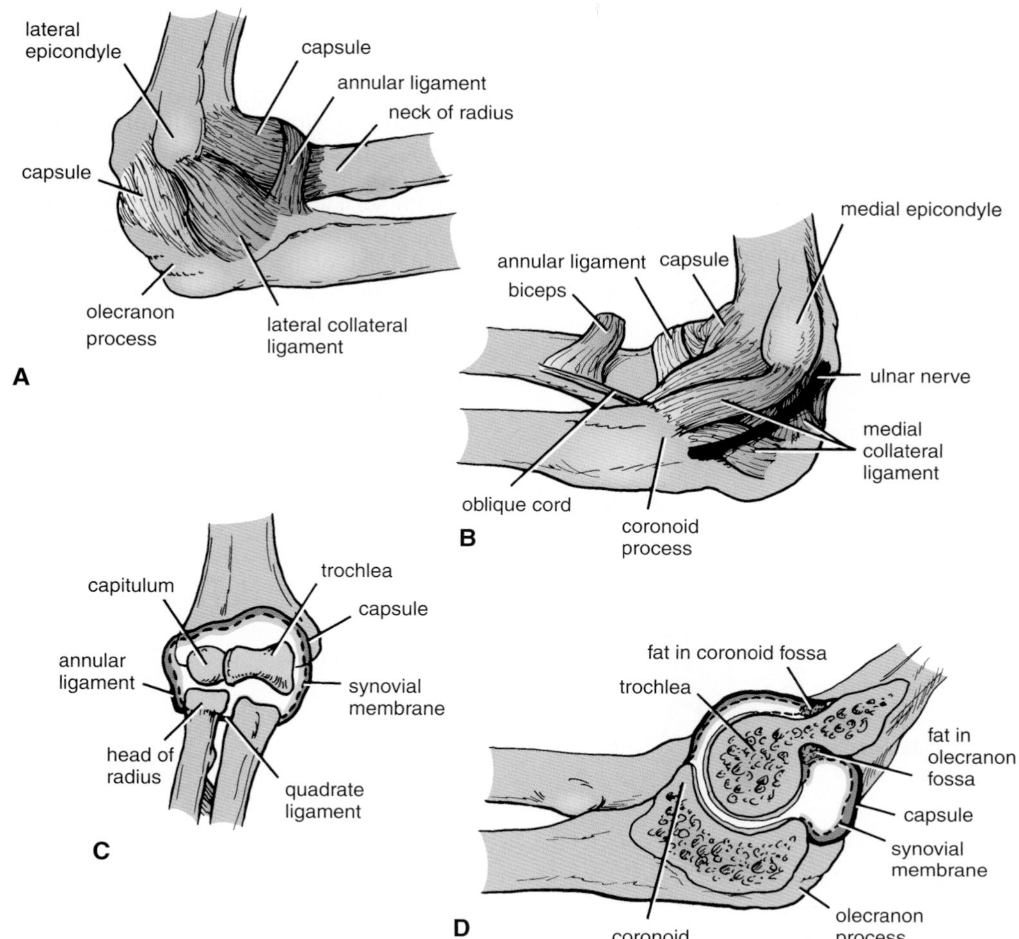

Figure 9-72 Right elbow joint. **A.** Lateral view. **B.** Medial view. **C.** Anterior view of the interior of the joint. **D.** Sagittal section.

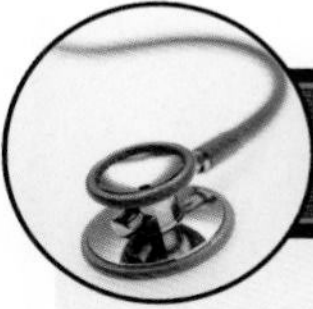

CLINICAL NOTES

Stability of Elbow Joint

The elbow joint is stable because of the wrench-shaped articular surface of the olecranon and the pulley-shaped trochlea of the humerus; it also has strong medial and lateral ligaments. When examining the elbow joint, the physician must remember the normal relations of the bony points. In extension, the medial and lateral epicondyles and the top of the olecranon process are in a straight line; in flexion, the bony points form the boundaries of an equilateral triangle.

Dislocations of the Elbow Joint

Elbow dislocations are common, and most are posterior. Posterior dislocation usually follows falling on the outstretched hand. Posterior dislocations of the joint are common in children because the parts of the bones that stabilize the joint are incompletely developed. Avulsion of the epiphysis of the medial epicondyle is also common in childhood because then the medial ligament is much stronger than the bond of union between the epiphysis and the diaphysis.

Arthrocentesis of the Elbow Joint

The anterior and posterior walls of the capsule are weak, and when the joint is distended with fluid, the posterior aspect of the joint becomes swollen. Aspiration of joint fluid can easily be performed through the back of the joint on either side of the olecranon process.

Damage to the Ulnar Nerve With Elbow Joint Injuries

The close relationship of the ulnar nerve to the medial side of the joint often results in its becoming damaged in dislocations of the joint or in fracture dislocations in this region. The nerve lesion can occur at the time of injury or weeks, months, or years later. The nerve can be involved in scar tissue formation or can become stretched owing to lateral deviation of the forearm in a badly reduced supracondylar fracture of the humerus. During movements of the elbow joint, the continued friction between the medial epicondyle and the stretched ulnar nerve eventually results in ulnar palsy.

Radiology of the Elbow Region after Injury

In examining lateral radiographs of the elbow region, it is important to remember that the lower end of the humerus is normally angulated forward 45° on the shaft; when examining a patient, the physician should see that the medial epicondyle, in the anatomic position, is directed medially and posteriorly and faces in the same direction as the head of the humerus.

Proximal Radioulnar Joint

- **Articulation:** Between the circumference of the head of the radius and the anular ligament and the radial notch on the ulna (Figs. 9-72 and 9-73)
- **Type:** Synovial pivot joint
- **Capsule:** The capsule encloses the joint and is continuous with that of the elbow joint.
- **Ligament:** The **anular ligament** is attached to the anterior and posterior margins of the radial notch on the ulna and forms a collar around the head of the radius (Fig. 9-73). It is continuous above with the capsule of the elbow joint. It is not attached to the radius.
- **Synovial membrane:** This is continuous above with that of the elbow joint. Below it is attached to the inferior margin of the articular surface of the radius and the lower margin of the radial notch of the ulna.
- **Nerve supply:** Branches of the median, ulnar, musculocutaneous, and radial nerves

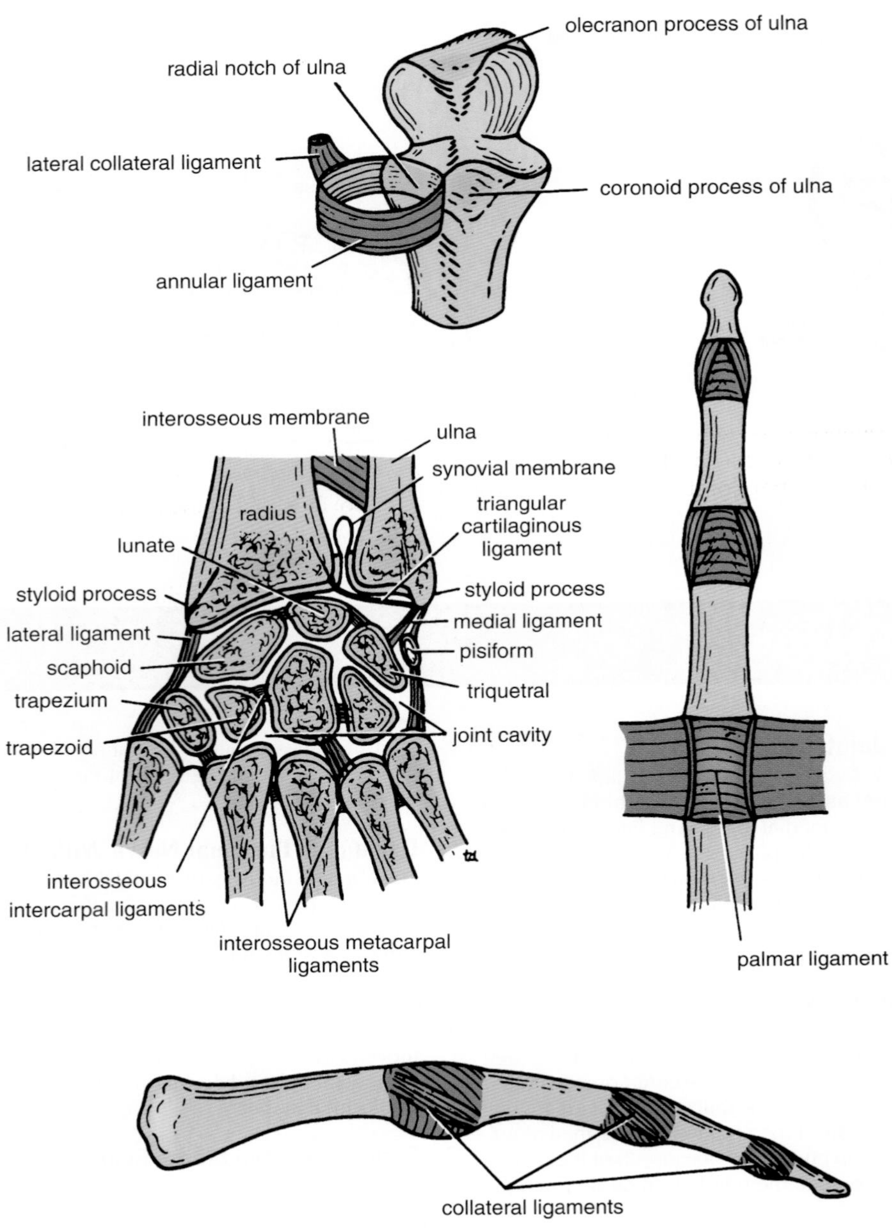

Figure 9-73 Ligaments of the proximal and distal radioulnar joints, wrist joint, carpal joints, and joints of the fingers.

Movements

Pronation and supination of the forearm (see below)

Important Relations

- **Anteriorly:** Supinator muscle and the radial nerve
- **Posteriorly:** Supinator muscle and the common extensor tendon

Distal Radioulnar Joint

- **Articulation:** Between the rounded head of the ulna and the ulnar notch on the radius (Fig. 9-73)
- **Type:** Synovial pivot joint
- **Capsule:** The capsule encloses the joint but is deficient superiorly.
- **Ligaments:** Weak **anterior** and **posterior** ligaments strengthen the capsule.
- **Articular disc:** This is triangular and composed of fibrocartilage. It is attached by its apex to the lateral side of the base of the styloid process of the ulna and by its base to the lower border of the ulnar notch of the radius (Figs. 9-73 and 9-74). It shuts off the distal radioulnar joint from the wrist and strongly unites the radius to the ulna.
- **Synovial membrane:** This lines the capsule passing from the edge of one articular surface to that of the other.
- **Nerve supply:** Anterior interosseous nerve and the deep branch of the radial nerve

Movements

The movements of pronation and supination of the forearm involve a rotary movement around a vertical axis at the proximal and distal radioulnar joints. The axis passes through the head of the radius above and the attachment of the apex of the triangular articular disc below.

In the movement of pronation, the head of the radius rotates within the anular ligament, whereas the distal end of the radius with the hand moves bodily forward, the ulnar notch of the radius moving around the circumference of the head of the ulna (Fig. 9-75). In addition, the distal end of the ulna moves laterally so that the hand remains in line with the upper limb and is not displaced medially. This movement of the ulna is important when using an instrument such as a screwdriver because it prevents side-to-side movement of the hand during the repetitive movements of supination and pronation.

The movement of pronation results in the hand's rotating medially in such a manner that the palm comes to face posteriorly and the thumb lies on the medial side. The movement of supination is a reversal of this process so that the hand returns to the anatomic position and the palm faces anteriorly.

Pronation is performed by the pronator teres and the pronator quadratus.

Supination is performed by the biceps brachii and the supinator. Supination is the more powerful of the two movements because of the strength of the biceps muscle. Because supination is the more powerful movement, screw threads and the spiral of corkscrews are made so that the screw and corkscrews are driven inward by the movement of supination in right-handed people.

Important Relations

- **Anteriorly:** The tendons of flexor digitorum profundus
- **Posteriorly:** The tendon of extensor digiti minimi

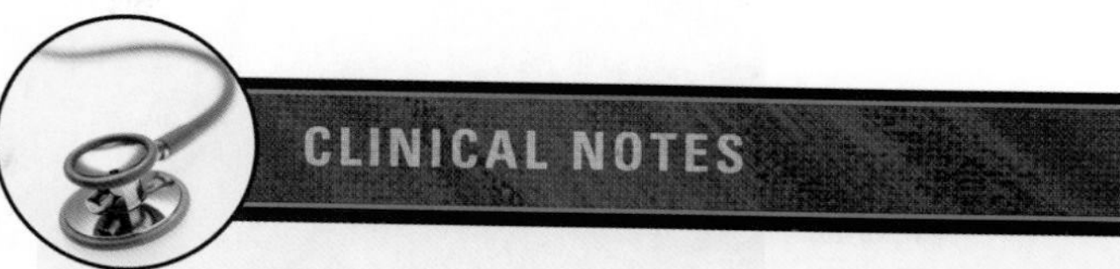

Radioulnar Joint Disease

The proximal radioulnar joint communicates with the elbow joint, whereas the distal radioulnar joint does not communicate with the wrist joint. In practical terms, this means that infection of the elbow joint invariably involves the proximal radioulnar joint. The strength of the proximal radioulnar joint depends on the integrity of the strong anular ligament. Rupture of this ligament occurs in cases of anterior dislocation of the head of the radius on the capitulum of the humerus. In young children, in whom the head of the radius is still small and undeveloped, a sudden jerk on the arm can pull the radial head down through the anular ligament.

Wrist Joint (Radiocarpal Joint)

- **Articulation:** Between the distal end of the radius and the articular disc above and the scaphoid, lunate, and triquetral bones below (Figs. 9-73 and 9-74). The proximal articular surface forms an ellipsoid concave surface, which is adapted to the distal ellipsoid convex surface.
- **Type:** Synovial ellipsoid joint
- **Capsule:** The capsule encloses the joint and is attached above to the distal ends of the radius and ulna and below to the proximal row of carpal bones.
- **Ligaments: Anterior** and **posterior ligaments** strengthen the capsule. The **medial ligament** is attached to the styloid process of the ulna and to the triquetral bone (Figs. 9-73 and 9-74). The **lateral ligament** is attached to the styloid process of the radius and to the scaphoid bone (Figs. 9-73 and 9-74).
- **Synovial membrane:** This lines the capsule and is attached to the margins of the articular surfaces. The joint cavity does not communicate with that of the distal radioulnar joint or with the joint cavities of the intercarpal joints.
- **Nerve supply:** Anterior interosseous nerve and the deep branch of the radial nerve

Movements

The following movements are possible: flexion, extension, abduction, adduction, and circumduction. Rotation is **not** possible because the articular surfaces are ellipsoid shaped. The lack of rotation is compensated for by the movements of pronation and supination of the forearm.

Flexion is performed by the flexor carpi radialis, the flexor carpi ulnaris, and the palmaris longus. These muscles are assisted by the flexor digitorum superficialis, the flexor digitorum profundus, and the flexor pollicis longus.

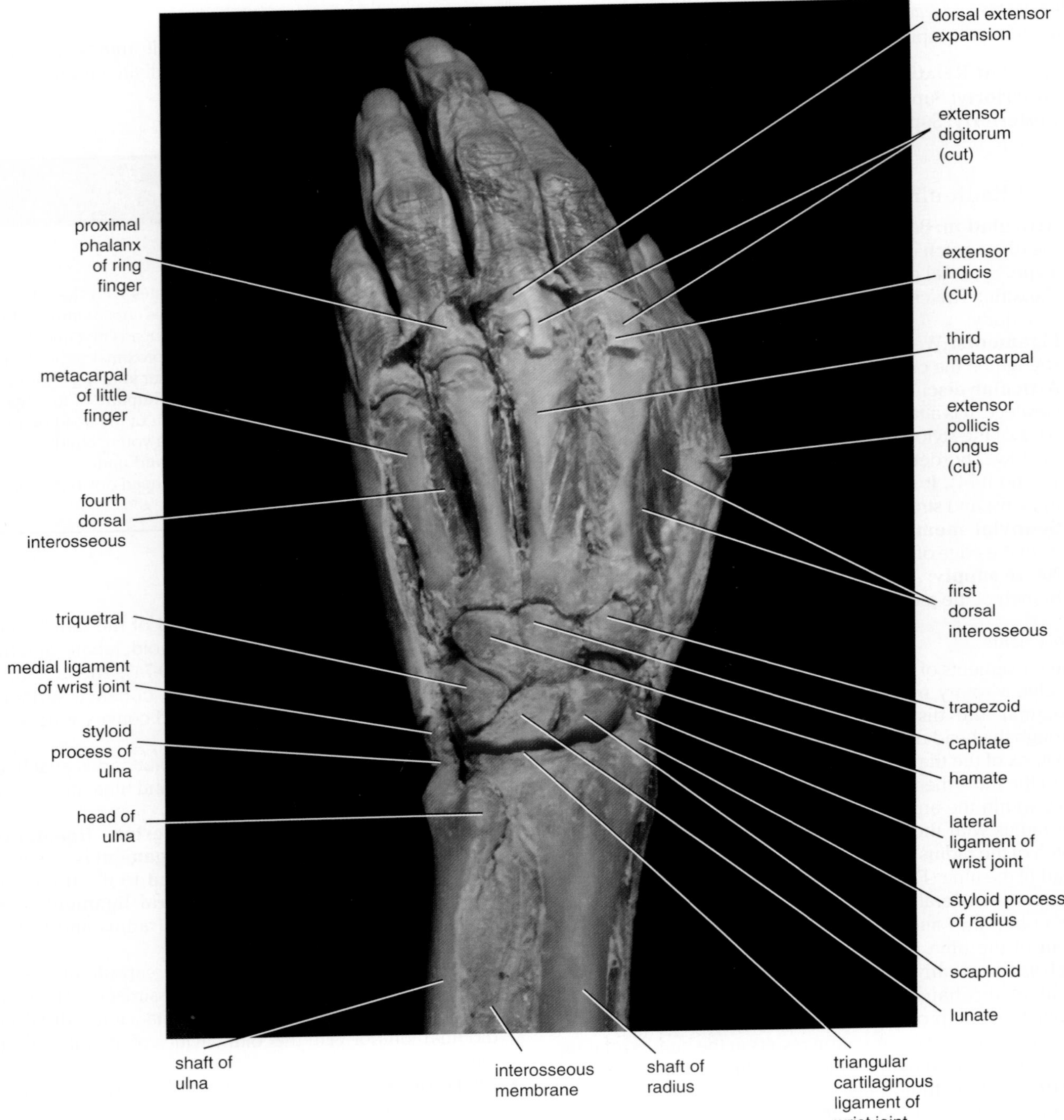

Figure 9-74 Dissection of the dorsal surface of the left hand and distal end of the forearm. Note the carpal bones and the intercarpal joints; note also the wrist (radiocarpal) joint.

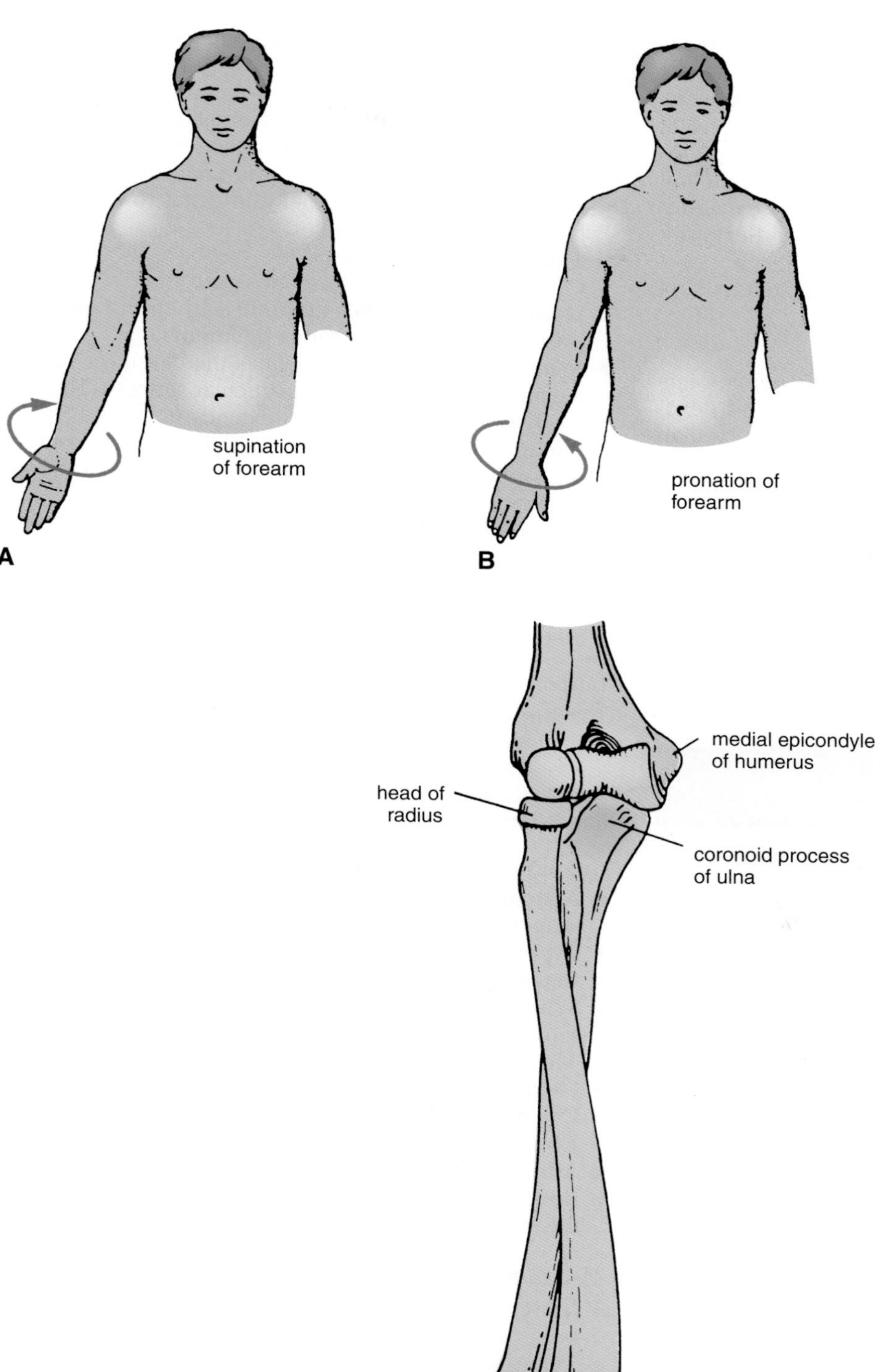

Figure 9-75 Movements of supination (**A**) and pronation (**B**) of the forearm that take place at the proximal and distal radioulnar joints. **C.** Relative positions of the radius and ulna when the forearm is fully pronated.

Extension is performed by the extensor carpi radialis longus, the extensor carpi radialis brevis, and the extensor carpi ulnaris. These muscles are assisted by the extensor digitorum, the extensor indicis, the extensor digiti minimi, and the extensor pollicis longus.

Abduction is performed by the flexor carpi radialis and the extensor carpi radialis longus and brevis. These muscles are assisted by the abductor pollicis longus and extensor pollicis longus and brevis.

Adduction is performed by the flexor and extensor carpi ulnaris.

Important Relations

- **Anteriorly:** The tendons of the flexor digitorum profundus and superficialis, the flexor pollicis longus, the flexor carpi radialis, the flexor carpi ulnaris, and the median and ulnar nerves
- **Posteriorly:** The tendons of the extensor carpi ulnaris, the extensor digiti minimi, the extensor digitorum, the extensor indicis, the extensor carpi radialis longus and brevis, the extensor pollicis longus and brevis, and the abductor pollicis longus
- **Medially:** The posterior cutaneous branch of the ulnar nerve
- **Laterally:** The radial artery

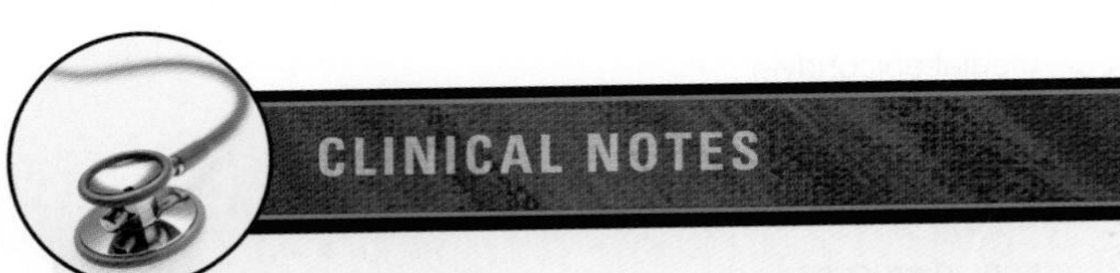

Wrist Joint Injuries

The wrist joint is essentially a synovial joint between the distal end of the radius and the proximal row of carpal bones. The head of the ulna is separated from the carpal bones by the strong triangular fibrocartilaginous ligament, which separates the wrist joint from the distal radioulnar joint. The joint is stabilized by the strong medial and lateral ligaments.

Because the styloid process of the radius is longer than that of the ulna, abduction of the wrist joint is less extensive than adduction. In flexion–extension movements, the hand can be flexed about 80° but extended to only about 45°. The range of flexion is increased by movement at the midcarpal joint.

A fall on the outstretched hand can strain the anterior ligament of the wrist joint, producing synovial effusion, joint pain, and limitation of movement. These symptoms and signs must not be confused with those produced by a fractured scaphoid or dislocation of the lunate bone, which are similar.

Falls on the Outstretched Hand

In falls on the outstretched hand, forces are transmitted from the scaphoid to the distal end of the radius, from the radius across the interosseous membrane to the ulna, and from the ulna to the humerus; thence, through the glenoid fossa of the scapula to the coracoclavicular ligament and the clavicle; and finally, to the sternum. If the forces are excessive, different parts of the upper limb give way under the strain. The area affected seems to be related to age. In a young child, for example, there may be a posterior displacement of the distal radial epiphysis; in the teenager the clavicle might fracture; in the young adult the scaphoid is commonly fractured; and in the elderly the distal end of the radius is fractured about 1 in. (2.5 cm) proximal to the wrist joint (Colles' fracture) (Fig. 9-50).

Joints of the Hand and Fingers

Intercarpal Joints

- **Articulation:** Between the individual bones of the proximal row of the carpus; between the individual bones of the distal row of the carpus; and finally, the midcarpal joint, between the proximal and distal rows of carpal bones (Figs. 9-73 and 9-74)
- **Type:** Synovial plane joints
- **Capsule:** The capsule surrounds each joint.
- **Ligaments:** The bones are united by strong **anterior, posterior,** and **interosseous ligaments.**
- **Synovial membrane:** This lines the capsule and is attached to the margins of the articular surfaces. The joint cavity of the midcarpal joint extends not only between the two rows of carpal bones but also upward between the individual bones forming the proximal row and downward between the bones of the distal row.
- **Nerve supply:** Anterior interosseous nerve, deep branch of the radial nerve, and deep branch of the ulnar nerve

Movements

A small amount of gliding movement is possible.

Carpometacarpal and Intermetacarpal Joints

The carpometacarpal and intermetacarpal joints are synovial plane joints possessing anterior, posterior, and interosseous ligaments. They have a common joint cavity. A small amount of gliding movement is possible (Figs. 9-73 and 9-74).

Carpometacarpal Joint of the Thumb

- **Articulation:** Between the trapezium and the saddle-shaped base of the first metacarpal bone (Fig. 9-73)
- **Type:** Synovial saddle-shaped joint
- **Capsule:** The capsule surrounds the joint.
- **Synovial membrane:** This lines the capsule and forms a separate joint cavity.

Movements The following movements are possible:

- **Flexion:** Flexor pollicis brevis and opponens pollicis
- **Extension:** Extensor pollicis longus and brevis
- **Abduction:** Abductor pollicis longus and brevis
- **Adduction:** Adductor pollicis
- **Rotation (opposition):** The thumb is rotated medially by the opponens pollicis.

Metacarpophalangeal Joints

- **Articulation:** Between the heads of the metacarpal bones and the bases of the proximal phalanges (Fig. 9-73)
- **Type:** Synovial condyloid joints
- **Capsule:** The capsule surrounds the joint.
- **Ligaments:** The **palmar ligaments** are strong and contain some fibrocartilage. They are firmly attached to the phalanx but less so to the metacarpal bone (Fig. 9-73). The palmar ligaments of the second, third, fourth, and fifth joints are united by the **deep transverse metacarpal ligaments,** which hold the heads of the metacarpal bones together. The **collateral ligaments** are cordlike bands present on each side of the joints (Fig. 9-73). Each passes downward and forward from the head of the metacarpal bone to the base of the phalanx. The

collateral ligaments are taut when the joint is in flexion and lax when the joint is in extension.

- **Synovial membrane:** This lines the capsule and is attached to the margins of the articular surfaces.

Movements

The following movements are possible:

- **Flexion:** The lumbricals and the interossei, assisted by the flexor digitorum superficialis and profundus
- **Extension:** Extensor digitorum, extensor indicis, and extensor digiti minimi
- **Abduction:** Movement away from the midline of the third finger is performed by the dorsal interossei.
- **Adduction:** Movement toward the midline of the third finger is performed by the palmar interossei. In the case of the metacarpophalangeal joint of the thumb, **flexion** is performed by the flexor pollicis longus and brevis and **extension** is performed by the extensor pollicis longus and brevis. The movements of abduction and adduction are performed at the carpometacarpal joint.

Interphalangeal Joints

Interphalangeal joints are synovial hinge joints that have a structure similar to that of the metacarpophalangeal joints (Fig. 9-73).

The Hand as a Functional Unit

The upper limb is a multijointed lever freely movable on the trunk at the shoulder joint. At the distal end of the upper limb is the important prehensile organ—the hand. Much of the importance of the hand depends on the pincer action of the thumb, which enables one to grasp objects between the thumb and index finger. The extreme mobility of the first metacarpal bone makes the thumb functionally as important as all the remaining fingers combined.

To comprehend fully the important positioning and movements of the hand described in this section, the reader is strongly advised to closely observe the movements in his or her own hand.

Position of the Hand

For the hand to be able to perform delicate movements, such as those used in the holding of small instruments in watch repairing, the forearm is placed in the semiprone position and the wrist joint is partially extended. It is interesting to note that the forearm bones are most stable in the midprone position, when the interosseous membrane is taut; in other positions of the forearm bones, the interosseous membrane is lax. With the wrist partially extended, the long flexor and extensor tendons of the fingers are working to their best mechanical advantage; at the same time, the flexors and extensors of the carpus can exert a balanced fixator action on the wrist joint, ensuring a stable base for the movements of the fingers.

The **position of rest** is the posture adopted by the hand when the fingers are at rest and the hand is relaxed (Fig. 9-76). The forearm is in the semiprone position; the wrist joint is slightly extended; the second, third, fourth, and fifth fingers are partially flexed, although the index finger is not flexed as much as the others; and the plane of the thumbnail lies at a right angle to the plane of the other fingernails.

The **position of function** is the posture adopted by the hand when it is about to grasp an object between the thumb and index finger (Fig. 9-76). The forearm is in the semiprone position, the wrist joint is partially extended (more so than in the position of rest), and the fingers are partially flexed, the index finger being flexed as much as the others. The metacarpal bone of the thumb is rotated in such a manner that the plane of the thumbnail lies parallel with that of the index finger, and the pulp of the thumb and index finger are in contact.

The following movements are described with the hand in the anatomic position.

Movements of the Thumb

Flexion is the movement of the thumb across the palm in such a manner as to maintain the plane of the thumbnail at right angles to the plane of the other fingernails (Fig. 9-76). The movement takes place between the trapezium and the first metacarpal bone, at the metacarpophalangeal and interphalangeal joints. The muscles producing the movement are the flexor pollicis longus and brevis and the opponens pollicis.

Extension is the movement of the thumb in a lateral or coronal plane away from the palm in such a manner as to maintain the plane of the thumbnail at right angles to the plane of the other fingernails (Figs. 9-76 and 9-77A). The movement takes place between the trapezium and the first metacarpal bone, at the metacarpophalangeal and interphalangeal joints. The muscles producing the movement are the extensor pollicis longus and brevis.

Abduction is the movement of the thumb in an anteroposterior plane away from the palm, the plane of the thumbnail being kept at right angles to the plane of the other nails (Figs. 9-76 and 9-78A). The movement takes place mainly between the trapezium and the first metacarpal bone; a small amount of movement takes place at the metacarpophalangeal joint. The muscles producing the movement are the abductor pollicis longus and brevis.

Adduction is the movement of the thumb in an anteroposterior plane toward the palm, the plane of the thumbnail being kept at right angles to the plane of the other fingernails (Fig. 9-76 and 9-78B). The movement takes place between the trapezium and the first metacarpal bone. The muscle producing the movement is the adductor pollicis.

Opposition is the movement of the thumb across the palm in such a manner that the anterior surface of the tip comes into contact with the anterior surface of the tip of any of the other fingers (Figs. 9-76 and 9-77C). The movement is accomplished by the medial rotation of the first metacarpal bone and the attached phalanges on the trapezium. The plane of the thumbnail comes to lie parallel with the plane of the nail of the opposed finger. The muscle producing the movement is the opponens pollicis.

Movements of the Index, Middle, Ring, and Little Fingers

Flexion is the movement forward of the finger in an anteroposterior plane. The movement takes place at the interpha-

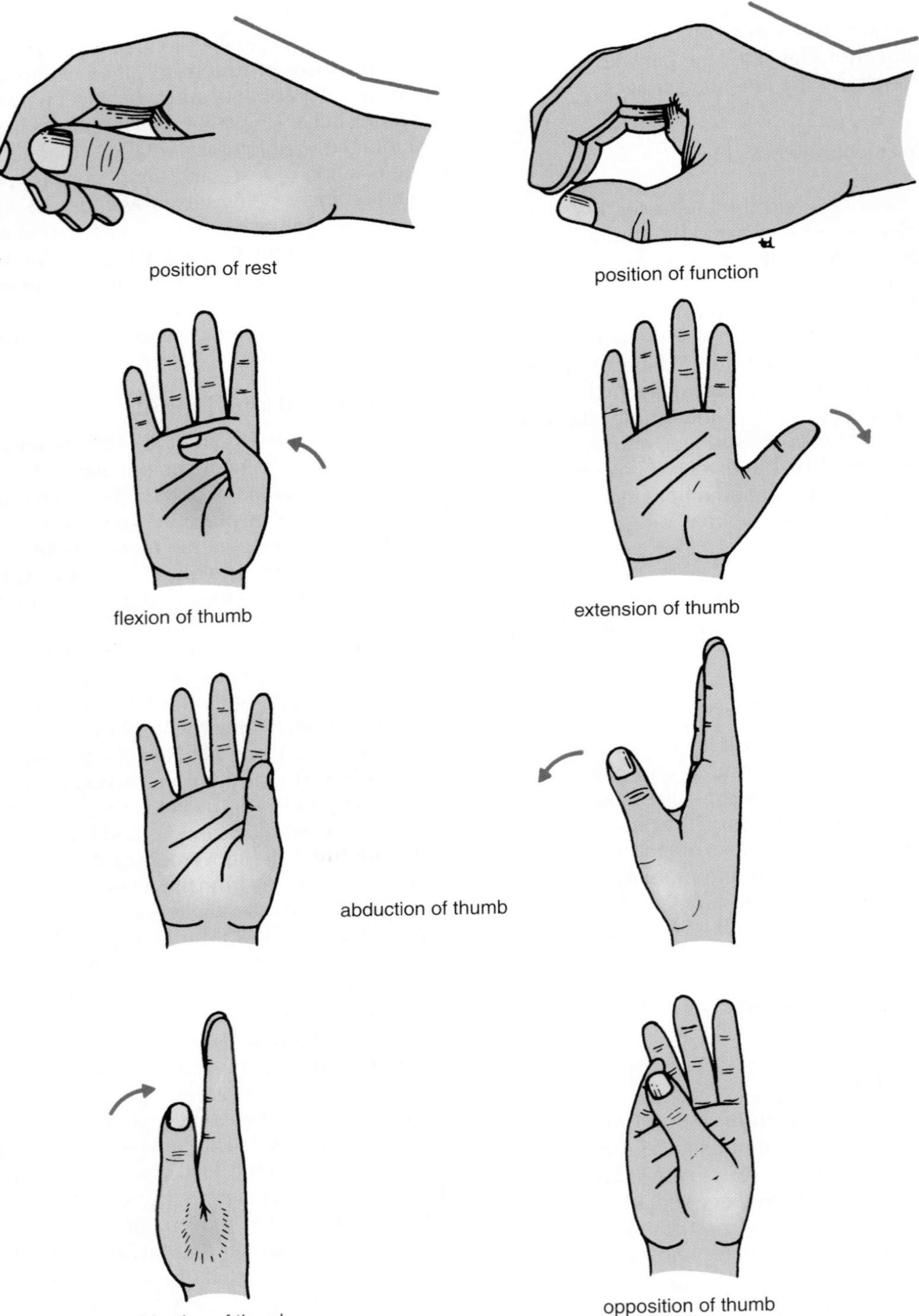

Figure 9-76 Various positions of the hand and movements of the thumb.

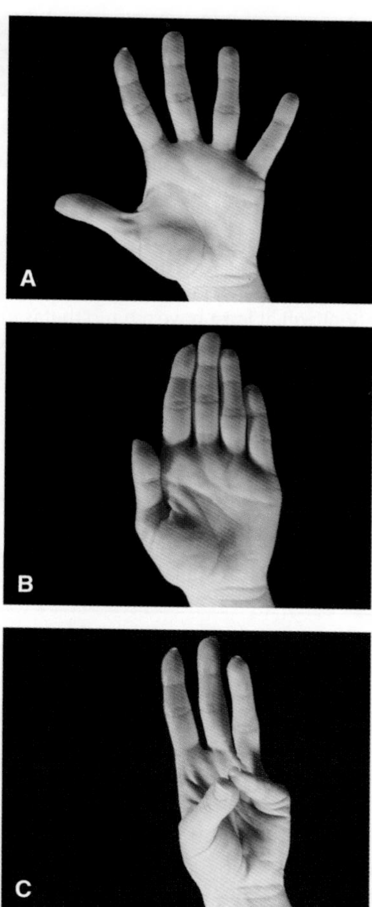

Figure 9-77 Left hand with the fingers abducted and the thumb extended (**A**), with the fingers adducted and the thumb adducted (**B**), and with the thumb in the position of opposition (**C**).

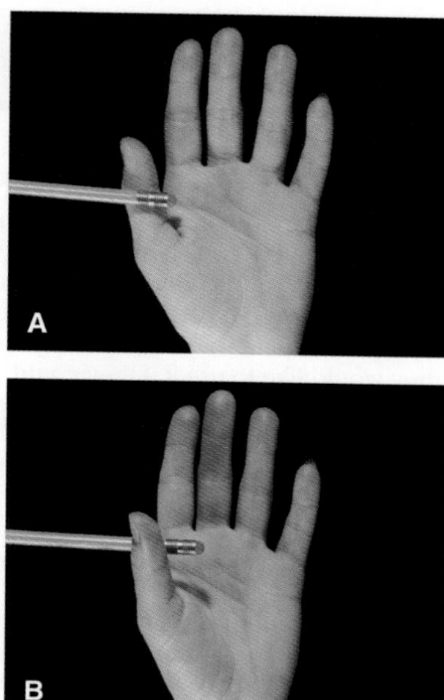

Figure 9-78 Left hand with the thumb about to move the pencil away from the palm to demonstrate abduction (**A**) and with the thumb about to move the pencil in the direction of the palm to demonstrate adduction (**B**).

langeal and metacarpophalangeal joints. The distal phalanx is flexed by the flexor digitorum profundus, the middle phalanx by the flexor digitorum superficialis, and the proximal phalanx by the lumbricals and the interossei.

Extension is the movement backward of the finger in an anteroposterior plane. The movements take place at the interphalangeal and metacarpophalangeal joints. The distal phalanx is extended by the lumbricals and interossei, the middle phalanx by the lumbricals and interossei, and the proximal phalanx by the extensor digitorum (in addition, by the extensor indicis for the index finger and the extensor digiti minimi for the little finger).

Abduction is the movement of the fingers (including the middle finger) away from the imaginary midline of the middle finger (Figs. 9-69 and 9-77A). The movement takes place at the metacarpophalangeal joint. The muscles producing the movement are the dorsal interossei; the abductor digiti minimi abducts the little finger.

Adduction is the movement of the fingers toward the midline of the middle finger (Fig. 9-77B). The movement takes place at the metacarpophalangeal joint. The muscles producing the movement are the palmar interossei.

Abduction and adduction of the fingers are possible only in the extended position. In the flexed position of the finger, the articular surface of the base of the proximal phalanx lies in contact with the flattened anterior surface of the head of the metacarpal bone. The two bones are held in close contact by the collateral ligaments, which are taut in this position. In the extended position of the metacarpophalangeal joint, the base of the phalanx is in contact with the rounded part of the metacarpal head, and the collateral ligaments are slack.

Cupping the Hand

In the cupped position, the palm of the hand is formed into a deep concavity. To achieve this, the thumb is abducted and placed in a partially opposed position and is also slightly flexed. This has the effect of drawing the thenar eminence forward.

The fourth and fifth metacarpal bones are flexed and slightly rotated at the carpometacarpal joints. This has the effect of drawing the hypothenar eminence forward. The palmaris brevis muscle contracts and pulls the skin over the hypothenar eminence medially; it also puckers the skin, which improves the gripping ability of the palm.

The index, middle, ring, and little fingers are partially flexed; the fingers are also rotated slightly at the metacarpophalangeal joints to increase the general concavity of the cupped hand.

Making a Fist

Making a fist is accomplished by flexing the metacarpophalangeal joints and the interphalangeal joints of the fingers and thumb. It is performed by the contraction of the long flexor muscles of the fingers and thumb. For this movement to be carried out efficiently a synergic contraction of the extensor carpi radialis longus and brevis and the extensor carpi ulnaris muscles must occur to extend the wrist joint. (Try to make a "strong fist" with the wrist joint flexed—it is very difficult.)

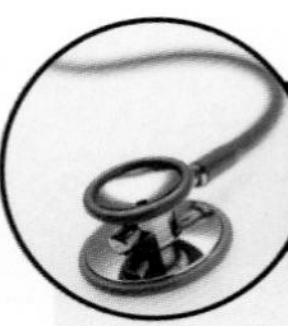

CLINICAL NOTES

Diseases of the Hand and Preservation of Function

From the clinical standpoint the hand is one of the most important organs of the body. Without a normally functioning hand the patient's livelihood is often in jeopardy. To students who doubt this statement, I would suggest that they place their right (or left) hand in a pocket for 24 hours. They will be astonished at the number of times they would like to use it if they could.

From the purely mechanical point of view, the hand can be regarded as a pincerlike mechanism between the thumb and fingers, situated at the end of a multijointed lever. The most important part of the hand is the thumb, and it is the physician's responsibility to preserve the thumb, or as much of it as possible, so that the pincerlike mechanism can be maintained. The pincerlike action of the thumb largely depends on its unique ability to be drawn across the palm and opposed to the other fingers. This movement alone, although important, is insufficient for the mechanism to work effectively. The opposing skin surfaces must have tactile sensation—and this explains why median nerve palsy is so much more disabling than ulnar nerve palsy.

If the hand requires immobilization for the treatment of disease of any part of the upper limb, it should be immobilized (if possible) in the **position of function.** This means that if loss of movement occurs at the wrist joint, or at the joints of the hand or fingers, the patient will at least have a hand that is in a position of mechanical advantage, and one that can serve a useful purpose.

Physicians should also remember that when a finger (excluding the thumb) is normally flexed into the palm, it points to the tubercle of the scaphoid; individual fingers requiring immobilization in flexion, on a splint or within a cast, should therefore always be placed in this position.

Always refer to the patient's fingers by name: thumb, index, middle, ring, and little finger. Numbering the fingers is confusing (is the thumb a finger?) and has led to such disastrous results as amputating the wrong finger.

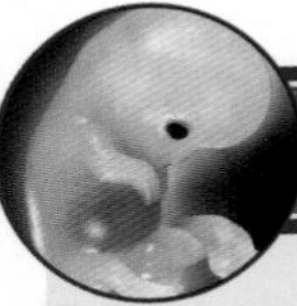

EMBRYOLOGIC NOTES

Development of the Upper Limb

The limb buds appear during the sixth week of development as the result of a localized proliferation of somatopleuric mesenchyme. This causes the overlying ectoderm to bulge from the trunk as two pairs of flattened paddles (Fig. 9-79). The arm buds develop before the leg buds and lie at the level of the lower six cervical and upper two thoracic segments. The flattened limb buds have a cephalic **preaxial border** and a caudal **postaxial border.** As the limb buds elongate, the anterior rami of the spinal nerves situated opposite the bases of the limb buds start to grow into the limbs. The mesenchyme situated along the preaxial border becomes associated and innervated with the lower five cervical nerves, whereas the mesenchyme of the postaxial border becomes associated with the eighth cervical and first thoracic nerves.

Later the mesenchymal masses divide into anterior and posterior groups, and the nerve trunks entering the base of each limb also divide into anterior and posterior divisions. The mesenchyme within the limbs differentiates into individual muscles that migrate within each limb. As a consequence of these two factors, the anterior rami of the spinal nerves become arranged in complicated plexuses that are found near the base of each limb so that the **brachial plexus** is formed.

Amelia

Absence of one or more limbs **(amelia)** or partial absence **(ectromelia)** may occur. A defective limb may possess a rudimentary hand at the extremity of the limb or a well-developed hand may spring from the shoulder with absence of the intermediate portion of the limb **(phocomelia)** (Fig. 9-80).

Congenital Absence of the Radius

Occasionally, the radius is congenitally absent and the growth of the ulna pushes the hand laterally (Fig. 9-81).

Syndactyly

In syndactyly, there is webbing of the fingers. It is usually bilateral and often familial (Fig. 9-82). Plastic repair of the fingers is carried out at the age of 5 years.

Lobster Hand

Lobster hand is a form of syndactyly that is associated with a central cleft dividing the hand into two parts. It is a heredofamilial disorder, for which plastic surgery is indicated where possible.

Brachydactyly

In brachydactyly, there is an absence of one or more phalanges in several fingers. Provided that the thumb is functioning normally, surgery is not indicated (Fig. 9-83).

Floating Thumb

A floating thumb results if the metacarpal bone of the thumb is absent but the phalanges are present. Plastic surgery is indicated where possible to improve the functional capabilities of the hand (Fig. 9-84).

Polydactyly

In polydactyly, one or more extra digits develop. It tends to run in families. The additional digits are removed surgically.

Local Gigantism

Macrodactyly affects one or more digits; these may be of adult size at birth, but the size usually diminishes with age (Fig. 9-85). Surgical removal may be necessary.

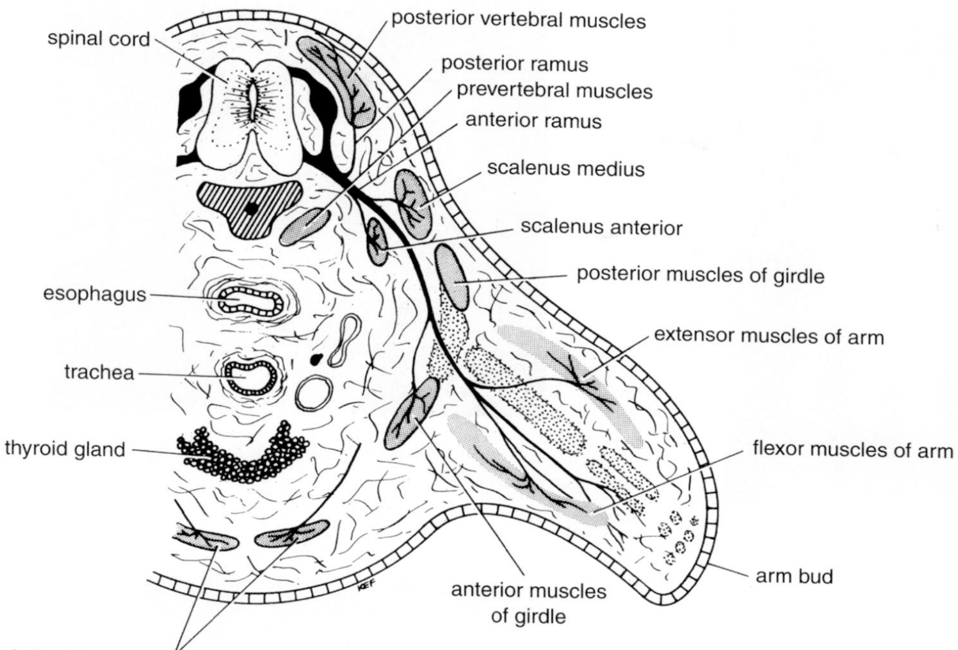

Figure 9-79 Section through the lower cervical region and the formation of the upper limb bud. Note the presence of the developing bones and muscles from the mesenchyme.

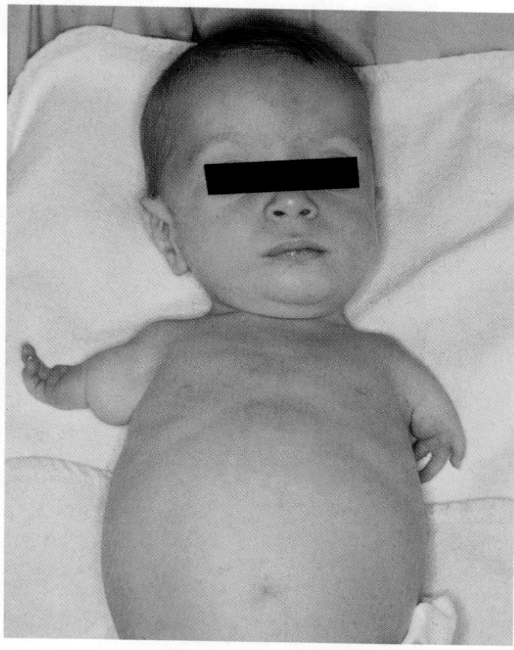

Figure 9-80 Ectromelia. (Courtesy of G. Avery.)

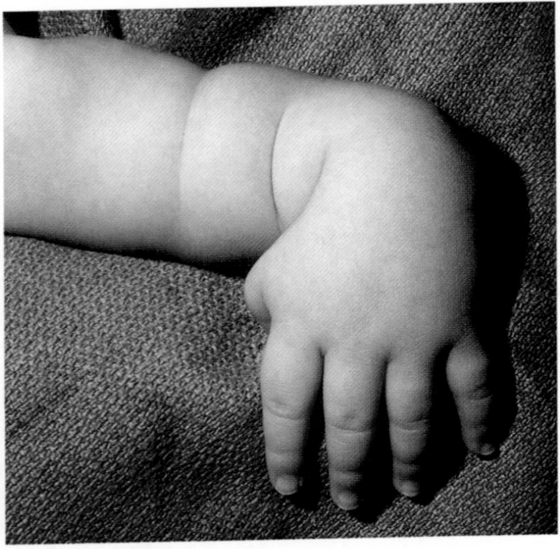

Figure 9-81 Congenital absence of the radius.

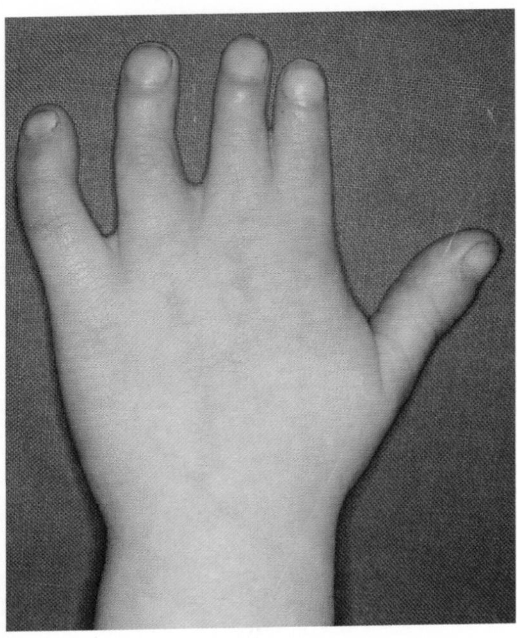

Figure 9-82 Partial syndactyly. (Courtesy of L. Thompson.)

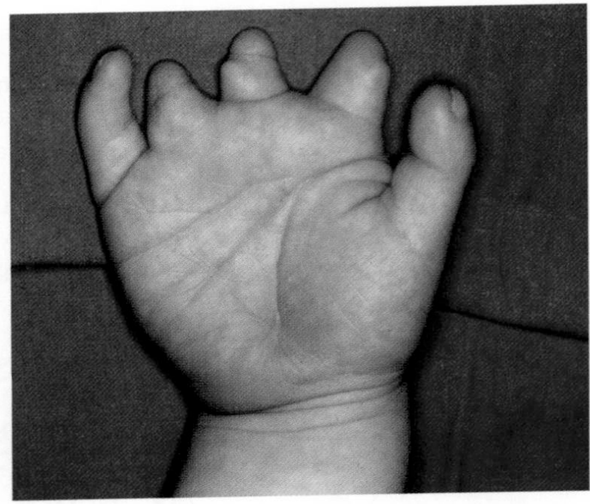

Figure 9-83 Brachydactyly due to defects of the phalanges. (Courtesy of L. Thompson.)

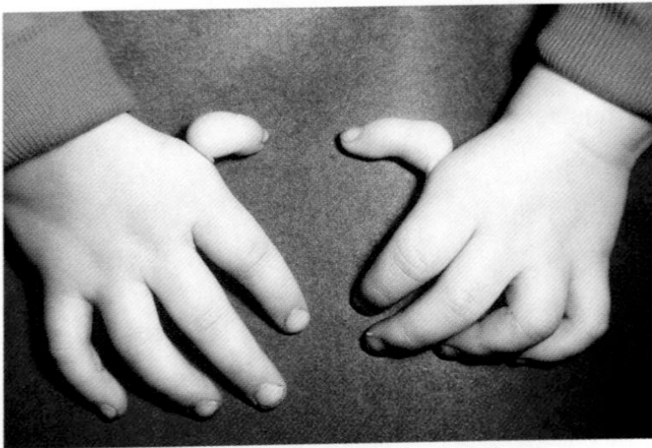

Figure 9-84 Floating thumb. The metacarpal bone of the thumb is absent, but the phalanges are present. (Courtesy of R. Chase.)

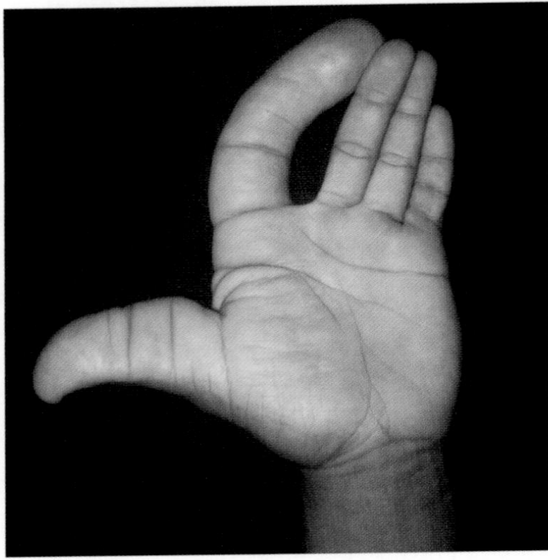

Figure 9-85 Macrodactyly affecting the thumb and index finger. (Courtesy of R. Neviaser.)

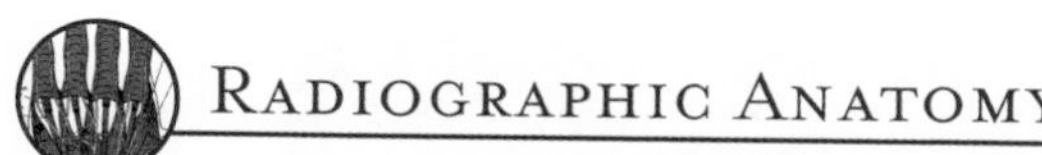

Radiographic Anatomy

Radiographic Appearances of the Upper Limb

Radiologic examination of the upper limb concentrates mainly on the bony structures because the muscles, tendons, and nerves blend into a homogeneous mass. The radiographic appearances of the upper limb are shown in Figures 9-86 through 9-93.

Magnetic resonance imaging of the upper limb can be useful to demonstrate the soft tissues around the bones (Fig. 9-94).

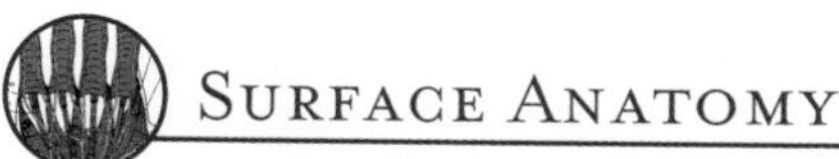

Surface Anatomy

Anterior Surface of the Chest

Suprasternal Notch

The suprasternal notch is the superior margin of the manubrium sterni and is easily palpated between the prominent medial ends of the clavicles in the midline (Figs. 9-95 and 9-96).

Sternal Angle (Angle of Louis)

The sternal angle is the angle between the manubrium and the body of the sternum (Fig. 9-95); at this level the second costal cartilage joins the lateral margin of the sternum.

Xiphisternal Joint

The xiphisternal joint is between the xiphoid process of the sternum and the body of the sternum (Fig. 9-97).

Costal Margin

The costal margin is the lower boundary of the thorax and is formed by the cartilages of the 7th, 8th, 9th, and 10th ribs and the ends of the 11th and 12th cartilages (Figs. 9-95, 9-96, and 9-97).

Clavicle

The clavicle is situated at the root of the neck and throughout its entire length lies just beneath the skin and can be easily palpated (Figs. 9-95, 9-96, and 9-97). The positions of the sternoclavicular and acromioclavicular joints can be easily identified. Note that the medial end of the clavicle projects above the margin of the manubrium sterni.

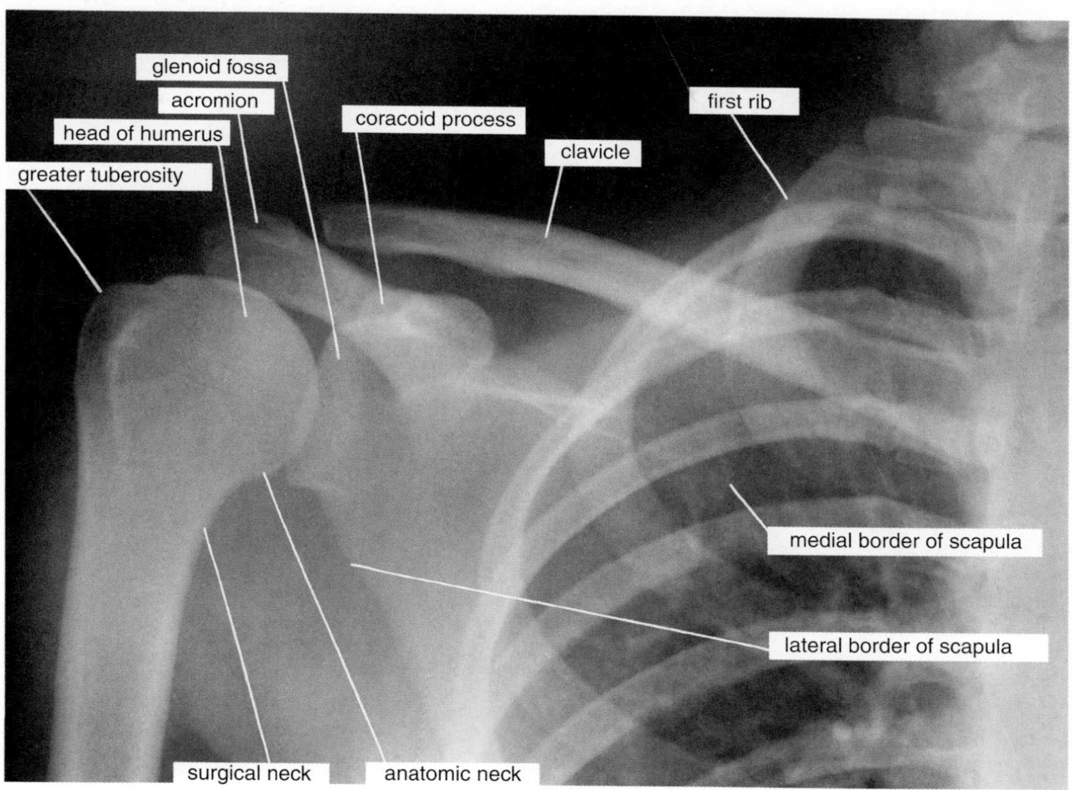

Figure 9-86 Anteroposterior radiograph of the shoulder region in the adult.

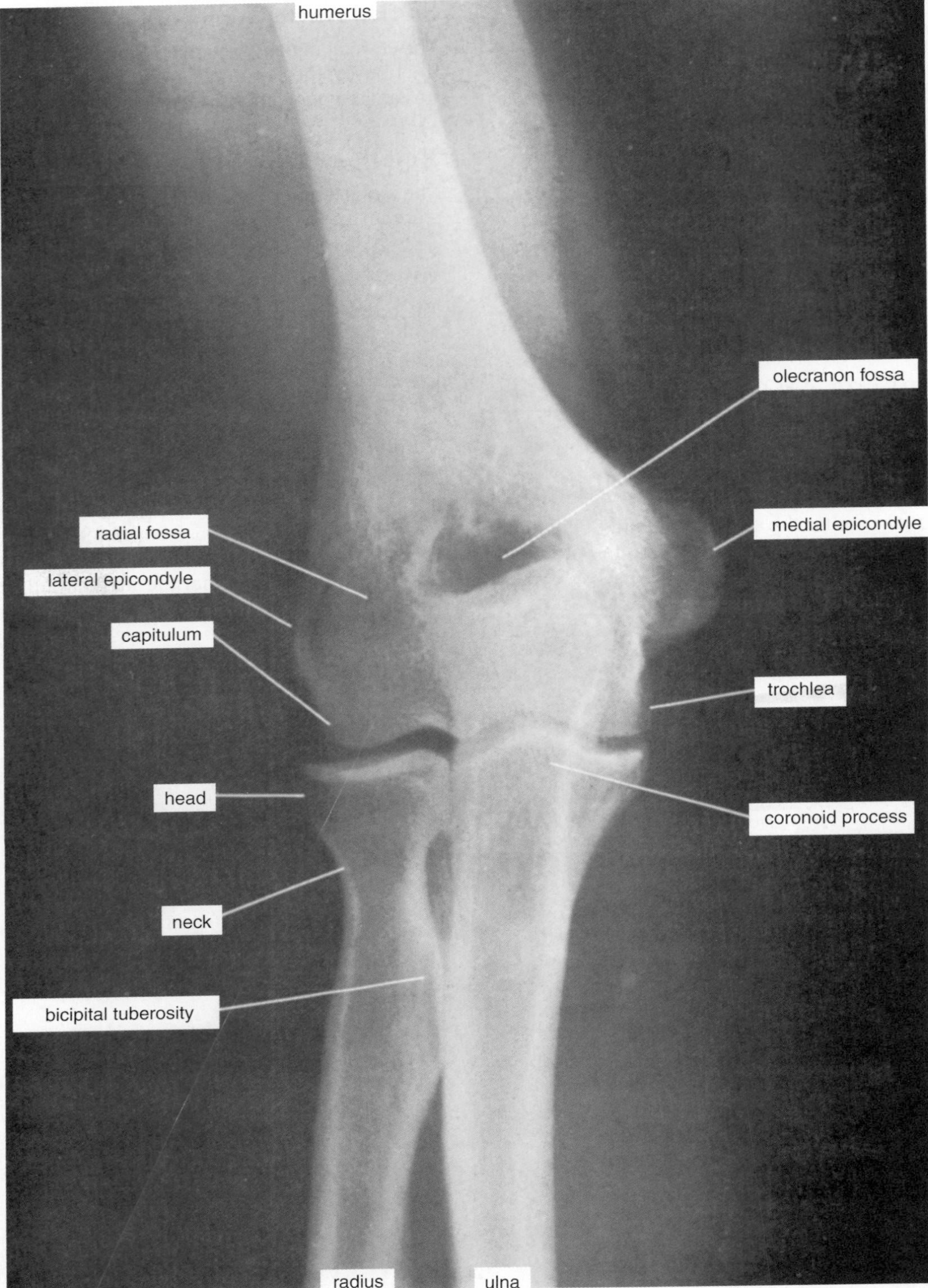

Figure 9-87 Anteroposterior radiograph of the elbow region in the adult.

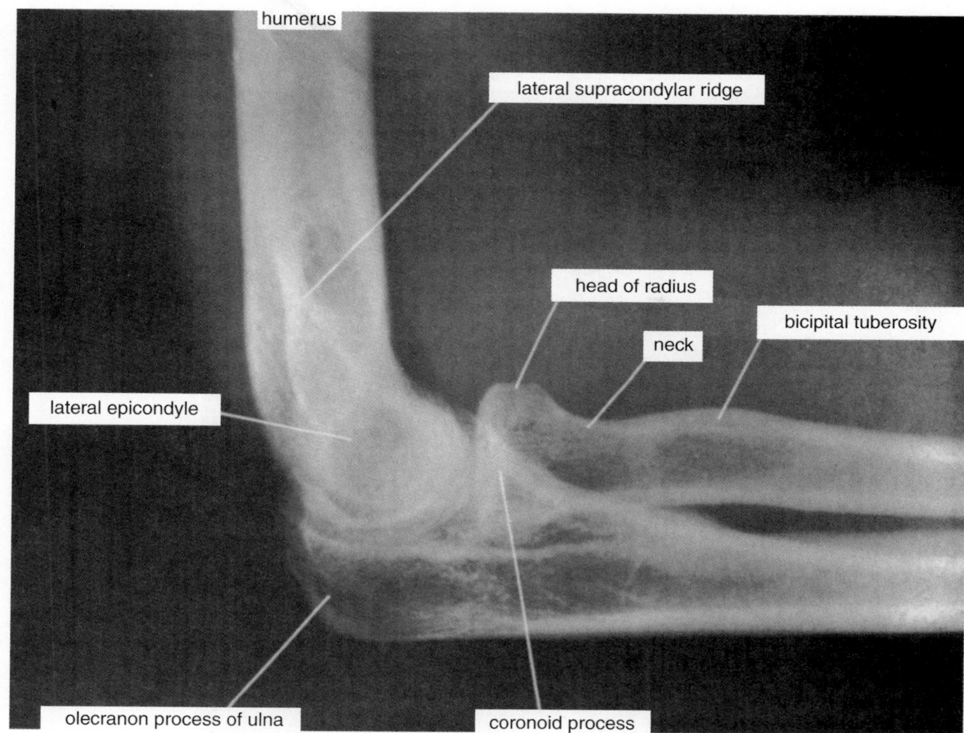

Figure 9-88 Lateral radiograph of the elbow region in the adult.

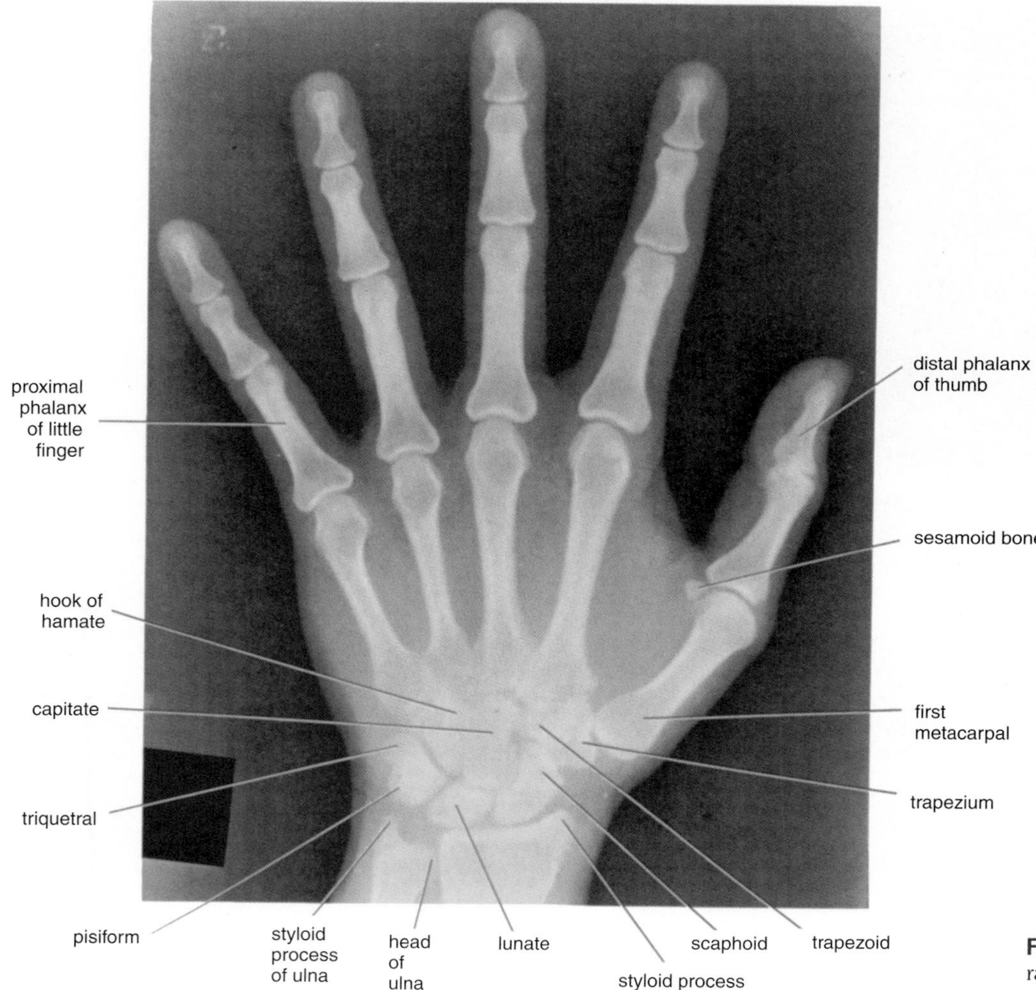

Figure 9-89 Posteroanterior radiograph of an adult wrist and hand.

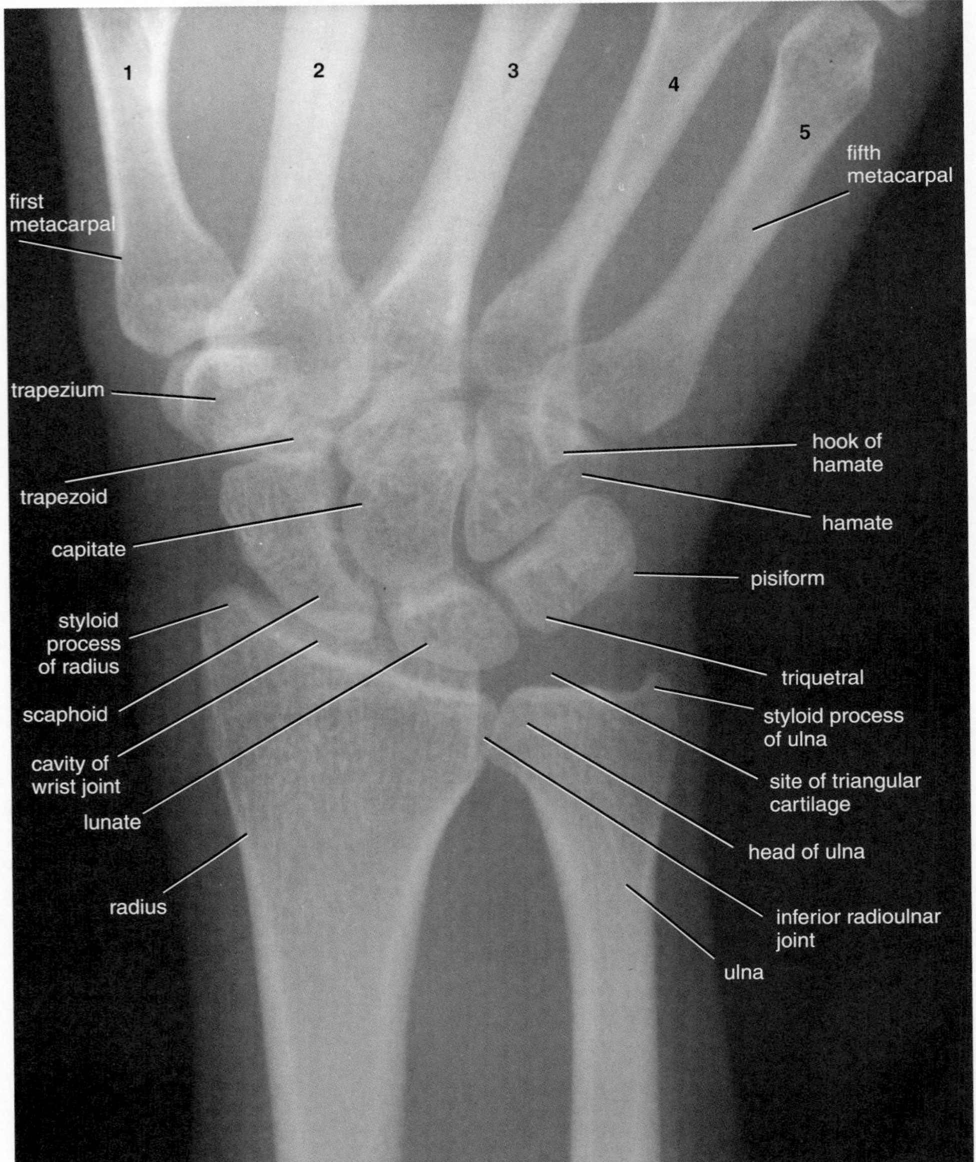

Figure 9-90 Posteroanterior radiograph of the wrist with the forearm pronated.

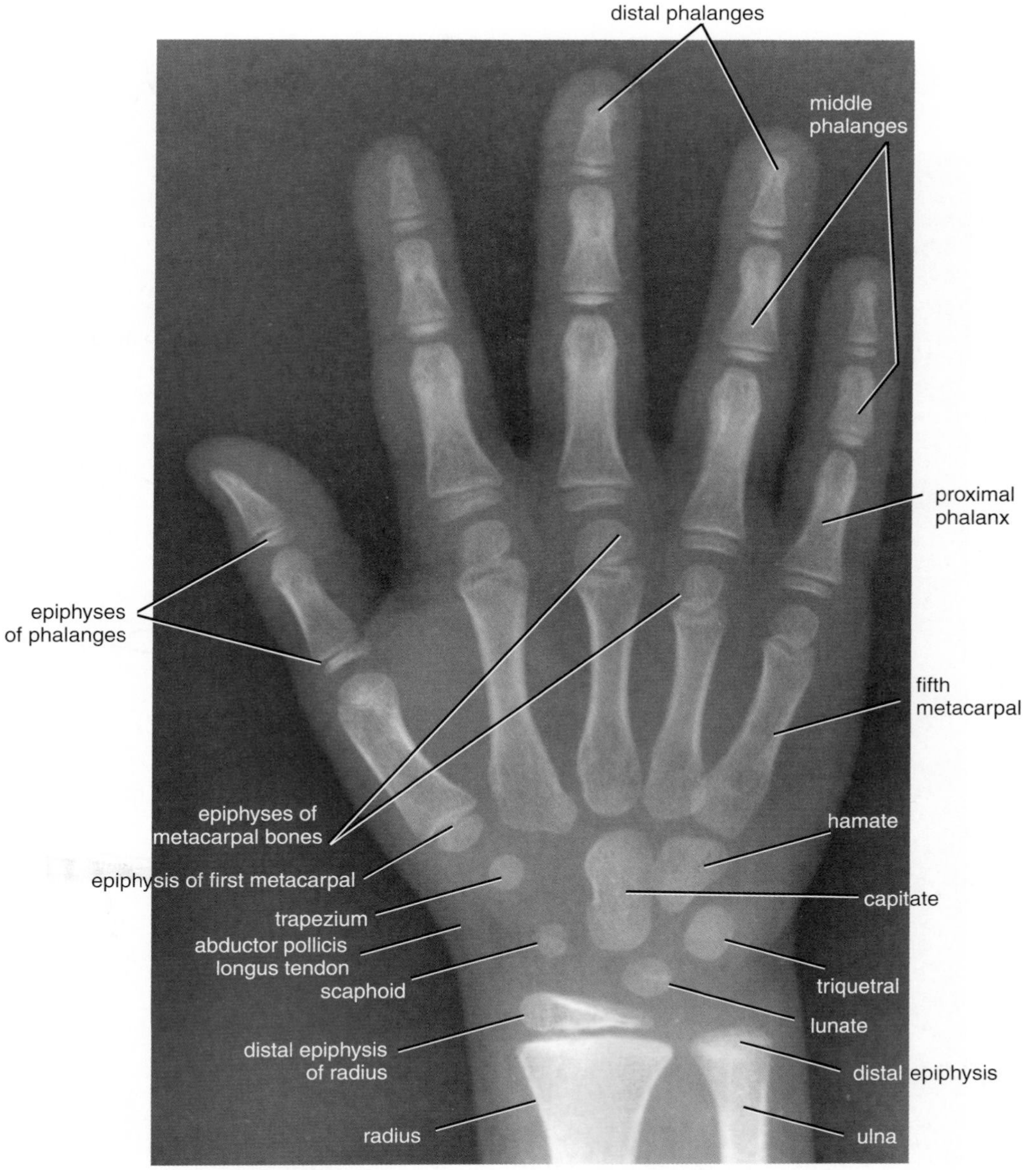

Figure 9-91 Posteroanterior radiograph of the wrist and hand of an 8-year-old boy.

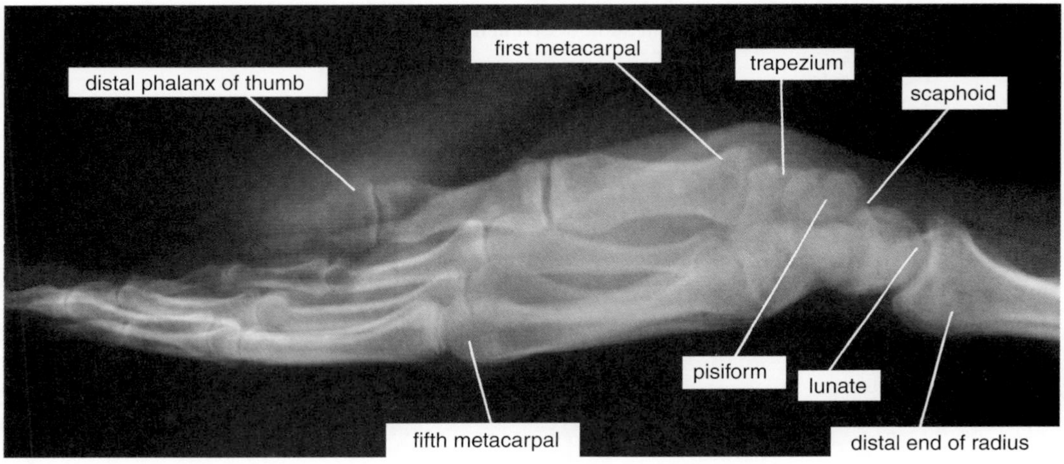

Figure 9-92 Lateral radiograph of an adult wrist and hand.

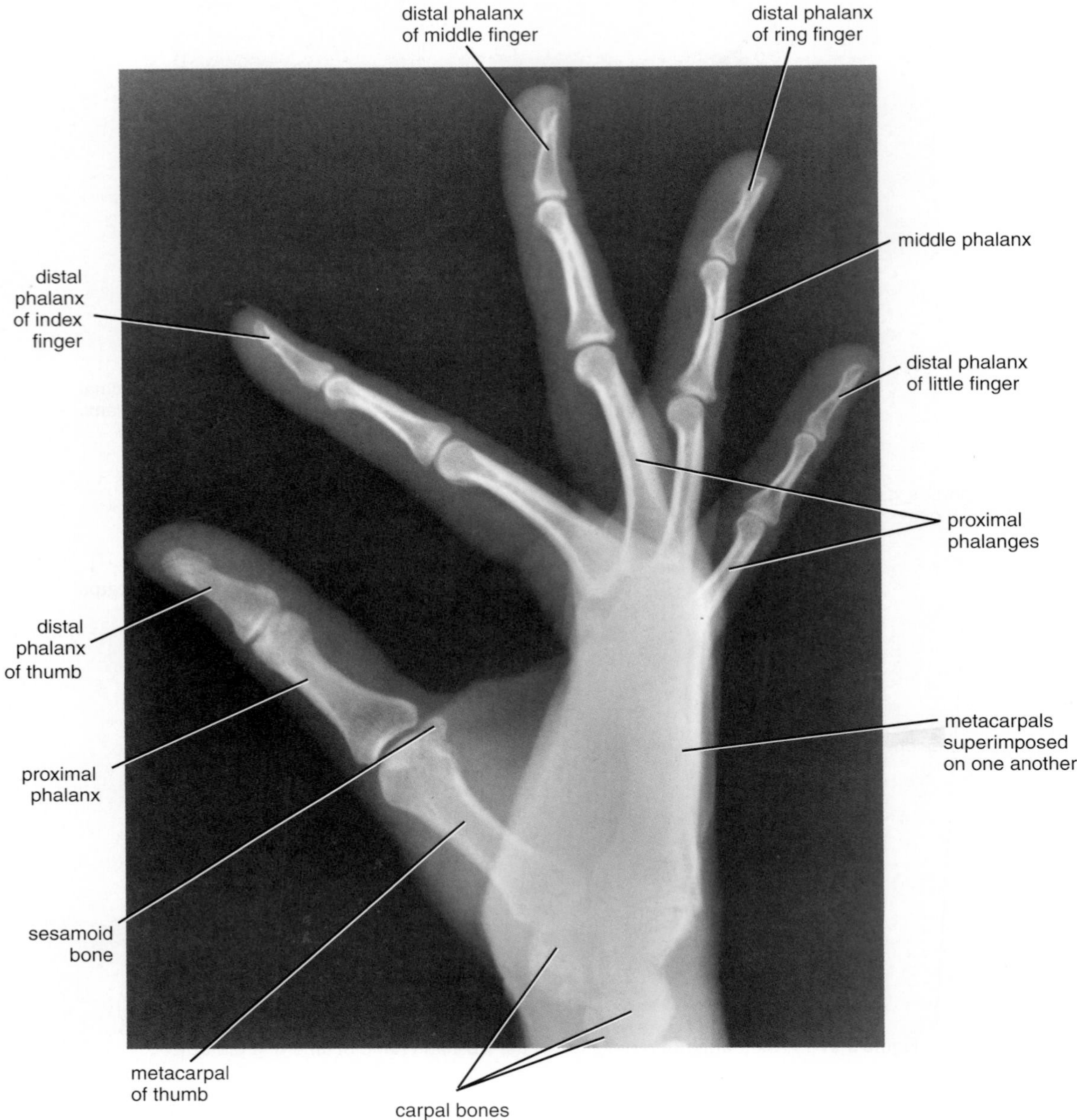

Figure 9-93 Lateral radiograph of an adult wrist and hand with the fingers at different degrees of flexion.

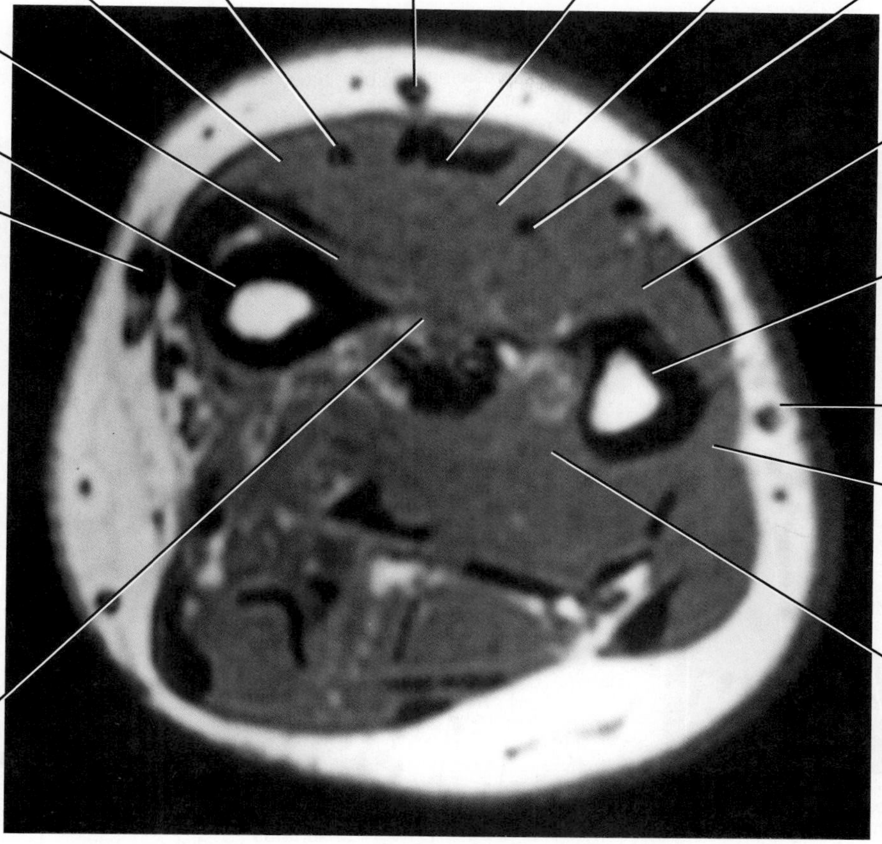

brachioradialis
radial artery and superficial branch of radial nerve
anterior median vein of forearm
flexor carpi radialis
flexor digitorum superficialis
median nerve
flexor pollicis longus
radius
cephalic vein
flexor digitorum profundus
ulna
basilic vein
extensor carpi ulnaris
extensor pollicis longus
interosseous membrane

Figure 9-94 Transverse (axial) magnetic resonance image of the upper part of the right forearm (as seen from below).

clavicle
acromion process
suprasternal notch
deltopectoral triangle
greater tuberosity of humerus
sternal angle (angle of Louis)
deltoid
pectoralis major
areola
anterior axillary fold
nipple
axillary tail of mammary gland
xiphoid process
costal margin
rectus abdominis
iliac crest
umbilicus

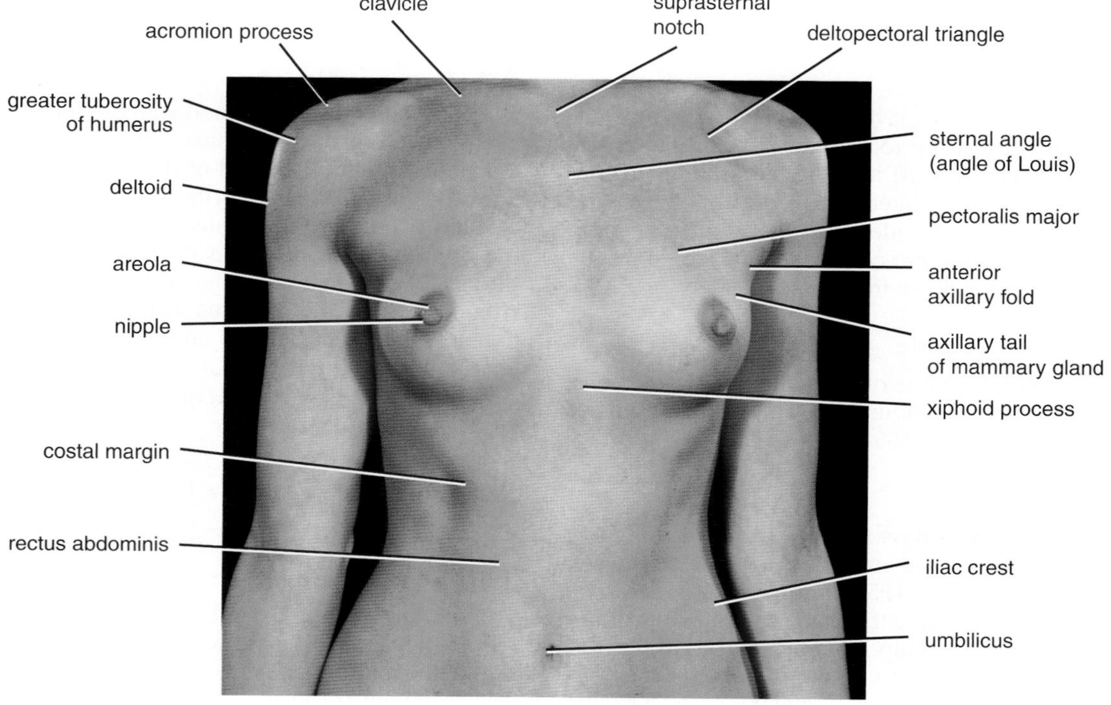

Figure 9-95 Anterior view of the thorax and abdomen in a 29-year-old woman.

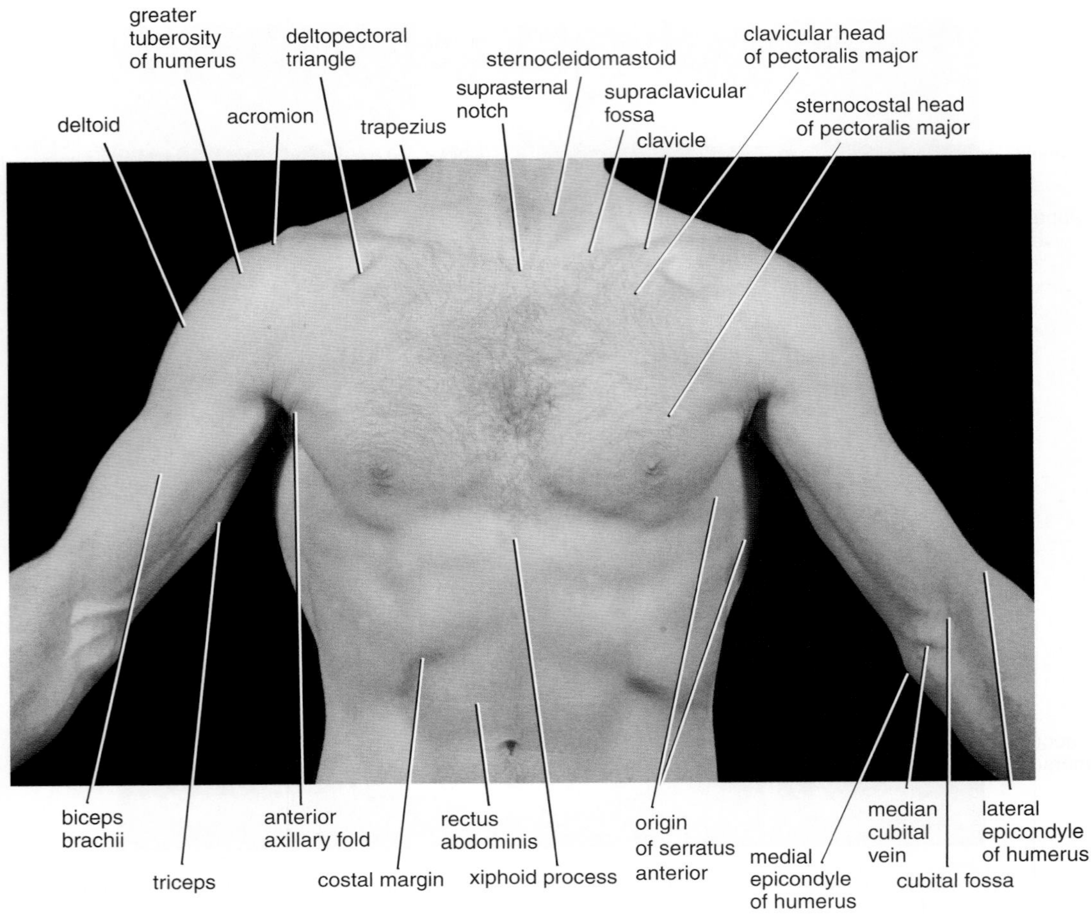

Figure 9-96 The pectoral region in a 27-year-old man.

Ribs

The first rib lies deep to the clavicle and cannot be palpated. The lateral surfaces of the remaining ribs can be felt by pressing the fingers upward into the axilla and drawing them downward over the lateral surface of the chest wall (Fig. 9-97). Each rib can be identified by first palpating the sternal angle and the second costal cartilage (see previous column) and counting down from there.

Deltopectoral Triangle

This small, triangular depression is situated below the outer third of the clavicle and is bounded by the pectoralis major and deltoid muscles (Figs. 9-95 and 9-96).

Axillary Folds

The **anterior axillary fold** is formed by the lower margin of the pectoralis major muscle and can be palpated between the finger and thumb (Figs. 9-95, 9-96, and 9-97). This can be made to stand out by asking the patient to press his or her hand against the ipsilateral hip. The **posterior axillary fold** is formed by the tendon of latissimus dorsi as it passes around the lower border of the teres major muscle. It can be easily palpated between the finger and thumb (Fig. 9-98).

Axilla

The axilla should be examined with the forearm supported and the pectoral muscles relaxed. With the arm by the side, the inferior part of the **head of the humerus** can be easily palpated through the floor of the axilla. The pulsations of the **axillary artery** can be felt high up in the axilla, and around the artery can be palpated the **cords of the brachial plexus.** The medial wall of the axilla is formed by the **upper ribs** covered by the **serratus anterior muscle,** the serrations of which can be seen and felt in a muscular subject (Fig. 9-96). The lateral wall is formed by the **coracobrachialis** and **biceps brachii muscles** and the bicipital groove of the humerus.

Posterior Surface of the Chest

Spinous Processes of Cervical and Thoracic Vertebrae

The spinous processes can be palpated in the midline posteriorly (Fig. 9-98). The index finger should be placed on the skin in the midline on the posterior surface of the neck and drawn downward in the nuchal groove. The first spinous process to be felt is that of the seventh cervical vertebra

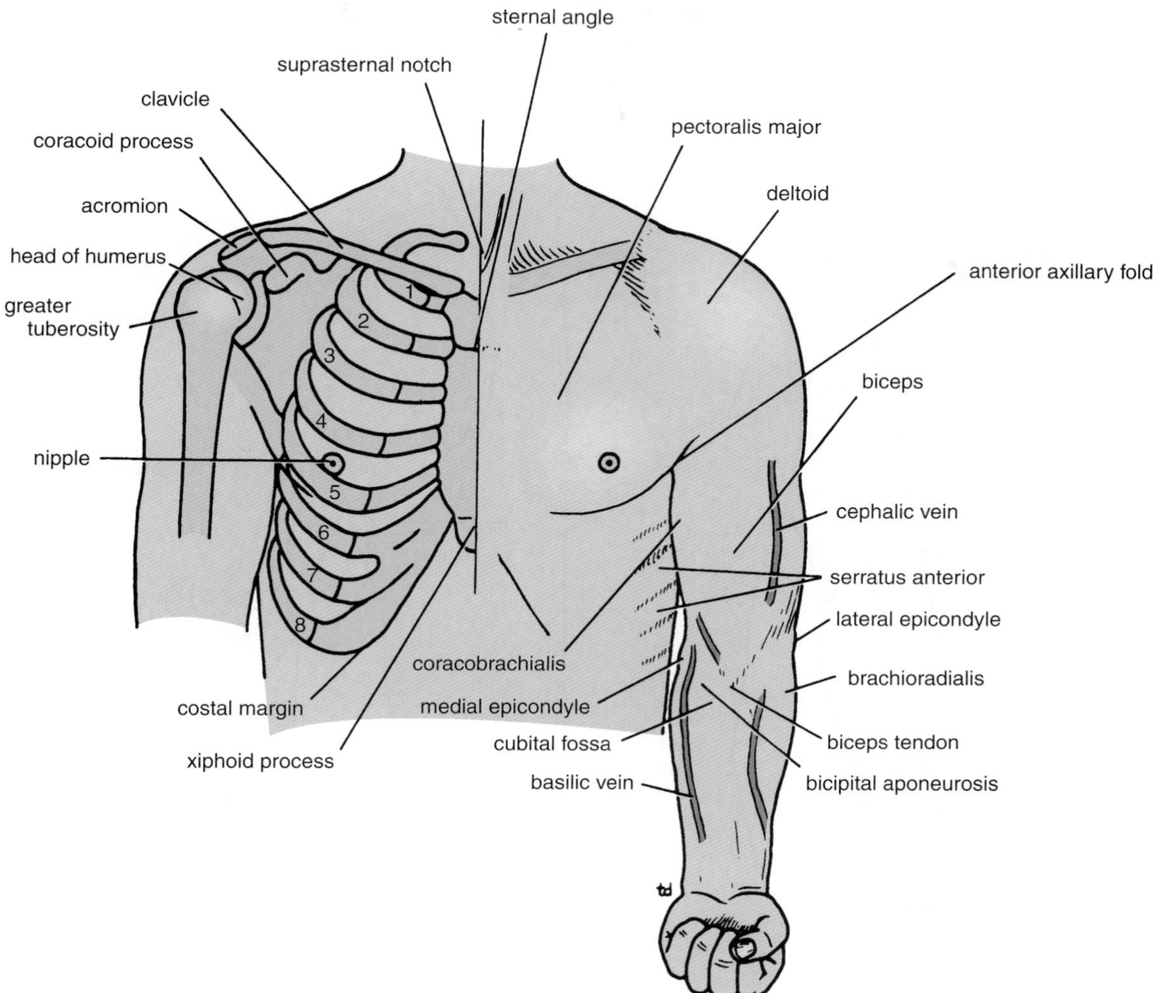

Figure 9-97 Surface anatomy of the chest, shoulder, and upper limb as seen anteriorly.

(vertebra prominens). Below this level are the overlapping spines of the thoracic vertebrae. The spines of the first through sixth cervical vertebrae are covered by the large ligament called the **ligamentum nuchae.**

Scapula

The tip of the **coracoid process** of the scapula (Fig. 9-97) can be felt on deep palpation in the lateral part of the deltopectoral triangle; it is covered by the anterior fibers of the deltoid muscle. The **acromion** forms the lateral extremity of the spine of the scapula. It is subcutaneous and easily located (Figs. 9-95 and 9-96).

Immediately below the lateral edge of the acromion is the smooth, rounded curve of the shoulder produced by the **deltoid muscle,** which covers the **greater tuberosity of the humerus** (Figs. 9-95 and 9-96).

The **crest of the spine of the scapula** can be palpated and traced medially to the medial border of the scapula, which it joins at the level of the third thoracic spine (Fig. 9-98).

The **superior angle of the scapula** can be felt through the trapezius muscle and lies opposite the second thoracic spine.

The **inferior angle of the scapula** can be palpated opposite the seventh thoracic spine (Figs. 9-98 and 9-99).

The Breast

In children and men, the breast anatomy is rudimentary and the glandular tissue is confined to a small area beneath the pigmented areola. In young women (Fig. 9-95) it is usually hemispherical and slightly pendulous, overlaps the second to the sixth ribs and their costal cartilages, and extends from the lateral margin of the sternum to the midaxillary line (Fig. 9-95). The greater part of the breast lies in the superficial fascia and can be moved freely in all directions. Its upper lateral edge **(axillary tail)** extends around the lower border of the pectoralis major and enters the axilla (Fig. 9-95), where it comes into close relationship with the axillary vessels. In middle-aged multiparous women the breast may be large and pendulous, and in older women the breast may be smaller.

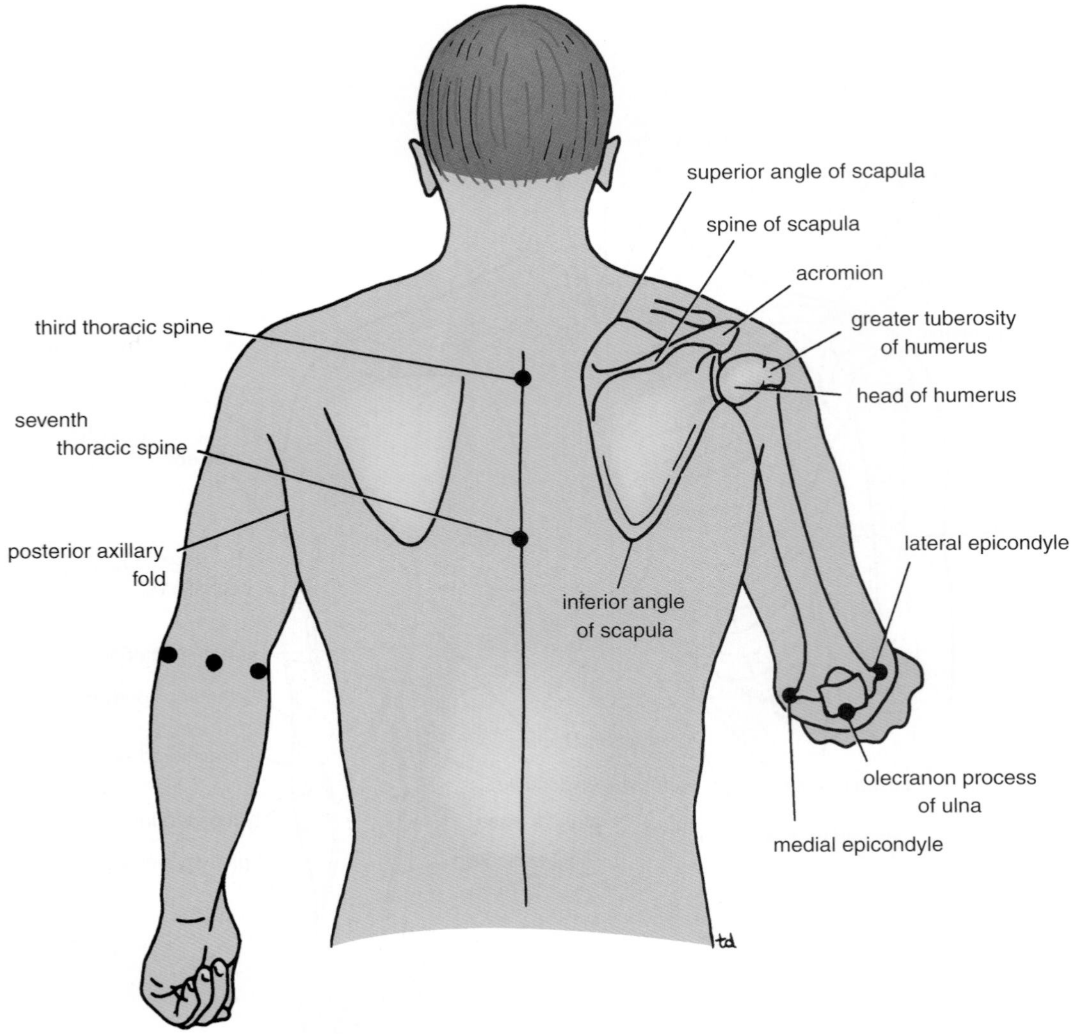

superior angle of scapula
spine of scapula
acromion
third thoracic spine
greater tuberosity
of humerus
head of humerus
seventh
thoracic spine
posterior axillary
fold
lateral epicondyle
inferior angle
of scapula
olecranon process
of ulna
medial epicondyle
td

Figure 9-98 Surface anatomy of the scapula, shoulder, and elbow regions as seen posteriorly.

acromion
deltoid
trapezius
infraspinatus
teres major
inferior angle
of scapula
spinous processes
of lumbar vertebrae
latissimus dorsi
iliac crest

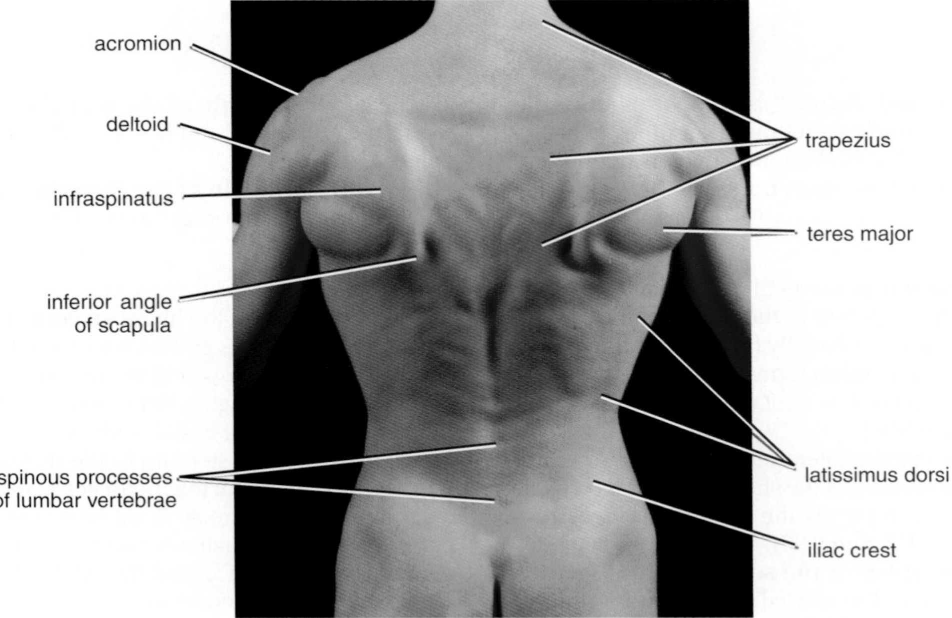

Figure 9-99 The back in a 27-year-old man.

In the living subject, the breast is soft because the fat contained within it is fluid. On careful palpation with the open hand, the breast has a firm, overall lobulated consistency, produced by its glandular tissue.

The **nipple** projects from the lower half of the breast (Fig. 9-95), but its position in relation to the chest wall varies greatly and depends on the development of the gland. In males and immature females, the nipples are small and usually lie over the fourth intercostal spaces about 4 in. (10 cm) from the midline. The base of the nipple is surrounded by a circular area of pigmented skin called the **areola** (Fig. 9-95). Pink in color in the young girl, the areola becomes darker in color in the second month of the first pregnancy and never regains its former tint. Tiny tubercles on the areola are produced by the underlying **areolar glands.**

The Elbow Region

The **medial** and **lateral epicondyles** of the humerus (Figs. 9-96 and 9-98) and the olecranon process of the ulna can be palpated (Fig. 9-98). When the elbow joint is extended, these bony points lie on the same straight line; when the elbow is flexed, these three points form the boundaries of an equilateral triangle.

The **head of the radius** can be palpated in a depression on the posterolateral aspect of the extended elbow, distal to the lateral epicondyle. The head of the radius can be felt to rotate during pronation and supination of the forearm.

The **cubital fossa** is a skin depression in front of the elbow (Figs. 9-48 and 9-97), and the boundaries can be seen and felt; the brachioradialis muscle forms the lateral boundary and the pronator teres forms the medial boundary. The **tendon of the biceps muscle** can be palpated as it passes downward into the fossa, and the **bicipital aponeurosis** can be felt as it leaves the tendon to join the deep fascia on the medial side of the forearm (Figs. 9-48 and 9-97). The tendon and aponeurosis are most easily felt if the elbow joint is flexed against resistance.

The **ulnar nerve** can be palpated where it lies behind the medial epicondyle of the humerus. It feels like a rounded cord, and when it is compressed, a "pins and needles" sensation is felt along the medial part of the hand.

The **brachial artery** can be felt to pulsate as it passes down the arm, overlapped by the medial border of the biceps muscle. In the cubital fossa, it lies beneath the bicipital aponeurosis, and, at a level just below the head of the radius, it divides into the radial and ulnar arteries.

The **posterior border of the ulna bone** is subcutaneous and can be palpated along its entire length.

The Wrist and Hand

At the wrist, the **styloid processes of the radius** (Fig. 9-100) and **ulna** can be palpated. The styloid process of the radius lies about 0.75 in. (1.9 cm) distal to that of the ulna.

The **dorsal tubercle of the radius** is palpable on the posterior surface of the distal end of the radius (Fig. 9-100).

The **head of the ulna** is most easily felt with the forearm pronated; the head then stands out prominently on the lateral side of the wrist (Fig. 9-75). The rounded head can be distinguished from the more distal pointed styloid process.

The **pisiform bone** can be felt on the medial side of the anterior aspect of the wrist between the two transverse creases (Figs. 9-48 and 9-100). The **hook of the hamate bone** can be felt on deep palpation of the hypothenar eminence, a fingerbreadth distal and lateral to the pisiform bone.

The **transverse creases** seen in front of the wrist are important landmarks (Fig. 9-100). The proximal transverse crease lies at the level of the wrist joint. The distal transverse crease corresponds to the proximal border of the flexor retinaculum.

Important Structures Lying in Front of the Wrist

Radial Artery

The pulsations of the radial artery can easily be felt anterior to the distal third of the radius (Figs. 9-48 and 9-100). Here it lies just beneath the skin and fascia lateral to the tendon of flexor carpi radialis muscle.

Tendon of Flexor Carpi Radialis

The tendon of the flexor carpi radialis lies medial to the pulsating radial artery.

Tendon of Palmaris Longus (If Present)

The tendon of the palmaris longus lies medial to the tendon of flexor carpi radialis and overlies the median nerve (Fig. 9-100).

Tendons of Flexor Digitorum Superficialis

The tendons of the flexor digitorum superficialis are a group of four that lie medial to the tendon of palmaris longus and can be seen moving beneath the skin when the fingers are flexed and extended.

Tendon of Flexor Carpi Ulnaris

The tendon of the flexor carpi ulnaris is the most medially placed tendon on the front of the wrist and can be followed distally to its insertion on the pisiform bone (Figs. 9-48 and 9-100). The tendon can be made prominent by asking the patient to clench the fist (the muscle contracts to assist in fixing and stabilizing the wrist joint).

Ulnar Artery

The pulsations of the ulnar artery can be felt lateral to the tendon of flexor carpi ulnaris (Fig. 9-100).

Ulnar Nerve

The ulnar nerve lies immediately medial to the ulnar artery (Fig. 9-100).

Important Structures Lying on the Lateral Side of the Wrist

Anatomic Snuffbox

The "anatomic snuffbox" is an important area. It is a skin depression that lies distal to the styloid process of the radius. It is bounded medially by the **tendon of extensor pollicis longus** and laterally by the **tendons of abductor pollicis**

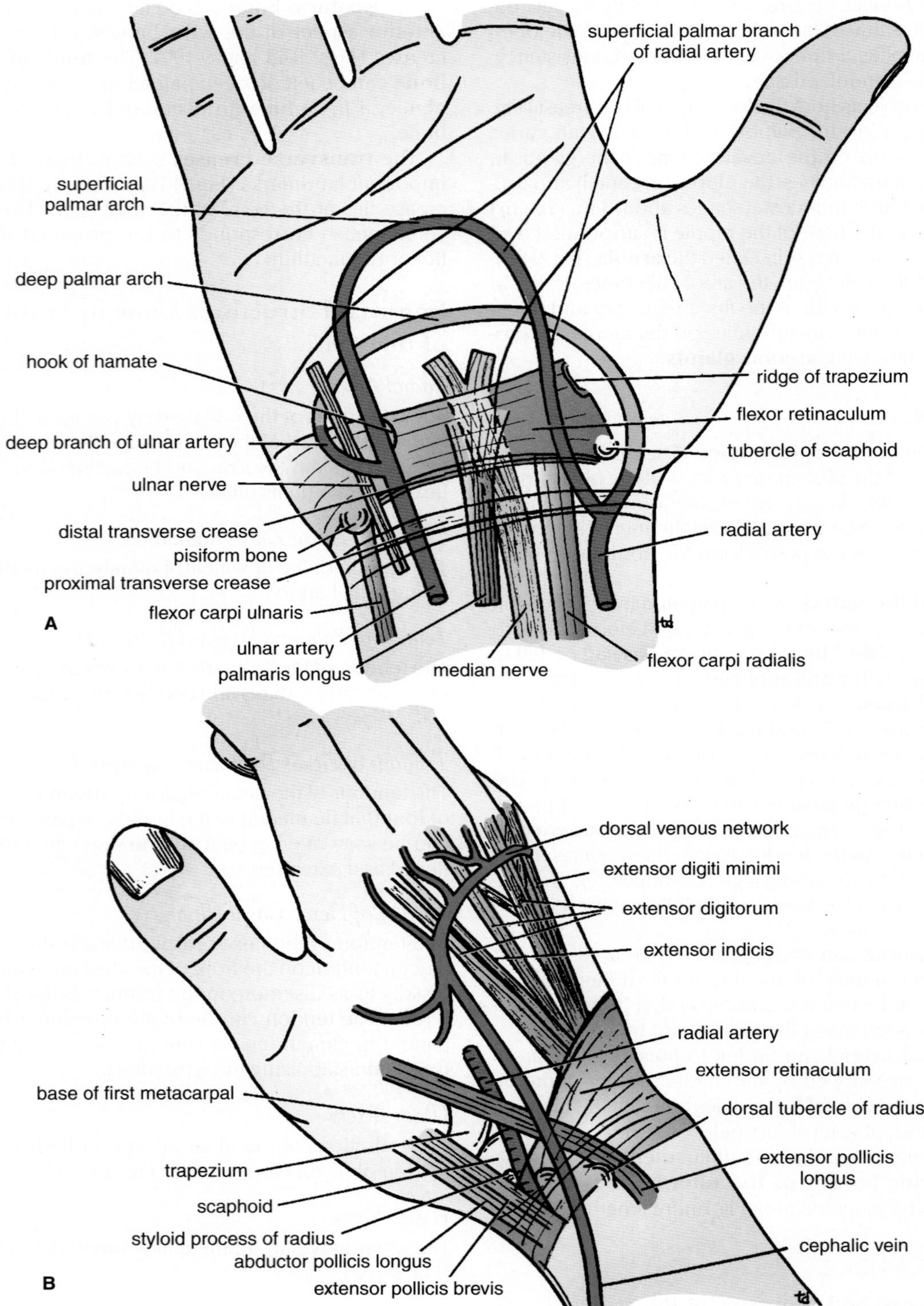

Figure 9-100 Surface anatomy of the wrist region.

longus and **extensor pollicis brevis** (Fig. 9-100). In its floor can be palpated the **styloid process of the radius** (proximally) and the **base of the first metacarpal bone** of the thumb (distally); between these bones beneath the floor lie the **scaphoid** and the **trapezium** (felt but not identifiable). The **radial artery** can be palpated within the snuffbox as the artery winds around the lateral margin of the wrist to reach the dorsum of the hand (Fig. 9-100). The **cephalic vein** can also sometimes be recognized crossing the snuffbox as it ascends the forearm.

Important Structures Lying on the Back of the Wrist

Lunate

The lunate lies in the proximal row of carpal bones. It can be palpated just distal to the dorsal tubercle of the radius when the wrist joint is flexed.

Important Structures Lying in the Palm

Recurrent Branch of the Median Nerve

The recurrent branch to the muscles of the thenar eminence curves around the lower border of the flexor retinaculum and lies about one fingerbreadth distal to the tubercle of the scaphoid (Fig. 9-62).

Superficial Palmar Arterial Arch

The superficial palmar arterial arch is located in the central part of the palm (Fig. 9-100) and lies on a line drawn across the palm at the level of the distal border of the fully extended thumb.

Deep Palmar Arterial Arch

The deep palmar arterial arch is also located in the central part of the palm (Fig. 9-100) and lies on a line drawn across the palm at the level of the proximal border of the fully extended thumb.

Metacarpophalangeal Joints

The metacarpophalangeal joints lie approximately at the level of the distal transverse palmar crease. The **interphalangeal joints** lie at the level of the middle and distal finger creases.

Important Structures Lying on the Dorsum of the Hand

The **tendons of extensor digitorum,** the **extensor indicis,** and the **extensor digiti minimi** can be seen and felt as they pass distally to the bases of the fingers (Fig. 9-100).

Dorsal Venous Network

The network of superficial veins can be seen on the dorsum of the hand (Fig. 9-100). The network drains upward into the lateral cephalic vein and a medial basilic vein.

The **cephalic vein** crosses the anatomic snuffbox and winds around onto the anterior aspect of the forearm. It then ascends into the arm and runs along the lateral border of the biceps (Fig. 9-39). It ends by piercing the deep fascia in the deltopectoral triangle and enters the axillary vein.

The **basilic vein** can be traced from the dorsum of the hand around the medial side of the forearm and reaches the anterior aspect just below the elbow (Fig. 9-39). It pierces the deep fascia at about the middle of the arm. The **median cubital vein** (or median cephalic and median basilic veins) links the cephalic and basilic veins in the cubital fossa (Fig. 9-39).

To identify these veins easily, apply firm pressure around the upper arm and repeatedly clench and relax the fist. By this means the veins become distended with blood.

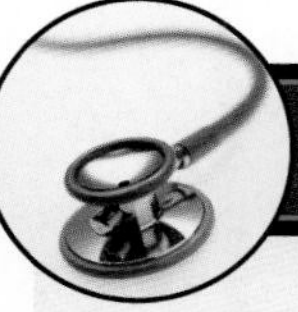

CLINICAL NOTES ON THE ARTERIES OF THE UPPER LIMB

Arterial Injury

The arteries of the upper limb can be damaged by penetrating wounds or may require ligation in amputation operations. Because of the existence of an adequate collateral circulation around the shoulder, elbow, and wrist joints, ligation of the main arteries of the upper limb is not followed by tissue necrosis or gangrene, provided, of course, that the arteries forming the collateral circulation are not diseased and the patient's general circulation is satisfactory. Nevertheless, it can take days or weeks for the collateral vessels to open sufficiently to provide the distal part of the limb with the same volume of blood as previously supplied by the main artery.

Palpation and Compression of Arteries

A clinician must know where the arteries of the upper limb can be palpated or compressed in an emergency. The subclavian artery, as it crosses the first rib to become the axillary artery, can be palpated in the root of the posterior triangle of the neck (Fig. 9-31). The artery can be compressed here against the first rib to stop a catastrophic hemorrhage. The third part of the axillary artery can be felt in the axilla as it lies in front of the teres major muscle (Fig. 9-17). The brachial artery can be palpated in the arm as it lies on the brachialis and is overlapped from the lateral side by the biceps brachii (Fig. 9-43).

The radial artery lies superficially in front of the distal end of the radius, between the tendons of the brachioradialis and flexor carpi radialis; it is here that the clinician takes the radial pulse (Fig. 9-58). If the pulse cannot be felt, try feeling for the radial artery on the other wrist; occasionally a congenitally abnormal radial artery can be difficult to feel. The radial artery can be less easily felt as it crosses the anatomic snuffbox (Fig. 9-100).

The ulnar artery can be palpated as it crosses anterior to the flexor retinaculum in company with the ulnar nerve. The artery lies lateral to the pisiform bone, separated from it by the ulnar nerve. The artery is commonly damaged here in laceration wounds in front of the wrist.

(continues)

Clinical Notes, *continued*

Allen Test

The Allen test is used to determine the patency of the ulnar and radial arteries. With the patient's hands resting in the lap, compress the radial arteries against the anterior surface of each radius and ask the patient to tightly clench the fists. The clenching of the fists closes off the superficial and deep palmar arterial arches. When the patient is asked to open the hands, the skin of the palms is at first white, and then normally the blood quickly flows into the arches through the ulnar arteries, causing the palms to promptly turn pink. This establishes that the ulnar arteries are patent. The patency of the radial arteries can be established by repeating the test but this time compressing the ulnar arteries as they lie lateral to the pisiform bones.

Arterial Innervation and Raynaud's Disease

The arteries of the upper limb are innervated by sympathetic nerves. The preganglionic fibers originate from cell bodies in the second to eighth thoracic segments of the spinal cord. They ascend in the sympathetic trunk and synapse in the middle cervical, inferior cervical, first thoracic, or stellate ganglia. The postganglionic fibers join the nerves that form the brachial plexus and are distributed to the arteries within the branches of the plexus. For example, the digital arteries of the fingers are supplied by postganglionic sympathetic fibers that run in the digital nerves. Vasospastic diseases involving digital arterioles, such as Raynaud's disease, may require a cervicodorsal preganglionic sympathectomy to prevent necrosis of the fingers. The operation is followed by arterial vasodilatation, with consequent increased blood flow to the upper limb.

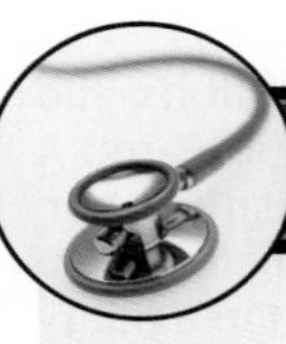

CLINICAL NOTES ON THE NERVES OF THE UPPER LIMB

Dermatomes and Cutaneous Nerves

The importance of the dermatomes and cutaneous nerves in the upper limb is discussed on page 467.

Tendon Reflexes and the Segmental Innervation of Muscles

The skeletal muscle receives a segmental innervation. Most muscles are innervated by several spinal nerves and therefore by several segments of the spinal cord. A physician should know the segmental innervation of the following muscles because it is possible to test them by eliciting simple muscle reflexes in the patient:

Biceps brachii tendon reflex: C5 and **6** (flexion of the elbow joint by tapping the biceps tendon).

Triceps tendon reflex: C6, 7, and **8** (extension of the elbow joint by tapping the triceps tendon).

Brachioradialis tendon reflex: C5, 6, and 7 (supination of the radioulnar joints by tapping the insertion of the brachioradialis tendon).

Brachial Plexus Injuries

The roots, trunks, and divisions of the brachial plexus reside in the lower part of the posterior triangle of the neck, whereas the cords and most of the branches of the plexus lie in the axilla. Complete lesions involving all the roots of the plexus are rare. Incomplete injuries are common and are usually caused by traction or pressure; individual nerves can be divided by stab wounds.

Upper Lesions of the Brachial Plexus (Erb-Duchenne Palsy)

Upper lesions of the brachial plexus are injuries resulting from excessive displacement of the head to the opposite side and depression of the shoulder on the same side. This causes excessive traction or even tearing of C5 and 6 roots of the plexus. It occurs in infants during a difficult delivery or in adults after a blow to or fall on the shoulder. The suprascapular nerve, the nerve to the subclavius, and the musculocutaneous and axillary nerves all possess nerve fibers derived from C5 and 6 roots and will therefore be functionless. The following muscles will consequently be paralyzed: the supraspinatus (abductor of the shoulder) and infraspinatus (lateral rotator of the shoulder); the subclavius (depresses the clavicle); the biceps brachii (supinator of the forearm, flexor of the elbow, weak flexor of the shoulder) and the greater part of the brachialis (flexor of the elbow) and the coracobrachialis (flexes the shoulder); and the deltoid (abductor of the shoulder) and the teres minor (lateral rotator of the shoulder).

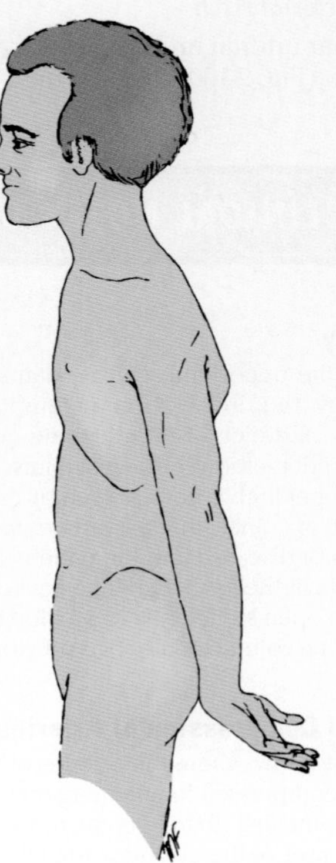

Figure 9-101 Erb-Duchenne palsy (waiter's tip).

(continues)

Clinical Notes, *continued*

Thus, the limb will hang limply by the side, medially rotated by the unopposed sternocostal part of the pectoralis major; the forearm will be pronated because of loss of the action of the biceps. The position of the upper limb in this condition has been likened to that of a porter or waiter hinting for a tip (Fig. 9-101). In addition, there will be a loss of sensation down the lateral side of the arm.

Lower Lesions of the Brachial Plexus (Klumpke Palsy)

Lower lesions of the brachial plexus are usually traction injuries caused by excessive abduction of the arm, as occurs in the case of a person falling from a height clutching at an object to save himself or herself. The first thoracic nerve is usually torn. The nerve fibers from this segment run in the ulnar and median nerves to supply **all the small muscles of the hand.** The hand has a clawed appearance caused by hyperextension of the metacarpophalangeal joints and flexion of the interphalangeal joints. The extensor digitorum is unopposed by the lumbricals and interossei and extends the metacarpophalangeal joints; the flexor digitorum superficialis and profundus are unopposed by the lumbricals and interossei and flex the middle and terminal phalanges, respectively. In addition, loss of sensation will occur along the medial side of the arm. If the eighth cervical nerve is also damaged, the extent of anesthesia will be greater and will involve the medial side of the forearm, hand, and medial two fingers.

Lower lesions of the brachial plexus can also be produced by the presence of a cervical rib or malignant metastases from the lungs in the lower deep cervical lymph nodes.

Long Thoracic Nerve

The long thoracic nerve, which arises from C5, 6, and 7 and supplies the serratus anterior muscle, can be injured by blows to or pressure on the posterior triangle of the neck or during the surgical procedure of radical mastectomy. Paralysis of the serratus anterior results in the inability to rotate the scapula during the movement of abduction of the arm above a right angle. The patient therefore experiences difficulty in raising the arm above the head. The vertebral border and inferior angle of the scapula will no longer be kept closely applied to the chest wall and will protrude posteriorly, a condition known as **"winged scapula"** (Fig. 9-8).

Axillary Nerve

The axillary nerve (Fig. 9-24), which arises from the posterior cord of the brachial plexus (C5 and 6), can be injured by the pressure of a badly adjusted crutch pressing upward into the armpit. The passage of the axillary nerve backward from the axilla through the quadrangular space makes it particularly vulnerable here to downward displacement of the humeral head in shoulder dislocations or fractures of the surgical neck of the humerus. Paralysis of the deltoid and teres minor muscles results. The cutaneous branches of the axillary nerve, including the upper lateral cutaneous nerve of the arm, are functionless, and consequently there is a loss of skin sensation over the **lower half** of the deltoid muscle. The paralyzed deltoid wastes rapidly, and the underlying greater tuberosity can be readily palpated. Because the supraspinatus is the only other abductor of the shoulder, this movement is much impaired. Paralysis of the teres minor is not recognizable clinically.

Radial Nerve

The radial nerve (Fig. 9-25), which arises from the posterior cord of the brachial plexus, characteristically gives off its branches some distance proximal to the part to be innervated.

In the axilla it gives off three branches: the posterior cutaneous nerve of the arm, which supplies the skin on the back of the arm down to the elbow; the nerve to the long head of the triceps; and the nerve to the medial head of the triceps.

In the spiral groove of the humerus it gives off four branches: the lower lateral cutaneous nerve of the arm, which supplies the lateral surface of the arm down to the elbow; the posterior cutaneous nerve of the forearm, which supplies the skin down the middle of the back of the forearm as far as the wrist; the nerve to the lateral head of the triceps; and the nerve to the medial head of the triceps and the anconeus.

In the anterior compartment of the arm above the lateral epicondyle it gives off three branches: the nerve to a small part of the brachialis, the nerve to the brachioradialis, and the nerve to the extensor carpi radialis longus.

In the cubital fossa it gives off the deep branch of the radial nerve and continues as the superficial radial nerve. The deep branch supplies the extensor carpi radialis brevis and the supinator in the cubital fossa and all the extensor muscles in the posterior compartment of the forearm. The superficial radial nerve is sensory and supplies the skin over the lateral part of the dorsum of the hand and the dorsal surface of the lateral three and a half fingers proximal to the nail beds (Fig. 9-102). (The ulnar nerve supplies the medial part of the dorsum of the hand and the dorsal surface of the medial one and a half fingers; the exact cutaneous areas innervated by the radial and ulnar nerves on the hand are subject to variation.)

The radial nerve is commonly damaged in the axilla and in the spiral groove.

Injuries to the Radial Nerve in the Axilla

In the axilla the nerve can be injured by the pressure of the upper end of a badly fitting crutch pressing up into the armpit or by a drunkard falling asleep with one arm over the back of a chair. It can also be badly damaged in the axilla by fractures and dislocations of the proximal end of the humerus. When the humerus is displaced downward in dislocations of the shoulder, the radial nerve, which is wrapped around the back of the shaft of the bone, is pulled downward, stretching the nerve in the axilla excessively.

The clinical findings in injury to the radial nerve in the axilla are as follows.

Motor

The triceps, the anconeus, and the long extensors of the wrist are paralyzed. The patient is unable to extend the elbow joint, the wrist joint, and the fingers. Wristdrop, or flexion of the wrist (Fig. 9-103), occurs as a result of the action of the unopposed flexor muscles of the wrist. Wristdrop is very disabling because one is unable to flex the fingers strongly for the purpose of firmly gripping an object with the wrist fully flexed. (Try it on yourself.) If the wrist and proximal phalanges are passively extended by holding them in position with the opposite hand, the middle and distal phalanges of the fingers can be extended by the action of the lumbricals and interossei, which are inserted into the extensor expansions.

The brachioradialis and supinator muscles are also paralyzed, but supination is still performed well by the biceps brachii.

Sensory

A small loss of skin sensation occurs down the posterior surface of the lower part of the arm and down a narrow strip on the back of the forearm. A variable area of sensory loss is present on the lateral part of the dorsum of the hand and on the dorsal surface of the

(continues)

Clinical Notes, *continued*

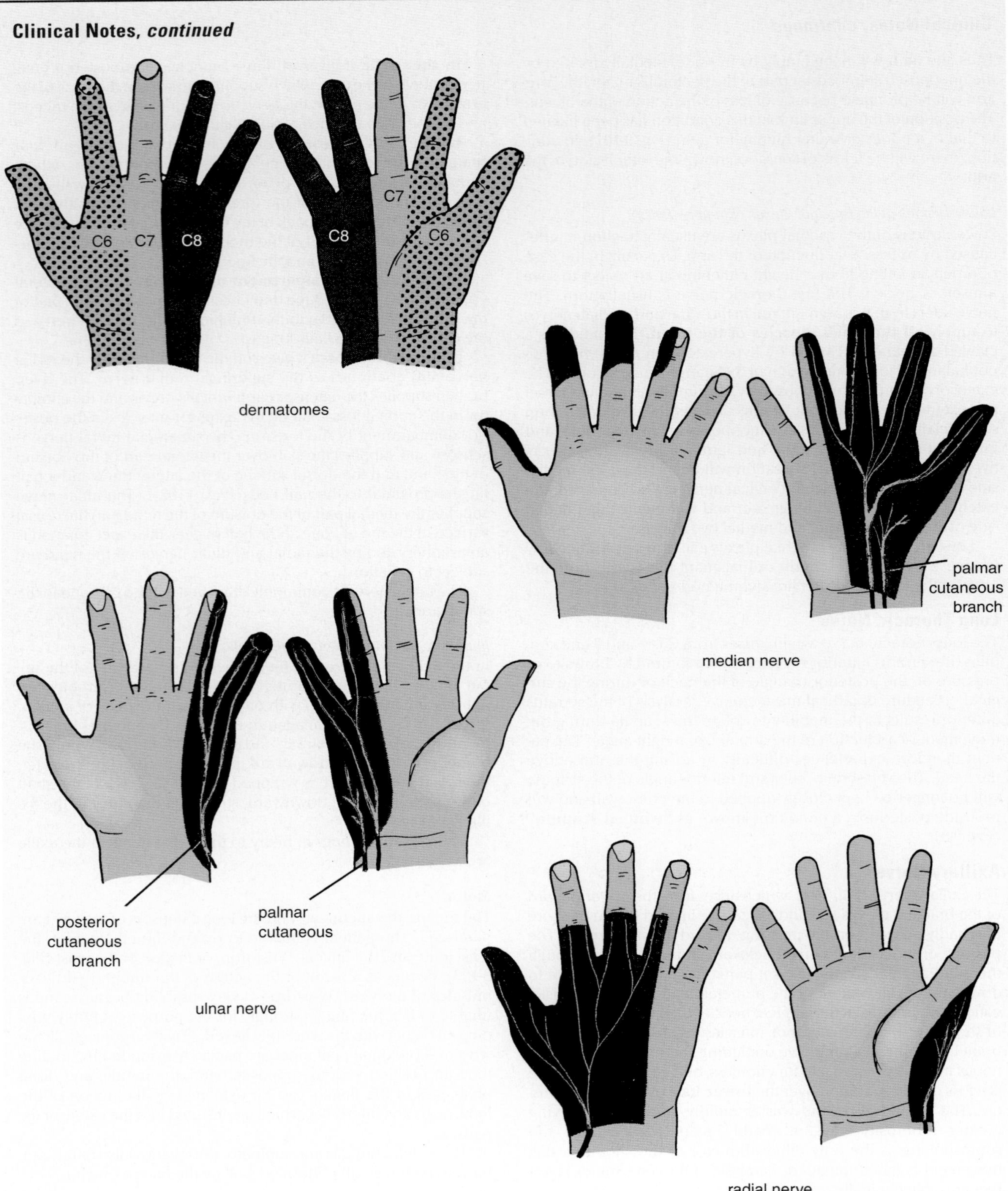

Figure 9-102 Sensory innervation of the skin of the volar (palmar) and dorsal aspects of the hand; the arrangement of the dermatomes is also shown.

(continues)

Clinical Notes, *continued*

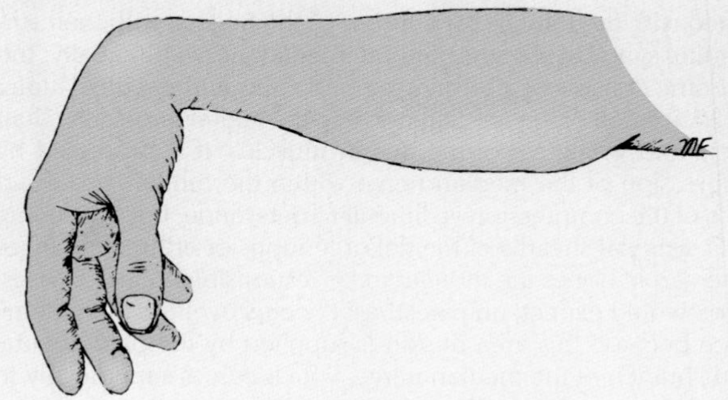

Figure 9-103 Wristdrop.

roots of the lateral three and a half fingers. The area of total anesthesia is relatively small because of the overlap of sensory innervation by adjacent nerves.

Trophic Changes

Trophic changes are slight.

Injuries to the Radial Nerve in the Spiral Groove

In the spiral groove of the humerus, the radial nerve can be injured at the time of fracture of the shaft of the humerus, or subsequently involved during the formation of the callus. The pressure of the back of the arm on the edge of the operating table in an unconscious patient has also been known to injure the nerve at this site. The prolonged application of a tourniquet to the arm in a person with a slender triceps muscle is often followed by temporary radial palsy.

The clinical findings in injury to the radial nerve in the spiral groove are as follows.

The injury to the radial nerve occurs most commonly in the distal part of the groove, beyond the origin of the nerves to the triceps and the anconeus and beyond the origin of the cutaneous nerves.

- **Motor:** The patient is unable to extend the wrist and the fingers, and wristdrop occurs (see page 537).
- **Sensory:** A variable small area of anesthesia is present over the dorsal surface of the hand and the dorsal surface of the roots of the lateral three and a half fingers.
- **Trophic changes:** These are very slight or absent.

Injuries to the Deep Branch of the Radial Nerve

The deep branch of the radial nerve is a motor nerve to the extensor muscles in the posterior compartment of the forearm. It can be damaged in fractures of the proximal end of the radius or during dislocation of the radial head. The nerve supply to the supinator and the extensor carpi radialis longus will be undamaged, and because the latter muscle is powerful, it will keep the wrist joint extended, and wristdrop will not occur. No sensory loss occurs because this is a motor nerve.

Injuries to the Superficial Radial Nerve

Division of the superficial radial nerve, which is sensory, as in a stab wound, results in a variable small area of anesthesia over the dorsum of the hand and the dorsal surface of the roots of the lateral three and a half fingers.

Musculocutaneous Nerve

The musculocutaneous nerve (Fig. 9-22) is rarely injured because of its protected position beneath the biceps brachii muscle. If it is injured high up in the arm, the biceps and coracobrachialis are paralyzed and the brachialis muscle is weakened (the latter muscle is also supplied by the radial nerve). Flexion of the forearm at the elbow joint is then produced by the remainder of the brachialis muscle and the flexors of the forearm. When the forearm is in the prone position, the extensor carpi radialis longus and the brachioradialis muscles assist in flexion of the forearm. There is also sensory loss along the lateral side of the forearm. Wounds or cuts of the forearm can sever the lateral cutaneous nerve of the forearm, a continuation of the musculocutaneous nerve beyond the cubital fossa, resulting in sensory loss along the lateral side of the forearm.

Median Nerve

The median nerve (Fig. 9-22), which arises from the medial and lateral cords of the brachial plexus, gives off no cutaneous or motor branches in the axilla or in the arm. In the proximal third of the front of the forearm, by unnamed branches or by its anterior interosseous branch, it supplies all the muscles of the front of the forearm except the flexor carpi ulnaris and the medial half of the flexor digitorum profundus, which are supplied by the ulnar nerve. In the distal third of the forearm, it gives rise to a palmar cutaneous branch, which crosses in front of the flexor retinaculum and supplies the skin on the lateral half of the palm (Fig. 9-102). In the palm the median nerve supplies the muscles of the thenar eminence and the first two lumbricals and gives sensory innervation to the skin of the palmar aspect of the lateral three and a half fingers, including the nail beds on the dorsum.

From a clinical standpoint, the median nerve is injured occasionally in the elbow region in supracondylar fractures of the humerus. It is most commonly injured by stab wounds or broken glass just proximal to the flexor retinaculum; here it lies in the interval between the tendons of the flexor carpi radialis and flexor digitorum superficialis, overlapped by the palmaris longus.

The clinical findings in injury to the median nerve are as follows.

Injuries to the Median Nerve at the Elbow

Motor

The pronator muscles of the forearm and the long flexor muscles of the wrist and fingers, with the exception of the flexor carpi ulnaris and the medial half of the flexor digitorum profundus, will be paralyzed. As a result, the forearm is kept in the supine position; wrist flexion is weak and is accompanied by adduction. The latter deviation is caused by the paralysis of the flexor carpi radialis and the strength of the flexor carpi ulnaris and the medial half of the flexor digitorum profundus. No flexion is possible at the interphalangeal joints of the index and middle fingers, although weak flexion of the metacarpophalangeal joints of these fingers is attempted by the interossei. When the patient tries to make a fist, the index and to a lesser extent the middle fingers tend to remain straight, whereas the ring and little fingers flex (Fig. 9-104). The latter two fingers are, however, weakened by the loss of the flexor digitorum superficialis.

Flexion of the terminal phalanx of the thumb is lost because of paralysis of the flexor pollicis longus. The muscles of the thenar eminence are paralyzed and wasted so that the eminence is flattened. The thumb is laterally rotated and adducted. The hand looks flattened and "apelike."

(continues)

Clinical Notes, *continued*

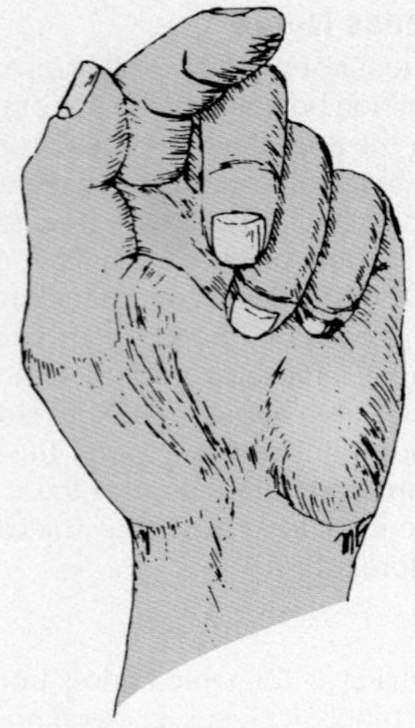

Figure 9-104 Median nerve palsy.

Sensory

Skin sensation is lost on the lateral half or less of the palm of the hand and the palmar aspect of the lateral three and a half fingers. Sensory loss also occurs on the skin of the distal part of the dorsal surfaces of the lateral three and a half fingers. The area of total anesthesia is considerably less because of the overlap of adjacent nerves.

Vasomotor Changes

The skin areas involved in sensory loss are warmer and drier than normal because of the arteriolar dilatation and absence of sweating resulting from loss of sympathetic control.

Trophic Changes

In long-standing cases, changes are found in the hand and fingers. The skin is dry and scaly, the nails crack easily, and atrophy of the pulp of the fingers is present.

Injuries to the Median Nerve at the Wrist

- **Motor:** The muscles of the thenar eminence are paralyzed and wasted so that the eminence becomes flattened. The thumb is laterally rotated and adducted. The hand looks flattened and "apelike." Opposition movement of the thumb is impossible. The first two lumbricals are paralyzed, which can be recognized clinically when the patient is asked to make a fist slowly, and the index and middle fingers tend to lag behind the ring and little fingers.
- **Sensory, vasomotor, and trophic changes:** These changes are identical to those found in the elbow lesions.

Perhaps the most serious disability of all in median nerve injuries is the loss of the ability to oppose the thumb to the other fingers and the loss of sensation over the lateral fingers. The delicate pincerlike action of the hand is no longer possible.

Carpal Tunnel Syndrome

The carpal tunnel, formed by the concave anterior surface of the carpal bones and closed by the flexor retinaculum, is tightly packed with the long flexor tendons of the fingers, with their surrounding synovial sheaths, and the median nerve. Clinically, the syndrome consists of a burning pain or "pins and needles" along the distribution of the median nerve to the lateral three and a half fingers and weakness of the thenar muscles. It is produced by compression of the median nerve within the tunnel. The exact cause of the compression is difficult to determine, but thickening of the synovial sheaths of the flexor tendons or arthritic changes in the carpal bones are thought to be responsible in many cases. As you would expect, no paresthesia occurs over the thenar eminence because this area of skin is supplied by the palmar cutaneous branch of the median nerve, which passes superficially to the flexor retinaculum. The condition is dramatically relieved by decompressing the tunnel by making a longitudinal incision through the flexor retinaculum.

Ulnar Nerve

The ulnar nerve (Fig. 9-23), which arises from the medial cord of the brachial plexus (C8 and T1), gives off no cutaneous or motor branches in the axilla or in the arm. As it enters the forearm from behind the medial epicondyle, it supplies the flexor carpi ulnaris and the medial half of the flexor digitorum profundus. In the distal third of the forearm, it gives off its palmar and posterior cutaneous branches. The palmar cutaneous branch supplies the skin over the hypothenar eminence; the posterior branch supplies the skin over the medial third of the dorsum of the hand and the medial one and a half fingers. Not uncommonly, the posterior branch supplies two and a half instead of one and a half fingers. It does not supply the skin over the distal part of the dorsum of these fingers.

Having entered the palm by passing in **front of the flexor retinaculum,** the **superficial branch** of the ulnar nerve supplies the skin of the palmar surface of the medial one and a half fingers (Fig. 9-102), including their nail beds; it also supplies the palmaris brevis muscle. The **deep branch** supplies all the small muscles of the hand except the muscles of the thenar eminence and the first two lumbricals, which are supplied by the median nerve.

The ulnar nerve is most commonly injured at the elbow, where it lies behind the medial epicondyle, and at the wrist, where it lies with the ulnar artery in front of the flexor retinaculum. The injuries at the elbow are usually associated with fractures of the medial epicondyle. The superficial position of the nerve at the wrist makes it vulnerable to damage from cuts and stab wounds.

The clinical findings in injury to the ulnar nerve are as follows.

Injuries to the Ulnar Nerve at the Elbow

Motor

The flexor carpi ulnaris and the medial half of the flexor digitorum profundus muscles are paralyzed. The paralysis of the flexor carpi ulnaris can be observed by asking the patient to make a tightly clenched fist. Normally, the synergistic action of the flexor carpi ulnaris tendon can be observed as it passes to the pisiform bone; the tightening of the tendon will be absent if the muscle is paralyzed. The profundus tendons to the ring and little fingers will be functionless, and the terminal phalanges of these fingers are therefore not capable of being markedly flexed. Flexion of the wrist joint will result in abduction, owing to paralysis of the flexor carpi ulnaris. The medial border of the front of the forearm will show flattening owing to the wasting of the underlying ulnaris and profundus muscles.

(continues)

Clinical Notes, *continued*

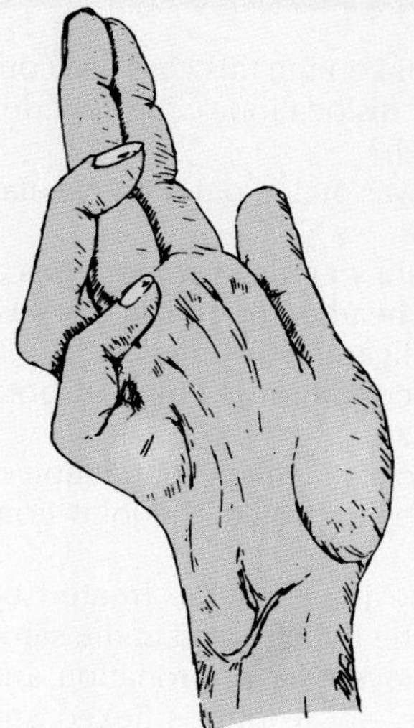

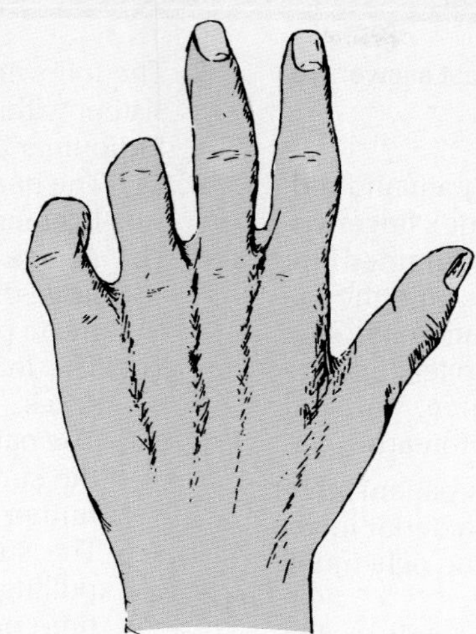

Figure 9-105 Ulnar nerve palsy.

The small muscles of the hand will be paralyzed, except the muscles of the thenar eminence and the first two lumbricals, which are supplied by the median nerve. The patient is unable to adduct and abduct the fingers and consequently is unable to grip a piece of paper placed between the fingers. Remember that the extensor digitorum can abduct the fingers to a small extent, but only when the metacarpophalangeal joints are hyperextended.

It is impossible to adduct the thumb because the adductor pollicis muscle is paralyzed. If the patient is asked to grip a piece of paper between the thumb and the index finger, he or she does so by strongly contracting the flexor pollicis longus and flexing the terminal phalanx **(Froment's sign).**

The metacarpophalangeal joints become hyperextended because of the paralysis of the lumbrical and interosseous muscles, which normally flex these joints. Because the first and second lumbricals are not paralyzed (they are supplied by the median nerve), the hyperextension of the metacarpophalangeal joints is most prominent in the fourth and fifth fingers. The interphalangeal joints are flexed, owing again to the paralysis of the lumbrical and interosseous muscles, which normally extend these joints through the extensor expansion. The flexion deformity at the interphalangeal joints of the fourth and fifth fingers is obvious because the first and second lumbrical muscles of the index and middle fingers are not paralyzed. In long-standing cases the hand assumes the characteristic "claw" deformity (main en griffe). Wasting of the paralyzed muscles results in flattening of the hypothenar eminence and loss of the convex curve to the medial border of the hand. Examination of the dorsum of the hand will show hollowing between the metacarpal bones caused by wasting of the dorsal interosseous muscles (Fig. 9-105).

Sensory

Loss of skin sensation will be observed over the anterior and posterior surfaces of the medial third of the hand and the medial one and a half fingers.

Vasomotor Changes

The skin areas involved in sensory loss are warmer and drier than normal because of the arteriolar dilatation and absence of sweating resulting from loss of sympathetic control.

Injuries to the Ulnar Nerve at the Wrist

- **Motor:** The small muscles of the hand will be paralyzed and show wasting, except for the muscles of the thenar eminence and the first two lumbricals, as described (see previous column). The clawhand is much more obvious in wrist lesions because the flexor digitorum profundus muscle is not paralyzed, and marked flexion of the terminal phalanges occurs.
- **Sensory:** The main ulnar nerve and its palmar cutaneous branch are usually severed; the posterior cutaneous branch, which arises from the ulnar nerve trunk about 2.5 in. (6.25 cm) above the pisiform bone, is usually unaffected. The sensory loss will therefore be confined to the palmar surface of the medial third of the hand and the medial one and a half fingers and to the dorsal aspects of the middle and distal phalanges of the same fingers.
- **Vasomotor and trophic changes:** These are the same as those described for injuries at the elbow. It is important to remember that with ulnar nerve injuries, the higher the lesion, the less obvious the clawing deformity of the hand.

Unlike median nerve injuries, lesions of the ulnar nerve leave a relatively efficient hand. The sensation over the lateral part of the hand is intact, and the pincerlike action of the thumb and index finger is reasonably good, although there is some weakness owing to loss of the adductor pollicis.

CLINICAL PROBLEM SOLVING

Study the following case histories and select the best answers to the question following them.

An 18-year-old woman complaining of severe pain and redness around the base of the nail of the right index finger visited her physician. She stated that she had trimmed the cuticle (eponychium) of her nail with scissors, and the following day the pain commenced. On examination, the skin folds around the root of the nail were red, swollen, and extremely tender. The index finger was swollen, and red streaks were seen coursing up the front of the forearm.

1. The following symptoms and signs in this patient were consistent with a diagnosis of an acute bacterial infection under the nail folds (paronychia) of the right index finger except which?
   (a) Some tender lymph nodules could be palpated in the infraclavicular fossa.
   (b) The patient's temperature was raised.
   (c) The infection had spread into the lymph vessels draining the finger.
   (d) The red streaks on the front of the forearm were caused by the local vasodilatation of the blood vessels along the course of the lymph vessels.
   (e) The lymph vessels from the index finger drain into the supratrochlear node, which was inflamed and enlarged.

A 20-year-old man, riding pillion on a snowmobile, was involved in an accident. The machine was traveling at high speed when it hit a tree stump buried in snow. The man was thrown 12 ft. and landed on his right shoulder and the right side of his head. After 3 weeks of hospitalization, it was noticed that he kept his right arm internally rotated by his side with the forearm pronated. An area of anesthesia was present along the lateral side of the upper part of the arm.

2. The following statements concerning this patient are correct except which?
   (a) A diagnosis of damage to the upper part of the brachial plexus (Erb-Duchenne palsy) was made.
   (b) A lesion of the fifth and sixth cervical roots of the brachial plexus was present.
   (c) The median radial ulnar nerve was made functionless.
   (d) The supraspinatus, infraspinatus, subclavius, biceps brachii, greater part of the brachialis, coracobrachialis, deltoid, and teres minor were paralyzed.
   (e) The loss of sensation down the lateral side of the right arm was caused by the lesion involving the fifth and sixth cervical dermatomes.

A father, seeing his 3-year-old son playing in the garden, ran up and picked him up by both hands and swung him around in a circle. The child's enjoyment suddenly turned to tears, and he said his left elbow hurt. On examination, the child held his left elbow joint semiflexed and his forearm pronated.

3. The following statements concerning this case are consistent with the diagnosis of dislocation of the superior radioulnar joint except which?
   (a) The head of the radius was pulled out of the anular ligament.
   (b) At age 3 years, the child's anular ligament has a large diameter and the head of the radius can easily be pulled out of the ligament by traction.
   (c) The incidence of this condition is equal in both sexes.
   (d) The pain from the joint caused reflex contraction of the surrounding muscles to protect the joint from further movement.
   (e) The subluxation of the joint can be treated by pulling downward on the forearm and at the same time performing the movement of pronation and supination. Finally, the elbow joint is flexed and held in that position.

A 60-year-old woman fell down the stairs and was admitted to the emergency department with severe right shoulder pain. On examination, the patient was sitting up with her right arm by her side and her right elbow joint supported by the left hand. Inspection of the right shoulder showed loss of the normal rounded curvature and evidence of a slight swelling below the right clavicle. Any attempt at active or passive movement of the shoulder joint was stopped by severe pain in the shoulder. A diagnosis of dislocation of the right shoulder joint was made.

4. The following statements concerning this patient are consistent with the diagnosis except which?
   (a) This patient had a subcoracoid dislocation of the right shoulder joint.
   (b) The head of the humerus was dislocated downward through the weakest part of the capsule of the joint.
   (c) The pull of the pectoralis major and subscapularis muscles had displaced the upper end of the humerus medially.
   (d) The greater tuberosity of the humerus no longer displaced the deltoid muscle laterally, and the curve of the shoulder was lost.
   (e) The integrity of the axillary nerve should always be tested by touching the skin over the upper half of the deltoid muscle.

A 45-year-old woman having her yearly physical examination was found the have a hard, painless lump in the upper lateral quadrant of the left breast. On examination with her arms at her sides, the left nipple was seen to be higher than the right, and a small dimple of skin was noted over the lump. On examination of the left axilla, three small, hard discrete nodules could be palpated below the lower border of the pectoralis major muscle. The right breast was normal. A diagnosis of carcinoma of the left breast was made, with secondary deposits in the axilla.

5. The following statements concerning this patient are correct except which?
   (a) The contracting fibrous tissue of the malignant tumor had pulled on the lactiferous ducts of the nipple, raising it above the level of the opposite nipple.
   (b) The dimpling of the skin was caused by the fibrous tissue pulling on the suspensory ligaments of the breast.
   (c) The upper lateral quadrant of the breast is drained into the pectoral or anterior axillary lymph nodes.
   (d) The enlarged pectoral lymph nodes could be palpated against the surgical neck of the humerus.
   (e) The malignant tumor had spread by way of the lymph vessels to the pectoral lymph nodes.

A young secretary, running from her office, had a glass door swing back in her face. To protect herself, she held out her left hand, which smashed through the glass. On admission to the hospital, she was bleeding profusely from a superficial laceration in front of her left wrist. She had sensory loss over the palmar aspect of the medial one and a half fingers but normal sensation of the back of these fingers over the middle and proximal phalanges. She had difficulty in grasping a piece of paper between her left index and middle fingers. All her long flexor tendons were intact.

6. The following statements concerning this patient are correct except which?
   (a) The radial artery was cut in front of the flexor retinaculum, and this accounted for the profuse bleeding.
   (b) The loss of skin sensation on the palmar aspect of the medial one and a half fingers was caused by the severance of the ulnar nerve as it crossed in front of the flexor retinaculum.
   (c) The normal sensation on the back of the medial one and a half fingers over the proximal phalanges was caused by the fact that the posterior cutaneous branch of the ulnar nerve arises about 2.5 in. (6.25 cm) proximal to the flexor retinaculum and was spared.
   (d) The inability to hold the piece of paper was caused by the paralysis of the second palmar interosseous muscle, which is supplied by the deep branch of the ulnar nerve.
   (e) There was no sensory loss on the palm of the hand because the palmar cutaneous branch of the ulnar nerve was not cut.

A 50-year-old woman complaining of severe "pins and needles" in her right hand and lateral fingers visited her physician. She said that she had experienced difficulty in buttoning up her clothes when dressing. On physical examination the patient pointed to her thumb and index, middle, and ring fingers as the areas where she felt discomfort. No objective impairment of sensation was found in these areas. The muscles of the thenar eminence appeared to be functioning normally, although there was some loss of power compared with the activity of the muscles of the left thenar eminence.

7. The following statements concerning this patient are correct except which?
   (a) Altered skin sensation was felt in the skin areas supplied by the digital branches of the median nerve.
   (b) The muscles of the thenar eminence showed some evidence of wasting as seen by flattening of the thenar eminence.
   (c) The muscles of the thenar eminence are supplied by the recurrent muscular branch of the median nerve.
   (d) The median nerve enters the palm through the carpal tunnel.
   (e) The median nerve occupies a large space between the tendons behind the flexor retinaculum.
   (f) This patient has carpal tunnel syndrome.

A 64-year-old man consulted his physician because he had noticed during the past 6 months a thickening of the skin at the base of his left ring finger. As he described it: "There appears to be a band of tissue that is pulling my ring finger into the palm." On examination of the palms of both hands, a localized thickening of subcutaneous tissue could be felt at the base of the left ring and little fingers. The metacarpophalangeal joint of the ring finger could not be fully extended, either actively or passively.

8. The following statements concerning this patient are correct except which?
   (a) The deep fascia beneath the skin of the palm is thickened to form the palmar aponeurosis.
   (b) The distal end of the aponeurosis gives rise to five slips to the five fingers.
   (c) Each slip is attached to the base of the proximal phalanx and to the fibrous flexor sheath of each finger.
   (d) Fibrous contraction of the slip to the ring finger resulted in permanent flexion of the metacarpophalangeal joint.
   (e) The patient had Dupuytren's contracture.

A 15-year-old girl, while demonstrating to her friends her proficiency at standing on her hands, suddenly went off balance and put all her body weight on her left outstretched hand. A distinctive cracking noise was heard, and she felt a sudden pain in her left shoulder region. On examination in the emergency department, the smooth contour of her left shoulder was absent. The clavicle was obviously fractured, and the edges of the bony fragments could be palpated.

9. The following statements concerning this case are correct except which?
   (a) The clavicle is one of the most common bones in the body to be fractured.
   (b) Anatomically, the weakest part of the clavicle is the junction of the medial and middle thirds, and this is where the fracture commonly occurs.
   (c) The lateral bony fragment is depressed downward by the weight of the arm.
   (d) The lateral fragment is pulled forward and medially by the pectoral muscles.
   (e) The medial fragment is elevated by the sternocleidomastoid muscle.
   (f) The supraclavicular nerves or a communicating vein between the cephalic and internal jugular vein may be damaged by the bone fragments.

A 63-year-old man fell down a flight of stairs and sustained a fracture of the lower end of the left radius. On examination the distal end of the radius was displaced posteriorly. This patient had sustained a Colles' fracture.

10. The following statements concerning this case are correct except which?
    (a) Occasionally the styloid process of the ulna is also fractured.
    (b) The median nerve may be injured at the time of the fall.
    (c) When the fracture is reduced, the styloid process of the radius should come to lie about 0.75 in. (1.9 cm) proximal to that of the ulna.
    (d) The fracture produces posterior angulation of the distal fragment of the radius.
    (e) On reduction of the fracture the distal end of the radius should lie at an angle of 15° anteriorly.
    (f) The hand should always be splinted in the position of function.

A 22-year-old medical student fell off her bicycle onto her outstretched hand. She thought she had sprained her right wrist joint and treated herself by binding her wrist with an elastic bandage. But 3 weeks later, she was still experiencing pain on moving her wrist and so decided to visit the emergency department. On examination of the dorsal surfaces of both hands, with the fingers and thumbs fully extended, a localized tenderness could be felt in the anatomic snuffbox of her right hand. A diagnosis of fracture of the right scaphoid bone was made.

11. The following statements concerning this patient are correct except which?
    (a) The fracture line on the scaphoid bone may deprive the proximal fragment of its arterial supply.
    (b) A bony fragment deprived of its blood supply may undergo ischemic necrosis.
    (c) Because the scaphoid bone articulates with other bones, the fracture line may enter a joint cavity and become bathed in synovial fluid, which would inhibit repair.
    (d) The scaphoid bone is an easy bone to immobilize because of its small size.
    (e) Fractures of the scaphoid bone have a high incidence of nonunion.

A 6-year-old boy, running along a concrete path with a glass jam jar in his hand, slipped and fell. The glass from the broken jar pierced the skin on the front of his left wrist. On examination a small wound was present on the front of the left wrist and the palmaris longus tendon had been severed. The thumb was laterally rotated and adducted, and the boy was unable to oppose his thumb to the other fingers. There was loss of skin sensation over the lateral half of the palm and the palmar aspect of the lateral three and a half fingers.

12. The following facts concerning this patient are correct except which?
    (a) Sensory loss of the distal part of the dorsal surfaces of the lateral three and a half fingers was experienced.
    (b) The median nerve lies superficial to the palmaris longus proximal to the flexor retinaculum and was severed by the piece of glass.
    (c) The median nerve lies in the interval between the tendons of flexor digitorum superficialis and the flexor carpi radialis muscles just proximal to the wrist joint.
    (d) Adduction of the thumb was produced by the contraction of the adductor pollicis muscle, which is supplied by the ulnar nerve.
    (e) The palmar cutaneous branch of the median nerve had been severed.

ANSWERS TO CLINICAL PROBLEMS

1. E. The lymph vessels from the index finger drain into the infraclavicular nodes.
2. C. The suprascapular nerve, the nerve to the subclavius, the musculocutaneous nerve, and the axillary nerve were made functionless.
3. B. Under age 6 years, the child's head of the radius is of a relatively small size and may easily be pulled out of the anular ligament by traction on the forearm.
4. E. The integrity of the axillary nerve is tested by touching the skin over the lower half of the deltoid muscle. The skin of the curve of the shoulder, including the skin covering the upper half of the deltoid muscle, is supplied by the supraclavicular nerves.
5. D. The enlarged pectoral lymph nodes can be palpated against the posterior surface of the contracted pectoralis major muscle.
6. A. The radial artery does not enter the palm by passing in front of the flexor retinaculum; it does so by passing forward between the two heads of the first dorsal interosseous muscles between the first and second metacarpal bones. It was the ulnar artery that was cut with the ulnar nerve in front of the flexor retinaculum.
7. E. The median nerve occupies a small restricted space in the carpal tunnel.
8. B. The distal end of the palmar aponeurosis gives rise to four slips, which pass to the four medial fingers.
9. B. Anatomically, the weakest part of the clavicle is the junction of the middle and lateral thirds, and that is where the fracture occurred in this patient.
10. C. The normal position of the tip of the styloid process of the radius is about 0.75 in. (1.9 cm) distal to that of the ulna.
11. D. The scaphoid bone is a difficult bone to immobilize because of its position and small size.
12. B. The median nerve lies deep to the palmaris longus tendon proximal to the flexor retinaculum.

REVIEW QUESTIONS

Multiple-Choice Questions

Select the best answer for each question.

1. The following structures pass posterior to the flexor retinaculum except which?
   (a) Flexor digitorum superficialis tendons
   (b) Median nerve
   (c) Flexor pollicis longus tendon
   (d) Ulnar nerve
   (e) Anterior interosseous nerve
2. The following tendons are inserted into the base of the proximal phalanx of the thumb except which?
   (a) Extensor pollicis brevis
   (b) Abductor pollicis longus
   (c) Oblique head of adductor pollicis
   (d) Flexor pollicis brevis
   (e) First palmar interosseous
3. The following muscles abduct the hand at the wrist joint except which?
   (a) Flexor carpi radialis
   (b) Abductor pollicis longus
   (c) Extensor carpi radialis longus
   (d) Extensor digiti minimi
   (e) Extensor pollicis longus
4. The following bones form the proximal row of carpal bones except which?
   (a) Lunate
   (b) Pisiform
   (c) Scaphoid
   (d) Triquetral
   (e) Trapezium
5. The tendons of the following muscles form the rotator cuff except which?
   (a) Teres minor
   (b) Supraspinatus
   (c) Subscapularis
   (d) Teres major
   (e) Infraspinatus
6. The quadrangular space is bounded by the following structures except which?
   (a) Surgical neck of the humerus
   (b) Long head of triceps
   (c) Deltoid
   (d) Teres major
   (e) Teres minor
7. The radial nerve gives off the following branches in the posterior compartment of the arm except which?
   (a) Lateral head of the triceps
   (b) Lower lateral cutaneous nerve of the arm
   (c) Medial head of the triceps
   (d) Brachioradialis
   (e) Anconeus
8. All the following statements concerning the brachial plexus are correct except which?
   (a) The roots C8 and T1 join to form the lower trunk.
   (b) The cords are named according to their position relative to the first part of the axillary artery.
   (c) The nerve that innervates the levator scapulae is a branch of the upper trunk.
   (d) The roots, trunks, and divisions are not located in the axilla.
   (e) No nerves originate as branches from the individual divisions of the brachial plexus.
9. The anterior fascial compartment of the forearm contains the following arteries except which?
   (a) Brachial
   (b) Anterior interosseous
   (c) Radial
   (d) Ulnar
   (e) Profunda
10. The boundaries of the anatomic snuffbox include the following except which?
    (a) Abductor pollicis brevis
    (b) Extensor pollicis longus
    (c) Extensor pollicis brevis
    (d) Abductor pollicis longus
11. The following structures are attached to the greater tuberosity of the humerus except which?
    (a) Supraspinatus muscle
    (b) Coracohumeral ligament
    (c) Teres minor muscle
    (d) Infraspinatus muscle
    (e) Subscapularis muscle
12. The following structures form the boundaries to the superior entrance into the axilla except which?
    (a) Clavicle
    (b) Coracoid process
    (c) Upper border of the scapula
    (d) Outer border of the first rib
13. The carpal tunnel contains the following important structures except which?
    (a) Flexor pollicis longus tendon
    (b) Flexor digitorum profundus tendons
    (c) Median nerve
    (d) Flexor carpi radialis tendon
    (e) Flexor digitorum superficialis tendons

Completion Questions

Select the phrase that best completes each statement.

14. Hyperextension of the proximal phalanges of the little and ring fingers (i.e., claw hand) can result from damage to the ________ nerve.
    (a) ulnar
    (b) axillary
    (c) radial
    (d) median
    (e) anterior interosseous
15. Wrist drop can result from damage to the ________ nerve.
    (a) median

(b) ulnar
(c) radial
(d) anterior interosseous
(e) axillary

16. An inability to oppose the thumb to the little finger can result from damage to the ________ nerve.
(a) anterior interosseous
(b) posterior interosseous
(c) radial
(d) ulnar
(e) median

17. The sensory innervation of the nail bed of the index finger is the
(a) median nerve.
(b) radial nerve.
(c) dorsal cutaneous branch of the ulnar nerve.
(d) superficial branch of the ulnar nerve.
(e) palmar cutaneous branch of the ulnar nerve.

18. The sensory innervation of the medial side of the palm is the
(a) radial nerve.
(b) palmar cutaneous branch of the ulnar nerve.
(c) dorsal cutaneous branch of the ulnar nerve.
(d) median nerve.
(e) superficial branch of the ulnar nerve.

19. The sensory innervation of the dorsal surface of the root of the thumb is the
(a) median nerve.
(b) radial nerve.
(c) superficial branch of the ulnar nerve.
(d) dorsal cutaneous branch of the ulnar nerve.
(e) posterior interosseous nerve.

20. The sensory innervation of the medial side of the palmar aspect of the ring finger is the
(a) radial nerve.
(b) posterior interosseous nerve.
(c) dorsal cutaneous branch of the ulnar nerve.
(d) median nerve.
(e) superficial branch of the ulnar nerve.

21. The musculocutaneous nerve originates from the ________ of the brachial plexus.
(a) posterior cord
(b) lateral cord
(c) both medial and lateral cords
(d) upper trunk
(e) medial cord

22. The suprascapular nerve originates from the ________ of the brachial plexus.
(a) medial cord
(b) lower trunk
(c) posterior cord
(d) lateral cord
(e) upper trunk

23. The median nerve originates from the ________ of the brachial plexus.
(a) medial and lateral cords
(b) medial cord
(c) posterior cord
(d) upper and lower trunk
(e) lateral cord

24. The thoracodorsal nerve originates from the ________ of the brachial plexus.
(a) lateral cord
(b) posterior cord
(c) medial cord
(d) medial and posterior cords
(e) lower trunk

25. The axillary nerve originates from the ________ of the brachial plexus.
(a) posterior cord
(b) middle trunk
(c) lateral cord
(d) lower trunk
(e) medial cord

26. The lymph from the upper lateral quadrant of the breast drains mainly into the
(a) lateral axillary nodes
(b) internal thoracic nodes
(c) posterior axillary nodes
(d) anterior axillary nodes
(e) deltopectoral group of nodes

27. The medial collateral ligament of the elbow joint is closely related to the
(a) brachial artery
(b) radial nerve
(c) ulnar nerve
(d) basilic vein
(e) ulnar artery

Multiple-Choice Questions

Read the case histories and select the best answer to the question following them.

A patient was seen in the emergency department with a laceration of the skin over the middle phalanx of the right index finger. After carefully examining the patient, the physician decided to suture the wound under a digital nerve block.

28. The site of the anesthetic injection depended on the following statements except which?
(a) The skin of the right index finger over the middle phalanx is innervated anteriorly by two digital branches of the median nerve.
(b) The skin of the right index finger over the middle phalanx is innervated posteriorly by two digital branches of the superficial radial nerve.
(c) These nerves can easily be blocked by injecting small volumes of anesthetic solution around the base of the finger.
(d) The digital nerves to the fingers are difficult to inject because they are imbedded in tough deep fascia.
(e) Provided that the wound was clean and did not become infected, the healing process should take place without any complications and full return of skin sensation should occur.

A 46-year-old man was involved in an automobile accident and sustained a tear of the capsule of the carpometacarpal joint of his right thumb. In view of his history of lung disease, it was decided to repair the laceration under a brachial plexus nerve block. The orthopedic surgeon decided to inject the anesthetic into the brachial plexus below the clavicle.

29. The injection procedure depended on the following statements except which?
    (a) The brachial plexus lies in the axilla and is formed from the anterior rami of C5 through C8 and T1 spinal nerves.
    (b) The axillary sheath is formed of deep fascia and surrounds the axillary artery and the brachial plexus.
    (c) The arm is abducted to an angle greater than 90° so that the axillary artery could be palpated high up in the axilla.
    (d) The anesthetic blocking needle is inserted into the sheath.
    (e) The cords and branches of the brachial plexus, including the musculocutaneous nerve, lie within the sheath, and all the branches are blocked by the anesthetic using this approach.

ANSWERS TO REVIEW QUESTIONS

1. D. The ulnar nerve passes superficial to the flexor retinaculum just lateral to the pisiform bone.
2. B. The abductor pollicis longus is inserted into the base of the first metacarpal bone.
3. D. The extensor digiti minimi extends the metacarpophalangeal joint of the little finger and adducts the hand at the wrist joint.
4. E. The trapezium is in the distal row of carpal bones.
5. D. The teres major tendon is inserted into the medial lip of the bicipital groove of the humerus.
6. C
7. D. The branch from the radial nerve to the brachioradialis muscle leaves the nerve after it has left the posterior compartment of the arm by piercing the lateral intermuscular septum.
8. B. The cords are named according to their relative position to the second part of the axillary artery as it lies behind the pectoralis minor muscle.
9. E. The profunda artery runs through the posterior fascial compartment of the arm accompanied by the radial nerve.
10. A. The abductor pollicis brevis is a muscle of the thenar eminence and is not near the anatomic snuffbox.
11. E. The subscapularis muscle is inserted into the lesser tuberosity of the humerus.
12. B
13. D. The flexor carpi radialis tendon enters the palm through a split in the flexor retinaculum in a groove on the trapezium.
14. A. The ulnar nerve supplies the lumbrical and interossei muscles, which normally flex the proximal phalanges and extend the middle and distal phalanges of the little and ring fingers.
15. C. See page 537 and Figure 9-103.
16. E. The opponens pollicis muscle, which is responsible for pulling the thumb medially and forward across the palm so that the palmar surface of the tip of the thumb may come into contact with the palmar surface of the tips of the other fingers, is supplied by the median nerve.
17. A
18. B
19. B
20. E
21. B
22. E
23. A
24. B
25. A
26. D
27. C
28. D. The digital nerves at the root of the fingers are relatively easy to inject and are not imbedded in tough deep fascia.
29. E. The disadvantage of the axillary approach to the brachial plexus nerve block is the difficulty sometimes experienced in blocking the musculocutaneous nerve. This nerve is a branch of the lateral cord of the plexus and the anesthetic agent may not reach high enough up in the sheath to block this nerve. To overcome this disadvantage, the axillary artery and the sheath are compressed distal to the point of injection, so that the sheath may be closed off below. By using this maneuver, the anesthetic agent rises in the sheath to the level of the musculocutaneous nerve. It is the terminal branches of the musculocutaneous nerve (lateral cutaneous nerve of the forearm) that supply the skin over the carpometacarpal joint of the thumb.

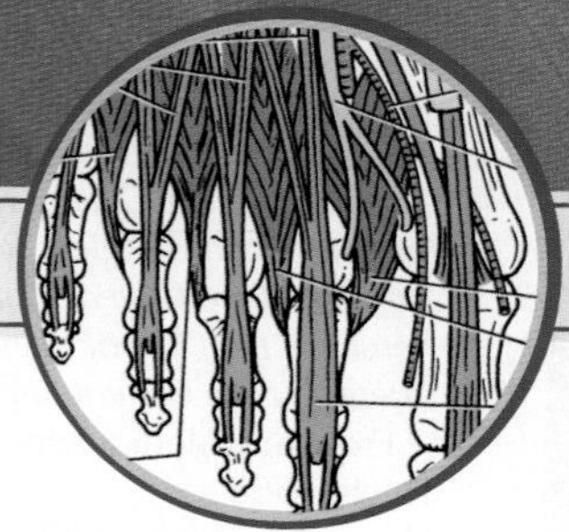

CHAPTER 10

THE LOWER LIMB

An 18-year-old student was doing part-time work delivering pizzas on his motorcycle. His boss insisted on quick delivery, so the student tended to weave in and out of traffic whenever there was a holdup. On one occasion, he misjudged the gap between two vehicles, and the outer surface of his left knee hit a car bumper. On examination in the emergency department, he was found to have extensive paralysis of the muscles of the anterior and lateral compartments of the left leg. As a result, the patient was unable to dorsiflex the ankle joint (which showed footdrop) and evert the foot. In addition, there was evidence of diminished sensation down the anterior and lateral sides of the leg and dorsum of the foot and toes, including the medial side of the big toe. A series of radiographs of the knee region showed no evidence of bone fractures.

The physician made the diagnosis of paralysis of the common peroneal nerve secondary to blunt trauma to the lateral side of the left fibula. The radiographic examination ruled out the possibility of fracture of the neck of the fibula.

To be in a position to make such a diagnosis, physicians must be cognizant of the detailed anatomy of the course of the common peroneal nerve as it winds around the outer side of the neck of the fibula. Knowledge of the distribution of the branches of this nerve enables physicians to eliminate other nerve injuries. Moreover, they are able to assess the degree of nerve damage by testing the strength of the various muscles supplied by this nerve and conducting suitable tests to assess the sensory deficits.

CHAPTER OUTLINE

Basic Anatomy 550
Organization of the Lower Limb 550
The Gluteal Region 551
The Skin of the Buttock 551
Fascia of the Buttock 553
Bones of the Gluteal Region 555
Ligaments of the Gluteal Region 562
Foramina of the Gluteal Region 562
Muscles of the Gluteal Region 562
Nerves of the Gluteal Region 565
Arteries of the Gluteal Region 566
The Front and Medial Aspects of the Thigh 568
Skin of the Thigh 568
Superficial Fascia of the Thigh 573
Deep Fascia of the Thigh (Fascia Lata) 573
Fascial Compartments of the Thigh 573
Contents of the Anterior Fascial Compartment of the Thigh 573
Contents of the Medial Fascial Compartment of the Thigh 583
The Back of the Thigh 587
Skin 587
Contents of the Posterior Fascial Compartment of the Thigh 587
Hip Joint 587
Bones of the Leg 592
Bones of the Foot 596
Popliteal Fossa 600
Boundaries 600
Popliteus Muscle 600
Popliteal Artery 600
Popliteal Vein 604
Arterial Anastomosis Around the Knee Joint 604
Popliteal Lymph Nodes 604
Tibial Nerve 604
Common Peroneal Nerve 604
Posterior Cutaneous Nerve of the Thigh 605
Obturator Nerve 605
Fascial Compartments of the Leg 605
The Front of the Leg 609
Skin 609
Contents of the Anterior Fascial Compartment of the Leg 609
Contents of the Lateral Fascial Compartment of the Leg 614
The Back of the Leg 615
Skin 615
Contents of the Posterior Fascial Compartment of the Leg 615
The Region of the Ankle 618
Anterior Aspect of the Ankle 618
Posterior Aspect of the Ankle 619
The Foot 619
The Sole of the Foot 619
Skin 619
Deep Fascia 619
Muscles of the Sole of the Foot 619
Arteries of the Sole of the Foot 624
Veins of the Sole of the Foot 626
Nerves of the Sole of the Foot 626
The Dorsum of the Foot 627
Skin 627
Dorsal Venous Arch (or Network) 627
Muscles of the Dorsum of the Foot 627
Artery of the Dorsum of the Foot 627
Nerve Supply of the Dorsum of the Foot 629
Joints of the Lower Limb 629
Knee Joint 629
Proximal Tibiofibular Joint 632
Distal Tibiofibular Joint 632
Ankle Joint 634
Tarsal Joints 637
Tarsometatarsal and Intermetatarsal Joints 638
Metatarsophalangeal and Interphalangeal Joints 638
The Foot as a Functional Unit 638
Radiographic Anatomy 644
Radiographic Appearances of the Lower Limb 644
Surface Anatomy 644
Gluteal Region 644
Inguinal Region 650
Femoral Triangle 650
Adductor Canal 654
Knee Region 654
Tibia 657
Ankle Region and Foot 657
Clinical Notes on the Arteries of the Lower Limb 658
Clinical Notes on the Nerves of the Lower Limb 659
Clinical Problem Solving 661
Answers to Clinical Problems 663
Review Questions 663
Answers to Review Questions 666

CHAPTER OBJECTIVES

- Lower limb problems are some of the most common dealt with by health professionals, whether working in general practice, surgery, or an emergency department.
- Arthritis, varicose veins, vascular deficiencies, fractures, dislocations, sprains, lacerations, knee effusions, leg pain, ankle injuries, and peripheral nerve injuries are just a few of the conditions that physicians see.
- The anatomy of the lower limb is discussed in relation to common clinical conditions.
- A general description of the bones, joints, and actions of muscles is given. Emphasis is placed on the functions of the muscles, and only the briefest coverage of their attachments is provided.
- The basic anatomy of the vascular supply, lymphatic drainage, and distribution of the nerves is reviewed.

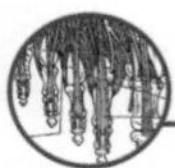

Basic Anatomy

The primary function of the lower limbs is to support the weight of the body and to provide a stable foundation in standing, walking, and running; they have become specialized for locomotion.

Organization of the Lower Limb

The lower limbs are divided into the gluteal region, the thigh, the knee, the leg, the ankle, and the foot. The thigh and the leg are compartmentalized, each compartment having its own muscles that perform group functions and its own distinct nerve and blood supply.

The Gluteal Region

The gluteal region, or buttock, is bounded superiorly by the iliac crest and inferiorly by the fold of the buttock. The region is largely made up of the gluteal muscles and a thick layer of superficial fascia.

The Skin of the Buttock

The **cutaneous nerves** (Figs. 10-1 and 10-2) are derived from posterior and anterior rami of spinal nerves, as follows:

- The upper medial quadrant is supplied by the posterior rami of the upper three lumbar nerves and the upper three sacral nerves.
- The upper lateral quadrant is supplied by the lateral branches of the iliohypogastric (L1) and 12th thoracic nerves (anterior rami).
- The lower lateral quadrant is supplied by branches from the lateral cutaneous nerve of the thigh (L2 and 3, anterior rami).
- The lower medial quadrant is supplied by branches from the posterior cutaneous nerve of the thigh (S1, 2, and 3, anterior rami).

The skin over the coccyx in the floor of the cleft between the buttocks is supplied by small branches of the lower sacral and coccygeal nerves.

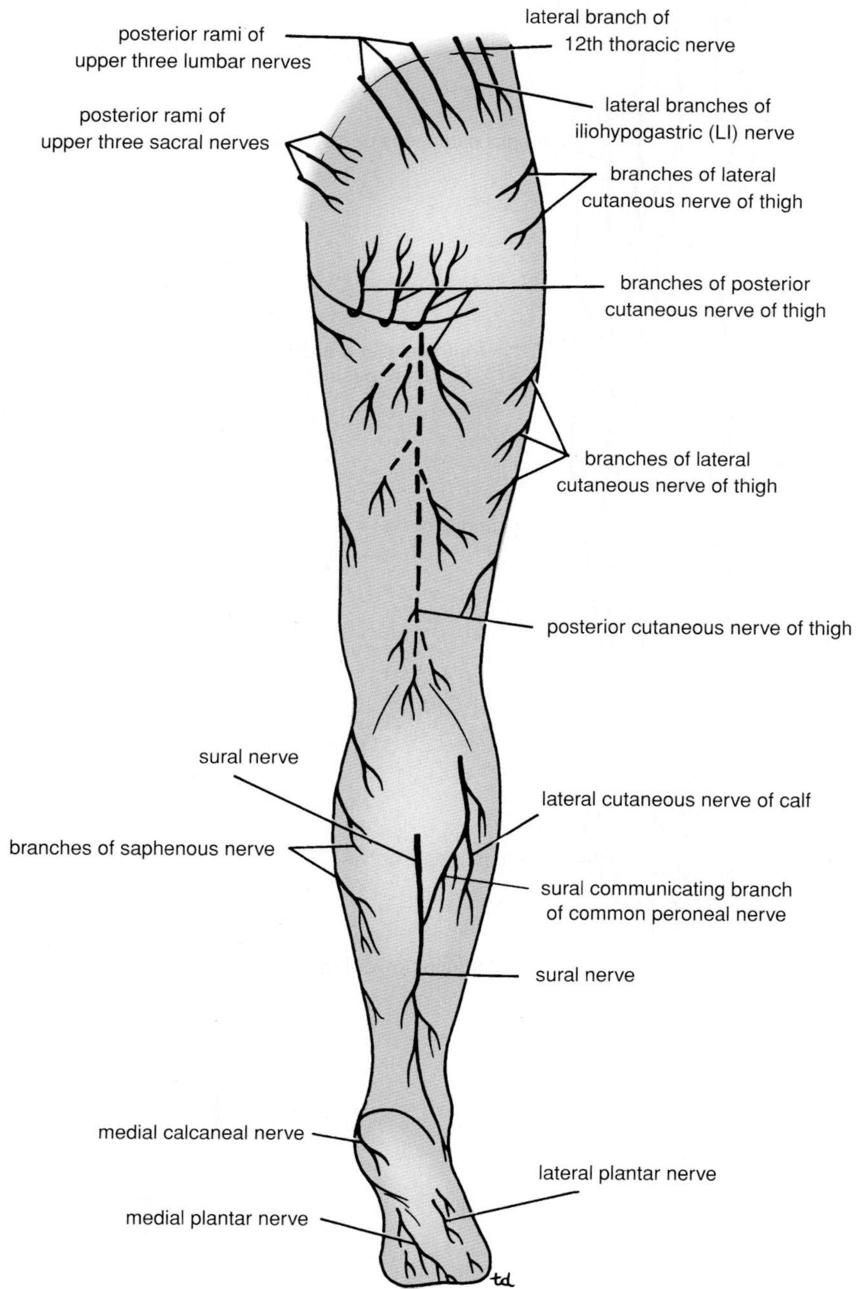

Figure 10-1 Cutaneous nerves of the posterior surface of the right lower limb.

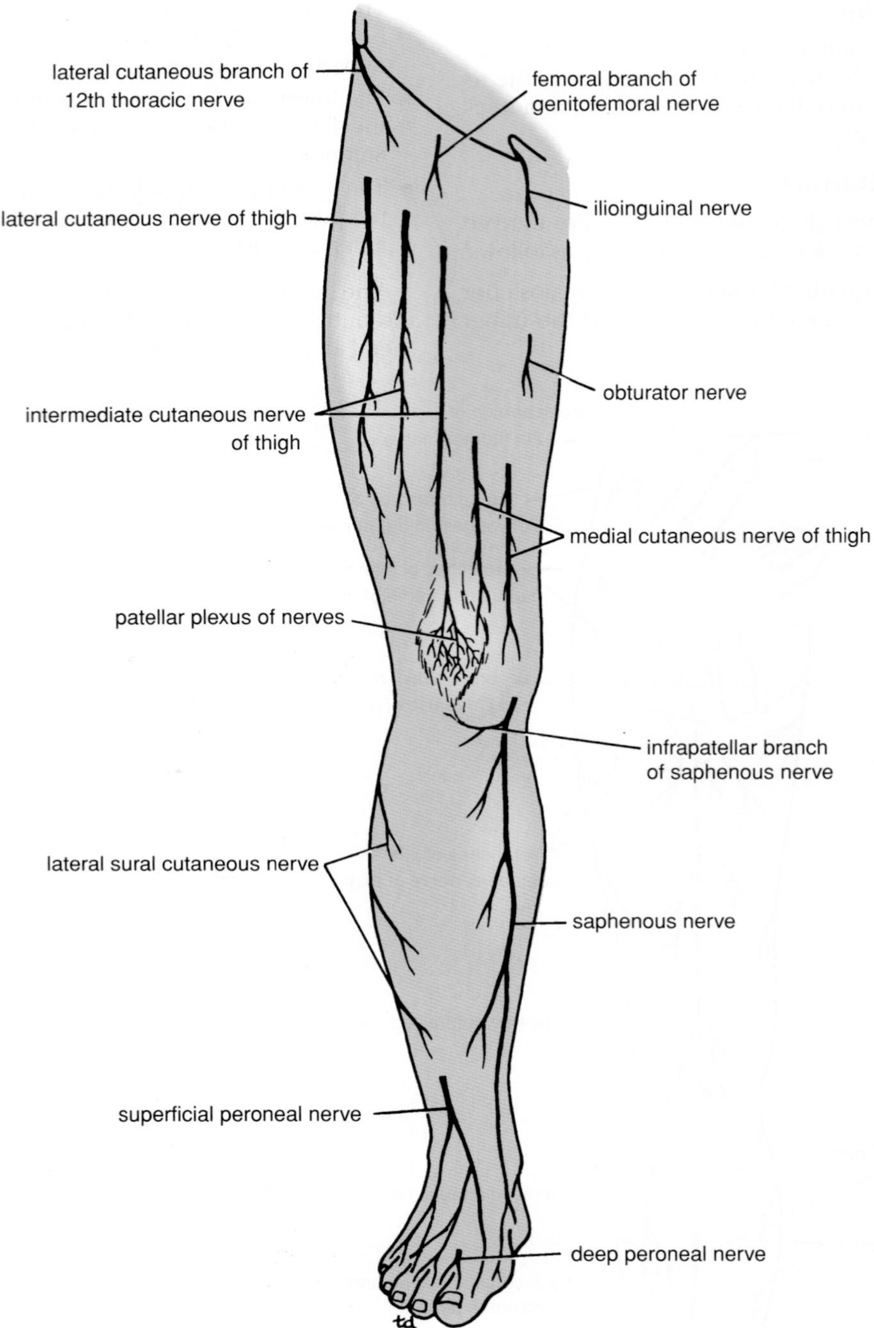

Figure 10-2 Cutaneous nerves of the anterior surface of the right lower limb.

The **lymph vessels** drain into the lateral group of the superficial inguinal nodes (Figs. 10-3 and 10-4).

Fascia of the Buttock

The **superficial fascia** is thick, especially in women, and is impregnated with large quantities of fat. It contributes to the prominence of the buttock.

The **deep fascia** is continuous below with the **deep fascia,** or **fascia lata,** of the thigh. In the gluteal region, it splits to enclose the gluteus maximus muscle (Fig. 10-5). Above the gluteus maximus, it continues as a single layer that covers the outer surface of the gluteus medius and is attached to the iliac crest. On the lateral surface of the thigh, the fascia is thickened to form a strong, wide band, the **iliotibial**

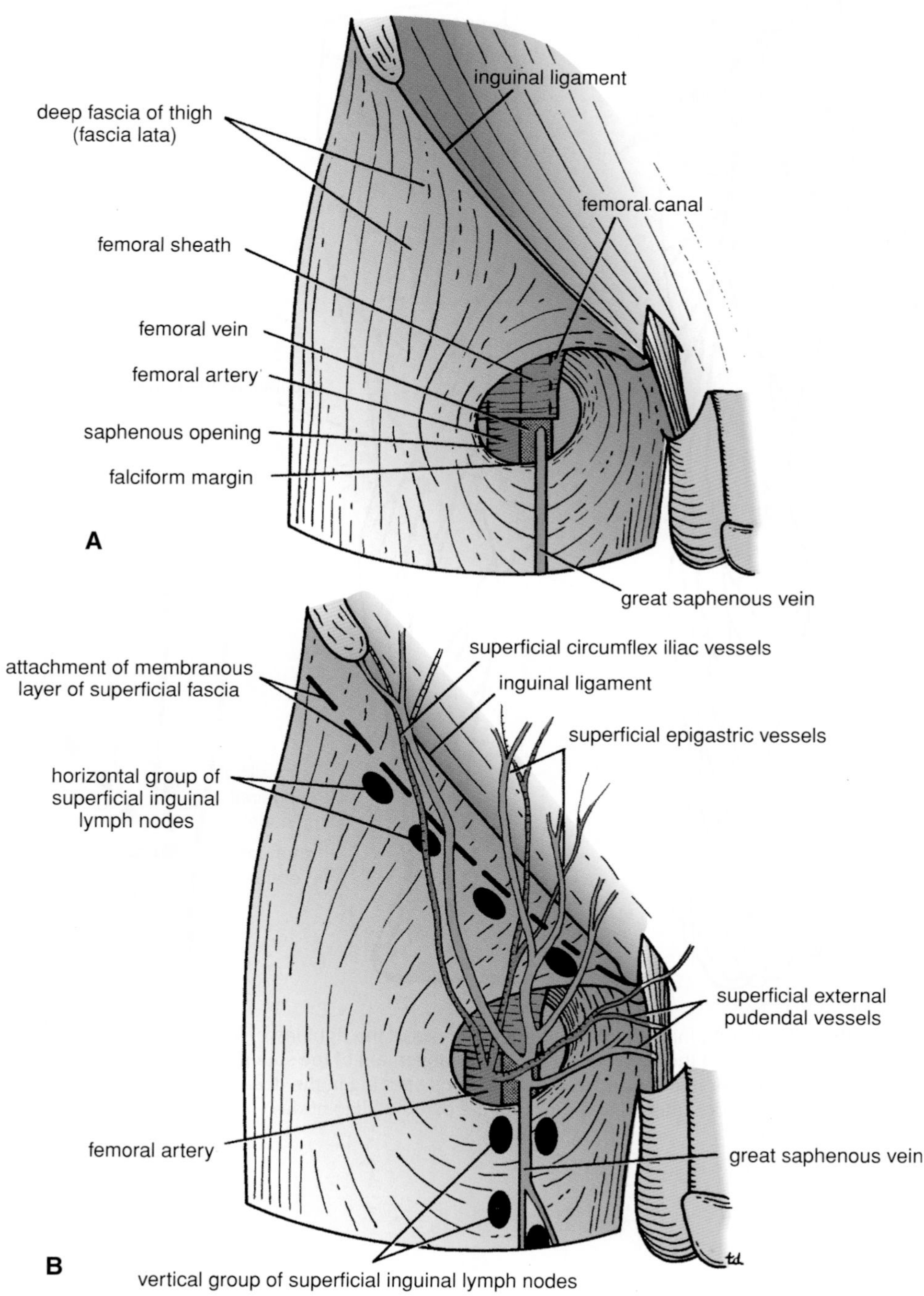

Figure 10-3 **A, B.** Superficial veins, arteries, and lymph nodes over the right femoral triangle. Note the saphenous opening in the deep fascia and its relationship to the femoral sheath. Note also the line of attachment of the membranous layer of superficial fascia to the deep fascia, about a fingerbreadth below the inguinal ligament.

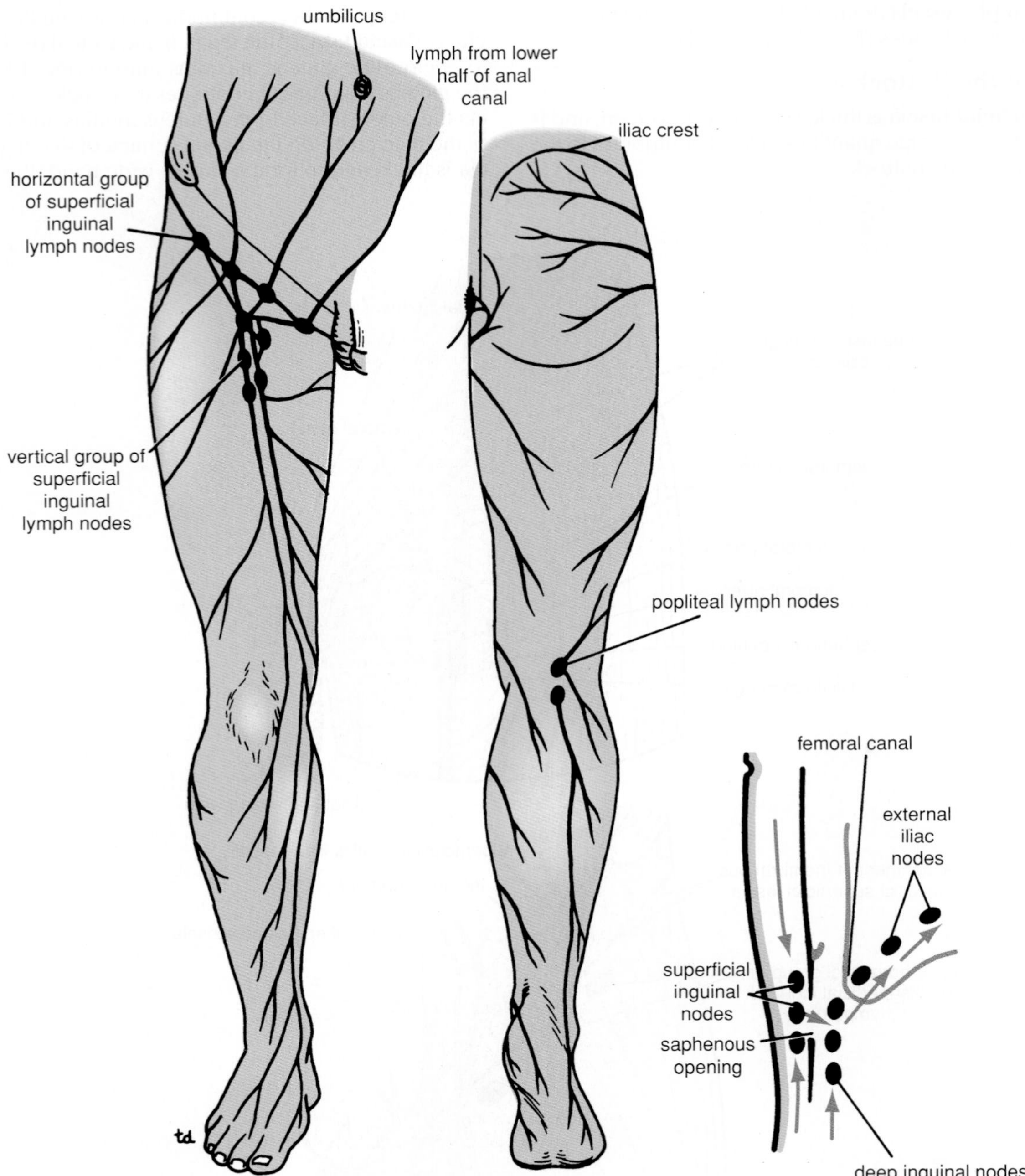

Figure 10-4 Lymph drainage for the superficial tissues of the right lower limb and the abdominal walls below the level of the umbilicus. Note the arrangement of the superficial and deep inguinal lymph nodes and their relationship to the saphenous opening in the deep fascia. Note also that all lymph from these nodes ultimately drains into the external iliac nodes via the femoral canal.

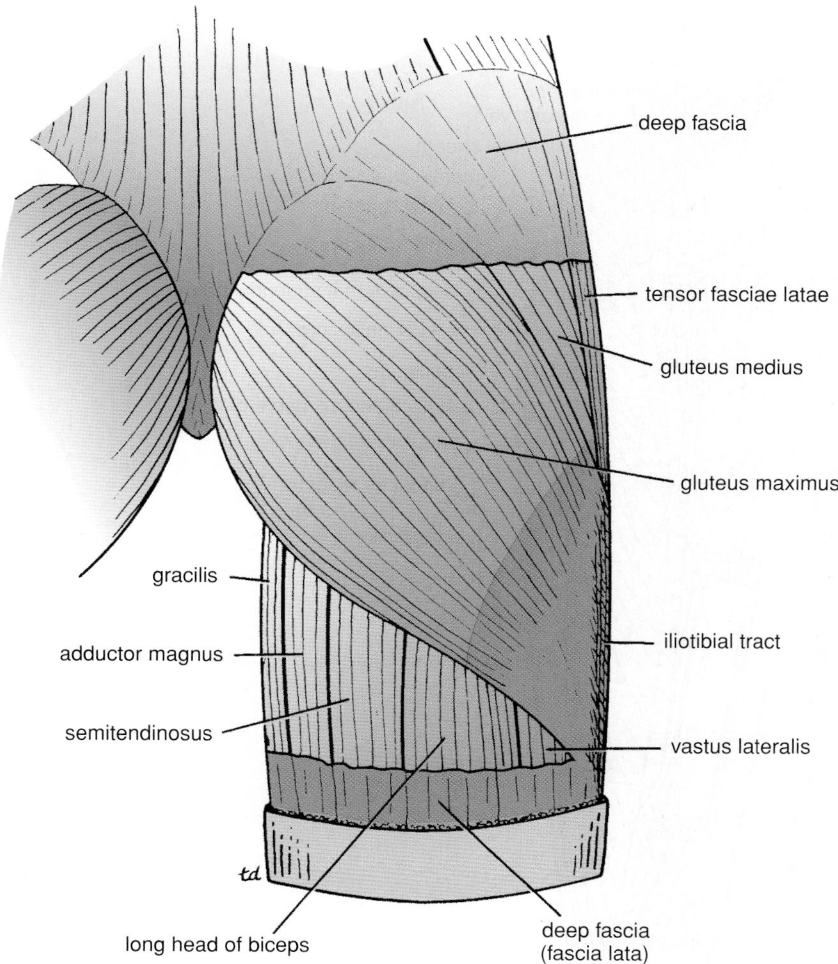

Figure 10-5 Right gluteus maximus muscle.

tract (Fig. 10-6). This is attached above to the tubercle of the iliac crest and below to the lateral condyle of the tibia. The iliotibial tract forms a sheath for the tensor fasciae latae muscle and receives the greater part of the insertion of the gluteus maximus.

Bones of the Gluteal Region

Hip Bone

The ilium, ischium, and pubis form the hip bone (Figs. 10-7 and 10-8). They meet one another at the acetabulum. The hip bones articulate with the sacrum at the sacroiliac joints and form the anterolateral walls of the pelvis; they also articulate with one another anteriorly at the symphysis pubis. The detailed structure of the internal aspect of the bony pelvis is considered on page 308.

The important features found on the outer surface of the hip bone in the gluteal region are as follows.

The **ilium,** which is the upper flattened part of the bone, possesses the **iliac crest** (Fig. 10-8). This can be felt through the skin along its entire length; it ends in front at the **anterior superior iliac spine** and behind at the **posterior superior iliac spine.** The **iliac tubercle** lies about 2 in. (5 cm) behind the anterior superior spine. Below the anterior superior iliac spine is a prominence, the **anterior inferior iliac spine;** a similar prominence, the **posterior inferior iliac spine,** is located below the posterior superior iliac spine. Above and behind the acetabulum, the ilium possesses a large notch, the **greater sciatic notch** (Figs. 10-7 and 10-8).

The **ischium** is L shaped, possessing an upper thicker part, the **body,** and a lower thinner part, the **ramus** (Figs. 10-7 and 10-8). The **ischial spine** projects from the posterior border of the ischium and intervenes between the **greater** and **lesser sciatic notches.** The **ischial tuberosity** forms the posterior aspect of the lower part of the body of the bone. The greater and lesser sciatic notches are converted into **greater** and **lesser sciatic foramina** by the presence of the sacrospinous and sacrotuberous ligaments (see page 318).

The **pubis** can be divided into a **body,** a **superior ramus,** and an **inferior ramus** (Fig. 10-8). The bodies of the two pubic bones articulate with each other in the midline anteriorly at the **symphysis pubis;** the superior ramus joins the ilium and ischium at the acetabulum, and the inferior ramus joins the ischial ramus below the **obturator foramen.** The obturator foramen in life is filled in by the **obturator membrane** (see page 318). The **pubic crest** forms the upper border of the body of the pubis, and it ends laterally as the **pubic tubercle** (Figs. 10-7 and 10-8).

On the outer surface of the hip bone is a deep depression, called the **acetabulum,** that articulates with the

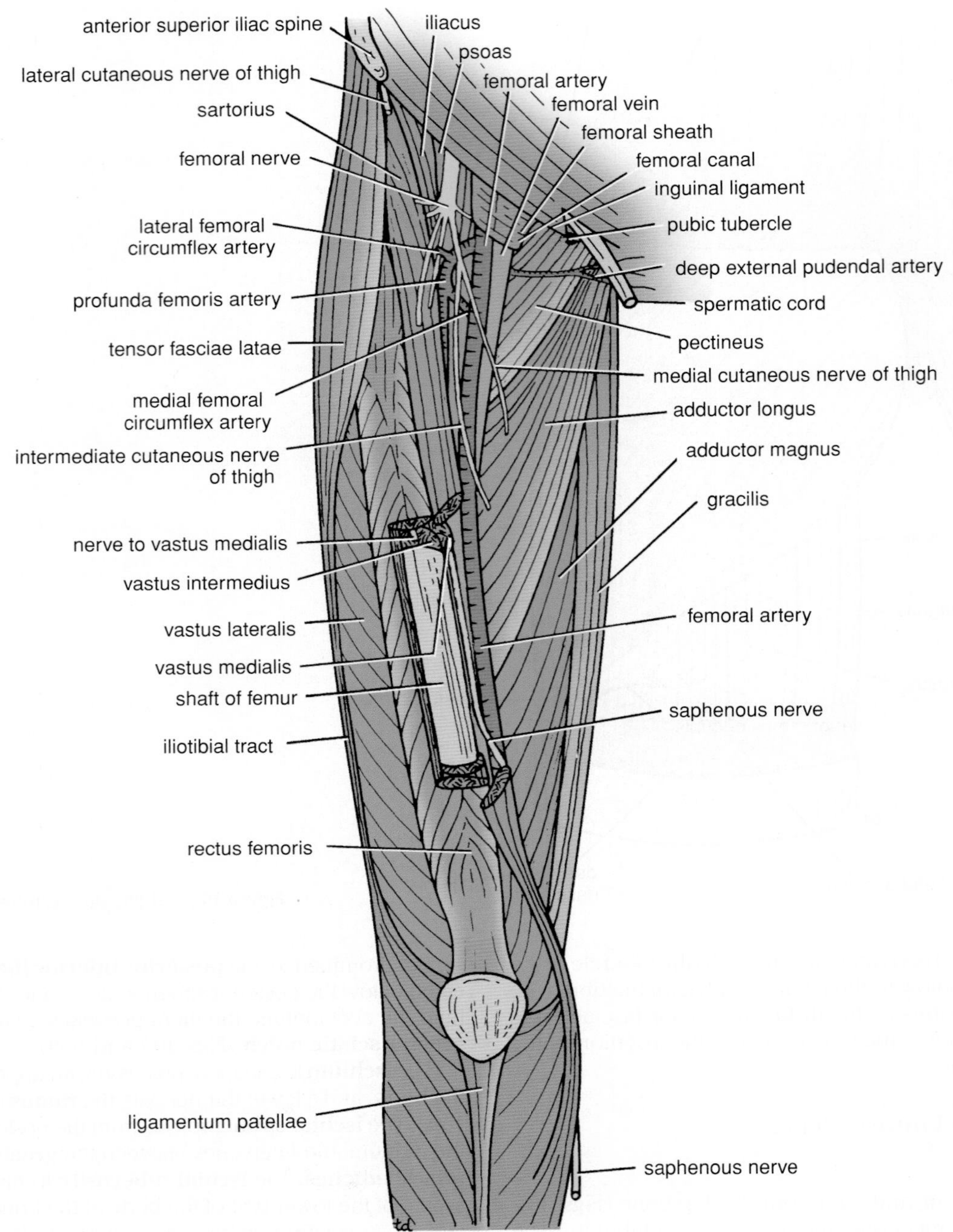

Figure 10-6 Femoral triangle and adductor (subsartorial) canal in the right lower limb.

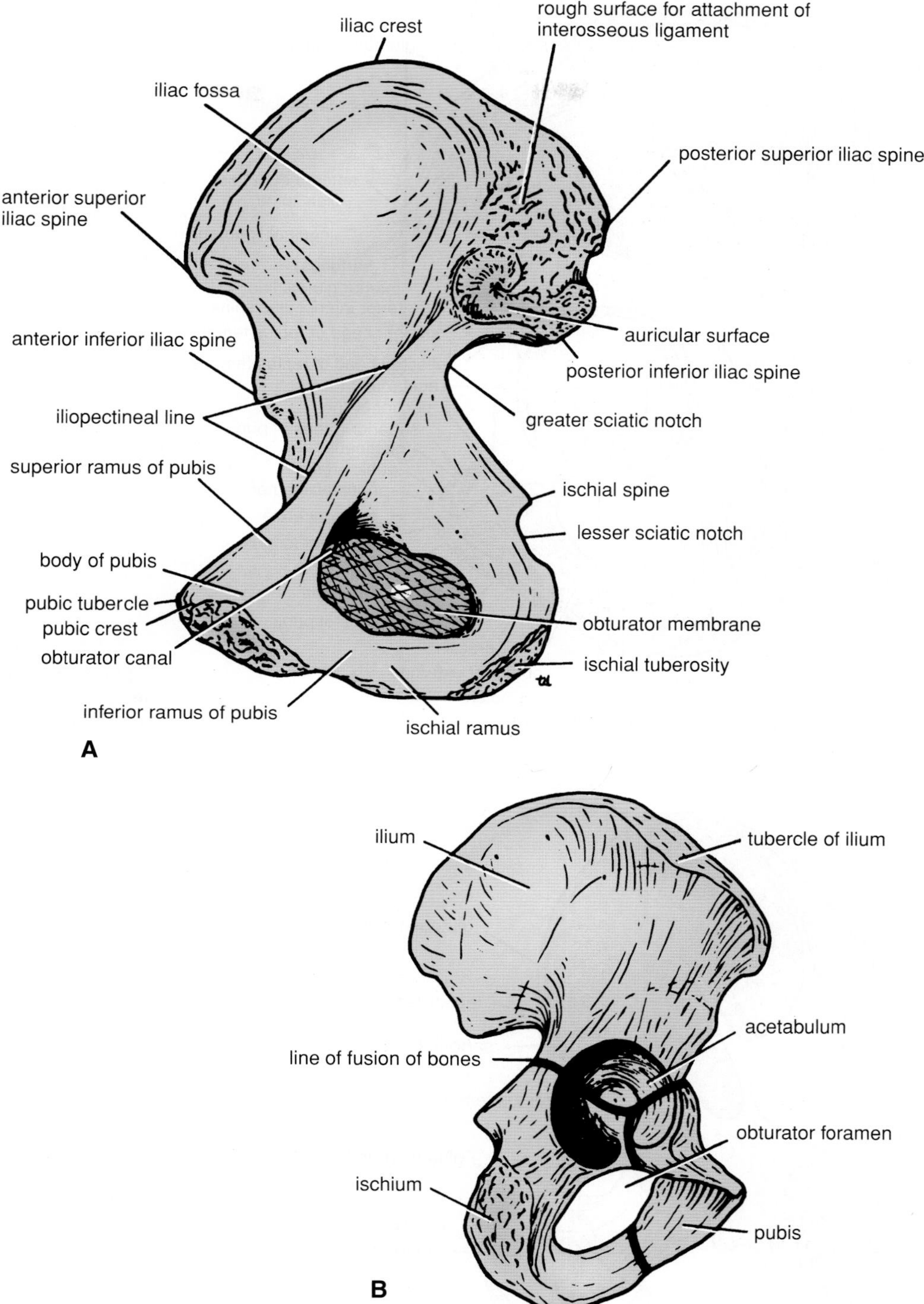

Figure 10-7 Medial surface (**A**) and lateral surface (**B**) of the right hip bone. Note the lines of fusion between the three bones (the ilium, the ischium, and the pubis).

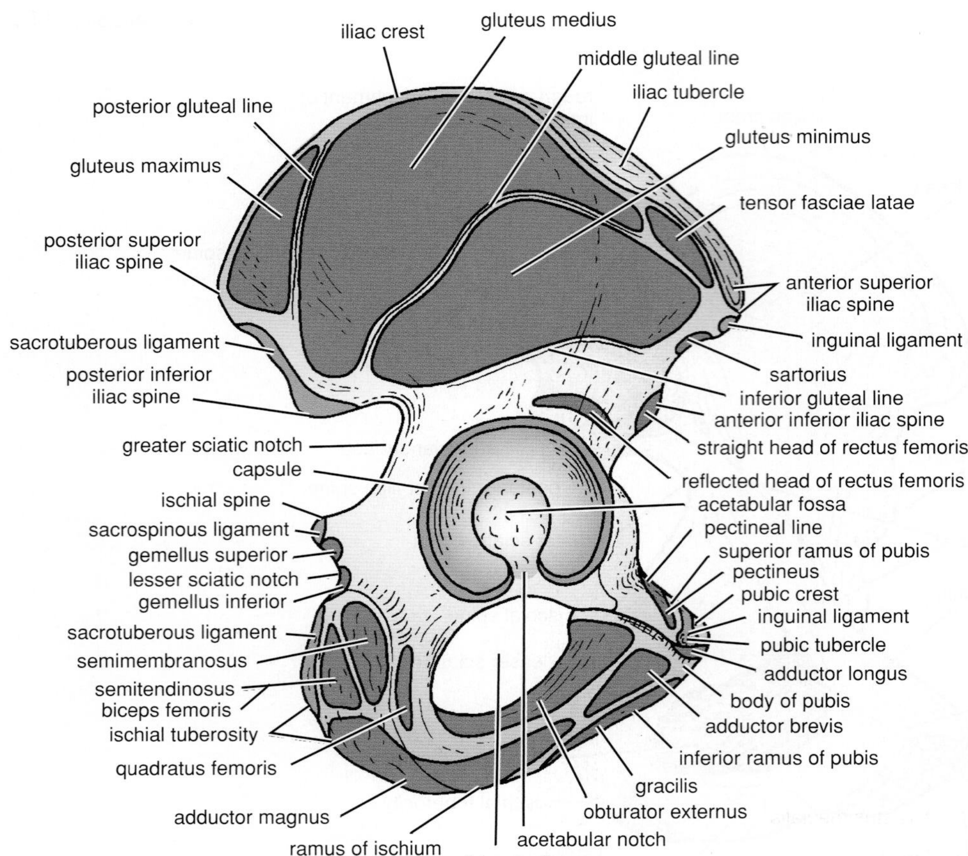

Figure 10-8 Muscles and ligaments attached to the external surface of the right hip bone.

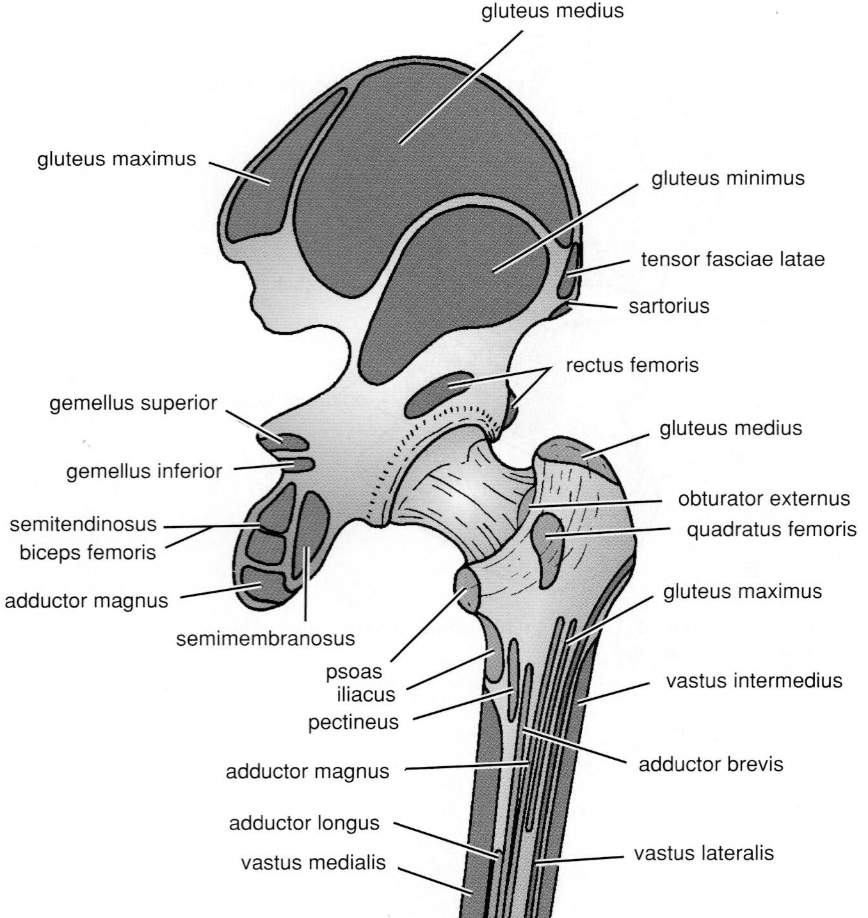

Figure 10-9 Muscles attached to the external surface of the right hip bone and the posterior surface of the femur.

almost spherical head of the femur to form the hip joint (Figs. 10-8 and 10-9). The inferior margin of the acetabulum is deficient and is marked by the **acetabular notch** (Fig. 10-8). The articular surface of the acetabulum is limited to a horseshoe-shaped area and is covered with hyaline cartilage. The floor of the acetabulum is nonarticular and is called the **acetabular fossa** (Fig. 10-8).

In the anatomic position, the front of the symphysis pubis and the anterior superior iliac spines lie in the same vertical plane. This means that the pelvic surface of the symphysis pubis faces upward and backward and the anterior surface of the sacrum is directed forward and downward.

The important muscles and ligaments attached to the outer surface of the hip bone are shown in Figure 10-8.

Femur

The femur articulates above with the acetabulum to form the hip joint and below with the tibia and the patella to form the knee joint.

The upper end of the femur has a head, a neck, and greater and lesser trochanters (Figs. 10-10 and 10-11). The **head** forms about two thirds of a sphere and articulates with the acetabulum of the hip bone to form the hip joint (Fig. 10-9). In the center of the head is a small depression, called the

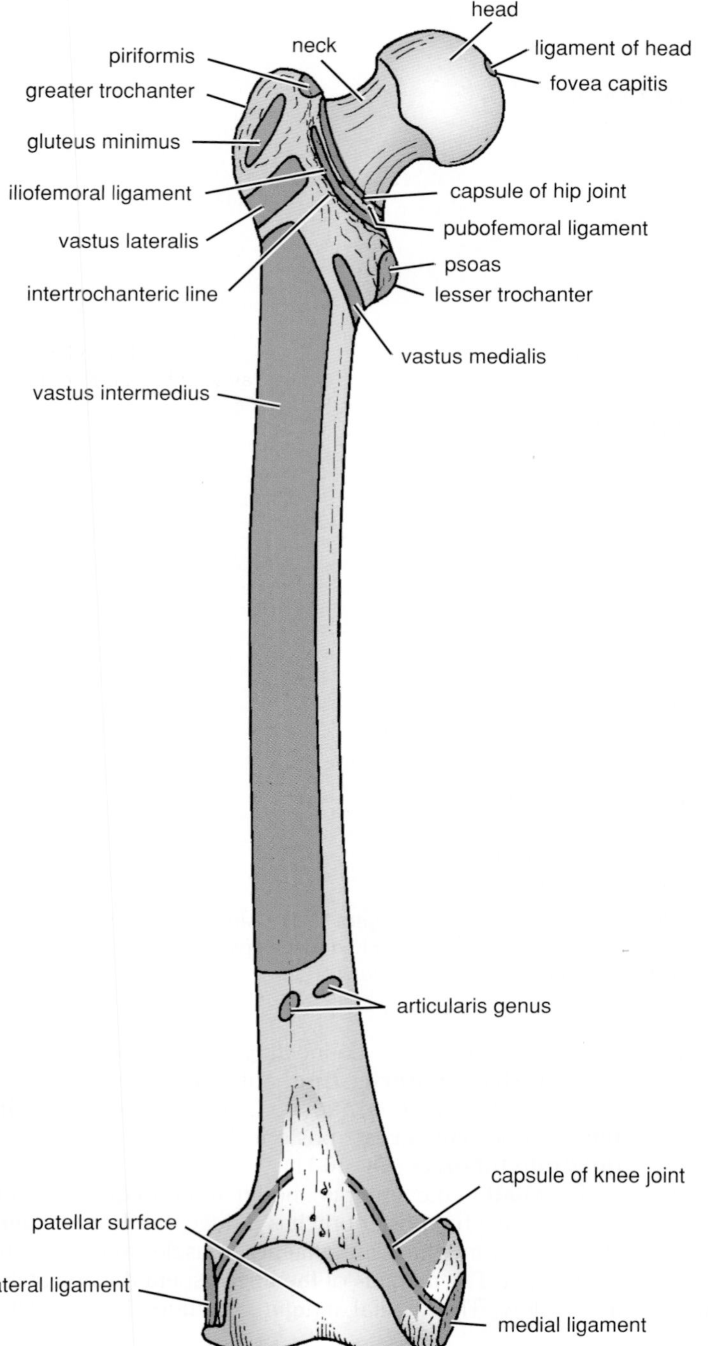

Figure 10-10 Muscles and ligaments attached to the anterior surface of the right femur.

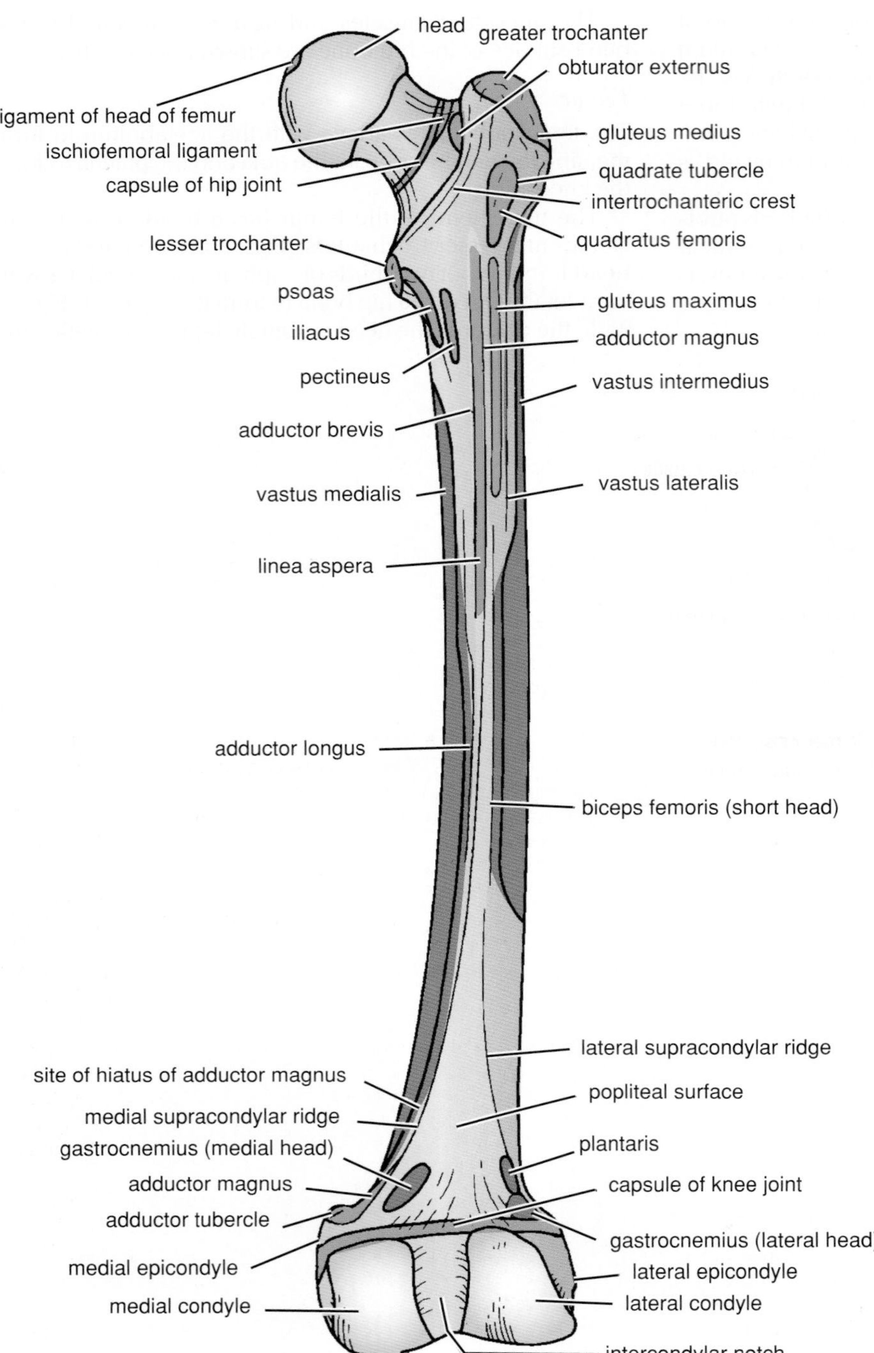

Figure 10-11 Muscles and ligaments attached to the posterior surface of the right femur.

fovea capitis, for the attachment of the ligament of the head. Part of the blood supply to the head of the femur from the obturator artery is conveyed along this ligament and enters the bone at the fovea.

The **neck,** which connects the head to the shaft, passes downward, backward, and laterally and makes an angle of about 125° (slightly less in the female) with the long axis of the shaft. The size of this angle can be altered by disease.

The **greater** and **lesser trochanters** are large eminences situated at the junction of the neck and the shaft (Figs. 10-10 and 10-11). Connecting the two trochanters are the **intertrochanteric line** anteriorly, where the iliofemoral ligament is attached, and a prominent **intertrochanteric crest** posteriorly, on which is the **quadrate tubercle** (Fig. 10-11).

The **shaft** of the femur is smooth and rounded on its anterior surface but posteriorly has a ridge, the **linea aspera** (Fig. 10-11), to which are attached muscles and intermuscular septa. The margins of the linea aspera diverge above and below. The medial margin continues below as the

medial supracondylar ridge to the **adductor tubercle** on the medial condyle (Fig. 10-11). The lateral margin becomes continuous below with the **lateral supracondylar ridge.** On the posterior surface of the shaft below the greater trochanter is the **gluteal tuberosity** for the attachment of the gluteus maximus muscle. The shaft becomes broader toward its distal end and forms a flat, triangular area on its posterior surface called the **popliteal surface** (Fig. 10-11).

The lower end of the femur has **lateral** and **medial** condyles, separated posteriorly by the **intercondylar notch.** The anterior surfaces of the condyles are joined by an articular surface for the patella. The two condyles take part in the formation of the knee joint. Above the condyles are the **medial** and **lateral epicondyles** (Fig. 10-11). The adductor tubercle is continuous with the medial epicondyle.

The important muscles and ligaments attached to the femur are shown in Figures 10-10 and 10-11.

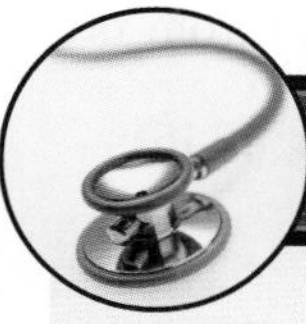

CLINICAL NOTES

Tenderness of the Head of the Femur and Arthritis of the Hip Joint

The head of the femur—that is, that part that is not intra-acetabular—can be palpated on the anterior aspect of the thigh just inferior to the inguinal ligament and just lateral to the pulsating femoral artery. Tenderness over the head of the femur usually indicates the presence of arthritis of the hip joint.

Blood Supply to the Femoral Head and Neck Fractures

Anatomic knowledge of the blood supply to the femoral head explains why avascular necrosis of the head can occur after fractures of the neck of the femur. In the young, the epiphysis of the head is supplied by a small branch of the obturator artery, which passes to the head along the ligament of the femoral head. The upper part of the neck of the femur receives a profuse blood supply from the medial femoral circumflex artery. These branches pierce the capsule and ascend the neck deep to the synovial membrane. As long as the epiphyseal cartilage remains, no communication occurs between the two sources of blood. In the adult, after the epiphyseal cartilage disappears, an anastomosis between the two sources of blood supply is established. Fractures of the femoral neck interfere with or completely interrupt the blood supply from the root of the femoral neck to the femoral head. The scant blood flow along the small artery that accompanies the round ligament may be insufficient to sustain the viability of the femoral head, and ischemic necrosis gradually takes place.

The Neck of the Femur and Coxa Valga and Coxa Vara

The neck of the femur is inclined at an angle with the shaft; the angle is about 160° in the young child and about 125° in the adult. An increase in this angle is referred to as **coxa valga,** and it occurs, for example, in cases of congenital dislocation of the hip. In this condition, adduction of the hip joint is limited. A decrease in this angle is referred to as **coxa vara,** and it occurs in fractures of the neck of the femur and in slipping of the femoral epiphysis. In this condition, abduction of the hip joint is limited. Shenton's line is a useful means of assessing the angle of the femoral neck on a radiograph of the hip region (see Figure 10-72).

Fractures of the Femur

Fractures of the neck of the femur are common and are of two types, subcapital and trochanteric. The **subcapital fracture** occurs in the elderly and is usually produced by a minor trip or stumble. Subcapital femoral neck fractures are particularly common in women after menopause. This gender predisposition is because of a thinning of the cortical and trabecular bone caused by estrogen deficiency. Avascular necrosis of the head is a common complication. If the fragments are not impacted, considerable displacement occurs. The strong muscles of the thigh (Fig. 10-12), including the rectus femoris, the adductor muscles, and the hamstring muscles, pull the distal fragment upward, so that the leg is shortened (as measured from the anterior superior iliac spine to the adductor tubercle or medial malleolus). The gluteus maximus, the piriformis, the obturator internus, the gemelli, and the quadratus femoris rotate the distal fragment laterally, as seen by the toes pointing laterally.

Trochanteric fractures commonly occur in the young and middle-aged as a result of direct trauma. The fracture line is extracapsular, and both fragments have a profuse blood supply. If the bone fragments are not impacted, the pull of the strong muscles will produce shortening and lateral rotation of the leg, as previously explained.

Fractures of the shaft of the femur usually occur in young and healthy persons. In **fractures of the upper third of the shaft** of the femur, the proximal fragment is flexed by the iliopsoas; abducted by the gluteus medius and minimus; and laterally rotated by the gluteus maximus, the piriformis, the obturator internus, the gemelli, and the quadratus femoris (Fig. 10-13). The lower fragment is adducted by the adductor muscles, pulled upward by the hamstrings and quadriceps, and laterally rotated by the adductors and the weight of the foot (Fig. 10-13).

In **fractures of the middle third of the shaft** of the femur, the distal fragment is pulled upward by the hamstrings and the quadriceps (Fig. 10-13), resulting in considerable shortening. The distal fragment is also rotated backward by the pull of the two heads of the gastrocnemius (Fig. 10-13).

In **fractures of the distal third of the shaft** of the femur, the same displacement of the distal fragment occurs as seen in fractures of the middle third of the shaft. However, the distal fragment is smaller and is rotated backward by the gastrocnemius muscle (Fig. 10-13) to a greater degree and may exert pressure on the popliteal artery and interfere with the blood flow through the leg and foot.

From these accounts it is clear that knowledge of the different actions of the muscles of the leg is necessary to understand the displacement of the fragments of a fractured femur. Considerable traction on the distal fragment is usually required to overcome the powerful muscles and restore the limb to its correct length before manipulation and operative therapy to bring the proximal and distal fragments into correct alignment.

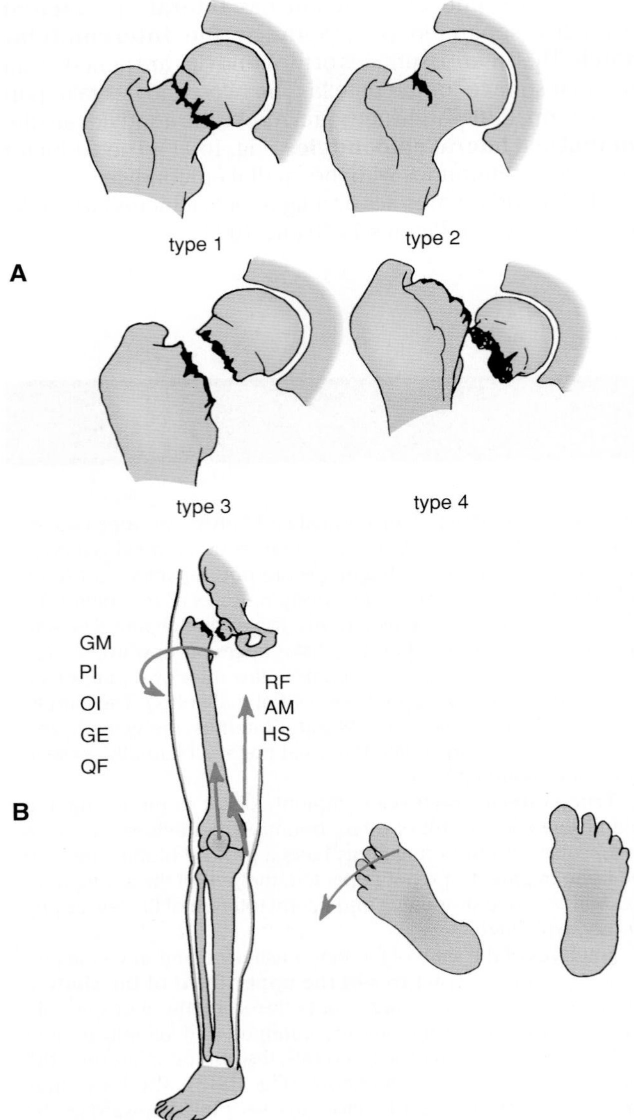

Figure 10-12 **A.** Fractures of the neck of the femur. **B.** Displacement of the lower bone fragment caused by the pull of the powerful muscles. Note in particular the outward rotation of the leg so that the foot characteristically points laterally. GM, gluteus maximus; PI, piriformis; OI, obturator internus; GE, gemelli; QF, quadratus femoris; RF, rectus femoris; AM, adductor muscles; HS, hamstring muscles.

Ligaments of the Gluteal Region

The two important ligaments in the gluteal region are the sacrotuberous and sacrospinous ligaments. The function of these ligaments is to stabilize the sacrum and prevent its rotation at the sacroiliac joint by the weight of the vertebral column.

Sacrotuberous Ligament

The sacrotuberous ligament connects the back of the sacrum to the ischial tuberosity (Fig. 10-14; see Fig. 6-1).

Sacrospinous Ligament

The sacrospinous ligament connects the back of the sacrum to the spine of the ischium (Fig. 10-14; see Fig. 6-1).

Foramina of the Gluteal Region

The two important foramina in the gluteal region are the greater sciatic foramen and the lesser sciatic foramen.

Greater Sciatic Foramen

The greater sciatic foramen (see Fig. 6-11) is formed by the greater sciatic notch of the hip bone and the sacrotuberous and sacrospinous ligaments. It provides an exit from the pelvis into the gluteal region.

The following structures exit the foramen (Fig. 10-15):

- Piriformis
- Sciatic nerve
- Posterior cutaneous nerve of the thigh
- Superior and inferior gluteal nerves
- Nerves to the obturator internus and quadratus femoris
- Pudendal nerve
- Superior and inferior gluteal arteries and veins
- Internal pudendal artery and vein

Lesser Sciatic Foramen

The lesser sciatic foramen (see Fig. 6-11) is formed by the lesser sciatic notch of the hip bone and the sacrotuberous and sacrospinous ligaments. It provides an entrance into the perineum from the gluteal region. Its presence enables nerves and blood vessels that have left the pelvis through the greater sciatic foramen above the pelvic floor to enter the perineum below the pelvic floor.

The following structures pass through the foramen (Fig. 10-14):

- Tendon of obturator internus muscle
- Nerve to obturator internus
- Pudendal nerve
- Internal pudendal artery and vein

Muscles of the Gluteal Region

The muscles of the gluteal region include the gluteus maximus, the gluteus medius, the gluteus minimus, the tensor fasciae latae, the piriformis, the obturator internus, the superior and inferior gemelli, and the quadratus femoris. The muscles are shown in Figures 10-5, 10-14, and 10-15 and described in Table 10-1.

Note the following:

- The gluteus maximus (Fig. 10-5) is the largest muscle in the body. It lies superficial in the gluteal region and is largely responsible for the prominence of the buttock.
- The tensor fasciae latae runs downward and backward to its insertion in the iliotibial tract and thus assists the gluteus maximus muscle in maintaining the knee in the extended position

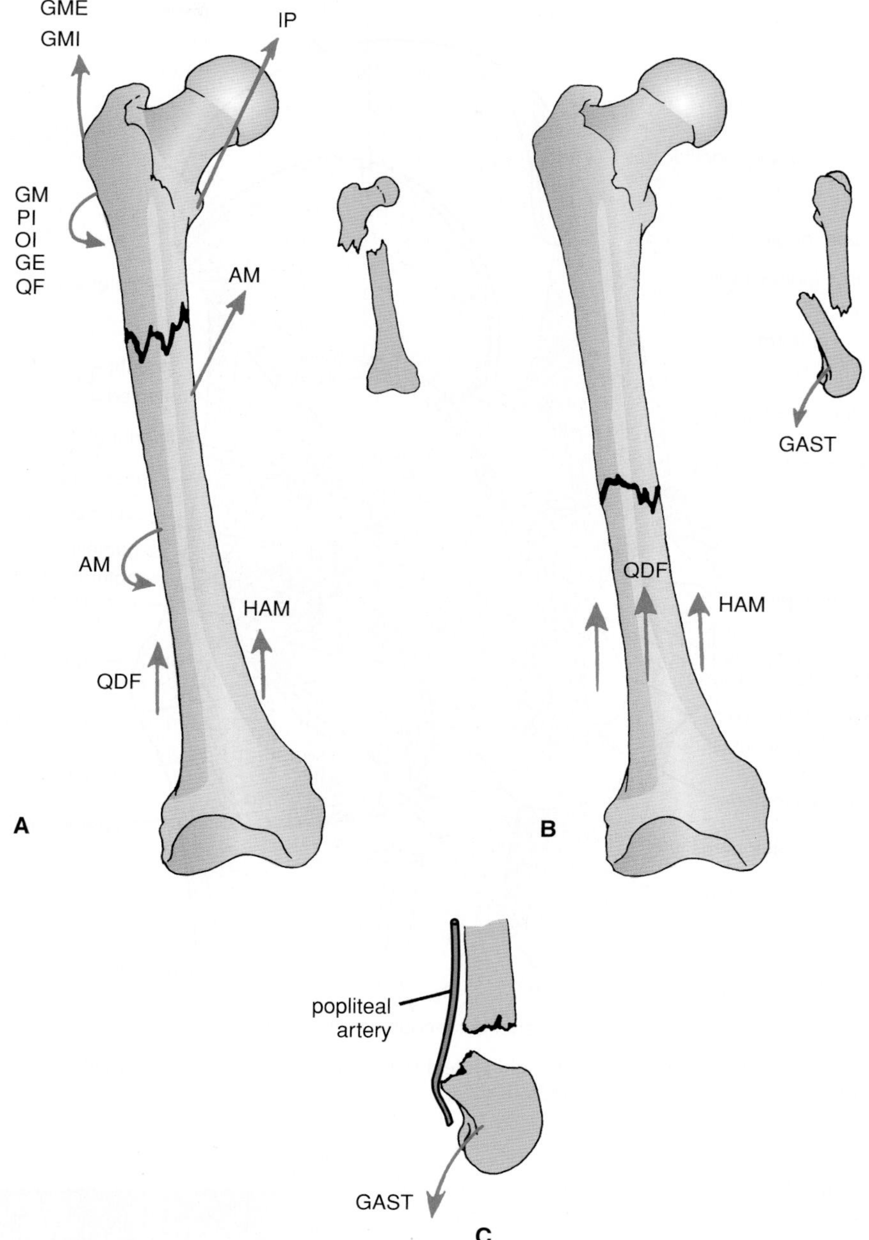

Figure 10-13 Fractures of the shaft of the femur. **A.** Upper third of the femoral shaft. Note the displacement caused by the pull of the powerful muscles. **B.** Middle third of the femoral shaft. Note the posterior displacement of the lower fragment caused by the gastrocnemius muscle. **C.** Lower third of the femoral shaft. Note the excessive displacement of the lower fragment caused by the pull of the gastrocnemius muscle, threatening the integrity of the popliteal artery. IP, iliopsoas; GME, gluteus medius; GMI, gluteus minimus; GM, gluteus maximus; PI, piriformis; OI, obturator internus; GE, gemelli; QF, quadratus femoris; AM, adductor muscles; QDF, quadriceps femoris; HAM, hamstrings; GAST, gastrocnemius.

- The piriformis (Fig.10-15) lies partly within the pelvis at its origin. It emerges through the greater sciatic foramen to enter the gluteal region. Its position serves to separate the superior gluteal vessels and nerves from the inferior gluteal vessels and nerves (Fig.10-15).
- The obturator internus is a fan-shaped muscle that lies within the pelvis at its origin. It emerges through the lesser sciatic foramen to enter the gluteal region. The tendon is joined by the superior and inferior gemelli and is inserted into the greater trochanter of the femur.

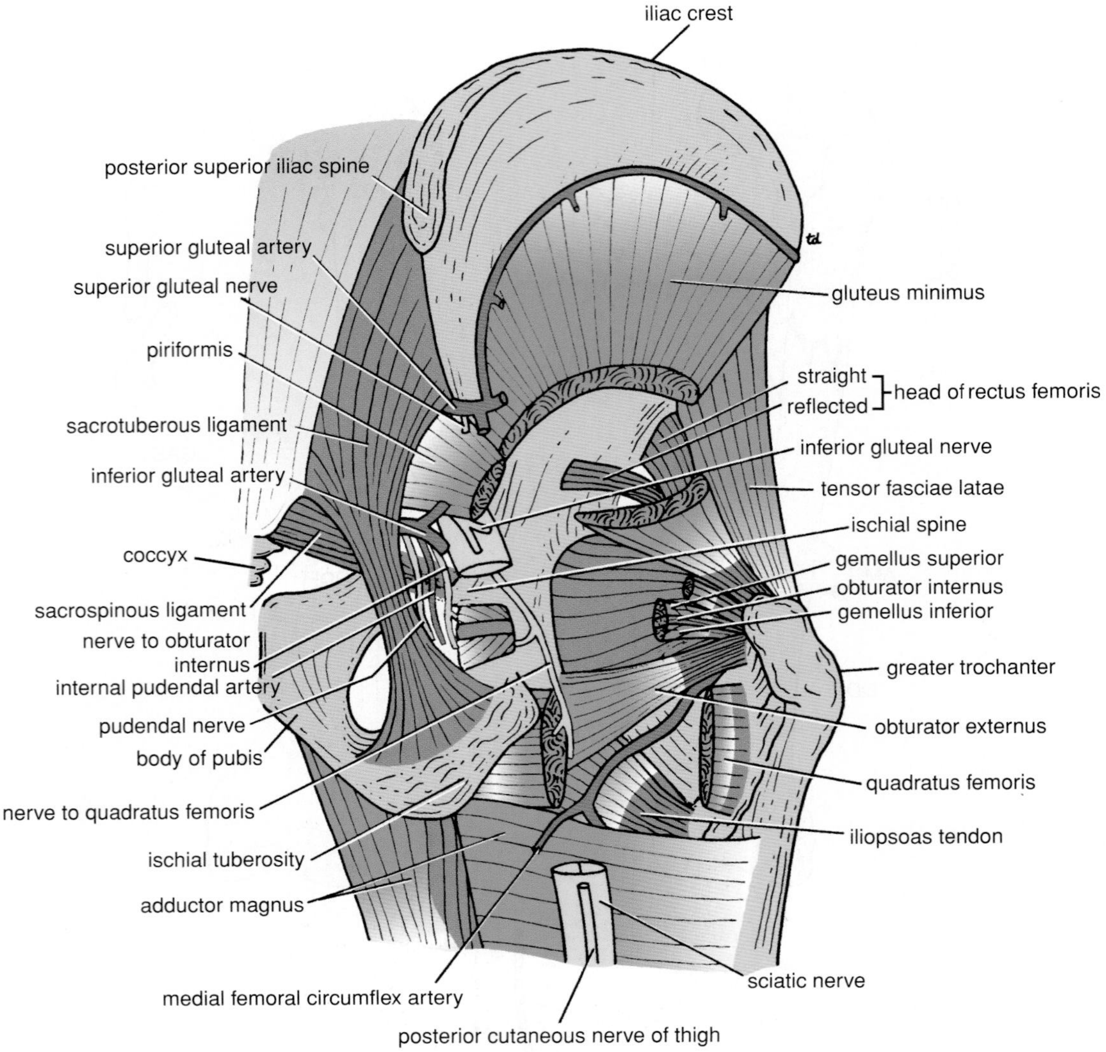

Figure 10-14 Deep structures in the right gluteal region; the gluteus maximus and gluteus medius muscles have been completely removed.

- Three bursae are usually associated with the gluteus maximus: between the tendon of insertion and the greater trochanter, between the tendon of insertion and the vastus lateralis, and overlying the ischial tuberosity.

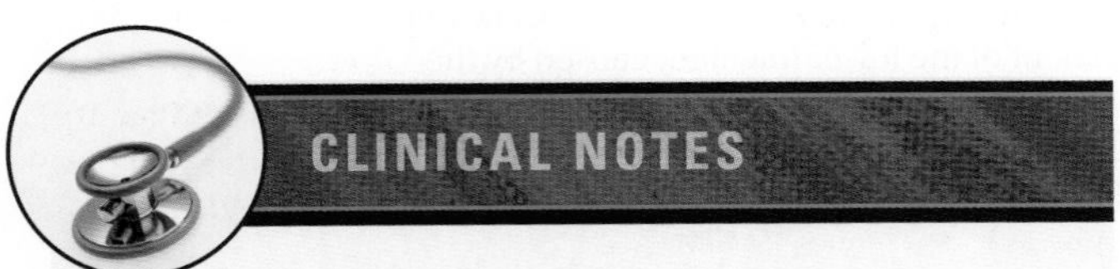

Gluteus Medius and Minimus and Poliomyelitis

The gluteus medius and minimus muscles may be paralyzed when poliomyelitis involves the lower lumbar and sacral segments of the spinal cord. They are supplied by the superior gluteal nerve (L4 and 5 and S1). Paralysis of these muscles seriously interferes with the ability of the patient to tilt the pelvis when walking.

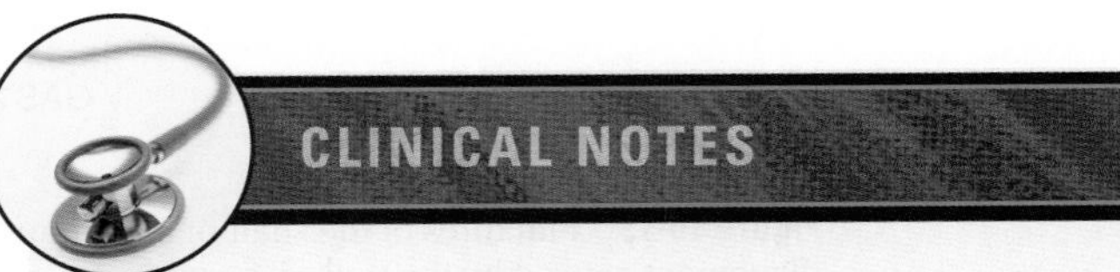

Gluteus Maximus and Intramuscular Injections

The gluteus maximus is a large, thick muscle with coarse fasciculi that can be easily separated without damage. The great thickness of this muscle makes it ideal for intramuscular injections. To avoid injury to the underlying sciatic nerve, the injection should be given well forward on the **upper outer quadrant of the buttock.**

Gluteus Maximus and Bursitis

Bursitis, or inflammation of a bursa, can be caused by acute or chronic trauma. An inflamed bursa becomes distended with excessive amounts of fluid and can be extremely painful. The bursae associated with the gluteus maximus are prone to inflammation.

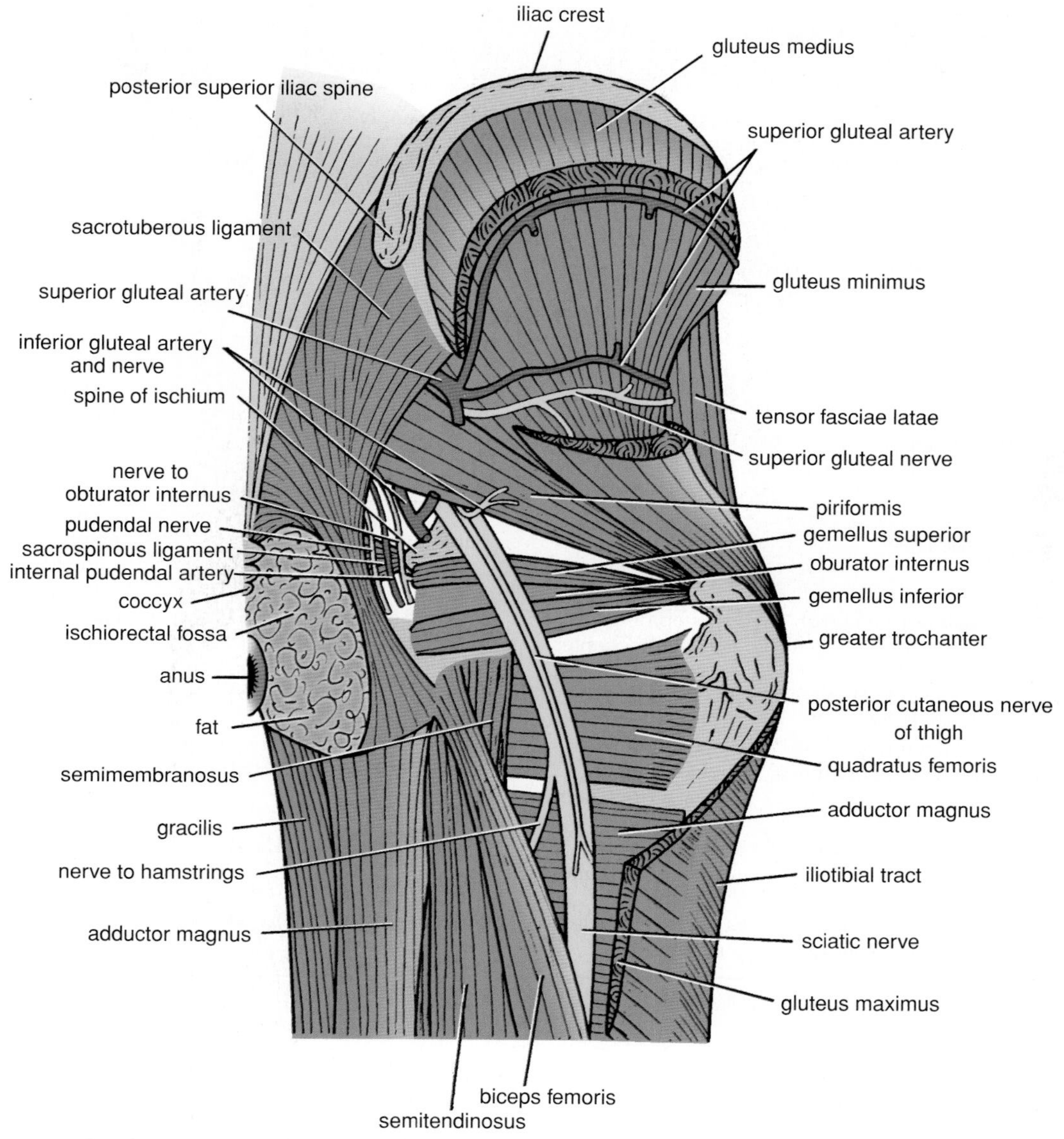

Figure 10-15 Structures in the right gluteal region. The greater part of the gluteus maximus and part of the gluteus medius have been removed.

Nerves of the Gluteal Region

Sciatic Nerve

The sciatic nerve, a branch of the sacral plexus (L4 and 5; S1, 2, and 3), emerges from the pelvis through the lower part of the greater sciatic foramen (Figs. 10-14 and 10-15). It is the largest nerve in the body and consists of the tibial and common peroneal nerves bound together with fascia (Figs. 10-16 and 10-17). The nerve appears below the piriformis muscle and curves downward and laterally, lying successively on the root of the ischial spine, the superior gemellus, the obturator internus, the inferior gemellus, and the quadratus femoris to reach the back of the adductor magnus muscle (Fig. 10-15). It is related posteriorly to the posterior cutaneous nerve of the thigh and the gluteus maximus. It leaves the buttock region by passing deep to the long head of the biceps femoris to enter the back of the thigh (see page 587).

Occasionally, the common peroneal nerve leaves the sciatic nerve high in the pelvis and appears in the gluteal region by passing above or through the piriformis muscle.

The sciatic nerve usually gives no branches in the gluteal region.

Posterior Cutaneous Nerve of the Thigh

The posterior cutaneous nerve of the thigh, a branch of the sacral plexus, enters the gluteal region through the lower part of the greater sciatic foramen below the piriformis muscle (Fig. 10-14). It passes downward on the posterior surface of the sciatic nerve and runs down the back of the thigh beneath the deep fascia. In the popliteal fossa it supplies the skin.

Table 10-1 Muscles of the Gluteal Region

Muscle	Origin	Insertion	Nerve Supply	Nerve Root[a]	Action
Gluteus maximus	Outer surface of ilium, sacrum, coccyx, sacrotuberous ligament	Iliotibial tract and gluteal tuberosity of femur	Inferior gluteal nerve	L5; **S1, 2**	Extends and laterally rotates hip joint; through iliotibial tract, it extends knee joint
Gluteus medius	Outer surface of ilium	Lateral surface of greater trochanter of femur	Superior gluteal nerve	**L5;** S1	Abducts thigh at hip joint; tilts pelvis when walking to permit opposite leg to clear ground
Gluteus minimus	Outer surface of ilium	Anterior surface of greater trochanter of femur	Superior gluteal nerve	**L5;** S1	Abducts thigh at hip joint; tilts pelvis when walking to permit opposite leg to clear ground
Tensor fasciae latae	Iliac crest	Iliotibial tract	Superior gluteal nerve	L4; 5	Assists gluteus maximus in extending the knee joint
Piriformis	Anterior surface of sacrum	Upper border of greater trochanter of femur	First and second sacral nerves	L5; **S1,** 2	Lateral rotator of thigh at hip joint
Obturator internus	Inner surface of obturator membrane	Upper border of greater trochanter of femur	Sacral plexus	L5; **S1**	Lateral rotator of thigh at hip joint
Gemellus superior	Spine of ischium	Upper border of greater trochanter of femur	Sacral plexus	L5; S1	Lateral rotator of thigh at hip joint
Gemellus inferior	Ischial tuberosity	Upper border of greater trochanter of femur	Sacral plexus	L5; S1	Lateral rotator of thigh at hip joint
Quadratus femoris	Lateral border of ischial tuberosity	Quadrate tubercle of femur	Sacral plexus	L5; S1	Lateral rotator of thigh at hip joint

[a] The predominant nerve root supply is indicated by boldface type.

Branches

- **Gluteal branches** to the skin over the lower medial quadrant of the buttock (Fig. 10-1)
- **Perineal branch** to the skin of the back of the scrotum or labium majus
- **Cutaneous branches** to the back of the thigh and the upper part of the leg (Fig. 10-1)

Superior Gluteal Nerve

The superior gluteal nerve, a branch of the sacral plexus, leaves the pelvis through the upper part of the greater sciatic foramen above the piriformis (Fig. 10-15). It runs forward between the gluteus medius and minimus, supplies both, and ends by supplying the tensor fasciae latae.

Inferior Gluteal Nerve

The inferior gluteal nerve, a branch of the sacral plexus, leaves the pelvis through the lower part of the greater sciatic foramen below the piriformis (Figs. 10-14 and 10-15). It supplies the gluteus maximus muscle.

Nerve to the Quadratus Femoris

A branch of the sacral plexus, the nerve to the quadratus femoris leaves the pelvis through the lower part of the greater sciatic foramen (Fig. 10-15). It ends by supplying the quadratus femoris and the inferior gemellus.

Pudendal Nerve and the Nerve to the Obturator Internus

Branches of the sacral plexus, the pudendal nerve, and nerve to the obturator internus leave the pelvis through the lower part of the greater sciatic foramen, below the piriformis (Figs. 10-14 and 10-15). They cross the ischial spine with the internal pudendal artery and immediately re-enter the pelvis through the lesser sciatic foramen; they then lie in the ischiorectal fossa (see page 394). The pudendal nerve supplies structures in the perineum. The nerve to the obturator internus supplies the obturator internus muscle on its pelvic surface.

Arteries of the Gluteal Region

Superior Gluteal Artery

The superior gluteal artery is a branch from the internal iliac artery and enters the gluteal region through the upper part of the greater sciatic foramen above the piriformis (Figs. 10-14 and 10-15). It divides into branches that are distributed throughout the gluteal region.

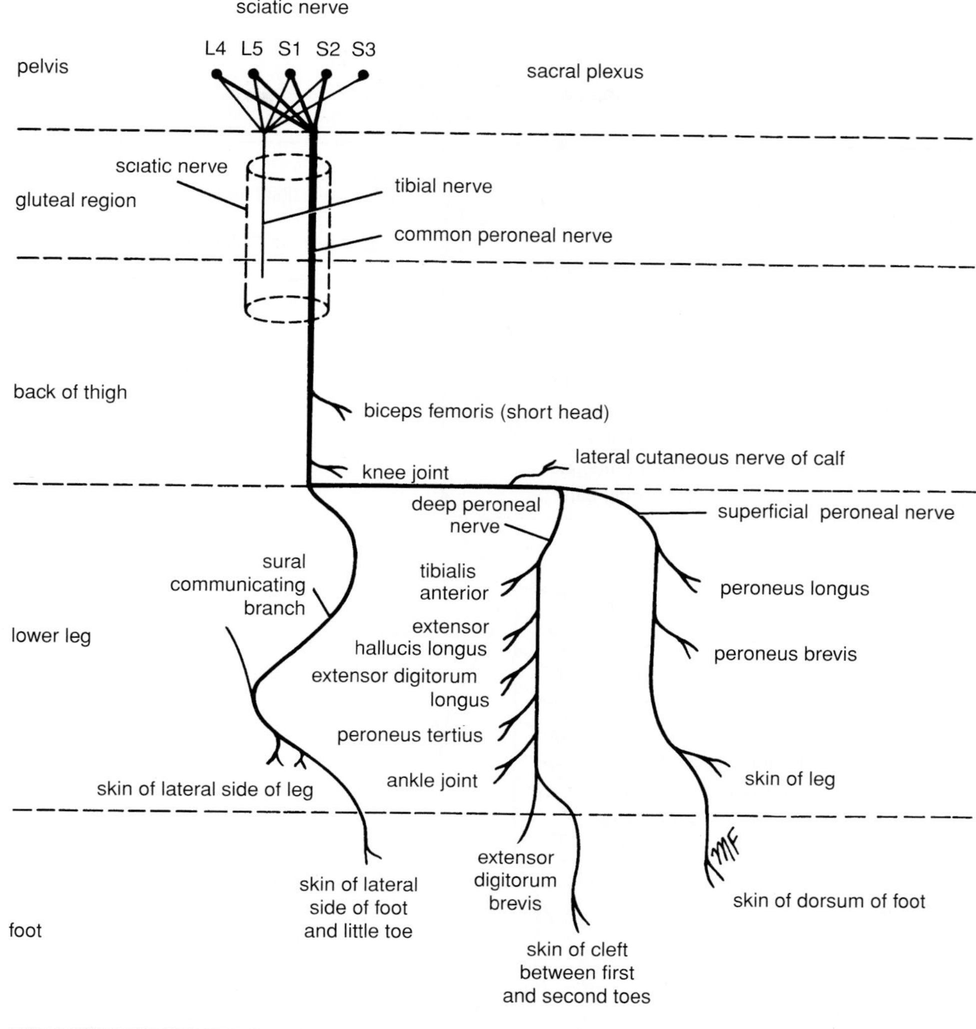

Figure 10-16 Summary of the origin of the sciatic nerve and the main branches of the common peroneal nerve.

Inferior Gluteal Artery

The inferior gluteal artery is a branch of the internal iliac artery and enters the gluteal region through the lower part of the greater sciatic foramen, below the piriformis (Figs. 10-14 and 10-15). It divides into numerous branches that are distributed throughout the gluteal region.

The Trochanteric Anastomosis

The trochanteric anastomosis provides the main blood supply to the head of the femur. The nutrient arteries pass along the femoral neck beneath the capsule (Fig. 10-18). The following arteries take part in the anastomosis: the superior gluteal artery, the inferior gluteal artery, the medial femoral circumflex artery, and the lateral femoral circumflex artery.

The Cruciate Anastomosis

The cruciate anastomosis is situated at the level of the lesser trochanter of the femur and, together with the trochanteric anastomosis, provides a connection between the internal iliac and the femoral arteries. The following arteries take part in the anastomosis: the inferior gluteal artery, the medial femoral circumflex artery, the lateral femoral circumflex artery, and the first perforating artery, a branch of the profunda artery.

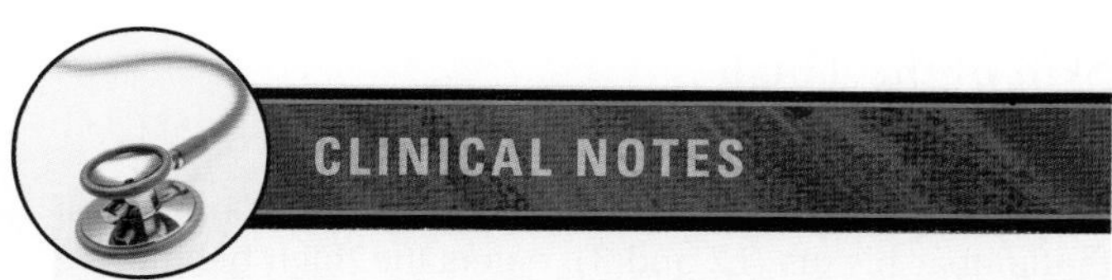

Arterial Anastomoses and Femoral Artery Occlusion

The importance of the trochanteric and cruciate anastomoses in femoral artery occlusion is discussed on page 658.

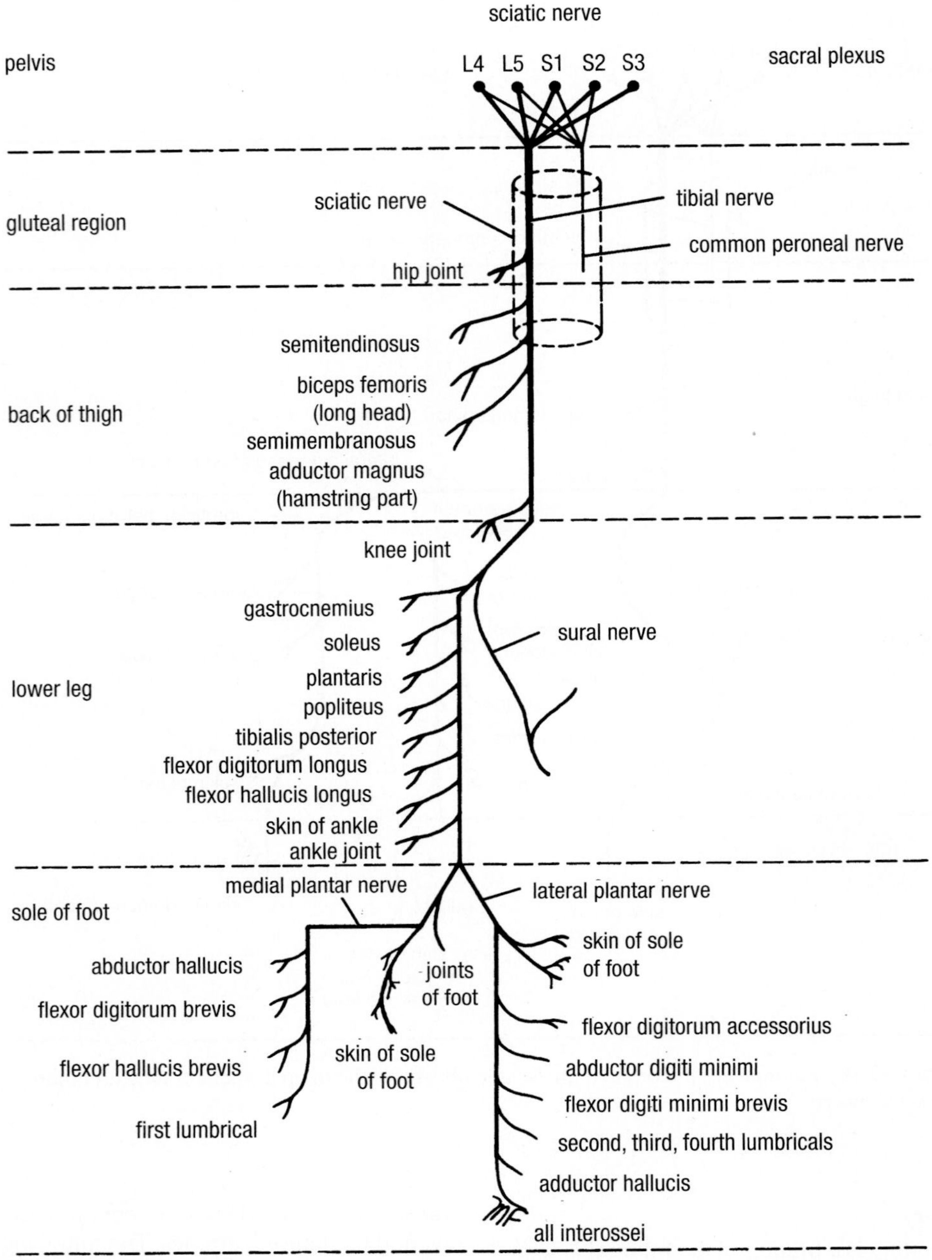

Figure 10-17 Summary of the origin of the sciatic nerve and the main branches of the tibial nerve.

The Front and Medial Aspects of the Thigh

Skin of the Thigh

Cutaneous Nerves

The **lateral cutaneous nerve of the thigh,** a branch of the lumbar plexus (L2 and 3), enters the thigh behind the lateral end of the inguinal ligament (Fig. 10-2). Having divided into anterior and posterior branches, it supplies the skin of the lateral aspect of the thigh and knee. It also supplies the skin of the lower lateral quadrant of the buttock (Fig. 10-1).

The **femoral branch of the genitofemoral nerve,** a branch of the lumbar plexus (L1 and 2), enters the thigh behind the middle of the inguinal ligament and supplies a small area of skin (Fig. 10-2). The genital branch supplies the cremaster muscle (see page 279).

The **ilioinguinal nerve,** a branch of the lumbar plexus (L1), enters the thigh through the superficial inguinal ring (Fig. 10-2). It is distributed to the skin of the root of the penis

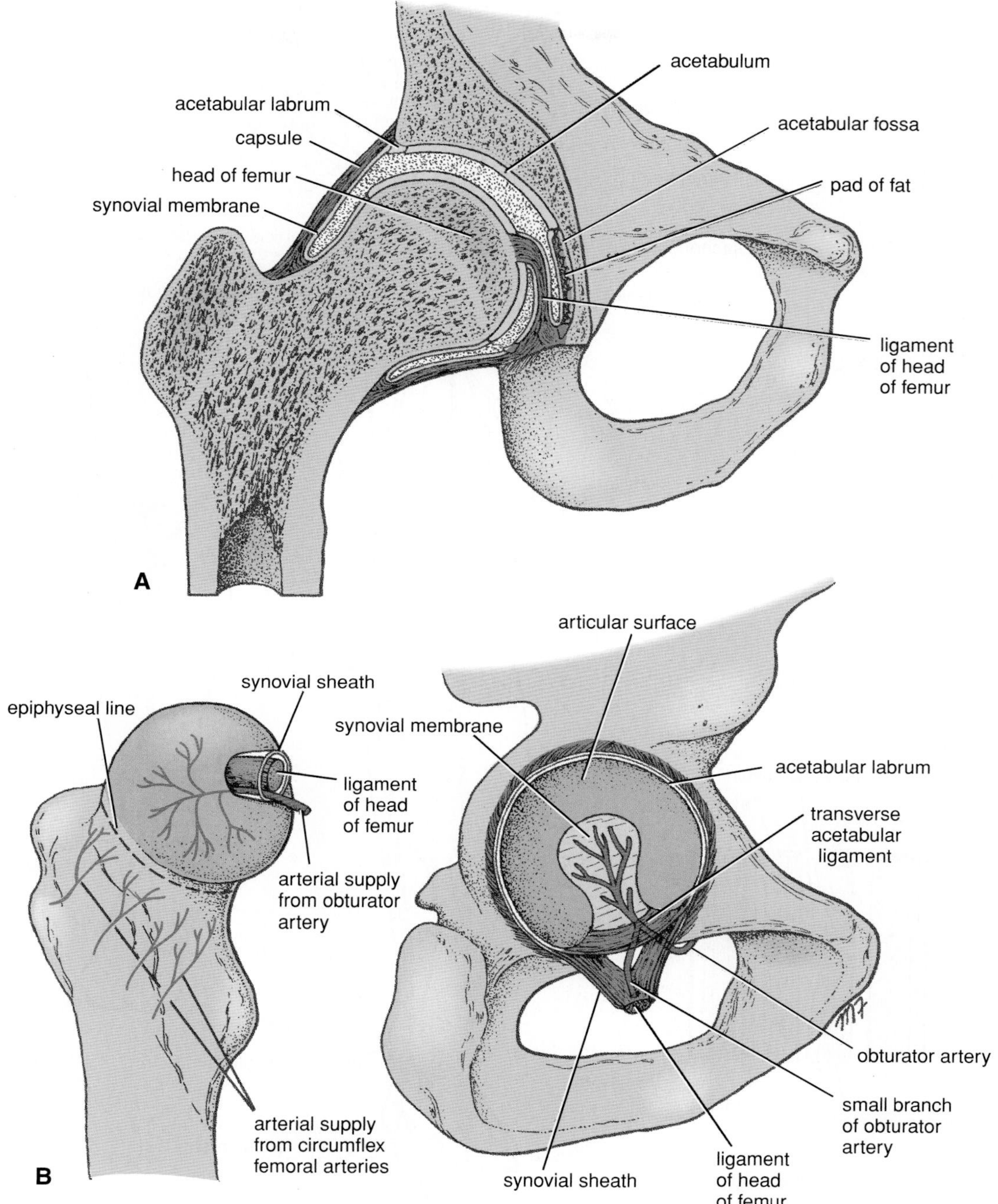

Figure 10-18 Coronal section of the right hip joint (**A**) and articular surfaces of the right hip joint and arterial supply of the head of the femur (**B**).

and adjacent part of the scrotum (or root of the clitoris and adjacent part of the labium majus in the female) and to a small skin area below the medial part of the inguinal ligament.

The **medial cutaneous nerve of the thigh,** a branch of the femoral nerve, supplies the medial aspect of the thigh and joins the patellar plexus (Fig. 10-2).

The **intermediate cutaneous nerve of the thigh,** a branch of the femoral nerve, divides into two branches that supply the anterior aspect of the thigh and joins the patellar plexus (Fig. 10-2).

Branches from the anterior division of the **obturator nerve** supply a variable area of skin on the medial aspect of the thigh (Fig. 10-2).

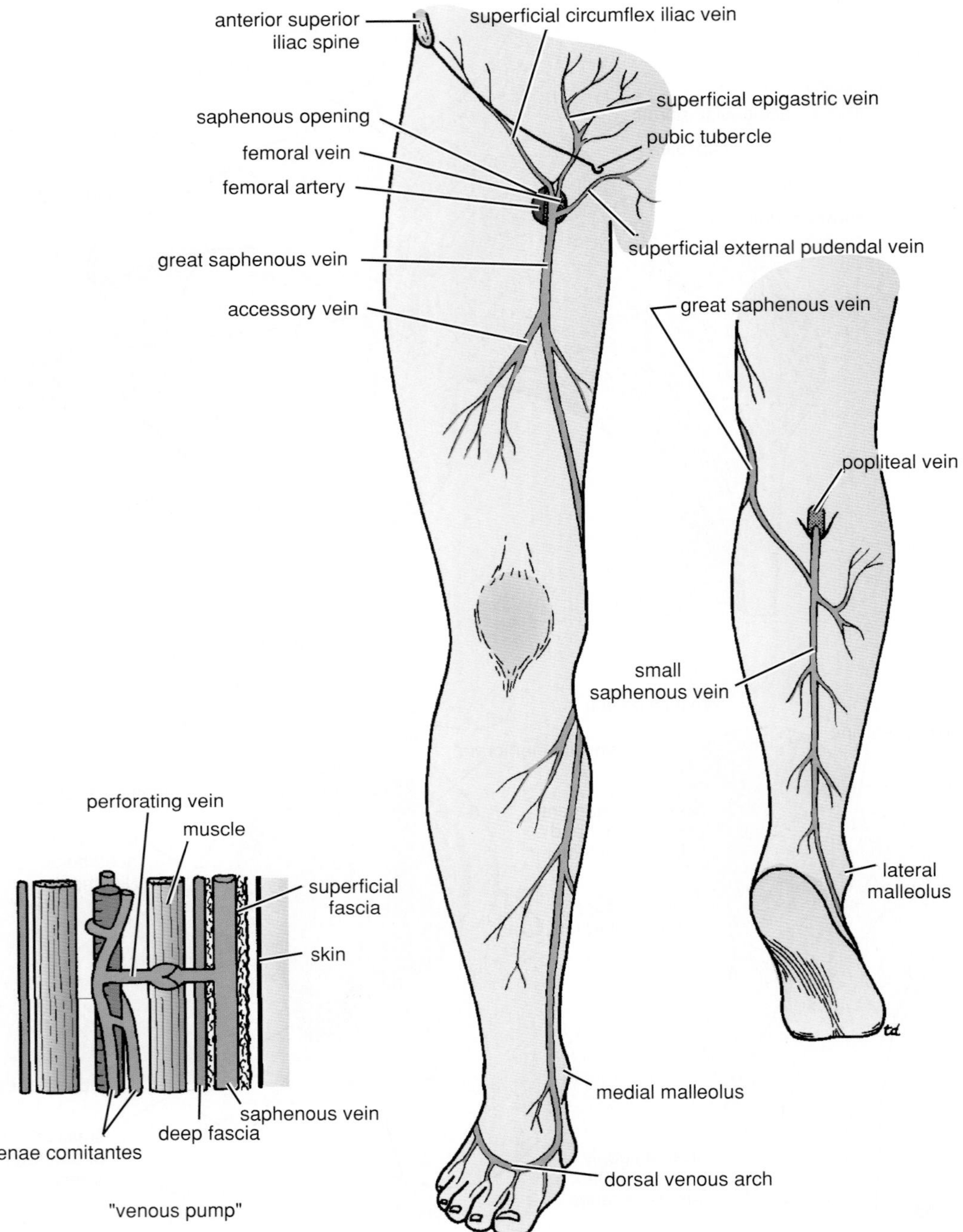

Figure 10-19 Superficial veins of the right lower limb. Note the importance of the valved perforating veins in the "venous pump."

The **patellar plexus** lies in front of the knee and is formed from the terminal branches of the lateral, intermediate, and medial cutaneous nerves of the thigh and the infrapatellar branch of the saphenous nerve (Fig. 10-2).

Superficial Veins

The superficial veins of the leg are the great and small saphenous veins and their tributaries (Fig. 10-19). They are of great clinical importance.

The **great saphenous vein** drains the medial end of the dorsal venous arch of the foot and passes upward **directly in front of** the medial malleolus (Fig. 10-19). It then ascends in company with the saphenous nerve in the superficial fascia over the medial side of the leg. The vein passes behind the knee and curves forward around the medial side of the thigh. It passes through the lower part of the saphenous opening in the deep fascia and joins the femoral vein about 1.5 in. (4 cm) below and lateral to the pubic tubercle (Figs. 10-3 and 10-19).

The great saphenous vein possesses numerous valves and is connected to the small saphenous vein by one or two branches that pass behind the knee. Several **perforating veins** connect the great saphenous vein with the deep veins along the medial side of the calf (Fig. 10-19).

At the saphenous opening in the deep fascia, the great saphenous vein usually receives three tributaries that are variable in size and arrangement (Figs. 10-3 and 10-19): the **superficial circumflex iliac vein,** the **superficial epigastric vein,** and the **superficial external pudendal vein.** These veins correspond with the three branches of the femoral artery found in this region.

An additional vein, known as the **accessory vein,** usually joins the main vein about the middle of the thigh or higher up at the saphenous opening.

The **small saphenous vein** is described on page 615.

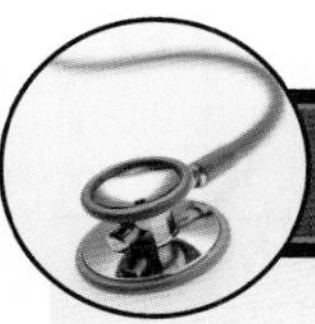

CLINICAL NOTES

Veins of the Lower Limb

The veins of the lower limb can be divided into three groups: superficial, deep, and perforating. The **superficial veins** consist of the great and small saphenous veins and their tributaries, which are situated beneath the skin in the superficial fascia. The constant position of the great saphenous vein in front of the medial malleolus should be remembered for patients requiring emergency blood transfusion. The **deep veins** are the venae comitantes to the anterior and posterior tibial arteries, the popliteal vein, and the femoral veins and their tributaries. The **perforating veins** are communicating vessels that run between the superficial and deep veins. Many of these veins are found particularly in the region of the ankle and the medial side of the lower part of the leg. They possess valves that are arranged to prevent the flow of blood from the deep to the superficial veins.

Venous Pump of the Lower Limb

Within the closed fascial compartments of the lower limb, the thin-walled, valved venae comitantes are subjected to intermittent pressure at rest and during exercise. The pulsations of the adjacent arteries help move the blood up the limb. However, the contractions of the large muscles within the compartments during exercise compress these deeply placed veins and force the blood up the limb.

The superficial saphenous veins, except near their termination, lie within the superficial fascia and are not subject to these compression forces. The valves in the perforating veins prevent the high-pressure venous blood from being forced outward into the low-pressure superficial veins. Moreover, as the muscles within the closed fascial compartments relax, venous blood is sucked from the superficial into the deep veins.

Varicose Veins

A varicosed vein is one that has a larger diameter than normal and is elongated and tortuous. Varicosity of the esophageal and rectal veins is described elsewhere (see pages 129 and 395). This condition commonly occurs in the superficial veins of the lower limb and, although not life-threatening, is responsible for considerable discomfort and pain.

Varicosed veins have many causes, including hereditary weakness of the vein walls and incompetent valves; elevated intra-abdominal pressure as a result of multiple pregnancies or abdominal tumors; and thrombophlebitis of the deep veins, which results in the superficial veins becoming the main venous pathway for the lower limb. It is easy to understand how this condition can be produced by incompetence of a valve in a perforating vein. Every time the patient exercises, high-pressure venous blood escapes from the deep veins into the superficial veins and produces a varicosity, which might be localized to begin with but becomes more extensive later.

The successful operative treatment of varicosed veins depends on the ligation and division of all the main tributaries of the great or small saphenous veins, to prevent a collateral venous circulation from developing, and the ligation and division of all the perforating veins responsible for the leakage of high-pressure blood from the deep to the superficial veins. It is now common practice to remove or strip the superficial veins in addition. Needless to say, it is imperative to ascertain that the deep veins are patent before operative measures are taken.

Great Saphenous Vein Cutdown

Exposure of the great saphenous vein through a skin incision (a "cutdown") is usually performed at the ankle (Fig. 10-20). This site has the disadvantage that phlebitis (inflammation of the vein wall) is a potential complication. The great saphenous vein also can be entered at the groin in the femoral triangle, where phlebitis is relatively rare; the larger diameter of the vein at this site permits the use of large-diameter catheters and the rapid infusion of large volumes of fluids.

Anatomy of Ankle Vein Cutdown

The procedure is as follows:

1. The sensory nerve supply to the skin immediately in front of the medial malleolus of the tibia is from branches of the saphenous nerve, a branch of the femoral nerve. The saphenous nerve branches are blocked with local anesthetic.
2. A transverse incision is made through the skin and subcutaneous tissue across the long axis of the vein just anterior and superior to the medial malleolus (Fig. 10-20). Although the vein may not be visible through the skin, it is **constantly** found at this site.
3. The vein is easily identified, and the **saphenous nerve** should be recognized; the nerve usually lies just anterior to the vein (Fig. 10-20).

Anatomy of Groin Vein Cutdown

1. The area of thigh skin below and lateral to the scrotum or labium majus is supplied by branches of the ilioinguinal nerve and the intermediate cutaneous nerve of the thigh. The branches of these nerves are blocked with local anesthetic.
2. A transverse incision is made through the skin and subcutaneous tissue centered on a point about 1.5 in. (4 cm) below and lateral to the pubic tubercle (Fig. 10-20). If the femoral pulse can be felt (may be absent in patients with severe

(continues)

Clinical Notes, *continued*

shock), the incision is carried medially just medial to the pulse.

3. The great saphenous vein lies in the subcutaneous fat and passes posteriorly through the saphenous opening in the deep fascia to join the femoral vein about 1.5 in. (4 cm), or two fingerbreadths below and lateral to the pubic tubercle. It is important to understand that the great saphenous vein passes through the saphenous opening to gain entrance to the femoral vein. However, the size and shape of the opening are subject to variation.

The Great Saphenous Vein in Coronary Bypass Surgery

In patients with occlusive coronary disease caused by atherosclerosis, the diseased arterial segment can be bypassed by inserting a graft consisting of a portion of the great saphenous vein. The venous segment is reversed so that its valves do not obstruct the arterial flow. Following removal of the great saphenous vein at the donor site, the superficial venous blood ascends the lower limb by passing through perforating veins and entering the deep veins.

The great saphenous vein can also be used to bypass obstructions of the brachial or femoral arteries.

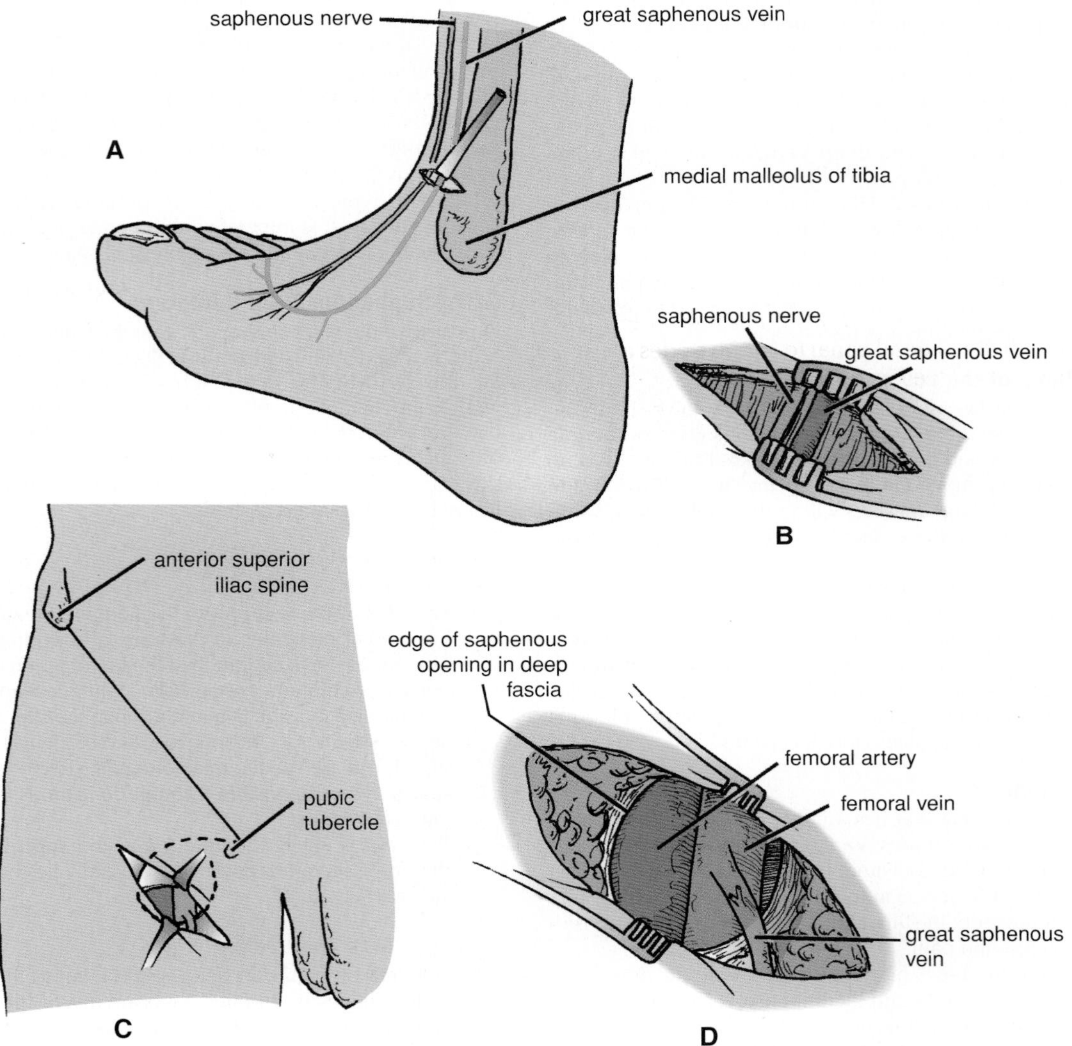

Figure 10-20 Great saphenous vein cutdown. **A, B.** At the ankle. The great saphenous vein is constantly found in front of the medial malleolus of the tibia. **C, D.** At the groin. The great saphenous vein drains into the femoral vein two fingerbreadths below and lateral to the pubic tubercle.

Inguinal Lymph Nodes

The inguinal lymph nodes are divided into superficial and deep groups.

Superficial Inguinal Lymph Nodes

The superficial nodes lie in the superficial fascia below the inguinal ligament and can be divided into a horizontal and a vertical group (Figs. 10-3 and 10-4).

The **horizontal group** lies just below and parallel to the inguinal ligament (Figs. 10-3 and 10-4). The medial members of the group receive superficial lymph vessels from the anterior abdominal wall below the level of the umbilicus and from the perineum (Fig. 10-4). The lymph vessels from the urethra, the external genitalia of both sexes (but not the testes), and the lower half of the anal canal are drained by this route. The lateral members of the group receive superficial lymph vessels from the back below the level of the iliac crests (Fig. 10-4).

The **vertical group** lies along the terminal part of the great saphenous vein and receives most of the superficial lymph vessels of the lower limb (Figs. 10-3 and 10-4).

The efferent lymph vessels from the superficial inguinal nodes pass through the saphenous opening in the deep fascia and join the deep inguinal nodes.

Deep Inguinal Lymph Nodes

The deep nodes are located beneath the deep fascia and lie along the medial side of the femoral vein (Fig. 10-21); the efferent vessels from these nodes enter the abdomen by passing through the femoral canal to lymph nodes along the external iliac artery (see Fig. 5-76).

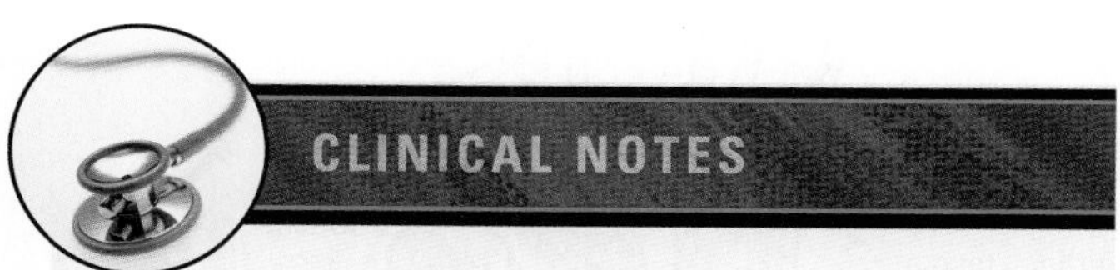

Lymphatics of the Lower Limb

The superficial and deep inguinal lymph nodes not only drain all the lymph from the lower limb, but also drain lymph from the skin and superficial fascia of the anterior and posterior abdominal walls below the level of the umbilicus; lymph from the external genitalia and the mucous membrane of the lower half of the anal canal also drains into these nodes. Remember the large distances the lymph has had to travel in some instances before it reaches the inguinal nodes. For example, a patient may present with an enlarged, painful inguinal lymph node caused by lymphatic spread of pathogenic organisms that entered the body through a small scratch on the undersurface of the big toe.

Superficial Fascia of the Thigh

The **membranous layer of the superficial fascia** of the anterior abdominal wall extends into the thigh and is attached to the deep fascia (fascia lata) about a fingerbreadth below the inguinal ligament (Figs. 10-3 and 10-21). The importance of this fact in connection with extravasation of urine after a rupture of the urethra is fully described in Chapter 4.

The **fatty layer of the superficial fascia** on the anterior abdominal wall extends into the thigh and continues down over the lower limb without interruption (Fig. 10-21).

Deep Fascia of the Thigh (Fascia Lata)

The deep fascia encloses the thigh like a trouser leg (Fig. 10-22) and at its upper end is attached to the pelvis and the inguinal ligament. On its lateral aspect, it is thickened to form the **iliotibial tract** (Figs. 10-6 and 10-22), which is attached above to the iliac tubercle and below to the lateral condyle of the tibia. The iliotibial tract receives the insertion of the tensor fasciae latae and the greater part of the gluteus maximus muscle (see Figures 10-5 and 10-6). In the gluteal region, the deep fascia forms sheaths, which enclose the tensor fasciae latae and the gluteus maximus muscles.

The **saphenous opening** is a gap in the deep fascia in the front of the thigh just below the inguinal ligament. It transmits the great saphenous vein, some small branches of the femoral artery, and lymph vessels (Fig. 10-3). The saphenous opening is situated about 1.5 in. (4 cm) below and lateral to the pubic tubercle. The **falciform margin** is the lower lateral border of the opening, which lies anterior to the femoral vessels (Fig. 10-3). The border of the opening then curves upward and medially, and then laterally behind the femoral vessels, to be attached to the pectineal line of the superior ramus of the pubis.

The saphenous opening is filled with loose connective tissue called the **cribriform fascia.**

Fascial Compartments of the Thigh

Three fascial septa pass from the inner aspect of the deep fascial sheath of the thigh to the linea aspera of the femur (Fig. 10-22). By this means, the thigh is divided into three compartments, each having muscles, nerves, and arteries. The compartments are anterior, medial, and posterior in position.

Contents of the Anterior Fascial Compartment of the Thigh

- **Muscles:** Sartorius, iliacus, psoas, pectineus, and quadriceps femoris
- **Blood supply:** Femoral artery
- **Nerve supply:** Femoral nerve

Muscles of the Anterior Fascial Compartment of the Thigh

The muscles are seen in Figures 10-6, 10-23, and 10-24 and are described in Table 10-2.

Note the following:

Action of Quadriceps Femoris Muscle (Quadriceps Mechanism)

The quadriceps femoris muscle, consisting of the rectus femoris, the vastus intermedius, the vastus lateralis, and

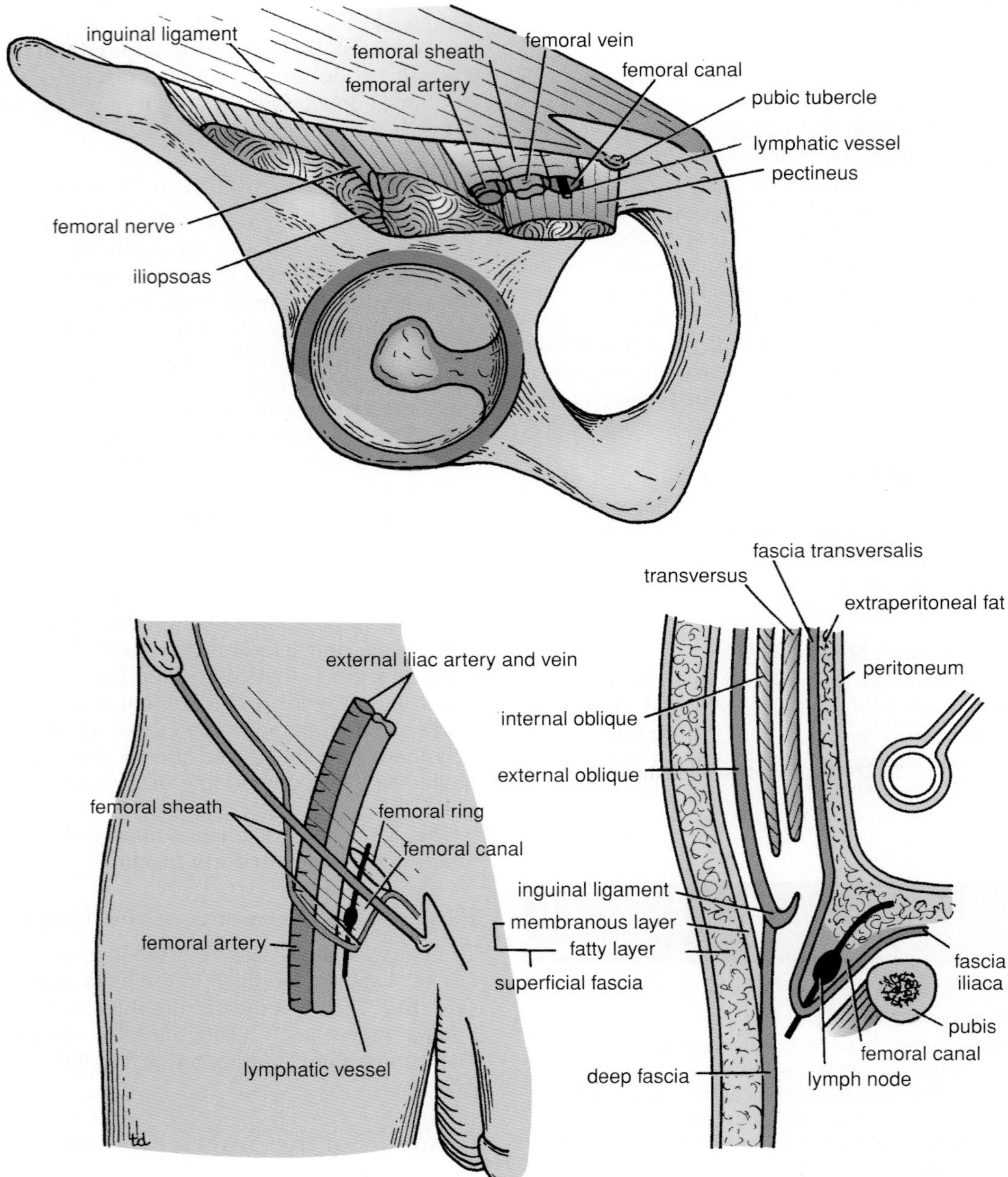

Figure 10-21 Right femoral sheath and its contents.

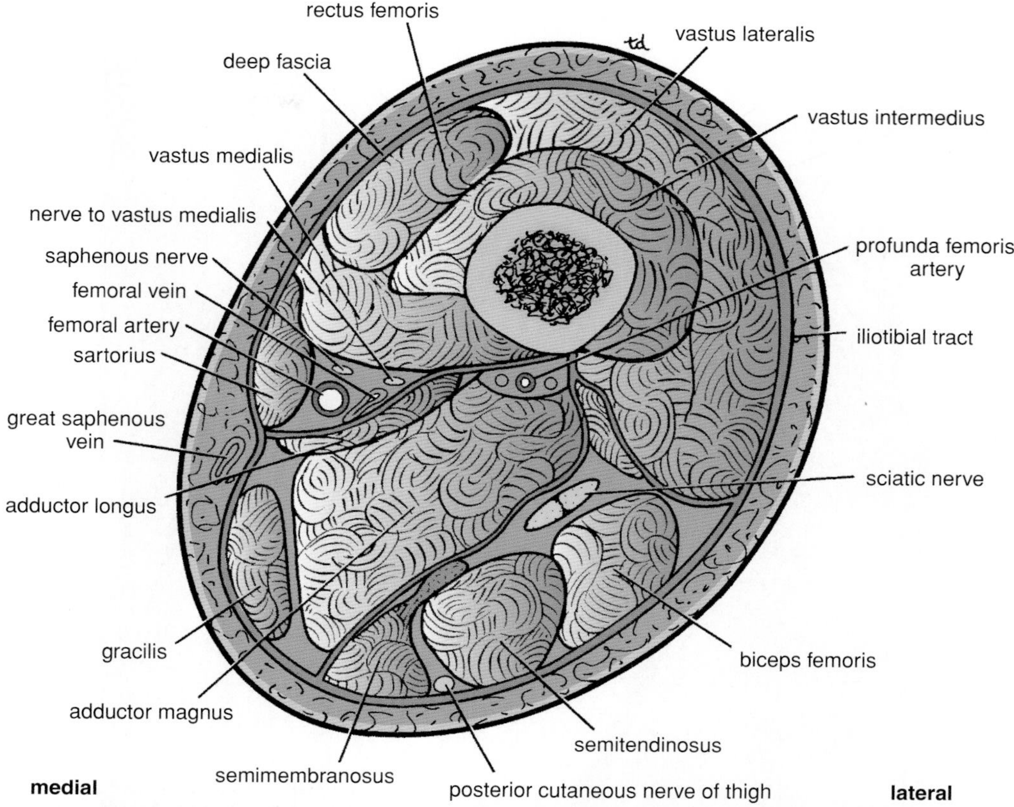

Figure 10-22 Transverse section through the middle of the right thigh as seen from above.

the vastus medialis, is inserted into the patella and, via the ligamentum patellae, is attached to the tibial tuberosity (Fig. 10-25). Together they provide a powerful extensor of the knee joint. Some of the tendinous fibers of the vastus lateralis and vastus medialis form bands, or **retinacula,** that join the capsule of the knee joint and strengthen it. The lowest muscle fibers of the vastus medialis are almost horizontal and prevent the patella from being pulled laterally during contraction of the quadriceps muscle. The tone of the quadriceps muscle greatly strengthens the knee joint.

The rectus femoris muscle also flexes the hip joint.

Femoral Triangle

The femoral triangle is a triangular depressed area situated in the upper part of the medial aspect of the thigh just below the inguinal ligament (Fig. 10-6). Its boundaries are as follows:

- **Superiorly:** The inguinal ligament
- **Laterally:** The sartorius muscle
- **Medially:** The adductor longus muscle

Its **floor** is gutter shaped and formed from lateral to medial by the iliopsoas, the pectineus, and the adductor longus. Its **roof** is formed by the skin and fasciae of the thigh.

The femoral triangle contains the terminal part of the femoral nerve and its branches, the femoral sheath, the femoral artery and its branches, the femoral vein and its tributaries, and the deep inguinal lymph nodes.

Adductor (Subsartorial) Canal

The adductor canal is an intermuscular cleft situated on the medial aspect of the middle third of the thigh beneath the sartorius muscle (Figs. 10-6 and 10-22). It commences above at the apex of the femoral triangle and ends below at the opening in the adductor magnus. In cross section it is triangular, having an anteromedial wall, a posterior wall, and a lateral wall.

- The **anteromedial wall** is formed by the sartorius muscle and fascia.
- The **posterior wall** is formed by the adductor longus and magnus.
- The **lateral wall** is formed by the vastus medialis.

The adductor canal contains the terminal part of the femoral artery, the femoral vein, the deep lymph vessels, the saphenous nerve, the nerve to the vastus medialis, and the terminal part of the obturator nerve.

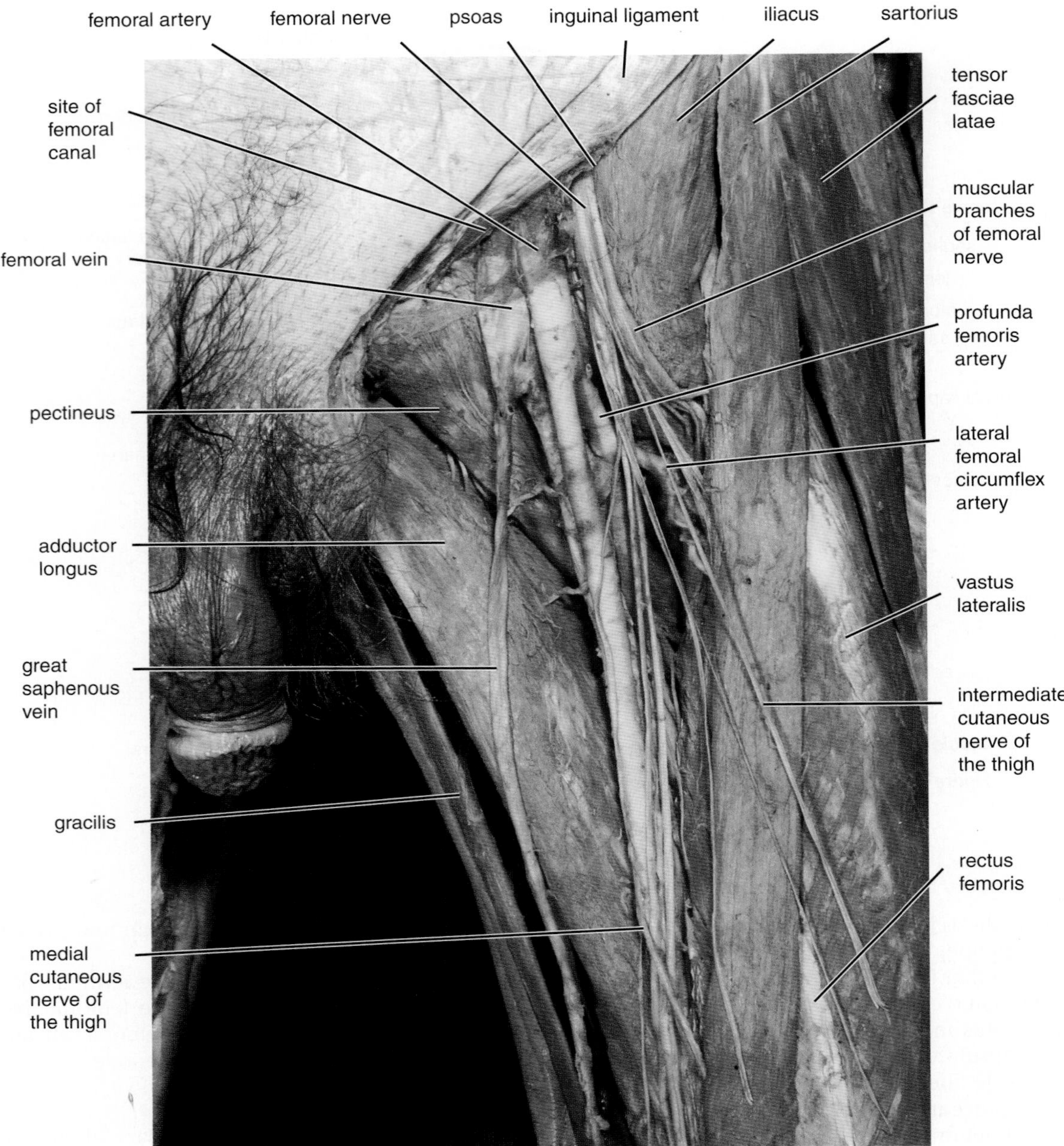

Figure 10-23 Dissection of the femoral triangle in the left lower limb

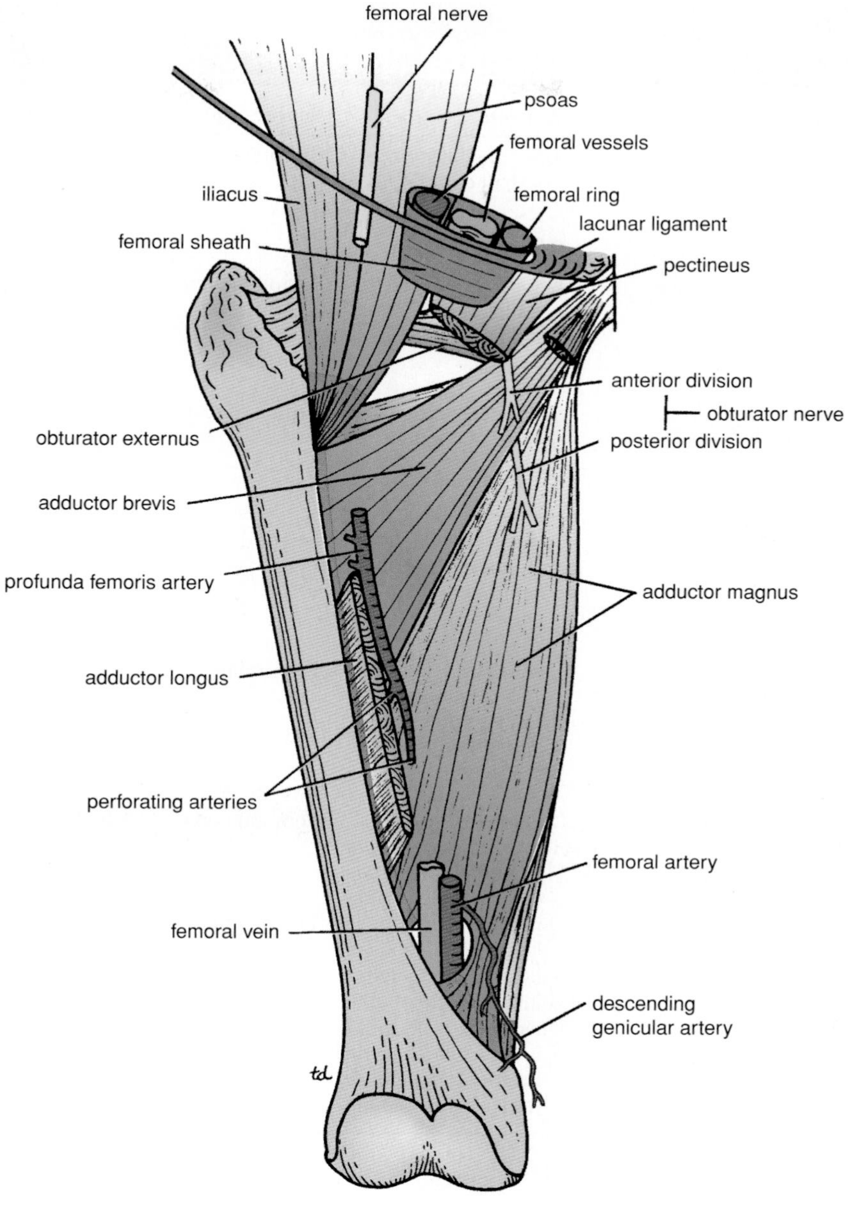

Figure 10-24 Relationship between the obturator nerve and the adductor muscles in the right lower limb.

Table 10-2 Muscles of the Anterior Fascial Compartment of the Thigh

Muscle	Origin	Insertion	Nerve Supply	Nerve Root[a]	Action
Sartorius	Anterior superior iliac spine	Upper medial surface of shaft of tibia	Femoral nerve	L2, 3	Flexes, abducts, laterally rotates thigh at hip joint; flexes and medially rotates leg at knee joint
Iliacus	Iliac fossa of hip bone	With psoas into lesser trochanter of femur	Femoral nerve	**L2,** 3	Flexes thigh on trunk; if thigh is fixed, it flexes the trunk on the thigh as in sitting up from lying down
Psoas	Transverse processes, bodies, and intervertebral discs of the 12th thoracic and five lumbar vertebrae	With iliacus into lesser trochanter of femur	Lumbar plexus	**L1, 2,** 3	Flexes thigh on trunk; if thigh is fixed, it flexes the trunk on thigh as in sitting up from lying down
Pectineus	Superior ramus of pubis	Upper end of linea aspera of shaft of femur	Femoral nerve	**L2,** 3	Flexes and adducts thigh at hip joint
Quadriceps femoris					
Rectus femoris	Straight head: anterior inferior iliac spine	Quadriceps tendon into patella, then via ligamentum patellae into tubercle of tibia	Femoral nerve	L2, **3, 4**	Extension of leg at knee joint; flexes thigh at hip joint
	Reflected head: ilium above acetabulum				
Vastus lateralis	Upper end and shaft of femur	Quadriceps tendon into patella, then via ligamentum patellae into tubercle of tibia	Femoral nerve	L2, **3, 4**	Extension of leg at knee joint
Vastus medialis	Upper end and shaft of femur	Quadriceps tendon into patella, then via ligamentum patellae into tubercle of tibia	Femoral nerve	L2, **3, 4**	Extension of leg at knee joint; stabilizes patella
Vastus intermedius	Anterior and lateral surfaces of shaft of femur	Quadriceps tendon into patella, then via ligamentum patellae into tubercle of tibia	Femoral nerve	L2, **3, 4**	Extension of leg at knee joint; articularis genus retracts synovial membrane

[a] The predominant nerve root supply is indicated by boldface type.

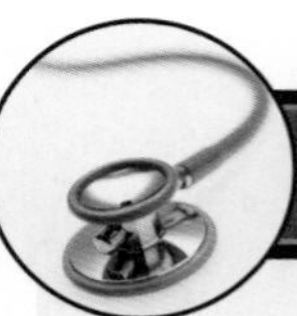

CLINICAL NOTES

Quadriceps Femoris as a Knee Joint Stabilizer

The quadriceps femoris is a most important extensor muscle for the knee joint. Its tone greatly strengthens the joint; therefore, this muscle mass must be carefully examined when disease of the knee joint is suspected. Both thighs should be examined, and the size, consistency, and strength of the quadriceps muscles should be tested. Reduction in size caused by muscle atrophy can be tested by measuring the circumference of each thigh a fixed distance above the superior border of the patella.

The vastus medialis muscle extends farther distally than the vastus lateralis. Remember that the vastus medialis is the first part of the quadriceps muscle to atrophy in knee joint disease and the last to recover.

Rupture of the Rectus Femoris

The rectus femoris muscle can rupture in sudden violent extension movements of the knee joint. The muscle belly retracts proximally, leaving a gap that may be palpable on the anterior surface of the thigh. In complete rupture of the muscle, surgical repair is indicated.

Rupture of the Ligamentum Patellae

This can occur when a sudden flexing force is applied to the knee joint when the quadriceps femoris muscle is actively contracting

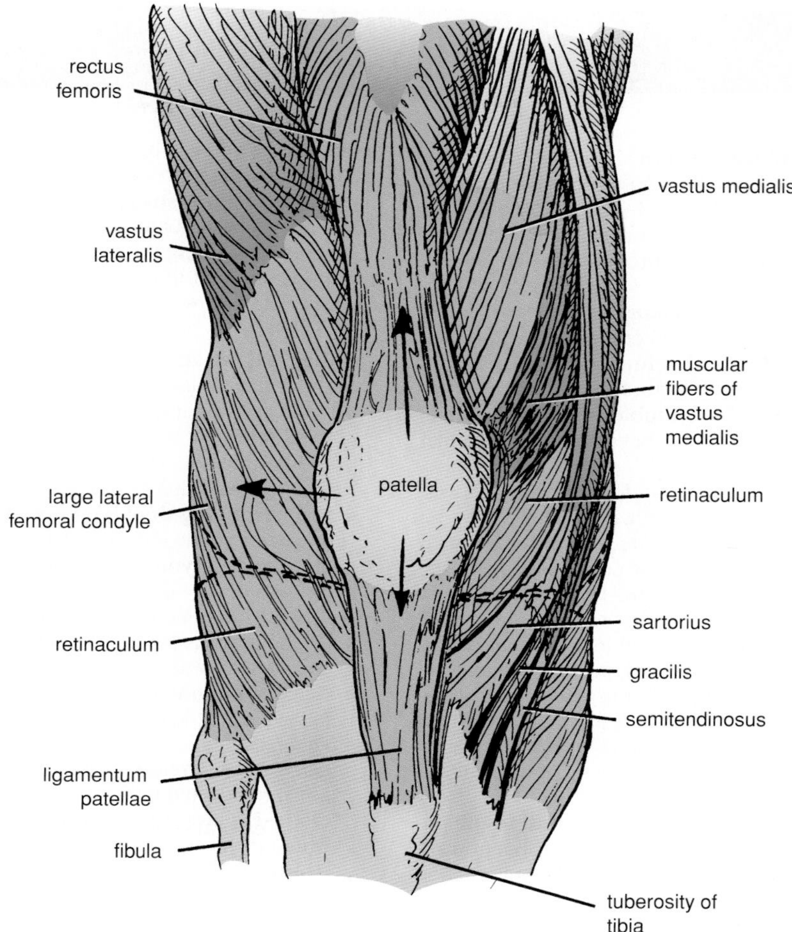

Figure 10-25 The quadriceps femoris mechanism. The lateral and upward pull of the powerful rectus femoris and the vastus lateralis muscles on the patella is counteracted by the lowest horizontal muscular fibers of the vastus medialis and the large lateral condyle of the femur, which projects forward.

Femoral Sheath

The femoral sheath (Figs. 10-3, 10-6, 10-21, and 10-24) is a downward protrusion into the thigh of the fascial envelope lining the abdominal walls (see page 177). Its anterior wall is continuous above with the fascia transversalis, and its posterior wall with the fascia iliaca. The sheath surrounds the femoral vessels and lymphatics for about 1 in. (2.5 cm) below the inguinal ligament. The **femoral artery,** as it enters the thigh beneath the inguinal ligament, occupies the **lateral compartment** of the sheath. The **femoral vein,** as it leaves the thigh, lies on its medial side and is separated from it by a fibrous septum and occupies the **intermediate compartment.** The lymph vessels, as they leave the thigh, are separated from the vein by a fibrous septum and occupy the most **medial compartment** (Fig. 10-21).

The **femoral canal** is the small medial compartment for the lymph vessels (Fig. 10-21). It is about 0.5 in. (1.3 cm) long, and its upper opening is called the **femoral ring.** The **femoral septum,** which is a condensation of extraperitoneal tissue, closes the ring. The femoral canal contains fatty connective tissue, all the efferent lymph vessels from the deep inguinal lymph nodes, and one of the deep inguinal lymph nodes.

The femoral sheath is adherent to the walls of the blood vessels and inferiorly blends with the tunica adventitia of these vessels. The part of the femoral sheath that forms the medially located femoral canal is not adherent to the walls of the small lymph vessels; it is this site that forms a potentially weak area in the abdomen. A protrusion of peritoneum could be forced down the femoral canal, pushing the femoral septum before it. Such a condition is known as a **femoral hernia** and is described below.

The femoral ring (Fig. 10-21) has the following important relations: anteriorly, the inguinal ligament; posteriorly, the superior ramus of the pubis; medially, the lacunar ligament; and laterally, the femoral vein.

The lower end of the canal is normally closed by the adherence of its medial wall to the tunica adventitia of the femoral vein. It lies close to the saphenous opening in the deep fascia of the thigh (Fig. 10-3).

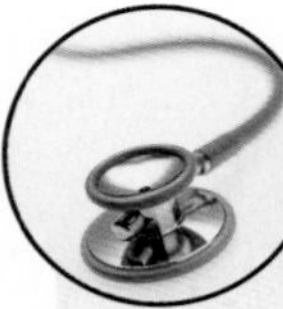

CLINICAL NOTES

Femoral Sheath and Femoral Hernia

The hernial sac descends through the femoral canal within the femoral sheath.

The femoral sheath is a prolongation downward into the thigh of the fascial lining of the abdomen. It surrounds the femoral vessels and lymphatic vessels for about 1 in. (2.5 cm) below the inguinal ligament (see Fig. 10-21). The **femoral artery,** as it enters the thigh below the inguinal ligament, occupies the lateral compartment of the sheath. The **femoral vein,** which lies on its medial side and is separated from it by a fibrous septum, occupies the intermediate compartment. The **lymphatics,** which are separated from the vein by a fibrous septum, occupy the most medial compartment.

The **femoral canal,** the compartment for the lymphatic vessels, occupies the medial part of the sheath. It is about 0.5 in. (1.3 cm) long, and its upper opening is referred to as the **femoral ring.** The **femoral septum,** which is a condensation of extraperitoneal tissue, plugs the opening of the femoral ring.

A **femoral hernia** is more common in women than in men (possibly because of their wider pelvis and femoral canal). The hernial sac passes down the femoral canal, pushing the femoral septum before it. On escaping through the lower end of the femoral canal, it expands to form a swelling in the upper part of the thigh deep to the deep fascia (see page 184). With further expansion, the hernial sac may turn upward to cross the anterior surface of the inguinal ligament.

The neck of the sac always lies **below and lateral to the pubic tubercle** (see page 185). This serves to distinguish it from an inguinal hernia, which lies above and medial to the pubic tubercle. The neck of the sac is narrow and lies at the femoral ring. The ring is related anteriorly to the inguinal ligament, posteriorly to the pectineal ligament and the superior ramus of the pubis, medially to the sharp free edge of the lacunar ligament, and laterally to the femoral vein. Because of these anatomic structures, the neck of the sac is unable to expand. Once an abdominal viscus has passed through the neck into the body of the sac, it may be difficult to push it up and return it to the abdominal cavity **(irreducible hernia).** Furthermore, after the patient strains or coughs, a piece of bowel may be forced through the neck, and its blood vessels may be compressed by the femoral ring, seriously impairing its blood supply **(strangulated hernia).** A femoral hernia is a dangerous condition and should always be treated surgically.

When considering the differential diagnosis of a femoral hernia, it is important to consider diseases that may involve other anatomic structures close to the inguinal ligament. For example:

- **Inguinal canal:** The swelling of an inguinal hernia lies above the medial end of the inguinal ligament. Should the hernial sac emerge through the superficial inguinal ring to start its descent into the scrotum, the swelling will lie above and medial to the pubic tubercle. The sac of a femoral hernia lies below and lateral to the pubic tubercle.
- **Superficial inguinal lymph nodes:** Usually, more than one lymph node is enlarged. In patients with inflammation of the nodes **(lymphadenitis),** carefully examine the entire area of the body that drains its lymph into these nodes. A small, unnoticed skin abrasion may be found. Never forget the mucous membrane of the lower half of the anal canal—it may have an undiscovered carcinoma.
- **Great saphenous vein:** A localized dilatation of the terminal part of the great saphenous vein, a **saphenous varix,** can cause confusion, especially because a hernia and a varix increase in size when the patient is asked to cough. (Elevated intra-abdominal pressure drives the blood downward.) The presence of varicose veins elsewhere in the leg should help in the diagnosis.
- **Psoas sheath:** Tuberculous infection of a lumbar vertebra can result in the extravasation of pus down the psoas sheath into the thigh. The presence of a swelling above and below the inguinal ligament, together with clinical signs and symptoms referred to the vertebral column, should make the diagnosis obvious.
- **Femoral artery:** An expansile swelling lying along the course of the femoral artery that fluctuates in time with the pulse rate should make the diagnosis of **aneurysm of the femoral artery** certain.

Blood Supply of the Anterior Fascial Compartment of the Thigh

Femoral Artery

The femoral artery enters the thigh from behind the inguinal ligament, as a continuation of the external iliac artery (Figs. 10-6, 10-23, and 10-26). Here, it lies midway between the anterior superior iliac spine and the symphysis pubis. The femoral artery is the main arterial supply to the lower limb. It descends almost vertically toward the adductor tubercle of the femur and ends at the opening in the adductor magnus muscle by entering the popliteal space as the popliteal artery (Fig. 10-24).

Relations

- **Anteriorly:** In the upper part of its course, it is superficial and is covered by skin and fascia. In the lower part of its course, it passes behind the sartorius muscle (Fig. 10-6).
- **Posteriorly:** The artery lies on the psoas, which separates it from the hip joint, the pectineus, and the adductor longus (Fig. 10-6). The femoral vein intervenes between the artery and the adductor longus.
- **Medially:** It is related to the femoral vein in the upper part of its course (Figs. 10-6 and 10-23).
- **Laterally:** The femoral nerve and its branches (Fig. 10-6)

Branches

- The **superficial circumflex iliac artery** is a small branch that runs up to the region of the anterior superior iliac spine (Fig. 10-3).
- The **superficial epigastric artery** is a small branch that crosses the inguinal ligament and runs to the region of the umbilicus (Fig. 10-3).
- The **superficial external pudendal artery** (Fig. 10-3) is a small branch that runs medially to supply the skin of the scrotum (or labium majus).
- The **deep external pudendal artery** (Fig. 10-6) runs medially and supplies the skin of the scrotum (or labium majus).
- The **profunda femoris artery** is a large and important branch that arises from the lateral side of the femoral artery about 1.5 in. (4 cm) below the inguinal ligament

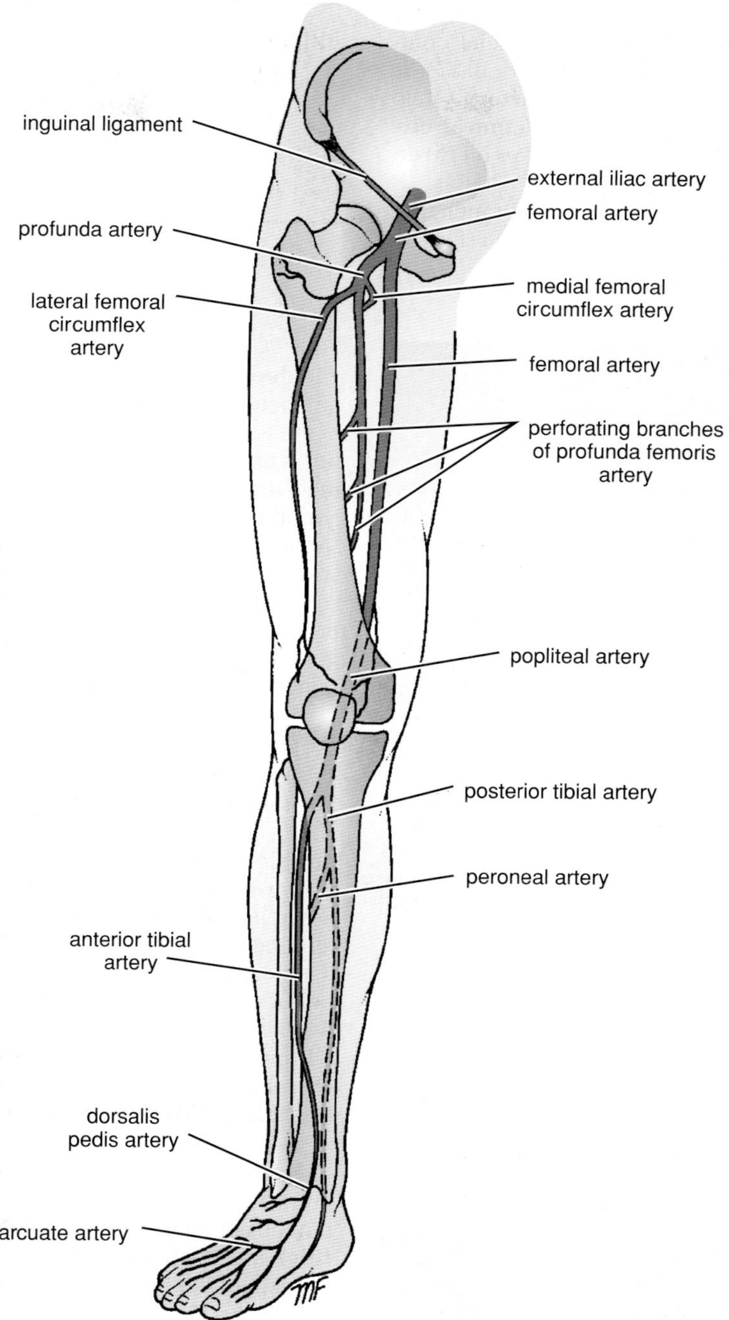

Figure 10-26 Major arteries of the lower limb.

(Figs. 10-6, 10-23, and 10-26). It passes medially behind the femoral vessels and enters the medial fascial compartment of the thigh (Figs. 10-23, 10-24, and 10-27). It ends by becoming the **fourth perforating artery.** At its origin, it gives off the **medial** and **lateral femoral circumflex arteries,** and during its course it gives off **three perforating arteries** (Fig. 10-27).

- The **descending genicular artery** is a small branch that arises from the femoral artery near its termination (Fig. 10-24). It assists in supplying the knee joint.

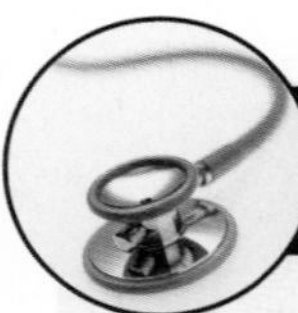

CLINICAL NOTES

Femoral Artery Catheterization

A long, fine catheter can be inserted into the femoral artery as it descends through the femoral triangle. The catheter is guided under fluoroscopic view along the external and common iliac arteries into the aorta. The catheter can then be passed into the inferior mesenteric, superior mesenteric, celiac, or renal arteries. Contrast medium can then be injected into the artery under examination and a permanent record obtained by taking a radiograph. Pressure records can also be obtained by guiding the catheter through the aortic valve into the left ventricle.

Femoral Vein

The femoral vein enters the thigh by passing through the opening in the adductor magnus as a continuation of the popliteal vein (Figs. 10-23 and 10-24). It ascends through the thigh, lying at first on the lateral side of the artery, then posterior to it, and finally on its medial side (Fig. 10-6). It leaves the thigh in the intermediate compartment of the femoral sheath and passes behind the inguinal ligament to become the external iliac vein.

Tributaries The tributaries of the femoral vein are the **great saphenous vein** and veins that correspond to the branches of the femoral artery (Fig. 10-3). The superficial circumflex iliac vein, the superficial epigastric vein, and the external pudendal veins drain into the great saphenous vein.

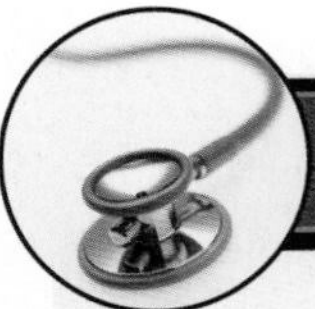

CLINICAL NOTES

Femoral Vein Catheterization

Femoral vein catheterization is used when rapid access to a large vein is needed. The femoral vein has a constant relationship to the medial side of the femoral artery just below the inguinal ligament and is easily cannulated. However, because of the high incidence of thrombosis with the possibility of fatal pulmonary embolism, the catheter should be removed once the patient is stabilized.

Anatomy of the Procedure

1. The skin of the thigh below the inguinal ligament is supplied by the genitofemoral nerve; this nerve is blocked with a local anesthetic.

(continues)

Clinical Notes, *continued*

2. The femoral pulse is palpated midway between the anterior superior iliac spine and the symphysis pubis, and the femoral vein lies immediately medial to it.
3. At a site about two fingerbreadths below the inguinal ligament, the needle is inserted into the femoral vein.

Lymph Nodes of the Anterior Fascial Compartment of the Thigh

The **deep inguinal lymph nodes** are variable in number, but there are commonly three. They lie along the medial side of the terminal part of the femoral vein, and the most superior is usually located in the femoral canal (Fig. 10-21). They receive all the lymph from the superficial inguinal nodes via lymph vessels that pass through the cribriform fascia of the saphenous opening. They also receive lymph from the deep structures of the lower limb that have ascended in lymph vessels alongside the arteries, some having passed through the popliteal nodes. The efferent lymph vessels from the deep inguinal nodes ascend into the abdominal cavity through the femoral canal and drain into the external iliac nodes.

Nerve Supply of the Anterior Fascial Compartment of the Thigh

Femoral Nerve

The femoral nerve is the largest branch of the lumbar plexus (L2, 3, and 4). It emerges from the lateral border of the psoas muscle within the abdomen (see page 278) and passes downward in the interval between the psoas and iliacus. It lies behind the fascia iliaca and enters the thigh lateral to the femoral artery and the femoral sheath, behind the inguinal ligament (Figs. 10-6, 10-21, and 10-23). About 1.5 in. (4 cm) below the inguinal ligament, it terminates by dividing into anterior and posterior divisions. The femoral nerve supplies all the muscles of the anterior compartment of the thigh (Fig. 10-6). **Note that the femoral nerve does not enter the thigh within the femoral sheath.**

Branches

Anterior Division: The anterior division (Fig. 10-28) gives off two cutaneous and two muscular branches. The cutaneous branches are the **medial cutaneous nerve of the thigh** and the **intermediate cutaneous nerves** that supply the skin of the medial and anterior surfaces of the thigh, respectively (Figs. 10-2 and 10-6). The muscular branches supply the sartorius and the pectineus.

Posterior Division: The posterior division (Fig. 10-28) gives off one cutaneous branch, the saphenous nerve, and muscular branches to the quadriceps muscle. The **saphenous nerve** runs downward and medially and crosses the femoral artery from its lateral to its medial side (Fig. 10-6). It emerges on the medial side of the knee between the tendons of sartorius and gracilis (Fig. 10-2). It then runs down the medial side of the leg in company with the great saphenous vein. It passes in front of the medial malleolus and along the medial border of the foot, where it terminates in the region of the ball of the big toe.

The **muscular branch** of the rectus femoris also supplies the hip joint; the branches to the three vasti muscles also supply the knee joint.

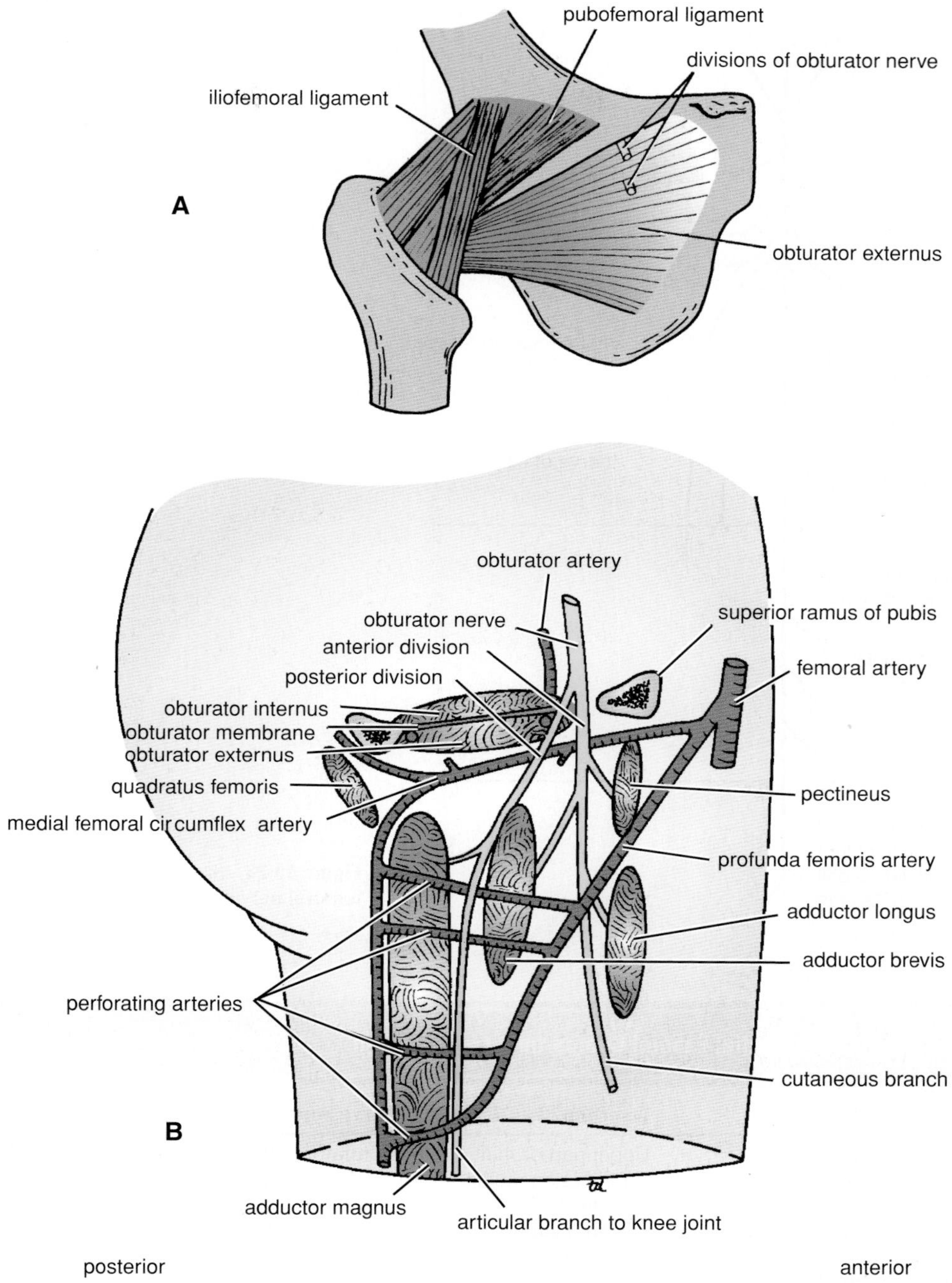

Figure 10-27 Obturator externus muscle (**A**) and vertical section of the medial compartment of the thigh (**B**). Note the courses taken by the obturator nerve and its divisions and the profunda femoris artery and its branches. Note also the anastomosis between the perforating arteries and the medial femoral circumflex artery.

Contents of the Medial Fascial Compartment of the Thigh

- **Muscles:** Gracilis, adductor longus, adductor brevis, adductor magnus, and obturator externus
- **Blood supply:** Profunda femoris artery and obturator artery
- **Nerve supply:** Obturator nerve

Muscles of the Medial Fascial Compartment of the Thigh

The muscles of the medial fascial compartment are seen in Figures 10-22, 10-23, 10-24, and 10-27 and are described in Table 10-3.

Note the following:

- The adductor magnus (Figs. 10-24, 10-27, and 10-29) is a large, triangular muscle consisting of adductor and ham-

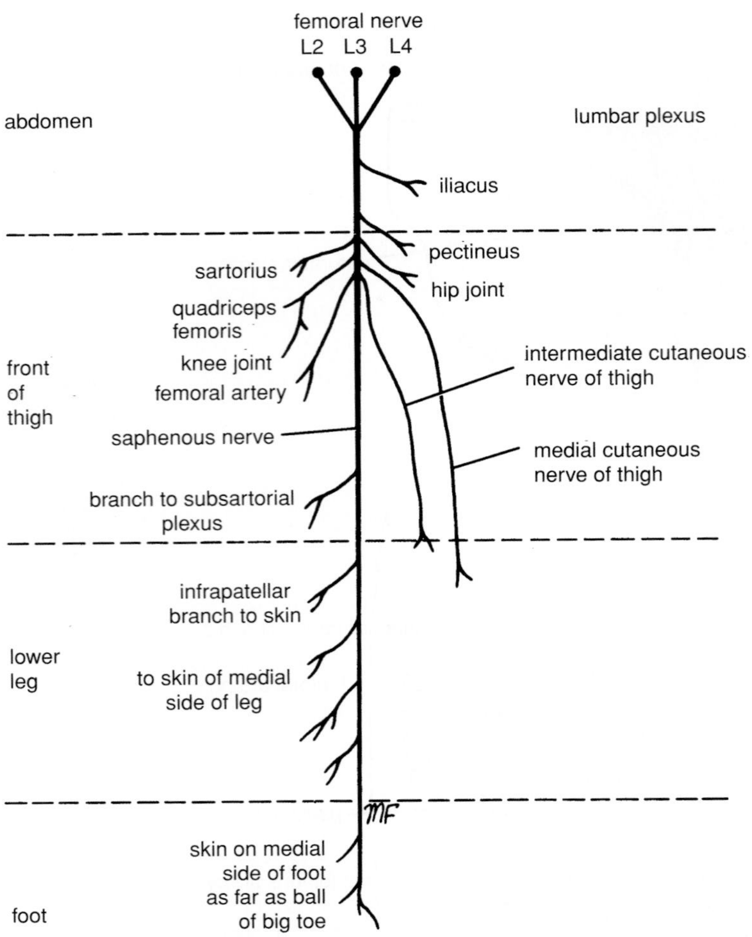

Figure 10-28 Summary of the main branches of the femoral nerve.

Table 10-3 Muscles of the Medial Fascial Compartment of the Thigh

Muscle	Origin	Insertion	Nerve Supply	Nerve Root[a]	Action
Gracilis	Inferior ramus of pubis, ramus of ischium	Upper part of shaft of tibia on medial surface	Obturator nerve	**L2,** 3	Adducts thigh at hip joint; flexes leg at knee joint
Adductor longus	Body of pubis, medial to pubic tubercle	Posterior surface of shaft of femur (linea aspera)	Obturator nerve	L2, **3, 4**	Adducts thigh at hip joint and assists in lateral rotation
Adductor brevis	Inferior ramus of pubis	Posterior surface of shaft of femur (linea aspera)	Obturator nerve	L2, **3, 4**	Adducts thigh at hip joint and assists in lateral rotation
Adductor magnus	Inferior ramus of pubis, ramus of ischium, ischial tuberosity	Posterior surface of shaft of femur, adductor tubercle of femur	Adductor portion: obturator nerve Hamstring portion: sciatic nerve	L2, **3, 4**	Adducts thigh at hip joint and assists in lateral rotation; hamstring portion extends thigh at hip joint
Obturator externus	Outer surface of obturator membrane and pubic and ischial rami	Medial surface of greater trochanter	Obturator nerve	L3, **4**	Laterally rotates thigh at hip joint

[a] The predominant nerve root supply is indicated by boldface type.

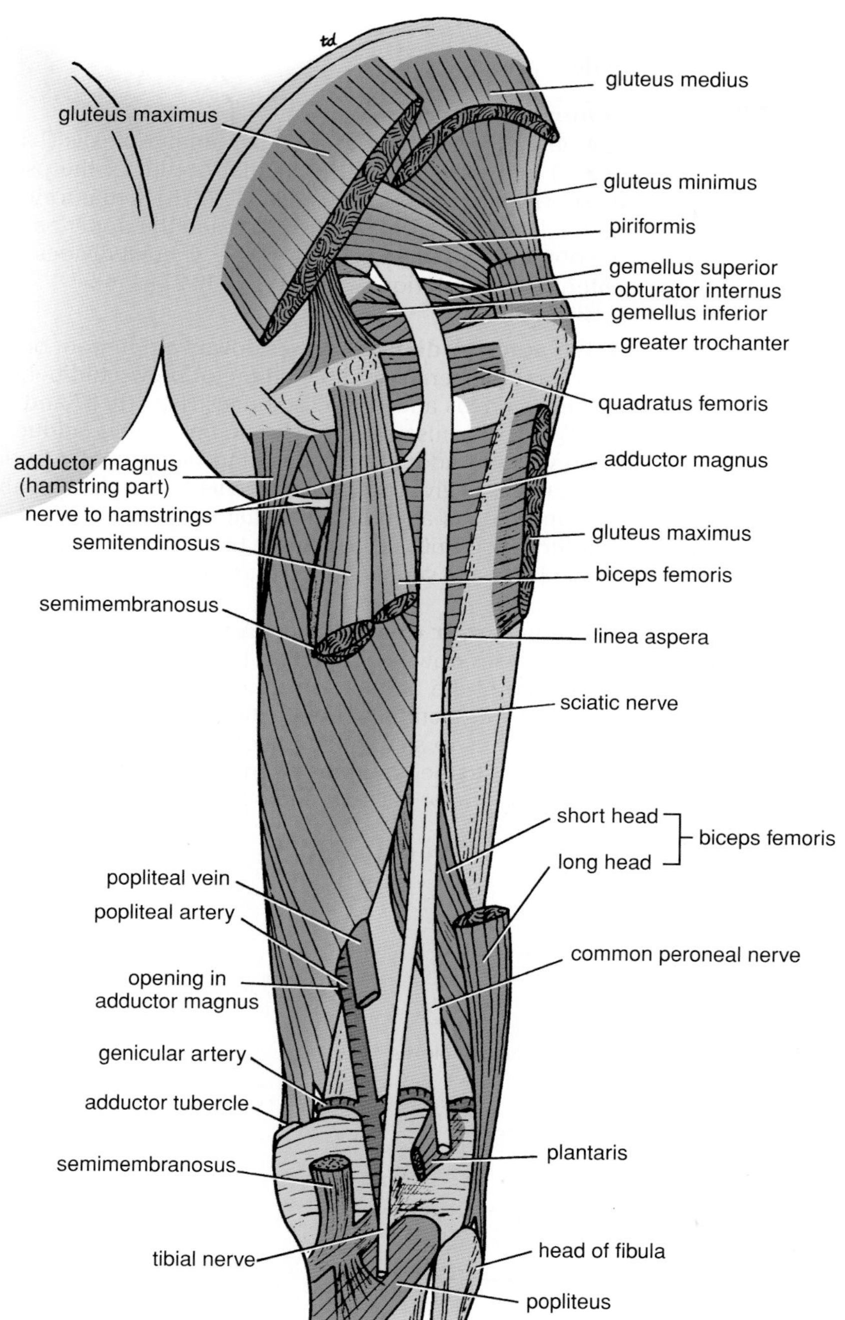

Figure 10-29 Deep structures in the posterior aspect of the right thigh.

string portions. The **adductor hiatus** is a gap in the attachment of this muscle to the femur, which permits the femoral vessels to pass from the adductor canal downward into the popliteal space.

Blood Supply of the Medial Fascial Compartment of the Thigh

Profunda Femoris Artery

The profunda femoris is a large artery that arises from the lateral side of the femoral artery in the femoral triangle, about 1.5 in. (4 cm) below the inguinal ligament (Figs. 10-6, 10-24, and 10-26). It descends in the interval between the adductor longus and adductor brevis and then lies on the adductor magnus, where it ends as the fourth perforating artery (Fig. 10-27).

Branches

- **Medial femoral circumflex artery:** This passes backward between the muscles that form the floor of the femoral triangle and gives off muscular branches in the medial fascial compartment of the thigh (Fig. 10-27). It takes part in the formation of the cruciate anastomosis.
- **Lateral femoral circumflex artery:** This passes laterally between the terminal branches of the femoral nerve (Fig.

10-6). It breaks up into branches that supply the muscles of the region and takes part in the formation of the cruciate anastomosis.

- **Four perforating arteries:** Three of these arise as branches of the profunda femoris artery; the fourth perforating artery is the terminal part of the profunda artery (Fig. 10-27). The perforating arteries run backward, piercing the various muscle layers as they go. They supply the muscles and terminate by anastomosing with one another and with the inferior gluteal artery and the circumflex femoral arteries above and the muscular branches of the popliteal artery below.

Profunda Femoris Vein

The profunda femoris vein receives tributaries that correspond to the branches of the artery. It drains into the femoral vein.

Obturator Artery

The obturator artery is a branch of the internal iliac artery (see page 328). It passes forward on the lateral wall of the pelvis and accompanies the obturator nerve through the obturator canal (i.e., the upper part of the obturator foramen) (Fig. 10-27). On entering the medial fascial compartment of the thigh, it divides into medial and lateral branches, which pass around the margin of the outer surface of the obturator membrane. It gives off muscular branches and an articular branch to the hip joint.

Obturator Vein

The obturator vein receives tributaries that correspond to the branches of the artery. It drains into the internal iliac vein.

Nerve Supply of the Medial Fascial Compartment of the Thigh

Obturator Nerve

The obturator nerve arises from the lumbar plexus (L2, 3, and 4) and emerges on the medial border of the psoas muscle within the abdomen (see page 278). It runs forward on the lateral wall of the pelvis to reach the upper part of the obturator foramen (see Fig. 6-12), where it divides into anterior and posterior divisions (Fig. 10-27).

Branches

- The **anterior division** passes downward in front of the obturator externus and the adductor brevis and behind the pectineus and adductor longus (Figs. 10-27 and 10-30). It gives muscular branches to the gracilis, adductor brevis, and adductor longus, and occasionally to the pectineus. It gives articular branches to the hip joint and terminates as a small nerve that supplies the femoral artery. It contributes a variable branch to the subsartorial plexus and supplies the skin on the medial side of the thigh.
- The **posterior division** pierces the obturator externus and passes downward behind the adductor brevis and in front of the adductor magnus (Fig. 10-27). It terminates by descending through the opening in the adductor magnus to supply the knee joint. It gives muscular branches to the obturator externus, to the adductor part of the adductor magnus, and occasionally to the adductor brevis.

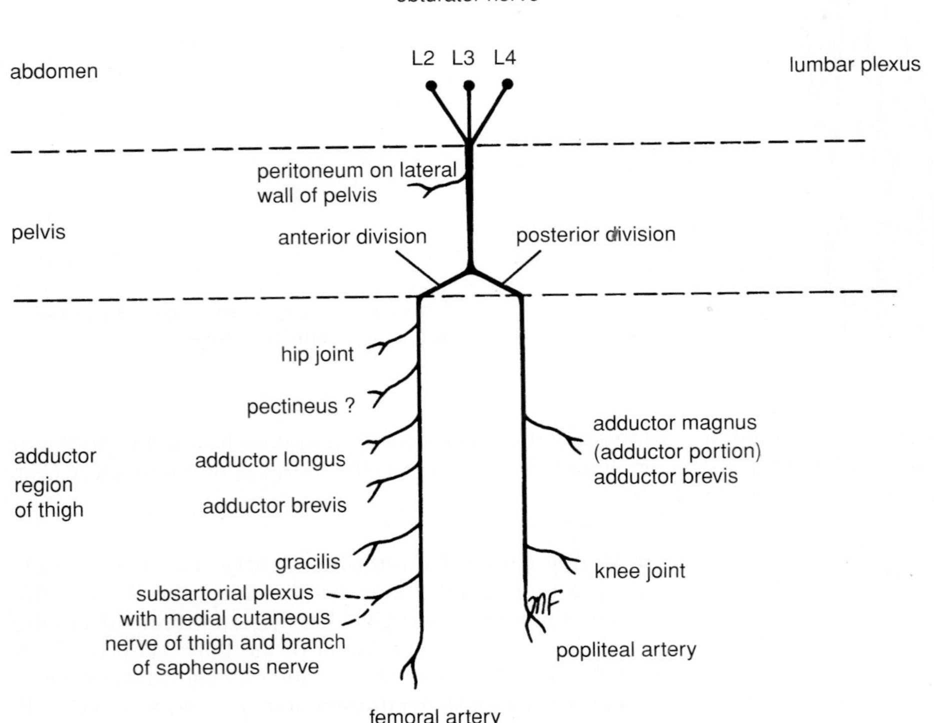

Figure 10-30 Summary of the main branches of the obturator nerve.

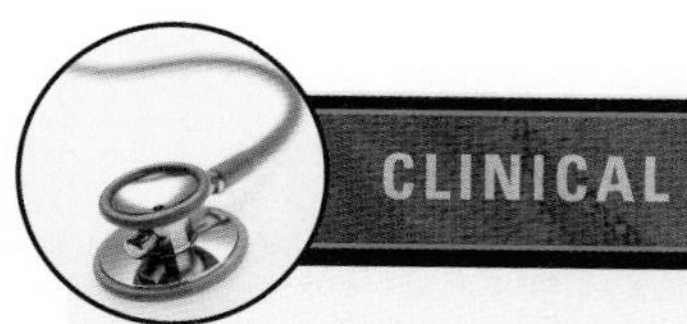

Adductor Muscles and Cerebral Palsy

In patients with cerebral palsy who have marked spasticity of the adductor group of muscles, it is common practice to perform a tenotomy of the adductor longus tendon and to divide the anterior division of the obturator nerve. In addition, in some severe cases the posterior division of the obturator nerve is crushed. This operation overcomes the spasm of the adductor group of muscles and permits slow recovery of the muscles supplied by the posterior division of the obturator nerve.

The Back of the Thigh

Skin

Cutaneous Nerves

The **posterior cutaneous nerve of the thigh,** a branch of the sacral plexus, leaves the gluteal region by emerging from beneath the lower border of the gluteus maximus muscle (Fig. 10-1). It descends on the back of the thigh, and in the popliteal fossa it pierces the deep fascia and supplies the skin. It gives off numerous branches to the skin on the back of the thigh and the upper part of the leg (Fig. 10-1).

Superficial Veins

Many small veins curve around the medial and lateral aspects of the thigh and ultimately drain into the great saphenous vein (Fig. 10-19). Superficial veins from the lower part of the back of the thigh join the small saphenous vein in the popliteal fossa.

Lymph Vessels

Lymph from the skin and superficial fascia on the back of the thigh drains upward and forward into the vertical group of superficial inguinal lymph nodes (Fig. 10-4).

Contents of the Posterior Fascial Compartment of the Thigh

- **Muscles:** Biceps femoris, semitendinosus, semimembranosus, and a small part of the adductor magnus (hamstring muscles)
- **Blood supply:** Branches of the profunda femoris artery
- **Nerve supply:** Sciatic nerve

The muscles of the posterior fascial compartment are seen in Figure 10-31 and are described in Table 10-4.

Note the following:

- The biceps femoris muscle receives its nerve supply from the sciatic nerve, the long head from the tibial portion and the short head from the common peroneal portion.
- The hamstring part of the adductor magnus muscle receives its nerve supply from the tibial portion of the sciatic nerve and the adductor part from the obturator nerve.
- The semimembranosus insertion sends a fibrous expansion upward and laterally, which reinforces the capsule on the back of the knee joint; the expansion is called the **oblique popliteal ligament.**

Blood Supply of the Posterior Compartment of the Thigh

The four perforating branches of the profunda femoris artery provide a rich blood supply to this compartment (Fig. 10-27). The profunda femoris vein drains the greater part of the blood from the compartment.

Nerve Supply of the Posterior Compartment of the Thigh

Sciatic Nerve

The sciatic nerve, a branch of the sacral plexus (L4 and 5; S1, 2, and 3), leaves the gluteal region as it descends in the midline of the thigh (Fig. 10-31). It is overlapped posteriorly by the adjacent margins of the biceps femoris and semimembranosus muscles. It lies on the posterior aspect of the adductor magnus muscle. In the lower third of the thigh it ends by dividing into the tibial and common peroneal nerves (Figs. 10-29 and 10-31). Occasionally, the sciatic nerve divides into its two terminal parts at a higher level—in the upper part of the thigh, the gluteal region, or even inside the pelvis.

Branches

- The **tibial nerve,** a terminal branch of the sciatic nerve (Figs. 10-17, 10-29, and 10-31), enters the popliteal fossa. Its further course is described on page 604.
- The **common peroneal nerve,** a terminal branch of the sciatic nerve (Figs. 10-29 and 10-31), enters the popliteal fossa on the lateral side of the tibial nerve. Its further course is described on page 604.
- **Muscular branches** to the long head of the biceps femoris, the semitendinosus, the semimembranosus, and the hamstring part of the adductor magnus. These branches arise from the tibial component of the sciatic nerve and run medially to supply the muscles (Figs. 10-29 and 10-31).

Hip Joint

Articulation

The hip joint is the articulation between the hemispherical head of the femur and the cup-shaped acetabulum of the hip bone (Fig. 10-18). The articular surface of the acetabulum is horseshoe shaped and is deficient inferiorly at the **acetabular notch.** The cavity of the acetabulum is deepened by the presence of a fibrocartilaginous rim called the **acetabular labrum.** The labrum bridges across the acetabular notch and is here called the **transverse acetabular ligament** (Fig. 10-18).

The articular surfaces are covered with hyaline cartilage.

Type

The hip joint is a synovial ball-and-socket joint.

Capsule

The capsule encloses the joint and is attached to the acetabular labrum medially (Fig. 10-18). Laterally, it is at-

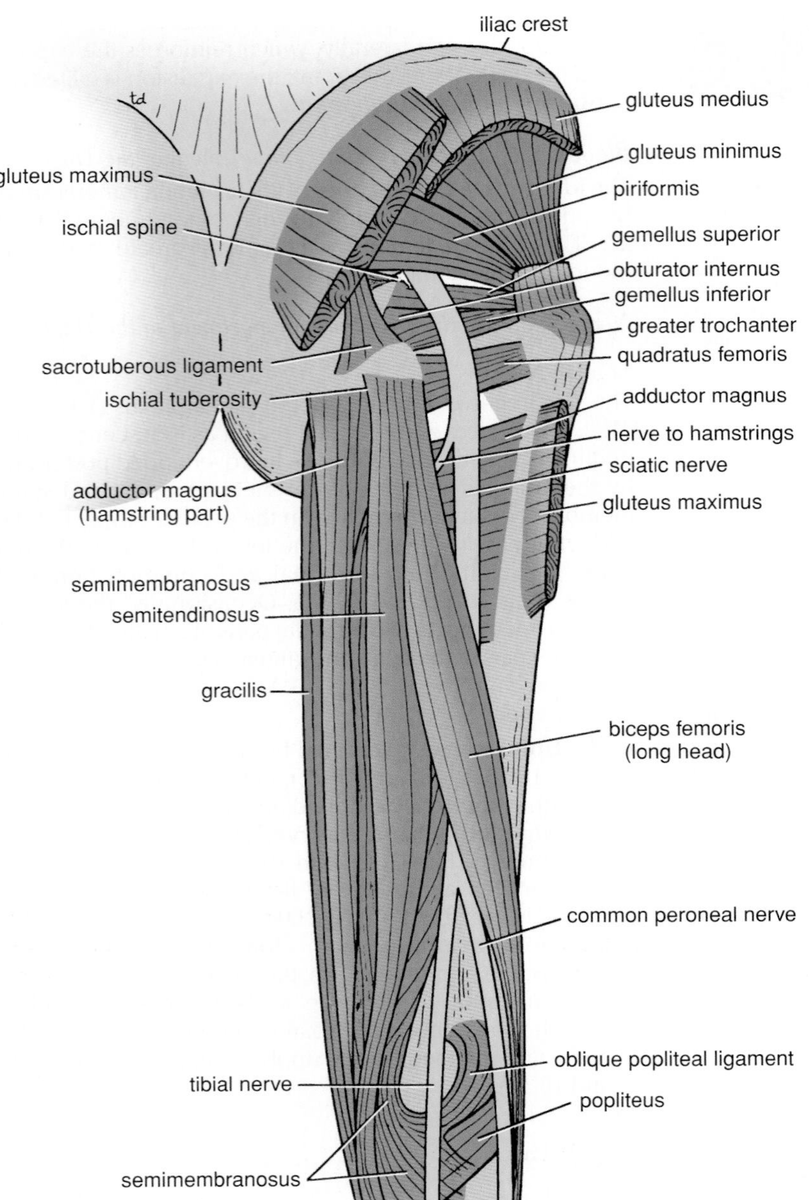

Figure 10-31 Structures in the posterior aspect of the right thigh.

tached to the intertrochanteric line of the femur in front and halfway along the posterior aspect of the neck of the bone behind. At its attachment to the intertrochanteric line in front, some of its fibers, accompanied by blood vessels, are reflected upward along the neck as bands called **retinacula.** These blood vessels supply the head and neck of the femur.

Ligaments

The **iliofemoral ligament** is a strong, inverted Y-shaped ligament (Fig. 10-32). Its base is attached to the anterior inferior iliac spine above; below, the two limbs of the Y are attached to the upper and lower parts of the intertrochanteric line of the femur. This strong ligament prevents overextension during standing.

The **pubofemoral ligament** is triangular (Fig. 10-32). The base of the ligament is attached to the superior ramus of the pubis, and the apex is attached below to the lower part of the intertrochanteric line. This ligament limits extension and abduction.

The **ischiofemoral ligament** is spiral shaped and is attached to the body of the ischium near the acetabular margin (Fig. 10-32). The fibers pass upward and laterally and are attached to the greater trochanter. This ligament limits extension.

The **transverse acetabular ligament** is formed by the acetabular labrum as it bridges the acetabular notch (Fig.

Table 10-4 Muscles of the Posterior Fascial Compartment of the Thigh

Muscle	Origin	Insertion	Nerve Supply	Nerve Root[a]	Action
Biceps femoris	Long head: ischial tuberosity	Head of fibula	Long head: tibial portion of sciatic nerve	L5; **S1,** 2	Flexes and laterally rotates leg at knee joint; long head also extends thigh at hip joint
	Short head: linea aspera, lateral supracondylar ridge of shaft of femur		Short head: common peroneal portion of sciatic nerve		
Semitendinosus	Ischial tuberosity	Upper part of medial surface of shaft of tibia	Tibial portion of sciatic nerve	**L5; S1,** 2	Flexes and medially rotates leg at knee joint; extends thigh at hip joint
Semimembranosus	Ischial tuberosity	Medial condyle of tibia	Tibial portion of sciatic nerve	**L5; S1,** 2	Flexes and medially rotates leg at knee joint; extends thigh at hip joint
Adductor magnus (hamstring portion)	Ischial tuberosity	Adductor tubercle of femur	Tibial portion of sciatic nerve	L2, **3, 4**	Extends thigh at hip joint

[a] The predominant nerve root supply is indicated by boldface type.

10-18). The ligament converts the notch into a tunnel through which the blood vessels and nerves enter the joint.

The **ligament of the head of the femur** is flat and triangular (Fig. 10-18). It is attached by its apex to the pit on the head of the femur (fovea capitis) and by its base to the transverse ligament and the margins of the acetabular notch. It lies within the joint and is ensheathed by synovial membrane (Fig. 10-18).

Synovial Membrane

The synovial membrane lines the capsule and is attached to the margins of the articular surfaces (Fig. 10-18). It covers the portion of the neck of the femur that lies within the joint capsule. It ensheathes the ligament of the head of the femur and covers the pad of fat contained in the acetabular fossa. A pouch of synovial membrane frequently protrudes through a gap in the anterior wall of the capsule, between the pubofemoral and iliofemoral ligaments, and forms the **psoas bursa** beneath the psoas tendon (Figs. 10-32 and 10-33).

Nerve Supply

Femoral, obturator, and sciatic nerves and the nerve to the quadratus femoris supply the area.

Movements

The hip joint has a wide range of movement. The strength of the joint depends largely on the shape of the bones taking part in the articulation and on the strong ligaments. When the knee is flexed, flexion is limited by the anterior surface of the thigh coming into contact with the anterior abdominal wall. When the knee is extended, flexion is limited by the tension of the hamstring group of muscles. Extension, which is the movement of the flexed thigh backward to the anatomic position, is limited by the tension of the iliofemoral, pubofemoral, and ischiofemoral ligaments. Abduction is limited by the tension of the pubofemoral ligament, and adduction is limited by contact with the opposite limb and by the tension in the ligament of the head of the femur. Lateral rotation is limited by the tension in the iliofemoral and pubofemoral ligaments, and medial rotation is limited by the ischiofemoral ligament. The following movements take place:

- **Flexion** is performed by the iliopsoas, rectus femoris, and sartorius and also by the adductor muscles.
- **Extension** (a backward movement of the flexed thigh) is performed by the gluteus maximus and the hamstring muscles.
- **Abduction** is performed by the gluteus medius and minimus, assisted by the sartorius, tensor fasciae latae, and piriformis.
- **Adduction** is performed by the adductor longus and brevis and the adductor fibers of the adductor magnus. These muscles are assisted by the pectineus and the gracilis.
- **Lateral rotation** is performed by the piriformis, obturator internus and externus, superior and inferior gemelli, and quadratus femoris, assisted by the gluteus maximus.

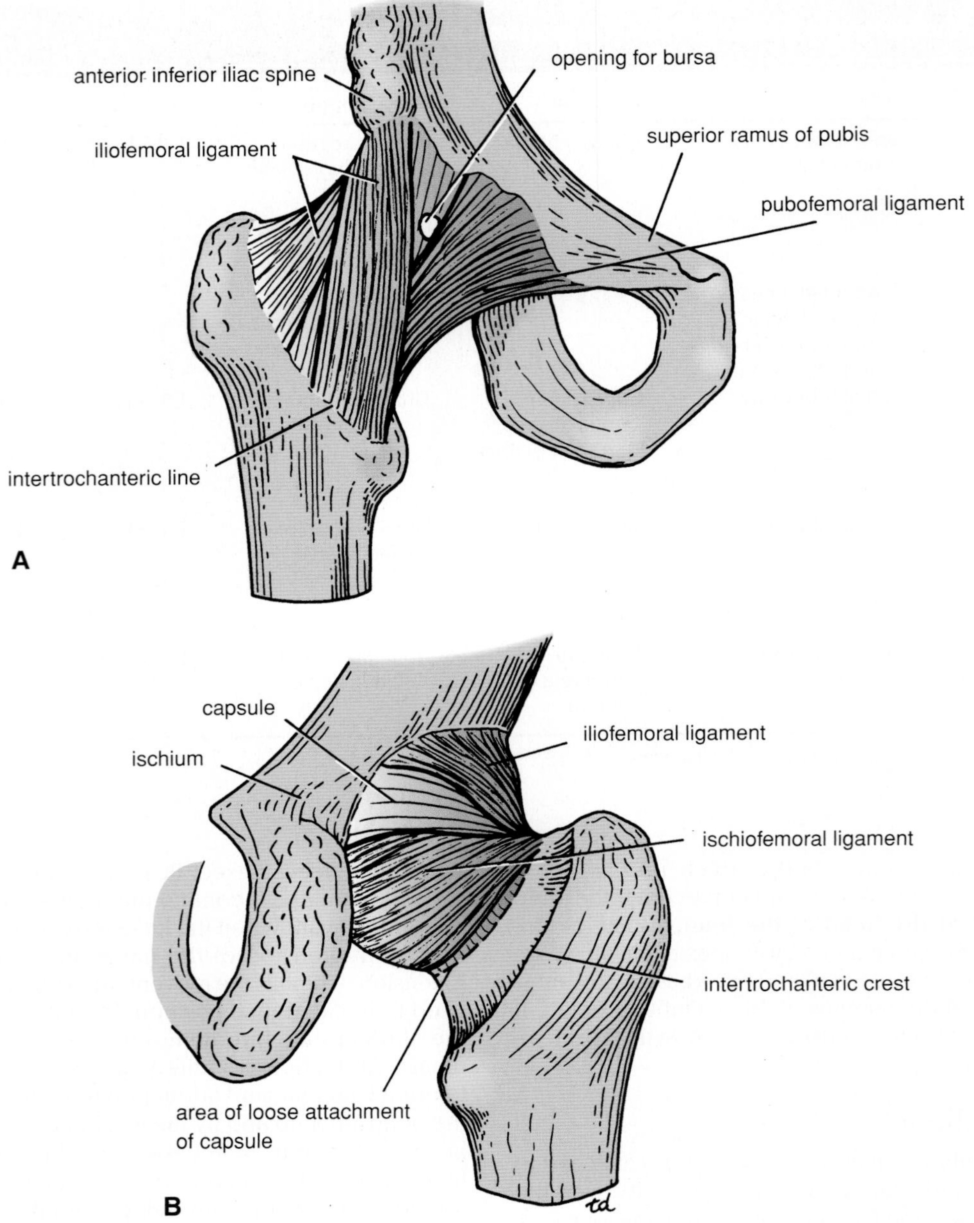

Figure 10-32 Anterior aspect (**A**) and posterior aspect (**B**) of the right hip joint.

- **Medial rotation** is performed by the anterior fibers of the gluteus medius and gluteus minimus and the tensor fasciae latae.
- **Circumduction** is a combination of the previous movements.

The extensor group of muscles is more powerful than the flexor group, and the lateral rotators are more powerful than the medial rotators.

Important Relations

- **Anteriorly:** Iliopsoas, pectineus, and rectus femoris muscles. The iliopsoas and pectineus separate the femoral vessels and nerve from the joint (Fig. 10-33).
- **Posteriorly:** The obturator internus, the gemelli, and the quadratus femoris muscles separate the joint from the sciatic nerve (Fig. 10-32).
- **Superiorly:** Piriformis and gluteus minimus (Fig. 10-33)
- **Inferiorly:** Obturator externus tendon (Fig. 10-33)

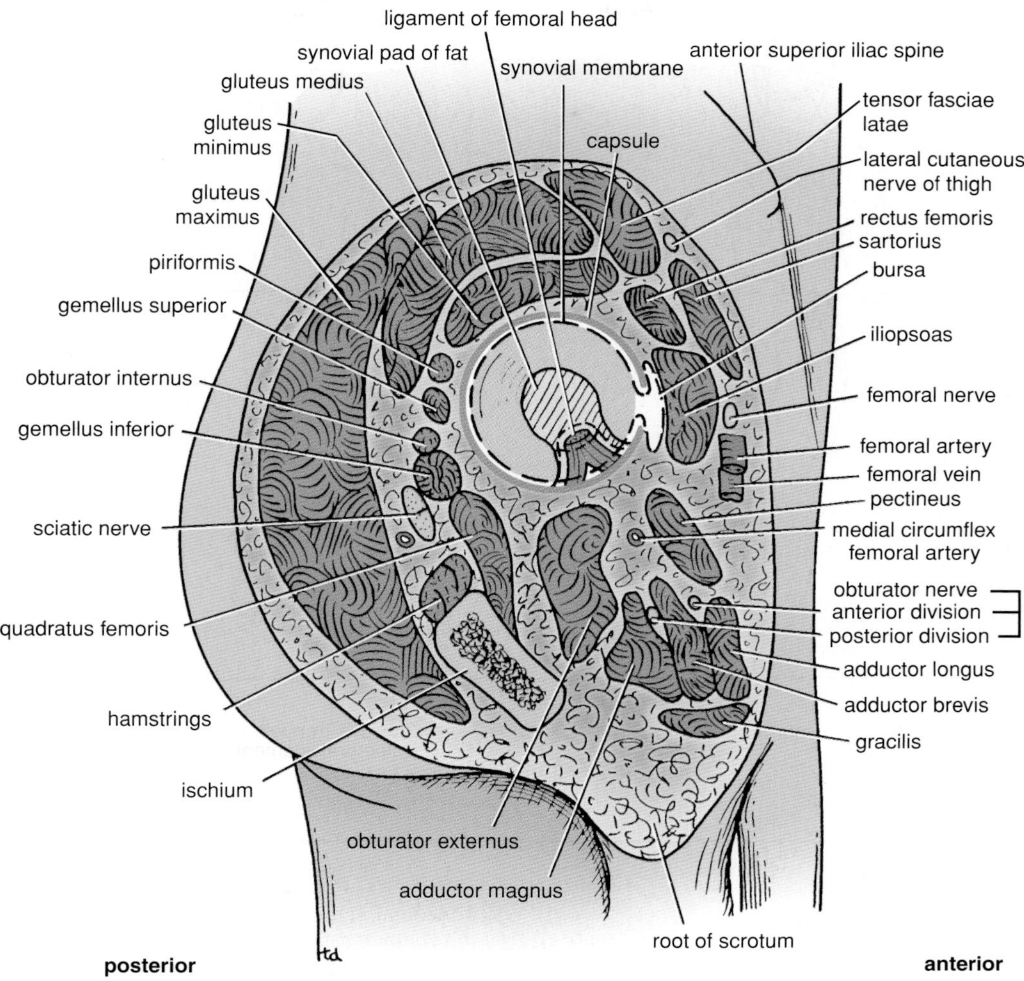

Figure 10-33 Structures surrounding the right hip joint.

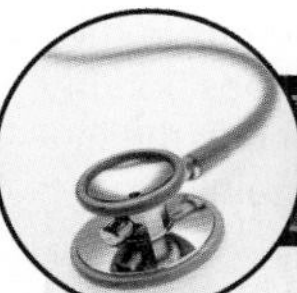

CLINICAL NOTES

Referred Pain From the Hip Joint

The femoral nerve not only supplies the hip joint but, via the intermediate and medial cutaneous nerves of the thigh, also supplies the skin of the front and medial side of the thigh. It is not surprising, therefore, for pain originating in the hip joint to be referred to the front and medial side of the thigh. The posterior division of the obturator nerve supplies both the hip and knee joints. This would explain why hip joint disease sometimes gives rise to pain in the knee joint.

Congenital Dislocation of the Hip

The stability of the hip joint depends on the ball-and-socket arrangement of the articular surfaces and the strong ligaments. In congenital dislocation of the hip (see page 643), the upper lip of the acetabulum fails to develop adequately, and the head of the femur, having no stable platform under which it can lodge, rides up out of the acetabulum onto the gluteal surface of the ilium.

Traumatic Dislocation of the Hip

Traumatic dislocation of the hip is rare because of its strength; it is usually caused by motor vehicle accidents. However, should it occur, it usually does so when the joint is flexed and adducted. The head of the femur is displaced posteriorly out of the acetabulum, and it comes to rest on the gluteal surface of the ilium (posterior dislocation). The close relation of the sciatic nerve to the posterior surface of the joint makes it prone to injury in posterior dislocations.

Hip Joint Stability and Trendelenburg's Sign

The stability of the hip joint when a person stands on one leg with the foot of the opposite leg raised above the ground depends on three factors:

- The gluteus medius and minimus must be functioning normally.
- The head of the femur must be located normally within the acetabulum.

(continues)

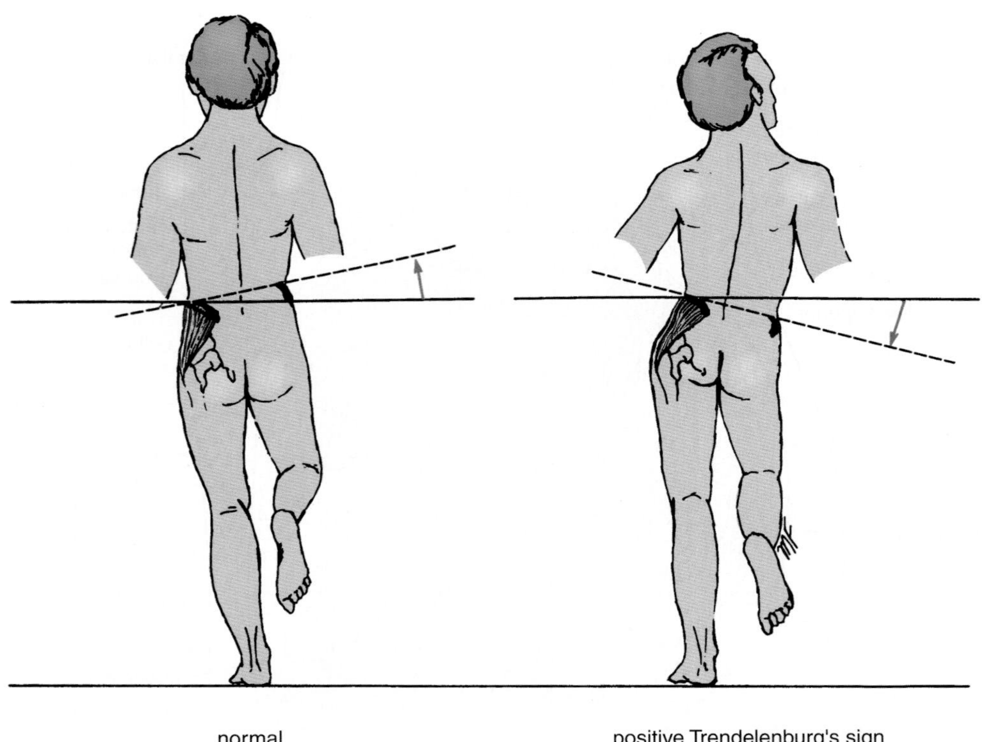

Figure 10-34 Trendelenburg's test.

Clinical Notes, *continued*

- The neck of the femur must be intact and must have a normal angle with the shaft of the femur.

If any one of these factors is defective, then the pelvis will sink downward on the opposite, unsupported side. The patient is then said to exhibit a positive **Trendelenburg's sign** (Fig. 10-34).

Normally, when walking, a person alternately contracts the gluteus medius and minimus, first on one side and then on the other. By this means he or she is able to raise the pelvis first on one side and then on the other, allowing the leg to be flexed at the hip joint and moved forward—that is, the leg is raised clear of the ground before it is thrust forward in taking the forward step. A patient with a right-sided congenital dislocation of the hip, when asked to stand on the right leg and raise the opposite leg clear off the ground, will exhibit a positive Trendelenburg's sign, and the unsupported side of the pelvis will sink below the horizontal. If the patient is asked to walk, he or she will show the characteristic "dipping" gait. In patients with bilateral congenital dislocation of the hip, the gait is typically "waddling" in nature.

Arthritis of the Hip Joint

A patient with an inflamed hip joint will place the femur in the position that gives minimum discomfort—that is, the position in which the joint cavity has the greatest capacity to contain the increased amount of synovial fluid secreted. The hip joint is partially flexed, abducted, and externally rotated.

Osteoarthritis, the most common disease of the hip joint in the adult, causes pain, stiffness, and deformity. The pain may be in the hip joint itself or referred to the knee (the obturator nerve supplies both joints). The stiffness is caused by the pain and reflex spasm of the surrounding muscles. The deformity is flexion, adduction, and external rotation and is produced initially by muscle spasm and later by muscle contracture.

Bones of the Leg

The leg is the part of the lower limb between the knee joint and the ankle joint.

Patella

The patella (Fig. 10-35) is the largest sesamoid bone (i.e., a bone that develops within the tendon of the quadriceps femoris muscle in front of the knee joint). It is triangular, and its apex lies inferiorly; the apex is connected to the tuberosity of the tibia by the ligamentum patellae. The posterior surface articulates with the condyles of the femur. The patella is situated in an exposed position in front of the knee joint and can easily be palpated through the skin. It is separated from the skin by an important subcutaneous bursa (Fig. 10-36).

The upper, lateral, and medial margins give attachment to the different parts of the quadriceps femoris muscle. It is prevented from being displaced laterally during the action

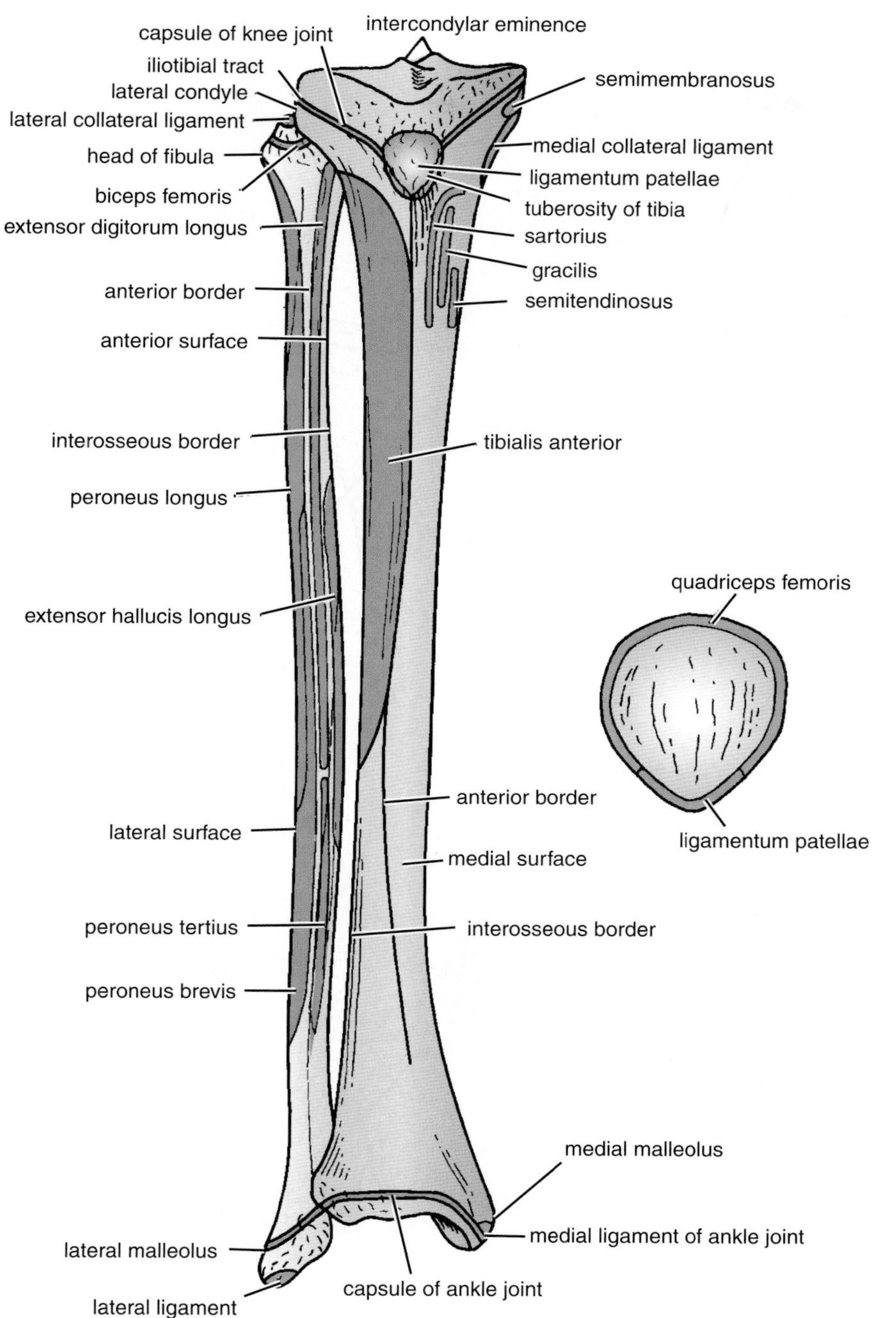

Figure 10-35 Muscles and ligaments attached to the anterior surfaces of the right tibia and fibula. Attachments to the patella are also shown.

of the quadriceps muscle by the lower horizontal fibers of the vastus medialis and by the large size of the lateral condyle of the femur.

Tibia

The tibia is the large weight-bearing medial bone of the leg (Figs. 10-35 and 10-37). It articulates with the condyles of the femur and the head of the fibula above and with the talus and the distal end of the fibula below. It has an expanded upper end, a smaller lower end, and a shaft.

At the upper end are the **lateral** and **medial condyles** (sometimes called lateral and medial **tibial plateaus),** which articulate with the lateral and medial condyles of the femur and the **lateral** and **medial menisci** intervening. Separating the upper articular surfaces of the tibial condyles are **anterior** and **posterior intercondylar areas;** lying between these areas is the **intercondylar eminence** (Fig. 10-35).

The lateral condyle possesses on its lateral aspect a small **circular articular facet for the head of the fibula.** The medial condyle has on its posterior aspect the insertion of the semimembranosus muscle (Fig. 10-37).

The **shaft of the tibia** is triangular in cross section, presenting three borders and three surfaces. Its anterior and medial borders, with the medial surface between them, are subcutaneous. The anterior border is prominent and forms

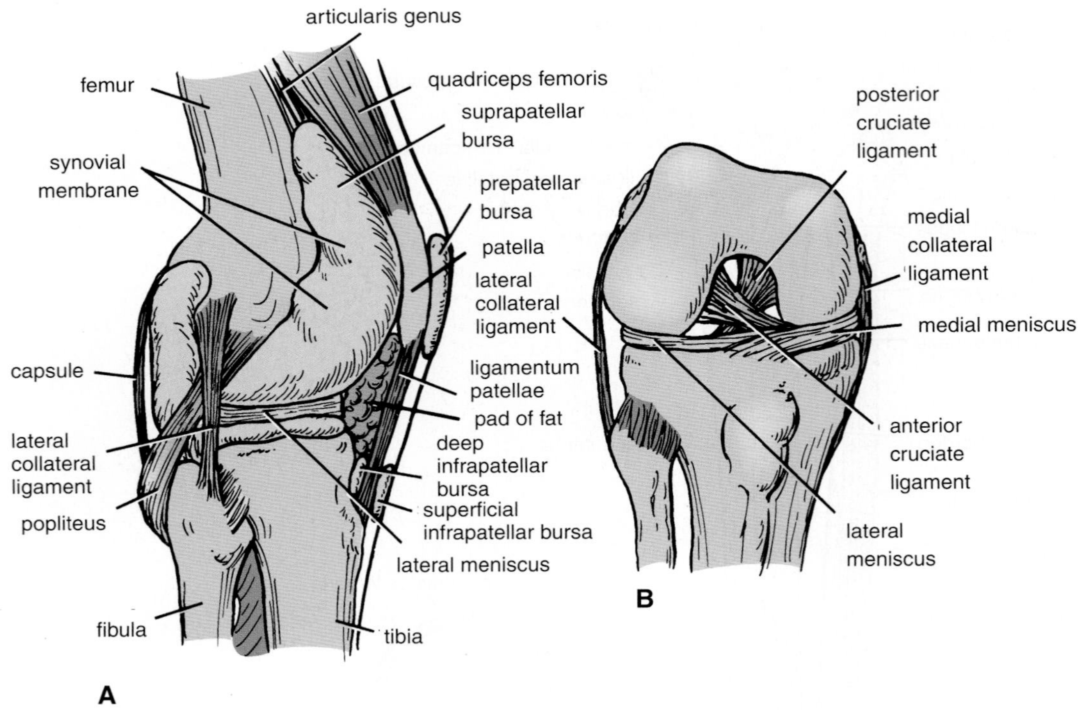

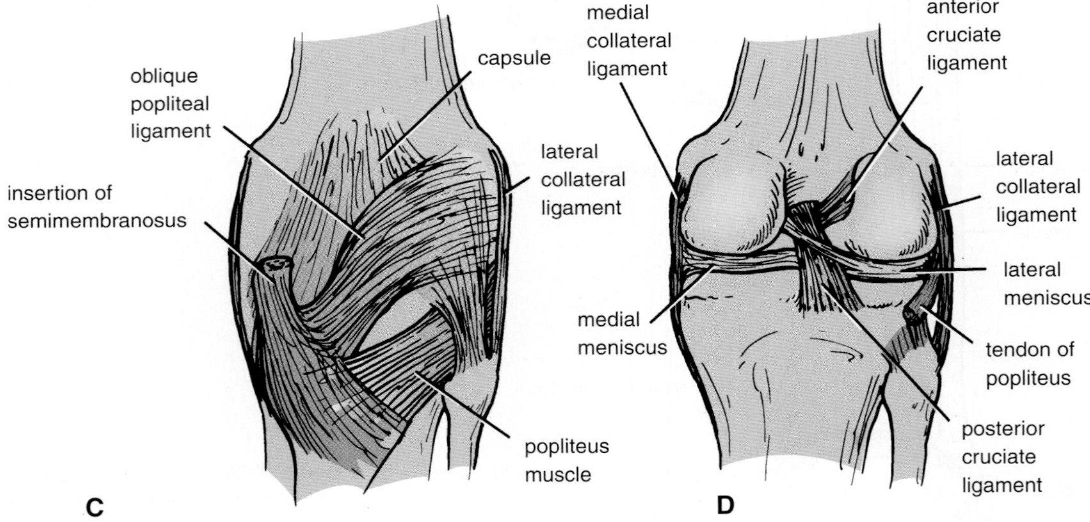

Figure 10-36 **A.** The right knee joint as seen from the lateral aspect. **B.** The anterior aspect, with the joint flexed. **C, D.** The posterior aspect.

the shin. At the junction of the anterior border with the upper end of the tibia is the **tuberosity,** which receives the attachment of the ligamentum patellae. The anterior border becomes rounded below, where it becomes continuous with the medial malleolus. The lateral or interosseous border gives attachment to the interosseous membrane.

The posterior surface of the shaft shows an oblique line, the **soleal line** (Fig. 10-37), for the attachment of the soleus muscle.

The lower end of the tibia is slightly expanded and on its inferior aspect shows a saddle-shaped articular surface for the talus. The lower end is prolonged downward medially to form the **medial malleolus.** The lateral surface of the medial malleolus articulates with the talus. The lower end of the tibia shows a wide, rough depression on its lateral surface for articulation with the fibula.

The important muscles and ligaments attached to the tibia are shown in Figures 10-35 and 10-37.

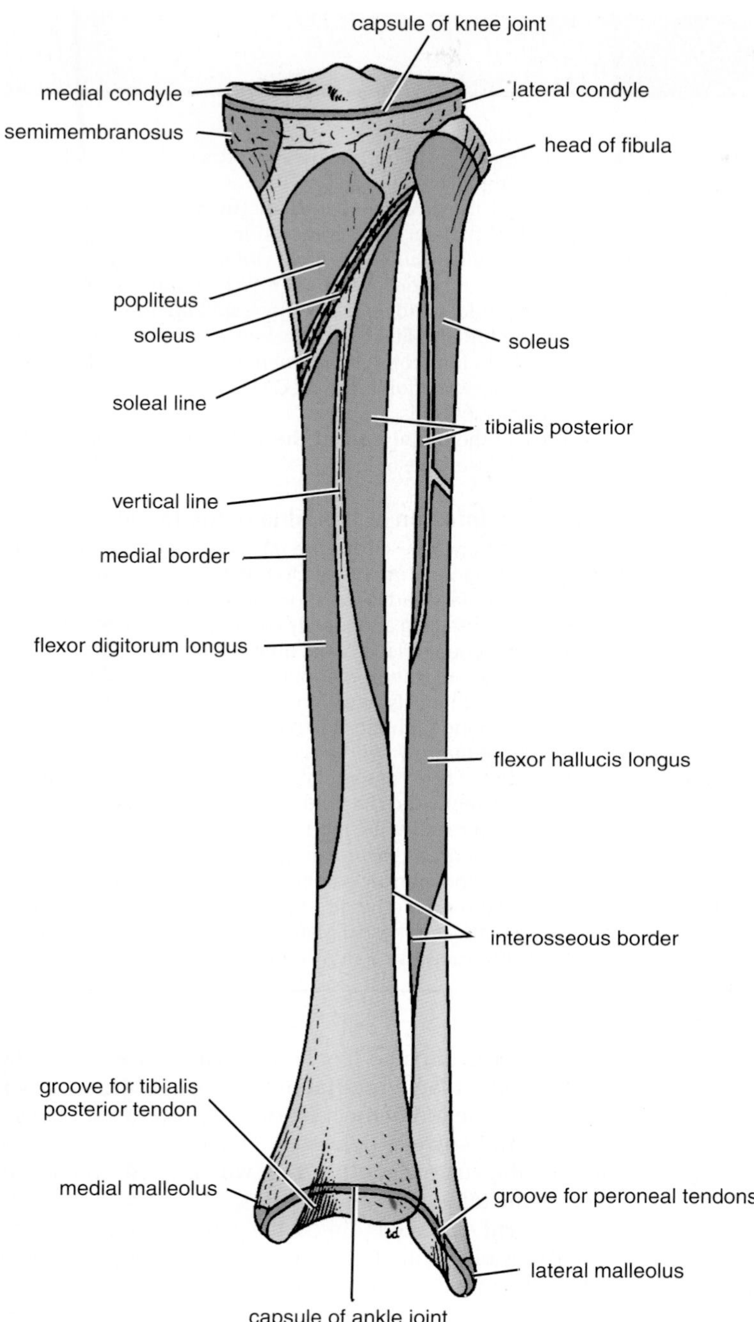

Figure 10-37 Muscles and ligaments attached to the posterior surfaces of the right tibia and the fibula.

Fibula

The fibula is the slender lateral bone of the leg (Figs. 10-35 and 10-37). It takes no part in the articulation at the knee joint, but below it forms the lateral malleolus of the ankle joint. It takes no part in the transmission of body weight, but it provides attachment for muscles. The fibula has an expanded upper end, a shaft, and a lower end.

The **upper end,** or **head,** is surmounted by a **styloid process.** It possesses an **articular surface** for articulation with the lateral condyle of the tibia.

The **shaft of the fibula** is long and slender. Typically, it has four borders and four surfaces. The medial or interosseous border gives attachment to the interosseous membrane.

The **lower end of the fibula** forms the triangular lateral malleolus, which is subcutaneous. On the medial surface of the lateral malleolus is a triangular **articular facet** for articulation with the lateral aspect of the talus. Below and behind the articular facet is a depression called the **malleolar fossa.**

The important muscles and ligaments attached to the fibula are shown in Figures 10-35 and 10-37.

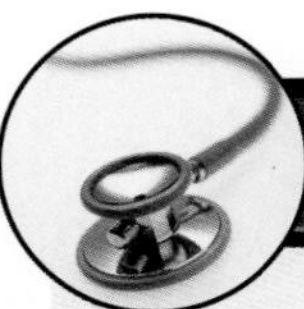

CLINICAL NOTES

Patellar Dislocations

The patella is a sesamoid bone lying within the quadriceps tendon. The importance of the lower horizontal fibers of the vastus medialis and the large size of the lateral condyle of the femur in preventing lateral displacement of the patella has been emphasized. Congenital recurrent dislocations of the patella are caused by underdevelopment of the lateral femoral condyle. Traumatic dislocation of the patella results from direct trauma to the quadriceps attachments of the patella (especially the vastus medialis), with or without fracture of the patella.

Patellar Fractures

A patella fractured as a result of direct violence, as in an automobile accident, is broken into several small fragments. Because the bone lies within the quadriceps femoris tendon, little separation of the fragments takes place. The close relationship of the patella to the overlying skin may result in the fracture being open. Fracture of the patella as a result of indirect violence is caused by the sudden contraction of the quadriceps snapping the patella across the front of the femoral condyles. The knee is in the semiflexed position, and the fracture line is transverse. Separation of the fragments usually occurs.

Fractures of the Tibia and Fibula

Fractures of the tibia and fibula are common. If only one bone is fractured, the other acts as a splint and displacement is minimal. Fractures of the shaft of the tibia are often open because the entire length of the medial surface is covered only by skin and superficial fascia. Fractures of the distal third of the shaft of the tibia are prone to delayed union or nonunion. This can be because the nutrient artery is torn at the fracture line, with a consequent reduction in blood flow to the distal fragment; it is also possible that the splint-like action of the intact fibula prevents the proximal and distal fragments from coming into apposition.

Fractures of the **proximal end of the tibia,** at the tibial condyles (tibial plateau), are common in the middle-aged and elderly; they usually result from direct violence to the lateral side of the knee joint, as when a person is hit by the bumper of an automobile. The tibial condyle may show a split fracture or be broken up, or the fracture line may pass between both condyles in the region of the intercondylar eminence. As a result of forced abduction of the knee joint, the medial collateral ligament can also be torn or ruptured.

Fractures of the **distal end of the tibia** are considered with the ankle joint (see page 637).

Intraosseous Infusion of the Tibia in the Infant

The technique may be used for the infusion of fluids and blood when it has been found impossible to obtain an intravenous line. The procedure is easy and rapid to perform, as follows:

1. With the distal leg adequately supported, the anterior subcutaneous surface of the tibia is palpated.
2. The skin is anesthetized about 1 in. (2.5 cm) distal to the tibial tuberosity, thus blocking the infrapatellar branch of the saphenous nerve.
3. The bone marrow needle is directed at right angles through the skin, superficial fascia, deep fascia, and tibial periosteum and the cortex of the tibia. Once the needle tip reaches the medulla and bone marrow, the operator senses a feeling of "give." The position of the needle in the marrow can be confirmed by aspiration. The needle should be directed slightly caudad to avoid injury to the epiphyseal plate of the proximal end of the tibia. The transfusion may then commence.

Bones of the Foot

The bones of the foot are the **tarsal bones,** the **metatarsals,** and the **phalanges.**

Tarsal Bones

The tarsal bones are the calcaneum, the talus, the navicular, the cuboid, and the three cuneiform bones. Only the talus articulates with the tibia and the fibula at the ankle joint.

Calcaneum

The calcaneum is the largest bone of the foot and forms the prominence of the heel (Figs. 10-38, 10-39, and 10-40). It articulates above with the talus and in front with the cuboid. It has six surfaces.

- The **anterior surface** is small and forms the articular facet that articulates with the cuboid bone.
- The **posterior surface** forms the prominence of the heel and gives attachment to the tendo calcaneus (Achilles tendon).
- The **superior surface** is dominated by two articular facets for the talus, separated by a roughened groove, the **sulcus calcanei.**
- The **inferior surface** has an **anterior tubercle** in the midline and a large **medial** and a smaller **lateral** tubercle at the junction of the inferior and posterior surfaces.
- The **medial surface** possesses a large, shelflike process, termed the **sustentaculum tali,** which assists in the support of the talus.
- The **lateral surface** is almost flat. On its anterior part is a small elevation called the **peroneal tubercle,** which separates the tendons of the peroneus longus and brevis muscles.

The important muscles and ligaments attached to the calcaneum are shown in Figures 10-39 and 10-40.

Talus

The talus articulates above at the ankle joint with the tibia and fibula, below with the calcaneum, and in front with the navicular bone. It possesses a head, a neck, and a body (Figs. 10-38 and 10-39).

The **head** of the talus is directed distally and has an oval convex articular surface for articulation with the navicular bone. This articular surface is continued on its inferior surface, where it rests on the sustentaculum tali behind and the calcaneonavicular ligament in front.

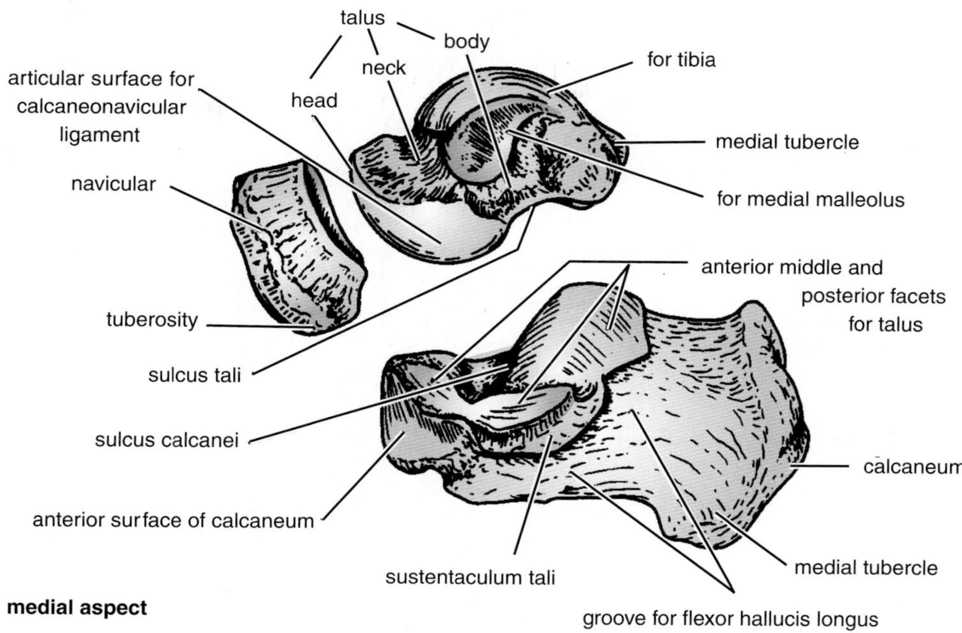

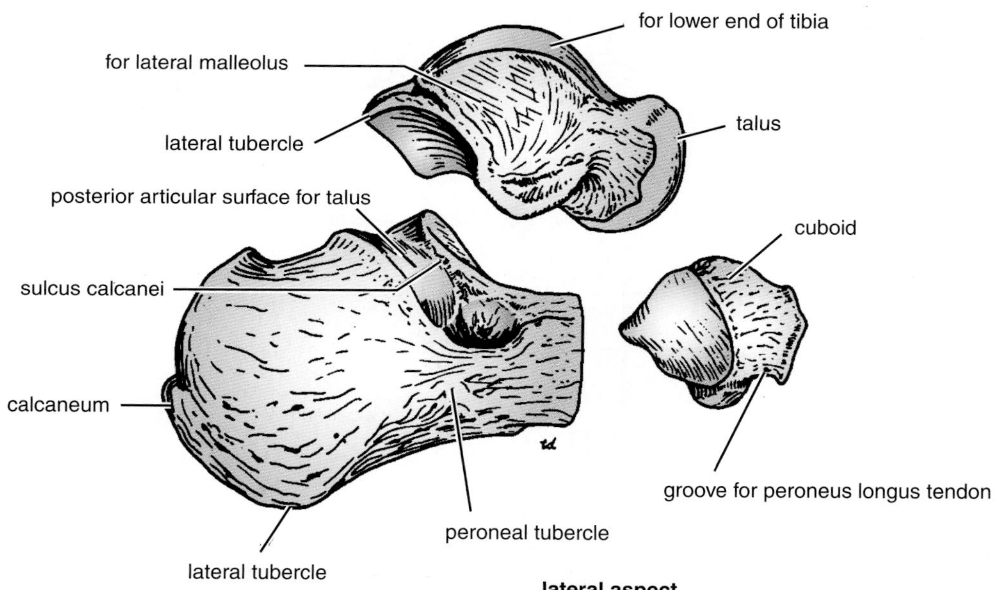

Figure 10-38 Calcaneum, talus, navicular, and cuboid bones.

The **neck** of the talus lies posterior to the head and is slightly narrowed. Its upper surface is roughened and gives attachment to ligaments, and its lower surface shows a deep groove, the **sulcus tali.** The sulcus tali and the sulcus calcanei in the articulated foot form a tunnel, the **sinus tarsi,** which is occupied by the strong **interosseous talocalcaneal ligament.**

The **body** of the talus is cuboidal. Its superior surface articulates with the distal end of the tibia; it is convex from before backward and slightly concave from side to side. Its lateral surface presents a triangular **articular facet** for articulation with the lateral malleolus of the fibula. Its medial surface has a small, comma-shaped **articular facet** for articulation with the medial malleolus of the tibia. The posterior surface is marked by two small **tubercles,** separated by a groove for the flexor hallucis longus tendon.

Numerous important ligaments are attached to the talus, but no muscles are attached to this bone.

The remaining tarsal bones should be identified and the following important features noted.

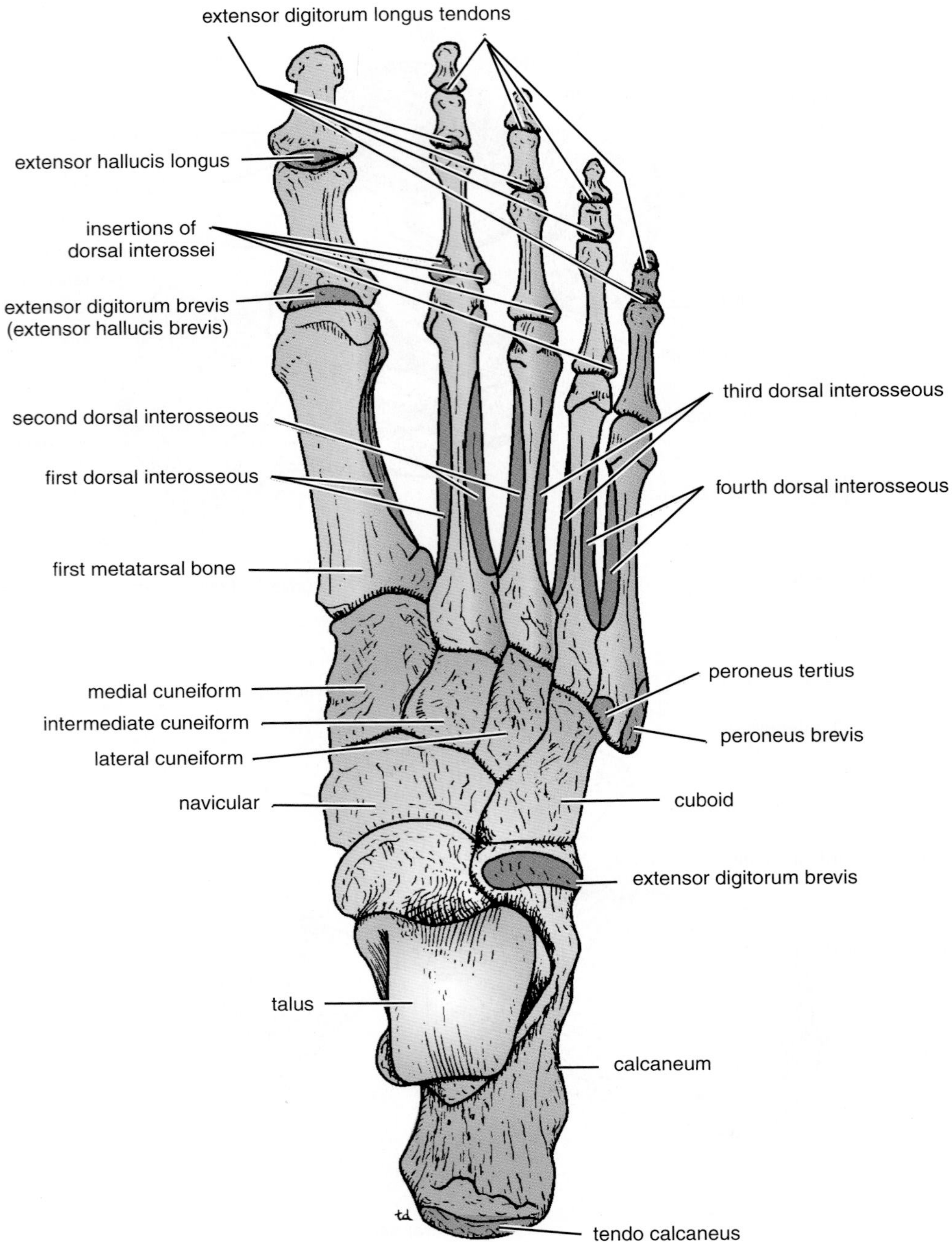

Figure 10-39 Muscle attachments on the dorsal aspect of the bones of the right foot.

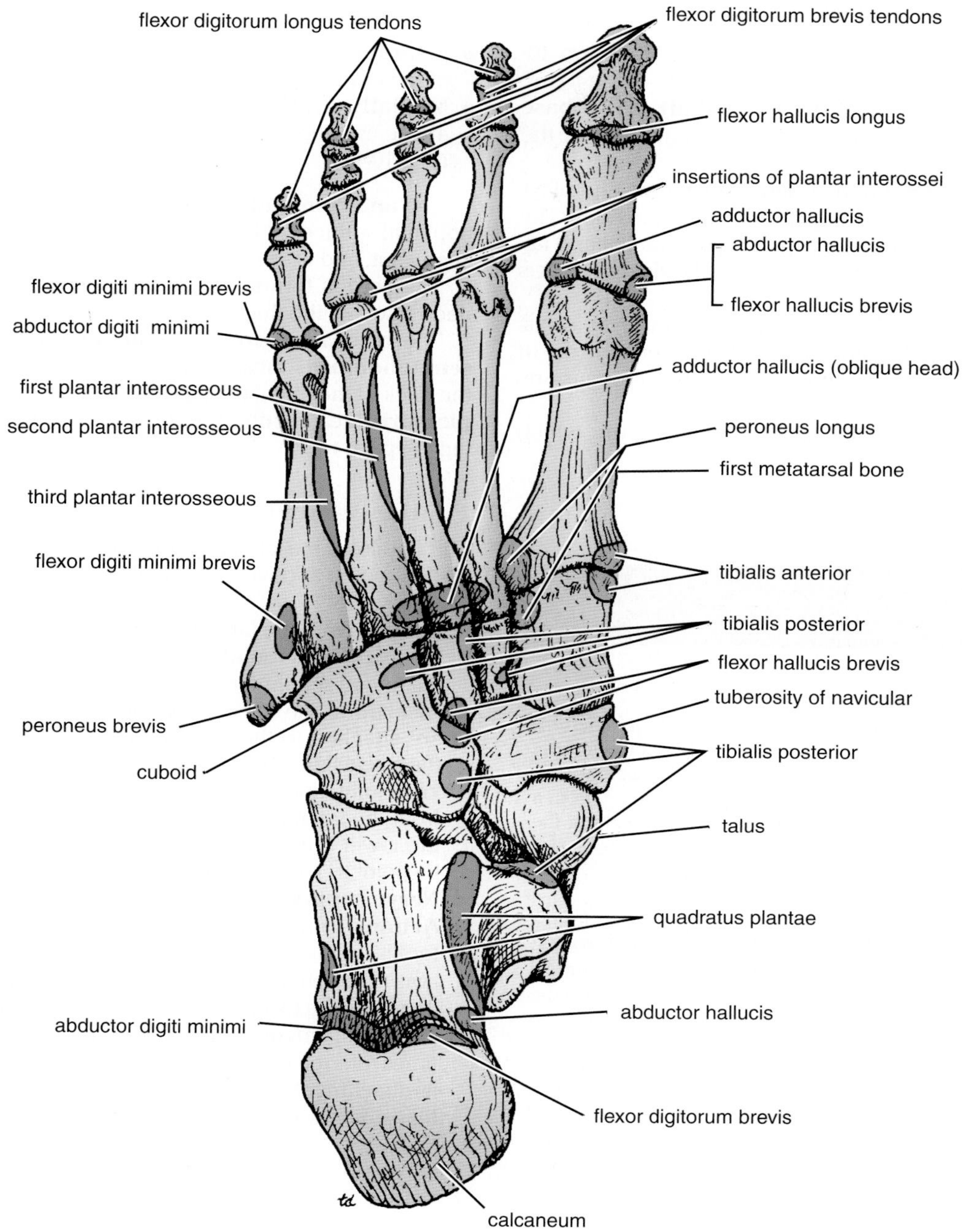

Figure 10-40 Muscle attachments on the plantar aspect of the bones of the right foot.

Navicular Bone

The **tuberosity** of the navicular bone (Figs. 10-38, 10-39, and 10-40) can be seen and felt on the medial border of the foot 1 in. (2.5 cm) in front of and below the medial malleolus; it gives attachment to the main part of the tibialis posterior tendon.

Cuboid Bone

A deep **groove** on the inferior aspect of the cuboid bone (Figs. 10-38, 10-39, and 10-40) lodges the tendon of the peroneus longus muscle.

Cuneiform Bones

The three small, wedge-shaped cuneiform bones (Figs. 10-39 and 10-40) articulate proximally with the navicular bone and distally with the first three metatarsal bones. Their wedge shape contributes greatly to the formation and maintenance of the transverse arch of the foot (see page 642).

The tarsal bones, unlike those of the carpus, start to ossify before birth. Centers of ossification for the calcaneum and the talus, and often for the cuboid, are present at birth. By the fifth year, ossification is taking place in all the tarsal bones.

Metatarsal Bones and Phalanges

The metatarsal bones and phalanges (Figs. 10-39 and 10-40) resemble the metacarpals and phalanges of the hand, and each possesses a **head** distally, a **shaft,** and a **base** proximally. The five metatarsals are numbered from the medial to the lateral side.

The **first metatarsal** bone is large and strong and plays an important role in supporting the weight of the body. The head is grooved on its inferior aspect by the medial and lateral **sesamoid bones** in the tendons of the flexor hallucis brevis.

The **fifth metatarsal** has a prominent **tubercle** on its base that can be easily palpated along the lateral border of the foot. The tubercle gives attachment to the peroneus brevis tendon.

Each toe has three phalanges except the big toe, which possesses only two.

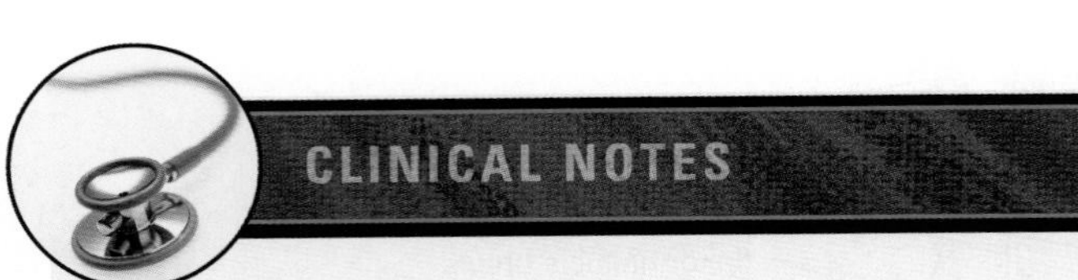

CLINICAL NOTES

Fractures of the Talus

Fractures occur at the neck or body of the talus. Neck fractures occur during violent dorsiflexion of the ankle joint when the neck is driven against the anterior edge of the distal end of the tibia. The body of the talus can be fractured by jumping from a height, although the two malleoli prevent displacement of the fragments.

Fractures of the Calcaneum

Compression fractures of the calcaneum result from falls from a height. The weight of the body drives the talus downward into the calcaneum, crushing it in such a way that it loses vertical height and becomes wider laterally. The posterior portion of the calcaneum above the insertion of the tendo calcaneus can be fractured by posterior displacement of the talus. The sustentaculum tali can be fractured by forced inversion of the foot.

Fractures of the Metatarsal Bones

The base of the fifth metatarsal can be fractured during forced inversion of the foot, at which time the tendon of insertion of the peroneus brevis muscle pulls off the base of the metatarsal.

Stress fracture of a metatarsal bone is common in joggers and in soldiers after long marches; it can also occur in nurses and hikers. It occurs most frequently in the distal third of the second, third, or fourth metatarsal bone. Minimal displacement occurs because of the attachment of the interosseous muscles.

Popliteal Fossa

The popliteal fossa is a diamond-shaped intermuscular space situated at the back of the knee (Fig. 10-41). The fossa is most prominent when the knee joint is flexed. It contains the popliteal vessels, the small saphenous vein, the common peroneal and tibial nerves, the posterior cutaneous nerve of the thigh, the genicular branch of the obturator nerve, connective tissue, and lymph nodes.

Boundaries

- **Laterally:** The biceps femoris above and the lateral head of the gastrocnemius and plantaris below (Fig. 10-41)
- **Medially:** The semimembranosus and semitendinosus above and the medial head of the gastrocnemius below (Fig. 10-41)

The **anterior wall** or **floor** of the fossa is formed by the popliteal surface of the femur, the posterior ligament of the knee joint, and the popliteus muscle (Figs. 10-41 and 10-42).

The **roof** is formed by skin, superficial fascia, and the deep fascia of the thigh.

The **biceps femoris,** the **semimembranosus,** and the **semitendinosus** muscles are described in the section on the back of the thigh, on page 587. The **gastrocnemius** and **plantaris** are described in the section on the back of the leg, on page 615.

Popliteus Muscle

The popliteus muscle plays a key role in the movements of the knee joint and will be described in detail.

- **Origin:** From the lateral surface of the lateral condyle of the femur by a rounded tendon and by a few fibers from the lateral semilunar cartilage (Figs. 10-42 and 10-43)
- **Insertion:** The fibers pass downward and medially and are attached to the posterior surface of the tibia, above the soleal line. The muscle arises within the capsule of the knee joint, and its tendon separates the lateral meniscus from the lateral ligament of the joint. It emerges through the lower part of the posterior surface of the capsule of the joint to pass to its insertion.
- **Nerve supply:** Tibial nerve
- **Action:** Medial rotation of the tibia on the femur or, if the foot is on the ground, lateral rotation of the femur on the tibia. The latter action occurs at the commencement of flexion of the extended knee, and its rotatory action slackens the ligaments of the knee joint; this action is sometimes referred to as "unlocking the knee joint." Because of its attachment to the lateral meniscus, it also pulls the cartilage backward at the commencement of flexion of the knee.

Popliteal Artery

The popliteal artery is deeply placed and enters the popliteal fossa through the opening in the adductor magnus, as a continuation of the femoral artery (Fig. 10-42). It ends at the level of the lower border of the popliteus muscle by dividing into anterior and posterior tibial arteries.

Relations

- **Anteriorly:** The popliteal surface of the femur, the knee joint, and the popliteus muscle (Fig. 10-42)
- **Posteriorly:** The popliteal vein and the tibial nerve, fascia, and skin (Figs. 10-41 and 10-42)

Branches

The popliteal artery has **muscular branches** and **articular branches** to the knee.

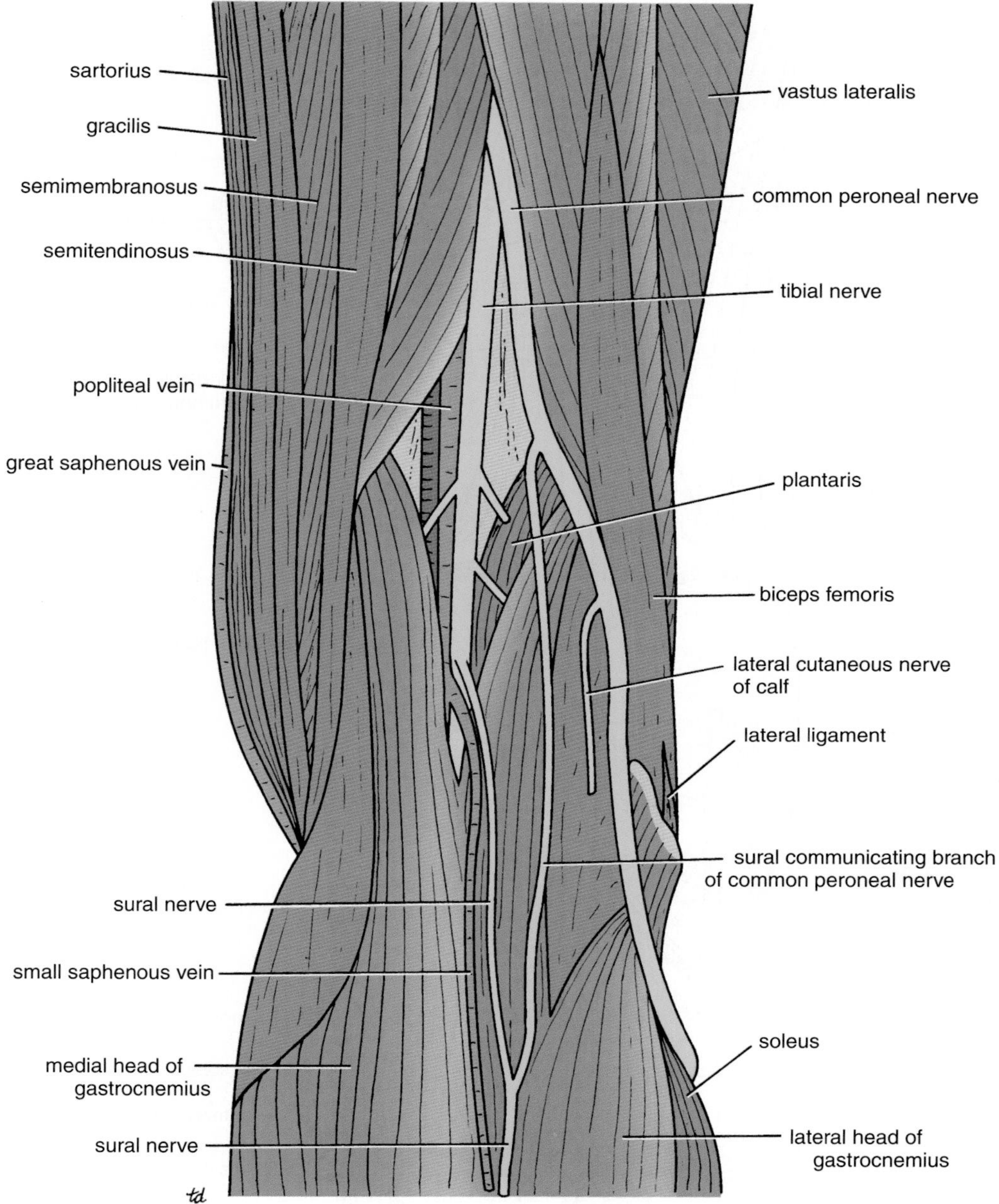

Figure 10-41 Boundaries and contents of the right popliteal fossa.

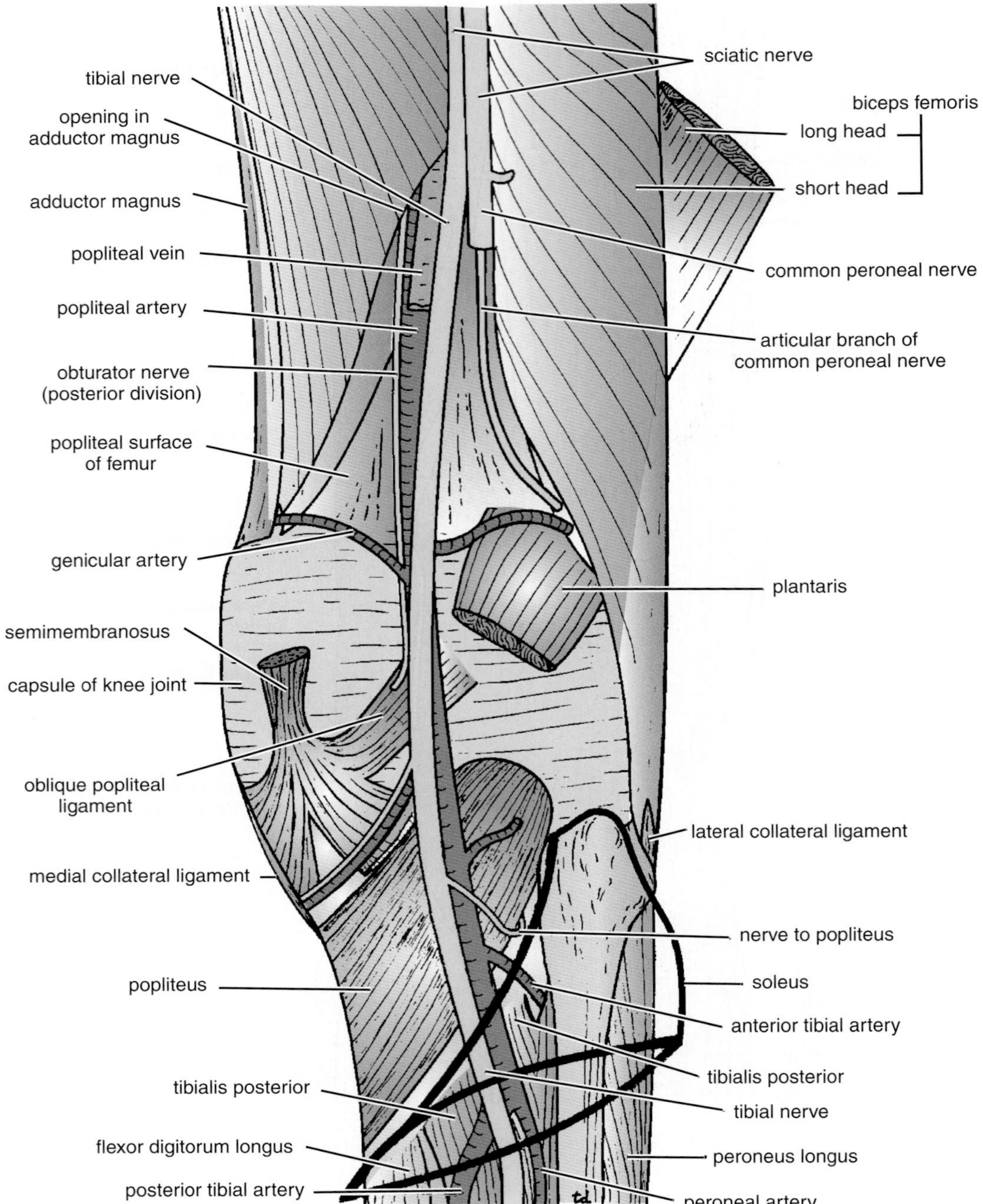

Figure 10-42 Deep structures in the right popliteal fossa. The proximal end of the soleus muscle is shown in outline only.

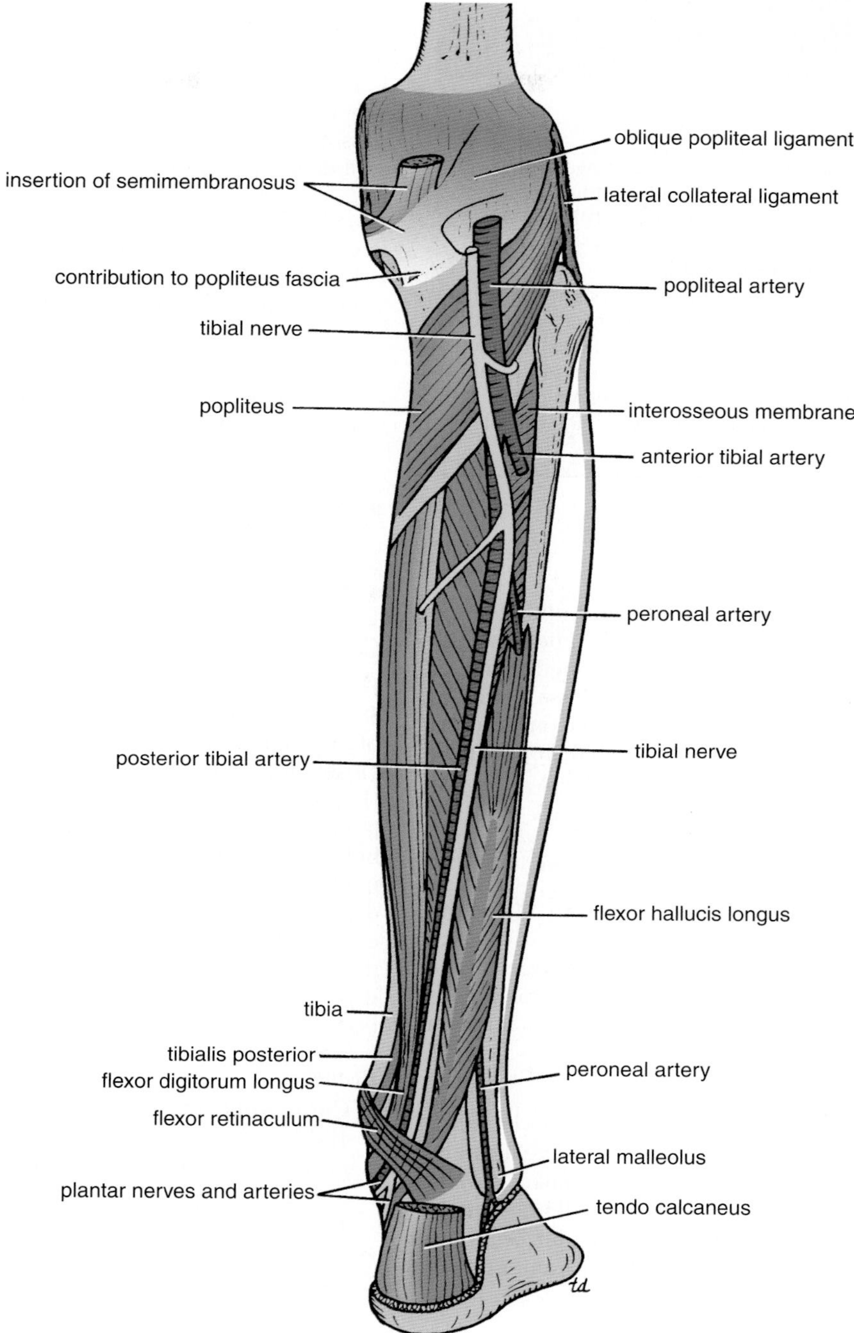

Figure 10-43 Deep structures in the posterior aspect of the right leg.

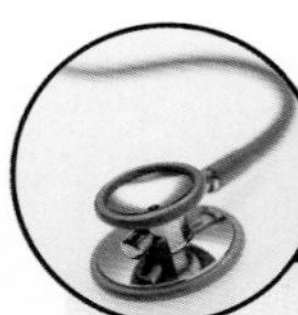

CLINICAL NOTES

Popliteal Aneurysm

The pulsations of the wall of the femoral artery against the tendon of adductor magnus at the opening of the adductor magnus is thought to contribute to the cause of popliteal aneurysms.

Semimembranosus Bursa Swelling

Semimembranosus bursa swelling is the most common swelling found in the popliteal space. It is made tense by extending the knee joint and becomes flaccid when the joint is flexed. It should be distinguished from a Baker's cyst, which is centrally located and arises as a pathologic (osteoarthritis) diverticulum of the synovial membrane through a hole in the back of the capsule of the knee joint.

Popliteal Vein

The popliteal vein is formed by the junction of the venae comitantes of the anterior and posterior tibial arteries at the lower border of the popliteus muscle on the medial side of the popliteal artery. As it ascends through the fossa, it crosses behind the popliteal artery so that it comes to lie on its lateral side (Figs. 10-41 and 10-42). It passes through the opening in the adductor magnus to become the femoral vein.

Tributaries

The tributaries of the popliteal vein are as follows:

- Veins that correspond to branches given off by the popliteal artery
- **Small saphenous vein,** which perforates the deep fascia and passes between the two heads of the gastrocnemius muscle to end in the popliteal vein. The origin of this vein is described on page 615.

Arterial Anastomosis Around the Knee Joint

To compensate for the narrowing of the popliteal artery, which occurs during extreme flexion of the knee, around the knee joint is a profuse anastomosis of small branches of the femoral artery with muscular and articular branches of the popliteal artery and with branches of the anterior and posterior tibial arteries.

Popliteal Lymph Nodes

About six lymph nodes are embedded in the fatty connective tissue of the popliteal fossa (Fig. 10-4). They receive superficial lymph vessels from the lateral side of the foot and leg; these accompany the small saphenous vein into the popliteal fossa. They also receive lymph from the knee joint and from deep lymph vessels accompanying the anterior and posterior tibial arteries.

Tibial Nerve

The larger terminal branch of the sciatic nerve (see page 587), the tibial nerve arises in the lower third of the thigh. It runs downward through the popliteal fossa, lying first on the lateral side of the popliteal artery, then posterior to it, and finally medial to it (Figs. 10-41 and 10-42). The popliteal vein lies between the nerve and the artery throughout its course. The nerve enters the posterior compartment of the leg by passing beneath the soleus muscle. Its further course is described on page 618.

Branches

- **Cutaneous:** The **sural nerve** descends between the two heads of the gastrocnemius muscle and is usually joined by the **sural communicating** branch of the common peroneal nerve (Figs. 10-41 and 10-17). Numerous small branches arise from the sural nerve to supply the skin of the calf and the back of the leg. The sural nerve accompanies the small saphenous vein behind the lateral malleolus and is distributed to the skin along the lateral border of the foot and the lateral side of the little toe.
- **Muscular** branches supply both heads of the gastrocnemius and the plantaris, soleus, and popliteus (Figs. 10-41 and 10-42).
- **Articular** branches supply the knee joint.

Common Peroneal Nerve

The smaller terminal branch of the sciatic nerve (see page 587), the common peroneal nerve arises in the lower third of the thigh. It runs downward through the popliteal fossa, closely following the medial border of the biceps muscle (Fig. 10-42). It leaves the fossa by crossing superficially the lateral head of the gastrocnemius muscle. It then passes behind the head of the fibula, winds laterally around the neck of the bone, pierces the peroneus longus muscle, and divides into two terminal branches: the superficial peroneal nerve and the deep peroneal nerve (Fig. 10-44). As the nerve lies on the lateral aspect of the neck of the fibula, it is subcutaneous and can easily be rolled against the bone.

Branches

- **Cutaneous:** The **sural communicating branch** (Figs. 10-16 and 10-41) runs downward and joins the sural nerve. The **lateral cutaneous nerve of the calf** supplies the skin on the lateral side of the back of the leg (Figs. 10-1 and 10-41).
- **Muscular** branch to the short head of the biceps femoris muscle, which arises high up in the popliteal fossa (Fig. 10-42)
- **Articular** branches to the knee joint

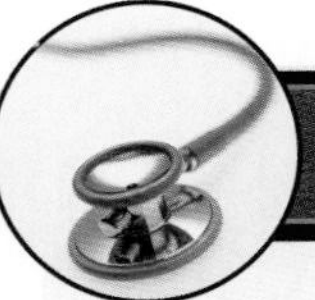

CLINICAL NOTES

Common Peroneal Nerve Injury

The common peroneal nerve is extremely vulnerable to injury as it winds around the neck of the fibula. At this site, it is exposed to direct trauma or is involved in fractures of the upper part of the fibula. Injury to the common peroneal nerve causes **footdrop.**

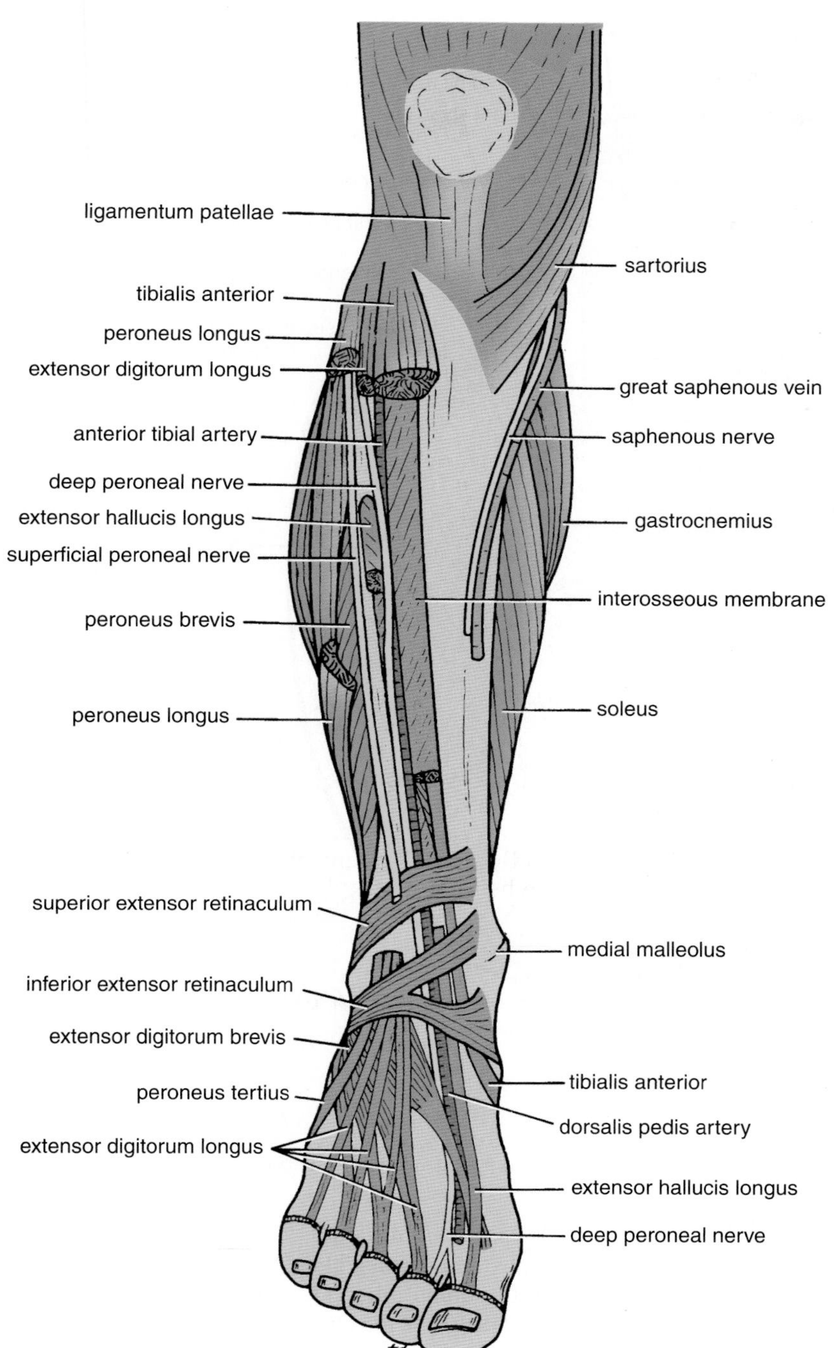

Figure 10-44 Deep structures in the anterior and lateral aspects of the right leg and the dorsum of the foot.

Posterior Cutaneous Nerve of the Thigh

The course of the posterior cutaneous nerve of the thigh through the gluteal region and the back of the thigh is described on page 565. It terminates by supplying the skin over the popliteal fossa (Fig. 10-1).

Obturator Nerve

The course of the posterior division of the obturator nerve in the medial compartment of the thigh is described on page 586. It leaves the subsartorial canal with the femoral artery by passing through the opening in the adductor magnus (Fig. 10-42). The nerve terminates by supplying the knee joint.

Fascial Compartments of the Leg

The deep fascia surrounds the leg and is continuous above with the deep fascia of the thigh. Below the tibial condyles it is attached to the periosteum on the anterior and medial borders of the tibia (Fig. 10-45). Two intermuscular septa

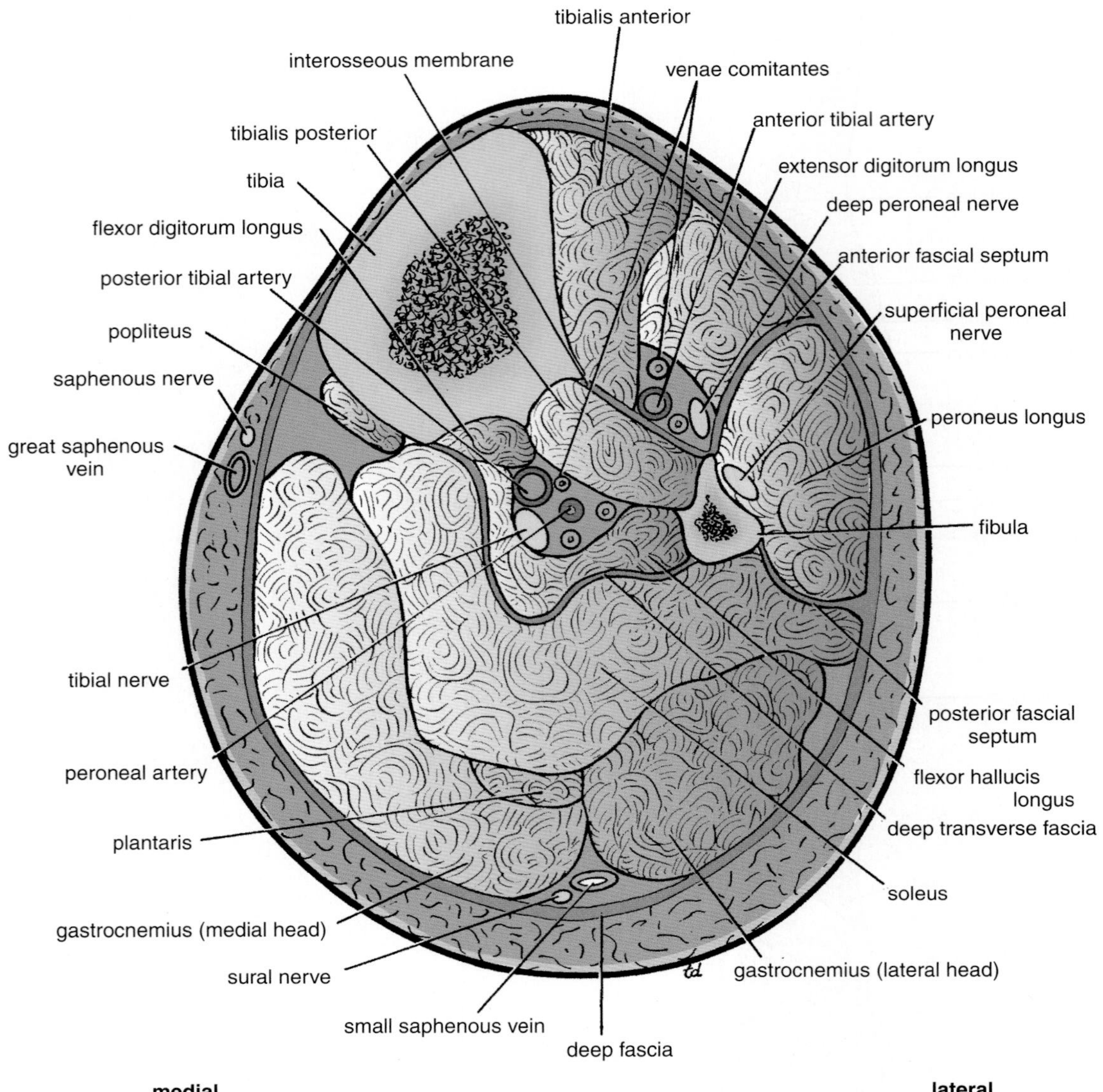

Figure 10-45 Transverse section through the middle of the right leg as seen from above.

pass from its deep aspect to be attached to the fibula. These, together with the interosseous membrane, divide the leg into three compartments—anterior, lateral, and posterior—each having its own muscles, blood supply, and nerve supply.

Interosseous Membrane

The interosseous membrane binds the tibia and fibula together and provides attachment for neighboring muscles (Figs. 10-44 and 10-45).

Retinacula of the Ankle

The retinacula are thickenings of the deep fascia that keep the long tendons around the ankle joint in position and act as pulleys.

Superior Extensor Retinaculum

The superior extensor retinaculum is attached to the distal ends of the anterior borders of the fibula and tibia (Figs. 10-46, 10-47, and 10-50).

Inferior Extensor Retinaculum

The inferior extensor retinaculum is a Y-shaped band located in front of the ankle joint (Figs. 10-44, 10-46, and 10-47). Fibrous bands separate the tendons into compartments (Figs. 10-48 and 10-50), each of which is lined by a synovial sheath.

Flexor Retinaculum

The flexor retinaculum extends from the medial malleolus downward and backward to be attached to the medial surface of the calcaneum (Fig. 10-49). It binds the tendons of the deep muscles of the back of the leg to the back of the medial malleolus as they pass forward to enter the sole. The tendons lie in compartments (Fig. 10-48), each of which is lined by a synovial sheath.

Superior Peroneal Retinaculum

The superior peroneal retinaculum connects the lateral malleolus to the lateral surface of the calcaneum (Fig. 10-49). It binds the tendons of the peroneus longus and brevis

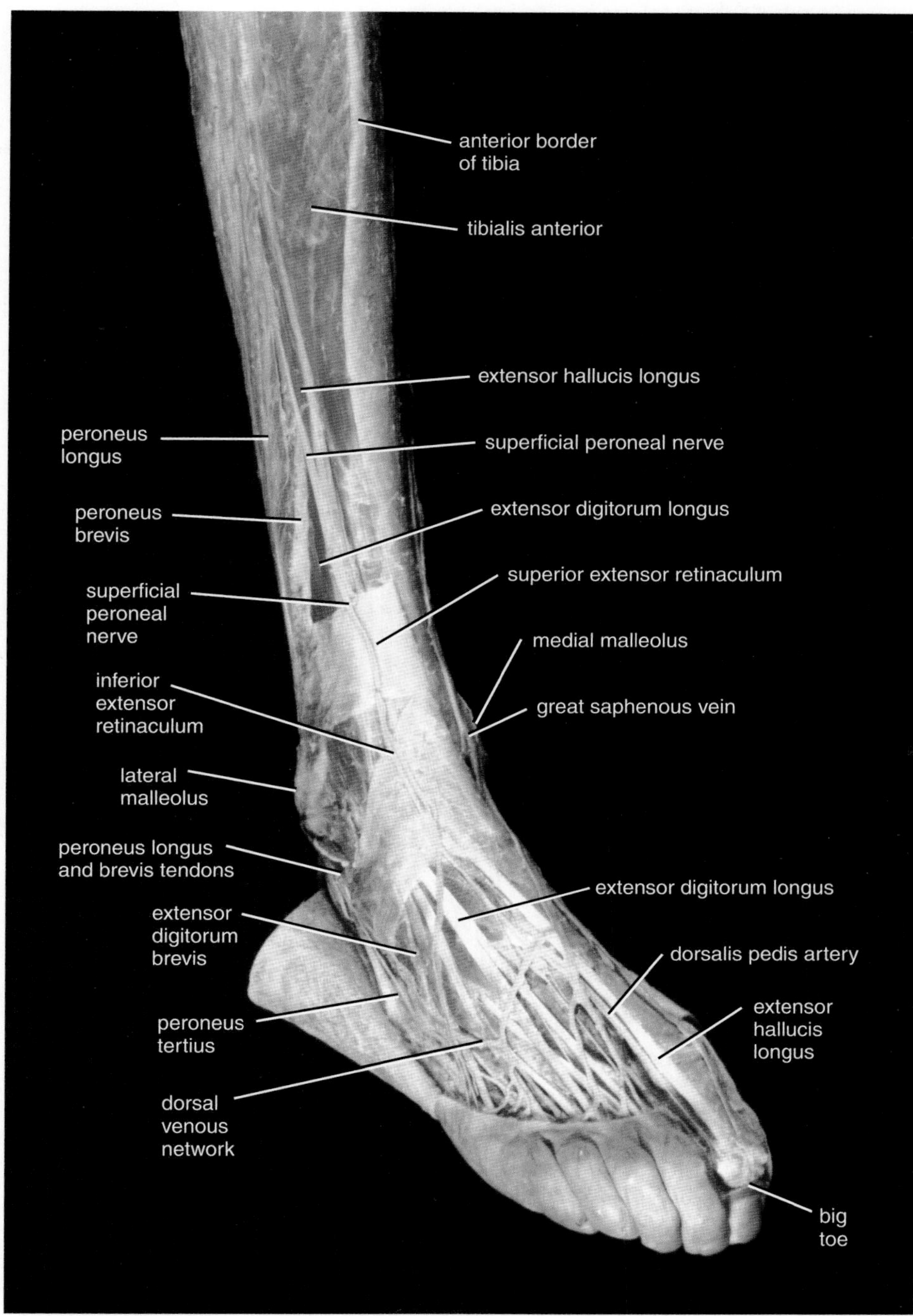

Figure 10-46 Dissection of the front of the right leg and dorsum of the foot.

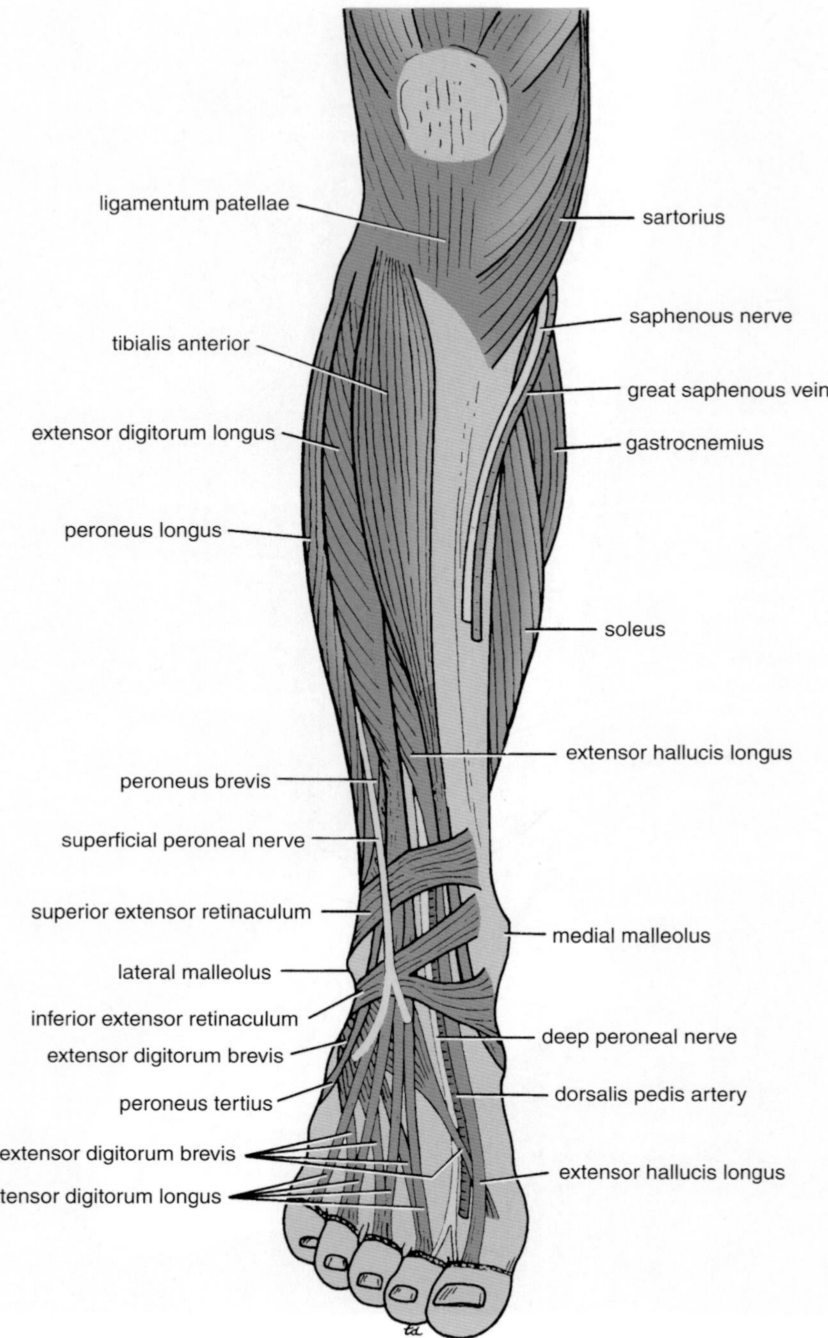

Figure 10-47 Structures in the anterior and lateral aspects of the right leg and the dorsum of the foot.

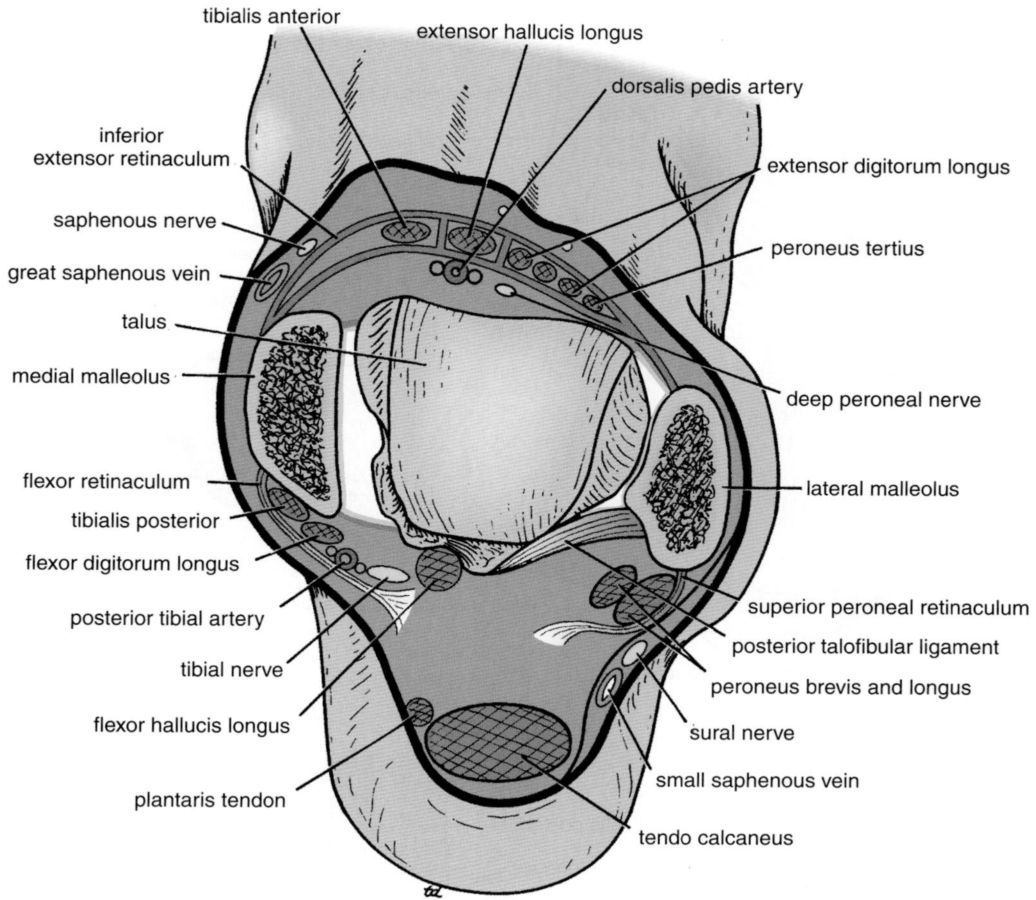

Figure 10-48 Relations of the right ankle joint.

to the back of the lateral malleolus. The tendons are provided with a common synovial sheath.

Inferior Peroneal Retinaculum

The inferior peroneal retinaculum binds the tendons of the peroneus longus and brevis muscles to the lateral side of the calcaneum (Fig. 10-49). The tendons each possess a synovial sheath, which is continuous above with the common sheath.

The arrangement of the tendons beneath the different retinacula is described on pages 618 and 619.

The Front of the Leg

Skin

Cutaneous Nerves

The **lateral cutaneous nerve of the calf,** a branch of the common peroneal nerve (see page 604), supplies the skin on the upper part of the lateral surface of the leg (Fig. 10-1).

The **superficial peroneal nerve,** a branch of the common peroneal nerve (see page 604), supplies the skin of the lower part of the anterolateral surface of the leg (Fig. 10-2).

The **saphenous nerve,** a branch of the femoral nerve (see page 582), supplies the skin on the anteromedial surface of the leg (Fig. 10-2).

Superficial Veins

Numerous small veins curve around the medial aspect of the leg and ultimately drain into the great saphenous vein (Fig. 10-51).

Lymph Vessels

The greater part of the lymph from the skin and superficial fascia on the front of the leg drains upward and medially in vessels that follow the great saphenous vein, to end in the vertical group of superficial inguinal lymph nodes (Fig. 10-4). A small amount of lymph from the upper lateral part of the front of the leg may pass via vessels that accompany the small saphenous vein and drain into the popliteal nodes (Fig. 10-4).

Contents of the Anterior Fascial Compartment of the Leg

- **Muscles:** The tibialis anterior, extensor digitorum longus, peroneus tertius, and extensor hallucis longus
- **Blood supply:** Anterior tibial artery
- **Nerve supply:** Deep peroneal nerve

Muscles of the Anterior Fascial Compartment of the Leg

The muscles are seen in Figures 10-44, 10-45, 10-46, 10-47, 10-48, and 10-50 and are described in Table 10-5.

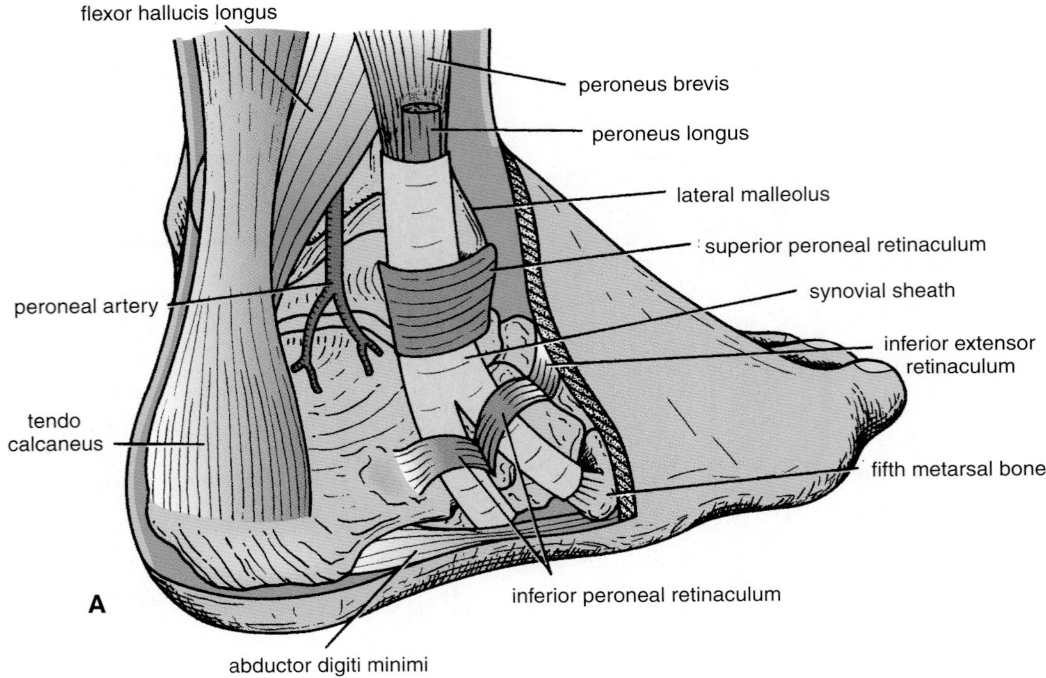

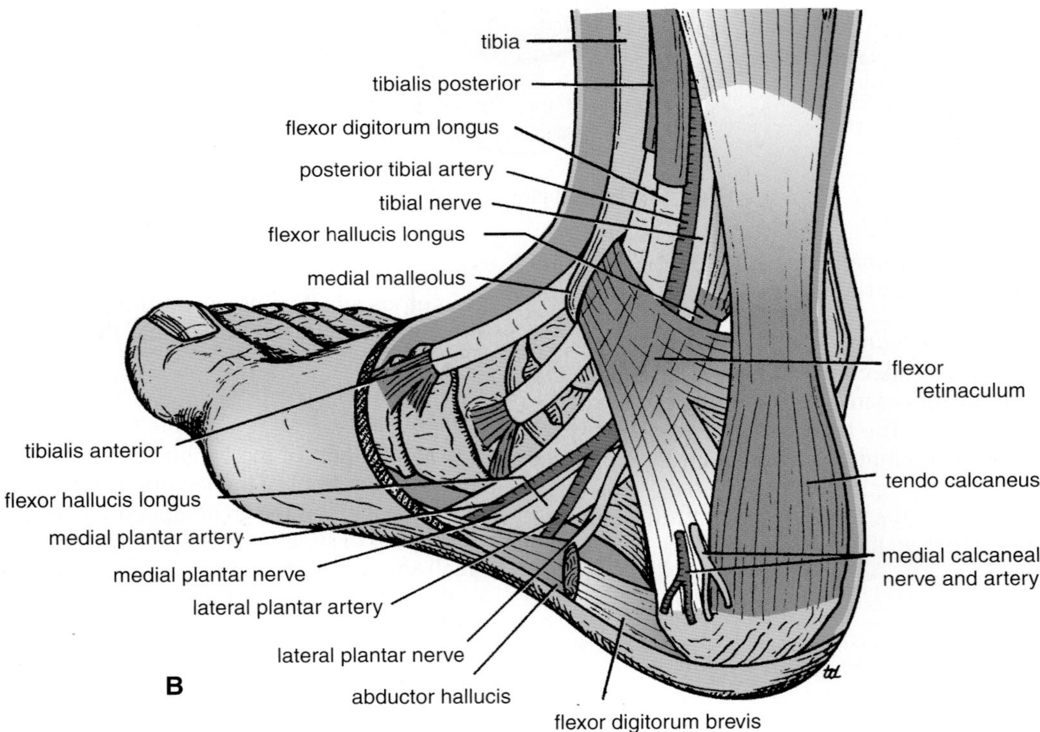

Figure 10-49 Structures passing behind the lateral malleolus (**A**) and the medial malleolus (**B**). Synovial sheaths of the tendons are shown in blue. Note the positions of the retinacula.

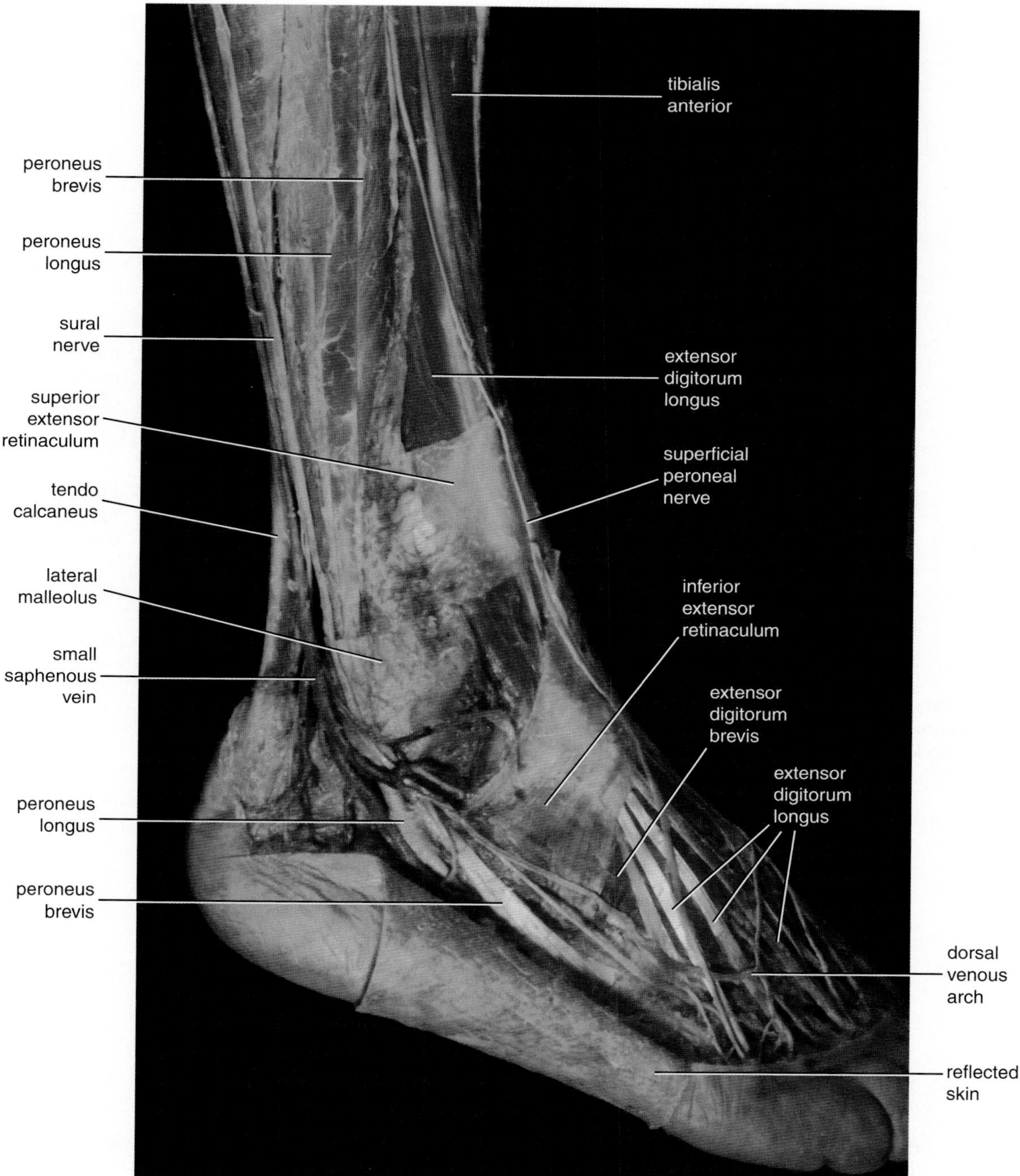

Figure 10-50 Dissection of the right ankle region showing the structures passing behind the lateral malleolus. Note the position of the retinacula.

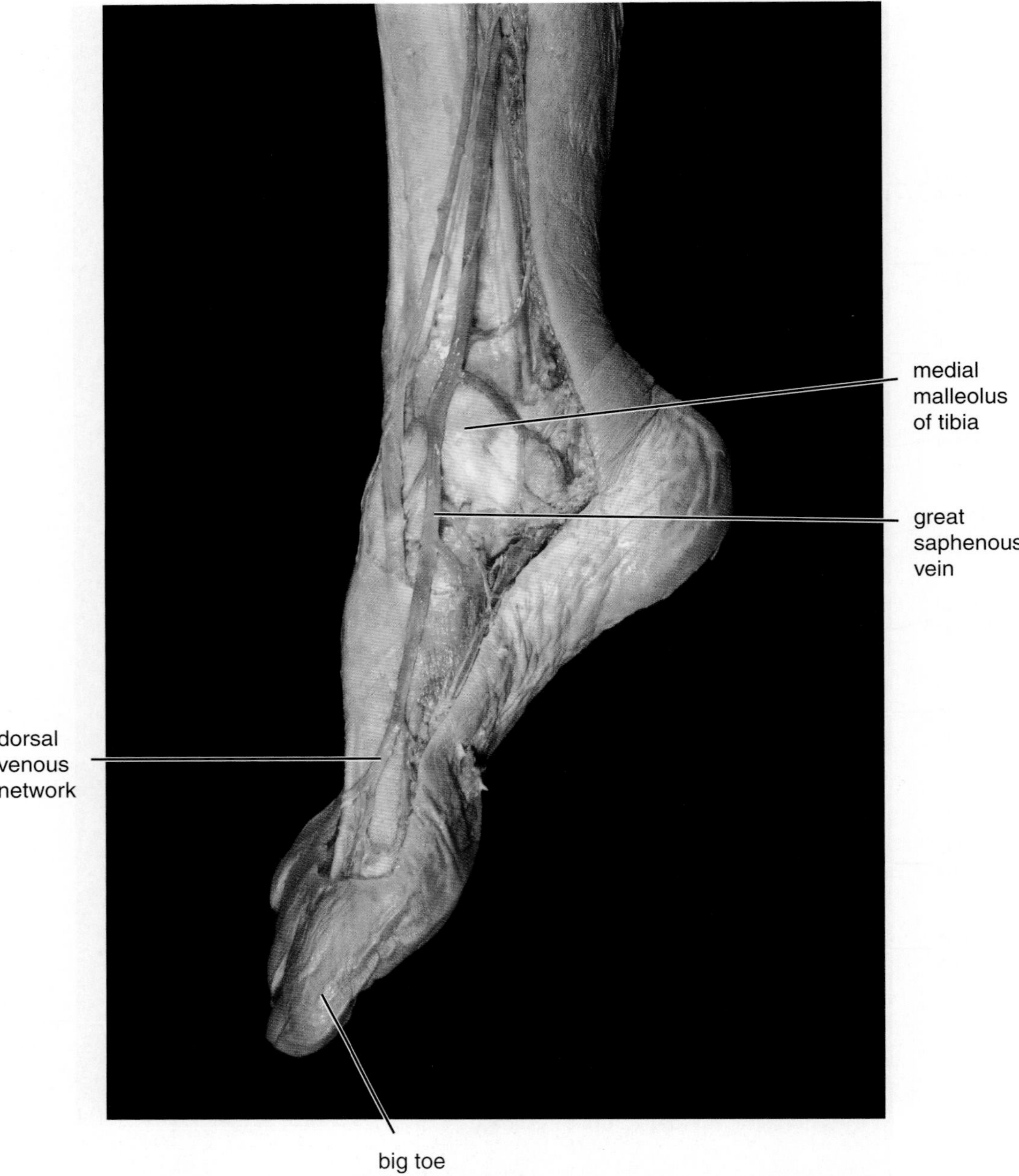

Figure 10-51 Dissection of the right ankle region showing the origin of the great saphenous vein from the dorsal venous arch. Note that the great saphenous vein ascends in front of the medial malleolus of the tibia.

Note the following:

- Extension, or dorsiflexion of the ankle, is the movement of the foot away from the ground.
- The peroneus tertius muscle extends the foot at the ankle joint along with the other muscles in this compartment and is supplied by the deep peroneal nerve. The muscle also everts the foot at the subtalar and transverse tarsal joints along with the peroneus longus and brevis muscles but receives no innervation from the superficial peroneal nerve.
- The extensor digitorum longus tendons on the dorsal surface of each toe become incorporated into a fascial expansion called the **extensor expansion.** The central part of the expansion is inserted into the base of the middle phalanx, and the two lateral parts converge to be inserted into the base of the distal phalanx. (Compare with the insertion of extensor digitorum in the hand.)

Artery of the Anterior Fascial Compartment of the Leg

Anterior Tibial Artery

The anterior tibial artery is the smaller of the terminal branches of the popliteal artery. It arises at the level of the lower border of the popliteus muscle (see page 600) and passes forward into the anterior compartment of the leg through an opening in the upper part of the interosseous

Table 10-5 Muscles of the Anterior Fascial Compartment of the Leg

Muscle	Origin	Insertion	Nerve Supply	Nerve Root[a]	Action
Tibialis anterior	Lateral surface of shaft of tibia and interosseous membrane	Medial cuneiform and base of first metatarsal bone	Deep peroneal nerve	**L4,** 5	Extends[b] foot at ankle joint; inverts foot at subtalar and transverse tarsal joints; holds up medial longitudinall arch of foot
Extensor digitorum longus	Anterior surface of shaft of fibula	Extensor expansion of lateral four toes	Deep peroneal nerve	L5; S1	Extends toes; extends foot at ankle joint
Peroneus tertius	Anterior surface of shaft of fibula	Base of fifth metatarsal bone	Deep peroneal nerve	L5; S1	Extends foot at ankle joint; everts foot at subtalar and transverse tarsal joints
Extensor hallucis longus	Anterior surface of shaft of fibula	Base of distal phalanx of great toe	Deep peroneal nerve	L5; S1	Extends big toe; extends foot at ankle joint; inverts foot at subtalar and transverse tarsal joints
Extensor digitorum brevis	Calcaneum	By four tendons into the proximal phalanx of big toe and long extensor tendons to second, third, and fourth toes	Deep peroneal nerve	S1, 2	Extends toes

[a] The predominant nerve root supply is indicated by boldface type.
[b] Extension, or dorsiflexion, of the ankle is the movement of the foot away from the ground.

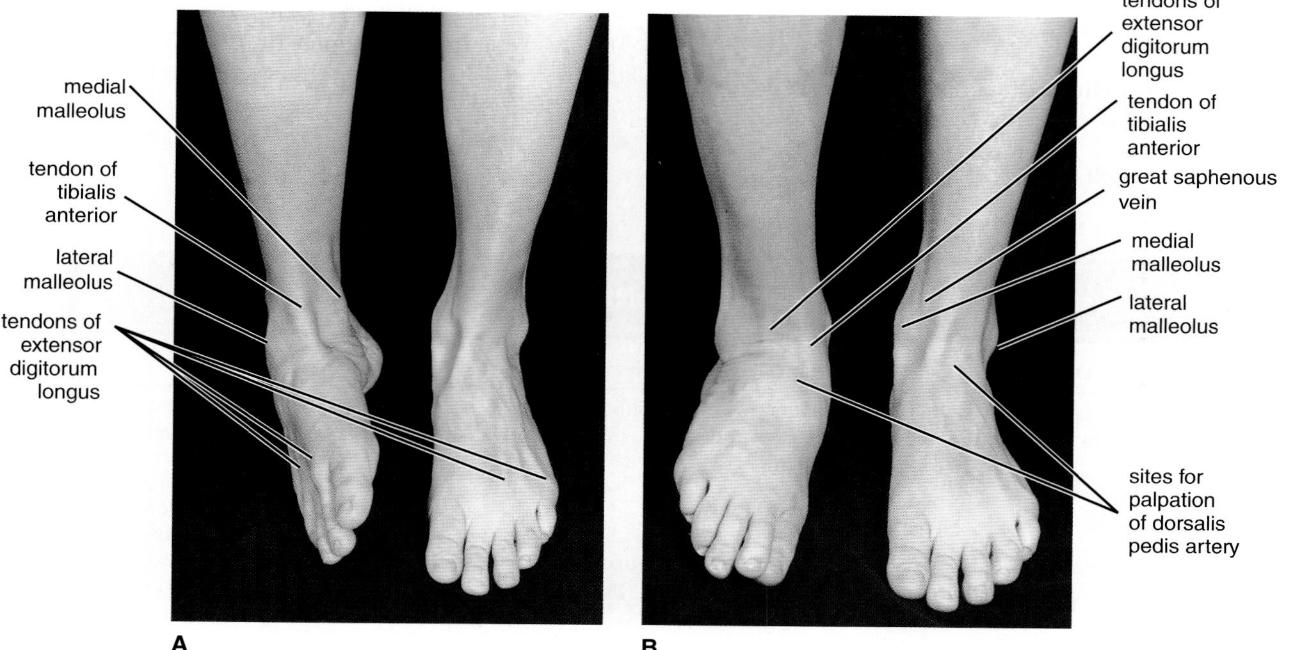

Figure 10-52 Anterior view of the ankles and feet of a 29-year-old woman showing inversion (**A**) and eversion (**B**) of the right foot.

membrane (Fig. 10-42). It descends on the anterior surface of the interosseous membrane, accompanied by the deep peroneal nerve (Fig. 10-44). In the upper part of its course, it lies deep beneath the muscles of the compartment. In the lower part of its course, it lies superficial in front of the lower end of the tibia (Figs. 10-44 and 10-47). Having passed behind the superior extensor retinaculum, it has the tendon of the extensor hallucis longus on its medial side and the deep peroneal nerve and the tendons of extensor digitorum longus on its lateral side. It is here that its pulsations can easily be felt in the living subject. In front of the ankle joint, the artery becomes the dorsalis pedis artery (see page 625).

Branches

- **Muscular branches** to neighboring muscles
- **Anastomotic branches** that anastomose with branches of other arteries around the knee and ankle joints

Venae comitantes of the anterior tibial artery join those of the posterior tibial artery in the popliteal fossa to form the popliteal vein.

Nerve Supply of the Anterior Fascial Compartment of the Leg

Deep Peroneal Nerve

The deep peroneal nerve is one of the terminal branches of the common peroneal nerve (see page 604). It arises in the substance of the peroneus longus muscle on the lateral side of the neck of the fibula (Fig. 10-44). The nerve enters the anterior compartment by piercing the anterior fascial septum. It then descends deep to the extensor digitorum longus muscle, first lying lateral, then anterior, and finally lateral to the anterior tibial artery (Fig. 10-44). The nerve passes behind the extensor retinacula. Its further course in the foot is described on page 629.

Branches

- **Muscular branches** to the tibialis anterior, the extensor digitorum longus, the peroneus tertius, and the extensor hallucis longus
- **Articular branch** to the ankle joint

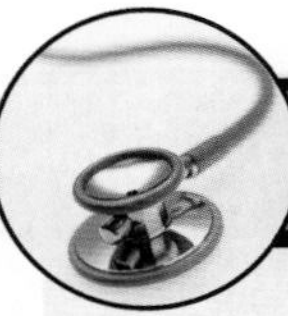

CLINICAL NOTES

Anterior Compartment of the Leg Syndrome

The anterior compartment syndrome is produced by an increase in the intracompartmental pressure that results from an increased production of tissue fluid. Soft tissue injury associated with bone fractures is a common cause, and early diagnosis is critical. The deep, aching pain in the anterior compartment of the leg that is characteristic of this syndrome can become severe. Dorsiflexion of the foot at the ankle joint increases the severity of the pain. Stretching of the muscles that pass through the compartment by passive plantar flexion of the ankle also increases the pain. As the pressure rises, the venous return is diminished, thus producing a further rise in pressure. In severe cases, the arterial supply is eventually cut off by compression, and the dorsalis pedis arterial pulse disappears. The tibialis anterior, the extensor digitorum longus, and the extensor hallucis longus muscles are paralyzed. Loss of sensation is limited to the area supplied by the deep peroneal nerve—that is, the skin cleft between the first and second toes. The surgeon can open the anterior compartment of the leg by making a longitudinal incision through the deep fascia and thus decompress the area and prevent anoxic necrosis of the muscles.

Contents of the Lateral Fascial Compartment of the Leg

- **Muscles:** Peroneus longus and peroneus brevis
- **Blood supply:** Branches from the peroneal artery
- **Nerve supply:** Superficial peroneal nerve

Muscles of the Lateral Fascial Compartment of the Leg

The muscles are seen in Figures 10-44, 10-45, 10-46, 10-47, 10-48, 10-49, and 10-50 and described in Table 10-6.

Note the following:

- The peroneus longus and brevis muscles both flex the foot at the ankle joint and evert the foot at the subtalar

Table 10-6 Muscles of the Lateral Fascial Compartment of the Leg

Muscle	Origin	Insertion	Nerve Supply	Nerve Root[a]	Action
Peroneus longus	Lateral surface of shaft of fibula	Base of first metatarsal and the medial cuneiform	Superficial peroneal nerve	**L5; S1,** 2	Plantar flexes foot at ankle joint; everts foot at subtalar and transverse tarsal joints; supports lateral longitudinal and transverse arches of foot
Peroneus brevis	Lateral surface of shaft of fibula	Base of fifth metatarsal bone	Superficial peroneal nerve	**L5; S1,** 2	Plantar flexes foot at ankle joint; everts foot at subtalar and transverse tarsal joint; supports lateral longitudinal arch of foot

[a] The predominant nerve root supply is indicated by boldface type.

and transverse tarsal joints. They also play an important role in holding up the lateral longitudinal arch in the foot. In addition, the peroneus longus tendon serves as a tie to the transverse arch of the foot.

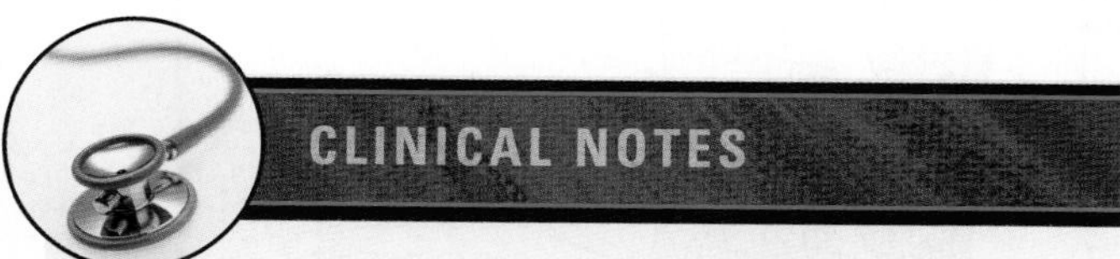

Tenosynovitis and Dislocation of the Peroneus Longus and Brevis Tendons

Tenosynovitis (inflammation of the synovial sheaths) can affect the tendon sheaths of the peroneus longus and brevis muscles as they pass posterior to the lateral malleolus. Treatment consists of immobilization, heat, and physiotherapy. Tendon dislocation can occur when the tendons of peroneus longus and brevis dislocate forward from behind the lateral malleolus. For this condition to occur, the superior peroneal retinaculum must be torn. It usually occurs in older children and is caused by trauma.

Artery of the Lateral Fascial Compartment of the Leg

Numerous branches from the peroneal artery (see page 618), which lies in the posterior compartment of the leg, pierce the posterior fascial septum and supply the peroneal muscles.

Nerve of the Lateral Fascial Compartment of the Leg

Superficial Peroneal Nerve

The superficial peroneal nerve is one of the terminal branches of the common peroneal nerve (see page 604). It arises in the substance of the peroneus longus muscle on the lateral side of the neck of the fibula (Figs. 10-44, 10-46, and 10-50). It descends between the peroneus longus and brevis muscles, and in the lower part of the leg it becomes cutaneous (Figs. 10-47 and 10-50).

Branches

- **Muscular** branches to the peroneus longus and brevis (Fig. 10-44)
- **Cutaneous:** Medial and lateral branches are distributed to the skin on the lower part of the front of the leg and the dorsum of the foot. In addition, branches supply the dorsal surfaces of the skin of all the toes, except the adjacent sides of the first and second toes and the lateral side of the little toe (see page 627).

The Back of the Leg

Skin

Cutaneous Nerves

The **posterior cutaneous nerve** of the thigh descends on the back of the thigh (see page 587). In the popliteal fossa, it supplies the skin over the popliteal fossa and the upper part of the back of the leg (Fig. 10-1).

The **lateral cutaneous nerve of the calf,** a branch of the common peroneal nerve (see page 604), supplies the skin on the upper part of the posterolateral surface of the leg (Fig. 10-1).

The **sural nerve,** a branch of the tibial nerve (see page 604), supplies the skin on the lower part of the posterolateral surface of the leg (Fig. 10-1).

The **saphenous nerve,** a branch of the femoral nerve (see page 582), gives off branches that supply the skin on the posteromedial surface of the leg (Fig. 10-1).

Superficial Veins

The **small saphenous vein** arises from the lateral part of the dorsal venous arch of the foot (Fig. 10-19). It ascends **behind** the lateral malleolus in company with the sural nerve. It follows the lateral border of the tendo calcaneus and then runs up the middle of the back of the leg. The vein pierces the deep fascia and passes between the two heads of the gastrocnemius muscle in the lower part of the popliteal fossa (Figs. 10-19 and 10-40); it ends in the popliteal vein (see page 604). The small saphenous vein has numerous valves along its course.

Tributaries

- Numerous **small veins** from the back of the leg
- **Communicating veins** with the deep veins of the foot
- Important **anastomotic branches** that run upward and medially and join the great saphenous vein (Fig. 10-19)

The mode of termination of the small saphenous vein is subject to variation: It may join the popliteal vein; it may join the great saphenous vein; or it may split in two, one division joining the popliteal and the other joining the great saphenous vein.

Lymph Vessels

Lymph vessels from the skin and superficial fascia on the back of the leg drain upward and either pass forward around the medial side of the leg to end in the vertical group of superficial inguinal nodes or drain into the popliteal nodes (Fig. 10-4).

Contents of the Posterior Fascial Compartment of the Leg

The **deep transverse fascia** of the leg is a septum that divides the muscles of the posterior compartment into superficial and deep groups (Fig. 10-45).

- **Superficial group of muscles:** Gastrocnemius, plantaris, and soleus
- **Deep group of muscles:** Popliteus, flexor digitorum longus, flexor hallucis longus, and tibialis posterior
- **Blood supply:** Posterior tibial artery
- **Nerve supply:** Tibial nerve

Muscles of the Posterior Fascial Compartment of the Leg: Superficial Group

The muscles are seen in Figures 10-45 and 10-53 and are described in Table 10-7.

Note the following:

- Together, the soleus, gastrocnemius, and plantaris act as powerful plantar flexors of the ankle joint. They provide the main forward propulsive force in walking and running by using the foot as a lever and raising the heel off the ground.

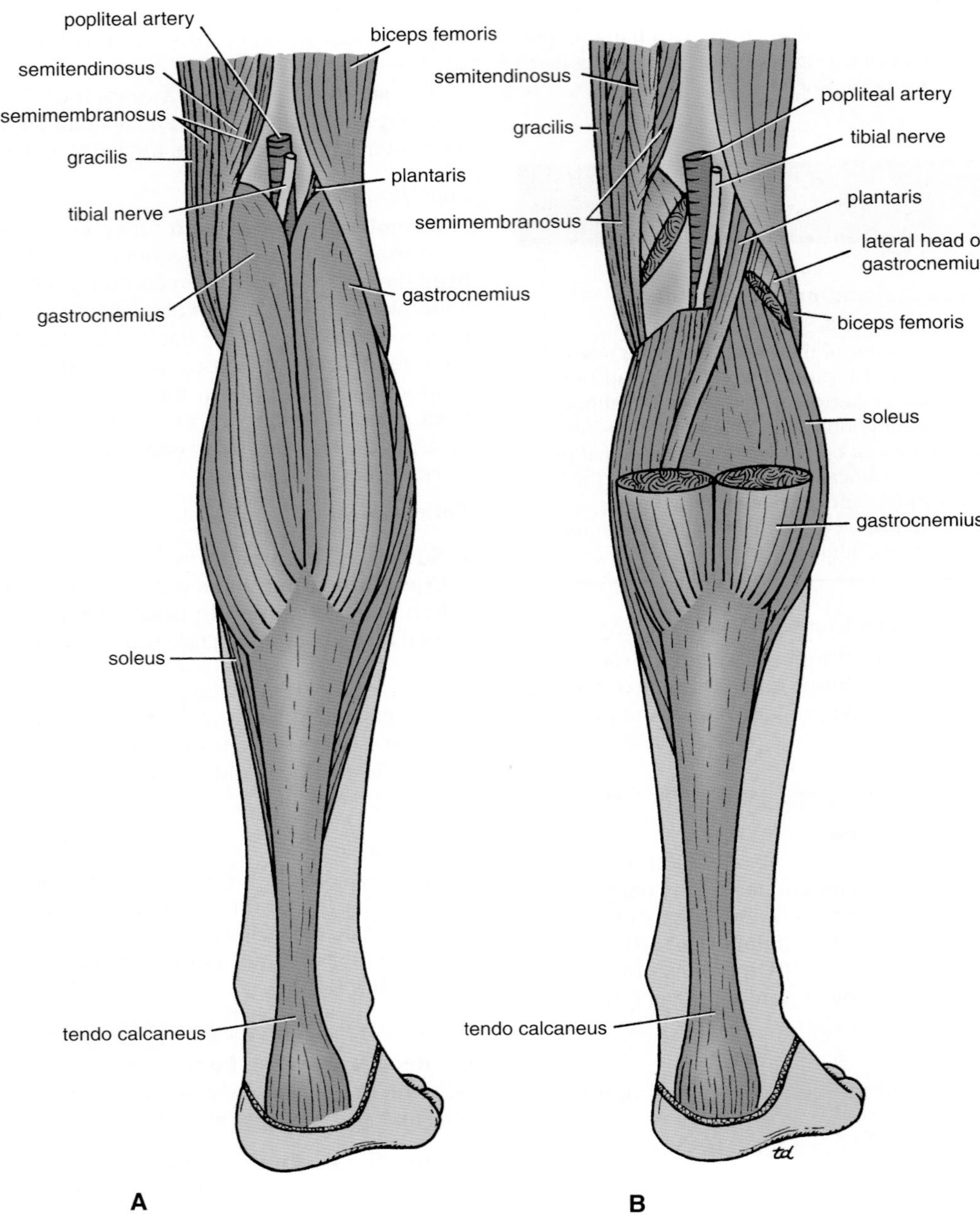

Figure 10-53 Structures in the posterior aspect of the right leg. In **B,** part of the gastrocnemius has been removed.

Table 10-7 Muscles of the Posterior Fascial Compartment of the Leg

Muscle	Origin	Insertion	Nerve Supply	Nerve Root[a]	Action
Superficial Group					
Gastrocnemius	Lateral head from lateral condyle of femur and medial head from above medial condyle	Via tendo calcaneus into posterior surface of calcaneum	Tibial nerve	**S1,** 2	Plantar flexes foot at ankle joint; flexes knee joint
Plantaris	Lateral supracondylar ridge of femur	Posterior surface of calcaneum	Tibial nerve	**S1,** 2	Plantar flexes foot at ankle joint; flexes knee joint
Soleus	Shafts of tibia and fibula	Via tendo calcaneus into posterior surface of calcaneum	Tibial nerve	S1, **2**	Together with gastrocnemius and plantaris is powerful plantar flexor of ankle joint; provides main propulsive force in walking and running
Deep Group					
Popliteus	Lateral surface of lateral condyle of femur	Posterior surface of shaft of tibia above soleal line	Tibial nerve	L4, 5; S1	Flexes leg at knee joint; unlocks knee joint by lateral rotation of femur on tibia and slackens ligaments of joint
Flexor digitorum longus	Posterior surface of shaft of tibia	Bases of distal phalanges of lateral four toes	Tibial nerve	**S2,** 3	Flexes distal phalanges of lateral four toes; plantar flexes foot at ankle joint; supports medial and lateral longitudinal arches of foot
Flexor hallucis longus	Posterior surface of shaft of fibula	Base of distal phalanx of big toe	Tibial nerve	**S2,** 3	Flexes distal phalanx of big toe; plantar flexes foot at ankle joint; supports medial longitudinal arch of foot
Tibialis posterior	Posterior surface of shafts of tibia and fibula and interosseous membrane	Tuberosity of navicular bone and other neighboring bones	Tibial nerve	L4, 5	Plantar flexes foot at ankle joint; inverts foot at subtalar and transverse tarsal joints; supports medial longitudinal arch of foot

[a] The predominant nerve root supply is indicated by boldface type.

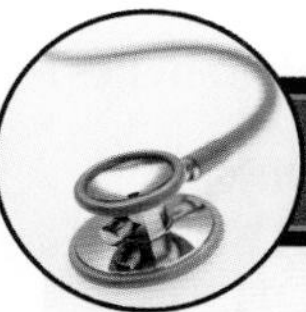

CLINICAL NOTES

Gastrocnemius and Soleus Muscle Tears

Tearing of the gastrocnemius or soleus muscles will produce severe localized pain over the damaged muscle. Swelling may be present.

Ruptured Tendo Calcaneus

Rupture of the tendo calcaneus is common in middle-aged men and frequently occurs in tennis players. The rupture occurs at its narrowest part, about 2 in. (5 cm) above its insertion. A sudden, sharp pain is felt, with immediate disability. The gastrocnemius and soleus muscles retract proximally, leaving a palpable gap in the tendon. It is impossible for the patient to actively plantar flex the foot. The tendon should be sutured as soon as possible and the leg immobilized with the ankle joint plantar flexed and the knee joint flexed.

Rupture of the Plantaris Tendon

Rupture of the plantaris tendon is rare, although tearing of the fibers of the soleus or partial tearing of the tendo calcaneus is frequently diagnosed as such a rupture.

Plantaris Tendon and Autografts

The plantaris muscle, which is often missing, can be used for tendon autografts in repairing severed flexor tendons to the fingers; the tendon of the palmaris longus muscle can also be used for this purpose.

Muscles of the Posterior Fascial Compartment of the Leg: Deep Group

The muscles are seen in Figures 10-43, 10-45, 10-48, and 10-49 and are described in Table 10-7.

Note the following:

- The popliteus muscle arises inside the capsule of the knee joint and is inserted into the upper part of the posterior surface of the tibia. The tendon separates the lateral ligament of the knee joint from the lateral meniscus so that the meniscus is not tethered to the ligament and is freer to move and adapt to the surfaces of the condyle of the femur and the tibia.
- The popliteus muscle is responsible for "unlocking" the knee joint.

Artery of the Posterior Fascial Compartment of the Leg

Posterior Tibial Artery

The posterior tibial artery is one of the terminal branches of the popliteal artery (see page 600). It begins at the level of the lower border of the popliteus muscle and passes downward deep to the gastrocnemius and soleus and the deep transverse fascia of the leg (Figs. 10-41, 10-42, and 10-44). It lies on the posterior surface of the tibialis posterior muscle above and on the posterior surface of the tibia below. In the lower part of the leg the artery is covered only by skin and fascia. The artery passes behind the medial malleolus deep to the flexor retinaculum and terminates by dividing into medial and lateral plantar arteries (Fig. 10-49).

Branches

- **Peroneal artery,** which is a large artery that arises close to the origin of the posterior tibial artery (Fig. 10-44). It descends behind the fibula, either within the substance of the flexor hallucis longus muscle or posterior to it. The peroneal artery gives off numerous **muscular branches** and a **nutrient artery to the fibula** and ends by taking part in the anastomosis around the ankle joint. A **perforating branch** pierces the interosseous membrane to reach the lower part of the front of the leg.
- **Muscular branches** are distributed to muscles in the posterior compartment of the leg.
- **Nutrient artery to the tibia**
- **Anastomotic branches,** which join other arteries around the ankle joint
- **Medial and lateral plantar arteries** (see pages 624 and 625). **Venae comitantes** of the posterior tibial artery join those of the anterior tibial artery in the popliteal fossa to form the popliteal vein.

Nerve of the Posterior Fascial Compartment of the Leg

Tibial Nerve

The tibial nerve is the larger terminal branch of the sciatic nerve (Fig. 10-17) in the lower third of the back of the thigh (see page 604). It descends through the popliteal fossa and passes deep to the gastrocnemius and soleus muscles (Figs. 10-43 and 10-53). It lies on the posterior surface of the tibialis posterior and, lower down the leg, on the posterior surface of the tibia (Fig. 10-43). The nerve accompanies the posterior tibial artery and lies at first on its medial side, then crosses posterior to it, and finally lies on its lateral side. The nerve, with the artery, passes behind the medial malleolus, between the tendons of the flexor digitorum longus and the flexor hallucis longus (Fig. 10-49). It is covered here by the flexor retinaculum and divides into the medial and lateral plantar nerves.

Branches in the Leg (Below the Popliteal Fossa)

- **Muscular branches** to the soleus, flexor digitorum longus, flexor hallucis longus, and tibialis posterior
- **Cutaneous:** The **medial calcaneal branch** supplies the skin over the medial surface of the heel (Fig. 10-49).
- **Articular branch** to the ankle joint
- **Medial and lateral plantar nerves:** See pages 626 and 627.

The Region of the Ankle

Before learning the anatomy of the foot, it is essential that a student have a sound knowledge of the arrangement of the tendons, arteries, and nerves in the region of the ankle joint. From the clinical standpoint, the ankle is a common site for fractures, sprains, and dislocations.

A transverse section through the ankle joint is shown in Figure 10-48; on it, identify the structures from medial to lateral. At the same time, examine your own ankle and identify as many of the structures as possible.

Anterior Aspect of the Ankle

Structures That Pass Anterior to the Extensor Retinacula From Medial to Lateral (Fig. 10-48)

- Saphenous nerve and great saphenous vein **(in front of the medial malleolus)**
- Superficial peroneal nerve (medial and lateral branches)

Structures That Pass Beneath or Through the Extensor Retinacula From Medial to Lateral (Fig. 10-48)

- Tibialis anterior tendon
- Extensor hallucis longus tendon
- Anterior tibial artery with venae comitantes

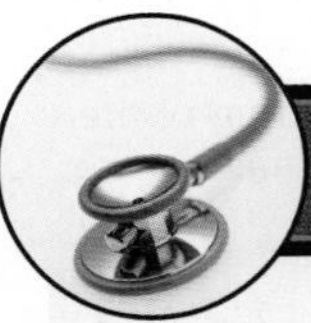

CLINICAL NOTES

Deep Vein Thrombosis and Long-Distance Air Travel

Passengers who sit immobile for hours on long-distance flights are very prone to deep vein thrombosis in the legs. Thrombosis of the veins of the soleus muscle gives rise to mild pain or tightness in the calf and calf muscle tenderness. However, deep vein thrombosis can also occur with no signs or symptoms. Should the thrombus become dislodged, it passes rapidly to the heart and lungs, causing pulmonary embolism, which is often fatal. Preventative measures include stretching of the legs every hour to improve the venous circulation

- Deep peroneal nerve
- Extensor digitorum longus tendons
- Peroneus tertius

As each of the above tendons passes beneath or through the extensor retinacula, it is surrounded by a synovial sheath. The tendons of extensor digitorum longus and the peroneus tertius share a common synovial sheath.

Structures That Pass in Front of the Medial Malleolus (Figs. 10-48 and 10-51)

- Great saphenous vein
- Saphenous nerve

Posterior Aspect of the Ankle

Structures That Pass Behind the Medial Malleolus Beneath the Flexor Retinaculum From Medial to Lateral (Figs. 10-48 and 10-49)

- Tibialis posterior tendon
- Flexor digitorum longus
- Posterior tibial artery with venae comitantes
- Tibial nerve
- Flexor hallucis longus

As each of these tendons passes beneath the flexor retinaculum, it is surrounded by a synovial sheath.

Structures That Pass Behind the Lateral Malleolus Superficial to the Superior Peroneal Retinaculum (Fig. 10-48)

- The sural nerve
- Small saphenous vein

Structures That Pass Behind the Lateral Malleolus Beneath the Superior Peroneal Retinaculum

The peroneus longus and brevis tendons (Figs. 10-48 and 10-49) share a common synovial sheath. Lower down, beneath the inferior peroneal retinaculum, they have separate sheaths.

Structures That Lie Directly Behind the Ankle

The fat and the large tendo calcaneus lie behind the ankle (Fig. 10-48).

The Foot

The foot supports the body weight and provides leverage for walking and running. It is unique in that it is constructed in the form of arches, which enable it to adapt its shape to uneven surfaces. It also serves as a resilient spring to absorb shocks, such as in jumping.

The Sole of the Foot

Skin

The skin of the sole of the foot is thick and hairless. It is firmly bound down to the underlying deep fascia by numerous fibrous bands. The skin shows a few flexure creases at the sites of skin movement. Sweat glands are present in large numbers.

The **sensory nerve supply** to the skin of the sole of the foot is derived from the **medial calcaneal branch** of the tibial nerve, which innervates the medial side of the heel; branches from the **medial plantar nerve,** which innervate the medial two thirds of the sole; and branches from the **lateral plantar nerve,** which innervate the lateral third of the sole (Figs. 10-1 and 10-54).

Deep Fascia

The **plantar aponeurosis** is a triangular thickening of the deep fascia that protects the underlying nerves, blood vessels, and muscles (Fig. 10-54). Its apex is attached to the medial and lateral tubercles of the calcaneum. The base of the aponeurosis divides into five slips that pass into the toes.

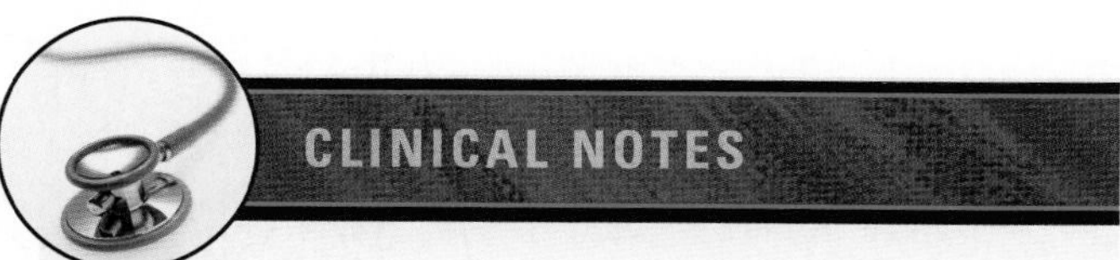

Plantar Fasciitis

Plantar fasciitis, which occurs in individuals who do a great deal of standing or walking, causes pain and tenderness of the sole of the foot. It is believed to be caused by repeated minor trauma. Repeated attacks of this condition induce ossification in the posterior attachment of the aponeurosis, forming a **calcaneal spur.**

Muscles of the Sole of the Foot

The muscles of the sole are conveniently described in four layers from the inferior layer superiorly.

- **First layer:** Abductor hallucis, flexor digitorum brevis, abductor digiti minimi
- **Second layer:** Quadratus plantae, lumbricals, flexor digitorum longus tendon, flexor hallucis longus tendon
- **Third layer:** Flexor hallucis brevis, adductor hallucis, flexor digiti minimi brevis
- **Fourth layer:** Interossei, peroneus longus tendon, tibialis posterior tendon

Unlike the small muscles of the hand, the sole muscles have few delicate functions and are chiefly concerned with supporting the arches of the foot. Although their names would suggest control of individual toes, this function is rarely used in most people.

The muscles of the sole are seen in Figures 10-55 through 10-59 and are described in Table 10-8.

Long Tendons of the Sole of the Foot

Flexor Digitorum Longus Tendon

The flexor digitorum longus tendon enters the sole by passing behind the medial malleolus beneath the flexor retinaculum (Figs. 10-47 and 10-56). It passes forward across the medial surface of the sustentaculum tali and then crosses the tendon of flexor hallucis longus, from which it receives a strong slip. It is here that it receives on its lateral border the insertion of the quadratus plantae muscle. The tendon now

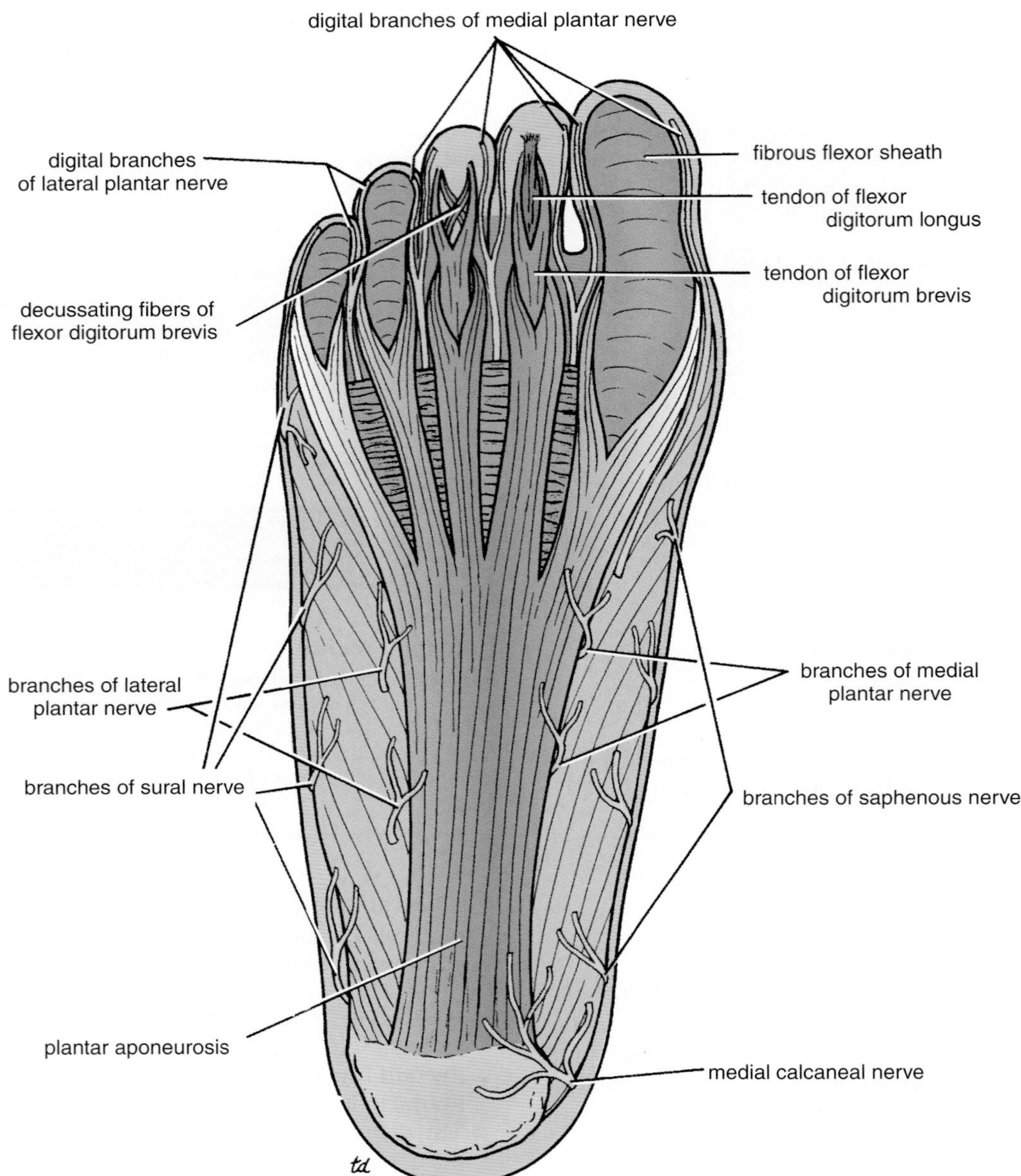

Figure 10-54 Plantar aponeurosis and cutaneous nerves of the sole of the right foot.

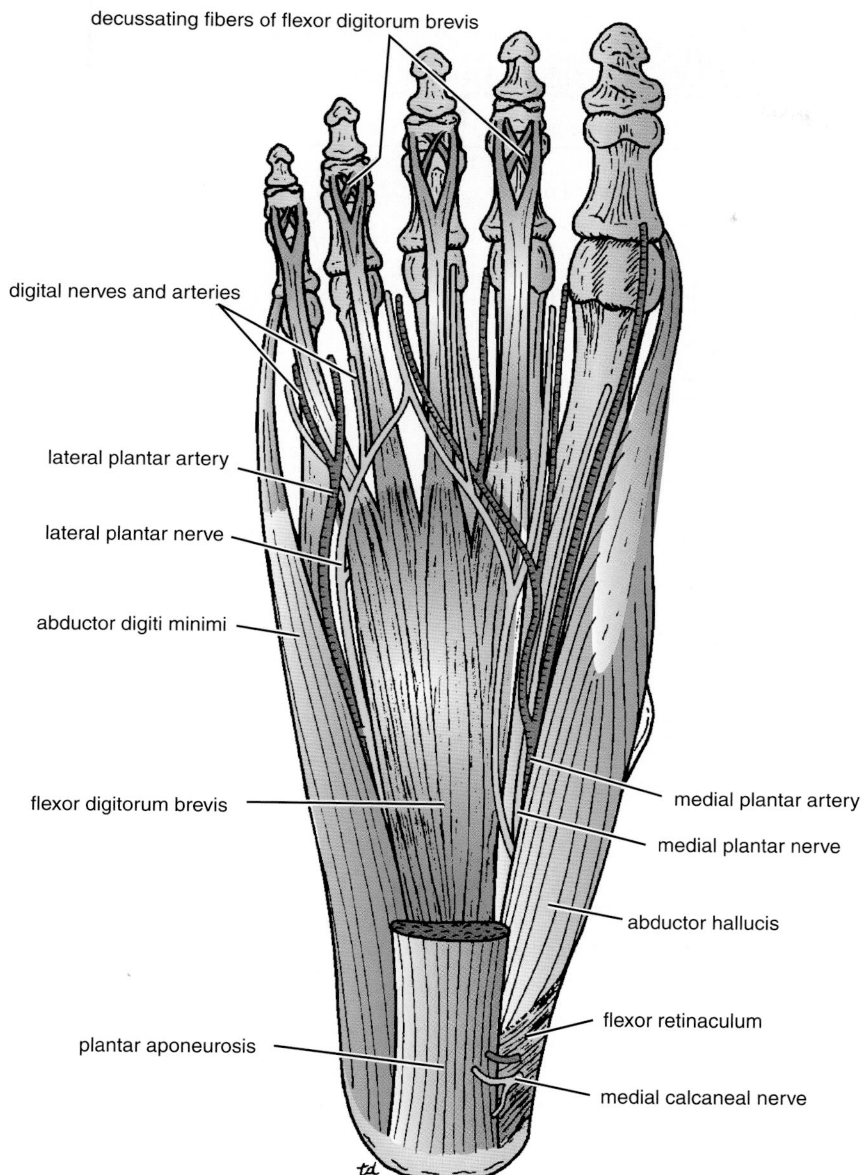

Figure 10-55 First layer of the plantar muscles of the right foot. Medial and lateral plantar arteries and nerves are also shown.

divides into its four tendons of insertion, which pass forward, giving origin to the lumbrical muscles. The tendons then enter the fibrous sheaths of the lateral four toes (Fig. 10-54). Each tendon perforates the corresponding tendon of flexor digitorum brevis and passes on to be inserted into the base of the distal phalanx. It should be noted that the method of insertion is similar to that found for the flexor digitorum profundus in the hand (see page 502).

Flexor Hallucis Longus Tendon

The flexor hallucis longus tendon (Fig. 10-56) enters the sole by passing behind the medial malleolus beneath the flexor retinaculum. It runs forward below the sustentaculum tali and crosses deep to the flexor digitorum longus tendon, to which it gives a strong slip. It then enters the fibrous sheath of the big toe and is inserted into the base of the distal phalanx.

Fibrous Flexor Sheaths: The inferior surface of each toe, from the head of the metatarsal bone to the base of the distal phalanx, is provided with a strong fibrous sheath, which is attached to the sides of the phalanges (Fig. 10-54). The arrangement is similar to that found in the fingers (see page 500). The fibrous sheath, together with the inferior surfaces of the phalanges and the interphalangeal joints, forms a blind tunnel in which lie the flexor tendons of the toe (Fig. 10-57).

Synovial Flexor Sheaths: The tendons of the flexor hallucis longus and the flexor digitorum longus are surrounded by synovial sheaths (Fig. 10-49 and 10-57).

Peroneus Longus Tendon

The peroneus longus tendon (Fig. 10-59) enters the foot from behind the lateral malleolus and runs obliquely across the sole to be inserted into the base of the first metatarsal

Table 10-8 Muscles of the Sole of the Foot

Muscle	Origin	Insertion	Nerve Supply	Nerve Root[a]	Action
First Layer					
Abductor hallucis	Medial tuberosity of calcaneum and flexor retinaculum	Base of proximal phalanx of big toe	Medial plantar nerve	S2, **3**	Flexes and abducts big toe; braces medial longitudinal arch
Flexor digitorum brevis	Medial tubercle of calcaneum	Four tendons to four lateral toes—inserted into borders of middle phalanx; tendons perforated by those of flexor digitorum longus	Medial plantar nerve	S2, **3**	Flexes lateral four toes; braces medial and lateral longitudinal arches
Abductor digiti minimi	Medial and lateral tubercles of calcaneum	Base of proximal phalanx of fifth toe	Lateral plantar nerve	S2, **3**	Flexes and abducts fifth toe; braces lateral longitudinal arch
Second Layer					
Quadratus plantae	Medial and lateral sides of calcaneum	Tendon of flexor digitorum longus	Lateral plantar nerve	S2, **3**	Assists flexor digitorum longus in flexing lateral four toes
Lumbricals (4)	Tendons of flexor digitorum longus	Dorsal extensor expansion; bases of proximal phalanges of lateral four toes	First lumbrical: medial plantar nerve; remainder: lateral plantar nerve	S2, **3**	Extends toes at interphalangeal joints
Flexor digitorum longus tendon	See Table 10-7				
Flexor hallucis longus tendon	See Table 10-7				
Third Layer					
Flexor hallucis brevis	Cuboid, lateral cuneiform, tibialis posterior insertion	Medial tendon into medial side of base of proximal phalanx of big toe; lateral tendon into lateral side of base of proximal phalanx of big toe	Medial plantar nerve	S2, **3**	Flexes metatarsophalangeal joint of big toe; supports medial longitudinal arch
Adductor hallucis	Oblique head bases of second, third, and fourth metatarsal bones; transverse head from plantar ligaments	Lateral side of base of proximal phalanx of big toe	Deep branch lateral plantar nerve	S2, **3**	Flexes metatarsophalangeal joint of big toe; holds together metatarsal bones
Flexor digiti minimi brevis	Base of fifth metatarsal bone	Lateral side of base of proximal phalanx of little toe	Lateral plantar nerve	S2, **3**	Flexes metatarsophalangeal joint of little toe
Fourth Layer					
Interossei Dorsal (4)	Adjacent sides of metatarsal bones	Bases of proximal phalanges—first: medial side of second toe; remainder: lateral sides of second, third, and fourth toes—also dorsal extensor expansion	Lateral plantar nerve	S2, **3**	Abduction of toes; flexes metatarsophalangeal joints and extends interphalangeal joints

(continues)

Table 10-8 Muscles of the Sole of the Foot *(continued)*

Muscle	Origin	Insertion	Nerve Supply	Nerve Root[a]	Action
Fourth Layer *(continued)*					
Plantar (3)	Inferior surfaces of third, fourth, and fifth metatarsal bones	Medial side of bases of proximal phalanges of lateral three toes	Lateral plantar nerve	S2, **3**	Adduction of toes; flexes metatarsophalangeal joints and extends interphalangeal joints
Peroneus longus tendon	See Table 10-6				
Tibialis posterior tendon	See Table 10-7				

[a] The predominant nerve root supply is indicated by boldface type.

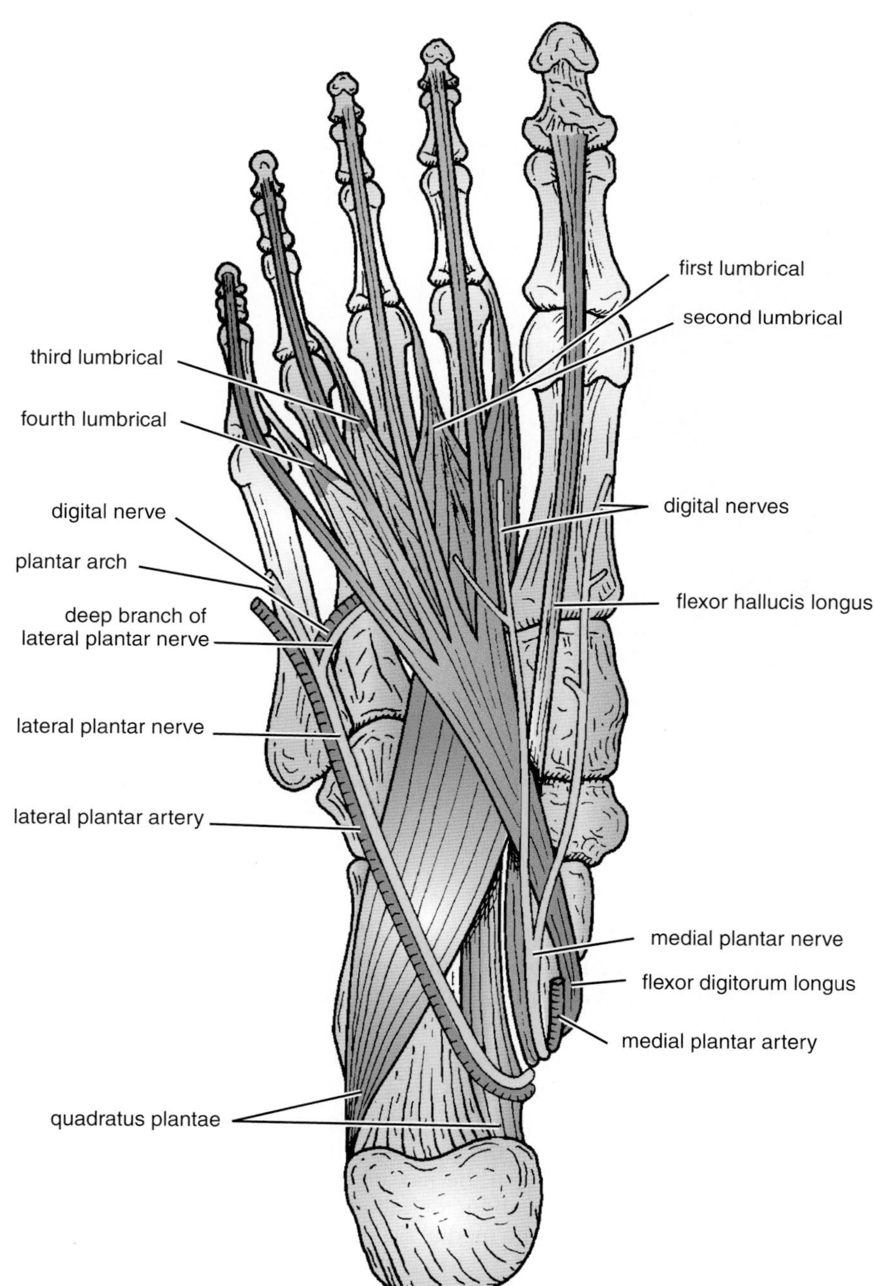

Figure 10-56 Second layer of the plantar muscles of the right foot. Medial and lateral plantar arteries and nerves are also shown.

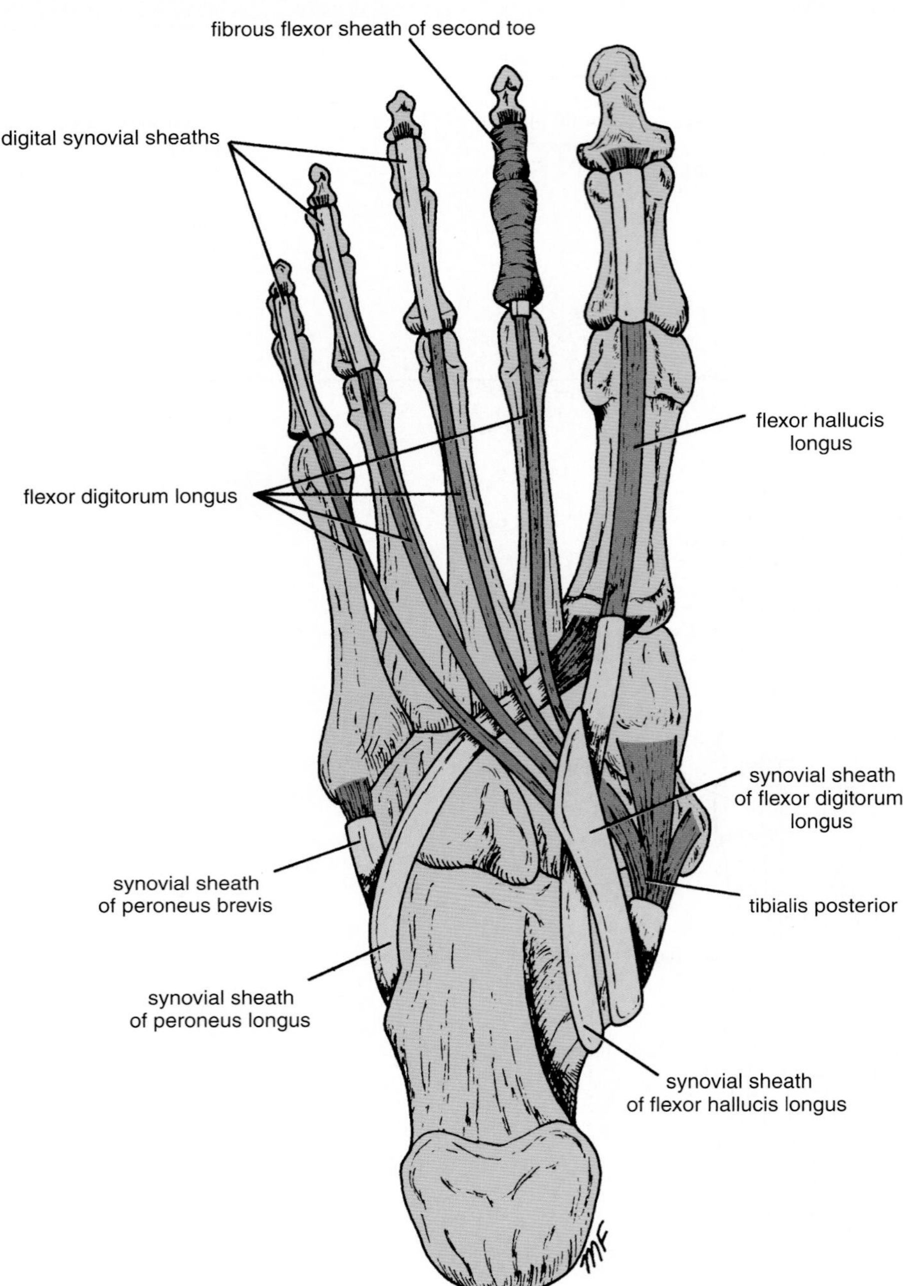

Figure 10-57 Synovial sheaths of the tendons seen on the sole of the right foot.

bone and the adjacent part of the medial cuneiform. The tendon grooves the inferior surface of the cuboid where it is held in position by the long plantar ligament and is surrounded by a synovial sheath (Fig.10-57).

Tibialis Posterior Tendon

The tibialis posterior tendon (Fig. 10-59) enters the foot from behind the medial malleolus. It passes beneath the flexor retinaculum and runs downward and forward above the sustentaculum tali to be inserted mainly into the tuberosity of the navicular. Small tendinous slips pass to the cuboid and the cuneiforms and to the bases of the second, third, and fourth metatarsals. The tendon is surrounded by a synovial sheath.

Arteries of the Sole of the Foot

Medial Plantar Artery

The medial plantar artery is the smaller of the terminal branches of the posterior tibial artery (see page 618). It arises beneath the flexor retinaculum and passes forward deep to the abductor hallucis muscle (Fig. 10-49). It ends by supplying the medial side of the big toe (Fig. 10-55). During

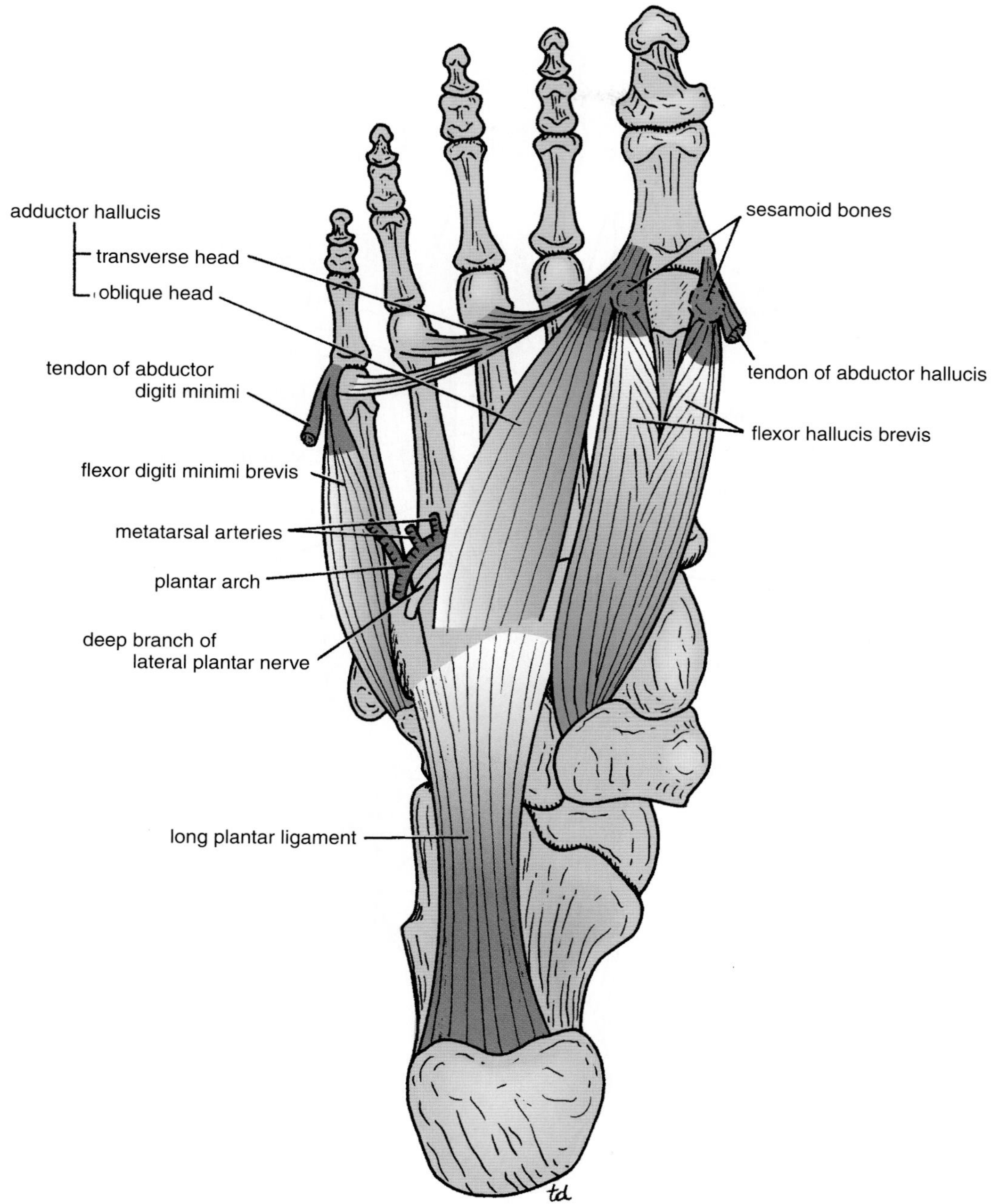

Figure 10-58 Third layer of the plantar muscles of the right foot. The deep branch of the lateral plantar nerve and the plantar arterial arch are also shown.

its course it gives off numerous muscular, cutaneous, and articular branches.

Lateral Plantar Artery

The lateral plantar artery is the larger of the terminal branches of the posterior tibial artery (see page 618). It arises beneath the flexor retinaculum and passes forward deep to the abductor hallucis and the flexor digitorum brevis (Figs. 10-49, 10-55, and 10-56). On reaching the base of the fifth metatarsal bone, the artery curves medially to form the **plantar arch** (Fig. 10-58) and at the proximal end of the first intermetatarsal space joins the dorsalis pedis artery (Fig. 10-59). During its course, it gives off numerous muscular, cutaneous, and articular branches. The plantar arch gives off plantar digital arteries to the toes.

Dorsalis Pedis Artery (the Dorsal Artery of the Foot)

On entering the sole between the two heads of the first dorsal interosseous muscle, the dorsalis pedis artery immediately joins the lateral plantar artery (Fig. 10-59).

Branches The first plantar metatarsal artery, which supplies the cleft between the big and second toes

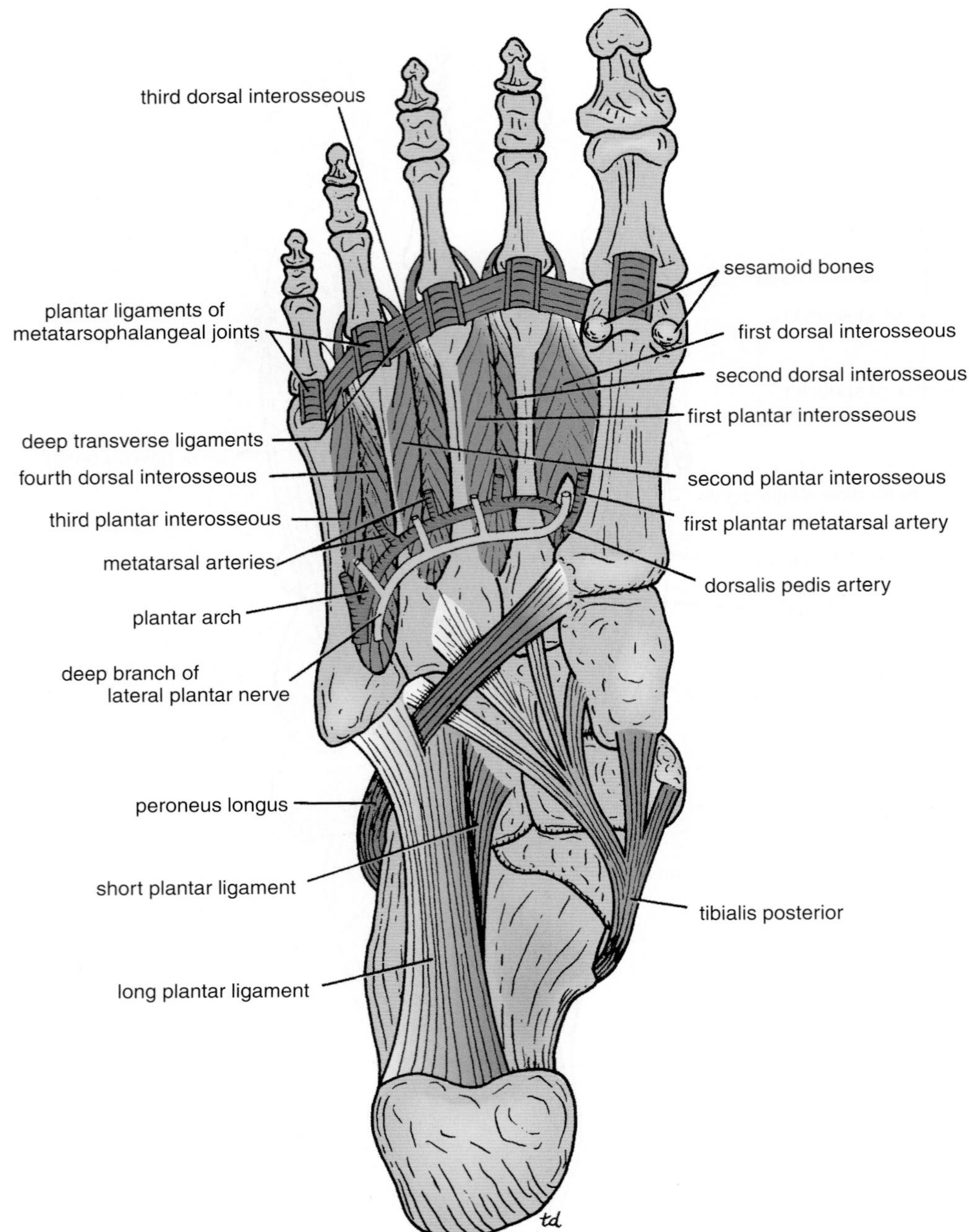

Figure 10-59 Fourth layer of the plantar muscles of the right foot. The deep branch of the lateral plantar nerve and the plantar arterial arch are also shown. Note the deep transverse ligaments.

Veins of the Sole of the Foot

Medial and **lateral plantar veins** accompany the corresponding arteries, and they unite behind the medial malleolus to form the posterior tibial venae comitantes.

Nerves of the Sole of the Foot

Medial Plantar Nerve

The medial plantar nerve is a terminal branch of the tibial nerve (see page 618). It arises beneath the flexor retinaculum (Fig. 10-49) and runs forward deep to the abductor hallucis, with the medial plantar artery (Fig. 10-55). It comes to lie in the interval between the abductor hallucis and the flexor digitorum brevis.

Branches

- **Muscular branches** to the abductor hallucis, the flexor digitorum brevis, the flexor hallucis brevis, and the first lumbrical muscle
- **Cutaneous branches: Plantar digital nerves** run to the sides of the medial three and a half toes (Fig. 10-54). The nerves extend onto the dorsum and supply the nail beds and the tips of the toes.

Compare with the distribution of the median nerve in the palm of the hand.

Lateral Plantar Nerve

The lateral plantar nerve is a terminal branch of the tibial nerve (see page 618). It arises beneath the flexor retinaculum (Fig. 10-49) and runs forward deep to the abductor hallucis and the flexor digitorum brevis, in company with the lateral plantar artery (Fig. 10-56). On reaching the base of the fifth metatarsal bone, it divides into superficial and deep branches (Fig. 10-56).

Branches

- **From the main trunk** to the quadratus plantae and abductor digiti minimi; cutaneous branches to the skin of the lateral part of the sole
- **From the superficial terminal branch** to the flexor digiti minimi and the interosseous muscles of the fourth intermetatarsal space. Plantar digital branches pass to the sides of the lateral one and a half toes. The nerves extend onto the dorsum and supply the nail beds and tips of the toes.
- **From the deep terminal branch** (Fig. 10-59). This branch curves medially with the lateral plantar artery and supplies the adductor hallucis; the second, third, and fourth lumbricals; and all the interossei, except those in the fourth intermetatarsal space (see superficial branch above).

Compare with the distribution of the ulnar nerve in the palm of the hand.

The Dorsum of the Foot

Skin

The skin on the dorsum of the foot is thin, hairy, and freely mobile on the underlying tendons and bones.

The **sensory nerve supply** (Fig. 10-2) to the skin on the dorsum of the foot is derived from the superficial peroneal nerve, assisted by the deep peroneal, saphenous, and sural nerves.

The **superficial peroneal nerve** emerges from between the peroneus brevis and the extensor digitorum longus muscle in the lower part of the leg (see page 615). It now divides into medial and lateral cutaneous branches that supply the skin on the dorsum of the foot; the medial side of the big toe; and the adjacent sides of the second, third, fourth, and fifth toes.

The **deep peroneal nerve** supplies the skin of the adjacent sides of the big and second toes (Fig. 10-2).

The **saphenous nerve** passes onto the dorsum of the foot in front of the medial malleolus (Fig. 10-2). It supplies the skin along the medial side of the foot as far forward as the head of the first metatarsal bone.

The **sural nerve** (Fig. 10-1) enters the foot behind the lateral malleolus and supplies the skin along the lateral margin of the foot and the lateral side of the little toe.

The nail beds and the skin covering the dorsal surfaces of the terminal phalanges are supplied by the medial and lateral plantar nerves (see above).

Dorsal Venous Arch (or Network)

The dorsal venous arch lies in the subcutaneous tissue over the heads of the metatarsal bones and drains on the medial side into the great saphenous vein and on the lateral side into the small saphenous vein (Fig. 10-19). The great saphenous vein leaves the dorsum of the foot by ascending into the leg in front of the medial malleolus. Its further course is described on page 570. The small saphenous vein ascends into the leg behind the lateral malleolus. Its course in the back of the leg is described on page 615. The greater part of the blood from the whole foot drains into the arch via digital veins and communicating veins from the sole, which pass through the interosseous spaces.

Muscles of the Dorsum of the Foot

Extensor Digitorum Brevis

The muscle is seen in Figure 10-60 and described in Table 10-9.

The Insertion of the Long Extensor Tendons

The tendon of extensor digitorum longus passes beneath the superior extensor retinaculum and through the inferior extensor retinaculum, in company with the peroneus tertius muscle (Fig. 10-60). The tendon divides into four, which fan out over the dorsum of the foot and pass to the lateral four toes. Opposite the metatarsophalangeal joints of the second, third, and fourth toes, each tendon is joined on its lateral side by a tendon of extensor digitorum brevis (Fig. 10-60).

On the dorsal surface of each toe, the extensor tendon joins the fascial expansion called the **extensor expansion.** Near the proximal interphalangeal joint, the extensor expansion splits into three parts: a central part, which is inserted into the base of the middle phalanx, and two lateral parts, which converge to be inserted into the base of the distal phalanx (Fig. 10-60).

The dorsal expansion, as in the fingers, receives the tendons of insertion of the interosseous and lumbrical muscles.

Synovial Sheath of the Tendon of Extensor Digitorum Longus

The extensor digitorum longus and peroneus tertius tendons are surrounded by a common synovial sheath as they pass beneath the extensor retinacula (Fig. 10-60). The sheath extends proximally for a short distance above the malleoli and distally to the level of the base of the fifth metatarsal bone.

Artery of the Dorsum of the Foot

Dorsalis Pedis Artery (the Dorsal Artery of the Foot)

The dorsalis pedis artery begins in front of the ankle joint as a continuation of the anterior tibial artery (see page 612). It terminates by passing downward into the sole between the two heads of the first dorsal interosseous muscle, where it joins the lateral plantar artery and completes the plantar arch (Fig. 10-59). It is superficial in position and is crossed by the inferior extensor retinaculum and the first tendon of

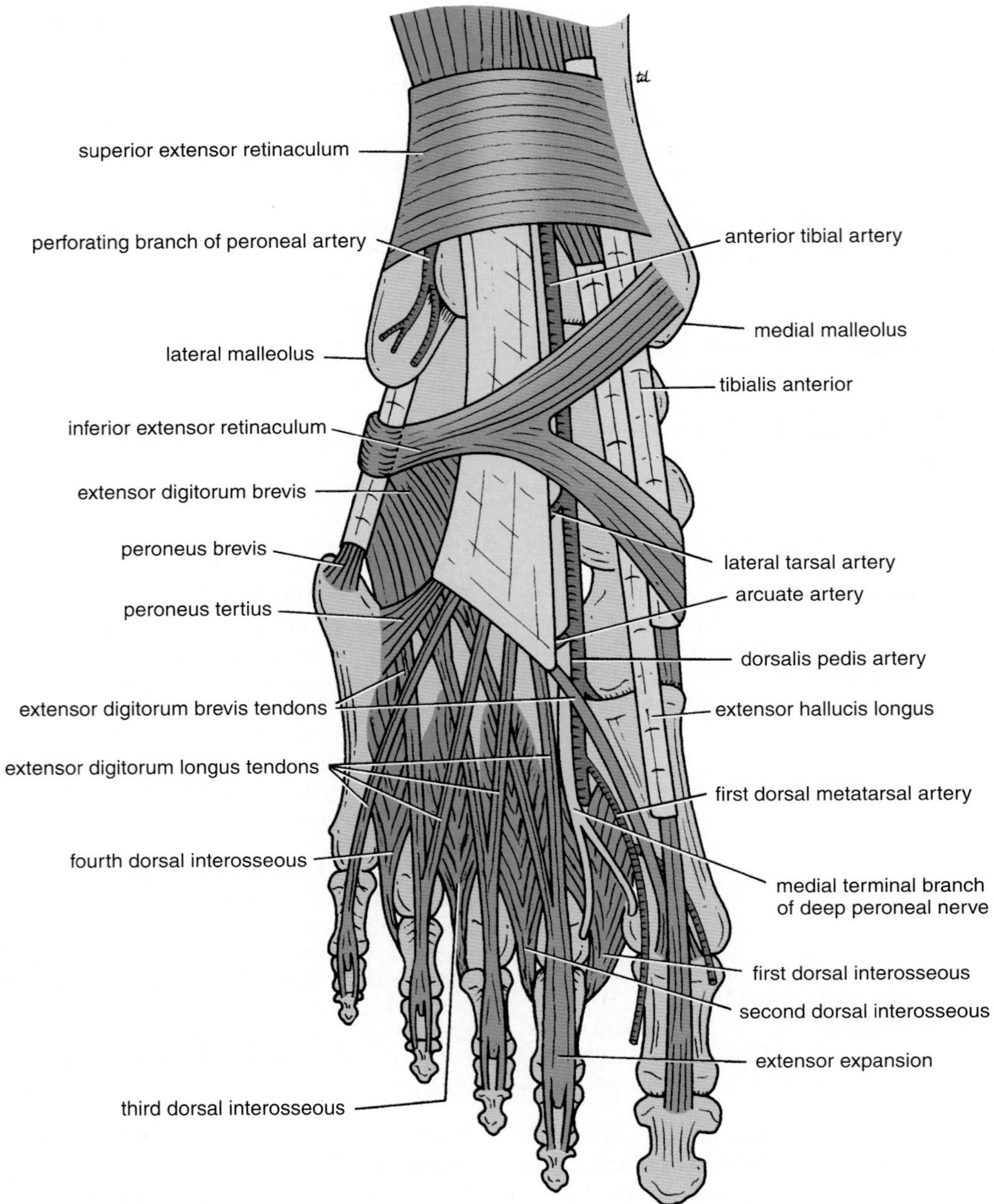

Figure 10-60 Structures in the dorsal aspect of the right foot.

Table 10-9 Muscle of the Dorsum of the Foot

Muscle	Origin	Insertion	Nerve Supply	Nerve Root	Action
Extensor digitorum brevis	Anterior part of upper surface of the calcaneum and from the inferior extensor retinaculum	By four tendons into the proximal phalanx of big toe and long extensor tendons to second, third, and fourth toes	Deep peroneal nerve	S1, S2	Extends toes

extensor digitorum brevis (Fig. 10-60). On its lateral side lie the terminal part of the deep peroneal nerve and the extensor digitorum longus tendons. On the medial side lies the tendon of extensor hallucis longus (Fig. 10-60). **Its pulsations can easily be felt.**

Branches

- **Lateral tarsal artery,** which crosses the dorsum of the foot just below the ankle joint (Fig. 10-60)
- **Arcuate artery,** which runs laterally under the extensor tendons opposite the bases of the metatarsal bones (Fig. 10-60). It gives off metatarsal branches to the toes.
- **First dorsal metatarsal artery,** which supplies both sides of the big toe (Fig. 10-60)

Nerve Supply of the Dorsum of the Foot

Deep Peroneal Nerve

The deep peroneal nerve enters the dorsum of the foot by passing deep to the extensor retinacula on the lateral side of the dorsalis pedis artery (see page 614). It divides into terminal, medial, and lateral branches. The medial branch supplies the skin of the adjacent sides of the big and second toes (Fig. 10-60). The lateral branch supplies the extensor digitorum brevis muscle. Both terminal branches give articular branches to the joints of the foot.

Joints of the Lower Limb

The hip joint is fully described on page 587.

Knee Joint

The knee joint is the largest and most complicated joint in the body. Basically, it consists of two condylar joints between the medial and lateral condyles of the femur and the corresponding condyles of the tibia, and a gliding joint, between the patella and the patellar surface of the femur. Note that the fibula is not directly involved in the joint.

Articulation

Above are the rounded condyles of the femur; below are the condyles of the tibia and their cartilaginous menisci (Fig. 10-35); in front is the articulation between the lower end of the femur and the patella.

The articular surfaces of the femur, tibia, and patella are covered with hyaline cartilage. Note that the articular surfaces of the medial and lateral condyles of the tibia are often referred to clinically as the medial and lateral **tibial plateaus.**

Type

The joint between the femur and tibia is a synovial joint of the hinge variety, but some degree of rotatory movement is possible. The joint between the patella and femur is a synovial joint of the plane gliding variety.

Capsule

The capsule is attached to the margins of the articular surfaces and surrounds the sides and posterior aspect of the joint. On the front of the joint, the capsule is absent, permitting the synovial membrane to pouch upward beneath the quadriceps tendon, forming the **suprapatellar bursa** (Fig. 10-35). On each side of the patella, the capsule is strengthened by expansions from the tendons of vastus lateralis and medialis. Behind the joint, the capsule is strengthened by an expansion of the semimembranous muscle called the **oblique popliteal ligament** (Fig. 10-35). An opening in the capsule behind the lateral tibial condyle permits the tendon of the popliteus to emerge (Fig. 10-35).

Ligaments

The ligaments may be divided into those that lie outside the capsule and those that lie within the capsule.

Extracapsular Ligaments

The **ligamentum patellae** is attached above to the lower border of the patella and below to the tuberosity of the tibia (Fig. 10-35). It is, in fact, a continuation of the central portion of the common tendon of the quadriceps femoris muscle.

The **lateral collateral ligament** is cordlike and is attached above to the lateral condyle of the femur and below to the head of the fibula (Fig. 10-35). The tendon of the popliteus muscle intervenes between the ligament and the lateral meniscus (Fig. 10-61).

The **medial collateral ligament** is a flat band and is attached above to the medial condyle of the femur and below to the medial surface of the shaft of the tibia (Fig. 10-35). **It is firmly attached to the edge of the medial meniscus** (Fig. 10-61).

The **oblique popliteal ligament** is a tendinous expansion derived from the semimembranosus muscle. It strengthens the posterior aspect of the capsule (Fig. 10-35).

Intracapsular Ligaments

The **cruciate ligaments** are two strong intracapsular ligaments that cross each other within the joint cavity (Fig. 10-35). They are named anterior and posterior, according to their tibial attachments (Fig. 10-61). These important ligaments are the main bond between the femur and the tibia throughout the joint's range of movement.

Anterior Cruciate Ligament The anterior cruciate ligament is attached to the anterior intercondylar area of the tibia and passes upward, backward, and laterally, to be attached to the posterior part of the medial surface of the lateral femoral condyle (Figs. 10-35 and 10-61). The anterior cruciate ligament prevents posterior displacement of the femur on the tibia. With the knee joint flexed, the anterior cruciate ligament prevents the tibia from being pulled anteriorly.

Posterior Cruciate Ligament The posterior cruciate ligament is attached to the posterior intercondylar area of the tibia and passes upward, forward, and medially to be attached to the anterior part of the lateral surface of the medial femoral condyle (Figs. 10-35 and 10-61). The posterior cruciate ligament prevents anterior displacement of the femur on the tibia. With the knee joint flexed, the posterior cruciate ligament prevents the tibia from being pulled posteriorly.

Menisci The menisci are C-shaped sheets of fibrocartilage. The peripheral border is thick and attached to the capsule, and the inner border is thin and concave and forms a free edge (Figs. 10-35 and 10-61). The upper surfaces are in contact with the femoral condyles. The lower surfaces are in

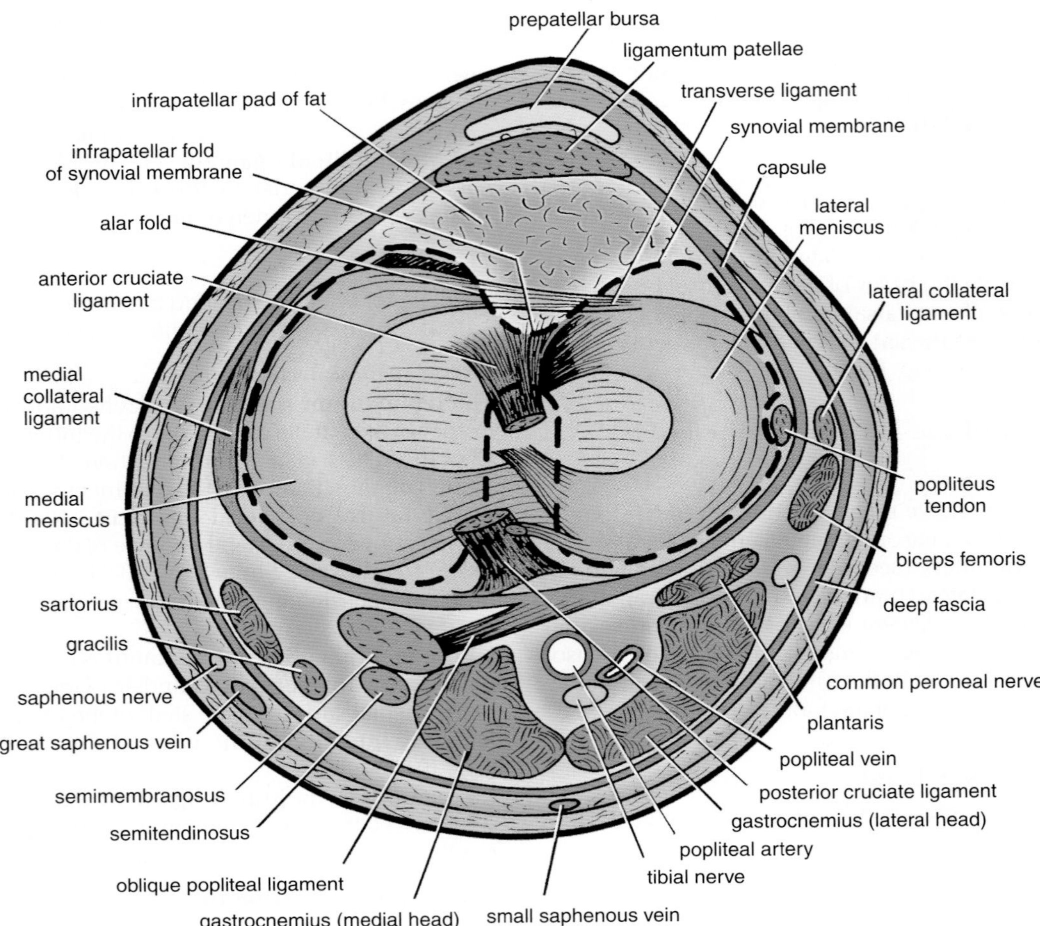

Figure 10-61 Relations of the right knee joint.

contact with the tibial condyles. Their function is to deepen the articular surfaces of the tibial condyles to receive the convex femoral condyles; they also serve as cushions between the two bones.

Each meniscus is attached to the upper surface of the tibia by anterior and posterior horns. Because the medial meniscus is also attached to the medial collateral ligament, it is relatively immobile.

Synovial Membrane

The synovial membrane lines the capsule and is attached to the margins of the articular surfaces (Figs. 10-35 and 10-61). On the front and above the joint, it forms a pouch, which extends up beneath the quadriceps femoris muscle for three fingerbreadths above the patella, forming the **suprapatellar bursa.** This is held in position by the attachment of a small portion of the vastus intermedius muscle, called the **articularis genus** muscle (Fig. 10-35).

At the back of the joint, the synovial membrane is prolonged downward on the deep surface of the tendon of the popliteus, forming the **popliteal bursa.** A bursa is interposed between the medial head of the gastrocnemius and the medial femoral condyle and the semimembranosus tendon; this is termed the **semimembranosus bursa,** and it frequently communicates with the synovial cavity of the joint.

The synovial membrane is reflected forward from the posterior part of the capsule around the front of the cruciate ligaments (Fig. 10-61). As a result, the cruciate ligaments lie behind the synovial cavity and are not bathed in synovial fluid.

In the anterior part of the joint, the synovial membrane is reflected backward from the posterior surface of the ligamentum patellae to form the **infrapatellar fold;** the free borders of the fold are termed the **alar folds** (Fig. 10-61).

Bursae Related to the Knee Joint

Numerous bursae are related to the knee joint. They are found wherever skin, muscle, or tendon rubs against bone. Four are situated in front of the joint and six are found behind the joint. The **suprapatellar bursa** and the **popliteal bursa** always communicate with the joint, and the **semimembranosus bursa** may communicate with the joint.

Anterior Bursae

- The **suprapatellar bursa** lies beneath the quadriceps muscle and communicates with the joint cavity (Fig. 10-35). It is described above.

- The **prepatellar bursa** lies in the subcutaneous tissue between the skin and the front of the lower half of the patella and the upper part of the ligamentum patellae (Figs. 10-35 and 10-61).
- The **superficial infrapatellar bursa** lies in the subcutaneous tissue between the skin and the front of the lower part of the ligamentum patellae (Fig. 10-35).
- The **deep infrapatellar bursa** lies between the ligamentum patellae and the tibia (Fig. 10-35).

Posterior Bursae

- The **popliteal bursa** is found in association with the tendon of the popliteus and communicates with the joint cavity. It was described previously.
- The **semimembranosus bursa** is found related to the insertion of the semimembranosus muscle and may communicate with the joint cavity. It was described previously.

The remaining four bursae are found related to the tendon of insertion of the biceps femoris; related to the tendons of the sartorius, gracilis, and semitendinosus muscles as they pass to their insertion on the tibia; beneath the lateral head of origin of the gastrocnemius muscle; and beneath the medial head of origin of the gastrocnemius muscle.

Nerve Supply

The femoral, obturator, common peroneal, and tibial nerves supply the knee joint.

Movements

The knee joint can flex, extend, and rotate. As the knee joint assumes the position of full extension,* medial rotation of the femur results in a twisting and tightening of all the major ligaments of the joint, and the knee becomes a mechanically rigid structure; the cartilaginous menisci are compressed like rubber cushions between the femoral and tibial condyles. The extended knee is said to be in the locked position.

Before flexion of the knee joint can occur, it is essential that the major ligaments be untwisted and slackened to permit movements between the joint surfaces. This unlocking or untwisting process is accomplished by the popliteus muscle, which laterally rotates the femur on the tibia. Once again, the menisci have to adapt their shape to the changing contour of the femoral condyles. The attachment of the popliteus to the lateral meniscus results in that structure being pulled backward also.

When the knee joint is flexed to a right angle, a considerable range of rotation is possible. In the flexed position, the tibia can also be moved passively forward and backward on the femur. This is possible because the major ligaments, especially the cruciate ligaments, are slack in this position. The following muscles produce movements of the knee joint.

Flexion

The biceps femoris, semitendinosus, and semimembranosus muscles, assisted by the gracilis, sartorius, and popliteus muscles, produce flexion. Flexion is limited by the contact of the back of the leg with the thigh.

Extension

The quadriceps femoris produces extension. Extension is limited by the tension of all the major ligaments of the joint.

Medial Rotation

The sartorius, gracilis, and semitendinosus produce medial rotation.

Lateral Rotation

The biceps femoris produces lateral rotation.

The stability of the knee joint depends on the tone of the strong muscles acting on the joint and the strength of the ligaments. Of these factors, the tone of the muscles is the most important, and it is the job of the physiotherapist to build up the strength of these muscles, especially the quadriceps femoris, after injury to the knee joint.

Important Relations

- **Anteriorly:** The prepatellar bursa (Fig. 10-61)
- **Posteriorly:** The popliteal vessels; tibial and common peroneal nerves; lymph nodes; and the muscles that form the boundaries of the popliteal fossa, namely, the semimembranosus, the semitendinosus, the biceps femoris, the two heads of the gastrocnemius, and the plantaris (Fig. 10-61)
- **Medially:** Sartorius, gracilis, and semitendinosus muscles (Fig. 10-61)
- **Laterally:** Biceps femoris and common peroneal nerve (Fig. 10-61)

* Note that when the foot is firmly planted on the ground when a person is standing, the femur is medially rotated on the tibia to lock and stabilize the knee joint. However, if the foot is raised off the ground, the tibia may be laterally rotated on the femur to lock the knee joint.

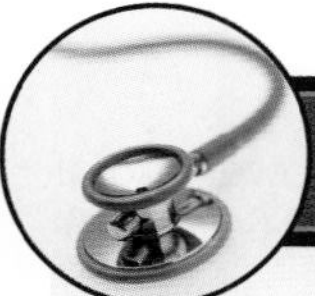

CLINICAL NOTES

Strength of the Knee Joint

The strength of the knee joint depends on the strength of the ligaments that bind the femur to the tibia and on the tone of the muscles acting on the joint. The most important muscle group is the quadriceps femoris; provided that this is well developed, it is capable of stabilizing the knee in the presence of torn ligaments.

Knee Injury and the Synovial Membrane

The synovial membrane of the knee joint is extensive, and if the articular surfaces, menisci, or ligaments of the joint are damaged, the large synovial cavity becomes distended with fluid. The wide communication between the suprapatellar bursa and the joint cavity results in this structure becoming distended also. The

(continues)

Clinical Notes, *continued*

swelling of the knee extends three or four fingerbreadths above the patella and laterally and medially beneath the aponeuroses of insertion of the vastus lateralis and medialis, respectively.

Ligamentous Injury of the Knee Joint

Four ligaments—the medial collateral ligament, the lateral collateral ligament, the anterior cruciate ligament, and the posterior cruciate ligament—are commonly injured in the knee. Sprains or tears occur depending on the degree of force applied.

Medial Collateral Ligament

Forced abduction of the tibia on the femur can result in partial tearing of the medial collateral ligament, which can occur at its femoral or tibial attachments. It is useful to remember that tears of the menisci result in localized tenderness on the joint line, whereas sprains of the medial collateral ligament result in tenderness over the femoral or tibial attachments of the ligament.

Lateral Collateral Ligament

Forced adduction of the tibia on the femur can result in injury to the lateral collateral ligament (less common than medial ligament injury).

Cruciate Ligaments

Injury to the cruciate ligaments can occur when excessive force is applied to the knee joint. Tears of the anterior cruciate ligament are common; tears of the posterior cruciate ligament are rare. The injury is always accompanied by damage to other knee structures; the collateral ligaments are commonly torn or the capsule may be damaged. The joint cavity quickly fills with blood **(hemarthrosis)** so that the joint is swollen. Examination of patients with a ruptured anterior cruciate ligament shows that the tibia can be pulled excessively forward on the femur; with rupture of the posterior cruciate ligament, the tibia can be made to move excessively backward on the femur (Fig. 10-62). Because the stability of the knee joint depends largely on the tone of the quadriceps femoris muscle and the integrity of the collateral ligaments, operative repair of isolated torn cruciate ligaments is not always attempted. The knee is immobilized in slight flexion in a cast, and active physiotherapy on the quadriceps femoris muscle is begun at once. Should, however, the capsule of the joint and the collateral ligaments be torn in addition, early operative repair is essential.

Meniscal Injury of the Knee Joint

Injuries of the menisci are common. The medial meniscus is damaged much more frequently than the lateral, and this is probably because of its strong attachment to the medial collateral ligament of the knee joint, which restricts its mobility. The injury occurs when the femur is rotated on the tibia, or the tibia is rotated on the femur, with the knee joint partially flexed and taking the weight of the body. The tibia is usually abducted on the femur, and the medial meniscus is pulled into an abnormal position between the femoral and tibial condyles (Fig. 10-62A). A sudden movement between the condyles results in the meniscus being subjected to a severe grinding force, and it splits along its length (Fig. 10-63). When the torn part of the meniscus becomes wedged between the articular surfaces, further movement is impossible, and the joint is said to "lock."

Injury to the lateral meniscus is less common, probably because it is not attached to the lateral collateral ligament of the knee joint and is consequently more mobile. The popliteus muscle sends a few of its fibers into the lateral meniscus, and these can pull the meniscus into a more favorable position during sudden movements of the knee joint.

Pneumoarthrography

Air can be injected into the synovial cavity of the knee joint so that soft tissues can be studied. This technique is based on the fact that air is less radiopaque than structures such as the medial and lateral menisci, so their outline can be visualized on a radiograph (Fig. 10-76).

Arthroscopy

Arthroscopy involves the introduction of a lighted instrument into the synovial cavity of the knee joint through a small incision. This technique permits the direct visualization of structures, such as the cruciate ligaments and the menisci, for diagnostic purposes.

Proximal Tibiofibular Joint

Articulation

Articulation is between the lateral condyle of the tibia and the head of the fibula (Fig. 10-35). The articular surfaces are flattened and covered by hyaline cartilage.

Type

This is a synovial, plane, gliding joint.

Capsule

The capsule surrounds the joint and is attached to the margins of the articular surfaces.

Ligaments

Anterior and **posterior ligaments** strengthen the capsule. The **interosseous membrane,** which connects the shafts of the tibia and fibula together, also greatly strengthens the joint.

Synovial Membrane

The synovial membrane lines the capsule and is attached to the margins of the articular surfaces.

Nerve Supply

The common peroneal nerve supplies the joint.

Movements

A small amount of gliding movement takes place during movements at the ankle joint.

Distal Tibiofibular Joint

Articulation

Articulation is between the fibular notch at the lower end of the tibia and the lower end of the fibula (Figs. 10-64 and 10-65). The opposed bony surfaces are roughened.

Type

The distal tibiofibular joint is a fibrous joint.

Capsule

There is no capsule.

Ligaments

The **interosseous ligament** is a strong, thick band of fibrous tissue that binds the two bones together. The

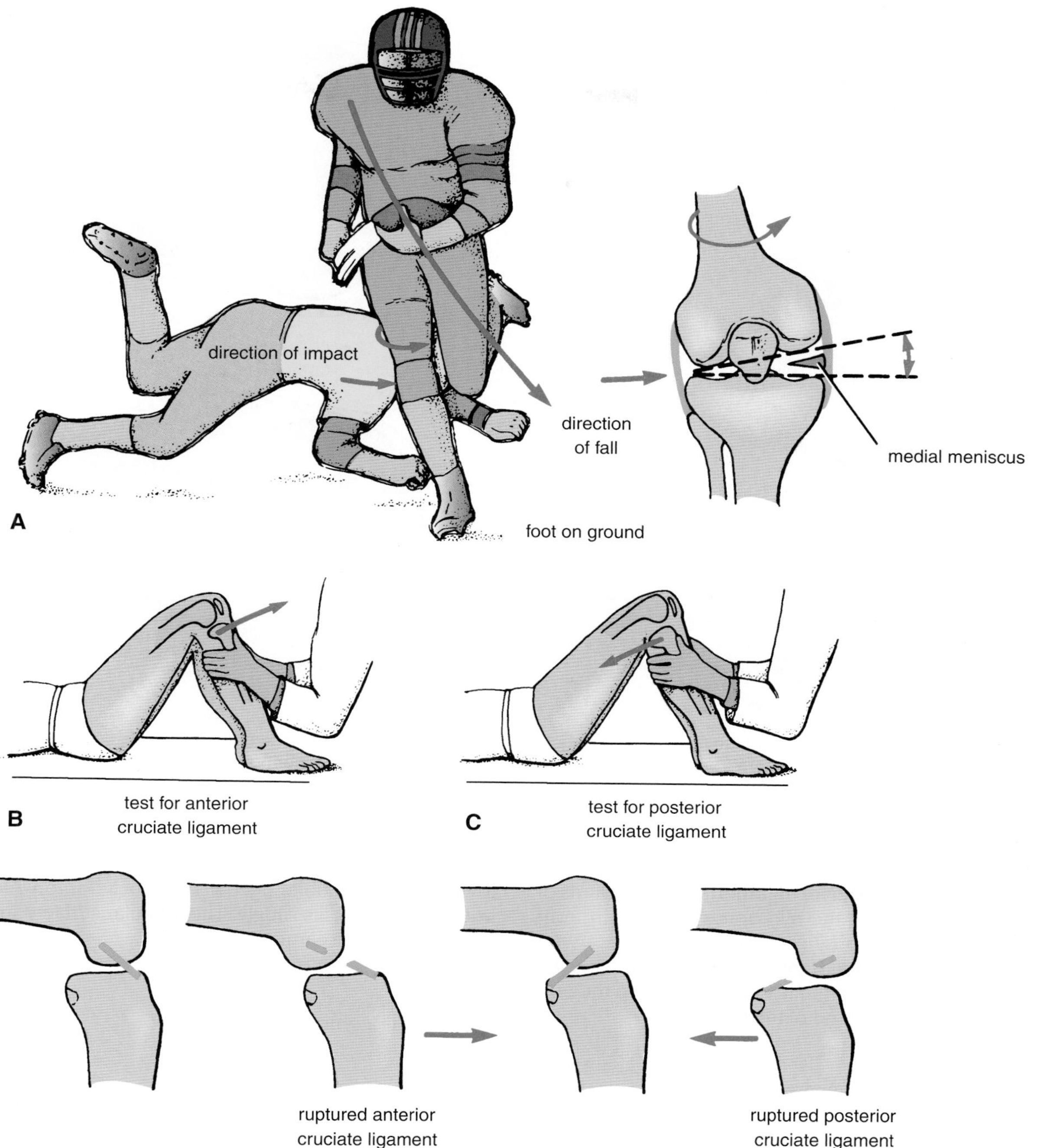

Figure 10-62 **A.** Mechanism involved in damage to the medial meniscus of the knee joint from playing football. Note that the right knee joint is semiflexed and that medial rotation of the femur on the tibia occurs. The impact causes forced abduction of the tibia on the femur, and the medial meniscus is pulled into an abnormal position. The cartilaginous meniscus is then ground between the femur and the tibia. **B.** Test for integrity of the anterior cruciate ligament. **C.** Test for integrity of the posterior cruciate ligament.

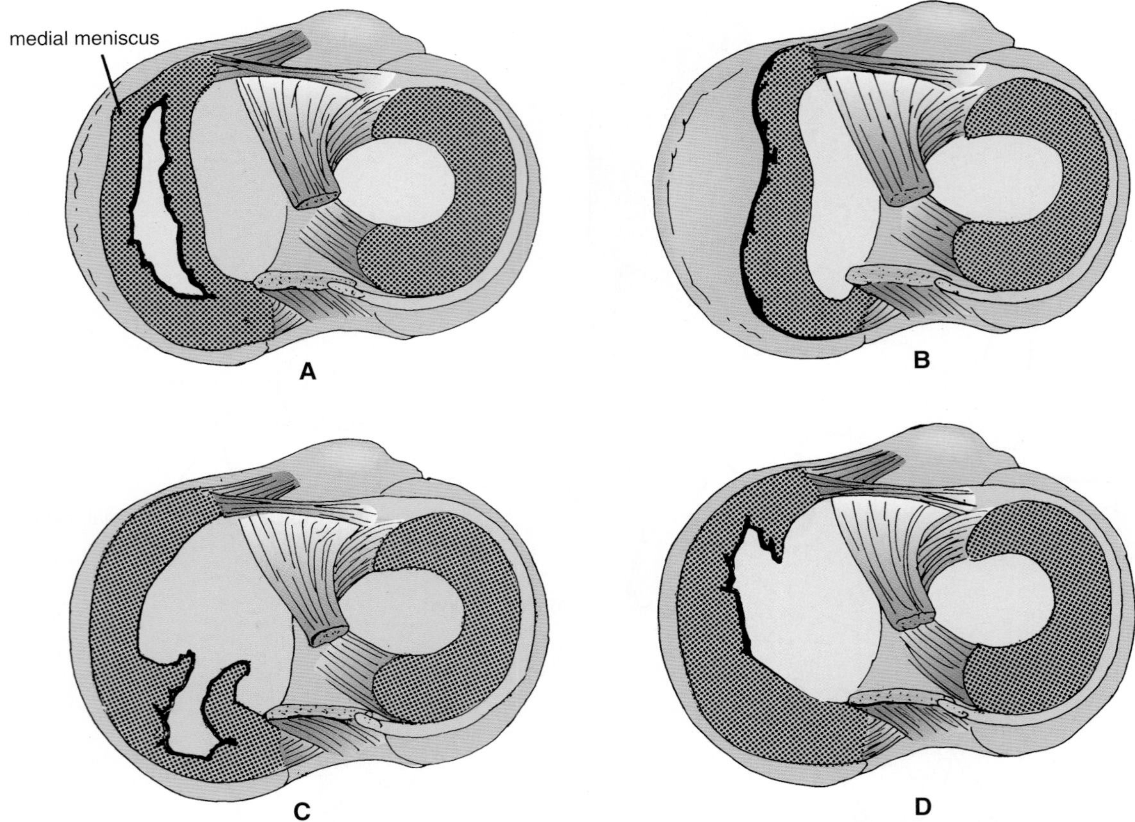

Figure 10-63 Tears of the medial meniscus of the knee joint. **A.** Complete bucket handle tear. **B.** The meniscus is torn from its peripheral attachment. **C.** Tear of the posterior portion of the meniscus. **D.** Tear of the anterior portion of the meniscus.

interosseous membrane, which connects the shafts of the tibia and fibula together, also greatly strengthens the joint.

The **anterior** and **posterior ligaments** are flat bands of fibrous tissue connecting the two bones together in front and behind the interosseous ligament.

The **inferior transverse ligament** runs from the medial surface of the upper part of the lateral malleolus to the posterior border of the lower end of the tibia.

Nerve Supply

Deep peroneal and tibial nerves supply the joint.

Movements

A small amount of movement takes place during movements at the ankle joint.

Ankle Joint

The ankle joint consists of a deep socket formed by the lower ends of the tibia and fibula, into which is fitted the upper part of the body of the talus. The talus is able to move on a transverse axis in a hingelike manner. The shape of the bones and the strength of the ligaments and the surrounding tendons make this joint strong and stable.

Articulation

Articulation is between the lower end of the tibia, the two malleoli, and the body of the talus (Figs. 10-64 and 10-65). The inferior transverse tibiofibular ligament, which runs between the lateral malleolus and the posterior border of the lower end of the tibia, deepens the socket into which the body of the talus fits snugly. The articular surfaces are covered with hyaline cartilage.

Type

The ankle is a synovial hinge joint.

Capsule

The capsule encloses the joint and is attached to the bones near their articular margins.

Ligaments

The **medial,** or **deltoid, ligament** is strong and is attached by its apex to the tip of the medial malleolus (Fig. 10-65). Below, the deep fibers are attached to the nonarticular area on the medial surface of the body of the talus; the superficial fibers are attached to the medial side of the talus, the sustentaculum tali, the plantar calcaneonavicular ligament, and the tuberosity of the navicular bone.

The **lateral ligament** is weaker than the medial ligament and consists of three bands.

The **anterior talofibular ligament** (Fig. 10-64) runs from the lateral malleolus to the lateral surface of the talus.

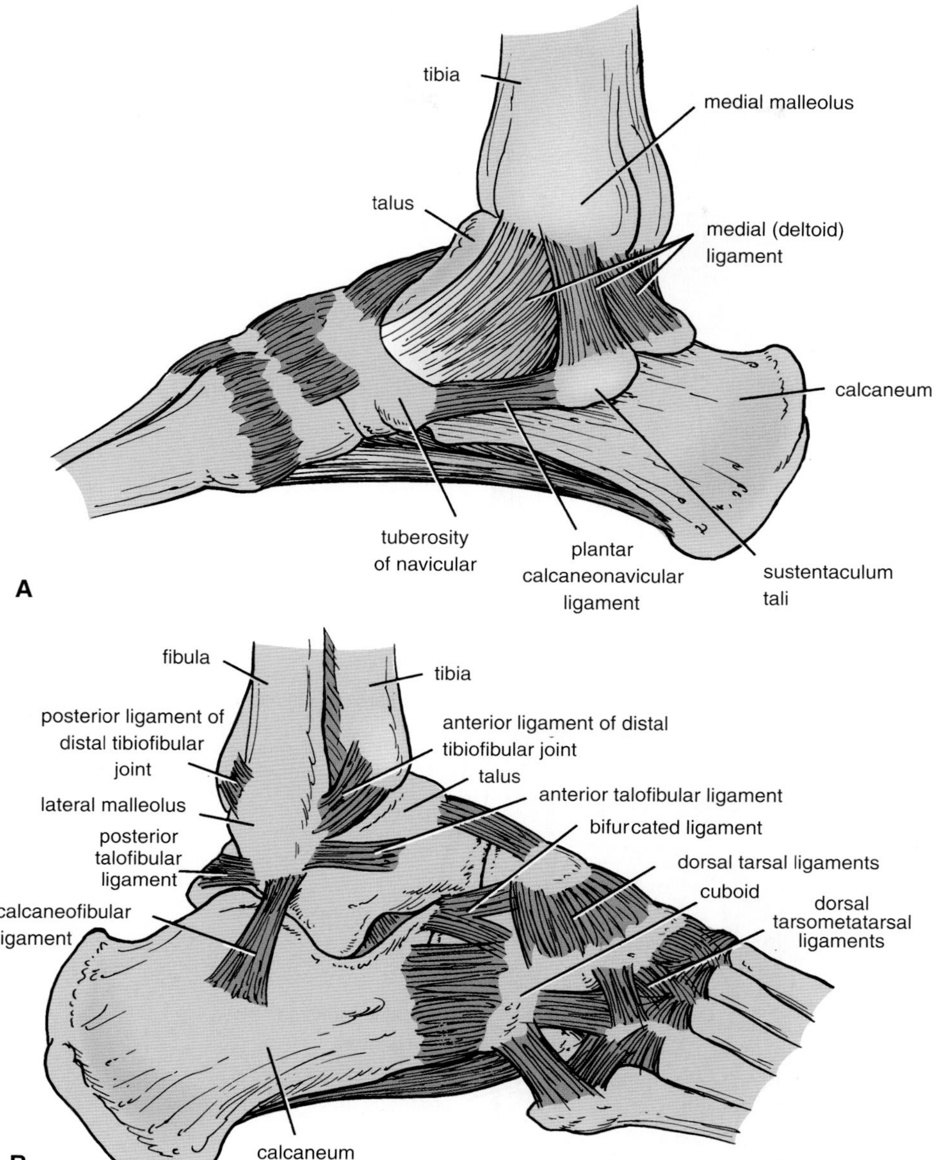

Figure 10-64 The right ankle joint as seen from the medial aspect (**A**) and the lateral aspect (**B**).

The **calcaneofibular ligament** (Fig. 10-64) runs from the tip of the lateral malleolus downward and backward to the lateral surface of the calcaneum.

The **posterior talofibular ligament** (Fig. 10-64) runs from the lateral malleolus to the posterior tubercle of the talus.

Synovial Membrane

The synovial membrane lines the capsule.

Nerve Supply

Deep peroneal and tibial nerves supply the ankle joint.

Movements

Dorsiflexion (toes pointing upward) and plantar flexion (toes pointing downward) are possible. The movements of inversion and eversion take place at the tarsal joints and **not at the ankle joint.**

Dorsiflexion is performed by the tibialis anterior, extensor hallucis longus, extensor digitorum longus, and peroneus tertius. It is limited by the tension of the tendo calcaneus, the posterior fibers of the medial ligament, and the calcaneofibular ligament.

Plantar flexion is performed by the gastrocnemius, soleus, plantaris, peroneus longus, peroneus brevis, tibialis posterior, flexor digitorum longus, and flexor hallucis longus. It is limited by the tension of the opposing muscles, the anterior fibers of the medial ligament, and the anterior talofibular ligament.

Note that during dorsiflexion of the ankle joint, the wider anterior part of the articular surface of the talus is forced between the medial and lateral malleoli, causing them to sep-

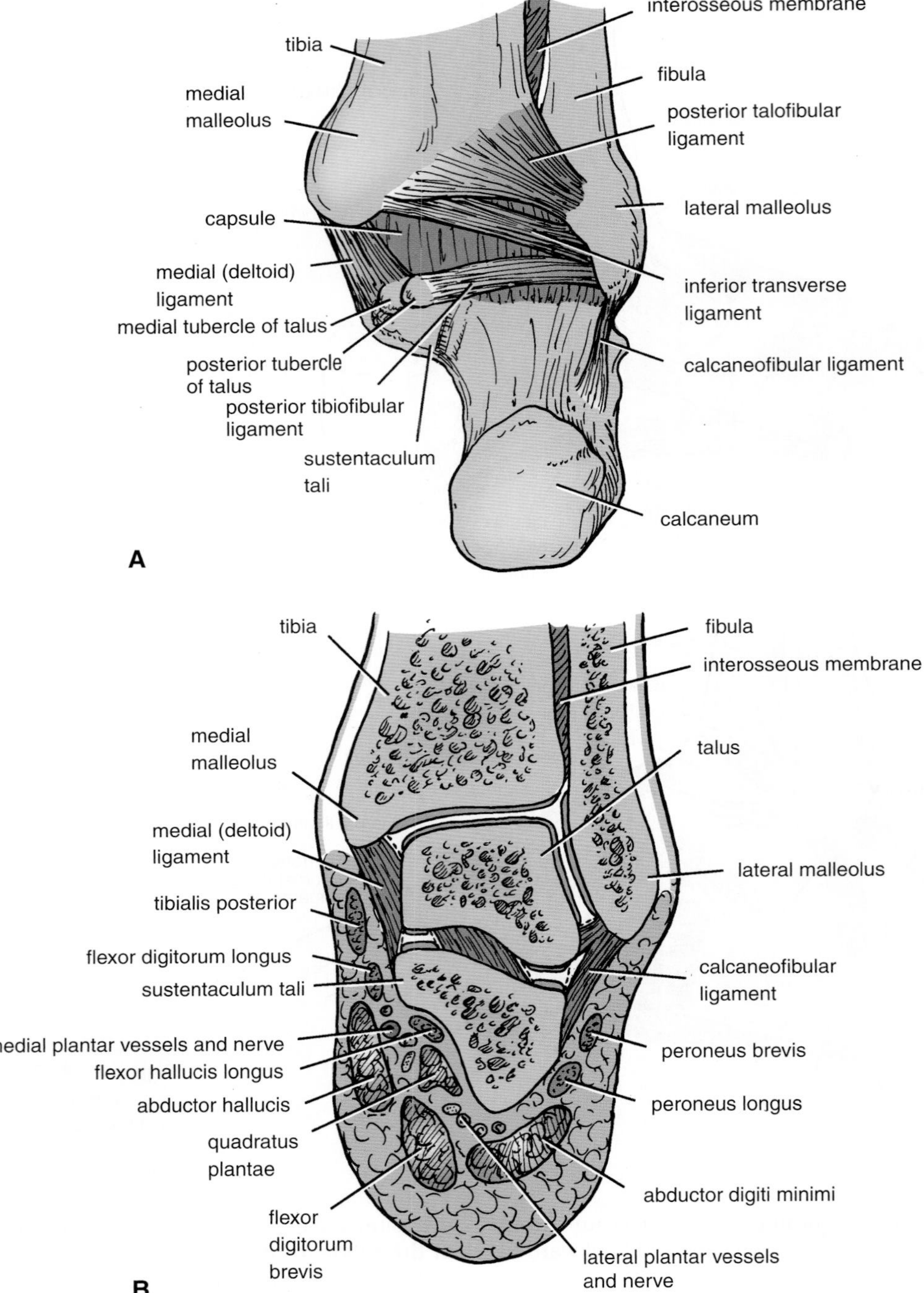

Figure 10-65 The right ankle joint as seen from the posterior aspect (**A**) and in coronal section (**B**).

arate slightly and tighten the ligaments of the distal tibiofibular joint. This arrangement greatly increases the stability of the ankle joint when the foot is in the initial position for major thrusting movements in walking, running, and jumping.

Note also that when the ankle joint is fully plantar flexed, the ligaments of the distal tibiofibular joint are less taut and small amounts of rotation, abduction, and adduction are possible.

Important Relations

- **Anteriorly:** The tibialis anterior, the extensor hallucis longus, the anterior tibial vessels, the deep peroneal nerve, the extensor digitorum longus, and the peroneus tertius (Fig. 10-48)
- **Posteriorly:** The tendo calcaneus and plantaris (Fig. 10-48)
- **Posterolaterally (behind the lateral malleolus):** The peroneus longus and brevis (Fig. 10-46)
- **Posteromedially (behind the medial malleolus):** The tibialis posterior, the flexor digitorum longus, the posterior tibial vessels, the tibial nerve, and the flexor hallucis longus (Fig. 10-48)

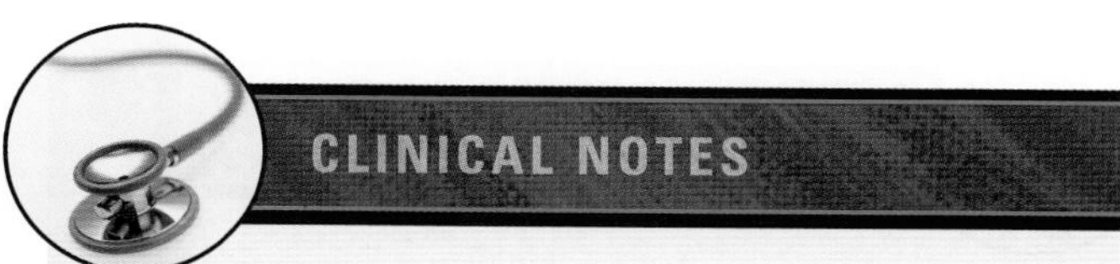

Ankle Joint Stability

The ankle joint is a hinge joint possessing great stability. The deep mortise formed by the lower end of the tibia and the medial and lateral malleoli securely holds the talus in position.

Acute Sprains of the "Lateral Ankle"

Acute sprains of the lateral ankle are usually caused by excessive inversion of the foot with plantar flexion of the ankle. The anterior talofibular ligament and the calcaneofibular ligament are partially torn, giving rise to great pain and local swelling.

Acute Sprains of the "Medial Ankle"

Acute sprains of the medial ankle are similar to but less common than those of the lateral ankle. They may occur to the medial or deltoid ligament as a result of excessive eversion. The great strength of the medial ligament usually results in the ligament pulling off the tip of the medial malleolus.

Fracture Dislocations of the Ankle Joint

Fracture dislocations of the ankle are common and are caused by forced external rotation and overeversion of the foot. The talus is externally rotated forcibly against the lateral malleolus of the fibula. The torsion effect on the lateral malleolus causes it to fracture spirally. If the force continues, the talus moves laterally, and the medial ligament of the ankle joint becomes taut and pulls off the tip of the medial malleolus. If the talus is forced to move still farther, its rotary movement results in its violent contact with the posterior inferior margin of the tibia, which shears off.

Other less common types of fracture dislocation are caused by forced overeversion (without rotation), in which the talus presses the lateral malleolus laterally and causes it to fracture transversely. Overinversion (without rotation), in which the talus presses against the medial malleolus, produces a vertical fracture through the base of the medial malleolus.

Tarsal Joints

Subtalar Joint

The subtalar joint is the posterior joint between the talus and the calcaneum.

Articulation

Articulation is between the inferior surface of the body of the talus and the facet on the middle of the upper surface of the calcaneum (Fig. 10-37). The articular surfaces are covered with hyaline cartilage.

Type

These joints are synovial, of the plane variety.

Capsule

The capsule encloses the joint and is attached to the margins of the articular areas of the two bones.

Ligaments

Medial and **lateral (talocalcaneal) ligaments** strengthen the capsule. The **interosseous (talocalcaneal) ligament** (Fig. 10-65) is strong and is the main bond of union between the two bones. It is attached above to the sulcus tali and below to the sulcus calcanei.

Synovial Membrane

The synovial membrane lines the capsule.

Movements

Gliding and rotatory movements are possible.

Talocalcaneonavicular Joint

The talocalcaneonavicular joint is the anterior joint between the talus and the calcaneum and also involves the navicular bone (Fig. 10-37).

Articulation

Articulation is between the rounded head of the talus, the upper surface of the sustentaculum tali, and the posterior concave surface of the navicular bone. The articular surfaces are covered with hyaline cartilage.

Type

The joint is a synovial joint.

Capsule

The capsule incompletely encloses the joint.

Ligaments

The **plantar calcaneonavicular ligament** is strong and runs from the anterior margin of the sustentaculum tali to the inferior surface and tuberosity of the navicular bone. The superior surface of the ligament is covered with fibrocartilage and supports the head of the talus.

Synovial Membrane

The synovial membrane lines the capsule.

Movements

Gliding and rotatory movements are possible.

Calcaneocuboid Joint

Articulation

Articulation is between the anterior end of the calcaneum and the posterior surface of the cuboid (Fig. 10-37). The articular surfaces are covered with hyaline cartilage.

Type
The calcaneocuboid joint is synovial, of the plane variety.

Capsule
The capsule encloses the joint.

Ligaments
The **bifurcated ligament** is a strong ligament on the upper surface of the joint (Fig. 10-64). It is Y shaped, and the stem is attached to the upper surface of the anterior part of the calcaneum. The lateral limb is attached to the upper surface of the cuboid, and the medial limb to the upper surface of the navicular bone.

The **long plantar ligament** is a strong ligament on the lower surface of the joint (Figs. 10-58 and 10-59). It is attached to the undersurface of the calcaneum behind and to the undersurface of the cuboid and the bases of the third, fourth, and fifth metatarsal bones in front. It bridges over the groove for the peroneus longus tendon, converting it into a tunnel.

The **short plantar ligament** is a wide, strong ligament that is attached to the anterior tubercle on the undersurface of the calcaneum and to the adjoining part of the cuboid bone (Fig. 10-59).

Synovial Membrane
The synovial membrane lines the capsule.

Movements in the Subtalar, Talocalcaneonavicular, and Calcaneocuboid Joints

The talocalcaneonavicular and the calcaneocuboid joints are together referred to as the **midtarsal** or **transverse tarsal joints.**

The important movements of inversion and eversion of the foot take place at the subtalar and transverse tarsal joints. **Inversion** is the movement of the foot so that the sole faces medially. **Eversion** is the opposite movement of the foot so that the sole faces in the lateral direction. The movement of inversion is more extensive than eversion.

Inversion is performed by the tibialis anterior, the extensor hallucis longus, and the medial tendons of extensor digitorum longus; the tibialis posterior also assists.

Eversion is performed by the peroneus longus, peroneus brevis, and peroneus tertius; the lateral tendons of the extensor digitorum longus also assist.

Cuneonavicular Joint

The cuneonavicular joint is the **articulation** between the navicular bone and the three cuneiform bones. It is a synovial joint of the gliding variety. The **capsule** is strengthened by dorsal and plantar ligaments. The **joint cavity** is continuous with those of the intercuneiform and cuneocuboid joints and also with the cuneometatarsal and intermetatarsal joints, between the bases of the second and third and the third and fourth metatarsal bones.

Cuboideonavicular Joint

The cuboideonavicular joint is usually a fibrous joint, with the two bones connected by dorsal, plantar, and interosseous ligaments.

Intercuneiform and Cuneocuboid Joints

The intercuneiform and cuneocuboid joints are synovial joints of the plane variety. Their joint cavities are continuous with that of the cuneonavicular joint. The bones are connected by dorsal, plantar, and interosseous ligaments.

Tarsometatarsal and Intermetatarsal Joints

The tarsometatarsal and intermetatarsal joints are synovial joints of the plane variety. The bones are connected by dorsal, plantar, and interosseous ligaments. The tarsometatarsal joint of the big toe has a separate joint cavity.

Metatarsophalangeal and Interphalangeal Joints

The metatarsophalangeal and interphalangeal joints closely resemble those of the hand (see pages 516 and 517). The deep transverse ligaments connect the joints of the five toes.

The movements of abduction and adduction of the toes, performed by the interossei muscles, are minimal and take place from the midline of the second digit and not the third, as in the hand.

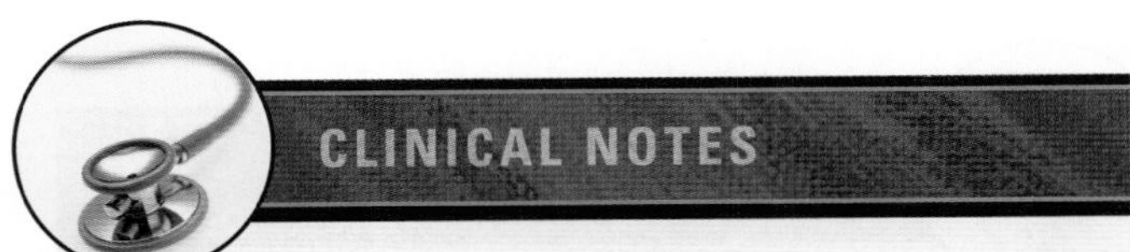

Metatarsophalangeal Joint of the Big Toe
Hallux valgus, which is a lateral deviation of the great toe at the metatarsophalangeal joint, is a common condition. Its incidence is greater in women than in men and is associated with badly fitting shoes. It is often accompanied by the presence of a short first metatarsal bone. Once the deformity is established, it is progressively worsened by the pull of the flexor hallucis longus and extensor hallucis longus muscles. Later, osteoarthritic changes occur in the metatarsophalangeal joint, which then becomes stiff and painful; the condition is then known as **hallux rigidus.**

The Foot as a Functional Unit

The Foot as a Weight-Bearer and a Lever

The foot has two important functions: to support the body weight and to serve as a lever to propel the body forward in walking and running. If the foot possessed a single strong bone instead of a series of small bones, it could sustain the body weight and serve well as a rigid lever for forward propulsion (Fig. 10-66). However, with such an arrangement, the foot could not adapt itself to uneven surfaces, and the forward propulsive action would depend entirely on the activities of the gastrocnemius and soleus muscles. Because the lever is segmented with multiple joints, the foot is pliable and can adapt itself to uneven surfaces. Moreover, the long flexor muscles and the small muscles of the foot can exert their action on the bones of the forepart of the foot and toes (i.e., the takeoff point of the foot) and greatly assist the forward propulsive action of the gastrocnemius and soleus muscles (Fig. 10-66).

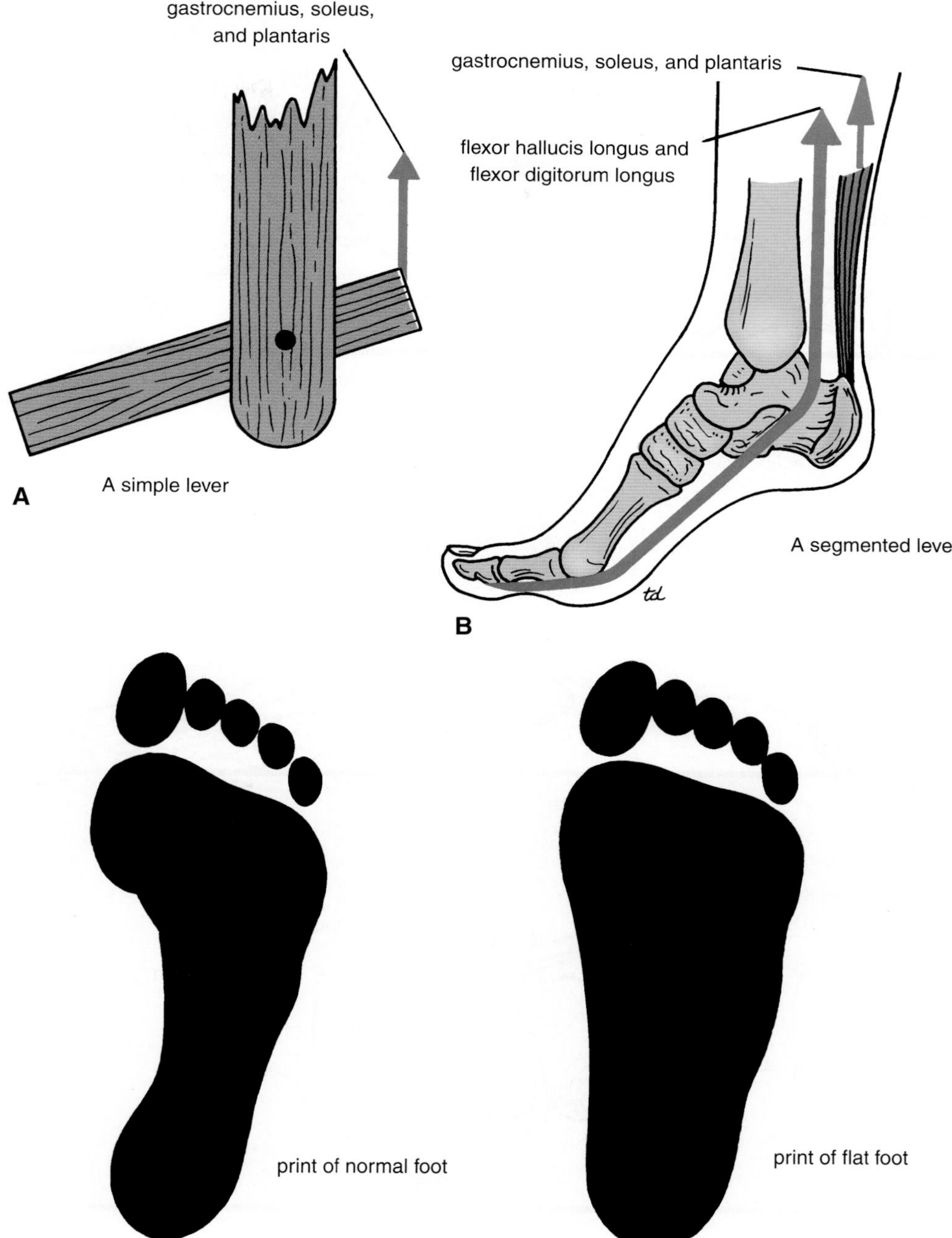

Figure 10-66 The foot as a simple lever (**A**) and as a segmented lever (**B**). Floor prints of a normal foot and a flat foot are also shown.

The Arches of the Foot

A segmented structure can hold up weight only if it is built in the form of an arch. The foot has three such arches, which are present at birth: the **medial longitudinal, lateral longitudinal,** and **transverse arches** (Fig. 10-67). In the young child, the foot appears to be flat because of the presence of a large amount of subcutaneous fat on the sole of the foot.

On examination of the imprint of a wet foot on the floor made with the person in the standing position, one can see that the heel, the lateral margin of the foot, the pad under the metatarsal heads, and the pads of the distal phalanges are in contact with the ground (Fig. 10-67). The medial margin of the foot, from the heel to the first metatarsal head, is arched above the ground because of the important medial longitudinal arch. The pressure exerted on the ground by the lateral

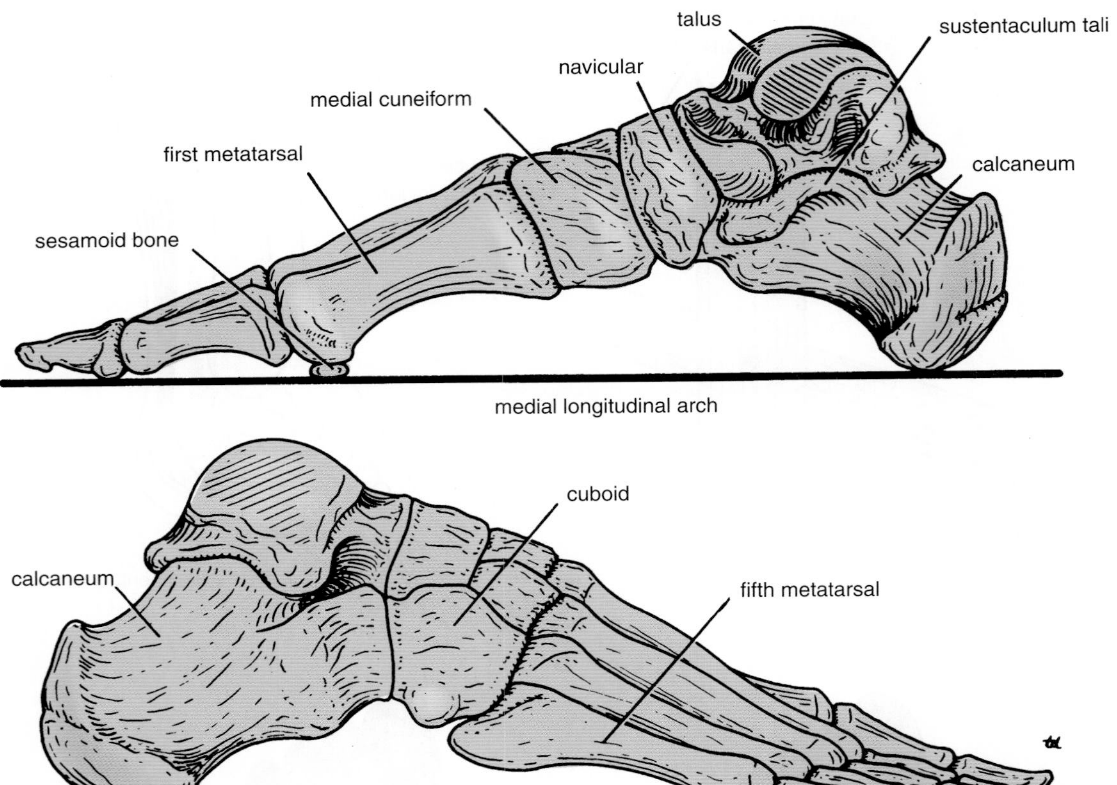

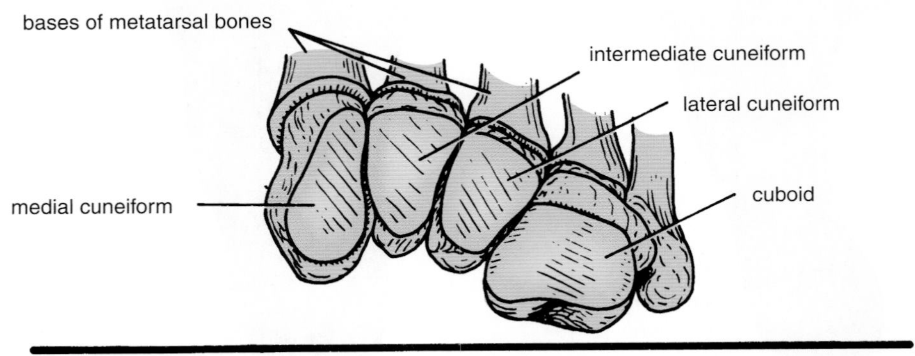

Figure 10-67 Bones forming the medial longitudinal, lateral longitudinal, and transverse arches of the right foot.

margin of the foot is greatest at the heel and the fifth metatarsal head and least between these areas because of the presence of the low-lying lateral longitudinal arch. The transverse arch involves the bases of the five metatarsals and the cuboid and cuneiform bones. This is, in fact, only half an arch, with its base on the lateral border of the foot and its summit on the foot's medial border. The foot has been likened to a half-dome, so that when the medial borders of the two feet are placed together, a complete dome is formed.

From this description, it can be understood that the body weight on standing is distributed through a foot via the heel behind and six points of contact with the ground in front, namely, the two sesamoid bones under the head of the first metatarsal and the heads of the remaining four metatarsals.

The Bones of the Arches

An examination of an articulated foot or a lateral radiograph of the foot shows the bones that form the arches.

- **Medial longitudinal arch:** This consists of the calcaneum, the talus, the navicular bone, the three cuneiform bones, and the first three metatarsal bones (Fig. 10-63).

- **Lateral longitudinal arch:** This consists of the calcaneum, the cuboid, and the fourth and fifth metatarsal bones (Fig. 10-67).
- **Transverse arch:** This consists of the bases of the metatarsal bones and the cuboid and the three cuneiform bones (Fig. 10-67).

Mechanisms of Arch Support

Examination of the design of any stone bridge reveals the following engineering methods used for its support (Fig. 10-68):

- **The shape of the stones:** The most effective way of supporting the arch is to make the stones wedge shaped, with the thin edge of the wedge lying inferiorly. This applies particularly to the important stone that occupies the center of the arch and is referred to as the "keystone."
- **The inferior edges of the stones are tied together:** This is accomplished by interlocking the stones or binding their lower edges together with metal staples. This method effectively counteracts the tendency of the lower edges of the stones to separate when the arch is weightbearing.
- **The use of the tie beams:** When the span of the bridge is large and the foundations at either end are insecure, a tie beam connecting the ends effectively prevents separation of the pillars and consequent sagging of the arch.

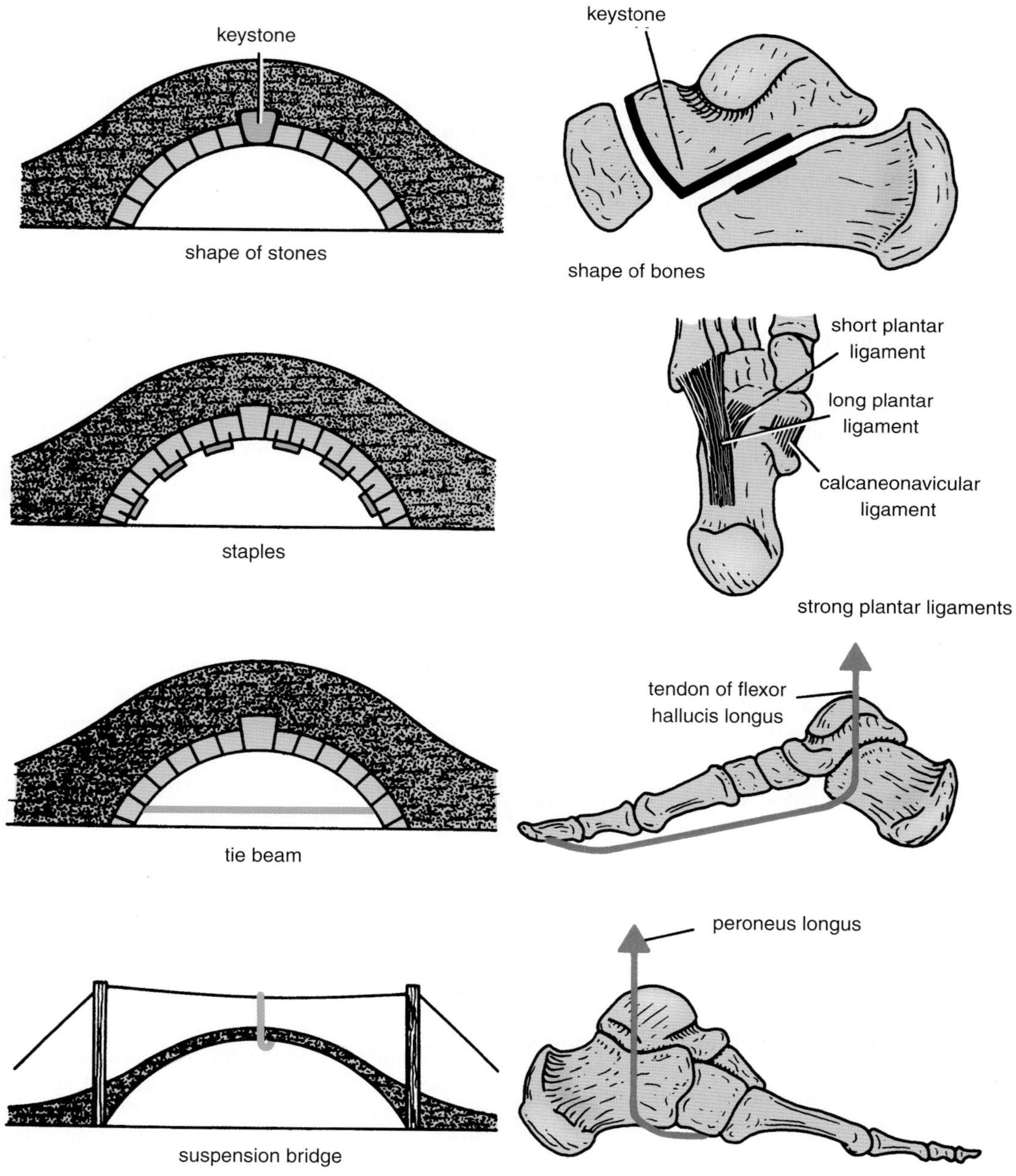

Figure 10-68 Different methods by which the arches of the foot may be supported.

- **A suspension bridge:** Here, the maintenance of the arch depends on multiple supports suspending the arch from a cable above the level of the bridge.

Using the bridge analogy, one can now examine the methods used to support the arches of the feet (Fig. 10-68).

Maintenance of the Medial Longitudinal Arch

- **Shape of the bones:** The sustentaculum tali holds up the talus; the concave proximal surface of the navicular bone receives the rounded head of the talus; the slight concavity of the proximal surface of the medial cuneiform bone receives the navicular. The rounded head of the talus is the keystone in the center of the arch (Fig. 10-68).
- **The inferior edges of the bones are tied together** by the plantar ligaments, which are larger and stronger than the dorsal ligaments. The most important ligament is the plantar calcaneonavicular ligament (Fig. 10-68). The tendinous extensions of the insertion of the tibialis posterior muscle play an important role in this respect.
- **Tying the ends of the arch together** are the plantar aponeurosis, the medial part of the flexor digitorum brevis, the abductor hallucis, the flexor hallucis longus, the medial part of the flexor digitorum longus, and the flexor hallucis brevis (Fig. 10-68).
- **Suspending the arch from above** are the tibialis anterior and posterior and the medial ligament of the ankle joint.

Maintenance of the Lateral Longitudinal Arch

- **Shape of the bones:** Minimal shaping of the distal end of the calcaneum and the proximal end of the cuboid. The cuboid is the keystone.
- **The inferior edges of the bones are tied together** by the long and short plantar ligaments and the origins of the short muscles from the forepart of the foot (Fig. 10-68).
- **Tying the ends of the arch together** are the plantar aponeurosis, the abductor digiti minimi, and the lateral part of the flexor digitorum longus and brevis.
- **Suspending the arch from above** are the peroneus longus and the brevis (Fig. 10-68).

Maintenance of the Transverse Arch

- **Shape of the bones:** The marked wedge shaping of the cuneiform bones and the bases of the metatarsal bones (Fig. 10-67)
- **The inferior edges of the bones are tied together** by the deep transverse ligaments, the strong plantar ligaments, and the origins of the plantar muscles from the forepart of the foot; the dorsal interossei and the transverse head of the adductor hallucis are particularly important in this respect.
- **Tying the ends of the arch together** is the peroneus longus tendon.
- **Suspending the arch from above** are the peroneus longus tendon and the peroneus brevis.

The arches of the feet are maintained by the shape of the bones, strong ligaments, and muscle tone. Which of these factors is the most important? Basmajian and Stecko demonstrated electromyographically that the tibialis anterior, the peroneus longus, and the small muscles of the foot play no important role in the normal static support of the arches. They are commonly totally inactive. However, during walking and running all these muscles become active. Standing immobile for long periods, especially if the person is overweight, places excessive strain on the bones and ligaments of the feet and results in fallen arches or flat feet. Athletes, route-marching soldiers, and nurses are able to sustain their arches provided that they receive adequate training to develop their muscle tone.

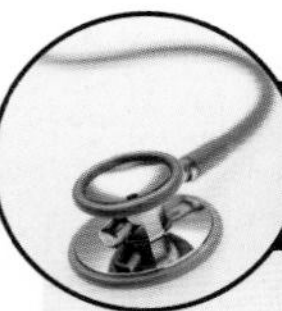

CLINICAL NOTES

Clinical Problems Associated With the Arches of the Foot

Of the three arches, the medial longitudinal is the largest and clinically the most important. The shape of the bones, the strong ligaments, especially those on the plantar surface of the foot, and the tone of muscles all play an important role in supporting the arches. It has been shown that in the active foot the tone of muscles is an important factor in arch support. When the muscles are fatigued by excessive exercise (a long-route march by an army recruit), by standing for long periods (waitress or nurse), by overweight, or by illness, the muscular support gives way, the ligaments are stretched, and pain is produced.

Pes planus (flat foot) is a condition in which the medial longitudinal arch is depressed or collapsed. As a result, the forefoot is displaced laterally and everted. The head of the talus is no longer supported, and the body weight forces it downward and medially between the calcaneum and the navicular bone. When the deformity has existed for some time, the plantar, calcaneonavicular, and medial ligaments of the ankle joint become permanently stretched, and the bones change shape. The muscles and tendons are also permanently stretched. The causes of flat foot are both congenital and acquired.

Pes cavus (clawfoot) is a condition in which the medial longitudinal arch is unduly high. Most cases are caused by muscle imbalance, in many instances resulting from poliomyelitis.

The Propulsive Action of the Foot

Standing Immobile The body weight is distributed via the heel behind and the heads of the metatarsal bones in front (including the two sesamoid bones under the head of the first metatarsal).

Walking As the body weight is thrown forward, the weight is born successively on the lateral margin of the foot and the heads of the metatarsal bones. As the heel rises, the toes are extended at the metatarsophalangeal joints, and the plantar aponeurosis is pulled on, thus shortening the tie beams and heightening the longitudinal arches. The "slack" in the long flexor tendons is taken up, thereby increasing their efficiency. The body is then thrown forward by the actions of the gastrocnemius and soleus (and plantaris) on the ankle joint, using the foot as a lever, and by the toes being strongly flexed by the long and short flexors of the foot, providing the final thrust forward. The lumbricals and interossei contract and keep the toes extended so that they do not fold under because of the strong action of the flexor digitorum longus. In this action, the long flexor tendons also assist in plantar flexing the ankle joint.

Running When a person runs, the weight is borne on the forepart of the foot, and the heel does not touch the ground. The forward thrust to the body is provided by the mechanisms described for walking (above).

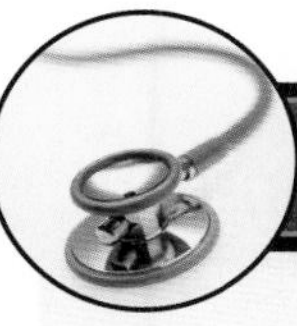

CLINICAL NOTES

Bursae and Bursitis in the Lower Limb

A variety of bursae are found in the lower limb where skin, tendons, ligaments, or muscles repeatedly rub against bony points or ridges.

Bursitis, or inflammation of a bursa, can be caused by acute or chronic trauma, crystal disease, infection, or disease of a neighboring joint that communicates with the bursa. An inflamed bursa becomes distended with excessive amounts of fluid. The following bursae are prone to inflammation: the bursa over the ischial tuberosity; the greater trochanter bursa; the prepatellar and superficial infrapatellar bursae; the bursa between the tendons of insertion of the sartorius, gracilis, and semitendinosus muscles on the medial proximal aspect of the tibia; and the bursa between the tendo calcaneus and the upper part of the calcaneum (long-distance runner's ankle).

Two important bursae communicate with the knee joint, and they can become distended if excessive amounts of synovial fluid accumulate within the joint. The suprapatellar bursa extends proximally about three fingerbreadths above the patella beneath the quadriceps femoris muscle. The bursa, which is associated with the insertion of the semimembranosus muscle, may enlarge in patients with osteoarthritis of the knee joint.

The anatomic bursae described should not be confused with **adventitious bursae,** which develop in response to abnormal and excessive friction. For example, a subcutaneous bursa sometimes develops over the tendo calcaneus in response to badly fitting shoes. A **bunion** is an adventitial bursa located over the medial side of the head of the first metatarsal bone.

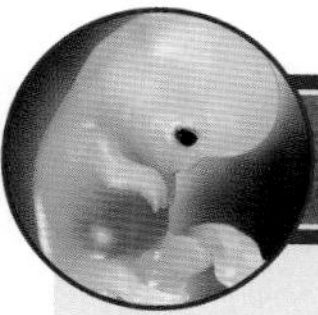

EMBRYOLOGIC NOTES

Development of the Lower Limb

The limb buds appear during the sixth week of development as the result of a localized proliferation of the somatopleuric mesenchyme. This causes the overlying ectoderm to bulge from the trunk as two pairs of flattened paddles. The leg buds develop after the arm buds and arise at the level of the lower four lumbar and upper three sacral segments.

The flattened limb buds have a cephalic **preaxial border** and a caudal **postaxial border.** As the limb buds elongate, the mesenchyme along the preaxial border becomes innervated by the second lumbar nerve to the first sacral nerve and that of the postaxial border becomes innervated by the first to the third sacral nerves. Later, the mesenchymal masses divide into anterior and posterior groups, and the nerve trunks entering the base of each limb also divide into anterior and posterior divisions. As development continues and the limbs further elongate, their attachment to the trunk moves caudally. At the same time, the mesenchyme within the limbs differentiates into individual muscles that migrate within each limb. As a consequence of these two factors, the anterior rami of the spinal nerves become arranged near the base of the limb into the complicated lumbosacral plexus.

It is interesting to note that the dermatomal pattern in the lower limb appears to be more complicated than that of the upper limb (see Figs. 1-26 and 1-27). This can be explained embryologically, since during fetal development, the lower limb bud undergoes medial rotation as it grows out from the trunk. This results in the big toe coming to lie on the medial side of the foot and accounts for the spiraling pattern of the dermatomes.

Ectromelia

In ectromelia, there is a partial absence of a lower limb (Fig. 10-69). The condition in the upper limb is described on page 521.

Congenital Dislocation of the Hip

Congenital dislocation of the hip is 10 times more common in female children than in male children, and it is particularly common in northern Italy (Fig. 10-70). Three possible causes have been suggested:

- **Generalized joint laxity:** Excessive laxity of the ligaments of the hip joint may predispose to this condition.
- **Breech position:** The flexed hip and extended knees of the breech position may alter the normal pressure of the head of the femur on the acetabulum, and this may result in a failure of the upper part of the acetabulum to develop adequately.
- **Shallow acetabulum:** If the acetabulum is poorly developed, the upper lip offers an insufficient shelf under which the head of the femur can lodge. The condition of shallow acetabulum tends to run in families.

(continues)

Embryologic Notes, *continued*

Congenital dislocation of the hip should be diagnosed at birth and is treated by splinting the joint in the position of abduction.

Genu Recurvatum

Hyperextension of the knee joint is found in babies who have had a breech presentation with extended legs. No treatment is required, because the legs return to normal within a few weeks.

Talipes

Talipes (club foot) often is caused by abnormal position or restricted movement of the fetus in utero. A small number of cases may be caused by muscle paralysis associated with spina bifida. The different types are named according to the position of the foot. **Talipes calcaneovalgus** is a form of club foot in which the foot is dorsiflexed at the ankle joint and everted at the midtarsal joints. In **talipes equinovarus** the foot is plantar flexed at the ankle joint and inverted at the midtarsal joints (Fig. 10-71). The conditions may be unilateral or bilateral, and they require orthopedic treatment.

Metatarsus Varus

Metatarsus varus is a common condition in which the forefoot is adducted on the rear part of the foot. Correction may be accomplished by manipulation followed by splinting.

Overriding Toes

Overriding toes most commonly involves the fourth and fifth toes. The fourth toe is depressed and overridden by the fifth toe. This may be corrected by the application of splints.

Curly Toes

Curly toes most often affects the fourth and fifth toes; the condition commonly runs in families. The affected toe lies flexed under its medial neighbor. In mild cases, there is no treatment; in severe cases, the flexor digitorum longus tendon is transplanted into the extensor tendon.

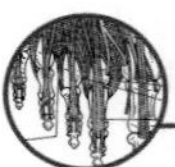

Radiographic Anatomy

Radiographic Appearances of the Lower Limb

Radiologic examination of the lower limb concentrates mainly on the bony structures, because most of the muscles, tendons, and nerves blend into a homogeneous mass. Examples of radiographs of the different regions of the lower limb are shown in Figures 10-72 through 10-80.

Magnetic resonance imaging of the lower limb can be useful to demonstrate the soft tissues around the bones (Fig. 10-81).

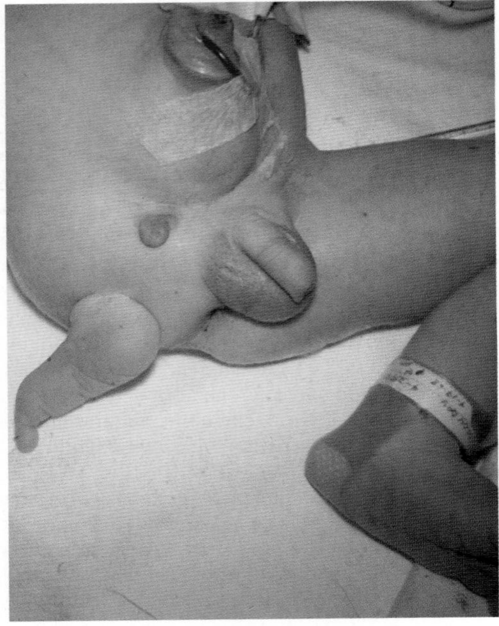

Figure 10-69 Ectromelia. (Courtesy of G. Avery.)

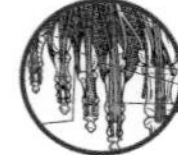

Surface Anatomy

The following information should be verified on the living body. An adequate physical examination of the lower limb of a patient requires a sound knowledge of the surface anatomy of the region.

Gluteal Region

The **iliac crests** are easily palpable along their entire length (Figs. 10-82 and 10-83). Each crest ends in front at the **anterior superior iliac spine** (Figs. 10-79 and 10-80) and behind at the **posterior superior iliac spine** (Fig. 10-82); the latter lies beneath a skin dimple at the level of the second sacral vertebra and the middle of the sacroiliac joint. The **iliac tubercle** is a prominence felt on the outer surface of the iliac crest about 2 in. (5 cm) posterior to the anterior superior iliac spine (Fig. 10-83).

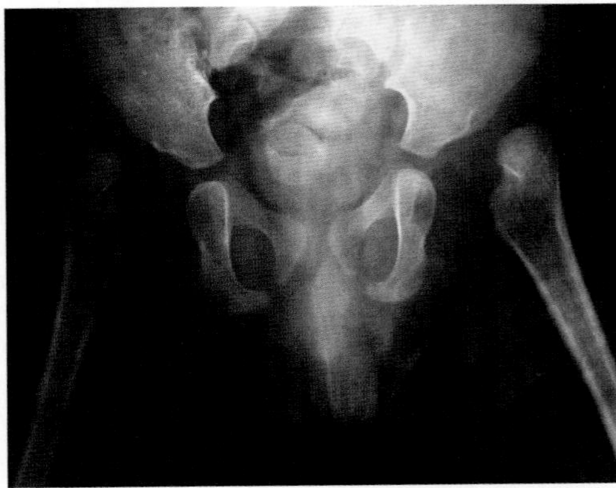

Figure 10-70 Radiograph of bilateral congenital dislocation of the hip showing that the femoral heads are not within the shallow acetabular fossae. (Courtesy of J. Adams.)

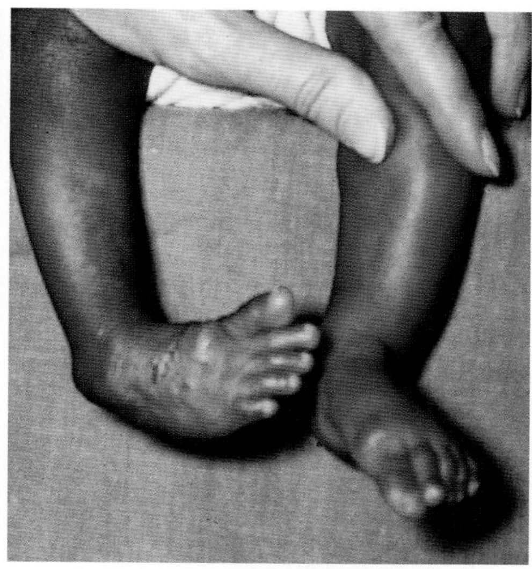

Figure 10-71 Talipes equinovarus. (Courtesy of J. Adams.)

The **ischial tuberosity** can be palpated in the lower part of the buttock (Figs. 10-82 and 10-83). In the standing position, the tuberosity is covered by the gluteus maximus. In the sitting position, the ischial tuberosity emerges from beneath the lower border of the gluteus maximus and supports the weight of the body; in this position, the tuberosity is separated from the skin by only a bursa and a pad of fat.

The **greater trochanter** of the femur can be felt on the lateral surface of the thigh (Figs. 10-82 and 10-83) and moves beneath the examining finger as the hip joint is flexed and extended. It is important to verify that, in the normal hip joint, the upper border of the greater trochanter lies on a line connecting the anterior superior iliac spine to the ischial tuberosity (Fig. 10-83).

The **spinous processes** of the sacrum (Fig. 10-79) are fused with each other to form the **median sacral crest.** The crest can be felt beneath the skin in the upper part of the cleft between the buttocks.

The tip of the **coccyx** can be palpated beneath the skin in the cleft between the buttocks about 1 in. (2.5 cm)

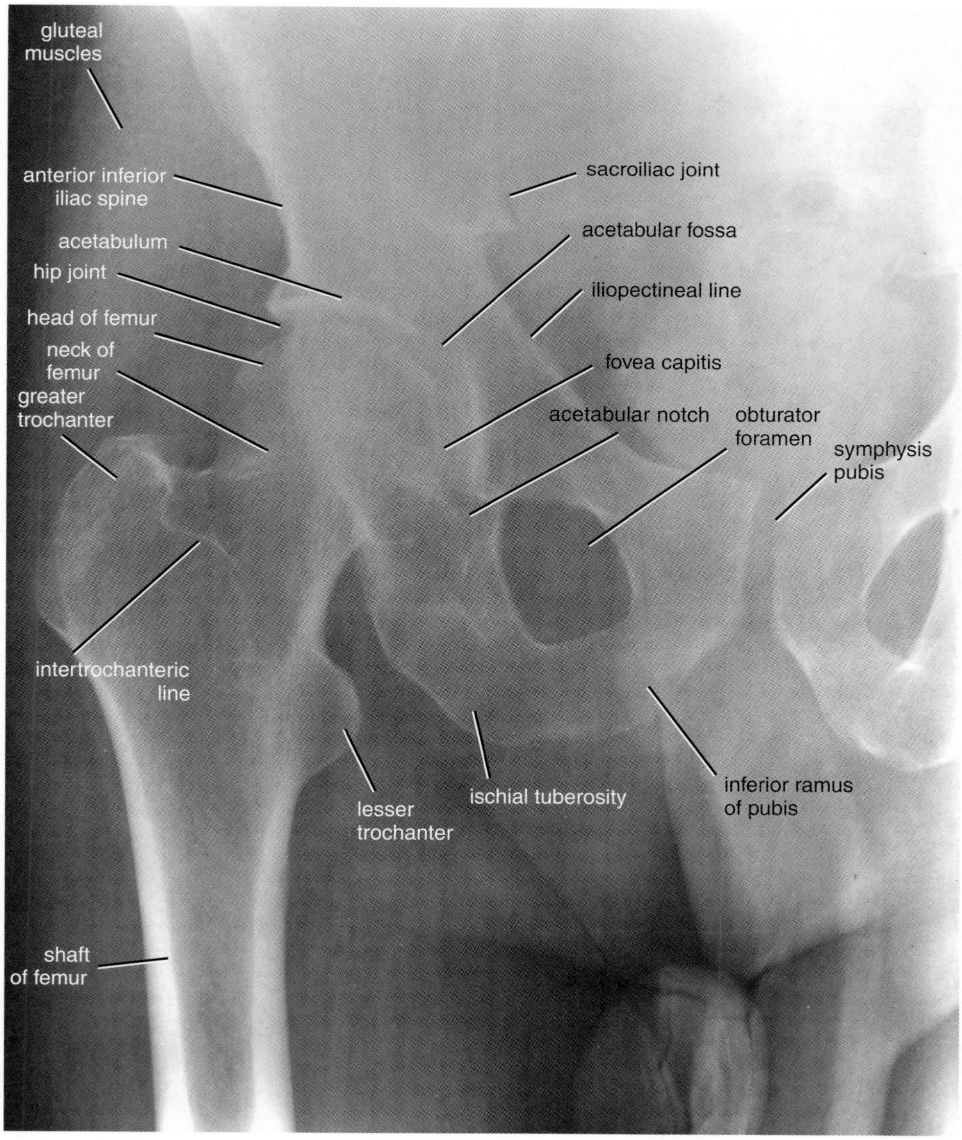

Figure 10-72 Anteroposterior radiograph of the hip joint. Note that the inferior margin of the neck of the femur should form a continuous curve with the upper margin of the obturator foramen **(Shenton's line).**

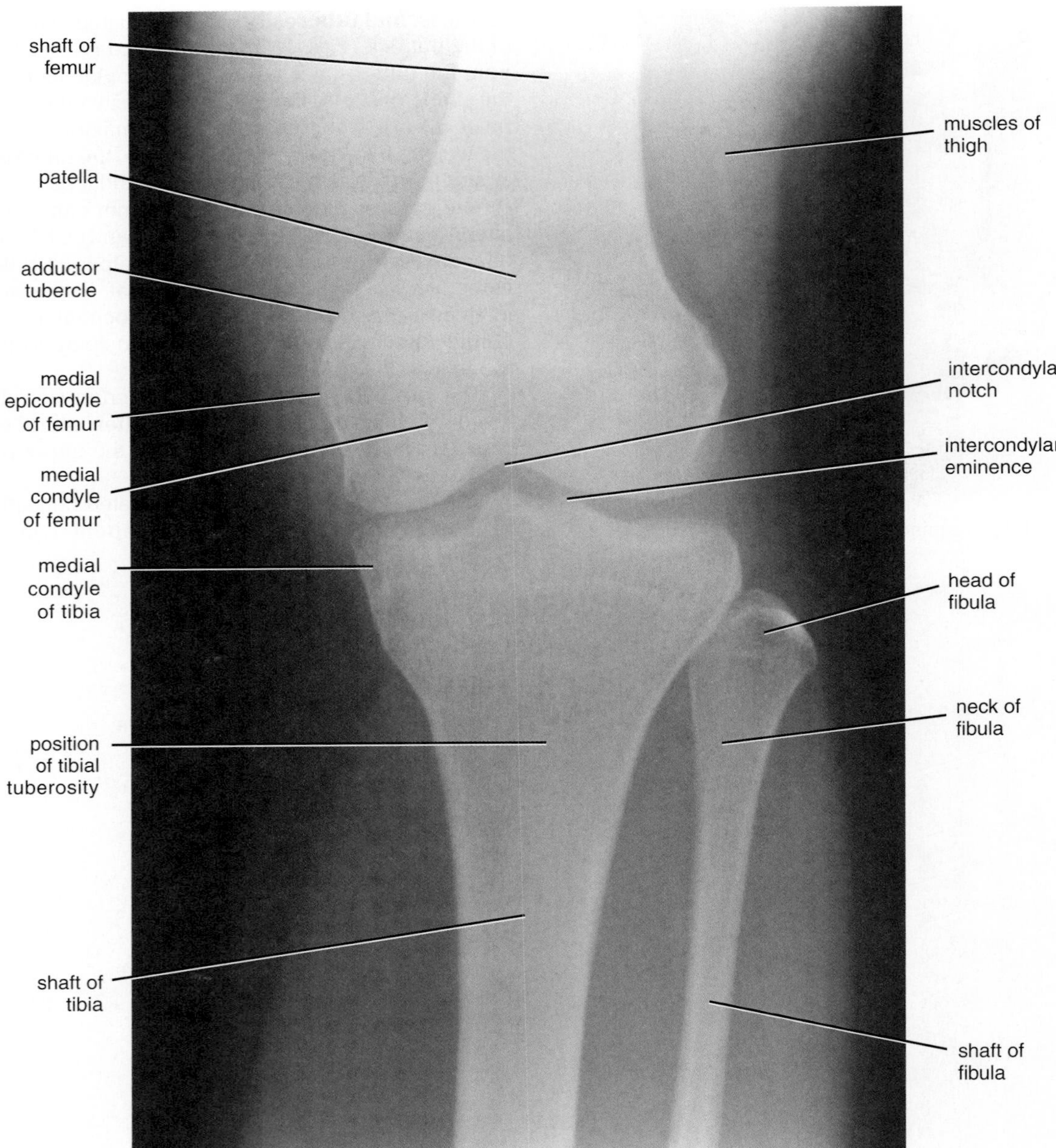

Figure 10-73 Anteroposterior radiograph of the adult knee.

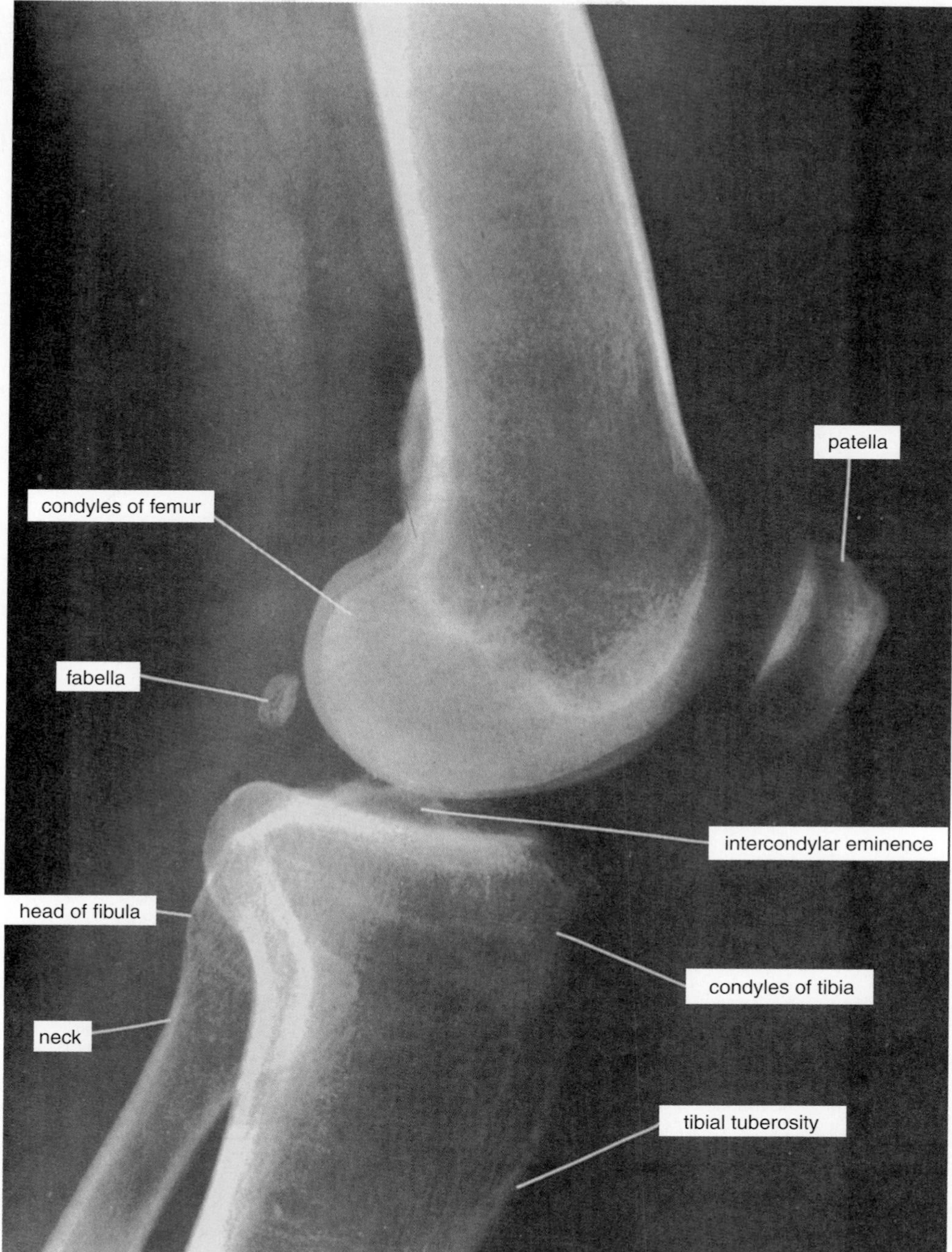

Figure 10-74 Lateral radiograph of the adult knee.

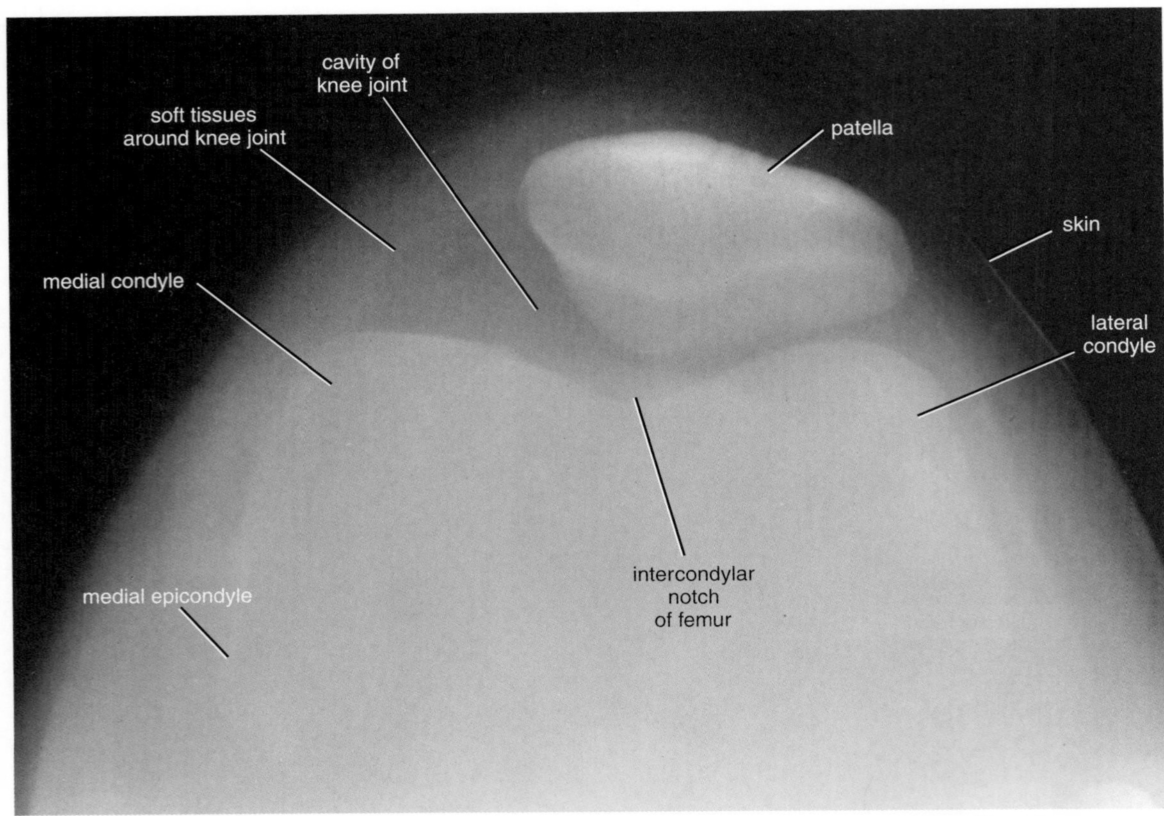

Figure 10-75 Tangential view of the patella.

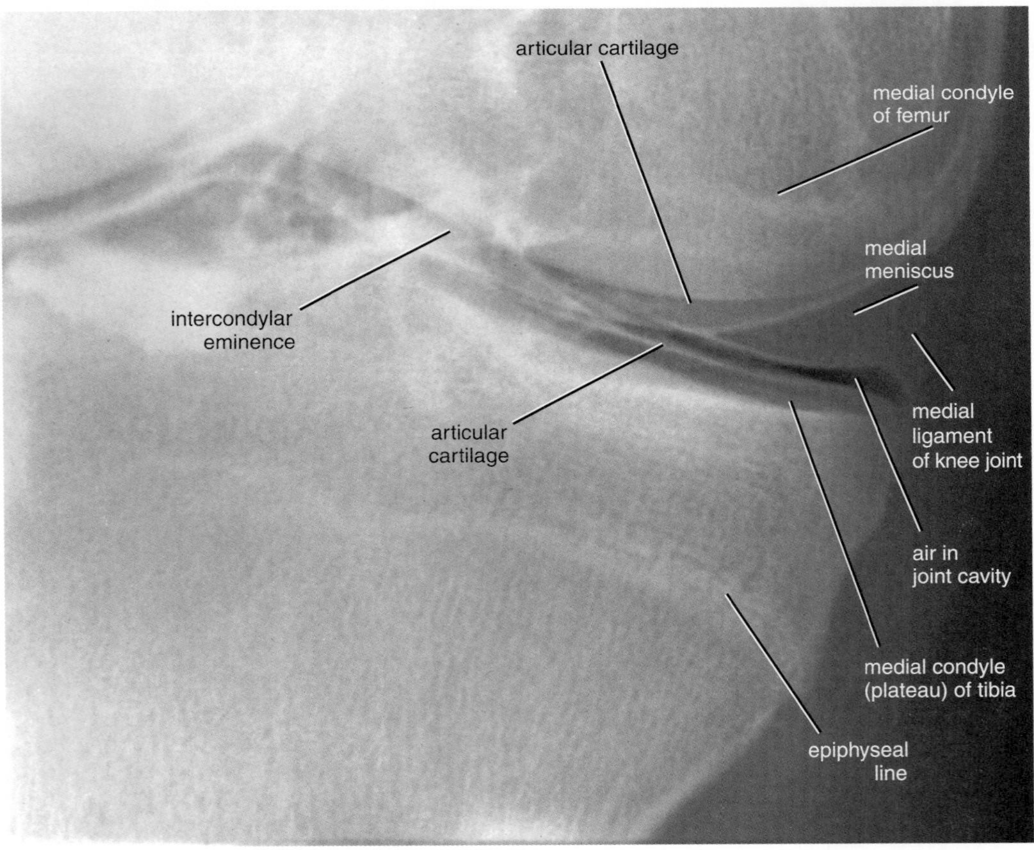

Figure 10-76 Pneumoarthrography of the knee.

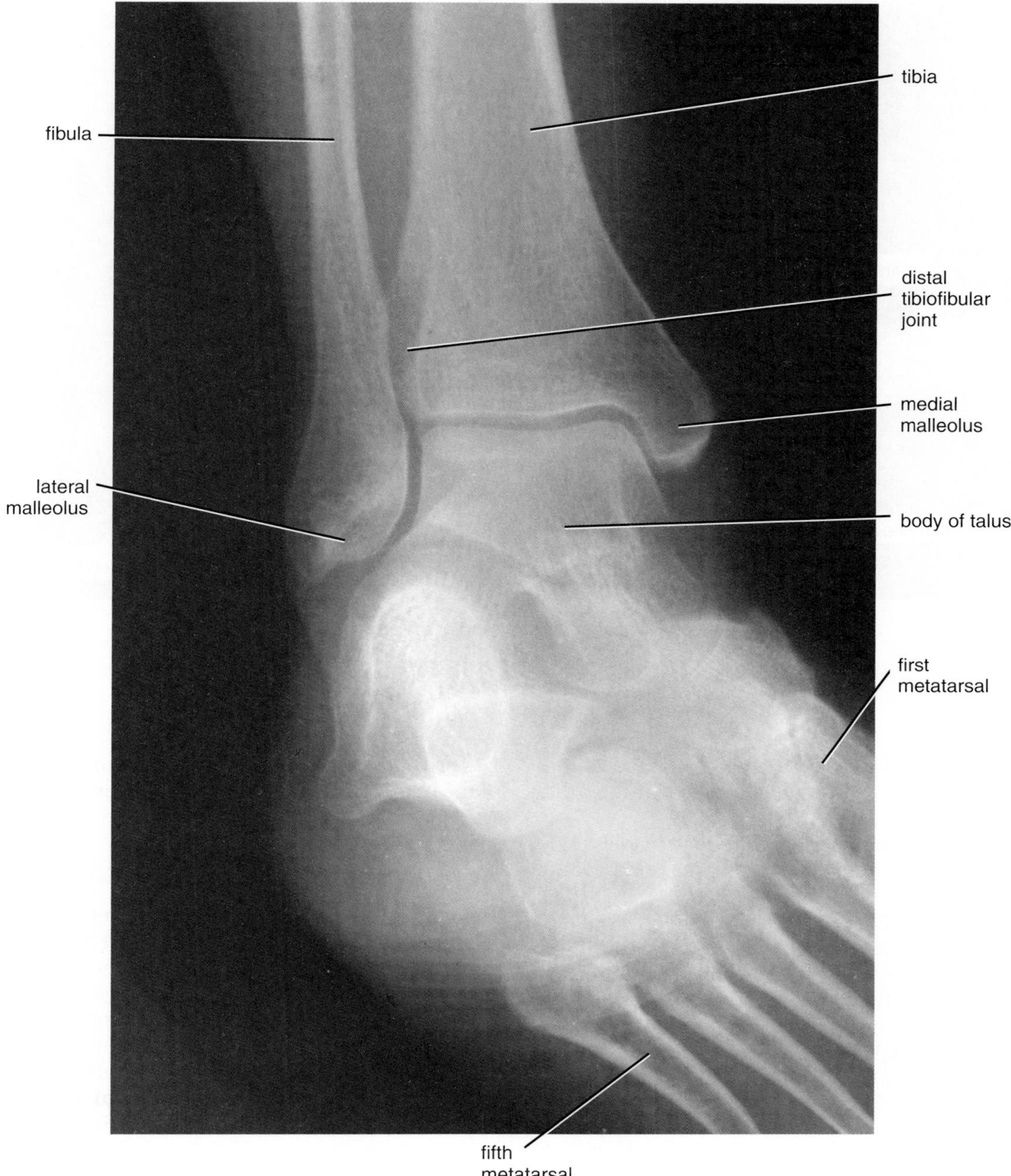

Figure 10-77 Anteroposterior radiograph of the adult ankle.

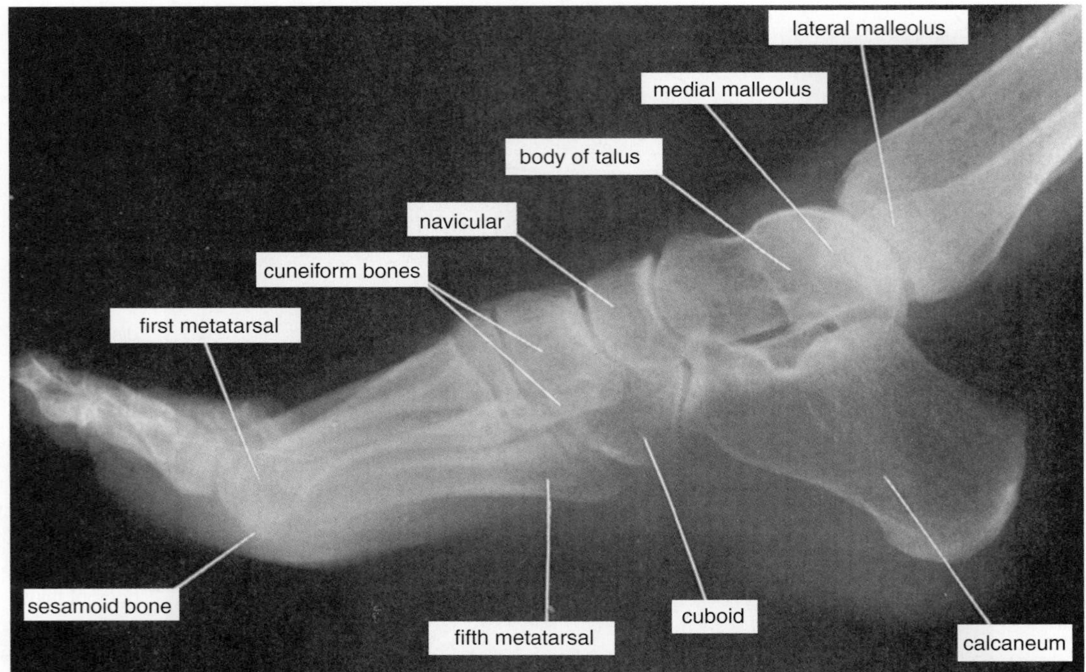

Figure 10-78 Lateral radiograph of the adult ankle.

behind the anus (Fig. 10-83). The anterior surface of the coccyx can be palpated with a gloved finger in the anal canal.

The **fold of the buttocks** is most prominent in the standing position; its lower border does not correspond to the lower border of the gluteus maximus muscle.

The **sciatic nerve** in the buttock lies under cover of the gluteus maximus muscle. As it curves laterally and downward, it is situated at first midway between the posterior superior iliac spine and the ischial tuberosity and, lower down, midway between the tip of the greater trochanter and the ischial tuberosity (Figs. 10-82 and 10-83).

Inguinal Region

The **inguinal ligament** lies beneath the skin fold in the groin and can be felt along its length. It is attached laterally to the anterior superior iliac spine and medially to the pubic tubercle (Figs. 10-83 and 10-84).

The **symphysis pubis** is a cartilaginous joint that lies in the midline between the bodies of the pubic bones (Fig. 10-80). The **upper margin of the symphysis pubis** and the bodies of the pubic bones can be felt on palpation through the lower part of the anterior abdominal wall.

The **pubic tubercle** can be felt on the upper border of the pubis (Figs. 10-83 and 10-84). Attached to it is the medial end of the inguinal ligament. The tubercle is easily palpated in the male by invaginating the scrotum with the examining finger. In the female, it can be palpated through the lateral margin of the labium majus.

The **pubic crest** is the ridge of bone on the upper surface of the body of the pubis, medial to the pubic tubercle (Figs. 10-7 and 10-8).

Femoral Triangle

The femoral triangle can be seen as a depression below the fold of the groin in the upper part of the thigh (Figs. 10-83 and 10-84). In a thin, muscular subject, the boundaries of the triangle can be identified when the thigh is flexed, abducted, and laterally rotated. The **base** of the triangle is formed by the inguinal ligament, the **lateral border** by the sartorius muscle, and the **medial border** by the adductor longus muscle.

The horizontal group of **superficial inguinal lymph nodes** can be palpated in the superficial fascia just below and parallel to the inguinal ligament (Fig. 10-3).

The **femoral artery** enters the thigh behind the inguinal ligament (Fig. 10-6) at the midpoint of a line joining the symphysis pubis to the anterior superior iliac spine; its pulsations are easily felt (Fig. 10-84).

The **femoral vein** leaves the thigh by passing behind the inguinal ligament medial to the pulsating femoral artery (Fig. 10-6).

The lower opening of the **femoral canal** lies below and lateral to the pubic tubercle (Figs. 10-3 and 10-6).

The **femoral nerve** enters the thigh behind the midpoint of the inguinal ligament—that is, lateral to the pulsating femoral artery (Fig. 10-6).

The **great saphenous vein** pierces the saphenous opening in the deep fascia (fascia lata) of the thigh and joins the

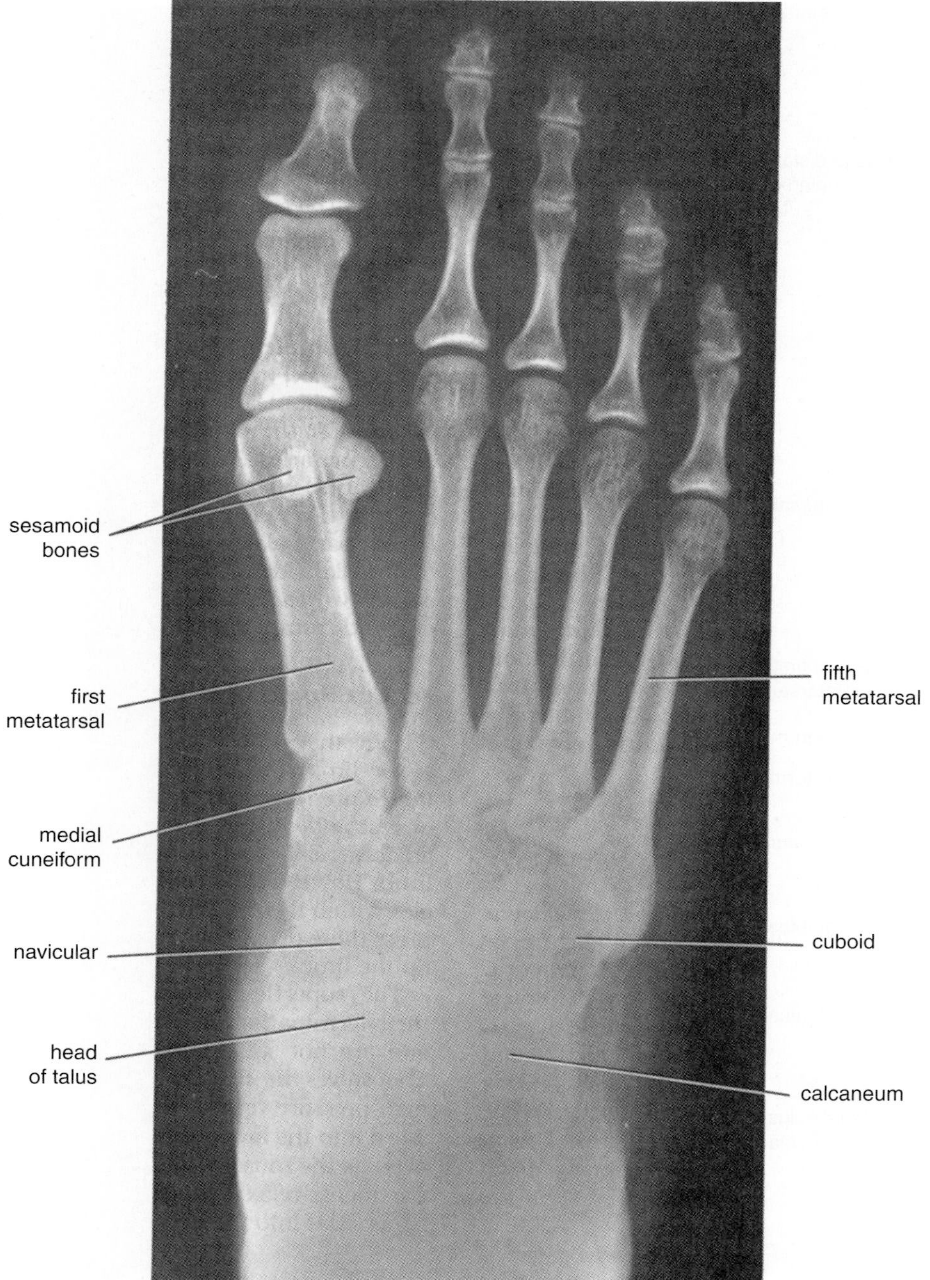

Figure 10-79 Anteroposterior radiograph of the adult foot.

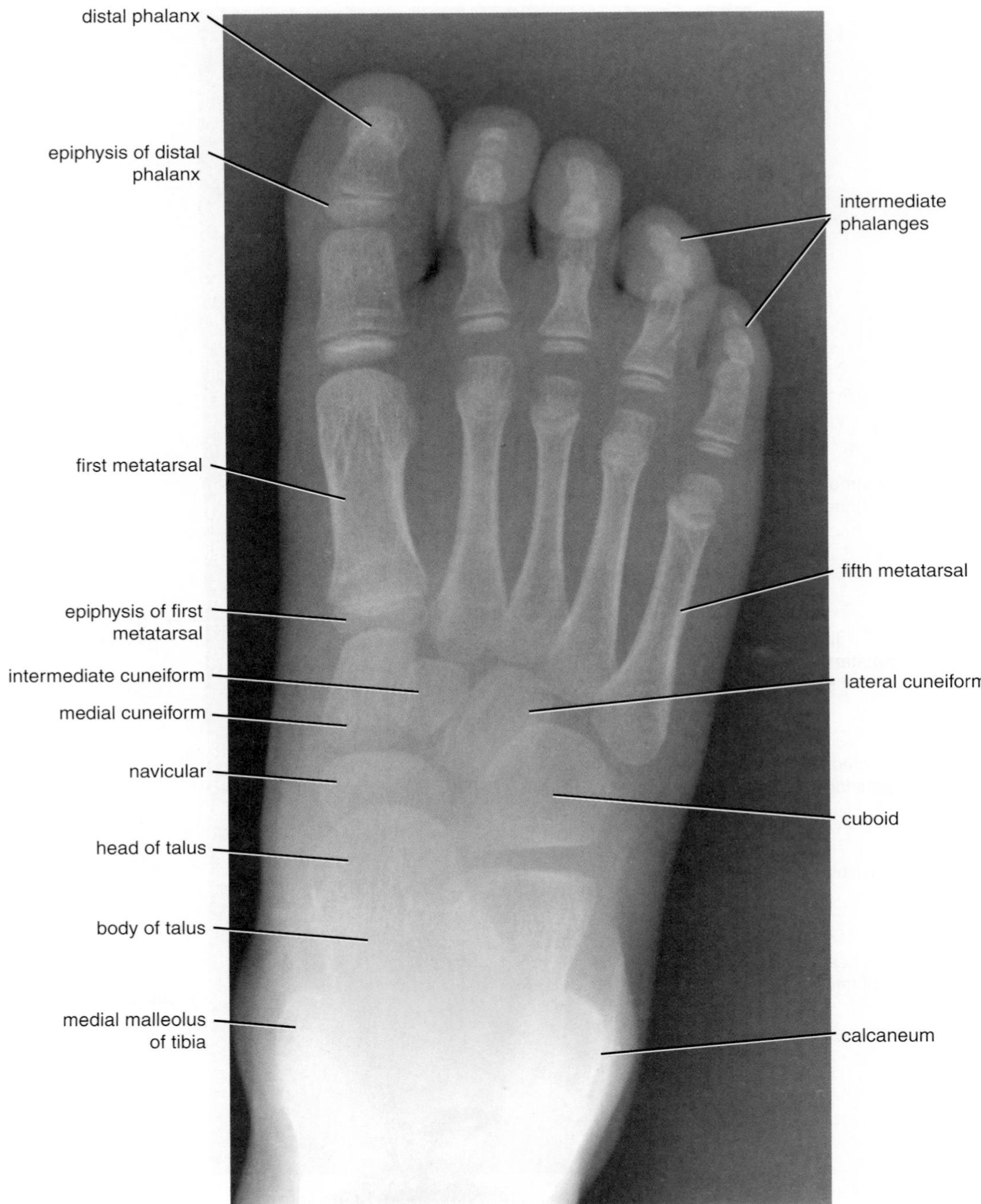

Figure 10-80 Anteroposterior radiograph of the foot showing the epiphyses of the phalanges and metatarsal bones (10-year-old boy).

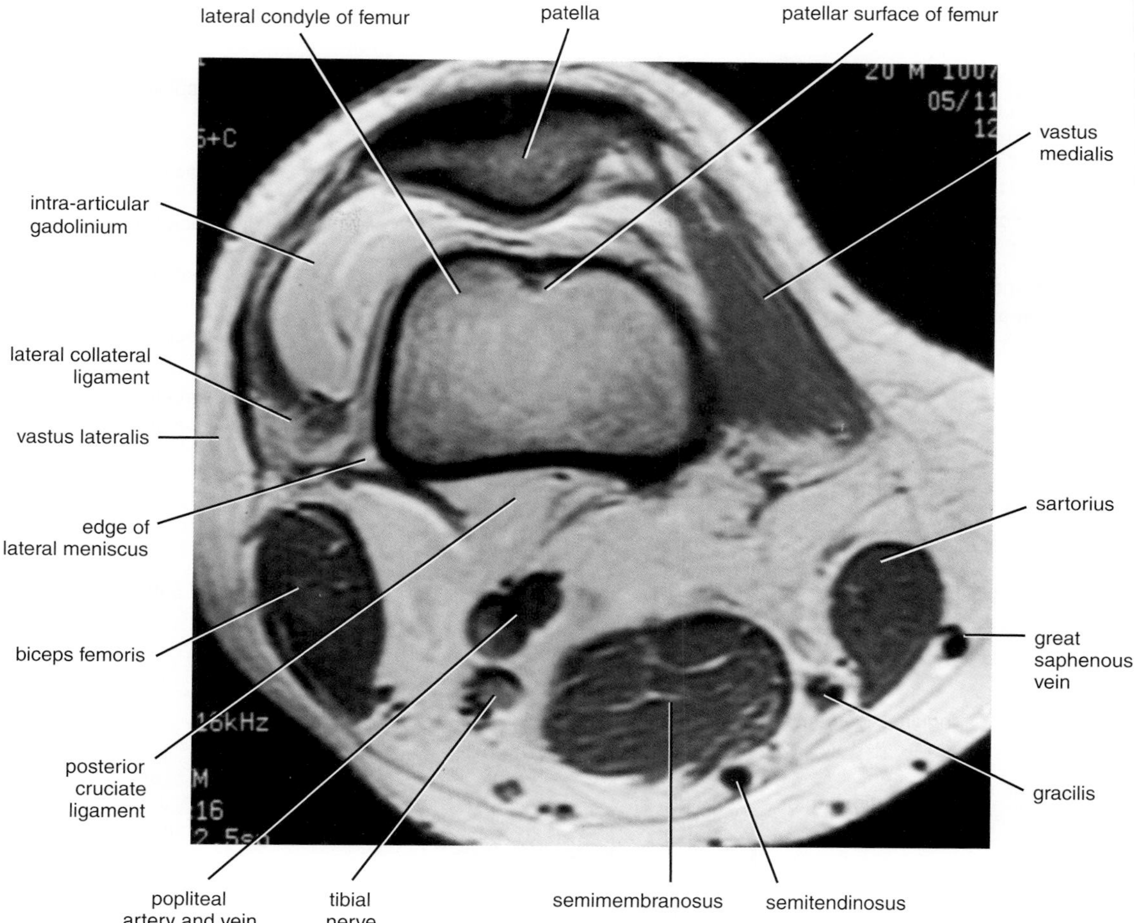

Figure 10-81 Transverse (axial) proton density magnetic resonance image of the right knee with intra-articular gadolinium–saline solution (as seen from below).

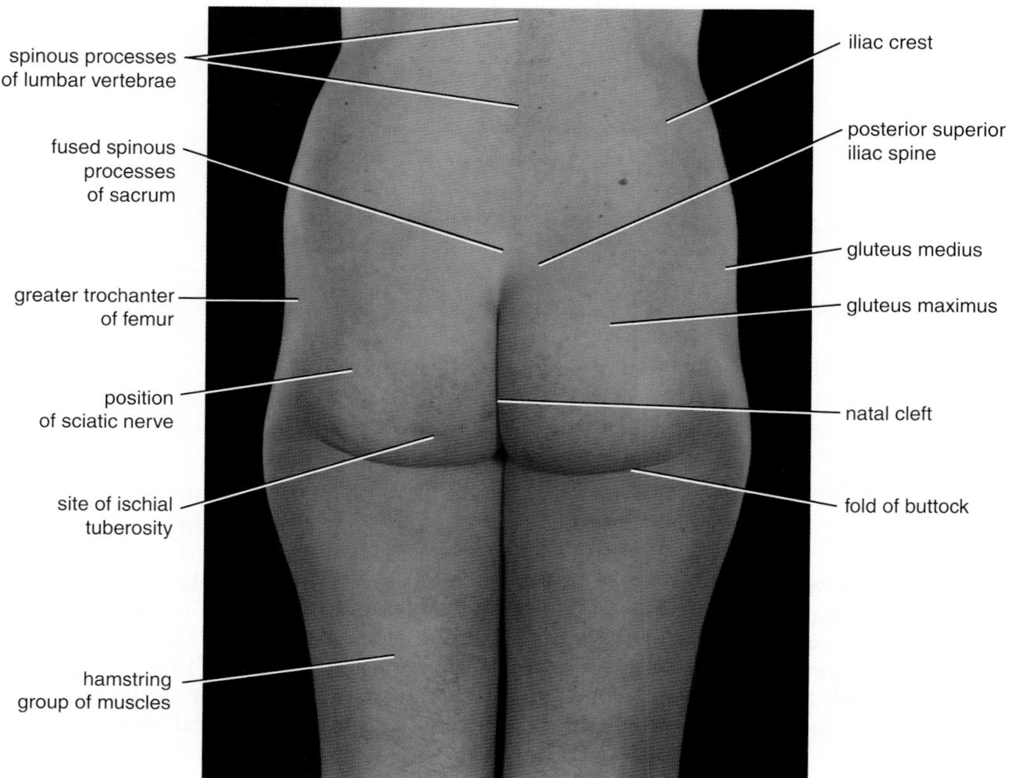

Figure 10-82 The gluteal region and the posterior aspect of the thigh of a 25-year-old woman.

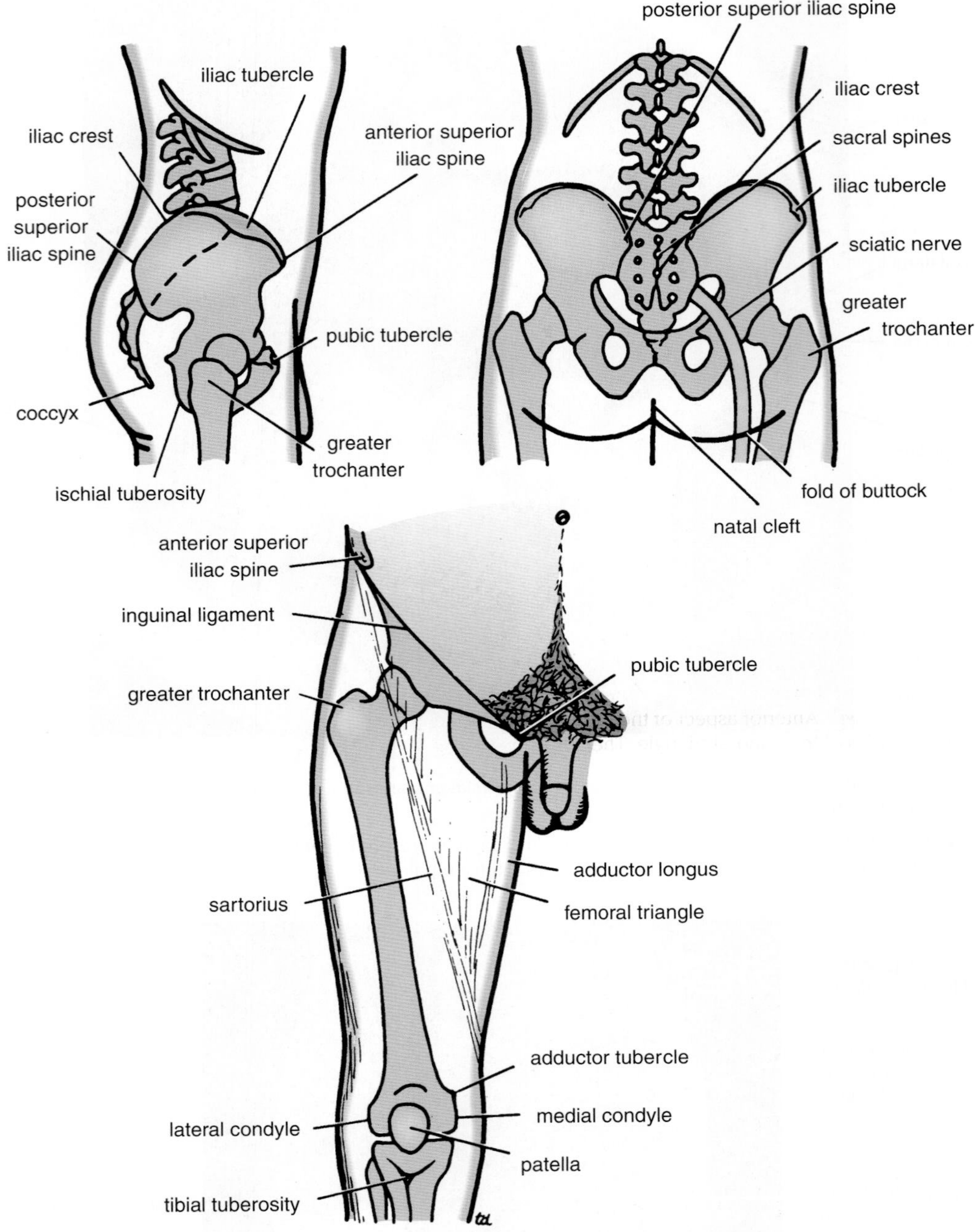

Figure 10-83 Surface markings in the gluteal region and the front of the thigh.

femoral vein 1.5 in. (4 cm) below and lateral to the pubic tubercle (Figs. 10-3 and 10-19).

Adductor Canal

The **adductor (subsartorial) canal** lies in the middle third of the thigh (Fig. 10-84), immediately distal to the apex of the femoral triangle. It is an intermuscular cleft situated beneath the sartorius muscle and is bounded laterally by the vastus medialis muscle and posteriorly by the adductor longus and magnus muscles. It contains the femoral vessels and the saphenous nerve.

Knee Region

In front of the knee joint the **patella** and the **ligamentum patellae** can be easily palpated (Fig. 10-85). The ligamentum patellae can be traced downward to its attachment to the **tuberosity of the tibia.**

The **condyles of the femur and tibia** can be recognized on the sides of the knee and the joint line can be identified between them (Fig. 10-85).

The bandlike **medial collateral ligament** and the rounded **lateral collateral ligament** can be palpated on the sides of the joint line; they can be followed above and

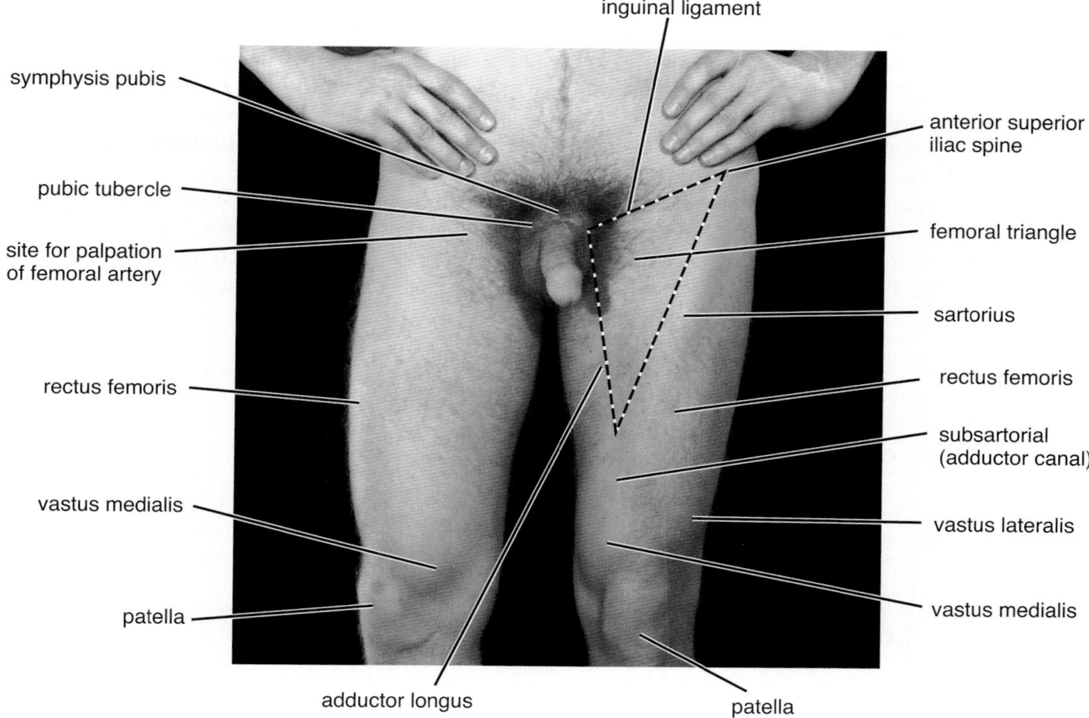

Figure 10-84 Anterior aspect of the thigh of a 27-year-old man. The broken lines indicate the boundaries of the femoral triangle. The right leg is laterally rotated at the hip joint.

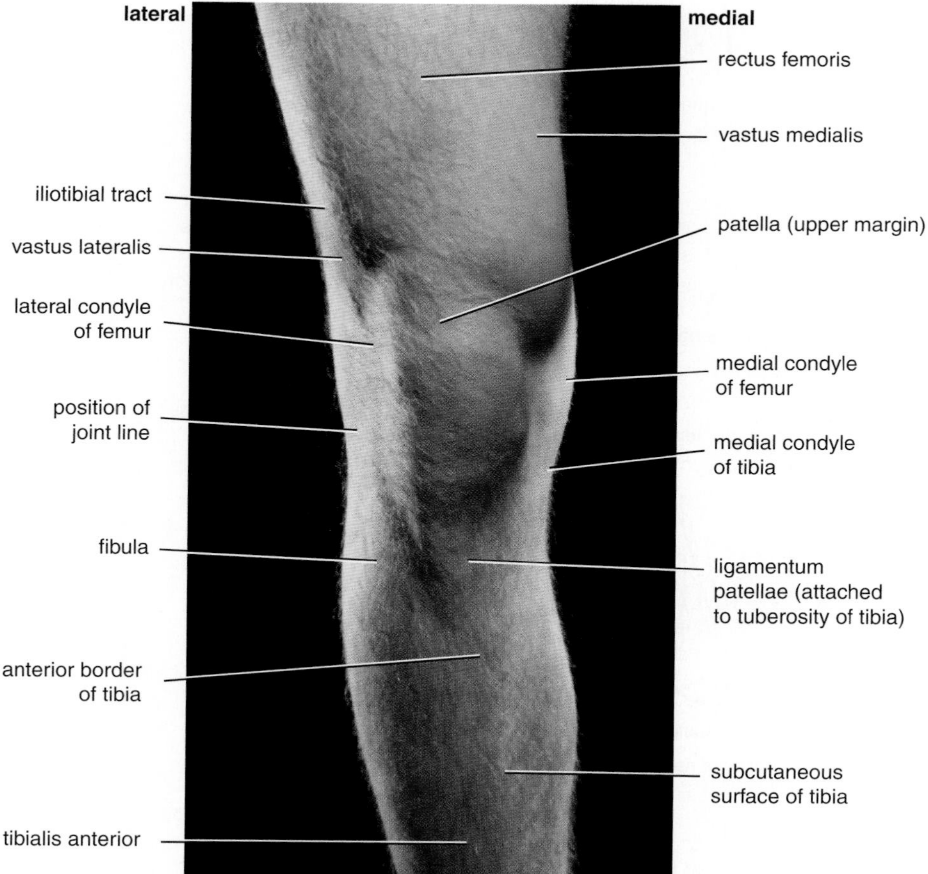

Figure 10-85 Anterior aspect of the right knee of a 27-year-old man.

below to their bony attachments. Because the ligaments cover the joint line, the joint line cannot be palpated at the sites of the collateral ligaments (Fig. 10-61).

The **menisci** are located in the interval between the femoral and tibial condyles. Although not recognizable, the outer edges of the medial and lateral menisci can be palpated on the joint line between the ligamentum patellae and the medial and lateral collateral ligaments, respectively.

The **tendon of biceps** can be felt as a rounded structure on the lateral aspect of the knee and can be traced down to the **head of the fibula** (Fig. 10-85).

The **common peroneal nerve** can be rolled beneath the examining finger just below the head of the fibula (Fig. 10-86); here it passes forward around the lateral side of the bone.

The **adductor tubercle** can be palpated on the medial aspect of the femur just above the medial condyle; the hamstring part of the **adductor magnus** can be felt passing to it (Fig. 10-86).

Behind the knee joint is a diamond-shaped skin depression called the **popliteal fossa** (Fig. 10-86). When the knee is flexed, the deep fascia, which roofs over the fossa, is relaxed and the boundaries are easily defined. Its upper part is

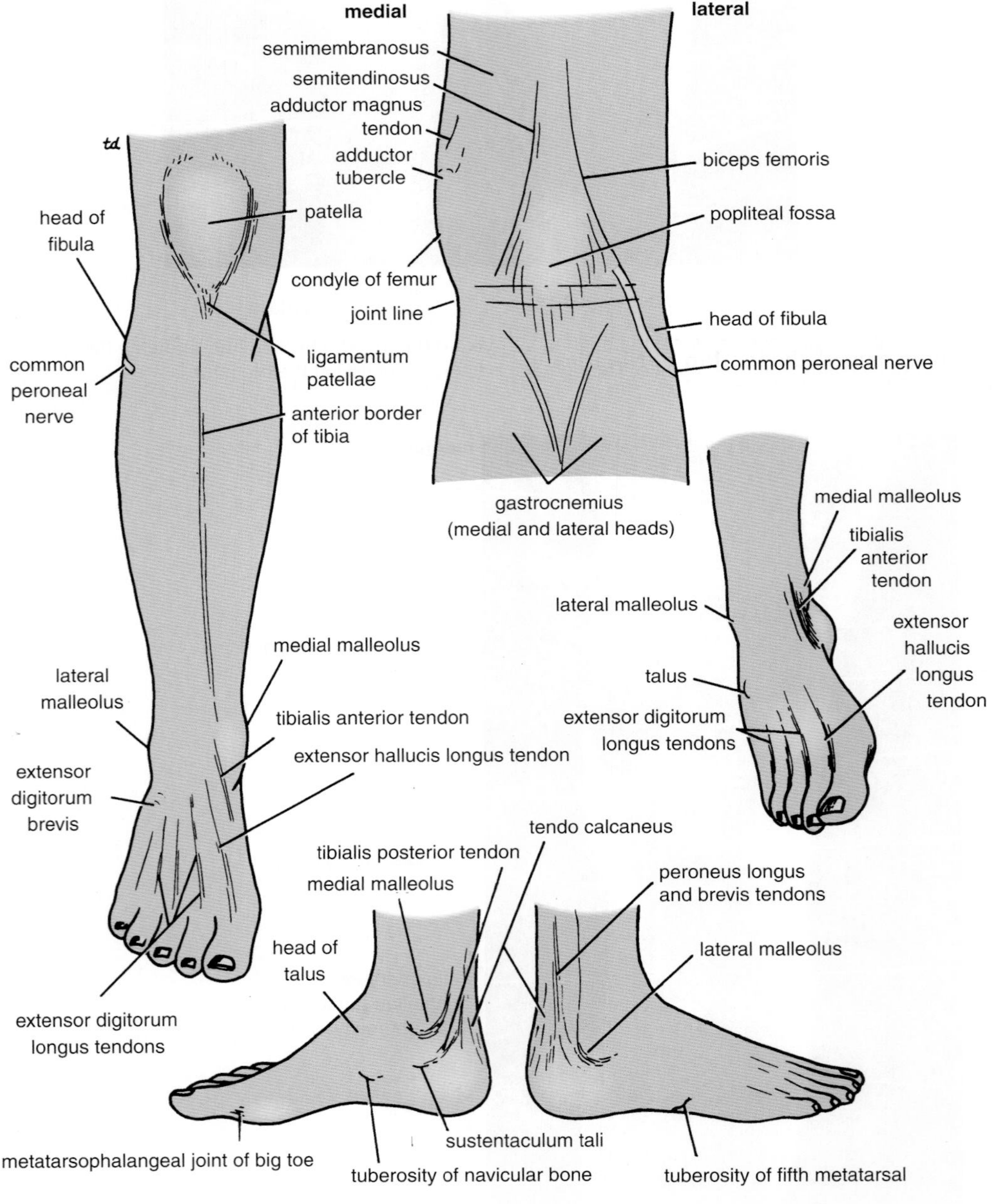

Figure 10-86 Surface markings in the popliteal fossa, the front of the leg, and the foot.

bounded **laterally** by the tendon of the biceps femoris muscle and **medially** by the tendons of the semimembranosus and semitendinosus muscles. Its lower part is bounded on each side by one of the heads of the gastrocnemius muscle.

The **common peroneal nerve** can be palpated on the medial side of the tendon of the biceps femoris (Fig. 10-86), as the latter passes to its insertion on the head of the fibula. With the knee joint partially flexed, the nerve can be rolled beneath the finger.

The **popliteal artery** can be felt by gentle palpation in the depths of the popliteal fossa, provided that the deep fascia is fully relaxed by passively flexing the knee joint.

Tibia

The medial surface and anterior border of the **tibia** are subcutaneous and can be felt throughout their length (Fig. 10-85).

Ankle Region and Foot

In the region of the ankle, the fibula is subcutaneous and can be followed downward to form the **lateral malleolus** (Figs. 10-86 and 10-87). The tip of the **medial malleolus** of the tibia lies about 0.5 in. (1.3 cm) proximal to the level of the tip of the lateral malleolus (Figs. 10-86 and 10-87).

In the interval behind the medial malleolus (Fig. 10-86) and the medial surface of the calcaneum lie the following structures, in the order named: the **tendon of tibialis posterior,** the **tendon of flexor digitorum longus,** the **posterior tibial vessels,** the **posterior tibial nerve,** and the **tendon of flexor hallucis longus.** The pulsations of the **posterior tibial artery** can be felt halfway between the medial malleolus and the heel (Fig. 10-88). Behind the lateral malleolus are the **tendons of peroneus brevis** and **longus** (Figs. 10-87 and 10-88).

On the anterior surface of the ankle joint, the **tendon of tibialis anterior** can be seen when the foot is dorsiflexed and inverted (Figs. 10-86 and 10-88). The **tendon of extensor hallucis longus** lies lateral to it and can be made to stand out by extending the big toe (Figs. 10-86 and 10-88). Lateral to the extensor hallucis longus lie the **tendons of extensor digitorum longus** and **peroneus tertius.** The pulsations of the **dorsalis pedis artery** can be felt between the tendons of extensor hallucis longus and extensor digitorum longus, midway between the two malleoli on the front of the ankle.

On the posterior surface of the ankle joint, the prominence of the heel is formed by the **calcaneum.** Above the heel is the **tendo calcaneus** (Achilles tendon) (Fig. 10-88).

On the dorsum of the foot, the **head of the talus** can be palpated just in front of the malleoli (Fig. 10-87). The **tendons of extensor digitorum longus** and **extensor hallucis longus** can be made prominent by dorsiflexing the toes (Fig. 10-86).

The **dorsal venous arch** or **plexus** can be seen on the dorsal surface of the foot proximal to the toes (Figs. 10-19 and 10-87). The **great saphenous vein** leaves the medial part of the plexus and passes upward **in front** of the medial malleolus (Fig. 10-87). The **small saphenous vein** drains the lateral part of the plexus and passes up **behind** the lateral malleolus (Fig. 10-19).

On the lateral aspect of the foot, the **peroneal tubercle** of the calcaneum can be palpated about 1 in. (2.5 cm) below and in front of the tip of the lateral malleolus (Fig. 10-86). Above the tubercle, the **tendon of peroneus brevis** passes forward to its insertion on the prominent tuberosity on the

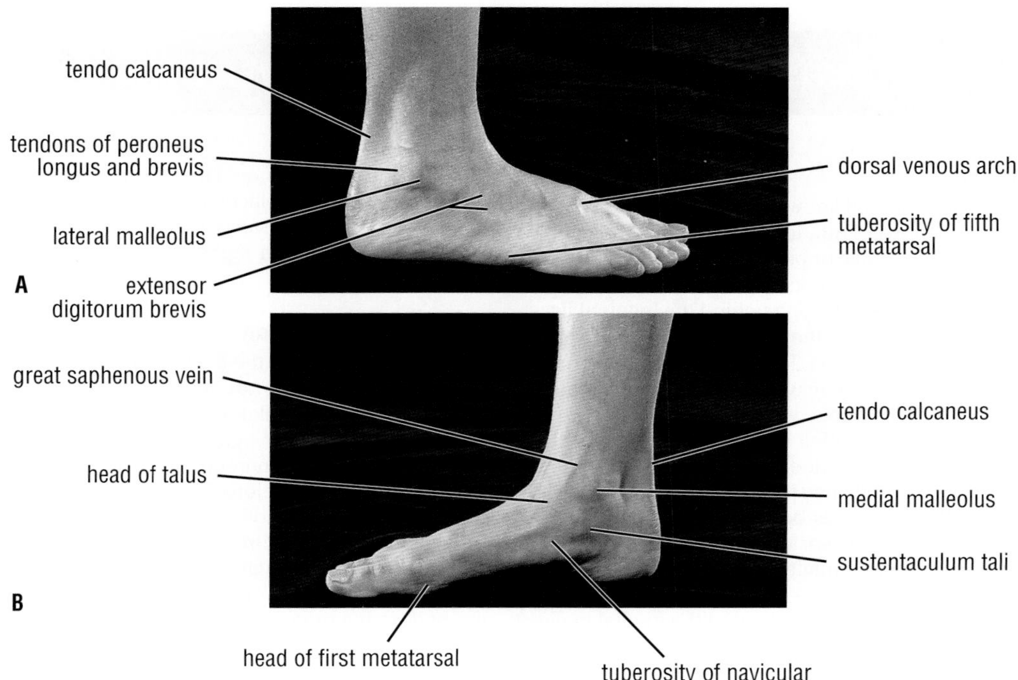

Figure 10-87 Lateral aspect (**A**) and medial aspect (**B**) of the right ankle of a 29-year-old woman.

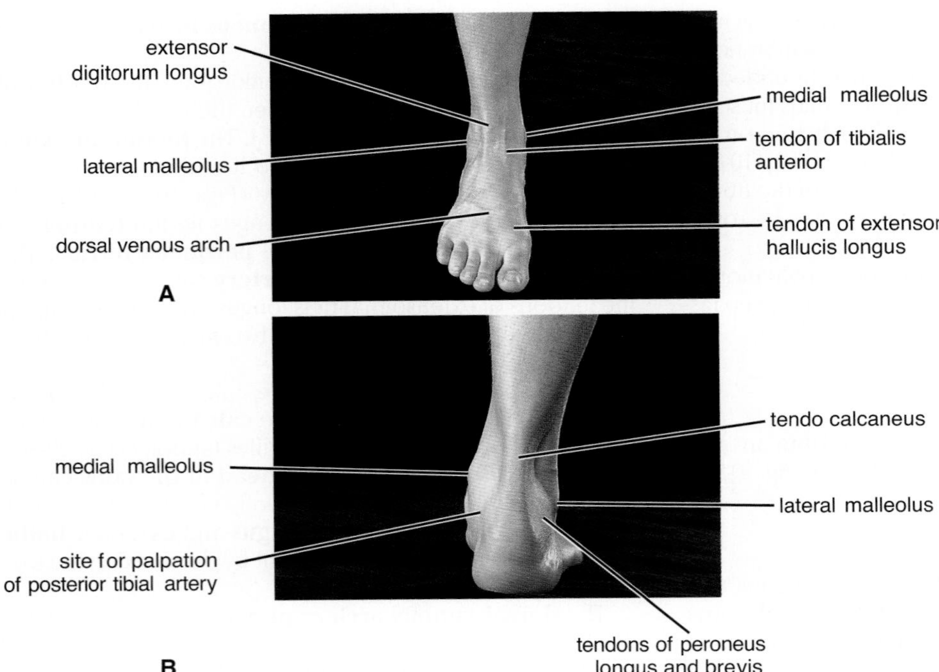

Figure 10-88 Anterior aspect (**A**) and posterior aspect (**B**) of the right foot and ankle of a 29-year-old woman.

base of the **fifth metatarsal bone** (Fig. 10-87). Below the tubercle, the **tendon of peroneus longus** passes forward to enter the groove on the under aspect of the cuboid bone.

On the medial aspect of the foot, the **sustentaculum tali** can be palpated about 1 in. (2.5 cm) below the tip of the medial malleolus (Fig. 10-87). The tendon of tibialis posterior lies immediately above the sustentaculum tali; the tendon of flexor digitorum longus crosses its medial surface; and the tendon of flexor hallucis longus winds around its lower surface.

In front of the sustentaculum tali, the **tuberosity of the navicular bone** can be seen and palpated (Fig. 10-87). It receives the main part of the tendon of insertion of the tibialis posterior muscle.

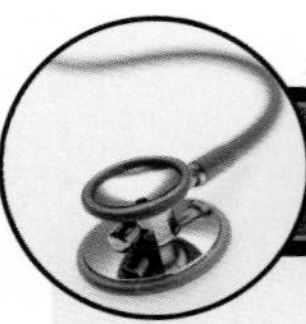

CLINICAL NOTES ON THE ARTERIES OF THE LOWER LIMB

Arterial Palpation

Every health professional should know the precise position of the main arteries within the lower limb, for he or she may be called on to arrest a severe hemorrhage or palpate different parts of the arterial tree in patients with arterial occlusion.

The **femoral artery** enters the thigh behind the inguinal ligament at a point midway between the anterosuperior iliac spine and the symphysis pubis (Fig. 10-84). The artery is easily palpated here because it can be pressed backward against the pectineus and the superior ramus of the pubis.

The **popliteal artery** can be felt by gentle palpation in the depths of the popliteal space provided that the deep fascia is fully relaxed by passively flexing the knee joint (Fig. 10-41).

The **dorsalis pedis artery** lies between the tendons of extensor hallucis longus and extensor digitorum longus, midway between the medial and lateral malleoli on the front of the ankle (Fig. 10-44).

The **posterior tibial artery** passes behind the medial malleolus, and beneath the flexor retinaculum; it lies between the tendons of flexor digitorum longus and flexor hallucis longus. The pulsations of the artery can be felt midway between the medial malleolus and the heel (Fig. 10-49).

It should be remembered that the dorsalis pedis artery is sometimes absent and is replaced by a large perforating branch of the peroneal artery. In the same manner, the peroneal artery may be larger than normal and replace the posterior tibial artery in the lower part of the leg.

Collateral Circulation

If the arterial supply to the leg is occluded, necrosis or gangrene will follow unless an adequate bypass to the obstruction is present—that is, a collateral circulation. Sudden occlusion of the femoral artery by ligature or embolism, for example, is usually followed by gangrene. However, gradual occlusion such as occurs in atherosclerosis is less likely to be followed by necrosis because the collateral blood vessels have time to dilate fully. The collateral circulation for the proximal part of the femoral artery is through the cruciate and trochanteric anastomoses; for the femoral artery in the adductor canal, it is through the perforating branches of the profunda femoris artery and the articular and muscular branches of the femoral and popliteal arteries.

(continues)

Clinical Notes, *continued*

Traumatic Injury

Injury to the large femoral artery can cause rapid exsanguination of the patient. Unlike in the upper extremity, arterial injuries of the lower limb do not have a good prognosis. The collateral circulations around the hip and knee joints, although present, are not as adequate as those around the shoulder and elbow. Damage to a neighboring large vein can further complicate the situation and causes further impairment of the circulation to the distal part of the limb.

Arterial Occlusive Disease of the Leg

Arterial occlusive disease of the leg is common in men. Ischemia of the muscles produces a cramplike pain with exercise. If the femoral artery is obstructed, the supply of blood to the calf muscles is inadequate; the patient is forced to stop walking after a limited distance because of the intensity of the pain. With rest, the oxygen depletion is corrected and the pain disappears. However, on resumption of walking, the pain recurs. This condition is known as **intermittent claudication.**

Sympathetic Innervation of the Arteries

Sympathetic innervation of the arteries to the leg is derived from the lower three thoracic and upper two or three lumbar segments of the spinal cord. The preganglionic fibers pass to the lower thoracic and upper lumbar ganglia via white rami. The fibers synapse in the lumbar and sacral ganglia, and the postganglionic fibers reach the blood vessels via branches of the lumbar and sacral plexuses. The femoral artery receives its sympathetic fibers from the femoral and obturator nerves. The more distal arteries receive their postganglionic fibers via the common peroneal and tibial nerves.

Lumbar Sympathectomy and Occlusive Arterial Disease

Lumbar sympathectomy may be advocated as a form of treatment for occlusive arterial disease of the lower limb to increase blood flow through the collateral circulation. Preganglionic sympathectomy is performed by removing the upper three lumbar ganglia and the intervening parts of the sympathetic trunk.

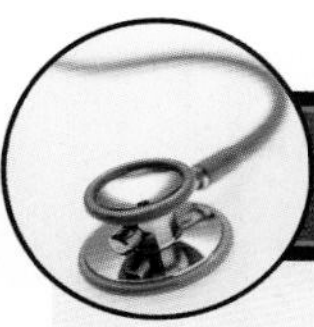

CLINICAL NOTES ON THE NERVES OF THE LOWER LIMB

Tendon Reflexes of the Lower Limb

Skeletal muscles receive a segmental innervation. Most muscles are innervated by two, three, or four spinal nerves and therefore by the same number of segments of the spinal cord. The segmental innervation of the following muscles in the lower limb should be known because it is possible to test them by eliciting simple muscle reflexes in the patient.

- **Patellar tendon reflex** (knee jerk) L2, **3,** and **4** (extension of the knee joint on tapping the patellar tendon)
- **Achilles tendon reflex** (ankle jerk) S**1** and S2 (plantar flexion of the ankle joint on tapping the Achilles tendon)

Femoral Nerve Injury

The femoral nerve (L2, 3, and 4) enters the thigh from behind the inguinal ligament, at a point midway between the anterior superior iliac spine and the pubic tubercle; it lies about a fingerbreadth lateral to the femoral pulse. About 2 in. (5 cm) below the inguinal ligament, the nerve splits into its terminal branches (Fig. 10-28).

The femoral nerve can be injured in stab or gunshot wounds, but a complete division of the nerve is rare. The following clinical features are present when the nerve is completely divided:

- **Motor:** The quadriceps femoris muscle is paralyzed, and the knee cannot be extended. In walking, this is compensated for to some extent by use of the adductor muscles.
- **Sensory:** Skin sensation is lost over the anterior and medial sides of the thigh, over the medial side of the lower part of the leg, and along the medial border of the foot as far as the ball of the big toe; this area is normally supplied by the saphenous nerve.

Sciatic Nerve Injury

The sciatic nerve (L4 and 5 and S1, 2, and 3) curves laterally and downward through the gluteal region, situated at first midway between the posterosuperior iliac spine and the ischial tuberosity, and lower down, midway between the tip of the greater trochanter and the ischial tuberosity. The nerve then passes downward in the midline on the posterior aspect of the thigh and divides into the common peroneal and tibial nerves, at a variable site above the popliteal fossa (Figs. 10-16 and 10-17).

Trauma

The nerve is sometimes injured by penetrating wounds, fractures of the pelvis, or dislocations of the hip joint. It is most frequently injured by badly placed intramuscular injections in the gluteal region. To avoid this injury, injections into the gluteus maximus or the gluteus medius should be made well forward on the upper outer quadrant of the buttock. Most nerve lesions are incomplete, and in 90% of injuries, the common peroneal part of the nerve is the most affected. This can probably be explained by the fact that the common peroneal nerve fibers lie most superficial in the sciatic nerve. The following clinical features are present:

- **Motor:** The hamstring muscles are paralyzed, but weak flexion of the knee is possible because of the action of the sartorius (femoral nerve) and gracilis (obturator nerve). All the muscles below the knee are paralyzed, and the weight of the foot causes it to assume the plantar-flexed position, or **footdrop** (Fig. 10-89).
- **Sensory:** Sensation is lost below the knee, except for a narrow area down the medial side of the lower part of the leg and along the medial border of the foot as far as the ball of the big toe, which is supplied by the saphenous nerve (femoral nerve).

(continues)

Clinical Notes, *continued*

The result of operative repair of a sciatic nerve injury is poor. It is rare for active movement to return to the small muscles of the foot, and sensory recovery is rarely complete. Loss of sensation in the sole of the foot makes the development of trophic ulcers inevitable.

Sciatica

Sciatica describes the condition in which patients have pain along the sensory distribution of the sciatic nerve. Thus, the pain is experienced in the posterior aspect of the thigh, the posterior and lateral sides of the leg, and the lateral part of the foot. Sciatica can be caused by prolapse of an intervertebral disc (see page 858), with pressure on one or more roots of the lower lumbar and sacral spinal nerves, pressure on the sacral plexus or sciatic nerve by an intrapelvic tumor, or inflammation of the sciatic nerve or its terminal branches.

Common Peroneal Nerve Injury

The common peroneal nerve (Fig. 10-16) is in an exposed position as it leaves the popliteal fossa and winds around the neck of the fibula to enter the peroneus longus muscle.

It is commonly injured in fractures of the neck of the fibula and by pressure from casts or splints. The following clinical features are present:

- **Motor:** The muscles of the anterior and lateral compartments of the leg are paralyzed, namely, the tibialis anterior, the extensor digitorum longus and brevis, the peroneus tertius, the extensor hallucis longus (supplied by the deep peroneal nerve), and the peroneus longus and brevis (supplied by the superficial peroneal nerve). As a result, the opposing muscles, the plantar flexors of the ankle joint and the invertors of the subtalar and transverse tarsal joints, cause the foot to be plantar flexed (foot drop) and inverted, an attitude referred to as **equinovarus** (Fig. 10-89).
- **Sensory:** Loss of sensation occurs down the anterior and lateral sides of the leg and dorsum of the foot and toes, including the medial side of the big toe. The lateral border of the foot and the lateral side of the little toe are virtually unaffected (sural nerve, mainly formed from tibial nerve). The medial border of the foot as far as the ball of the big toe is completely unaffected (saphenous nerve, a branch of the femoral nerve).

When the injury occurs distal to the site of origin of the lateral cutaneous nerve of the calf, the loss of sensibility is confined to the area of the foot and toes.

Tibial Nerve Injury

The tibial nerve (Fig. 10-17) leaves the popliteal fossa by passing deep to the gastrocnemius and soleus muscles. Because of its deep and protected position, it is rarely injured. Complete division results in the following clinical features:

- **Motor:** All the muscles in the back of the leg and the sole of the foot are paralyzed. The opposing muscles dorsiflex the foot at the ankle joint and evert the foot at the subtalar and transverse tarsal joints, an attitude referred to as **calcaneovalgus.**
- **Sensory:** Sensation is lost on the sole of the foot; later, trophic ulcers develop.

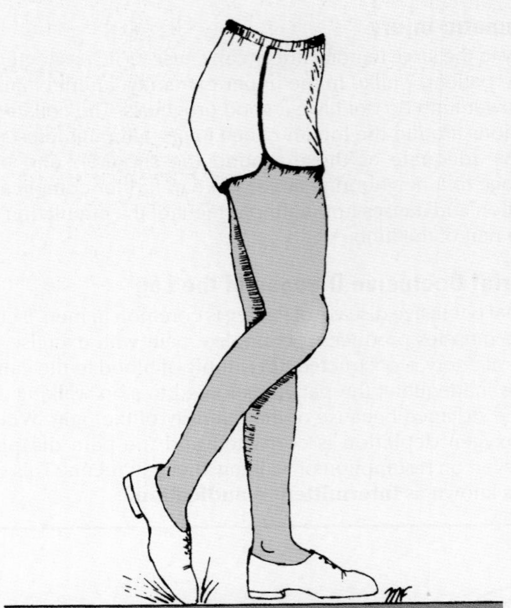

Figure 10-89 Footdrop. With this condition, the individual catches his or her toes on the ground when walking.

Obturator Nerve Injury

The obturator nerve (L2, 3, and 4) enters the thigh as anterior and posterior divisions through the upper part of the obturator foramen. The anterior division descends in front of the obturator externus and the adductor brevis, deep to the floor of the femoral triangle. The posterior division descends behind the adductor brevis and in front of the adductor magnus (Fig. 10-30).

It is rarely injured in penetrating wounds, in anterior dislocations of the hip joint, or in abdominal herniae through the obturator foramen. It may be pressed on by the fetal head during parturition. The following clinical features occur:

- **Motor:** All the adductor muscles are paralyzed except the hamstring part of the adductor magnus, which is supplied by the sciatic nerve.
- **Sensory:** The cutaneous sensory loss is minimal on the medial aspect of the thigh.

CLINICAL PROBLEM SOLVING

Study the following case histories and select the best answers to the question following them.

After a major abdominal operation, a patient was given a course of antibiotics by intramuscular injection. The nurse was instructed to give the injections into the right buttock. Later, when the patient left the hospital, he developed several symptoms and signs that suggested that the injections into the gluteus maximus muscle had been given over the course of the sciatic nerve and had caused a lesion of the common peroneal nerve.

1. The symptoms and signs displayed by this patient included the following except which?
   (a) He experienced numbness and tingling sensations down the anterior and lateral sides of the right leg and the dorsum of the foot.
   (b) His right foot tended to catch on steps and on the edges of the carpet.
   (c) On testing, he had impaired skin sensation on the lateral side of the right thigh.
   (d) The patient tended to hold the foot plantar flexed and slightly inverted.
   (e) Dorsiflexion of the right ankle joint was weaker than the same movement of the left ankle.
   (f) The everter muscles of the right midtarsal joints were weaker than those of the opposite side.

A 45-year-old man complaining of a lump in the groin was seen by his physician. The lump, which caused him no pain or discomfort, was first recognized 3 months previously. On examination, a large discrete hard lump was found about 2 in. (5 cm) below and lateral to the pubic tubercle on the front of the right thigh.

2. The following signs indicated that this patient had a melanoma of the right big toe with secondaries in the inguinal lymph nodes except which?
   (a) Two smaller hard swellings were found immediately below the large swelling.
   (b) On flexing the right knee joint, three small hard swellings could be palpated in the popliteal fossa.
   (c) The external genitalia were found to be normal.
   (d) Examination of the anal canal revealed nothing abnormal.
   (e) A small pigmented mole was discovered beneath the nail of the right big toe.

A 54-year-old woman complaining of abdominal pain and repeated vomiting was seen in the emergency department. On questioning, the patient stated that the pain was severe and colicky in nature and most intense in the region of the umbilicus. On examination, the abdomen was distended, and excessively loud bowel peristaltic sounds could be heard with the stethoscope. A diagnosis of acute intestinal obstruction was made secondary to a left femoral hernia.

3. The following statements concerning this case are correct except which?
   (a) A small, tender, tense swelling was found in the front of the left thigh.
   (b) When the patient was asked to cough, there was no expansion of the swelling in the left thigh.
   (c) The swelling in the left thigh was located below and medial to the left pubic tubercle.
   (d) The hernia had strangulated because of the unyielding nature of the femoral ring.
   (e) A loop of small intestine was forced into the femoral sac and the pain from the small bowel was referred to the umbilicus.
   (f) Venous congestion followed by arterial occlusion of the intestinal loop was responsible for the intestinal obstruction.

A 47-year-old woman complaining of a dull, aching pain in the lower part of both legs visited her physician. She stated that the pain was particularly severe at the end of a long day of standing at her work. On examination, the patient was found to have widespread varicosed veins in both legs.

4. The following symptoms and signs supported the diagnosis except which?
   (a) The patient stated that the skin down the medial side of the leg was irritated, especially in dry weather.
   (b) If the patient coughed in the standing position, a fluid thrill was transmitted from the abdomen to the hand palpating the veins.
   (c) The skin showed marked discoloration over the medial malleoli and was dry and scaly.
   (d) The patient had a large family of six children and the varicosed veins showed improvement during each pregnancy.
   (e) The great and small saphenous veins in both legs were enlarged and elongated.

A 25-year-old man was admitted to the emergency department after an automobile accident. Apart from other superficial injuries, he was found to have a fracture of the middle third of the right femur.

5. The following statements concerning this patient are possible except which?
   (a) The right leg was 2 in. (5 cm) shorter than the left leg.
   (b) A lateral radiograph showed overlap of the fragments, with the distal fragment rotated backward.
   (c) A large amount of force would be necessary to restore the leg to its original length.
   (d) The hamstrings and quadriceps femoris muscles were responsible for the leg shortening.
   (e) The soleus muscle was responsible for the backward rotation of the distal fragment.

A 65-year-old man told his physician that he could walk only about 50 yd. (46 m) before a cramplike pain in his left leg forced him to rest. After a thorough physical examination, a diagnosis of severe intermittent claudication of the left leg was made.

6. The following findings in this patient supported the diagnosis except which?
   (a) His femoral pulses were normal in both legs.

(b) The popliteal, posterior tibial, and dorsalis pedis pulses were present in the right leg and completely absent in the left leg.
(c) Arteriography revealed a blockage of the left femoral artery at the level of the adductor tubercle.
(d) The lower part of the left leg was receiving its blood supply through the muscular and genicular branches of the femoral artery and the muscular and genicular branches of the popliteal artery.
(e) The collateral circulation in the left leg was adequate to prevent gangrene but was insufficient to supply oxygen to the active leg muscles.
(f) The perforating branches of the profunda femoris artery did not participate in the collateral circulation around the blocked femoral artery.

A medical student, while playing football, collided with another player and fell to the ground. As he fell, the right knee, which was taking the weight of his body, was partially flexed; the femur was rotated medially; and the leg was abducted on the thigh. A sudden pain was felt in the right knee joint, and he was unable to extend it. The student was diagnosed as having a torn medial meniscus of the knee joint.

7. The following statements concerning this case confirmed the diagnosis except which?
   (a) The right knee joint quickly became swollen.
   (b) Severe local tenderness was felt along the medial side of the joint line.
   (c) The medial meniscus split along part of its length, and the detached portion became jammed between the articular surfaces, limiting further extension.
   (d) The trauma stimulated the production of synovial fluid, which filled the joint cavity.
   (e) The distention of the suprapatellar bursa was responsible for the large amount of swelling above the injured knee.
   (f) The pain sensation from the injured knee was confined to the femoral nerve as it ascended to the central nervous system.

A 27-year-old woman was found to have an unstable right knee joint following a severe automobile accident. On examination, it was possible to pull the tibia excessively forward on the femur. A diagnosis of ruptured anterior cruciate ligament was made.

8. The following statements concerning this patient are correct except which?
   (a) The anterior cruciate ligament is attached to the tibia in the anterior part of the intercondylar area.
   (b) The anterior cruciate ligament passes upward, backward, and laterally from its tibial attachment.
   (c) The anterior cruciate ligament is attached above to the posterior part of the medial surface of the lateral femoral condyle.
   (d) The anterior cruciate ligament is more commonly torn than is the posterior cruciate ligament.
   (e) Because the cruciate ligaments are located outside the synovial membrane, bleeding from a torn ligament does not enter the joint cavity.

An 18-year-old woman was running across some rough ground when she stumbled and overinverted her left foot. On examination in the emergency department of the local hospital, the lateral side of the left ankle was tender and swollen. A small area of great tenderness was found below and in front of the lateral malleolus. X-ray examination of the ankle joint was negative. A diagnosis of sprain of the left ankle was made.

9. The following statements concerning this patient are correct except which?
   (a) The movement of inversion of the foot takes place at the ankle joint.
   (b) Overinversion places a strain on the lateral ligaments of the ankle joint.
   (c) The localized tenderness felt below and in front of the lateral malleolus would indicate that some of the fibers of the anterior talofibular ligament had been torn.
   (d) The resulting hemorrhage from the torn ligament was responsible for the swelling in the area.
   (e) By immobilizing the ankle joint with adequate splinting, the torn fibers of the anterior talofibular ligament are repaired with new fibrous tissue.

A 25-year-old man was running across a field when he caught his right foot in a rabbit hole. As he fell, the right foot was violently rotated laterally and overeverted. On attempting to stand, he could place no weight on his right foot. On examination by a physician, the right ankle was considerably swollen, especially on the lateral side. After further examination, including a radiograph of the ankle, a diagnosis of severe fracture dislocation of the ankle joint was made.

10. The following statements concerning this patient are correct except which?
    (a) This type of fracture dislocation is caused by forced external rotation and overeversion of the foot.
    (b) The talus is externally rotated against the lateral malleolus of the fibula causing it to fracture.
    (c) The torsion effect on the lateral malleolus produces a spiral fracture.
    (d) The medial ligament of the ankle joint is strong and never ruptures.
    (e) If the talus is forced to move farther laterally and continues to rotate, the posterior inferior margin of the tibia will be sheared off.

A 54-year-old man was told by his physician to reduce his weight. He was prescribed a diet and was advised to exercise more. One morning while jogging, he heard a sharp snap and felt a sudden pain in his right lower calf. On examination in the emergency department, the physician noted that the upper part of the right calf was swollen and a gap was apparent between the swelling and the heel. A diagnosis of rupture of the right Achilles tendon was made.

11. The following statements concerning this patient are correct except which?
    (a) With the patient supine, gentle squeezing of the upper part of the right calf did not produce plantar flexion of the ankle joint.

(b) The Achilles tendon is the tendon of insertion of the gastrocnemius and soleus muscles.
(c) The Achilles tendon is inserted into the posterior surface of the talus.
(d) Rupture of the Achilles tendon results in the bellies of the gastrocnemius and soleus muscles retracting upward, leaving a gap between the divided ends of the tendon.
(e) Normally, the gastrocnemius and soleus muscles are the main muscles responsible for plantar flexion of the ankle joint.

A 17-year-old girl was dealing drugs on a street corner when she became involved in a fight. During the brawl she received a deep knife wound to the front of her right thigh. After a thorough examination in the emergency department of the local hospital, it was determined that the knife point had severed the trunk of the right femoral nerve just below the inguinal ligament.

12. This patient had the following signs and symptoms except which?
    (a) The right quadriceps femoris muscle failed to contract when the patient was asked to extend her right knee joint.
    (b) Skin sensation was lost over the anterior and medial sides of the thigh.
    (c) Skin sensation was lost along the medial border of the big toe.
    (d) Skin sensation was lost on the lower part of the leg and the medial border of the foot as far as the ball of the big toe.
    (e) Weak extension of the knee was possible when walking because of the use of the adductor muscles.

ANSWERS TO CLINICAL PROBLEMS

1. C. The skin on the lateral side of the thigh is innervated by the lateral cutaneous nerve of the thigh (L2 and L3), a branch of the lumbar plexus.
2. B. Melanomas, which are highly malignant tumors, tend to initially spread via the lymph vessels to the local lymph nodes. These become enlarged and firm on palpation. The lymphatic drainage of the big toe is into the vertical group of superficial inguinal lymph nodes.
3. C. The swelling of the femoral hernia is always located below and lateral to the pubic tubercle.
4. D. During the later months of pregnancy, the enlarged uterus presses on the inferior vena cava and impedes the venous return from the lower limbs. This condition results in a worsening of preexisting varicosed veins.
5. E. The gastrocnemius muscle is responsible for the backward rotation of the distal fragment of the fractured femur.
6. F. The profunda femoris artery arises from the femoral artery about 1.5 in. (3.8 cm) below the inguinal ligament. It plays a major role in the formation of the collateral circulation around the knee joint.
7. F. The sensation of pain from the knee joint ascends to the central nervous system via the femoral, obturator, common peroneal, and tibial nerves.
8. E. The synovial membrane covering the cruciate ligaments is torn along with the ligaments, and the joint cavity quickly fills with blood.
9. A. Normally, the movements of inversion and eversion of the foot take place at the subtalar and transverse tarsal joints of the foot.
10. D. Although the medial ligament of the ankle joint is strong, extreme force can result in rupture of the ligament, or the ligament can be torn from the medial malleolus, or the pull on the ligament can fracture the medial malleolus.
11. C. The Achilles tendon is inserted into the posterior surface of the calcaneum.
12. C. The skin covering the medial border of the big toe is innervated by the superficial peroneal nerve.

REVIEW QUESTIONS

Multiple-Choice Questions

Select the best answer for each question.

1. Which of the following nerves innervates at least one muscle that acts on both the hip and knee joints?
    (a) Ilioinguinal nerve
    (b) Femoral nerve
    (c) Saphenous nerve
    (d) Common peroneal nerve
    (e) Superficial peroneal nerve
2. In walking, the hip bone of the suspended leg is raised by which of the following muscles acting on the supported side of the body?
    (a) Gluteus maximus
    (b) Obturator internus
    (c) Gluteus medius
    (d) Obturator externus
    (e) Quadratus femoris
3. Which of the following muscles is a flexor of the thigh?
    (a) Superior gemellus
    (b) Adductor longus

(c) Gracilis
(d) Psoas
(e) Obturator internus

4. Which of the following muscles dorsiflexes the foot at the ankle joint?
(a) Peroneus longus
(b) Extensor digitorum brevis
(c) Tibialis posterior
(d) Extensor hallucis brevis
(e) Tibialis anterior

Completion Questions

Select the phrase that best completes each statement.

5. A femoral hernia descends through the femoral canal, and the neck of the sac lies
(a) below and lateral to the pubic tubercle.
(b) above and medial to the pubic tubercle.
(c) at the saphenous opening.
(d) in the obturator canal.
(e) lateral to the iliacus muscle.

6. The peroneal artery is a branch of the
(a) anterior tibial artery.
(b) popliteal artery.
(c) posterior tibial artery.
(d) arcuate artery.
(e) lateral plantar artery.

7. Unlocking of the knee joint to permit flexion is caused by the action of the
(a) vastus medialis muscle.
(b) articularis genu muscle.
(c) gastrocnemius muscle.
(d) biceps femoris muscle.
(e) popliteus muscle.

8. In the adult, the chief arterial supply to the head of the femur is from the
(a) superior circumflex iliac artery.
(b) obturator artery.
(c) branches from the medial and lateral circumflex femoral arteries.
(d) deep external pudendal artery.
(e) inferior gluteal artery.

9. The lymph drainage of the skin covering the ball of the big toe is into the
(a) vertical group of superficial inguinal nodes.
(b) popliteal nodes.
(c) horizontal group of superficial inguinal nodes.
(d) axillary nodes.
(e) internal iliac nodes.

10. The lymph drainage of the skin covering the medial side of the knee joint is into the
(a) popliteal nodes.
(b) internal iliac nodes.
(c) vertical group of superficial inguinal nodes.
(d) horizontal group of superficial inguinal nodes.
(e) obturator nodes.

11. The lymph drainage of the skin of the buttock is into the
(a) axillary nodes.
(b) superior gluteal nodes.
(c) vertical group of superficial inguinal nodes.
(d) horizontal group of superficial inguinal nodes.
(e) internal iliac nodes.

12. The lymph drainage of the skin of the calf is into the
(a) vertical group of superficial inguinal nodes.
(b) internal iliac nodes.
(c) horizontal group of superficial inguinal nodes.
(d) popliteal nodes.
(e) obturator nodes.

13. Hyperextension of the hip joint is prevented by the
(a) obturator internus tendon.
(b) ischiofemoral ligament.
(c) tensor fascia latae muscle.
(d) iliotibial tract.
(e) ligamentum teres.

Fill-in-the-Blank Questions

Fill in the blank with the best answer.

14. The ________ prevents dislocation of the femur backward at the knee joint.
(a) posterior cruciate ligament
(b) anterior cruciate ligament
(c) medial collateral ligament
(d) lateral collateral ligament
(e) tendon of the popliteus muscle

15. The ________ prevents abduction of the tibia at the knee joint.
(a) posterior cruciate ligament
(b) anterior cruciate ligament
(c) lateral collateral ligament
(d) lateral meniscus
(e) medial collateral ligament

16. The ________ is attached to the head of the fibula.
(a) lateral meniscus
(b) lateral collateral ligament
(c) anterior cruciate ligament
(d) posterior cruciate ligament
(e) medial meniscus

Multiple-Choice Questions

Select the best answer for each question.

17. The calcaneum participates in the formation of which arch(es) of the foot?
(a) Medial longitudinal arch only
(b) Medial and lateral longitudinal arches
(c) Transverse arch only
(d) Medial longitudinal and transverse arches
(e) Lateral longitudinal and transverse arches

18. The talus participates in the formation of which arch(es) of the foot?
(a) Transverse arch only
(b) Lateral longitudinal arch only
(c) Medial longitudinal arch only
(d) Medial and lateral longitudinal arches
(e) Transverse and medial longitudinal arches

19. The cuboid participates in the formation of which arch(es) of the foot?
(a) Medial longitudinal arch only
(b) Lateral longitudinal arch only

(c) Transverse arch only
(d) Medial longitudinal and transverse arches
(e) Lateral longitudinal and transverse arches

20. The sesamoid bones under the head of the first metatarsal bone participate in the formation of which arch(es) of the foot?
(a) Lateral longitudinal arch only
(b) Medial longitudinal arch only
(c) Medial longitudinal and transverse arches
(d) Transverse arch only
(e) Lateral longitudinal and transverse arches

21. The following statements concerning the dorsalis pedis artery are correct except which?
(a) It is a continuation of the anterior tibial artery.
(b) It enters the sole of the foot by passing between the two heads of the first dorsal interosseous muscle.
(c) It can be palpated on the foot between the tendons of tibialis anterior and the extensor hallucis longus muscles.
(d) It joins the lateral plantar artery.
(e) On its lateral side lies the terminal part of the deep peroneal nerve.

22. The following structures contribute to the boundaries of the popliteal fossa except which?
(a) The semimembranosus muscle
(b) The plantaris
(c) The biceps femoris muscle
(d) The medial head of the gastrocnemius muscle
(e) The soleus

23. The following structures pass through the greater sciatic foramen except which?
(a) The superior gluteal artery
(b) The sciatic nerve
(c) The obturator internus tendon
(d) The pudendal nerve
(e) The inferior gluteal vein

24. The femoral ring is bounded by the following structures except which?
(a) The femoral vein
(b) The lacunar ligament
(c) The superior ramus of the pubis
(d) The femoral artery
(e) The inguinal ligament

25. The following structures pass through the subsartorial canal except which?
(a) The posterior division of the obturator nerve
(b) The nerve to vastus lateralis
(c) The femoral artery
(d) The saphenous nerve
(e) The femoral vein

26. The floor of the femoral triangle is formed by the following muscles except which?
(a) The pectineus
(b) The adductor longus
(c) The iliacus
(d) The psoas
(e) The adductor brevis

27. The following statements concerning the ankle joint are correct except which?
(a) It is strengthened by the deltoid (medial collateral) ligament.
(b) It is a hinge joint.
(c) It is formed by the articulation of the talus and the distal ends of the tibia and the fibula.
(d) It is most stable in the fully plantar-flexed position.
(e) It is a synovial joint.

28. The foot is inverted by the following muscles except which?
(a) The tibialis anterior
(b) The extensor hallucis longus
(c) The extensor digitorum longus
(d) The peroneus tertius
(e) The tibialis posterior

Read the case histories and select the best answer to the question following them.

A 58-year-old businessman flew to Korea from New York by plane. Except for infrequent visits to the toilet, he remained in his seat sleeping or reading. Toward the end of the long flight, he experienced mild cramplike pain in his right calf. On feeling his leg, he found it to be tender but thought nothing more about it. On reaching his destination, he was walking down the ramp from the plane, when he suddenly collapsed with severe pain in his left chest and was experiencing extreme respiratory distress. The airport physician made the diagnosis of pulmonary embolism, secondary to deep vein thrombosis of the right calf.

29. The blood clot (embolus) reached the left lung via the following blood vessels except which?
(a) The right popliteal vein
(b) The right common iliac vein
(c) The inferior vena cava
(d) The pulmonary trunk
(e) The left pulmonary vein

A 65-year-old woman suddenly woke up in bed with excruciating pain in the left calf. After about 20 minutes, the pain diminished, leaving the calf very tender to touch. On placing her left foot on the ground, she experienced further pain in her calf. After conducting a thorough examination, her physician noted that the upper third of the left calf was very tender on deep palpation and that there was a blue skin discoloration in the lower third of the leg alongside the Achilles tendon. A diagnosis of torn muscle fibers in the left calf was made.

30. In view of the history and the clinical findings, the most likely muscle to have been torn in this patient was the
(a) soleus.
(b) flexor digitorum longus.
(c) flexor hallucis longus.
(d) popliteus.
(e) tibialis posterior.

ANSWERS TO REVIEW QUESTIONS

1. B. The femoral nerve innervates the rectus femoris muscle.
2. C. The gluteus medius muscle acts with the gluteus minimus muscle to raise the pelvis on the opposite side.
3. D
4. E
5. A
6. C
7. E. The rotatory action of the popliteus muscle slackens the ligaments of the extended knee joint, thus permitting flexion to take place.
8. C. Since the epiphyseal plate is no longer present in the neck of the femur, branches from the medial and lateral circumflex femoral arteries can ascend through the femoral neck to the head of the femur.
9. A. The lymphatic vessels follow the course of the great saphenous vein.
10. C
11. D
12. D. The lymphatic vessels follow the course of the small saphenous vein.
13. B
14. B
15. E
16. B
17. B
18. C
19. E
20. B
21. C. The dorsalis pedis artery can be palpated on the dorsum of the foot as it lies between the tendons of the extensor hallucis longus and the most medial tendon of the extensor digitorum longus muscle; it can also be palpated midway between the medial and lateral malleoli on the front of the ankle.
22. E
23. C
24. D
25. B
26. E
27. D
28. D
29. E
30. A

CHAPTER 11

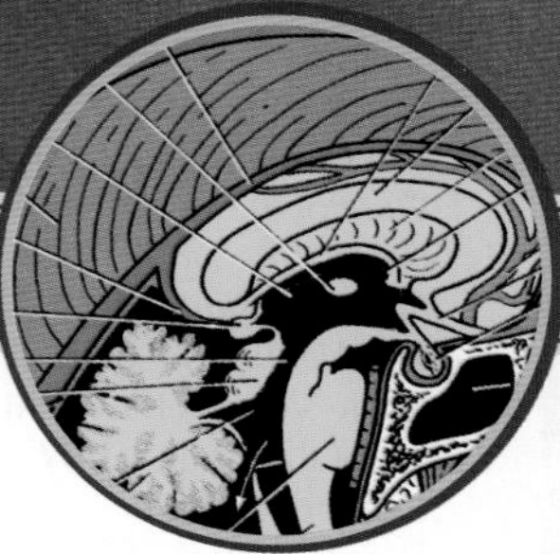

THE HEAD AND NECK

A 58-year-old woman woke up one morning to find that the right side of her face felt "peculiar and heavy." On looking in the mirror, she saw that the corner of her mouth on the right side was drooping and her right lower eyelid seemed to be lower than her left. When she attempted to smile, the right side of her face remained immobile and boardlike. While eating her breakfast, she noticed that her food tended to stick on the inside of her right cheek. On taking her dog for a walk, she found to her amazement that she could not whistle for his return to her side; her lips just would not pucker.

When examined by her physician, she was found to have paralysis of the muscles of the entire right side of the face. She talked with a slightly slurred speech and her blood pressure was very high. To make the diagnosis, the physician had to have knowledge of the facial muscles, the laryngeal muscles, and their nerve supply. The facial paralysis, slurred speech, high blood pressure, and absence of any other abnormal findings suggested a diagnosis of a left-sided cerebral hemorrhage (stroke), secondary to high blood pressure. However, because a left-sided cerebral hemorrhage would cause paralysis of only the muscles of the lower part of the right side of the face, this was not the diagnosis.

This patient had paralysis of the muscles of the entire right side of the face; this could only be caused by a lesion of the right facial nerve, which supplies the muscles. Fortunately, this patient was suffering from Bell's palsy, the prognosis was excellent, and she had a complete recovery.

CHAPTER OUTLINE

Basic Anatomy 669
The Head 669
Bones of the Skull 669
Composition 669
External Views of the Skull 670
The Cranial Cavity 674
Vault of the Skull 674
Base of the Skull 675
Neonatal Skull 677
The Meninges 681
The Venous Blood Sinuses 686
Parts of the Brain 687
Cerebrum 687
Diencephalon 687
Midbrain 689
Hindbrain 689
Ventricles of the Brain 690
Blood Supply of the Brain 690
The Cranial Nerves in the Cranial Cavity 691
The Orbital Region 691
Eyelids 691
Lacrimal Apparatus 694
The Orbit 695
Description 695
Openings Into the Orbital Cavity 696
Orbital Fascia 697
Nerves of the Orbit 697
Blood Vessels and Lymph Vessels of the Orbit 698
The Eye 699
Movements of the Eyeball 699
Extrinsic Muscles Producing Movement of the Eye 699
Intrinsic Muscles 702
Fascial Sheath of the Eyeball 702
Structure of the Eye 702
Coats of the Eyeball 703
Contents of the Eyeball 704
The Ear 706
External Ear 706
Middle Ear (Tympanic Cavity) 706
The Internal Ear, or Labyrinth 714
The Mandible 715
Temporomandibular Joint 715
The Scalp 722
The Face 727
Skin of the Face 727
Sensory Nerves of the Face 727
Arterial Supply of the Face 729
Venous Drainage of the Face 730
Lymph Drainage of the Face 730
Bones of the Face 731
Muscles of the Face (Muscles of Facial Expression) 731
Facial Nerve 732
Development of the Face 734
The Neck 735
Skin of the Neck 736
Superficial Fascia 737
Bones of the Neck 739
Cervical Vertebrae 739
Hyoid Bone 739
Muscles of the Neck 739
Deep Cervical Fascia 743
Cervical Ligaments 747
Muscular Triangles of the Neck 747
Arteries of the Head and Neck 747
Common Carotid Artery 747
Carotid Sinus 747
Carotid Body 747
External Carotid Artery 748
Internal Carotid Artery 750
Circle of Willis 751
Subclavian Arteries 751
Veins of the Head and Neck 752
Veins of the Brain 752
Venous Sinuses 752
Veins of the Face and Neck 752
Internal Jugular Vein 752
Subclavian Vein 753
Lymph Drainage of the Head and Neck 754
Cranial Nerves 757
Clinical Testing of the Cranial Nerves 769
Main Nerves of the Neck 771
Cervical Plexus 771
Brachial Plexus 771
The Autonomic Nervous System in the Head and Neck 773
The Digestive System in the Head and Neck 774
The Mouth 774
The Lips 774
The Mouth Cavity 774
Sensory Innervation of the Mouth 776
The Teeth 778
The Tongue 778
The Palate 781
Hard Palate 781
Soft Palate 781
The Salivary Glands 787
Parotid Gland 787
Submandibular Gland 789
Sublingual Gland 789
The Pharynx 789
Muscles of the Pharynx 789
Interior of the Pharynx 789
Sensory Nerve Supply of the Pharyngeal Mucous Membrane 793
Blood Supply of the Pharynx 793
Lymph Drainage of the Pharynx 793
The Process of Swallowing (Deglutition) 795
Palatine Tonsils 795
Waldeyer's Ring of Lymphoid Tissue 795
The Esophagus 795
The Respiratory System in the Head and Neck 795
The Nose 795
External Nose 795
Nasal Cavity 796
The Paranasal Sinuses 799
Crossing of Air and Food Pathways in the Pharynx 802
The Larynx 802
Cartilages of the Larynx 802
Membranes and Ligaments of the Larynx 802
Inlet of the Larynx 805
Laryngeal Folds 805
Cavity of the Larynx 805
Muscles of the Larynx 805
Movements of the Vocal Folds (Cords) 805
Sphincteric Function of the Larynx 806
Voice Production in the Larynx 806
Mucous Membrane of the Larynx 807
Nerve Supply of the Larynx 807
Blood Supply of the Larynx 807
Lymph Drainage of the Larynx 807
The Trachea 810
Description 810
Relations of the Trachea in the Neck 810
Nerve Supply of the Trachea 811
Blood Supply of the Trachea 811
Lymph Drainage of the Trachea 811
Endocrine Glands in the Head and Neck 815
Pituitary Gland (Hypophysis Cerebri) 815
Location and Description 815
Relations 815
Blood Supply 815
Pineal Gland 816
Location and Description 816
Thyroid Gland 817
Location and Description 817
Blood Supply 818
Lymph Drainage 818
Nerve Supply 818
Parathyroid Glands 821
Location and Description 821
Blood Supply 821
Lymph Drainage 821
Nerve Supply 821
The Root of the Neck 822
Muscles of the Root of the Neck 822
Subclavian Artery 822
Subclavian Vein 824
The Thoracic Duct 824

Radiographic Anatomy 824
Radiographic Appearance of the Head and Neck 824
Radiographic Appearance of the Skull 824
Cerebral Angiography 824
Computed Tomography Scans 824
Magnetic Resonance Imaging 824
Surface Anatomy 824
Surface Landmarks of the Head 824
Surface Landmarks of the Neck 839
Clinical Problem Solving 843
Answers to Clinical Problems 846
Review Questions 847
Answers to Review Questions 850

CHAPTER OBJECTIVES

- Head injuries from blunt trauma and penetrating missiles are associated with high mortality and severe disability. Headaches are usually caused by nonserious conditions such as sinusitis or neuralgia; however, they can represent the earliest manifestations of a life-threatening disease.
- Facial, scalp, and mouth injuries are commonly encountered in practice and vary in seriousness from a small skin laceration to major maxillofacial trauma. Even an untreated boil on the side of the nose can be life-threatening. Facial paralysis and unequal pupils may indicate the existence of a serious neurologic deficit.
- Many vital structures are present in the neck. Injuries or pressure on the larynx or trachea can compromise the airway. Swellings can indicate the existence of a tumor of the thyroid gland or the presence of a malignant secondary lesion in a lymph node.
- Clearly, many signs and symptoms related to the region of the head and neck are determined by the anatomic arrangement of the various structures. This chapter discusses the basic anatomy of this complicated region and highlights the clinical relevance of the structures considered. It specifically excludes consideration of the detailed structure of the brain, which is covered in a neurology text.

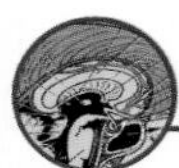

Basic Anatomy

The head and neck region of the body contains many important structures compressed into a relatively small area.

The Head

The head is formed mainly by the skull with the brain and its covering meninges enclosed in the cranial cavity. The special senses, the eye and the ear, lie within the skull bones or in the cavities bounded by them. The brain gives rise to 12 pairs of cranial nerves, which leave the brain and pass through foramina and fissures in the skull. All the cranial nerves are distributed to structures in the head and neck, except the 10th, which also supplies structures in the chest and abdomen.

Bones of the Skull

Composition

The skull is composed of several separate bones united at immobile joints called **sutures.** The connective tissue between the bones is called a **sutural ligament.** The mandible is an exception to this rule, for it is united to the skull by the mobile temporomandibular joint (see page 715).

The bones of the skull can be divided into those of the cranium and those of the face. The **vault** is the upper part of the cranium, and the **base of the skull** is the lowest part of the cranium (Fig. 11-1).

The skull bones are made up of **external** and **internal tables** of compact bone separated by a layer of spongy bone called the **diploë** (Fig. 11-2). The internal table is thinner and more brittle than the external table. The bones are covered on the outer and inner surfaces with periosteum.

The **cranium** consists of the following bones, two of which are paired (Figs. 11-3 and 11-4):

- Frontal bone: 1
- Parietal bones: 2
- Occipital bone: 1
- Temporal bones: 2
- Sphenoid bone: 1
- Ethmoid bone: 1

The **facial bones** consist of the following, two of which are single:

- Zygomatic bones: 2
- Maxillae: 2
- Nasal bones: 2
- Lacrimal bones: 2
- Vomer: 1
- Palatine bones: 2
- Inferior conchae: 2
- Mandible: 1

It is unnecessary for students of medicine to know the detailed structure of each individual skull bone. However,

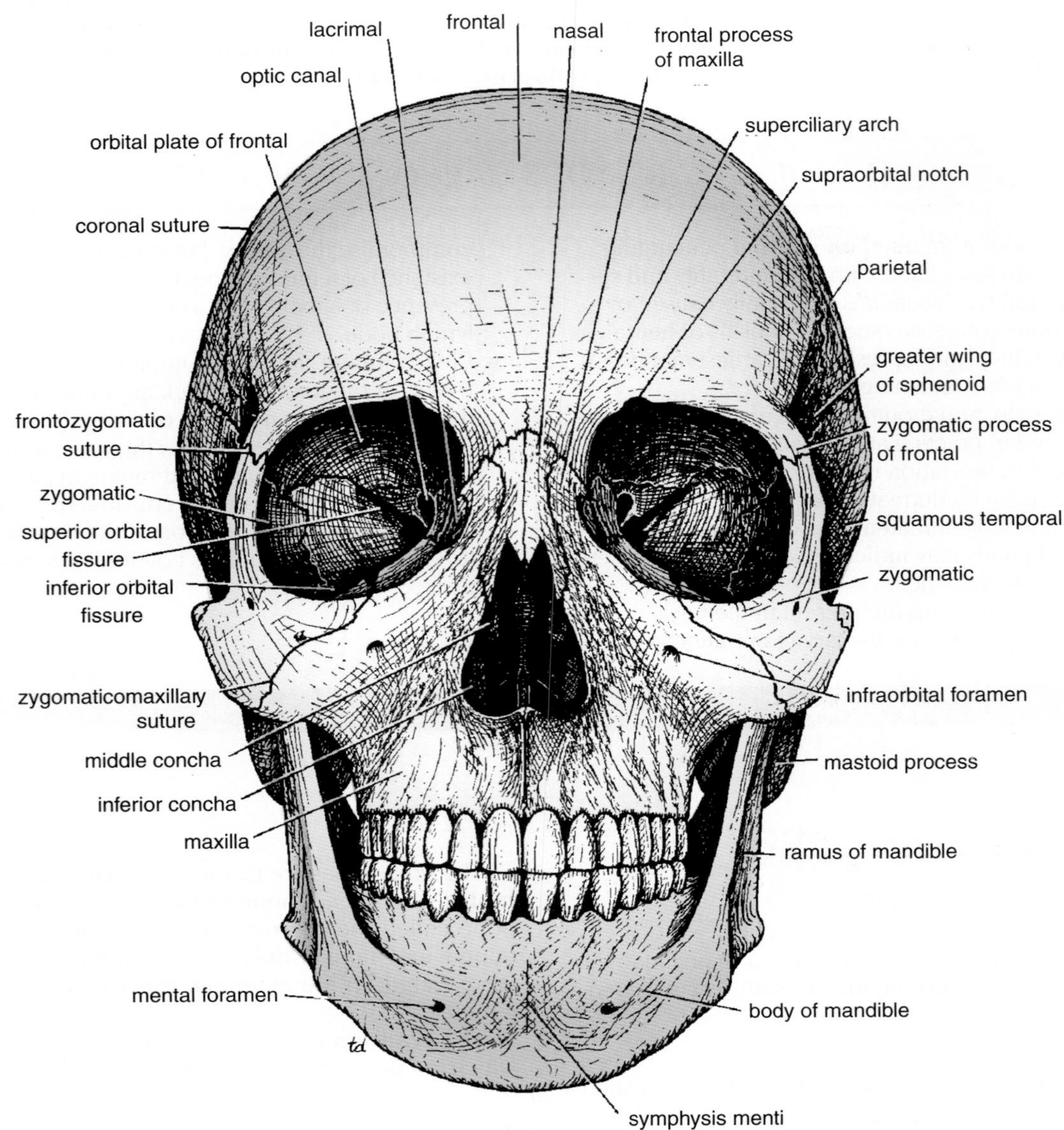

Figure 11-1 Bones of the anterior aspect of the skull.

students should be familiar with the skull as a whole and should have a dried skull available for reference as they read the following description.

External Views of the Skull

Anterior View of the Skull

The **frontal bone,** or forehead bone, curves downward to make the upper margins of the orbits (Fig. 11-1). The **superciliary arches** can be seen on either side, and the **supraorbital notch,** or **foramen,** can be recognized. Medially, the frontal bone articulates with the frontal processes of the maxillae and with the nasal bones. Laterally, the frontal bone articulates with the zygomatic bone.

The **orbital margins** are bounded by the frontal bone superiorly, the zygomatic bone laterally, the maxilla inferiorly, and the processes of the maxilla and frontal bone medially.

Within the **frontal bone,** just above the orbital margins, are two hollow spaces lined with mucous membrane called the **frontal air sinuses.** These communicate with the nose and serve as voice resonators.

The **two nasal bones** form the bridge of the nose. Their lower borders, with the maxillae, make the **anterior nasal aperture.** The nasal cavity is divided into two by the bony nasal septum, which is largely formed by the **vomer.** The **superior** and **middle conchae** are shelves of bone that project into the nasal cavity from the **ethmoid** on each side; the **inferior conchae** are separate bones.

The two **maxillae** form the upper jaw, the anterior part of the hard palate, part of the lateral walls of the nasal cavities, and part of the floors of the orbital cavities. The two bones meet in the midline at the **intermaxillary suture** and form the lower margin of the nasal aperture. Below the orbit, the maxilla is perforated by the **infraorbital foramen.** The

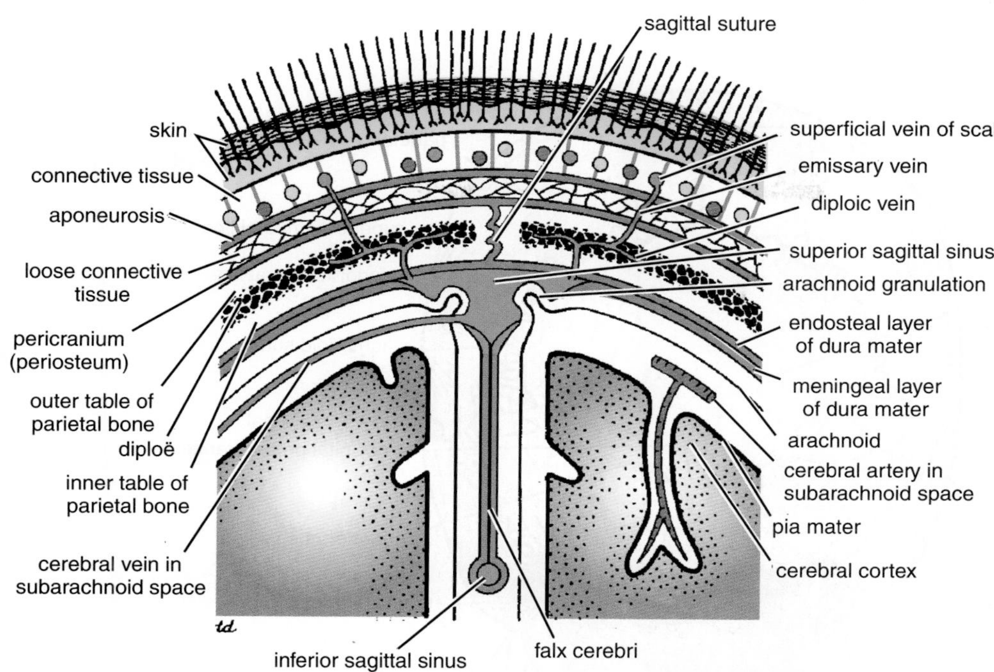

Figure 11-2 Coronal section of the upper part of the head showing the layers of the scalp, the sagittal suture of the skull, the falx cerebri, the superior and inferior sagittal venous sinuses, the arachnoid granulations, the emissary veins, and the relation of cerebral blood vessels to the subarachnoid space.

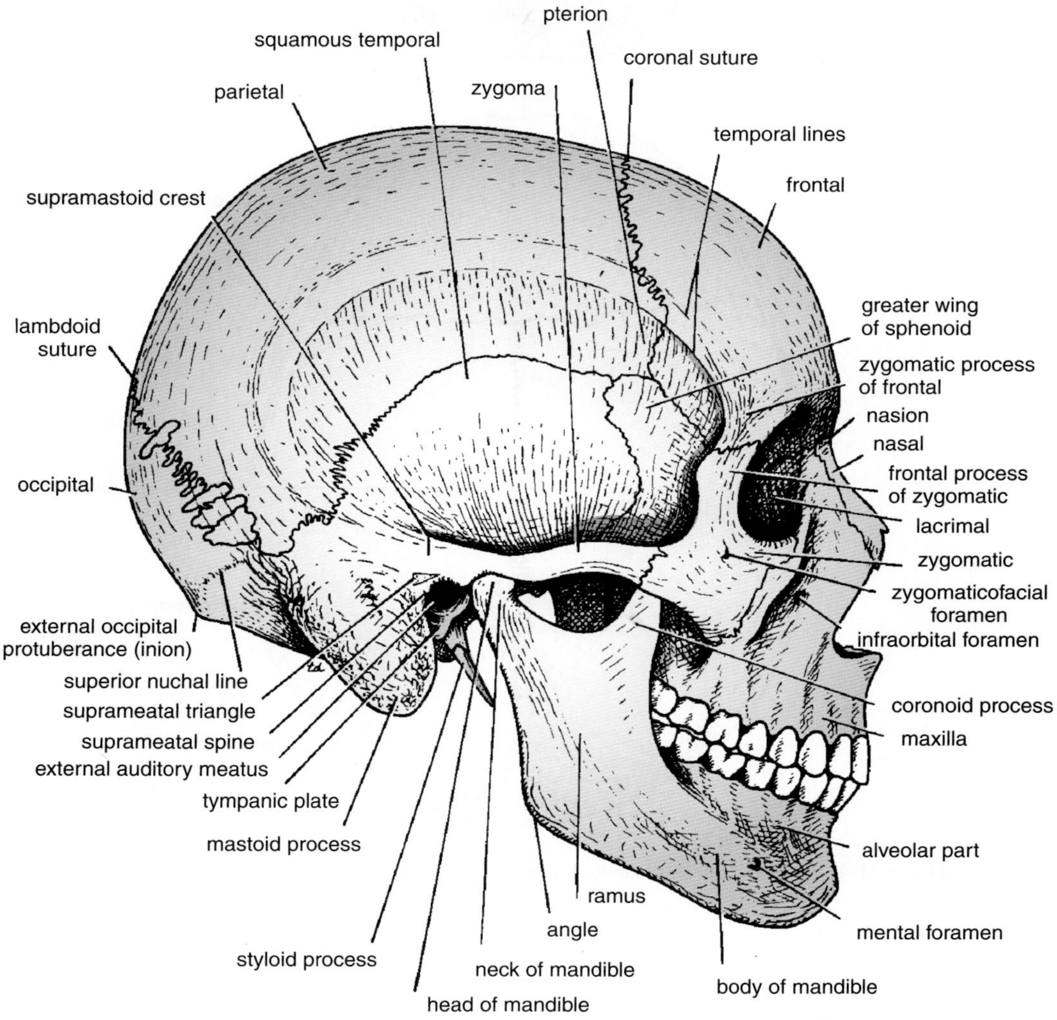

pterion
squamous temporal
coronal suture
parietal
zygoma
temporal lines
frontal
supramastoid crest
greater wing of sphenoid
lambdoid suture
zygomatic process of frontal
nasion
nasal
occipital
frontal process of zygomatic
lacrimal
zygomatic
zygomaticofacial foramen
external occipital protuberance (inion)
infraorbital foramen
superior nuchal line
td
suprameatal triangle
coronoid process
suprameatal spine
maxilla
external auditory meatus
tympanic plate
mastoid process
alveolar part
ramus
mental foramen
angle
styloid process
neck of mandible
body of mandible
head of mandible

Figure 11-3 Bones of the lateral aspect of the skull.

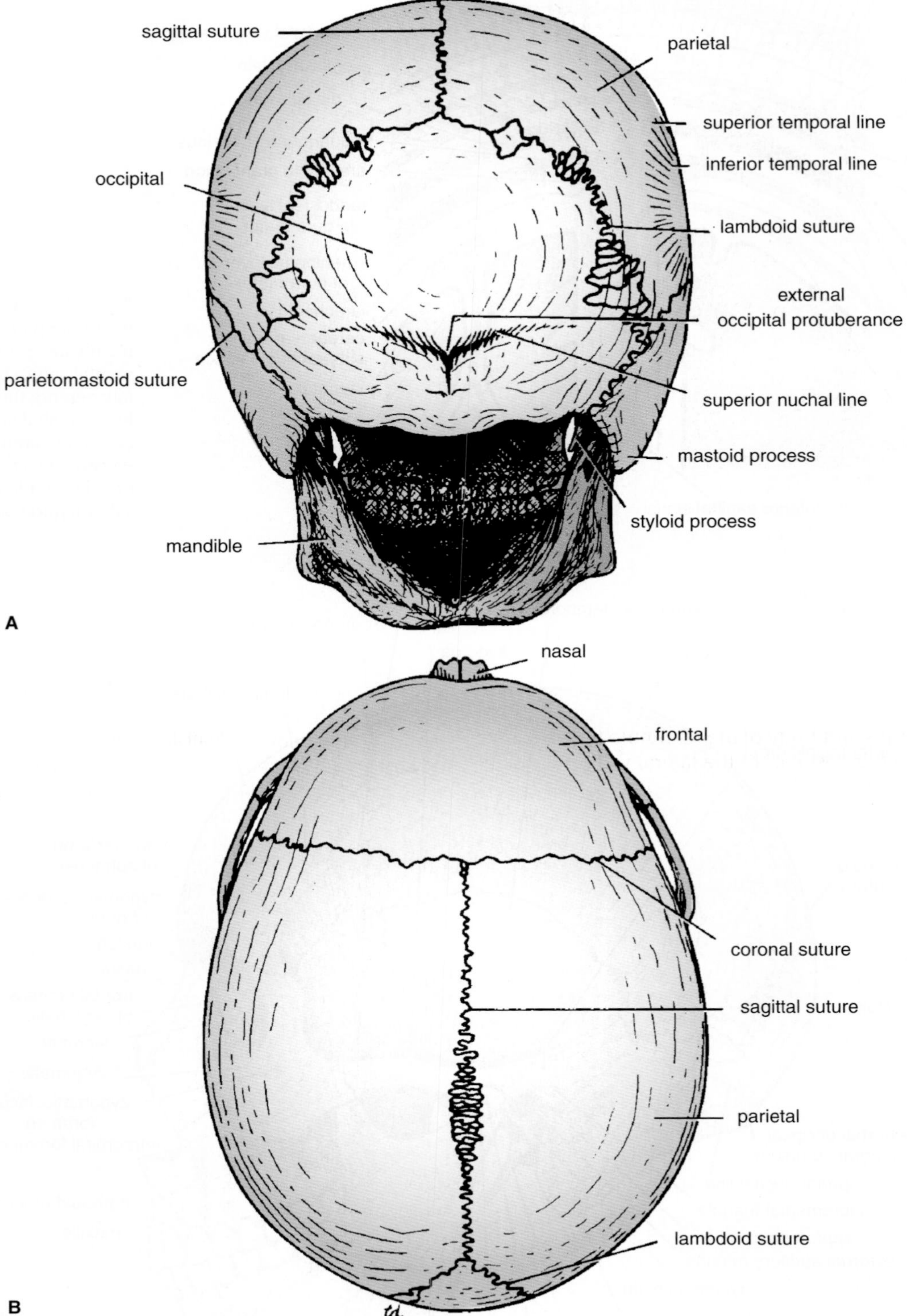

Figure 11-4 Bones of the skull viewed from the posterior (**A**) and superior (**B**) aspects.

alveolar process projects downward and, together with the fellow of the opposite side, forms the **alveolar arch,** which carries the upper teeth. Within each maxilla is a large, pyramid-shaped cavity lined with mucous membrane called the **maxillary sinus.** This communicates with the nasal cavity and serves as a voice resonator.

The **zygomatic bone** forms the prominence of the cheek and part of the lateral wall and floor of the orbital cavity. Medially, it articulates with the maxilla and laterally it articulates with the zygomatic process of the temporal bone to form the zygomatic arch. The zygomatic bone is perforated by two foramina for the zygomaticofacial and zygomaticotemporal nerves.

The **mandible,** or lower jaw, consists of a horizontal body and two vertical rami (for details, see page 715).

Lateral View of the Skull

The **frontal bone** forms the anterior part of the side of the skull and articulates with the parietal bone at the coronal suture (Fig. 11-3).

The **parietal bones** form the sides and roof of the cranium and articulate with each other in the midline at the **sagittal suture.** They articulate with the occipital bone behind, at the **lambdoid suture.**

The skull is completed at the side by the squamous part of the **occipital bone;** parts of the **temporal bone,** namely, the **squamous, tympanic, mastoid process, styloid process,** and **zygomatic process;** and the **greater wing of the sphenoid.** Note the position of the external auditory meatus. The ramus and body of the mandible lie inferiorly.

Note that the thinnest part of the lateral wall of the skull is where the anteroinferior corner of the parietal bone articulates with the greater wing of the sphenoid; this point is referred to as the **pterion.**

Clinically, the pterion is an important area because it overlies the anterior division of the **middle meningeal artery** and **vein.**

Identify the **superior** and **inferior temporal lines,** which begin as a single line from the posterior margin of the zygomatic process of the frontal bone and diverge as they arch backward. The **temporal fossa** lies below the inferior temporal line.

The **infratemporal fossa** lies below the **infratemporal crest** on the greater wing of the sphenoid. The **pterygomaxillary fissure** is a vertical fissure that lies within the fossa between the pterygoid process of the sphenoid bone and back of the maxilla. It leads medially into the **pterygopalatine fossa.**

The **inferior orbital fissure** is a horizontal fissure between the greater wing of the sphenoid bone and the maxilla. It leads forward into the orbit.

The **pterygopalatine fossa** is a small space behind and below the orbital cavity. It communicates laterally with the infratemporal fossa through the pterygomaxillary fissure, medially with the nasal cavity through the **sphenopalatine foramen,** superiorly with the skull through the foramen rotundum, and anteriorly with the orbit through the **inferior orbital fissure.**

Posterior View of the Skull

The posterior parts of the two parietal bones (Fig. 11-4) with the intervening **sagittal suture** are seen above. Below, the parietal bones articulate with the squamous part of the occipital bone at the **lambdoid suture.** On each side the occipital bone articulates with the temporal bone. In the midline of the occipital bone is a roughened elevation called the **external occipital protuberance,** which gives attachment to muscles and the ligamentum nuchae. On either side of the protuberance the **superior nuchal lines** extend laterally toward the temporal bone.

Superior View of the Skull

Anteriorly, the frontal bone (Fig. 11-4) articulates with the two parietal bones at the **coronal suture.** Occasionally, the two halves of the frontal bone fail to fuse, leaving a midline **metopic suture.** Behind, the two parietal bones articulate in the midline at the **sagittal suture.**

Inferior View of the Skull

If the mandible is discarded, the anterior part of this aspect of the skull is seen to be formed by the **hard palate** (Fig. 11-5).

The **palatal processes of the maxillae** and the **horizontal plates of the palatine bones** can be identified. In the midline anteriorly is the **incisive fossa** and **foramen.** Posterolaterally are the **greater** and **lesser palatine foramina.**

Above the posterior edge of the hard palate are the **choanae** (posterior nasal apertures). These are separated from each other by the posterior margin of the **vomer** and are bounded laterally by the **medial pterygoid plates** of the sphenoid bone. The inferior end of the **medial pterygoid plate** is prolonged as a curved spike of bone, the **pterygoid hamulus.**

Posterolateral to the **lateral pterygoid plate,** the greater wing of the sphenoid is pierced by the large **foramen ovale** and the small **foramen spinosum.** Posterolateral to the foramen spinosum is the **spine of the sphenoid.**

Behind the spine of the sphenoid, in the interval between the greater wing of the sphenoid and the petrous part of the temporal bone, is a groove for the cartilaginous part of the **auditory tube.** The opening of the bony part of the tube can be identified.

The **mandibular fossa** of the temporal bone and the **articular tubercle** form the upper articular surfaces for the temporomandibular joint. Separating the mandibular fossa from the tympanic plate posteriorly is the **squamotympanic fissure,** through the medial end of which the chorda tympani nerve exits from the tympanic cavity.

The **styloid process** of the temporal bone projects downward and forward from its inferior aspect. The opening of the **carotid canal** can be seen on the inferior surface of the petrous part of the temporal bone.

The medial end of the petrous part of the temporal bone is irregular and, together with the basilar part of the occipital bone and the greater wing of the sphenoid, forms the **foramen lacerum.** During life, the foramen lacerum is closed with fibrous tissue, and only a few small vessels pass through this foramen from the cavity of the skull to the exterior.

The **tympanic plate,** which forms part of the temporal bone, is C shaped on section and forms the bony part of the **external auditory meatus.** While examining this region, identify the **suprameatal crest** on the lateral surface of the squamous part of the temporal bone, the **suprameatal triangle,** and the **suprameatal spine.**

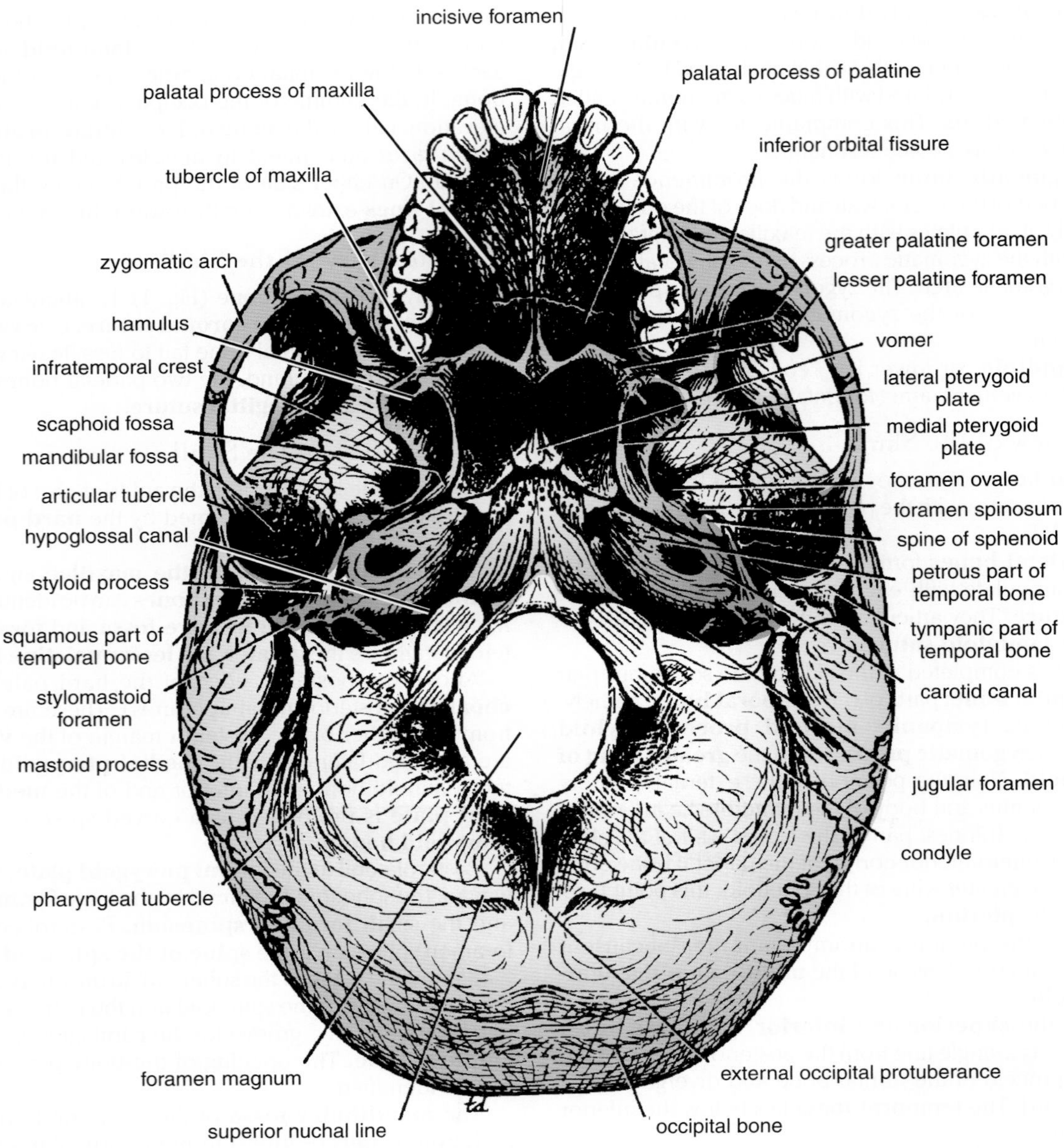

Figure 11-5 Inferior surface of the base of the skull.

In the interval between the styloid and mastoid processes, the **stylomastoid foramen** can be seen. Medial to the styloid process, the petrous part of the temporal bone has a deep notch, which, together with a shallower notch on the occipital bone, forms the **jugular foramen.**

Behind the posterior apertures of the nose and in front of the foramen magnum are the sphenoid bone and the basilar part of the occipital bone. The **pharyngeal tubercle** is a small prominence on the undersurface of the basilar part of the occipital bone in the midline.

The **occipital condyles** should be identified; they articulate with the superior aspect of the lateral mass of the first cervical vertebra, the atlas. Superior to the occipital condyle is the **hypoglossal canal** for transmission of the hypoglossal nerve (Fig. 11-6).

Posterior to the foramen magnum in the midline is the external occipital protuberance. The superior nuchal lines should be identified as they curve laterally on each side.

The Cranial Cavity

The cranial cavity contains the brain and its surrounding meninges, portions of the cranial nerves, arteries, veins, and venous sinuses.

Vault of the Skull

The internal surface of the vault shows the coronal, sagittal, and lambdoid sutures. In the midline is a shallow sagittal groove that lodges the **superior sagittal sinus.** On each side of the groove are several small pits, called **granular pits,**

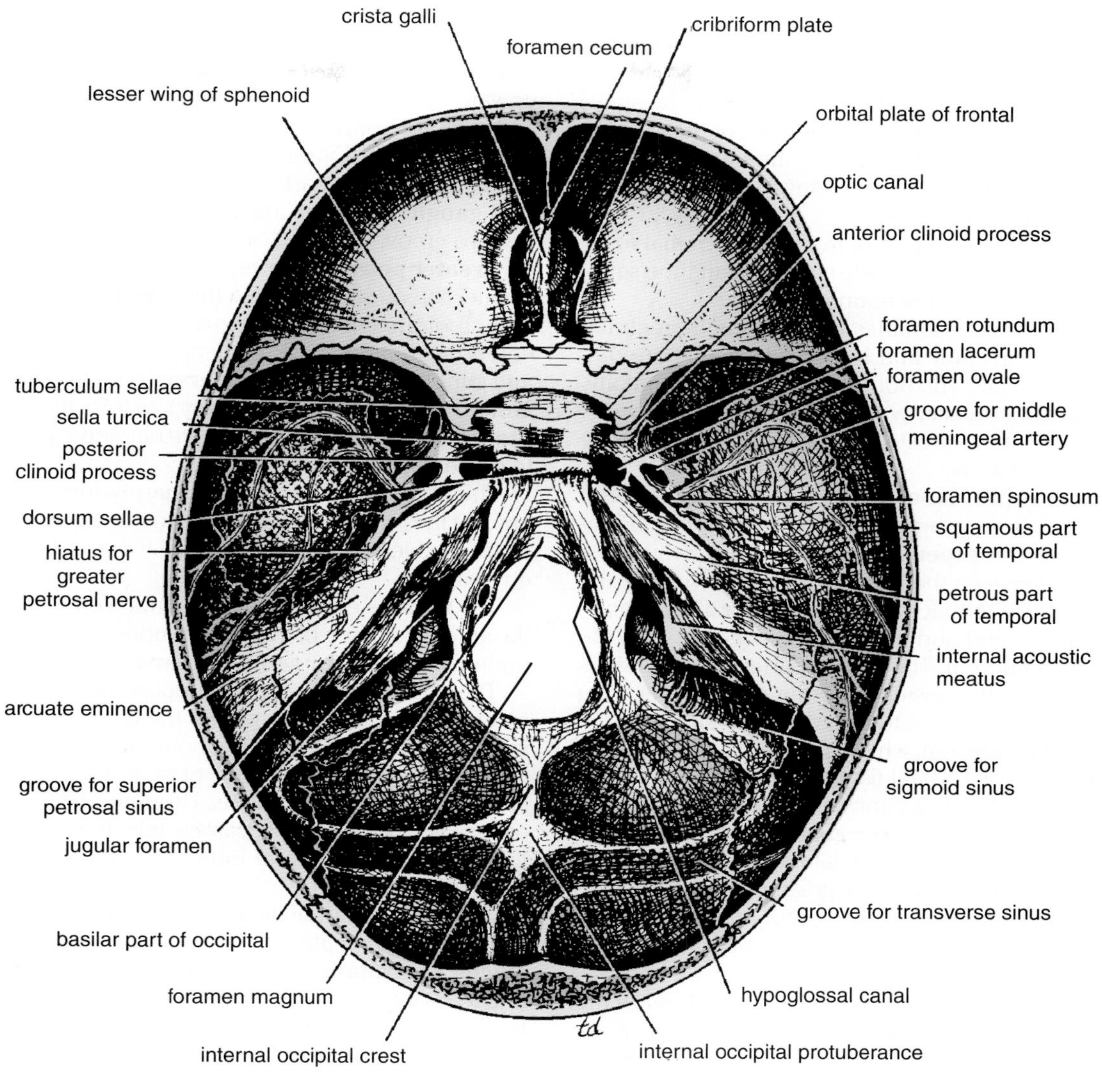

Figure 11-6 Internal surface of the base of the skull.

which lodge the **lateral lacunae** and **arachnoid granulations** (see page 683). Several narrow grooves are present for the anterior and posterior divisions of the **middle meningeal vessels** as they pass up the side of the skull to the vault.

Base of the Skull

The interior of the base of the skull (Fig. 11-6) is divided into three cranial fossae: anterior, middle, and posterior. The anterior cranial fossa is separated from the middle cranial fossa by the lesser wing of the sphenoid, and the middle cranial fossa is separated from the posterior cranial fossa by the petrous part of the temporal bone.

Anterior Cranial Fossa

The anterior cranial fossa lodges the frontal lobes of the cerebral hemispheres. It is bounded anteriorly by the inner surface of the frontal bone, and in the midline is a crest for the attachment of the **falx cerebri.** Its posterior boundary is the sharp lesser wing of the sphenoid, which articulates laterally with the frontal bone and meets the anteroinferior angle of the parietal bone, or the pterion. The medial end of the lesser wing of the sphenoid forms the **anterior clinoid process** on each side, which gives attachment to the **tentorium cerebelli.** The median part of the anterior cranial fossa is limited posteriorly by the groove for the optic chiasma.

The floor of the fossa is formed by the ridged orbital plates of the frontal bone laterally and by the **cribriform plate** of the ethmoid medially (Fig. 11-6). The **crista galli** is a sharp upward projection of the ethmoid bone in the midline for the attachment of the falx cerebri. Alongside the crista galli is a narrow slit in the cribriform plate for the passage of the **anterior ethmoidal nerve** into the nasal cavity. The upper surface of the cribriform plate supports the olfactory bulbs, and the small perforations in the cribriform plate are for the **olfactory nerves.**

Middle Cranial Fossa

The middle cranial fossa consists of a small median part and expanded lateral parts (Fig. 11-6). The median raised part is formed by the body of the sphenoid, and the expanded lateral parts form concavities on either side, which lodge the **temporal lobes** of the **cerebral hemispheres.**

It is bounded anteriorly by the lesser wings of the sphenoid and posteriorly by the superior borders of the petrous parts of the temporal bones. Laterally lie the squamous parts of the temporal bones, the greater wings of the sphenoid, and the parietal bones.

The floor of each lateral part of the middle cranial fossa is formed by the greater wing of the sphenoid and the squamous and petrous parts of the temporal bone.

The sphenoid bone resembles a bat having a centrally placed **body** with **greater** and **lesser wings** that are outstretched on each side. The body of the sphenoid contains the **sphenoid air sinuses,** which are lined with mucous membrane and communicate with the nasal cavity; they serve as voice resonators.

Anteriorly, the **optic canal** transmits the optic nerve and the ophthalmic artery, a branch of the internal carotid artery, to the orbit. The **superior orbital fissure,** which is a slitlike opening between the lesser and greater wings of the sphenoid, transmits the lacrimal, frontal, trochlear, oculomotor, nasociliary, and abducent nerves, together with the superior ophthalmic vein. The sphenoparietal venous sinus runs medially along the posterior border of the lesser wing of the sphenoid and drains into the cavernous sinus.

The **foramen rotundum,** which is situated behind the medial end of the superior orbital fissure, perforates the greater wing of the sphenoid and transmits the maxillary nerve from the trigeminal ganglion to the pterygopalatine fossa.

The **foramen ovale** lies posterolateral to the foramen rotundum (Fig. 11-6). It perforates the greater wing of the sphenoid and transmits the large sensory root and small motor root of the mandibular nerve to the infratemporal fossa; the lesser petrosal nerve also passes through it.

The small **foramen spinosum** lies posterolateral to the foramen ovale and also perforates the greater wing of the sphenoid. The foramen transmits the middle meningeal artery from the infratemporal fossa (see page 750) into the cranial cavity. The artery then runs forward and laterally in a groove on the upper surface of the squamous part of the temporal bone and the greater wing of the sphenoid (Fig. 11-20). After a short distance, the artery divides into anterior and posterior branches. The anterior branch passes forward and upward to the anteroinferior angle of the parietal bone (Fig. 11-131A). Here, the bone is deeply grooved or tunneled by the artery for a short distance before it runs backward and upward on the parietal bone. It is at this site that the artery may be damaged after a blow to the side of the head. The posterior branch passes backward and upward across the squamous part of the temporal bone to reach the parietal bone.

The large and irregularly shaped **foramen lacerum** lies between the apex of the petrous part of the temporal bone and the sphenoid bone (Fig. 11-6). The inferior opening of the foramen lacerum in life is filled by cartilage and fibrous tissue, and only small blood vessels pass through this tissue from the cranial cavity to the neck.

The **carotid canal** opens into the side of the foramen lacerum above the closed inferior opening. The internal carotid artery enters the foramen through the carotid canal and immediately turns upward to reach the side of the body of the sphenoid bone. Here, the artery turns forward in the cavernous sinus to reach the region of the anterior clinoid process. At this point, the internal carotid artery turns vertically upward, medial (Fig. 11-20) to the anterior clinoid process, and emerges from the cavernous sinus (see page 750).

Lateral to the foramen lacerum is an impression on the apex of the petrous part of the temporal bone for the **trigeminal ganglion.** On the anterior surface of the petrous bone are two grooves for nerves; the largest medial groove is for the **greater petrosal nerve,** a branch of the facial nerve; the smaller lateral groove is for the **lesser petrosal nerve,** a branch of the tympanic plexus. The greater petrosal nerve enters the foramen lacerum deep to the trigeminal ganglion and joins the **deep petrosal nerve** (sympathetic fibers from around the internal carotid artery), to form the **nerve of the pterygoid canal.** The lesser petrosal nerve passes forward to the foramen ovale.

The abducent nerve bends sharply forward across the apex of the petrous bone, medial to the trigeminal ganglion. Here, it leaves the posterior cranial fossa and enters the cavernous sinus.

The **arcuate eminence** is a rounded eminence found on the anterior surface of the petrous bone and is caused by the underlying **superior semicircular canal.**

The **tegmen tympani,** a thin plate of bone, is a forward extension of the petrous part of the temporal bone and adjoins the squamous part of the bone (Fig. 11-6). From behind forward, it forms the roof of the mastoid antrum, the tympanic cavity, and the auditory tube. This thin plate of bone is the only major barrier that separates infection in the tympanic cavity from the temporal lobe of the cerebral hemisphere (Fig. 11-30).

The median part of the middle cranial fossa is formed by the body of the sphenoid bone (Fig. 11-6). In front is the **sulcus chiasmatis,** which is related to the optic chiasma and leads laterally to the **optic canal** on each side. Posterior to the sulcus is an elevation, the **tuberculum sellae.** Behind the elevation is a deep depression, the **sella turcica,** which lodges the **pituitary gland.** The sella turcica is bounded posteriorly by a square plate of bone called the **dorsum sellae.** The superior angles of the dorsum sellae have two tubercles, called the **posterior clinoid processes,** which give attachment to the fixed margin of the tentorium cerebelli.

The cavernous sinus is directly related to the side of the body of the sphenoid (Figs. 11-9 and 11-10). It carries in its lateral wall the third and fourth cranial nerves and the ophthalmic and maxillary divisions of the fifth cranial nerve (Fig. 11-12). The internal carotid artery and the sixth cranial nerve pass forward through the sinus.

Posterior Cranial Fossa

The posterior cranial fossa is deep and lodges the parts of the hindbrain, namely, the **cerebellum, pons,** and **medulla oblongata.** Anteriorly the fossa is bounded by the superior border of the petrous part of the temporal bone, and posteriorly it is bounded by the internal surface of the squamous part of the occipital bone (Fig. 11-6). The floor of the posterior fossa is formed by the basilar, condylar, and squamous parts of the occipital bone and the mastoid part of the temporal bone.

The roof of the fossa is formed by a fold of dura, the **tentorium cerebelli,** which intervenes between the cerebellum below and the occipital lobes of the cerebral hemispheres above (Fig. 11-10).

The **foramen magnum** occupies the central area of the floor and transmits the medulla oblongata and its surrounding meninges, the ascending spinal parts of the accessory nerves, and the two vertebral arteries.

The **hypoglossal canal** is situated above the anterolateral boundary of the foramen magnum (Fig. 11-6) and transmits the **hypoglossal nerve.**

The **jugular foramen** lies between the lower border of the petrous part of the temporal bone and the condylar part of the occipital bone. It transmits the following structures from before backward: the **inferior petrosal sinus;** the **9th, 10th,** and **11th cranial nerves;** and the large **sigmoid sinus.** The inferior petrosal sinus descends in the groove on the lower border of the petrous part of the temporal bone to reach the foramen. The sigmoid sinus turns down through the foramen to become the **internal jugular vein.**

The **internal acoustic meatus** pierces the posterior surface of the petrous part of the temporal bone. It transmits the vestibulocochlear nerve and the motor and sensory roots of the facial nerve.

The **internal occipital crest** runs upward in the midline posteriorly from the foramen magnum to the **internal occipital protuberance;** to it is attached the small **falx cerebelli** over the **occipital sinus.**

On each side of the internal occipital protuberance is a wide groove for the **transverse sinus** (Fig. 11-6). This groove sweeps around on either side, on the internal surface of the occipital bone, to reach the posteroinferior angle or corner of the parietal bone. The groove now passes onto the mastoid part of the temporal bone, and here the transverse sinus becomes the **sigmoid sinus.** The **superior petrosal sinus** runs backward along the upper border of the petrous bone in a narrow groove and drains into the sigmoid sinus. As the sigmoid sinus descends to the jugular foramen, it deeply grooves the back of the petrous bone and the mastoid part of the temporal bone. Here, it lies directly posterior to the mastoid antrum.

Table 11-1 provides a summary of the more important openings in the base of the skull and the structures that pass through them.

Neonatal Skull

The newborn skull (Fig. 11-8), compared with the adult skull, has a disproportionately large cranium relative to the face. In childhood, the growth of the mandible, the maxillary sinuses, and the alveolar processes of the maxillae results in a great increase in length of the face.

The bones of the skull are smooth and unilaminar, there being no diploë present. Most of the skull bones are ossified at birth, but the process is incomplete, and the bones are mobile on each other, being connected by fibrous tissue or cartilage. The bones of the vault are ossified in membrane; the bones of the base are ossified in cartilage. The bones of the vault are not closely knit at sutures, as in the adult, but are separated by unossified membranous intervals called

Table 11-1 Summary of the More Important Openings in the Base of the Skull and the Structures That Pass Through Them

Opening in Skull	Bone of Skull	Structures Transmitted
Anterior Cranial Fossa		
Perforations in cribriform plate	Ethmoid	Olfactory nerves
Middle Cranial Fossa		
Optic canal	Lesser wing of sphenoid	Optic nerve, ophthalmic artery
Superior orbital fissure	Between lesser and greater wings of sphenoid	Lacrimal, frontal, trochlear, oculomotor, nasociliary, and abducent nerves; superior ophthalmic vein
Foramen rotundum	Greater wing of sphenoid	Maxillary division of the trigeminal nerve
Foramen ovale	Greater wing of sphenoid	Mandibular division of the trigeminal nerve, lesser petrosal nerve
Foramen spinosum	Greater wing of sphenoid	Middle meningeal artery
Foramen lacerum	Between petrous part of temporal and sphenoid	Internal carotid artery
Posterior Cranial Fossa		
Foramen magnum	Occipital	Medulla oblongata, spinal part of accessory nerve, and right and left vertebral arteries
Hypoglossal canal	Occipital	Hypoglossal nerve
Jugular foramen	Between petrous part of temporal and condylar part of occipital	Glossopharyngeal, vagus, and accessory nerves; sigmoid sinus becomes internal jugular vein
Internal acoustic meatus	Petrous part of temporal	Vestibulocochlear and facial nerves

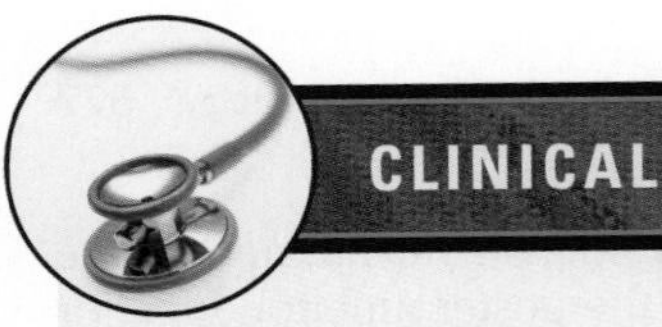

CLINICAL NOTES

Fractures of the Skull

Fractures of the skull are common in the adult but much less so in the young child. In the infant skull, the bones are more resilient than in the adult skull, and they are separated by fibrous sutural ligaments. In the adult, the inner table of the skull is particularly brittle. Moreover, the sutural ligaments begin to ossify during middle age.

The type of fracture that occurs in the skull depends on the age of the patient, the severity of the blow, and the area of skull receiving the trauma. The **adult skull** may be likened to an eggshell in that it possesses a certain limited resilience beyond which it splinters. A severe, localized blow produces a local indentation, often accompanied by splintering of the bone. Blows to the vault often result in a series of linear fractures, which radiate out through the thin areas of bone. The petrous parts of the temporal bones and the occipital crests strongly reinforce the base of the skull and tend to deflect linear fractures.

In the **young child,** the skull may be likened to a table-tennis ball in that a localized blow produces a depression without splintering. This common type of circumscribed lesion is referred to as a **"pond" fracture.**

Fractures of the Anterior Cranial Fossa

In fractures of the anterior cranial fossa, the cribriform plate of the ethmoid bone may be damaged. This usually results in tearing of the overlying meninges and underlying mucoperiosteum. The patient will have bleeding from the nose **(epistaxis)** and leakage of cerebrospinal fluid into the nose **(cerebrospinal rhinorrhea).** Fractures involving the orbital plate of the frontal bone result in hemorrhage beneath the conjunctiva and into the orbital cavity, causing **exophthalmos.** The frontal air sinus may be involved, with hemorrhage into the nose.

Fractures of the Middle Cranial Fossa

Fractures of the middle cranial fossa are common, because this is the weakest part of the base of the skull. Anatomically, this weakness is caused by the presence of numerous foramina and canals in this region; the cavities of the middle ear and the sphenoidal air sinuses are particularly vulnerable. The leakage of cerebrospinal fluid and blood from the external auditory meatus is common. The seventh and eighth cranial nerves may be involved as they pass through the petrous part of the temporal bone. The third, fourth, and sixth cranial nerves may be damaged if the lateral wall of the cavernous sinus is torn. Blood and cerebrospinal fluid may leak into the sphenoidal air sinuses and then into the nose.

Fractures of the Posterior Cranial Fossa

In fractures of the posterior cranial fossa, blood may escape into the nape of the neck deep to the postvertebral muscles. Some days later, it tracks between the muscles and appears in the posterior triangle, close to the mastoid process. The mucous membrane of the roof of the nasopharynx may be torn, and blood may escape there. In fractures involving the jugular foramen, the 9th, 10th, and 11th cranial nerves may be damaged. The strong bony walls of the hypoglossal canal usually protect the hypoglossal nerve from injury.

Fractures of Facial Bones

Bone Injuries and Skeletal Development

The developing bones of a child's face are more pliable than an adult's, and fractures may be incomplete or greenstick. In adults, the presence of well-developed, air-filled sinuses and the mucoperiosteal surfaces of the alveolar parts of the upper and lower jaws means that most facial fractures should be considered to be open fractures, susceptible to infection, and requiring antibiotic therapy.

Anatomy of Common Facial Fractures

Automobile accidents, fisticuffs, and falls are common causes of facial fractures. Fortunately, the upper part of the skull is developed from membrane (whereas the remainder is developed from cartilage); therefore, this part of the skull in children is relatively flexible and can absorb considerable force without resulting in a fracture.

Signs of fractures of the facial bones include deformity, ocular displacement, or abnormal movement accompanied by crepitation and malocclusion of the teeth. Anesthesia or paresthesia of the facial skin will follow fracture of bones through which branches of the trigeminal nerve pass to the skin.

The muscles of the face are thin and weak and cause little displacement of the bone fragments. Once a fracture of the maxilla has been reduced, for example, prolonged fixation is not needed. However, in the case of the mandible, the strong muscles of mastication can create considerable displacement, requiring long periods of fixation.

The most common facial fractures involve the nasal bones, followed by the zygomatic bone and then the mandible. To fracture the maxillary bones and the supraorbital ridges of the frontal bones, an enormous force is required.

Nasal Fractures

Fractures of the nasal bones, because of the prominence of the nose, are the most common facial fractures. Because the bones are lined with mucoperiosteum, the fracture is considered open; the overlying skin may also be lacerated. Although most are simple fractures and are reduced under local anesthesia, some are associated with severe injuries to the nasal septum and require careful treatment under general anesthesia.

Maxillofacial Fractures

Maxillofacial fractures usually occur as the result of massive facial trauma. There is extensive facial swelling, midface mobility of the underlying bone on palpation, malocclusion of the teeth with anterior open bite, and possibly leakage of cerebrospinal fluid (cerebrospinal rhinorrhea) secondary to fracture of the cribriform plate of the ethmoid bone. Double vision (diplopia) may be present, owing to orbital wall damage. Involvement of the infraorbital nerve with anesthesia or paresthesia of the skin of the cheek and upper gum may occur in fractures of the body of the maxilla. Nose bleeding may also occur in maxillary fractures. Blood enters the maxillary air sinus and then leaks into the nasal cavity.

The sites of the fractures were classified by Le Fort as type I, II, or III; these fractures are summarized in Figure 11-7.

Blowout Fractures of the Maxilla

A severe blow to the orbit (as from a baseball) may cause the contents of the orbital cavity to explode downward through the floor of the orbit into the maxillary sinus. Damage to the infraorbital nerve, resulting in altered sensation to the skin of the cheek, upper lip, and gum, may occur.

Fractures of the Zygoma or Zygomatic Arch

The zygoma or zygomatic arch can be fractured by a blow to the side of the face. Although it can occur as an isolated fracture, as from a blow from a clenched fist, it may be associated with multiple other fractures of the face, as often seen in automobile accidents.

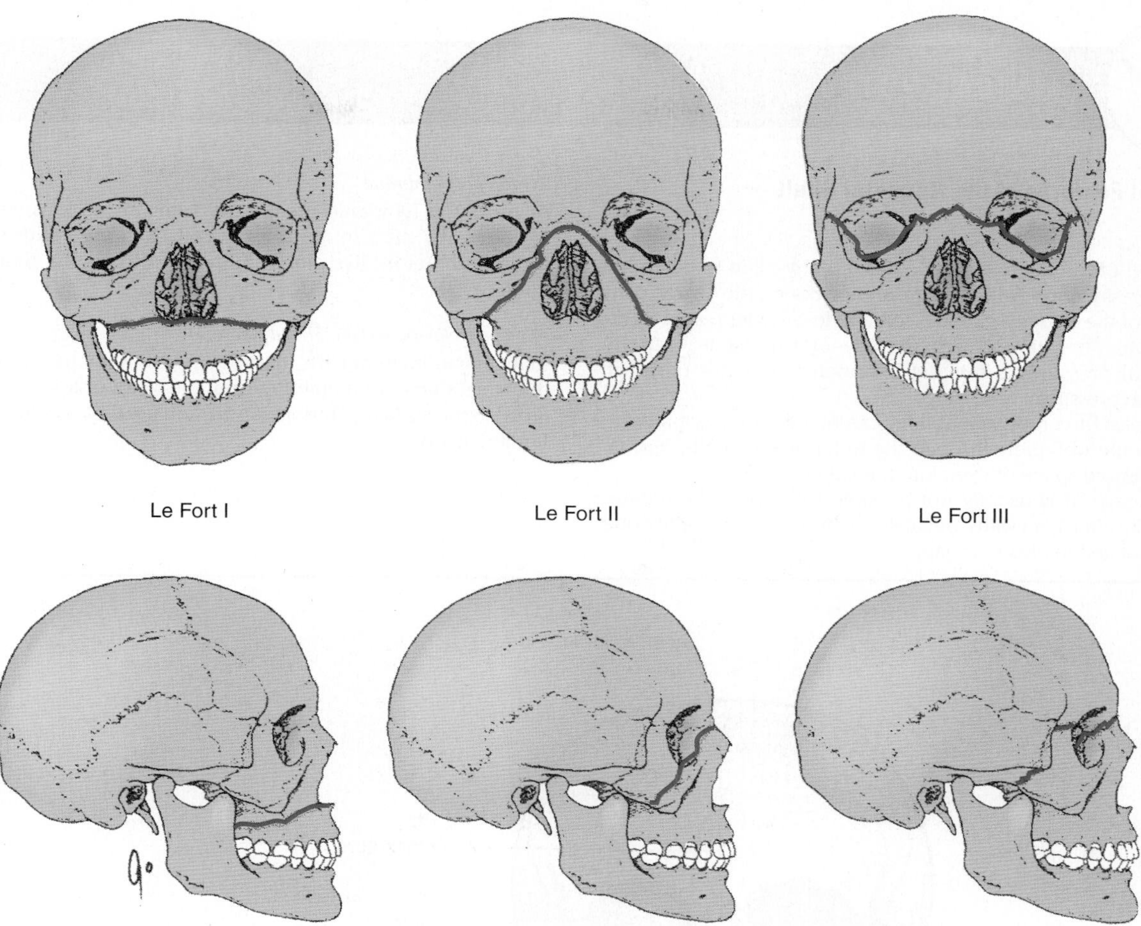

Figure 11-7 Le Fort classification of maxillofacial fractures. The red line denotes the fracture line.

fontanelles. Clinically, the anterior and posterior fontanelles are most important and are easily examined in the midline of the vault.

The **anterior fontanelle** is diamond shaped and lies between the two halves of the frontal bone in front and the two parietal bones behind (Fig. 11-8). The fibrous membrane forming the floor of the anterior fontanelle is replaced by bone and is closed by 18 months of age. The **posterior fontanelle** is triangular and lies between the two parietal bones in front and the occipital bone behind. By the end of the first year, the fontanelle is usually closed and can no longer be palpated.

The **tympanic part of the temporal bone** is merely a C-shaped ring at birth, compared with a C-shaped curved plate in the adult. This means that the external auditory meatus is almost entirely cartilaginous in the newborn, and the **tympanic membrane** is nearer the surface. Although the tympanic membrane is nearly as large as in the adult, it faces more inferiorly. During childhood the tympanic plate grows laterally, forming the bony part of the meatus, and the tympanic membrane comes to face more directly laterally.

The **mastoid process** is not present at birth (Fig. 11-8) and develops later in response to the pull of the sternocleidomastoid muscle when the child moves his or her head.

At birth, the mastoid antrum lies about 3 mm deep to the floor of the **suprameatal triangle.** As growth of the skull continues, the lateral bony wall thickens so that at puberty the antrum may lie as much as 15 mm from the surface.

The mandible has right and left halves at birth, united in the midline with fibrous tissue. The two halves fuse at the **symphysis menti** by the end of the first year.

The **angle of the mandible** at birth is obtuse (Fig. 11-8), the head being placed level with the upper margin of the body and the coronoid process lying at a superior level to the head. It is only after eruption of the permanent teeth that the angle of the mandible assumes the adult shape and the head and neck grow so that the head comes to lie higher than the coronoid process.

In old age, the size of the mandible is reduced when the teeth are lost. As the alveolar part of the bone becomes smaller, the ramus becomes oblique in position so that the head is bent posteriorly.

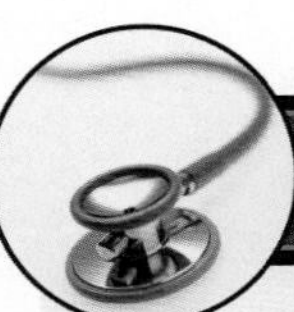

CLINICAL NOTES

Clinical Features of the Neonatal Skull

Fontanelles

Palpation of the fontanelles enables the physician to determine the progress of growth in the surrounding bones, the degree of hydration of the baby (e.g., if the fontanelles are depressed below the surface, the baby is dehydrated), and the state of the intracranial pressure (a bulging fontanelle indicates raised intracranial pressure).

Samples of cerebrospinal fluid can be obtained by passing a long needle obliquely through the anterior fontanelle into the subarachnoid space or even into the lateral ventricle.

Clinically, it is usually not possible to palpate the anterior fontanelle after 18 months, because the frontal and parietal bones have enlarged to close the gap.

Tympanic Membrane

At birth, the tympanic membrane faces more downward and less laterally than in maturity; when examined with the otoscope it therefore lies more obliquely in the infant than in the adult.

Forceps Delivery and the Facial Nerve

In the newborn infant, the mastoid process is not developed, and the facial nerve, as it emerges from the stylomastoid foramen, is close to the surface. Thus, it can be damaged by forceps in a difficult delivery.

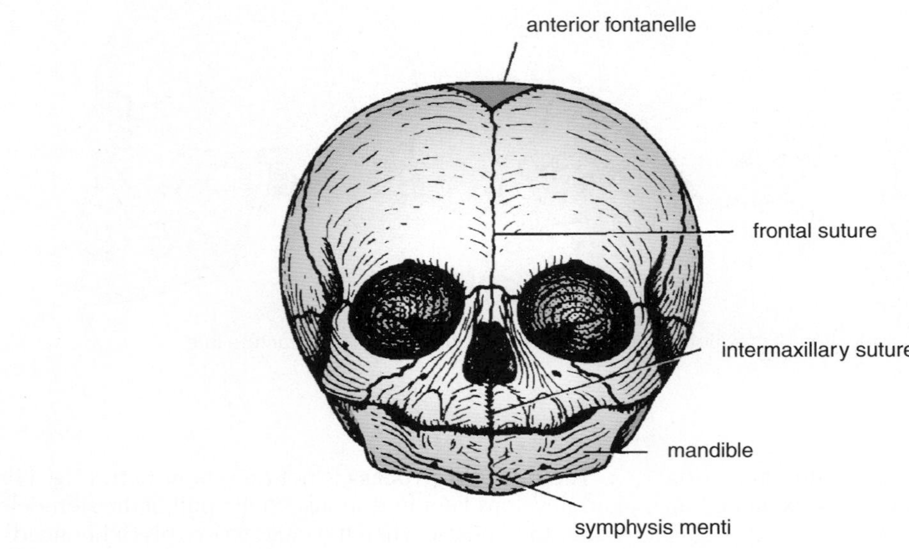

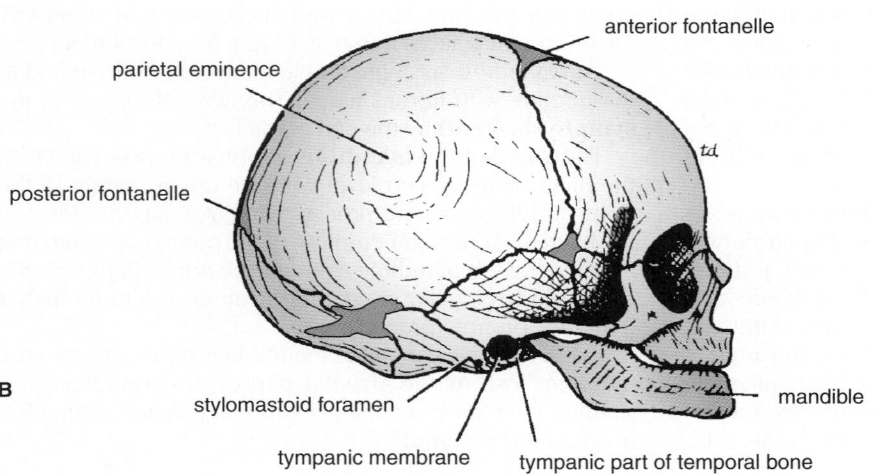

Figure 11-8 Neonatal skull as seen from the anterior (**A**) and lateral (**B**) aspects.

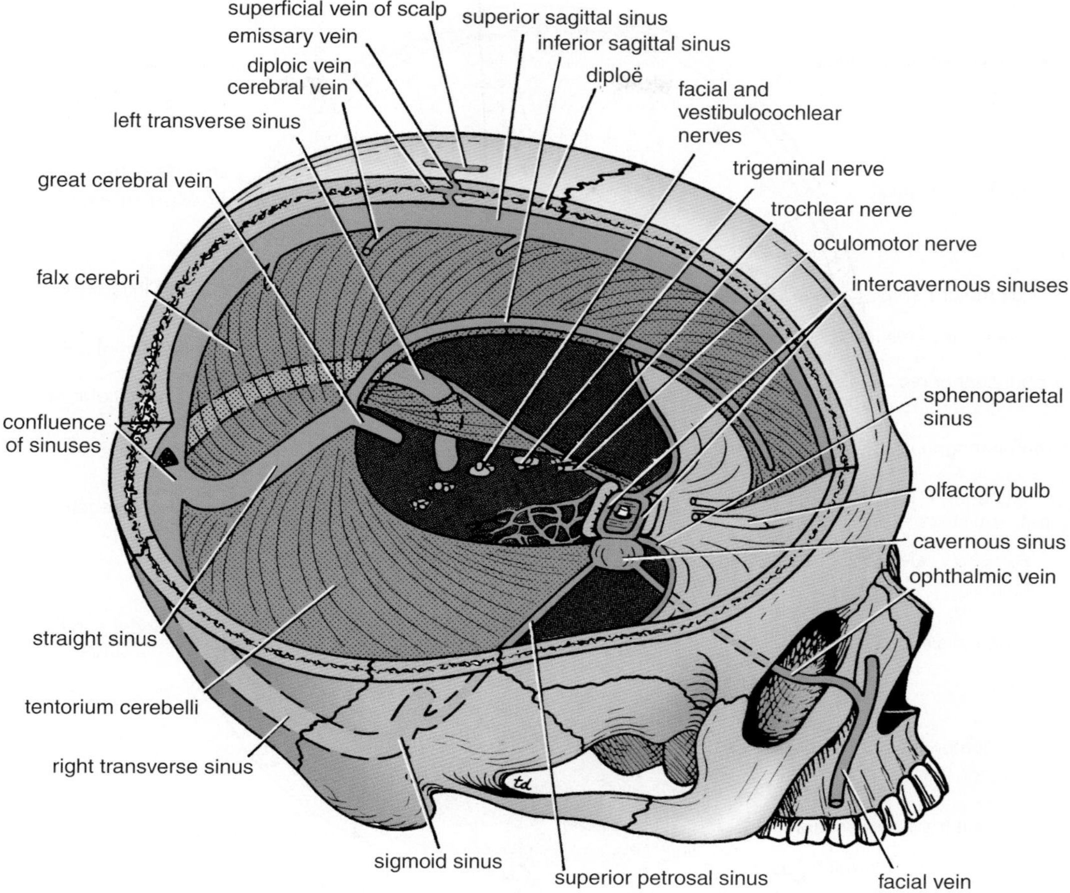

Figure 11-9 Interior of the skull showing the dura mater and its contained venous sinuses. Note the connections of the veins of the scalp and the veins of the face with the venous sinuses.

The Meninges

The brain in the skull is surrounded by three protective membranes, or meninges: the dura mater, the arachnoid mater, and the pia mater. (The spinal cord in the vertebral column is also surrounded by three meninges. See page 871.)

Dura Mater of the Brain

The dura mater is conventionally described as two layers: the endosteal layer and the meningeal layer (Fig. 11-2). These are closely united except along certain lines, where they separate to form venous sinuses.

The **endosteal layer** is nothing more than the ordinary periosteum covering the inner surface of the skull bones. **It does not extend** through the foramen magnum to become continuous with the dura mater of the spinal cord. Around the margins of all the foramina in the skull it becomes continuous with the periosteum on the outside of the skull bones. At the sutures it is continuous with the sutural ligaments. It is most strongly adherent to the bones over the base of the skull.

The **meningeal layer** is the dura mater proper. It is a dense, strong, fibrous membrane covering the brain and is continuous through the foramen magnum with the dura mater of the spinal cord. It provides tubular sheaths for the cranial nerves as the latter pass through the foramina in the skull. Outside the skull the sheaths fuse with the epineurium of the nerves.

The meningeal layer sends inward four septa that divide the cranial cavity into freely communicating spaces lodging the subdivisions of the brain. The function of these septa is to restrict the rotatory displacement of the brain.

The **falx cerebri** is a sickle-shaped fold of dura mater that lies in the midline between the two cerebral hemispheres (Figs. 11-9 and 11-13). Its narrow end in front is attached to the internal frontal crest and the crista galli. Its broad posterior part blends in the midline with the upper surface of the tentorium cerebelli. The superior sagittal sinus runs in its upper fixed margin, the inferior sagittal sinus runs in its lower concave free margin, and the straight sinus runs along its attachment to the tentorium cerebelli.

The **tentorium cerebelli** is a crescent-shaped fold of dura mater that roofs over the posterior cranial fossa (Figs. 11-9, 11-10, and 11-11). It covers the upper surface of the cerebellum and supports the occipital lobes of the cerebral hemispheres. In front is a gap, the **tentorial notch,** for the

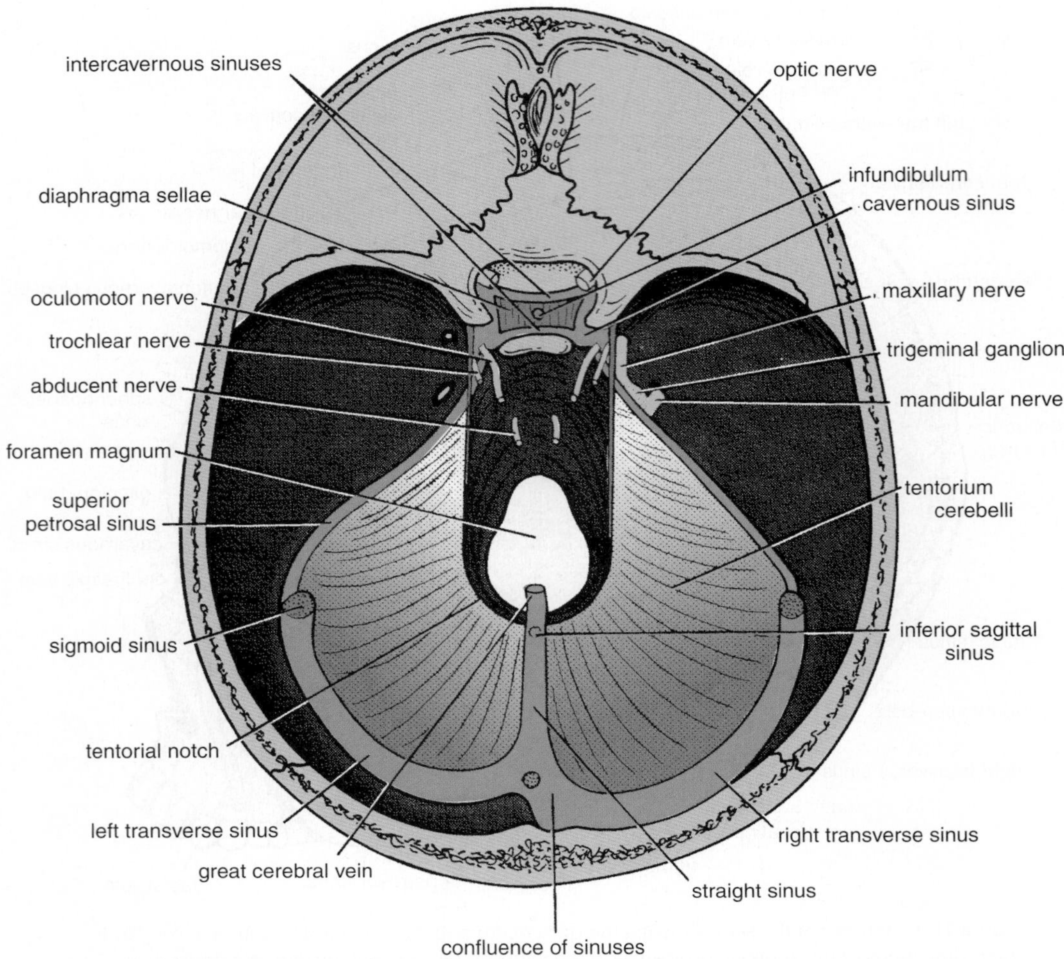

Figure 11-10 Diaphragma sellae and tentorium cerebelli. Note the position of the venous sinuses.

passage of the midbrain (Figs. 11-11 and 11-12), thus producing an inner free border and an outer attached or fixed border. The fixed border is attached to the posterior clinoid processes, the superior borders of the petrous bones, and the margins of the grooves for the transverse sinuses on the occipital bone. The free border runs forward at its two ends, crosses the attached border, and is affixed to the anterior clinoid process on each side. At the point where the two borders cross, the third and fourth cranial nerves pass forward to enter the lateral wall of the cavernous sinus (Figs. 11-11 and 11-12).

Close to the apex of the petrous part of the temporal bone, the lower layer of the tentorium is pouched forward beneath the superior petrosal sinus to form a recess for the trigeminal nerve and the trigeminal ganglion (Fig. 11-11).

The falx cerebri and the falx cerebelli are attached to the upper and lower surfaces of the tentorium, respectively. The straight sinus runs along its attachment to the falx cerebri, the superior petrosal sinus along its attachment to the petrous bone, and the transverse sinus along its attachment to the occipital bone (Fig. 11-10).

The **falx cerebelli** is a small, sickle-shaped fold of dura mater that is attached to the internal occipital crest and projects forward between the two cerebellar hemispheres. Its posterior fixed margin contains the occipital sinus.

The **diaphragma sellae** is a small circular fold of dura mater that forms the roof for the sella turcica (Fig. 11-6). A small opening in its center allows passage of the stalk of the pituitary gland (Fig. 11-12).

Dural Nerve Supply

Branches of the trigeminal, vagus, and first three cervical nerves and branches from the sympathetic system pass to the dura.

Numerous sensory endings are in the dura. The dura is sensitive to stretching, which produces the sensation of headache. Stimulation of the sensory endings of the trigeminal nerve above the level of the tentorium cerebelli produces referred pain to an area of skin on the same side of the head. Stimulation of the dural endings below the level of the tentorium produces referred pain to the back of the neck and back of the scalp along the distribution of the greater occipital nerve.

Dural Arterial Supply

Numerous arteries supply the dura mater from the internal carotid, maxillary, ascending pharyngeal, occipital, and

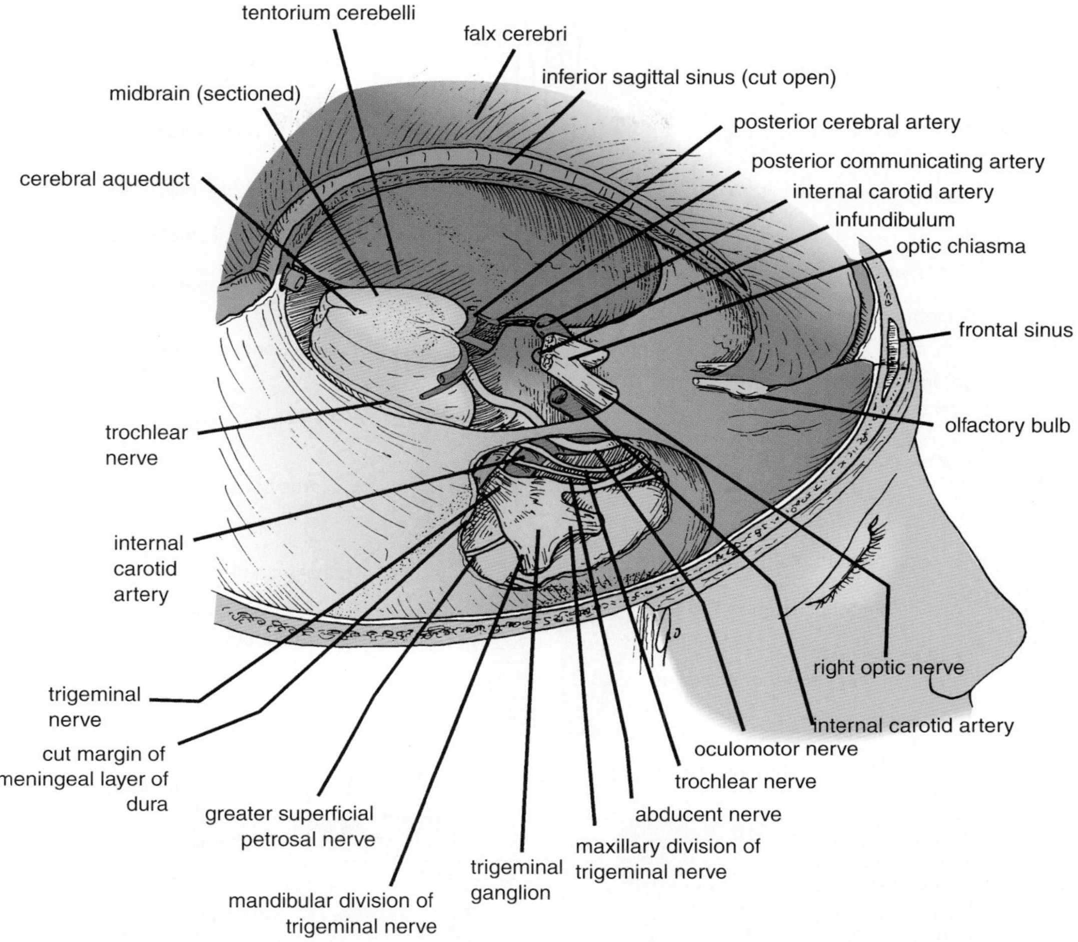

Figure 11-11 Lateral view of the skull showing the falx cerebri, tentorium cerebelli, brainstem, and trigeminal ganglion.

vertebral arteries. From a clinical standpoint, the most important is the middle meningeal artery, which is commonly damaged in head injuries.

The **middle meningeal artery** arises from the maxillary artery in the infratemporal fossa (see page 750). It enters the cranial cavity and runs forward and laterally in a groove on the upper surface of the squamous part of the temporal bone (Fig. 11-20). To enter the cranial cavity, it passes through the foramen spinosum to **lie between the meningeal and endosteal layers of dura.** Its further course in the middle cranial fossa is described on page 750. The anterior (frontal) branch deeply grooves or tunnels the anteroinferior angle of the parietal bone, and its course corresponds roughly to the line of the underlying precentral gyrus of the brain. The posterior (parietal) branch curves backward and supplies the posterior part of the dura mater.

Dural Venous Drainage

The **meningeal veins** lie in the endosteal layer of dura. The middle meningeal vein follows the branches of the middle meningeal artery and drains into the pterygoid venous plexus or the sphenoparietal sinus. The veins lie lateral to the arteries.

Arachnoid Mater of the Brain

The arachnoid mater is a delicate, impermeable membrane covering the brain and lying between the pia mater internally and the dura mater externally (Fig. 11-2). It is separated from the dura by a potential space, the **subdural space,** and from the pia by the **subarachnoid space,** which is filled with **cerebrospinal fluid.**

The arachnoid bridges over the sulci on the surface of the brain, and in certain situations the arachnoid and pia are widely separated to form the **subarachnoid cisternae.**

In certain areas the arachnoid projects into the venous sinuses to form **arachnoid villi.** The arachnoid villi are most numerous along the superior sagittal sinus. Aggregations of arachnoid villi are referred to as **arachnoid granulations** (Fig. 11-2). Arachnoid villi serve as sites where the cerebrospinal fluid diffuses into the bloodstream.

It is important to remember that structures passing to and from the brain to the skull or its foramina must pass through the subarachnoid space. All the cerebral arteries and veins lie in the space, as do the cranial nerves (Fig. 11-2). The arachnoid fuses with the epineurium of the nerves at their point of exit from the skull. In the case of the optic nerve, the

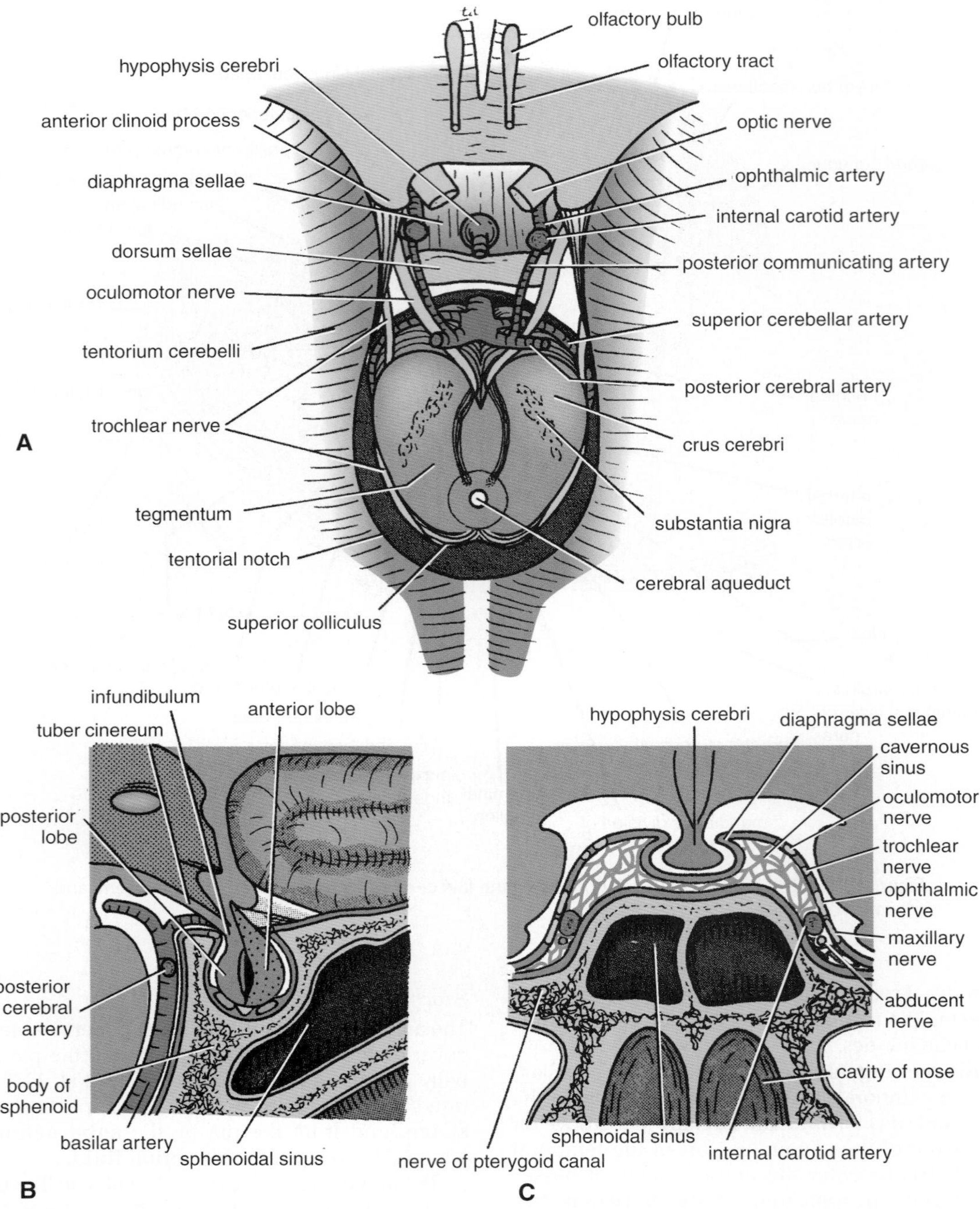

Figure 11-12 **A.** The forebrain has been removed, leaving the midbrain, the hypophysis cerebri, and the internal carotid and basilar arteries in position. **B.** Sagittal section through the sella turcica showing the hypophysis cerebri. **C.** Coronal section through the body of the sphenoid showing the hypophysis cerebri and the cavernous sinuses. Note the position of the cranial nerves.

arachnoid forms a sheath for the nerve that extends into the orbital cavity through the optic canal and fuses with the sclera of the eyeball (Fig. 11-25). Thus, the subarachnoid space extends around the optic nerve as far as the eyeball (see page 697).

The **cerebrospinal fluid** is produced by the **choroid plexuses** within the lateral, third, and fourth ventricles of the brain. It escapes from the ventricular system of the brain through the three foramina in the roof of the fourth ventricle and so enters the subarachnoid space. It now circulates both upward over the surfaces of the cerebral hemispheres and downward around the spinal cord. The spinal subarachnoid space extends down as far as the **second sacral vertebra** (see Fig. 12-7). Eventually, the fluid enters the

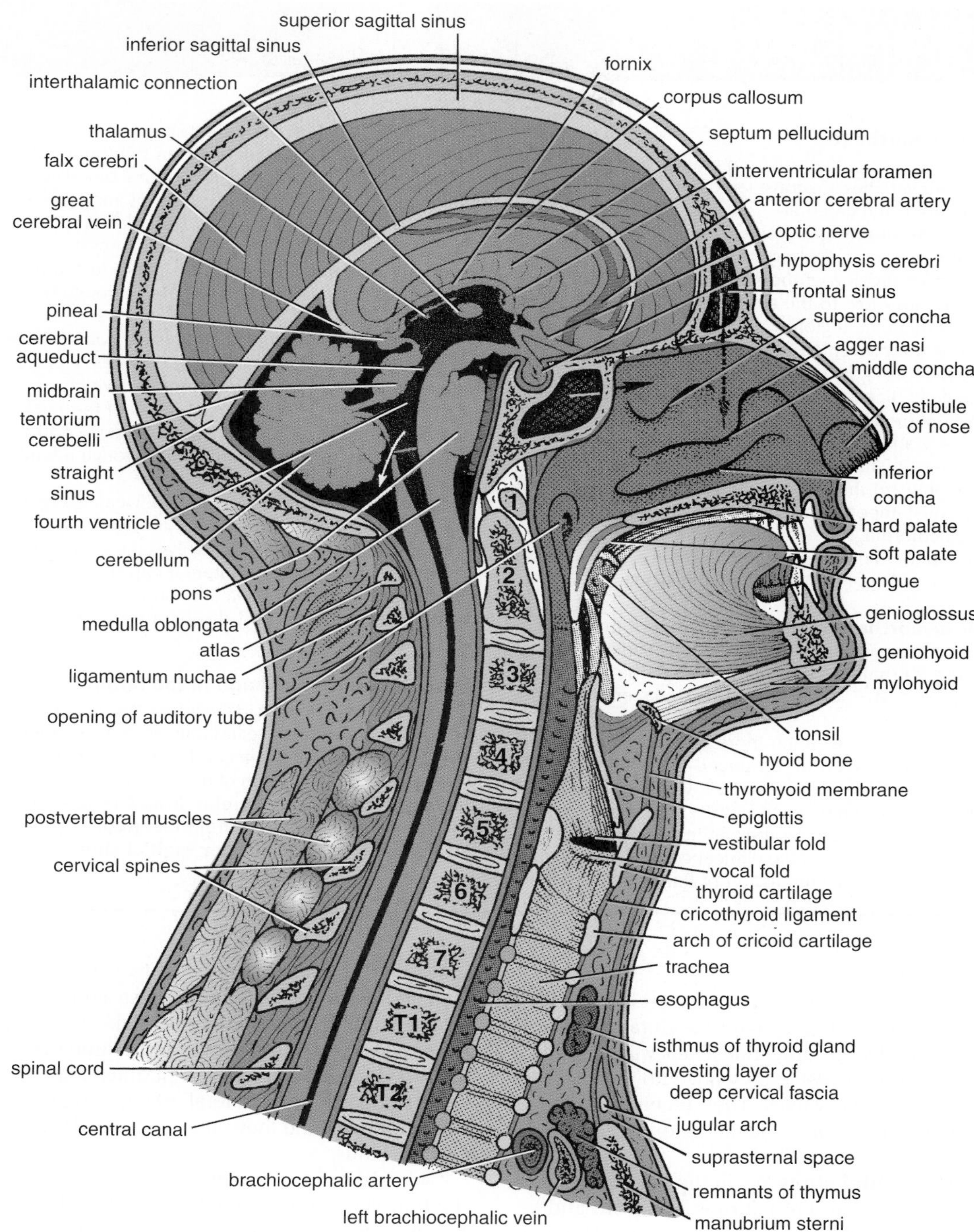

Figure 11-13 Sagittal section of the head and neck.

bloodstream by passing into the arachnoid villi and diffusing through their walls.

In addition to removing waste products associated with neuronal activity, the cerebrospinal fluid provides a fluid medium in which the brain floats. This mechanism effectively protects the brain from trauma.

Pia Mater of the Brain

The pia mater is a vascular membrane that closely invests the brain, covering the gyri and descending into the deepest sulci (Fig. 11-2). It extends over the cranial nerves and fuses with their epineurium. The cerebral arteries entering the substance of the brain carry a sheath of pia with them.

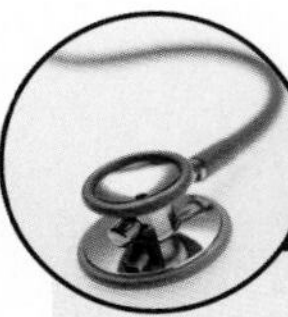

CLINICAL NOTES

Intracranial Hemorrhage

Intracranial hemorrhage may result from trauma or cerebral vascular lesions. Four varieties are considered here: extradural, subdural, subarachnoid, and cerebral.

Extradural hemorrhage results from injuries to the meningeal arteries or veins. The most common artery to be damaged is the anterior division of the middle meningeal artery. A comparatively minor blow to the side of the head, resulting in fracture of the skull in the region of the anteroinferior portion of the parietal bone, may sever the artery. The arterial or venous injury is especially liable to occur if the artery and vein enter a bony canal in this region. Bleeding occurs and strips up the meningeal layer of dura from the internal surface of the skull. The intracranial pressure rises, and the enlarging blood clot exerts local pressure on the underlying motor area in the precentral gyrus. Blood may also pass outward through the fracture line to form a soft swelling under the temporalis muscle.

To stop the hemorrhage, the torn artery or vein must be ligated or plugged. The burr hole through the skull wall should be placed about 1 to 1.5 in. (2.5 to 4 cm) above the midpoint of the zygomatic arch.

Subdural hemorrhage results from tearing of the superior cerebral veins at their point of entrance into the superior sagittal sinus. The cause is usually a blow on the front or the back of the head, causing excessive anteroposterior displacement of the brain within the skull.

This condition, which is much more common than middle meningeal hemorrhage, can be produced by a sudden minor blow. Once the vein is torn, blood under low pressure begins to accumulate in the potential space between the dura and the arachnoid. In about half the cases the condition is bilateral.

Acute and chronic forms of the clinical condition occur, depending on the speed of accumulation of fluid in the subdural space. For example, if the patient starts to vomit, the venous pressure will rise as a result of a rise in the intrathoracic pressure. Under these circumstances, the subdural blood clot will increase rapidly in size and produce acute symptoms. In the chronic form, over a course of several months, the small blood clot will attract fluid by osmosis so that a hemorrhagic cyst is formed, which gradually expands and produces pressure symptoms. In both forms the blood clot must be removed through burr holes in the skull.

Subarachnoid hemorrhage results from leakage or rupture of a congenital aneurysm on the circle of Willis or, less commonly, from an angioma. The symptoms, which are sudden in onset, include severe headache, stiffness of the neck, and loss of consciousness. The diagnosis is established by withdrawing heavily blood-stained cerebrospinal fluid through a lumbar puncture (spinal tap).

Cerebral hemorrhage is generally caused by rupture of the thin-walled lenticulostriate artery, a branch of the middle cerebral artery. The hemorrhage involves the vital corticobulbar and corticospinal fibers in the internal capsule and produces hemiplegia on the opposite side of the body. The patient immediately loses consciousness, and the paralysis is evident when consciousness is regained.

Intracranial Hemorrhage in the Infant

Intracranial hemorrhage in the infant may occur during birth and may result from excessive molding of the head. Bleeding may occur from the cerebral veins or the venous sinuses. Excessive anteroposterior compression of the head often tears the anterior attachment of the falx cerebri from the tentorium cerebelli. Bleeding then takes place from the **great cerebral veins,** the **straight sinus,** or the **inferior sagittal sinus.**

The Venous Blood Sinuses

The venous sinuses of the cranial cavity are blood-filled spaces situated between the layers of the dura mater (Fig. 11-2); they are lined by endothelium. Their walls are thick and composed of fibrous tissue; they have no muscular tissue. The sinuses have no valves. They receive tributaries from the brain, the diploë of the skull, the orbit, and the internal ear.

The **superior sagittal sinus** lies in the upper fixed border of the falx cerebri (Fig. 11-9). It runs backward and becomes continuous with the right transverse sinus. The sinus communicates on each side with the **venous lacunae.** Numerous arachnoid villi and granulations project into the lacunae (Fig. 11-2). The superior sagittal sinus receives the **superior cerebral veins.**

The **inferior sagittal sinus** lies in the free lower margin of the falx cerebri. It runs backward and joins the great cerebral vein to form the straight sinus (Fig. 11-9). It receives cerebral veins from the medial surface of the cerebral hemisphere.

The **straight sinus** lies at the junction of the falx cerebri with the tentorium cerebelli (Fig. 11-9). Formed by the union of the inferior sagittal sinus with the great cerebral vein, it drains into the left transverse sinus.

The **right transverse sinus** begins as a continuation of the superior sagittal sinus; the **left transverse sinus** is usually a continuation of the straight sinus (Figs. 11-9 and 11-10). Each sinus lies in the lateral attached margin of the tentorium cerebelli, and they end on each side by becoming the sigmoid sinus.

The **sigmoid sinuses** are a direct continuation of the transverse sinuses. Each sinus turns downward behind the mastoid antrum of the temporal bone and then leaves the skull through the jugular foramen to become the internal jugular vein (Fig. 11-30).

The **occipital sinus** lies in the attached margin of the falx cerebelli. It communicates with the vertebral veins through the foramen magnum and the transverse sinuses.

Each **cavernous sinus** lies on the lateral side of the body of the sphenoid bone (Fig. 11-9). Anteriorly, the sinus receives the inferior ophthalmic vein and the central vein of the retina. The sinus drains posteriorly into the transverse sinus through the superior petrosal sinus. Intercavernous sinuses connect the two cavernous sinuses through the sella turcica.

Important Structures Associated With the Cavernous Sinuses

- The internal carotid artery and the sixth cranial nerve, which travel through it (Fig. 11-12)
- In the lateral wall, the third and fourth cranial nerves, and the ophthalmic and maxillary divisions of the fifth cranial nerve (Fig. 11-12).
- The pituitary gland, which lies medially in the sella turcica (Fig.11-12)
- The veins of the face, which are connected with the cavernous sinus via the facial vein and inferior ophthalmic vein, and are an important route for the spread of infection from the face (Fig. 11-9)
- The **superior** and **inferior petrosal sinuses,** which run along the upper and lower borders of the petrous part of the temporal bone (Fig. 11-9)

Pituitary Gland (Hypophysis Cerebri)

The pituitary gland is a small, oval structure attached to the undersurface of the brain by the **infundibulum** (Fig. 11-12). The gland is well protected by virtue of its location in the sella turcica of the sphenoid bone. The pituitary gland is vital to life and is fully described on page 815.

Parts of the Brain

For a detailed description of the gross structure of the brain, a textbook of neuroanatomy should be consulted. In the following account, only the main parts of the brain are described.

Major Parts of the Brain		Cavities of the Brain
Forebrain	Cerebrum	Right and left lateral ventricles
	Diencephalon	Third ventricle
Midbrain		Cerebral aqueduct
Hindbrain	Pons Medulla oblongata Cerebellum	Fourth ventricle and central canal

The brain is that part of the central nervous system that lies inside the cranial cavity. It is continuous with the spinal cord through the foramen magnum.

Cerebrum

The **cerebrum** is the largest part of the brain and consists of two **cerebral hemispheres** connected by a mass of white matter called the **corpus callosum** (Fig. 11-13). Each hemisphere extends from the frontal to the occipital bones; above the anterior and middle cranial fossae; and, posteriorly, above the tentorium cerebelli. The hemispheres are separated by a deep cleft, the **longitudinal fissure,** into which projects the **falx cerebri** (Fig. 11-13).

The surface layer of each hemisphere is called the **cortex** and is composed of **gray matter** (Fig. 11-2). The cerebral cortex is thrown into folds, or **gyri,** separated by fissures, or **sulci.** By this means the surface area of the cortex is greatly increased. Several of the large sulci conveniently subdivide the surface of each hemisphere into **lobes.** The lobes are named for the bones of the cranium under which they lie (Fig. 11-14).

The **frontal lobe** is situated in front of the **central sulcus** (Fig. 11-14) and above the **lateral sulcus.** The **parietal lobe** is situated behind the central sulcus and above the lateral sulcus. The **occipital lobe** lies below the **parieto-occipital sulcus.** Below the lateral sulcus is situated the **temporal lobe.**

The **precentral gyrus** lies immediately anterior to the central sulcus and is known as the **motor area** (Fig. 11-14). The large motor nerve cells in this area control voluntary movements on the opposite side of the body. Most nerve fibers cross over to the opposite side in the medulla oblongata as they descend to the spinal cord.

In the motor area, the body is represented in an inverted position, with the nerve cells controlling the movements of the feet located in the upper part and those controlling the movements of the face and hands in the lower part (Fig. 11-14).

The **postcentral gyrus** lies immediately posterior to the central sulcus and is known as the **sensory area** (Fig. 11-14). The small nerve cells in this area receive and interpret sensations of pain, temperature, touch, and pressure from the opposite side of the body.

The **superior temporal gyrus** lies immediately below the lateral sulcus (Fig. 11-14). The middle of this gyrus is concerned with the reception and interpretation of sound and is known as the **auditory area.**

Broca's area, or the **motor speech area,** lies just above the lateral sulcus (Fig. 11-14). It controls the movements employed in speech. It is dominant in the left hemisphere in right-handed persons and in the right hemisphere in left-handed persons.

The **visual area** is situated on the posterior pole and medial aspect of the cerebral hemisphere in the region of the **calcarine sulcus** (Fig. 11-14). It is the receiving area for visual impressions.

The cavity present within each cerebral hemisphere is called the **lateral ventricle.** The lateral ventricles communicate with the third ventricle through the **interventricular foramina** (Fig. 11-13).

Diencephalon

The diencephalon is almost completely hidden from the surface of the brain. It consists of a dorsal **thalamus** (Fig. 11-13) and a ventral **hypothalamus.** The thalamus is a large mass of gray matter that lies on either side of the third ventricle. It is the great relay station on the afferent sensory pathway to the cerebral cortex.

The hypothalamus forms the lower part of the lateral wall and floor of the third ventricle. The following structures are found in the floor of the third ventricle from before backward: the **optic chiasma** (Fig. 11-15), the **tuber cinereum** and the **infundibulum,** the **mammillary bodies,** and the **posterior perforated substance.**

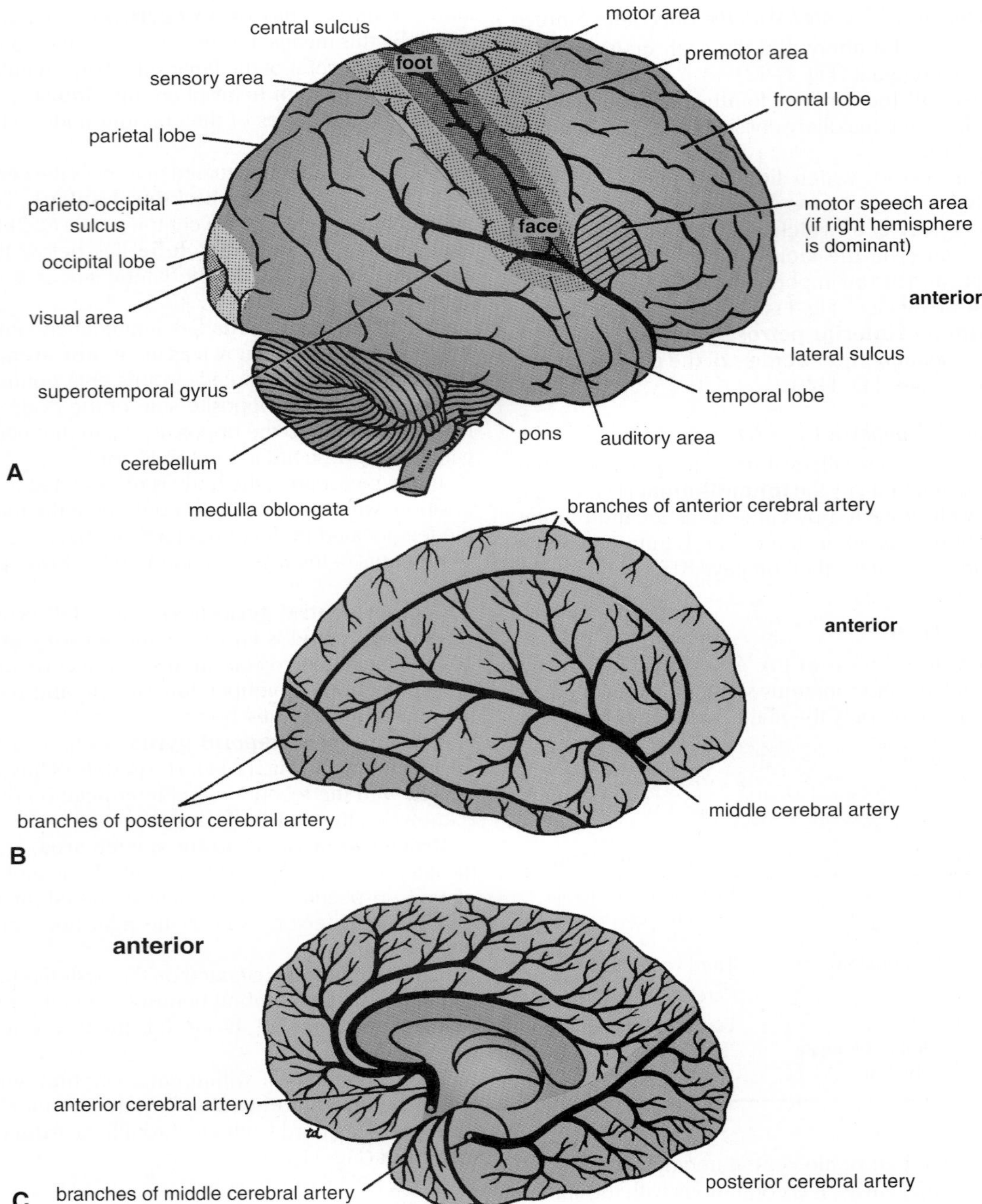

Figure 11-14 **A.** Right side of the brain showing some important localized areas of cerebral function. Note that the motor speech area is most commonly located in the left rather than the right cerebral hemisphere. **B.** Lateral surface of the cerebral hemisphere showing areas supplied by the cerebral arteries. In this and the next figure, areas colored blue are supplied by the anterior cerebral artery; those colored red, by the middle cerebral artery; and those colored green, by the posterior cerebral artery. **C.** Medial surface of the cerebral hemisphere showing the areas supplied by the cerebral arteries.

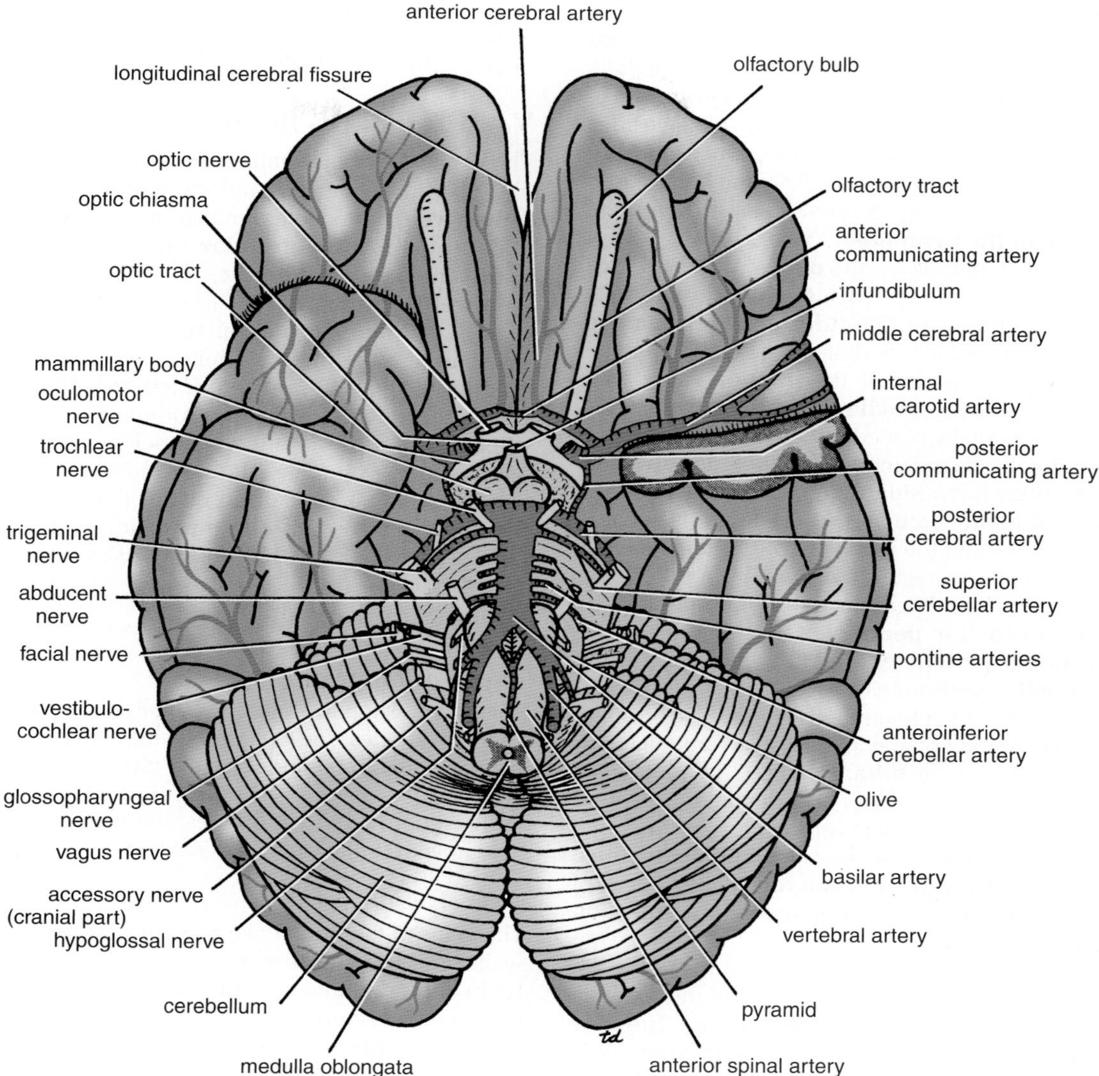

Figure 11-15 Arteries and cranial nerves seen on the inferior surface of the brain. To show the course of the middle cerebral artery, the anterior pole of the left temporal lobe has been removed.

Midbrain

The midbrain is the narrow part of the brain that passes through the tentorial notch and connects the forebrain to the hindbrain (Fig. 11-13).

The midbrain comprises two lateral halves called the **cerebral peduncles;** each of these is divided into an anterior part, the **crus cerebri,** and a posterior part, the **tegmentum,** by a pigmented band of gray matter, the **substantia nigra** (Fig. 11-12). The narrow cavity of the midbrain is the **cerebral aqueduct,** which connects the third and fourth ventricles. The **tectum** is the part of the midbrain posterior to the cerebral aqueduct; it has four small surface swellings, namely, the **two superior** (Fig. 11-12) and **two inferior colliculi.** The colliculi are deeply placed between the cerebellum and the cerebral hemispheres.

The **pineal body** is a small glandular structure that lies between the superior colliculi (Fig. 11-13). It is attached by a stalk to the region of the posterior wall of the third ventricle (see also page 816). The pineal commonly calcifies in middle age, and thus it can be visualized on radiographs.

Hindbrain

The **pons** is situated on the anterior surface of the cerebellum below the midbrain and above the medulla oblongata (Fig. 11-13). It is composed mainly of nerve fibers, which connect the two halves of the cerebellum. It also contains ascending and descending fibers connecting the forebrain, the midbrain, and the spinal cord. Some of the nerve cells within the pons serve as relay stations, whereas others form cranial nerve nuclei.

The **medulla oblongata** is conical in shape and connects the pons above to the spinal cord below (Fig. 11-13). A **median fissure** is present on the anterior surface of the medulla, and on each side of this is a swelling called the **pyramid** (Fig. 11-15). The pyramids are composed of bundles of nerve fibers that originate in large nerve cells in the precentral gyrus of the cerebral cortex. The pyramids taper below, and here most of the descending fibers cross over to the opposite side, forming the **decussation of the pyramids.**

Posterior to the pyramids are the **olives,** which are oval elevations produced by the underlying **olivary nuclei** (Fig. 11-15). Behind the olives are the **inferior cerebellar peduncles,** which connect the medulla to the cerebellum.

On the posterior surface of the inferior part of the medulla oblongata are the **gracile** and **cuneate tubercles,** produced by the medially placed underlying **nucleus gracilis** and the laterally placed underlying **nucleus cuneatus.**

The **cerebellum** lies within the posterior cranial fossa beneath the tentorium cerebelli (Fig. 11-13). It is situated posterior to the pons and the medulla oblongata. It consists of two hemispheres connected by a median portion, the **vermis.** The cerebellum is connected to the midbrain by the **superior cerebellar peduncles,** to the pons by the **middle cerebellar peduncles,** and to the medulla by the **inferior cerebellar peduncles.**

The surface layer of each cerebellar hemisphere, called the **cortex,** is composed of gray matter. The cerebellar cortex is thrown into folds, or **folia,** separated by closely set transverse fissures. Certain masses of gray matter are found in the interior of the cerebellum, embedded in the white matter; the largest of these is known as the **dentate nucleus.**

The cerebellum plays an important role in the control of muscle tone and the coordination of muscle movement on the same side of the body.

The cavity of the hindbrain is the fourth ventricle (Fig. 11-13). This is bounded in front by the pons and the medulla oblongata and behind by the **superior** and **inferior medullary vela** and the cerebellum. The fourth ventricle is connected above to the third ventricle by the cerebral aqueduct, and below it is continuous with the central canal of the spinal cord. It communicates with the subarachnoid space through three openings in the lower part of the roof: a median and two lateral openings.

Ventricles of the Brain

The ventricles of the brain consist of the two lateral ventricles, the third ventricle, and the fourth ventricle. The two **lateral ventricles** communicate with the **third ventricle** through the **interventricular foramina** (Fig. 11-13); the third ventricle communicates with the fourth ventricle by the **cerebral aqueduct.** The fourth ventricle, in turn, is continuous with the narrow **central canal** of the spinal cord and, through the three foramina in its roof, with the subarachnoid space. The ventricles are filled with cerebrospinal fluid, which is produced by the **choroid plexuses** of the two lateral ventricles, the third ventricle, and the fourth ventricle. The size and shape of the cerebral ventricles may be visualized clinically using computed tomography (CT) scans and magnetic resonance imaging (MRI) (Figs. 11-127, 11-128, and 11-129).

Blood Supply of the Brain

Arteries of the Brain

The brain is supplied by the two internal carotid and the two vertebral arteries. The four arteries anastomose on the inferior surface of the brain and form the **circle of Willis** (circulus arteriosus).

The internal carotid arteries, the vertebral arteries, and the circle of Willis are fully described on page 750 and 751.

Veins of the Brain

The veins of the brain have no muscular tissue in their thin walls, and they possess no valves. They emerge from the brain and drain into the cranial venous sinuses (Fig. 11-2). Cerebral and cerebellar veins and veins of the brainstem are present. The **great cerebral vein** is formed by the union of the two **internal cerebral veins** and drains into the straight sinus (Fig. 11-9).

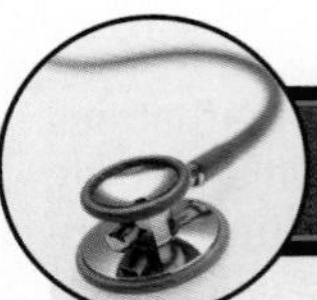

CLINICAL NOTES

Brain Injuries

Injuries of the brain are produced by displacement and distortion of the neuronal tissues at the moment of impact. The brain may be likened to a log soaked with water floating submerged in water. The brain is floating in the cerebrospinal fluid in the subarachnoid space and is capable of a certain amount of anteroposterior movement, which is limited by the attachment of the superior cerebral veins to the superior sagittal sinus. Lateral displacement of the brain is limited by the falx cerebri. The tentorium cerebelli and the falx cerebelli also restrict displacement of the brain.

It follows from these anatomic facts that blows on the front or back of the head lead to displacement of the brain, which may produce severe cerebral damage, stretching and distortion of the brainstem, and stretching and even tearing of the commissures of the brain. The terms **concussion, contusion,** and **laceration** are used clinically to describe the degrees of brain injury.

Blows on the side of the head produce less cerebral displacement, and the injuries to the brain consequently tend to be less severe.

The Cranial Nerves in the Cranial Cavity

The 12 pairs of cranial nerves are named as follows:

- I. Olfactory (sensory)
- II. Optic (sensory)
- III. Oculomotor (motor)
- IV. Trochlear (motor)
- V. Trigeminal (mixed)
- VI. Abducent (motor)
- VII. Facial (mixed)
- VIII. Vestibulocochlear (sensory)
- IX. Glossopharyngeal (mixed)
- X. Vagus (mixed)
- XI. Accessory (motor)
- XII. Hypoglossal (motor)

The nerves emerge from the brain and are transmitted through foramina and fissures in the base of the skull. All the nerves are distributed in the head and neck except the vagus, which also supplies structures in the thorax and abdomen. The olfactory, optic, and vestibulocochlear nerves are entirely sensory; the oculomotor, trochlear, abducent, accessory, and hypoglossal nerves are entirely motor; and the remaining nerves are mixed. The origins and courses of the cranial nerves are described on page 757.

The cranial nerves, their component parts, their function, and the openings through which they exit from the skull are summarized in Table 11-6.

The Orbital Region

The orbits are a pair of bony cavities that contain the eyeballs; their associated muscles, nerves, vessels, and fat; and most of the lacrimal apparatus. The orbital opening is guarded by two thin, movable folds, the eyelids.

Eyelids

The eyelids protect the eye from injury and excessive light by their closure (Fig. 11-16). The upper eyelid is larger and more mobile than the lower, and they meet each other at the **medial** and **lateral angles.** The **palpebral fissure** is the elliptical opening between the eyelids and is the entrance into the conjunctival sac. When the eye is closed, the upper eyelid completely covers the cornea of the eye. When the eye is open and looking straight ahead, the upper lid just covers the upper margin of the cornea. The lower lid lies just below the cornea when the eye is open and rises only slightly when the eye is closed.

The superficial surface of the eyelids is covered by skin, and the deep surface is covered by a mucous membrane, called the **conjunctiva.** The **eyelashes** are short, curved hairs on the free edges of the eyelids (Figs. 11-16 and 11-17). They are arranged in double or triple rows at the mucocutaneous junction. The sebaceous glands (glands of Zeis) open directly into the eyelash follicles. The **ciliary glands** (glands of Moll) are modified sweat glands that open separately between adjacent lashes. The **tarsal glands** are long, modified sebaceous glands that pour their oily secretion onto the margin of the lid; their openings lie behind the eyelashes (Fig. 11-16). This oily material prevents the overflow of tears and helps make the closed eyelids airtight.

The more rounded medial angle is separated from the eyeball by a small space, the **lacus lacrimalis,** in the center of which is a small, reddish yellow elevation, the **caruncula lacrimalis** (Figs. 11-16 and 11-17). A reddish semilunar fold, called the **plica semilunaris,** lies on the lateral side of the caruncle.

Near the medial angle of the eye a small elevation, the **papilla lacrimalis,** is present. On the summit of the papilla is a small hole, the **punctum lacrimale,** which leads into the **canaliculus lacrimalis** (Figs. 11-16 and 11-17). The papilla lacrimalis projects into the lacus, and the punctum and canaliculus carry tears down into the nose (see page 694).

The **conjunctiva** is a thin mucous membrane that lines the eyelids and is reflected at **the superior** and **inferior fornices** onto the anterior surface of the eyeball (Fig. 11-16). Its epithelium is continuous with that of the cornea. The upper lateral part of the superior fornix is pierced by the ducts of the lacrimal gland (see below). The conjunctiva thus forms a potential space, the **conjunctival sac,** which is open at the **palpebral fissure.** Beneath the eyelid is a groove, the **subtarsal sulcus,** which runs close to and parallel with the margin of the lid (Fig. 11-16). The sulcus tends to trap small foreign particles introduced into the conjunctival sac and is thus clinically important.

The framework of the eyelids is formed by a fibrous sheet, the **orbital septum** (Fig. 11-16). This is attached to the periosteum at the orbital margins. The orbital septum is thickened at the margins of the lids to form the superior and inferior **tarsal plates.** The lateral ends of the plates are attached by a band, the **lateral palpebral ligament,** to a bony tubercle just within the orbital margin. The medial ends of the plates are attached by a band, the **medial palpebral ligament,** to the crest of the lacrimal bone (Fig. 11-16). The tarsal glands are embedded in the posterior surface of the tarsal plates.

The superficial surface of the tarsal plates and the orbital septum are covered by the palpebral fibers of the **orbicularis oculi muscle** (Table 11-16). The aponeurosis of insertion of the **levator palpebrae superioris muscle** pierces the orbital septum to reach the anterior surface of the superior tarsal plate and the skin (Fig. 11-16).

Movements of the Eyelids

The position of the eyelids at rest depends on the tone of the **orbicularis oculi** and the **levator palpebrae superioris muscles** and the position of the eyeball. The eyelids are closed by the contraction of the orbicularis oculi and the relaxation of the levator palpebrae superioris muscles. The eye is opened by the levator palpebrae superioris raising the upper lid. On looking upward, the levator palpebrae superioris contracts, and the upper lid moves with the eyeball. On looking downward, both lids move, the upper lid continues to cover the upper part of the cornea, and the lower lid is pulled downward slightly by the conjunctiva, which is attached to the sclera and the lower lid.

The origins and insertions of the muscles of the eyelids are summarized in Table 11-2.

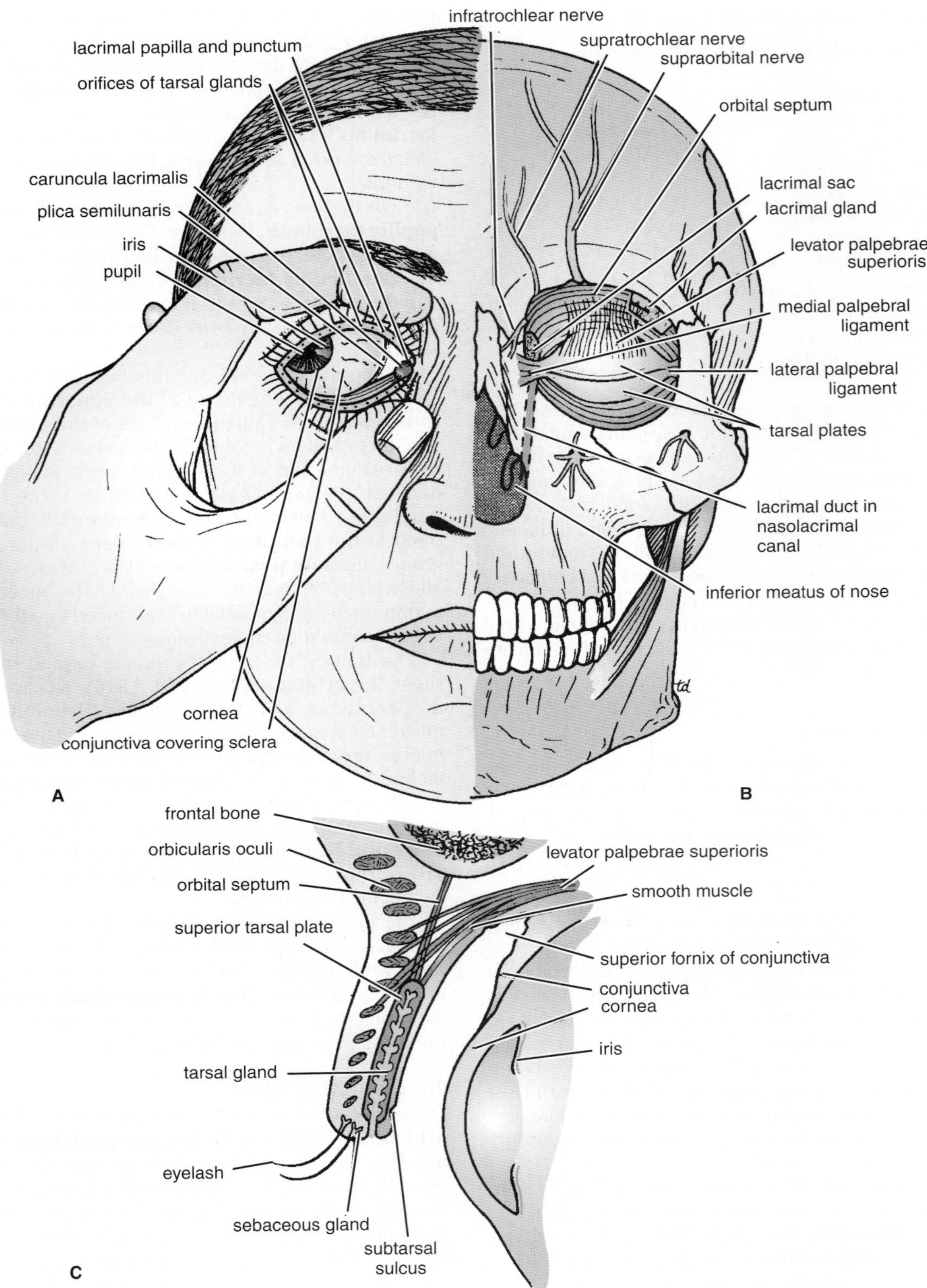

Figure 11-16 **A.** Right eye, with the eyelids separated to show the openings of the tarsal glands, plica semilunaris, caruncula lacrimalis, and puncta lacrimalis. **B.** Left eye, showing the superior and inferior tarsal plates and the lacrimal gland, sac, and duct. Note that a small window has been cut in the orbital septum to show the underlying lacrimal gland and fat (*yellow*). **C.** Sagittal section through the upper eyelid, and the superior fornix of the conjunctiva. Note the presence of smooth muscle in the levator palpebrae superioris.

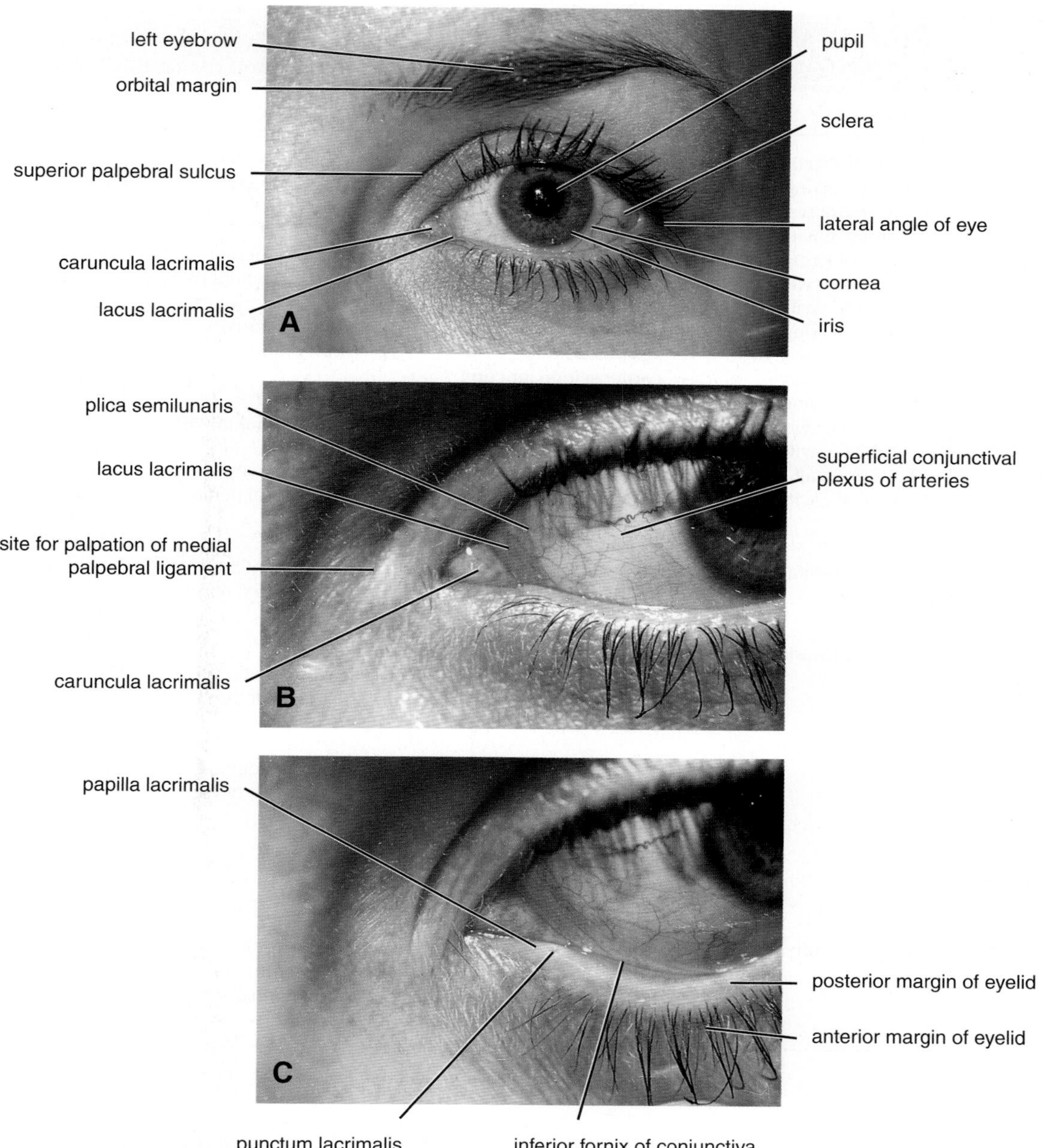

Figure 11-17 Left eye of a 29-year-old woman. **A.** The names of structures seen in the examination of the eye. **B.** An enlarged view of the medial angle between the eyelids. **C.** The lower eyelid pulled downward and slightly everted to reveal the punctum lacrimale.

Table 11-2 Muscles of the Eyeball and Eyelids

Muscle	Origin	Insertion	Nerve Supply	Action
Extrinsic Muscles of Eyeball (Striated Skeletal Muscle)				
Superior rectus	Tendinous ring on posterior wall of orbital cavity	Superior surface of eyeball just posterior to corneoscleral junction	Oculomotor nerve (third cranial nerve)	Raises cornea upward and medially
Inferior rectus	Tendinous ring on posterior wall of orbital cavity	Inferior surface of eyeball just posterior to corneoscleral junction	Oculomotor nerve (third cranial nerve)	Depresses cornea downward and medially
Medial rectus	Tendinous ring on posterior wall of orbital cavity	Medial surface of eyeball just posterior to corneoscleral junction	Oculomotor nerve (third cranial nerve)	Rotates eyeball so that cornea looks medially
Lateral rectus	Tendinous ring on posterior wall of orbital cavity	Lateral surface of eyeball just posterior to corneoscleral junction	Abducent nerve (sixth cranial nerve)	Rotates eyeball so that cornea looks laterally
Superior oblique	Posterior wall of orbital cavity	Passes through pulley and is attached to superior surface of eyeball beneath superior rectus	Trochlear nerve (fourth cranial nerve)	Rotates eyeball so that cornea looks downward and laterally
Inferior oblique	Floor of orbital cavity	Lateral surface of eyeball deep to lateral rectus	Oculomotor nerve (third cranial nerve)	Rotates eyeball so that cornea looks upward and laterally
Intrinsic Muscles of Eyeball (Smooth Muscle)				
Sphincter pupillae of iris			Parasympathetic via oculomotor nerve	Constricts pupil
Dilator pupillae of iris			Sympathetic	Dilates pupil
Ciliary muscle			Parasympathetic via oculomotor nerve	Controls shape of lens; in accommodation, makes lens more globular
Muscles of Eyelids				
Orbicularis oculi (Table 11-4)				
Levator palpebrae superioris	Back of orbital cavity	Anterior surface and upper margin of superior tarsal plate	Striated muscle oculomotor nerve, smooth muscle sympathetic	Raises upper lid

Lacrimal Apparatus

Lacrimal Gland

The lacrimal gland consists of a large **orbital part** and a small **palpebral part,** which are continuous with each other around the lateral edge of the aponeurosis of the levator palpebrae superioris. It is situated above the eyeball in the anterior and upper part of the orbit posterior to the orbital septum (Fig. 11-16). The gland opens into the lateral part of the superior fornix of the conjunctiva by 12 ducts.

The **parasympathetic secretomotor nerve supply** is derived from the **lacrimal nucleus** of the facial nerve. The preganglionic fibers reach the pterygopalatine ganglion (sphenopalatine ganglion) via the nervus intermedius and its great petrosal branch and via the nerve of the pterygoid canal. The postganglionic fibers leave the ganglion and join the maxillary nerve. They then pass into its zygomatic branch and the zygomaticotemporal nerve. They reach the lacrimal gland within the lacrimal nerve.

The **sympathetic postganglionic nerve supply** is from the internal carotid plexus and travels in the deep petrosal nerve, the nerve of the pterygoid canal, the maxillary nerve, the zygomatic nerve, the zygomaticotemporal nerve, and finally the lacrimal nerve.

Lacrimal Ducts

The tears circulate across the cornea and accumulate in the **lacus lacrimalis.** From here, the tears enter the **canaliculi lacrimales** through the **puncta lacrimalis.** The canaliculi lacrimales pass medially and open into the **lacrimal sac** (Fig. 11-16), which lies in the lacrimal groove behind the medial palpebral ligament and is the upper blind end of the nasolacrimal duct.

The **nasolacrimal duct** is about 0.5 in. (1.3 cm) long and emerges from the lower end of the lacrimal sac (Fig. 11-16). The duct descends downward, backward, and laterally in a bony canal and opens into the inferior meatus of the nose. The opening is guarded by a fold of mucous membrane known as the **lacrimal fold.** This prevents air from being forced up the duct into the lacrimal sac on blowing the nose.

The Orbit

Description

The orbit is a pyramidal cavity with its base in front and its apex behind (Fig. 11-18). The **orbital margin** is formed above by the frontal bone, the lateral margin is formed by the processes of the frontal and zygomatic bones, the inferior margin is formed by the zygomatic bone and the maxilla, and the medial margin is formed by the processes of the maxilla and the frontal bone.

The orbital walls are shown in Figure 11-18.

Roof: Formed by the orbital plate of the frontal bone, which separates the orbital cavity from the anterior cranial fossa and the frontal lobe of the cerebral hemisphere

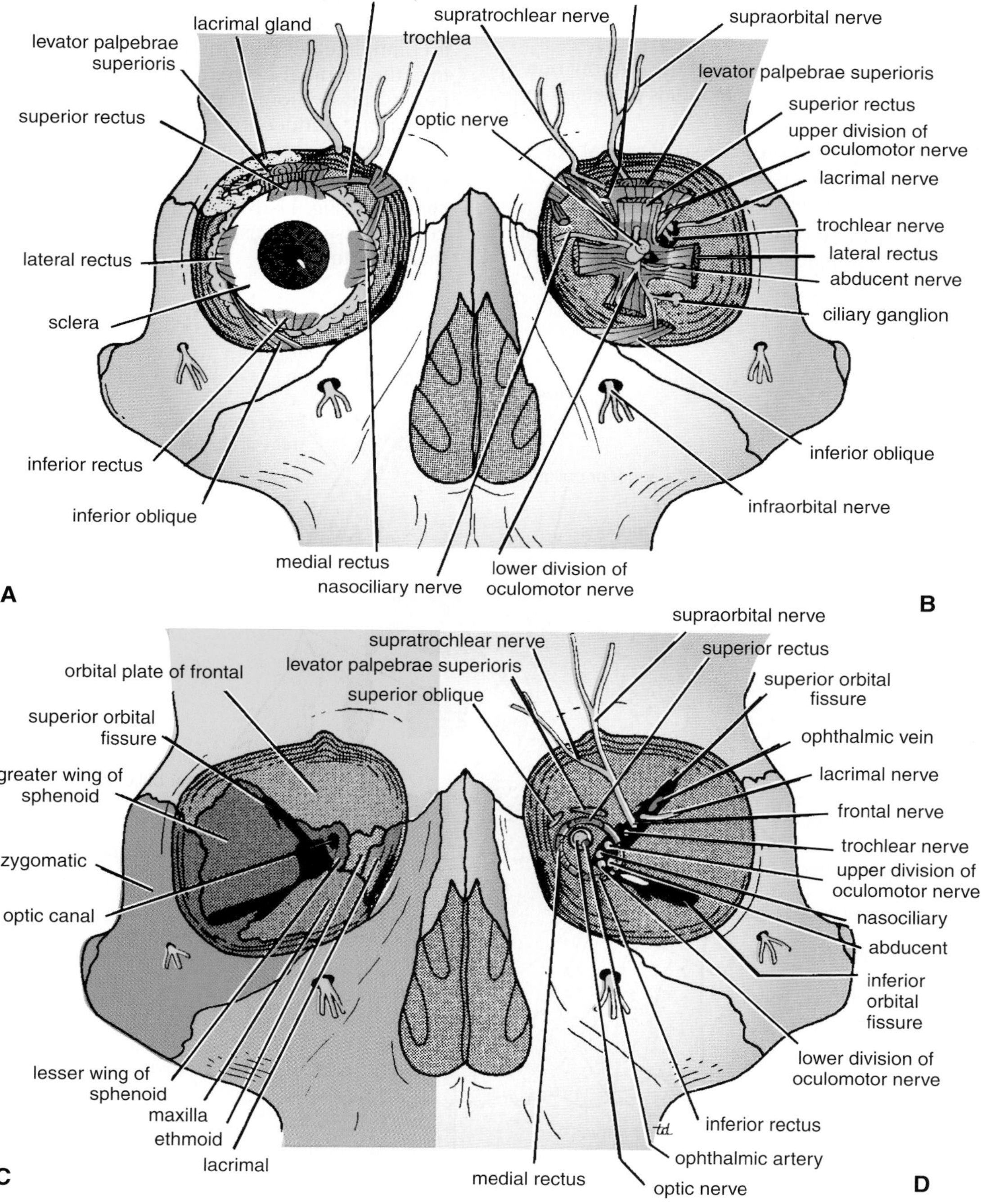

Figure 11-18 **A.** Right eyeball exposed from in front. **B.** Muscles and nerves of the left orbit as seen from in front. **C.** Bones forming the walls of the right orbit. **D.** The optic canal and the superior and inferior orbital fissures on the left side.

Lateral wall: Formed by the zygomatic bone and the greater wing of the sphenoid (Fig. 11-18)

Floor: Formed by the orbital plate of the maxilla, which separates the orbital cavity from the maxillary sinus

Medial wall: Formed from before backward by the frontal process of the maxilla, the lacrimal bone, the orbital plate of the ethmoid (which separates the orbital cavity from the ethmoid sinuses), and the body of the sphenoid

Openings Into the Orbital Cavity

The openings into the orbital cavity are shown in Figure 11-18.

Orbital opening: Lies anteriorly (Fig. 11-18). About one-sixth of the eye is exposed; the remainder is protected by the walls of the orbit.

Supraorbital notch (Foramen): The supraorbital notch is situated on the superior orbital margin (Fig. 11-18). It transmits the supraorbital nerve and blood vessels.

Infraorbital groove and canal: Situated on the floor of the orbit in the orbital plate of the maxilla (Fig. 11-19); they transmit the infraorbital nerve (a continuation of the maxillary nerve) and blood vessels.

Nasolacrimal canal: Located anteriorly on the medial wall; it communicates with the inferior meatus of the nose (Fig. 11-16). It transmits the nasolacrimal duct.

Inferior orbital fissure: Located posteriorly between the maxilla and the greater wing of the sphenoid (Fig. 11-18); it communicates with the pterygopalatine fossa. It transmits the maxillary nerve and its zygomatic branch, the inferior ophthalmic vein, and sympathetic nerves.

Superior orbital fissure: Located posteriorly between the greater and lesser wings of the sphenoid (Fig. 11-18); it communicates with the middle cranial fossa. It transmits the lacrimal nerve, the frontal nerve, the trochlear nerve, the oculomotor nerve (upper and lower divisions), the abducent nerve, the nasociliary nerve, and the superior ophthalmic vein.

Optic canal: Located posteriorly in the lesser wing of the sphenoid (Fig. 11-18); it communicates with the middle cranial fossa. It transmits the optic nerve and the ophthalmic artery.

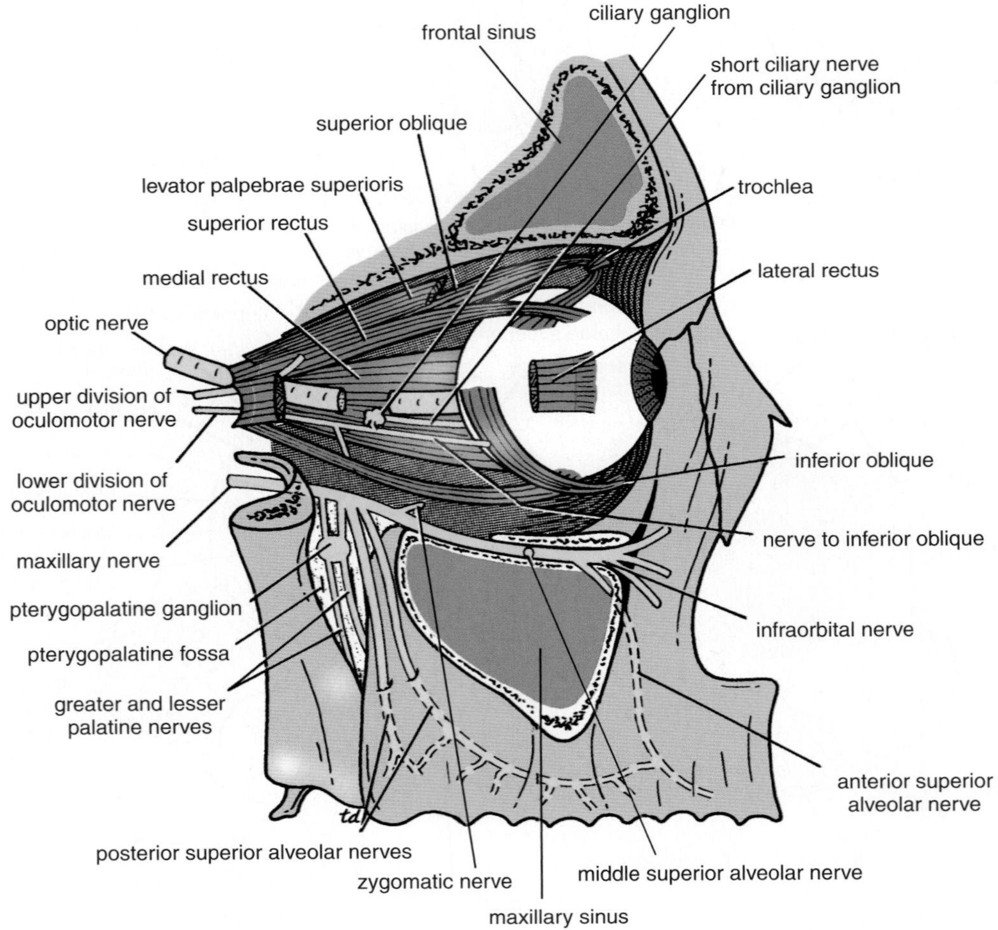

Figure 11-19 Muscles and nerves of the right orbit viewed from the lateral side. The maxillary nerve and the pterygopalatine ganglion are also shown.

Orbital Fascia

The orbital fascia is the periosteum of the bones that form the walls of the orbit. It is loosely attached to the bones and is continuous through the foramina and fissures with the periosteum covering the outer surfaces of the bones. The **muscle of Müller,** or **orbitalis muscle,** is a thin layer of smooth muscle that bridges the inferior orbital fissure. It is supplied by sympathetic nerves, and its function is unknown.

Nerves of the Orbit

Optic Nerve

The optic nerve enters the orbit from the middle cranial fossa by passing through the optic canal (Fig. 11-20). It is accompanied by the ophthalmic artery, which lies on its lower lateral side. The nerve is surrounded by sheaths of pia mater, arachnoid mater, and dura mater (Fig. 11-25). It runs forward and laterally within the cone of the recti muscles and pierces the sclera at a point medial to the posterior pole of the eyeball. Here, the meninges fuse with the sclera so that the subarachnoid space with its contained cerebrospinal fluid extends forward from the middle cranial fossa, around the optic nerve, and through the optic canal, as far as the eyeball. A rise in pressure of the cerebrospinal fluid within the cranial cavity therefore is transmitted to the back of the eyeball.

Lacrimal Nerve

The lacrimal nerve arises from the ophthalmic division of the trigeminal nerve. It enters the orbit through the upper part of the superior orbital fissure (Fig. 11-18) and passes forward along the upper border of the lateral rectus muscle (Fig. 11-20). It is joined by a branch of the zygomaticotemporal nerve, which later leaves it to enter the lacrimal gland

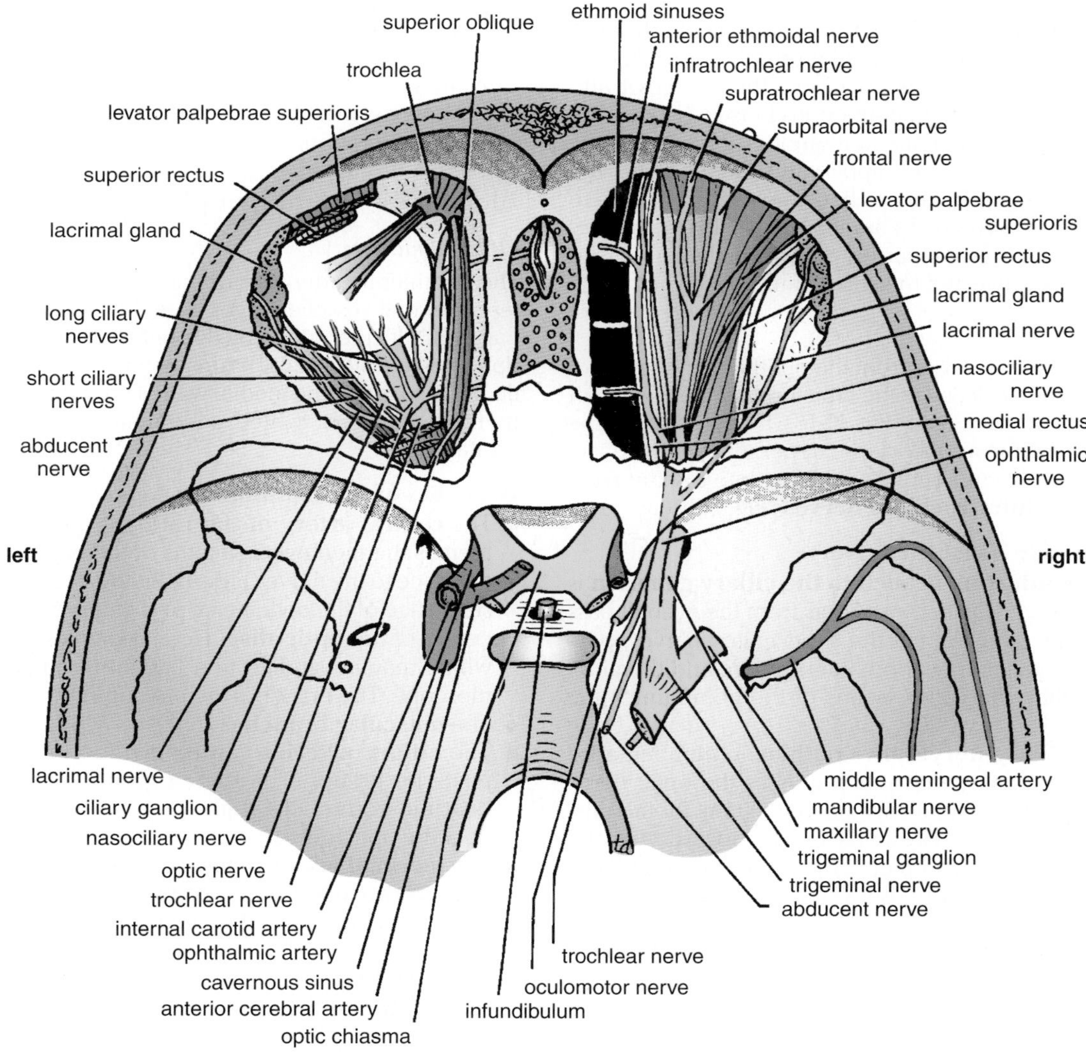

Figure 11-20 Right and left orbital cavities viewed from above. The roof of the orbit, formed by the orbital plate of the frontal bone, has been removed from both sides. On the left side, the levator palpebrae superioris and the superior rectus muscles have also been removed to expose the underlying structures.

(parasympathetic secretomotor fibers). The lacrimal nerve ends by supplying the skin of the lateral part of the upper lid.

Frontal Nerve

The frontal nerve arises from the ophthalmic division of the trigeminal nerve. It enters the orbit through the upper part of the superior orbital fissure (Fig. 11-18) and passes forward on the upper surface of the levator palpebrae superioris beneath the roof of the orbit (Fig. 11-20). It divides into the **supratrochlear** and **supraorbital nerves** that wind around the upper margin of the orbital cavity to supply the skin of the forehead; the supraorbital nerve also supplies the mucous membrane of the frontal air sinus.

Trochlear Nerve

The trochlear nerve enters the orbit through the upper part of the superior orbital fissure (Fig. 11-18). It runs forward and supplies the superior oblique muscle (Fig. 11-20).

Oculomotor Nerve

The **superior ramus** of the oculomotor nerve enters the orbit through the lower part of the superior orbital fissure (Fig. 11-18). It supplies the superior rectus muscle, then pierces it, and supplies the levator palpebrae superioris muscle (Fig. 11-18).

The **inferior ramus** of the oculomotor nerve enters the orbit in a similar manner and supplies the inferior rectus, the medial rectus, and the inferior oblique muscles. The nerve to the inferior oblique gives off a branch (Fig. 11-19) that passes to the ciliary ganglion and carries parasympathetic fibers to the sphincter pupillae and the ciliary muscle (see below).

Nasociliary Nerve

The nasociliary nerve arises from the ophthalmic division of the trigeminal nerve. It enters the orbit through the lower part of the superior orbital fissure (Fig. 11-18). It crosses above the optic nerve, runs forward along the upper margin of the medial rectus muscle, and ends by dividing into the **anterior ethmoidal** and **infratrochlear nerves** (Fig. 11-20).

Branches of the Nasociliary Nerve

- The **communicating branch to the ciliary ganglion** is a sensory nerve. The sensory fibers from the eyeball pass to the ciliary ganglion via the short ciliary nerves, pass through the ganglion without interruption, and then join the nasociliary nerve by means of the communicating branch.
- The **long ciliary nerves,** two or three in number, arise from the nasociliary nerve as it crosses the optic nerve (Fig. 11-20). They contain sympathetic fibers for the dilator pupillae muscle. The nerves pass forward with the short ciliary nerves and pierce the sclera of the eyeball. They continue forward between the sclera and the choroid to reach the iris.
- The **posterior ethmoidal nerve** supplies the ethmoidal and sphenoidal air sinuses (Fig. 11-20).
- The **infratrochlear nerve** passes forward below the pulley of the superior oblique muscle and supplies the skin of the medial part of the upper eyelid and the adjacent part of the nose (Fig. 11-16).
- The **anterior ethmoidal nerve** passes through the anterior ethmoidal foramen and enters the anterior cranial fossa on the upper surface of the cribriform plate of the ethmoid (Fig. 11-20). It enters the nasal cavity through a slitlike opening alongside the crista galli. After supplying an area of mucous membrane, it appears on the face as the **external nasal branch** at the lower border of the nasal bone, and supplies the skin of the nose down as far as the tip (see page 729).

Abducent Nerve

The abducent nerve enters the orbit through the lower part of the superior orbital fissure (Fig. 11-18). It supplies the lateral rectus muscle.

Ciliary Ganglion

The ciliary ganglion is a parasympathetic ganglion about the size of a pinhead (Fig. 11-19) and situated in the posterior part of the orbit. It receives its preganglionic parasympathetic fibers from the oculomotor nerve via the nerve to the inferior oblique. The postganglionic fibers leave the ganglion in the **short ciliary nerves,** which enter the back of the eyeball and supply the sphincter pupillae and the ciliary muscle.

A number of sympathetic fibers pass from the internal carotid plexus into the orbit and run through the ganglion without interruption.

Blood Vessels and Lymph Vessels of the Orbit

Ophthalmic Artery

The ophthalmic artery is a branch of the internal carotid artery after that vessel emerges from the cavernous sinus (see page 750). It enters the orbit through the optic canal with the optic nerve (Fig. 11-20). It runs forward and crosses the optic nerve to reach the medial wall of the orbit. It gives off numerous branches, which accompany the nerves in the orbital cavity.

Branches of the Ophthalmic Artery

- The **central artery of the retina** is a small branch that pierces the meningeal sheaths of the optic nerve to gain entrance to the nerve (Figs. 11-25 and 11-26). It runs in the substance of the optic nerve and enters the eyeball at the center of the **optic disc.** Here, it divides into branches, which may be studied in a patient through an ophthalmoscope. The branches are end arteries.
- The **muscular branches**
- The **ciliary arteries** can be divided into anterior and posterior groups. The former group enters the eyeball near the corneoscleral junction; the latter group enters near the optic nerve.
- The **lacrimal artery** to the lacrimal gland
- The **supratrochlear** and **supraorbital arteries** are distributed to the skin of the forehead (see page 729).

Ophthalmic Veins

The **superior ophthalmic vein** communicates in front with the facial vein (Fig. 11-9). The **inferior ophthalmic vein** communicates through the inferior orbital fissure with the pterygoid venous plexus. Both veins pass backward through the superior orbital fissure and drain into the cavernous sinus.

Lymph Vessels

No lymph vessels or nodes are present in the orbital cavity.

The Eye

Movements of the Eyeball

Terms Used in Describing Eye Movements

The center of the cornea or the center of the pupil is used as the anatomic "anterior pole" of the eye. All movements of the eye are then related to the direction of the movement of the anterior pole as it rotates on any one of the three axes (horizontal, vertical, and sagittal). The terminology then becomes as follows: **Elevation** is the rotation of the eye upward, **depression** is the rotation of the eye downward, **abduction** is the rotation of the eye laterally, and **adduction** is the rotation of the eye medially. Rotatory movements of the eyeball use the upper rim of the cornea (or pupil) as the marker. The eye rotates either medially or laterally.

Extrinsic Muscles Producing Movement of the Eye

There are six voluntary muscles that run from the posterior wall of the orbital cavity to the eyeball (Fig. 11-18). These are the **superior rectus,** the **inferior rectus,** the **medial rectus,** the **lateral rectus,** and the **superior** and **inferior oblique muscles.**

Because the superior and the inferior recti are inserted on the medial side of the vertical axis of the eyeball, they not only raise and depress the cornea, respectively, but also **rotate it medially** (Fig. 11-21). For the superior rectus muscle to raise the cornea directly upward, the inferior oblique muscle must assist; for the inferior rectus to depress the cornea directly downward, the superior oblique muscle must assist (Figs. 11-21 and 11-22). Note that the tendon of

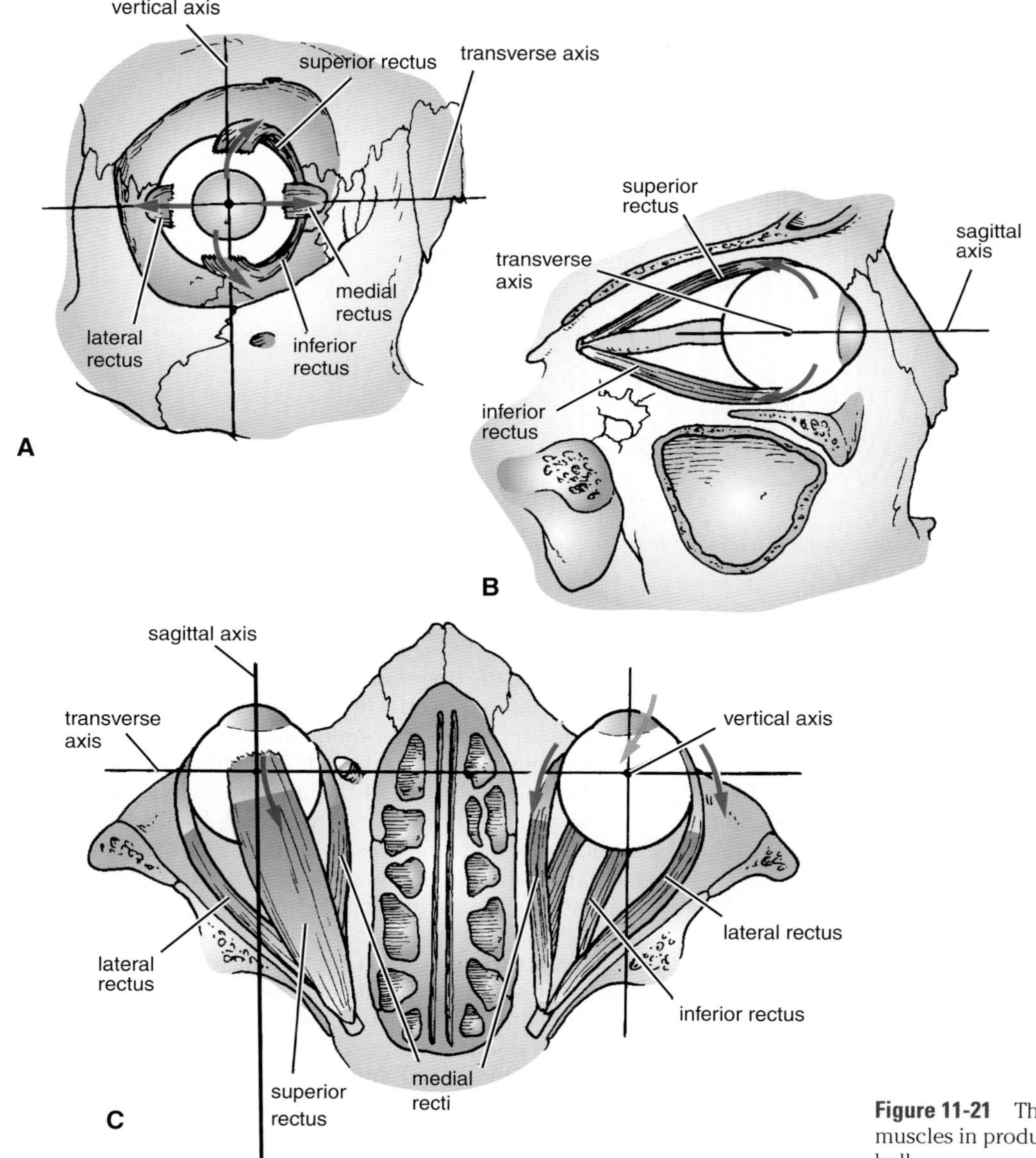

Figure 11-21 The actions of the four recti muscles in producing movements of the eyeball.

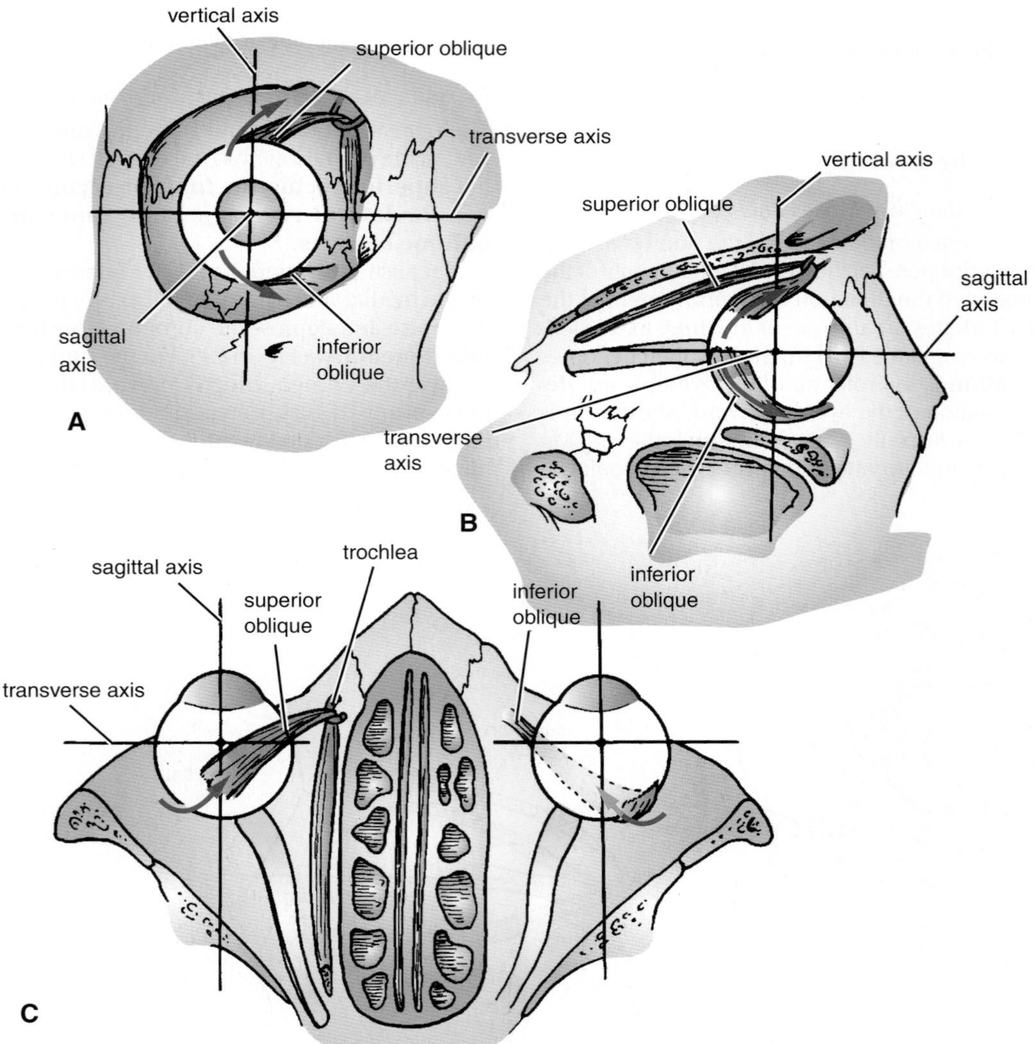

Figure 11-22 The actions of the superior and inferior oblique muscles in producing movements of the eyeball.

the superior oblique muscle passes through a fibrocartilaginous pulley (trochlea) attached to the frontal bone. The tendon now turns backward and laterally and is inserted into the sclera beneath the superior rectus muscle.

The origins, insertions, nerve supply, and actions of the muscles of the eyeball are summarized in Table 11-2. Study carefully Figure 11-24.

Clinical Testing for the Actions of the Superior and Inferior Recti and the Superior and Inferior Oblique Muscles

Because the actions of the superior and inferior recti and the superior and inferior oblique muscles are complicated when a patient is asked to look vertically upward or vertically downward, the physician tests the eye movements where the single action of each muscle predominates.

The origins of the superior and inferior recti are situated about 23° medial to their insertions, and, therefore, when the patient is asked to turn the cornea laterally, these muscles are placed in the optimum position to raise (superior rectus) or lower (inferior rectus) the cornea.

Using the same rationale, the superior and inferior oblique muscles can be tested. The pulley of the superior oblique and the origin of the inferior oblique muscles lie medial and anterior to their insertions. The physician tests the action of these muscles by asking the patient first to look medially, thus placing these muscles in the optimum position to lower (superior oblique) or raise (inferior oblique) the cornea. In other words, when you ask a patient to look medially and downward at the tip of his or her nose, you are testing the superior oblique at its best position. Conversely, by asking the patient to look medially and upward, you are testing the inferior oblique at its best position.

Because the lateral and medial recti are simply placed relative to the eyeball, asking the patient to turn his or her cornea directly laterally tests the lateral rectus and turning the cornea directly medially tests the medial rectus.

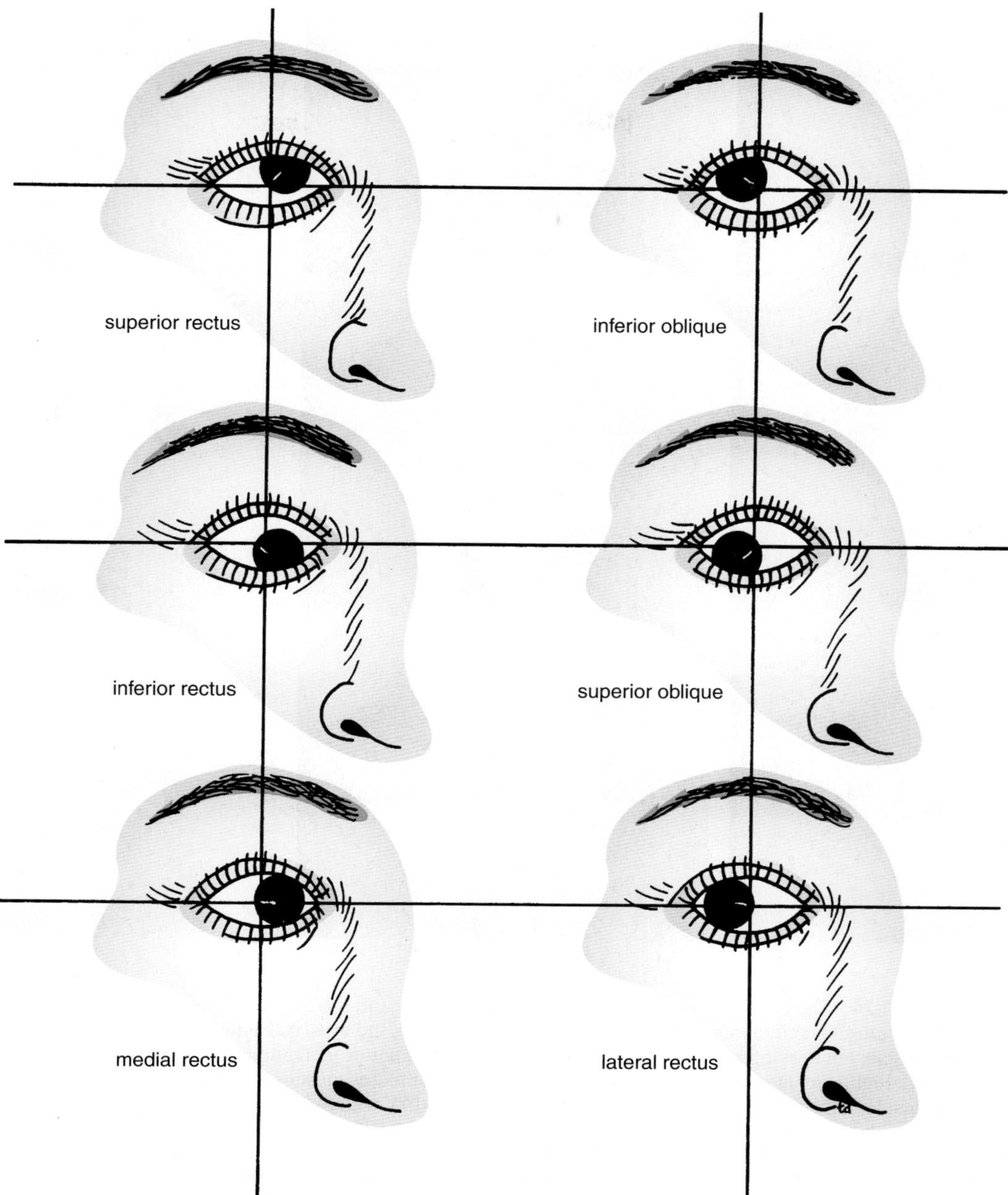

Figure 11-23 Actions of the four recti and two oblique muscles of the right orbit, assuming that each muscle is acting alone. The position of the pupil in relation to the vertical and horizontal planes should be noted in each case. The actions of the superior and inferior recti and the oblique muscles in the living intact eye are tested clinically, as described on page 700.

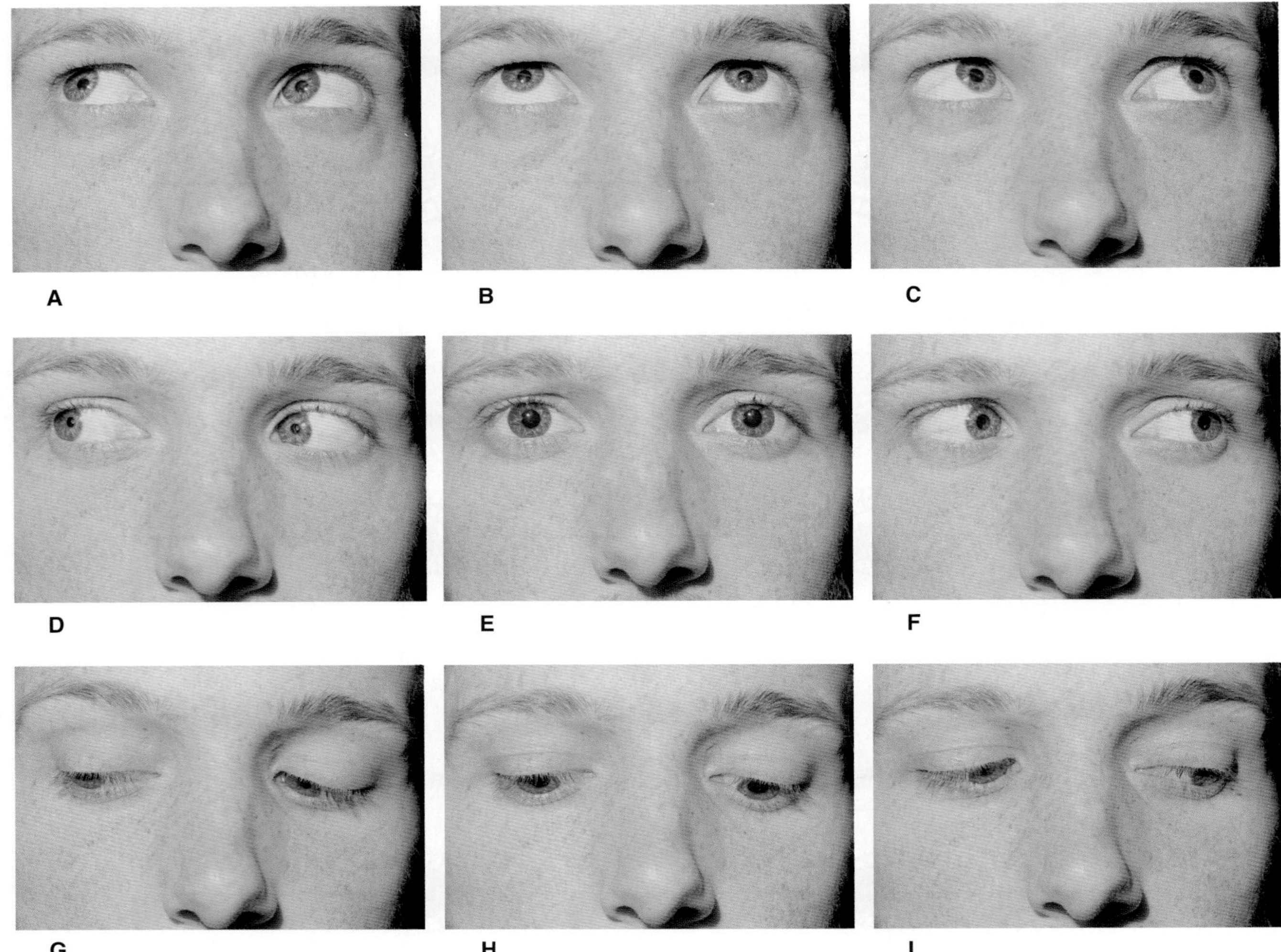

Figure 11-24 The cardinal positions of the right and left eyes and the actions of the recti and oblique muscles principally responsible for the movements of the eyes. **A.** Right eye, superior rectus muscle; left eye, inferior oblique muscle. **B.** Both eyes, superior recti and inferior oblique muscles. **C.** Right eye, inferior oblique muscle; left eye, superior rectus muscle. **D.** Right eye, lateral rectus muscle; left eye, medial rectus muscle. **E.** Primary position, with the eyes fixed on a distant fixation point. **F.** Right eye, medial rectus muscle; left eye, lateral rectus muscle. **G.** Right eye, inferior rectus muscle; left eye, superior oblique muscle. **H.** Both eyes, inferior recti and superior oblique muscles. **I.** Right eye, superior oblique muscle; left eye, inferior rectus muscle.

The cardinal positions of the eyes and the actions of the recti and oblique muscles are shown in Figure 11-24.

Intrinsic Muscles

The involuntary intrinsic muscles are the **ciliary muscle** and the **constrictor,** and the **dilator pupillae of the iris** take no part in the movement of the eyeball and are discussed later.

Fascial Sheath of the Eyeball

The fascial sheath surrounds the eyeball from the optic nerve to the corneoscleral junction (Fig. 11-25). It separates the eyeball from the orbital fat and provides it with a socket for free movement. It is perforated by the tendons of the orbital muscles and is reflected onto each of them as a tubular sheath. The sheaths for the tendons of the medial and lateral recti are attached to the medial and lateral walls of the orbit by triangular ligaments called the **medial** and **lateral check ligaments.** The lower part of the fascial sheath, which passes beneath the eyeball and connects the check ligaments, is thickened and serves to suspend the eyeball; it is called the **suspensory ligament of the eye** (Fig. 11-25). By this means the eye is suspended from the medial and lateral walls of the orbit, as if in a hammock.

Structure of the Eye

The eyeball (Fig. 11-25) is embedded in orbital fat but is separated from it by the fascial sheath of the eyeball. The eyeball

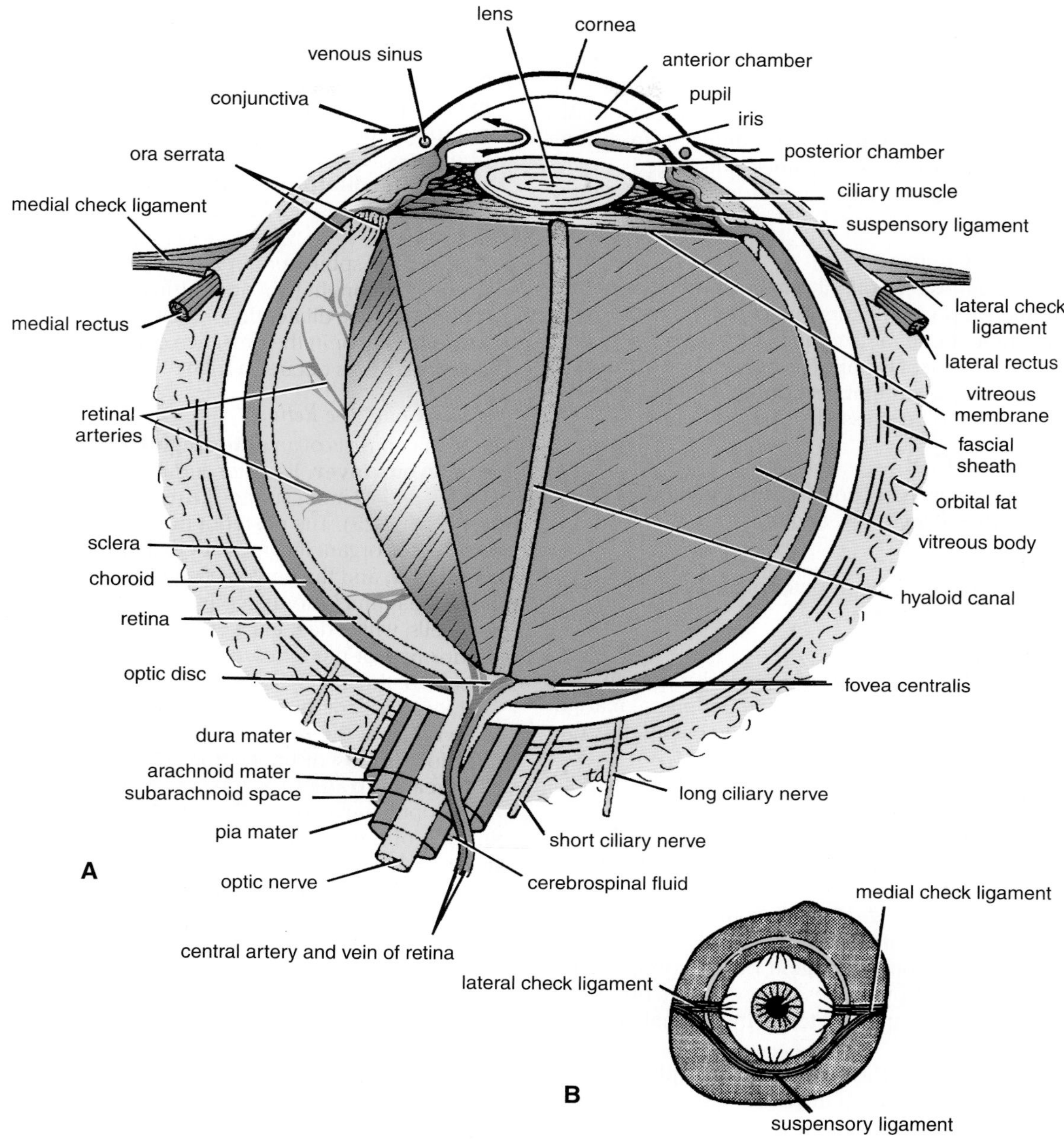

Figure 11-25 **A.** Horizontal section through the eyeball and the optic nerve. Note that the central artery and vein of the retina cross the subarachnoid space to reach the optic nerve. **B.** Check ligaments and suspensory ligament of the eyeball.

consists of three coats, which, from without inward, are the fibrous coat, the vascular pigmented coat, and the nervous coat.

Coats of the Eyeball

Fibrous Coat

The fibrous coat is made up of a posterior opaque part, the sclera, and an anterior transparent part, the cornea (Fig. 11-25).

The Sclera

The opaque sclera is composed of dense fibrous tissue and is white. Posteriorly, it is pierced by the optic nerve and is fused with the dural sheath of that nerve (Fig. 11-25). The **lamina cribrosa** is the area of the sclera that is pierced by the nerve fibers of the optic nerve.

The sclera is also pierced by the ciliary arteries and nerves and their associated veins, the venae vorticosae. The sclera is directly continuous in front with the cornea at the corneoscleral junction, or limbus.

The Cornea

The transparent **cornea** is largely responsible for the refraction of the light entering the eye (Fig. 11-25). It is in contact posteriorly with the aqueous humor.

Blood Supply The cornea is avascular and devoid of lymphatic drainage. It is nourished by diffusion from the aqueous humor and from the capillaries at its edge.

Nerve Supply Long ciliary nerves from the ophthalmic division of the trigeminal nerve

Function of the Cornea

The cornea is the most important refractive medium of the eye. This refractive power occurs on the anterior surface of the cornea, where the refractive index of the cornea (1.38) differs greatly from that of the air. The importance of the tear film in maintaining the normal environment for the corneal epithelial cells should be stressed.

Vascular Pigmented Coat

The vascular pigmented coat consists, from behind forward, of the choroid, the ciliary body, and the iris.

The Choroid

The choroid is composed of an outer pigmented layer and an inner, highly vascular layer.

The Ciliary Body

The **ciliary body** is continuous posteriorly with the choroid, and anteriorly it lies behind the peripheral margin of the iris (Fig. 11-25). It is composed of the ciliary ring, the ciliary processes, and the ciliary muscle.

The **ciliary ring** is the posterior part of the body, and its surface has shallow grooves, the **ciliary striae.**

The **ciliary processes** are radially arranged folds, or ridges, to the posterior surfaces of which are connected the suspensory ligaments of the lens.

The **ciliary muscle** (Fig. 11-25) is composed of meridianal and circular fibers of smooth muscle. The meridianal fibers run backward from the region of the corneoscleral junction to the ciliary processes. The circular fibers are fewer in number and lie internal to the meridianal fibers.

- **Nerve supply:** The **ciliary muscle** is supplied by the parasympathetic fibers from the oculomotor nerve. After synapsing in the ciliary ganglion, the postganglionic fibers pass forward to the eyeball in the short ciliary nerves.
- **Action:** Contraction of the ciliary muscle, especially the meridianal fibers, pulls the ciliary body forward. This relieves the tension in the suspensory ligament, and the elastic lens becomes more convex. This increases the refractive power of the lens.

The Iris and Pupil

The iris is a thin, contractile, pigmented diaphragm with a central aperture, the pupil (Fig. 11-25). It is suspended in the aqueous humor between the cornea and the lens. The periphery of the iris is attached to the anterior surface of the ciliary body. It divides the space between the lens and the cornea into an **anterior** and a **posterior chamber.**

The muscle fibers of the iris are involuntary and consist of circular and radiating fibers. The circular fibers form the **sphincter pupillae** and are arranged around the margin of the pupil. The radial fibers form the **dilator pupillae** and consist of a thin sheet of radial fibers that lie close to the posterior surface.

- **Nerve supply:** The **sphincter pupillae** is supplied by parasympathetic fibers from the oculomotor nerve. After synapsing in the ciliary ganglion, the postganglionic fibers pass forward to the eyeball in the short ciliary nerves. The **dilator pupillae** is supplied by sympathetic fibers, which pass forward to the eyeball in the long ciliary nerves.
- **Action:** The sphincter pupillae constricts the pupil in the presence of bright light and during accommodation. The dilator pupillae dilates the pupil in the presence of light of low intensity or in the presence of excessive sympathetic activity such as occurs in fright.

Nervous Coat: The Retina

The retina consists of an **outer pigmented layer** and an **inner nervous layer.** Its outer surface is in contact with the choroid, and its inner surface is in contact with the vitreous body (Fig. 11-25). The posterior three fourths of the retina is the receptor organ. Its anterior edge forms a wavy ring, the **ora serrata,** and the nervous tissues end here. The anterior part of the retina is nonreceptive and consists merely of pigment cells, with a deeper layer of columnar epithelium. This anterior part of the retina covers the ciliary processes and the back of the iris.

At the center of the posterior part of the retina is an oval, yellowish area, the **macula lutea,** which is the area of the retina for the most distinct vision. It has a central depression, the **fovea centralis** (Figs. 11-25 and 11-26).

The optic nerve leaves the retina about 3 mm to the medial side of the macula lutea by the optic disc. The **optic disc** is slightly depressed at its center, where it is pierced by the **central artery of the retina.** At the optic disc is a complete absence of **rods** and **cones** so that it is insensitive to light and is referred to as the **"blind spot."** On ophthalmoscopic examination, the optic disc is seen to be pale pink in color, much paler than the surrounding retina.

Contents of the Eyeball

The contents of the eyeball consist of the refractive media, the aqueous humor, the vitreous body, and the lens.

Aqueous Humor

The aqueous humor is a clear fluid that fills the anterior and posterior chambers of the eyeball (Fig. 11-25). It is believed to be a secretion from the ciliary processes, from which it enters the posterior chamber. It then flows into the anterior chamber through the pupil and is drained away through the spaces at the iridocorneal angle into the **canal of Schlemm.** Obstruction to the draining of the aqueous humor results in a rise in intraocular pressure called **glaucoma.** This can produce degenerative changes in the retina, with consequent blindness.

The function of the aqueous humor is to support the wall of the eyeball by exerting internal pressure and thus maintaining its optical shape. It also nourishes the cornea and the lens and removes the products of metabolism; these functions are important because the cornea and the lens do not possess a blood supply.

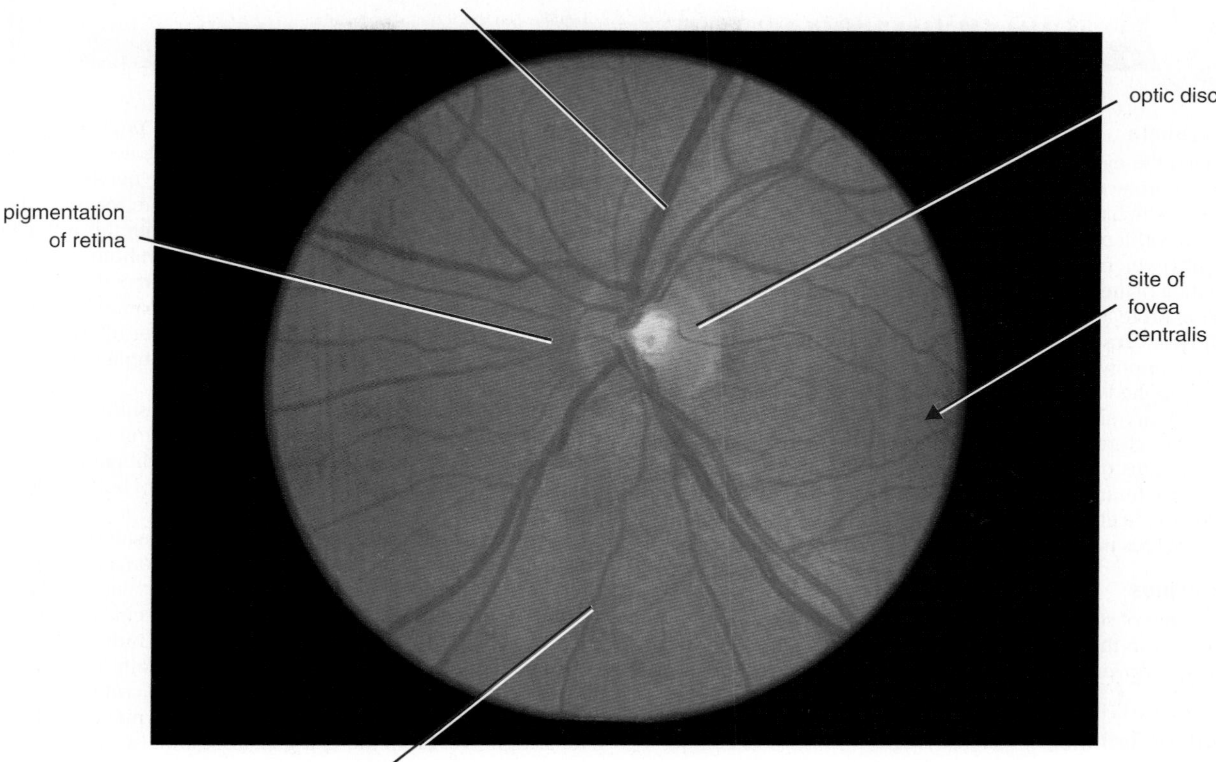

Figure 11-26 The left ocular fundus as seen with an ophthalmoscope.

Vitreous Body

The vitreous body fills the eyeball behind the lens (Fig. 11-25) and is a transparent gel. The **hyaloid canal** is a narrow channel that runs through the vitreous body from the optic disc to the posterior surface of the lens; in the fetus, it is filled by the hyaloid artery, which disappears before birth.

The function of the vitreous body is to contribute slightly to the magnifying power of the eye. It supports the posterior surface of the lens and assists in holding the neural part of the retina against the pigmented part of the retina.

The Lens

The lens (Fig. 11-25) is a transparent, biconvex structure enclosed in a transparent capsule. It is situated behind the iris and in front of the vitreous body and is encircled by the ciliary processes.

The lens consists of an elastic **capsule,** which envelops the structure; a **cuboidal epithelium,** which is confined to the anterior surface of the lens; and **lens fibers,** which are formed from the cuboidal epithelium at the equator of the lens. The lens fibers make up the bulk of the lens.

The elastic lens capsule is under tension, causing the lens constantly to endeavor to assume a globular rather than a disc shape. The equatorial region, or circumference, of the lens is attached to the ciliary processes of the ciliary body by the **suspensory ligament.** The pull of the radiating fibers of the suspensory ligament tends to keep the elastic lens flattened so that the eye can be focused on distant objects.

Accommodation of the Eye

To accommodate the eye for close objects, the ciliary muscle contracts and pulls the ciliary body forward and inward so that the radiating fibers of the suspensory ligament are relaxed. This allows the elastic lens to assume a more globular shape.

With advancing age, the lens becomes denser and less elastic, and, as a result, the ability to accommodate is lessened (presbyopia). This disability can be overcome by the use of an additional lens in the form of glasses to assist the eye in focusing on nearby objects.

Constriction of the Pupil During Accommodation of the Eye

To ensure that the light rays pass through the central part of the lens so spherical aberration is diminished during accommodation for near objects, the sphincter pupillae muscle contracts so the pupil becomes smaller

Convergence of the Eyes During Accommodation of the Lens

In humans, the retinae of both eyes focus on only one set of objects (single binocular vision). When an object moves from a distance toward an individual, the eyes converge so that a single object, not two, is seen. Convergence of the eyes results from the coordinated contraction of the medial rectus muscles.

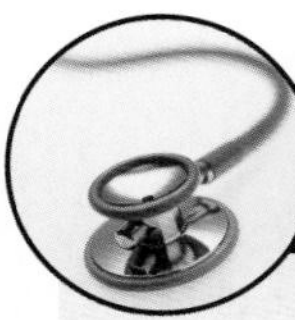

CLINICAL NOTES

Eye Trauma

Although the eyeball is well protected by the surrounding bony orbit, it is protected anteriorly only from large objects, such as tennis balls, which tend to strike the orbital margin but not the globe. The bony orbit provides no protection from small objects, such as golf balls, which can cause severe damage to the eye. Careful examination of the eyeball relative to the orbital margins shows that it is least protected from the lateral side.

Blowout fractures of the orbital floor involving the maxillary sinus commonly occur as a result of blunt force to the face. If the force is applied to the eye, the orbital fat explodes inferiorly into the maxillary sinus, fracturing the orbital floor. Not only can blowout fractures cause displacement of the eyeball, with resulting symptoms of double vision (diplopia), but also the fracture can injure the infraorbital nerve, producing loss of sensation of the skin of the cheek and the gum on that side. Entrapment of the inferior rectus muscle in the fracture may limit upward gaze.

Strabismus

Many cases of strabismus are nonparalytic and are caused by an imbalance in the action of opposing muscles. This type of strabismus is known as **concomitant strabismus** and is common in infancy.

Pupillary Reflexes

The pupillary reflexes—that is, the reaction of the pupils to light and accommodation—depend on the integrity of nervous pathways. In the **direct light reflex,** the normal pupil reflexly contracts when a light is shone into the patient's eye. The nervous impulses pass from the retina along the optic nerve to the optic chiasma and then along the optic tract. Before reaching the lateral geniculate body, the fibers concerned with this reflex leave the tract and pass to the oculomotor nuclei on both sides via the pretectal nuclei. From the parasympathetic part of the nucleus, efferent fibers leave the midbrain in the oculomotor nerve and reach the ciliary ganglion via the nerve to the inferior oblique. Postganglionic fibers pass to the constrictor pupillae muscles via the short ciliary nerves.

The **consensual light reflex** is tested by shining the light in one eye and noting the contraction of the pupil in the opposite eye. This reflex is possible because the afferent pathway just described travels to the parasympathetic nuclei of both oculomotor nerves.

The **accommodation reflex** is the contraction of the pupil that occurs when a person suddenly focuses on a near object after having focused on a distant object. The nervous impulses pass from the retina via the optic nerve, the optic chiasma, the optic tract, the lateral geniculate body, the optic radiation, and the cerebral cortex of the occipital lobe of the brain. The visual cortex is connected to the eye field of the frontal cortex. From here, efferent pathways pass to the parasympathetic nucleus of the oculomotor nerve. From there, the efferent impulses reach the constrictor pupillae via the oculomotor nerve, the ciliary ganglion, and the short ciliary nerves.

The Ear

The ear consists of the external ear; the middle ear, or tympanic cavity; and the internal ear, or labyrinth, which contains the organs of hearing and balance.

External Ear

The external ear has an auricle and an external auditory meatus.

The **auricle** has a characteristic shape (Fig. 11-27A) and collects air vibrations. It consists of a thin plate of elastic cartilage covered by skin. It possesses both extrinsic and intrinsic muscles, which are supplied by the facial nerve.

The **external auditory meatus** is a curved tube that leads from the auricle to the tympanic membrane (Figs. 11-27 and 11-28). It conducts sound waves from the auricle to the tympanic membrane.

The framework of the outer third of the meatus is elastic cartilage, and the inner two thirds is bone, formed by the tympanic plate. The meatus is lined by skin, and its outer third is provided with **hairs** and **sebaceous** and **ceruminous glands.** The latter are modified sweat glands that secrete a yellowish brown wax. The hairs and the wax provide a sticky barrier that prevents the entrance of foreign bodies.

The **sensory nerve** supply of the lining skin is derived from the auriculotemporal nerve and the auricular branch of the vagus nerve.

The **lymph drainage** is to the superficial parotid, mastoid, and superficial cervical lymph nodes.

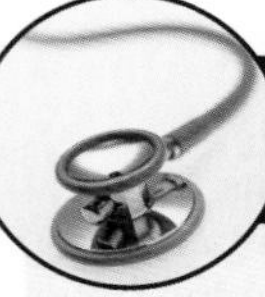

CLINICAL NOTES

Tympanic Membrane Examination

Otoscopic examination of the tympanic membrane is facilitated by first straightening the external auditory meatus by gently pulling the auricle upward and backward in the adult, and straight backward or backward and downward in the infant. Normally, the tympanic membrane is pearly gray and concave. Remember that in the adult the external meatus is about 1 in. (2.5 cm) long and is narrowest about 0.2 in. (5 mm) from the tympanic membrane.

Middle Ear (Tympanic Cavity)

The middle ear is an air-containing cavity in the petrous part of the temporal bone (Fig. 11-28) and is lined with mucous membrane. It contains the auditory ossicles, whose function is to transmit the vibrations of the tympanic membrane (eardrum) to the perilymph of the internal ear. It is a narrow, oblique, slitlike cavity whose long axis lies approximately parallel to the plane of the tympanic membrane. It communicates in front through the auditory tube with the nasopharynx and behind with the mastoid antrum.

The middle ear has a roof, floor, anterior wall, posterior wall, lateral wall, and medial wall.

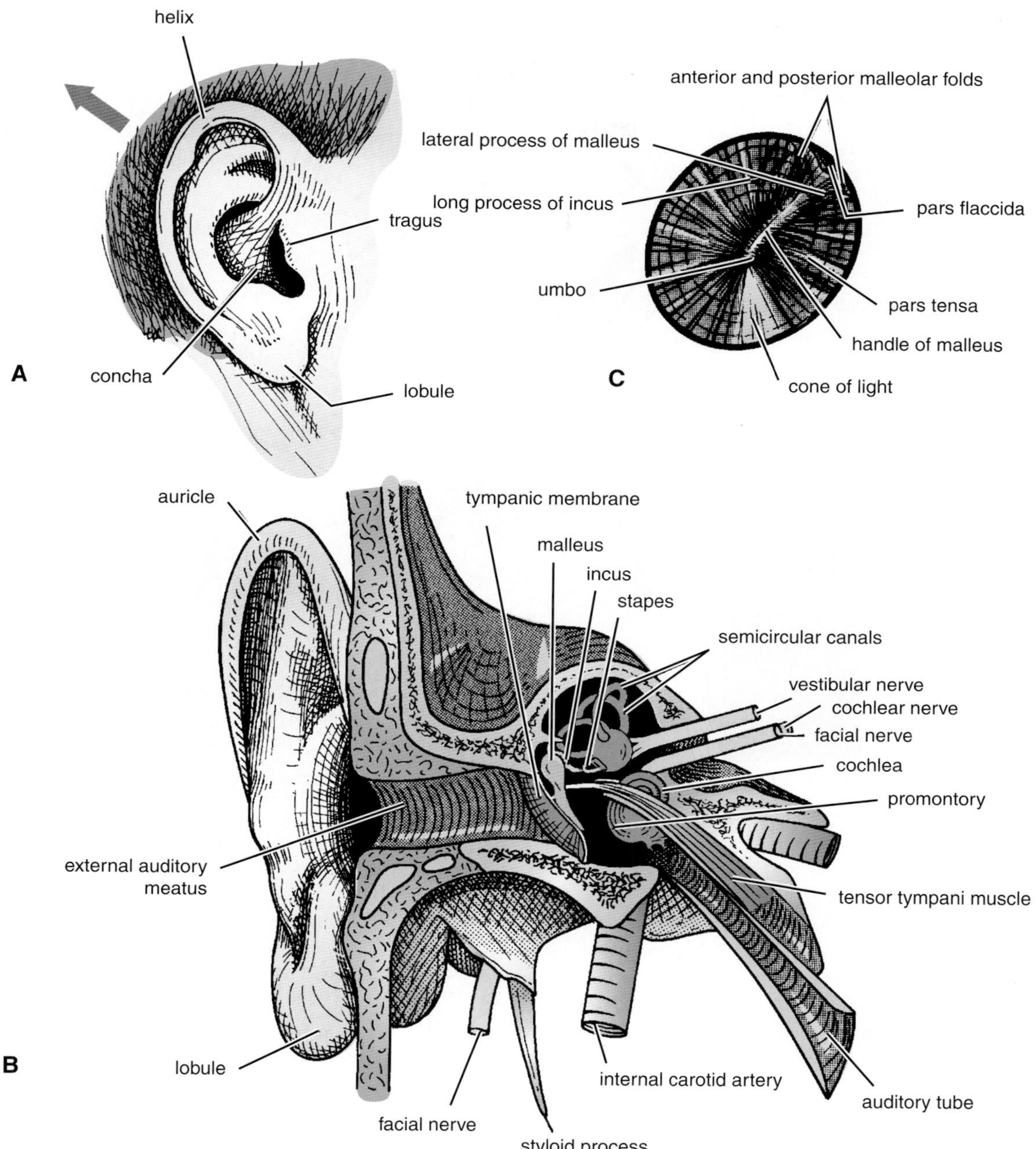

Figure 11-27 **A.** Different parts of the auricle of the external ear. The arrow indicates the direction that the auricle should be pulled to straighten the external auditory meatus before insertion of the otoscope in the adult. **B.** External and middle portions of the right ear viewed from in front. **C.** The right tympanic membrane as seen through the otoscope.

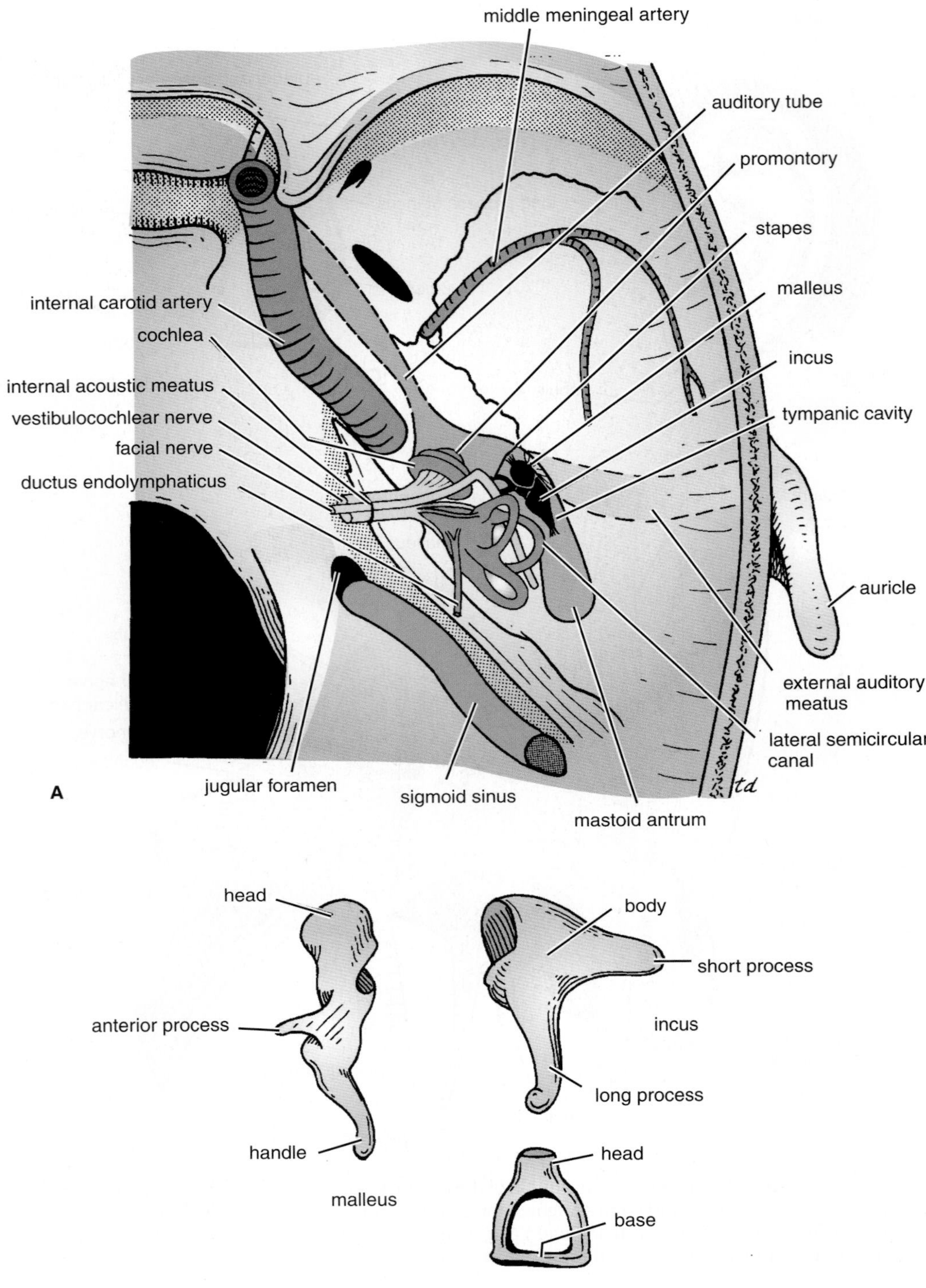

Figure 11-28 **A.** Parts of the right ear in relation to the temporal bone viewed from above. **B.** The auditory ossicles.

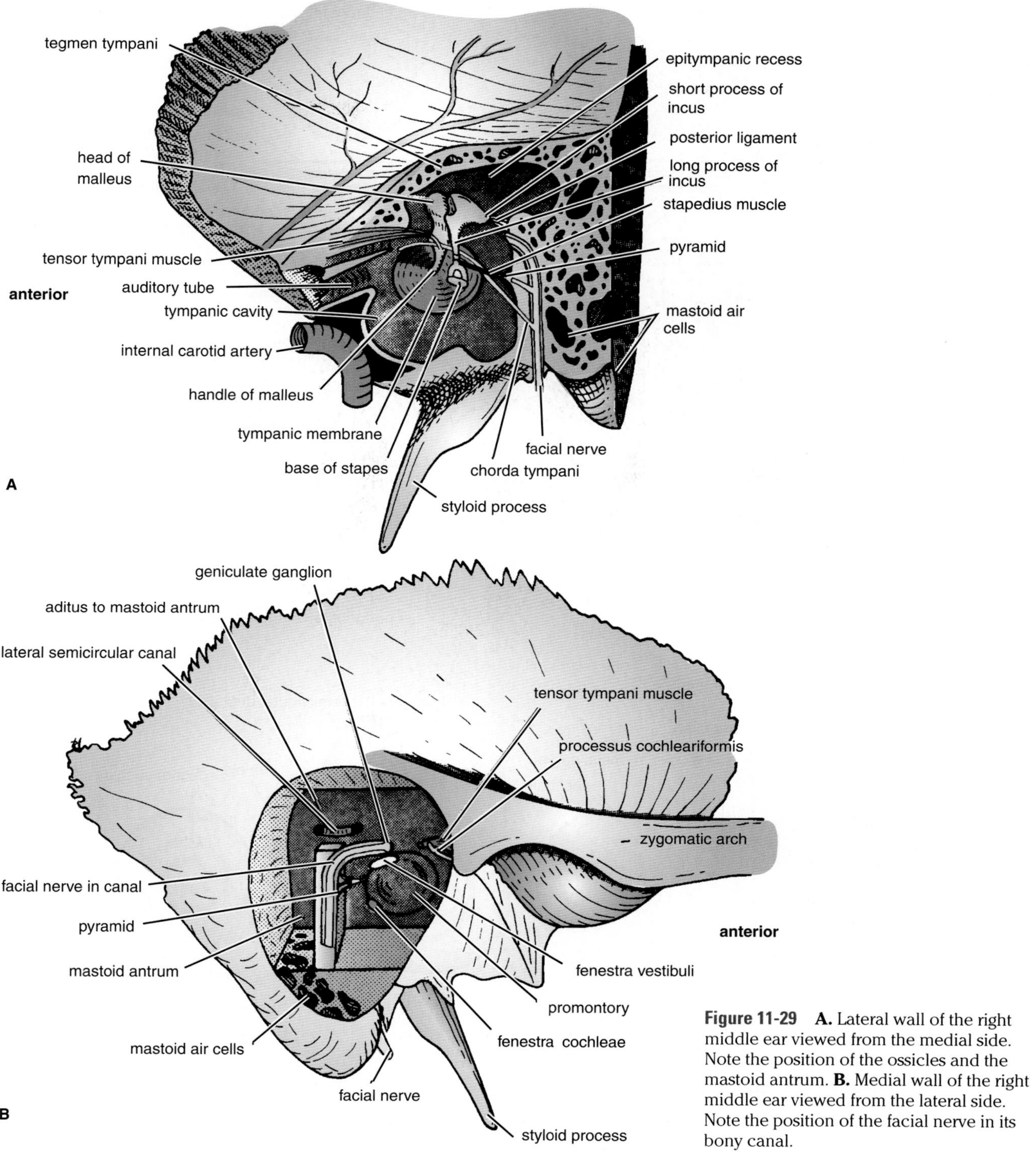

Figure 11-29 **A.** Lateral wall of the right middle ear viewed from the medial side. Note the position of the ossicles and the mastoid antrum. **B.** Medial wall of the right middle ear viewed from the lateral side. Note the position of the facial nerve in its bony canal.

The **roof** is formed by a thin plate of bone, the **tegmen tympani,** which is part of the petrous temporal bone (Figs. 11-29 and 11-30). It separates the tympanic cavity from the meninges and the temporal lobe of the brain in the middle cranial fossa.

The **floor** is formed by a thin plate of bone, which may be partly replaced by fibrous tissue. It separates the tympanic cavity from the superior bulb of the internal jugular vein (Fig. 11-30).

The **anterior wall** is formed below by a thin plate of bone that separates the tympanic cavity from the internal carotid artery (Fig. 11-30). At the upper part of the anterior wall are the openings into two canals. The lower and larger of these leads into the auditory tube, and the upper and

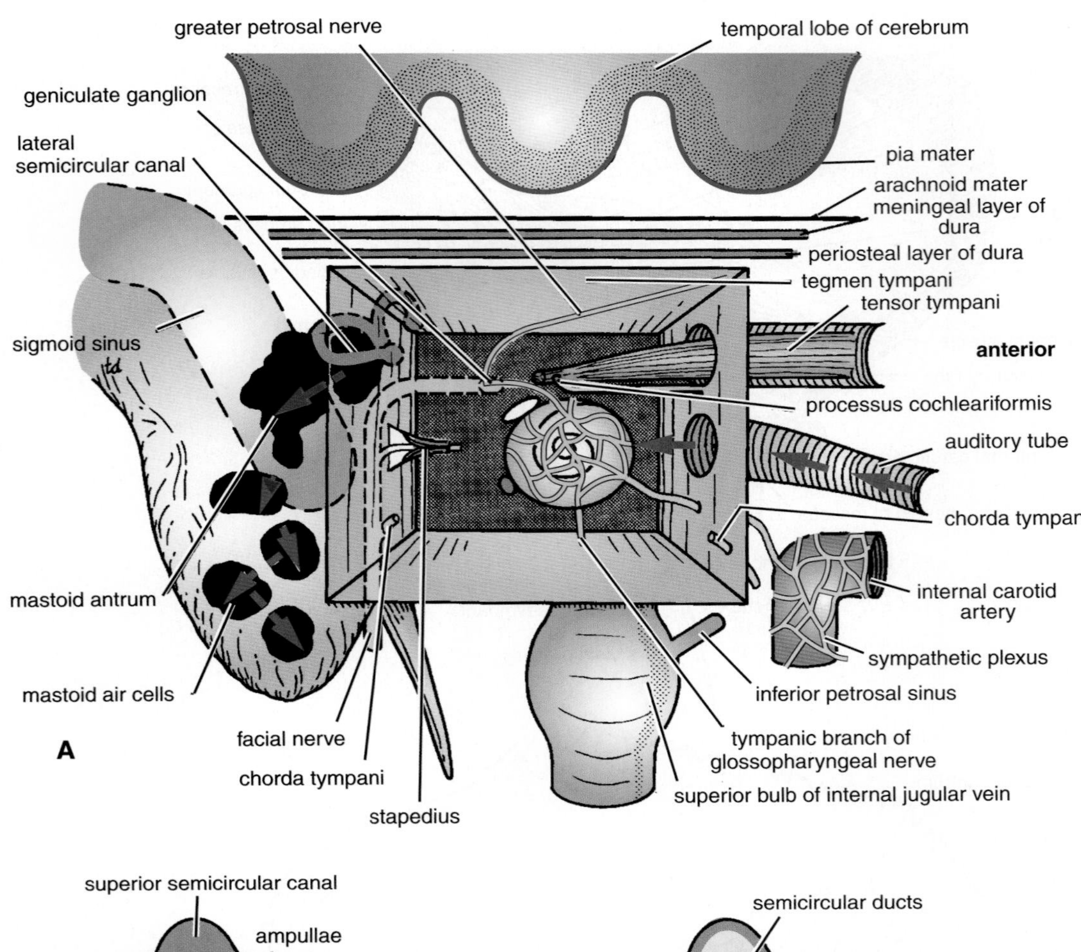

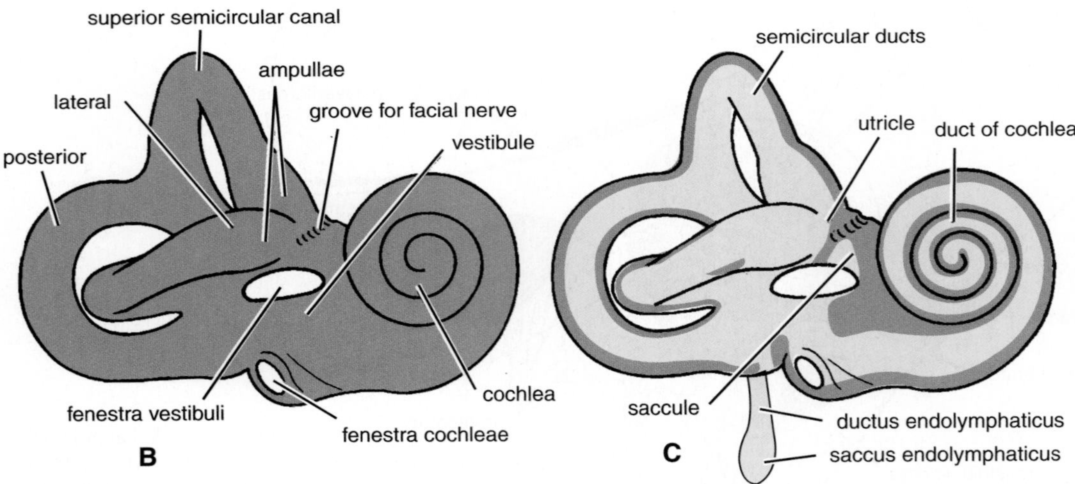

Figure 11-30 **A.** The middle ear and its relations. Bony (**B**) and membranous (**C**) labyrinths.

smaller is the entrance into the canal for the tensor tympani muscle (Fig. 11-29). The thin, bony septum, which separates the canals, is prolonged backward on the medial wall, where it forms a shelflike projection.

The **posterior wall** has in its upper part a large, irregular opening, the **aditus to the mastoid antrum** (Figs. 11-29 and 11-30). Below this is a small, hollow, conical projection, the **pyramid,** from whose apex emerges the tendon of the **stapedius muscle.**

The **lateral wall** is largely formed by the tympanic membrane (Figs. 11-27 and 11-29).

The **medial wall** is formed by the lateral wall of the inner ear. The greater part of the wall shows a rounded projection, called the **promontory,** which results from the underlying first turn of the cochlea (Figs. 11-27 and 11-29). Above and behind the promontory lies the **fenestra vestibuli,** which is oval shaped and closed by the base of the stapes. On the medial side of the window is the perilymph of the scala vestibuli of the internal ear. Below the posterior end of the promontory lies the **fenestra cochleae,** which is round and closed by the **secondary tympanic membrane.** On the medial side of this window is the perilymph of the blind end of the scala tympani (see page 714).

The bony shelf derived from the anterior wall extends backward on the medial wall above the promontory and above the fenestra vestibuli. It supports the tensor tympani muscle. Its posterior end is curved upward and forms a pulley, the **processus cochleariformis,** around which the tendon of the tensor tympani bends laterally to reach its insertion on the handle of the malleus (Fig. 11-29).

A rounded ridge runs horizontally backward above the promontory and the fenestra vestibuli and is known as the **prominence of the facial nerve canal.** On reaching the posterior wall, it curves downward behind the pyramid.

The **tympanic membrane** (Fig. 11-27) is a thin, fibrous membrane that is pearly gray. The membrane is obliquely placed, facing downward, forward, and laterally. It is concave laterally, and at the depth of the concavity is a small depression, the **umbo,** produced by the tip of the handle of the malleus. When the membrane is illuminated through an otoscope, the concavity produces a "cone of light," which radiates anteriorly and inferiorly from the umbo.

The tympanic membrane is circular and measures about 1 cm in diameter. The circumference is thickened and is slotted into a groove in the bone. The groove, or **tympanic sulcus,** is deficient superiorly, which forms a notch. From the sides of the notch, two bands, termed the **anterior** and **posterior malleolar folds,** pass to the lateral process of the malleus. The small triangular area on the tympanic membrane that is bounded by the folds is slack and is called the **pars flaccida** (Fig. 11-27). The remainder of the membrane is tense and is called the **pars tensa.** The handle of the malleus is bound down to the inner surface of the tympanic membrane by the mucous membrane.

The tympanic membrane is extremely sensitive to pain and is innervated on its outer surface by the auriculotemporal nerve and the auricular branch of the vagus.

Auditory Ossicles

The auditory ossicles are the malleus, incus, and stapes (Figs. 11-28 and 11-29).

The **malleus** is the largest ossicle and possesses a head, a neck, a long process or handle, an anterior process, and a lateral process.

The **head** is rounded and articulates posteriorly with the incus. The **neck** is the constricted part below the head. The **handle** passes downward and backward and is firmly attached to the medial surface of the tympanic membrane. It can be seen through the tympanic membrane on otoscopic examination. The **anterior process** is a spicule of bone that is connected to the anterior wall of the tympanic cavity by a ligament. The lateral process projects laterally and is attached to the anterior and posterior malleolar folds of the tympanic membrane.

The **incus** possesses a large body and two processes (Fig. 11-29).

The **body** is rounded and articulates anteriorly with the head of the malleus.

The **long process** descends behind and parallel to the handle of the malleus. Its lower end bends medially and articulates with the head of the stapes. Its shadow on the tympanic membrane can sometimes be recognized on otoscopic examination.

The **short process** projects backward and is attached to the posterior wall of the tympanic cavity by a ligament.

The **stapes** has a head, a neck, two limbs, and a base (Fig. 11-28).

The **head** is small and articulates with the long process of the incus. The **neck** is narrow and receives the insertion of the stapedius muscle. The **two limbs** diverge from the neck and are attached to the oval **base.** The edge of the base is attached to the margin of the fenestra vestibuli by a ring of fibrous tissue, the **anular ligament.**

Muscles of the Ossicles

These are the **tensor tympani** and the **stapedius muscles.**

The muscles of the ossicles, their nerve supply, and their actions are summarized in Table 11-3.

Table 11-3 Muscles of the Middle Ear

Muscle	Origin	Insertion	Nerve Supply	Action
Tensor tympani	Wall of auditory tube and wall of its own canal	Handle of malleus	Mandibular division of trigeminal nerve	Dampens down vibrations of tympanic membrane
Stapedius	Pyramid (bony projection on posterior wall of middle ear)	Neck of stapes	Facial nerve	Dampens down vibrations of stapes

Movements of the Auditory Ossicles

The malleus and incus rotate on an anteroposterior axis that runs through the ligament connecting the anterior process of the malleus to the anterior wall of the tympanic cavity, the anterior process of the malleus and the short process of the incus, and the ligament connecting the short process of the incus to the posterior wall of the tympanic cavity.

When the tympanic membrane moves medially (Fig. 11-31), the handle of the malleus also moves medially. The head of the malleus and the body of the incus move laterally. The long process of the incus moves medially with the stapes. The base of the stapes is pushed medially in the fenestra vestibuli, and the motion is communicated to the perilymph in the scala vestibuli. Liquid being incompressible, the perilymph causes an outward bulging of the secondary tympanic membrane in the fenestra cochleae at the lower end of the scala tympani (Fig. 11-31). The above movements are reversed if the tympanic membrane moves laterally. Excessive lateral movements of the head of the malleus cause a temporary separation of the articular surfaces between the malleus and incus so that the base of the stapes is not pulled laterally out of the fenestra vestibuli.

During passage of the vibrations from the tympanic membrane to the perilymph via the small ossicles, the leverage increases at a rate of 1.3 to 1. Moreover, the area of the tympanic membrane is about 17 times greater than that of the base of the stapes, causing the effective pressure on the perilymph to increase by a total of 22 to 1.

Auditory Tube

The auditory tube connects the anterior wall of the tympanic cavity to the nasal pharynx (Fig. 11-27). Its posterior third is bony, and its anterior two thirds is cartilaginous. As the tube descends it passes over the upper border of the superior constrictor muscle (Fig. 11-80). It serves to equalize air pressures in the tympanic cavity and the nasal pharynx.

Mastoid Antrum

The mastoid antrum lies behind the middle ear in the petrous part of the temporal bone (Fig. 11-28). It communicates with the middle ear by the aditus (Fig. 11-29).

Relations of the Mastoid Antrum

These are important in understanding the spread of infection.

Anterior wall is related to the middle ear and contains the aditus to the mastoid antrum (Fig. 11-30).

Posterior wall separates the antrum from the sigmoid venous sinus and the cerebellum (Fig. 11-30).

Lateral wall is (1.5 cm) thick and forms the floor of the suprameatal triangle (see page 838).

Medial wall is related to the posterior semicircular canal (Fig. 11-30).

Superior wall is the thin plate of bone, the tegmen tympani, which is related to the meninges of the middle cranial fossa and the temporal lobe of the brain (Fig. 11-30).

Inferior wall is perforated with holes, through which the antrum communicates with the mastoid air cells (Fig. 11-30).

Mastoid Air Cells

The mastoid process begins to develop during the second year of life. The mastoid air cells are a series of communicating cavities within the process that are continuous above with the antrum and the middle ear (Fig. 11-30). They are lined with mucous membrane.

Facial Nerve

The entire course of the facial nerve is described on page 763. On reaching the bottom of the internal acoustic meatus (see page 764), the facial nerve enters the facial canal (Fig. 11-28). The nerve runs laterally above the vestibule of the internal ear until it reaches the medial wall of the middle ear. Here, the nerve expands to form the sensory **geniculate ganglion** (Figs. 11-29 and 11-30). The nerve then bends sharply backward above the promontory.

On arriving at the posterior wall of the middle ear, it curves downward on the medial side of the aditus of the mastoid antrum (Fig. 11-30). It descends in the posterior wall of the middle ear, behind the pyramid, and finally emerges through the stylomastoid foramen into the neck.

Important Branches of the Intrapetrous Part of the Facial Nerve

- The **greater petrosal nerve** arises from the facial nerve at the geniculate ganglion (Fig. 11-30). It contains preganglionic parasympathetic fibers that pass to the pterygopalatine ganglion and are there relayed through the zygomatic and lacrimal nerves to the lacrimal gland; other postganglionic fibers pass through the nasal and palatine nerves to the glands of the mucous membrane of the nose and palate. It also contains many taste fibers from the mucous membrane of the palate.

The nerve emerges on the superior surface of the petrous part of the temporal bone and is eventually joined by the deep petrosal nerve from the sympathetic plexus on the internal carotid artery and forms the **nerve of the pterygoid canal.** This passes forward and enters the pterygopalatine fossa, where it ends in the pterygopalatine ganglion.

- The **nerve to the stapedius** arises from the facial nerve as it descends in the facial canal behind the pyramid (Fig. 11-30). It supplies the muscle within the pyramid.
- The **chorda tympani** arises from the facial nerve just above the stylomastoid foramen (Fig. 11-29). It enters the middle ear close to the posterior border of the tympanic membrane. It then runs forward over the tympanic membrane and crosses the root of the handle of the malleus (Fig. 11-29). It lies in the interval between the mucous membrane and the fibrous layers of the tympanic membrane. The nerve leaves the middle ear through the petrotympanic fissure and enters the infratemporal fossa, where it joins the lingual nerve (see page 765).

The chorda tympani contains:

Taste fibers from the mucous membrane covering the anterior two thirds of the tongue (not the vallate papillae) and the floor of the mouth. The taste fibers are the peripheral processes of the cells in the geniculate ganglion.

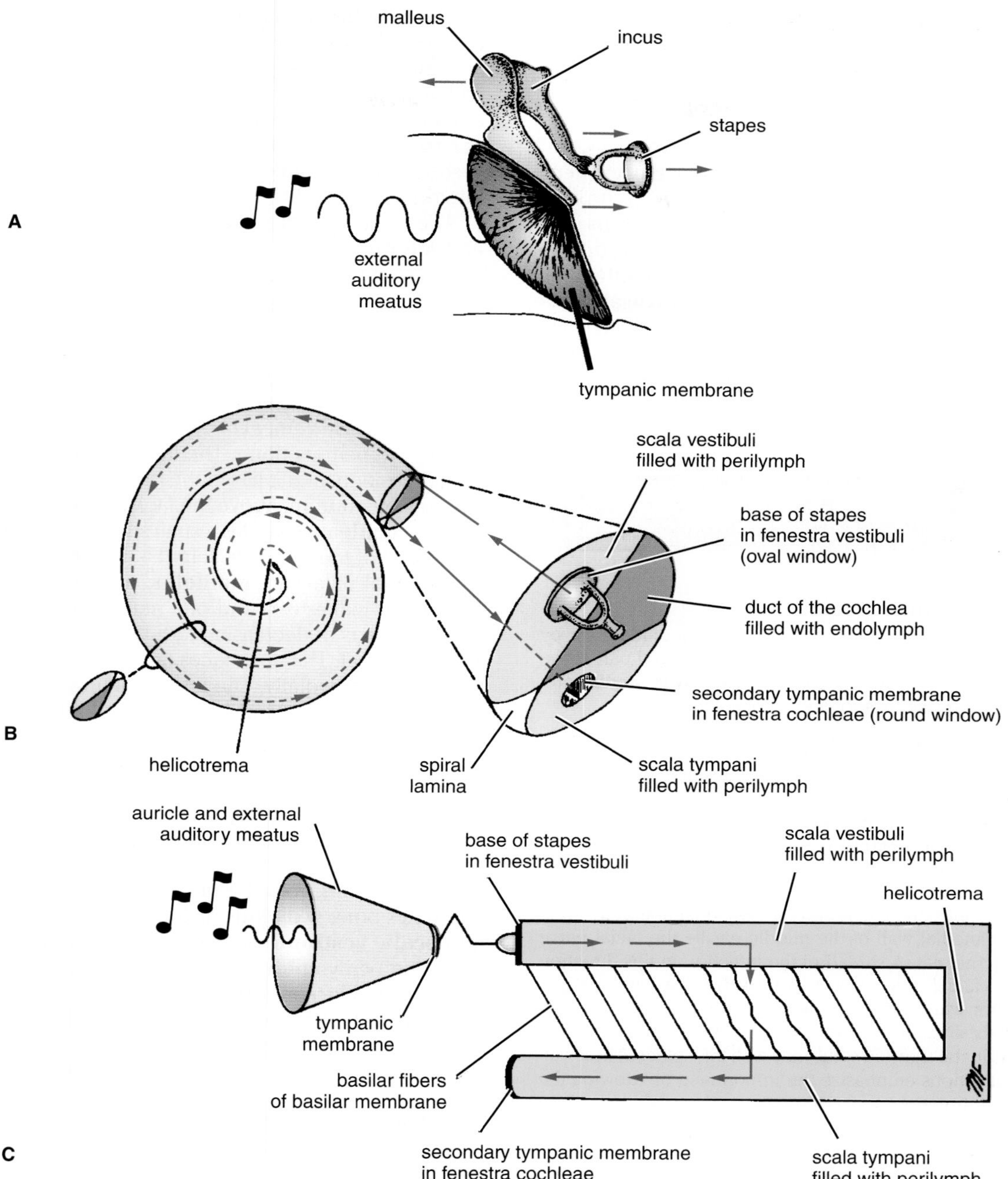

Figure 11-31 **A.** Vibrations of music passing into the external auditory meatus cause the tympanic membrane to move medially; the head of the malleus and incus move laterally, and the long process of the incus, with the stapes, moves laterally. **B.** The medial movement of the base of the stapes in the fenestra vestibuli causes motion (*arrows*) in the perilymph in the scala vestibuli. At the apex of the cochlea (the helicotrema), the compression wave in the perilymph passes down the scala tympani, causing a lateral bulging of the secondary tympanic membrane in the fenestra cochleae. **C.** Movement of the perilymph (*arrows*) after movement of the base of the stapes. Note the position of the basilar fibers of the basilar membrane.

Preganglionic parasympathetic secretomotor fibers that reach the submandibular ganglion and are there relayed to the submandibular and sublingual salivary glands

Tympanic Nerve

The tympanic nerve arises from the glossopharyngeal nerve, just below the jugular foramen (see page 765). It passes through the floor of the middle ear and onto the promontory (Fig. 11-30). Here it splits into branches, which form the **tympanic plexus.** The tympanic plexus supplies the lining of the middle ear and gives off the **lesser petrosal nerve,** which sends secretomotor fibers to the parotid gland via the otic ganglion (see page 787). It leaves the skull through the foramen ovale and joins the otic ganglion.

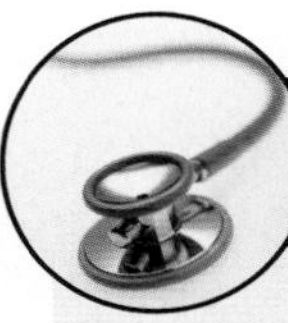

CLINICAL NOTES

Infections and Otitis Media

Pathogenic organisms can gain entrance to the middle ear by ascending through the auditory tube from the nasal part of the pharynx. Acute infection of the middle ear **(otitis media)** produces bulging and redness of the tympanic membrane.

Complications of Otitis Media

Inadequate treatment of otitis media can result in the spread of the infection into the mastoid antrum and the mastoid air cells **(acute mastoiditis).** Acute mastoiditis may be followed by the further spread of the organisms beyond the confines of the middle ear. The meninges and the temporal lobe of the brain lie superiorly. A spread of the infection in this direction could produce a meningitis and a cerebral abscess in the temporal lobe. Beyond the medial wall of the middle ear lie the facial nerve and the internal ear. A spread of the infection in this direction can cause a facial nerve palsy and **labyrinthitis** with **vertigo.** The posterior wall of the mastoid antrum is related to the sigmoid venous sinus. If the infection spreads in this direction, a thrombosis in the sigmoid sinus may well take place. These various complications emphasize the importance of knowing the anatomy of this region.

The Internal Ear, or Labyrinth

The labyrinth is situated in the petrous part of the temporal bone, medial to the middle ear (Fig. 11-28). It consists of the bony labyrinth, comprising a series of cavities within the bone, and the membranous labyrinth, comprising a series of membranous sacs and ducts contained within the bony labyrinth.

Bony Labyrinth

The bony labyrinth consists of three parts: the vestibule, the semicircular canals, and the cochlea (Fig. 11-30). These are cavities situated in the substance of dense bone. They are lined by endosteum and contain a clear fluid, the **perilymph,** in which is suspended the membranous labyrinth.

The **vestibule,** the central part of the bony labyrinth, lies posterior to the cochlea and anterior to the semicircular canals. In its lateral wall are the **fenestra vestibuli,** which is closed by the base of the stapes and its anular ligament, and the **fenestra cochleae,** which is closed by the **secondary tympanic membrane.** Lodged within the vestibule are the **saccule** and **utricle** of the membranous labyrinth (Fig. 11-30).

The three **semicircular canals—superior, posterior,** and **lateral**—open into the posterior part of the vestibule. Each canal has a swelling at one end called the **ampulla.** The canals open into the vestibule by five orifices, one of which is common to two of the canals. Lodged within the canals are the **semicircular ducts** (Fig. 11-30).

The superior semicircular canal is vertical and placed at right angles to the long axis of the petrous bone. The posterior canal is also vertical but is placed parallel with the long axis of the petrous bone. The lateral canal is set in a horizontal position, and it lies in the medial wall of the aditus to the mastoid antrum, above the facial nerve canal.

The **cochlea** resembles a snail shell. It opens into the anterior part of the vestibule (Fig. 11-30). Basically, it consists of a central pillar, the **modiolus,** around which a hollow bony tube makes two and one half spiral turns. Each successive turn is of decreasing radius so that the whole structure is conical. The apex faces anterolaterally and the base faces posteromedially. The first basal turn of the cochlea is responsible for the promontory seen on the medial wall of the middle ear.

The modiolus has a broad base, which is situated at the bottom of the internal acoustic meatus. It is perforated by branches of the cochlear nerve. A spiral ledge, the **spiral lamina,** winds around the modiolus and projects into the interior of the canal and partially divides it. The **basilar membrane** stretches from the free edge of the spiral lamina to the outer bony wall, thus dividing the cochlear canal into the **scala vestibuli** above and the **scala tympani** below. The perilymph within the scala vestibuli is separated from the middle ear by the base of the stapes and the anular ligament at the fenestra vestibuli. The perilymph in the scala tympani is separated from the middle ear by the secondary tympanic membrane at the fenestra cochleae.

Membranous Labyrinth

The membranous labyrinth is lodged within the bony labyrinth (Fig. 11-30). It is filled with endolymph and surrounded by perilymph. It consists of the utricle and saccule, which are lodged in the bony vestibule; the three semicircular ducts, which lie within the bony semicircular canals; and the duct of the cochlea, which lies within the bony cochlea. All these structures freely communicate with one another.

The **utricle** is the larger of the two vestibular sacs. It is indirectly connected to the saccule and the ductus endolymphaticus by the **ductus utriculosaccularis.**

The **saccule** is globular and is connected to the utricle, as described previously. The ductus endolymphaticus, after being joined by the ductus utriculosaccularis, passes on to end in a small blind pouch, the **saccus endolymphaticus** (Fig. 11-30). This lies beneath the dura on the posterior surface of the petrous part of the temporal bone.

Located on the walls of the utricle and saccule are specialized sensory receptors, which are sensitive to the orientation of the head to gravity or other acceleration forces.

The **semicircular ducts,** although much smaller in diameter than the semicircular canals, have the same configuration. They are arranged at right angles to each other so that all three planes are represented. Whenever the head begins or ceases to move, or whenever a movement of the head accelerates or decelerates, the endolymph in the semicircular ducts changes its speed of movement relative to that of the walls of the semicircular ducts. This change is detected in the sensory receptors in the ampullae of the semicircular ducts.

The **duct of the cochlea** is triangular in cross section and is connected to the saccule by the **ductus reuniens.** The highly specialized epithelium that lies on the **basilar membrane** forms the spiral organ of Corti and contains the sensory receptors for hearing. For a detailed description of the spiral organ, a textbook of histology should be consulted.

Vestibulocochlear Nerve

On reaching the bottom of the internal acoustic meatus (see page 765), the nerve divides into vestibular and cochlear portions (Fig. 11-28).

The **vestibular nerve** is expanded to form the **vestibular ganglion.** The branches of the nerve then pierce the lateral end of the internal acoustic meatus and gain entrance to the membranous labyrinth, where they supply the utricle, the saccule, and the ampullae of the semicircular ducts.

The **cochlear nerve** divides into branches, which enter foramina at the base of the modiolus. The sensory ganglion of this nerve takes the form of an elongated **spiral ganglion** that is lodged in a canal winding around the modiolus in the base of the spiral lamina. The peripheral branches of this nerve pass from the ganglion to the **spiral organ of Corti.**

The Mandible

The mandible or lower jaw is the largest and strongest bone of the face, and it articulates with the skull at the temporomandibular joint.

The mandible consists of a horseshoe-shaped **body** and a pair of **rami.** The body of the mandible meets the ramus on each side at the **angle of the mandible** (Fig. 11-32).

The **body of the mandible,** on its external surface in the midline, has a faint ridge indicating the line of fusion of the two halves during development at the **symphysis menti.** The **mental foramen** can be seen below the second premolar tooth; it transmits the terminal branches of the inferior alveolar nerve and vessels.

On the medial surface of the body of the mandible in the median plane are seen the **mental spines;** these give origin to the genioglossus muscles above and the geniohyoid muscles below (Fig. 11-31). The **mylohyoid line** can be seen as an oblique ridge that runs backward and laterally from the area of the mental spines to an area below and behind the third molar tooth. The **submandibular fossa,** for the superficial part of the submandibular salivary gland, lies below the posterior part of the mylohyoid line. The **sublingual fossa,** for the sublingual gland, lies above the anterior part of the mylohyoid line (Fig. 11-32).

The upper border of the body of the mandible is called the **alveolar part;** in the adult it contains 16 sockets for the roots of the teeth.

The lower border of the body of the mandible is called the **base.** The **digastric fossa** is a small, roughened depression on the base, on either side of the symphysis menti (Fig. 11-32). It is in these fossae that the anterior bellies of the digastric muscles are attached.

The **ramus of the mandible** is vertically placed and has an anterior **coronoid process** and a posterior **condyloid process,** or **head;** the two processes are separated by the **mandibular notch** (Fig. 11-32).

On the lateral surface of the ramus are markings for the attachment of the masseter muscle. On the medial surface is the **mandibular foramen** for the inferior alveolar nerve and vessels. In front of the foramen is a projection of bone, called the **lingula,** for the attachment of the **sphenomandibular ligament** (Figs. 11-32 and 11-33). The foramen leads into the **mandibular canal,** which opens on the lateral surface of the body of the mandible at the **mental foramen** (see above). The **incisive canal** is a continuation forward of the mandibular canal beyond the mental foramen and below the incisor teeth.

The **coronoid process** receives on its medial surface the attachment of the temporalis muscle. Below the **condyloid process,** or **head,** is a short **neck** (Fig. 11-32).

The important muscles and ligaments attached to the mandible are shown in Figure 11-32.

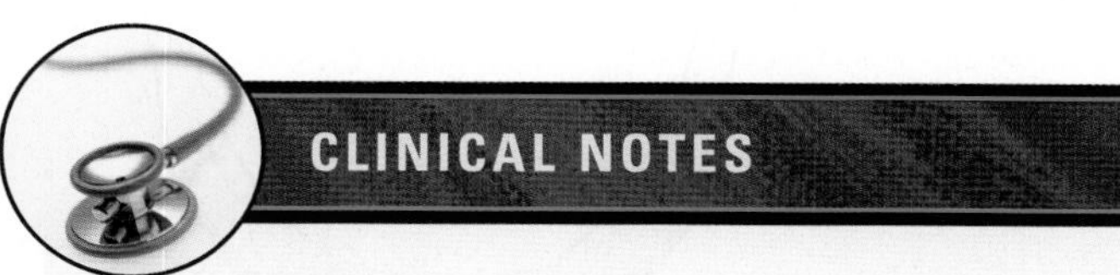

Fractures of the Mandible

The mandible is horseshoe shaped and forms part of a bony ring with the two temporomandibular joints and the base of the skull. Traumatic impact is transmitted around the ring, causing a single fracture or multiple fractures of the mandible, often far removed from the point of impact.

Temporomandibular Joint

Articulation

Articulation occurs between the articular tubercle and the anterior portion of the mandibular fossa of the temporal bone above and the head (condyloid process) of the mandible below (Figs. 11-33 and 11-34). The articular surfaces are covered with fibrocartilage.

Type of Joint

The temporomandibular joint is synovial. The articular disc divides the joint into upper and lower cavities (Fig. 11-35).

Capsule

The capsule surrounds the joint and is attached above to the articular tubercle and the margins of the mandibular fossa and below to the neck of the mandible.

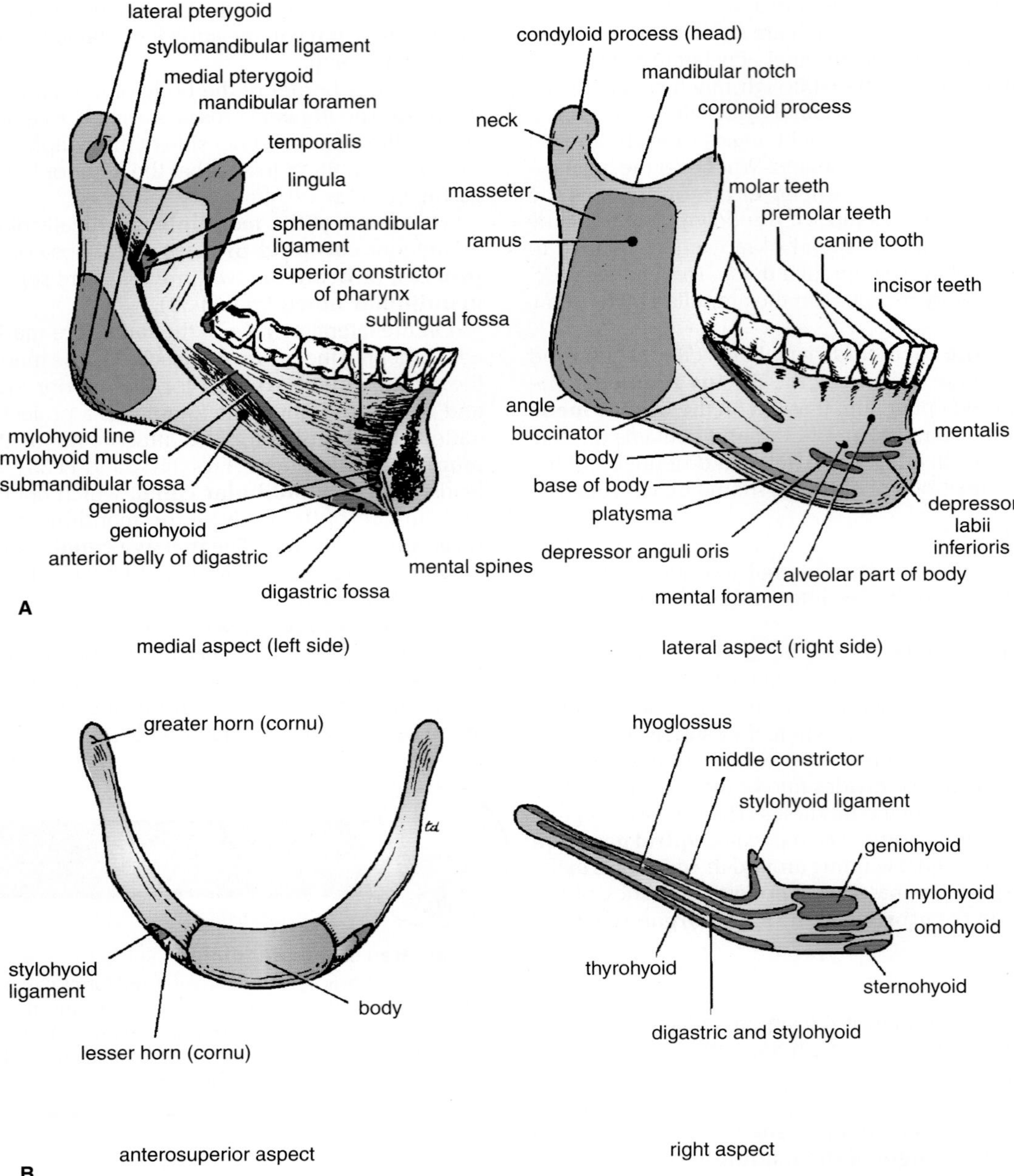

Figure 11-32 **A.** Mandible. **B.** Hyoid bone.

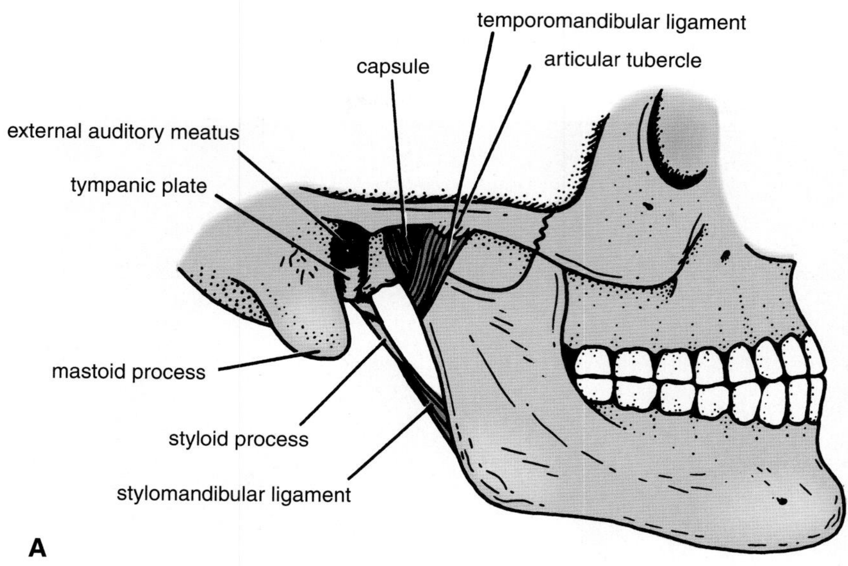

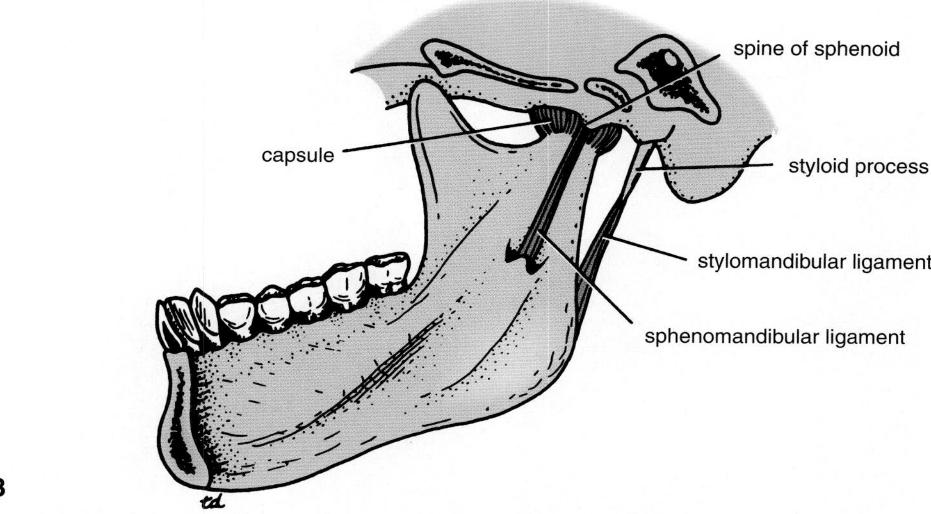

Figure 11-33 Temporomandibular joint as seen from the lateral (**A**) and medial (**B**) aspects.

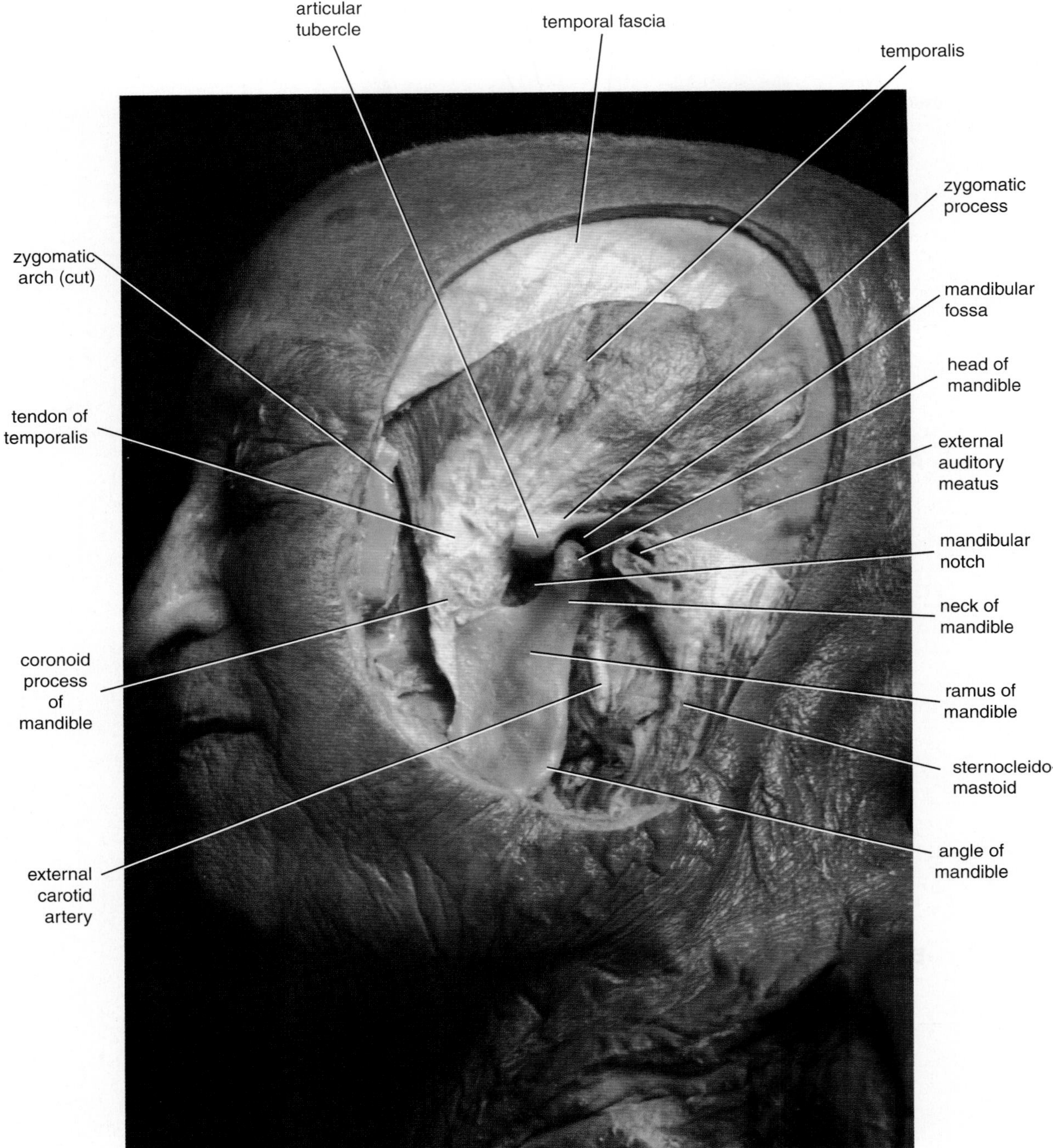

Figure 11-34 A dissection of the left temporomandibular joint. The capsule and lateral temporomandibular ligament have been removed to reveal the interior of the joint. Note the articular tubercle and mandibular fossa of the temporal bone and the head of the mandible. The articular disc is present within the joint cavity on the upper surface of the head of the mandible.

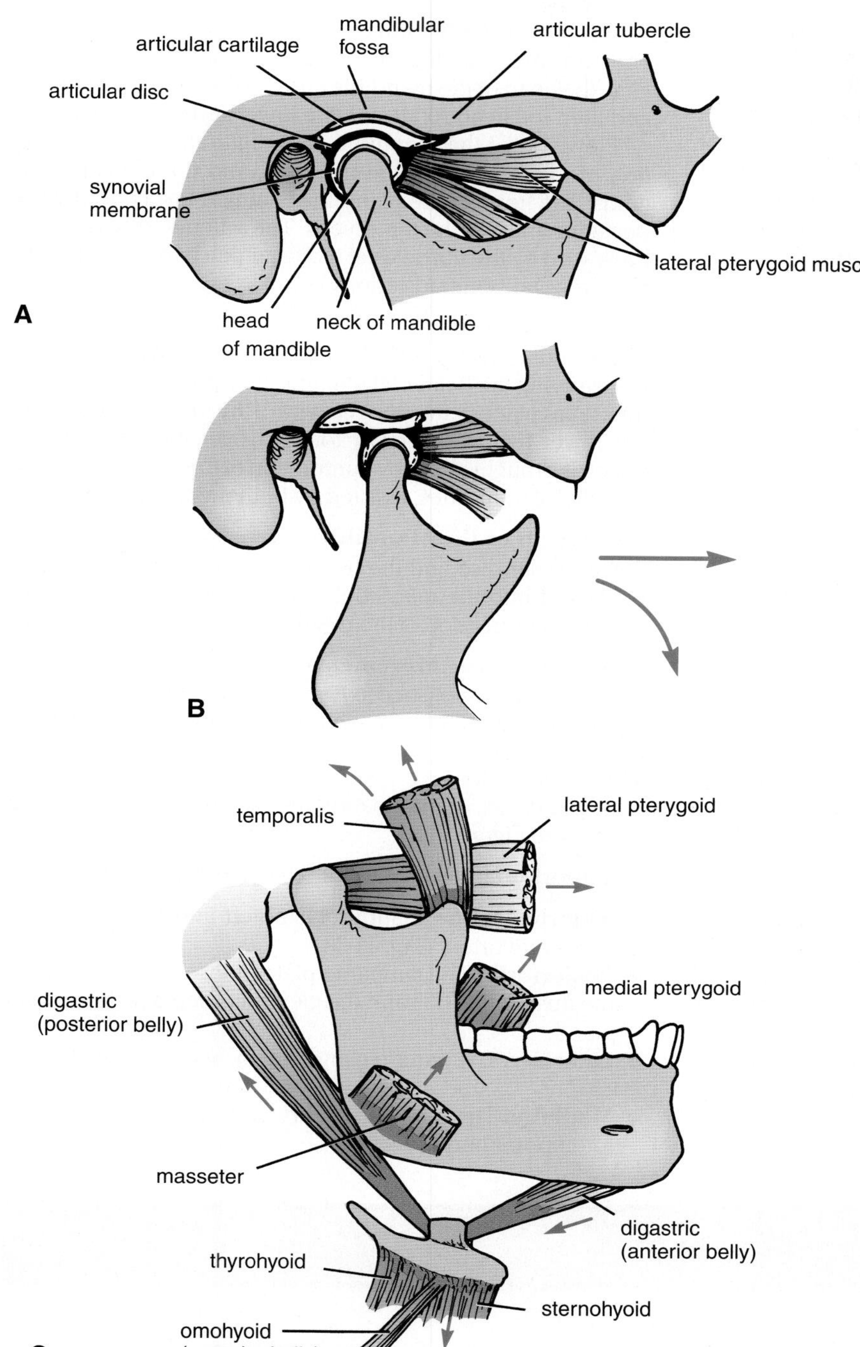

Figure 11-35 Temporomandibular joint with mouth closed (**A**) and with the mouth open (**B**). Note the position of the head of the mandible and articular disc in relation to the articular tubercle in each case. **C.** The attachment of the muscles of mastication to the mandible. The arrows indicate the direction of their actions.

Ligaments

The **lateral temporomandibular ligament** strengthens the lateral aspect of the capsule, and its fibers run downward and backward from the tubercle on the root of the zygoma to the lateral surface of the neck of the mandible (Fig. 11-33). This ligament limits the movement of the mandible in a posterior direction and thus protects the external auditory meatus.

The **sphenomandibular ligament** lies on the medial side of the joint (Fig. 11-33). It is a thin band that is attached above to the spine of the sphenoid bone and below to the lingula of the mandibular foramen. It represents the remains of the first pharyngeal arch in this region.

The **stylomandibular ligament** lies behind and medial to the joint and some distance from it. It is merely a band of thickened deep cervical fascia that extends from the apex of the styloid process to the angle of the mandible (Fig. 11-33).

The **articular disc** divides the joint into upper and lower cavities (Fig. 11-35). It is an oval plate of fibrocartilage that is attached circumferentially to the capsule. It is also attached in front to the tendon of the lateral pterygoid muscle and by fibrous bands to the head of the mandible. These bands ensure that the disc moves forward and backward with the head of the mandible during protraction and retraction of the mandible. The upper surface of the disc is concavoconvex from before backward to fit the shape of the articular tubercle and the mandibular fossa; the lower surface is concave to fit the head of the mandible.

Synovial Membrane

This lines the capsule in the upper and lower cavities of the joint (Fig. 11-35).

Nerve Supply

Auriculotemporal and masseteric branches of the mandibular nerve

Movements

The mandible can be depressed or elevated, protruded or retracted. Rotation can also occur, as in chewing. In the position of rest, the teeth of the upper and lower jaws are slightly apart. On closure of the jaws, the teeth come into contact.

Depression of the Mandible

As the mouth is opened, the head of the mandible rotates on the undersurface of the articular disc around a horizontal axis. To prevent the angle of the jaw impinging unnecessarily on the parotid gland and the sternocleidomastoid muscle, the mandible is pulled forward. This is accomplished by the contraction of the lateral pterygoid muscle, which pulls forward the neck of the mandible and the articular disc so that the latter moves onto the articular tubercle (Fig. 11-35). The forward movement of the disc is limited by the tension of the fibroelastic tissue, which tethers the disc to the temporal bone posteriorly.

Depression of the mandible is brought about by contraction of the digastrics, the geniohyoids, and the mylohyoids; the lateral pterygoids play an important role by pulling the mandible forward.

Elevation of the Mandible

The movements in depression of the mandible are reversed. First, the head of the mandible and the disc move backward, and then the head rotates on the lower surface of the disc.

Elevation of the mandible is brought about by contraction of the temporalis, the masseter, and the medial pterygoids. The head of the mandible is pulled backward by the posterior fibers of the temporalis. The articular disc is pulled backward by the fibroelastic tissue, which tethers the disc to the temporal bone posteriorly.

Protrusion of the Mandible

The articular disc is pulled forward onto the anterior tubercle, carrying the head of the mandible with it. All movement thus takes place in the upper cavity of the joint. In protrusion, the lower teeth are drawn forward over the upper teeth, which is brought about by contraction of the lateral pterygoid muscles of both sides, assisted by both medial pterygoids.

Retraction of the Mandible

The articular disc and the head of the mandible are pulled backward into the mandibular fossa. Retraction is brought about by contraction of the posterior fibers of the temporalis.

Lateral Chewing Movements

These are accomplished by alternately protruding and retracting the mandible on each side. For this to take place, a certain amount of rotation occurs, and the muscles responsible on both sides work alternately and not in unison.

The muscles of mastication are summarized in Table 11-4. See also Figure 11-35.

Important Relations of the Temporomandibular Joint

- **Anteriorly:** The mandibular notch and the masseteric nerve and artery (Fig. 11-36)
- **Posteriorly:** The tympanic plate of the external auditory meatus (Fig. 11-33) and the glenoid process of the parotid gland
- **Laterally:** The parotid gland, fascia, and skin (see Fig. 11-85)
- **Medially:** The maxillary artery and vein and the auriculotemporal nerve

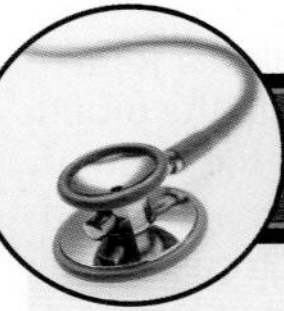

CLINICAL NOTES

Clinical Significance of the Temporomandibular Joint

The temporomandibular joint lies immediately in front of the external auditory meatus. The great strength of the lateral temporomandibular ligament prevents the head of the mandible from passing backward and fracturing the tympanic plate when a severe blow falls on the chin.

The **articular disc** of the temporomandibular joint may become partially detached from the capsule, and this results in its movement becoming noisy and producing an audible click during movements at the joint.

Dislocation of the Temporomandibular Joint

Dislocation sometimes occurs when the mandible is depressed. In this movement, the head of the mandible and the articular disc both move forward until they reach the summit of the articular tubercle. In this position, the joint is unstable, and a minor blow on the chin or a sudden contraction of the lateral pterygoid muscles, as in yawning, may be sufficient to pull the disc forward beyond the summit. In bilateral cases the mouth is fixed in an open position, and both heads of the mandible lie in front of the articular tubercles. Reduction of the dislocation is easily achieved by pressing the gloved thumbs downward on the lower molar teeth and pushing the jaw backward. The downward pressure overcomes the tension of the temporalis and masseter muscles, and the backward pressure overcomes the spasm of the lateral pterygoid muscles.

Table 11-4 Muscles of the Head

Muscle	Origin	Insertion	Nerve Supply	Action
Muscle of Scalp				
Occipitofrontalis				
Occipital belly	Highest nuchal line of occipital bone	Epicranial aponeurosis	Facial nerve	Moves scalp on skull and raises eyebrows
Frontal belly	Skin and superficial fascia of eyebrows			
Muscles of Facial Expression				
Orbicularis oculi				
Palpebral part	Medial palpebral ligament	Lateral palpebral raphe	Facial nerve	Closes eyelids and dilates lacrimal sac
Orbital part	Medial palpebral ligament and adjoining bone	Loops return to origin	Facial nerve	Throws skin around orbit into folds to protect eyeball
Corrugator supercilii	Superciliary arch	Skin of eyebrow	Facial nerve	Vertical wrinkles of forehead, as in frowning
Compressor nasi	Frontal process of maxilla	Aponeurosis of bridge of nose	Facial nerve	Compresses mobile nasal cartilages
Dilator naris	Maxilla	Ala of nose	Facial nerve	Widens nasal aperture
Procerus	Nasal bone	Skin between eyebrows	Facial nerve	Wrinkles skin of nose
Orbicularis oris	Maxilla, mandible, and skin	Encircles oral orifice	Facial nerve	Compresses lips together
Dilator Muscles of Lips				
Levator labii superioris alaeque nasi; Levator labii superioris; Zygomaticus minor; Zygomaticus major; Levator anguli oris; Risorius; Depressor anguli oris; Depressor labii inferioris; Mentalis	Arise from bones and fascia around oral aperture and insert into substance of lips		Facial nerve	Separate lips
Buccinator	Outer surface of alveolar margins of maxilla and mandible and pterygomandibular ligament		Facial nerve	Compresses cheeks and lips against teeth
Platysma	See Table 11-5			
Muscles of Mastication				
Masseter	Zygomatic arch	Lateral surface ramus of mandible	Mandibular division of trigeminal nerve	Elevates mandible to occlude teeth
Temporalis	Floor of temporal fossa	Coronoid process of mandible	Mandibular division of trigeminal nerve	Anterior and superior fibers elevate mandible; posterior fibers retract mandible
Lateral pterygoid (two heads)	Greater wing of sphenoid and lateral pterygoid plate	Neck of mandible and articular disc	Mandibular division of trigeminal nerve	Pulls neck of mandible forward
Medial pterygoid (two heads)	Tuberosity of maxilla and lateral pterygoid plate	Medial surface of angle of mandible	Mandibular division of trigeminal nerve	Elevates mandible

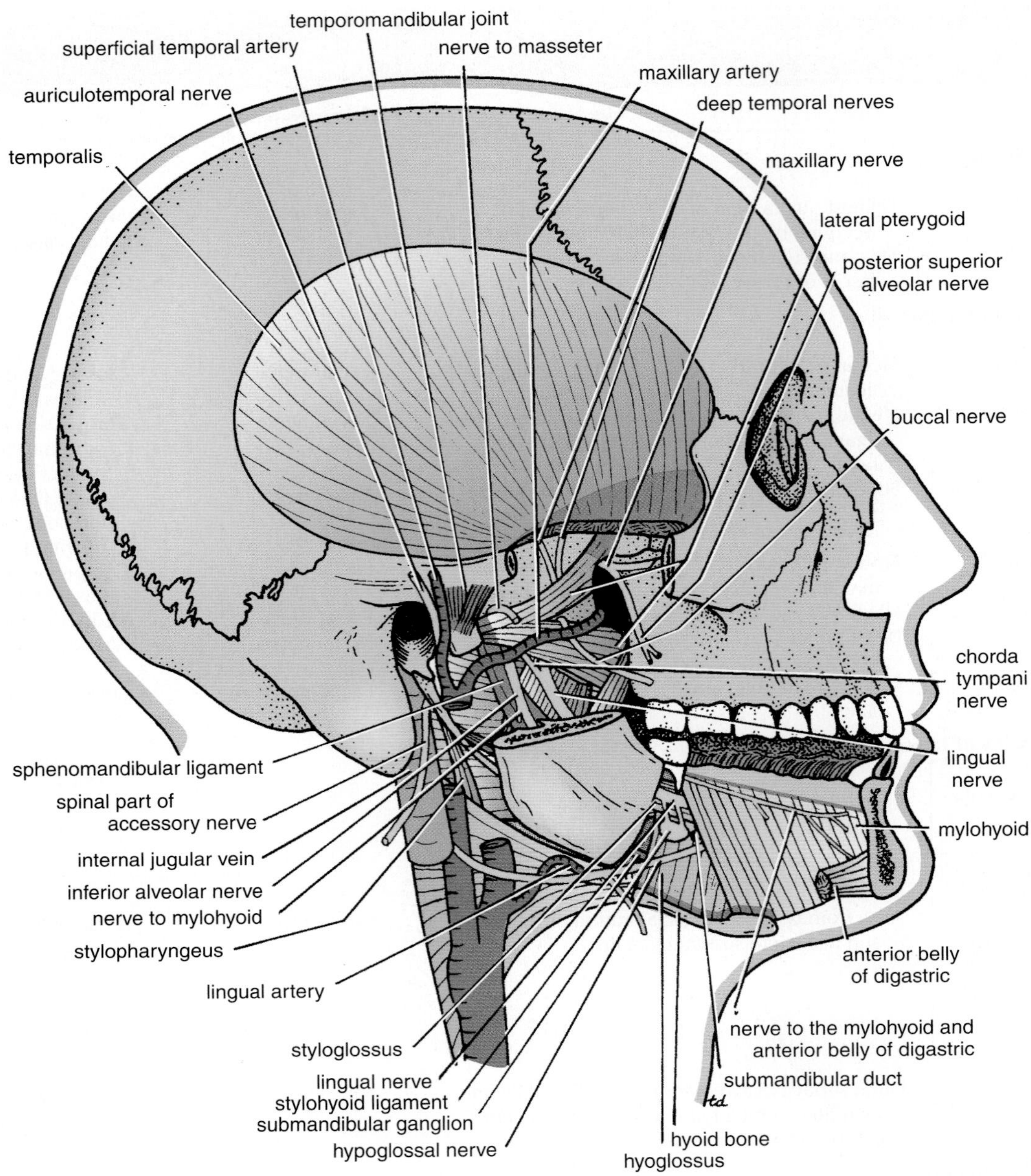

Figure 11-36 Infratemporal and submandibular regions. Parts of the zygomatic arch, the ramus, and the body of the mandible have been removed to display deeper structures.

The Scalp

Structure

The scalp consists of five layers, the first three of which are intimately bound together and move as a unit (Fig. 11-37). To assist one in memorizing the names of the five layers of the scalp, use each letter of the word **SCALP** to denote the layer of the scalp.

- **S**kin, which is thick and hair bearing and contains numerous sebaceous glands
- **C**onnective tissue beneath the skin, which is fibrofatty, the fibrous septa uniting the skin to the underlying aponeurosis of the occipitofrontalis muscle (Fig. 11-37). Numerous arteries and veins are found in this layer. The arteries are branches of the external and internal carotid arteries, and a free anastomosis takes place between them.
- **A**poneurosis (epicranial), which is a thin, tendinous sheet that unites the occipital and frontal bellies of the occipitofrontalis muscle (Figs. 11-37 and 11-38). The lateral margins of the aponeurosis are attached to the temporal fascia. The subaponeurotic space is the potential space

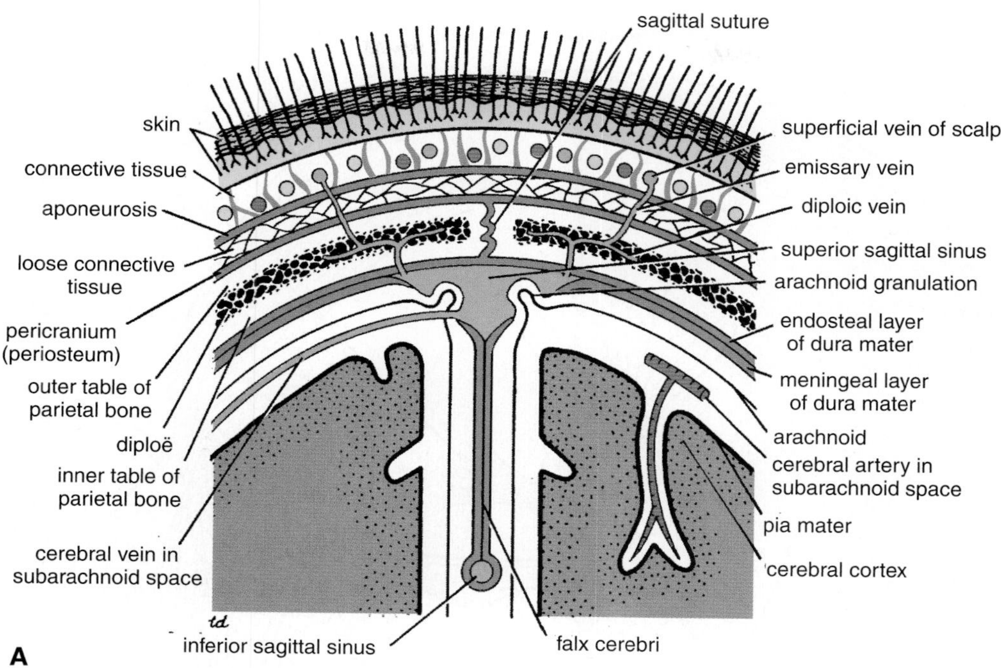

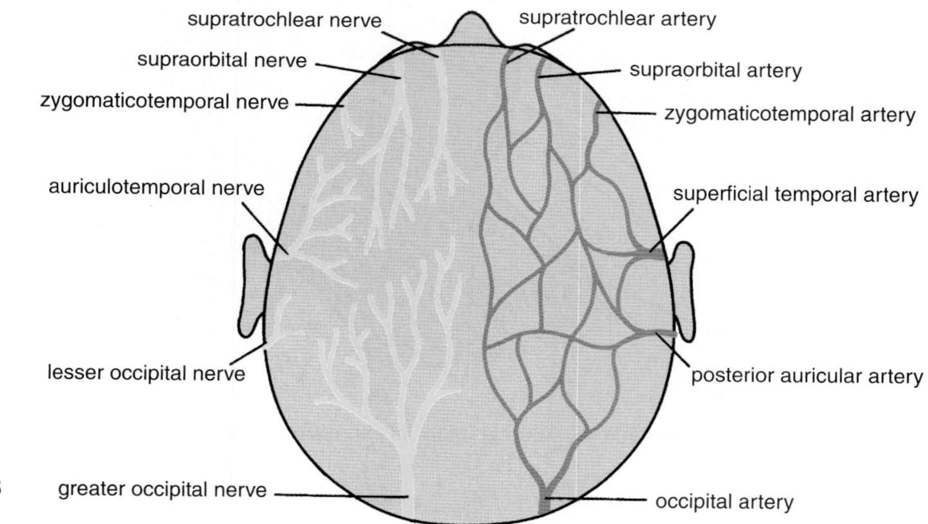

Figure 11-37 **A.** Coronal section of the upper part of the head showing the layers of the scalp, the sagittal suture of the skull, the falx cerebri, the superior and inferior sagittal venous sinuses, the arachnoid granulations, the emissary veins, and the relation of cerebral blood vessels to the subarachnoid space. **B.** Sensory nerve supply and arterial supply to the scalp.

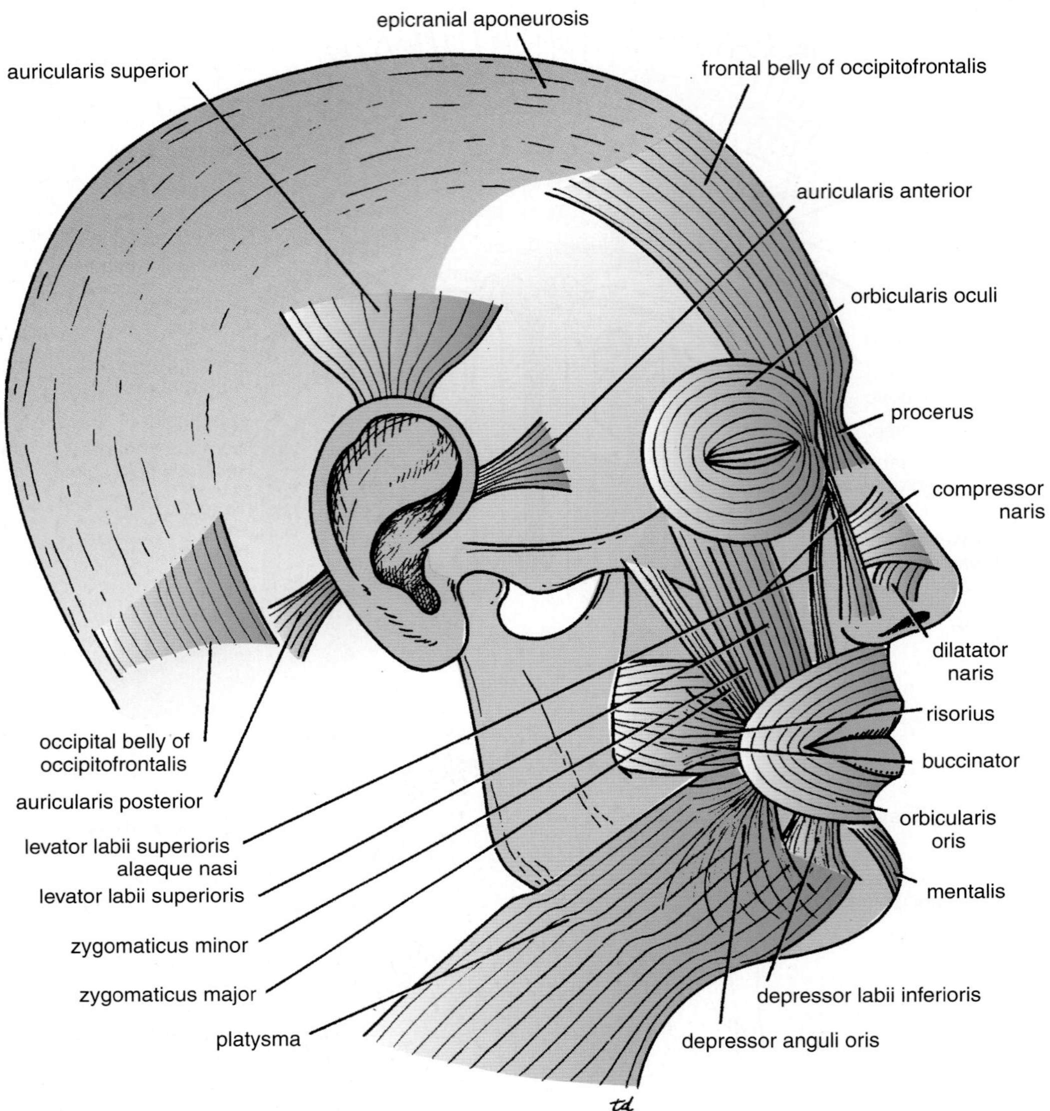

Figure 11-38 Muscles of facial expression.

beneath the epicranial aponeurosis. It is limited in front and behind by the origins of the occipitofrontalis muscle, and it extends laterally as far as the attachment of the aponeurosis to the temporal fascia.

- **L**oose areolar tissue, which occupies the subaponeurotic space (Fig. 11-37) and loosely connects the epicranial aponeurosis to the periosteum of the skull (the pericranium). The areolar tissue contains a few small arteries, but it also contains some important emissary veins. The emissary veins are valveless and connect the superficial veins of the scalp with the diploic veins of the skull bones and with the intracranial venous sinuses (Fig. 11-37).
- **P**ericranium, which is the periosteum covering the outer surface of the skull bones. It is important to remember that at the sutures between individual skull bones, the periosteum on the outer surface of the bones becomes continuous with the periosteum on the inner surface of the skull bones (Fig. 11-37).

Muscles of the Scalp

Occipitofrontalis

The origin, insertion, nerve supply, and action of this muscle are described in Table 11-4.

Note that when this muscle contracts, the first three layers of the scalp move forward or backward, the loose areolar tissue of the fourth layer of the scalp allowing the aponeurosis to move on the pericranium. The frontal bellies of the occipitofrontalis can raise the eyebrows in expressions of surprise or horror.

Sensory Nerve Supply of the Scalp

The main trunks of the sensory nerves lie in the superficial fascia. Moving laterally from the midline anteriorly, the following nerves are present:

The **supratrochlear nerve,** a branch of the ophthalmic division of the trigeminal nerve, winds around the superior orbital margin and supplies the scalp (Fig. 11-37). It passes backward close to the median plane and reaches nearly as far as the vertex of the skull.

The **supraorbital nerve,** a branch of the ophthalmic division of the trigeminal nerve, winds around the superior orbital margin and ascends over the forehead (Fig. 11-37). It supplies the scalp as far backward as the vertex.

The **zygomaticotemporal nerve,** a branch of the maxillary division of the trigeminal nerve, supplies the scalp over the temple (Fig. 11-37).

The **auriculotemporal nerve,** a branch of the mandibular division of the trigeminal nerve, ascends over the side of the head from in front of the auricle (Fig. 11-37). Its terminal branches supply the skin over the temporal region.

The **lesser occipital nerve,** a branch of the cervical plexus (C2), supplies the scalp over the lateral part of the occipital region (Fig. 11-37) and the skin over the medial surface of the auricle.

The **greater occipital nerve,** a branch of the posterior ramus of the second cervical nerve, ascends over the back of the scalp and supplies the skin as far forward as the vertex of the skull (Fig. 11-37).

Arterial Supply of the Scalp

The scalp has a rich supply of blood to nourish the hair follicles, and, for this reason, the smallest cut bleeds profusely. The arteries lie in the superficial fascia. Moving laterally from the midline anteriorly, the following arteries are present:

The **supratrochlear** and the **supraorbital arteries,** branches of the ophthalmic artery, ascend over the forehead in company with the supratrochlear and supraorbital nerves (Fig. 11-37).

The **superficial temporal artery,** the smaller terminal branch of the external carotid artery, ascends in front of the auricle in company with the auriculotemporal nerve (Fig. 11-37). It divides into anterior and posterior branches, which supply the skin over the frontal and temporal regions.

The **posterior auricular artery,** a branch of the external carotid artery, ascends behind the auricle to supply the scalp above and behind the auricle (Fig. 11-37).

The **occipital artery,** a branch of the external carotid artery, ascends from the apex of the posterior triangle, in company with the greater occipital nerve (Fig. 11-37). It supplies the skin over the back of the scalp and reaches as high as the vertex of the skull.

Venous Drainage of the Scalp

The **supratrochlear** and **supraorbital veins** unite at the medial margin of the orbit to form the facial vein.

The **superficial temporal vein** unites with the maxillary vein in the substance of the parotid gland to form the retromandibular vein (Fig. 11-39).

The **posterior auricular vein** unites with the posterior division of the retromandibular vein, just below the parotid gland, to form the external jugular vein (Fig. 11-39).

The **occipital vein** drains into the suboccipital venous plexus, which lies beneath the floor of the upper part of the posterior triangle; the plexus in turn drains into the vertebral veins or the internal jugular vein.

The veins of the scalp freely anastomose with one another and are connected to the diploic veins of the skull bones and the intracranial venous sinuses by the valveless **emissary veins** (Fig. 11-37).

Lymph Drainage of the Scalp

Lymph vessels in the anterior part of the scalp and forehead drain into the submandibular lymph nodes (Fig. 11-40). Drainage from the lateral part of the scalp above the ear is into the superficial parotid (preauricular) nodes; lymph vessels in the part of the scalp above and behind the ear drain into the mastoid nodes. Vessels in the back of the scalp drain into the occipital nodes.

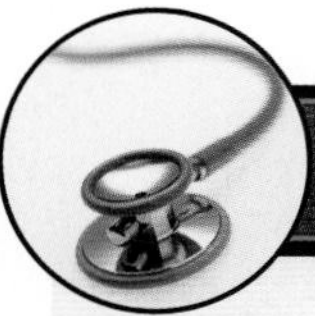

CLINICAL NOTES

Clinical Significance of the Scalp Structure

It is important to realize that the skin, the subcutaneous tissue, and the epicranial aponeurosis are closely united to one another and are separated from the periosteum by loose areolar tissue.

The skin of the scalp possesses numerous sebaceous glands, the ducts of which are prone to infection and damage by combs. For this reason, **sebaceous cysts** of the scalp are common.

Lacerations of the Scalp

The **scalp has a profuse blood supply** to nourish the hair follicles. Even a small laceration of the scalp can cause severe blood loss. It is often difficult to stop the bleeding of a scalp wound because the arterial walls are attached to fibrous septa in the subcutaneous tissue and are unable to contract or retract to allow blood clotting to take place. Local pressure applied to the scalp is the only satisfactory method of stopping the bleeding (see below).

In automobile accidents, it is common for large areas of the scalp to be cut off the head as a person is projected forward through the windshield. Because of the profuse blood supply, it is often possible to replace large areas of scalp that are only hanging to the skull by a narrow pedicle. Suture them in place, and necrosis will not occur.

(continues)

Clinical Notes, *continued*

The tension of the **epicranial aponeurosis,** produced by the tone of the occipitofrontalis muscles, is important in all deep wounds of the scalp. If the aponeurosis has been divided, the wound will gape open. For satisfactory healing to take place, the opening in the aponeurosis must be closed with sutures.

Often a wound caused by a blunt object such as a baseball bat closely resembles an incised wound. This is because the scalp is split against the unyielding skull, and the pull of the occipitofrontalis muscles causes a gaping wound. This anatomic fact may be of considerable forensic importance.

Life-Threatening Scalp Hemorrhage

Anatomically, it is useful to remember in an emergency that all the superficial arteries supplying the scalp ascend from the face and the neck. Thus, in an emergency situation, encircle the head just above the ears and eyebrows with a tie, shoelaces, or even a piece of string and tie it tight. Then insert a pen, pencil, or stick into the loop and rotate it so that the tourniquet exerts pressure on the arteries.

Scalp Infections

Infections of the scalp tend to remain localized and are usually painful because of the abundant fibrous tissue in the subcutaneous layer.

Occasionally, an infection of the scalp spreads by the emissary veins, which are valveless, to the skull bones, causing osteomyelitis. Infected blood in the diploic veins may travel by the emissary veins farther into the venous sinuses and produce venous sinus thrombosis.

Blood or pus may collect in the potential space beneath the epicranial aponeurosis. It tends to spread over the skull, being limited in front by the orbital margin, behind by the nuchal lines, and laterally by the temporal lines. On the other hand, subperiosteal blood or pus is limited to one bone because of the attachment of the periosteum to the sutural ligaments.

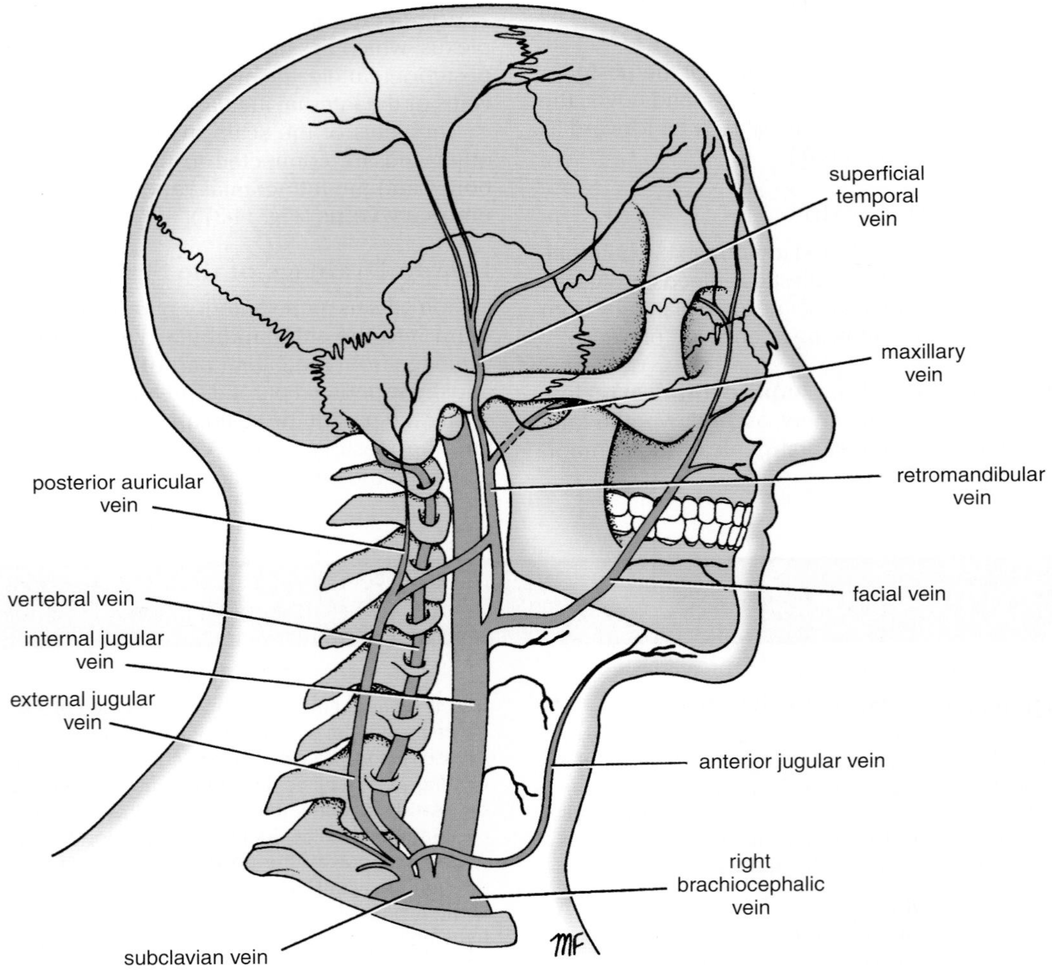

Figure 11-39 Main veins of the head and neck.

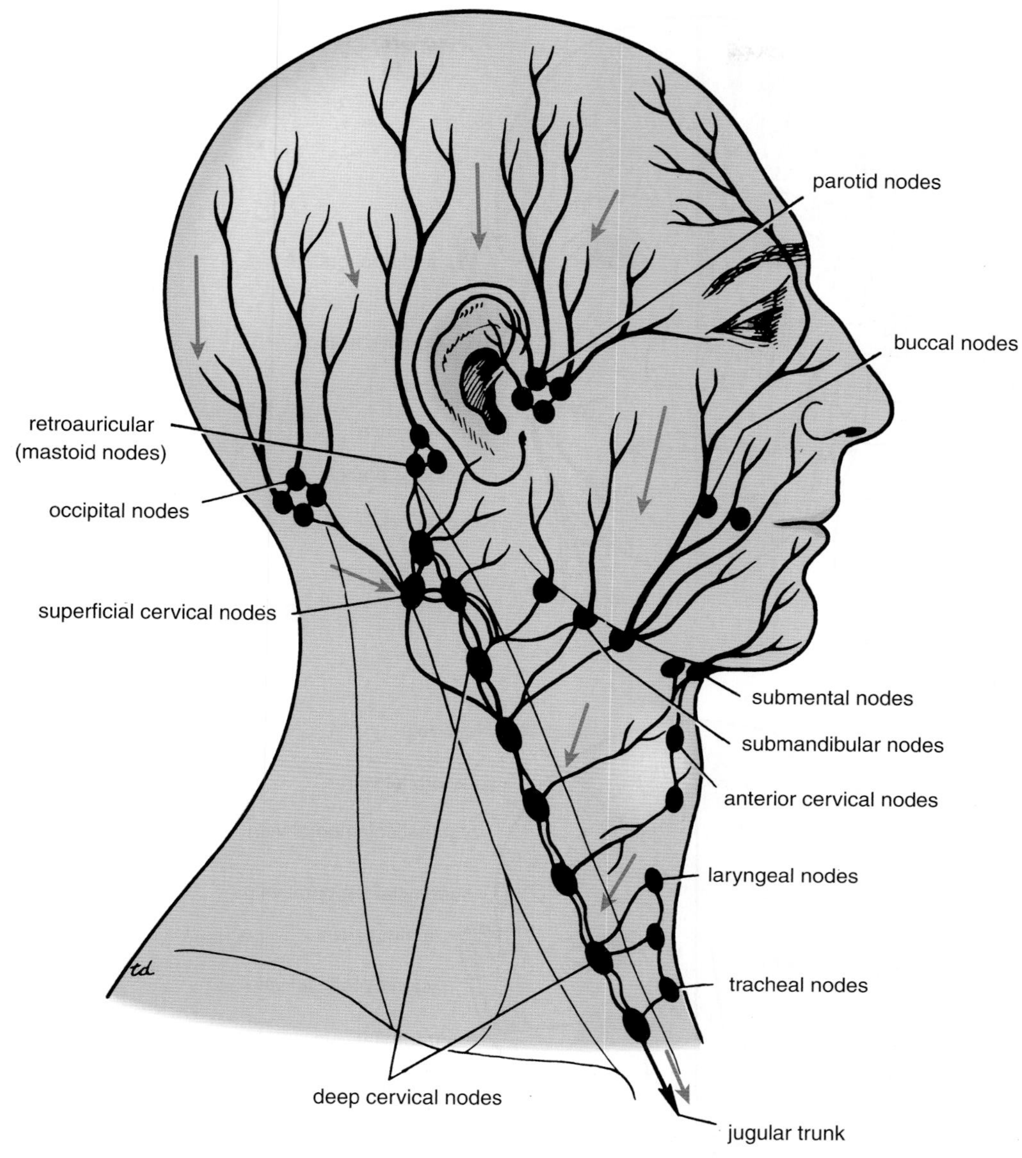

Figure 11-40 Lymph drainage of the head and neck.

The Face

Skin of the Face

The skin of the face possesses numerous sweat and sebaceous glands. It is connected to the underlying bones by loose connective tissue, in which are embedded the muscles of facial expression. **No deep fascia is present in the face.**

Wrinkle lines of the face result from the repeated folding of the skin perpendicular to the long axis of the underlying contracting muscles, coupled with the loss of youthful skin elasticity. Surgical scars of the face are less conspicuous if they follow the wrinkle lines.

Sensory Nerves of the Face

The skin of the face is supplied by branches of the three divisions of the trigeminal nerve, except for the small area over the angle of the mandible and the parotid gland (Fig. 11-41), which is supplied by the great auricular nerve (C2 and 3). The overlap of the three divisions of the trigeminal nerve is slight compared with the considerable overlap of dermatomes of the trunk and limbs. The ophthalmic nerve supplies the region developed from the frontonasal process; the maxillary nerve serves the region developed from the maxillary process of the first pharyngeal arch; and the mandibular nerve serves the region developed from the mandibular process of the first pharyngeal arch.

These nerves not only supply the skin of the face, but also supply proprioceptive fibers to the underlying muscles of facial expression. They are, in addition, the sensory nerve supply to the mouth, teeth, nasal cavities, and paranasal air sinuses.

Ophthalmic Nerve

The ophthalmic nerve supplies the skin of the forehead, the upper eyelid, the conjunctiva, and the side of the nose down

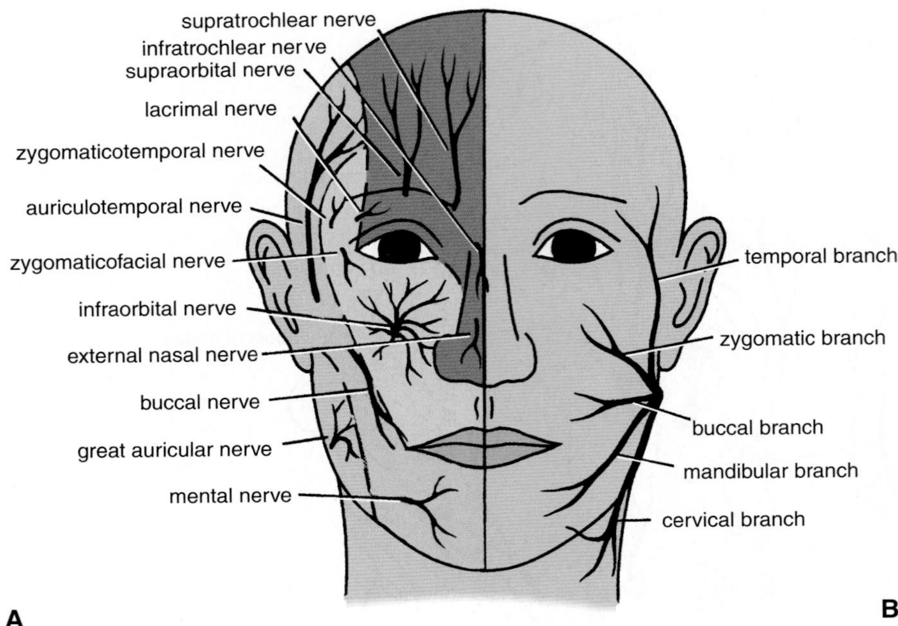

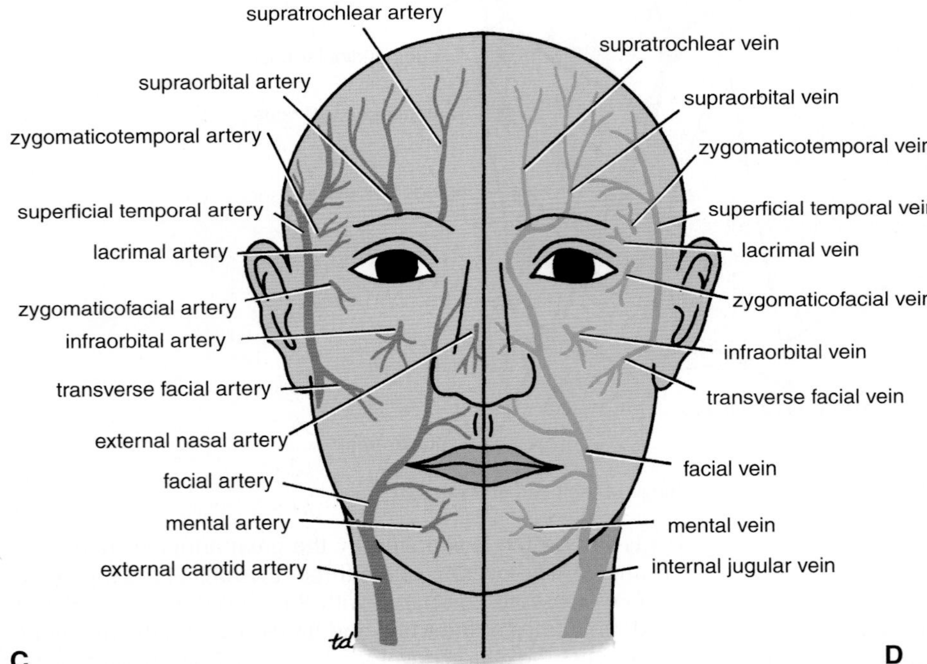

Figure 11-41 **A.** Sensory nerve supply to the skin of the face. **B.** Branches of the seventh cranial nerve to muscles of facial expression. **C.** Arterial supply of the face. **D.** Venous drainage of the face.

to and including the tip. Five branches of the nerve pass to the skin.

- The **lacrimal nerve** supplies the skin and conjunctiva of the lateral part of the upper eyelid (Fig. 11-41).
- The **supraorbital nerve** winds around the upper margin of the orbit at the supraorbital notch (Fig. 11-41). It divides into branches that supply the skin and conjunctiva on the central part of the upper eyelid; it also supplies the skin of the forehead.
- The **supratrochlear nerve** winds around the upper margin of the orbit medial to the supraorbital nerve (Fig. 11-41). It divides into branches that supply the skin and conjunctiva on the medial part of the upper eyelid and the skin over the lower part of the forehead, close to the median plane.
- The **infratrochlear nerve** leaves the orbit below the pulley of the superior oblique muscle. It supplies the skin and conjunctiva on the medial part of the upper eyelid and the adjoining part of the side of the nose (Fig. 11-41).

- The **external nasal nerve** leaves the nose by emerging between the nasal bone and the upper nasal cartilage. It supplies the skin on the side of the nose down as far as the tip (Fig. 11-41).

Maxillary Nerve

The maxillary nerve supplies the skin on the posterior part of the side of the nose, the lower eyelid, the cheek, the upper lip, and the lateral side of the orbital opening. Three branches of the nerve pass to the skin.

- The **infraorbital nerve** is a direct continuation of the maxillary nerve. It enters the orbit and appears on the face through the infraorbital foramen. It immediately divides into numerous small branches, which radiate out from the foramen and supply the skin of the lower eyelid and cheek, the side of the nose, and the upper lip (Fig. 11-41).
- The **zygomaticofacial nerve** passes onto the face through a small foramen on the lateral side of the zygomatic bone. It supplies the skin over the prominence of the cheek (Fig. 11-41).
- The **zygomaticotemporal nerve** emerges in the temporal fossa through a small foramen on the posterior surface of the zygomatic bone. It supplies the skin over the temple (Fig. 11-41).

Mandibular Nerve

The mandibular nerve supplies the skin of the lower lip, the lower part of the face, the temporal region, and part of the auricle. It then passes upward to the side of the scalp. Three branches of the nerve pass to the skin.

- The **mental nerve** emerges from the mental foramen of the mandible and supplies the skin of the lower lip and chin (Fig. 11-41).
- The **buccal nerve** emerges from beneath the anterior border of the masseter muscle and supplies the skin over a small area of the cheek (Fig. 11-41).
- The **auriculotemporal nerve** ascends from the upper border of the parotid gland between the superficial temporal vessels and the auricle. It supplies the skin of the auricle, the external auditory meatus, the outer surface of the tympanic membrane, and the skin of the scalp above the auricle (Fig. 11-41).

Arterial Supply of the Face

The face receives a rich blood supply from two main vessels: the facial and superficial temporal arteries, which are supplemented by several small arteries that accompany the sensory nerves of the face.

The **facial artery** arises from the external carotid artery (Figs. 11-55 and 11-59). Having arched upward and over the submandibular salivary gland, it curves around the inferior margin of the body of the mandible at the anterior border of the masseter muscle. **It is here that the pulse can be easily felt** (Fig. 11-135). It runs upward in a tortuous course toward the angle of the mouth and is covered by the platysma and the risorius muscles. It then ascends deep to the zygomaticus muscles and the levator labii superioris muscle and runs along the side of the nose to the medial angle of the eye, where it anastomoses with the terminal branches of the ophthalmic artery (Fig. 11-41).

Branches

- The **submental artery** arises from the facial artery at the lower border of the body of the mandible. It supplies the skin of the chin and lower lip.
- The **inferior labial artery** arises near the angle of the mouth. It runs medially in the lower lip and anastomoses with its fellow of the opposite side.
- The **superior labial artery** arises near the angle of the mouth. It runs medially in the upper lip and gives branches to the septum and ala of the nose.
- The **lateral nasal artery** arises from the facial artery alongside the nose. It supplies the skin on the side and dorsum of the nose.
- The **superficial temporal artery** (Fig. 11-41), the smaller terminal branch of the external carotid artery, commences in the parotid gland. It ascends in front of the auricle to supply the scalp (see page 725).
- The **transverse facial artery,** a branch of the superficial temporal artery, arises within the parotid gland. It runs forward across the cheek just above the parotid duct (Fig. 11-41).
- The **supraorbital** and **supratrochlear arteries,** branches of the ophthalmic artery, supply the skin of the forehead (Fig. 11-41).

CLINICAL NOTES

Sensory Innervation and Trigeminal Neuralgia

The facial skin receives its sensory nerve supply from the three divisions of the trigeminal nerve. Remember that a small area of skin over the angle of the jaw is supplied by the great auricular nerve (C2 and 3). **Trigeminal neuralgia** is a relatively common condition in which the patient experiences excruciating pain in the distribution of the mandibular or maxillary division, with the ophthalmic division usually escaping. A physician should be able to map out accurately on a patient's face the distribution of each of the divisions of the trigeminal nerve.

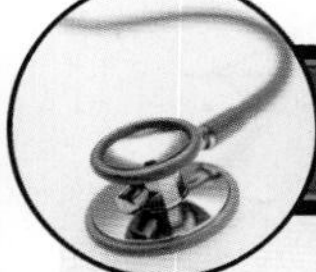

CLINICAL NOTES

Blood Supply of the Facial Skin

The blood supply to the skin of the face is profuse so that it is rare in plastic surgery for skin flaps to necrose in this region.

Facial Arteries and Taking the Patient's Pulse

The superficial temporal artery, as it crosses the zygomatic arch in front of the ear, and the facial artery, as it winds around the lower margin of the mandible level with the anterior border of the masseter, are commonly used by the anesthetist to take the patient's pulse.

Venous Drainage of the Face

The **facial vein** is formed at the medial angle of the eye by the union of the supraorbital and supratrochlear veins (Fig. 11-41). It is connected to the superior ophthalmic vein directly through the supraorbital vein. By means of the superior ophthalmic vein, the facial vein is connected to the cavernous sinus (Fig. 11-9); this connection is of great clinical importance because it provides a pathway for the spread of infection from the face to the cavernous sinus. The facial vein descends behind the facial artery to the lower margin of the body of the mandible. It crosses superficial to the submandibular gland and is joined by the anterior division of the retromandibular vein. The facial vein ends by draining into the internal jugular vein.

Tributaries

The facial vein receives tributaries that correspond to the branches of the facial artery. It is joined to the pterygoid venous plexus by the **deep facial vein** and to the cavernous sinus by the superior ophthalmic vein.

The **transverse facial vein** joins the superficial temporal vein within the parotid gland.

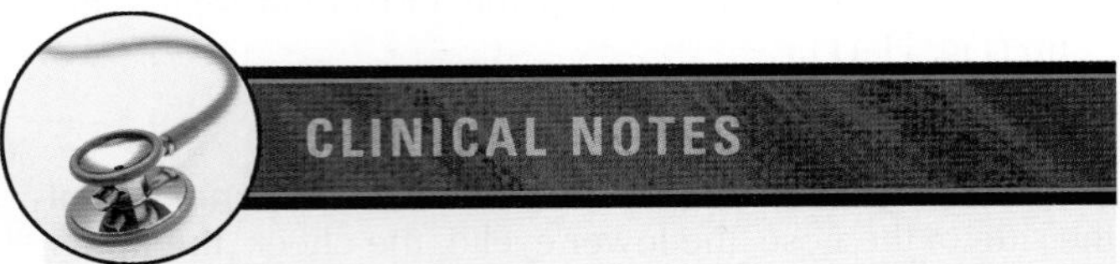

Facial Infections and Cavernous Sinus Thrombosis

The area of facial skin bounded by the nose, the eye, and the upper lip is a potentially dangerous zone to have an infection. For example, a boil in this region can cause thrombosis of the facial vein, with spread of organisms through the inferior ophthalmic veins to the cavernous sinus. The resulting cavernous sinus thrombosis may be fatal unless adequately treated with antibiotics.

Lymph Drainage of the Face

Lymph from the forehead and the anterior part of the face drains into the submandibular lymph nodes (Fig. 11-42). A

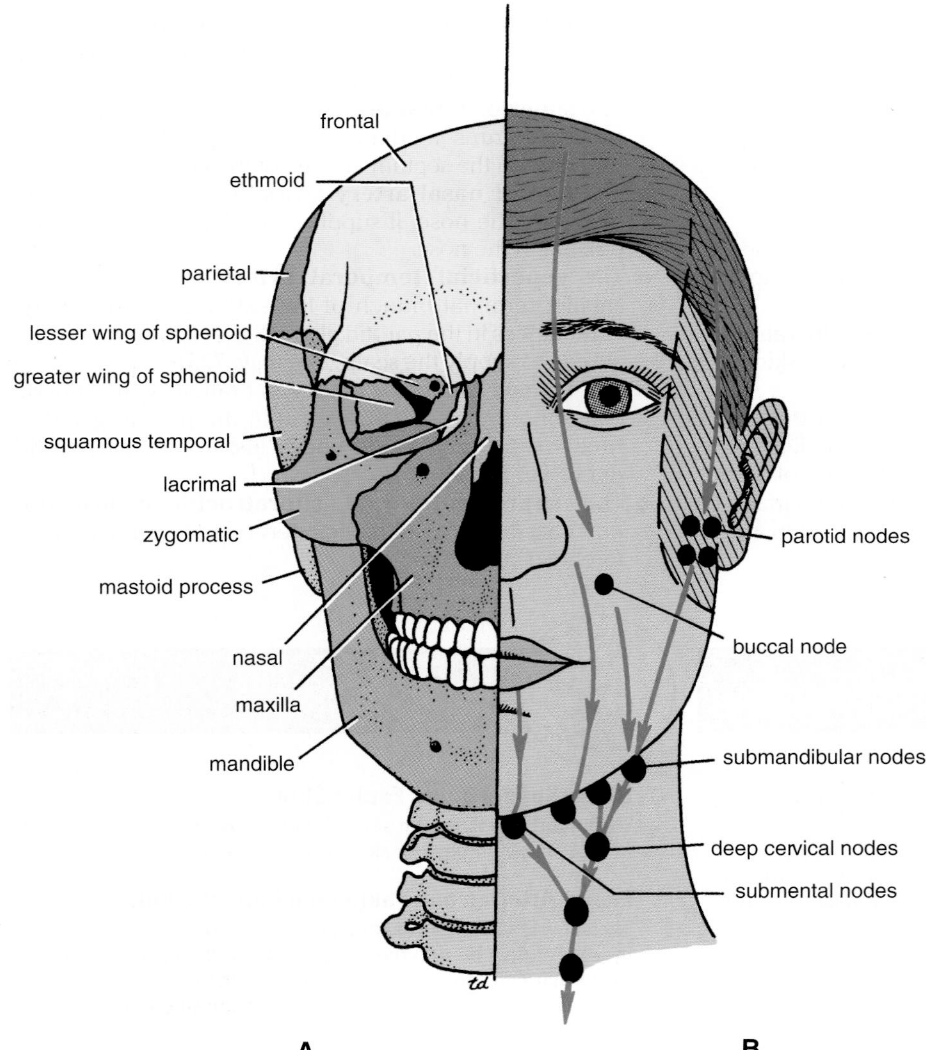

Figure 11-42 **A.** Bones of the front of the skull. **B.** Lymph drainage of the face.

few buccal lymph nodes may be present along the course of these lymph vessels. The lateral part of the face, including the lateral parts of the eyelids, is drained by lymph vessels that end in the parotid lymph nodes. The central part of the lower lip and the skin of the chin are drained into the submental lymph nodes.

Bones of the Face

The bones that form the front of the skull are shown in Figure 11-42. The superior orbital margins and the area above them are formed by the **frontal bone,** which contains the **frontal air sinuses.** The lateral orbital margin is formed by the **zygomatic bone** and the inferior orbital margin is formed by the **zygomatic bone** and the **maxilla.** The medial orbital margin is formed above the maxillary process of the frontal bone and below by the frontal process of the **maxilla.**

The root of the nose is formed by the **nasal bones,** which articulate below with the maxilla and above with the frontal bones. Anteriorly, the nose is completed by upper and lower plates of hyaline cartilage and small cartilages of the ala nasi.

The important central bone of the middle third of the face is the maxilla, containing its teeth and the maxillary air sinus. The bone of the lower third of the face is the mandible, with its teeth. A more detailed account of the bones of the face is given in the discussion of the skull (see page 669).

Muscles of the Face (Muscles of Facial Expression)

The muscles of the face are embedded in the superficial fascia, and most arise from the bones of the skull and are inserted into the skin (Fig. 11-38). The orifices of the face, namely, the orbit, nose, and mouth, are guarded by the eyelids, nostrils, and lips, respectively. It is the function of the facial muscles to serve as sphincters or dilators of these structures. A secondary function of the facial muscles is to modify the expression of the face. All the muscles of the face are developed from the second pharyngeal arch and are supplied by the facial nerve.

Muscles of the Eyelids

The sphincter muscle of the eyelids is the orbicularis oculi, and the dilator muscles are the levator palpebrae superioris and the occipitofrontalis (Fig. 11-38). The levator palpebrae superioris is described on page 691. The occipitofrontalis forms part of the scalp and is described on page 724.

The origin, insertion, nerve supply, and action of the orbicularis oculi and the corrugator supercilii are described in Table 11-4.

Muscles of the Nostrils

The sphincter muscle is the compressor naris and the dilator muscle is the dilator naris (Fig. 11-38).

The origin, insertion, nerve supply, and action of the compressor naris, the dilator naris, and the procerus are shown in Table 11-4.

Muscles of the Lips and Cheeks

The sphincter muscle is the orbicularis oris. The dilator muscles consist of a series of small muscles that radiate out from the lips.

Sphincter Muscle of the Lips: Orbicularis Oris

- **Origin and insertion:** The fibers encircle the oral orifice within the substance of the lips (Fig. 11-38). Some of the fibers arise near the midline from the maxilla above and the mandible below. Other fibers arise from the deep surface of the skin and pass obliquely to the mucous membrane lining the inner surface of the lips. Many of the fibers are derived from the buccinator muscle.
- **Nerve supply:** Buccal and mandibular branches of the facial nerve
- **Action:** Compresses the lips together

Dilator Muscles of the Lips

The dilator muscles (Fig. 11-38) radiate out from the lips, and their action is to separate the lips; this movement is usually accompanied by separation of the jaws.

The muscles arise from the bones and fascia around the oral aperture and converge to be inserted into the substance of the lips. Traced from the side of the nose to the angle of the mouth and then below the oral aperture, the muscles are named as follows:

- Levator labii superioris alaeque nasi
- Levator labii superioris
- Zygomaticus minor
- Zygomaticus major
- Levator anguli oris (deep to the zygomatic muscles)
- Risorius
- Depressor anguli oris
- Depressor labii inferioris
- Mentalis

Nerve Supply Buccal and mandibular branches of the facial nerve

Muscle of the Cheek

Buccinator

- **Origin:** From the outer surface of the alveolar margins of the maxilla and mandible opposite the molar teeth and from the pterygomandibular ligament (Fig. 11-38)
- **Insertion:** The muscle fibers pass forward, forming the muscle layer of the cheek. The muscle is pierced by the parotid duct. At the angle of the mouth the central fibers decussate, those from below entering the upper lip and those from above entering the lower lip; the highest and lowest fibers continue into the upper and lower lips, respectively, without intersecting. The buccinator muscle thus blends and forms part of the orbicularis oris muscle.
- **Nerve supply:** Buccal branch of the facial nerve
- **Action:** Compresses the cheeks and lips against the teeth

The origin, insertion, nerve supply, and action of the muscles of the lips and cheeks are shown in Table 11-4.

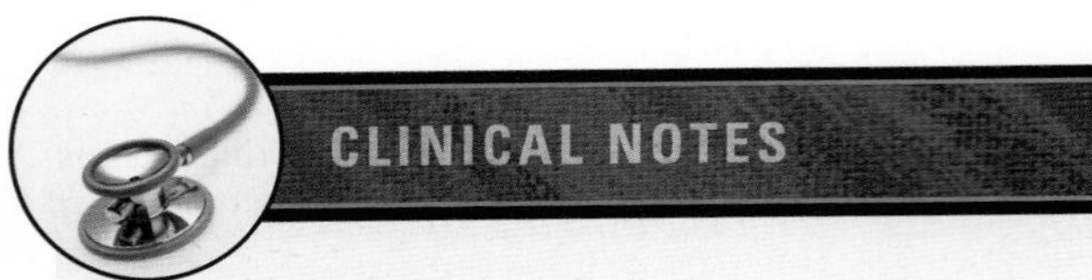

Facial Muscle Paralysis

The facial muscles are innervated by the facial nerve. Damage to the facial nerve in the internal acoustic meatus (by a tumor), in the middle ear (by infection or operation), in the facial nerve canal (perineuritis, **Bell's palsy),** or in the parotid gland (by a tumor) or caused by lacerations of the face will cause distortion of the face, with drooping of the lower eyelid, and the angle of the mouth will sag on the affected side. This is essentially a lower motor neuron lesion. An upper motor neuron lesion (involvement of the pyramidal tracts) will leave the upper part of the face normal because the neurons supplying this part of the face receive corticobulbar fibers from both cerebral cortices.

Facial Nerve

As the facial nerve runs forward within the substance of the parotid salivary gland (see page XXX), it divides into its five terminal branches (Fig. 11-41).

- The **temporal branch** emerges from the upper border of the gland and supplies the anterior and superior auricular muscles, the frontal belly of the occipitofrontalis, the orbicularis oculi, and the corrugator supercilii.
- The **zygomatic branch** emerges from the anterior border of the gland and supplies the orbicularis oculi.
- The **buccal branch** emerges from the anterior border of the gland below the parotid duct and supplies the buccinator muscle and the muscles of the upper lip and nostril.

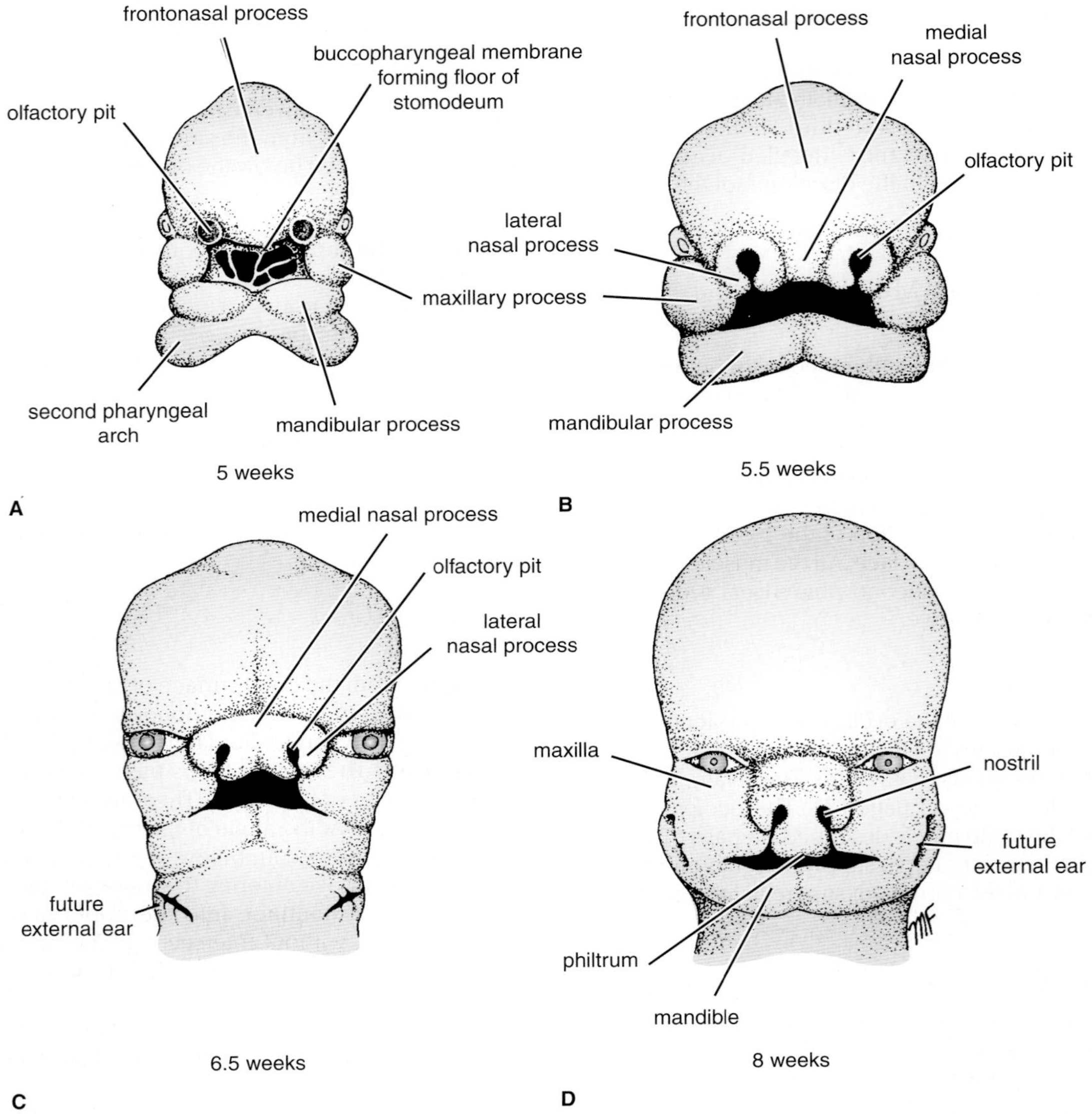

Figure 11-43 Different stages in development of the face.

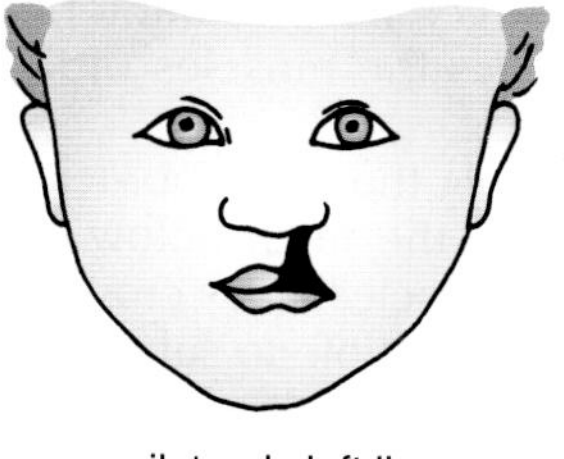

unilateral cleft lip

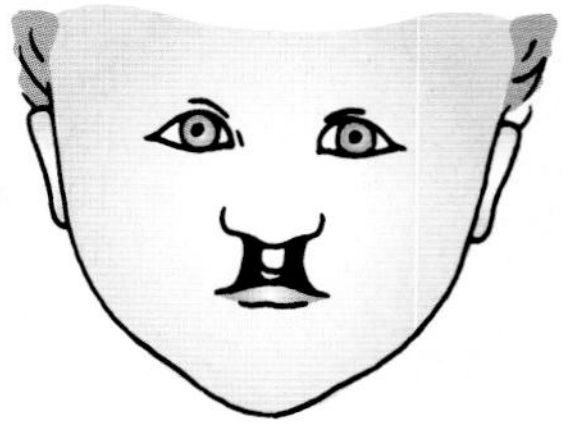

bilateral cleft lip

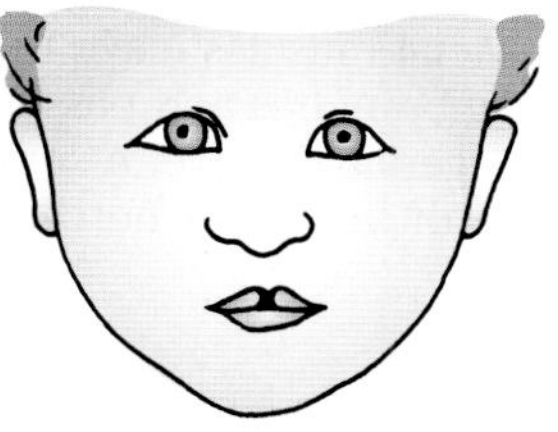

median cleft upper lip

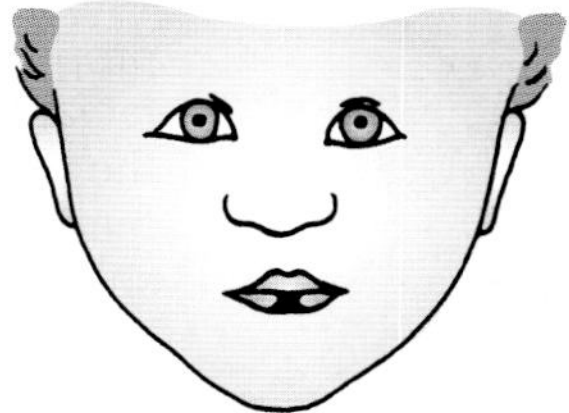

median cleft lower lip

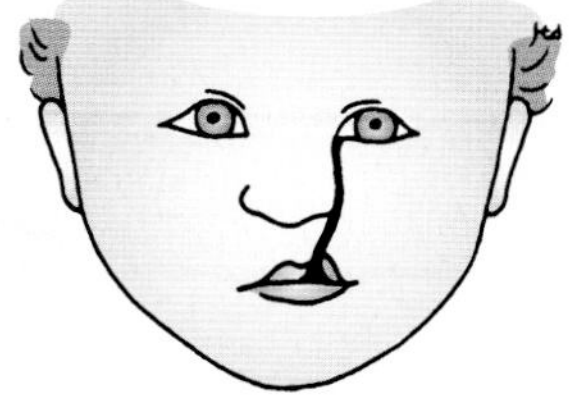

oblique facial cleft

Figure 11-44 Various forms of cleft lip.

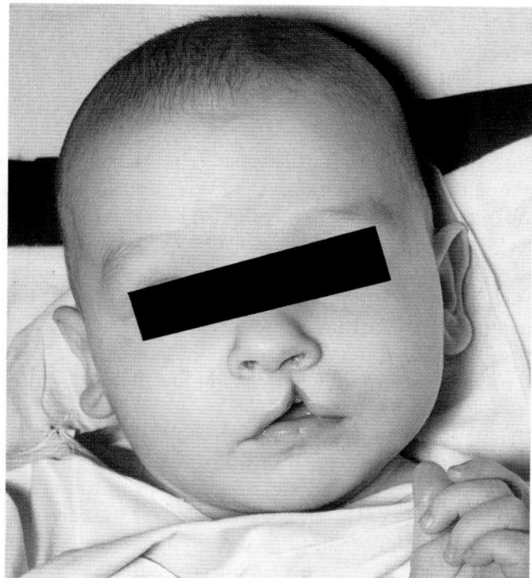

Figure 11-45 Unilateral cleft upper lip. (Courtesy of R. Chase.)

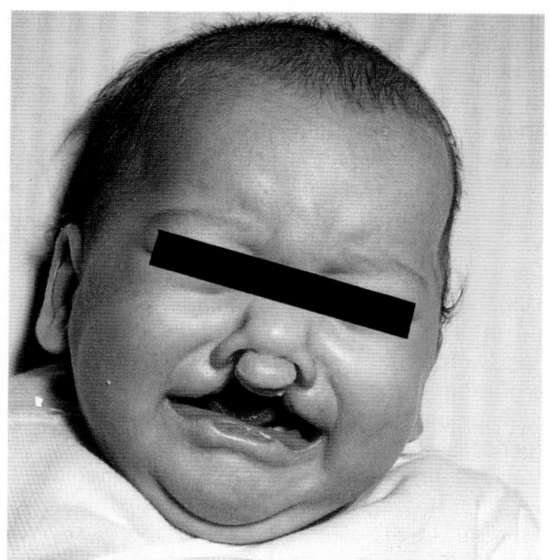

Figure 11-46 Bilateral cleft upper lip and palate. (Courtesy of R. Chase.)

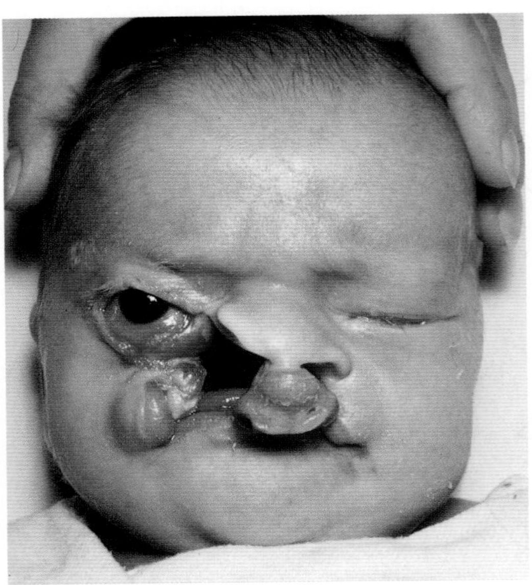

Figure 11-47 Right-sided oblique facial cleft and left-sided cleft upper lip. There also is total bilateral cleft palate. (Courtesy of R. Chase.)

- The **mandibular branch** emerges from the anterior border of the gland and supplies the muscles of the lower lip.
- The **cervical branch** emerges from the lower border of the gland and passes forward in the neck below the mandible to supply the platysma muscle; it may cross the lower margin of the body of the mandible to supply the depressor anguli oris muscle.

The facial nerve is the nerve of the second pharyngeal arch and supplies all the muscles of facial expression. **It does not supply the skin,** but its branches communicate with branches of the trigeminal nerve. It is believed that the proprioceptive nerve fibers of the facial muscles leave the facial nerve in these communicating branches and pass to the central nervous system via the trigeminal nerve. A summary of the origin and distribution of the facial nerve is shown in Figure 11-67.

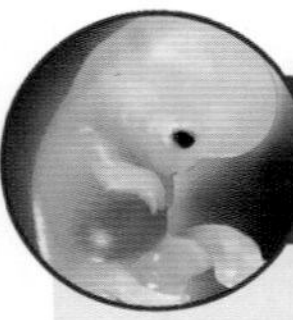

EMBRYOLOGIC NOTES

Development of the Face

Early in development, the face of the embryo is represented by an area bounded cranially by the neural plate, caudally by the pericardium, and laterally by the mandibular process of the first pharyngeal arch on each side (Fig. 11-43). In the center of this area is a depression in the ectoderm known as the **stomodeum.** In the floor of the depression is the **buccopharyngeal membrane.** By the fourth week, the buccopharyngeal membrane breaks down so that the stomodeum communicates with the foregut.

The further development of the face depends on the coming together and fusion of several important processes, namely, the **frontonasal process,** the **maxillary processes,** and the **mandibular processes** (Fig. 11-43). The frontonasal process begins as a proliferation of mesenchyme on the ventral surface of the developing brain, and this grows toward the stomodeum. Meanwhile, the maxillary process grows out from the upper end of each first arch and passes medially, forming the lower border of the developing orbit. The mandibular processes of the first arches now approach one another in the midline below the stomodeum and fuse to form the lower jaw and lower lip (Fig. 11-43).

The **olfactory pits** appear as depressions in the lower edge of the advancing frontonasal process, dividing it into a **medial nasal process** and two **lateral nasal processes.** With further development, the maxillary processes grow medially and fuse with the lateral nasal processes and with the medial nasal process (Fig. 11-43). The medial nasal process forms the **philtrum** of the upper lip and the **premaxilla.** The maxillary processes extend medially, forming the upper jaw and the cheek, and finally bury the premaxilla and fuse in the midline. The various processes that ultimately form the face unite during the second month.

The **upper lip** is formed by the growth medially of the maxillary processes of the first pharyngeal arch on each side. Ultimately, the maxillary processes meet in the midline and fuse with each other and with the medial nasal process (Fig. 11-43). Thus, the lateral parts of the upper lip are formed from the maxillary processes, and the medial part, or philtrum, from the medial nasal process, with contributions from the maxillary processes.

The **lower lip** is formed from the mandibular process of the first pharyngeal arch on each side (Fig. 11-43). These processes grow medially below the stomodeum and fuse in the midline to form the entire lower lip.

Each lip separates from its respective gum as the result of the appearance of a linear thickening of ectoderm, the **labiogingival lamina,** which grows down into the underlying mesenchyme and later degenerates. A deep groove thus forms between the lips and the gums. In the midline, a short area of the labiogingival lamina remains and tethers each lip to the gum, thus forming the **frenulum.**

At first, the **mouth** has a broad opening, but later this diminishes in extent because of fusion of the lips at the lateral angles.

Sensory Nerve Supply to the Skin of the Developing Face

The area of skin overlying the frontonasal process and its derivatives receives its sensory nerve supply from the ophthalmic division of the trigeminal nerve, whereas the maxillary division of the trigeminal nerve supplies the area of skin overlying the maxillary process. The area of skin overlying the mandibular process is supplied by the mandibular division of the trigeminal nerve.

(continues)

Embryologic Notes, *continued*

Muscles of the Developing Face (Muscles of Facial Expression)

The muscles of the face are derived from the mesenchyme of the second pharyngeal arch. The nerve supply of these muscles is the nerve of the second pharyngeal arch—namely, the seventh cranial nerve.

Cleft Upper Lip

Cleft upper lip may be confined to the lip or may be associated with a cleft palate. The anomaly is usually **unilateral cleft lip** and is caused by a failure of the maxillary process to fuse with the medial nasal process (Figs. 11-44 and 11-45). **Bilateral cleft lip** is caused by a failure of both maxillary processes to fuse with the medial nasal process, which then remains as a central flap of tissue (Figs. 11-46 and 11-48). **Median cleft upper lip** is very rare and is caused by the failure of the rounded swellings of the medial nasal process to fuse in the midline.

Oblique Facial Cleft

Oblique facial cleft is a rare condition in which the cleft lip on one side extends to the medial margin of the orbit (Figs. 11-44 and 11-47). This is caused by the failure of the maxillary process to fuse with the lateral and medial nasal processes.

Cleft Lower Lip

Cleft lower lip is a rare condition. The cleft is exactly central and is caused by incomplete fusion of the mandibular processes (Fig. 11-44).

Treatment of Isolated Cleft Lip

The condition of isolated cleft lip usually is treated by plastic surgery no later than 2 months after birth, provided the baby's condition permits. The surgeon strives to approximate the vermilion border and to form a normal-looking lip (Fig. 11-48A–C).

Macrostomia and Microstomia

The normal size of the mouth shows considerable individual variation. Rarely, there is incomplete fusion of the maxillary with the mandibular processes, producing an excessively large mouth or macrostomia. Very rarely, there is excessive fusion of these processes, producing a small mouth or microstomia. These conditions can easily be corrected surgically.

The Neck

The neck is the region of the body that lies between the lower margin of the mandible above and the suprasternal notch and the upper border of the clavicle below. It is strengthened by the cervical part of the vertebral column, which is convex forward and supports the skull. Behind the vertebrae is a mass of extensor muscles and in front is a smaller group of flexor muscles (Fig. 11-49). In the central region of the neck are parts of the respiratory system, namely, the larynx and the trachea, and behind are parts of the alimentary system, the pharynx and the esophagus. At the sides of these structures are the vertically running carotid arteries, internal jugular veins, the vagus nerve, and the deep cervical lymph nodes (Fig. 11-49).

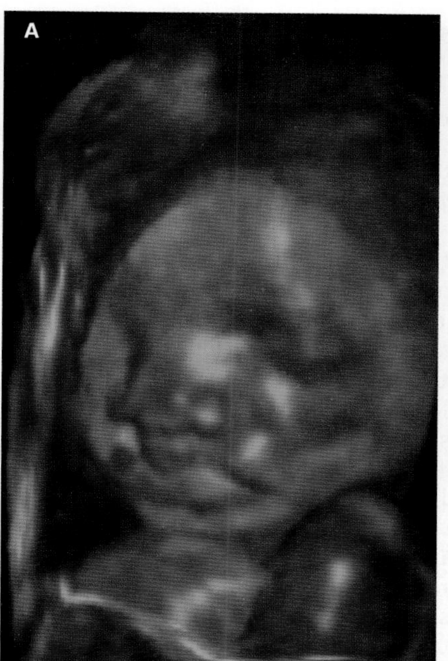

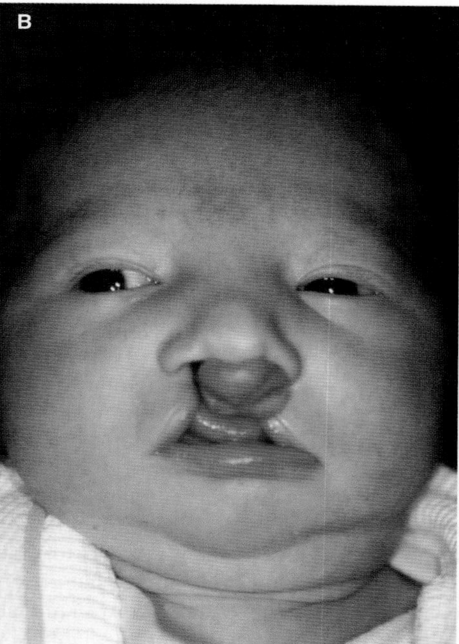

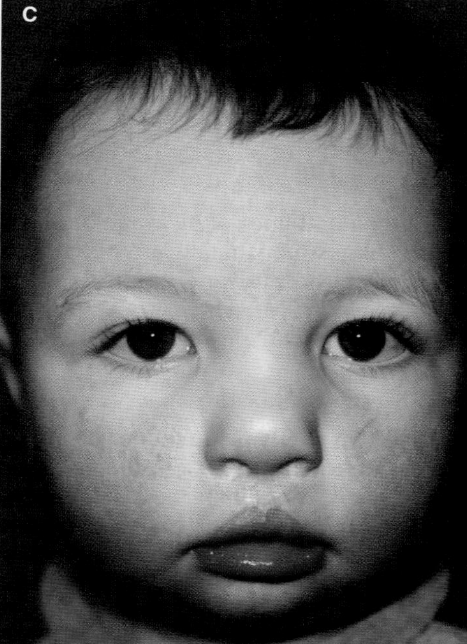

Figure 11-48 Cleft lip and palate. **A.** A three-dimensional ultrasonograph reveals bilateral cleft lip at 22 weeks of gestation. (Courtesy of Dr. B. Benacerraf.) **B.** An infant with bilateral complete cleft lip and palate. **C.** Shows the same child at 18 months of age, after synchronous nasolabial repair and palatal closure performed at a second stage. (Courtesy of Dr. J. B. Mulliken. *N Engl J Med* 351;8:769.)

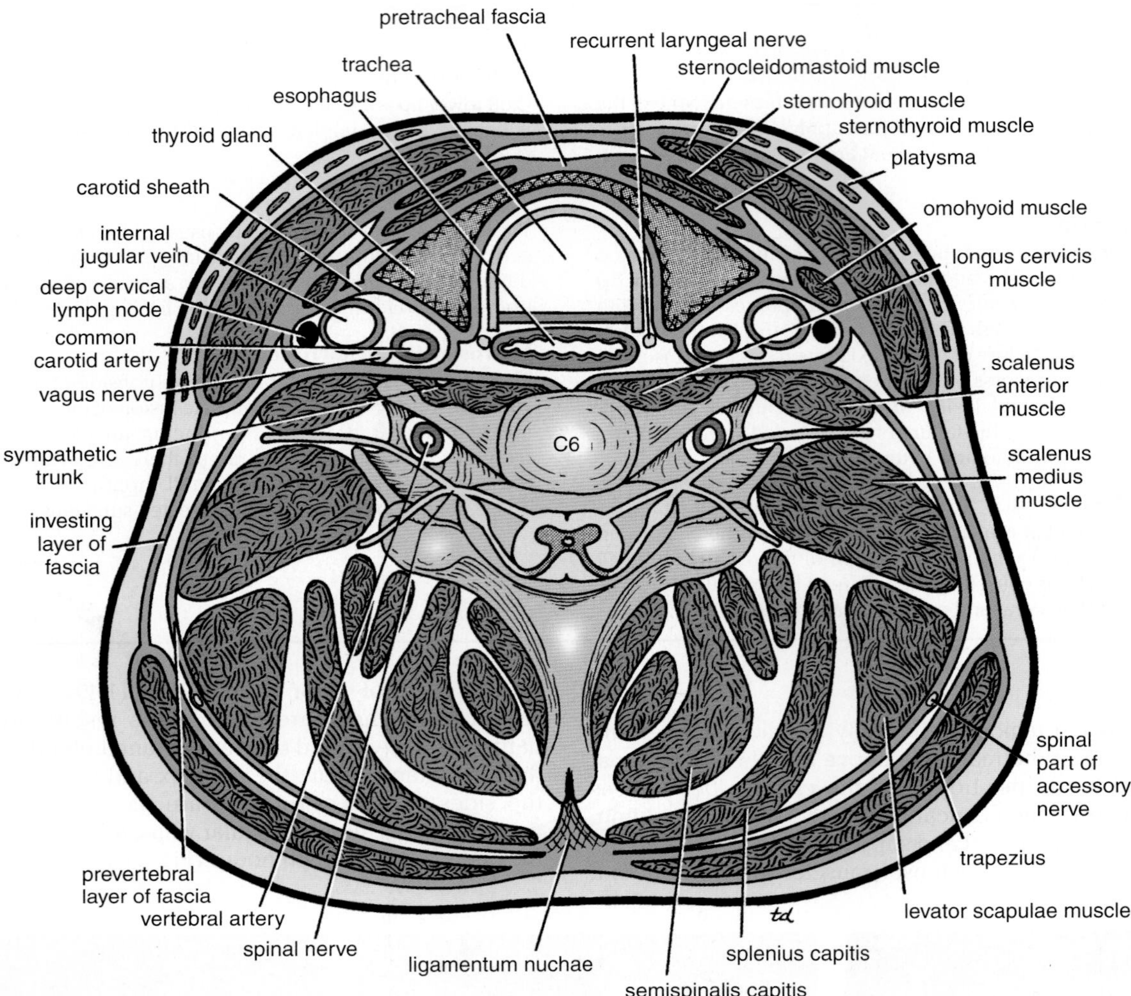

Figure 11-49 Cross section of the neck at the level of the sixth cervical vertebra.

Skin of the Neck

The natural lines of cleavage of the skin are constant and run almost horizontally around the neck. This is important clinically because an incision along a cleavage line will heal as a narrow scar, whereas one that crosses the lines will heal as a wide or heaped-up scar.

Cutaneous Nerves

The skin overlying the trapezius muscle on the back of the neck and on the back of the scalp as high as the vertex is supplied segmentally by posterior rami of cervical nerves 2 to 5 (Fig. 11-50). The **greater occipital nerve** is a branch of the posterior ramus of the second cervical nerve. The first cervical nerve has no cutaneous branch.

The skin of the front and sides of the neck is supplied by anterior rami of cervical nerves 2 to 4 through branches of the cervical plexus. The branches emerge from beneath the posterior border of the sternocleidomastoid muscle (Fig. 11-50).

The **lesser occipital nerve** (C2) hooks around the accessory nerve and ascends along the posterior border of the sternocleidomastoid muscle to supply the skin over the lateral part of the occipital region and the medial surface of the auricle (Fig. 11-50).

The **great auricular nerve** (C2 and 3) ascends across the sternocleidomastoid muscle and divides into branches that supply the skin over the angle of the mandible, the parotid gland, and on both surfaces of the auricle (Fig. 11-50).

The **transverse cutaneous nerve** (C2 and 3) emerges from behind the middle of the posterior border of the sternocleidomastoid muscle. It passes forward across that muscle and divides into branches that supply the skin on the anterior and lateral surfaces of the neck, from the body of the mandible to the sternum (Fig. 11-50).

The **supraclavicular nerves** (C3 and 4) emerge from beneath the posterior border of the sternocleidomastoid muscle and descend across the side of the neck. They pass onto the chest wall and shoulder region, down to the level of the second rib (Fig. 11-50). The **medial supraclavicular nerve** crosses the medial end of the clavicle and supplies the skin as far as the median plane. The **intermediate supraclavicular nerve** crosses the middle of the clavicle and supplies the skin of the chest wall. The **lateral supraclavicular nerve** crosses the lateral end of the clavicle and supplies the

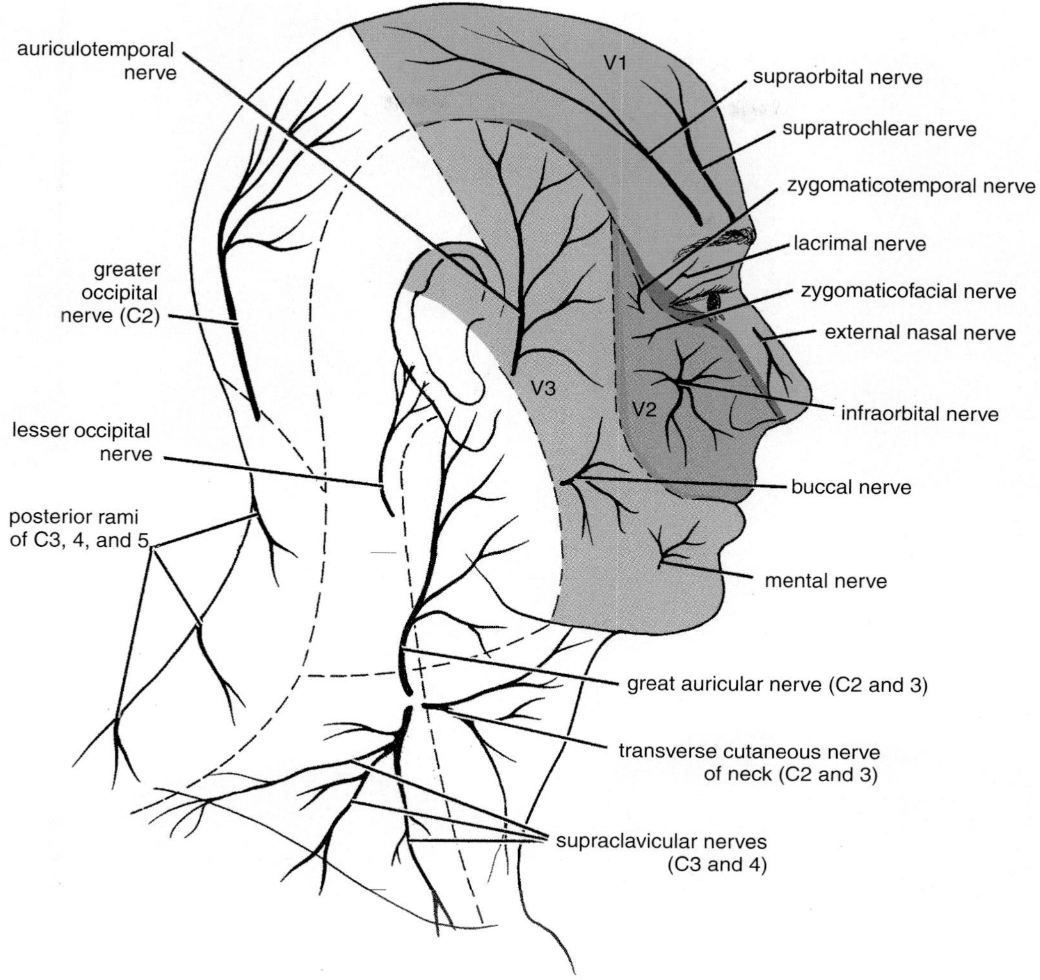

Figure 11-50 Sensory nerve supply to skin of the head and neck. Note that the skin over the angle of the jaw is supplied by the great auricular nerve (C2 and 3) and not by branches of the trigeminal nerve.

skin over the shoulder and the upper half of the deltoid muscle; this nerve also supplies the posterior aspect of the shoulder as far down as the spine of the scapula.

Superficial Fascia

The superficial fascia of the neck forms a thin layer that encloses the platysma muscle. Also embedded in it are the cutaneous nerves referred to in the previous section, the superficial veins, and the superficial lymph nodes.

Platysma

The platysma muscle (Figs. 11-38 and 11-51) is a thin but clinically important muscular sheet embedded in the superficial fascia. It is described in Table 11-5, page 742.

Superficial Veins

External Jugular Vein

The external jugular vein begins just behind the angle of the mandible by the union of the posterior auricular vein with the posterior division of the retromandibular vein (Fig. 11-52). It descends obliquely across the sternocleidomastoid muscle and, just above the clavicle in the posterior triangle, pierces the deep fascia and drains into the subclavian vein (Fig. 11-53). It varies considerably in size, and its course extends from the angle of the mandible to the middle of the clavicle.

Tributaries

The external jugular vein (Fig. 11-52) has the following tributaries:

- Posterior auricular vein
- Posterior division of the retromandibular vein
- Posterior external jugular vein, a small vein that drains the posterior part of the scalp and neck and joins the external jugular vein about halfway along its course
- Transverse cervical vein
- Suprascapular vein
- Anterior jugular vein

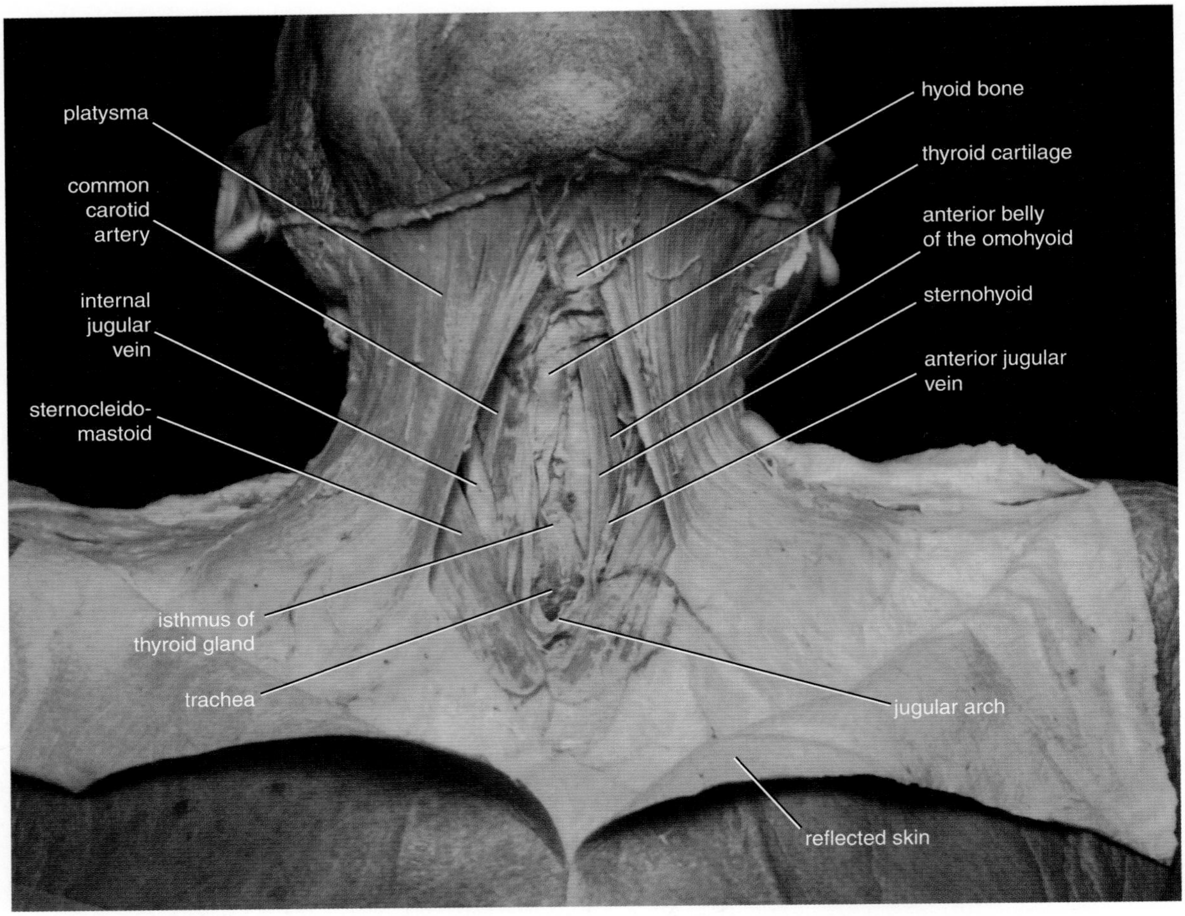

Figure 11-51 Dissection of the anterior aspect of the neck showing the platysma muscles and the lower ends of the sternocleidomastoid muscles on both sides. The skin has been reflected downward.

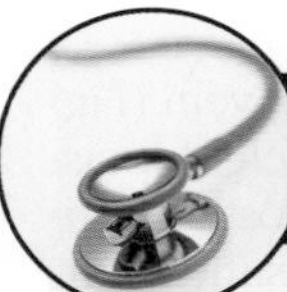

CLINICAL NOTES

Visibility of the External Jugular Vein

The external jugular vein is less obvious in children and women because their subcutaneous tissue tends to be thicker than the tissue of men. In obese individuals, the vein may be difficult to identify even when they are asked to hold their breath, which impedes the venous return to the right side of the heart and distends the vein.

The superficial veins of the neck tend to be enlarged and often tortuous in professional singers because of prolonged periods of raised intrathoracic pressure.

The External Jugular Vein as a Venous Manometer

The external jugular vein serves as a useful venous manometer. Normally, when the patient is lying at a horizontal angle of 30°, the level of the blood in the external jugular veins reaches about one third of the way up the neck. As the patient sits up, the blood level falls until it is no longer visible behind the clavicle.

External Jugular Vein Catheterization

The external jugular vein can be used for catheterization, but the presence of valves or tortuosity may make the passage of the catheter difficult. Because the right external jugular vein is in the most direct line with the superior vena cava, it is the one most commonly used (Fig. 11-54).

The vein is catheterized about halfway between the level of the cricoid cartilage and the clavicle. The passage of the catheter should be performed during inspiration when the valves are open.

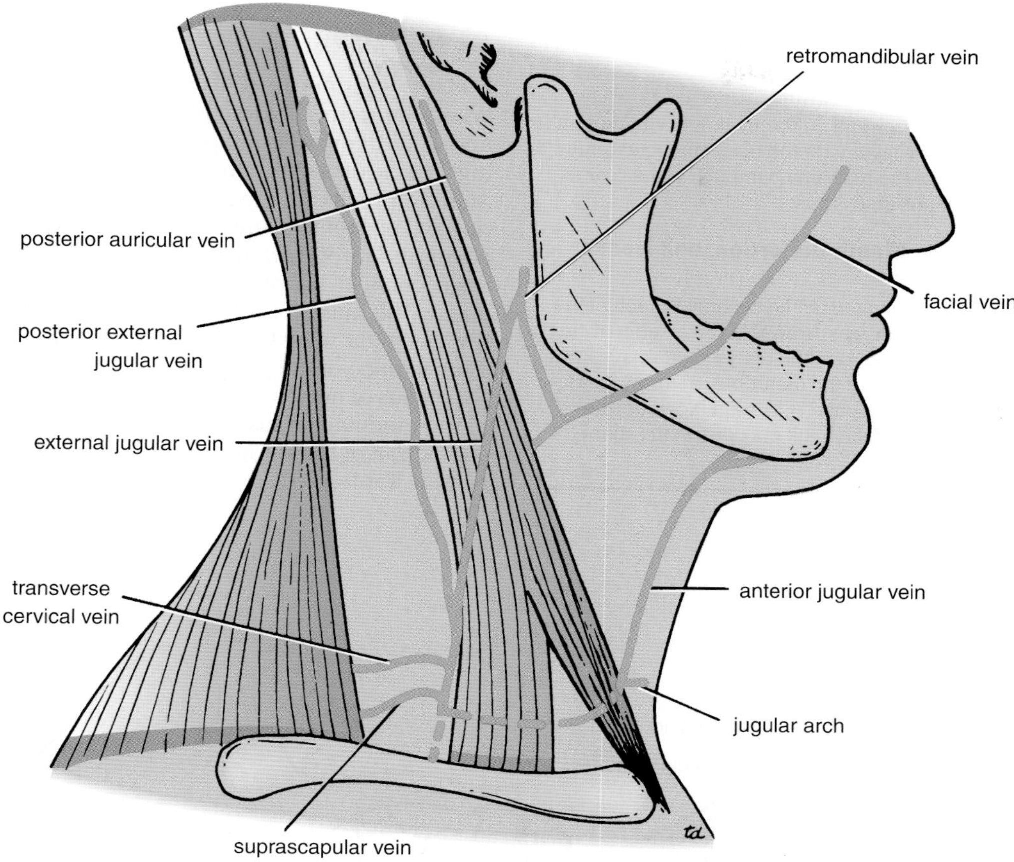

Figure 11-52 Major superficial veins of the face and neck.

Anterior Jugular Vein

The anterior jugular vein begins just below the chin, by the union of several small veins (Fig. 11-52). It runs down the neck close to the midline. Just above the suprasternal notch, the veins of the two sides are united by a transverse trunk called the jugular arch. The vein then turns sharply laterally and passes deep to the sternocleidomastoid muscle to drain into the external jugular vein.

Superficial Lymph Nodes

The superficial cervical lymph nodes lie along the external jugular vein superficial to the sternocleidomastoid muscle (Fig. 11-40). They receive lymph vessels from the occipital and mastoid lymph nodes (see page 755) and drain into the deep cervical lymph nodes.

Bones of the Neck

Cervical Vertebrae

The cervical part of the vertebral column is described on page 855.

Hyoid Bone

The hyoid bone is a mobile single bone found in the midline of the neck below the mandible and abides the larynx. It does not articulate with any other bones. The hyoid bone is U shaped and consists of a body and two greater and two lesser cornua (Fig. 11-32). It is attached to the skull by the stylohyoid ligament and to the thyroid cartilage by the thyrohyoid membrane. The hyoid bone forms a base for the tongue and is suspended in position by muscles that connect it to the mandible, to the styloid process of the temporal bone, to the thyroid cartilage, to the sternum, and to the scapula.

The important muscles attached to the hyoid bone are shown in Figure 11-32.

Muscles of the Neck

The superficial muscles of the side of the neck (Figs. 11-38 and 11-51) are described in Table 11-5. The suprahyoid and infrahyoid muscles and the anterior and lateral vertebral muscles are also described in Table 11-5.

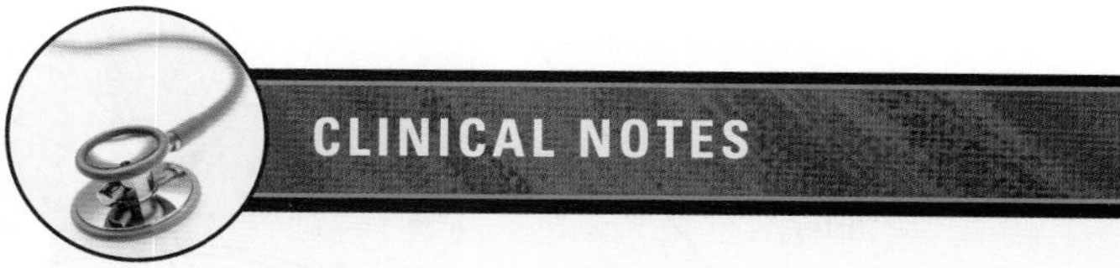

Clinical Identification of the Platysma

The platysma can be seen as a thin sheet of muscle just beneath the skin by having the patient clench his or her jaws firmly. The muscle extends from the body of the mandible downward over the clavicle onto the anterior chest wall.

(continues)

Clinical Notes, *continued*

Platysma Tone and Neck Incisions

In lacerations or surgical incisions in the neck it is very important that the subcutaneous layer with the platysma be carefully sutured, since the tone of the platysma can pull on the scar tissue, resulting in broad, unsightly scars.

Platysma Innervation, Mouth Distortion, and Neck Incisions

The platysma muscle is innervated by the cervical branch of the facial nerve. This nerve emerges from the lower end of the parotid gland and travels forward to the platysma; it then sometimes crosses the lower border of the mandible to supply the depressor anguli oris muscle (see page 765). Skin lacerations over the mandible or upper part of the neck may distort the shape of the mouth.

Key Neck Muscles

Sternocleidomastoid Muscle

When the sternocleidomastoid muscle (Figs. 11-51, 11-53, and 11-55) contracts, it appears as an oblique band crossing the side of the neck from the sternoclavicular joint to the mastoid process of the skull. It divides the neck into anterior and posterior triangles (Fig. 11-56). The anterior border covers the carotid arteries, the internal jugular vein, and the deep cervical lymph nodes; it also overlaps the thyroid gland. The muscle is covered superficially by skin, fascia, the platysma muscle, and the external jugular vein. The deep surface of the posterior border is related to the cervical plexus of nerves, the phrenic nerve, and the upper part of the brachial plexus. The origin, insertion, nerve supply, and action of the sternocleidomastoid muscle are summarized in Table 11-5.

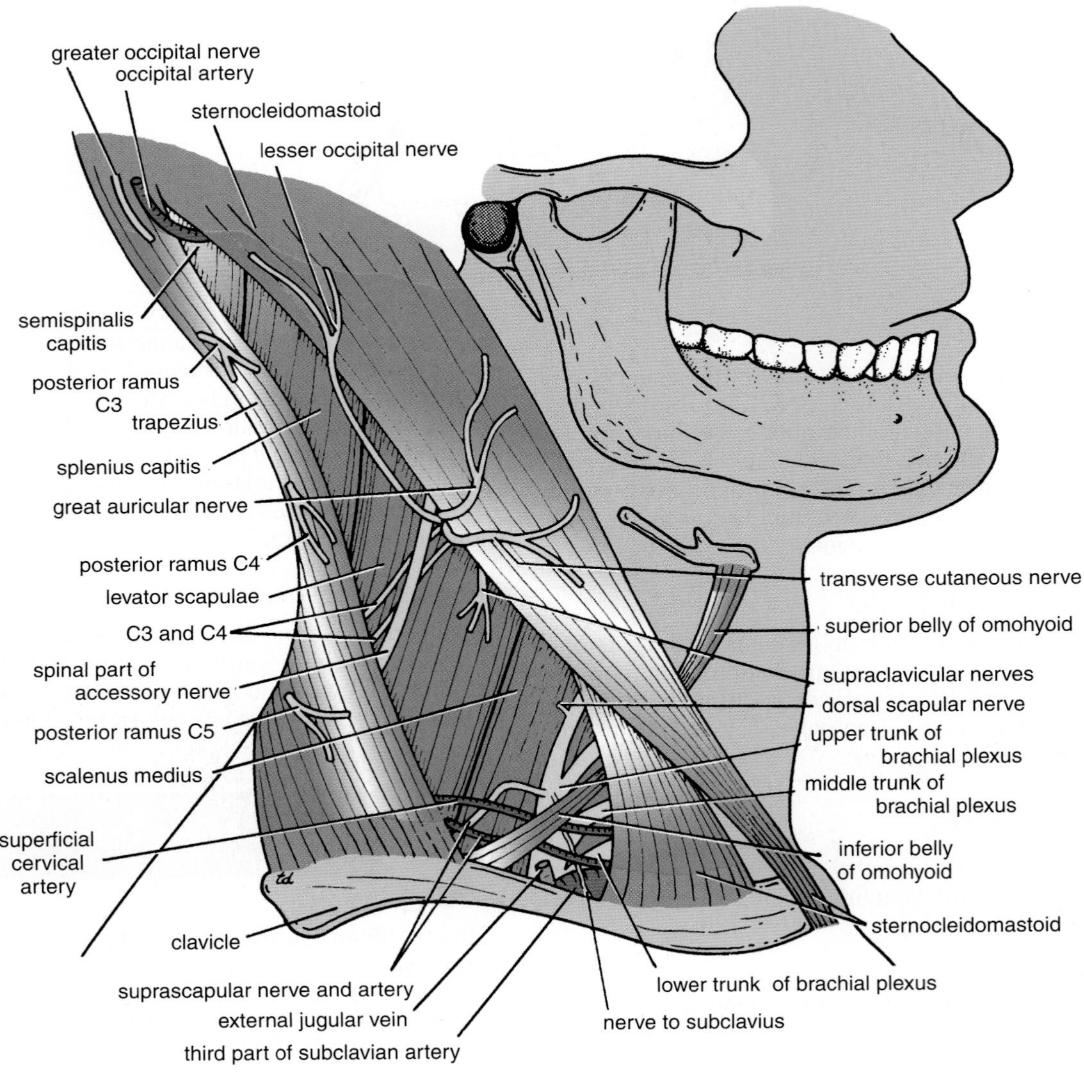

Figure 11-53 Posterior triangle of the neck.

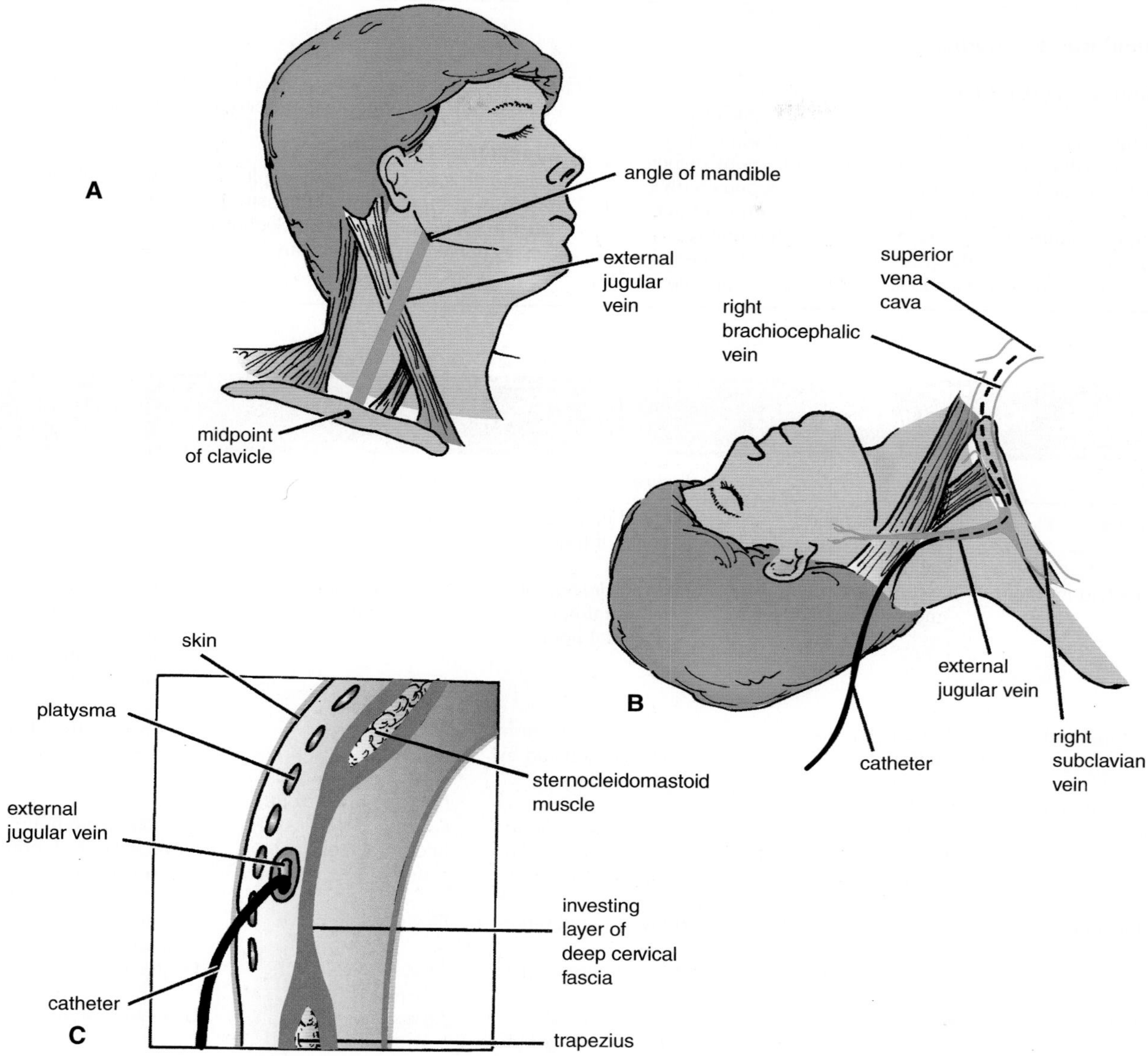

Figure 11-54 Catheterization of the right external jugular vein. **A.** Surface marking of the vein. **B.** Site of catheterization. Note how the external jugular vein joins the subclavian vein at a right angle. **C.** Cross section of the neck showing the relationships of the external jugular vein as it crosses the posterior triangle of the neck.

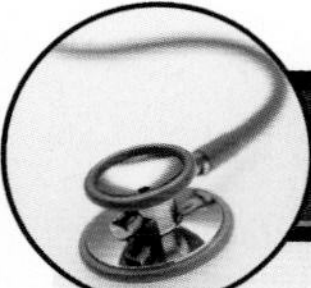

CLINICAL NOTES

Sternocleidomastoid Muscle and Protection From Trauma

The sternocleidomastoid, a strong, thick muscle crossing the side of the neck, protects the underlying soft structures from blunt trauma. Suicide attempts by cutting one's throat often fail because the individual first extends the neck before making several horizontal cuts with a knife. Extension of the cervical part of the vertebral column and extension of the head at the atlanto-occipital joint cause the carotid sheath with its contained large blood vessels to slide posteriorly beneath the sternocleidomastoid muscle. To achieve the desired result with the head and neck fully extended, some individuals have to make several attempts and only succeed when the larynx and the greater part of the sternocleidomastoid muscles have been severed. The common sites for the wounds are immediately above and below the hyoid bone.

(continues)

Clinical Notes, *continued*

Congenital Torticollis

Most cases of congenital torticollis are a result of excessive stretching of the sternocleidomastoid muscle during a difficult labor. Hemorrhage occurs into the muscle and may be detected as a small, rounded "tumor" during the early weeks after birth. Later, this becomes invaded by fibrous tissue, which contracts and shortens the muscle. The mastoid process is thus pulled down toward the sternoclavicular joint of the same side, the cervical spine is flexed, and the face looks upward to the opposite side. If left untreated, asymmetrical growth changes occur in the face, and the cervical vertebrae may become wedge shaped.

Spasmodic Torticollis

Spasmodic torticollis, which results from repeated chronic contractions of the sternocleidomastoid and trapezius muscles, is usually psychogenic in origin. Section of the spinal part of the accessory nerve may be necessary in severe cases.

Table 11-5 Muscles of the Neck

Muscle	Origin	Insertion	Nerve Supply	Action
Platysma	Deep fascia over pectoralis major and deltoid	Body of mandible and angle of mouth	Facial nerve cervical branch	Depresses mandible and angle of mouth
Sternocleidomastoid	Manubrium sterni and medial third of clavicle	Mastoid process of temporal bone and occipital bone	Spinal part of accessory nerve and C2 and 3	Two muscles acting together extend head and flex neck; one muscle rotates head to opposite side
Digastric				
Posterior belly	Mastoid process of temporal bone	Intermediate tendon is held to hyoid by fascial sling	Facial nerve	Depresses mandible or elevates hyoid bone
Anterior belly	Body of mandible		Nerve to mylohyoid	
Stylohyoid	Styloid process	Body of hyoid bone	Facial nerve	Elevates hyoid bone
Mylohyoid	Mylohyoid line of body of mandible	Body of hyoid bone and fibrous raphe	Inferior alveolar nerve	Elevates floor of mouth and hyoid bone or depresses mandible
Geniohyoid	Inferior mental spine of mandible	Body of hyoid bone	First cervical nerve	Elevates hyoid bone or depresses mandible
Sternohyoid	Manubrium sterni and clavicle	Body of hyoid bone	Ansa cervicalis; C1, 2, and 3	Depresses hyoid bone
Sternothyroid	Manubrium sterni	Oblique line on lamina of thyroid cartilage	Ansa cervicalis; C1, 2, and 3	Depresses larynx
Thyrohyoid	Oblique line on lamina of thyroid cartilage	Lower border of body of hyoid bone	First cervical nerve	Depresses hyoid bone or elevates larynx
Omohyoid				
Inferior belly	Upper margin of scapula and suprascapular ligament	Intermediate tendon is held to clavicle and first rib by fascial sling	Ansa cervicalis; C1, 2, and 3	Depresses hyoid bone
Superior belly	Lower border of body of hyoid bone			
Scalenus anterior	Transverse processes of third, fourth, fifth, and sixth cervical vertebrae	First rib	C4, 5, and 6	Elevates first rib; laterally flexes and rotates cervical part of vertebral column
Scalenus medius	Transverse processes of upper six cervical vertebrae	First rib	Anterior rami of cervical nerves	Elevates first rib; laterally flexes and rotates cervical part of vertebral column
Scalenus posterior	Transverse processes of lower cervical vertebrae	Second rib	Anterior rami of cervical nerves	Elevates second rib; laterally flexes and rotates cervical part of vertebral column

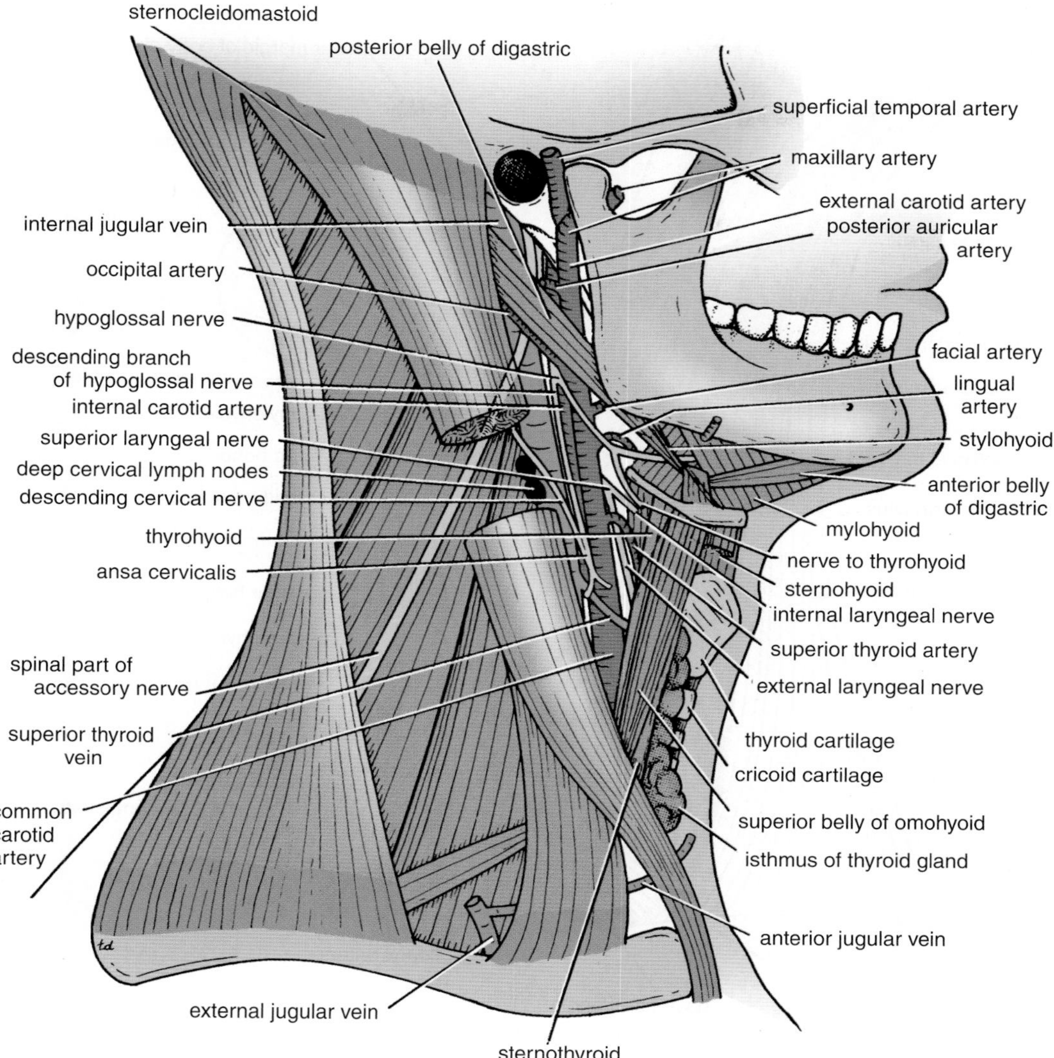

Figure 11-55 Anterior triangle of the neck.

Scalenus Anterior Muscle

The scalenus anterior muscle is a key muscle in understanding the root of the neck (Fig. 11-57). It is deeply placed and it descends almost vertically from the vertebral column to the first rib.

Important Relations

- **Anteriorly:** Related to the carotid arteries, the vagus nerve, the internal jugular vein, and the deep cervical lymph nodes (Fig. 11-49). The transverse cervical and suprascapular arteries and the prevertebral layer of deep cervical fascia bind the phrenic nerve to the muscle.
- **Posteriorly:** Related to the pleura, the origin of the brachial plexus, and the second part of the subclavian artery (Fig. 11-57). The scalenus medius muscle lies behind the scalenus anterior muscle.
- **Medially:** Related to the vertebral artery and vein and the sympathetic trunk (Fig. 11-57). On the left side, the medial border is related to the thoracic duct.
- **Laterally:** Related to the emerging branches of the cervical plexus, the roots of the brachial plexus, and the third part of the subclavian artery (Fig. 11-57)

The origin, insertion, nerve supply, and action of the scalenus anterior muscle are summarized in Table 11-5.

Deep Cervical Fascia

The deep cervical fascia supports the muscles, the vessels, and the viscera of the neck (Fig. 11-49). In certain areas, it is condensed to form well-defined, fibrous sheets called the investing layer, the pretracheal layer, and the prevertebral layer. It is also condensed to form the carotid sheath (Fig. 11-49).

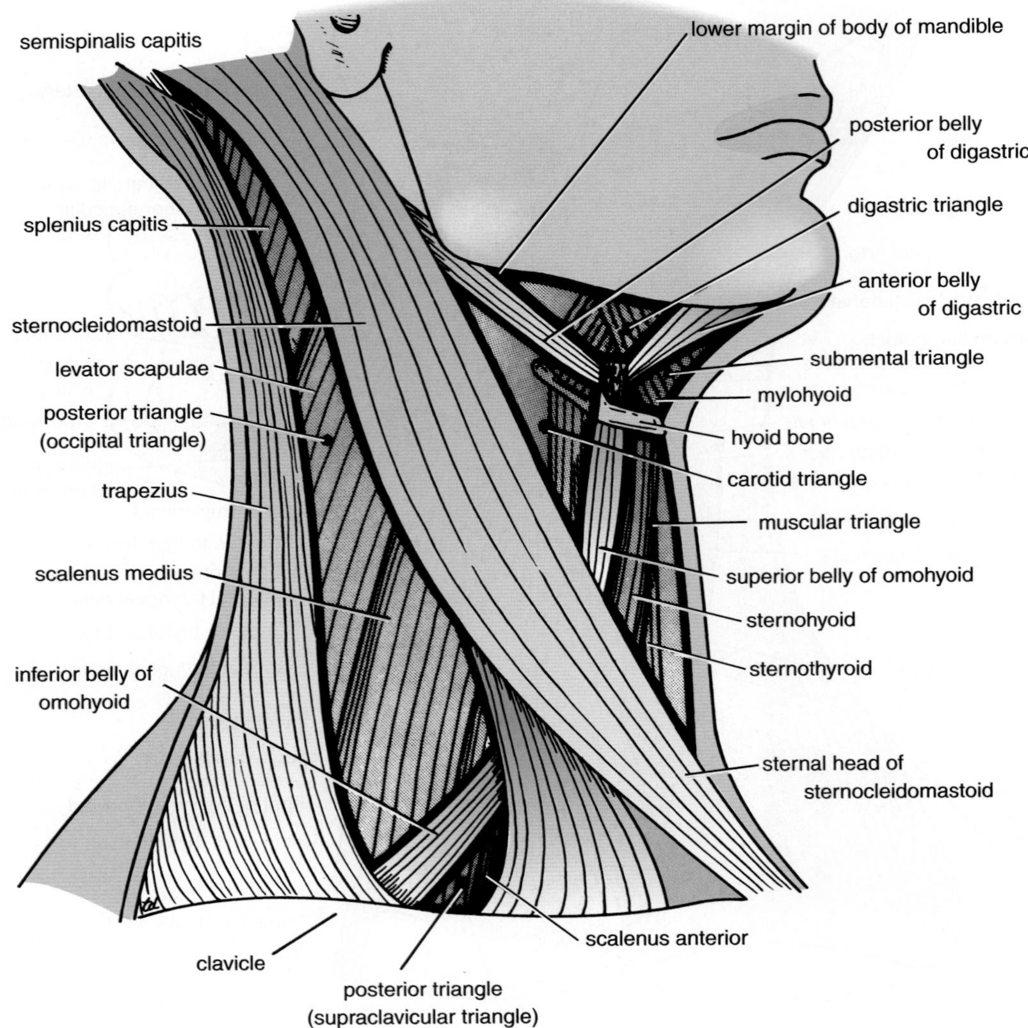

Figure 11-56 Muscular triangles of the neck.

Investing Layer

The investing layer is a thick layer that encircles the neck. It splits to enclose the trapezius and the sternocleidomastoid muscles (Fig. 11-49).

Pretracheal Layer

The pretracheal layer is a thin layer that is attached above to the laryngeal cartilages (Fig. 11-49). It surrounds the thyroid and the parathyroid glands, forming a sheath for them, and encloses the infrahyoid muscles.

Prevertebral Layer

The prevertebral layer is a thick layer that passes like a septum across the neck behind the pharynx and the esophagus and in front of the prevertebral muscles and the vertebral column (Fig. 11-49). It forms the fascial floor of the posterior triangle, and it extends laterally over the first rib into the axilla to form the important **axillary sheath** (see page 747).

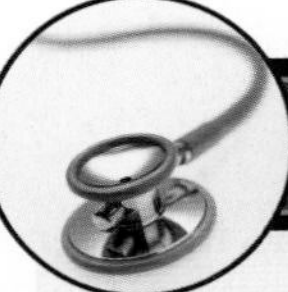

CLINICAL NOTES

Clinical Significance of the Deep Fascia of the Neck

As previously described, the deep fascia in certain areas forms distinct sheets called the investing, pretracheal, and prevertebral layers. These fascial layers are easily recognizable to the surgeon at operation.

Fascial Spaces

Between the more dense layers of deep fascia in the neck is loose connective tissue that forms potential spaces that are clinically important. Among the more important spaces are the visceral, retropharyngeal, submandibular, and masticatory spaces (Fig. 11-58).

(continues)

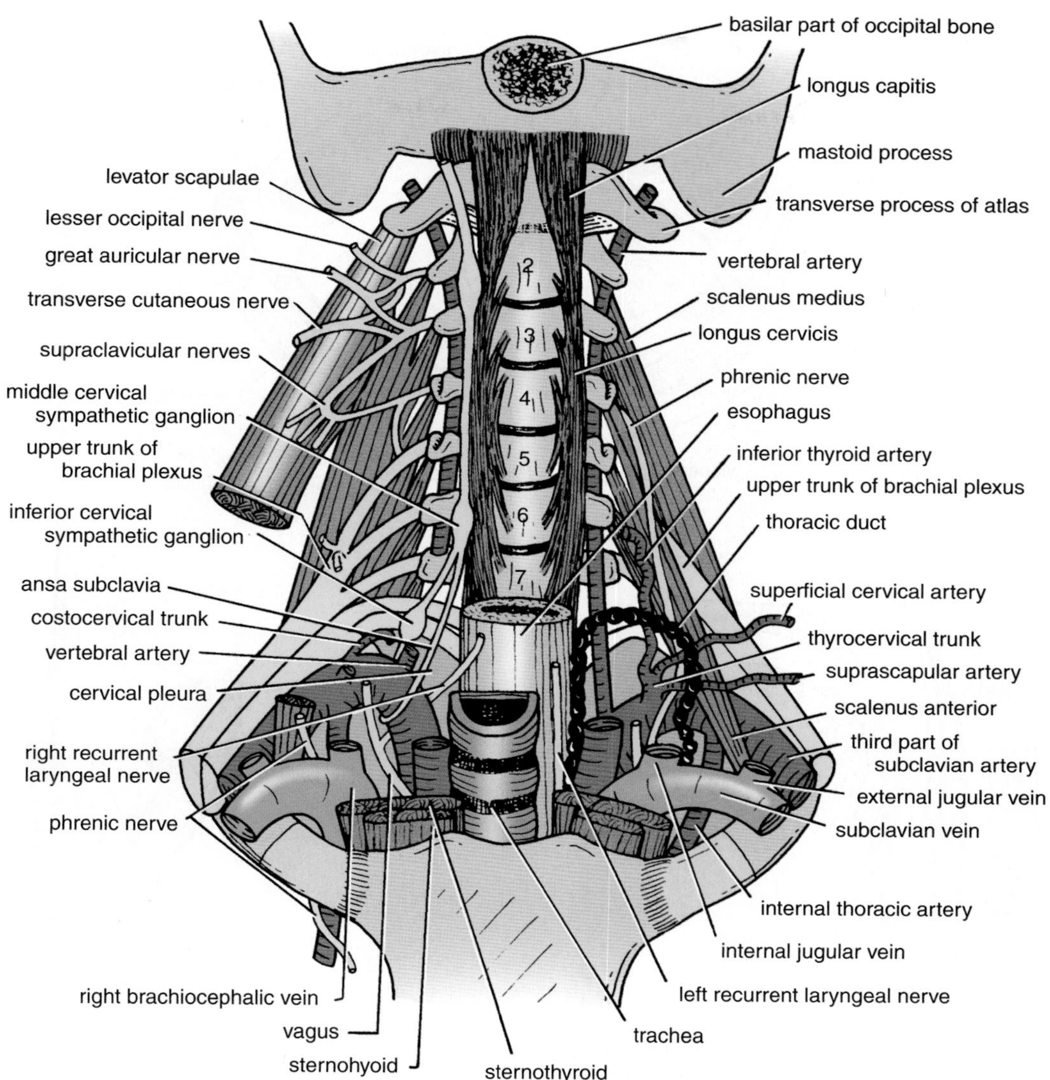

Figure 11-57 Prevertebral region and the root of the neck.

Clinical Notes, *continued*

The deep fascia and the fascial spaces are important because organisms originating in the mouth, teeth, pharynx, and esophagus can spread among the fascial planes and spaces, and the tough fascia can determine the direction of spread of infection and the path taken by pus. It is possible for blood, pus, or air in the retropharyngeal space to spread downward into the superior mediastinum of the thorax.

Acute Infections of the Fascial Spaces of the Neck

Dental infections most commonly involve the lower molar teeth. The infection spreads medially from the mandible into the submandibular and masticatory spaces and pushes the tongue forward and upward. Further spread downward may involve the visceral space and lead to edema of the vocal cords and airway obstruction.

Ludwig's angina is an acute infection of the submandibular fascial space and is commonly secondary to dental infection.

Chronic Infection of the Fascial Spaces of the Neck

Tuberculous infection of the deep cervical lymph nodes can result in liquefaction and destruction of one or more of the nodes. The pus is at first limited by the investing layer of the deep fascia. Later, this becomes eroded at one point, and the pus passes into the less restricted superficial fascia. A dumbbell or collar-stud abscess is now present. The clinician is aware of the superficial abscess but must not forget the existence of the deeply placed abscess.

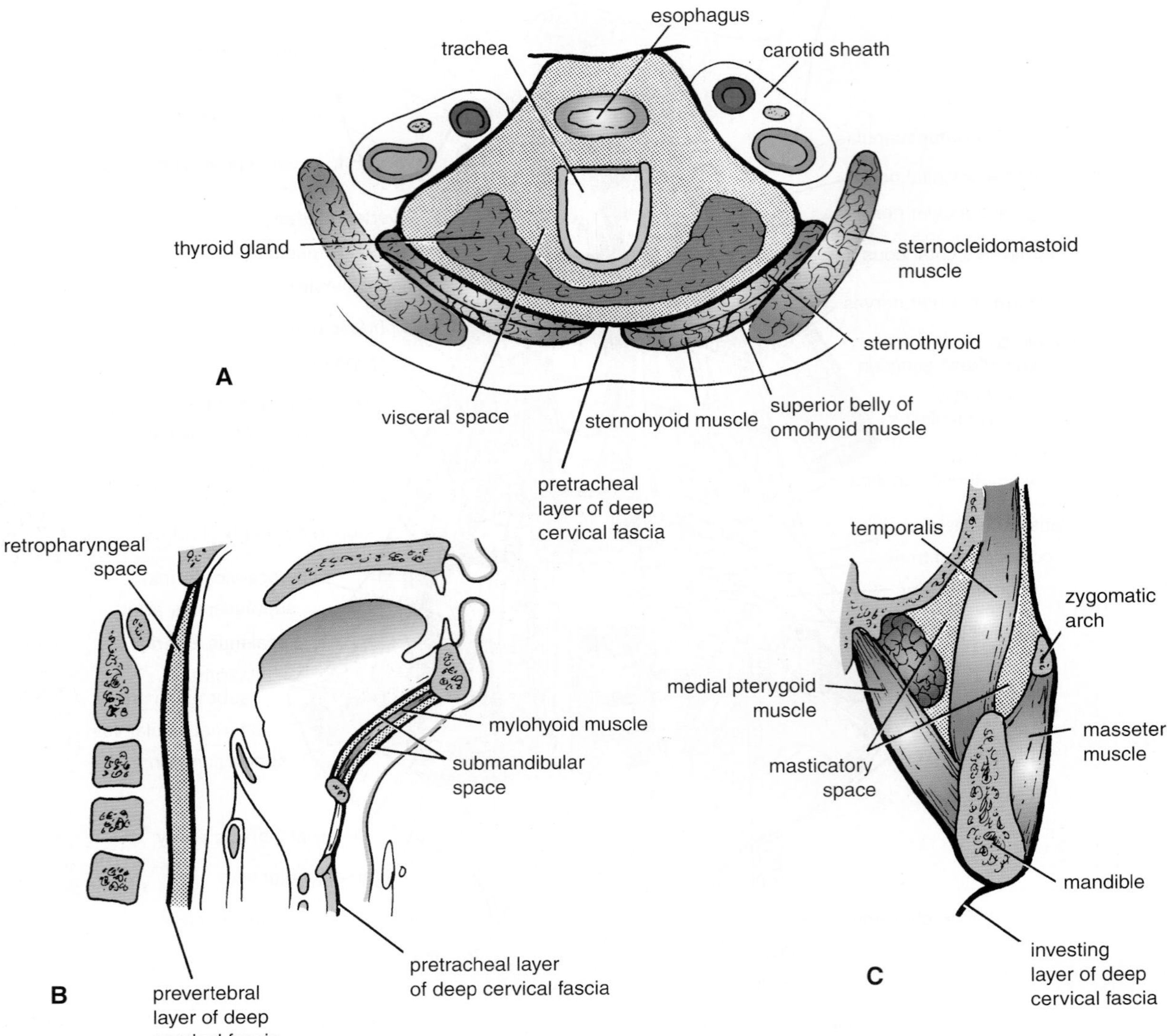

Figure 11-58 **A.** Cross section of the neck showing the visceral space. **B.** Sagittal section of the neck showing the positions of the retropharyngeal and submandibular spaces. **C.** Vertical section of the body of the mandible close to the angle showing the masticatory space.

Carotid Sheath

The carotid sheath is a local condensation of the prevertebral, the pretracheal, and the investing layers of the deep fascia that surround the common and internal carotid arteries, the internal jugular vein, the vagus nerve, and the deep cervical lymph nodes (Fig. 11-49).

Axillary Sheath

All the anterior rami of the cervical nerves that emerge in the interval between the scalenus anterior and scalenus medius muscles lie at first deep to the prevertebral fascia. As the subclavian artery and the brachial plexus emerge in the interval between the scalenus anterior and the scalenus medius muscles, they carry with them a sheath of the fascia, which extends into the axilla and is called the axillary sheath.

Cervical Ligaments

Stylohyoid ligament: Connects the styloid process to the lesser cornu of the hyoid bone (Fig. 11- 80)

Stylomandibular ligament: Connects the styloid process to the angle of the mandible (Fig. 11-33)

Sphenomandibular ligament: Connects the spine of the sphenoid bone to the lingula of the mandible (Fig. 11-33)

Pterygomandibular ligament: Connects the hamular process of the medial pterygoid plate to the posterior end of the mylohyoid line of the mandible. It gives attachment to the superior constrictor and the buccinator muscles (Fig. 11-80).

Muscular Triangles of the Neck

The sternocleidomastoid muscle divides the neck into the anterior and the posterior triangles (Fig. 11-56).

Anterior Triangle

The anterior triangle is bounded above by the body of the mandible, posteriorly by the sternocleidomastoid muscle, and anteriorly by the midline (Fig. 11-56). It is further subdivided into the **carotid triangle,** the **digastric triangle,** the **submental triangle,** and the **muscular triangle** (Fig. 11-56).

Posterior Triangle

The posterior triangle is bounded posteriorly by the trapezius muscle, anteriorly by the sternocleidomastoid muscle, and inferiorly by the clavicle (Fig. 11-56). The posterior triangle of the neck is further subdivided by the **inferior belly of the omohyoid muscle** into a large **occipital triangle** above and a small **supraclavicular triangle** below (Fig. 11-56).

The suprahyoid and infrahyoid muscles and the anterior and lateral vertebral muscles are described in Table 11-5.

Arteries of the Head and Neck

Common Carotid Artery

The right common carotid artery arises from the brachiocephalic artery behind the right sternoclavicular joint (Figs. 11-57 and 11-59). The left artery arises from the arch of the aorta in the superior mediastinum (see page 125). The common carotid artery runs upward through the neck under cover of the anterior border of the sternocleidomastoid muscle, from the sternoclavicular joint to the upper border of the thyroid cartilage. Here it divides into the external and internal carotid arteries (Figs. 11-55 and 11-60).

Carotid Sinus

At its point of division, the terminal part of the common carotid artery or the beginning of the internal carotid artery shows a localized dilatation, called the carotid sinus (Fig. 11-60). The tunica media of the sinus is thinner than elsewhere, but the adventitia is relatively thick and contains numerous nerve endings derived from the glossopharyngeal nerve. The carotid sinus serves as a reflex pressoreceptor mechanism: A rise in blood pressure causes a slowing of the heart rate and vasodilatation of the arterioles.

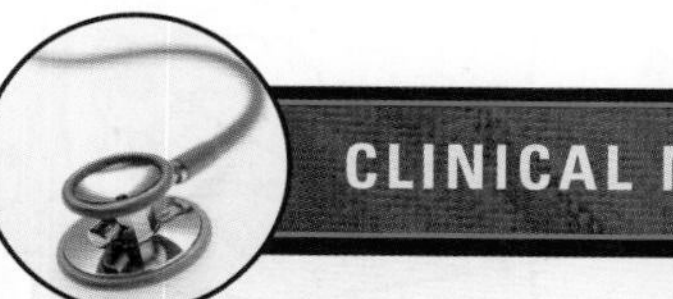

CLINICAL NOTES

Carotid Sinus Hypersensitivity

In cases of carotid sinus hypersensitivity, pressure on one or both carotid sinuses can cause excessive slowing of the heart rate, a fall in blood pressure, and cerebral ischemia with fainting.

Carotid Body

The carotid body is a small structure that lies posterior to the point of bifurcation of the common carotid artery (Fig. 11-60). It is innervated by the glossopharyngeal nerve. The carotid body is a chemoreceptor, being sensitive to excess carbon dioxide and reduced oxygen tension in the blood. Such a stimulus reflexly produces a rise in blood pressure and heart rate and an increase in respiratory movements.

The common carotid artery is embedded in a connective tissue sheath, called the carotid sheath, throughout its course and is closely related to the internal jugular vein and vagus nerve (Fig. 11-49).

Relations of the Common Carotid Artery

- **Anterolaterally:** The skin, the fascia, the sternocleidomastoid, the sternohyoid, the sternothyroid, and the superior belly of the omohyoid (Fig. 11-55)
- **Posteriorly:** The transverse processes of the lower four cervical vertebrae, the prevertebral muscles, and the sympathetic trunk (Fig. 11-57). In the lower part of the neck are the vertebral vessels.
- **Medially:** The larynx and pharynx and, below these, the trachea and esophagus (Fig. 11-49). The lobe of the thyroid gland also lies medially.
- **Laterally:** The internal jugular vein and, posterolaterally, the vagus nerve (Fig. 11-49)

Branches of the Common Carotid Artery

Apart from the two terminal branches, the common carotid artery gives off no branches.

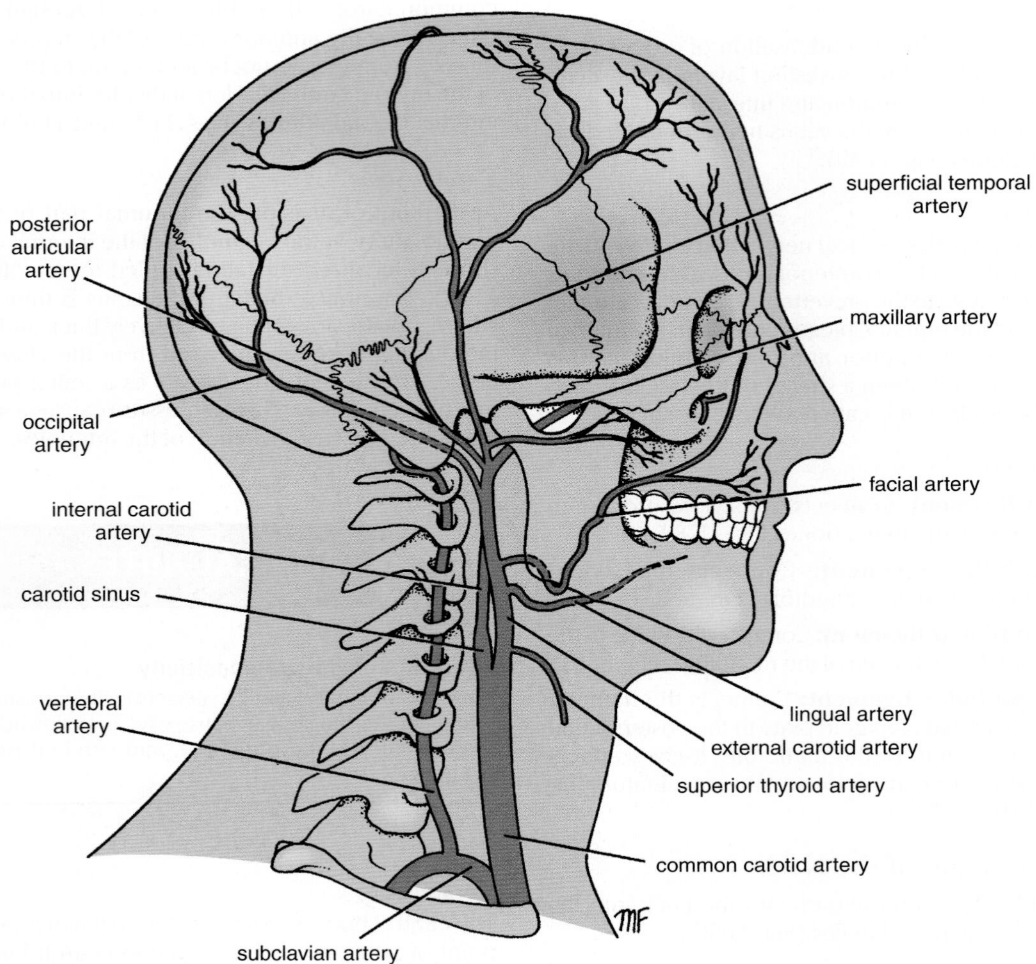

Figure 11-59 Main arteries of the head and neck. Note that for clarity the thyrocervical trunk, the costocervical trunk, and the internal thoracic artery—branches of the subclavian artery—are not shown.

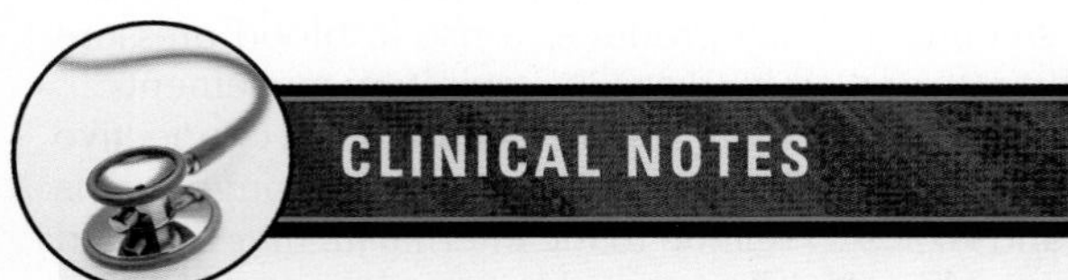

Taking the Carotid Pulse

The bifurcation of the common carotid artery into the internal and external carotid arteries can be easily palpated just beneath the anterior border of the sternocleidomastoid muscle at the level of the superior border of the thyroid cartilage. This is a convenient site to take the carotid pulse.

External Carotid Artery

The external carotid artery is one of the terminal branches of the common carotid artery (Fig. 11-59). It supplies structures in the neck, face, and scalp; it also supplies the tongue and the maxilla. The artery begins at the level of the upper border of the thyroid cartilage and terminates in the substance of the parotid gland behind the neck of the mandible by dividing into the superficial temporal and maxillary arteries.

Close to its origin, the artery emerges from undercover of the sternocleidomastoid muscle, where its pulsations can be felt. At first, it lies medial to the internal carotid artery, but as it ascends in the neck, it passes backward and lateral to it. It is crossed by the posterior belly of the digastric and the stylohyoid (Fig. 11-55).

Relations of the External Carotid Artery

- **Anterolaterally:** The artery is overlapped at its beginning by the anterior border of the sternocleidomastoid. Above this level, the artery is comparatively superficial, being covered by skin and fascia. It is crossed by the hypoglossal nerve (Fig. 11-55), the posterior belly of the digastric muscle, and the stylohyoid muscles. Within the parotid gland, it is crossed by the facial nerve (Fig. 11-85). The internal jugular vein first lies lateral to the artery and then posterior to it.
- **Medially:** The wall of the pharynx and the internal carotid artery. The stylopharyngeus muscle, the glossopharyngeal nerve, and the pharyngeal branch of the vagus pass between the external and internal carotid arteries (Fig. 11-60).

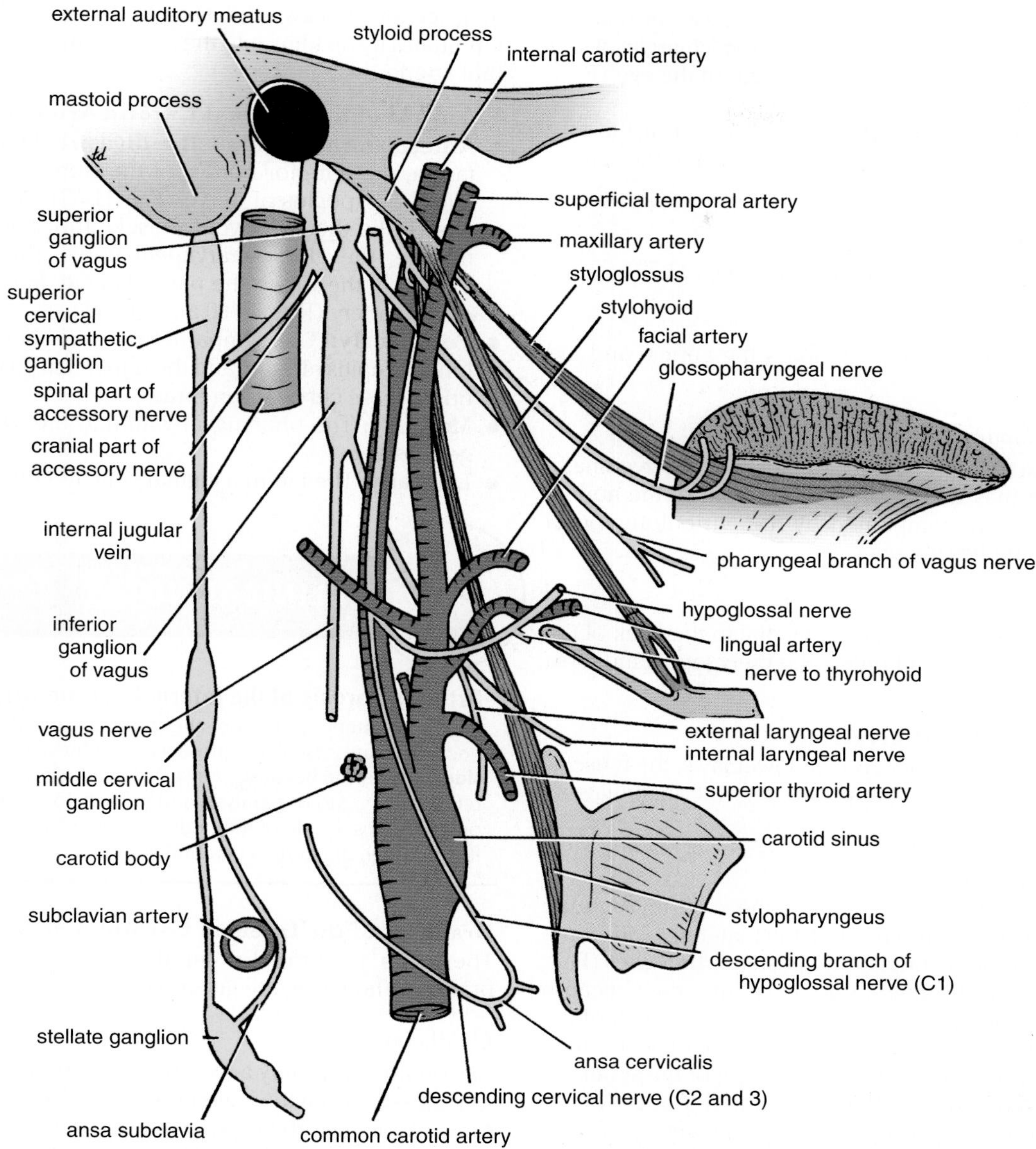

Figure 11-60 Styloid muscles, vessels, and nerves of the neck.

For the relations of the external carotid artery in the parotid gland, see Figure 11-85B.

Branches of the External Carotid Artery

- Superior thyroid artery
- Ascending pharyngeal artery
- Lingual artery
- Facial artery
- Occipital artery
- Posterior auricular artery
- Superficial temporal artery
- Maxillary artery

Superior Thyroid Artery

The superior thyroid artery curves downward to the upper pole of the thyroid gland (Figs. 11-55 and 11-60). It is accompanied by the external laryngeal nerve, which supplies the cricothyroid muscle.

Ascending Pharyngeal Artery

The ascending pharyngeal artery ascends along and supplies the pharyngeal wall.

Lingual Artery

The lingual artery loops upward and forward and supplies the tongue (Figs. 11-55 and 11-60).

Facial Artery

The facial artery loops upward close to the outer surface of the pharynx and the tonsil. It lies deep to the submandibular salivary gland and emerges and bends around the lower border of the mandible. It then ascends over the face close to the anterior border of the masseter muscle. The artery then ascends around the lateral margin of the mouth and terminates at the medial angle of the eye (Figs. 11-55 and 11-59).

Branches of the facial artery supply the tonsil, the submandibular salivary gland, and the muscles and the skin of the face.

Occipital Artery

The artery supplies the back of the scalp (Fig. 11-59).

Posterior Auricular Artery

The posterior auricular artery supplies the auricle and the scalp (Fig. 11-59).

Superficial Temporal Artery

The superficial temporal artery ascends over the zygomatic arch, where it may be palpated just in front of the auricle (Fig. 11-59). It is accompanied by the auriculotemporal nerve, and it supplies the scalp.

Maxillary Artery

The maxillary artery runs forward medial to the neck of the mandible (Fig. 11-59) and enters the pterygopalatine fossa of the skull.

Branches of the Maxillary Artery

Branches supply the upper and the lower jaws, the muscles of mastication, the nose, the palate, and the meninges inside the skull.

Middle Meningeal Artery

The middle meningeal artery enters the skull through the foramen spinosum (Fig. 11-66). It runs laterally within the skull and divides into anterior and posterior branches (Figs. 11-20 and 11-131). The anterior branch is important because it lies close to the motor area of the cerebral cortex of the brain. Accompanied by its vein, it grooves (or tunnels) through the upper part of the greater wing of the sphenoid bone of the skull and the thin anteroinferior angle of the parietal bone, where it is prone to damage after a blow to the head.

The origin and distribution of the branches of the external carotid artery are shown in Figure 11-59.

Internal Carotid Artery

The internal carotid artery begins at the bifurcation of the common carotid artery at the level of the upper border of the thyroid cartilage (Figs. 11-55 and 11-59). It supplies the brain, the eye, the forehead, and part of the nose. The artery ascends in the neck embedded in the carotid sheath with the internal jugular vein and vagus nerve. At first it lies superficially; it then passes deep to the parotid salivary gland (Figs. 11-60 and 11-85B).

The internal carotid artery leaves the neck by passing into the cranial cavity through the carotid canal in the petrous part of the temporal bone. It then passes upward and forward in the cavernous venous sinus (without communicating with it). The artery then leaves the sinus and passes upward again medial to the anterior clinoid process of the sphenoid bone. The internal carotid artery then inclines backward, lateral to the optic chiasma, and terminates by dividing into the anterior and the middle cerebral arteries.

Relations of the Internal Carotid Artery in the Neck

- **Anterolaterally: Below the digastric** lie the skin, the fascia, the anterior border of the sternocleidomastoid, and the hypoglossal nerve (Fig. 11-55). **Above the digastric** lie the stylohyoid muscle, the stylopharyngeus muscle, the glossopharyngeal nerve, the pharyngeal branch of the vagus, the parotid gland, and the external carotid artery (Figs. 11-60 and 11-85B).
- **Posteriorly:** The sympathetic trunk (Fig. 11-60), the longus capitis muscle, and the transverse processes of the upper three cervical vertebrae
- **Medially:** The pharyngeal wall and the superior laryngeal nerve
- **Laterally:** The internal jugular vein and the vagus nerve

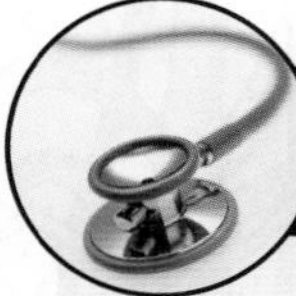

CLINICAL NOTES

Arteriosclerosis of the Internal Carotid Artery

Extensive arteriosclerosis of the internal carotid artery in the neck can cause visual impairment or blindness in the eye on the side of the lesion because of insufficient blood flow through the retinal artery. Motor paralysis and sensory loss may also occur on the opposite side of the body because of insufficient blood flow through the middle cerebral artery.

Branches of the Internal Carotid Artery

There are no branches in the neck. Many important branches, however, are given off in the skull.

Ophthalmic Artery

The ophthalmic artery arises from the internal carotid artery as it emerges from the cavernous sinus (Fig. 11-20). It passes forward into the orbital cavity through the optic canal, and it gives off the central artery of the retina, which enters the optic nerve and runs forward to enter the eyeball. The central artery is an end artery and the only blood supply to the retina.

Posterior Communicating Artery

The posterior communicating artery runs backward to join the posterior cerebral artery (Fig. 11-15).

Anterior Cerebral Artery

The anterior cerebral artery is a terminal branch of the internal carotid artery (Fig. 11-15). It passes forward between the cerebral hemispheres and then winds around the corpus callosum of the brain to supply the medial and the superolateral surfaces of the cerebral hemisphere. It is joined to the artery of the opposite side by the **anterior communicating artery.**

Middle Cerebral Artery

The middle cerebral artery is the largest terminal branch of the internal carotid artery (Fig. 11-15), and it runs laterally in the lateral cerebral sulcus of the brain. It supplies the entire lateral surface of the cerebral hemisphere except the narrow strip along the superolateral margin (which is supplied by the anterior cerebral artery) and the occipital pole and inferolateral surface of the hemisphere (both of which are supplied by the posterior cerebral artery). The middle cerebral artery thus supplies all the motor area of the cerebral cortex except the leg area. It also gives off central branches that supply central masses of gray matter and the internal capsule of the brain.

Circle of Willis

The circle of Willis lies in the subarachnoid space (see page 683) at the base of the brain. It is formed by the anastomosis between the branches of the two internal carotid arteries and the two vertebral arteries (Fig. 11-15). The anterior communicating, posterior cerebral, and basilar (formed by the junction of the two vertebral arteries) are all arteries that contribute to the circle. Cortical and central branches arise from the circle and supply the brain.

Subclavian Arteries

Right Subclavian Artery

The right subclavian artery arises from the brachiocephalic artery, behind the right sternoclavicular joint (Figs. 11-57 and 11-59). It arches upward and laterally over the pleura and between the scalenus anterior and medius muscles. At the outer border of the first rib, it becomes the axillary artery.

Left Subclavian Artery

The left subclavian artery arises from the arch of the aorta in the thorax. It ascends to the root of the neck and then arches laterally in a manner similar to that of the right subclavian artery (Fig. 11-57).

The scalenus anterior muscle passes anterior to the artery on each side and divides it into three parts.

First Part of the Subclavian Artery

The first part of the subclavian artery extends from the origin of the subclavian artery to the medial border of the scalenus anterior muscle (Fig. 11-57). This part gives off the vertebral artery, the thyrocervical trunk, and the internal thoracic artery.

Branches The **vertebral artery** ascends in the neck through the foramina in the transverse processes of the upper six cervical vertebrae (Fig. 11-57). It passes medially above the posterior arch of the atlas and then ascends through the foramen magnum into the skull. On reaching the anterior surface of the medulla oblongata of the brain at the level of the lower border of the pons, it joins the vessel of the opposite side to form the basilar artery.

The **basilar artery** (Fig. 11-15) ascends in a groove on the anterior surface of the pons. It gives off branches to the pons, the cerebellum, and the internal ear. It finally divides into the two posterior cerebral arteries.

On each side, the **posterior cerebral artery** (Fig. 11-15) curves laterally and backward around the midbrain. Cortical branches supply the inferolateral surfaces of the temporal lobe and the visual cortex on the lateral and the medial surfaces of the occipital lobe.

Branches in the neck: Spinal and muscular arteries

Branches in the skull: Meningeal, anterior and posterior spinal, posterior inferior cerebellar, medullary arteries

The **thyrocervical trunk** is a short trunk that gives off three terminal branches (Fig. 11-57).

The **inferior thyroid artery** ascends to the posterior surface of the thyroid gland, where it is closely related to the recurrent laryngeal nerve. It supplies the thyroid and the inferior parathyroid glands.

The **superficial cervical artery** is a small branch that crosses the brachial plexus (Fig. 11-57).

The **suprascapular artery** runs laterally over the brachial plexus and follows the suprascapular nerve onto the back of the scapula (Fig. 11-57).

The **internal thoracic artery** descends into the thorax behind the first costal cartilage and in front of the pleura (Fig. 11-57). It descends vertically one fingerbreadth lateral to the sternum; in the sixth intercostal space, it divides into the superior epigastric and the musculophrenic arteries.

Second Part of the Subclavian Artery

The second part of the subclavian artery lies behind the scalenus anterior muscle (Fig. 11-57).

Branches The **costocervical trunk** runs backward over the dome of the pleura and divides into the **superior intercostal artery,** which supplies the first and the second intercostal spaces, and the **deep cervical artery,** which supplies the deep muscles of the neck.

Third Part of the Subclavian Artery

The third part of the subclavian artery extends from the lateral border of the scalenus anterior muscle (Fig. 11-57) across the posterior triangle of the neck to the lateral border of the first rib, where it becomes the axillary artery. Here, in the root of the neck, it is closely related to the nerves of the brachial plexus.

Branches The third part of the subclavian artery usually has no branches. Occasionally, however, the superficial cervical arteries, the suprascapular arteries, or both arise from this part.

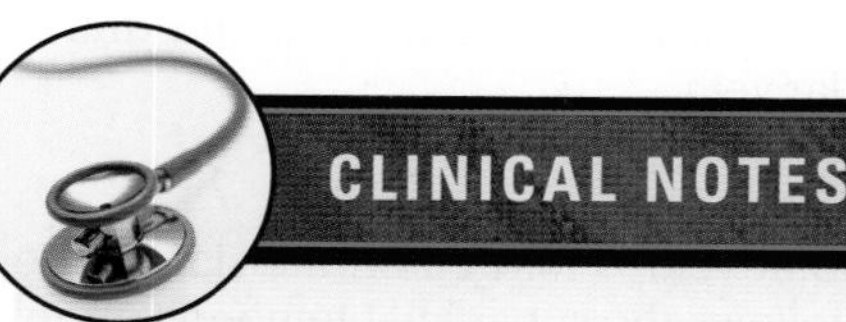

Palpation and Compression of the Subclavian Artery in Patients With Upper Limb Hemorrhage

In severe traumatic accidents to the upper limb involving laceration of the brachial or axillary arteries, it is important to remember that the hemorrhage can be stopped by exerting strong pressure downward and backward on the third part of the subclavian artery. The use of a blunt object to exert the pressure is of great help, and the artery is compressed against the upper surface of the first rib.

Veins of the Head and Neck

The veins of the head and neck may be divided into:

- The veins of the brain, venous sinuses, diploic veins, and emissary veins
- The veins of the scalp, face, and neck

Veins of the Brain

The veins of the brain are thin walled and have no valves. They consist of the cerebral veins, the cerebellar veins, and the veins of the brainstem, all of which drain into the neighboring venous sinuses.

Venous Sinuses

The venous sinuses are situated between the periosteal and the meningeal layer of the dura mater (Fig. 11-37A; see also page 686). They have thick, fibrous walls, but they possess no valves. They receive tributaries from the brain, the skull bones, the orbit, and the internal ear. The venous sinuses include the superior and inferior sagittal sinuses, the straight sinus, the transverse sinuses, the sigmoid sinuses, the occipital sinus, the cavernous sinuses, and the superior and inferior petrosal sinuses (Fig. 11-9). All these sinuses are described on page 686 and 687.

Diploic Veins

The diploic veins occupy channels within the bones of the vault of the skull (Fig. 11-9).

Emissary Veins

The emissary veins are valveless veins that pass through the skull bones (Fig. 11-9). They connect the veins of the scalp to the venous sinuses (and are an important route for the spread of infection).

Veins of the Face and the Neck

Facial Vein

The facial vein is formed at the medial angle of the eye by the union of the supraorbital and **supratrochlear veins** (Fig. 11-39). It is connected through the ophthalmic veins with the cavernous sinus. The facial vein descends down the face with the facial artery and passes around the lateral side of the mouth. It then crosses the mandible, is joined by the anterior division of the retromandibular vein, and drains into the internal jugular vein.

Superficial Temporal Vein

The superficial temporal vein is formed on the side of the scalp (Fig. 11-39). It follows the superficial temporal artery and the auriculotemporal nerve and then enters the parotid salivary gland, where it joins the maxillary vein to form the retromandibular vein.

Maxillary Vein

The maxillary vein is formed in the infratemporal fossa from the pterygoid venous plexus (Fig. 11-39). The maxillary vein joins the superficial temporal vein to form the retromandibular vein.

Retromandibular Vein

The retromandibular vein is formed by the union of the superficial temporal and the maxillary veins (Fig. 11-39). On leaving the parotid salivary gland, it divides into an anterior branch, which joins the facial vein, and a posterior branch, which joins the posterior auricular vein to form the external jugular vein.

External Jugular Vein

The external jugular vein is formed behind the angle of the jaw by the union of the posterior auricular vein with the posterior division of the retromandibular vein (Fig. 11-39). It descends across the sternocleidomastoid muscle and beneath the platysma muscle, and it drains into the subclavian vein behind the middle of the clavicle.

Tributaries

Posterior external jugular vein from the back of the scalp

Transverse cervical vein from the skin and the fascia over the posterior triangle

Suprascapular vein from the back of the scapula

Anterior jugular vein

Anterior Jugular Vein

The anterior jugular vein descends in the front of the neck close to the midline (Fig. 11-39). Just above the sternum, it is joined to the opposite vein by the jugular arch. The anterior jugular vein joins the external jugular vein deep to the sternocleidomastoid muscle.

Internal Jugular Vein

The internal jugular vein is a large vein that receives blood from the brain, face, and neck (Fig. 11-39). It starts as a continuation of the sigmoid sinus and leaves the skull through the jugular foramen. It then descends through the neck in the carotid sheath lateral to the vagus nerve and the internal and common carotid arteries. It ends by joining the subclavian vein behind the medial end of the clavicle to form the brachiocephalic vein (Figs. 11-39 and 11-57). Throughout its course, it is closely related to the **deep cervical lymph nodes.**

The vein has a dilatation at its upper end called the **superior bulb** and another near its termination called the **inferior bulb.** Directly above the inferior bulb is a bicuspid valve.

Relations of the Internal Jugular Vein

- **Anterolaterally:** The skin, the fascia, the sternocleidomastoid, and the parotid salivary gland. Its lower part is covered by the sternothyroid, sternohyoid, and omohyoid muscles, which intervene between the vein and the sternocleidomastoid (Fig. 11-55). Higher up, it is crossed by the stylohyoid, the posterior belly of the digastric, and the spinal part of the accessory nerve. The chain of deep cervical lymph nodes runs alongside the vein.
- **Posteriorly:** The transverse processes of the cervical vertebrae, the levator scapulae, the scalenus medius, the scalenus anterior, the cervical plexus, the phrenic nerve,

the thyrocervical trunk, the vertebral vein, and the first part of the subclavian artery (Fig. 11-57). On the left side it passes in front of the thoracic duct.

- **Medially:** Above lie the internal carotid artery and the 9th, 10th, 11th, and 12th cranial nerves. Below lie the common carotid artery and the vagus nerve.

Tributaries of the Internal Jugular Vein

- **Inferior petrosal sinus** (Fig. 11-30)
- **Facial vein** (Fig. 11-39)
- **Pharyngeal veins**
- **Lingual vein**
- **Superior thyroid vein** (Fig. 11-55)
- **Middle thyroid vein** (Fig. 11-110)

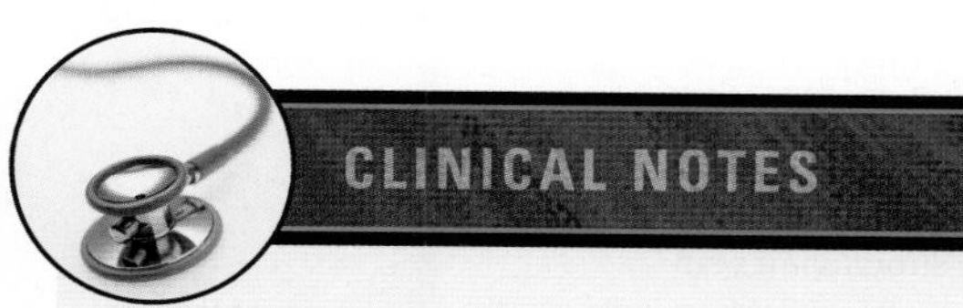

CLINICAL NOTES

Penetrating Wounds of the Internal Jugular Vein

The hemorrhage of low-pressure venous blood into the loose connective tissue beneath the investing layer of deep cervical fascia may present as a large, slowly expanding hematoma. Air embolism is a serious complication of a lacerated wall of the internal jugular vein. Because the wall of this large vein contains little smooth muscle, its injury is not followed by contraction and retraction (as occurs with arterial injuries). Moreover, the adventitia of the vein wall is attached to the deep fascia of the carotid sheath, which hinders the collapse of the vein. Blind clamping of the vein is prohibited because the vagus and hypoglossal nerves are in the vicinity.

(continues)

Clinical Notes, *continued*

Internal Jugular Vein Catheterization

The internal jugular vein is remarkably constant in position. It descends through the neck from a point halfway between the tip of the mastoid process and the angle of the jaw to the sternoclavicular joint. Above, it is overlapped by the anterior border of the sternocleidomastoid muscle, and below, it is covered laterally by this muscle. Just above the sternoclavicular joint the vein lies beneath a skin depression between the sternal and clavicular heads of the sternocleidomastoid muscle. In the posterior approach, the tip of the needle and the catheter are introduced into the vein about two fingerbreadths above the clavicle at the posterior border of the sternocleidomastoid muscle (Fig. 11-61). In the anterior approach, with the patient's head turned to the opposite side, the triangle formed by the sternal and clavicular heads of the sternocleidomastoid muscle and the medial end of the clavicle are identified. A shallow skin depression usually overlies the triangle. The needle and catheter are inserted into the vein at the apex of the triangle in a caudal direction (Fig. 11-61).

Subclavian Vein

The subclavian vein is a continuation of the axillary vein at the outer border of the first rib (Fig. 11-57). It joins the internal jugular vein to form the brachiocephalic vein, and it receives the external jugular vein. In addition, it often receives the thoracic duct on the left side and the right lymphatic duct on the right.

Relations

- **Anteriorly:** The clavicle
- **Posteriorly:** The scalenus anterior muscle and the phrenic nerve
- **Inferiorly:** The upper surface of the first rib

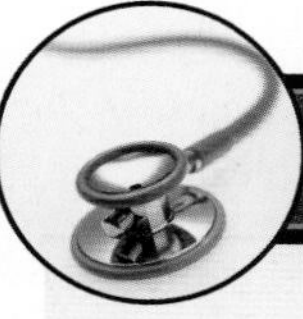

CLINICAL NOTES

Subclavian Vein Thrombosis

Spontaneous thrombosis of the subclavian and/or axillary veins occasionally occurs after excessive and unaccustomed use of the arm at the shoulder joint. The close relationship of these veins to the first rib and the clavicle and the possibility of repeated minor trauma from these structures is probably a factor in its development.

Secondary thrombosis of subclavian and/or axillary veins is a common complication of an indwelling venous catheter. Rarely, the condition may follow a radical mastectomy with a block dissection of the lymph nodes of the axilla. Persistent pain, heaviness, or edema of the upper limb, especially after exercise, is a complication of this condition.

Anatomy of Subclavian Vein Catheterization

The subclavian vein is located in the lower anterior corner of the posterior triangle of the neck (Fig. 11-62), where it lies immediately posterior to the medial third of the clavicle.

Infraclavicular Approach

Since the subclavian vein lies close to the undersurface of the medial third of the clavicle (Fig. 11-62), this is a relatively safe site for catheterization. The vein is slightly more medially placed on the left side than on the right side.

Anatomy of Procedure

The needle should be inserted through the skin just below the lower border of the clavicle at the junction of the medial third and outer two thirds, coinciding with the posterior border of the origin of the clavicular head of the sternocleidomastoid muscle on the upper border of the clavicle (Fig. 11-62). The needle pierces the following structures:

- Skin
- Superficial fascia
- Pectoralis major muscle (clavicular head)
- Clavipectoral fascia and subclavius muscle
- Wall of subclavian vein

(continues)

Clinical Notes, *continued*

The needle is pointed upward and posteriorly toward the middle of the suprasternal notch.

Anatomy of Problems

- **Hitting the clavicle:** The needle may be "walked" along the lower surface of the clavicle until its posterior edge is reached.
- **Hitting the first rib:** The needle may hit the first rib, if the needle is pointed downward and not upward.
- **Hitting the subclavian artery:** A pulsatile resistance and bright red blood flow indicate that the needle has passed posterior to the scalenus anterior muscle and perforated the subclavian artery.

Anatomy of Complications

Refer to Figure 11-62.

- **Pneumothorax:** The needle may pierce the cervical dome of the pleura, permitting air to enter the pleural cavity. This complication is more common in children, in whom the pleural reflection is higher than in adults.
- **Hemothorax:** The catheter may pierce the posterior wall of the subclavian vein and the pleura.
- **Subclavian artery puncture:** The needle pierces the wall of the artery during its insertion.
- **Internal thoracic artery injury:** Hemorrhage may occur into the superior mediastinum.
- **Diaphragmatic paralysis:** This occurs when the needle damages the phrenic nerve.

The Procedure in Children

The needle pierces the skin in the deltopectoral groove about 2 cm from the clavicle. The catheter is tunneled beneath the skin to enter the subclavian vein at the point where the clavicle and the first rib cross. The more oblique approach in children minimizes the possibility of entering the subclavian artery.

Supraclavicular Approach

This approach (Fig. 11-62) is preferred by many for the following anatomic reasons.

- The site of penetration of the vein wall is larger, since it lies at the junction of the internal jugular vein and the subclavian vein, which makes the procedure easier.
- The needle is pointed downward and medially toward the mediastinum, away from the pleura, avoiding the complication of pneumothorax.
- The catheter is inserted along a more direct course into the brachiocephalic vein and superior vena cava.

Anatomy of the Procedure

With the patient in the Trendelenburg position (patient supine with head tilted downward) or simple supine position and the head turned to the opposite side, the posterior border of the clavicular origin of sternocleidomastoid muscle is palpated (Fig. 11-62). The needle is inserted through the skin at the site where the posterior border of the clavicular origin of sternocleidomastoid is attached to the upper border of the clavicle. At this point, the needle lies lateral to the lateral border of scalenus anterior muscle and above the first rib. The needle pierces the following structures (Fig. 11-62):

- Skin
- Superficial fascia and platysma
- Investing layer of deep cervical fascia
- Wall of the subclavian vein

The needle is directed downward in the direction of the opposite nipple. The needle enters the junction of the internal jugular vein and the subclavian vein. It is important that the operator understands that the pleura is not being penetrated and that it is possible for the needle to lie in a zone between the chest wall and the cervical dome of the parietal pleura but outside the pleural space (cavity).

Anatomic Complications

The following complications may occur as the result of damage to neighboring anatomic structures (Fig. 11-62):

- **Paralysis of the diaphragm:** This is caused by injury to the phrenic nerve as it descends posterior to the internal jugular vein on the surface of the scalenus anterior muscle.
- **Pneumothorax or hemothorax:** This is caused by damage to the pleura and/or internal thoracic artery by the needle passing posteriorly and downward.
- **Brachial plexus injury:** This is caused by the needle passing posteriorly into the roots or trunks of the plexus.

Lymph Drainage of the Head and Neck

The lymph nodes of the head and neck (Fig. 11-40) are arranged as a regional collar that extends from below the chin to the back of the head and as a deep vertical terminal group that is embedded in the carotid sheath in the neck (Fig. 11-55).

Regional Nodes

The regional nodes are arranged as follows:

- **Occipital nodes:** These are situated over the occipital bone on the back of the skull. They receive lymph from the back of the scalp.
- **Retroauricular (mastoid) nodes:** These lie behind the ear over the mastoid process. They receive lymph from the scalp above the ear, the auricle, and the external auditory meatus.
- **Parotid nodes:** These are situated on or within the parotid salivary gland. They receive lymph from the scalp above the parotid gland, the eyelids, the parotid gland, the auricle, and the external auditory meatus.
- **Buccal (facial) nodes:** One or two nodes lie in the cheek over the buccinator muscle. They drain lymph that ultimately passes into the submandibular nodes.
- **Submandibular nodes:** These lie superficial to the submandibular salivary gland just below the lower margin of the jaw. They receive lymph from the front of the scalp; the nose; the cheek; the upper lip and the lower lip (except the central part); the frontal, maxillary, and ethmoid sinuses; the upper and lower teeth (except the lower incisors); the anterior two thirds of the tongue (except the tip); the floor of the mouth and vestibule; and the gums.

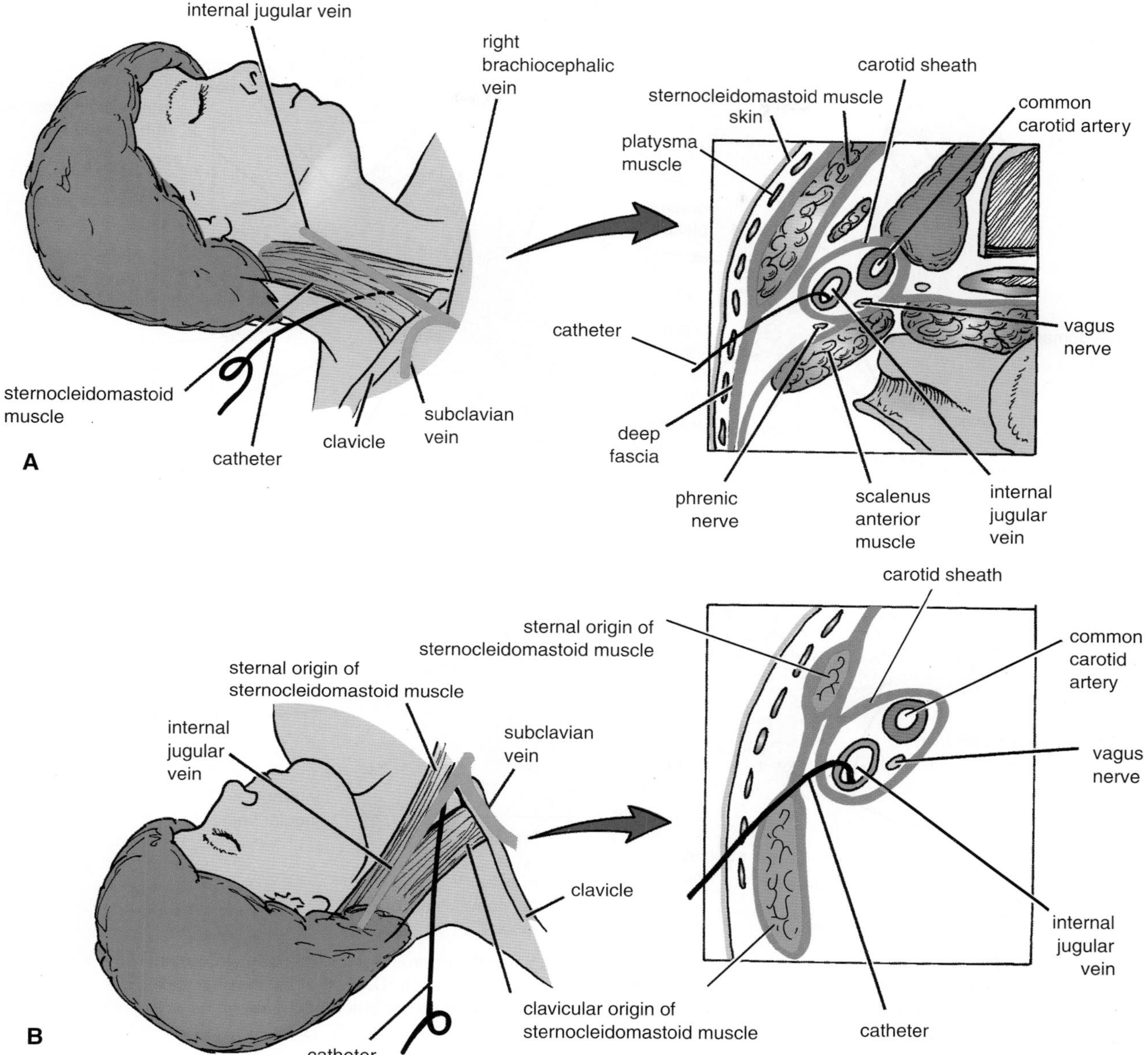

Figure 11-61 Catheterization of the right internal jugular vein. **A.** Posterior approach. Note the position of the catheter relative to the sternocleidomastoid muscle and the common carotid artery. **B.** Anterior approach. Note that the catheter is inserted into the vein close to the apex of the triangle formed by the sternal and clavicular heads of the sternocleidomastoid muscle and the clavicle.

- **Submental nodes:** These lie in the submental triangle just below the chin. They drain lymph from the tip of the tongue, the floor of the anterior part of the mouth, the incisor teeth, the center part of the lower lip, and the skin over the chin.
- **Anterior cervical nodes:** These lie along the course of the anterior jugular veins in the front of the neck. They receive lymph from the skin and superficial tissues of the front of the neck.
- **Superficial cervical nodes:** These lie along the course of the external jugular vein on the side of the neck. They drain lymph from the skin over the angle of the jaw, the skin over the lower part of the parotid gland, and the lobe of the ear.
- **Retropharyngeal nodes:** These lie behind the pharynx and in front of the vertebral column. They receive lymph from the nasal pharynx, the auditory tube, and the vertebral column.
- **Laryngeal nodes:** These lie in front of the larynx. They receive lymph from the larynx.
- **Tracheal (paratracheal) nodes:** These lie alongside the trachea. They receive lymph from neighboring structures, including the thyroid gland.

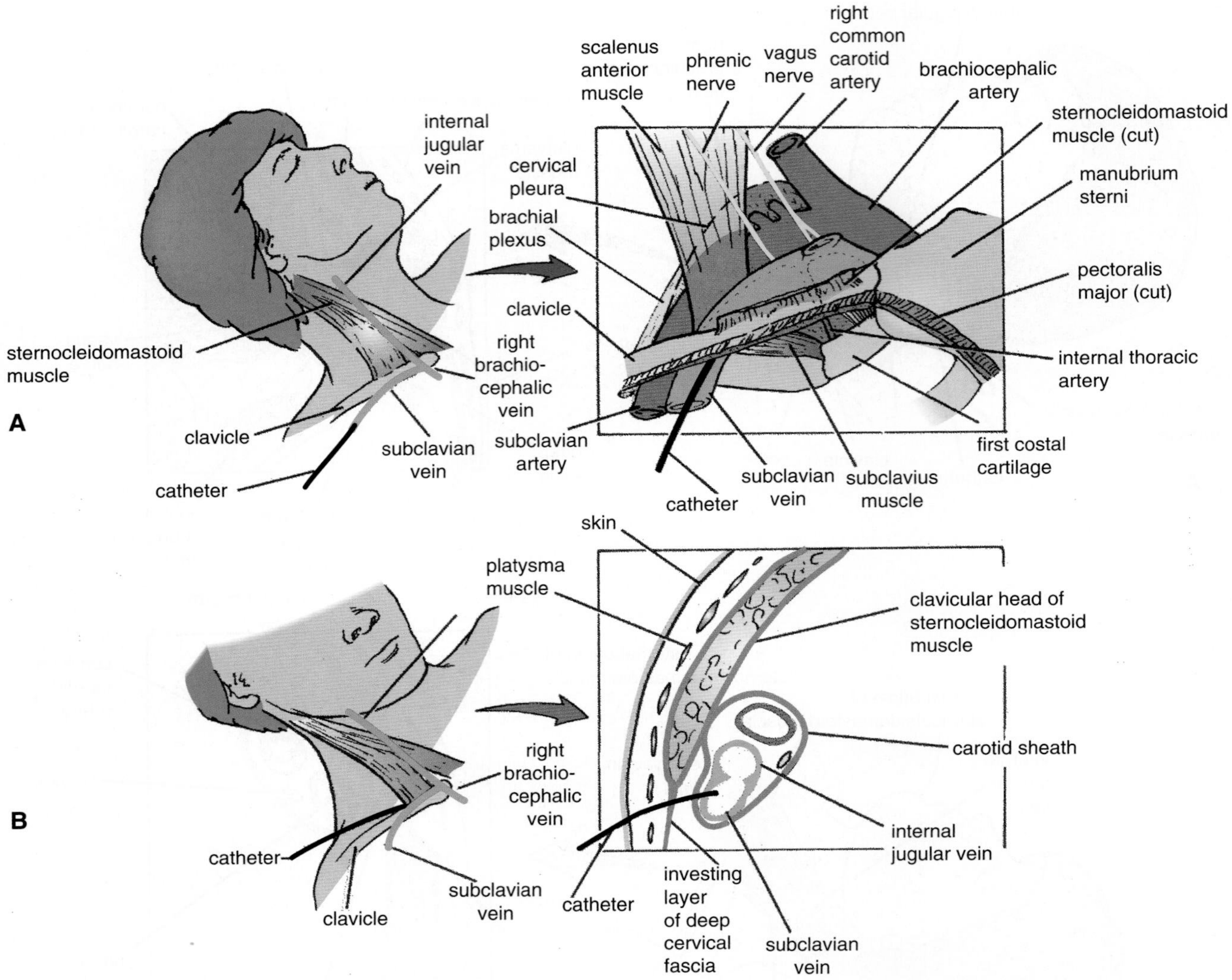

Figure 11-62 Subclavian vein catheterization. **A.** Infraclavicular approach. Note the many important anatomic structures located in this region. **B.** Supraclavicular approach. The catheter enters the subclavian vein close to its junction with the internal jugular vein to form the brachiocephalic vein.

Deep Cervical Nodes

The deep cervical nodes form a vertical chain along the course of the internal jugular vein within the carotid sheath (Fig. 11-49). They receive lymph from all the groups of regional nodes. The **jugulodigastric node,** which is located below and behind the angle of the jaw, is mainly concerned with drainage of the tonsil and the tongue. The **jugulo-omohyoid node,** which is situated close to the omohyoid muscle, is mainly associated with drainage of the tongue.

The efferent lymph vessels from the deep cervical lymph nodes join to form the jugular trunk, which drains into the thoracic duct or the right lymphatic duct (Fig. 11-40).

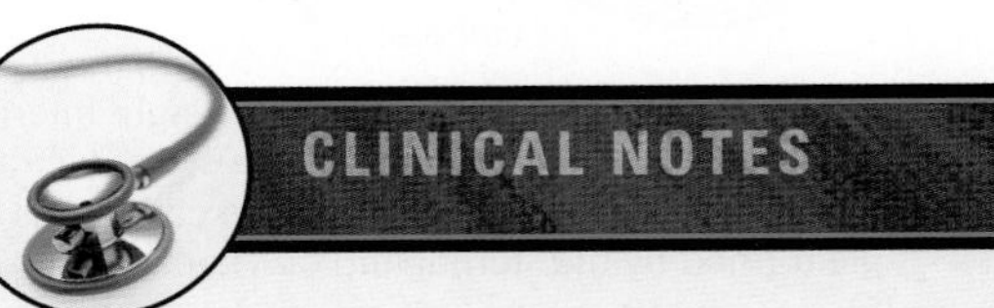

Clinical Significance of the Cervical Lymph Nodes

Knowledge of the lymph drainage of an organ or region is of great clinical importance. Examination of a patient may reveal an enlarged lymph node. It is the physician's responsibility to determine the cause and be knowledgeable about the area of the body that drains its lymph into a particular node. For example, an enlarged submandibular node can be caused by a pathologic condition in the scalp, the face, the maxillary sinus, or the tongue. An infected tooth of the upper or lower jaw may be responsible. Often a physician has to search systematically the various areas known to drain into a node to discover the cause.

(continues)

Clinical Notes, *continued*

Examination of the Deep Cervical Lymph Nodes

Lymph nodes in the neck should be examined from behind the patient. The examination is made easier by asking the patient to flex the neck slightly to reduce the tension of the muscles. The groups of nodes should be examined in a definite order to avoid omitting any.

After the identification of enlarged lymph nodes, possible sites of infection or neoplastic growth should be examined, including the face, scalp, tongue, mouth, tonsil, and pharynx.

Carcinoma Metastases in the Deep Cervical Lymph Node

In the head and neck, all the lymph ultimately drains into the deep cervical group of nodes. Secondary carcinomatous deposits in these nodes are common. The primary growth may be easy to find. On the other hand, at certain anatomic sites the primary growth may be small and overlooked, for example, in the larynx, the pharynx, the cervical part of the esophagus, and the external auditory meatus. The bronchi, breast, and stomach are sometimes the site of the primary tumor. In these cases, the secondary growth has spread far beyond the local lymph nodes.

When cervical metastases occur, the surgeon usually decides to perform a block dissection of the cervical nodes. This procedure involves the removal en bloc of the internal jugular vein, the fascia, the lymph nodes, and the submandibular salivary gland. The aim of the operation is removal of all the lymph tissues on the affected side of the neck. The carotid arteries and the vagus nerve are carefully preserved. It is often necessary to sacrifice the hypoglossal and vagus nerves, which may be involved in the cancerous deposits. In patients with bilateral spread, a bilateral block dissection may be necessary. An interval of 3 to 4 weeks is necessary before removing the second internal jugular vein.

Cranial Nerves

Organization of the Cranial Nerves

The cranial nerves are named as follows:

- I. Olfactory
- II. Optic
- III. Oculomotor
- IV. Trochlear
- V. Trigeminal
- VI. Abducent
- VII. Facial
- VIII. Vestibulocochlear
- IX. Glossopharyngeal
- X. Vagus
- XI. Accessory
- XII. Hypoglossal

The olfactory, optic, and vestibulocochlear nerves are entirely sensory; the oculomotor, trochlear, abducent, accessory, and hypoglossal nerves are entirely motor; and the remaining nerves are mixed. The different components of the cranial nerves, their functions, and the openings in the skull through which the nerves leave the cranial cavity are summarized in Table 11-6.

Olfactory Nerves

The olfactory nerves arise from **olfactory receptor nerve cells** in the olfactory mucous membrane. The olfactory mucous membrane is situated in the upper part of the nasal cavity above the level of the superior concha (Fig. 11-63). Bundles of these olfactory nerve fibers pass through the openings of the cribriform plate of the ethmoid bone to enter the **olfactory bulb** in the cranial cavity. The olfactory bulb is connected to the olfactory area of the cerebral cortex by the **olfactory tract.**

Optic Nerve

The optic nerve is composed of the axons of the cells of the **ganglionic layer** of the retina. The optic nerve emerges from the back of the eyeball and leaves the orbital cavity through the optic canal to enter the cranial cavity (Fig. 11-11). The optic nerve then unites with the optic nerve of the opposite side to form the optic chiasma (Fig. 11-63).

In the chiasma, the fibers from the medial half of each retina cross the midline and enter the **optic tract** of the opposite side, whereas the fibers from the lateral half of each retina pass posteriorly in the optic tract of the same side. Most of the fibers of the optic tract terminate by synapsing with nerve cells in the **lateral geniculate body** (Fig. 11-63). A few fibers pass to the pretectal nucleus and the superior colliculus and are concerned with light reflexes.

The axons of the nerve cells of the lateral geniculate body pass posteriorly as the **optic radiation** and terminate in the **visual cortex** of the cerebral hemisphere (Fig. 11-63).

Oculomotor Nerve

The oculomotor nerve emerges on the anterior surface of the midbrain (Fig. 11-64). It passes forward between the posterior cerebral and superior cerebellar arteries (Fig. 11-11). It then continues into the middle cranial fossa in the lateral wall of the cavernous sinus. Here, it divides into a **superior** and an **inferior ramus,** which enter the orbital cavity through the superior orbital fissure (Fig. 11-18).

The oculomotor nerve supplies the following:

- **The extrinsic muscles of the eye:** the levator palpebrae superioris, superior rectus, medial rectus, inferior rectus, and inferior oblique (Fig. 11-64; see also Figs. 11-18 and 11-19)
- **The intrinsic muscles of the eye:** the constrictor pupillae of the iris and the ciliary muscles are supplied by the parasympathetic component of the oculomotor nerve. These fibers synapse in the **ciliary ganglion** and reach the eyeball in the **short ciliary nerves** (Fig. 11-19).

The oculomotor nerve, therefore, is entirely motor. It is responsible for lifting the upper eyelid; turning the eye upward, downward, and medially; constricting the pupil; and accommodation of the eye.

Table 11-6 Cranial Nerves

Nerve		Components	Function	Opening in Skull
I.	Olfactory	Sensory	Smell	Openings in cribriform plate of ethmoid
II.	Optic	Sensory	Vision	Optic canal
III.	Oculomotor	Motor	Lifts upper eyelid, turns eyeball upward, downward, and medially; constricts pupil; accommodates eye	Superior orbital fissure
IV.	Trochlear	Motor	Assists in turning eyeball downward and laterally	Superior orbital fissure
V.	Trigeminal			
	Ophthalmic division	Sensory	Cornea, skin of forehead, scalp, eyelids, and nose; also mucous membrane of paranasal sinuses and nasal cavity	Superior orbital fissure
	Maxillary division	Sensory	Skin of face over maxilla and the upper lip; teeth of upper jaw; mucous membrane of nose, the maxillary air sinus, and palate	Foramen rotundum
	Mandibular division	Motor	Muscles of mastication, mylohyoid, anterior belly of digastric, tensor veli palatini, and tensor tympani	Foramen ovale
		Sensory	Skin of cheek, skin over mandible, lower lip, and side of head; teeth of lower jaw and temporomandibular joint; mucous membrane of mouth and anterior two thirds of tongue	
VI.	Abducent	Motor	Lateral rectus muscle: turns eyeball laterally	Superior orbital fissure
VII.	Facial	Motor	Muscles of face, cheek, and scalp; stapedius muscle of middle ear; stylohyoid; and posterior belly of digastric	Internal acoustic meatus, facial canal, stylomastoid foramen
		Sensory	Taste from anterior two thirds of tongue, floor of mouth, and palate	
		Secretomotor parasympathetic	Submandibular and sublingual salivary glands, lacrimal gland, and glands of nose and palate	
VIII.	Vestibulocochlear			
	Vestibular	Sensory	Position and movement of head	Internal acoustic meatus
	Cochlear	Sensory	Hearing	
IX.	Glossopharyngeal	Motor	Stylopharyngeus muscle: assists swallowing	
		Secretomotor parasympathetic	Parotid salivary gland	Jugular foramen
		Sensory	General sensation and taste from posterior third of tongue and pharynx; carotid sinus and carotid body	
X.	Vagus	Motor	Constrictor muscles of pharynx and intrinsic muscles of larynx; involuntary muscle of trachea and bronchi, heart, alimentary tract from pharynx to splenic flexure of colon; liver and pancreas	Jugular foramen
		Sensory	Taste from epiglottis and vallecula and afferent fibers from structures named above	
XI.	Accessory			
	Cranial root	Motor	Muscles of soft palate, pharynx, and larynx	Jugular foramen
	Spinal root	Motor	Sternocleidomastoid and trapezius muscles	
XII.	Hypoglossal	Motor	Muscles of tongue controlling its shape and movement (except palatoglossus)	Hypoglossal canal

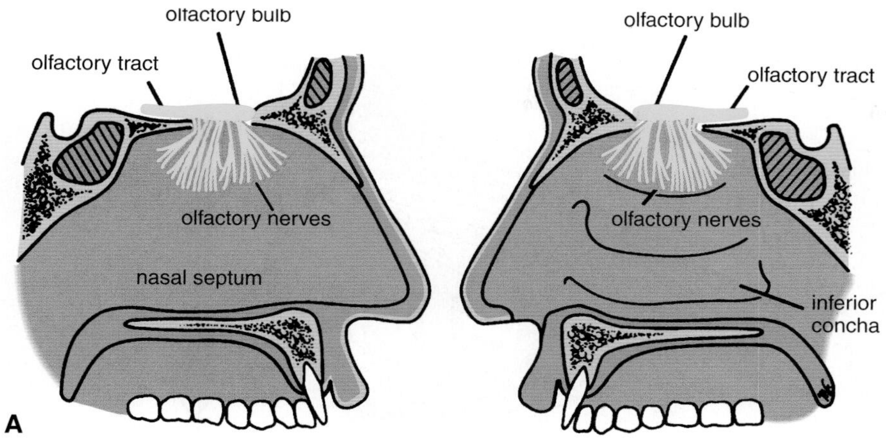

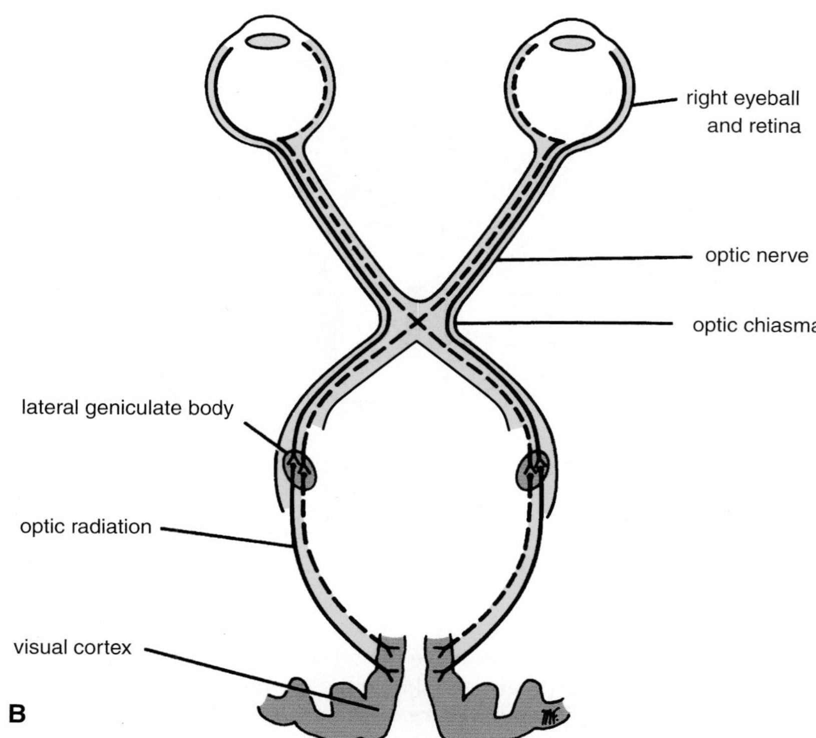

Figure 11-63 **A.** Distribution of the olfactory nerves on the nasal septum and the lateral wall of the nose. **B.** The optic nerve and its connections.

Trochlear Nerve

The trochlear nerve is the most slender of the cranial nerves. Having crossed the nerve of the opposite side, it leaves the posterior surface of the midbrain (Fig. 11-64). It then passes forward through the middle cranial fossa in the lateral wall of the cavernous sinus and enters the orbit through the superior orbital fissure (Figs. 11-11 and 11-18).

The trochlear nerve supplies:

The superior oblique muscle of the eyeball (extrinsic muscle) (Fig. 11-20)

The trochlear nerve is entirely motor and assists in turning the eye downward and laterally.

Trigeminal Nerve

The trigeminal nerve is the largest cranial nerve (Fig. 11-65). It leaves the anterior aspect of the pons as a small **motor root** and a large **sensory root,** and it passes forward, out of the posterior cranial fossa, to reach the apex of the petrous part of the temporal bone in the middle cranial fossa. Here, the large sensory root expands to form the **trigeminal ganglion** (Figs. 11-11 and 11-65). The trigeminal ganglion lies within a pouch of dura mater called the **trigeminal cave.** The motor root of the trigeminal nerve is situated below the sensory ganglion and is completely separate from it. The ophthalmic (V1), maxillary (V2), and mandibular (V3) nerves arise from the anterior border of the ganglion (Figs. 11-11 and 11-65).

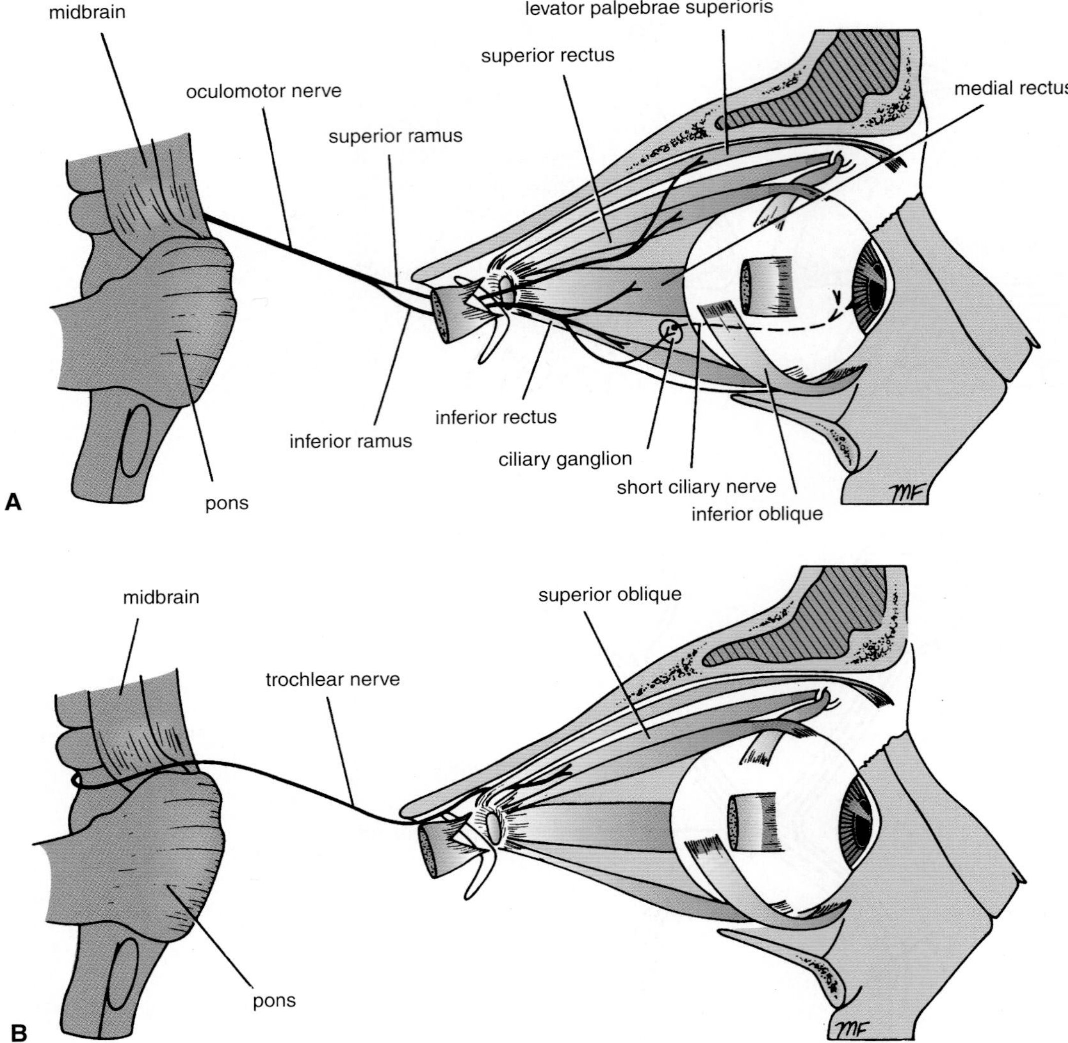

Figure 11-64 **A.** Origin and distribution of the oculomotor nerve. **B.** Origin and distribution of the trochlear nerve.

Ophthalmic Nerve (V1)

The ophthalmic nerve is purely sensory (Figs. 11-65 and 11-50). It runs forward in the lateral wall of the cavernous sinus in the middle cranial fossa and divides into three branches, the lacrimal, frontal, and nasociliary nerves, which enter the orbital cavity through the superior orbital fissure.

Branches

The **lacrimal nerve** runs forward on the upper border of the lateral rectus muscle (Fig. 11-18). It is joined by the zygomaticotemporal branch of the maxillary nerve, which contains the parasympathetic secretomotor fibers to the lacrimal gland. The lacrimal nerve then enters the lacrimal gland and gives branches to the conjunctiva and the skin of the upper eyelid.

The **frontal nerve** runs forward on the upper surface of the levator palpebrae superioris muscle and divides into the **supraorbital** and **supratrochlear nerves** (Fig. 11-20). These nerves leave the orbital cavity and supply the frontal air sinus and the skin of the forehead and the scalp.

The **nasociliary nerve** crosses the optic nerve, runs forward on the upper border of the medial rectus muscle (Fig. 11-20), and continues as the **anterior ethmoid nerve** through the anterior ethmoidal foramen to enter the cranial cavity. It then descends through a slit at the side of the crista galli to enter the nasal cavity. It gives off two **internal nasal branches** and it then supplies the skin of the tip of the nose with the **external nasal nerve.** Its branches include the following:

- **Sensory fibers** to the ciliary ganglion (Fig. 11-20)
- **Long ciliary nerves** that contain sympathetic fibers to the dilator pupillae muscle and sensory fibers to the cornea (Fig. 11-20)
- **Infratrochlear nerve** that supplies the skin of the eyelids
- **Posterior ethmoidal nerve** that is sensory to the ethmoid and sphenoid sinuses

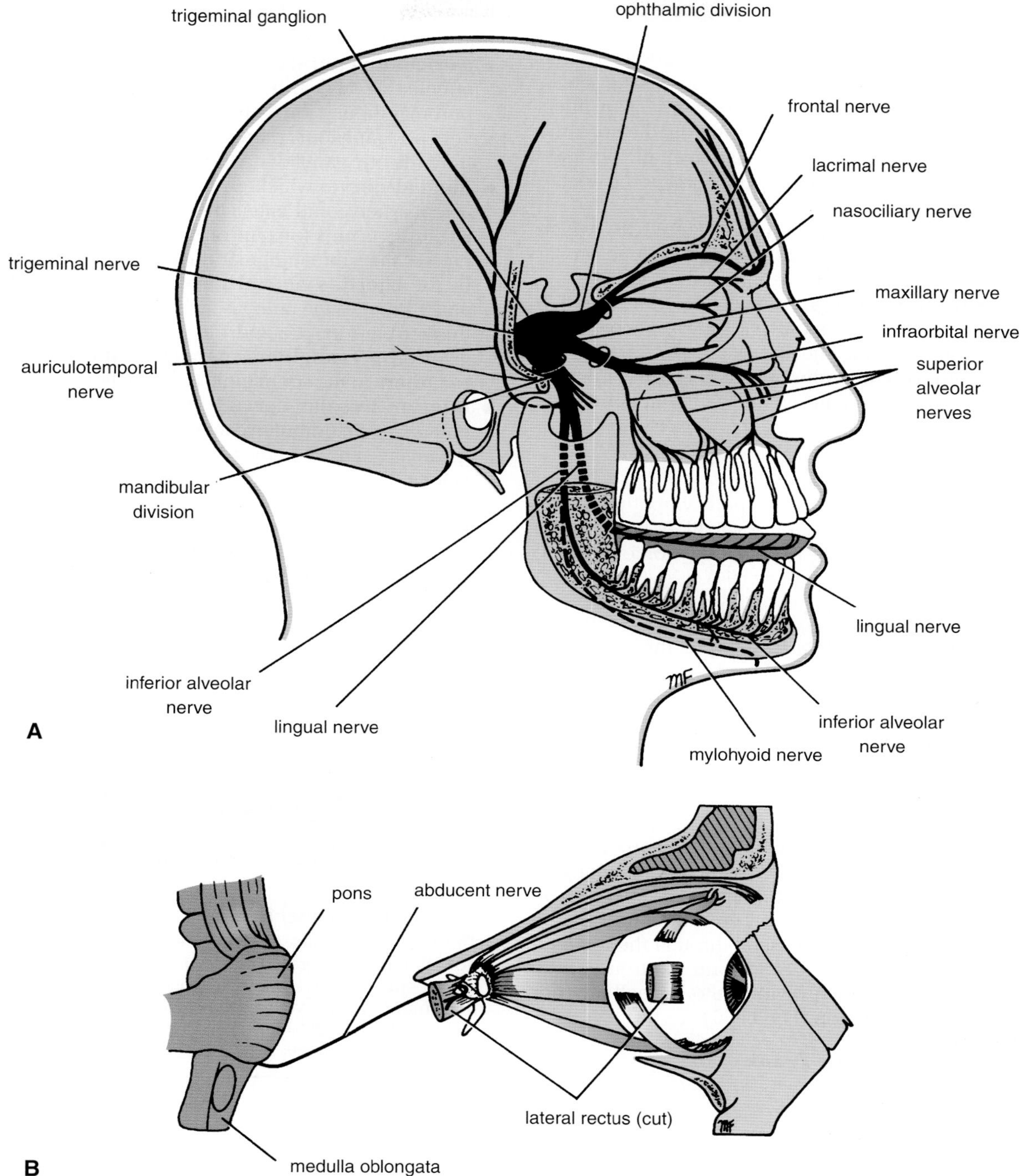

Figure 11-65 **A.** Distribution of the trigeminal nerve. **B.** Origin and distribution of the abducent nerve.

Maxillary Nerve (V2)

The maxillary nerve arises from the trigeminal ganglion in the middle cranial fossa. It passes forward in the lateral wall of the cavernous sinus and leaves the skull through the foramen rotundum (Fig. 11-11) and crosses the pterygopalatine fossa to enter the orbit through the inferior orbital fissure (Fig. 11-19). It then continues as the infraorbital nerve in the infraorbital groove, and it emerges on the face through the infraorbital foramen. It gives sensory fibers to the skin of the face and the side of the nose.

Branches

- **Meningeal branches**
- **Zygomatic branch** (Fig. 11-19), which divides into the zygomaticotemporal and the zygomaticofacial nerves that supply the skin of the face. The zygomaticotemporal

branch gives parasympathetic secretomotor fibers to the lacrimal gland via the lacrimal nerve.

- **Ganglionic branches,** which are two short nerves that suspend the pterygopalatine ganglion in the pterygopalatine fossa (Fig. 11-19). They contain sensory fibers that have passed through the ganglion from the nose, the palate, and the pharynx. They also contain postganglionic parasympathetic fibers that are going to the lacrimal gland.
- **Posterior superior alveolar nerve** (Fig. 11-19), which supplies the maxillary sinus as well as the upper molar teeth and adjoining parts of the gum and the cheek
- **Middle superior alveolar nerve** (Fig. 11-19), which supplies the maxillary sinus as well as the upper premolar teeth, the gums, and the cheek
- **Anterior superior alveolar nerve** (Fig. 11-19), which supplies the maxillary sinus as well as the upper canine and the incisor teeth

Pterygopalatine Ganglion

The pterygopalatine ganglion is a parasympathetic ganglion, which is suspended from the maxillary nerve in the pterygopalatine fossa (Fig. 11-19). It is secretomotor to the lacrimal and nasal glands (see page 694).

Branches

- **Orbital branches,** which enter the orbit through the inferior orbital fissure
- **Greater and lesser palatine nerves** (Fig. 11-19), which supply the palate, the tonsil, and the nasal cavity
- **Pharyngeal branch,** which supplies the roof of the nasopharynx

Mandibular Nerve (V3)

The mandibular nerve is both motor and sensory (Figs. 11-11 and 11-65). The sensory root leaves the trigeminal ganglion and passes out of the skull through the foramen ovale to enter the infratemporal fossa. The motor root of the trigeminal nerve also leaves the skull through the foramen ovale and joins the sensory root to form the trunk of the mandibular nerve, and then divides into a small anterior and a large posterior division (Fig. 11-66).

Branches From the Main Trunk of the Mandibular Nerve

- **Meningeal branch**
- **Nerve to the medial pterygoid muscle,** which supplies not only the medial pterygoid, but also the tensor veli palatini muscle.

Branches From the Anterior Division of the Mandibular Nerve

- **Masseteric nerve** to the masseter muscle (Fig. 11-36)
- **Deep temporal nerves** to the temporalis muscle (Fig. 11-36)
- **Nerve to the lateral pterygoid muscle**
- **Buccal nerve** to the skin and the mucous membrane of the cheek (Fig. 11-36). The buccal nerve **does not supply the buccinator muscle** (which is supplied by the facial nerve), and it is the **only sensory branch** of the anterior division of the mandibular nerve.

Branches From the Posterior Division of the Mandibular Nerve

- **Auriculotemporal nerve,** which supplies the skin of the auricle (Fig. 11-66), the external auditory meatus, the temporomandibular joint, and the scalp. This nerve also conveys postganglionic parasympathetic secretomotor fibers from the otic ganglion to the parotid salivary gland.
- **Lingual nerve,** which descends in front of the inferior alveolar nerve and enters the mouth (Figs. 11-36 and 11-66). It then runs forward on the side of the tongue and crosses the submandibular duct. In its course, it is joined by the **chorda tympani nerve** (Figs. 11-36 and 11-66), and it supplies the mucous membrane of the anterior two thirds of the tongue and the floor of the mouth. It also gives off **preganglionic parasympathetic secretomotor fibers** to the submandibular ganglion.
- **Inferior alveolar nerve** (Figs. 11-36 and 11-66), which enters the mandibular canal to supply the teeth of the lower jaw and emerges through the mental foramen (mental nerve) to supply the skin of the chin (Fig. 11-50). Before entering the canal, it gives off the **mylohyoid nerve** (Fig. 11-36), which supplies the mylohyoid muscle and the anterior belly of the digastric muscle.
- **Communicating branch,** which frequently runs from the inferior alveolar nerve to the lingual nerve

The branches of the posterior division of the mandibular nerve are sensory (except the nerve to the mylohyoid muscle).

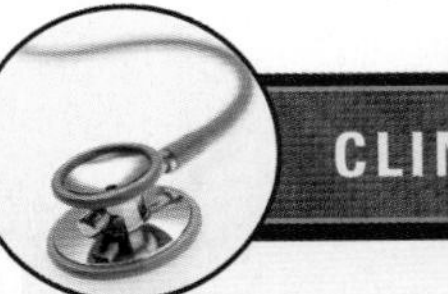

CLINICAL NOTES

Injury to the Lingual Nerve

The lingual nerve passes forward into the submandibular region from the infratemporal fossa by running beneath the origin of the superior constrictor muscle, which is attached to the posterior border of the mylohyoid line on the mandible. Here, it is closely related to the last molar tooth and is liable to be damaged in cases of clumsy extraction of an impacted third molar.

Otic Ganglion

The otic ganglion is a parasympathetic ganglion that is located medial to the mandibular nerve just below the skull, and it is adherent to the nerve to the medial pterygoid muscle. The preganglionic fibers originate in the glossopharyngeal nerve, and they reach the ganglion via the lesser petrosal nerve (see page 765). The postganglionic secretomotor fibers reach the parotid salivary gland via the auriculotemporal nerve.

Submandibular Ganglion

The submandibular ganglion is a parasympathetic ganglion that lies deep to the submandibular salivary gland and is attached to the lingual nerve by small nerves (Figs. 11-36 and 11-66). Preganglionic parasympathetic fibers reach the gan-

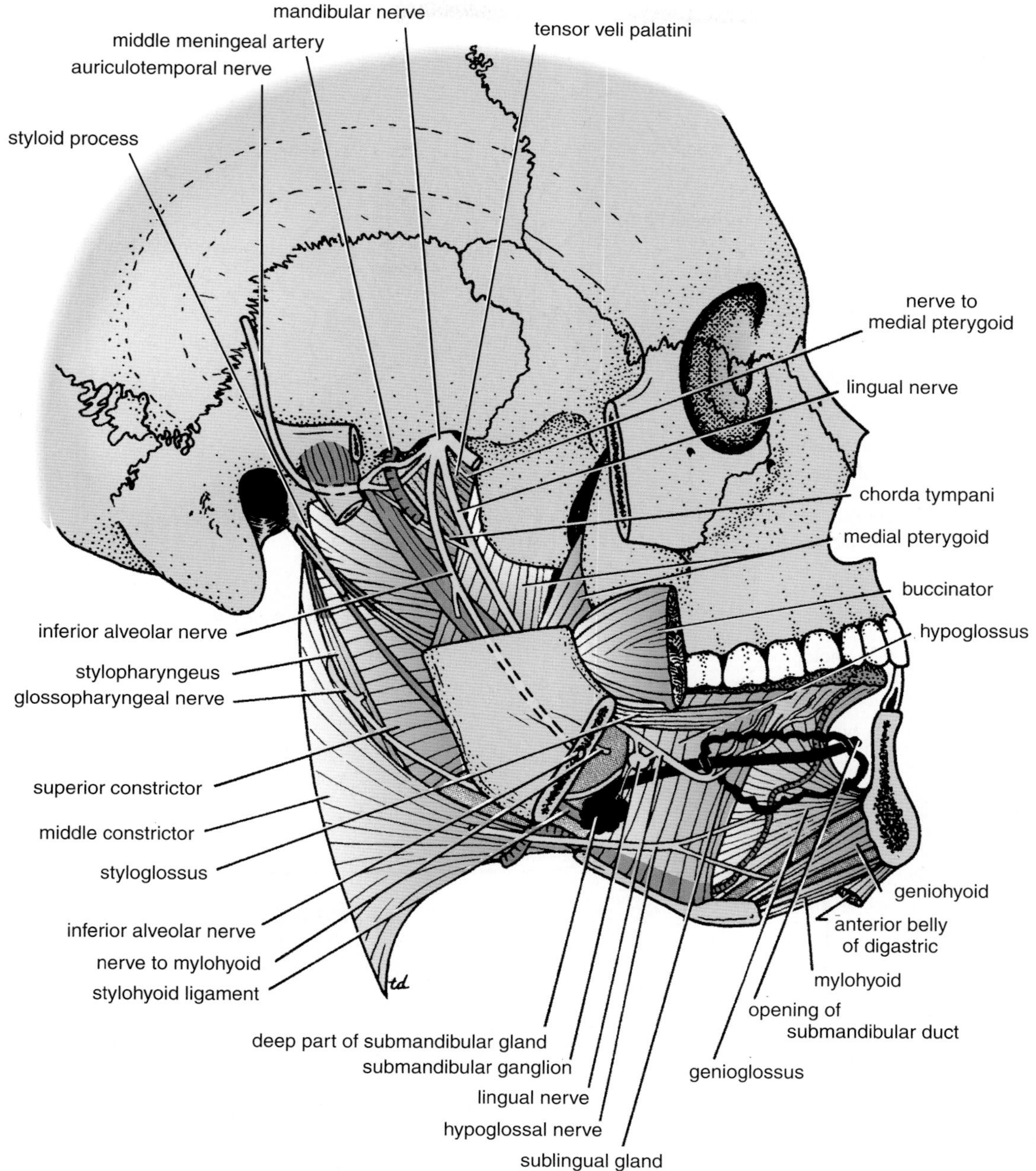

Figure 11-66 Infratemporal and submandibular regions. Parts of the zygomatic arch, the ramus, and the body of the mandible have been removed. Mylohyoid and lateral pterygoid muscles have also been removed to display deeper structures. The outline of the sublingual gland is shown as a solid black wavy line.

glion from the facial nerve via the chorda tympani and the lingual nerves. Postganglionic secretomotor fibers pass to the submandibular and the sublingual salivary glands.

The trigeminal nerve is thus the main sensory nerve of the head and innervates the muscles of mastication. It also tenses the soft palate and the tympanic membrane.

Abducent Nerve

This small nerve emerges from the anterior surface of the hindbrain between the pons and the medulla oblongata (Figs. 11-11 and 11-65). It passes forward with the internal carotid artery through the cavernous sinus in the middle cranial fossa and enters the orbit through the superior orbital fissure (Fig. 11-18). The abducent nerve supplies the lateral rectus muscle (Fig. 11-65) and is therefore responsible for turning the eye laterally.

Facial Nerve

The facial nerve has a motor root and a sensory root **(nervus intermedius)** (Fig. 11-67). The nerve emerges on

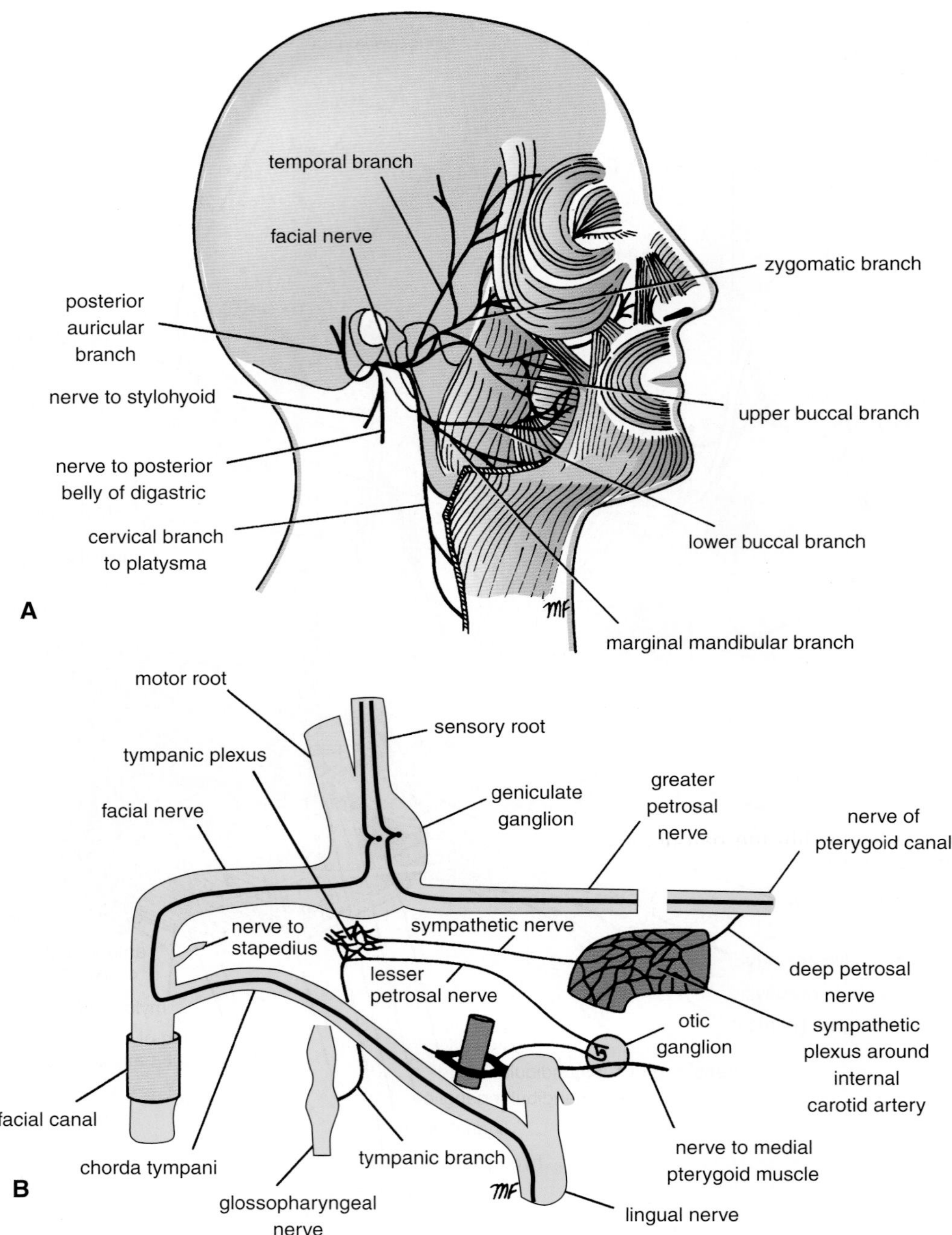

Figure 11-67 **A.** Distribution of the facial nerve. **B.** Branches of the facial nerve within the petrous part of the temporal bone; the taste fibers are shown in black. The glossopharyngeal nerve is also shown.

the anterior surface of the hindbrain between the pons and the medulla oblongata. The roots pass laterally in the posterior cranial fossa with the vestibulocochlear nerve and enter the internal acoustic meatus in the petrous part of the temporal bone (Fig. 11-28). At the bottom of the meatus, the nerve enters the facial canal that runs laterally through the inner ear. On reaching the medial wall of the middle ear (tympanic cavity), the nerve swells to form the sensory **geniculate ganglion** (Fig. 11-67; see also Figs. 11-29 and 11-30). The nerve then bends sharply backward above the promontory and, at the posterior wall of the middle ear, bends down on the medial side of the aditus of the mastoid antrum (see page 712). The nerve descends behind the pyramid and it emerges from the temporal bone through the stylomastoid foramen. The facial nerve now passes forward through the parotid gland to its distribution (Fig. 11-67).

Important Branches of the Facial Nerve

- **Greater petrosal nerve** arises from the nerve at the geniculate ganglion (Fig. 11-67). It contains preganglionic parasympathetic fibers that synapse in the pterygopalatine ganglion. The postganglionic fibers are secretomotor to the lacrimal gland and the glands of the nose and the palate. The greater petrosal nerve also contains taste fibers from the palate.
- **Nerve to stapedius** supplies the stapedius muscle in the middle ear (Fig. 11-67).
- **Chorda tympani** arises from the facial nerve in the facial canal in the posterior wall of the middle ear (Fig. 11-67). It runs forward over the medial surface of the upper part of the tympanic membrane (Fig. 11-29) and leaves the middle ear through the **petrotympanic fissure,** thus entering the infratemporal fossa and joining the lingual nerve. The chorda tympani contains preganglionic parasympathetic secretomotor fibers to the submandibular and the sublingual salivary glands. It also contains taste fibers from the anterior two thirds of the tongue and floor of the mouth.
- **Posterior auricular,** the posterior belly of the digastric, and the stylohyoid nerves (Fig. 11-67) are **muscular branches given off by the facial nerve as it emerges from the stylomastoid foramen.**
- **Five terminal branches to the muscles of facial expression.** These are the **temporal,** the **zygomatic,** the **buccal,** the **mandibular,** and the **cervical branches** (Fig. 11-67).

The facial nerve lies within the parotid salivary gland (Fig. 11-85B) after leaving the stylomastoid foramen, and it is located between the superficial and the deep parts of the gland (see page 787). Here, it gives off the terminal branches that emerge from the anterior border of the gland and pass to the muscles of the face and the scalp. **The buccal branch supplies the buccinator muscle, and the cervical branch supplies the platysma and the depressor anguli oris muscles.**

The facial nerve thus controls facial expression, salivation, and lacrimation and is a pathway for taste sensation from the anterior part of the tongue and floor of the mouth and from the palate.

Vestibulocochlear Nerve

The vestibulocochlear nerve is a sensory nerve that consists of two sets of fibers: **vestibular** and **cochlear.** They leave the anterior surface of the brain between the pons and the medulla oblongata (Fig. 11-68). They cross the posterior cranial fossa and enter the internal acoustic meatus with the facial nerve (Fig. 11-28).

Vestibular Fibers

The vestibular fibers are the central processes of the nerve cells of the vestibular ganglion situated in the internal acoustic meatus (Fig. 11-68). The vestibular fibers originate from the vestibule and the semicircular canals; therefore, they are concerned with the sense of position and with movement of the head.

Cochlear Fibers

The cochlear fibers are the central processes of the nerve cells of the **spiral ganglion of the cochlea** (Fig. 11-68). The cochlear fibers originate in the **spiral organ of Corti** and are therefore concerned with hearing.

Glossopharyngeal Nerve

The glossopharyngeal nerve is a motor and sensory nerve (Fig. 11-68). It emerges from the anterior surface of the medulla oblongata between the olive and the inferior cerebellar peduncle. It passes laterally in the posterior cranial fossa and leaves the skull by passing through the jugular foramen. The **superior** and **inferior sensory ganglia** are located on the nerve as it passes through the foramen. The glossopharyngeal nerve then descends through the upper part of the neck to the back of the tongue (Fig. 11-68).

Important Branches of the Glossopharyngeal Nerve

- **Tympanic branch** passes to the tympanic plexus in the middle ear (Fig. 11-68). Preganglionic parasympathetic fibers for the parotid salivary gland now leave the plexus as the **lesser petrosal nerve,** and they synapse in the otic ganglion.
- **Carotid branch** contains sensory fibers from the carotid sinus (pressoreceptor mechanism for the regulation of blood pressure and the carotid body and chemoreceptor mechanism for the regulation of heart rate and respiration) (Fig. 11-68).
- **Nerve to the stylopharyngeus muscle**
- **Pharyngeal branches** (Fig. 11-68) run to the **pharyngeal plexus** and also receive branches from the vagus nerve and the sympathetic trunk.
- **Lingual branch** (Fig. 11-68) passes to the mucous membrane of the posterior third of the tongue (including the vallate papillae).

The glossopharyngeal nerve thus assists swallowing and promotes salivation. It also conducts sensation from the pharynx and the back of the tongue and carries impulses, which influence the arterial blood pressure and respiration, from the carotid sinus and carotid body.

Vagus Nerve

The vagus nerve is composed of motor and sensory fibers (Fig. 11-69). It emerges from the anterior surface of the medulla oblongata between the olive and the inferior cerebellar peduncle. The nerve passes laterally through the posterior cranial fossa and leaves the skull through the jugular foramen. The vagus nerve has both **superior and inferior sensory ganglia.** Below the inferior ganglion, the **cranial root of the accessory nerve** joins the vagus nerve and is distributed mainly in its pharyngeal and recurrent laryngeal branches.

The vagus nerve descends through the neck alongside the carotid arteries and internal jugular vein within the carotid sheath (Fig. 11-49). It passes through the mediastinum of the thorax (Fig. 11-69), passing behind the root of the lung, and enters the abdomen through the esophageal opening in the diaphragm.

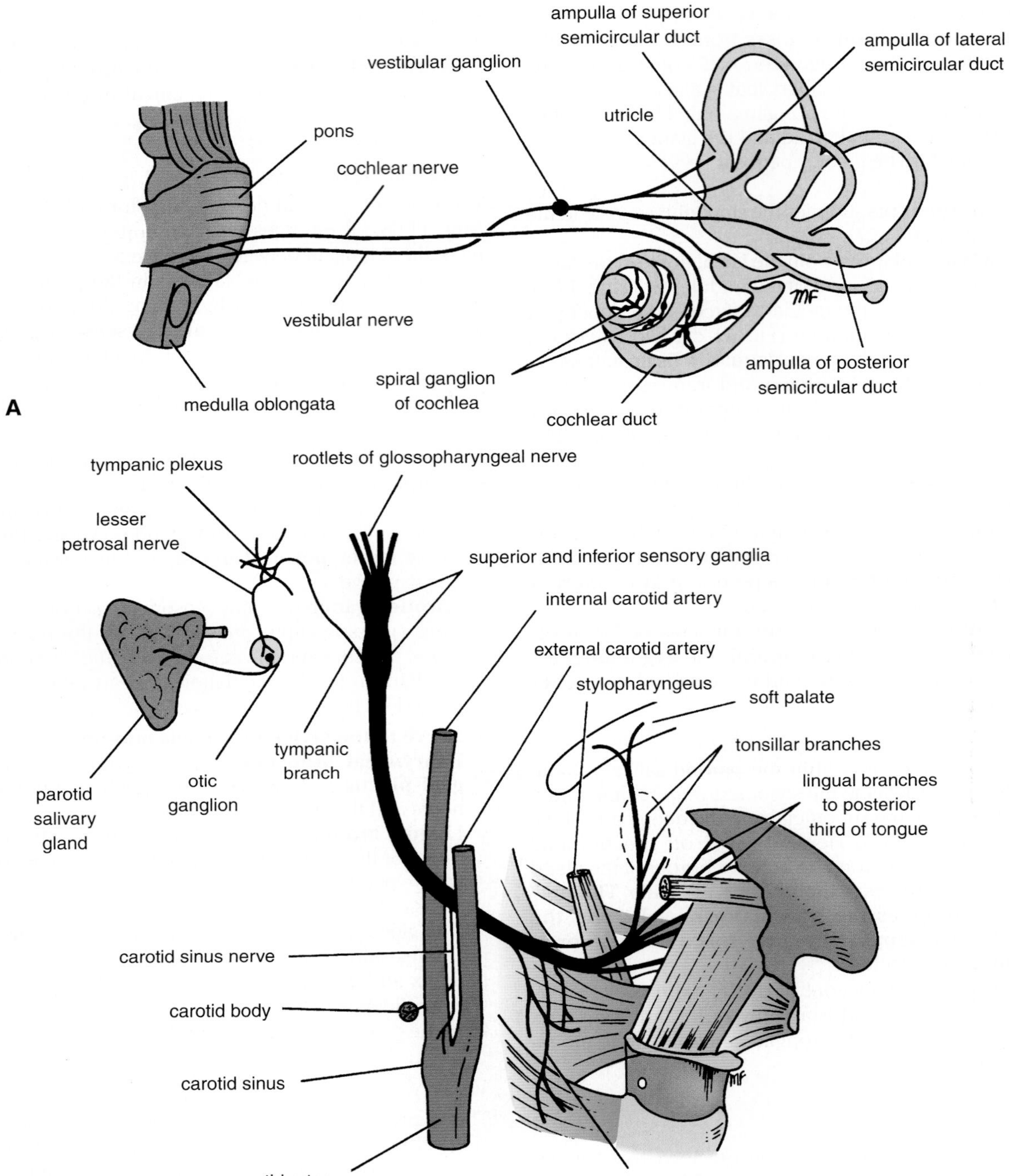

Figure 11-68 **A.** Origin and distribution of the vestibulocochlear nerve. **B.** Distribution of the glossopharyngeal nerve.

Important Branches of the Vagus Nerve in the Neck

- **Meningeal and auricular branches**
- **Pharyngeal branch** contains nerve fibers from the cranial part of the accessory nerve. This branch joins the pharyngeal plexus and supplies all the muscles of the pharynx (except the stylopharyngeus) and of the soft palate (except the tensor veli palatini).
- **Superior laryngeal nerve** (Fig. 11-69) divides into the internal and the external laryngeal nerves. The **internal laryngeal nerve** is sensory to the mucous membrane of the piriform fossa and the larynx down as far as the vocal cords. The **external laryngeal nerve** is motor and is located close to the superior thyroid artery; it supplies the cricothyroid muscle.

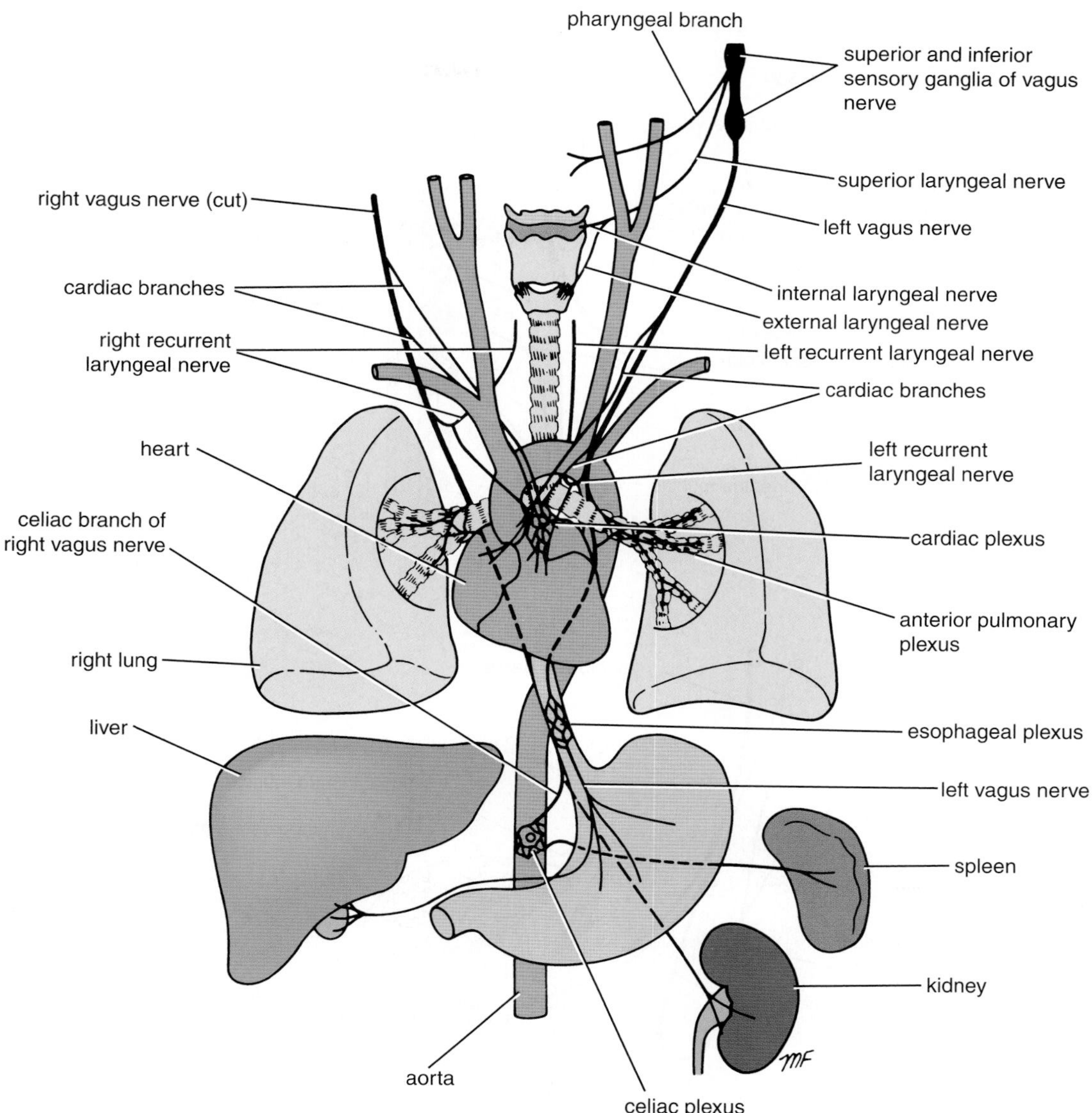

Figure 11-69 Distribution of the vagus nerve.

- **Recurrent laryngeal nerve** (Fig. 11-69). On the right side, the nerve hooks around the **first part of the subclavian artery** and then ascends in the groove between the trachea and the esophagus. On the left side, the nerve hooks around the **arch of the aorta** and then ascends into the neck between the trachea and the esophagus. The nerve is closely related to the inferior thyroid artery, and it supplies all the muscles of the larynx, except the cricothyroid muscle, the mucous membrane of the larynx below the vocal cords, and the mucous membrane of the upper part of the trachea.
- **Cardiac branches** (two or three) arise in the neck, descend into the thorax, and end in the cardiac plexus (Fig. 11-69).

The vagus nerve thus innervates the heart and great vessels within the thorax; the larynx, trachea, bronchi, and lungs; and much of the alimentary tract from the pharynx to the splenic flexure of the colon. It also supplies glands associated with the alimentary tract, such as the liver and pancreas.

The vagus nerve has the most extensive distribution of all the cranial nerves and supplies the aforementioned structures with afferent and efferent fibers.

Accessory Nerve

The accessory nerve is a motor nerve. It consists of a cranial root (part) and a spinal root (part) (Fig. 11-70).

Cranial Root

The cranial root emerges from the anterior surface of the medulla oblongata between the olive and the inferior cerebellar peduncle (Fig. 11-70). The nerve runs laterally in the posterior cranial fossa and joins the spinal root.

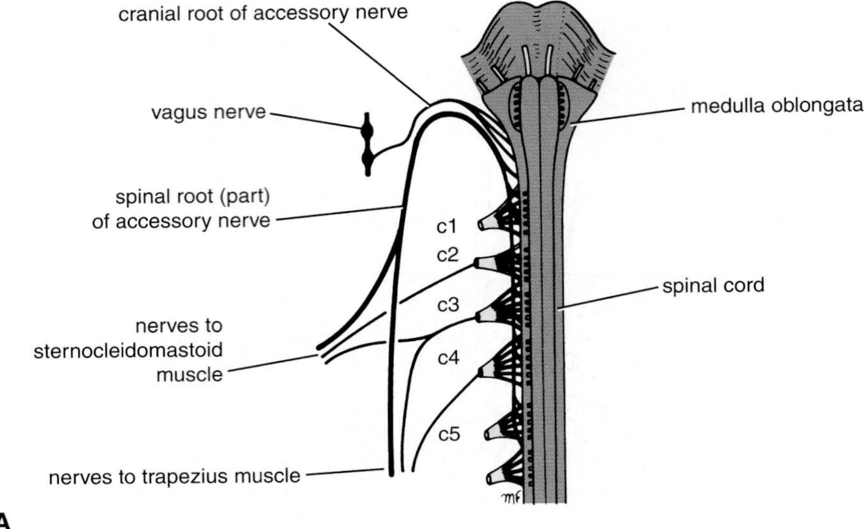

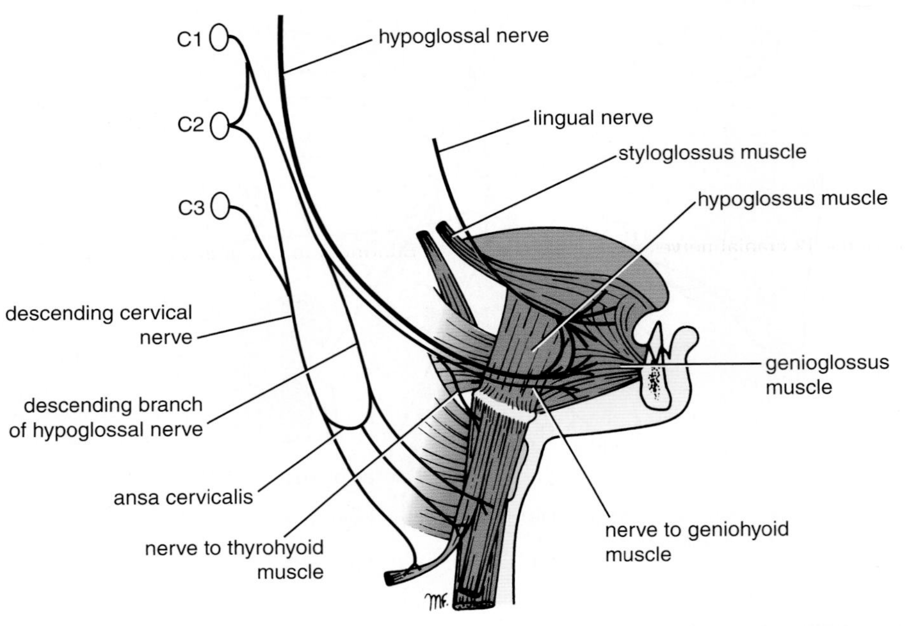

Figure 11-70 **A.** Origin and distribution of the accessory nerve. **B.** Distribution of the hypoglossal nerve.

Spinal Root

The spinal root arises from nerve cells in the anterior gray column (horn) of the upper five segments of the cervical part of the spinal cord (Fig. 11-70). The nerve ascends alongside the spinal cord and enters the skull through the foramen magnum. It then turns laterally to join the cranial root.

The two roots unite and leave the skull through the jugular foramen. The roots then separate: The cranial root joins the vagus nerves and is distributed in its branches to the muscles of the soft palate and pharynx (via the pharyngeal plexus) and to the muscles of the larynx (except the cricothyroid muscle). The spinal root runs downward and laterally and enters the deep surface of the sternocleidomastoid muscle, which it supplies, and then crosses the posterior triangle of the neck to supply the trapezius muscle (Fig. 11-55).

The accessory nerve thus brings about movements of the soft palate, pharynx, and larynx and controls the movements of the sternocleidomastoid and trapezius muscles, two large muscles in the neck.

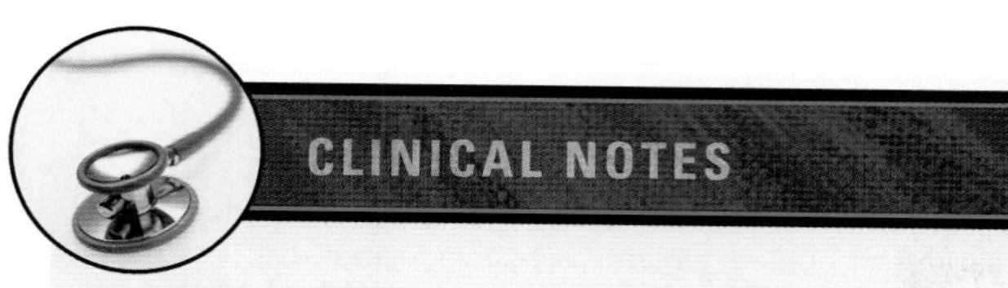

CLINICAL NOTES

Injury to the Spinal Part of the Accessory Nerve

The spinal part of the accessory nerve crosses the posterior triangle in a relatively superficial position. It can be injured at operation or from penetrating wounds. The trapezius muscle is paralyzed, the muscle will show wasting, and the shoulder will drop. The patient will experience difficulty in elevating the arm above the head, having abducted it to a right angle by using the deltoid muscle.

Clinical examination of this nerve involves asking the patient to rotate the head to one side against resistance, causing the sternocleidomastoid of the opposite side to come into action. Then the patient is asked to shrug the shoulders, causing the trapezius muscles to come into action.

Hypoglossal Nerve

The hypoglossal nerve is a motor nerve. It emerges on the anterior surface of the medulla oblongata between the pyramid and the olive, crosses the posterior cranial fossa, and leaves the skull through the hypoglossal canal. The nerve then passes downward and forward in the neck and crosses the internal and external carotid arteries to reach the tongue (Fig. 11-70). In the upper part of its course, it is joined by C1 fibers from the cervical plexus.

Important Branches of the Hypoglossal Nerve

- **Meningeal branch**
- **Descending branch** (C1 fibers) passes downward and joins the **descending cervical nerve** (C2 and 3) to form the **ansa cervicalis.** Branches from this loop supply the omohyoid, the sternohyoid, and the sternothyroid muscles.
- **Nerve to the thyrohyoid muscle (C1)**
- **Muscular branches to all the muscles of the tongue** except the palatoglossus (pharyngeal plexus)
- **Nerve to the geniohyoid muscle (C1).** The hypoglossal nerve thus innervates the muscles of the tongue (ex-

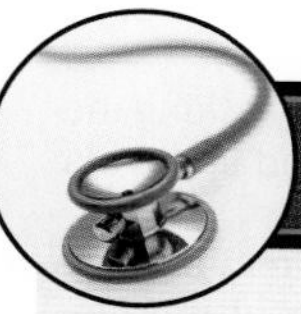

CLINICAL NOTES

Clinical Testing of the Cranial Nerves

Systematic examination of the 12 cranial nerves is an important part of the examination of every neurologic patient. It may reveal a lesion of a cranial nerve nucleus or its central connections, or it may show an interruption of the lower motor neurons.

Testing the Integrity of the Olfactory Nerve

The olfactory nerve can be tested by applying substances with different odors to each nostril in turn. It should be remembered that food flavors depend on the sense of smell and not on the sense of taste. Fractures of the anterior cranial fossa or cerebral tumors of the frontal lobes may produce lesions of the olfactory nerves, with consequent loss of the sense of smell **(anosmia).**

Testing the Integrity of the Optic Nerve

The optic nerve is evaluated by first asking the patient whether any changes in eyesight have been noted. The acuity of vision is then tested by using charts with lines of print of varying size. The retinas and optic discs should then be examined with an ophthalmoscope. When examining the optic disc, it should be remembered that the intracranial subarachnoid space extends forward around the optic nerve to the back of the eyeball. The retinal artery and vein run in the optic nerve and cross the subarachnoid space of the nerve sheath a short distance behind the eyeball. A rise in cerebrospinal fluid pressure in the subarachnoid space will compress the thin walls of the retinal vein as it crosses the space, resulting in congestion of the retinal veins, edema of the retina, and bulging of the optic disc **(papilledema).**

The visual fields should then be tested. The patient is asked to gaze straight ahead at a fixed object with the eye under test, the opposite eye being covered. A small object is then moved in an arc around the periphery of the field of vision, and the patient is asked whether he or she can see the object. It is important not to miss loss or impairment of vision in the central area of the field **(central scotoma).**

Blindness in one half of each visual field is called **hemianopia.** Lesions of the optic tract and optic radiation produce the same hemianopia for both eyes, that is, **homonymous hemianopia. Bitemporal hemianopia** is a loss of the lateral halves of the fields of vision of both eyes (i.e., loss of function of the medial half of both retinas). This condition is most commonly produced by a tumor of the pituitary gland exerting pressure on the optic chiasma.

Testing the Integrity of the Oculomotor, Trochlear, and Abducent Nerves

The oculomotor, trochlear, and abducent nerves innervate the muscles that move the eyeball. The oculomotor nerve supplies all the orbital muscles except the superior oblique and the lateral rectus. It also supplies the levator palpebrae superioris and the smooth muscles concerned with accommodation—namely, the sphincter pupillae and the ciliary muscle. The trochlear nerve supplies the superior oblique muscle, and the abducent nerve supplies the lateral rectus.

To examine the ocular muscles, the patient's head is fixed and he or she is asked to move the eyes in turn to the left, to the right, upward, and downward, as far as possible in each direction.

In **complete third nerve paralysis** the eye cannot be moved upward, downward, or inward. At rest the eye looks laterally **(external strabismus)** because of the activity of the lateral rectus and downward because of the activity of the superior oblique. The patient sees double **(diplopia).** Drooping of the upper eyelid **(ptosis)** occurs because of paralysis of the levator palpebrae superioris. The pupil is widely dilated and nonreactive to light because of the paralysis of the sphincter pupillae and the unopposed action of the dilator pupillae (supplied by the sympathetic). Accommodation of the eye is paralyzed.

(continues)

Clinical Notes, *continued*

In **fourth nerve paralysis** the patient complains of double vision on looking straight downward. This is because the superior oblique is paralyzed and the eye turns medially as the inferior rectus pulls the eye downward.

In **sixth nerve paralysis** the patient cannot turn the eyeball laterally. When looking straight ahead, the lateral rectus is paralyzed, and the unopposed medial rectus pulls the eyeball medially, causing internal strabismus.

Testing the Integrity of the Trigeminal Nerve

The trigeminal nerve has sensory and motor roots. The sensory root passes to the trigeminal ganglion, from which emerge the ophthalmic (V1), maxillary (V2), and mandibular (V3) divisions. The motor root joins the mandibular division.

The sensory function can be tested by using a cotton wisp over each area of the face supplied by the divisions of the trigeminal nerve (Fig. 11-50).

The motor function can be tested by asking the patient to clench the teeth. The masseter and the temporalis muscles, which are innervated by the mandibular division of the trigeminal nerve, can be palpated and felt to harden as they contract.

Testing the Integrity of the Facial Nerve

The facial nerve supplies the muscles of facial expression; supplies the anterior two thirds of the tongue with taste fibers; and is secretomotor to the lacrimal, submandibular, and sublingual glands.

The anatomic relationship of this nerve to other structures enables a physician to localize lesions of the nerve accurately. If the sixth and seventh nerves are not functioning, this would suggest a lesion within the pons of the brain. If the eighth and seventh nerves are not functioning, this would suggest a lesion in the internal acoustic meatus. If the patient is excessively sensitive to sound in one ear, the lesion probably involves the nerve to the stapedius. Loss of taste over the anterior two thirds of the tongue implies that the seventh nerve is damaged proximal to the point where it gives off the chorda tympani.

To test the facial nerve, the patient is asked to show the teeth by separating the lips with the teeth clenched, and then to close the eyes. Taste on each half of the anterior two thirds of the tongue can be tested with sugar, salt, vinegar, and quinine for the sweet, salt, sour, and bitter sensations, respectively.

It should be remembered that the part of the facial nerve nucleus that controls the muscles of the upper part of the face receives corticobulbar fibers from both cerebral cortices. Therefore, in patients with an upper motor neuron lesion, only the muscles of the lower part of the face will be paralyzed. However, in patients with a lower motor neuron lesion, all the muscles on the affected side of the face will be paralyzed. The lower eyelid will droop, and the angle of the mouth will sag. Tears will flow over the lower eyelid, and saliva will dribble from the corner of the mouth. The patient will be unable to close the eye and cannot expose the teeth fully on the affected side.

Testing the Integrity of the Vestibulocochlear Nerve

The vestibulocochlear nerve innervates the utricle and saccule, which are sensitive to static changes in equilibrium; the semicircular canals, which are sensitive to changes in dynamic equilibrium; and the cochlea, which is sensitive to sound.

Disturbances of vestibular function include dizziness **(vertigo)** and **nystagmus.** The latter is an uncontrollable pendular movement of the eyes. Disturbances of cochlear function reveal themselves as deafness and ringing in the ears **(tinnitus).** The patient's ability to hear a voice or a tuning fork should be tested, with each ear tested separately.

Testing the Integrity of the Glossopharyngeal Nerve

The glossopharyngeal nerve supplies the stylopharyngeus muscle and sends secretomotor fibers to the parotid gland. Sensory fibers innervate the posterior one third of the tongue.

The integrity of this nerve may be evaluated by testing the patient's general sensation and that of taste on the posterior third of the tongue.

Testing the Integrity of the Vagus Nerve

The vagus nerve innervates many important organs, but the examination of this nerve depends on testing the function of the branches to the pharynx, soft palate, and larynx. The pharyngeal reflex may be tested by touching the lateral wall of the pharynx with a spatula. This should immediately cause the patient to gag—that is, the pharyngeal muscles will contract.

The innervation of the soft palate can be tested by asking the patient to say "ah." Normally, the soft palate rises and the uvula moves backward in the midline.

All the muscles of the larynx are supplied by the recurrent laryngeal branch of the vagus, except the cricothyroid muscle, which is supplied by the external laryngeal branch of the superior laryngeal branch of the vagus. Hoarseness or absence of the voice may occur. Laryngoscopic examination may reveal abductor paralysis (see page 807).

Testing the Integrity of the Accessory Nerve

The accessory nerve supplies the sternocleidomastoid and the trapezius muscles by means of its spinal part. The patient should be asked to rotate the head to one side against resistance, causing the sternocleidomastoid of the opposite side to come into action. Then the patient should be asked to shrug the shoulders, causing the trapezius muscles to come into action.

Testing the Integrity of the Hypoglossal Nerve

The hypoglossal nerve supplies the muscles of the tongue. The patient is asked to put out the tongue, and if a lesion of the nerve is present, it will be noted that the tongue deviates toward the paralyzed side (Fig. 11-78). This can be explained as follows. One of the genioglossus muscles, which pull the tongue forward, is paralyzed on the affected side. The other, normal genioglossus muscle pulls the unaffected side of the tongue forward, leaving the paralyzed side of the tongue stationary. The result is the tip of the tongue's deviation toward the paralyzed side. In patients with long-standing paralysis, the muscles on the affected side are wasted, and the tongue is wrinkled on that side.

Table 11-7 Summary of the Branches of the Cervical Plexus and Their Distribution

Branches	Distribution
Cutaneous	
Lesser occipital	Skin of scalp behind ear
Greater auricular	Skin over parotid salivary gland, auricle, and angle of jaw
Transverse cutaneous	Skin over side and front of neck
Supraclavicular	Skin over upper part of chest and shoulder
Muscular	
Segmental	Prevertebral muscles, levator scapulae
Ansa cervicalis (C1, 2, 3)	Omohyoid, sternohyoid, sternothyroid
C1 fibers via hypoglossal nerve	Thyrohyoid, geniohyoid
Phrenic nerve (C3, 4, 5)	Diaphragm (most important muscle of respiration)
Sensory	
Phrenic nerve (C3, 4, 5)	Pericardium, mediastinal parietal pleura, and pleura and peritoneum covering central diaphragm

cept the palatoglossus) and therefore controls the shape and movements of the tongue.

Main Nerves of the Neck

Cervical Plexus

The cervical plexus is formed by the anterior rami of the first four cervical nerves. The rami are joined by connecting branches, which form loops that lie in front of the origins of the levator scapulae and the scalenus medius muscles (Fig. 11-57). The plexus is covered in front by the prevertebral layer of deep cervical fascia and is related to the internal jugular vein within the carotid sheath. The cervical plexus supplies the skin and the muscles of the head, the neck, and the shoulders.

Branches

- **Cutaneous branches**
  The **lesser occipital nerve** (C2), which supplies the back of the scalp and the auricle
  The **greater auricular nerve** (C2 and3), which supplies the skin over the angle of the mandible
  The **transverse cervical nerve** (C2 and 3), which supplies the skin over the front of the neck
  The **supraclavicular nerves** (C3 and 4). The medial, and intermediate, and lateral branches supply the skin over the shoulder region. These nerves are important clinically, because pain may be referred along them from the phrenic nerve (gallbladder disease).
- **Muscular branches to the neck muscles.** Prevertebral muscles, sternocleidomastoid (proprioceptive, C2 and 3), levator scapulae (C3 and 4), and trapezius (proprioceptive, C3 and 4). A branch from C1 joins the hypoglossal nerve. Some of these C1 fibers later leave the hypoglossal as the descending branch, which unites with the **descending cervical nerve** (C2 and 3), to form the **ansa cervicalis** (Fig. 11-60). The first, second, and third cervical nerve fibers within the ansa cervicalis supply the omohyoid, sternohyoid, and sternothyroid muscles. Other C1 fibers within the hypoglossal nerve leave it as the nerve to the thyrohyoid and geniohyoid.
- **Muscular branch to the diaphragm.** Phrenic nerve

Phrenic Nerve

The phrenic nerve arises in the neck from the third, fourth, and fifth cervical nerves of the cervical plexus. It runs vertically downward across the front of the scalenus anterior muscle (Fig. 11-57) and enters the thorax by passing in front of the subclavian artery. Its further course in the thorax is described on page 127.

The phrenic nerve is the only motor nerve supply to the diaphragm. It also sends sensory branches to the pericardium, the mediastinal parietal pleura, and the pleura and peritoneum covering the upper and lower surfaces of the central part of the diaphragm.

Table 11-7 summarizes the branches of the cervical plexus and their distribution.

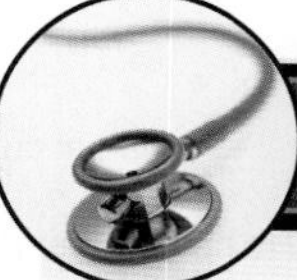

CLINICAL NOTES

Phrenic Nerve Injury and Paralysis of the Diaphragm

The phrenic nerve, which arises from the anterior rami of the third, fourth, and fifth cervical nerves, is of considerable clinical importance because it is the sole nerve supply to the muscle of the diaphragm. Each phrenic nerve supplies the corresponding half of the diaphragm.

The phrenic nerve can be injured by penetrating wounds in the neck. If that occurs, the paralyzed half of the diaphragm relaxes and is pushed up into the thorax by the positive abdominal pressure. Consequently, the lower lobe of the lung on that side may collapse.

About one third of persons have an **accessory phrenic nerve.** The root from the fifth cervical nerve may be incorporated in the nerve to the subclavius and may join the main phrenic nerve trunk in the thorax.

Brachial Plexus

The brachial plexus is formed in the posterior triangle of the neck by the union of the anterior rami of the fifth, sixth, seventh, and eighth cervical and the first thoracic spinal nerves (Fig. 11-71). This plexus is divided into **roots, trunks, divisions,** and **cords.** The roots of C5 and 6 unite to form the **upper trunk,** the root of C7 continues as the **middle trunk,** and the roots of C8 and T1 unite to form the **lower trunk.** Each trunk then divides into **anterior** and **posterior divisions.** The anterior divisions of the upper and middle trunks unite to form the **lateral cord,** the anterior division of the lower trunk continues as the **medial cord,** and the posterior divisions of all three trunks join to form the **posterior cord.**

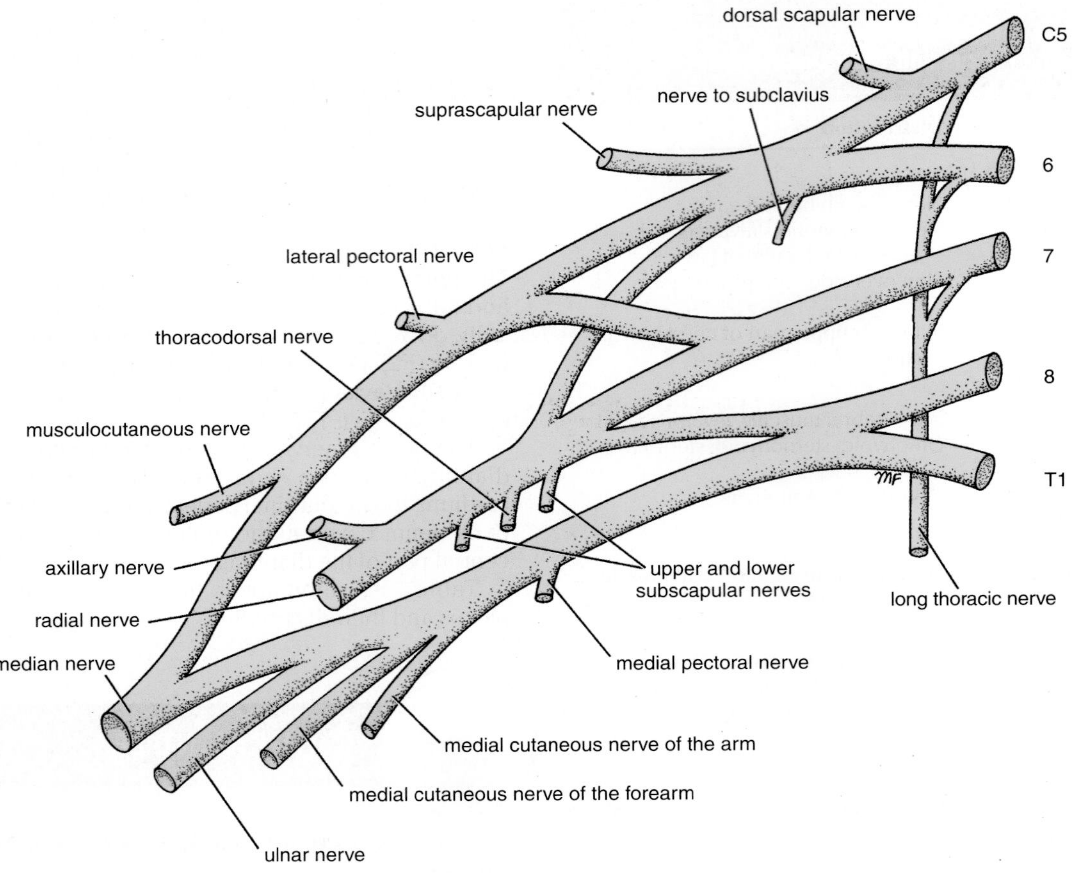

Figure 11-71 Brachial plexus and its branches.

The roots of the brachial plexus enter the base of the neck between the scalenus anterior and the scalenus medius muscles (Fig. 11-57). The trunks and divisions cross the posterior triangle of the neck, and the cords become arranged around the axillary artery in the axilla (see Fig. 9-20). Here, the brachial plexus and the axillary artery and vein are enclosed in the **axillary sheath.**

Branches

The branches of the brachial plexus and their distribution are summarized in Table 9-4.

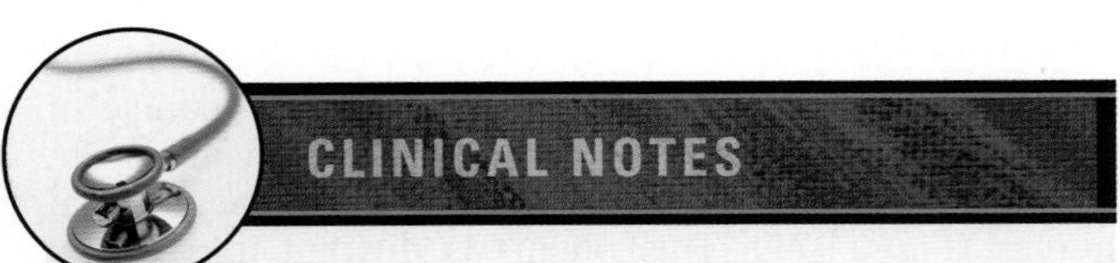

Injury to the Brachial Plexus

The roots and trunks of the brachial plexus occupy the anteroinferior angle of the posterior triangle of the neck. Incomplete lesions can result from stab or bullet wounds, traction, or pressure injuries. The clinical findings in the Erb-Duchenne and the Klumpke's lesions are fully described on pages 536 and 537.

(continues)

Clinical Notes, *continued*

Brachial Plexus Nerve Block

It will be remembered that the axillary sheath, formed from the prevertebral layer of deep cervical fascia, encloses the brachial plexus and the axillary artery. A brachial plexus nerve block can easily be obtained by closing the distal part of the sheath in the axilla with finger pressure, inserting a syringe needle into the proximal part of the sheath, and then injecting a local anesthetic. The anesthetic solution is massaged along the sheath, producing a nerve block. The syringe needle may be inserted into the axillary sheath in the lower part of the posterior triangle of the neck or in the axilla.

Compression of the Brachial Plexus and the Subclavian Artery

At the root of the neck, the brachial plexus and the subclavian artery enter the posterior triangle through a narrow muscular–bony triangle. The boundaries of the narrow triangle are formed in front by the scalenus anterior, behind by the scalenus medius, and below by the first rib. In the presence of a cervical rib (see page 50), the first thoracic nerve and the subclavian artery are raised and angulated as they pass over the rib. Partial or complete occlusion of the artery causes ischemic muscle pain in the arm, which is worsened by exercise. Rarely, pressure on the first thoracic nerve causes symptoms of pain in the forearm and hand and wasting of the small muscles of the hand.

The Autonomic Nervous System in the Head and Neck

Sympathetic Part

Cervical Part of the Sympathetic Trunk

The cervical part of the sympathetic trunk extends upward to the base of the skull and below to the neck of the first rib, where it becomes continuous with the thoracic part of the sympathetic trunk. It lies directly behind the internal and common carotid arteries (i.e., medial to the vagus) and is embedded in deep fascia between the carotid sheath and the prevertebral layer of deep fascia (Fig. 11-49).

The sympathetic trunk possesses three ganglia: the superior, middle, and inferior cervical ganglia.

Superior Cervical Ganglion

The superior cervical ganglion lies immediately below the skull (Fig. 11-60).

Branches

- The **internal carotid nerve,** consisting of postganglionic fibers, accompanies the internal carotid artery into the carotid canal in the temporal bone. It divides into branches around the artery to form the internal carotid plexus.
- **Gray rami communicantes** to the upper four anterior rami of the cervical nerves
- **Arterial branches** to the common and external carotid arteries. These branches form a plexus around the arteries and are distributed along the branches of the external carotid artery.
- **Cranial nerve branches,** which join the 9th, 10th, and 12th cranial nerves
- **Pharyngeal branches,** which unite with the pharyngeal branches of the glossopharyngeal and vagus nerves to form the pharyngeal plexus
- The **superior cardiac branch,** which descends in the neck and ends in the cardiac plexus in the thorax (see page 116)

Middle Cervical Ganglion

The middle cervical ganglion lies at the level of the cricoid cartilage (Fig. 11-57).

Branches

- **Gray rami communicantes** to the anterior rami of the fifth and sixth cervical nerves
- **Thyroid branches,** which pass along the inferior thyroid artery to the thyroid gland
- **The middle cardiac branch,** which descends in the neck and ends in the cardiac plexus in the thorax (see page 116)

Inferior Cervical Ganglion

The inferior cervical ganglion in most people is fused with the first thoracic ganglion to form the **stellate ganglion.** It lies in the interval between the transverse process of the seventh cervical vertebra and the neck of the first rib, behind the vertebral artery (Fig. 11-57).

Branches

- **Gray rami communicantes** to the anterior rami of the seventh and eighth cervical nerves
- **Arterial branches** to the subclavian and vertebral arteries
- The **inferior cardiac branch,** which descends to join the cardiac plexus in the thorax (see page 116)

The part of the sympathetic trunk connecting the middle cervical ganglion to the inferior or stellate ganglion is represented by two or more nerve bundles. The most anterior bundle crosses in front of the first part of the subclavian artery and then turns upward behind it. This anterior bundle is referred to as the **ansa subclavia** (Figs. 11-57 and 11-60).

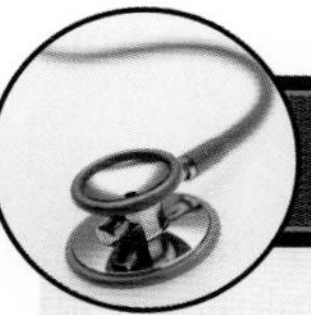

CLINICAL NOTES

Sympathectomy for Arterial Insufficiency of the Upper Limb

The sympathetic innervation of the upper limb is as follows: The preganglionic fibers leave the spinal cord in the second to the eighth thoracic nerves. On reaching the sympathetic trunk via the white rami, they ascend within the trunk and are relayed in the second thoracic, stellate, and middle cervical ganglia. Postganglionic fibers then join the roots of the brachial plexus as gray rami. Sympathectomy of the upper limb is a relatively common procedure for the treatment of arterial insufficiency. From this information, it is clear that the stellate and the second thoracic ganglia should be removed to block the sympathetic pathway to the arm completely.

Removal of the stellate ganglion also removes the sympathetic nerve supply to the head and neck on that side. This produces not only vasodilatation of the skin vessels, but also anhidrosis, nasal congestion, and Horner's syndrome. For this reason the stellate ganglion is usually left intact in sympathectomies of the upper limb.

Horner's Syndrome

Horner's syndrome includes constriction of the pupil, ptosis (drooping of the upper eyelid), and enophthalmos (depression of the eyeball into the orbital cavity). It is caused by an interruption of the sympathetic nerve supply to the orbit. Pathologic causes include lesions of the brainstem or cervical part of the spinal cord; traumatic injury to the cervical part of the sympa-

(continues)

Clinical Notes, *continued*

thetic trunk; traction of the stellate ganglion caused by a cervical rib; and involvement of the ganglion in cancerous growth, which may interrupt the peripheral part of the sympathetic pathway to the orbit.

Stellate Ganglion Block

A stellate ganglion block is performed by first palpating the large anterior tubercle (carotid tubercle) of the transverse process of the sixth cervical vertebra, which lies about a fingerbreadth lateral to the cricoid cartilage. The carotid sheath and the sternocleidomastoid muscle are pushed laterally and the needle of the anesthetic syringe is inserted through the skin over the tubercle. The local anesthetic is then injected beneath the prevertebral layer of deep cervical fascia. This procedure effectively blocks the ganglion and its rami communicantes.

Parasympathetic Part

The cranial portion of the craniosacral outflow of the parasympathetic part of the autonomic nervous system is located in the nuclei of the **oculomotor (3rd), facial (7th), glossopharyngeal (9th),** and **vagus (10th) cranial nerves.**

The parasympathetic nucleus of the oculomotor nerve is called the **Edinger-Westphal nucleus;** those of the facial nerve the **lacrimatory** and the **superior salivary nuclei;** that of the glossopharyngeal nerve the **inferior salivary nucleus;** and that of the vagus nerve the **dorsal nucleus of the vagus.** The axons of these connector nerve cells are myelinated preganglionic fibers that emerge from the brain within the cranial nerves.

These preganglionic fibers synapse in peripheral ganglia located close to the viscera they innervate. The cranial parasympathetic ganglia are the **ciliary,** the **pterygopalatine,** the **submandibular,** and the **otic.** In certain locations, the ganglion cells are placed in nerve plexuses, such as the **cardiac plexus,** the **pulmonary plexus,** the **myenteric plexus (Auerbach's plexus),** and the **mucosal plexus (Meissner's plexus).** The last two plexuses are found in the gastrointestinal tract. The postganglionic fibers are nonmyelinated, and they are short in length.

The Digestive System in the Head and Neck

The Mouth

The Lips

The lips are two fleshy folds that surround the oral orifice (Fig. 11-72). They are covered on the outside by skin and are lined on the inside by mucous membrane. The substance of the lips is made up by the orbicularis oris muscle and the muscles that radiate from the lips into the face (Fig. 11-73). Also included are the labial blood vessels and nerves, connective tissue, and many small salivary glands. The **philtrum** is the shallow vertical groove seen in the midline on the outer surface of the upper lip. Median folds of mucous membrane—the **labial frenulae**—connect the inner surface of the lips to the gums.

The Mouth Cavity

The mouth extends from the lips to the pharynx. The entrance into the pharynx, the **oropharyngeal isthmus,** is formed on each side by the palatoglossal fold (Fig. 11-72).

The mouth is divided into the vestibule and the mouth cavity proper.

Vestibule

The vestibule lies between the lips and the cheeks externally and the gums and the teeth internally. This slitlike space communicates with the exterior through the oral fissure between the lips. When the jaws are closed, it communicates with the mouth proper behind the third molar tooth on each side. The vestibule is limited above and below by the reflection of the mucous membrane from the lips and cheeks to the gums.

The lateral wall of the vestibule is formed by the cheek, which is made up by the buccinator muscle and is lined with mucous membrane. The tone of the buccinator muscle and that of the muscles of the lips keeps the walls of the vestibule in contact with one another. The **duct of the parotid salivary gland** opens on a small papilla into the vestibule opposite the upper second molar tooth (Fig. 11-72).

Mouth Proper

The mouth proper has a roof and a floor.

Roof of Mouth

The roof of the mouth is formed by the hard palate in front and the soft palate behind (Fig. 11-72).

Floor of Mouth

The floor is formed largely by the anterior two thirds of the tongue and by the reflection of the mucous membrane from the sides of the tongue to the gum of the mandible. A fold of mucous membrane called the **frenulum of the tongue** connects the undersurface of the tongue in the midline to the floor of the mouth (Fig. 11-72). Lateral to the frenulum, the mucous membrane forms a fringed fold, the **plica fimbriata** (Fig. 11-72).

The submandibular duct of the submandibular gland opens onto the floor of the mouth on the summit of a small papilla on either side of the frenulum of the tongue (Fig. 11-72). The sublingual gland projects up into the mouth, producing a low fold of mucous membrane, the **sublingual fold.** Numerous ducts of the gland open on the summit of the fold.

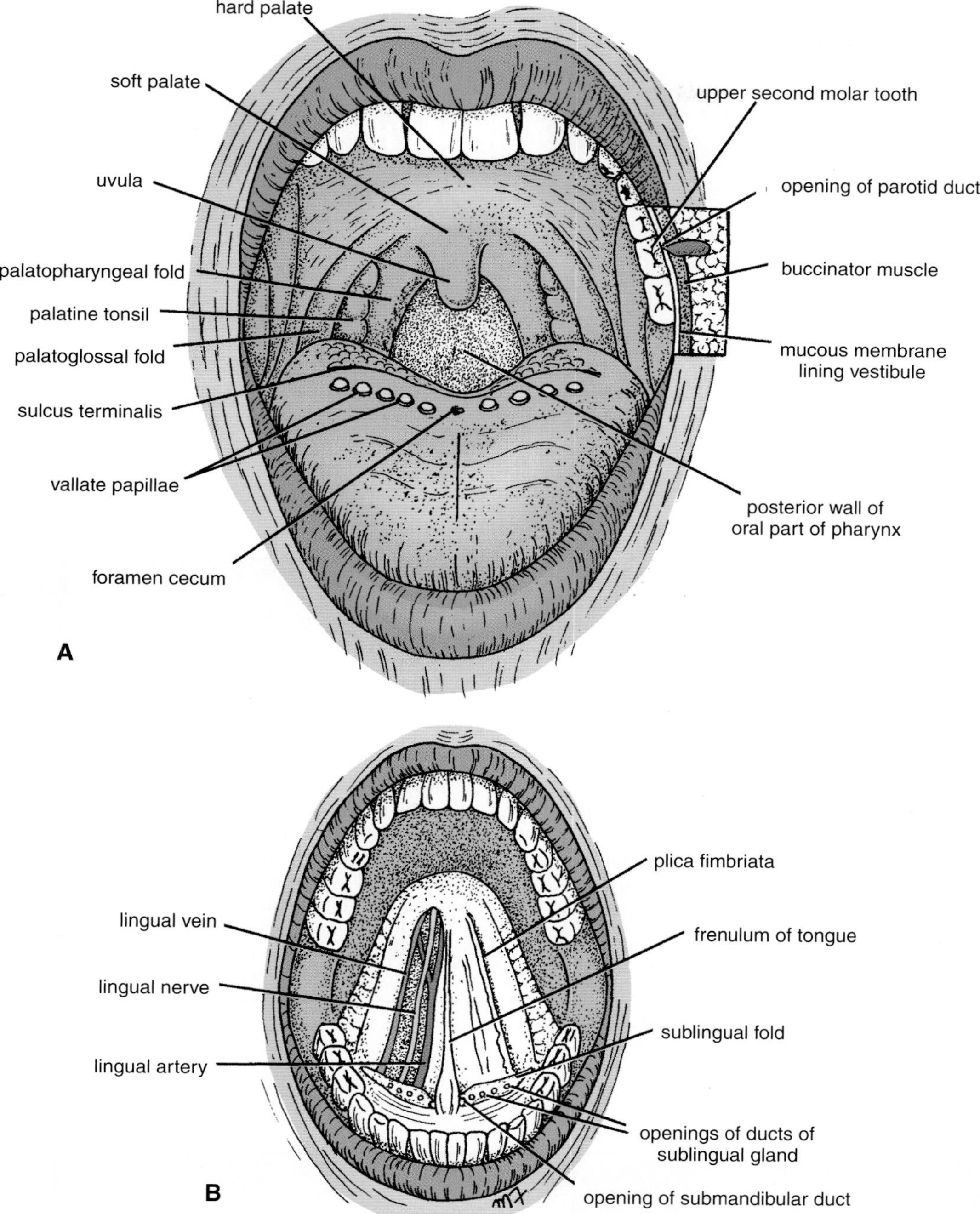

Figure 11-72 **A.** Cavity of the mouth. Cheek on the left side of the face has been cut away to show the buccinator muscle and the parotid duct. **B.** Undersurface of the tongue.

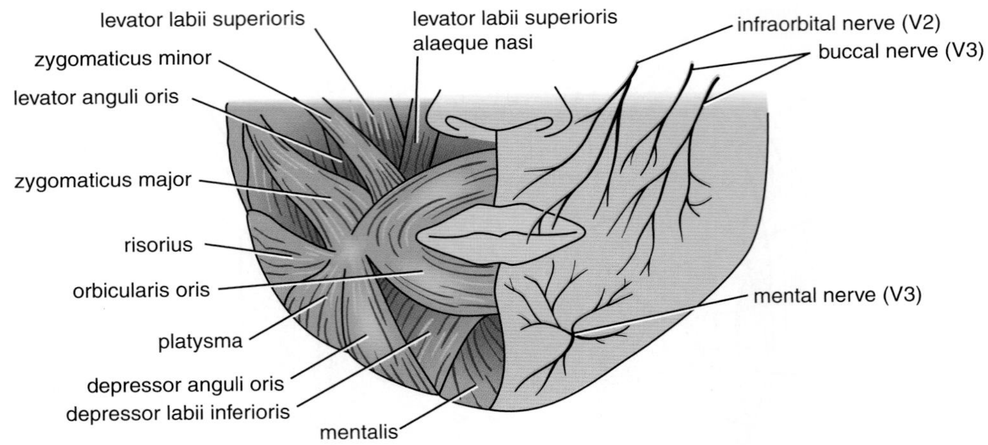

Figure 11-73 Arrangement of the facial muscles around the lips; the sensory nerve supply of the lips is shown.

Mucous Membrane of the Mouth

In the vestibule the mucous membrane is tethered to the buccinator muscle by elastic fibers in the submucosa that prevent redundant folds of mucous membrane from being bitten between the teeth when the jaws are closed. The mucous membrane of the gingiva, or gum, is strongly attached to the alveolar periosteum.

Sensory Innervation of the Mouth

Roof: The greater palatine and nasopalatine nerves (Fig.11-74) from the maxillary division of the trigeminal nerve

Floor: The lingual nerve (common sensation), a branch of the mandibular division of the trigeminal nerve. The taste fibers travel in the chorda tympani nerve, a branch of the facial nerve.

Cheek: The buccal nerve, a branch of the mandibular division of the trigeminal nerve (the buccinator muscle is innervated by the buccal branch of the facial nerve)

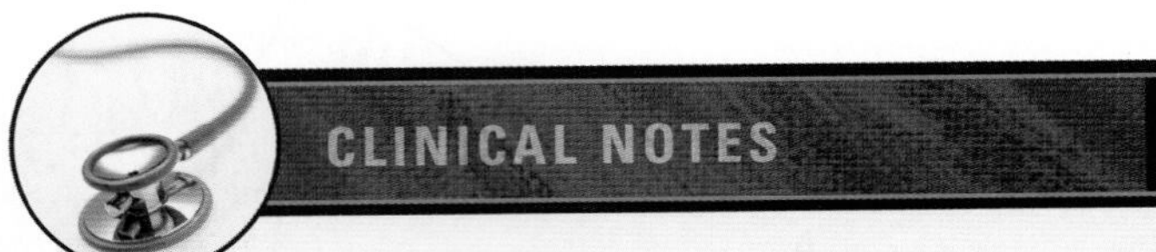

Clinical Significance of the Examination of the Mouth

The mouth is one of the important areas of the body that the medical professional is called on to examine. Needless to say, the physician must be able to recognize all the structures visible in the mouth and be familiar with the normal variations in the color of the mucous membrane covering underlying structures. The sensory nerve supply and lymph drainage of the mouth cavity should be known. The close relation of the lingual nerve to the lower third molar tooth should be remembered. The close relation of the submandibular duct to the floor of the mouth may enable one to palpate a calculus in cases of periodic swelling of the submandibular salivary gland.

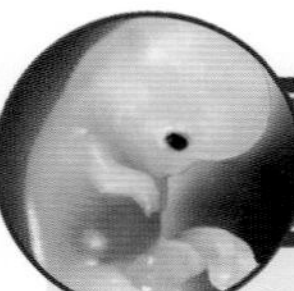

EMBRYOLOGIC NOTES

Development of the Mouth

The cavity of the mouth is formed from two sources: a depression from the exterior, called the stomodeum, which is lined with ectoderm, and a part immediately posterior to this, derived from the cephalic end of the foregut and lined with entoderm. These two parts at first are separated by the **buccopharyngeal membrane,** but this breaks down and disappears during the third week of development (Fig. 11-75). If this membrane were to persist into adult life, it would occupy an imaginary plane extending obliquely from the region of the body of the sphenoid, through the soft palate, and down to the inner surface of the mandible inferior to the incisor teeth. This means that the structures that are situated in the mouth anterior to this plane are derived from ectoderm. Thus, the epithelium of the hard palate, sides of the mouth, lips, and enamel of the teeth are ectodermal structures. The secretory epithelium and cells lining the ducts of the parotid salivary gland also are derived from ectoderm. On the other hand, the epithelium of the tongue, the floor of the mouth, the palatoglossal and palatopharyngeal folds, and most of the soft palate are entodermal in origin. The secretory and duct epithelia of the sublingual and submandibular salivary glands also are believed to be of entodermal origin.

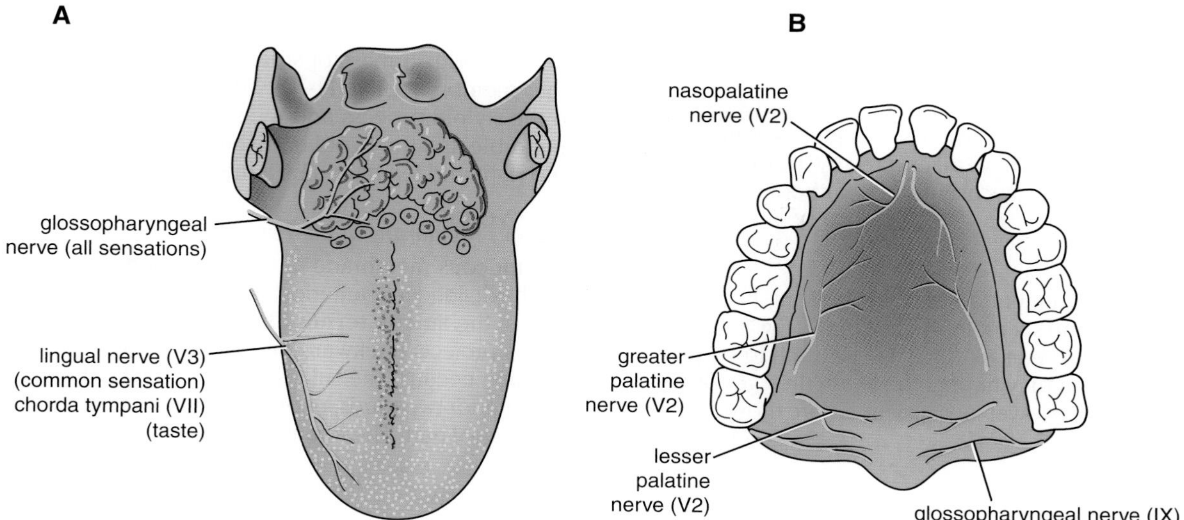

Figure 11-74 **A.** Sensory nerve supply to the mucous membrane of the tongue. **B.** Sensory nerve supply to the mucous membrane of the hard and soft palate; taste fibers run with branches of the maxillary nerve (V2) and join the greater petrosal branch of the facial nerve.

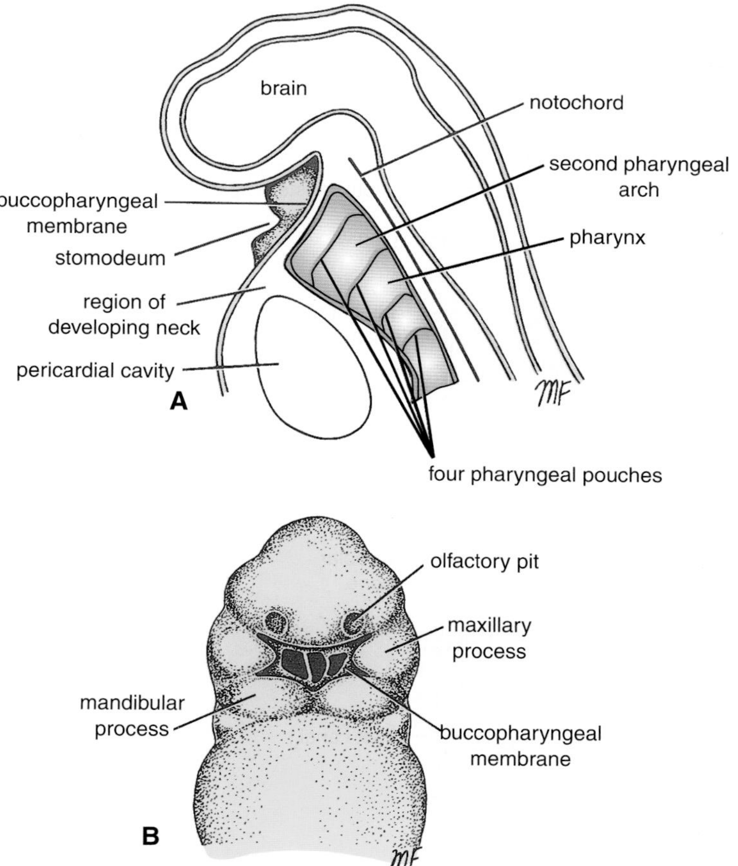

Figure 11-75 **A.** Sagittal section of the embryo showing the position of the buccopharyngeal membrane. **B.** The face of the developing embryo showing the buccopharyngeal membrane breaking down.

The Teeth

Deciduous Teeth

There are 20 deciduous teeth: four incisors, two canines, and four molars in each jaw. They begin to erupt about 6 months after birth and have all erupted by the end of 2 years. The teeth of the lower jaw usually appear before those of the upper jaw.

Permanent Teeth

There are 32 permanent teeth: four incisors, two canines, four premolars, and six molars in each jaw (Fig. 11-76). They begin to erupt at 6 years of age. The last tooth to erupt is the third molar, which may happen between the ages of 17 and 30. The teeth of the lower jaw appear before those of the upper jaw.

The Tongue

The tongue is a mass of striated muscle covered with mucous membrane (Fig. 11-77). The muscles attach the tongue to the styloid process and the soft palate above and to the mandible and the hyoid bone below. The tongue is divided into right and left halves by a median **fibrous septum.**

Mucous Membrane of the Tongue

The mucous membrane of the upper surface of the tongue can be divided into anterior and posterior parts by a V-shaped sulcus, the **sulcus terminalis** (Fig. 11-77). The apex of the sulcus projects backward and is marked by a small pit, the foramen cecum. The sulcus serves to divide the tongue into the anterior two thirds, or oral part, and the posterior third, or pharyngeal part. The foramen cecum is an embryologic rem-

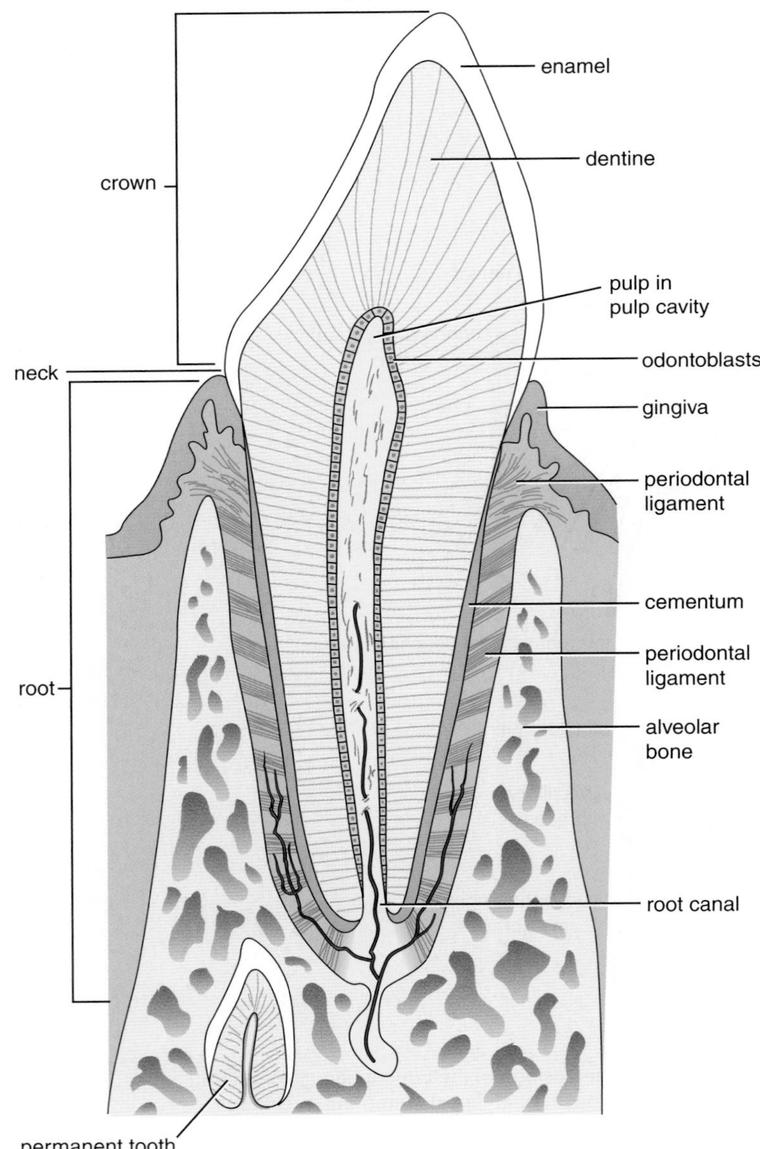

Figure 11-76 Sagittal section through the lower jaw and gum showing an erupted temporary incisor tooth and a developing permanent tooth.

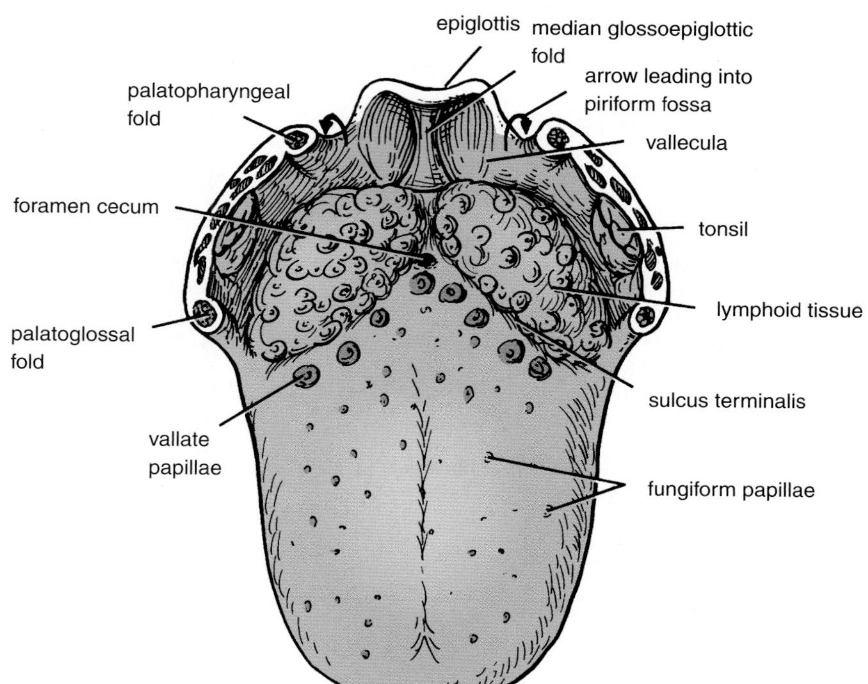

Figure 11-77 Dorsal surface of the tongue showing the valleculae, the epiglottis, and the entrance into the piriform fossa on each side (*arrows*).

nant and marks the site of the upper end of the thyroglossal duct (see page 819).

Three types of papillae are present on the upper surface of the anterior two thirds of the tongue: the **filiform papillae,** the **fungiform papillae,** and the **vallate papillae.**

The mucous membrane covering the posterior third of the tongue is devoid of papillae but has an irregular surface (Fig. 11-77), caused by the presence of underlying lymph nodules, the **lingual tonsil.**

The mucous membrane on the inferior surface of the tongue is reflected from the tongue to the floor of the mouth. In the midline anteriorly, the undersurface of the tongue is connected to the floor of the mouth by a fold of mucous membrane, the **frenulum of the tongue.** On the lateral side of the frenulum, the deep lingual vein can be seen through the mucous membrane. Lateral to the lingual vein, the mucous membrane forms a fringed fold called the **plica fimbriata** (Fig. 11-72).

Muscles of the Tongue

The muscles of the tongue are divided into two types: intrinsic and extrinsic.

Intrinsic Muscles

These muscles are confined to the tongue and are not attached to bone. They consist of longitudinal, transverse, and vertical fibers.

Nerve supply: Hypoglossal nerve

Action: Alter the shape of the tongue

Extrinsic Muscles

These muscles are attached to bones and the soft palate. They are the genioglossus, the hyoglossus, the styloglossus, and the palatoglossus.

Nerve supply: Hypoglossal nerve

The origin, insertion, nerve supply, and action of the tongue muscles are summarized in Table 11-8.

Blood Supply

The lingual artery, the tonsillar branch of the facial artery, and the ascending pharyngeal artery supply the tongue. The veins drain into the internal jugular vein.

Lymph Drainage

Tip: Submental lymph nodes

Sides of the anterior two thirds: Submandibular and deep cervical lymph nodes

Posterior third: Deep cervical lymph nodes

Sensory Innervation

Anterior two thirds: Lingual nerve branch of mandibular division of trigeminal nerve (general sensation) and chorda tympani branch of the facial nerve (taste)

Posterior third: Glossopharyngeal nerve (general sensation and taste)

Movements of the Tongue

Protrusion: The genioglossus muscles on both sides acting together (Fig. 11-78)

Retraction: Styloglossus and hyoglossus muscles on both sides acting together

Depression: Hyoglossus muscles on both sides acting together

Retraction and elevation of the posterior third: Styloglossus and palatoglossus muscles on both sides acting together

Shape changes: Intrinsic muscles

Table 11-8	Muscles of Tongue			
Muscle	**Origin**	**Insertion**	**Nerve Supply**	**Action**
Intrinsic Muscles				
Longitudinal	Median septum and submucosa	Mucous membrane	Hypoglossal nerve	Alters shape of tongue
Transverse				
Vertical				
Extrinsic Muscles				
Genioglossus	Superior genial spine of mandible	Blends with other muscles of tongue	Hypoglossal nerve	Protrudes apex of tongue through mouth
Hyoglossus	Body and greater cornu of hyoid bone	Blends with other muscles of tongue	Hypoglossal nerve	Depresses tongue
Styloglossus	Styloid process of temporal bone	Blends with other muscles of tongue	Hypoglossal nerve	Draws tongue upward and backward
Palatoglossus	Palatine aponeurosis	Side of tongue	Pharyngeal plexus	Pulls roots of tongue upward and backward, narrows oropharyngeal isthmus

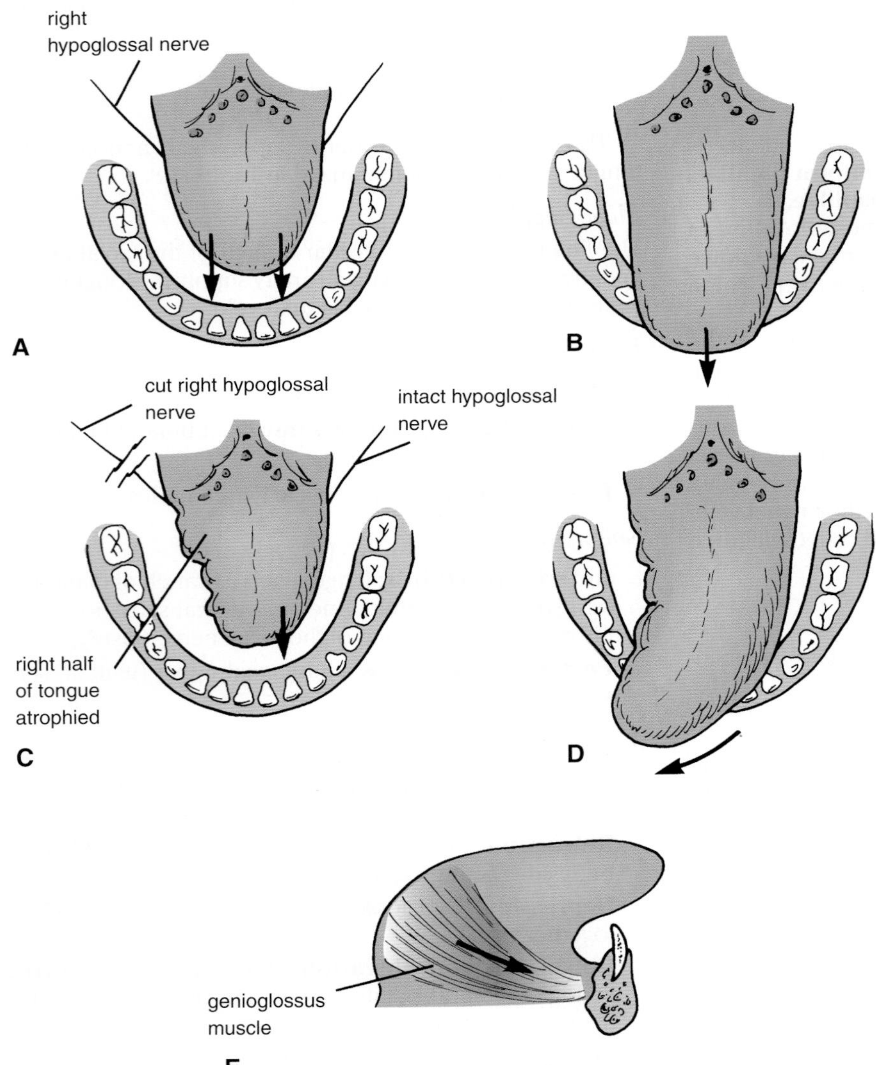

Figure 11-78 Diagrammatic representation of the action of the right and left genioglossus muscles of the tongue. **A.** The right and left muscles contract equally together and as a result (**B**) the tip of the tongue is protruded in the midline. **C.** The right hypoglossal nerve (which innervates the genioglossus muscle and the intrinsic tongue muscles on the same side) is cut and as a result the right side of the tongue is atrophied and wrinkled. **D.** When the patient is asked to protrude the tongue, the tip points to the side of the nerve lesion. **E.** The origin and insertion and direction of pull of the genioglossus muscle.

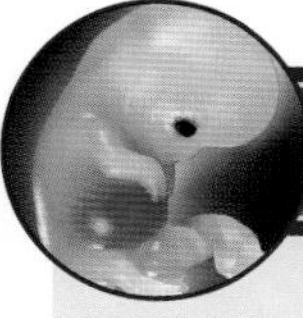

EMBRYOLOGIC NOTES

Development of the Tongue

At about the fourth week, a median swelling called the **tuberculum impar** appears in the entodermal ventral wall or floor of the pharynx (Fig. 11-79). A little later, another swelling, called the **lateral lingual swelling** (derived from the anterior end of each first pharyngeal arch), appears on each side of the tuberculum impar. The lateral lingual swellings now enlarge, grow medially, and fuse with each other and the tuberculum impar. The lingual swellings thus form the anterior two thirds of the body of the tongue, and since they are derived from the first pharyngeal arches, the mucous membrane on each side will be innervated by the lingual nerve, a branch of the mandibular division of the fifth cranial nerve (common sensation). The chorda tympani from the seventh cranial nerve (taste) also supplies this area.

Meanwhile, a second median swelling, called the **copula,** appears in the floor of the pharynx behind the tuberculum impar. The copula extends forward on each side of the tuberculum impar and becomes V shaped. At about this time, the anterior ends of the second, third, and fourth pharyngeal arches are entering this region. The anterior ends of the third arch on each side overgrow the other arches and extend into the copula, fusing in the midline. The copula now disappears. Thus, the mucous membrane of the posterior third of the tongue is formed from the third pharyngeal arches and is innervated by the ninth cranial nerve (common sensation and taste).

The anterior two thirds of the tongue is separated from the posterior third by a groove, the **sulcus terminalis,** which represents the interval between the lingual swellings of the first pharyngeal arches and the anterior ends of the third pharyngeal arches. Around the edge of the anterior two thirds of the tongue, the entodermal cells proliferate and grow inferiorly into the underlying mesenchyme. Later, these cells degenerate so that this part of the tongue becomes free. Some of the entodermal cells remain in the midline and help form the **frenulum of the tongue.**

Remember that the **circumvallate papillae** are situated on the mucous membrane just anterior to the sulcus terminalis, and that their taste buds are innervated by the ninth cranial nerve. It is presumed that during development the mucous membrane of the posterior third of the tongue becomes pulled anteriorly slightly, so that fibers of the ninth cranial nerve cross the succus terminalis to supply these taste buds (Fig. 11-79).

The muscles of the tongue are derived from the occipital myotomes, which at first are closely related to the developing hindbrain and later migrate inferiorly and anteriorly around the pharynx and enter the tongue. The migrating myotomes carry with them their innervation, the 12th cranial nerve, and this explains the long curving course taken by the 12th cranial nerve as it passes downward and forward in the carotid triangle of the neck (see page 769).

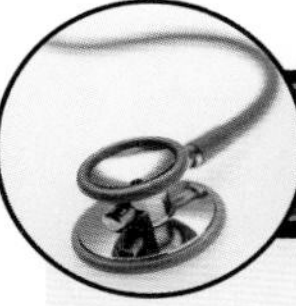

CLINICAL NOTES

Laceration of the Tongue

A wound of the tongue is often caused by the patient's teeth following a blow on the chin when the tongue is partly protruded from the mouth. It can also occur when a patient accidentally bites the tongue while eating, during recovery from an anesthetic, or during an epileptic attack. Bleeding is halted by grasping the tongue between the finger and thumb posterior to the laceration, thus occluding the branches of the lingual artery.

The Palate

The palate forms the roof of the mouth and the floor of the nasal cavity. It is divided into two parts: the hard palate in front and the soft palate behind.

Hard Palate

The hard palate is formed by the palatine processes of the maxillae and the horizontal plates of the palatine bones (Fig. 11-80). It is continuous behind with the soft palate.

Soft Palate

The soft palate is a mobile fold attached to the posterior border of the hard palate (Fig. 11-81). Its free posterior border presents in the midline a conical projection called the **uvula**. The soft palate is continuous at the sides with the lateral wall of the pharynx.

The soft palate is composed of mucous membrane, palatine aponeurosis, and muscles.

Mucous Membrane

The mucous membrane covers the upper and lower surfaces of the soft palate.

Palatine Aponeurosis

The palatine aponeurosis is a fibrous sheet attached to the posterior border of the hard palate. It is the expanded tendon of the tensor veli palatini muscle.

Muscles of the Soft Palate

The muscles of the soft palate are the tensor veli palatini, the levator veli palatini, the palatoglossus, the palatopharyngeus, and the musculus uvulae (Fig. 11-81).

The muscle fibers of the tensor veli palatini converge as they descend from their origin to form a narrow tendon, which turns medially around the pterygoid hamulus. The tendon, together with the tendon of the opposite side, expands to form the palatine aponeurosis. When the muscles of the two sides contract, the soft palate is tightened so that the soft palate may be moved upward or downward as a tense sheet.

The muscles of the soft palate, their origins, insertions, nerve supply, and actions are summarized in Table 11-9.

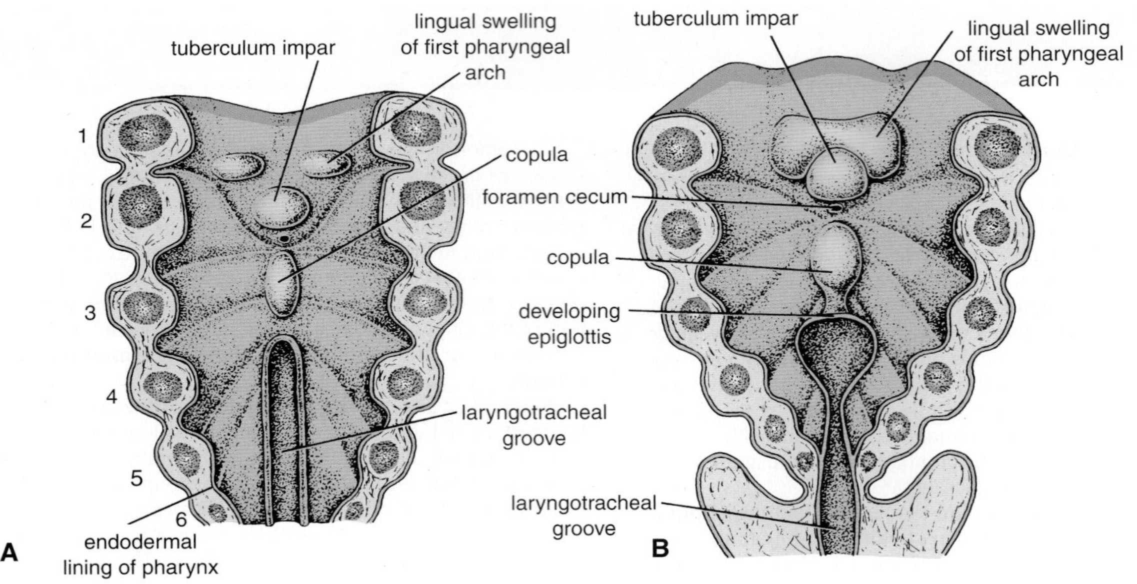

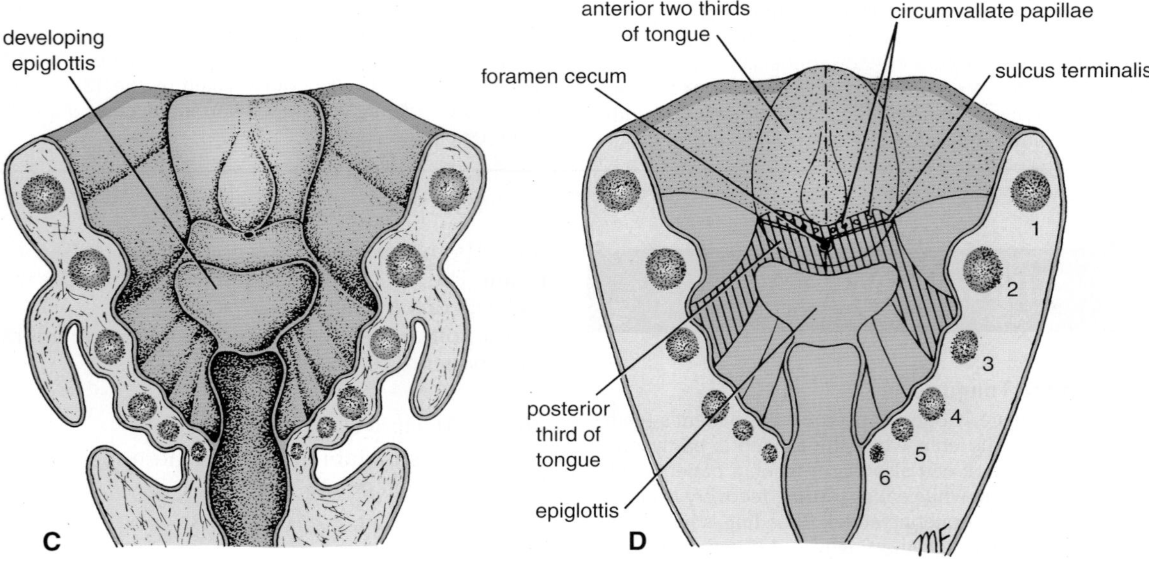

Figure 11-79 The floor of the pharynx showing the stages in the development of the tongue.

Nerve Supply of the Palate

The greater and lesser palatine nerves from the maxillary division of the trigeminal nerve enter the palate through the greater and lesser palatine foramina (Fig. 11-74). The nasopalatine nerve, also a branch of the maxillary nerve, enters the front of the hard palate through the incisive foramen. The glossopharyngeal nerve also supplies the soft palate.

Blood Supply of the Palate

The greater palatine branch of the maxillary artery, the ascending palatine branch of the facial artery, and the ascending pharyngeal artery

Lymph Drainage of the Palate

Deep Cervical Lymph Nodes

Palatoglossal Arch The palatoglossal arch is a fold of mucous membrane containing the **palatoglossus muscle,** which extends from the soft palate to the side of the tongue (Figs. 11-72 and 11-81). **The palatoglossal arch marks where the mouth becomes the pharynx.**

Palatopharyngeal Arch The palatopharyngeal arch is a fold of mucous membrane behind the palatoglossal arch (Figs. 11-72 and 11-81) that runs downward and laterally to join the pharyngeal wall. The muscle contained within the fold is the **palatopharyngeus muscle.** The **palatine tonsils,** which are masses of lymphoid tissue, are located between the palatoglossal and palatopharyngeal arches (Fig. 11-81).

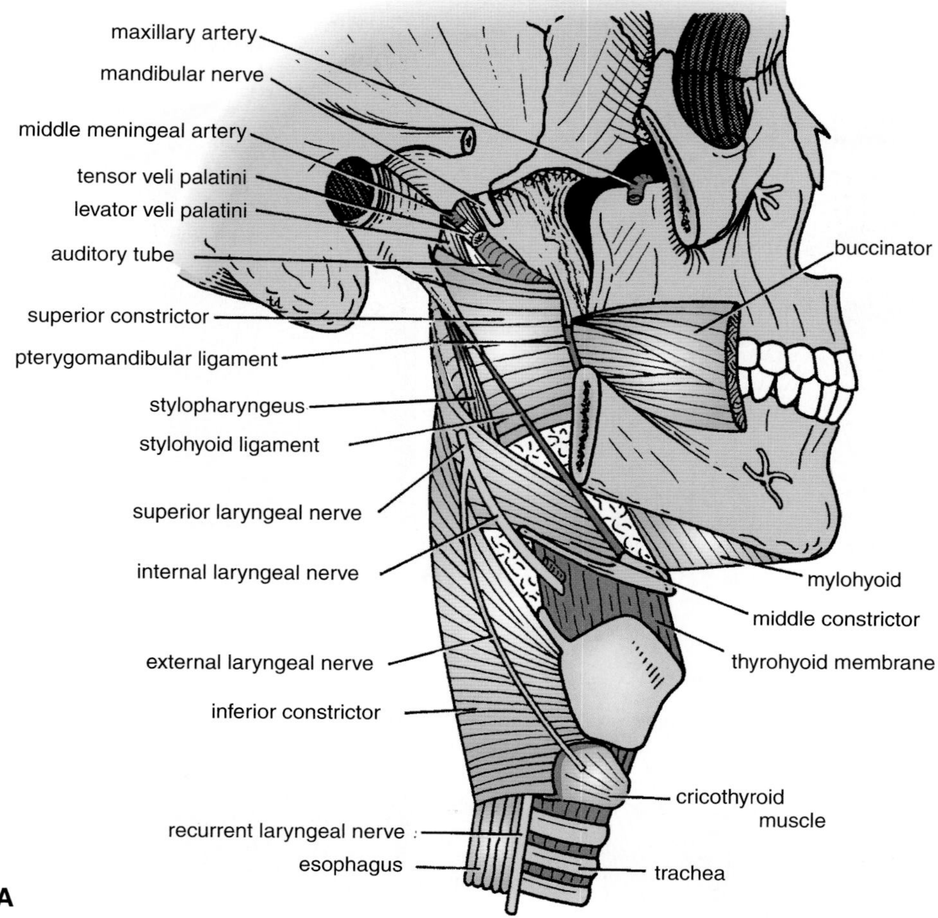

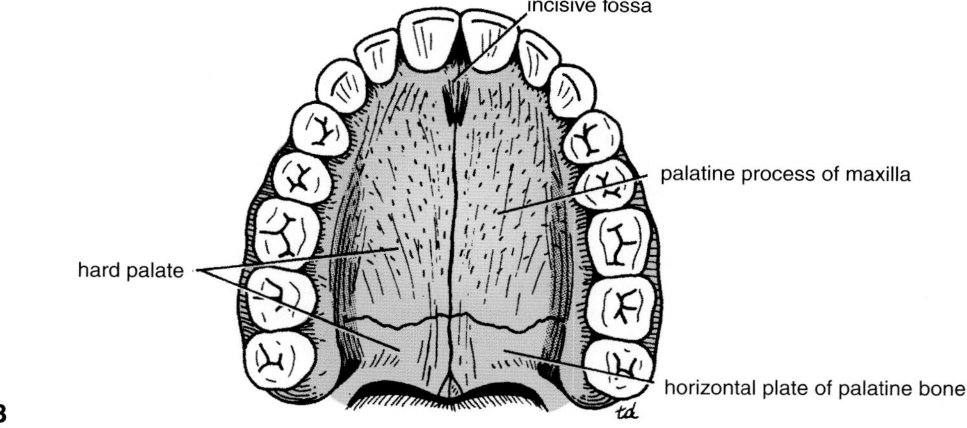

Figure 11-80 **A.** Three constrictor muscles of the pharynx. The superior and recurrent laryngeal nerves are also shown. **B.** Hard palate.

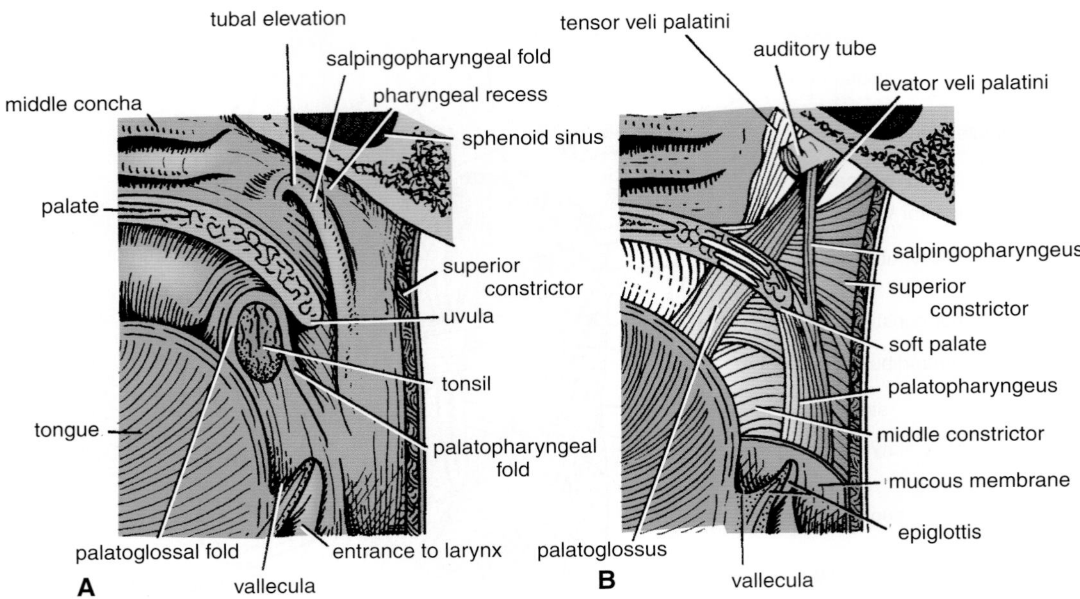

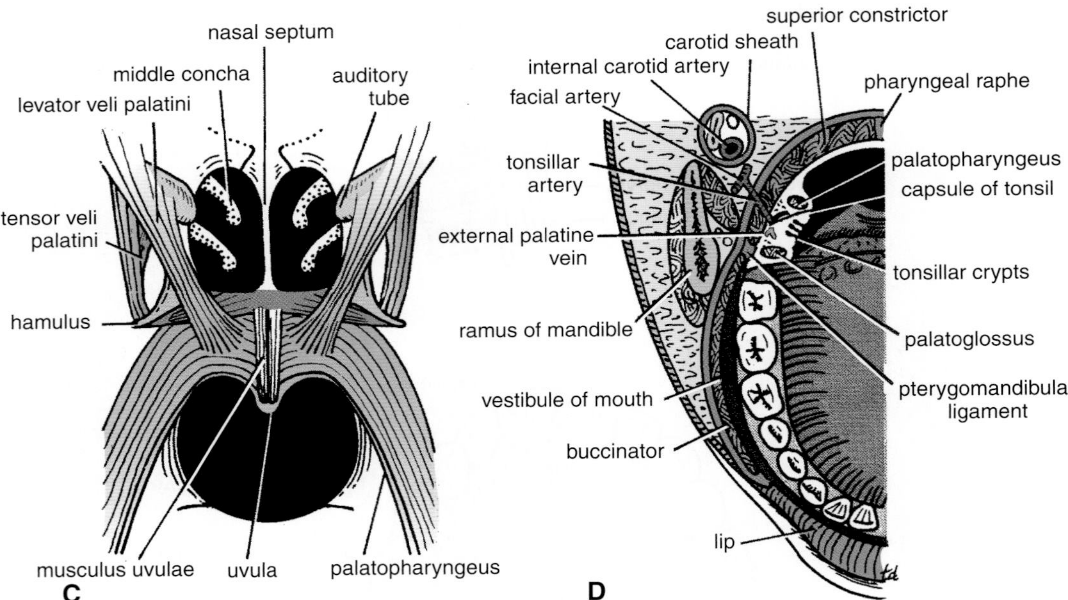

Figure 11-81 **A.** Junction of the nose with the nasal part of the pharynx and the mouth with the oral part of the pharynx. Note the position of the tonsil and the opening of the auditory tube. **B.** Muscles of the soft palate and the upper part of the pharynx. **C.** Muscles of the soft palate seen from behind. **D.** Horizontal section through the mouth and the oral part of the pharynx showing the relations of the tonsil.

Table 11-9 Muscles of the Soft Palate

Muscle	Origin	Insertion	Nerve Supply	Action
Tensor veli palatini	Spine of sphenoid, auditory tube	With muscle of other side, forms palatine aponeurosis	Nerve to medial pterygoid from mandibular nerve	Tenses soft palate
Levator veli palatini	Petrous part of temporal bone, auditory tube	Palatine aponeurosis	Pharyngeal plexus	Raises soft palate
Palatoglossus	Palatine aponeurosis	Side of tongue	Pharyngeal plexus	Pulls root of tongue upward and backward, narrows oropharyngeal isthmus
Palatopharyngeus	Palatine aponeurosis	Posterior border of thyroid cartilage	Pharyngeal plexus	Elevates wall of pharynx, pulls palatopharyngeal folds medially
Musculus uvulae	Posterior border of hard palate	Mucous membrane of uvula	Pharyngeal plexus	Elevates uvula

Movements of the Soft Palate

The pharyngeal isthmus (the communicating channel between the nasal and oral parts of the pharynx) is closed by raising the soft palate. Closure occurs during the production of explosive consonants in speech.

The soft palate is raised by the contraction of the levator veli palatini on each side. At the same time, the upper fibers of the superior constrictor muscle contract and pull the posterior pharyngeal wall forward. The palatopharyngeus muscles on both sides also contract so that the palatopharyngeal arches are pulled medially, like side curtains. By this means the nasal part of the pharynx is closed off from the oral part.

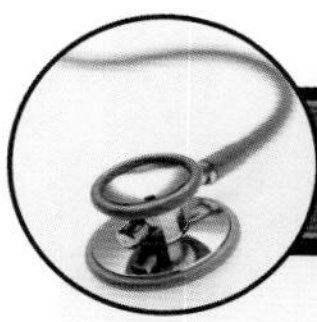

CLINICAL NOTES

Angioedema of the Uvula (Quincke's Uvula)

The uvula has a core of voluntary muscle, the musculus uvulae, that is attached to the posterior border of the hard palate. Surrounding the muscle is the loose connective tissue of the submucosa that is responsible for the great swelling of this structure secondary to angioedema.

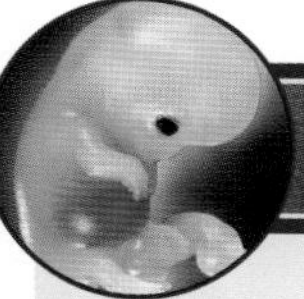

EMBRYOLOGIC NOTES

Development of the Palate

In early fetal life, the nasal and mouth cavities are in communication, but later they become separated by the development of the palate (Fig. 11-82). The **primary palate,** which carries the four incisor teeth, is formed by the medial nasal process. Posterior to the primary palate, the maxillary process on each side sends medially a horizontal plate called the **palatal process;** these plates fuse to form the **secondary palate** and also unite with the primary palate and the developing nasal septum. The fusion takes place from the anterior to the posterior region. The primary and secondary palates later will form the **hard palate.** Two folds grow posteriorly from the posterior edge of the palatal processes to create the **soft palate,** so that the **uvula** is the last structure to be formed (Fig. 11-82). The union of the two folds of the soft palate occurs during the eighth week. The two parts of the uvula fuse in the midline during the 11th week. The interval between the primary palate and secondary palate is represented in the midline by the **incisive foramen.**

Cleft Palate

Cleft palate is commonly associated with cleft upper lip. All degrees of cleft palate occur and are caused by failure of the palatal processes of the maxilla to fuse with each other in the midline; in severe cases, these processes also fail to fuse with the primary palate (premaxilla) (Figs. 11-83 and 11-84). The first degree of severity is cleft uvula, and the second degree is ununited palatal processes. The third degree is ununited palatal processes and a cleft on one side of the primary palate. This type is usually associated with unilateral cleft lip. The fourth degree of severity, which is rare, consists of ununited palatal processes and a cleft on both sides of the primary palate. This type is usually associated with bilateral cleft lip. A rare form may occur in which a bilateral cleft lip and failure of the primary palate to fuse with the palatal processes of the maxilla on each side are present.

A baby born with a severe cleft palate presents a difficult feeding problem, since he or she is unable to suck efficiently. Such a baby often receives in the mouth some milk, which then is regurgitated through the nose or aspirated into the lungs, leading to respiratory infection. For this reason, careful artificial feeding is required until the baby is strong enough to undergo surgery. Plastic surgery is recommended usually between 1 and 2 years of age, before improper speech habits have been acquired.

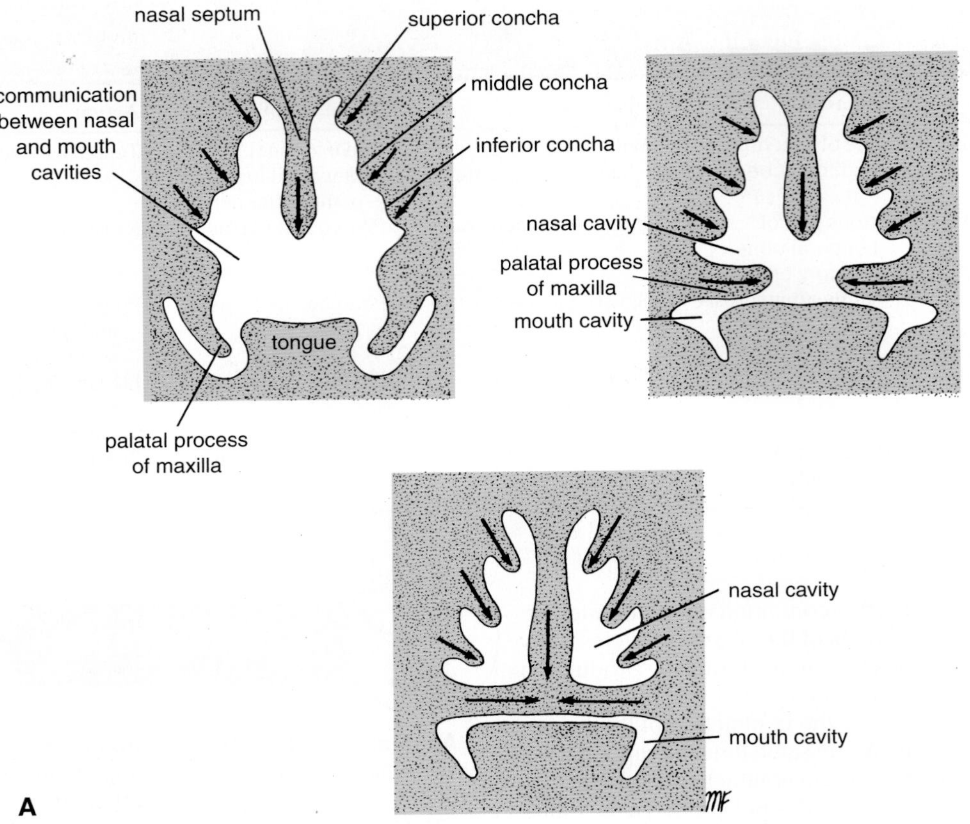

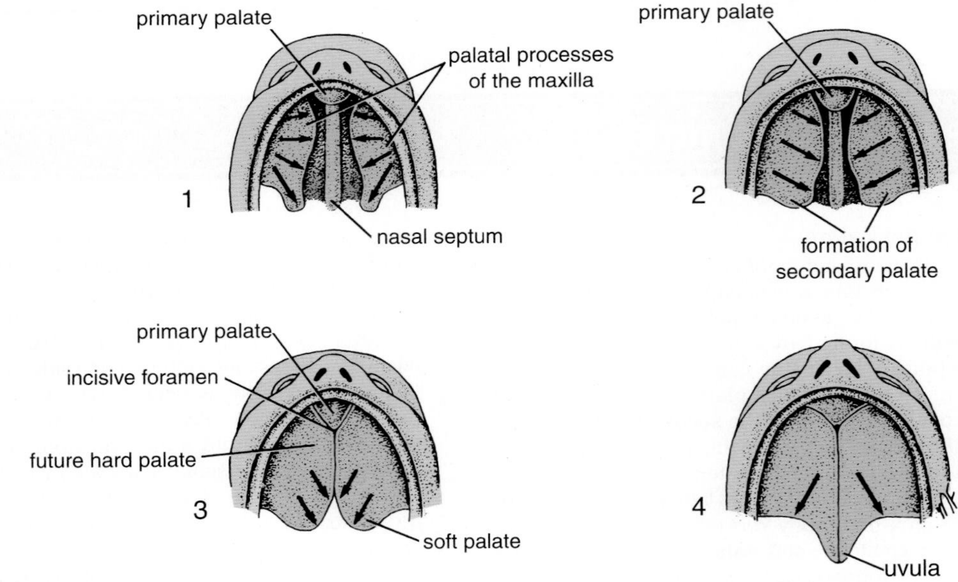

Figure 11-82 **A.** The formation of the palate and the nasal septum (coronal section). **B.** The different stages in the formation of the palate.

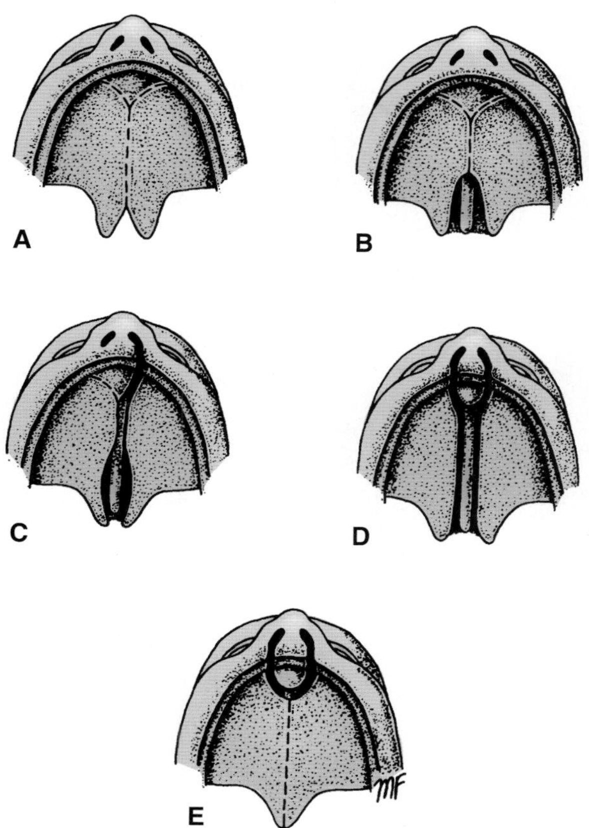

Figure 11-83 Different forms of cleft palate: cleft uvula (**A**), cleft soft and hard palate (**B**), total unilateral cleft palate and cleft lip (**C**), total bilateral cleft palate and cleft lip (**D**), and bilateral cleft lip and jaw (**E**).

The Salivary Glands

Parotid Gland

The parotid gland is the largest salivary gland and is composed mostly of serous acini. It lies in a deep hollow below the external auditory meatus, behind the ramus of the mandible (Fig. 11-85), and in front of the sternocleidomastoid muscle. The facial nerve divides the gland into **superficial** and **deep lobes.** The parotid duct emerges from the anterior border of the gland and passes forward over the lateral surface of the masseter. It enters the vestibule of the mouth upon a small papilla opposite the upper second molar tooth (Fig. 11-72).

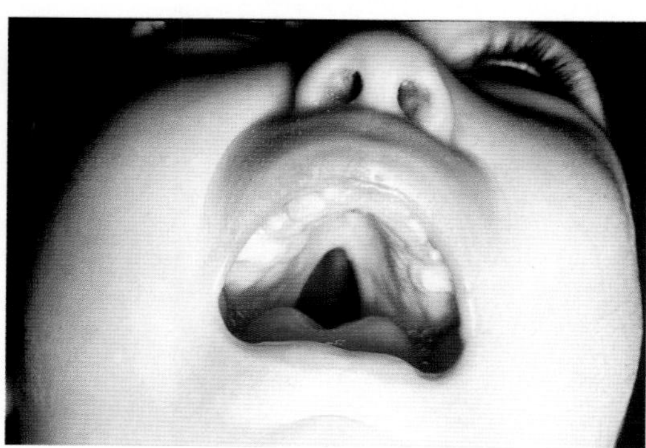

Figure 11-84 Cleft hard and soft palate. (Courtesy of R. Chase.)

Nerve Supply

Parasympathetic secretomotor supply arises from the glossopharyngeal nerve. The nerves reach the gland via the tympanic branch, the lesser petrosal nerve, the otic ganglion, and the auriculotemporal nerve.

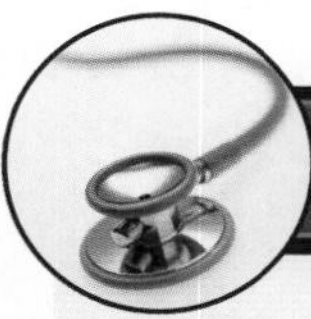

CLINICAL NOTES

Parotid Duct Injury

The parotid duct, which is a comparatively superficial structure on the face, may be damaged in injuries to the face or may be inadvertently cut during surgical operations on the face. The duct is about 2 in. (5 cm) long and passes forward across the masseter about a fingerbreadth below the zygomatic arch. It then pierces the buccinator muscle to enter the mouth opposite the upper second molar tooth.

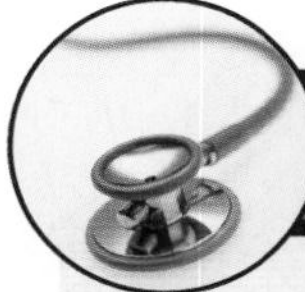

CLINICAL NOTES

Parotid Salivary Gland and Lesions of the Facial Nerve

The parotid salivary gland consists essentially of superficial and deep parts, and the important facial nerve lies in the interval between these parts. A benign parotid neoplasm rarely, if ever, causes facial palsy. A malignant tumor of the parotid is usually highly invasive and quickly involves the facial nerve, causing unilateral facial paralysis.

Parotid Gland Infections

The parotid gland may become acutely inflamed as a result of retrograde bacterial infection from the mouth via the parotid duct. The gland may also become infected via the bloodstream, as in mumps. In both cases the gland is swollen; it is painful because the fascial capsule derived from the investing layer of deep cervical fascia is strong and limits the swelling of the gland. The swollen glenoid process, which extends medially behind the temporomandibular joint, is responsible for the pain experienced in acute parotitis when eating.

Frey's Syndrome

Frey's syndrome is an interesting complication that sometimes develops after penetrating wounds of the parotid gland. When the patient eats, beads of perspiration appear on the skin covering the parotid. This condition is caused by damage to the auriculotemporal and great auricular nerves. During the process of healing, the parasympathetic secretomotor fibers in the auriculotemporal nerve grow out and join the distal end of the great auricular nerve. Eventually, these fibers reach the sweat glands in the facial skin. By this means, a stimulus intended for saliva production produces sweat secretion instead.

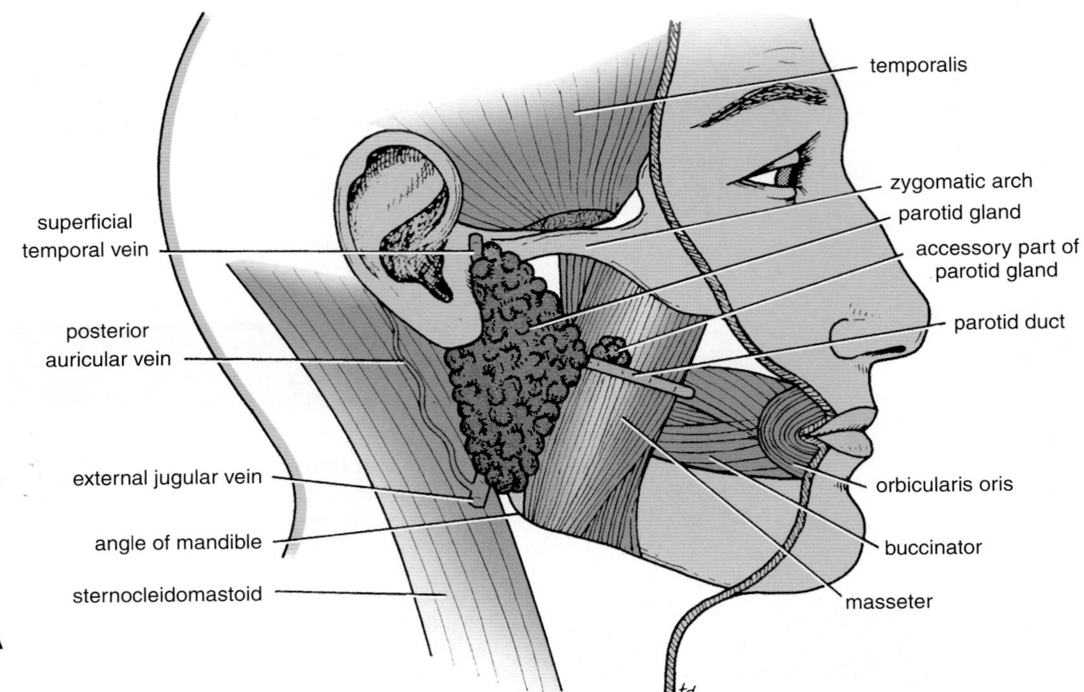

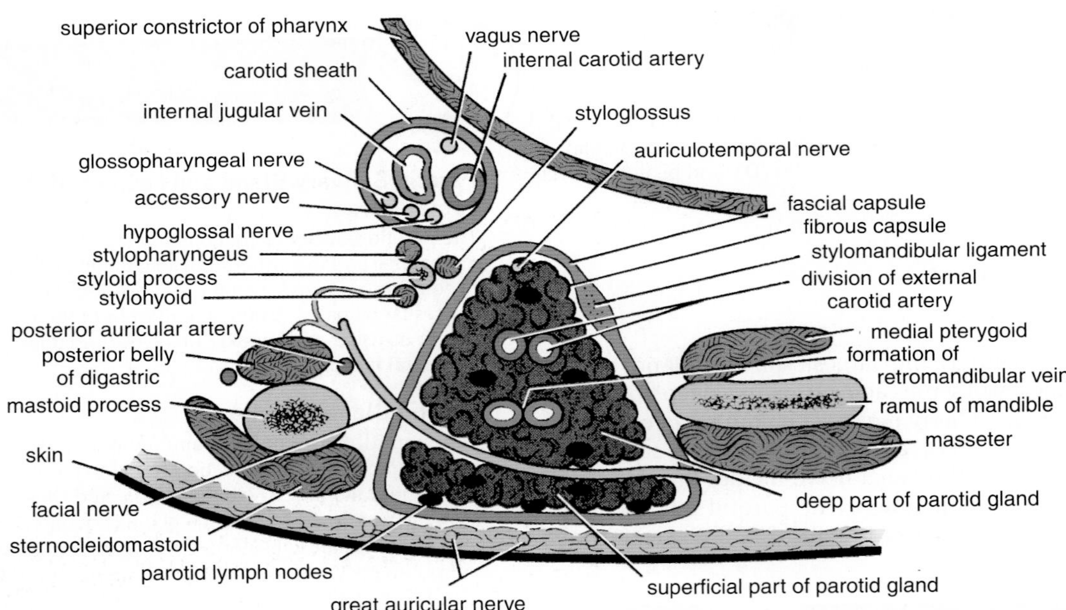

Figure 11-85 Parotid gland and its relations. **A.** Lateral surface of the gland and the course of the parotid duct. **B.** Horizontal section of the parotid gland.

Submandibular Gland

The submandibular gland consists of a mixture of serous and mucous acini. It lies beneath the lower border of the body of the mandible (Fig. 11-86) and is divided into superficial and deep parts by the mylohyoid muscle. The deep part of the gland lies beneath the mucous membrane of the mouth on the side of the tongue. The submandibular duct emerges from the anterior end of the deep part of the gland and runs forward beneath the mucous membrane of the mouth. It opens into the mouth on a small papilla, which is situated at the side of the frenulum of the tongue (Fig. 11-72).

Nerve Supply

Parasympathetic secretomotor supply is from the facial nerve via the chorda tympani, and the submandibular ganglion. The postganglionic fibers pass directly to the gland.

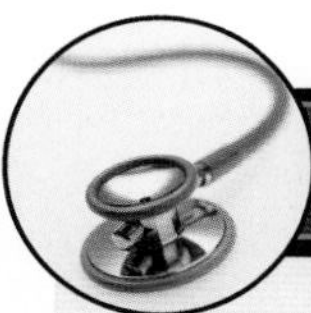

CLINICAL NOTES

Submandibular Salivary Gland: Calculus Formation

The submandibular salivary gland is a common site of calculus formation. This condition is rare in the other salivary glands. The presence of a tense swelling below the body of the mandible, which is greatest before or during a meal and is reduced in size or absent between meals, is diagnostic of the condition. Examination of the floor of the mouth will reveal absence of ejection of saliva from the orifice of the duct of the affected gland. Frequently, the stone can be palpated in the duct, which lies below the mucous membrane of the floor of the mouth.

Enlargement of the Submandibular Lymph Nodes and Swelling of the Submandibular Salivary Gland

The submandibular lymph nodes are commonly enlarged as a result of a pathologic condition of the scalp, face, maxillary sinus, or mouth cavity. One of the most common causes of painful enlargement of these nodes is acute infection of the teeth. Enlargement of these nodes should not be confused with pathologic swelling of the submandibular salivary gland.

Sublingual Gland

The sublingual gland lies beneath the mucous membrane (sublingual fold) of the floor of the mouth, close to the frenulum of the tongue (Fig. 11-86). It has both serous and mucous acini, with the latter predominating. The **sublingual ducts** (8 to 20 in number) open into the mouth on the summit of the sublingual fold (Fig. 11-72).

Nerve Supply

Parasympathetic secretomotor supply is from the facial nerve via the chorda tympani, and the submandibular ganglion. Postganglionic fibers pass directly to the gland.

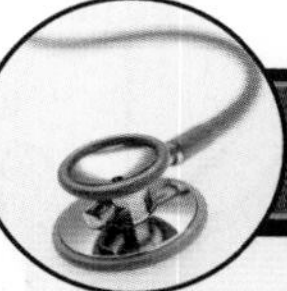

CLINICAL NOTES

Sublingual Salivary Gland and Cyst Formation

The sublingual salivary gland, which lies beneath the sublingual fold of the floor of the mouth, opens into the mouth by numerous small ducts. Blockage of one of these ducts is believed to be the cause of cysts under the tongue.

The Pharynx

The pharynx is situated behind the nasal cavities, the mouth, and the larynx (Fig. 11-87) and may be divided into **nasal, oral,** and **laryngeal parts.** The pharynx is funnel shaped, its upper, wider end lying under the skull and its lower, narrow end becoming continuous with the esophagus opposite the sixth cervical vertebra. The pharynx has a musculomembranous wall, which is deficient anteriorly. Here, it is replaced by the posterior openings into the nose (choanae), the opening into the mouth, and the inlet of the larynx. By means of the auditory tube, the mucous membrane is also continuous with that of the tympanic cavity.

Muscles of the Pharynx

The muscles in the wall of the pharynx consist of the **superior, middle, and inferior constrictor muscles** (Fig. 11-80A), whose fibers run in a somewhat circular direction, and the **stylopharyngeus** and **salpingopharyngeus muscles,** whose fibers run in a somewhat longitudinal direction.

The three constrictor muscles extend around the pharyngeal wall to be inserted into a fibrous band or raphe that extends from the pharyngeal tubercle on the basilar part of the occipital bone of the skull down to the esophagus. The three constrictor muscles overlap each other so that the middle constrictor lies on the outside of the lower part of the superior constrictor and the inferior constrictor lies outside the lower part of the middle constrictor (Fig. 11-88).

The lower part of the inferior constrictor, which arises from the cricoid cartilage, is called the **cricopharyngeus muscle** (Fig. 11-88). The fibers of the cricopharyngeus pass horizontally around the lowest and narrowest part of the pharynx and act as a sphincter. **Killian's dehiscence** is the area on the posterior pharyngeal wall between the upper propulsive part of the inferior constrictor and the lower sphincteric part, the cricopharyngeus.

The details of the origins, insertions, nerve supply, and actions of the pharyngeal muscles are summarized in Table 11-10.

Interior of the Pharynx

The pharynx is divided into three parts: the nasal pharynx, the oral pharynx, and the laryngeal pharynx.

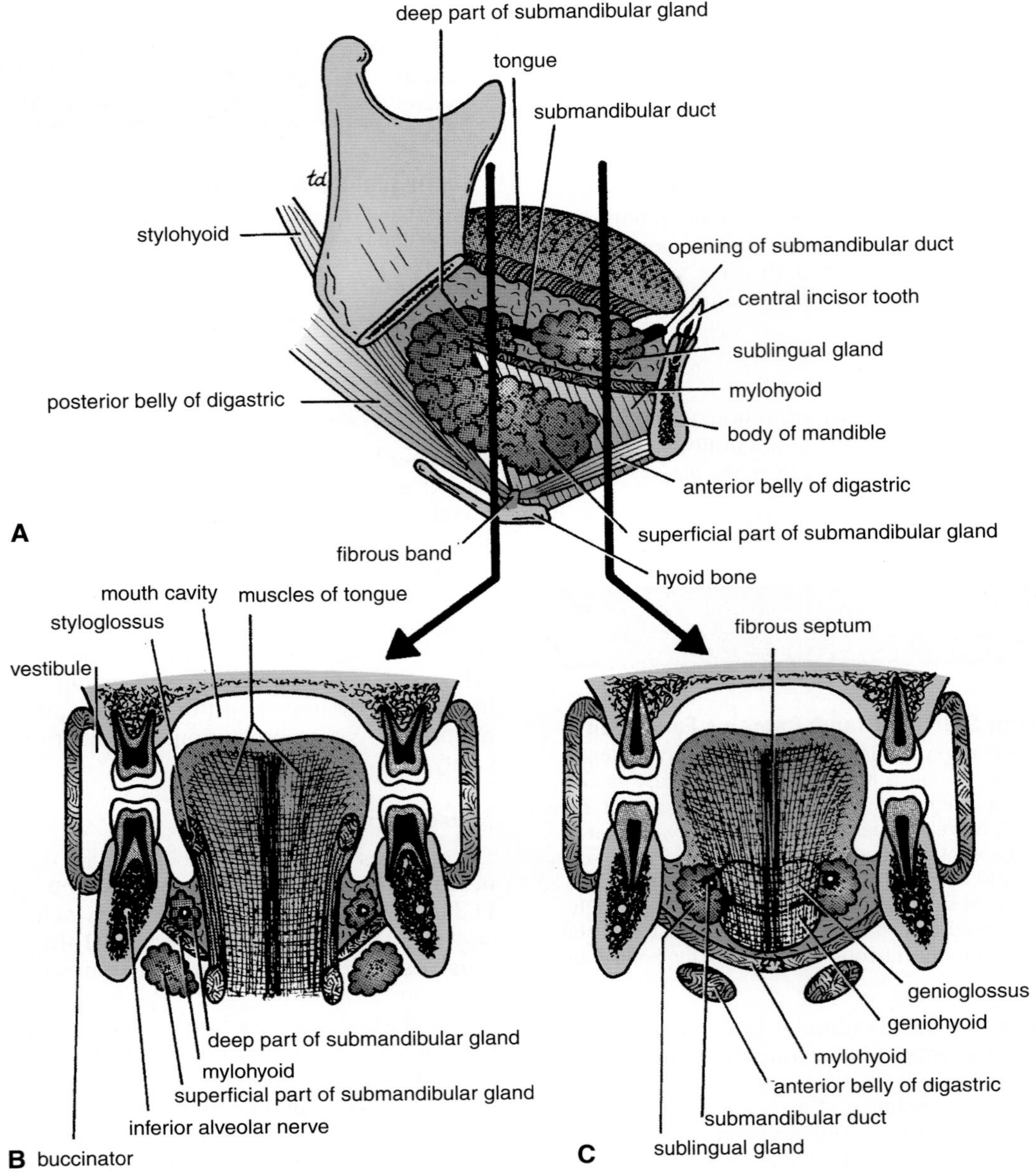

Figure 11-86 **A.** Submandibular and sublingual salivary glands (lateral view). **B.** Coronal section through the superficial and deep parts of the submandibular salivary glands. **C.** Coronal section (anterior to B) through the sublingual salivary glands and the ducts of the submandibular salivary glands.

Nasal Pharynx

This lies above the soft palate and behind the nasal cavities (Fig. 11-87). In the submucosa of the roof is a collection of lymphoid tissue called the **pharyngeal tonsil** (Fig. 11-89). The pharyngeal isthmus is the opening in the floor between the soft palate and the posterior pharyngeal wall. On the lateral wall is the opening of the **auditory tube,** the elevated ridge of which is called the **tubal elevation** (Fig. 11-89). The **pharyngeal recess** is a depression in the pharyngeal wall behind the tubal elevation. The **salpingopharyngeal fold** is a vertical fold of mucous membrane covering the salpingopharyngeus muscle.

Oral Pharynx

This lies behind the oral cavity (Fig. 11-87). The floor is formed by the posterior one third of the tongue and the interval between the tongue and epiglottis. In the midline is the **median glossoepiglottic fold** (Fig. 11-77), and on each side the **lateral glossoepiglottic fold.** The depression on each side of the median glossoepiglottic fold is called the **vallecula** (Fig. 11-77).

On the lateral wall on each side are the palatoglossal and the palatopharyngeal arches or folds and the palatine tonsils between them (Fig. 11-89). The palatoglossal arch is a fold of mucous membrane covering the palatoglossus muscle. The

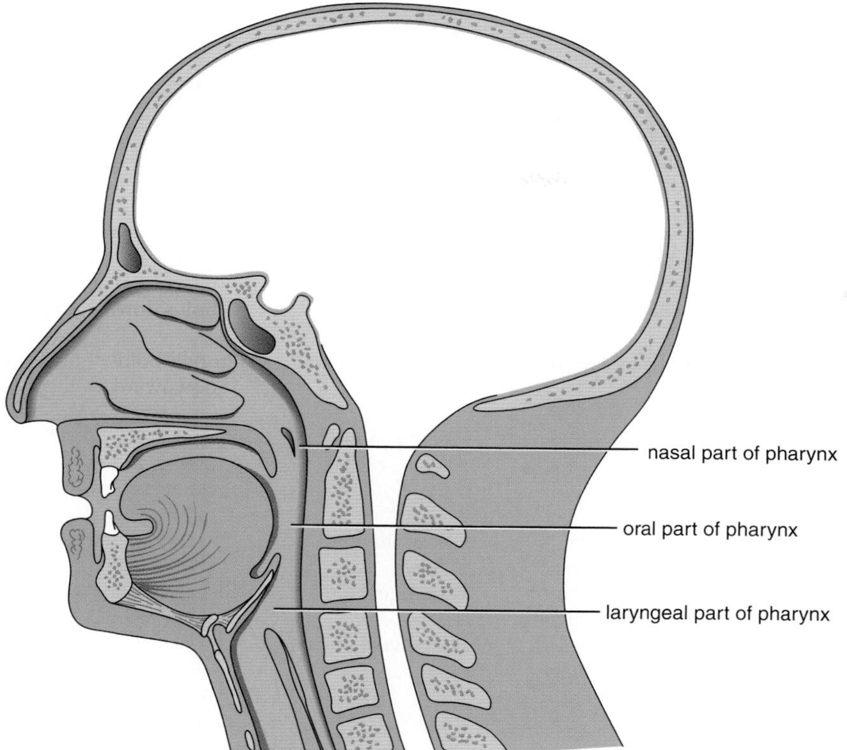

Figure 11-87 Sagittal section through the nose, mouth, pharynx, and larynx to show the subdivisions of the pharynx.

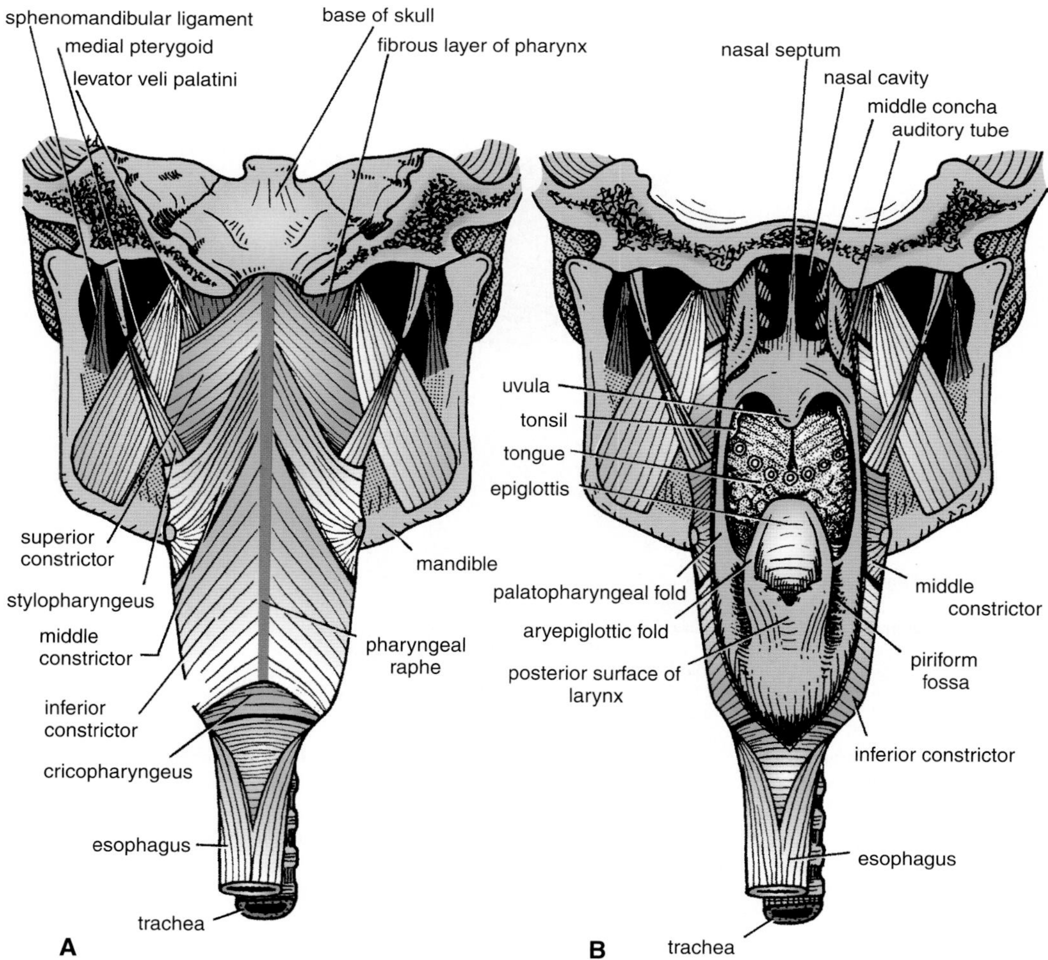

Figure 11-88 The pharynx seen from behind. **A.** Note the three constrictor muscles and the position of the stylopharyngeus muscles. **B.** The greater part of the posterior wall of the pharynx has been removed to display the nasal, oral, and laryngeal parts of the pharynx.

Table 11-10 Muscles of the Pharynx

Muscle	Origin	Insertion	Nerve Supply	Action
Superior constrictor	Medial pterygoid plate, pterygoid hamulus, pterygomandibular ligament, mylohyoid line of mandible	Pharyngeal tubercle of occipital bone, raphe in midline posteriorly	Pharyngeal plexus	Aids soft palate in closing off nasal pharynx, propels bolus downward
Middle constrictor	Lower part of stylohyoid ligament, lesser and greater cornu of hyoid bone	Pharyngeal raphe	Pharyngeal plexus	Propels bolus downward
Inferior constrictor	Lamina of thyroid cartilage, cricoid cartilage	Pharyngeal raphe	Pharyngeal plexus	Propels bolus downward
Cricopharyngeus	Lowest fibers of inferior constrictor muscle			Sphincter at lower end of pharynx
Stylopharyngeus	Styloid process of temporal bone	Posterior border of thyroid cartilage	Glossopharyngeal nerve	Elevates larynx during swallowing
Salpingopharyngeus	Auditory tube	Blends with palatopharyngeus	Pharyngeal plexus	Elevates pharynx
Palatopharyngeus	Palatine aponeurosis	Posterior border of thyroid cartilage	Pharyngeal plexus	Elevates wall of pharynx, pulls palatopharyngeal arch medially

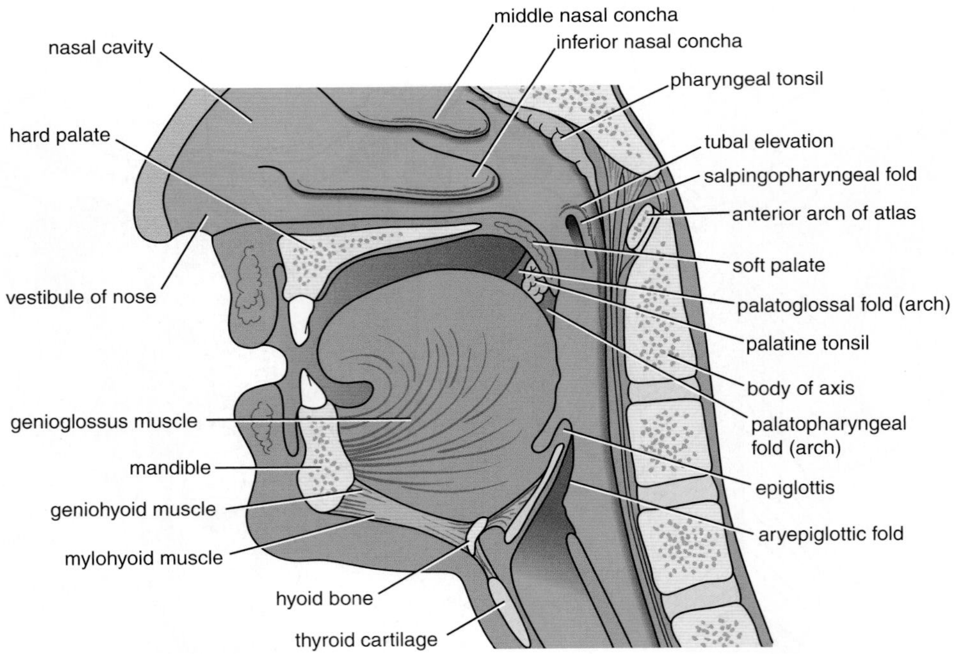

Figure 11-89 Sagittal section of the head and neck, showing the relations of the nasal cavity, mouth, pharynx, and larynx.

interval between the two palatoglossal arches is called the **oropharyngeal isthmus** and marks the boundary between the mouth and pharynx. The palatopharyngeal arch is a fold of mucous membrane covering the palatopharyngeus muscle. The recess between the palatoglossal and palatopharyngeal arches is occupied by the **palatine tonsil.**

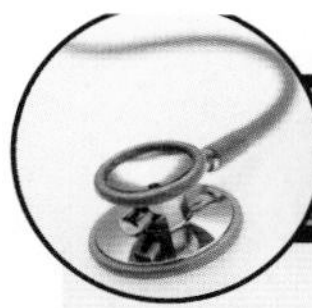

CLINICAL NOTES

The Lymphoid Tissue of the Pharynx

At the junction of the mouth with the oral part of the pharynx, and the nose with the nasal part of the pharynx, are collections of lymphoid tissue of considerable clinical importance. The palatine tonsils and the nasopharyngeal tonsils are the most important.

Tonsils and Tonsillitis

The palatine tonsils reach their maximum normal size in early childhood. After puberty, together with other lymphoid tissues in the body, they gradually atrophy. The palatine tonsils are a common site of infection, producing the characteristic sore throat and pyrexia. The deep cervical lymph node situated below and behind the angle of the mandible, which drains lymph from this organ, is usually enlarged and tender. Recurrent attacks of tonsillitis are best treated by tonsillectomy. After tonsillectomy, the external palatine vein, which lies lateral to the tonsil, may be the source of troublesome postoperative bleeding.

Quinsy

A **peritonsillar abscess** (quinsy) is caused by spread of infection from the palatine tonsil to the loose connective tissue outside the capsule (Fig. 11-90).

The nasopharyngeal tonsil or pharyngeal tonsil consists of a collection of lymphoid tissue beneath the epithelium of the roof of the nasal part of the pharynx. Like the palatine tonsil, it is largest in early childhood and starts to atrophy after puberty.

Adenoids

Excessive hypertrophy of the lymphoid tissue, usually associated with infection, causes the pharyngeal tonsils to become enlarged; they are then commonly referred to as adenoids. Marked hypertrophy blocks the posterior nasal openings and causes the patient to snore loudly at night and to breathe through the open mouth. The close relationship of the infected lymphoid tissue to the auditory tube may be the cause of deafness and recurrent otitis media. Adenoidectomy is the treatment of choice for hypertrophied adenoids with infection.

The nasal part of the pharynx may be viewed clinically by a mirror passed through the mouth (Fig. 11-91).

Laryngeal Pharynx

This lies behind the opening into the larynx (Fig. 11-87). The lateral wall is formed by the thyroid cartilage and the thyrohyoid membrane. The **piriform fossa** is a depression in the mucous membrane on each side of the laryngeal inlet (Fig. 11-88).

Sensory Nerve Supply of the Pharyngeal Mucous Membrane

Nasal pharynx: The maxillary nerve (V2)

Oral pharynx: The glossopharyngeal nerve

Laryngeal pharynx (around the entrance into the larynx): The internal laryngeal branch of the vagus nerve

Blood Supply of the Pharynx

Ascending pharyngeal, tonsillar branches of facial arteries, and branches of maxillary and lingual arteries

Lymph Drainage of the Pharynx

Directly into the deep cervical lymph nodes or indirectly via the retropharyngeal or paratracheal nodes into the deep cervical nodes

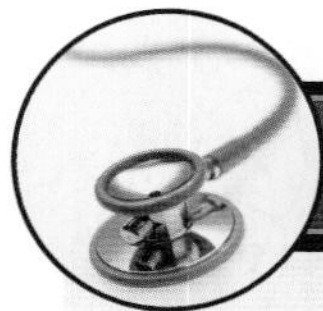

CLINICAL NOTES

Piriform Fossa and Foreign Bodies

The piriform fossa is a recess of mucous membrane situated on either side of the entrance of the larynx. It is bounded medially by the aryepiglottic folds and laterally by the thyroid cartilage. Clinically, it is important because it is a common site for the lodging of sharp ingested bodies such as fish bones. The presence of such a foreign body immediately causes the patient to gag violently. Once the object has become jammed, it is difficult for the patient to remove it without a physician's assistance.

Pharyngeal Pouch

Examination of the lower part of the posterior surface of the inferior constrictor muscle reveals a potential gap between the upper oblique and the lower horizontal fibers **(cricopharyngeus).** This area is marked by a dimple in the lining mucous membrane. It is believed that the function of the cricopharyngeus is to prevent the entry of air into the esophagus. Should the cricopharyngeus fail to relax during swallowing, the internal pharyngeal pressure may rise and force the mucosa and submucosa of the dimple posteriorly, to produce a diverticulum. Once the diverticulum has been formed, it may gradually enlarge and fill with food with each meal. Unable to expand posteriorly because of the vertebral column, it turns downward, usually on the left side. The presence of the pouch filled with food causes difficulty in swallowing **(dysphagia).**

Cervical Tuberculous Osteomyelitis and the Pharynx

Pus arising from tuberculosis of the upper cervical vertebrae is limited in front by the prevertebral layer of deep fascia. A midline swelling is formed and bulges forward in the posterior wall of the pharynx. The pus then tracks laterally and downward behind the carotid sheath to reach the posterior triangle. Here, the fascia, which forms a covering to the muscular floor of the triangle, is weaker, and the abscess points behind the sternocleidomastoid. Rarely, the abscess may track downward behind the prevertebral fascia to reach the superior and posterior mediastina in the thorax.

It is important to distinguish this condition from an abscess involving the **retropharyngeal lymph nodes.** These nodes lie in front of the prevertebral layer of fascia but behind the fascia, which covers the outer surface of the constrictor muscles. Such an abscess usually points on the posterior pharyngeal wall and, if untreated, ruptures into the pharyngeal cavity.

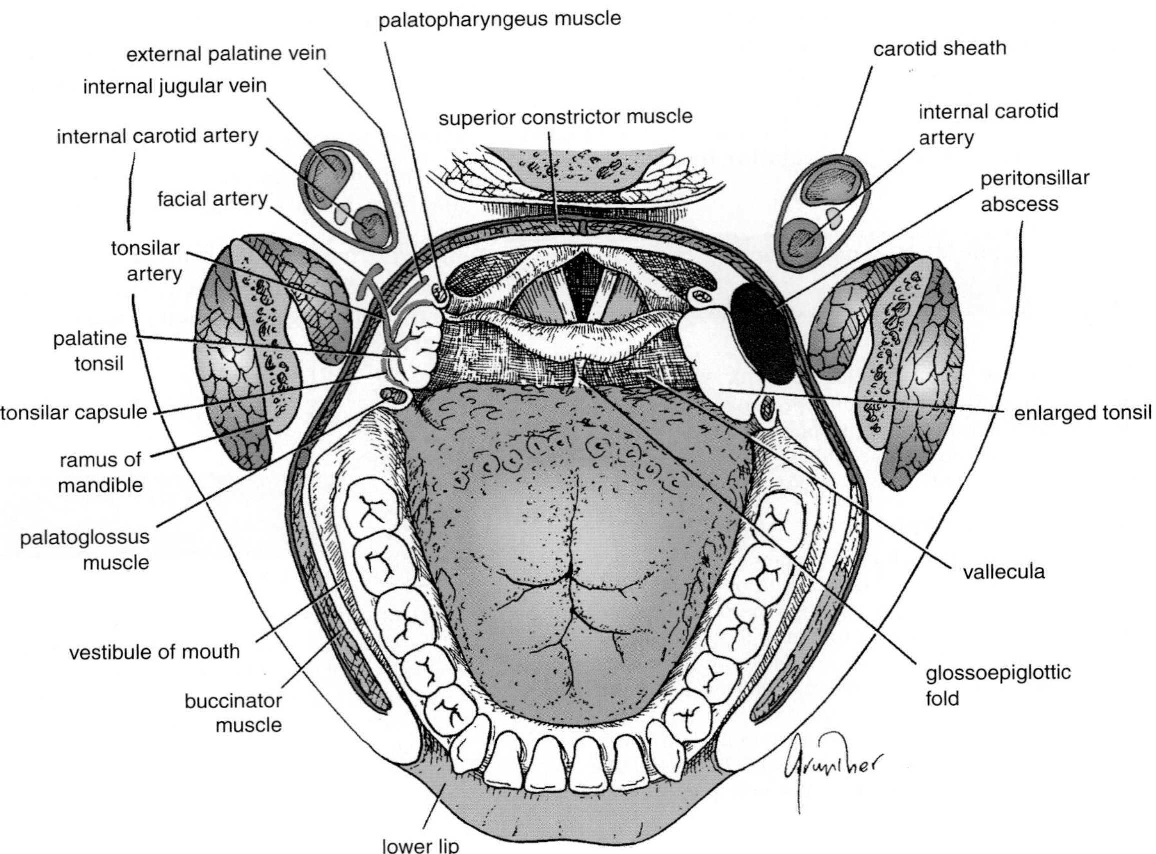

Figure 11-90 Horizontal section through the mouth and the oral pharynx. **Left,** the normal palatine tonsil and its relationships. **Right,** the position of a peritonsillar abscess. Note the relationship of the abscess to the superior constrictor muscle and the carotid sheath. The opening into the larynx can also be seen below and behind the tongue.

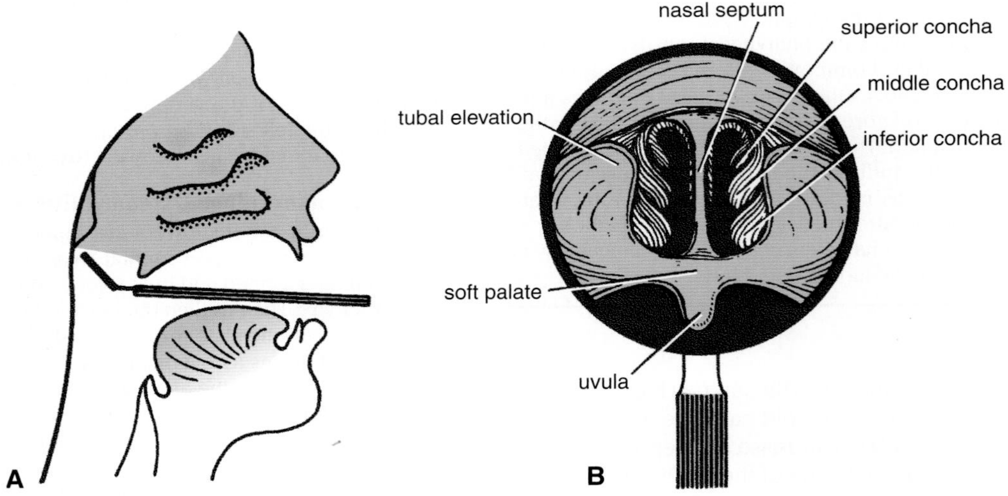

Figure 11-91 **A.** Sagittal section through the nose, mouth, larynx, and pharynx showing the position of the mirror in posterior rhinoscopy. **B.** Structures seen in posterior rhinoscopy.

The Process of Swallowing (Deglutition)

Masticated food is formed into a ball or bolus on the dorsum of the tongue and voluntarily pushed upward and backward against the undersurface of the hard palate. This is brought about by the contraction of the styloglossus muscles on both sides, which pull the root of the tongue upward and backward. The palatoglossus muscles then squeeze the bolus backward into the pharynx. From this point onward the process of swallowing becomes an involuntary act.

The nasal part of the pharynx is now shut off from the oral part of the pharynx by the elevation of the soft palate, the pulling forward of the posterior wall of the pharynx by the upper fibers of the superior constrictor muscle, and the contraction of the palatopharyngeus muscles. This prevents the passage of food and drink into the nasal cavities.

The larynx and the laryngeal part of the pharynx are pulled upward by the contraction of the stylopharyngeus, salpingopharyngeus, thyrohyoid, and palatopharyngeus muscles. The main part of the larynx is thus elevated to the posterior surface of the epiglottis, and the entrance into the larynx is closed. The laryngeal entrance is made smaller by the approximation of the aryepiglottic folds, and the arytenoid cartilages are pulled forward by the contraction of the aryepiglottic, oblique arytenoid, and thyroarytenoid muscles.

The bolus moves downward over the epiglottis, the closed entrance into the larynx, and reaches the lower part of the pharynx as the result of the successive contraction of the superior, middle, and inferior constrictor muscles. Some of the food slides down the groove on either side of the entrance into the larynx, that is, down through the **piriform fossae.** Finally, the lower part of the pharyngeal wall (the cricopharyngeus muscle) relaxes and the bolus enters the esophagus.

Palatine Tonsils

The palatine tonsils are two masses of lymphoid tissue, each located in the depression on the lateral wall of the oral part of the pharynx between the palatoglossal and palatopharyngeal arches (Fig. 11-90). Each tonsil is covered by mucous membrane, and its free medial surface projects into the pharynx. The surface is pitted by numerous small openings that lead into the **tonsillar crypts.**

The tonsil is covered on its lateral surface by a **fibrous capsule** (Fig. 11-90). The capsule is separated from the superior constrictor muscle by loose areolar tissue (Fig. 11-90) and the external palatine vein descends from the soft palate in this tissue to join the pharyngeal venous plexus. Lateral to the superior constrictor muscle lie the styloglossus muscle, the loop of the facial artery, and the internal carotid artery.

The tonsil reaches its maximum size during early childhood, but after puberty it diminishes considerably in size.

Blood Supply

The tonsillar branch of the facial artery. The veins pierce the superior constrictor muscle and join the external palatine, the pharyngeal, or the facial veins.

Lymph Drainage of the Tonsil

The upper deep cervical lymph nodes, just below and behind the angle of the mandible

Waldeyer's Ring of Lymphoid Tissue

The lymphoid tissue that surrounds the opening into the respiratory and digestive systems forms a ring. The lateral part of the ring is formed by the palatine tonsils and tubal tonsils (lymphoid tissue around the opening of the auditory tube in the lateral wall of the nasopharynx). The pharyngeal tonsil in the roof of the nasopharynx forms the upper part, and the lingual tonsil on the posterior third of the tongue forms the lower part.

The Esophagus

The esophagus is a muscular tube about 10 in. (25 cm) long, extending from the pharynx to the stomach (Figs. 11-13 and 11-88). It begins at the level of the cricoid cartilage, opposite the body of the sixth cervical vertebra. It commences in the midline, but as it descends through the neck, it inclines to the left side. Its further course in the thorax is described on page 128.

Relations in the Neck

- **Anteriorly:** The trachea; the recurrent laryngeal nerves ascend one on each side, in the groove between the trachea and the esophagus (Fig. 11-49).
- **Posteriorly:** The prevertebral layer of deep cervical fascia, the longus colli, and the vertebral column (Fig. 11-49)
- **Laterally:** On each side lie the lobe of the thyroid gland and the carotid sheath (Fig. 11-49)

Blood Supply in the Neck

The **arteries** of the esophagus in the neck are derived from the inferior thyroid arteries. The **veins** drain into the inferior thyroid veins.

Lymph Drainage in the Neck

The lymph vessels drain into the deep cervical lymph nodes.

Nerve Supply in the Neck

The nerves are derived from the recurrent laryngeal nerves and from the sympathetic trunks.

The Respiratory System in the Head and Neck

The Nose

The nose consists of the external nose and the nasal cavity, both of which are divided by a septum into right and left halves.

External Nose

The external nose has two elliptical orifices called the **nostrils,** which are separated from each other by the **nasal septum** (Fig. 11-92). The lateral margin, the **ala nasi,** is rounded and mobile.

The framework of the external nose is made up above by the nasal bones, the frontal processes of the maxillae, and the nasal part of the frontal bone. Below, the framework is formed of plates of hyaline cartilage (Fig. 11-92).

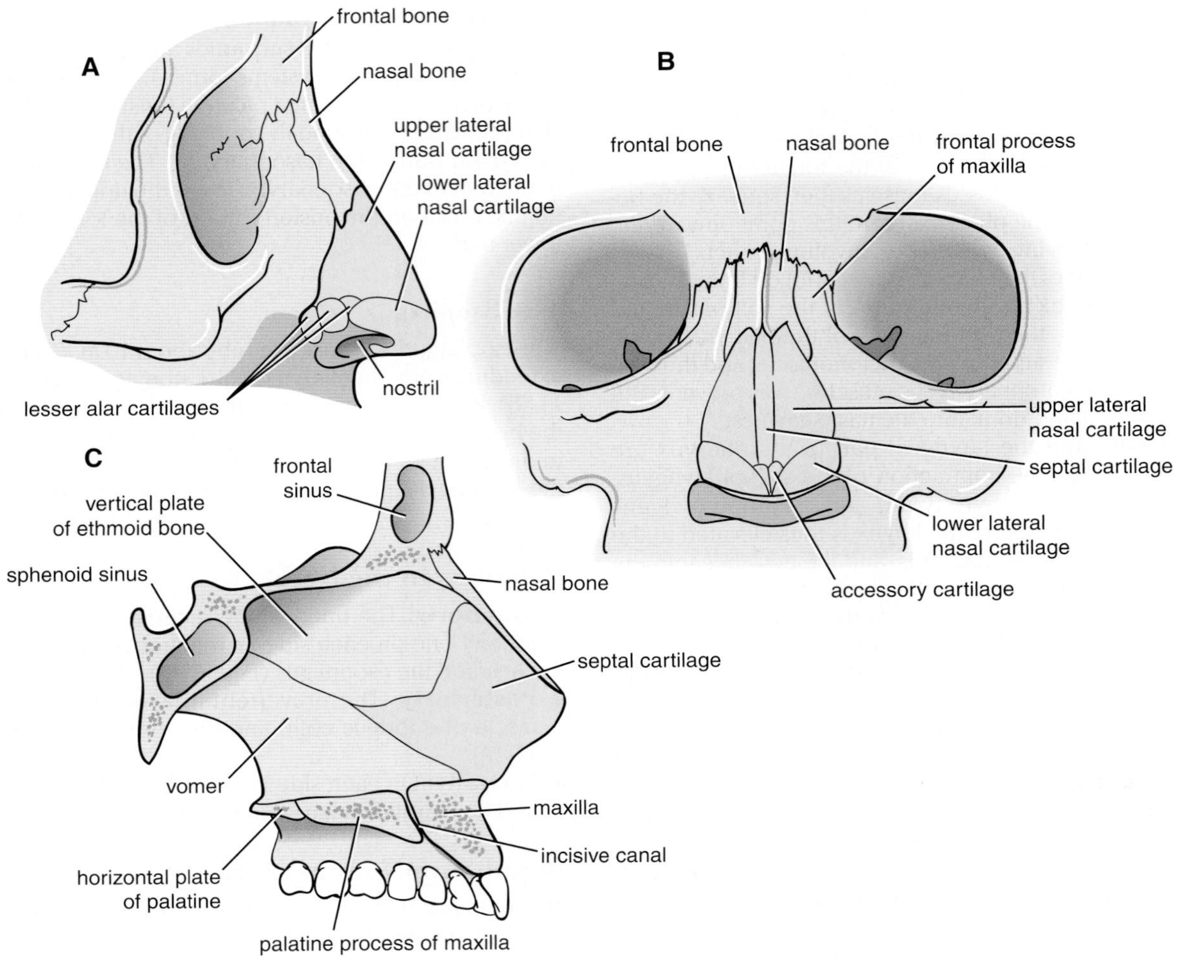

Figure 11-92 External nose and nasal septum. **A.** Lateral view of bony and cartilaginous skeleton of external nose. **B.** Anterior view of bony and cartilaginous skeleton of external nose. **C.** Bony and cartilaginous skeleton of nasal septum.

Blood Supply of the External Nose

The skin of the external nose is supplied by branches of the ophthalmic and the maxillary arteries (see page 750). The skin of the ala and the lower part of the septum are supplied by branches from the facial artery.

Nerve Supply of the External Nose

The infratrochlear and external nasal branches of the ophthalmic nerve (CN V) and the infraorbital branch of the maxillary nerve (CN V) (see pages 760 and 761).

Nasal Cavity

The nasal cavity extends from the nostrils in front to the **posterior nasal apertures** or **choanae** behind, where the nose opens into the nasopharynx. The **nasal vestibule** is the area of the nasal cavity lying just inside the nostril (Fig. 11-93). The nasal cavity is divided into right and left halves by the **nasal septum** (Fig. 11-92). The septum is made up of the **septal cartilage,** the **vertical plate of the ethmoid,** and the **vomer.**

Walls of the Nasal Cavity

Each half of the nasal cavity has a floor, a roof, a lateral wall, and a medial or septal wall.

Floor

The palatine process of the maxilla and the horizontal plate of the palatine bone (Fig. 11-92)

Roof

The roof is narrow and is formed anteriorly beneath the bridge of the nose by the nasal and frontal bones, in the middle by the cribriform plate of the ethmoid, located beneath the anterior cranial fossa, and posteriorly by the downward sloping body of the sphenoid (Fig. 11-93).

Lateral Wall

The lateral wall has three projections of bone called the **superior, middle,** and **inferior nasal conchae** (Fig. 11-93). The space below each concha is called a **meatus.**

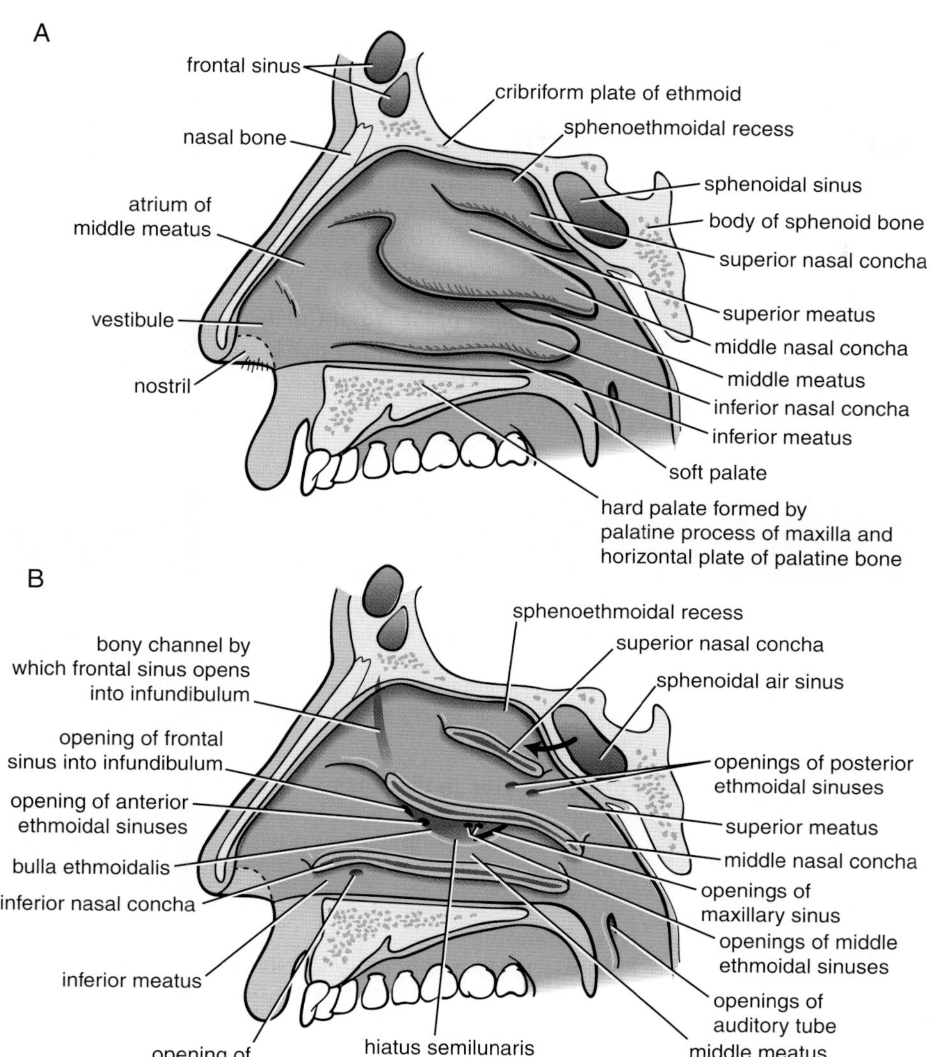

Figure 11-93 **A.** Lateral wall of the right nasal cavity. **B.** Lateral wall of the right nasal cavity; the superior, middle, and inferior conchae have been partially removed to show openings of the paranasal sinuses and the nasolacrimal duct into the meati.

Sphenoethmoidal Recess The sphenoethmoidal recess is a small area above the superior concha. It receives the opening of the **sphenoid air sinus** (Fig. 11-93).

Superior Meatus The superior meatus lies below the superior concha (Fig. 11-93). It receives the openings of the **posterior ethmoid sinuses.**

Middle Meatus The middle meatus lies below the middle concha. It has a rounded swelling called the **bulla ethmoidalis** that is formed by the **middle ethmoidal air sinuses,** which open on its upper border. A curved opening, the **hiatus semilunaris,** lies just below the bulla (Fig. 11-93). The anterior end of the hiatus leads into a funnel-shaped channel called the **infundibulum,** which is continuous with the **frontal sinus.** The **maxillary sinus** opens into the middle meatus through the **hiatus semilunaris.**

Inferior Meatus The inferior meatus lies below the inferior concha and receives the opening of the lower end of the **nasolacrimal duct,** which is guarded by a fold of mucous membrane (Fig. 11-93).

Medial Wall

The medial wall is formed by the nasal septum. The upper part is formed by the vertical plate of the ethmoid and the vomer (Fig. 11-92). The anterior part is formed by the septal cartilage. The septum rarely lies in the midline, thus increasing the size of one half of the nasal cavity and decreasing the size of the other.

Mucous Membrane of the Nasal Cavity

The vestibule is lined with modified skin and has coarse hairs. The area above the superior concha is lined with olfactory mucous membrane and contains nerve endings sensitive to the reception of smell. The lower part of the nasal cavity is lined with respiratory mucous membrane. A large plexus of veins in the submucous connective tissue is present in the respiratory region.

Function of Warm Blood and Mucus of Mucous Membrane

The presence of warm blood in the venous plexuses serves to heat up the inspired air as it enters the respiratory system. The presence of mucus on the surfaces of the conchae traps foreign particles and organisms in the inspired air, which are then swallowed and destroyed by gastric acid.

Nerve Supply of the Nasal Cavity.

The olfactory nerves from the olfactory mucous membrane ascend through the cribriform plate of the ethmoid bone to the olfactory bulbs (Fig. 11-94). The nerves of ordinary sensation are branches of the ophthalmic division (V1) and the maxillary division (V2) of the trigeminal nerve (Fig. 11-94).

Blood Supply to the Nasal Cavity

The arterial supply to the nasal cavity is from branches of the maxillary artery, one of the terminal branches of the external carotid artery. The most important branch is the sphenopalatine artery (Fig. 11-95). The sphenopalatine artery anastomoses with the septal branch of the superior labial branch of the facial artery in the region of the vestibule. The submucous venous plexus is drained by veins that accompany the arteries.

Lymph Drainage of the Nasal Cavity

The lymph vessels draining the vestibule end in the submandibular nodes. The remainder of the nasal cavity is drained by vessels that pass to the upper deep cervical nodes.

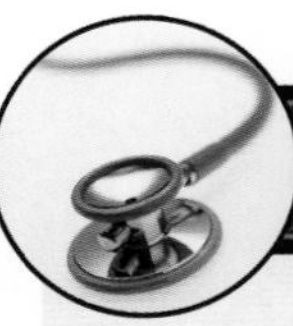

CLINICAL NOTES

Examination of the Nasal Cavity

Examination of the nasal cavity may be carried out by inserting a speculum through the external nares or by means of a mirror in the pharynx. In the latter case, the choanae and the posterior border of the septum can be visualized (Fig. 11-91).

It should be remembered that the nasal septum is rarely situated in the midline. A severely deviated septum may interfere with drainage of the nose and the paranasal sinuses.

Trauma to the Nose

Fractures involving the nasal bones are common. Blows directed from the front may cause one or both nasal bones to be displaced downward and inward. Lateral fractures also occur in which one nasal bone is driven inward and the other outward; the nasal septum is usually involved.

Infection of the Nasal Cavity

Infection of the nasal cavity can spread in a variety of directions. The paranasal sinuses are especially prone to infection. Organisms may spread via the nasal part of the pharynx and the auditory tube to the middle ear. It is possible for organisms to ascend to the meninges of the anterior cranial fossa, along the sheaths of the olfactory nerves through the cribriform plate, and produce meningitis.

Foreign Bodies in the Nose

Foreign bodies in the nose are common in children. The presence of the nasal septum and the existence of the folded, shelflike conchae make impaction and retention of balloons, peas, and small toys relatively easy.

Nose Bleeding

Epistaxis, or bleeding from the nose, is a frequent condition. The most common cause is nose picking. The bleeding may be arterial or venous, and most episodes occur on the anteroinferior portion of the septum and involve the septal branches of the sphenopalatine and facial vessels.

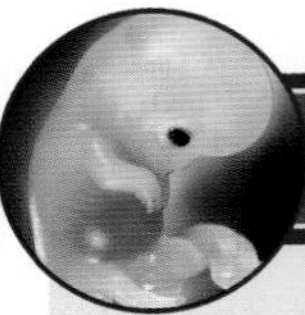

EMBRYOLOGIC NOTES

Development of the Nose

The roof of the nose is formed from the lateral nasal processes, from which the lateral walls also are formed, with the assistance of the maxillary processes (Fig. 11-43). The anterior openings of the nose begin as olfactory pits in the frontonasal process. Each olfactory pit is bounded medially by the medial nasal process, laterally by the lateral nasal process, and inferiorly by the maxillary process. As these processes fuse, the olfactory pits become deeper and form well-defined blind sacs, the opening into each of which is the nostril.

The floor of the nose at first is very short and consists of the medial nasal process and the anterior part of the maxillary process on each side. At this stage, the floors of the olfactory pits rupture so that the nasal cavities communicate with the developing mouth (Fig. 11-82). Meanwhile, the nasal septum is forming as a downgrowth from the medial nasal process (Fig. 11-82). Later, the palatal processes of the maxilla grow medially and fuse with each other and with the nasal septum, thus completing the floor of the nose. Each nasal cavity therefore communicates anteriorly with the exterior through the nostril and posteriorly through the choana with the nasopharynx.

In the early stages of development, the nose is a much-flattened structure and gains its recognizable form only after the facial development is complete.

Median Nasal Furrow

In median nasal furrow, the nasal septum is split, separating the two halves of the nose (Fig. 11-96A).

Lateral Proboscis

In lateral proboscis, a skin-covered process develops, usually with a dimple at its lower end (Fig. 11-96B).

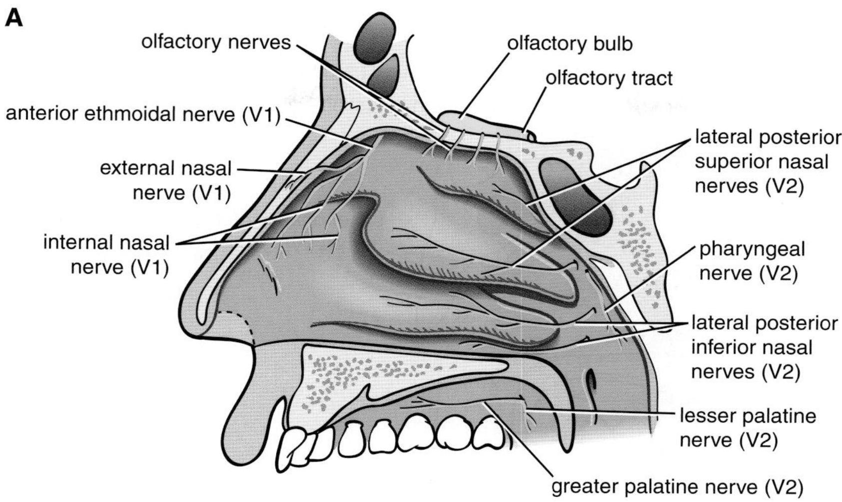

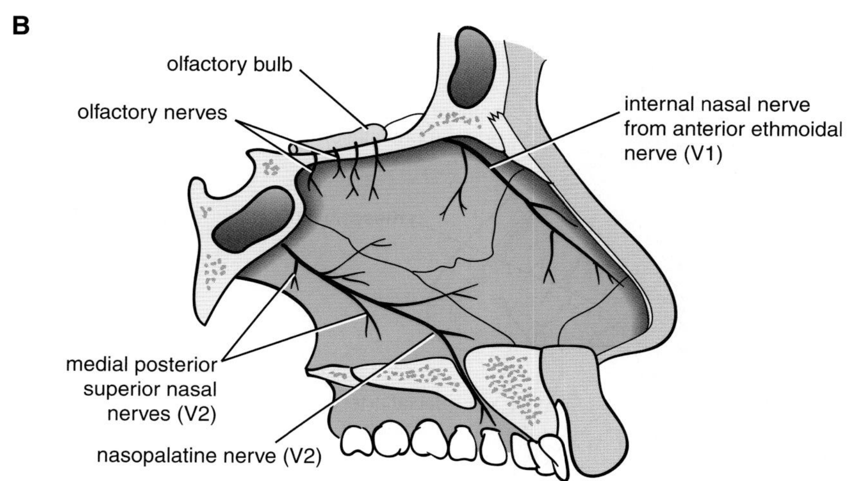

Figure 11-94 **A.** Lateral wall of nasal cavity showing sensory innervation of mucous membrane. **B.** Nasal septum showing sensory innervation of mucous membrane.

The Paranasal Sinuses

The paranasal sinuses are cavities found in the interior of the maxilla, frontal, sphenoid, and ethmoid bones (Fig. 11-97). They are lined with mucoperiosteum and filled with air; they communicate with the nasal cavity through relatively small apertures. The maxillary and sphenoidal sinuses are present in a rudimentary form at birth; they enlarge appreciably after the eighth year and become fully formed in adolescence.

Drainage of Mucus and Function of Paranasal Sinuses

The mucus produced by the mucous membrane is moved into the nose by ciliary action of the columnar cells. Drainage of the mucus is also achieved by the siphon action created during the blowing of the nose. The function of the sinuses is to act as resonators to the voice; they also reduce the weight of the skull. When the apertures of the sinuses are blocked or they become filled with fluid, the quality of the voice is markedly changed.

Maxillary Sinus

The maxillary sinus is pyramidal in shape and located within the body of the maxilla behind the skin of the cheek (Fig. 11-97). The roof is formed by the floor of the orbit, and the floor is related to the roots of the premolars and molar teeth. The maxillary sinus opens into the middle meatus of the nose through the hiatus semilunaris (Fig. 11-97).

Frontal Sinuses

The two frontal sinuses are contained within the frontal bone (Fig. 11-97). They are separated from each other by a bony septum. Each sinus is roughly triangular, extending upward above the medial end of the eyebrow and backward into the medial part of the roof of the orbit.

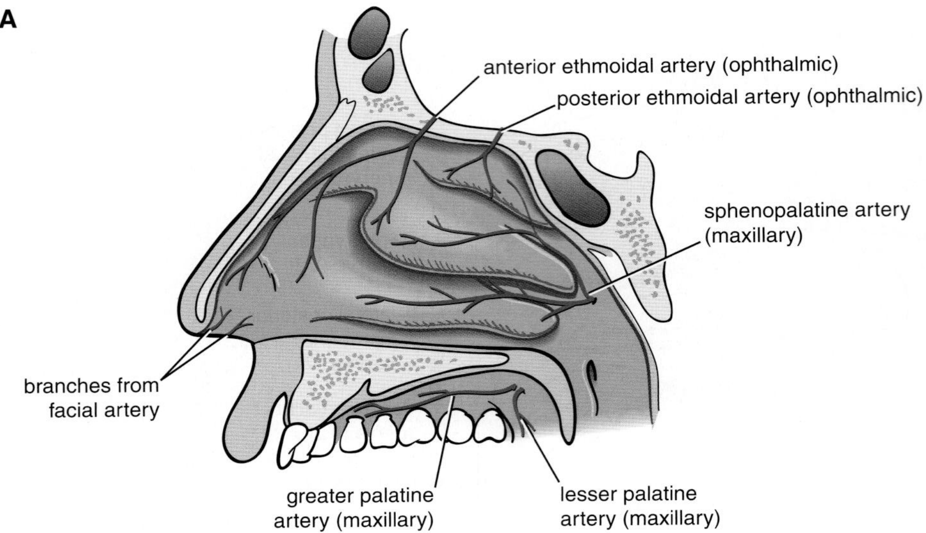

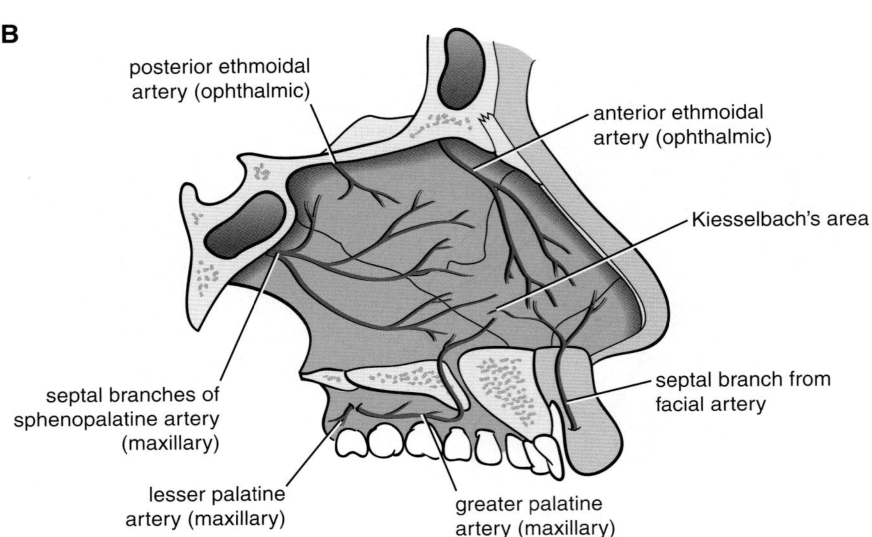

Figure 11-95 **A.** Lateral wall of nasal cavity showing the arterial supply of the mucous membrane. **B.** Nasal septum showing the arterial supply of the mucous membrane.

Each frontal sinus opens into the middle meatus of the nose through the infundibulum (Fig. 11-93).

Sphenoidal Sinuses

The two sphenoidal sinuses lie within the body of the sphenoid bone (Fig. 11-97). Each sinus opens into the sphenoethmoidal recess above the superior concha.

Ethmoid Sinuses

The ethmoidal sinuses are anterior, middle, and posterior and they are contained within the ethmoid bone, between the nose and the orbit (Fig. 11-97). They are separated from the latter by a thin plate of bone so that infection can readily spread from the sinuses into the orbit. The anterior sinuses open into the infundibulum; the middle sinuses open into the middle meatus, on or above the bulla ethmoidalis; and the posterior sinuses open into the superior meatus.

The various sinuses and their openings into the nose are summarized in Table 11-11.

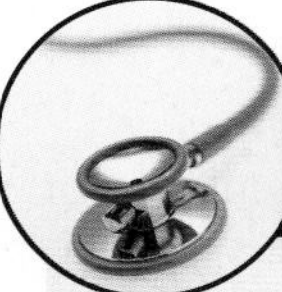

CLINICAL NOTES

Sinusitis and the Examination of the Paranasal Sinuses

Infection of the paranasal sinuses is a common complication of nasal infections. Rarely, the cause of maxillary sinusitis is extension from an apical dental abscess. The frontal, ethmoidal, and maxillary sinuses can be palpated clinically for areas of tenderness. The frontal sinus can be examined by pressing the finger upward beneath the medial end of the superior orbital margin. Here the floor of the frontal sinus is closest to the surface.

The ethmoidal sinuses can be palpated by pressing the finger medially against the medial wall of the orbit. The maxillary sinus can be examined for tenderness by pressing the finger against the

(continues)

Clinical Notes, *continued*

anterior wall of the maxilla below the inferior orbital margin; pressure over the infraorbital nerve may reveal increased sensitivity.

Directing the beam of a flashlight either through the roof of the mouth or through the cheek in a darkened room will often enable a physician to determine whether the maxillary sinus is full of inflammatory fluid rather than air. This method of transillumination is simple and effective. Radiologic examination of the sinuses is also most helpful in making a diagnosis. One should always compare the clinical findings of each sinus on the two sides of the body.

The frontal sinus is innervated by the supraorbital nerve, which also supplies the skin of the forehead and scalp as far back as the vertex. It is, therefore, not surprising that patients with frontal sinusitis have pain referred over this area. The maxillary sinus is innervated by the infraorbital nerve and, in this case, pain is referred to the upper jaw, including the teeth.

The frontal sinus drains into the hiatus semilunaris, via the infundibulum, close to the orifice of the maxillary sinus on the lateral wall of the nose. It is thus not unexpected to find that a patient with frontal sinusitis nearly always has a maxillary sinusitis. The maxillary sinus is particularly prone to infection because its drainage orifice through the hiatus semilunaris is badly placed near the roof of the sinus. In other words, the sinus has to fill up with fluid before it can effectively drain with the person in the upright position. The relation of the apices of the roots of the teeth in the maxilla to the floor of the maxillary sinus was already emphasized.

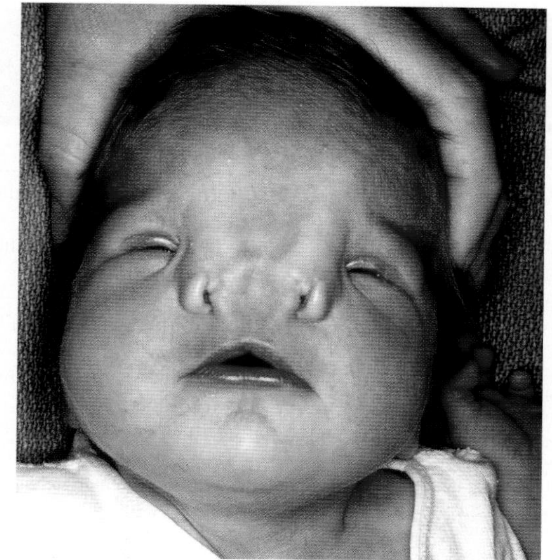

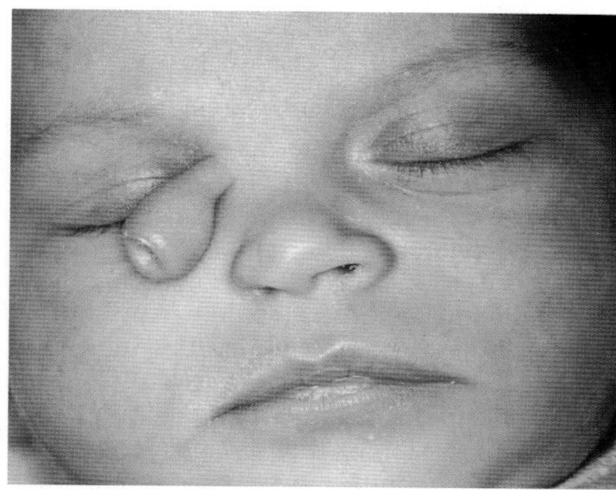

Figure 11-96 **A.** Median nasal furrow in which the nasal septum has completely split, separating the two halves of the nose. Note that the external nares are separated by a wide furrow. (Courtesy of L. Thompson.) **B.** Lateral proboscis. (Courtesy of R. Chase.)

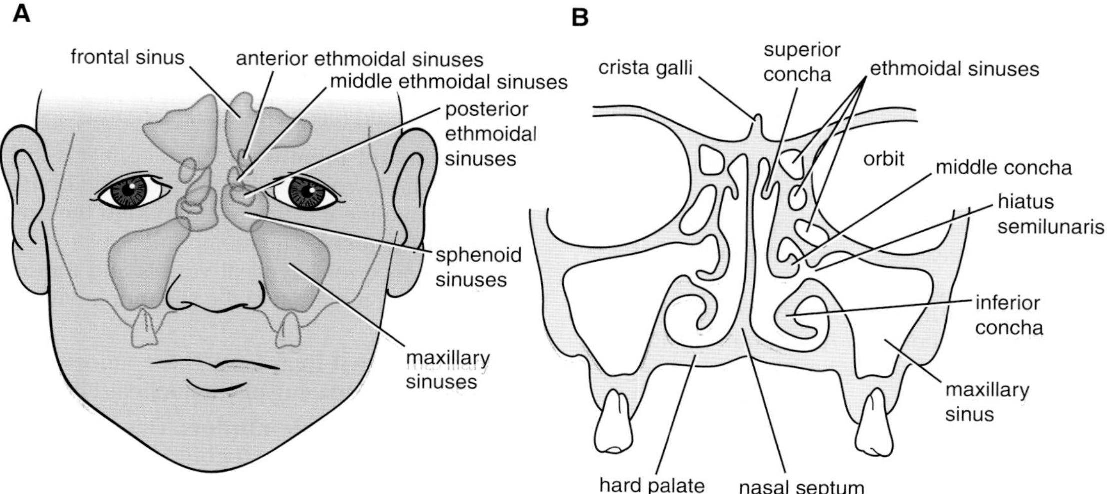

Figure 11-97 **A.** The position of the paranasal sinuses in relation to the face. **B.** Coronal section through the nasal cavity showing the ethmoidal and the maxillary sinuses.

Table 11-11 Paranasal Sinuses and Their Site of Drainage Into the Nose[a]

Sinus	Site of Drainage
Maxillary sinus	Middle meatus through hiatus semilunaris
Frontal sinuses	Middle meatus via infundibulum
Sphenoidal sinuses	Sphenoethmoidal recess
Ethmoidal sinuses	
Anterior group	Infundibulum and into middle meatus
Middle group	Middle meatus on or above bulla ethmoidalis
Posterior group	Superior meatus

[a] Note that maxillary and sphenoidal sinuses are present in rudimentary form at birth, enlarge appreciably after the eighth year, and are fully formed in adolescence.

Crossing of Air and Food Pathways in the Pharynx

It is in the pharynx that the air and food pathways cross. This is made possible by the presence of the soft palate, which serves as a flap-valve. This flap shuts off the mouth from the oropharynx, for example, during the process of chewing food so that breathing may continue unaffected. The completely raised soft palate can shut off the nasopharynx from the oropharynx, thus preventing food entering the nasopharynx in swallowing (see page 795). When it is desirable to direct the maximum amount of air in and out of the larynx, the soft palate is raised to direct air through the mouth rather than the narrow cavities of the nose. Such an arrangement permits the expectoration of mucus from the respiratory system through the mouth. It also allows the maximum expiration of air through the mouth as in the use of wind instruments such as the trumpet.

The Larynx

The larynx is an organ that provides a protective sphincter at the inlet of the air passages and is responsible for voice production. It is situated below the tongue and hyoid bone and between the great blood vessels of the neck and lies at the level of the fourth, fifth, and sixth cervical vertebrae (Fig. 11-87). It opens above into the laryngeal part of the pharynx, and below is continuous with the trachea. The larynx is covered in front by the infrahyoid strap muscles and at the sides by the thyroid gland.

The framework of the larynx is formed of cartilages that are held together by ligaments and membranes, moved by muscles, and lined by mucous membrane.

Cartilages of the Larynx

Thyroid cartilage: This is the largest cartilage of the larynx (Fig. 11-98) and consists of two laminae of hyaline cartilage that meet in the midline in the prominent V angle (the so-called Adam's apple). The posterior border extends upward into a **superior cornu** and downward into an **inferior cornu.** On the outer surface of each lamina is an oblique line for the attachment of muscles.

Cricoid cartilage: This cartilage is formed of hyaline cartilage and shaped like a signet ring, having a broad plate behind and a shallow arch in front (Fig. 11-98). The cricoid cartilage lies below the thyroid cartilage, and on each side of the lateral surface is a facet for articulation with the inferior cornu of the thyroid cartilage. Posteriorly, the lamina has on its upper border on each side a facet for articulation with the arytenoid cartilage. All these joints are synovial.

Arytenoid cartilages: There are two arytenoid cartilages, which are small and pyramid shaped and located at the back of the larynx (Fig. 11-98). They articulate with the upper border of the lamina of the cricoid cartilage. Each cartilage has an **apex** above that articulates with the small corniculate cartilage, a **base** below that articulates with the lamina of the cricoid cartilage, and a **vocal process** that projects forward and gives attachment to the vocal ligament. A **muscular process** that projects laterally gives attachment to the posterior and lateral cricoarytenoid muscles.

Corniculate cartilages: Two small conical-shaped cartilages articulate with the arytenoid cartilages (Fig. 11-99). They give attachment to the aryepiglottic folds.

Cuneiform cartilages: These two small rod-shaped cartilages are found in the aryepiglottic folds and serve to strengthen them (Fig. 11-99).

Epiglottis: This leaf-shaped lamina of elastic cartilage lies behind the root of the tongue (Fig. 11-98). Its stalk is attached to the back of the thyroid cartilage. The sides of the epiglottis are attached to the arytenoid cartilages by the aryepiglottic folds of mucous membrane. The upper edge of the epiglottis is free. The covering of mucous membrane passes forward onto the posterior surface of the tongue as the **median glossoepiglottic fold;** the depression on each side of the fold is called the **vallecula** (Fig. 11-90). Laterally the mucous membrane passes onto the wall of the pharynx as the lateral glossoepiglottic fold.

Membranes and Ligaments of the Larynx

Thyrohyoid membrane: This connects the upper margin of the thyroid cartilage to the hyoid bone (Fig. 11-98). In the midline it is thickened to form the **median thyrohyoid ligament.** The membrane is pierced on each side by the superior laryngeal vessels and the internal laryngeal nerve, a branch of the superior laryngeal nerve (Fig. 11-80).

Cricotracheal ligament: This connects the cricoid cartilage to the first ring of the trachea (Fig. 11-98).

Quadrangular membrane: This extends between the epiglottis and the arytenoid cartilages (Fig. 11-99). Its thickened inferior margin forms the **vestibular ligament,** and the vestibular ligaments form the interior of the **vestibular folds** (Fig. 11-99).

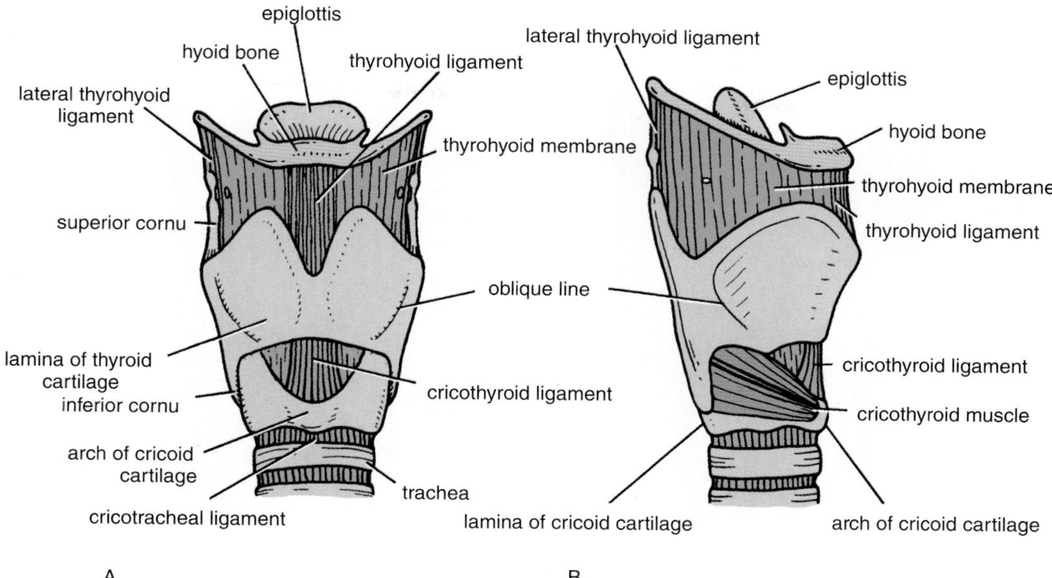

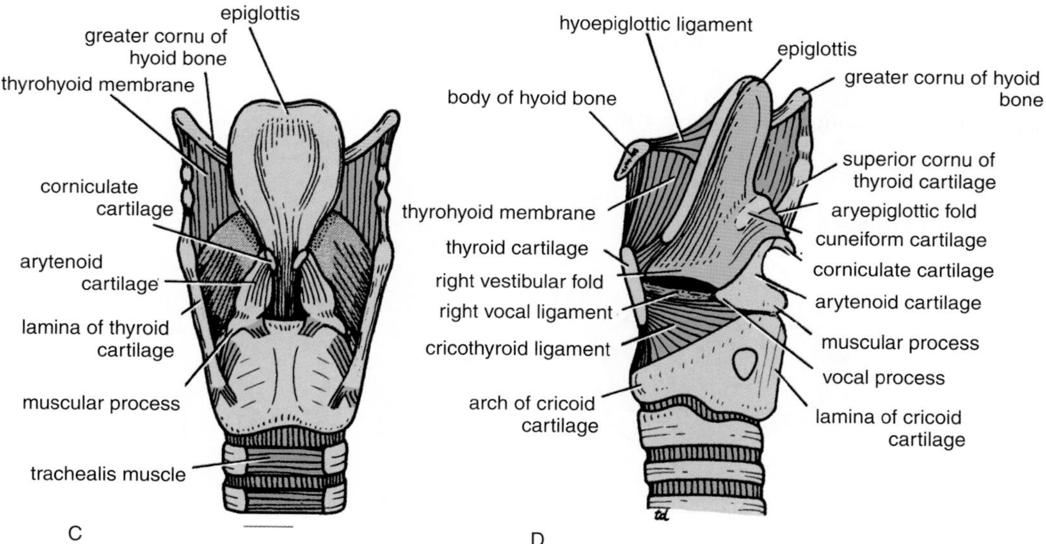

Figure 11-98 The larynx and its ligaments from the front (**A**), from the lateral aspect (**B**), and from behind (**C**). **D.** The left lamina of thyroid cartilage has been removed to display the interior of the larynx.

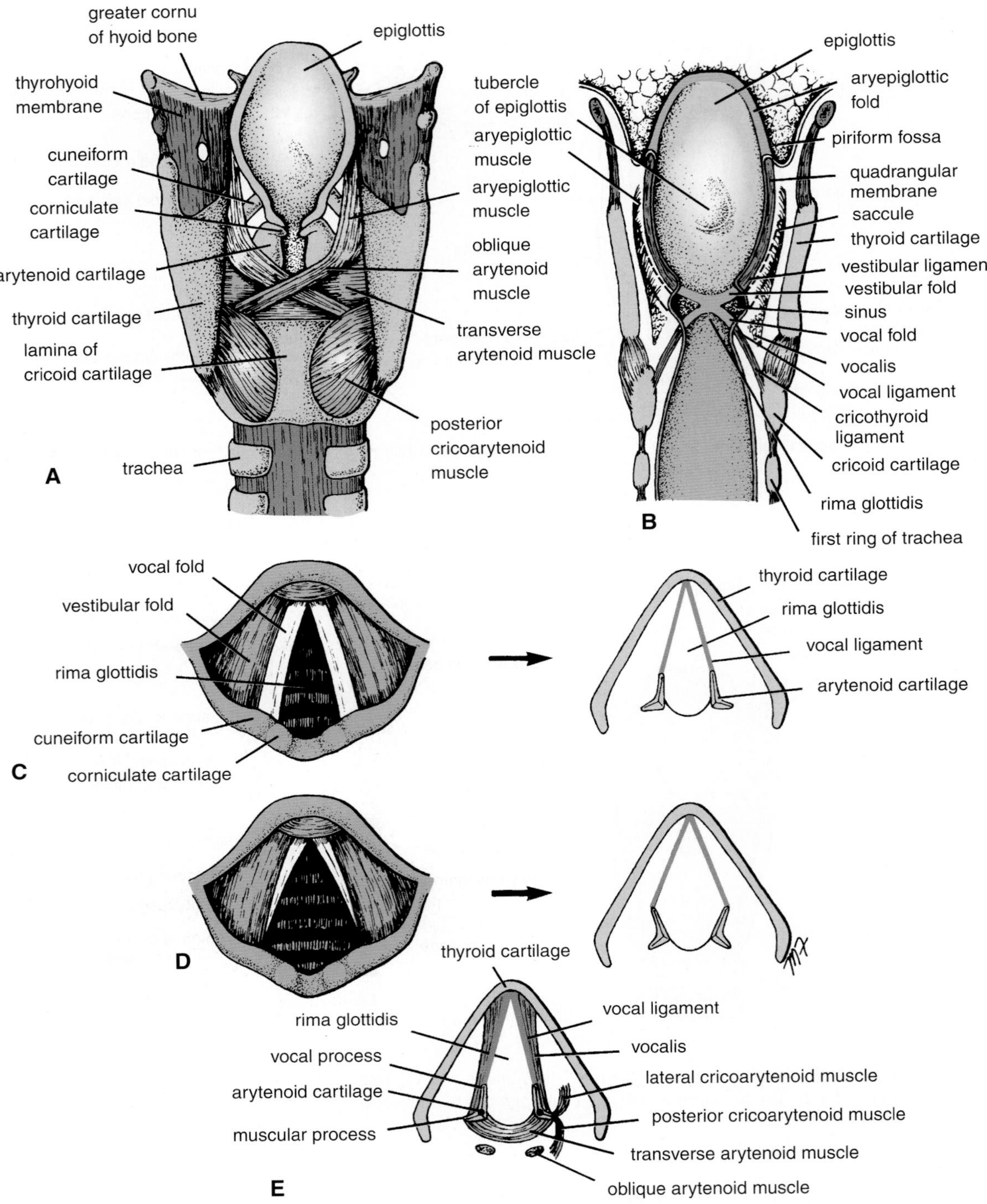

Figure 11-99 **A.** Muscles of the larynx seen from behind. **B.** Coronal section through the larynx. **C.** Rima glottidis partially open as in quiet breathing. **D.** Rima glottidis wide open as in deep breathing. **E.** Muscles that move vocal ligaments.

Cricothyroid ligament: The lower margin is attached to the upper border of the cricoid cartilage (Fig. 11-99). The superior margin of the ligament, instead of being attached to the thyroid cartilage, ascends on the medial surface of the thyroid cartilage. Its upper free margin, composed almost entirely of elastic tissue, forms the important **vocal ligament** on each side. The vocal ligaments form the interior of the **vocal folds (vocal cords)** (Fig. 11-99). The anterior end of each vocal ligament is attached to the thyroid cartilage, and the posterior end is attached to the vocal process of the arytenoid cartilage.

Inlet of the Larynx

The inlet of the larynx looks backward and upward into the laryngeal part of the pharynx (Fig. 11-88). The opening is wider in front than behind and is bounded in front by the epiglottis, laterally by the aryepiglottic fold of mucous membrane, and posteriorly by the arytenoid cartilages with the corniculate cartilages. The cuneiform cartilage lies within and strengthens the aryepiglottic fold and produces a small elevation on the upper border.

The Piriform Fossa

The piriform fossa is a recess on either side of the fold and inlet (Fig. 11-99). It is bounded medially by the aryepiglottic fold and laterally by the thyroid cartilage and the thyrohyoid membrane.

Laryngeal Folds

Vestibular Fold

The vestibular fold is a **fixed** fold on each side of the larynx (Fig. 11-98). It is formed by mucous membrane covering the vestibular ligament and is vascular and **pink** in color.

Vocal Fold (Vocal Cord)

The vocal fold is a **mobile** fold on each side of the larynx and is concerned with voice production. It is formed by mucous membrane covering the vocal ligament and is avascular and **white** in color. **The vocal fold moves with respiration and its white color is easily seen when viewed with a laryngoscope** (Fig. 11-99).

The gap between the vocal folds is called the **rima glottidis or glottis** (Fig. 11-99). The glottis is bounded in front by the vocal folds and behind by the medial surface of the arytenoid cartilages. The glottis is the narrowest part of the larynx and measures about 2.5 cm from front to back in the male adult and less in the female. In children the lower part of the larynx within the cricoid cartilage is the narrowest part.

Cavity of the Larynx

The cavity of the larynx extends from the inlet to the lower border of the cricoid cartilage, where it is continuous with the cavity of the trachea. It is divided into three regions:

The **vestibule,** which is situated between the inlet and the vestibular folds

The **middle region,** which is situated between the vestibular folds above and the vocal folds below

The **lower region,** which is situated between the vocal folds above and the lower border of the cricoid cartilage below

Sinus of the Larynx

The sinus of the larynx is a small recess on each side of the larynx situated between the vestibular and vocal folds. It is lined with mucous membrane (Fig. 11-99).

Saccule of the Larynx

The saccule of the larynx is a diverticulum of mucous membrane that ascends from the sinus (Fig. 11-99). The mucous secretion lubricates the vocal cords.

Muscles of the Larynx

The muscles of the larynx may be divided into two groups: extrinsic and intrinsic.

Extrinsic Muscles

These muscles move the larynx up and down during swallowing. Note that many of these muscles are attached to the hyoid bone, which is attached to the thyroid cartilage by the thyrohyoid membrane. It follows that movements of the hyoid bone are accompanied by movements of the larynx.

Elevation: The digastric, the stylohyoid, the mylohyoid, the geniohyoid, the stylopharyngeus, the salpingopharyngeus, and the palatopharyngeus muscles

Depression: The sternothyroid, the sternohyoid, and the omohyoid muscles

Intrinsic Muscles

Two muscles modify the laryngeal inlet (Fig. 11-99):

- **Narrowing the inlet:** The oblique arytenoid muscle
- **Widening the inlet:** The thyroepiglottic muscle

Five muscles move the vocal folds (cords) (Fig. 11-99):

- **Tensing the vocal cords:** The cricothyroid muscle
- **Relaxing the vocal cords:** The thyroarytenoid (vocalis) muscle
- **Adducting the vocal cords:** The lateral cricoarytenoid muscle
- **Abducting the vocal cords:** The posterior cricoarytenoid muscle
- **Approximates the arytenoid cartilages:** The transverse arytenoid muscle

The details of the origins, insertions, nerve supply, and action of the intrinsic muscles of the larynx are given in Table 11-12.

Movements of the Vocal Folds (Cords)

The movements of the vocal folds depend on the movements of the arytenoid cartilages, which rotate and slide up and down on the sloping shoulder of the superior border of the cricoid cartilage.

The rima glottidis is opened by the contraction of the posterior cricoarytenoid, which rotates the arytenoid cartilage and abducts the vocal process (Fig. 11-99). The elastic tissue in the capsules of the cricoarytenoid joints keeps the arytenoid cartilages apart so that the posterior part of the glottis is open.

Table 11-12 Intrinsic Muscles of the Larynx

Muscle	Origin	Insertion	Nerve Supply	Action
Muscles Controlling the Laryngeal Inlet				
Oblique arytenoid	Muscular process of arytenoid cartilage	Apex of opposite arytenoid cartilage	Recurrent laryngeal nerve	Narrows the inlet by bringing the aryepiglottic folds together
Thyroepiglottic	Medial surface of thyroid cartilage	Lateral margin of epiglottis and aryepiglottic fold	Recurrent laryngeal nerve	Widens the inlet by pulling the aryepiglottic folds apart
Muscles Controlling the Movements of the Vocal Folds (Cords)				
Cricothyroid	Side of cricoid cartilage	Lower border and inferior cornu of thyroid cartilage	External laryngeal nerve	Tenses vocal cords
Thyroarytenoid (vocalis)	Inner surface of thyroid cartilage	Arytenoid cartilage	Recurrent laryngeal nerve	Relaxes vocal cords
Lateral cricoarytenoid	Upper border of cricoid cartilage	Muscular process of arytenoid cartilage	Recurrent laryngeal nerve	Adducts the vocal cords by rotating arytenoid cartilage
Posterior cricoarytenoid	Back of cricoid cartilage	Muscular process of arytenoid cartilage	Recurrent laryngeal nerve	Abducts the vocal cords by rotating arytenoid cartilage
Transverse arytenoid	Back and medial surface of arytenoid cartilage	Back and medial surface of opposite arytenoid cartilage	Recurrent laryngeal nerve	Closes posterior part of rima glottidis by approximating arytenoid cartilages

The rima glottidis is closed by contraction of the lateral cricoarytenoid, which rotates the arytenoid cartilage and adducts the vocal process (Fig. 11-99). The posterior part of the glottis is narrowed when the arytenoid cartilages are drawn together by contraction of the transverse arytenoid muscles.

The vocal folds are stretched by contraction of the cricothyroid muscle (Fig. 11-100). The vocal folds are slackened by contraction of the vocalis, a part of the thyroarytenoid muscle (Fig. 11-99).

Movements of the Vocal Folds With Respiration On quiet inspiration, the vocal folds are abducted and the rima glottidis is triangular in shape with the apex in front (Fig. 11-99). On expiration the vocal folds are adducted, leaving a small gap between them (Fig. 11-99).

On deep inspiration, the vocal folds are maximally abducted and the triangular shape of the glottis becomes a diamond shape because of the maximal lateral rotation of the arytenoid cartilages (Fig. 11-99).

Sphincteric Function of the Larynx There are two sphincters in the larynx: one at the inlet and another at the rima glottidis.

The sphincter at the inlet is used only during swallowing. As the bolus of food is passed backward between the tongue and the hard palate, the larynx is pulled up beneath the back of the tongue. The inlet of the larynx is narrowed by the action of the oblique arytenoid and aryepiglottic muscles. The epiglottis is pulled backward by the tongue and serves as a cap over the laryngeal inlet. The bolus of food, or fluids, then enters the esophagus by passing over the epiglottis or moving down the grooves on either side of the laryngeal inlet, the piriform fossae.

In coughing or sneezing, the rima glottidis serves as a sphincter. After inspiration, the vocal folds are adducted, and the muscles of expiration are made to contract strongly. As a result, the intrathoracic pressure rises, and the vocal folds are suddenly abducted. The sudden release of the compressed air will often dislodge foreign particles or mucus from the respiratory tract and carry the material up into the pharynx, where the material is either swallowed or expectorated.

In the Valsalva maneuver, forced expiration takes place against a closed glottis. In abdominal straining associated with micturition, defecation, and parturition, air is often held temporarily in the respiratory tract by closing the rima glottidis. After deep inspiration the rima glottidis is closed. The muscles of the anterior abdominal wall now contract, and the upward movement of the diaphragm is prevented by the presence of compressed air within the respiratory tract. After a prolonged effort the person often releases some of the air by momentarily opening the rima glottidis, producing a grunting sound.

Voice Production in the Larynx The intermittent release of expired air between the adducted vocal folds results in their vibration and in the production of sound. The **frequency,** or **pitch,** of the sound is determined by changes in the length and tension of the vocal ligaments. The **quality** of the voice depends on the resonators above the larynx, namely, the pharynx, mouth, and paranasal sinuses. The quality of the voice is controlled by the muscles of the soft plate, tongue, floor of the mouth, cheeks, lips, and jaws. Normal speech depends on the modification of the sound into recognizable consonants and vowels by the use of the tongue, teeth, and lips. Vowel sounds are usually

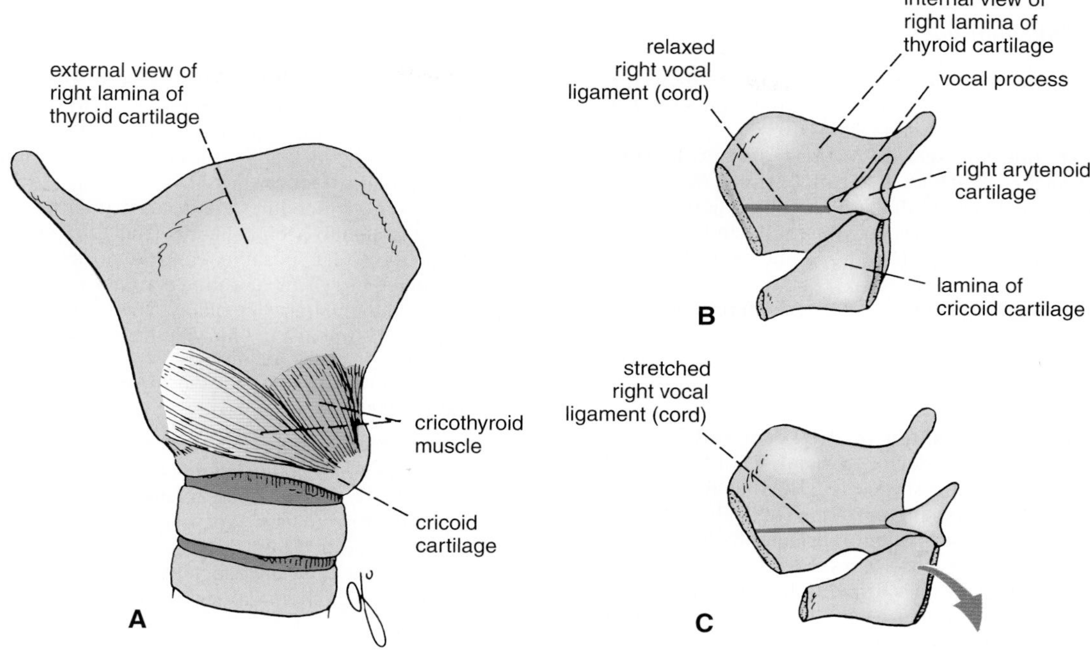

Figure 11-100 Diagrams showing the attachments and actions of the cricothyroid muscle. **A.** Right lateral view of the larynx and the cricothyroid muscle. **B.** Interior view of the larynx showing the relaxed right vocal ligament. **C.** Interior view of the larynx showing the right vocal ligament stretched as a result of the cricoid and arytenoid cartilages tilting backward by contraction of the cricothyroid muscles.

purely oral with the soft palate raised so that the air is channeled through the mouth rather than the nose.

Speech involves the intermittent release of expired air between the adducted vocal folds. **Singing** a note requires a more prolonged release of the expired air between the adducted vocal folds. In whispering, the vocal folds are adducted, but the arytenoid cartilages are separated; the vibrations are given to a constant stream of expired air that passes through the posterior part of the rima glottidis.

Mucous Membrane of the Larynx

The mucous membrane of the larynx lines the cavity and is covered with ciliated columnar epithelium. On the vocal cords, however, where the mucous membrane is subject to repeated trauma during phonation, the mucous membrane is covered with stratified squamous epithelium.

Nerve Supply of the Larynx

Sensory Nerves

- **Above the vocal cords:** The internal laryngeal branch of the superior laryngeal branch of the vagus
- **Below the level of the vocal cords**: The recurrent laryngeal nerve (Fig. 11-101)

Motor Nerves All the intrinsic muscles of the larynx except the cricothyroid muscle are supplied by the recurrent laryngeal nerve. The cricothyroid muscle is supplied by the external laryngeal branch of the superior laryngeal branch of the vagus.

Blood Supply of the Larynx

- **Upper half of the larynx:** The superior laryngeal branch of the superior thyroid artery
- **Lower half of the larynx:** The inferior laryngeal branch of the inferior thyroid artery

Lymph Drainage of the Larynx

The lymph vessels drain into the deep cervical group of nodes.

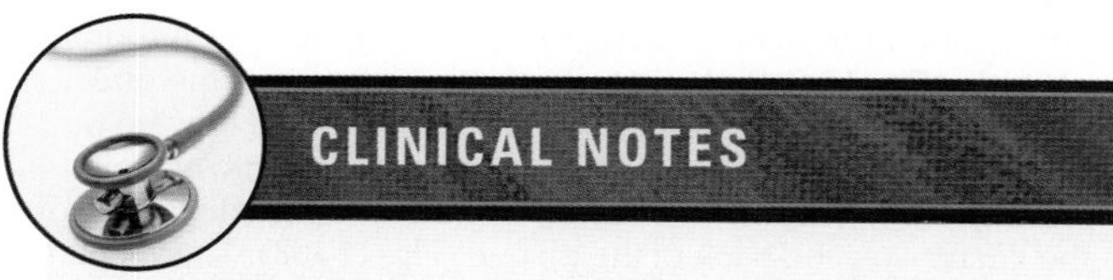

Lesions of the Laryngeal Nerves

The muscles of the larynx are innervated by the recurrent laryngeal nerves, with the exception of the cricothyroid muscle, which is supplied by the external laryngeal nerve. Both these nerves are vulnerable during operations on the thyroid gland because of the close relationship between them and the arteries of the gland. The left recurrent laryngeal nerve may be involved in a bronchial or esophageal carcinoma or in secondary metastatic deposits in the mediastinal lymph nodes. The right and left recurrent laryngeal nerves may be damaged by malignant involvement of the deep cervical lymph nodes.

(continues)

Clinical Notes, *continued*

Section of the external laryngeal nerve produces weakness of the voice because the vocal fold cannot be tensed. The cricothyroid muscle is paralyzed (Fig. 11-102).

Unilateral complete section of the recurrent laryngeal nerve results in the vocal fold on the affected side assuming the position midway between abduction and adduction. It lies just lateral to the midline. Speech is not greatly affected because the other vocal fold compensates to some extent and moves toward the affected vocal fold (Fig. 11-102).

Bilateral complete section of the recurrent laryngeal nerve results in both vocal folds assuming the position midway between abduction and adduction. Breathing is impaired because the rima glottidis is partially closed, and speech is lost (Fig. 11-102).

Unilateral partial section of the recurrent laryngeal nerve results in a greater degree of paralysis of the abductor muscles than of the adductor muscles. The affected vocal fold assumes the adducted midline position (Fig. 11-102). This phenomenon has not been explained satisfactorily. It must be assumed that the abductor muscles receive a greater number of nerves than the adductor muscles, and thus partial damage of the recurrent laryngeal nerve results in damage to relatively more nerve fibers to the abductor muscles. Another possibility is that the nerve fibers to the abductor muscles are traveling in a more exposed position in the recurrent laryngeal nerve and are therefore more prone to be damaged.

Bilateral partial section of the recurrent laryngeal nerve results in bilateral paralysis of the abductor muscles and the drawing together of the vocal folds (Fig. 11-102). Acute breathlessness (dyspnea) and stridor follow, and cricothyroidotomy or tracheostomy is necessary.

Edema of the Laryngeal Mucous Membrane

The mucous membrane of the larynx is loosely attached to the underlying structures by submucous connective tissue. In the region of the vocal folds, however, the mucous membrane is firmly attached to the vocal ligaments. This fact is of clinical importance in cases of edema of the larynx. The accumulation of tissue fluid causes the mucous membrane above the rima glottidis to swell and encroach on the airway. In severe cases, a cricothyroidotomy or tracheostomy may be necessary.

Laryngeal Mirror and Laryngoscope

The interior of the larynx can be inspected indirectly through a laryngeal mirror passed through the open mouth into the oral pharynx (Fig. 11-103). A more satisfactory method is the direct method using the laryngoscope. The neck is brought forward on a pillow and the head is fully extended at the atlanto-occipital joints. The illuminated instrument can then be introduced into the larynx over the back of the tongue (Fig. 11-103). The valleculae, the piriform fossae, the epiglottis, and the aryepiglottic folds are clearly seen. The two elevations produced by the corniculate and cuneiform cartilages can be recognized. Within the larynx, the vestibular folds and the vocal folds can be seen. The former are fixed, widely separated, and reddish in color; the latter move with respiration and are white in color. With quiet breathing, the rima glottidis is triangular, with the apex in front. With deep inspiration, the rima glottidis assumes a diamond shape because of the lateral rotation of the arytenoid cartilages.

If the patient is asked to breathe deeply, the vocal folds become widely abducted, and the inside of the trachea can be seen.

Important Anatomic Axes for Endotracheal Intubation

The upper airway has three axes that have to be brought into alignment if the glottis is to be viewed adequately through a laryngoscope—the axis of the mouth, the axis of the pharynx, and the axis of the trachea (Fig. 11-104).

The following procedures are necessary: First the head is extended at the atlanto-occipital joints. This brings the axis of the mouth into the correct position. Then the neck is flexed at cervical vertebrae C4 to C7 by elevating the back of the head off the table, often with the help of a pillow. This brings the axes of the pharynx and the trachea in line with the axis of the mouth.

Anatomy of the Visualization of the Vocal Cords With the Laryngoscope

- The pear-shaped epiglottis is attached by its stalk at its lower end to the interior of the thyroid cartilage (Fig. 11-98).
- The vocal cords (ligaments) are attached at their anterior ends to the thyroid cartilage just below the attachment of the epiglottis (Fig. 11-98).
- Because of the above two facts, it follows that manipulation of the epiglottis and possibly the thyroid cartilage will greatly assist the operator in visualizing the cords and the glottis.

The patient's head and neck are correctly positioned so that the three axes of the airway (noted above) have been established and the patient has assumed the "sniffing" position. The laryngoscope is inserted into the patient's mouth, and the blade is correctly placed alongside the right mandibular molar teeth. The blade can then be passed over the tongue and down into the esophagus. The tip of the blade must be fully inserted into the esophagus (so that you know where it is anatomically). The blade should by now have moved toward the midline and followed the anatomic curvature on the posterior surface of the tongue.

The laryngoscopic blade is then gently and slowly withdrawn. The tip of the blade is kept under direct vision at all times and is permitted to rise up out of the esophagus. Remember that the tip of the blade is at first in the esophagus and is, therefore, distal to the level of the vocal cords. Once the blade tip has left the esophagus, it is in the laryngeal part of the pharynx (Figs. 11-88 and 11-91), and a view of the glottis should immediately be apparent. This is the critical stage. If the glottis is not visualized, then the operator is viewing the posterior surface of the epiglottis. **Now use your anatomic knowledge.**

With the tip of the blade of the laryngoscope applied to the posterior surface of the epiglottis, gently lift up and elevate the epiglottis to expose the glottis. If the glottis is still not in view, **do not panic!** Again use your knowledge of anatomy. With the right free hand grasp the thyroid cartilage (to which the cords and the epiglottis are attached) between finger and thumb and apply firm backward, upward, rightward pressure **(BURP).** This maneuver realigns the box of the larynx relative to the laryngoscopic blade, and the visual axis of the operator and the glottis should immediately be seen.

Reflex Activity Secondary to Endotracheal Intubation

Stimulation of the mucous membrane of the upper airway during the process of intubation may produce cardiovascular changes such as bradycardia and hypertension. These changes are largely mediated through the branches of the vagus nerves.

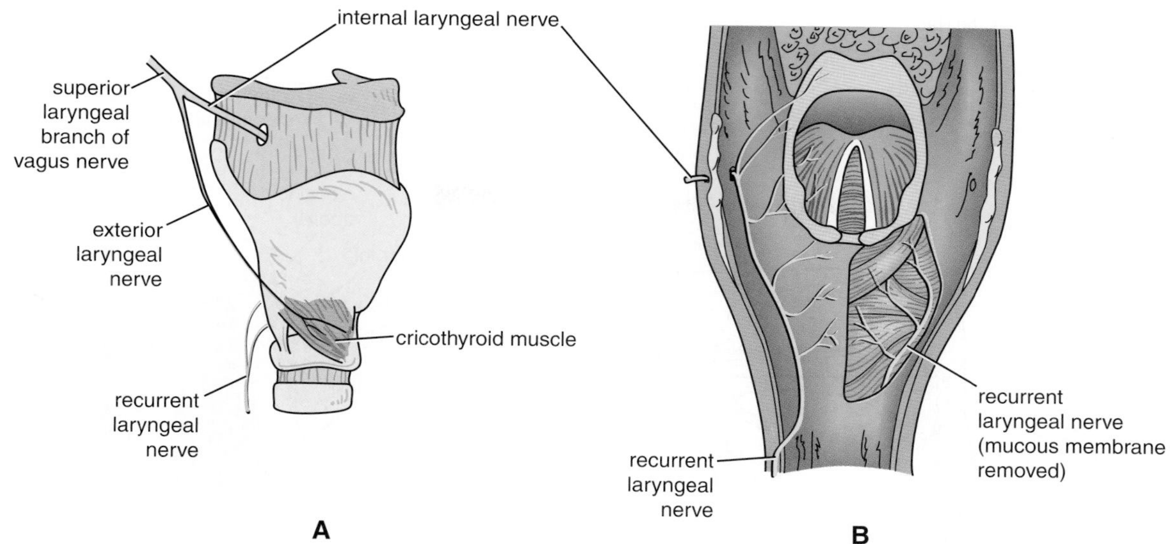

Figure 11-101 **A.** Lateral view of larynx showing the internal and external laryngeal branches of the superior laryngeal branch of the vagus nerve. **B.** The distribution of the terminal branches of the internal and recurrent laryngeal nerves. The larynx is viewed from above and posteriorly.

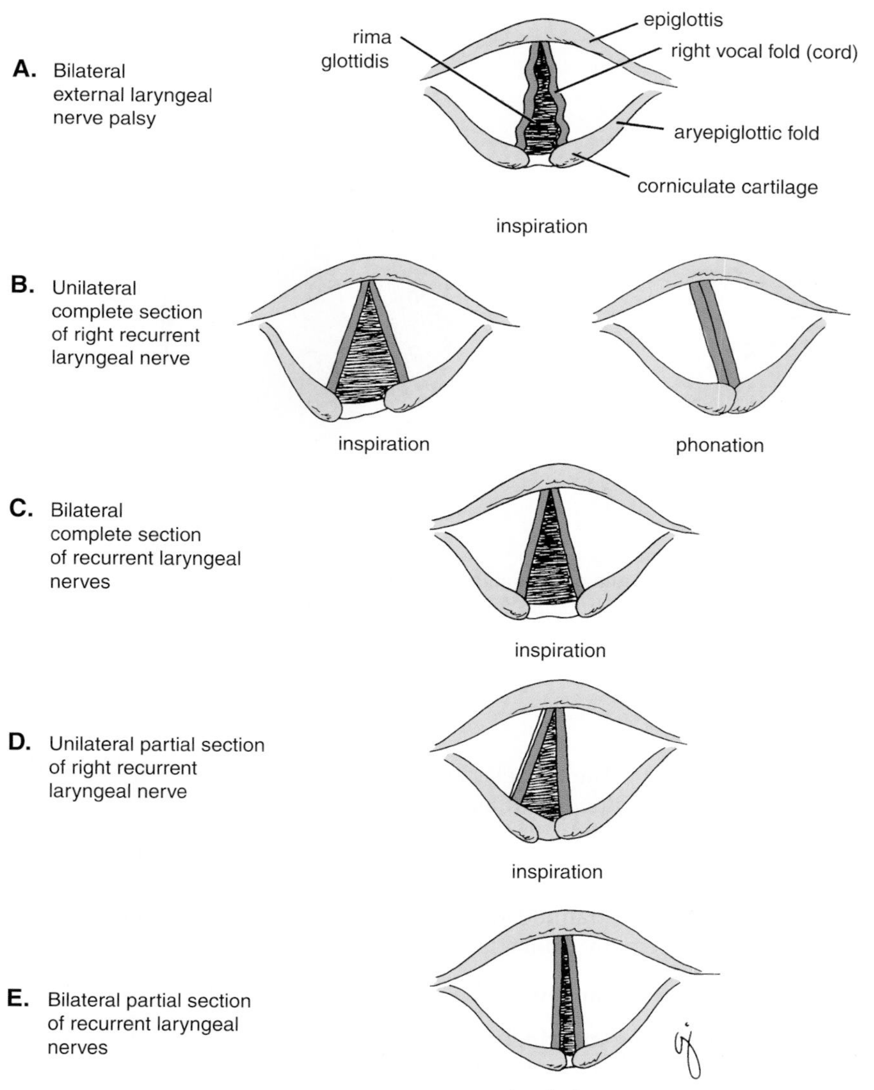

Figure 11-102 The position of the vocal folds (cords) after damage to the external and recurrent laryngeal nerves.

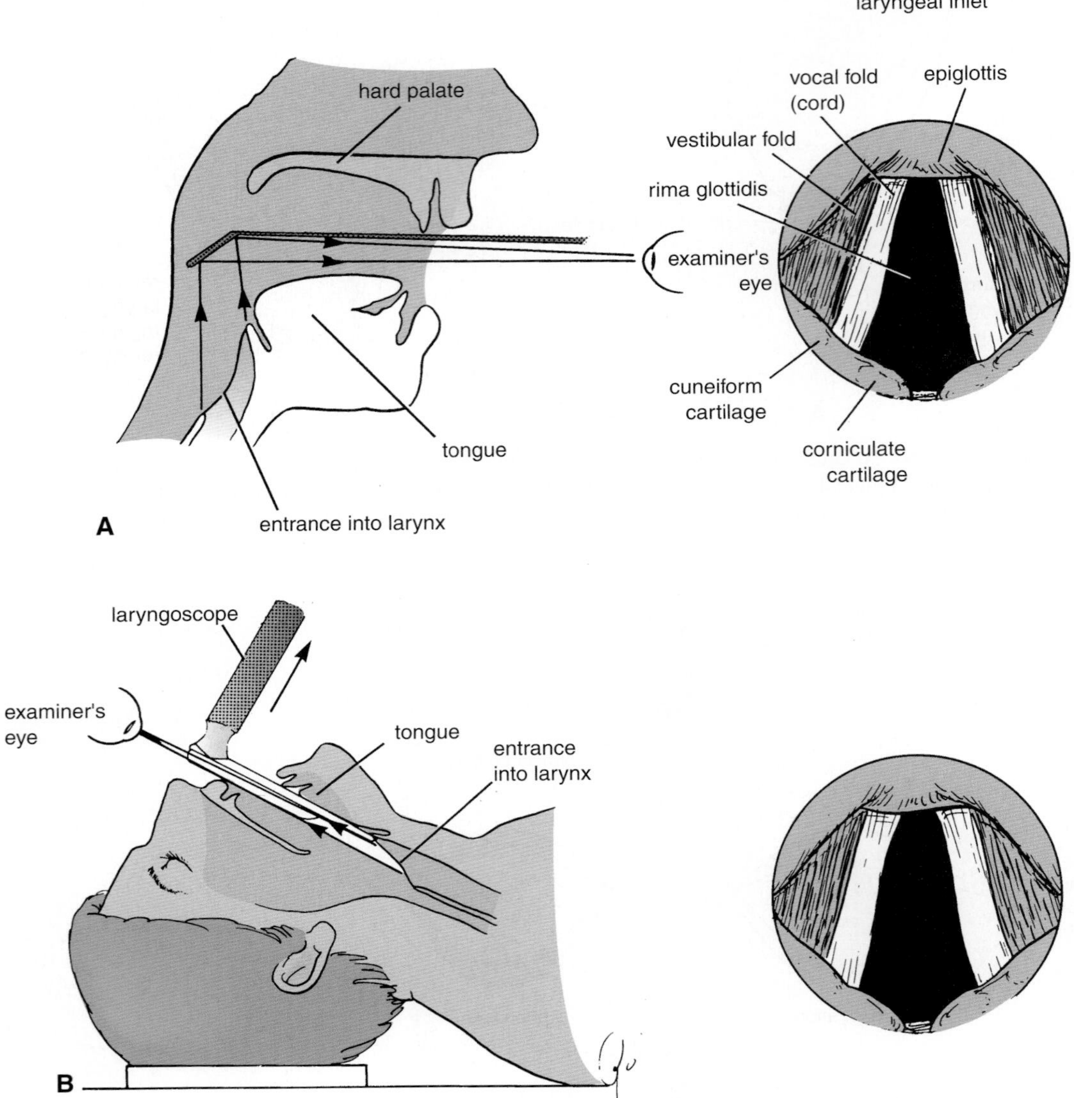

Figure 11-103 Inspection of the vocal folds (cords) indirectly through a laryngeal mirror (**A**) and through a laryngoscope (**B**). Note the orientation of the structures forming the laryngeal inlet.

The Trachea

Description

The trachea is a mobile cartilaginous and membranous tube (Fig. 11-105). It begins as a continuation of the larynx at the lower border of the cricoid cartilage at the level of the sixth cervical vertebra. It descends in the midline of the neck. In the thorax the trachea ends at the **carina** by dividing into right and left principal (main) bronchi at the level of the sternal angle (opposite the disc between the fourth and fifth thoracic vertebrae).

The fibroelastic tube is kept patent by the presence of U-shaped cartilaginous bar (rings) of hyaline cartilage embedded in its wall. The posterior free ends of the cartilage are connected by smooth muscle, the **trachealis muscle.**

The mucous membrane of the trachea is lined with pseudostratified ciliated columnar epithelium and contains many goblet cells and tubular mucous glands.

Relations of the Trachea in the Neck (Fig. 11-49)

- **Anteriorly:** Skin, fascia, isthmus of the thyroid gland (in front of the second, third, and fourth rings), inferior

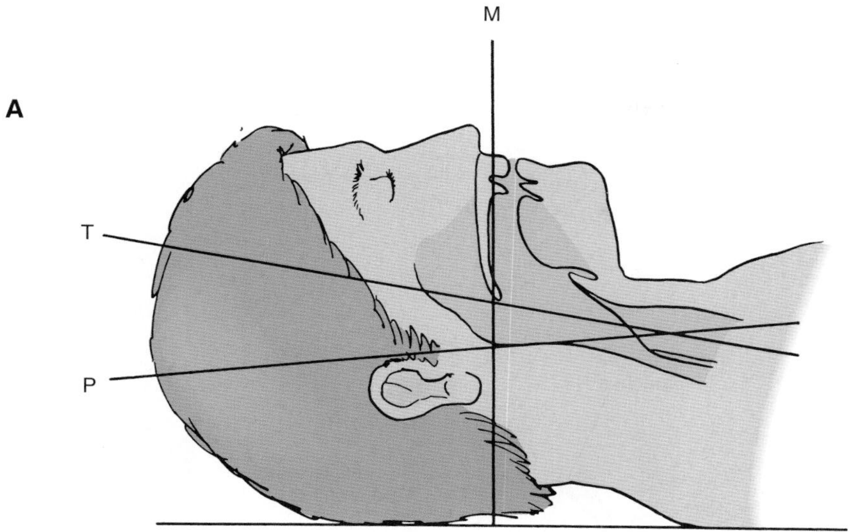

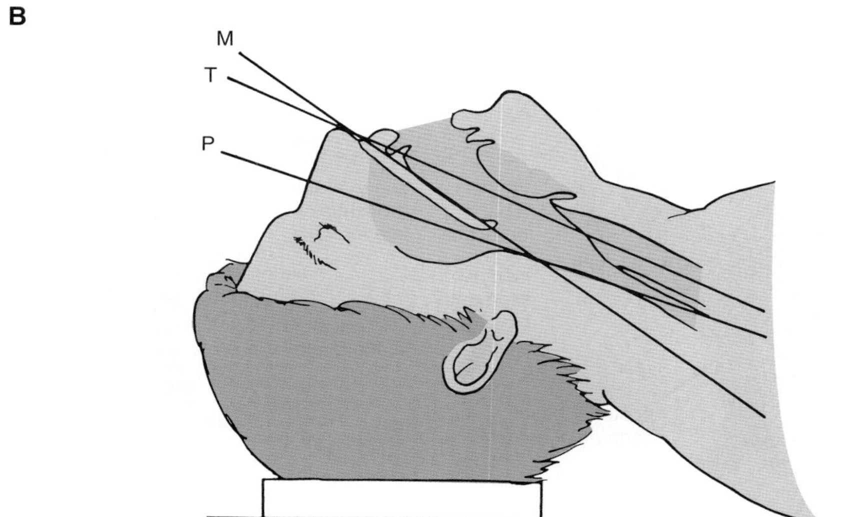

Figure 11-104 Anatomic axes for endotracheal intubation. **A.** With the head in the neutral position, the axis of the mouth (M), the axis of the trachea (T), and the axis of the pharynx (P) are not aligned with one another. **B.** If the head is extended at the atlanto-occipital joints, the axis of the mouth is correctly placed. If the back of the head is raised off the table with a pillow, thus flexing the cervical vertebral column, the axes of the trachea and pharynx are brought in line with the axis of the mouth.

thyroid vein, jugular arch, thyroidea ima artery (if present), and the left brachiocephalic vein in children, overlapped by the sternothyroid and sternohyoid muscles

- **Posteriorly:** Right and left recurrent laryngeal nerves and the esophagus
- **Laterally:** Lobes of the thyroid gland and the carotid sheath and contents

The relations of the trachea in the superior mediastinum of the thorax are described on page 87.

Nerve Supply of the Trachea

The sensory nerve supply is from the vagi and the recurrent laryngeal nerves.

Blood Supply of the Trachea

The upper two thirds is supplied by the inferior thyroid arteries and the lower third is supplied by the bronchial arteries.

Lymph Drainage of the Trachea

Into the pretracheal and paratracheal lymph nodes and the deep cervical nodes

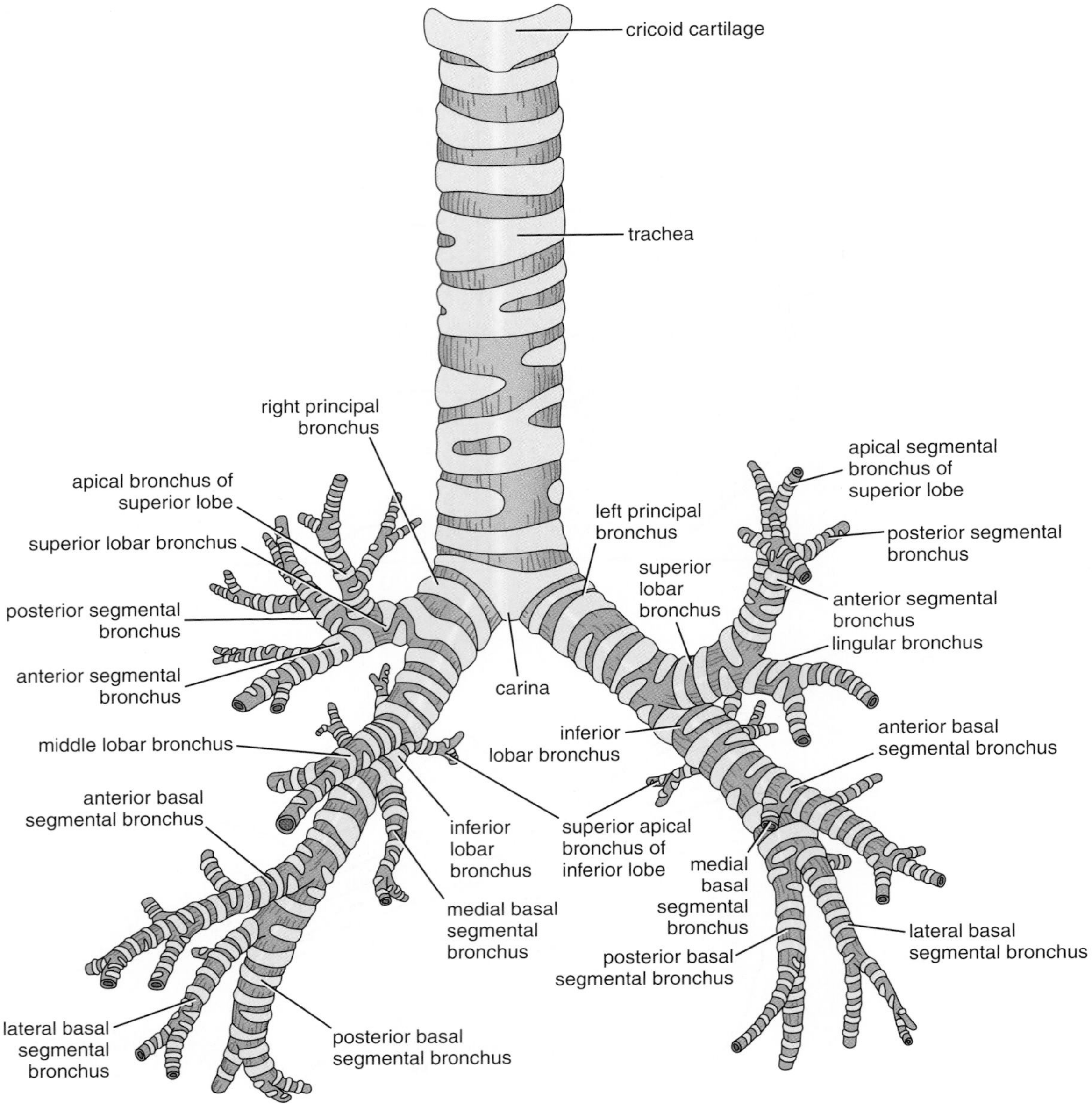

Figure 11-105 The trachea and the bronchi.

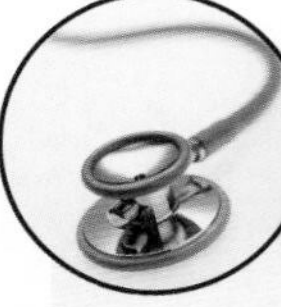

CLINICAL NOTES

Midline Structures in the Neck

The midline structures in the neck should be readily recognized as one passes an examining finger down the neck from the chin to the suprasternal notch (for details, see page 839). The physician commonly forgets that an enlarged submental lymph node may be caused by a pathologic condition anywhere between the tip of the tongue and the point of the chin.

Palpation of the Trachea

The trachea can be readily felt below the larynx. As it descends, it becomes deeply placed and may lie as much as 1.5 in. (4 cm) from the surface at the suprasternal notch. Remember that in the adult it may measure as much as 1 in. (2.5 cm) in diameter, but in a 3-year-old child it may measure only 0.5 in. in diameter. The trachea is a mobile elastic tube and is easily displaced by the enlargement of adjacent organs or the presence of tumors. Remember also that lateral displacement of the cervical part of the trachea may be caused by a pathologic lesion in the thorax.

Compromised Airway

No medical emergency quite produces the urgency and anxiety of the compromised airway. The physician has to institute almost immediate treatment. All techniques of airway management require a detailed knowledge of anatomy.

(continues)

Clinical Notes, *continued*

Cricothyroidotomy

In cricothyroidotomy, a tube is inserted in the interval between the cricoid cartilage and the thyroid cartilage. The trachea and larynx are steadied by extending the neck over a sandbag.

A vertical or transverse incision is made in the skin in the interval between the cartilages (Fig. 11-106). The incision is made through the following structures: the skin, the superficial fascia (beware of the anterior jugular veins, which lie close together on either side of the midline), the investing layer of deep cervical fascia, the pretracheal fascia (separate the sternohyoid muscles and incise the fascia), and the larynx. The larynx is incised through a horizontal incision through the cricothyroid ligament and the tube inserted.

Complications

- Esophageal perforation: Because the lower end of the pharynx and the beginning of the esophagus lie directly behind the cricoid cartilage, it is imperative that the scalpel incision through the cricothyroid membrane not be carried too far posteriorly. This is particularly important in young children, in whom the cross diameter of the larynx is so small.
- Hemorrhage: The small branches of the superior thyroid artery that occasionally cross the front of the cricothyroid membrane to anastomose with one another should be avoided.

Tracheostomy

Tracheostomy is rarely performed and is limited to patients with extensive laryngeal damage and infants with severe airway obstruction. Because of the presence of major vascular structures (carotid arteries and internal jugular vein), the thyroid gland, nerves (recurrent laryngeal branch of vagus and vagus nerve), the pleural cavities, and the esophagus, meticulous attention to anatomic detail has to be observed (Fig. 11-107).

The procedure is as follows:

1. The thyroid and cricoid cartilages are identified and the neck is extended to bring the trachea forward.

(continues)

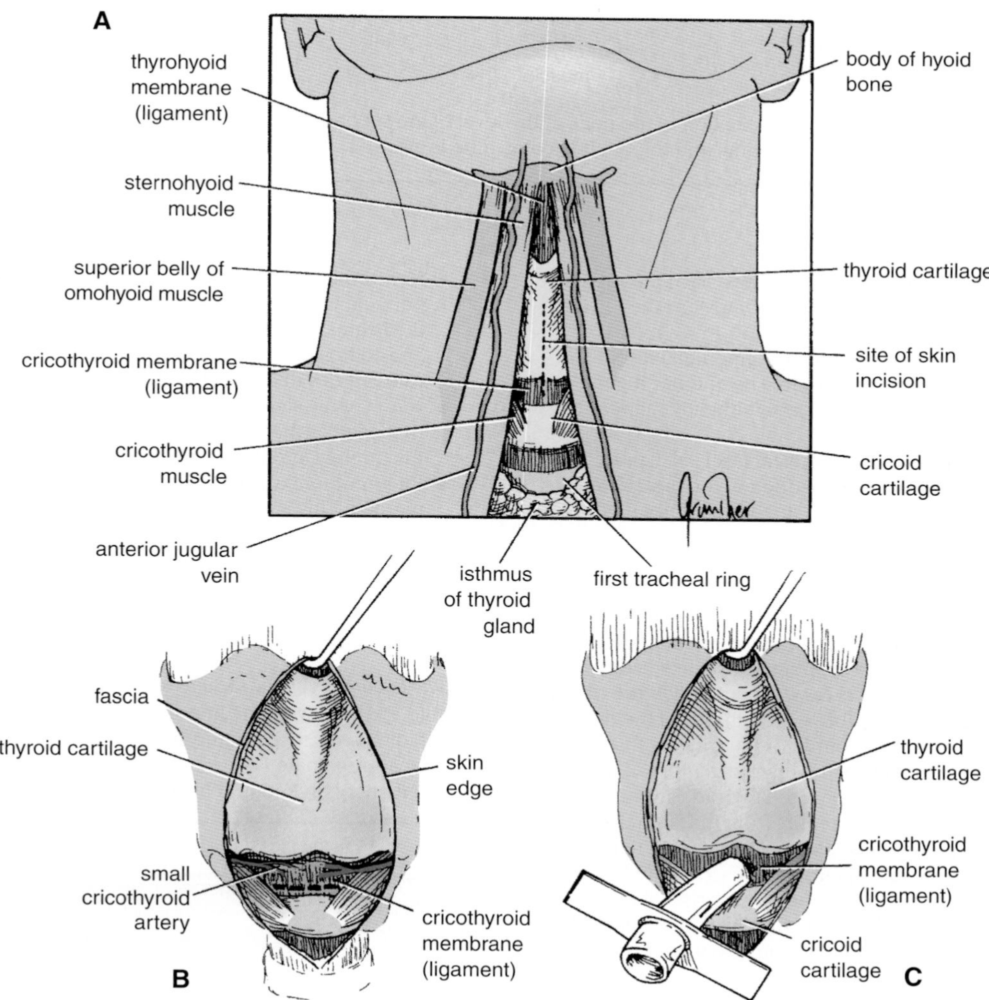

Figure 11-106 The anatomy of cricothyroidotomy. **A.** A vertical incision is made through the skin and superficial and deep cervical fasciae. **B.** The cricothyroid membrane (ligament) is incised through a horizontal incision close to the upper border of the cricoid cartilage. **C.** Insertion of the tube.

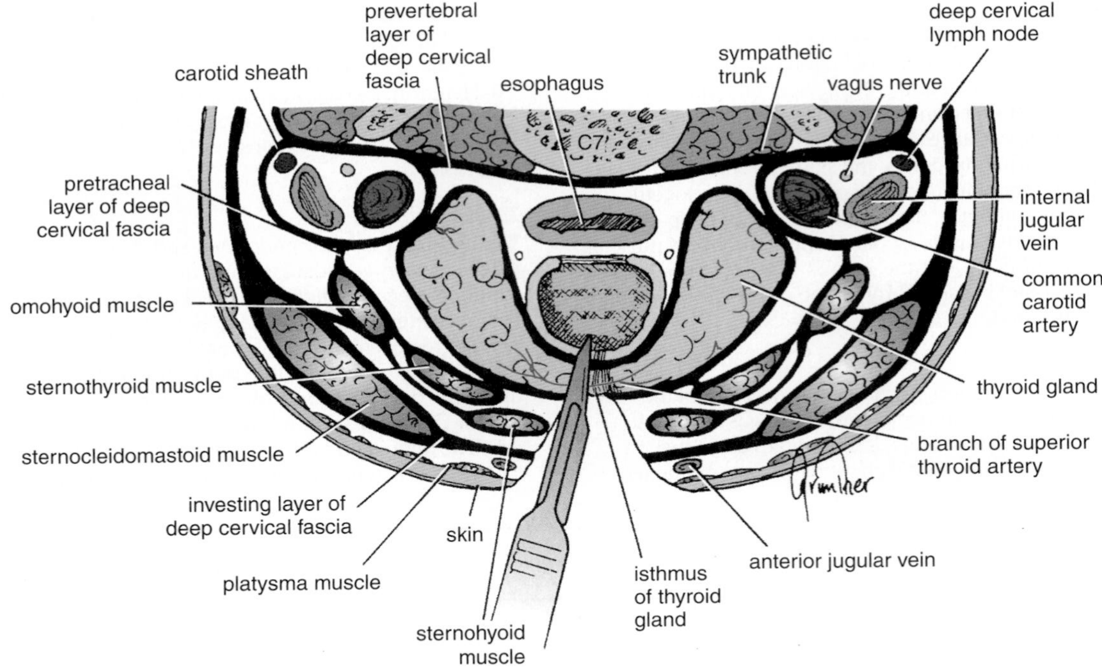

Figure 11-107 Cross section of the neck at the level of the second tracheal ring. A vertical incision is made through the ring, and the tracheostomy tube is inserted.

Clinical Notes, *continued*

2. A vertical midline skin incision is made from the region of the cricothyroid membrane inferiorly toward the suprasternal notch.
3. The incision is carried through the superficial fascia and the fibers of the platysma muscle. The anterior jugular veins in the superficial fascia are avoided by maintaining a midline position.
4. The investing layer of deep cervical fascia is incised.
5. The pretracheal muscles embedded in the pretracheal fascia are split in the midline two fingerbreadths superior to the sternal notch.
6. The tracheal rings are then palpable in the midline or the isthmus of the thyroid gland is visible. If a hook is placed under the lower border of the cricoid cartilage and traction is applied upward, the slack is taken out of the elastic trachea; this stops it from slipping from side to side.
7. A decision is then made as to whether to enter the trachea through the second ring above the isthmus of the thyroid gland; through the third, fourth, or fifth ring by first dividing the vascular isthmus of the thyroid gland; or through the lower tracheal rings below the thyroid isthmus. At the latter site, the trachea is receding from the surface of the neck, and the pretracheal fascia contains the inferior thyroid veins and possibly the thyroidea ima artery.
8. The preferred site is through the second ring of the trachea in the midline, with the thyroid isthmus retracted inferiorly. A vertical tracheal incision is made, and the tracheostomy tube is inserted.

Complications

Most complications result from not adequately palpating and recognizing the thyroid, cricoid, and tracheal cartilages and not confining the incision strictly to the midline.

- Hemorrhage: The anterior jugular veins located in the superficial fascia close to the midline should be avoided. If the isthmus of the thyroid gland is transected, secure the anastomosing branches of the superior and inferior thyroid arteries that cross the midline on the isthmus.
- Nerve paralysis: The recurrent laryngeal nerves may be damaged as they ascend the neck in the groove between the trachea and the esophagus.
- Pneumothorax: The cervical dome of the pleura may be pierced. This is especially common in children because of the high level of the pleura in the neck.
- Esophageal injury: Damage to the esophagus, which is located immediately posterior to the trachea, occurs most commonly in infants; it follows penetration of the small-diameter trachea by the point of the scalpel blade.

Some Important Airway Distances

Table 11-13 shows some important distances between the incisor teeth or nostrils to anatomic landmarks in the airway in the adult. These approximate figures are helpful in determining the correct placement of an endotracheal tube (see page 808).

Table 11-13 Important Airway Distances (Adult)[a]

Airway	Distances
Incisor teeth to the vocal cords	5.9 in. (15 cm)
Incisor teeth to the carina	7.9 in. (20 cm)
External nares to the carina	11.8 in. (30 cm)

[a]Average figures given ± 1–2 cm.

Endocrine Glands in the Head and Neck

Pituitary Gland (Hypophysis Cerebri)

Location and Description

The pituitary gland is a small, oval structure attached to the undersurface of the brain by the **infundibulum** (Figs. 11-13 and 11-108). The gland is well protected by virtue of its location in the sella turcica of the sphenoid bone. Because the hormones produced by the gland influence the activities of many other endocrine glands, the hypophysis cerebri is often referred to as the master endocrine gland. For this reason, it is vital to life.

The pituitary gland is divided into an **anterior lobe,** or **adenohypophysis,** and a **posterior lobe,** or **neurohypophysis.** The anterior lobe is subdivided into the **pars anterior** (sometimes called the pars distalis) and the **pars intermedia,** which may be separated by a cleft that is a remnant of an embryonic pouch. A projection from the pars anterior, the **pars tuberalis,** extends up along the anterior and lateral surfaces of the pituitary stalk.

Relations

- **Anteriorly:** The sphenoid sinus (Fig. 11-13)
- **Posteriorly:** The dorsum sellae, the basilar artery, and the pons
- **Superiorly:** The diaphragma sellae, which has a central aperture that allows the passage of the infundibulum. The diaphragma sellae separates the anterior lobe from the optic chiasma (Fig.11-108).
- **Inferiorly:** The body of the sphenoid, with its sphenoid air sinuses
- **Laterally:** The cavernous sinus and its contents (Fig. 11-108)

Blood Supply

The arteries are derived from the superior and **inferior hypophyseal arteries,** branches of the internal carotid artery. The veins drain into the intercavernous sinuses.

Functions of the Pituitary Gland

The pituitary gland influences the activities of many other endocrine glands. The pituitary gland is itself controlled by the hypothalamus and the activities of the hypothalamus are modified by information received along numerous nervous afferent pathways from different parts of the central nervous system and by the plasma levels of the circulating electrolytes and hormones.

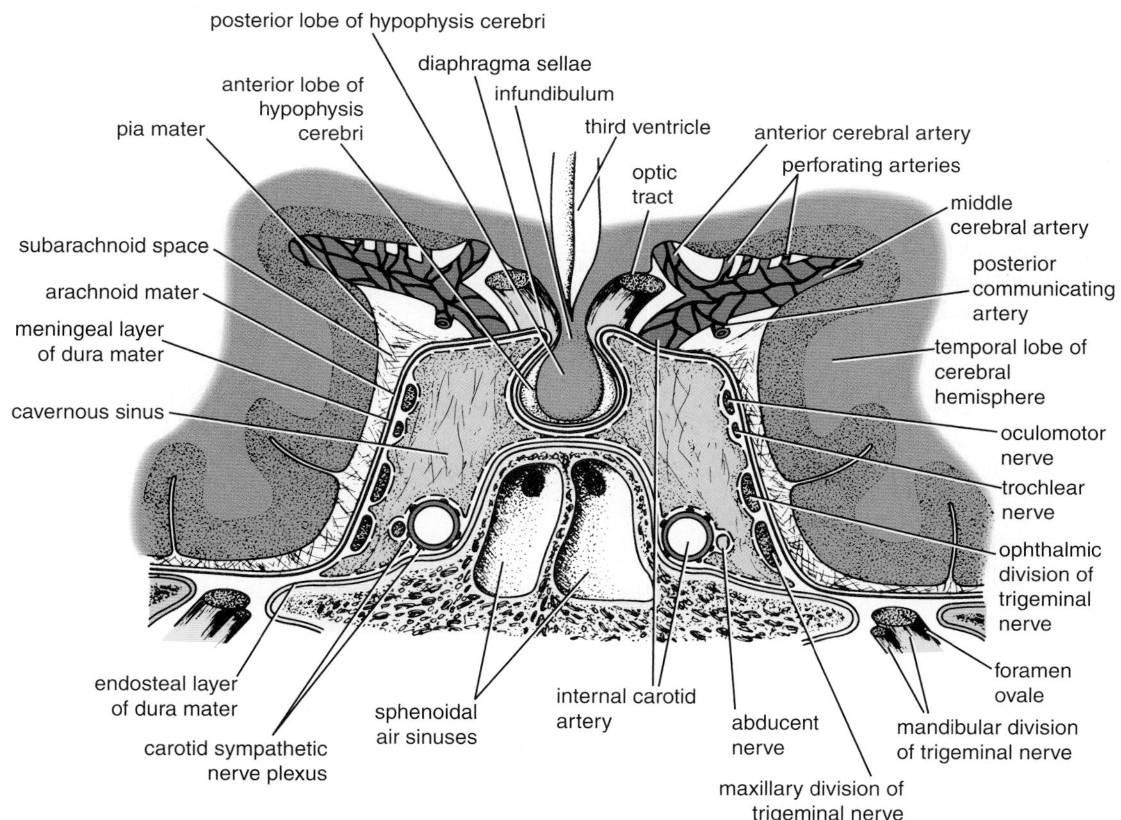

Figure 11-108 Coronal section through the body of the sphenoid bone, showing the pituitary gland and cavernous sinuses. Note the position of the internal carotid artery and the cranial nerves.

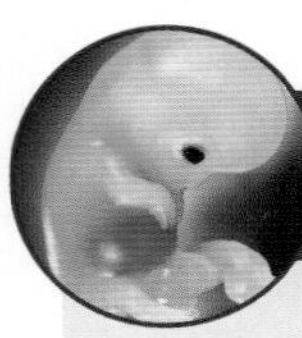

EMBRYOLOGIC NOTES

Development of the Pituitary Gland

The pituitary gland develops from two sources: a small ectodermal diverticulum (Rathke's pouch), which grows superiorly from the roof of the stomodeum immediately anterior to the buccopharyngeal membrane, and a small ectodermal diverticulum (the **infundibulum),** which grows inferiorly from the floor of the diencephalon of the brain (Fig. 11-109).

During the second month of development, Rathke's pouch comes into contact with the anterior surface of the infundibulum, and its connection with the oral epithelium elongates, narrows, and finally disappears (Fig. 11-109). Rathke's pouch now is a vesicle that flattens itself around the anterior and lateral surfaces of the infundibulum. The cells of the anterior wall of the vesicle proliferate and form the **pars anterior** of the pituitary; from the vesicle's upper part, there is a cellular extension that grows superiorly and around the stalk of the infundibulum, forming the **pars tuberalis.** The cells of the posterior wall of the vesicle never develop extensively; they form the **pars intermedia.** Some of the cells later migrate anteriorly into the pars anterior. The cavity of the vesicle is reduced to a narrow cleft, which may disappear completely. Meanwhile, the infundibulum has differentiated into the **stalk** and **pars nervosa** of the pituitary gland (Fig. 11-109).

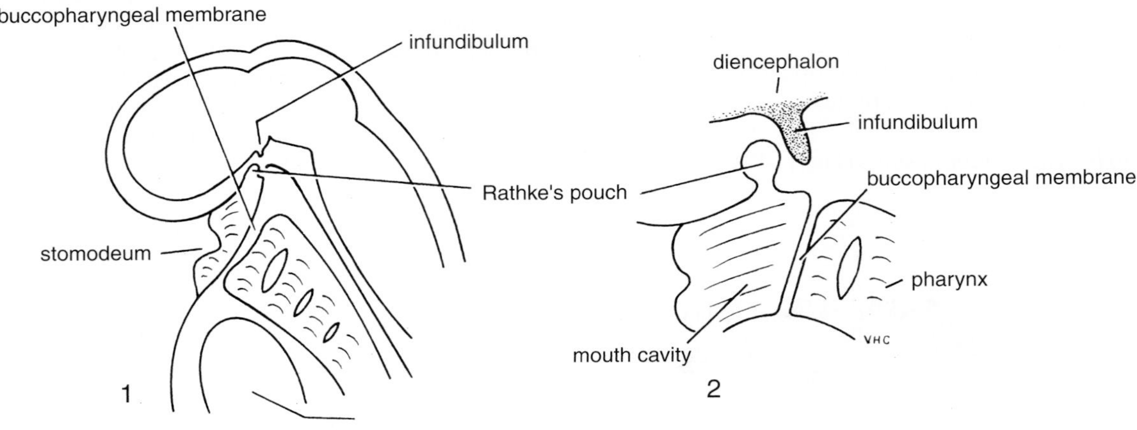

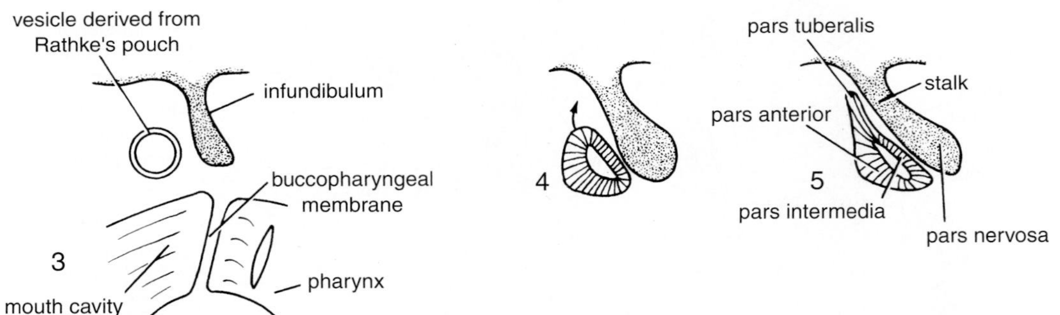

Figure 11-109 The different stages in the development of the pituitary gland shown in sagittal sections.

Pineal Gland

Location and Description

The pineal gland is a small cone-shaped body that projects posteriorly from the posterior end of the roof of the third ventricle of the brain (Fig. 11-13). The pineal consists essentially of groups of cells, the **pinealocytes,** supported by glial cells. The gland has a rich blood supply and is innervated by postganglionic sympathetic nerve fibers.

Functions of the Pineal Gland

The pineal gland can influence the activities of the pituitary gland, the islets of Langerhans of the pancreas, the parathyroids, the adrenals, and the gonads. The pineal secretions, produced by the pinealocytes, reach their target organs via the bloodstream or through the cerebrospinal fluid. Their actions are mainly inhibitory and either directly inhibit the production of hormones or indirectly inhibit the secretion of releasing factors by the hypothalamus.

Thyroid Gland

Location and Description

The thyroid gland consists of right and left lobes connected by a narrow isthmus (Fig. 11-110). It is a vascular organ surrounded by a sheath derived from the pretracheal layer of deep fascia. The sheath attaches the gland to the larynx and the trachea.

Each lobe is pear shaped, with its apex being directed upward as far as the oblique line on the lamina of the thyroid cartilage; its base lies below at the level of the fourth or fifth tracheal ring.

The **isthmus** extends across the midline in front of the second, third, and fourth tracheal rings (Fig. 11-110). A **pyramidal lobe** is often present, and it projects upward from the isthmus, usually to the left of the midline. A fibrous or

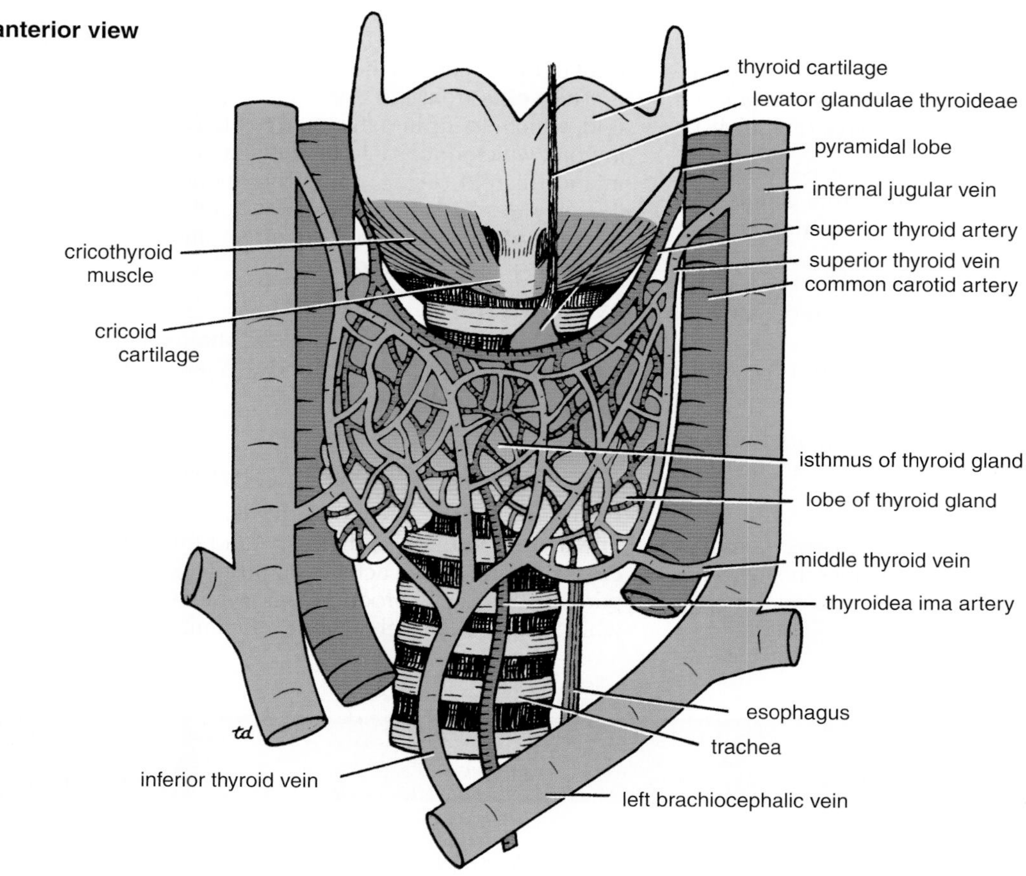

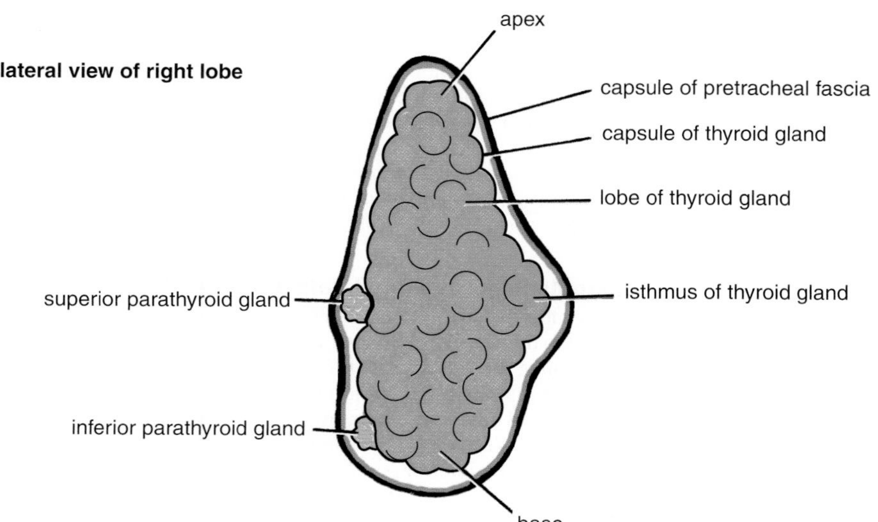

Figure 11-110 The blood supply and venous drainage of the thyroid gland.

muscular band frequently connects the pyramidal lobe to the hyoid bone; if it is muscular, it is referred to as the **levator glandulae thyroideae** (Fig. 11-110).

Relations of the Lobes

- **Anterolaterally:** The sternothyroid, the superior belly of the omohyoid, the sternohyoid, and the anterior border of the sternocleidomastoid (Fig. 11-49)
- **Posterolaterally:** The carotid sheath with the common carotid artery, the internal jugular vein, and the vagus nerve (Fig. 11-49)
- **Medially:** The larynx, the trachea, the pharynx, and the esophagus. Associated with these structures are the cricothyroid muscle and its nerve supply, the external laryngeal nerve. In the groove between the esophagus and the trachea is the recurrent laryngeal nerve (Fig. 11-49).

The rounded posterior border of each lobe is related posteriorly to the superior and inferior parathyroid glands (Fig. 11-110) and the anastomosis between the superior and inferior thyroid arteries.

Relations of the Isthmus

- **Anteriorly:** The sternothyroids, sternohyoids, anterior jugular veins, fascia, and skin
- **Posteriorly:** The second, third, and fourth rings of the trachea

The terminal branches of the superior thyroid arteries anastomose along its upper border.

Blood Supply

The **arteries** to the thyroid gland are the superior thyroid artery, the inferior thyroid artery, and sometimes the thyroidea ima. The arteries anastomose profusely with one another over the surface of the gland.

The **superior thyroid artery,** a branch of the external carotid artery, descends to the upper pole of each lobe, accompanied by the **external laryngeal nerve** (Fig. 11-110).

The **inferior thyroid artery,** a branch of the thyrocervical trunk, ascends behind the gland to the level of the cricoid cartilage. It then turns medially and downward to reach the posterior border of the gland. The **recurrent laryngeal nerve** crosses either in front of or behind the artery, or it may pass between its branches.

The **thyroidea ima,** if present, may arise from the brachiocephalic artery or the arch of the aorta. It ascends in front of the trachea to the isthmus (Fig. 11-110).

The **veins** from the thyroid gland are the superior thyroid, which drains into the internal jugular vein; the middle thyroid, which drains into the internal jugular vein; and the inferior thyroid (Fig. 11-110). The inferior thyroid veins of the two sides anastomose with one another as they descend in **front of the trachea.** They drain into the left brachiocephalic vein in the thorax.

Lymph Drainage

The lymph from the thyroid gland drains mainly laterally into the deep cervical lymph nodes. A few lymph vessels descend to the paratracheal nodes.

Nerve Supply

Superior, middle, and inferior cervical sympathetic ganglia

Functions of the Thyroid Gland

The thyroid hormones, thyroxine and triiodothyronine, increase the metabolic activity of most cells in the body. The parafollicular cells produce the hormone thyrocalcitonin, which lowers the level of blood calcium.

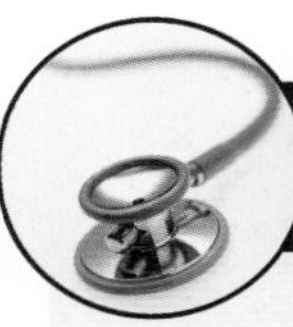

CLINICAL NOTES

Swellings of the Thyroid Gland and Movement on Swallowing

The thyroid gland is invested in a sheath derived from the pretracheal fascia. This tethers the gland to the larynx and the trachea and explains why the thyroid gland follows the movements of the larynx in swallowing. This information is important because any pathologic neck swelling that is part of the thyroid gland will move upward when the patient is asked to swallow.

The Thyroid Gland and the Airway

The close relationship between the trachea and the lobes of the thyroid gland commonly results in pressure on the trachea in patients with pathologic enlargement of the thyroid.

Retrosternal Goiter

The attachment of the sternothyroid muscles to the thyroid cartilage effectively binds down the thyroid gland to the larynx and limits upward expansion of the gland. There being no limitation to downward expansion, it is not uncommon for a pathologically enlarged thyroid gland to extend downward behind the sternum. A retrosternal goiter (any abnormal enlargement of the thyroid gland) can compress the trachea and cause dangerous dyspnea; it can also cause severe venous compression.

Thyroid Arteries and Important Nerves

It should be remembered that the two main arteries supplying the thyroid gland are closely related to important nerves that can be damaged during thyroidectomy operations. The superior thyroid artery on each side is related to the external laryngeal nerve, which supplies the cricothyroid muscle. The terminal branches of the inferior thyroid artery on each side are related to the recurrent laryngeal nerve. Damage to the external laryngeal nerve results in an inability to tense the vocal folds and in hoarseness. For the results of damage to the recurrent laryngeal nerve, see page 808.

Thyroidectomy and the Parathyroid Glands

The parathyroid glands are usually four in number and are closely related to the posterior surface of the thyroid gland. In partial thyroidectomy, the posterior part of the thyroid gland is left undisturbed so that the parathyroid glands are not damaged. The development of the inferior parathyroid glands is closely associated with the thymus. For this reason it is not uncommon for the surgeon to find the inferior parathyroid glands in the superior mediastinum because they have been pulled down into the thorax by the thymus.

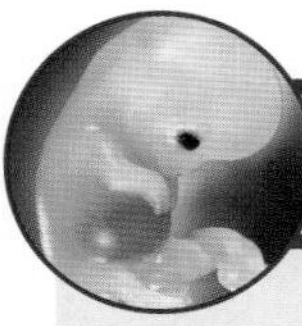

EMBRYOLOGIC NOTES

Development of the Thyroid Gland

The thyroid gland begins to develop during the third week as an entodermal thickening in the midline of the floor of the pharynx between the **tuberculum impar** and the **copula** (Fig. 11-111). Later, this thickening becomes a diverticulum that grows inferiorly into the underlying mesenchyme and is called the **thyroglossal duct.** As development continues, the duct elongates, and its distal end becomes bilobed. Soon, the duct becomes a solid cord of cells, and as a result of epithelial proliferation, the bilobed terminal swellings expand to form the thyroid gland.

The thyroid gland now migrates inferiorly in the neck and passes either anterior to, posterior to, or through the developing body of the hyoid bone. By the seventh week, it reaches its final position in relation to the larynx and trachea. Meanwhile, the solid cord connecting the thyroid gland to the tongue fragments and disappears. The site of origin of the thyroglossal duct on the tongue remains as a pit called the **foramen cecum.** The thyroid gland may now be divided into a small median **isthmus** and two large **lateral lobes** (Fig. 11-111).

In the earliest stages, the thyroid gland consists of a solid mass of cells. Later, as a result of invasion by surrounding vascular mesenchymal tissue, the mass becomes broken up into plates and cords and finally into small clusters of cells. By the third month, colloid starts to accumulate in the center of each cluster so that **follicles** are formed. The fibrous capsule and connective tissue develop from the surrounding mesenchyme.

The **ultimobranchial bodies** (from the fifth pharyngeal pouch) and neural crest cells are believed to be incorporated into the thyroid gland, where they form the **parafollicular cells,** which produce **calcitonin.**

Agenesis of the Thyroid

Failure of development of the thyroid gland may occur and is the commonest cause of **cretinism.**

Incomplete Descent of the Thyroid

The descent of the thyroid may be arrested at any point between the base of the tongue and the trachea (Fig. 11-112). **Lingual thyroid** is the most common form of incomplete descent (Fig. 11-113). The mass of tissue found just beneath the foramen cecum may be sufficiently large to obstruct swallowing in the infant.

Ectopic Thyroid Tissue

Ectopic thyroid tissue is occasionally found in the thorax in relation to the trachea or bronchi or even the esophagus. It is assumed that this thyroid tissue arises from entodermal cells displaced during the formation of the laryngotracheal tube or from entodermal cells of the developing esophagus

Persistent Thyroglossal Duct

Conditions related to a persistence of the thyroglossal duct usually appear in childhood, in adolescence, or in young adults.

(continues)

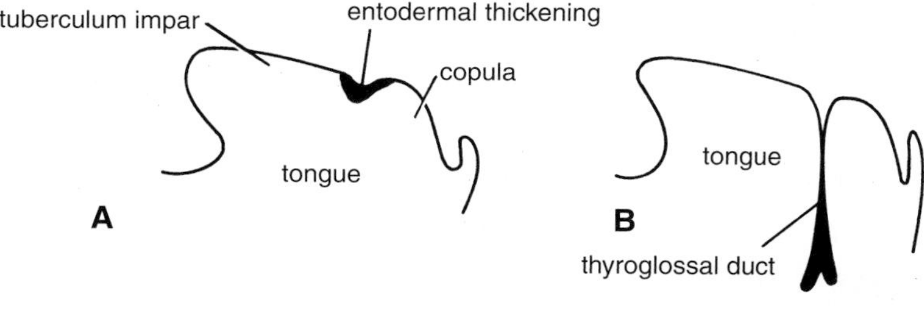

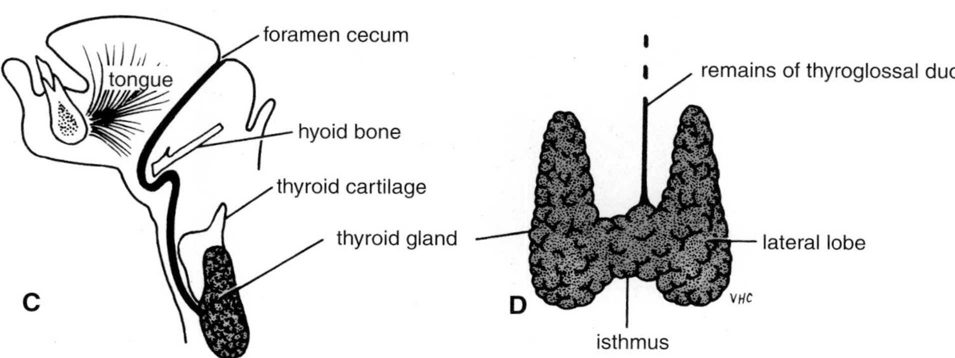

Figure 11-111 The different stages in the development of the thyroid gland. **A.** Sagittal section of the tongue showing an entodermal thickening between the tuberculum impar and the copula. **B.** Sagittal section of the tongue showing the development of the thyroglossal duct. **C.** Sagittal section of the tongue and neck showing the path taken by the thyroid gland as it migrates inferiorly. **D.** The fully developed thyroid gland as seen from in front. Note the remains of the thyroglossal duct above the isthmus.

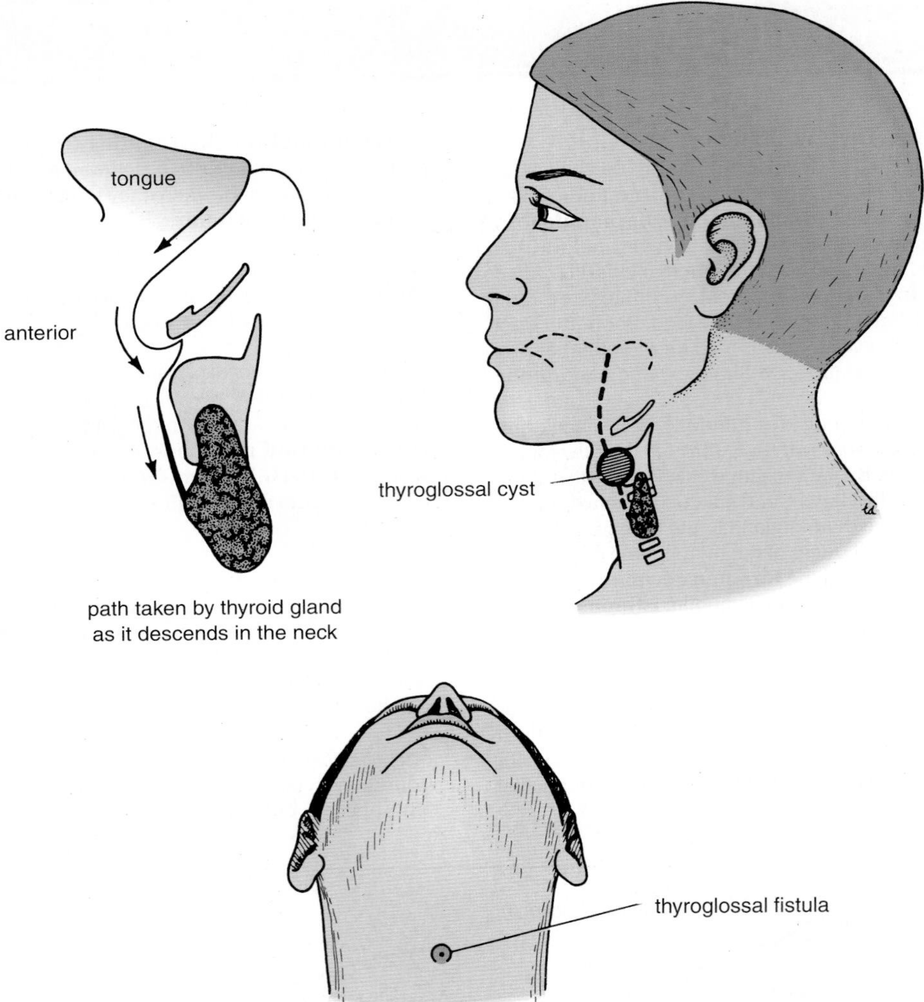

Figure 11-112 A thyroglossal cyst in the midline in the neck and a thyroglossal fistula.

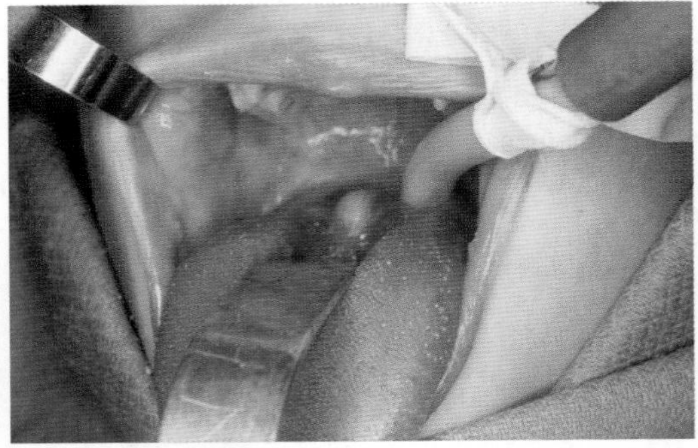

Figure 11-113 Lingual thyroid. (Courtesy of J. Randolph.)

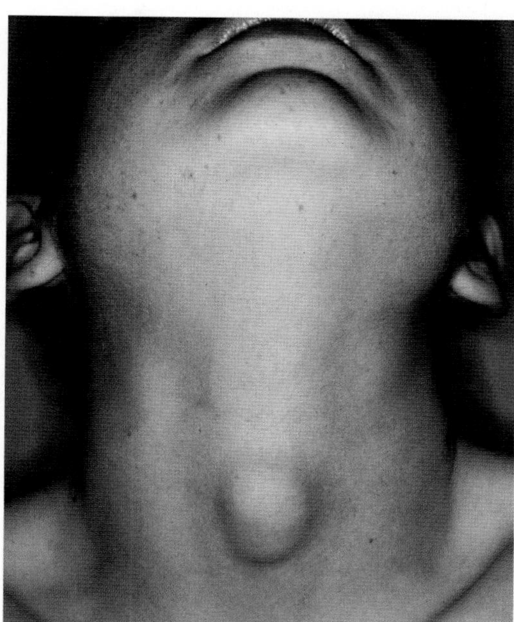

Figure 11-114 A thyroglossal cyst. (Courtesy of L. Thompson.)

Embryologic Notes, *continued*

Thyroglossal Cyst

Cysts may occur at any point along the thyroglossal tract (Figs. 11-112 and 11-114). They occur most commonly in the region below the hyoid bone. Such a cyst occupies the midline and develops as a result of persistence of a small amount of epithelium that continues to secrete mucus. As the cyst enlarges, it is prone to infection and so it should be removed surgically. Since remnants of the duct often traverse the body of the hyoid bone, this may have to be excised also to prevent recurrence.

Thyroglossal Sinus (Fistula)

Occasionally, a thyroglossal cyst ruptures spontaneously, producing a sinus (Fig. 11-112). Usually, this is a result of an infection of a cyst. All remnants of the thyroglossal duct should be removed surgically.

Parathyroid Glands

Location and Description

The parathyroid glands are ovoid bodies measuring about 6 mm long in their greatest diameter. They are four in number and are closely related to the posterior border of the thyroid gland, lying within its fascial capsule (Fig. 11-110).

The **two superior parathyroid glands** are the more constant in position and lie at the level of the middle of the posterior border of the thyroid gland.

The **two inferior parathyroid glands** usually lie close to the inferior poles of the thyroid gland. They may lie within the fascial sheath, embedded in the thyroid substance, or outside the fascial sheath. Sometimes they are found some distance caudal to the thyroid gland, in association with the inferior thyroid veins, or they may even reside in the superior mediastinum in the thorax.

Blood Supply

The arterial supply to the parathyroid glands is from the superior and inferior thyroid arteries. The venous drainage is into the superior, middle, and inferior thyroid veins.

Lymph Drainage

Deep cervical and paratracheal lymph nodes

Nerve Supply

Superior or middle cervical sympathetic ganglia

Functions of the Parathyroid Glands

The chief cells produce the **parathyroid hormone,** which stimulates osteoclastic activity in bones, thus mobilizing the bone calcium and increasing the calcium levels in the blood. The parathyroid hormone also stimulates the absorption of dietary calcium from the small intestine and the reabsorption of calcium in the proximal convoluted tubules of the kidney. It also strongly diminishes the reabsorption of phosphate in the proximal convoluted tubules of the kidney. The secretion of the parathyroid hormone is controlled by the calcium levels in the blood.

The Root of the Neck

The root of the neck can be defined as the area of the neck immediately above the inlet into the thorax (Fig. 11-16).

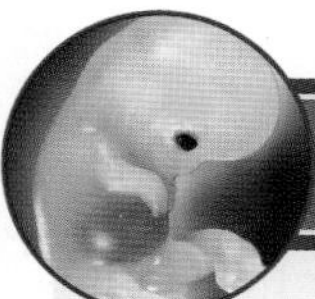

EMBRYOLOGIC NOTES

Development of the Parathyroid Glands

The pair of **inferior parathyroid glands,** known as **parathyroid III,** develop as the result of proliferation of entodermal cells in the third pharyngeal pouch on each side. As the thymic diverticulum on each side grows inferiorly in the neck, it pulls the inferior parathyroid with it, so that it finally comes to rest on the posterior surface of the lateral lobe of the thyroid gland near its lower pole and becomes completely separate from the thymus (Fig. 11-115).

(continues)

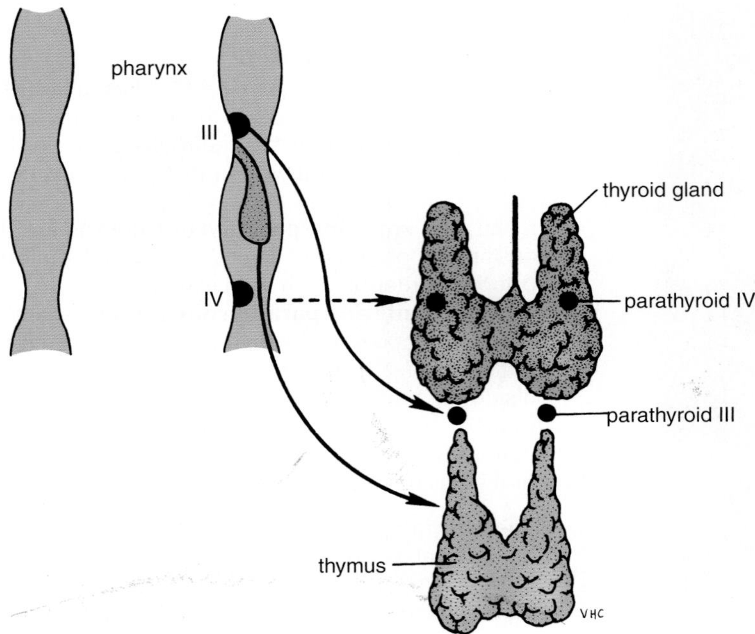

Figure 11-115 Parathyroid glands taking up their final positions in the neck.

Embryologic Notes, *continued*

The **pair of superior parathyroid glands, parathyroid IV,** develop as a proliferation of entodermal cells in the fourth pharyngeal pouch on each side. These loosen their connection with the pharyngeal wall and take up their final position on the posterior aspect of the lateral lobe of the thyroid gland on each side, at about the level of the isthmus (Fig. 11-115).

In the earliest stages, each gland consists of a solid mass of clear cells, the **chief cells.** In late childhood, acidophilic cells, the **oxyphil cells,** appear. The connective tissue and vascular supply are derived from the surrounding mesenchyme. It is believed that the parathyroid hormone is secreted early in fetal life by the chief cells, to regulate calcium metabolism. The oxyphil cells are thought to be nonfunctioning chief cells.

Absence and Hypoplasia of the Parathyroid Glands

Agenesis or incomplete development of the parathyroid glands has been demonstrated in individuals with idiopathic hypoparathyroidism.

Ectopic Parathyroid Glands

The close relationship between the parathyroid III and the developing thymus explains the frequent finding of parathyroid tissue in the superior mediastinum of the thorax (Fig. 11-115). If the parathyroid glands remain attached to the thymus, they may be pulled inferiorly into the lower part of the neck or thoracic cavity. Moreover, this also explains the variable position of the inferior parathyroid glands in relation to the lower poles of the lateral lobes of the thyroid gland.

Muscles of the Root of the Neck

Scalenus Anterior

The scalenus anterior muscle (Fig. 11-57) is a key muscle to the understanding of the root of the neck and has been fully described on page 743. It is deeply placed and descends almost vertically from the vertebral column to the first rib.

Because the muscle is an important landmark in the neck, its relations should be understood. See page 743.

Scalenus Medius

The scalenus medius lies behind the scalenus anterior and extends from the transverse process of the atlas and the transverse processes of the next five cervical vertebrae (Fig. 11-57) downward and laterally to be inserted into the upper surface of the first rib behind the groove for the subclavian artery. The muscle lies behind the roots of the brachial plexus and the subclavian artery.

For a summary of muscles of the neck, their nerve supply, and their action, see Table 11-5.

Subclavian Artery

The right subclavian artery arises from the brachiocephalic artery, behind the right sternoclavicular joint (Fig. 11-57). It passes upward and laterally as a gentle curve behind the scalenus anterior muscle, and at the outer border of the first rib it becomes the axillary artery. The left subclavian artery arises from the arch of the aorta in the thorax. It ascends to the root of the neck and then arches laterally in a manner similar to that of the right subclavian artery (Fig. 11-57). The relations and branches of the subclavian arteries have been described on page 751.

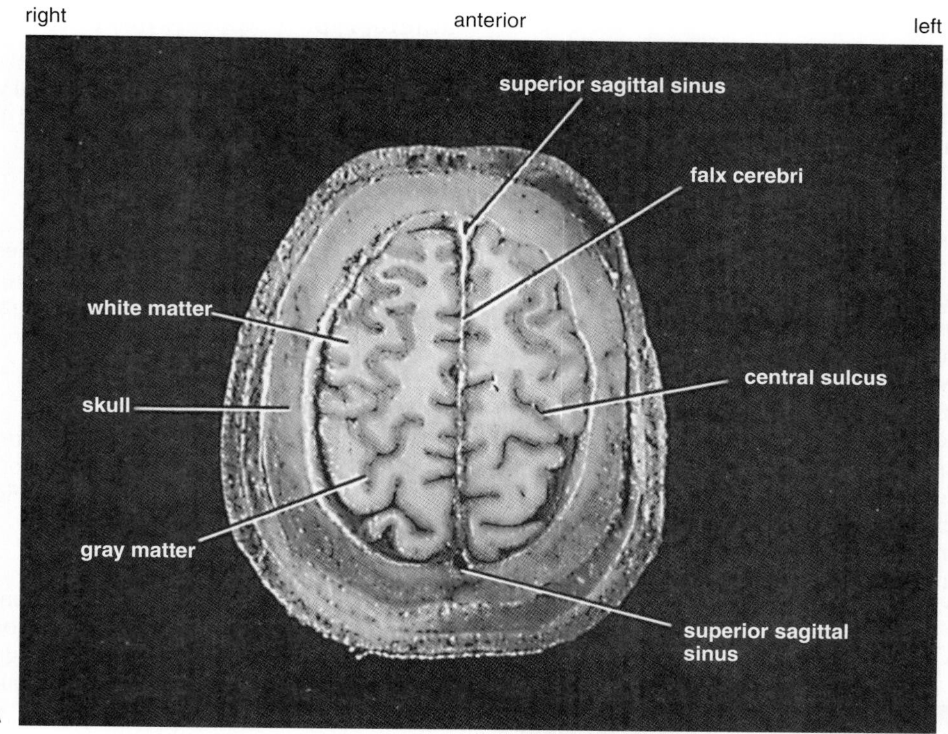

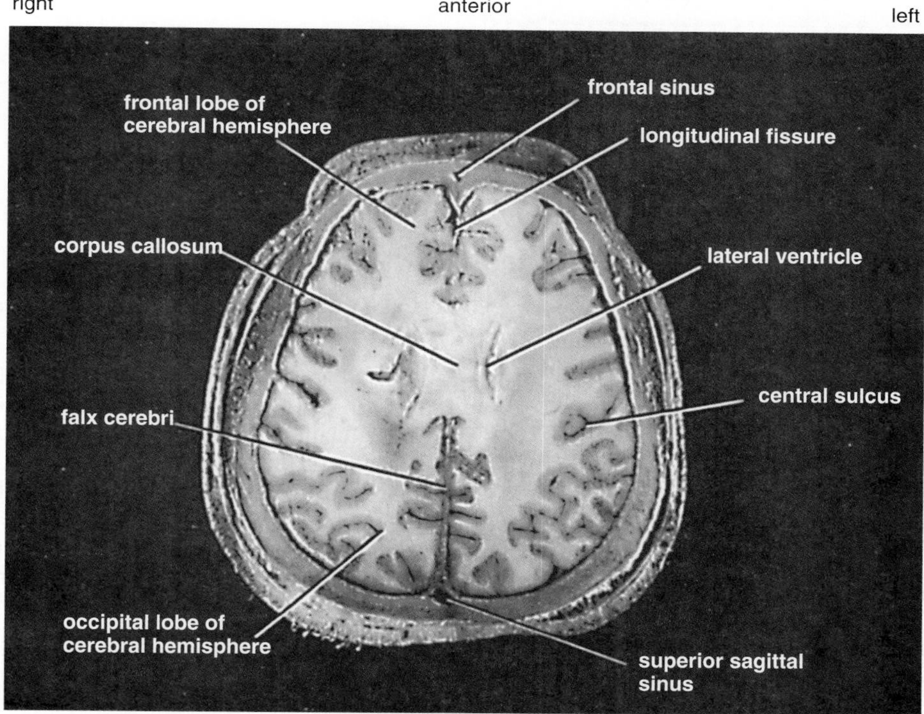

Figure 11-116 **A.** Cross section of the head a short distance beneath the vault of the skull viewed from below. **B.** Cross section of the head at the level of the corpus callosum viewed from below.

Subclavian Vein

The subclavian vein begins at the outer border of the first rib as a continuation of the axillary vein (Fig. 11-57). At the medial border of the scalenus anterior it joins the internal jugular vein to form the brachiocephalic vein.

The Thoracic Duct

The thoracic duct begins in the abdomen at the upper end of the cisterna chyli (see page 273). It enters the thorax through the aortic opening in the diaphragm and ascends through the posterior mediastinum, inclining gradually to the left. On reaching the superior mediastinum, it is found passing upward along the left margin of the esophagus. At the root of the neck, it continues to ascend along the left margin of the esophagus until it reaches the level of the transverse process of the seventh cervical vertebra. Here, it bends laterally behind the carotid sheath (Fig. 11-57). On reaching the medial border of the scalenus anterior, it turns downward and drains into the beginning of the left brachiocephalic vein. It may, however, end in the terminal part of the subclavian or internal jugular veins.

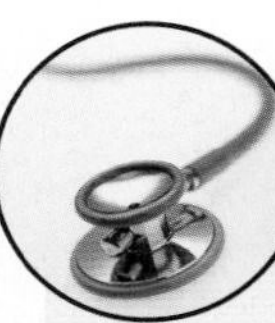

CLINICAL NOTES

Pleura and Lung Injuries in the Root of the Neck

The cervical dome of the pleura and the apex of the lung extend up into the root of the neck on each side. Covered by the suprapleural membrane, they lie behind the subclavian artery. A penetrating wound above the medial end of the clavicle may involve the apex of the lung.

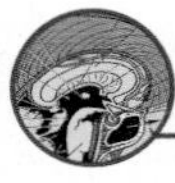

Radiographic Anatomy

Before studying the radiographic appearance of the head and neck, the student is encouraged to examine photographs of sections of the head and neck (Figs. 11-116, 11-117, and 11-118).

Radiographic Appearance of the Head and Neck

Routine radiologic examination of the head and neck concentrates mainly on the bony structures because the brain, muscles, tendons, and nerves blend into a homogeneous mass. However, a few normal structures within the skull become calcified in the adult, and the displacement of such structures may indirectly give evidence of a pathologic condition. The pineal gland, for example, is calcified in 50% of normal adults. It lies in the midline. The falx cerebri and the choroid plexuses also become calcified frequently.

The brain can be studied indirectly by the injection of contrast media into the arterial system leading to the brain **(cerebral arteriogram).** The introduction of CT and MRI scans has provided physicians with safe and accurate methods of studying the intracranial contents.

Radiographic Appearance of the Skull

The radiographic appearances of the skull as seen on straight posteroanterior views and lateral views can be studied in Figures 11-119, 11-120, 11-121, and 11-122.

Cerebral Arteriography

The technique of cerebral arteriography can be used to detect abnormalities of the cerebral arteries and localization of space-occupying lesions such as tumors, blood clots, or abscesses. Examples of cerebral arteriograms can be seen in Figures 11-123, 11-124, 11-125, and 11-126.

Computed Tomography Scans

CT is commonly used for the detection of intracranial lesions. It is safe and provides accurate information. Examples of CT scans of the head can be seen in Figure 11-127.

Magnetic Resonance Imaging

MRI is also commonly used for detection of intracranial lesions. MRI is absolutely safe to the patient, and because it provides better differentiation between gray and white matter in the brain, its use can be more revealing than a CT scan (Figs. 11-128, 11-129, and 11-130).

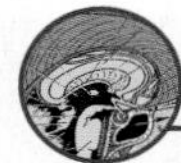

Surface Anatomy

Surface Landmarks of the Head

Nasion

The nasion is the depression in the midline at the root of the nose (Fig. 11-131).

External Occipital Protuberance

This is a bony prominence in the middle of the squamous part of the occipital bone (Fig. 11-131). It lies in the midline at the junction of the head and neck and gives attachment to the ligamentum nuchae, which is a large ligament that runs down the back of the neck, connecting the skull to the spinous processes of the cervical vertebrae. A line joining the nasion to the external occipital protuberance over the superior aspect of the head would indicate the position of the underlying **falx cerebri,** the **superior sagittal sinus,** and the **longitudinal cerebral fissure,** which separates the right and left cerebral hemispheres.

Vertex

The vertex is the highest point on the skull in the sagittal plane (Fig. 11-131).

Anterior Fontanelle

In the baby, the anterior fontanelle lies between the two halves of the frontal bone in front and the two parietal bones behind (Fig. 11-131). It is usually not palpable after 18 months.

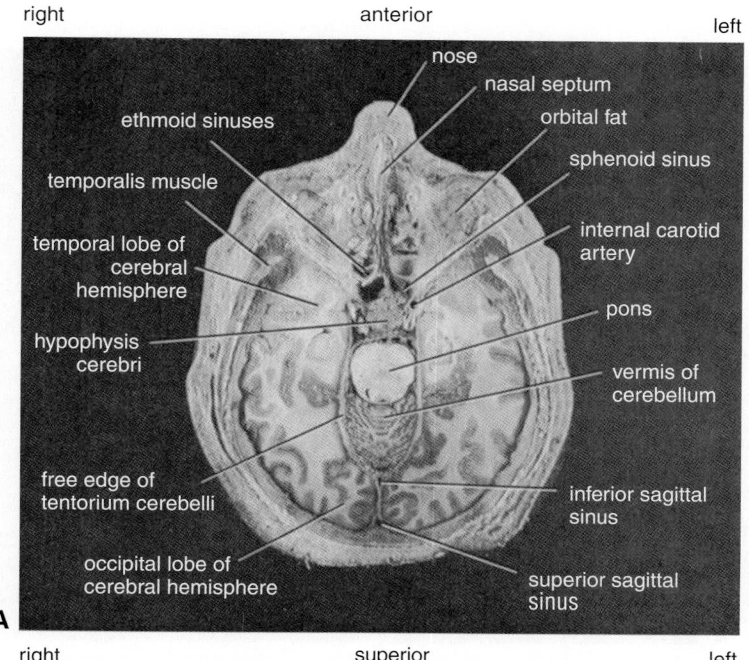

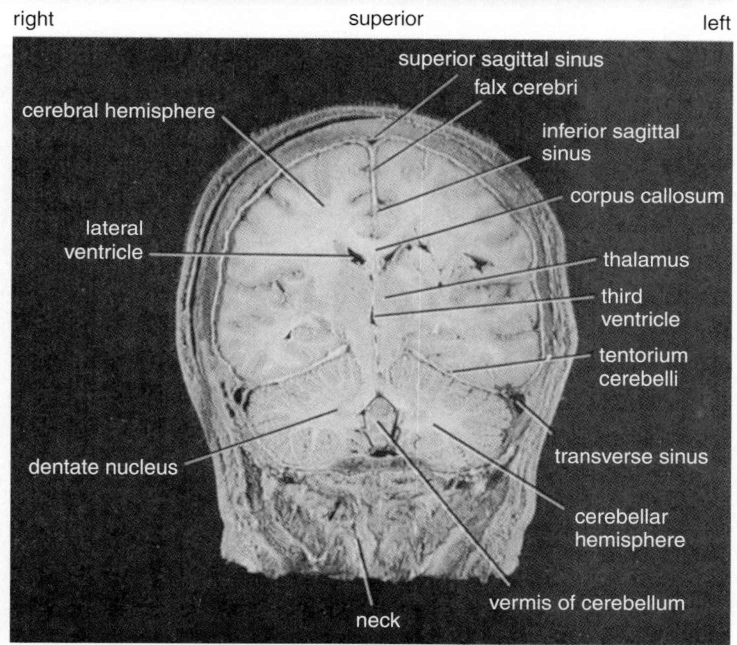

Figure 11-117 **A.** Cross section of the head viewed from below. **B.** Coronal section of the head and the upper part of the neck.

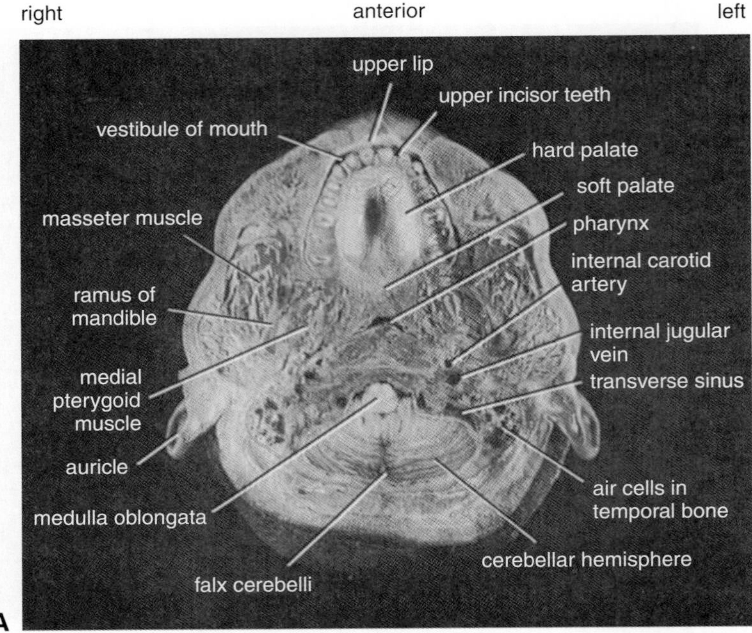

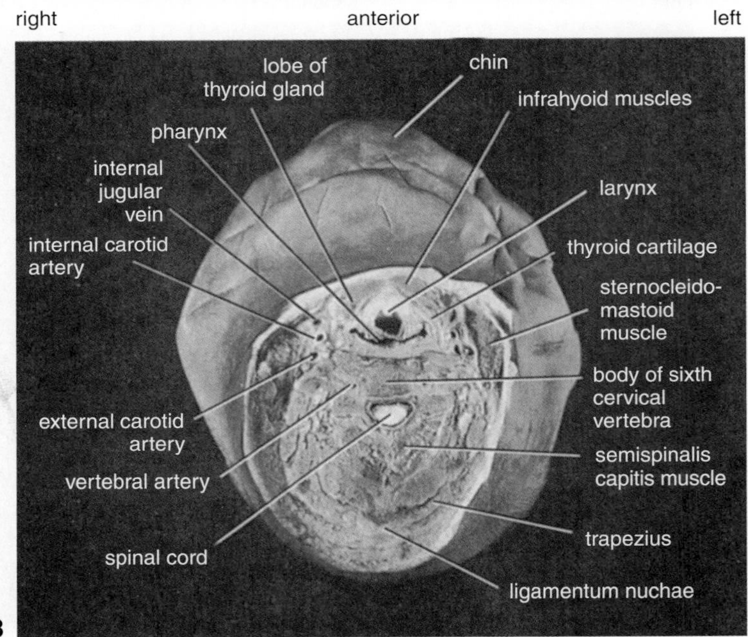

Figure 11-118 **A.** Cross section of the head just below the level of the hard palate viewed from below. **B.** Cross section of the neck at the level of the sixth cervical vertebra viewed from below.

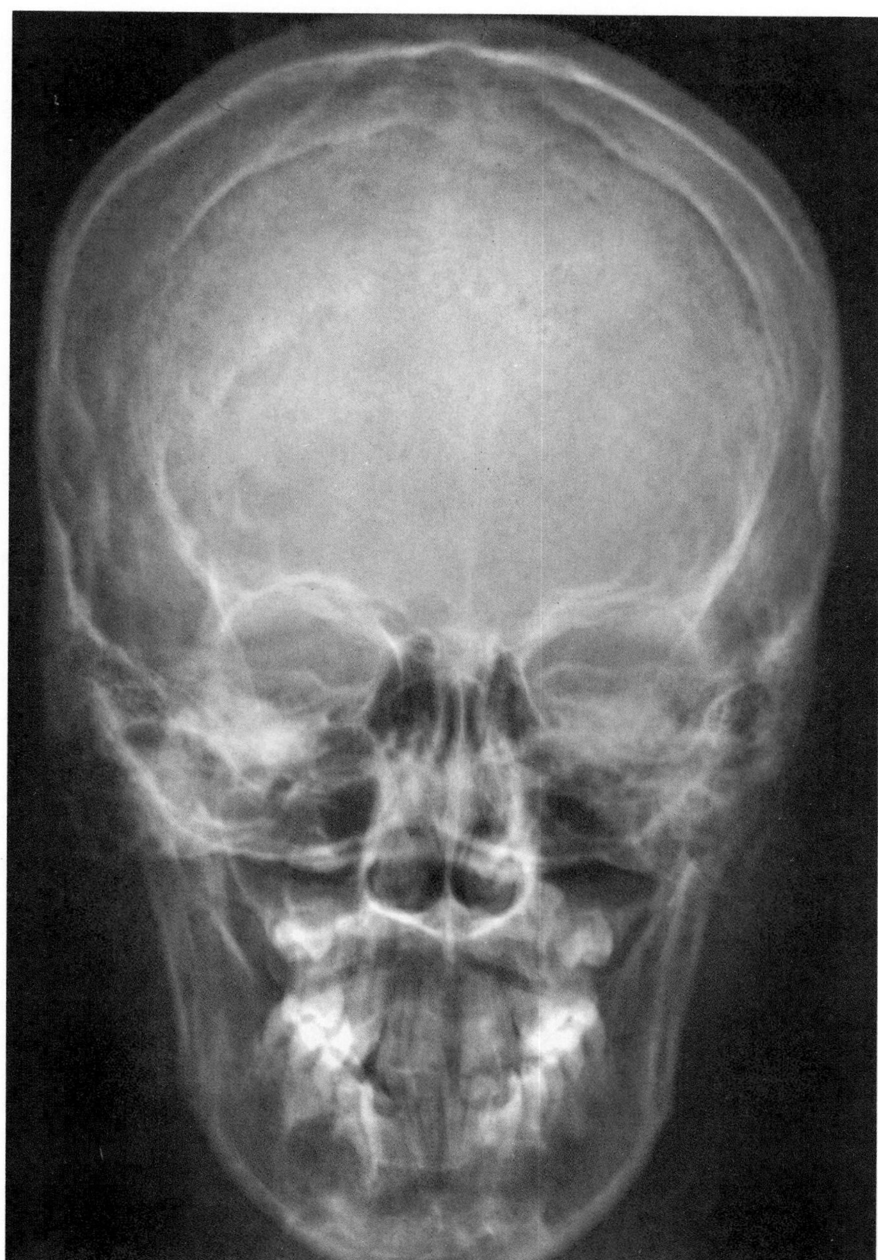

Figure 11-119 Posteroanterior radiograph of the skull.

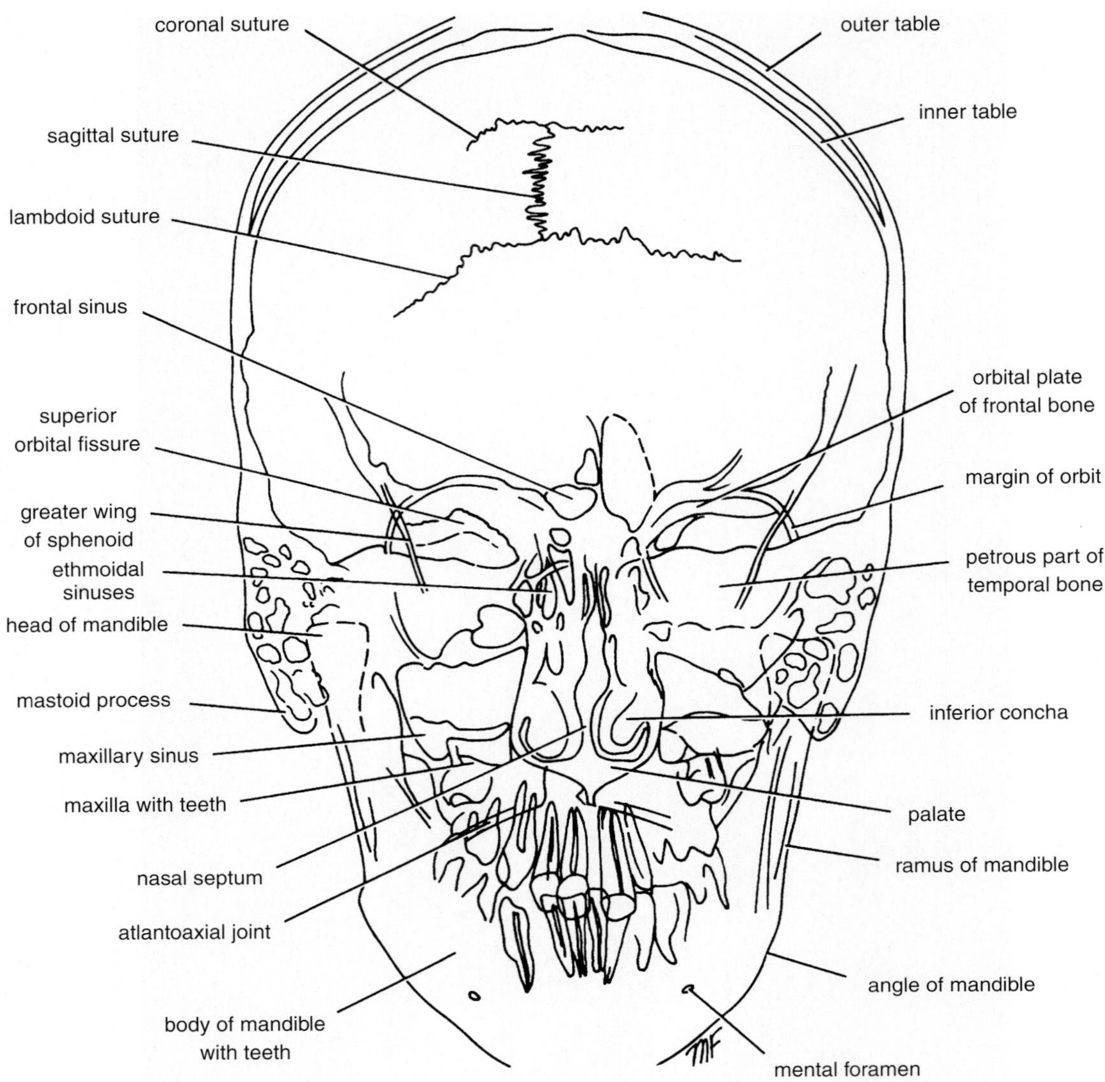

Figure 11-120 Main features that can be seen in the posteroanterior radiograph of the skull in Figure 11-119.

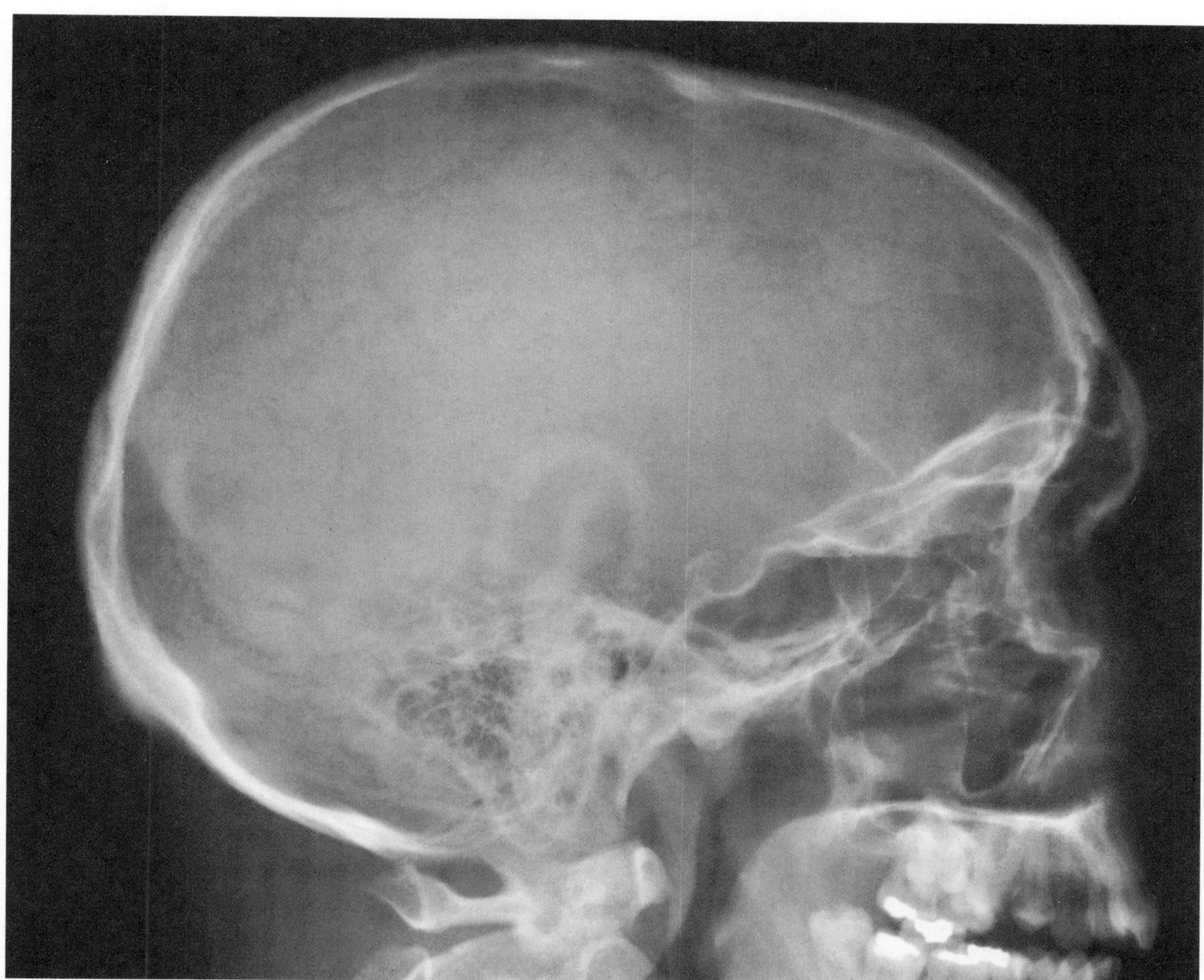

Figure 11-121 Lateral radiograph of the skull.

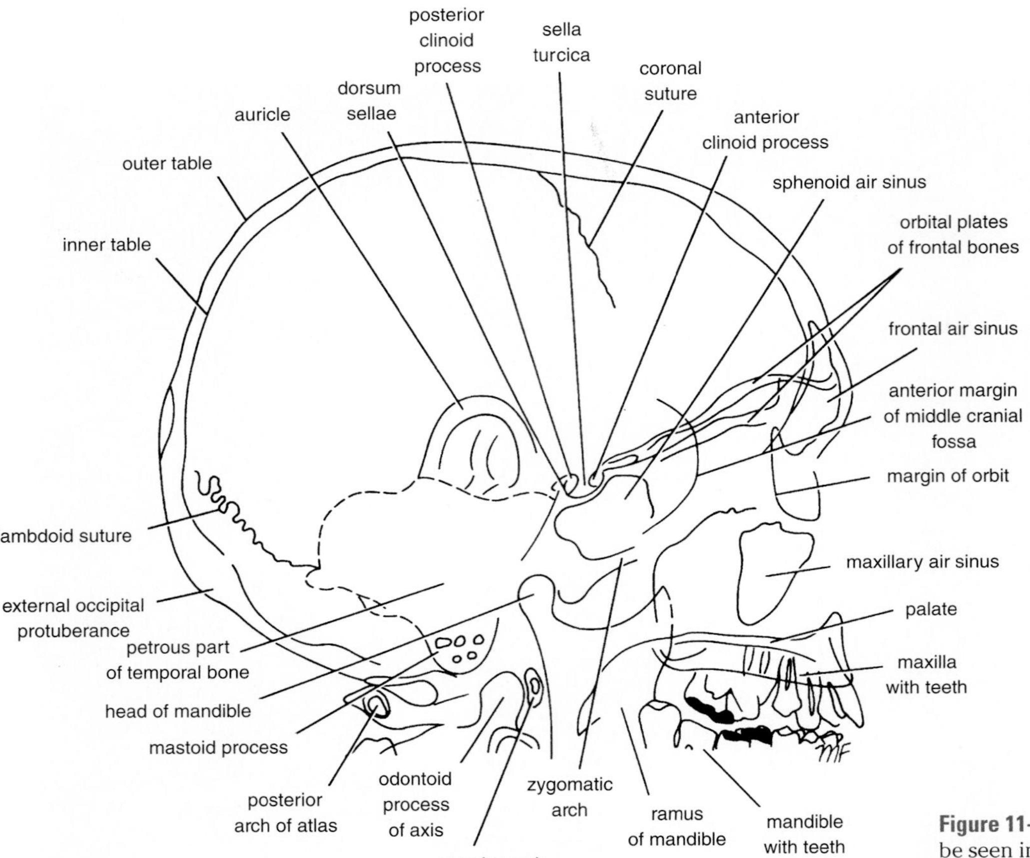

Figure 11-122 Main features that can be seen in the lateral radiograph of the skull in Figure 11-121.

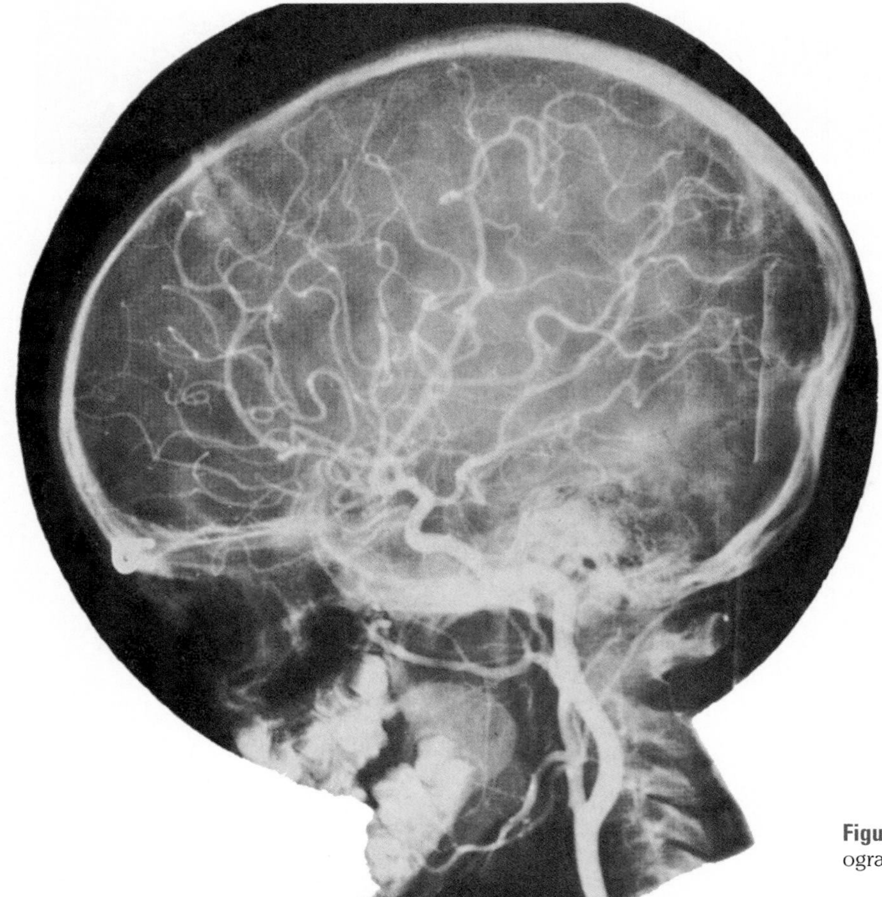

Figure 11-123 Lateral internal carotid arteriogram.

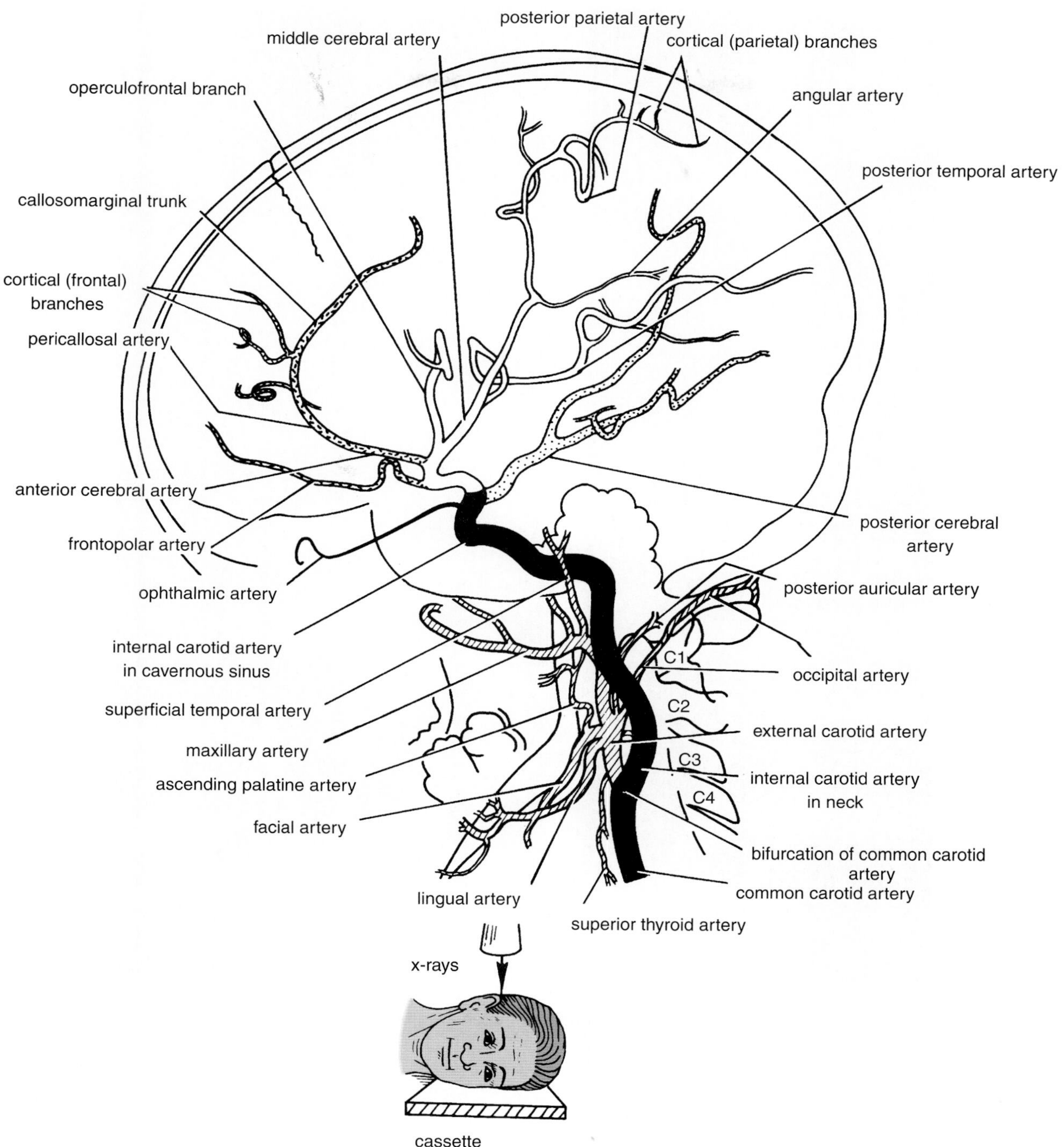

Figure 11-124 Main features that can be seen in the arteriogram in Figure 11-123.

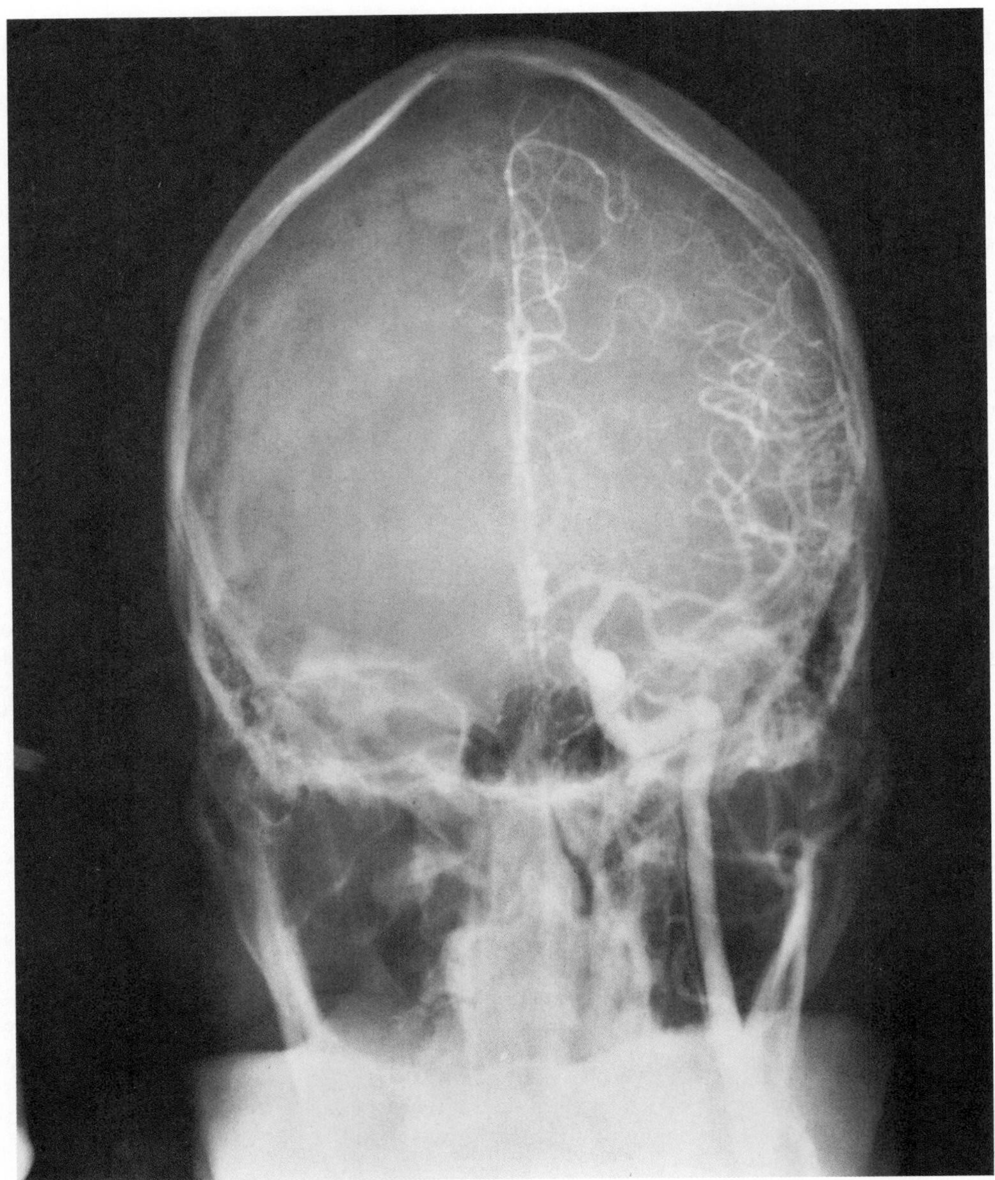

Figure 11-125 Anteroposterior internal carotid arteriogram.

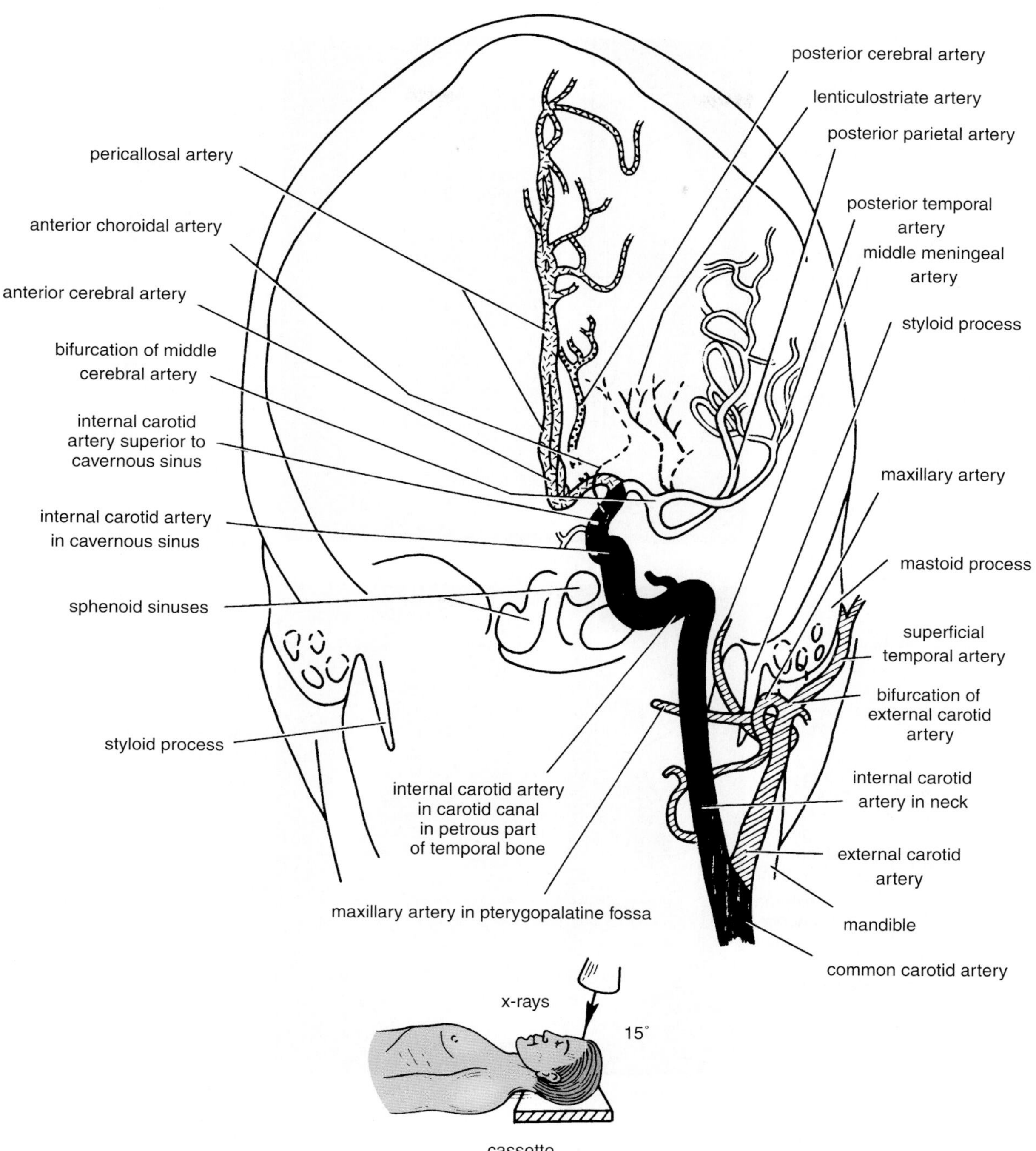

Figure 11-126 Main features that can be seen in the arteriogram in Figure 11-125.

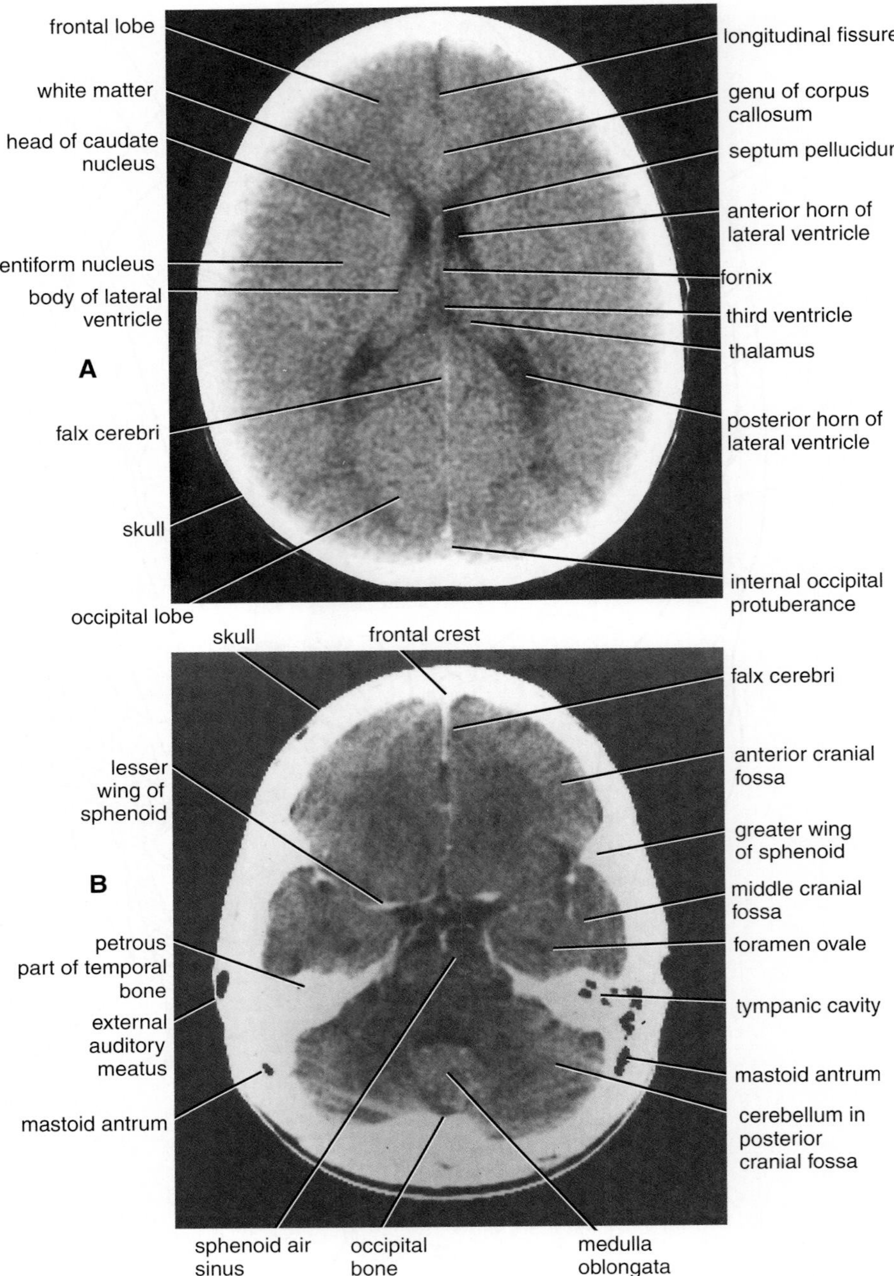

Figure 11-127 Axial (horizontal) computed tomography scans of the skull. **A.** The skull bones and the brain and the different parts of the lateral ventricles. **B.** A scan made at a lower level showing the three cranial fossae.

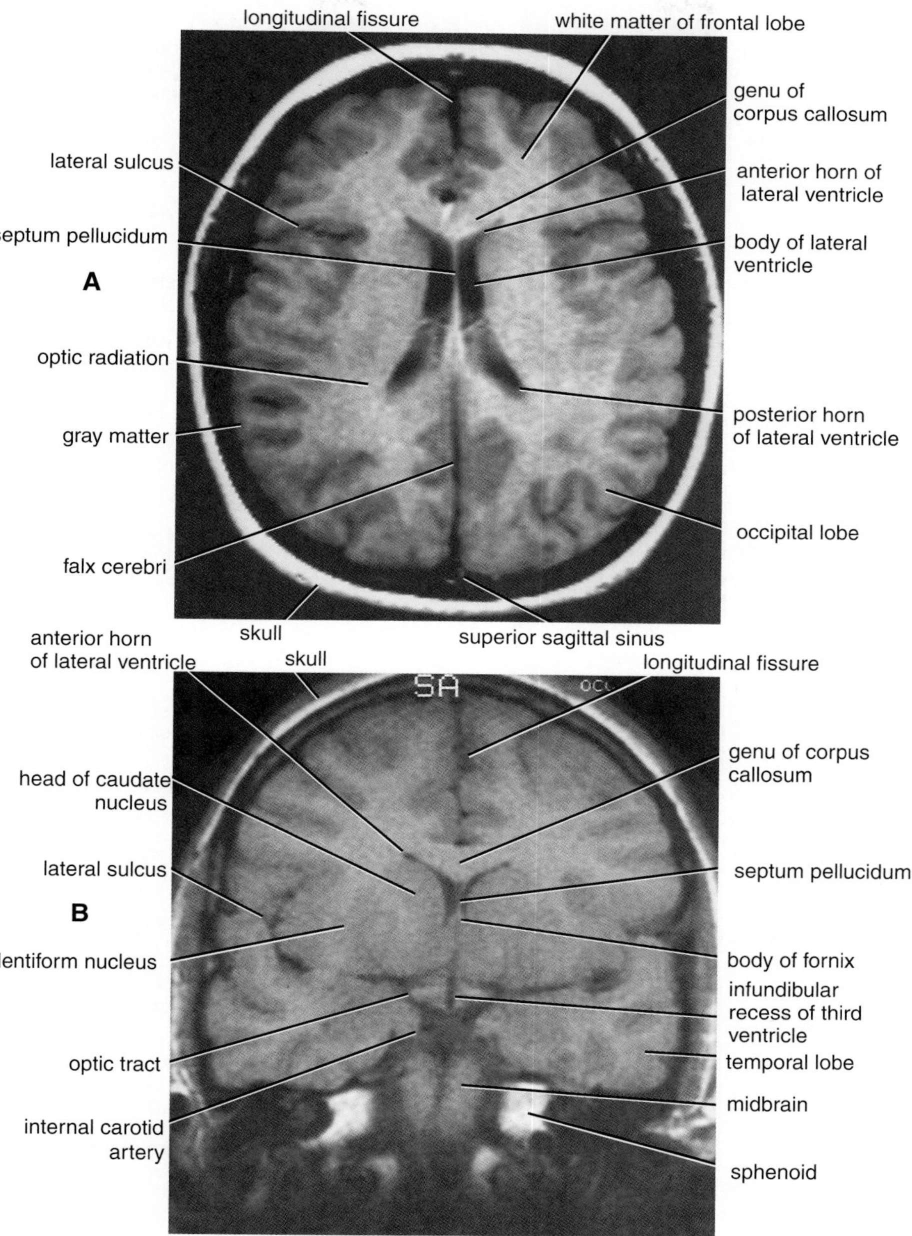

Figure 11-128 Magnetic resonance imaging of the skull. **A.** Axial image of the brain showing the different parts of the lateral ventricle and the lateral sulcus of the cerebral hemisphere. **B.** Coronal image through the frontal lobe of the brain showing the anterior horn of the lateral ventricle. Note the improved contrast between the gray and white matter compared with the computed tomography scans seen in Figure 11-127.

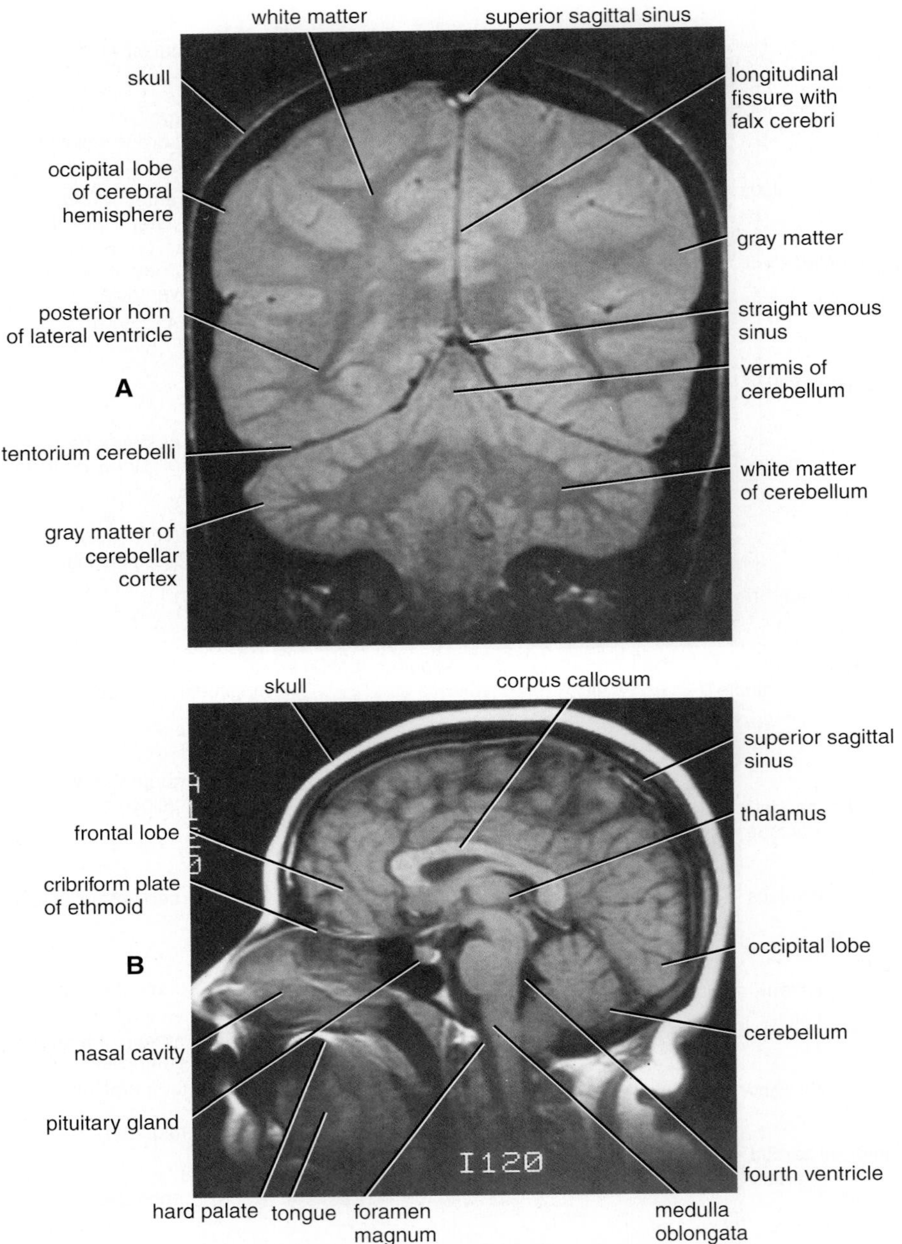

Figure 11-129 Magnetic resonance imaging of the skull. **A.** Coronal image through the occipital lobes of the brain showing the posterior horn of the lateral ventricle and the cerebellum. **B.** Sagittal image showing the different parts of the brain and the nasal and mouth cavities.

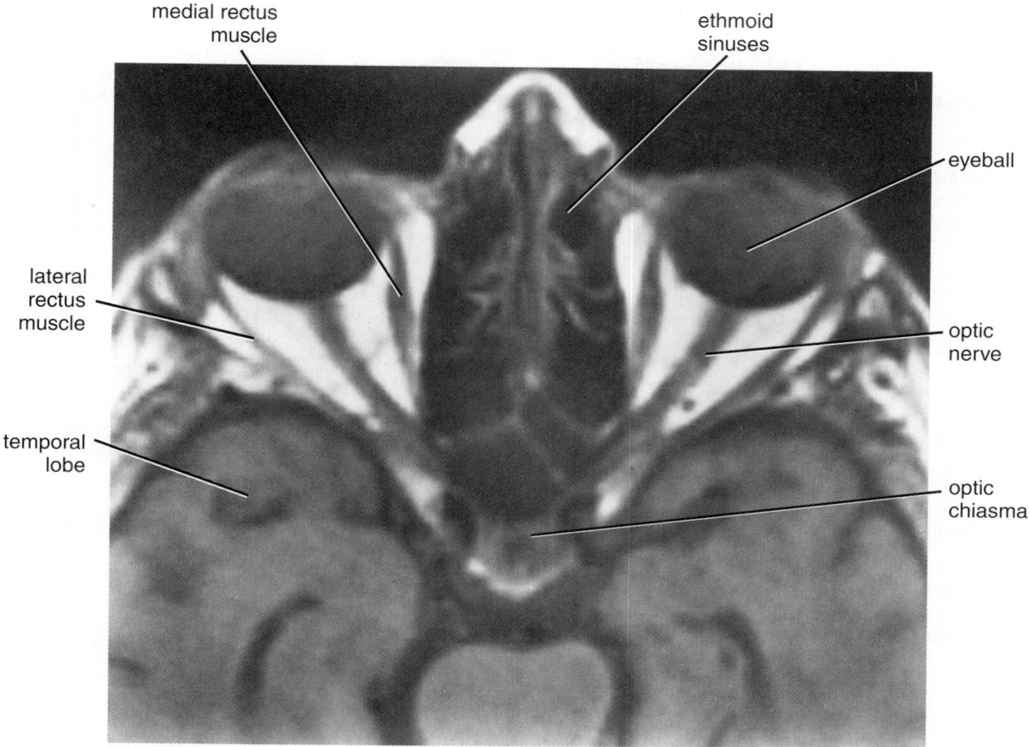

Figure 11-130 Axial (horizontal) magnetic resonance imaging showing the contents of the orbital and cranial cavities. Note that the eyeballs, the optic nerves, the optic chiasma, and the extraocular muscles can be identified.

Posterior Fontanelle

In the baby, the posterior fontanelle lies between the squamous part of the occipital bone and the posterior borders of the two parietal bones (Fig. 11-131). It is usually closed by the end of the first year.

Superciliary Ridges

The superciliary ridges are two prominent ridges on the frontal bones above the upper margin of the orbit (Fig. 11-131). Deep to these ridges on either side of the midline lie the **frontal air sinuses.**

Superior Nuchal Line

The superior nuchal line is a curved ridge that runs laterally from the external occipital protuberance to the mastoid process of the temporal bone. It gives attachment to the trapezius and sternocleidomastoid muscles.

Mastoid Process of the Temporal Bone

The mastoid process projects downward and forward from behind the ear (Figs. 11-131 and 11-134). It is undeveloped in the newborn child and grows only as the result of the pull of the sternocleidomastoid, as the child moves his or her head. It can be recognized as a bony projection at the end of the second year.

Auricle and External Auditory Meatus

These structures lie in front of the mastoid process (Fig. 11-27). The external auditory meatus is about 1 in. (2.5 cm) long and forms an S-shaped curve. To examine the outer surface of the tympanic membrane in the adult with an otoscope, the tube may be straightened by pulling the auricle upward and backward. In small children, the auricle is pulled straight back or downward and backward.

Tympanic Membrane

The tympanic membrane is normally pearly gray and is concave toward the meatus (Fig. 11-27). The most depressed part of the concavity is called the umbo and is caused by the attachment of the handle of the malleus on its medial surface.

Zygomatic Arch

The zygomatic arch extends forward in front of the ear and ends in front in the zygomatic bone (Fig. 11-131). Above the zygomatic arch is the **temporal fossa,** which is filled with

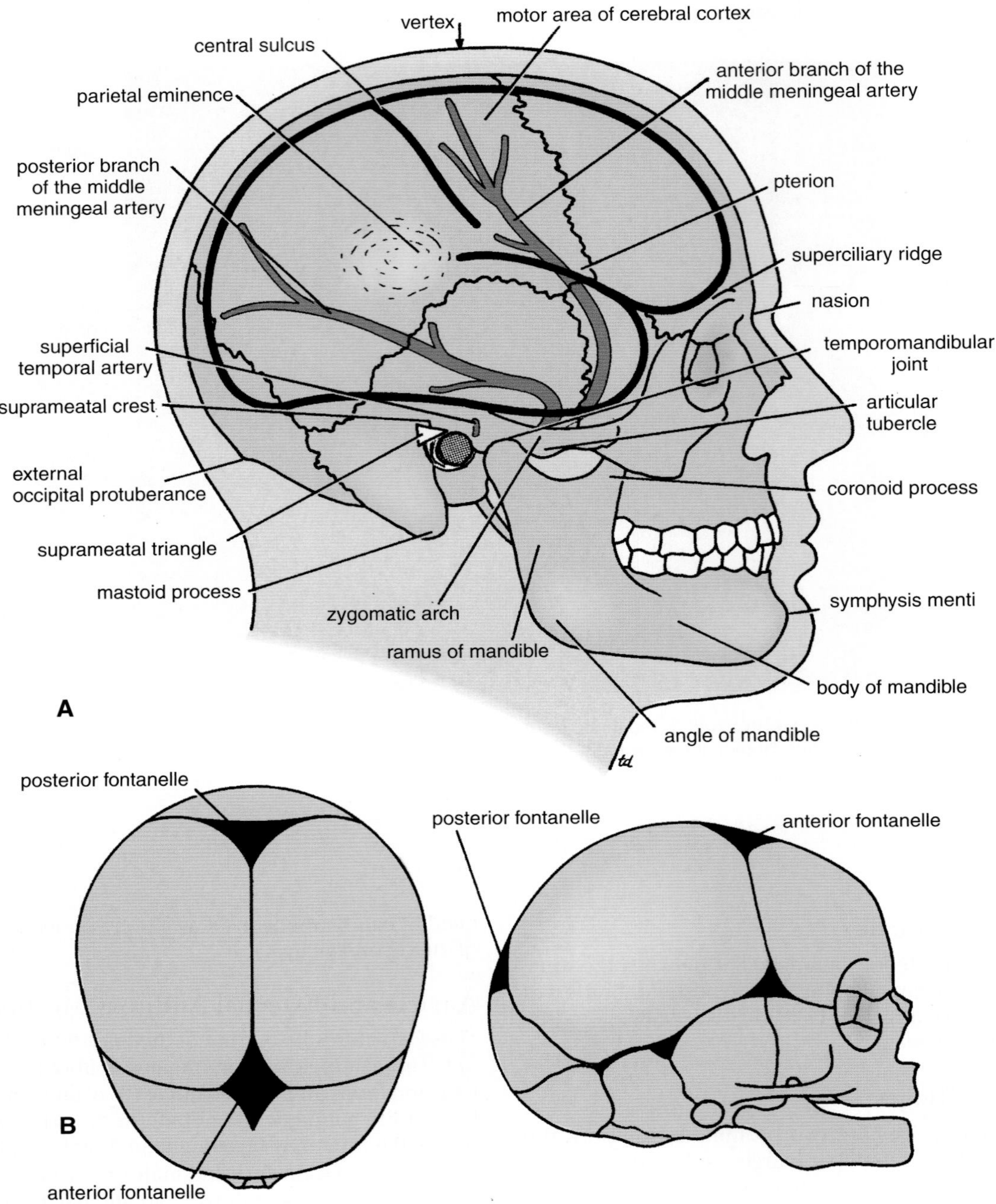

Figure 11-131 **A.** Right side of the head showing relations of the middle meningeal artery and the brain to the surface of the skull. **B.** Superior aspect and right side of the neonatal skull. Note the positions of the anterior and posterior fontanelles.

the **temporalis muscle.** Attached to the lower margin of the zygomatic arch is the **masseter muscle.** Contraction of both the temporalis and masseter muscles (Fig. 11-85) can be felt by clenching the teeth.

Superficial Temporal Artery

The pulsations of the superficial temporal artery can be felt as it crosses the zygomatic arch, immediately in front of the auricle (Fig. 11-131).

Pterion

The pterion is the point where the greater wing of the sphenoid meets the anteroinferior angle of the parietal bone. Lying 1.5 in. (4 cm) above the midpoint of the zygomatic arch (Fig. 11-131), it is not marked by an eminence or a depression, but it is important because beneath it lies the **anterior branch of the middle meningeal artery.**

Above and behind the external auditory meatus, deep to the auricle, can be felt a small depression, the **suprameatal**

triangle (Fig. 11-131). This is bounded behind by a line drawn vertically upward from the posterior margin of the external auditory meatus, above by the suprameatal crest of the temporal bone, and below by the external auditory meatus. The bony floor of the triangle forms the lateral wall of the **mastoid antrum.**

Temporomandibular Joint

The temporomandibular joint can be easily palpated in front of the auricle (Fig. 11-131). Note that as the mouth is opened, the head of the mandible rotates and moves forward below the tubercle of the zygomatic arch.

Anterior Border of the Ramus of the Mandible

The anterior border of the ramus can be felt deep to the masseter muscle. The coronoid process of the mandible can be felt with the gloved finger inside the mouth, and the pterygomandibular ligament can be palpated as a tense band on its medial side.

Posterior Border of the Ramus of the Mandible

The posterior border of the ramus is overlapped above by the parotid gland (Fig. 11-85), but below it is easily felt through the skin. The outer surface of the ramus of the mandible is covered by the masseter muscle and can be felt on deep palpation when this muscle is relaxed.

Body of the Mandible

The body of the mandible is best examined by having one finger inside the mouth and another on the outside. Thus, it is possible to examine the mandible from the symphysis menti, in the midline anteriorly, as far backward as the angle of the mandible (Fig. 11-131).

Facial Artery

The pulsations of the facial artery can be felt as it crosses the lower margin of the body of the mandible, at the anterior border of the masseter muscle (Fig. 11-135).

Anterior Border of the Masseter

The anterior border of the masseter can be easily felt by clenching the teeth.

Parotid Duct

The parotid duct runs forward from the parotid gland one fingerbreadth below the zygomatic arch (Fig. 11-135). It can be rolled beneath the examining finger at the anterior border of the masseter as it turns medially and opens into the mouth opposite the upper second molar tooth (Fig. 11-72).

Orbital Margin

The orbital margin is formed by the frontal, zygomatic, and maxillary bones (Fig. 11-18).

Supraorbital Notch

If present, the notch can be felt at the junction of the medial and intermediate thirds of the upper margin of the orbit. It transmits the **supraorbital nerve,** which can be rolled against the bone (Fig. 11-18).

Infraorbital Foramen

The infraorbital foramen lies 5 mm below the lower margin of the orbit (Fig. 11-1), on a line drawn downward from the supraorbital notch to the interval between the two lower premolar teeth.

Infraorbital Nerve

The infraorbital nerve emerges from the foramen and supplies the skin of the face.

Maxillary Air Sinus

The maxillary air sinus is situated within the maxillary bone and lies below the infraorbital foramen on each side (Fig. 11-97).

Frontal Air Sinus

The frontal air sinus is situated within the frontal bone and lies deep to the superciliary ridge on each side (Fig. 11-97).

Surface Landmarks of the Neck

Anterior Aspect

In the midline anteriorly, the following structures can be palpated from above downward:

- **Symphysis menti:** The lower margin can be felt where the two halves of the body of the mandible unite in the midline (Figs. 11-132 and 11-133).
- **Submental triangle:** This lies between the symphysis menti and the body of the hyoid bone (Fig. 11-56). It is bounded anteriorly by the midline of the neck, laterally by the anterior belly of the digastric muscle, and inferiorly by the body of the hyoid bone. The floor is formed by the mylohyoid muscle. The submental lymph nodes are located in this triangle.
- **Body of the hyoid bone:** This lies opposite the third cervical vertebra (Figs. 11-13 and 11-132).
- **Thyrohyoid membrane:** This fills in the interval between the hyoid bone and the thyroid cartilage (Fig. 11-133).
- **Upper border of the thyroid cartilage:** This notched structure lies opposite the fourth cervical vertebra (Figs. 11-13 and 11-132).
- **Cricothyroid ligament:** This structure fills in the interval between the cricoid cartilage and the thyroid cartilage (Fig. 11-133).
- **Cricoid cartilage:** An important landmark in the neck (Fig. 11-132), this lies at the level of the sixth cervical vertebra, at the junction of the larynx with the trachea, at the level of the junction of the pharynx with the esophagus, at the level of the middle cervical sympathetic ganglion, and at the level where the inferior thyroid artery enters the thyroid gland.

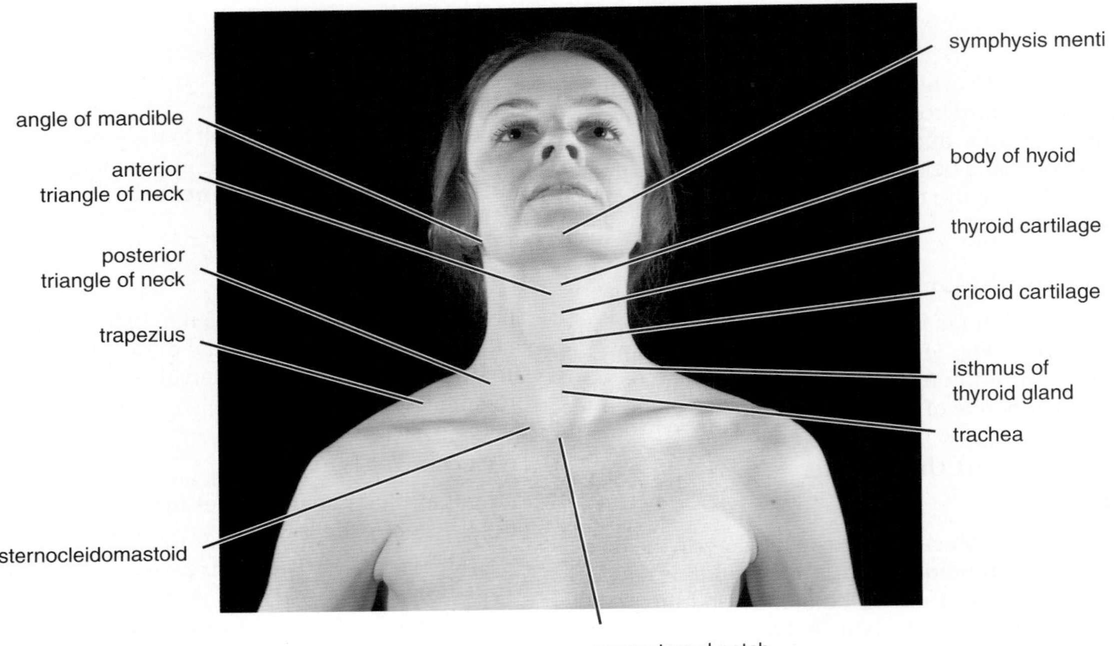

Figure 11-132 Anterior view of the head and neck of a 29-year-old woman. Note that the atlanto-occipital joints and the cervical part of the vertebral column are partially extended for full exposure of the front of the neck.

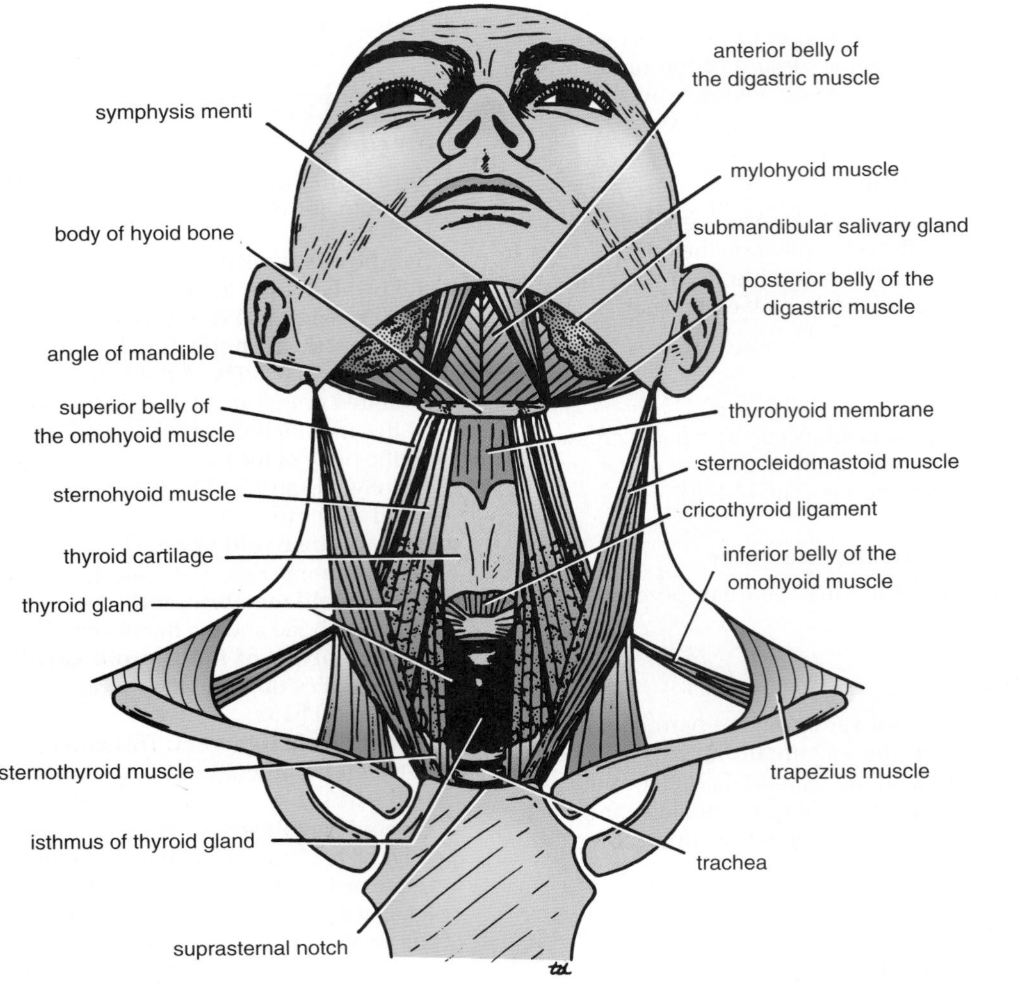

Figure 11-133 Surface anatomy of the neck from in front.

- **Cricotracheal ligament:** This structure fills in the interval between the cricoid cartilage and the first ring of the trachea (Fig. 11-98).
- **First ring of the trachea:** This can be felt by gentle palpation just above the isthmus of the thyroid gland.
- **Isthmus of the thyroid gland:** This lies in front of the second, third, and fourth rings of the trachea (Figs. 11-132 and 11-133).
- **Inferior thyroid veins:** The inferior thyroid veins lie in front of the fifth, sixth, and seventh rings of the trachea (Fig. 11-110).
- **Thyroidea ima artery:** When present, this artery ascends in front of the trachea to the isthmus of the thyroid gland, from the brachiocephalic artery (Fig. 11-110).
- **Jugular arch:** This vein connects the two anterior jugular veins just above the suprasternal notch (Fig. 11-13).
- **Suprasternal notch:** This can be felt between the anterior ends of the clavicles (Fig. 11-132). It is the superior border of the manubrium sterni and lies opposite the lower border of the body of the second thoracic vertebra.

In the adult the trachea may measure as much as 1 in. (2.5 cm) in diameter, whereas in a baby it may be narrower than a pencil. In young children, the thymus gland may extend above the suprasternal notch as far as the isthmus of the thyroid gland, and the brachiocephalic artery and the left brachiocephalic vein may protrude above the suprasternal notch.

Posterior Aspect

In the midline posteriorly, the following structures can be palpated from above downward.

The **external occipital protuberance** lies in the midline at the junction of the head and neck (Fig. 11-135). If the index finger is placed on the skin in the midline, it can be drawn downward in the **nuchal groove.** The first spinous process to be felt is that of the **seventh cervical vertebra (vertebra prominens).** Cervical spines one to six are covered by the **ligamentum nuchae.**

Lateral Aspect

Sternocleidomastoid Muscle

On the side of the neck, the sternocleidomastoid can be palpated throughout its length as it passes upward from the sternum and clavicle to the mastoid process (Figs. 11-134 and 11-135). The muscle can be made to stand out by asking the patient to approximate the ear to the shoulder of the same side and at the same time rotate the head so that the face looks upward toward the opposite side. If the movement is carried out against resistance, the muscle will be felt to contract, and its anterior and posterior borders will be defined.

The sternocleidomastoid divides the neck into anterior and posterior triangles. The anterior triangle of the neck is bounded by the body of the mandible, the sternocleidomastoid, and the midline (Fig. 11-56). The posterior triangle is bounded by the anterior border of the trapezius, the sternocleidomastoid, and the clavicle (Fig. 11-56).

Trapezius Muscle

The anterior border of the trapezius muscle (Fig. 11-132) can be felt by asking the patient to shrug the shoulders. It will be seen to extend from the superior nuchal line of the occipital bone, downward and forward to the posterior border of the lateral third of the clavicle.

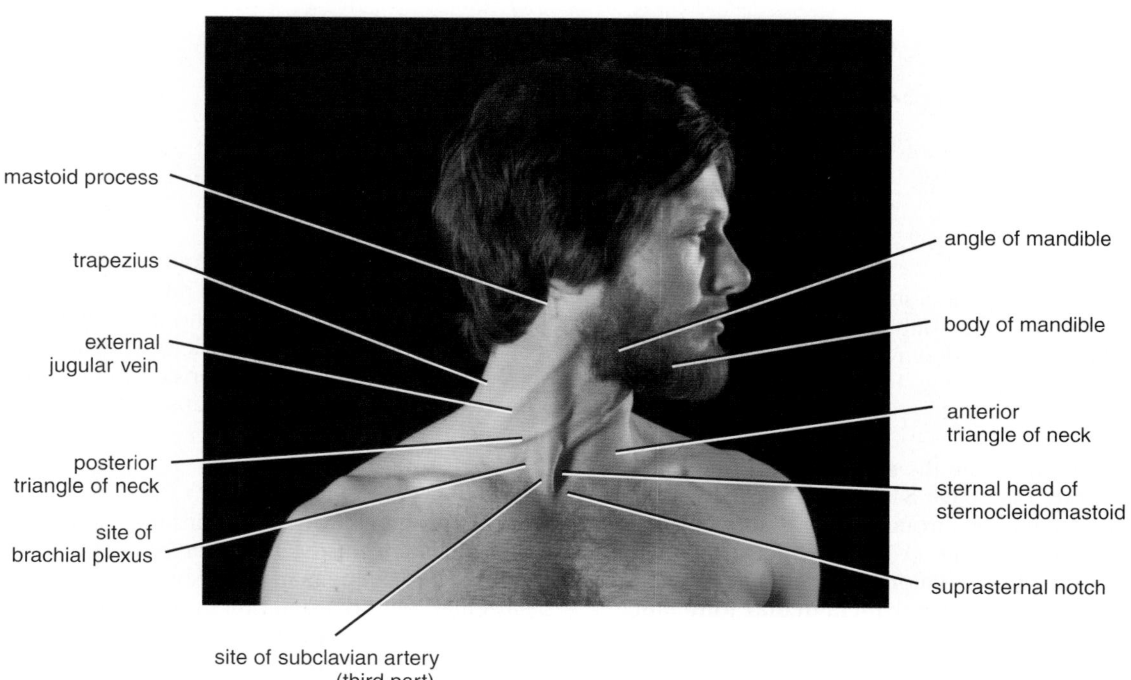

Figure 11-134 Anterior view of the neck of a 27-year-old man. Note that the head has been laterally rotated to the left at the atlantoaxial joints and at the joints of the cervical part of the vertebral column.

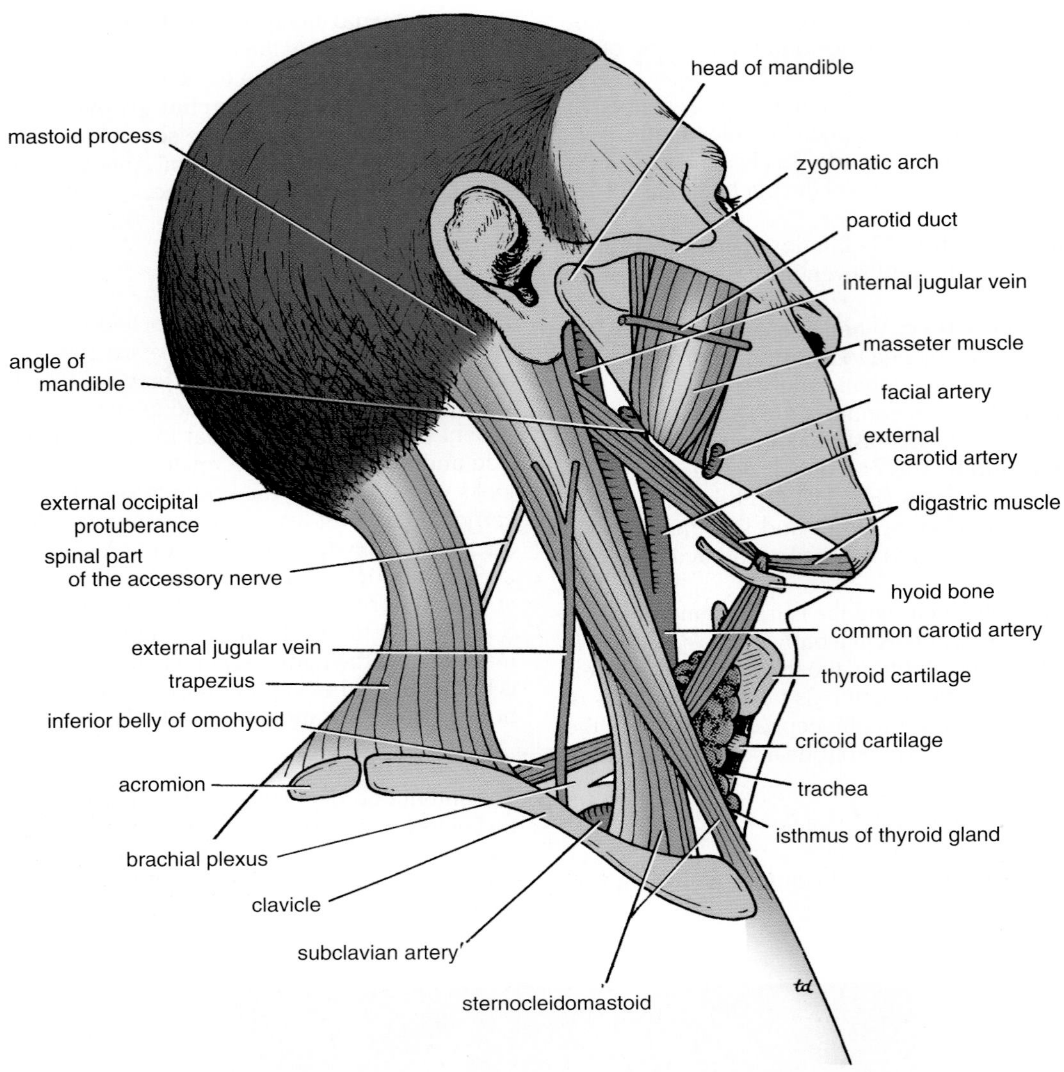

Figure 11-135 Surface anatomy of the neck from the lateral aspect.

Platysma Muscle

The platysma can be seen as a sheet of muscle by asking the patient to clench the jaws firmly. The muscle extends from the body of the mandible downward over the clavicle onto the anterior thoracic wall (Fig. 11-51).

Root of the Neck

At the root of the neck are the **suprasternal notch** in the midline anteriorly (see page 841) and the clavicles. Each clavicle is subcutaneous throughout its entire length and can be easily palpated (Fig. 11-135). It articulates at its lateral extremity with the acromion of the scapula. At the medial end of the clavicle, the **sternoclavicular joint** can be identified.

Anterior Triangle of the Neck

The isthmus of the thyroid gland lies in front of the second, third, and fourth rings of the trachea (Figs. 11-132 and 11-133). The lateral lobes of the thyroid gland can be palpated deep to the sternocleidomastoid muscles. This is most easily carried out by standing behind the seated patient and asking the patient to flex the neck forward and so relax the overlying muscles. The observer can then examine both lobes simultaneously with the tips of the fingers of both hands.

Carotid Sheath

The carotid sheath, which contains the carotid arteries, the internal jugular vein, the vagus nerve, and the deep cervical lymph nodes, can be marked out by a line joining the sternoclavicular joint to a point midway between the tip of the mastoid process and the angle of the mandible. At the level of the upper border of the thyroid cartilage, the common carotid artery bifurcates into the internal and external carotid arteries (Fig. 11-135). The pulsations of these arteries can be felt at this level.

Posterior Triangle of the Neck

At the posterior triangle of the neck, the spinal part of the **accessory nerve** is relatively superficial as it emerges from the posterior border of the sternocleidomastoid and runs downward and backward to pass beneath the anterior border of the trapezius (Fig. 11-135). The course of this nerve may be indicated as follows: Draw a line from the angle of the mandible to the tip of the mastoid process. Bisect this line at right angles and extend the second line downward across the posterior triangle; the second line indicates the course of the nerve.

Roots and Trunks of the Brachial Plexus

The roots and trunks of the brachial plexus occupy the lower anterior angle of the posterior triangle (Figs. 11-134 and 11-135). The upper limit of the plexus can be indicated by a line drawn from the cricoid cartilage downward to the middle of the clavicle.

Third Part of the Subclavian Artery

The third part of the subclavian artery also occupies the lower anterior angle of the posterior triangle (Figs. 11-134 and 11-135). Its course may be indicated by a curved line, which passes upward from the sternoclavicular joint for about 0.5 in. (1.3 cm) and then downward to the middle of the clavicle. It is here, where the artery lies on the upper surface of the first rib, that its pulsations can be felt easily. The subclavian vein lies behind the clavicle and does not enter the neck.

External Jugular Vein

The external jugular vein lies in the superficial fascia deep to the platysma. It passes downward from the region of the angle of the mandible to the middle of the clavicle (Figs. 11-134 and 11-135). It perforates the deep fascia just above the clavicle and drains into the subclavian vein.

Salivary Glands

The three large salivary glands can be palpated. The parotid gland lies below the ear in the interval between the mandible and the anterior border of the sternocleidomastoid muscle (Fig. 11-85). The surface marking of the parotid duct is given on page 787.

The submandibular gland can be divided into superficial and deep parts. The superficial part lies beneath the lower margin of the body of the mandible (Fig. 11-86). The deep part of the submandibular gland, the submandibular duct, and the sublingual gland can be palpated through the mucous membrane covering the floor of the mouth in the interval between the tongue and the lower jaw. The submandibular duct opens into the mouth on the side of the frenulum of the tongue (Fig. 11-72).

CLINICAL PROBLEM SOLVING

Study the following case histories and select the best answer to the questions following them.

An 8-year-old girl was taken to a pediatrician because her mother had noticed a small painless swelling below and behind the angle of the jaw on the right side. On examination, the swelling was superficial, cool to touch, and showed no redness. Careful palpation of the neck revealed two firm lumps matted together beneath the anterior border of the right sternocleidomastoid muscle. Examination of the palatine tonsils showed moderate hypertrophy on both sides with a few pustules exuding from the tonsillar crypts on the right side. The patient did not have a pyrexia.

1. The following statements concerning this case are consistent with the patient having chronic cervical lymphadenitis except which?
   (a) The lymph drains from the tonsil into the superficial cervical lymph nodes, which when enlarged produce a swelling below and behind the angle of the jaw.
   (b) Tuberculous cervical lymphadenitis is a chronic infection that can enter the tonsil and spread to the lymph nodes.
   (c) The investing layer of deep cervical fascia can limit the spread of infection in the neck.
   (d) Tuberculous infection of a lymph node commonly spreads to other nodes in the group and they become matted together.
   (e) Tuberculous infection results in the destruction of the node with the formation of pus that later erodes through the deep fascia, producing a large cold abscess beneath the skin.
   (f) Secondary infection of a cold abscess causes the abscess to break through the skin to form a discharging sinus.

A 25-year-old woman complaining of a swelling on the front of the neck and breathlessness visited her physician. On examination, a small, solitary swelling of firm consistency was found to the left of the midline of the neck below the thyroid cartilage of the larynx. The swelling was not attached to the skin but moved upward on swallowing. About 2 weeks previously the swelling had suddenly increased in size and become tender to touch; following this increase in size the patient became breathless.

2. The following statements concerning this case would suggest a diagnosis of adenoma of the thyroid gland except which?
   (a) The pretracheal layer of deep cervical fascia binds the thyroid gland to the larynx, which moves upward on swallowing.
   (b) Each lobe of the thyroid gland is closely related to the sides of the trachea.
   (c) The isthmus of the thyroid gland was found to cross in front of the third, fourth, and fifth rings of the trachea.

(d) The sudden increase in the size of the swelling can be explained by a hemorrhage into the adenoma.
(e) The swelling was located superficial to the left sternothyroid muscle.
(f) The breathlessness was caused by the adenoma pressing on the trachea, partially occluding the lumen.

A 70-year-old man complaining of a small painless swelling below his chin visited his physician. On questioning, he said that he had first noticed the swelling 4 months earlier and that it was gradually increasing in size. Because it had not caused any discomfort, he had chosen to ignore it. On examination, a single, small, hard swelling could be palpated in the submental triangle. It was mobile on the deep tissues and not attached to the skin.

3. The following statements suggest that the hard swelling was a secondary malignant deposit in a lymph node except which?
   (a) The submental lymph nodes are located in the submental triangle just below the chin.
   (b) The submental lymph nodes drain the tip of the tongue, the floor of the mouth in the region of the frenulum of the tongue, the gums and incisor teeth, the middle third of the lower lip, and the skin over the chin.
   (c) A small, hard-based carcinomatous ulcer was found on the right side of the tongue near the tip.
   (d) The deep cervical group of lymph nodes beneath the sternocleidomastoid muscle receive lymph from the submental lymph nodes.
   (e) The submental lymph nodes lie deep to the superficial part of the submandibular salivary gland.

A 45-year-old man with extensive maxillofacial injuries after an automobile accident was brought to the emergency department. Evaluation of the airway revealed partial obstruction. Despite an obvious fractured mandible, an attempt was made to move the tongue forward from the posterior pharyngeal wall by pushing the angles of the mandible forward. This maneuver failed to move the tongue, and it became necessary to hold the tongue forward directly to pull it away from the posterior pharyngeal wall.

4. The most likely reason the physician was unable to pull the tongue forward in this patient is which?
   (a) The hypoglossal nerves were damaged on both sides of the neck.
   (b) Spasm of the styloglossus muscles
   (c) The mandibular origin of the genioglossus muscles was floating because of bilateral fractures of the body of the mandible.
   (d) The presence of a blood clot in the mouth
   (e) The resistance of the patient

Having passed a laryngoscope into a patient, the anesthetist viewed the following anatomic structures in order from the base of the tongue to the trachea.

5. All the following structures were correctly recognized except which?
   (a) The median glossoepiglottic fold and the valleculae
   (b) The two lateral glossoepiglottic folds
   (c) The upper edge of the epiglottis
   (d) The aryepiglottic folds
   (e) The rounded swellings of the cuneiform and corniculate cartilages
   (f) The mobile vestibular folds
   (g) The whitish vocal cords (folds) with the rima glottidis

A 17-year-old boy was seen in the emergency department after receiving a stab wound at the front of the neck. The knife entrance wound was located on the left side of the neck just lateral to the tip of the greater cornu of the hyoid bone. During the physical examination the patient was asked to protrude his tongue, which deviated to the left.

6. The following statements would explain the physical signs in this patient except which?
   (a) The genioglossus muscles are responsible for protruding the tongue.
   (b) The genioglossus muscle is supplied by the glossopharyngeal nerve.
   (c) Paralysis of the left genioglossus muscle permitted the right genioglossus to pull the tongue forward and turned the tip to the left side.
   (d) The hypoglossal nerve descends in the neck between the internal carotid artery and the internal jugular vein.
   (e) At about the level of the tip of the greater cornu of the hyoid bone the hypoglossal nerve turns forward and crosses the internal and external carotid arteries and the lingual artery to enter the tongue.
   (f) The point of the knife blade severed the left hypoglossal nerve.

A 43-year-old woman was seen in the emergency department with a large abscess in the middle of the right posterior triangle of the neck. The abscess was red, hot, and fluctuant. The abscess showed evidence that it was pointing and about to rupture. The physician decided to incise the abscess and insert a drain. The patient returned to the department for the dressings to be changed 5 days later. She stated that she felt much better and that her neck was no longer painful. However, there was one thing that she could not understand. She could no longer raise her right hand above her head to brush her hair.

7. The following statements explain the signs and symptoms in this case, suggesting that the spinal part of the accessory nerve had been incised, except which?
   (a) To raise the hand above the head, it is necessary for the trapezius muscle, assisted by the serratus anterior, to contract and rotate the scapula so that the glenoid cavity faces upward.
   (b) The trapezius muscle is innervated by the spinal part of the accessory nerve.
   (c) As the spinal part of the accessory nerve crosses the posterior triangle of the neck, it is deeply placed, being covered by the skin, the superficial fascia, the investing layer of deep cervical fascia, and the levator scapulae muscle.
   (d) The surface marking of the spinal part of the accessory nerve is as follows: Bisect at right angles a line joining the angle of the jaw to the tip of the mastoid process. Continue the second line downward and backward across the posterior triangle.

(e) The knife opening the abscess had cut the accessory nerve.

A 35-year-old woman had a partial thyroidectomy for the treatment of thyrotoxicosis. During the operation a ligature slipped off the right superior thyroid artery. To stop the hemorrhage, the surgeon blindly grabbed for the artery with artery forceps. The operation was completed without further incident. The following morning the patient spoke with a husky voice.

8. The following statements about this patient would explain the husky voice except which?
   (a) Laryngoscopic examination revealed that the right vocal cord was slack, causing the huskiness of the voice.
   (b) The vocal cord is tensed by the contraction of the cricothyroid muscle.
   (c) The cricothyroid muscle tilts back the cricoid cartilage and pulls forward the thyroid cartilage.
   (d) The cricothyroid muscle is innervated by the recurrent laryngeal nerve.
   (e) The superior thyroid artery is closely related to the external laryngeal nerve.

A 46-year-old man was seen in the emergency department after being knocked down in a street brawl. He had received a blow on the head with an empty bottle. On examination, the patient was conscious and had a large doughlike swelling over the back of the head that was restricted to the area over the occipital bone. The skin was intact, and the swelling fluctuated on palpation.

9. The following statements concerning this patient are correct except which?
   (a) The hematoma, although large, did not extend forward to the orbital margins and did not extend laterally as far as the temporal lines.
   (b) The hematoma was located just beneath the epicranial aponeurosis and was superficial to the periosteum of the occipital bone.
   (c) The swelling did not occupy the subcutaneous tissue of the scalp.
   (d) The hematoma is restricted to one skull bone and is situated beneath the periosteum.
   (e) The edge of the swelling is limited by the attachment of the periosteum to the sutural ligaments.

A 17-year-old girl visited her dermatologist because of severe acne of the face. On examination, it was found that a small abscess was present on the side of the nose. The patient was given antibiotics and was warned not to press the abscess.

10. The following facts concerning this patient emphasize why it is important to adequately treat this condition except which?
   (a) The skin area between the eye, the upper lip, and the side of the nose is a hazardous area to have an infection of the skin.
   (b) The danger area is drained by the facial vein.
   (c) Interference with a boil by squeezing or pricking it can lead to spread of the infection and thrombosis of the facial vein.
   (d) The facial vein communicates with the cavernous sinus via the superior and inferior ophthalmic veins.
   (e) Cavernous sinus thrombosis can occur by the spread of infection by the venous blood.
   (f) The blood in the facial vein is unable to spread upward because of valves.

A 7-year-old boy with right-sided otitis media was treated with antibiotics. The organisms did not respond to the treatment, and the infection spread to the mastoid antrum and the mastoid air cells. The surgeon decided to perform a radical mastoid operation. After the operation, it was noticed that the boy's face was distorted.

11. The following signs and symptoms suggest that the right facial nerve had been damaged during the operation except which?
   (a) The mouth was drawn upward to the right.
   (b) He was unable to close his right eye.
   (c) Saliva tended to accumulate in his right cheek.
   (d) The saliva tended to dribble from the corner of his mouth.
   (e) All the muscles of the right side of his face were paralyzed.

A 43-year-old woman visited her physician complaining of severe intermittent pain on the right side of her face. The pain was precipitated by exposing the right side of her face to a draft of cold air. The pain was stabbing in nature and lasted about 12 hours before finally disappearing. When asked to point out on her face the area where the pain was experienced, the patient mapped out the skin area over the right side of the lower jaw extending backward and upward over the side of the head to the vertex.

12. The following signs and symptoms in this patient strongly suggest a diagnosis of trigeminal neuralgia except which?
   (a) The skin area where the patient experienced the pain was innervated by the mandibular division of the trigeminal nerve.
   (b) The stabbing nature of the pain is characteristic of the disease.
   (c) The trigger mechanism, stimulation of an area that received its sensory innervation from the trigeminal nerve, is characteristic of trigeminal neuralgia.
   (d) Examination of the actions of the masseter and the temporalis muscles showed evidence of weakness on the right side.
   (e) The patient experienced hyperesthesia in the distribution of the right auriculotemporal nerve.

A 10-year-old boy was playing darts with his friends. He bent down to pick up a fallen dart when another dart fell from the dart board and hit him on the side of his face. On examination in the emergency department a small skin wound was found over the right parotid salivary gland. Then 6 months later, the boy's mother noticed that before mealtimes the boy began to sweat profusely on the facial skin close to the healed dart wound.

13. The following statements can explain this phenomenon except which?
   (a) The point of the dart had entered the parotid salivary gland and damaged the parasympathetic secretomotor fibers to the gland.

(b) The secretomotor fibers to the parotid gland arise in the otic ganglion.
(c) The preganglionic parasympathetic fibers originate in the superior salivatory nucleus of the facial nerve.
(d) The skin over the parotid salivary gland is innervated by the great auricular nerve, which was also damaged by the dart.
(e) On regeneration of the damaged nerves some of the parasympathetic nerves to the parotid salivary gland had crossed over and joined the sympathetic secretomotor nerves to the sweat glands in the distal end of the great auricular nerve.
(f) The patient has Frey's syndrome.

A 26-year-old baseball player was struck on the right side of the head with a ball. The player fell to the ground but did not lose consciousness. After resting for 1 hour and then getting up, he was seen to be confused and irritable. Later, he staggered and fell to the floor. On questioning, he was seen to be drowsy, and twitching of the lower left half of his face and left arm was noted.

14. A diagnosis of extradural hemorrhage was made based on the following statements except which?
    (a) A minor blow on the side of the head can easily fracture the thin anteroinferior part of the parietal bone.
    (b) The posterior branch of the middle meningeal artery may be sectioned at the site of the fracture.
    (c) Arterial hemorrhage outside the meningeal layer of the dura mater may occur.
    (d) A large blood clot outside the dura can exert pressure on the lower end of the precentral gyrus.
    (e) The lower end of the precentral gyrus or motor area supplies the facial muscles and the muscles of the upper limb.

A 49-year-old woman was found on ophthalmoscopic examination to have edema of both optic discs (bilateral papilledema) and congestion of both retinal veins. The cause of the condition was found to be a rapidly expanding intracranial tumor.

15. The following statements concerning this patient are correct except which?
    (a) An intracranial tumor causes a rise in cerebrospinal fluid pressure.
    (b) The optic nerves are surrounded by sheaths derived from the pia mater, arachnoid mater, and dura mater.
    (c) The intracranial subarachnoid space extends forward around the optic nerve for about half its length.
    (d) The thin walls of the retinal vein will be compressed as the vein crosses the extension of the subarachnoid space around the optic nerve.
    (e) Because both subarachnoid extensions are continuous with the intracranial subarachnoid space, both eyes will exhibit papilledema and congestion of the retinal veins.

A 52-year-old man was eating his dinner in a seafood restaurant when he suddenly choked on a piece of fish. He gasped that he had a bone stuck in his throat.

16. Assuming that the fish bone was stuck in the piriform fossa, the following statements are correct except which?
    (a) The piriform fossae lie on either side of the entrance into the larynx.
    (b) The mucous membrane lining the piriform fossae is sensitive and innervated by the recurrent laryngeal nerve.
    (c) The piriform fossa is bounded laterally by the thyroid cartilage and the thyrohyoid membrane.
    (d) The piriform fossa is bounded medially by the aryepiglottic fold.
    (e) The piriform fossa leads inferiorly into the esophagus.

ANSWERS TO CLINICAL PROBLEMS

1. A. The lymph drains from the tonsil into the jugulodigastric member of the deep cervical lymph nodes.
2. E. The thyroid gland lies deep to the sternothyroid muscles.
3. E. The submental lymph nodes are not covered by the superficial parts of the submandibular salivary glands.
4. C. The genioglossus muscles arise from the superior mental spines behind the symphysis menti of the mandible.
5. F. The vestibular folds of the larynx are fixed and reddish and the vocal folds are mobile and whitish.
6. B. The genioglossus muscle is supplied by the hypoglossal nerve.
7. C. The spinal part of the accessory nerve lies superficial to the levator scapulae muscle in the posterior triangle of the neck.
8. D. The cricothyroid muscle is innervated by the external laryngeal nerve, which was damaged in this patient.
9. B. The hematoma was located deep to the periosteum of the occipital bone.
10. F. The facial and ophthalmic veins do not possess valves so that infected blood from the face can spread to the cavernous sinus.
11. A. The facial muscles on the left side of the mouth on contraction pull the mouth upward and to the left because the muscles on the right side were paralyzed.
12. D. The motor portion of the trigeminal nerve is unaffected in patients with trigeminal neuralgia.
13. C. The secretomotor fibers to the parotid salivary gland originate in the inferior salivatory nucleus of the glossopharyngeal nerve.
14. B. The anterior branch of the middle meningeal artery may be sectioned at the site of the fracture.
15. C. The intracranial subarachnoid space extends forward around the optic nerve as far as the back of the eyeball.
16. B. The mucous membrane lining the piriform fossa is innervated by the internal laryngeal branch of the superior laryngeal nerve from the vagus.

REVIEW QUESTIONS

Completion Questions

Select the phrase that best completes each statement.

1. The levator palpebrae superioris muscle is innervated by the
   (a) facial nerve.
   (b) trochlear nerve.
   (c) trigeminal nerve.
   (d) oculomotor nerve.
   (e) abducent nerve.
2. The inferior oblique muscle of the eye is innervated by the
   (a) abducent nerve.
   (b) trigeminal nerve.
   (c) oculomotor nerve.
   (d) facial nerve.
   (e) trochlear.
3. The lateral rectus muscle of the eye is innervated by the
   (a) optic nerve.
   (b) trochlear nerve.
   (c) oculomotor nerve.
   (d) facial nerve.
   (e) abducent nerve.
4. The superior oblique muscle of the eye is innervated by the
   (a) trigeminal nerve.
   (b) trochlear nerve.
   (c) abducent nerve.
   (d) chorda tympani nerve.
   (e) oculomotor nerve.
5. The orbicularis oculi muscle is innervated by the
   (a) facial nerve.
   (b) lacrimal nerve.
   (c) maxillary nerve.
   (d) nasociliary nerve.
   (e) frontal nerve.
6. The mandibular division of the trigeminal nerve leaves the skull through the
   (a) superior orbital fissure.
   (b) foramen rotundum.
   (c) foramen ovale.
   (d) jugular foramen.
   (e) foramen magnum.
7. The vagus nerve leaves the skull through the
   (a) jugular foramen.
   (b) occipital foramen.
   (c) inferior orbital fissure.
   (d) foramen rotundum.
   (e) foramen spinosum.
8. The abducent nerve leaves the skull through the
   (a) foramen rotundum.
   (b) jugular foramen.
   (c) inferior orbital fissure.
   (d) superior orbital fissure.
   (e) foramen ovale.
9. The ophthalmic division of the trigeminal nerve leaves the skull through the
   (a) inferior orbital fissure.
   (b) foramen ovale.
   (c) foramen rotundum.
   (d) superior orbital fissure.
   (e) pterygopalatine foramen.
10. The maxillary division of the trigeminal nerve leaves the skull through the
    (a) foramen spinosum.
    (b) foramen rotundum.
    (c) superior orbital fissure.
    (d) foramen ovale.
    (e) jugular foramen.
11. The oculomotor nerve leaves the skull through the
    (a) inferior orbital fissure.
    (b) foramen rotundum.
    (c) superior orbital fissure.
    (d) foramen magnum.
    (e) foramen ovale.
12. The optic canal is an opening in the
    (a) lesser wing of the sphenoid bone.
    (b) occipital bone.
    (c) petrous part of the temporal bone.
    (d) frontal bone.
    (e) squamous part of the temporal bone.
13. The carotid canal is located in the
    (a) frontal bone.
    (b) occipital bone.
    (c) petrous part of the temporal bone.
    (d) greater wing of the sphenoid bone.
    (e) parietal bone.
14. The foramen spinosum is located in the
    (a) sphenoid bone.
    (b) occipital bone.
    (c) frontal bone.
    (d) petrous part of the temporal bone.
    (e) squamous part of the temporal bone.
15. The hypoglossal canal is located in the
    (a) squamous part of the temporal bone.
    (b) occipital bone.
    (c) frontal bone.
    (d) sphenoid bone.
    (e) parietal bone.
16. The foramen rotundum is located in the
    (a) lesser wing of the sphenoid bone.
    (b) frontal bone.
    (c) petrous part of the temporal bone.
    (d) occipital bone.
    (e) greater wing of the sphenoid bone.
17. The facial nerve canal is located in the
    (a) temporal bone.
    (b) greater wing of the sphenoid bone.
    (c) occipital bone.
    (d) mastoid process.
    (e) lacrimal bone.

18. The foramen magnum is located in the
    (a) sphenoid bone.
    (b) temporal bone.
    (c) parietal bone.
    (d) frontal bone.
    (e) occipital bone.
19. The genioglossus muscle ________ the tongue.
    (a) retracts
    (b) depresses
    (c) elevates
    (d) protrudes
    (e) changes the shape of
20. The hyoglossus muscle
    (a) changes the shape of the tongue.
    (b) elevates the tongue.
    (c) depresses the tongue.
    (d) protrudes the tongue.
    (e) retracts the tongue upward and backward.
21. The styloglossus muscle
    (a) protrudes the tongue.
    (b) depresses the tongue.
    (c) retracts the tongue upward and backward.
    (d) changes the shape of the tongue.
    (e) elevates the tongue.
22. The palatoglossus muscle
    (a) depresses the tongue.
    (b) elevates the tongue.
    (c) changes the shape of the tongue.
    (d) retracts the tongue upward and backward.
    (e) protrudes the tongue.

Multiple-Choice Questions

Select the best answer for each question.

23. The following muscles of the pharynx receive their motor innervation from the pharyngeal plexus via the cranial part of the accessory nerve except which?
    (a) Superior constrictor
    (b) Palatopharyngeus
    (c) Stylopharyngeus
    (d) Middle constrictor
    (e) Salpingopharyngeus
24. The following statements concerning the stellate ganglion are correct except which?
    (a) It is formed from a fusion of the inferior cervical ganglion with the first thoracic ganglion.
    (b) It has white and gray rami communicantes, which pass to spinal nerves.
    (c) It is located behind the vertebral artery.
    (d) It lies in the interval between the transverse process of the seventh cervical vertebra and the neck of the first rib.
    (e) The large anterior tubercle of the transverse process of the fifth cervical vertebra is an important surface landmark when performing a stellate ganglion block.
25. The following statements concerning the chorda tympani are correct except which?
    (a) It contains parasympathetic postganglionic fibers.
    (b) It contains special sensory (taste) fibers.
    (c) It joins the lingual nerve in the infratemporal fossa.
    (d) It is a branch of the facial nerve in the temporal bone.
    (e) It carries secretomotor fibers to the submandibular and sublingual salivary glands.
26. The following statements concerning the pituitary gland (hypophysis cerebri) are correct except which?
    (a) It is separated from the optic chiasma by the diaphragma sellae.
    (b) The sphenoid sinus is inferior to it.
    (c) It receives its arterial supply from the internal carotid artery.
    (d) It is suspended from the floor of the third ventricle by the pars anterior.
    (e) It is deeply placed within the sella turcica of the skull.
27. The following statements concerning the submandibular lymph nodes are correct except which?
    (a) They drain into the deep cervical lymph nodes.
    (b) They drain the tip of the tongue.
    (c) They drain the skin of the forehead.
    (d) They are situated on the superficial surface of the submandibular salivary gland.
    (e) They drain the mucous membrane lining the cheek.
28. The following statements concerning the cervical part of the esophagus are correct except which?
    (a) The sensory nerve supply is the recurrent laryngeal nerve.
    (b) The lymph drains into the deep cervical lymph nodes.
    (c) It is the site of an important portal–systemic anastomosis.
    (d) The lumen is narrowed at the junction with the pharynx.
    (e) It begins at the level of the cricoid cartilage, opposite the body of the sixth cervical vertebra.
29. The following statements concerning the parotid salivary gland are correct except which?
    (a) The facial nerve passes through it, dividing the gland into superficial and deep parts.
    (b) The secretomotor nerve supply is derived from the facial nerve.
    (c) The parotid duct pierces the buccinator muscle and opens into the mouth.
    (d) The external carotid artery divides within its substance to form the superficial temporal and maxillary arteries.
    (e) The retromandibular vein is formed within it by the union of the superficial temporal vein and the maxillary vein.
30. The following statements concerning the head and neck are correct except which?
    (a) The mastoid process of the temporal bone cannot be palpated in the newborn.
    (b) The deep cervical lymph nodes are situated in the neck along a line that extends from the midpoint between the tip of the mastoid process and the angle of the mandible down to the sternoclavicular joint.
    (c) The external jugular vein runs down the neck from the angle of the jaw to the middle of the clavicle.
    (d) The parotid duct opens into the mouth opposite the upper second molar tooth.

(e) The anterior fontanelle can be palpated in a baby between the squamous part of the temporal bone, the parietal bone, and the greater wing of the sphenoid.
(f) The roots of the brachial plexus emerge into the posterior triangle on the neck between the scalenus anterior and scalenus medius muscles.

31. The following facts concerning the tongue are correct except which?
    (a) The intrinsic muscles of the tongue are innervated by the hypoglossal nerve.
    (b) The taste buds of the vallate papillae are innervated by the glossopharyngeal nerve.
    (c) The posterior third of the tongue forms part of the anterior wall of the oral pharynx.
    (d) Lymphoid tissue is found on the anterior third of the dorsum of the tongue.
    (e) On either side of the frenulum of the tongue are situated the openings of the submandibular ducts.
32. Which of the following muscles elevates the soft palate during swallowing?
    (a) Tensor veli palatini
    (b) Palatoglossus
    (c) Palatopharyngeus
    (d) Levator veli palatini
    (e) Salpingopharyngeus
33. Which of the following muscles partially inserts on the articular disc of the temporomandibular joint?
    (a) Medial pterygoid
    (b) Anterior fibers of the temporalis
    (c) Masseter
    (d) Posterior fibers of the temporalis
    (e) Lateral pterygoid
34. Assuming that the patient's eyesight is normal, in which cranial nerve is there likely to be a lesion when the direct and consensual light reflexes are absent?
    (a) Trochlear nerve
    (b) Optic nerve
    (c) Abducent nerve
    (d) Oculomotor nerve
    (e) Trigeminal nerve
35. A patient is unable to taste a piece of sugar placed on the anterior part of the tongue. Which cranial nerve is likely to have a lesion?
    (a) Hypoglossal
    (b) Vagus
    (c) Glossopharyngeal
    (d) Facial
    (e) Maxillary division of the trigeminal
36. On asking a patient to say "ah," the uvula is seen to be drawn upward to the right. Which cranial nerve is likely to be damaged?
    (a) Left glossopharyngeal
    (b) Right hypoglossal
    (c) Left accessory (cranial part)
    (d) Right vagus
    (e) Right trigeminal
37. When testing the sensory innervation of the face, it is important to remember that the skin of the tip of the nose is supplied by which one of the following nerves?
    (a) Zygomatic branch of the facial nerve
    (b) Maxillary division of the trigeminal nerve
    (c) Ophthalmic division of the trigeminal nerve
    (d) External nasal branch of the facial nerve
    (e) Buccal branch of the mandibular division of the trigeminal nerve

Read the case histories and select the best answer to the question following them.

An 18-year-old woman went to her physician because she had noticed a swelling in the midline of her neck. She said she had first noticed this swelling 3 years previously, and it had gradually increased in size. On physical examination, a small swelling was found in the midline of the neck; it measured about 0.5 in. (1.25 cm) in diameter. It was situated just below the body of the hyoid bone, was soft and fluctuant, and moved upward on swallowing. Nothing else abnormal was discovered.

38. The physician made the diagnosis of thyroglossal cyst based on the following symptoms and signs except which?
    (a) The swelling was not hard.
    (b) The swelling was fluctuant.
    (c) The swelling was located in the midline of the neck.
    (d) It moved upward on swallowing, which indicated that it was tethered to tissue associated with the thyroid gland.
    (e) A thyroglossal cyst is always found below the hyoid bone.

A 4-week-old baby boy was examined by a pediatrician because of failure to gain weight and difficulty with feeding. The mother said that the child was breast-fed and eagerly accepted the milk when it was manually expressed from the breast, but obviously was having difficulty in sucking at the nipple. The physician carefully examined the baby and then made a diagnosis and advised appropriate treatment.

39. The following statements about this case are correct except which?
    (a) The condition is often associated with a cleft upper lip.
    (b) The baby had a median cleft palate.
    (c) The cleft in the palate involved the hard palate but not the soft palate or the uvula.
    (d) The difficulty with the feeding was that the cleft palate prevented the child from actively sucking milk from the breast.
    (e) Surgical repair of a cleft palate should be undertaken at or before 18 months.

ANSWERS TO REVIEW QUESTIONS

1. D. The smooth muscle fibers of the levator palpebrae superioris are innervated by the sympathetic nerves. The greater part of the muscle is made up of striated muscle, which receives its innervation from the oculomotor nerve. Division of the oculomotor nerve causes severe ptosis.
2. C
3. E
4. B
5. A. The orbicularis oculi muscle is a muscle of facial expression.
6. C. Both the motor and sensory divisions of the mandibular division of the trigeminal nerve leave the skull together and quickly unite beneath the foramen ovale.
7. A. The glossopharyngeal, vagus, and accessory (cranial part) nerves leave the skull through the jugular foramen; the sigmoid sinus passes through the posterior part of the same foramen to become the internal jugular vein.
8. D
9. D. The ophthalmic division of the trigeminal nerve leaves the skull through the superior orbital fissure as its three terminal branches—namely, the lacrimal, frontal, and nasociliary nerves.
10. B
11. C. The oculomotor nerve passes through the superior orbital fissure as upper and lower divisions.
12. A
13. C
14. A. The foramen spinosum is located in the greater wing of the sphenoid bone; the middle meningeal artery passes through this foramen into the middle cranial fossa from the infratemporal fossa.
15. B. The hypoglossal canal is situated above the anterolateral boundary of the foramen magnum.
16. E. The foramen rotundum transmits the maxillary division of the trigeminal nerve from the middle cranial fossa of the skull into the pterygopalatine fossa.
17. A
18. E. The foramen magnum transmits the medulla oblongata, the spinal part of the accessory nerve, and the right and left vertebral arteries.
19. D. Remember that contraction of the right genioglossus muscle (for example) points the tip of the tongue to the patient's left.
20. C
21. C
22. D
23. C
24. E. The large anterior tubercle of the transverse process of the sixth cervical vertebra is an important surface landmark when performing a stellate ganglion block.
25. A. It contains parasympathetic preganglionic fibers.
26. D. The pituitary is suspended from the floor of the third ventricle by the infundibulum.
27. B. The lymph from the tip of the tongue drains into the submental lymph nodes.
28. C. The important portal–systemic anastomosis is located in the lower third of the esophagus where it passes through the diaphragm and enters the stomach (see page 245).
29. B. The secretomotor nerve supply to the parotid salivary gland is from the inferior salivatory nucleus via the glossopharyngeal nerve.
30. E
31. D. The lymphoid tissue is found on the dorsum of the posterior third of the tongue (lingual tonsil) where it forms part of the ring of lymphoid tissue guarding the entrance into the pharynx.
32. D
33. E
34. D
35. D
36. C
37. C. The external nasal nerve is a continuation of the anterior ethmoidal branch of the nasociliary branch of the ophthalmic division of the trigeminal nerve.
38. E. A thyroglossal cyst occurs most commonly in the midline of the neck below the hyoid bone and above the isthmus of the thyroid gland. It should be emphasized that it can occur anywhere along the path of the thyroglossal tract, even as far superiorly as the foramen cecum of the tongue. As the cyst enlarges it is prone to infection so it should be removed surgically.
39. C. During development the palatal processes of the maxilla grow medially and fuse with each other and the nasal septum; the fusion of the processes takes place from anterior to posterior so that the uvula is the last part of the palate to fuse, and this occurs at about the 11th week. If the pediatrician had made a more thorough examination in a good light, he or she would have seen that the cleft in the hard palate extended all the way posteriorly to the tip of the uvula.

    Surgical repair of a cleft palate must be undertaken before the child starts to speak. In the meantime, the child should be fed with the mother's milk with a pipette or spoon, after careful manual expression. Because of the risk of aspiration pneumonia, great care must be taken to prevent the milk from pouring down the throat into the larynx.

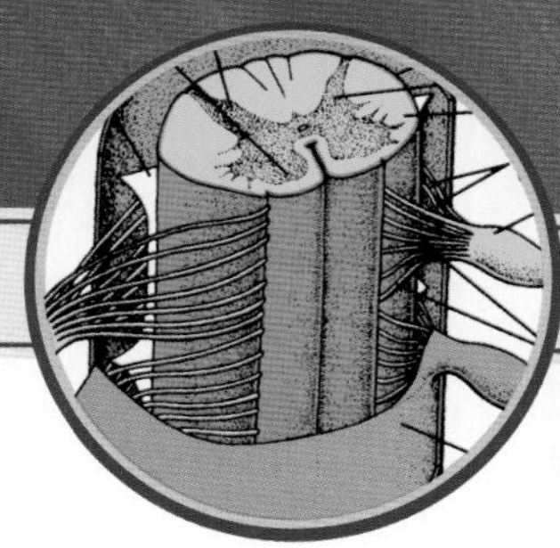

CHAPTER 12

THE BACK

A 35-year-old woman decided to help her neighbor move his car, which was stuck in a snowdrift. After much pushing, the car would not move. It was decided to make one last effort, and this time the back of the car was to be lifted by its bumper. Suddenly the woman experienced a sharp, shooting pain in the lower back. At the same time she felt a deep, sharp pain down the back of the right leg. She tried to walk but her back felt "locked," and any attempt to move intensified the pain.

On being questioned by her physician, the patient pointed to the lower back as the site of maximum pain and then ran her finger down the back of the thigh and the outer side of her right leg.

On physical examination a decrease in the range of motion of the lumbosacral region of the spine was noted. When asked to walk, she was reluctant to put her weight on the involved leg. The pain was made worse by sitting and coughing. Examination of the muscles of the legs revealed weakness in extension of the right big toe and slight weakness of the dorsiflexors of the foot. The muscle reflexes were normal in both lower limbs. Slight sensory deficit was present over the anterior part of the right leg and the dorsomedial aspect of the foot down to the big toe. Tension on the lumbar sacral nerve roots was created when the patient was in the supine position. With the pelvis stabilized, the right leg was slowly raised by the heel, with the knee extended. The patient experienced severe pain down the leg below the knee. Radiographic and computed tomography (CT) examination revealed nothing abnormal. A magnetic resonance imaging (MRI) study showed a herniated disc between the fourth and fifth lumbar vertebrae, which indicated that the nucleus pulposus was probably pressing on the fifth lumbar nerve root and would explain the symptoms and signs.

Low back pain is a common complaint in clinical practice and may be caused by a wide spectrum of diseases. The anatomy of the region is complex, and many structures have the potential to cause pain. Only by having a sound knowledge of the anatomy and the pathologic process involving the area can the physician identify the cause and start treatment.

CHAPTER OUTLINE

Basic Anatomy 852
The Vertebral Column 852
Composition of the Vertebral Column 852
General Characteristics of a Vertebra 852
Characteristics of a Typical Cervical Vertebra 855
Characteristics of a Typical Thoracic Vertebra 855
Characteristics of a Typical Lumbar Vertebra 855
Sacrum 856
Coccyx 856
Important Variations in the Vertebrae 857
Joints of the Vertebral Column 857
Nerve Supply of Vertebral Joints 860
Curves of the Vertebral Column 860
Movements of the Vertebral Column 860
Muscles of the Back 864
Deep Muscles of the Back (Postvertebral Muscles) 864
Splenius 865
Deep Fascia of the Back (Thoracolumbar Fascia) 865
Blood Supply of the Back 865
Lymph Drainage of the Back 867
Nerve Supply of the Back 867
Spinal Cord 867
Roots of the Spinal Nerves 867
Blood Supply of the Spinal Cord 870
Meninges of the Spinal Cord 871
Cerebrospinal Fluid 874
Radiographic Anatomy 876
Radiographic Appearances of the Vertebral Column 876
Spinal Subarachnoid Space 876
Computed Tomography and Magnetic Resonance Imaging Studies 876
Surface Anatomy 880
Midline Structures 880
External Occipital Protuberance 880
Cervical Vertebrae 880
Thoracic and Lumbar Vertebrae 881
Sacrum 881
Coccyx 881
Upper Lateral Part of the Thorax 881
Scapula 881
Lower Lateral Part of the Back 884
Iliac Crests 884
Spinal Cord and Subarachnoid Space 884
Symmetry of the Back 884
Clinical Problem Solving 894
Answers to Clinical Problems 896
Review Questions 896
Answers to Review Questions 898

CHAPTER OBJECTIVES

- Back injuries range from a simple muscular or ligamentous back strain to a catastrophic injury of the spinal cord or cauda equina.
- Automobile accidents, motorcycle accidents, gunshot wounds, and sports injuries are just some of the common causes of back injuries found in practice.
- Because of the anatomic configuration of this region, unprotected movement of the damaged vertebral column during initial medical care at the site of the accident can result in irreversible injury to the delicate spinal cord.
- Back pain provides the practicing physician with a challenge. The physician's task is to identify the likely source of the pain and the pathologic process causing it.
- The purpose of this chapter is to review the basic anatomy of the vertebral column and related soft nervous tissue structures so that the physician will feel reasonably confident to institute the appropriate treatment.

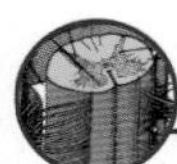

Basic Anatomy

The back, which extends from the skull to the tip of the coccyx, can be defined as the posterior surface of the trunk. Superimposed on the upper part of the posterior surface of the thorax are the scapulae and the muscles that connect the scapulae to the trunk.

The Vertebral Column

The vertebral column is the central bony pillar of the body. It supports the skull, pectoral girdle, upper limbs, and thoracic cage and, by way of the pelvic girdle, transmits body weight to the lower limbs. Within its cavity lie the spinal cord, the roots of the spinal nerves, and the covering meninges, to which the vertebral column gives great protection.

Composition of the Vertebral Column

The vertebral column (Figs. 12-1 and 12-2) is composed of 33 vertebrae—7 cervical, 12 thoracic, 5 lumbar, 5 sacral (fused to form the sacrum), and 4 coccygeal (the lower 3 are commonly fused). Because it is segmented and made up of vertebrae, joints, and pads of fibrocartilage called **intervertebral discs,** it is a flexible structure. The intervertebral discs form about one fourth the length of the column.

General Characteristics of a Vertebra

Although vertebrae show regional differences, they all possess a common pattern (Fig. 12-2).

A **typical vertebra** consists of a rounded **body** anteriorly and a **vertebral arch** posteriorly. These enclose a space called the **vertebral foramen,** through which run the spinal cord and its coverings. The vertebral arch consists

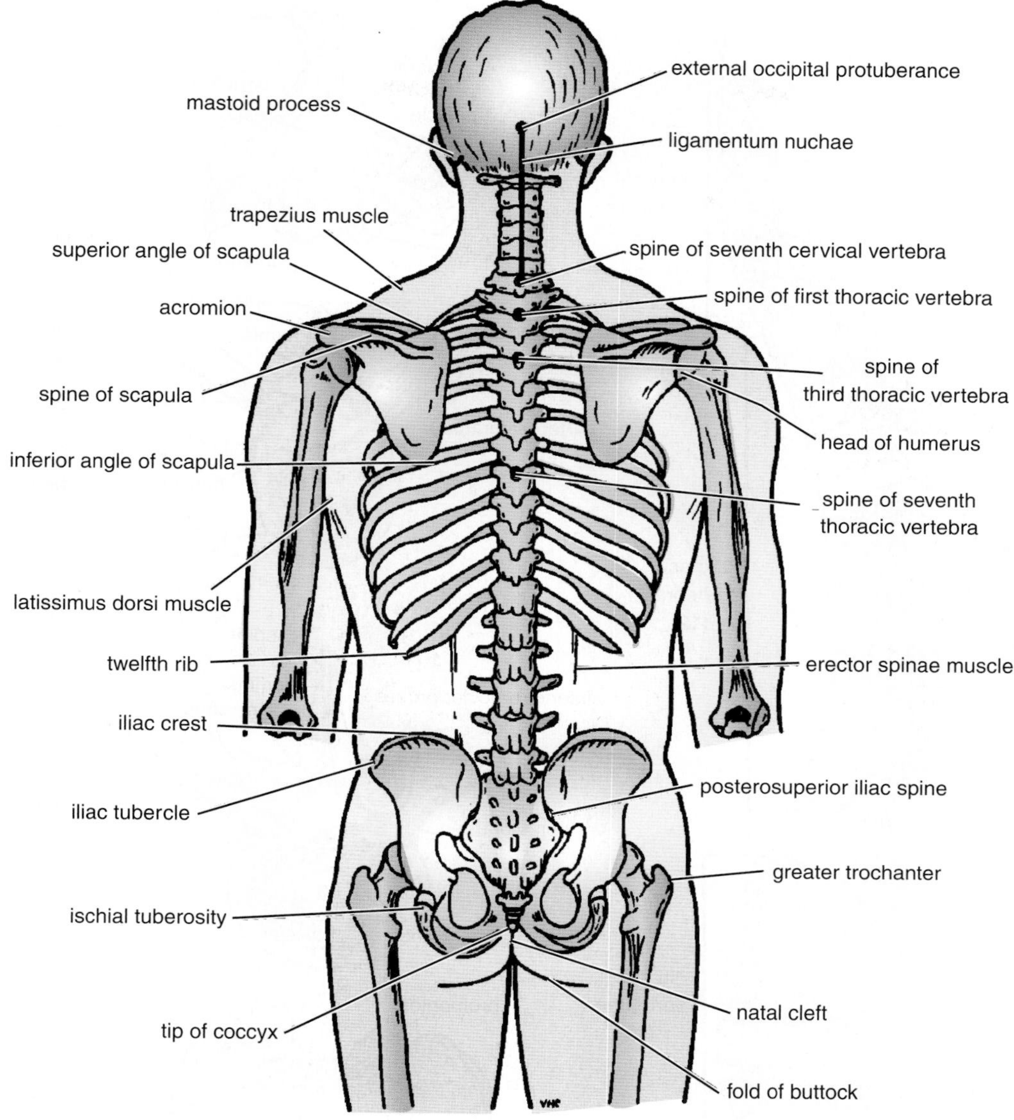

Figure 12-1 Posterior view of the skeleton showing the surface markings on the back.

of a pair of cylindrical **pedicles,** which form the sides of the arch, and a pair of flattened **laminae,** which complete the arch posteriorly.

The vertebral arch gives rise to seven processes: one spinous, two transverse, and four articular (Fig. 12-2).

The **spinous process,** or **spine,** is directed posteriorly from the junction of the two laminae. The transverse processes are directed laterally from the junction of the laminae and the pedicles. Both the spinous and transverse processes serve as levers and receive attachments of muscles and ligaments.

The **articular processes** are vertically arranged and consist of two superior and two inferior processes. They arise from the junction of the laminae and the pedicles, and their articular surfaces are covered with hyaline cartilage.

The two superior articular processes of one vertebral arch articulate with the two inferior articular processes of the arch above, forming two synovial joints.

The pedicles are notched on their upper and lower borders, forming the **superior** and **inferior vertebral notches.** On each side, the superior notch of one vertebra and the inferior notch of an adjacent vertebra together form an **intervertebral foramen.** These foramina, in an articulated skeleton, serve to transmit the spinal nerves and blood vessels. The anterior and posterior nerve roots of a spinal nerve unite within these foramina with their coverings of dura to form the segmental spinal nerves.

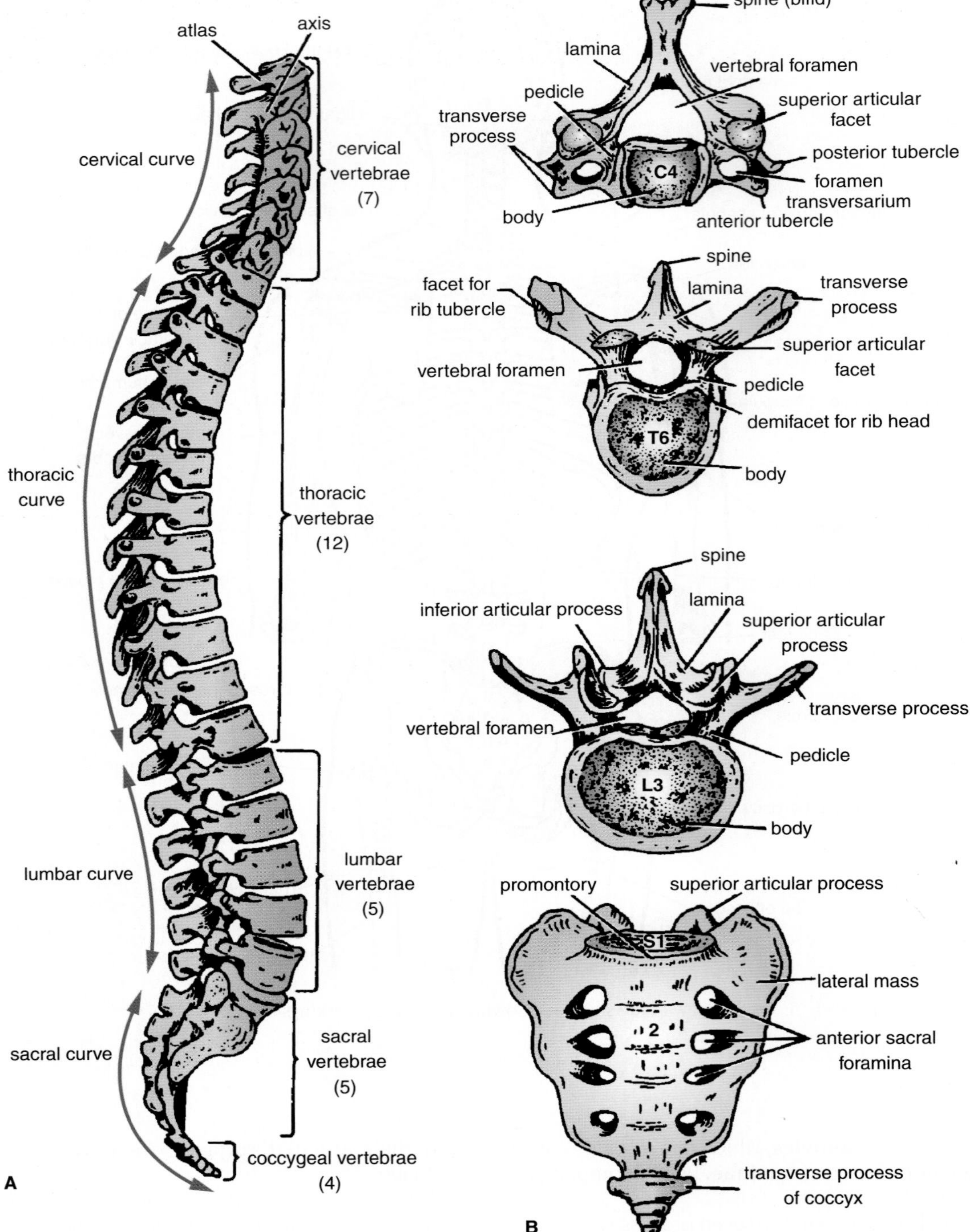

Figure 12-2 **A.** Lateral view of the vertebral column. **B.** General features of different kinds of vertebrae.

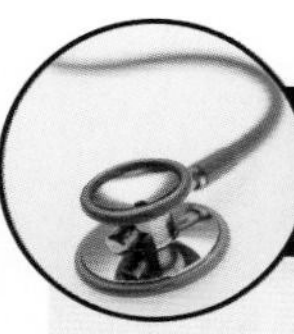

CLINICAL NOTES

Examination of the Back

It is important that the whole area of the back and legs be examined and that the shoes be removed. Unequal length of the legs or disease of the hip joints can lead to abnormal curvatures of the vertebral column. The patient should be asked to walk up and down the examination room so that the normal tilting movement of the pelvis can be observed. As one side of the pelvis is raised, a coronal lumbar convexity develops on the opposite side, with a compensatory thoracic convexity on the same side. When a person assumes the sitting position, it will be noted that the normal lumbar curvature becomes flattened, with an increase in the interval between the lumbar spines.

The normal range of movement of the different parts of the vertebral column should be tested. In the cervical region, flexion, extension, lateral rotation, and lateral flexion are possible. Remember that about half of the movement referred to as flexion is carried out at the atlanto-occipital joints. In flexion, the patient should be able to touch his or her chest with the chin, and in extension he or she should be able to look directly upward. In lateral rotation the patient should be able to place the chin nearly in line with the shoulder. Half of lateral rotation occurs between the atlas and the axis. In lateral flexion the head can normally be tilted 45° to each shoulder. It is important that the shoulder is not raised when this movement is being tested.

In the thoracic region the movements are limited by the presence of the ribs and sternum. When testing for rotation, make sure that the patient does not rotate the pelvis.

In the lumbar region, flexion, extension, lateral rotation, and lateral flexion are possible. Flexion and extension are fairly free. Lateral rotation, however, is limited by the interlocking of the articular processes. Lateral flexion in the thoracic and lumbar regions is tested by asking the patient to slide, in turn, each hand down the lateral side of the thigh.

Characteristics of a Typical Cervical Vertebra

A typical cervical vertebra has the following characteristics (Fig. 12-3):

- The transverse processes possess a **foramen transversarium** for the passage of the vertebral artery and veins (note that the vertebral artery passes through the transverse processes C1 to 6 and not through C7).
- The spines are small and bifid.
- The body is small and broad from side to side.
- The vertebral foramen is large and triangular.
- The superior articular processes have facets that face backward and upward; the inferior processes have facets that face downward and forward.

Characteristics of the Atypical Cervical Vertebrae

The first, second, and seventh cervical vertebrae are atypical.

The **first cervical vertebra,** or **atlas** (Fig. 12-3), does not possess a body or a spinous process. It has an anterior and posterior arch. It has a lateral mass on each side with articular surfaces on its upper surface for articulation with the occipital condyles **(atlanto-occipital joints)** and articular surfaces on its lower surface for articulation with the axis **(atlantoaxial joints).**

The **second cervical vertebra,** or **axis** (Fig. 12-3), has a peglike **odontoid process** that projects from the superior surface of the body (representing the body of the atlas that has fused with the body of the axis).

The **seventh cervical vertebra,** or **vertebra prominens** (Fig. 12-3), is so named because it has the longest spinous process, and the process is not bifid. The transverse process is large, but the foramen transversarium is small and transmits the vertebral vein or veins.

Characteristics of a Typical Thoracic Vertebra

A typical thoracic vertebra has the following characteristics (Fig. 12-2):

- The body is medium size and heart shaped.
- The vertebral foramen is small and circular.
- The spines are long and inclined downward.
- Costal facets are present on the sides of the bodies for articulation with the heads of the ribs.
- Costal facets are present on the transverse processes for articulation with the tubercles of the ribs (T11 and 12 have no facets on the transverse processes).
- The superior articular processes bear facets that face backward and laterally, whereas the facets on the inferior articular processes face forward and medially. The inferior articular processes of the 12th vertebra face laterally, as do those of the lumbar vertebrae.

Characteristics of a Typical Lumbar Vertebra

A typical lumbar vertebra has the following characteristics (Fig. 12-2):

- The body is large and kidney shaped.
- The pedicles are strong and directed backward.
- The laminae are thick.
- The vertebral foramina are triangular.
- The transverse processes are long and slender.
- The spinous processes are short, flat, and quadrangular and project backward.
- The articular surfaces of the superior articular processes face medially, and those of the inferior articular processes face laterally.

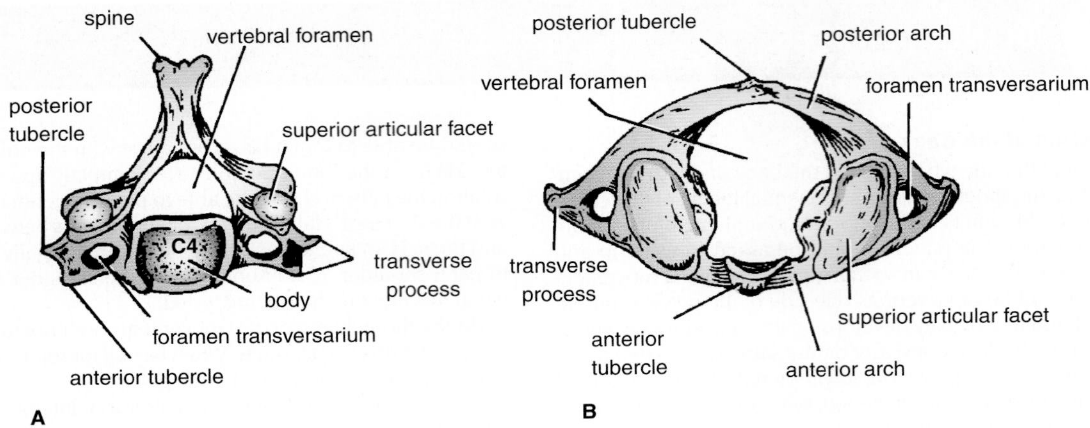

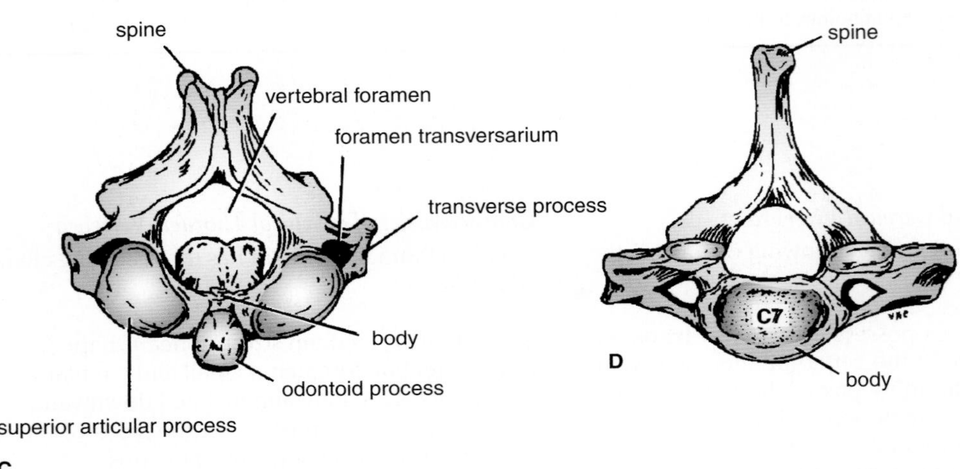

Figure 12-3 **A.** Typical cervical vertebra, superior aspect. **B.** Atlas, or first cervical vertebra, superior aspect. **C.** Axis, or second cervical vertebra, from above and behind. **D.** Seventh cervical vertebra, superior aspect; the foramen transversarium forms a passage for the vertebral vein but not for the vertebral artery.

Note that the lumbar vertebrae have no facets for articulation with ribs and no foramina in the transverse processes.

Sacrum

The sacrum (Fig. 12-2) consists of five rudimentary vertebrae fused together to form a wedge-shaped bone, which is concave anteriorly. The upper border, or base, of the bone articulates with the fifth lumbar vertebra. The narrow inferior border articulates with the coccyx. Laterally, the sacrum articulates with the two iliac bones to form the sacroiliac joints (see Fig. 6-1). The anterior and upper margin of the first sacral vertebra bulges forward as the posterior margin of the pelvic inlet and is known as the **sacral promontory.** The sacral promontory in the female is of considerable obstetric importance and is used when measuring the size of the pelvis.

The vertebral foramina are present and form the **sacral canal.** The laminae of the fifth sacral vertebra, and sometimes those of the fourth also, fail to meet in the midline, forming the **sacral hiatus** (see Fig. 6-8). The sacral canal contains the anterior and posterior roots of the sacral and coccygeal spinal nerves, the filum terminale, and fibrofatty material. It also contains the lower part of the subarachnoid space down as far as the lower border of the second sacral vertebra.

The anterior and posterior surfaces of the sacrum each have four foramina on each side for the passage of the anterior and posterior rami of the upper four sacral nerves.

Coccyx

The coccyx consists of four vertebrae fused together to form a single, small triangular bone that articulates at its base with the lower end of the sacrum (Fig. 12-2). The first coccygeal vertebra is usually not fused or is incompletely fused with the second vertebra.

Knowledge of the preceding basic anatomy of the vertebral column is important when interpreting radiographs and when noting the precise sites of bony pathologic features relative to soft tissue injury.

Important Variations in the Vertebrae

The number of cervical vertebrae is constant, but the seventh cervical vertebra may possess a **cervical rib** (see page 50). The thoracic vertebrae may be increased in number by the addition of the first lumbar vertebra, which may have a rib. The fifth lumbar vertebra may be incorporated into the sacrum; this is usually incomplete and may be limited to one side. The first sacral vertebra may remain partially or completely separate from the sacrum and resemble a sixth lumbar vertebra. A large extent of the posterior wall of the sacral canal may be absent because the laminae and spines fail to develop.

The coccyx, which usually consists of four fused vertebrae, may have three or five vertebrae. The first coccygeal vertebra may be separate. In this condition, the free vertebra usually projects downward and anteriorly from the apex of the sacrum.

Joints of the Vertebral Column

Atlanto-Occipital Joints

The atlanto-occipital joints are synovial joints that are formed between the occipital condyles, which are found on either side of the foramen magnum above and the facets on the superior surfaces of the lateral masses of the atlas below (Fig. 12-4). They are enclosed by a capsule.

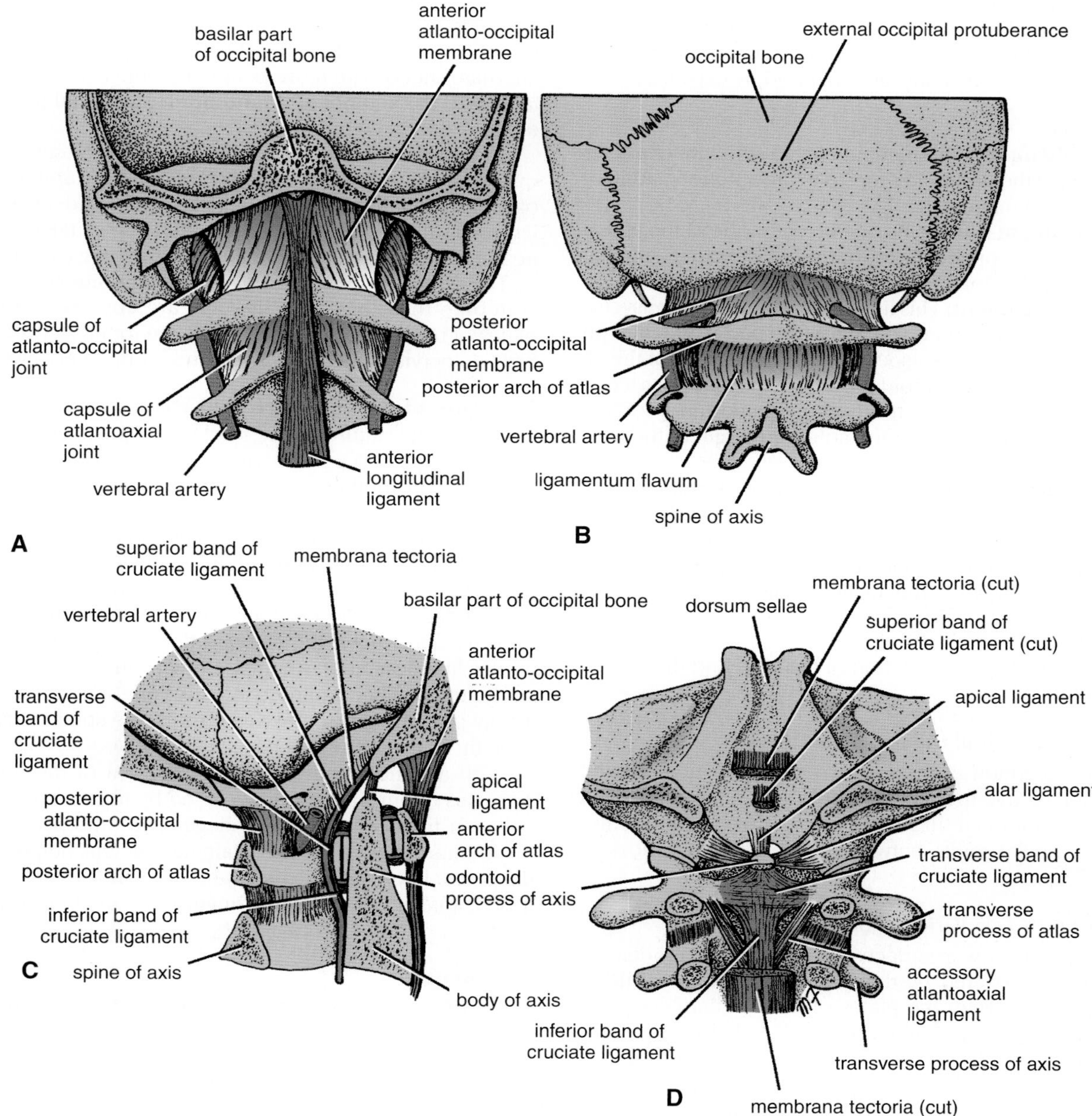

Figure 12-4 Anterior view (**A**) and posterior view (**B**) of the atlanto-occipital joints. Sagittal section (**C**) and posterior view (**D**) of the atlantoaxial joints. Note that the posterior arch of the atlas and the laminae and spine of the axis have been removed.

Ligaments

- **Anterior atlanto-occipital membrane:** This is a continuation of the anterior longitudinal ligament, which runs as a band down the anterior surface of the vertebral column. The membrane connects the anterior arch of the atlas to the anterior margin of the foramen magnum.
- **Posterior atlanto-occipital membrane:** This membrane is similar to the ligamentum flavum (see page 860) and connects the posterior arch of the atlas to the posterior margin of the foramen magnum.

Movements

Flexion, extension, and lateral flexion. No rotation is possible.

Atlantoaxial Joints

The atlantoaxial joints are three synovial joints: one is between the odontoid process and the anterior arch of the atlas, and the other two are between the lateral masses of the bones (Fig. 12-4). The joints are enclosed by capsules.

Ligaments

- **Apical ligament:** This median-placed structure connects the apex of the odontoid process to the anterior margin of the foramen magnum.
- **Alar ligaments:** These lie one on each side of the apical ligament and connect the odontoid process to the medial sides of the occipital condyles.
- **Cruciate ligament:** This ligament consists of a transverse part and a vertical part. The transverse part is attached on each side to the inner aspect of the lateral mass of the atlas and binds the odontoid process to the anterior arch of the atlas. The vertical part runs from the posterior surface of the body of the axis to the anterior margin of the foramen magnum.
- **Membrana tectoria:** This is an upward continuation of the posterior longitudinal ligament. It is attached above to the occipital bone just within the foramen magnum. It covers the posterior surface of the odontoid process and the apical, alar, and cruciate ligaments.

Movements

There can be extensive rotation of the atlas and thus of the head on the axis.

Joints of the Vertebral Column Below the Axis

With the exception of the first two cervical vertebrae, the remainder of the mobile vertebrae articulate with each other by means of cartilaginous joints between their bodies and by synovial joints between their articular processes (Fig. 12-5).

Joints Between Two Vertebral Bodies

The upper and lower surfaces of the bodies of adjacent vertebrae are covered by thin plates of hyaline cartilage. Sandwiched between the plates of hyaline cartilage is an intervertebral disc of fibrocartilage (Fig. 12-5). The collagen fibers of the disc strongly unite the bodies of the two vertebrae.

In the lower cervical region, small synovial joints are present at the sides of the intervertebral disc between the upper and lower surfaces of the bodies of the vertebrae.

Intervertebral Discs

The intervertebral discs are responsible for one fourth of the length of the vertebral column (Fig. 12-5). They are thickest in the cervical and lumbar regions, where the movements of the vertebral column are greatest. They may be regarded as semi-elastic discs, which lie between the rigid bodies of adjacent vertebrae (Fig. 12-5). Their physical characteristics permit them to serve as shock absorbers when the load on the vertebral column is suddenly increased, as when one is jumping from a height. Their elasticity allows the rigid vertebrae to move one on the other. Unfortunately, their resilience is gradually lost with advancing age.

Each disc consists of a peripheral part, the anulus fibrosus, and a central part, the nucleus pulposus (Fig. 12-5).

The **anulus fibrosus** is composed of fibrocartilage, in which the collagen fibers are arranged in concentric layers or sheets. The collagen bundles pass obliquely between adjacent vertebral bodies, and their inclination is reversed in alternate sheets. The more peripheral fibers are strongly attached to the anterior and posterior longitudinal ligaments of the vertebral column.

The **nucleus pulposus** in children and adolescents is an ovoid mass of gelatinous material containing a large amount of water, a small number of collagen fibers, and a few cartilage cells. It is normally under pressure and situated slightly nearer to the posterior than to the anterior margin of the disc.

The upper and lower surfaces of the bodies of adjacent vertebrae that abut onto the disc are covered with thin plates of hyaline cartilage. No discs are found between the first two cervical vertebrae or in the sacrum or coccyx.

Function of the Intervertebral Discs

The semifluid nature of the nucleus pulposus allows it to change shape and permits one vertebra to rock forward or backward on another, as in flexion and extension of the vertebral column.

A sudden increase in the compression load on the vertebral column causes the semifluid nucleus pulposus to become flattened. The outward thrust of the nucleus is accommodated by the resilience of the surrounding anulus fibrosus. Sometimes, the outward thrust is too great for the anulus fibrosus and it ruptures, allowing the nucleus pulposus to herniate and protrude into the vertebral canal, where it may press on the spinal nerve roots, the spinal nerve, or even the spinal cord (see page 867).

With advancing age, the water content of the nucleus pulposus diminishes and is replaced by fibrocartilage. The collagen fibers of the anulus degenerate and, as a result, the anulus cannot always contain the nucleus pulposus under stress. In old age the discs are thin and less elastic, and it is no longer possible to distinguish the nucleus from the anulus.

Ligaments

The **anterior** and **posterior longitudinal ligaments** run as continuous bands down the anterior and posterior surfaces of the vertebral column from the skull to the sacrum (Figs. 12-5 and 12-14). The anterior ligament is wide and is strongly attached to the front and sides of the vertebral bodies and to the intervertebral discs. The posterior ligament is weak and narrow and is attached to the posterior borders of

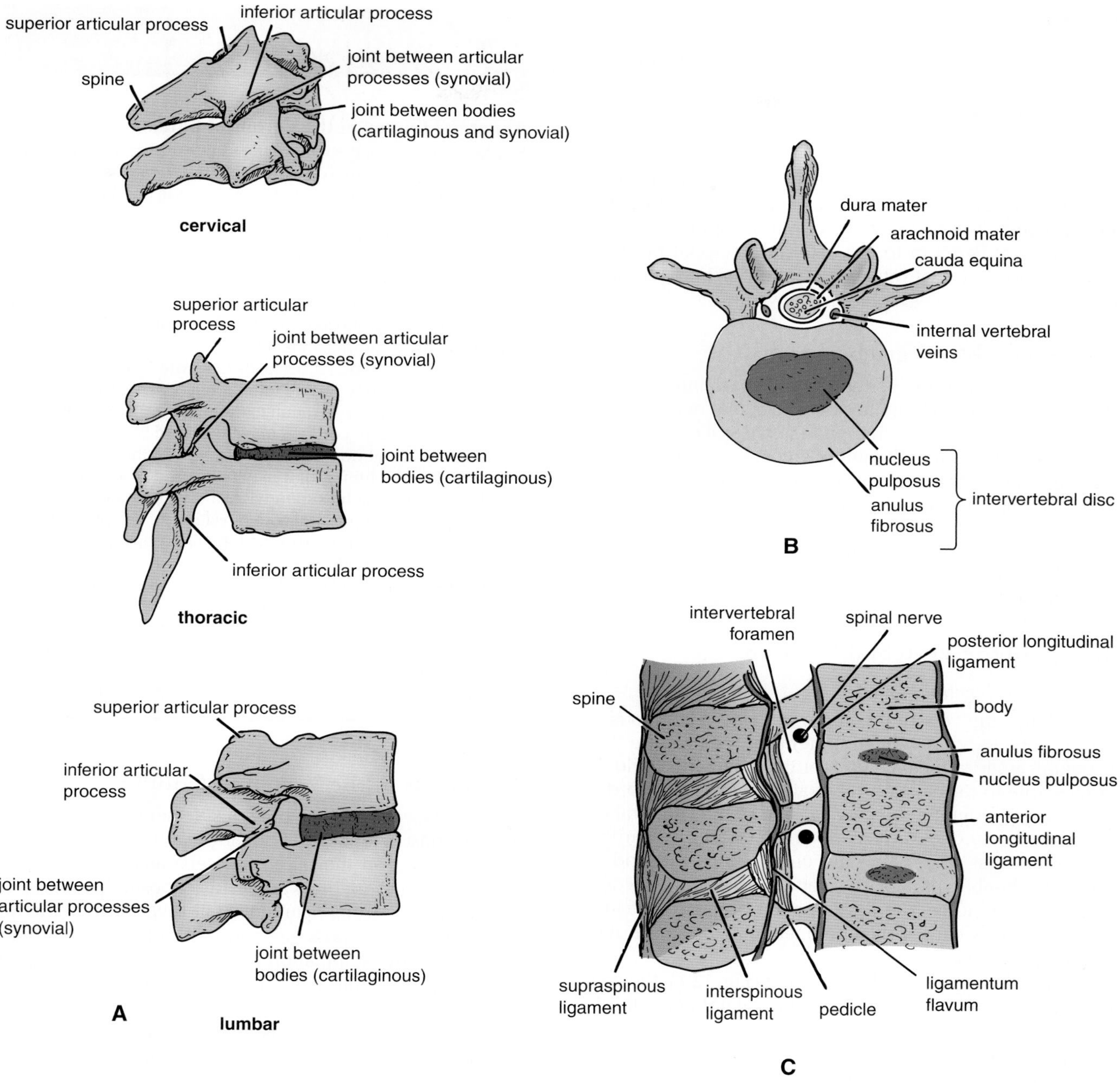

Figure 12-5 **A.** Joints in the cervical, thoracic, and lumbar regions of the vertebral column. **B.** Third lumbar vertebra seen from above showing the relationship between intervertebral disc and cauda equina. **C.** Sagittal section through three lumbar vertebrae showing ligaments and intervertebral discs. Note the relationship between the emerging spinal nerve in an intervertebral foramen and the intervertebral disc.

the discs. These ligaments hold the vertebrae firmly together but at the same time permit a small amount of movement to take place between them.

Joints Between Two Vertebral Arches

The joints between two vertebral arches consist of synovial joints between the superior and inferior articular processes of adjacent vertebrae (Fig. 12-5). The articular facets are covered with hyaline cartilage, and the joints are surrounded by a capsular ligament.

Ligaments

- **Supraspinous ligament** (Fig. 12-5): This runs between the tips of adjacent spines.

- **Interspinous ligament** (Fig. 12-5): This connects adjacent spines.
- **Intertransverse ligaments:** These run between adjacent transverse processes.
- **Ligamentum flavum** (Fig. 12-5): This connects the laminae of adjacent vertebrae.

In the cervical region, the supraspinous and interspinous ligaments are greatly thickened to form the strong **ligamentum nuchae.** The latter extends from the spine of the seventh cervical vertebra to the external occipital protuberance of the skull, with its anterior border being strongly attached to the cervical spines in between.

Nerve Supply of Vertebral Joints

The joints between the vertebral bodies are innervated by the small meningeal branches of each spinal nerve (Fig. 12-6). The nerve arises from the spinal nerve as it exits from the intervertebral foramen. It then re-enters the vertebral canal through the intervertebral foramen and supplies the meninges, ligaments, and intervertebral discs. The joints between the articular processes are innervated by branches from the posterior rami of the spinal nerves (Fig. 12-6). It should be noted that the joints of any particular level receive nerve fibers from two adjacent spinal nerves.

Curves of the Vertebral Column

Curves in the Sagittal Plane

In the fetus, the vertebral column has one continuous anterior concavity. As development proceeds, the lumbosacral angle appears. After birth, when the child becomes able to raise his or her head and keep it poised on the vertebral column, the cervical part of the vertebral column becomes concave posteriorly (Fig. 12-7). Toward the end of the first year, when the child begins to stand upright, the lumbar part of the vertebral column becomes concave posteriorly. The development of these secondary curves is largely caused by modification in the shape of the intervertebral discs.

In the adult in the standing position (Fig. 12-7), the vertebral column therefore exhibits in the sagittal plane the following regional curves: cervical, posterior concavity; thoracic, posterior convexity; lumbar, posterior concavity; and sacral, posterior convexity. During the later months of pregnancy, with the increase in size and weight of the fetus, women tend to increase the posterior lumbar concavity in an attempt to preserve their center of gravity. In old age, the intervertebral discs atrophy, resulting in a loss of height and a gradual return of the vertebral column to a continuous anterior concavity.

Curves in the Coronal Plane

In late childhood, it is common to find the development of minor lateral curves in the thoracic region of the vertebral column. This is normal and is usually caused by the predominant use of one of the upper limbs. For example, right-handed persons will often have a slight right-sided thoracic convexity. Slight compensatory curves are always present above and below such a curvature.

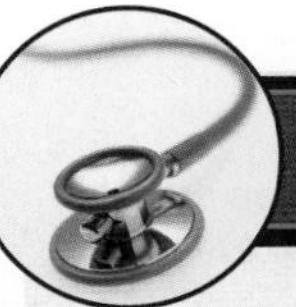

CLINICAL NOTES

Abnormal Curves of the Vertebral Column

Kyphosis is an exaggeration in the sagittal curvature present in the thoracic part of the vertebral column. It can be caused by muscular weakness or by structural changes in the vertebral bodies or by intervertebral discs. In sickly adolescents, for example, where the muscle tone is poor, long hours of study or work over a low desk can lead to a gently curved kyphosis of the upper thoracic region. The person is said to be "round-shouldered." Crush fractures or tuberculous destruction of the vertebral bodies leads to acute angular kyphosis of the vertebral column. In the aged, **osteoporosis** (abnormal rarefaction of bone) and/or degeneration of the intervertebral discs leads to **senile kyphosis,** involving the cervical, thoracic, and lumbar regions of the column.

Lordosis is an exaggeration in the sagittal curvature present in the lumbar region. Lordosis may be caused by an increase in the weight of the abdominal contents, as with the gravid uterus or a large ovarian tumor, or it may be caused by disease of the vertebral column such as spondylolisthesis (see page 862). The possibility that it is a postural compensation for a kyphosis in the thoracic region or a disease of the hip joint (congenital dislocation) must not be overlooked.

Scoliosis is a lateral deviation of the vertebral column. This is most commonly found in the thoracic region and may be caused by muscular or vertebral defects. Paralysis of muscles caused by poliomyelitis can cause severe scoliosis. The presence of a congenital hemivertebra can cause scoliosis. Often scoliosis is compensatory and may be caused by a short leg or hip disease.

Movements of the Vertebral Column

As has been seen in the previous sections, the vertebral column consists of several separate vertebrae accurately positioned one on the other and separated by intervertebral discs. The vertebrae are held in position relative to one another by strong ligaments that severely limit the degree of movement possible between adjacent vertebrae. Nevertheless, the summation of all these movements gives the vertebral column as a whole a remarkable degree of mobility.

The following movements are possible: flexion, extension, lateral flexion, rotation, and circumduction.

- **Flexion** is a forward movement, and **extension** is a backward movement. Both are extensive in the cervical and lumbar regions but restricted in the thoracic region.
- **Lateral flexion** is the bending of the body to one or the other side. It is extensive in the cervical and lumbar regions but restricted in the thoracic region.
- **Rotation** is a twisting of the vertebral column. This is least extensive in the lumbar region.
- **Circumduction** is a combination of all these movements.

The type and range of movements possible in each region of the column largely depend on the thickness of the intervertebral discs and the shape and direction of the articular processes. In the thoracic region, the ribs, the costal cartilages, and the sternum severely restrict the range of movement.

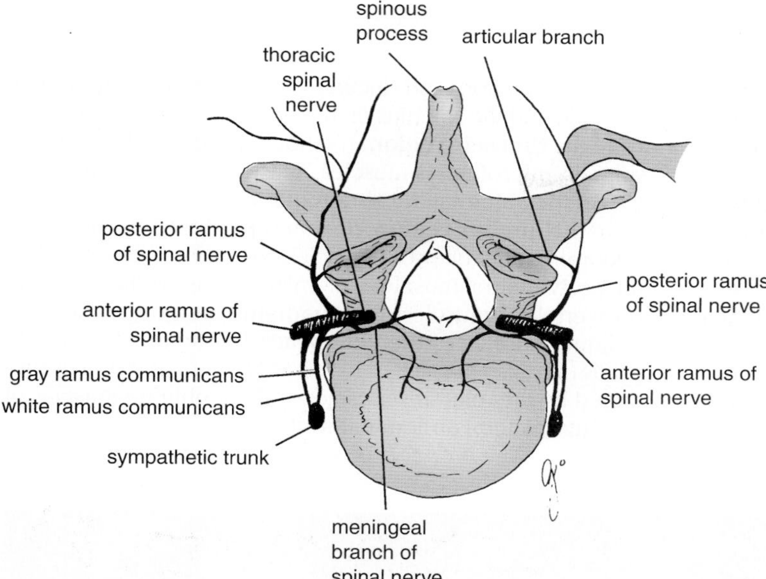

Figure 12-6 The innervation of vertebral joints. At any particular vertebral level, the joints receive nerve fibers from two adjacent spinal nerves.

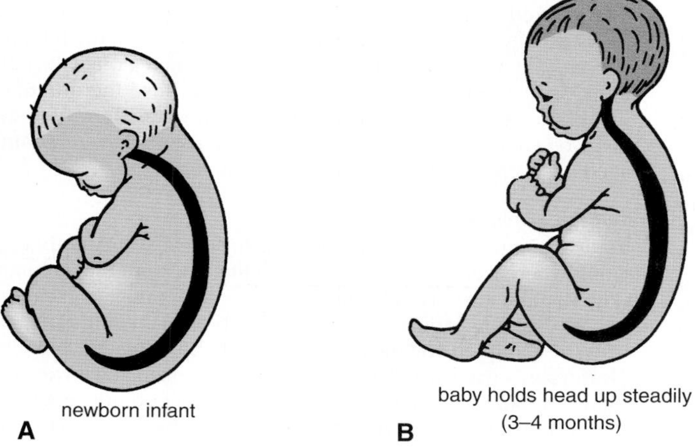

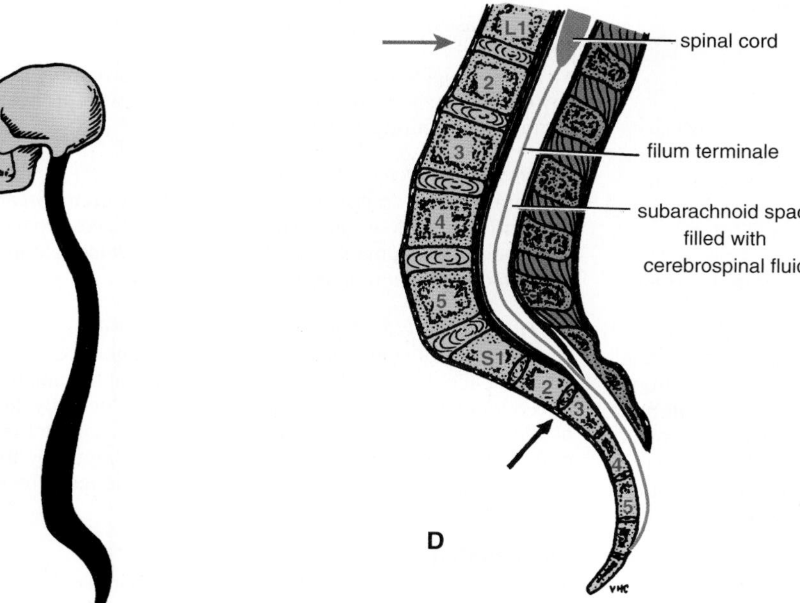

Figure 12-7 **A–C.** Curves of the vertebral column at different ages. **D.** In the adult, the lower end of the spinal cord lies at the level of the lower border of the body of the first lumbar vertebra (*top arrow*), and the subarachnoid space ends at the lower border of the body of the second sacral vertebra (*bottom arrow*).

The **atlanto-occipital joints** permit extensive flexion and extension of the head. The **atlantoaxial joints** allow a wide range of rotation of the atlas and thus of the head on the axis.

The vertebral column is moved by numerous muscles, many of which are attached directly to the vertebrae, whereas others, such as the sternocleidomastoid and the abdominal wall muscles, are attached to the skull or to the ribs or fasciae.

In the **cervical region,** flexion is produced by the longus cervicis, scalenus anterior, and sternocleidomastoid muscles. Extension is produced by the postvertebral muscles (see page 864). Lateral flexion is produced by the scalenus anterior and medius and the trapezius and sternocleidomastoid muscles. Rotation is produced by the sternocleidomastoid on one side and the splenius on the other side.

In the **thoracic region,** rotation is produced by the semispinalis and rotatores muscles, assisted by the oblique muscles of the anterolateral abdominal wall.

In the **lumbar region,** flexion is produced by the rectus abdominis and the psoas muscles. Extension is produced by the postvertebral muscles. Lateral flexion is produced by the postvertebral muscles, the quadratus lumborum, and the oblique muscles of the anterolateral abdominal wall. The psoas may also play a part in this movement. Rotation is produced by the rotatores muscles and the oblique muscles of the anterolateral abdominal wall.

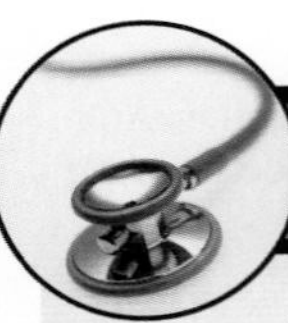

CLINICAL NOTES

Dislocations of the Vertebral Column

Dislocations without fracture occur only in the cervical region because the inclination of the articular processes of the cervical vertebrae permits dislocation to take place without fracture of the processes. In the thoracic and lumbar regions, dislocations can occur only if the vertically placed articular processes are fractured.

Dislocations commonly occur between the fourth and fifth or fifth and sixth cervical vertebrae, where mobility is greatest. In unilateral dislocations the inferior articular process of one vertebra is forced forward over the anterior margin of the superior articular process of the vertebra below. Because the articular processes normally overlap, they become locked in the dislocated position. The spinal nerve on the same side is usually nipped in the intervertebral foramen, producing severe pain. Fortunately, the large size of the vertebral canal allows the spinal cord to escape damage in most cases.

Bilateral cervical dislocations are almost always associated with severe injury to the spinal cord. Death occurs immediately if the upper cervical vertebrae are involved because the respiratory muscles, including the diaphragm (phrenic nerves C3 to 5), are paralyzed.

Fractures of the Vertebral Column

Fractures of the Spinous Processes, Transverse Processes, or Laminae

Fractures of the spinous processes, transverse processes, or laminae are caused by direct injury or, in rare cases, by severe muscular activity.

Anterior and Lateral Compression Fractures

Anterior compression fractures of the vertebral bodies are usually caused by an excessive flexion compression type of injury and take place at the sites of maximum mobility or at the junction of the mobile and fixed regions of the column. It is interesting to note that the body of a vertebra in such a fracture is crushed, whereas the strong posterior longitudinal ligament remains intact. The vertebral arches remain unbroken and the intervertebral ligaments remain intact so that vertebral displacement and spinal cord injury do not occur. When injury causes excessive lateral flexion in addition to excessive flexion, the lateral part of the body is also crushed.

Fracture Dislocations

Fracture dislocations are usually caused by a combination of a flexion and rotation type of injury; the upper vertebra is excessively flexed and twisted on the lower vertebra. Here again, the site is usually where maximum mobility occurs, as in the lumbar region, or at the junction of the mobile and fixed region of the column, as in the lower lumbar vertebrae. Because the articular processes are fractured and the ligaments are torn, the vertebrae involved are unstable, and the spinal cord is usually severely damaged or severed, with accompanying paraplegia.

Vertical Compression Fractures

Vertical compression fractures occur in the cervical and lumbar regions, where it is possible to fully straighten the vertebral column (Fig. 12-8). In the cervical region, with the neck straight, an excessive vertical force applied from above will cause the ring of the atlas to be disrupted and the lateral masses to be displaced laterally **(Jefferson's fracture).** If the neck is slightly flexed, the lower cervical vertebrae remain in a straight line and the compression load is transmitted to the lower vertebrae, causing disruption of the intervertebral disc and breakup of the vertebral body. Pieces of the vertebral body are commonly forced back into the spinal cord.

It is possible for nontraumatic compression fractures to occur in severe cases of osteoporosis and for pathologic fractures to take place.

In the straightened lumbar region, an excessive force from below can cause the vertebral body to break up, with protrusion of fragments posteriorly into the spinal canal.

Fractures of the Odontoid Process of the Axis

Fractures of the odontoid process are relatively common and result from falls or blows on the head (Fig. 12-8). Excessive mobility of the odontoid fragment or rupture of the transverse ligament can result in compression injury to the spinal cord.

Fracture of the Pedicles of the Axis (Hangman's Fracture)

Severe extension injury of the neck, such as might occur in an automobile accident or a fall, is the usual cause of hangman's fracture. Sudden overextension of the neck, as produced by the knot of a hangman's rope beneath the chin, is the reason for the common name. Because the vertebral canal is enlarged by the forward displacement of the vertebral body of the axis, the spinal cord is rarely compressed (Fig. 12-8).

Spondylolisthesis

In spondylolisthesis, the body of a lower lumbar vertebra, usually the fifth, moves forward on the body of the vertebra below and

(continues)

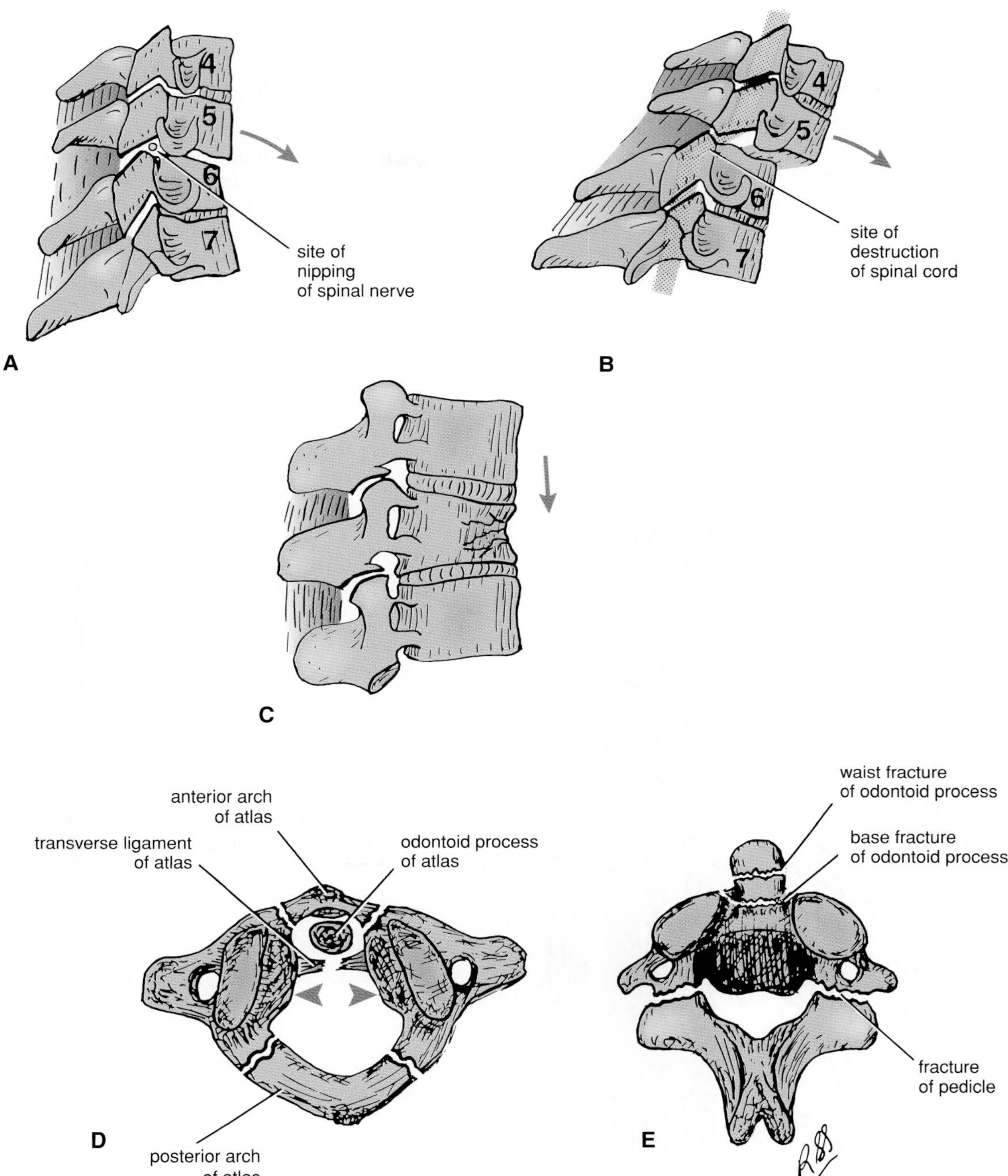

Figure 12-8 Dislocations and fractures of the vertebral column. **A.** Unilateral dislocation of the fifth or the sixth cervical vertebra. Note the forward displacement of the inferior articular process over the superior articular process of the vertebra below. **B.** Bilateral dislocation of the fifth or the sixth cervical vertebra. Note that 50% of the vertebral body width has moved forward on the vertebra below. **C.** Flexion compression–type fracture of the vertebral body in the lumbar region. **D.** Jefferson's-type fracture of the atlas. **E.** Fractures of the odontoid process and the pedicles (hangman's fracture) of the axis.

Clinical Notes, *continued*

carries with it the whole of the upper portion of the vertebral column. The essential defect is in the pedicles of the migrating vertebra. It is now generally believed that, in this condition, the pedicles are abnormally formed and accessory centers of ossification are present and fail to unite. The spine, laminae, and inferior articular processes remain in position, whereas the remainder of the vertebra, having lost the restraining influence of the inferior articular processes, slips forward. Because the laminae are left behind, the vertebral canal is not narrowed, but the nerve roots may be pressed on, causing low backache and sciatica. In severe cases the trunk becomes shortened, and the lower ribs contact the iliac crest.

Muscles of the Back

The muscles of the back may be divided into three groups:

- The **superficial muscles** connected with the shoulder girdle. They are described in Chapter 9.
- The **intermediate muscles** involved with movements of the thoracic cage. They are described with the thorax in Chapter 2.
- The **deep muscles** or **postvertebral muscles** belonging to the vertebral column

Deep Muscles of the Back (Postvertebral Muscles)

In the standing position, the line of gravity (Fig. 12-9) passes through the odontoid process of the axis, behind the centers of the hip joints, and in front of the knee and ankle joints. It follows that when the body is in this position, the greater part of its weight falls in front of the vertebral column. It is, therefore, not surprising to find that the postvertebral muscles of the back are well developed in humans. The postural tone of these muscles is the major

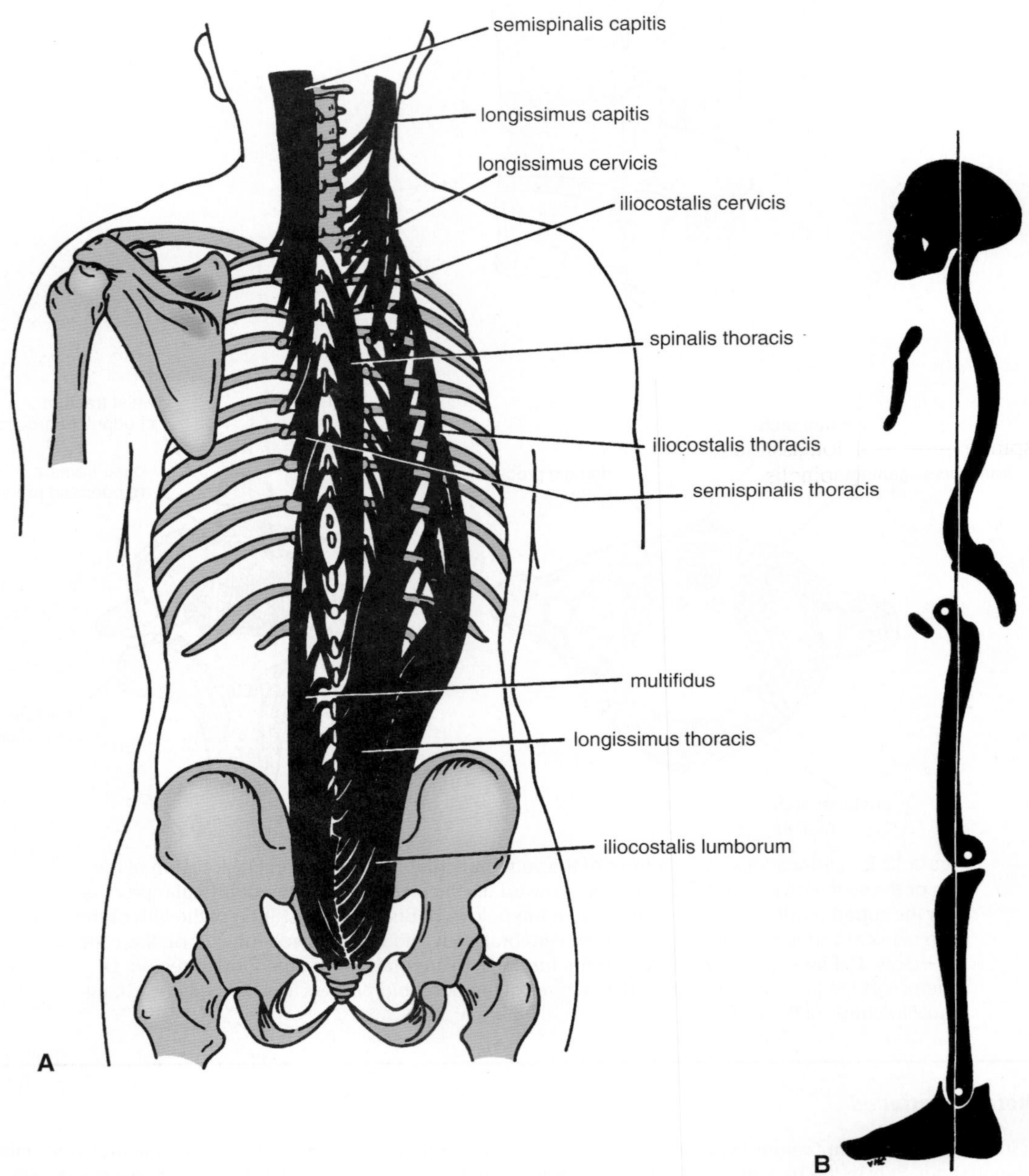

Figure 12-9 **A.** Arrangement of the deep muscles of the back. **B.** Lateral view of the skeleton showing the line of gravity. Because the greater part of the body weight lies anterior to the vertebral column, the deep muscles of the back are important in maintaining the normal postural curves of the vertebral column in the standing position.

factor responsible for the maintenance of the normal curves of the vertebral column.

The deep muscles of the back form a broad, thick column of muscle tissue, which occupies the hollow on each side of the spinous processes of the vertebral column (Fig. 12-9). They extend from the sacrum to the skull. It must be realized that this complicated muscle mass is composed of many separate muscles of varying length. Each individual muscle may be regarded as a string, which, when pulled on, causes one or several vertebrae to be extended or rotated on the vertebra below. Because the origins and insertions of the different groups of muscles overlap, entire regions of the vertebral column can be made to move smoothly.

The spines and transverse processes of the vertebrae serve as levers that facilitate the muscle actions. The muscles of longest length lie superficially and run vertically from the sacrum to the rib angles, the transverse processes, and the upper vertebral spines (Fig. 12-9). The muscles of intermediate length run obliquely from the transverse processes to the spines. The shortest and deepest muscle fibers run between the spines and between the transverse processes of adjacent vertebrae.

The deep muscles of the back may be classified as follows:

Superficial Vertically Running Muscles

- Erector spinae — iliocostalis, longissimus, spinalis

Intermediate Oblique Running Muscles

- Transversospinalis — semispinalis, multifidus, rotatores

Deepest Muscles

- Interspinales
- Intertransversarii

Knowledge of the detailed attachments of the various muscles of the back has no practical value to a clinical professional, and the attachments are therefore omitted in this text.

Splenius

The splenius is a detached part of the deep muscles of the back. It consists of two parts. The **splenius capitis** arises from the lower part of the ligamentum nuchae and the upper four thoracic spines and is inserted into the superior nuchal line of the occipital bone and the mastoid process of the temporal bone.

The **splenius cervicis** has a similar origin but is inserted into the transverse processes of the upper cervical vertebrae.

Nerve Supply

All the deep muscles of the back are innervated by the posterior rami of the spinal nerves.

Muscular Triangles of the Back

Auscultatory Triangle

The auscultatory triangle is the site on the back where breath sounds may be most easily heard with a stethoscope. The boundaries are the latissimus dorsi, the trapezius, and the medial border of the scapula.

Lumbar Triangle

The lumbar triangle is the site where pus may emerge from the abdominal wall. The boundaries are the latissimus dorsi, the posterior border of the external oblique muscle of the abdomen, and the iliac crest.

Deep Fascia of the Back (Thoracolumbar Fascia)

The lumbar part of the deep fascia is situated in the interval between the iliac crest and the 12th rib. It forms a strong aponeurosis and laterally gives origin to the middle fibers of the transversus and the upper fibers of the internal oblique muscles of the abdominal wall (see page 152).

Medially, the lumbar part of the deep fascia splits into three lamellae. The posterior lamella covers the deep muscles of the back and is attached to the lumbar spines. The middle lamella passes medially, to be attached to the tips of the transverse processes of the lumbar vertebrae; it lies in front of the deep muscles of the back and behind the quadratus lumborum. The anterior lamella passes medially and is attached to the anterior surface of the transverse processes of the lumbar vertebrae; it lies in front of the quadratus lumborum muscle.

Blood Supply of the Back

Arteries

- In the **cervical region,** branches arise from the occipital artery, a branch of the external carotid; from the vertebral artery, a branch of the subclavian; and from the deep cervical artery, a branch of the costocervical trunk.
- In the **thoracic region** branches arise from the posterior intercostal arteries.
- In the **lumbar region** branches arise from the subcostal and lumbar arteries.
- In the **sacral region** branches arise from the iliolumbar and lateral sacral arteries, branches of the internal iliac artery.

Veins

The veins draining the structures of the back form plexuses extending along the vertebral column from the skull to the coccyx.

- The **external vertebral venous plexus** lies external and surrounds the vertebral column.
- The **internal vertebral venous plexus** lies within the vertebral canal but outside the dura mater of the spinal cord (Fig. 12-10).

The external and internal vertebral plexuses form a capacious venous network whose walls are thin and whose channels have incompetent valves or are valveless. They communicate through the foramen magnum with the venous sinuses within the skull. Free venous blood flow may therefore take place between the skull, the neck, the thorax,

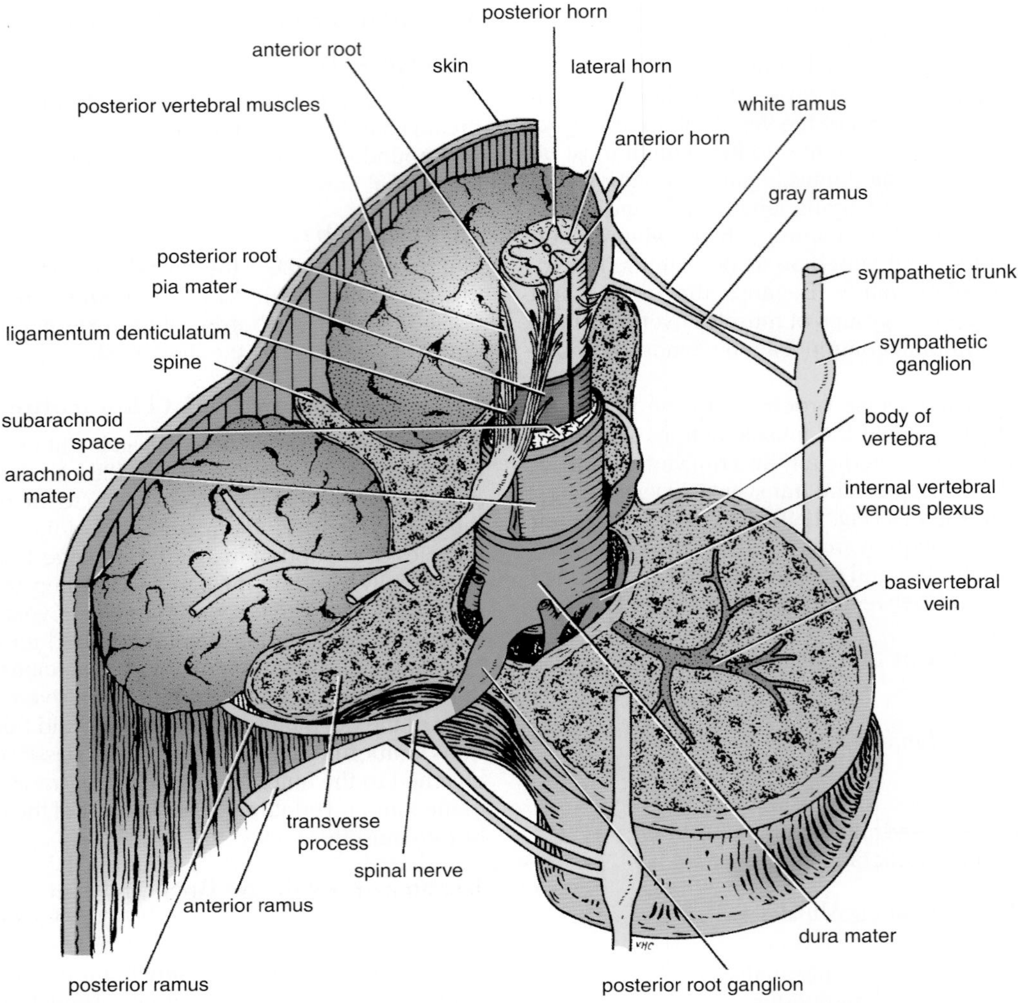

Figure 12-10 Oblique section through the first lumbar vertebra showing the spinal cord and its covering membranes. Note the relationship between the spinal nerve and sympathetic trunk on each side. Note also the important internal vertebral venous plexus.

the abdomen, the pelvis, and the vertebral plexuses, with the direction of flow depending on the pressure differences that exist at any given time between the regions. This fact is of considerable clinical significance.

The internal vertebral plexus receives tributaries from the vertebrae by way of the **basivertebral veins** (Fig. 12-10) and from the meninges and spinal cord. The internal plexus is drained by the **intervertebral veins,** which pass outward with the spinal nerves through the intervertebral foramina. Here, they are joined by tributaries from the external vertebral plexus and in turn drain into the vertebral, intercostal, lumbar, and lateral sacral veins.

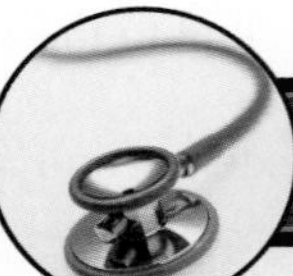

CLINICAL NOTES

Vertebral Venous Plexus and Carcinoma of the Prostate

Because the longitudinal, thin-walled, valveless vertebral venous plexus communicates above with the intracranial venous sinuses and segmentally with the veins of the thorax, abdomen, and pelvis, it is a clinically important structure. Pelvic venous blood enters not only the inferior vena cava, but also the vertebral venous plexus and by this route may also enter the skull. This is especially likely to occur if the intra-abdominal pressure is increased. The internal vertebral venous plexus is not subject to external pressures when the intra-abdominal pressure rises. A rise in pressure on the abdominal and pelvic veins would tend to force the blood backward out of the abdominal and pelvic cavities into the veins within the vertebral canal. The existence of this venous plexus explains how carcinoma of the prostate may metastasize to the vertebral column and the cranial cavity.

Lymph Drainage of the Back

The deep lymph vessels follow the veins and drain into the deep cervical, posterior mediastinal, lateral aortic, and sacral nodes. The lymph vessels from the skin of the neck drain into the cervical nodes, those from the trunk above the iliac crests drain into the axillary nodes, and those from below the level of the iliac crests drain into the superficial inguinal nodes (see page 163).

Nerve Supply of the Back

The skin and muscles of the back are supplied in a segmental manner by the posterior rami of the 31 pairs of spinal nerves. The posterior rami of the first, sixth, seventh, and eighth cervical nerves and the fourth and fifth lumbar nerves supply the deep muscles of the back and do not supply the skin. The posterior ramus of the second cervical nerve (the **greater occipital nerve)** ascends over the back of the head and supplies the skin of the scalp.

The posterior rami run downward and laterally and supply a band of skin at a lower level than the intervertebral foramen from which they emerge. Considerable overlap of skin areas supplied occurs so that section of a single nerve causes diminished, but not total, loss of sensation. Each posterior ramus divides into a medial and a lateral branch. For dermatomes of the back, see Figure 1-25.

Spinal Cord

The spinal cord is a cylindrical, grayish white structure that begins above at the foramen magnum, where it is continuous with the medulla oblongata of the brain. It terminates below in the adult at the level of the lower border of the first lumbar vertebra (Fig. 12-7). In the young child, it is relatively longer and ends at the upper border of the third lumbar vertebra. The spinal cord in the cervical region, where it gives origin to the brachial plexus, and in the lower thoracic and lumbar regions, where it gives origin to the lumbosacral plexus, has fusiform enlargements called **cervical** and **lumbar enlargements.**

Inferiorly, the spinal cord tapers off into the **conus medullaris,** from the apex of which a prolongation of the pia mater, the **filum terminale,** descends to be attached to the back of the coccyx (Figs. 12-7, 12-11, and 12-15). The cord possesses in the midline anteriorly a deep longitudinal fissure, the **anterior median fissure,** and on the posterior surface a shallow furrow, the **posterior median sulcus.**

Roots of the Spinal Nerves

Along the whole length of the spinal cord are attached 31 pairs of spinal nerves by the **anterior,** or **motor, roots** and the **posterior,** or **sensory, roots** (Figs. 12-11, 12-13, 12-14, and 12-15). Each root is attached to the cord by a series of rootlets, which extend the whole length of the corresponding segment of the cord. Each posterior nerve root possesses a posterior root ganglion, the cells of which give rise to peripheral and central nerve fibers.

The spinal nerve roots pass laterally from each spinal cord segment to the level of their respective intervertebral foramina, where they unite to form a **spinal nerve.** Here, the motor and sensory fibers become mixed so that a spinal nerve is made up of a mixture of motor and sensory fibers. Because of the disproportionate growth in length of the vertebral column during development compared to that of the spinal cord, the length of the roots increases progressively from above downward (Figs. 12-12 and 12-15). In the upper cervical region the spinal nerve roots are short and run almost horizontally, but the roots of the lumbar and sacral nerves below the level of the termination of the cord (lower border of the first lumbar vertebra in the adult) form a vertical leash of nerves around the filum terminale. The lower nerve roots together are called the **cauda equina** (Figs. 12-11 and 12-15).

After emergence from the intervertebral foramen, each spinal nerve immediately divides into a large **anterior ramus** and a smaller **posterior ramus,** which contain both motor and sensory fibers.

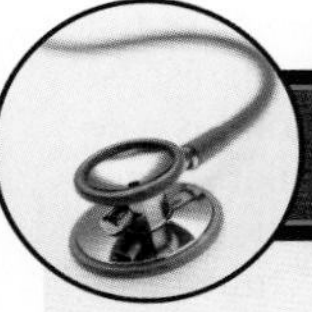

CLINICAL NOTES

Nerve Root Pain

Spinal nerve roots exit from the vertebral canal through the intervertebral foramina. Each foramen is bounded superiorly and inferiorly by the pedicles, anteriorly by the intervertebral disc and the vertebral body, and posteriorly by the articular processes and joints (Fig. 12-5). In the lumbar region, the largest foramen is between the first and second lumbar vertebrae and the smallest is between the fifth lumbar and first sacral vertebra.

One of the complications of osteoarthritis of the vertebral column is the growth of osteophytes, which commonly encroach on the intervertebral foramina, causing pain along the distribution of the segmental nerve. The fifth lumbar spinal nerve is the largest of the lumbar spinal nerves, and it exits from the vertebral column through the smallest intervertebral foramen. For this reason, it is the most vulnerable.

Osteoarthritis as a cause of root pain is suggested by the patient's age, its insidious onset, and a history of back pain of long duration; this diagnosis is made only when all other causes have been excluded. For example, a prolapsed disc usually occurs in a younger age group and often has an acute onset.

Herniated Intervertebral Discs

The structure and function of the intervertebral disc is described on page 858. The resistance of these discs to compression forces is substantial, as seen, for example, in circus acrobats who can support four or more of their colleagues on their shoulders. Nevertheless, the discs are vulnerable to sudden shocks, particularly if the vertebral column is flexed and the disc is undergoing degenerative changes that result in herniation of the nucleus pulposus.

(continues)

Clinical Notes, *continued*

The discs most commonly affected are those in areas where a mobile part of the column joins a relatively immobile part—that is, the cervicothoracic junction and the lumbosacral junction. In these areas, the posterior part of the anulus fibrosus ruptures, and the nucleus pulposus is forced posteriorly like toothpaste out of a tube. This is referred to as a **herniation of the nucleus pulposus.** This herniation can result either in a central protrusion in the midline under the posterior longitudinal ligament of the vertebrae or in a lateral protrusion at the side of the posterior ligament close to the intervertebral foramen (Fig. 12-16). The escape of the nucleus pulposus will produce narrowing of the space between the vertebral bodies, which may be visible on radiographs. Slackening of the anterior and posterior longitudinal ligaments results in abnormal mobility of the vertebral bodies, producing local pain and subsequent development of osteoarthritis.

Cervical disc herniations are less common than herniations in the lumbar region (Fig. 12-34). The discs most susceptible to this condition are those between the fifth and sixth or sixth and seventh vertebrae. Lateral protrusions cause pressure on a spinal nerve or its roots. Each spinal nerve emerges above the corresponding vertebra; thus, protrusion of the disc between the fifth and sixth cervical vertebrae can cause compression of the C6 spinal nerve or its roots (Fig. 12-16). Pain is felt near the lower part of the back of the neck and shoulder and along the area in the distribution of the spinal nerve involved. Central protrusions may press on the spinal cord and the anterior spinal artery and involve the various nerve tracts of the spinal cord.

Lumbar disc herniations are more common than cervical disc herniations (Fig. 12-16). The discs usually affected are those between the fourth and fifth lumbar vertebrae and between the fifth lumbar vertebra and the sacrum. In the lumbar region the roots of the cauda equina run posteriorly over several intervertebral discs (Fig. 12-16B). A lateral herniation may press on one or two roots and often involves the nerve root going to the intervertebral foramen just below. However, because C8 nerve roots exist and an eighth cervical vertebral body does not, the thoracic and lumbar roots **exit** below the vertebra of the corresponding number. Thus, the L5 nerve root exits between the fifth lumbar and first sacral vertebrae. Moreover, because the nerve roots move laterally as they pass toward their exit, the root corresponding to that disc space (L4 in the case of the L4 to 5 disc) is already too lateral to be pressed on by the herniated disc. Herniation of the L4 to 5 disc usually gives rise to symptoms referable to the L5 nerve roots, even though the L5 root exits between L5 and S1 vertebrae. The nucleus pulposus occasionally herniates directly backward, and if it is a large herniation, the whole cauda equina may be compressed, producing paraplegia.

An initial period of back pain is usually caused by the injury to the disc. The back muscles show spasm, especially on the side of the herniation, because of pressure on the spinal nerve root. As a consequence, the vertebral column shows a scoliosis, with its concavity on the side of the lesion. Pain is referred down the leg and foot in the distribution of the affected nerve. Since the sensory posterior roots most commonly pressed on are the fifth lumbar and the first sacral, pain is usually felt down the back and lateral side of the leg, radiating to the sole of the foot. This condition is often called **sciatica.** In severe cases paresthesia or actual sensory loss may be present.

Pressure on the anterior motor roots causes muscle weakness. Involvement of the fifth lumbar motor root produces weakness of dorsiflexion of the ankle, whereas pressure on the first sacral motor root causes weakness of plantar flexion, and the ankle jerk may be diminished or absent (Fig. 12-16).

A large, centrally placed protrusion may give rise to bilateral pain and muscle weakness in both legs. Acute retention of urine may also occur.

A correlation between the disc lesion, the nerve roots involved, the pain dermatome, the muscle weakness, and the missing or diminished reflex is shown in Table 12-1.

Disease and the Intervertebral Foramina

The intervertebral foramina (Fig. 12-5) transmit the spinal nerves and the small segmental arteries and veins, all of which are embedded in areolar tissue. Each foramen is bounded above and below by the pedicles of adjacent vertebrae, in front by the lower part of the vertebral body and by the intervertebral disc, and behind by the articular processes and the joint between them. In this situation, the spinal nerve is vulnerable and may be pressed on or irritated by disease of the surrounding structures. Herniation of the intervertebral disc, fractures of the vertebral bodies, and osteoarthritis involving the joints of the articular processes or the joints between the vertebral bodies can all result in pressure, stretching, or edema of the emerging spinal nerve. Such pressure would give rise to dermatomal pain, muscle weakness, and diminished or absent reflexes.

Narrowing of the Spinal Canal

After about the fourth decade of life the spinal canal becomes narrowed by aging. Osteoarthritic changes in the joints of the articular processes with the formation of osteophytes, together with degenerative changes in the intervertebral discs and the formation of large osteophytes between the vertebral bodies, can lead to narrowing of the spinal canal and intervertebral foramina. In persons in whom the spinal canal was originally small, significant stenosis in the cauda equina area can lead to neurologic compression. Symptoms vary from mild discomfort in the lower back to severe pain radiating down the leg with the inability to walk.

Sacroiliac Joint Disease

The sacroiliac joint is described on page 329. The clinical aspects of this joint are referred to again because disease of this joint can cause low back pain and may be confused with disease of the lumbosacral joints. Essentially, the sacroiliac joint is a synovial joint that has irregular elevations on one articular surface that fit into corresponding depressions on the other articular surface. It is a strong joint and is responsible for the transfer of weight from the vertebral column to the hip bones. The joint is innervated by the lower lumbar and sacral nerves so that disease in the joint may produce low back pain and sciatica.

The sacroiliac joint is inaccessible to clinical examination. However, a small area located just medial to and below the posterosuperior iliac spine is where the joint comes closest to the surface. In disease of the lumbosacral region, movements of the vertebral column in any direction cause pain in the lumbosacral part of the column. In sacroiliac disease, pain is extreme on rotation of the vertebral column and is worst at the end of forward flexion. The latter movement causes pain because the hamstring muscles hold the hip bones in position while the sacrum is rotating forward as the vertebral column is flexed.

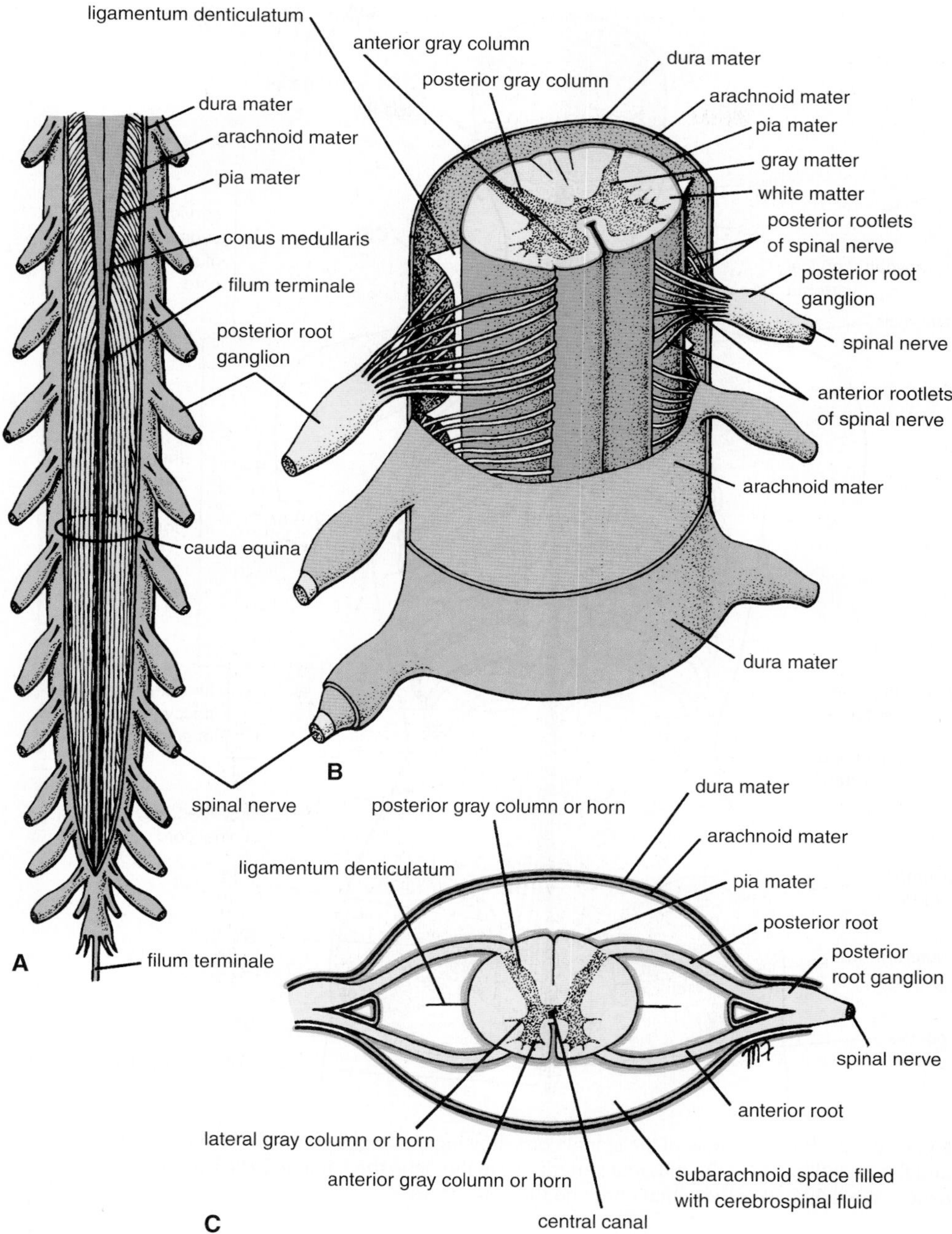

Figure 12-11 **A.** Lower end of the spinal cord and the cauda equina. **B.** Section through the thoracic part of the spinal cord showing the anterior and posterior roots of the spinal nerves and meninges. **C.** Transverse section through the spinal cord showing the meninges and the position of the cerebrospinal fluid.

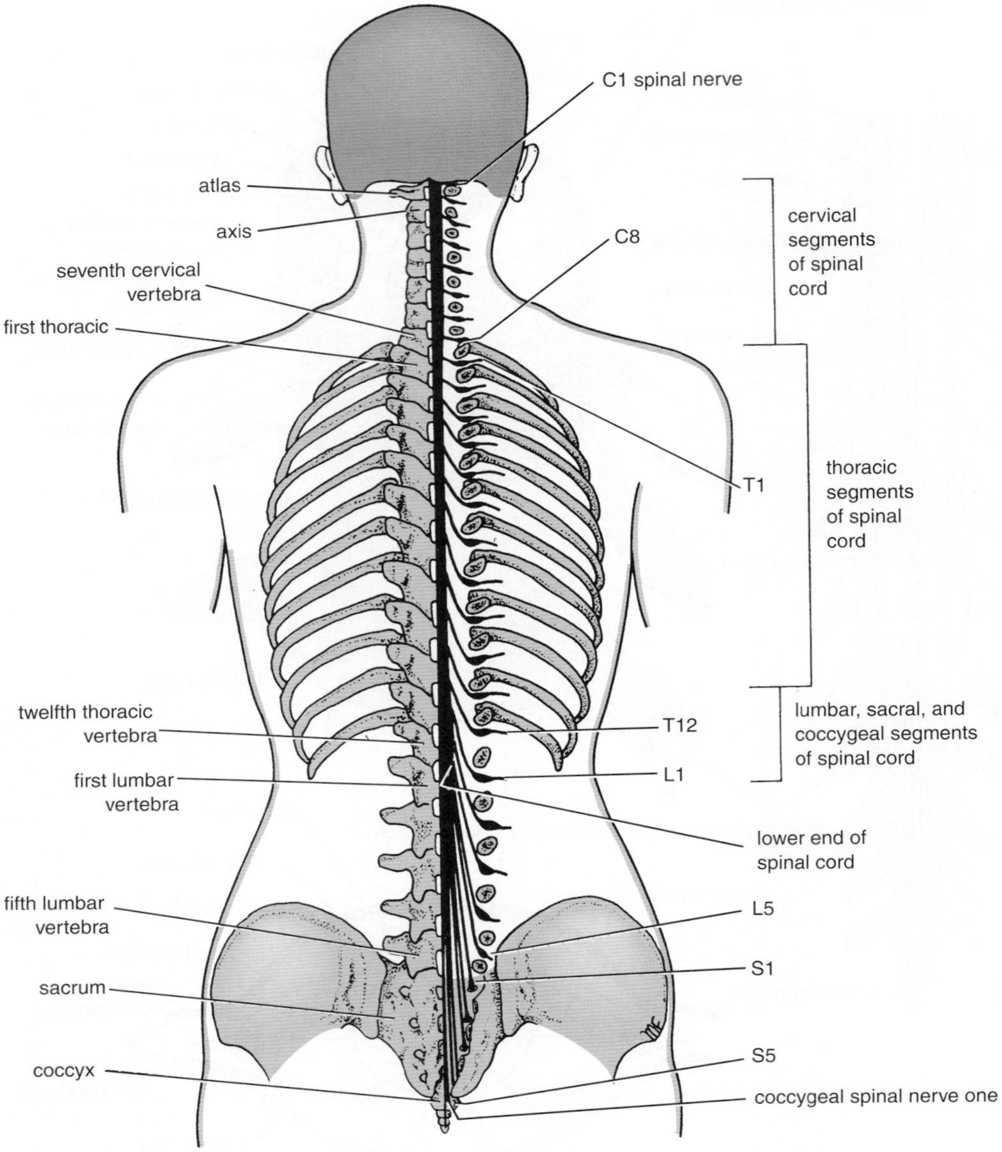

Figure 12-12 Posterior view of the spinal cord showing the origins of the roots of the spinal nerves and their relationship to the different vertebrae. On the right, the laminae have been removed to expose the right half of the spinal cord and the nerve roots.

Blood Supply of the Spinal Cord

The spinal cord receives its arterial supply from three small, longitudinally running arteries: the two posterior spinal arteries and one **anterior spinal artery.** The **posterior spinal arteries,** which arise either directly or indirectly from the vertebral arteries, run down the side of the spinal cord, close to the attachments of the posterior spinal nerve roots. The **anterior spinal arteries,** which arise from the vertebral arteries, unite to form a single artery, which runs down within the anterior median fissure.

The posterior and anterior spinal arteries are reinforced by **radicular arteries,** which enter the vertebral canal through the intervertebral foramina.

The **veins** of the spinal cord drain into the internal vertebral venous plexus.

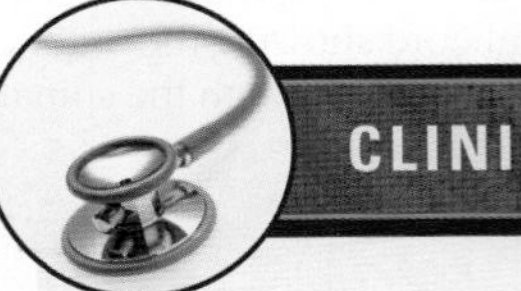

CLINICAL NOTES

Spinal Cord Ischemia

The blood supply to the spinal cord is surprisingly meager, considering the importance of this nervous tissue. The longitudinally running anterior and posterior spinal arteries are of small and variable diameter, and the reinforcing segmental arteries vary in number and in size. Ischemia of the spinal cord can easily follow minor damage to the arterial supply as a result of regional anesthesia, pain block procedures, or aortic surgery.

(continues)

Clinical Notes, *continued*

Spinal Cord Injuries

The degree of spinal cord injury at different vertebral levels is largely governed by anatomic factors. In the cervical region, dislocation or fracture dislocation is common, but the large size of the vertebral canal often results in the spinal cord escaping severe injury. However, when considerable displacement occurs, the cord is sectioned and death occurs immediately. Respiration ceases if the lesion occurs above the segmental origin of the phrenic nerves (C3, 4, and 5).

In fracture dislocations of the thoracic region, displacement is often considerable, and the small size of the vertebral canal results in severe injury to the spinal cord.

In fracture dislocations of the lumbar region, two anatomic facts aid the patient. First, the spinal cord in the adult extends only down as far as the level of the lower border of the first lumbar vertebra. Second, the large size of the vertebral foramen in this region gives the roots of the cauda equina ample room. Nerve injury may therefore be minimal in this region.

Injury to the spinal cord can produce partial or complete loss of function at the level of the lesion and partial or complete loss of function of afferent and efferent nerve tracts below the level of the lesion. The symptoms and signs of spinal shock and paraplegia in flexion and extension are beyond the scope of this book. For further information, a textbook of neurology should be consulted.

Relationships of Spinal Cord Segments to Vertebral Numbers

Because the spinal cord is shorter than the vertebral column, the spinal cord segments do not correspond numerically with the vertebrae that lie at the same level (Fig. 12-12). The following list helps determine which spinal segment is contiguous with a given vertebral body.

Vertebrae	Spinal Segment
Cervical	Add 1
Upper thoracic	Add 2
Lower thoracic (T7 to 9)	Add 3
Tenth thoracic	L1 and 2 cord segments
Eleventh thoracic	L3 and 4 cord segments
Twelfth thoracic	L5 cord segment
First lumbar	Sacral and coccygeal cord segments

Meninges of the Spinal Cord

The spinal cord, like the brain, is surrounded by three meninges: the dura mater, the arachnoid mater, and the pia mater (Figs. 12-11, 12-14, and 12-15).

Dura Mater

The dura mater is the most external membrane and is a dense, strong, fibrous sheet that encloses the spinal cord and cauda equina (Figs. 12-10, 12-11, 12-14, and 12-15). It is continuous above through the foramen magnum with the meningeal layer of dura covering the brain. Inferiorly, it ends on the filum terminale at the level of the lower border of the second sacral vertebra (Fig. 12-7). The dural sheath lies loosely in the vertebral canal and is separated from the walls of the canal by the **extradural space** (epidural space). This contains loose areolar tissue and the internal vertebral venous plexus. The dura mater extends along each nerve root and becomes continuous with connective tissue surrounding each spinal nerve **(epineurium)** at the intervertebral foramen. The inner surface of the dura mater is separated from the arachnoid mater by the potential **subdural space.**

Arachnoid Mater

The arachnoid mater is a delicate impermeable membrane covering the spinal cord and lying between the pia mater internally and the dura mater externally (Figs. 12-10 and 12-11). It is separated from the dura by the subdural space that contains a thin film of tissue fluid. The arachnoid is separated from the pia mater by a wide space, the **subarachnoid space,** which is filled with **cerebrospinal fluid** (Fig. 12-11). The arachnoid is continuous above through the foramen magnum with the arachnoid covering the brain. Inferiorly, it ends on the filum terminale at the level of the lower border of the second sacral vertebra (Figs. 12-7 and 12-15). Between the levels of the conus medullaris and the lower end of the subarachnoid space lie the nerve roots of the cauda equina bathed in cerebrospinal fluid (Figs. 12-11 and 12-15). The arachnoid mater is continued along the spinal nerve roots, forming small lateral extensions of the subarachnoid space.

Pia Mater

The pia mater is a vascular membrane that closely covers the spinal cord (Figs. 12-10 and 12-11). It is continuous above through the foramen magnum with the pia covering the brain; below it fuses with the filum terminale. The pia mater is thickened on either side between the nerve roots to form the **ligamentum denticulatum,** which passes laterally to be attached to the dura. It is by this means that the spinal cord is suspended in the middle of the dural sheath. The pia mater extends along each nerve root and becomes continuous with the connective tissue surrounding each spinal nerve (Fig. 12-11).

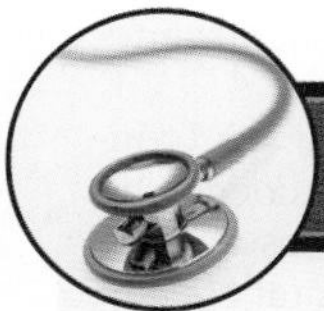

CLINICAL NOTES

Lumbar Puncture (Spinal Tap)

Lumbar puncture may be performed to withdraw a sample of cerebrospinal fluid for examination. Fortunately, the spinal cord terminates below at the level of the lower border of the first lumbar vertebra in the adult. (In the infant, it may reach as low as the third lumbar vertebra.) The subarachnoid space extends down as far as the lower border of the second sacral vertebra. The lower lumbar part of the vertebral canal is thus occupied by the subarachnoid space, which contains the cauda equina—that is, the lumbar and sacral nerve roots and the filum terminale. A needle

(continues)

Clinical Notes, *continued*

introduced into the subarachnoid space in this region usually pushes the nerve roots to one side without causing damage.

With the patient lying on the side with the vertebral column well flexed, the space between adjoining laminae in the lumbar region is opened to a maximum (Fig. 12-17). An imaginary line joining the highest points on the iliac crests passes over the fourth lumbar spine (Fig. 12-35). With a careful aseptic technique and under local anesthesia, the lumbar puncture needle, fitted with a stylet, is passed into the vertebral canal above or below the fourth lumbar spine (Fig. 12-17). The needle will pass through the following anatomic structures before it enters the subarachnoid space: skin, superficial fascia, supraspinous ligament, interspinous ligament, ligamentum flavum, areolar tissue (containing the internal vertebral venous plexus in the epidural space), dura mater, and arachnoid mater. The depth to which the needle will have to pass varies from 1 in. (2.5 cm) or less in a child to as much as 4 in. (10 cm) in obese adults.

As the stylet is withdrawn, a few drops of blood commonly escape. This usually indicates that the point of the needle is situated in one of the veins of the internal vertebral plexus and has not yet reached the subarachnoid space. If the entering needle should stimulate one of the nerve roots of the cauda equina, the patient will experience a fleeting discomfort in one of the dermatomes, or a muscle will twitch, depending on whether a sensory or a motor root was impaled. If the needle is pushed too far anteriorly, it may hit the body of the third or fourth lumbar vertebra (Fig. 12-17).

The cerebrospinal fluid pressure can be measured by attaching a manometer to the needle. In the recumbent position, the normal pressure is about 60 to 150 mm H_2O. It is interesting to note that the cerebrospinal fluid pressure normally fluctuates slightly with the heart beat and with each phase of respiration.

Anatomy of "Not Getting In"

If bone is encountered, the needle should be withdrawn as far as the subcutaneous tissue, and the angle of insertion should be changed. The most common bone encountered is the spinous process of the vertebra above or below the path of insertion. If the needle is directed laterally rather than in the midline, it may hit the lamina or an articular process.

Anatomy of Complications of Lumbar Puncture

- **Postlumbar puncture headache.** This headache starts after the procedure and lasts 24 to 48 hours. The cause is a leak of cerebrospinal fluid through the dural puncture, and it usually follows the use of a wide-bore needle. The leak reduces the volume of cerebrospinal fluid, which, in turn, causes a downward displacement of the brain and stretches the nerve-sensitive meninges—a headache follows. The headache is relieved by assuming the recumbent position. Using small-gauge styletted needles and avoiding multiple dural holes reduce the incidence of headache.
- **Brain herniation.** Lumbar puncture is contraindicated in cases in which intracranial pressure is significantly raised. A large tumor, for example, above the tentorium cerebelli with a high intracranial pressure may result in a caudal displacement of the uncus through the tentorial notch or a dangerous displacement of the medulla through the foramen magnum, when the lumbar cerebrospinal fluid pressure is reduced.

Block of the Subarachnoid Space

A block of the subarachnoid space in the vertebral canal, which may be caused by a tumor of the spinal cord or the meninges, can be detected by compressing the internal jugular veins in the neck. This raises the cerebral venous pressure and inhibits the absorption of cerebrospinal fluid in the arachnoid granulations, thus producing a rise in the manometric reading of the cerebrospinal fluid pressure. If this rise fails to occur, the subarachnoid space is blocked and the patient is said to exhibit a positive **Queckenstedt's** sign.

Caudal Anesthesia

Solutions of anesthetics may be injected into the sacral canal through the sacral hiatus. The solutions pass upward in the loose connective tissue and bathe the spinal nerves as they emerge from the dural sheath. Caudal anesthesia is used in operations in the sacral region, including anorectal surgery and culdoscopy. Obstetricians use this method of nerve block to relieve the pain during the first and second stages of labor. Its advantage is that, administered by this method, the anesthetic does not affect the infant.

The sacral hiatus is palpated as a distinct depression in the midline about 1.6 in. (4 cm) above the tip of the coccyx in the upper part of the cleft between the buttocks. The hiatus is triangular or U shaped and is bounded laterally by the sacral cornua (Fig. 12-18).

The size and shape of the hiatus depend on the number of laminae that fail to fuse in the midline posteriorly. The common arrangement is for the hiatus to be formed by the nonfusion of the fifth and sometimes the fourth sacral vertebrae.

With a careful aseptic technique and under local anesthesia, the needle, fitted with a stylet, is passed into the vertebral (sacral) canal through the sacral hiatus.

The needle pierces the skin and fascia and the sacrococcygeal membrane that fills in the sacral hiatus (Fig. 12-18). The membrane is formed of dense fibrous tissue and represents the fused supraspinous and interspinous ligaments as well as the ligamentum flavum. A distinct feeling of "give" is felt when the ligament is penetrated.

Note that the sacral canal is curved and follows the general curve of the sacrum (Fig. 12-20). The anterior wall, formed by the fusion of the bodies of the sacral vertebrae, is rough and ridged. The posterior wall, formed by the fusion of the laminae, is smooth. The average distance between the sacral hiatus and the lower end of the subarachnoid space at the second sacral vertebra is about 2 in. (5 cm) in adults.

Note also that the sacral canal contains the dural sac (containing the cauda equina), which is tethered to the coccyx by the filum terminale; the sacral and coccygeal nerves as they emerge from the dural sac surrounded by their dural sheath; and the thin-walled veins of the internal vertebral venous plexus.

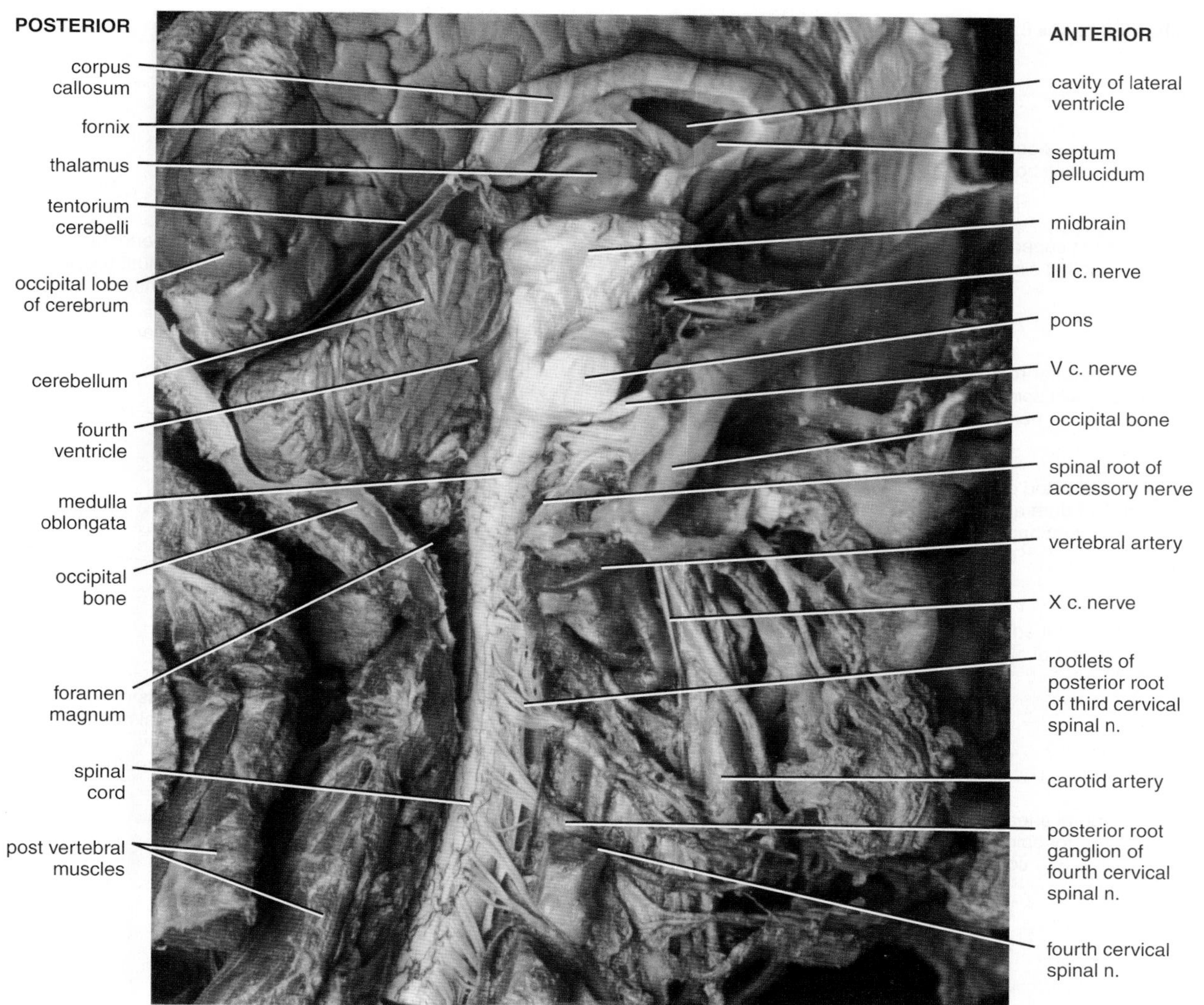

Figure 12-13 Dissection of the skull and the upper part of the cervical vertebral column showing the brain in sagittal section and the intact spinal cord in situ. Note the continuity of the medulla oblongata and the spinal cord at the foramen magnum. Note also the roots of the cervical spinal nerves and the trunks of the spinal nerves as they emerge through the dissected intervertebral foramina.

Table 12-1 Summary of Important Features Found in Cervical and Lumbosacral Root Syndromes

Root Injury	Dermatome Pain	Muscle Supplied	Movement Weakness	Reflex Involved
C5	Lower lateral aspect of upper arm	Deltoid and biceps	Shoulder abduction, elbow flexion	Biceps
C6	Lateral aspect of forearm	Extensor carpi radialis longus and brevis	Wrist extensors	Brachioradialis
C7	Middle finger	Triceps and flexor carpi radialis	Extension of elbow and flexion of wrist	Triceps
C8	Medial aspect of forearm	Flexor digitorum superficialis and profundus	Finger flexion	None
L1	Groin	Iliopsoas	Hip flexion	Cremaster
L2	Anterior aspect of thigh	Iliopsoas, sartorius, hip adductors	Hip flexion, hip adduction	Cremaster
L3	Medial aspect of knee	Iliopsoas, sartorius, quadriceps, hip adductors	Hip flexion, knee extension, hip adduction	Patellar
L4	Medial aspect of calf	Tibialis anterior, quadriceps	Foot inversion, knee extension	Patellar
L5	Lateral part of lower leg and dorsum of foot	Extensor hallucis longus, extensor digitorum longus	Toe extension, ankle dorsiflexion	None
S1	Lateral edge of foot	Gastrocnemius, soleus	Ankle plantar flexion	Ankle jerk
S2	Posterior part of thigh	Flexor digitorum longus, flexor hallucis longus	Ankle plantar flexion, toe flexion	None

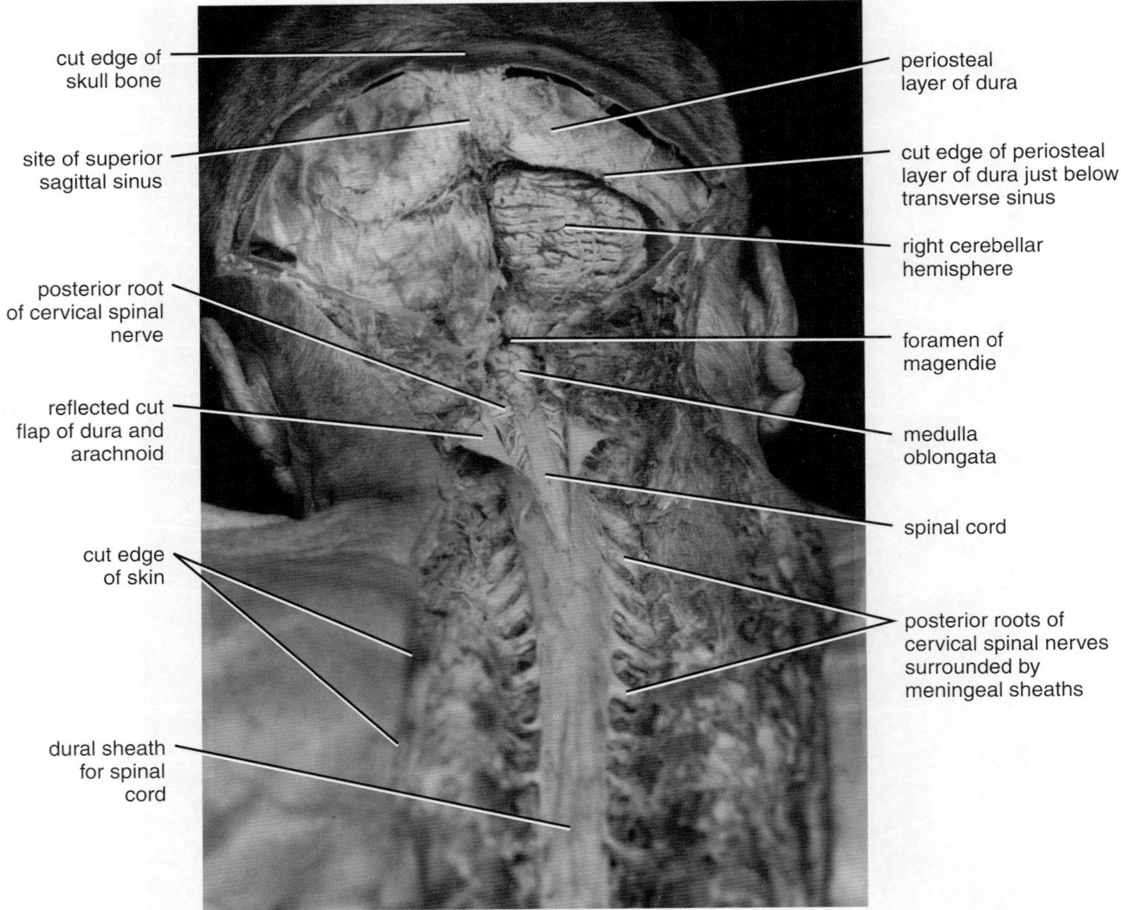

Figure 12-14 Dissection of the back of the head and neck. The greater part of the occipital bone has been removed exposing the periosteal layer of dura. On the right side a window has been made in the dura below the transverse venous sinus to expose the cerebellum and the medulla oblongata in the posterior cranial fossa. In the neck the dura and arachnoid have been incised in the midline to expose the spinal cord and rootlets of the cervical spinal nerves. Note the cervical spinal nerves leaving the vertebral canal enveloped in a meningeal sheath.

Cerebrospinal Fluid

The cerebrospinal fluid is a clear, colorless fluid formed mainly by the **choroid plexuses,** within the lateral, third, and fourth ventricles of the brain. The fluid circulates through the ventricular system and enters the subarachnoid space through the three foramina in the roof of the fourth ventricle (see page 690). It circulates both upward over the surface of the cerebral hemispheres and downward around the spinal cord. The spinal part of the subarachnoid space extends down as far as the lower border of the second sacral vertebra, where the arachnoid fuses with the filum terminale (Fig. 12-7). Eventually, the fluid enters the bloodstream by passing through the **arachnoid villi** into the dural venous sinuses, in particular the **superior sagittal venous sinus.**

In addition to removing waste products associated with neuronal activity, the cerebrospinal fluid provides a fluid medium that surrounds the spinal cord. This fluid, together with the bony and ligamentous walls of the vertebral canal, effectively protects the spinal cord from trauma.

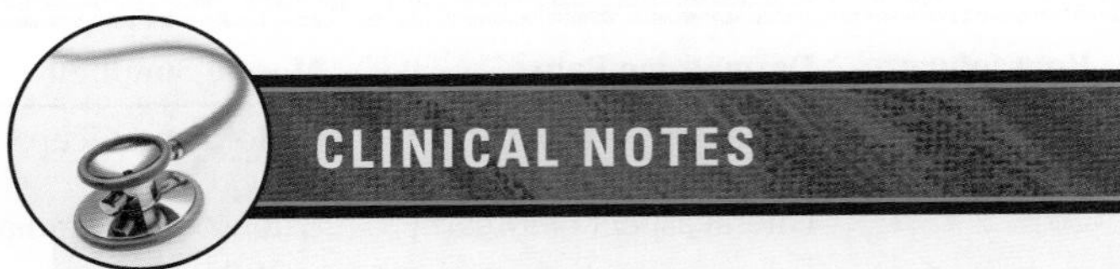

Relationship of the Vertebral Body to the Spinal Nerve

Since the fully developed vertebral body is intersegmental in position, each spinal nerve leaves the vertebral canal through the intervertebral foramen and is closely related to the intervertebral disc. This fact is of great clinical significance in cases with prolapse of an intervertebral disc (Fig. 12-16) (see page 867).

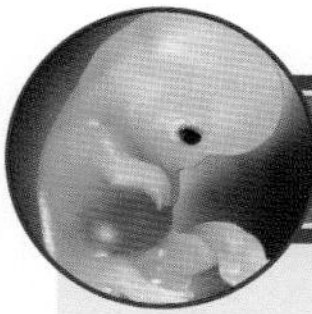

EMBRYOLOGIC NOTES

Development of the Vertebral Column

Early in development, the embryonic mesoderm becomes differentiated into three distinct regions: **paraxial mesoderm, intermediate mesoderm,** and **lateral mesoderm.** The paraxial mesoderm is a column of tissue situated on either side of the midline of the embryo, and at about the fourth week, it becomes divided into blocks of tissue called **somites.** Each somite becomes differentiated into a ventromedial part (the **sclerotome)** and a dorsolateral part (the **dermatomyotome).** The dermatomyotome now further differentiates into the **myotome** and the **dermatome** (Fig. 12-19)

The mesenchymal cells of the sclerotome rapidly divide and migrate medially during the fourth week of development and surround the **notochord** (Fig. 12-19). The caudal half of each sclerotome now fuses with the cephalic half of the immediately succeeding sclerotome to form the mesenchymal **vertebral body** (Figs. 12-19 and 12-20). Each vertebral body is thus an intersegmental structure. The notochord degenerates completely in the region of the vertebral body, but in the intervertebral region, it enlarges to form the **nucleus pulposus** of the **intervertebral discs** (Fig. 12-20). The surrounding fibrocartilage, the **anulus fibrosus,** of the intervertebral disc is derived from sclerotomic mesenchyme situated between adjacent vertebral bodies (Fig. 12-20).

Meanwhile, the mesenchymal vertebral body gives rise to dorsal and lateral outgrowths on each side. The dorsal outgrowths grow around the neural tube between the segmental nerves to fuse with their fellows of the opposite side and form the mesenchymal **neural arch** (Fig. 12-19). The lateral outgrowths pass between the myotomes to form the mesenchymal **costal processes,** or primordia of the **ribs.**

Two centers of chondrification appear in the middle of each mesenchymal vertebral body. These quickly fuse to form a cartilaginous **centrum** (Fig. 12-19). A chondrification center forms in each half of the mesenchymal neural arch and spreads dorsally to fuse behind the neural tube with its fellow of the opposite side. These centers also extend anteriorly to fuse with the cartilaginous centrum and laterally into the costal processes. The condensed mesenchymal or membranous vertebra has thus been converted into a **cartilaginous vertebra.**

In the thoracic region, each costal process forms a **cartilaginous rib.** The costal processes in the cervical region remain short and form the lateral and anterior boundaries of the **foramen transversarium** of each vertebra. In the lumbar region, the costal process forms part of the transverse process; in the sacral region, the costal processes fuse together to form the **lateral mass** of the **sacrum.**

At about the ninth week of development, primary ossification centers appear: two for each centum and one for each half of the neural arch (Fig. 12-19). The two centers for the centrum usually unite quickly, but the complete union of all the primary centers does not occur until several years after birth.

During adolescence, secondary centers appear in the cartilage covering the superior and inferior ends of the vertebral body, and the **epiphyseal plates** are formed. A secondary center also appears at the tip of each transverse process and at the tip of the spinous process. By the 25th year, all the secondary centers have fused with the rest of the vertebra.

The **atlas** and **axis** develop somewhat differently. The centrum of the atlas fuses with that of the axis and becomes the part of the axis vertebra known as the **odontoid process.** This leaves only the neural arch for the atlas, which grows anteriorly and finally fuses in the midline to form the characteristic ring shape of the atlas vertebra.

In the **sacral region,** the bodies of the individual vertebrae are separated from each other in early life by intervertebral discs. At about the 18th year, the bodies start to become united by bone; this process starts caudally. Usually by the 13th year all the sacral vertebrae are united. In the **coccygeal region,** segmental fusion also takes place, and in later life the coccyx often fuses with the sacrum.

Development of the Curves of the Vertebral Column

The embryonic vertebral column shows one continuous anterior (ventral) concavity. Later, the sacrovertebral angle develops. At birth, the cervical, thoracic, and lumbar regions show one continuous anterior (ventral) concavity. When the child begins to raise his or her head, the cervical curve, which is convex anteriorly, develops. Toward the end of the first year, when the child stands up, the lumbar curve, which is convex anteriorly, develops.

Development of the Muscles of the Vertebral Column

The prevertebral and postvertebral muscles develop from the segmental myotomes.

Scoliosis

Scoliosis results from a congenital hemivertebra. A hemivertebra is caused by a failure in development of one of the two ossification centers that appear in the centrum of the body of each vertebra (Fig. 12-21).

Spina Bifida

In spina bifida, the spines and arches of one or more adjacent vertebrae fail to develop. The condition occurs most frequently in the lower thoracic, lumbar, and sacral regions. Beneath this defect, the meninges and spinal cord may or may not be involved in varying degrees. This condition is a result of failure of the mesenchyme, which grows in between the neural tube and the surface ectoderm, to form the vertebral arches in the affected region. The types of spina bifida are shown in Figures 12-22 and 12-23.

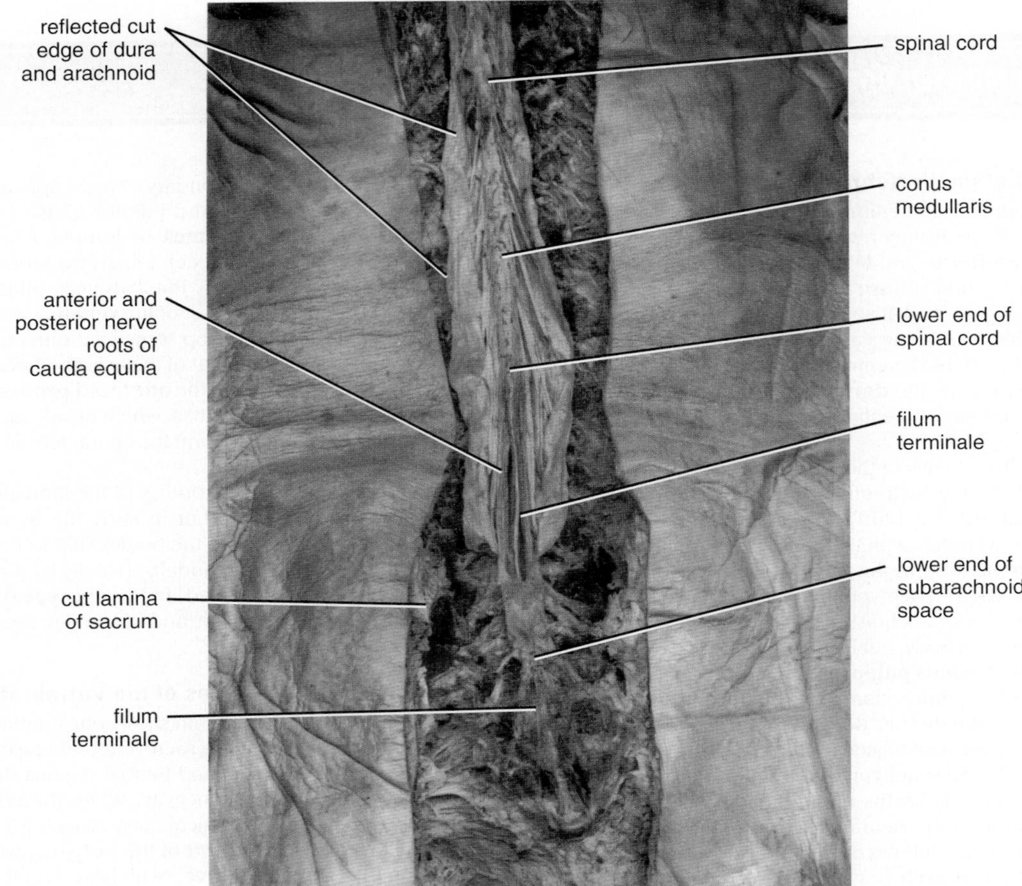

Figure 12-15 Dissection of the lower part of the back including a complete laminectomy of the lumbar and sacral regions of the vertebral column. The meningeal sheath has been incised and reflected laterally exposing the subarachnoid space, the lower end of the spinal cord, and the cauda equina. Note the filum terminale surrounded by the anterior and posterior nerve roots of the lumbar and sacral spinal nerves forming the cauda equina.

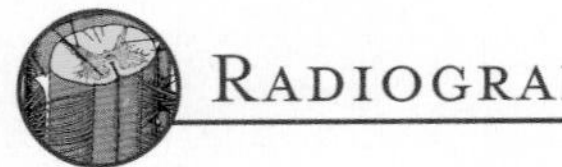

Radiographic Anatomy

Radiographic Appearances of the Vertebral Column

The views commonly used are the anteroposterior and the lateral. Examples of anteroposterior and lateral radiographs of the vertebral column can be seen in Figures 12-24 through 12-29.

Spinal Subarachnoid Space

The subarachnoid space can be studied radiographically by the injection of contrast media into the subarachnoid space by lumbar puncture. Iodized oil has been used with success. This technique is referred to as **myelography** (Figs. 12-30 and 12-31).

If the patient is sitting in the upright position, the oil sinks to the lower limit of the subarachnoid space at the level of the lower border of the second sacral vertebra. By placing the patient on a tilting table, the oil can be made to gravitate gradually to higher levels of the vertebral column.

A normal myelogram will show pointed lateral projections at regular intervals at the intervertebral space levels. This appearance is caused by the opaque medium filling the lateral extensions of the subarachnoid space around each spinal nerve. The presence of a tumor or a prolapsed intervertebral disc may obstruct the movement of the oil from one region to another when the patient is tilted.

Computed Tomography and Magnetic Resonance Imaging Studies

Computed tomography (CT) and magnetic resonance imaging (MRI) are extensively used to detect lesions of the vertebral column, especially those involving the soft tissues. CT scans can concentrate on the intervertebral spaces and reveal the intervertebral disc in transverse slices (Figs. 12-32 and 12-33). The disc has a higher density than the cerebrospinal fluid in the subarachnoid space and the

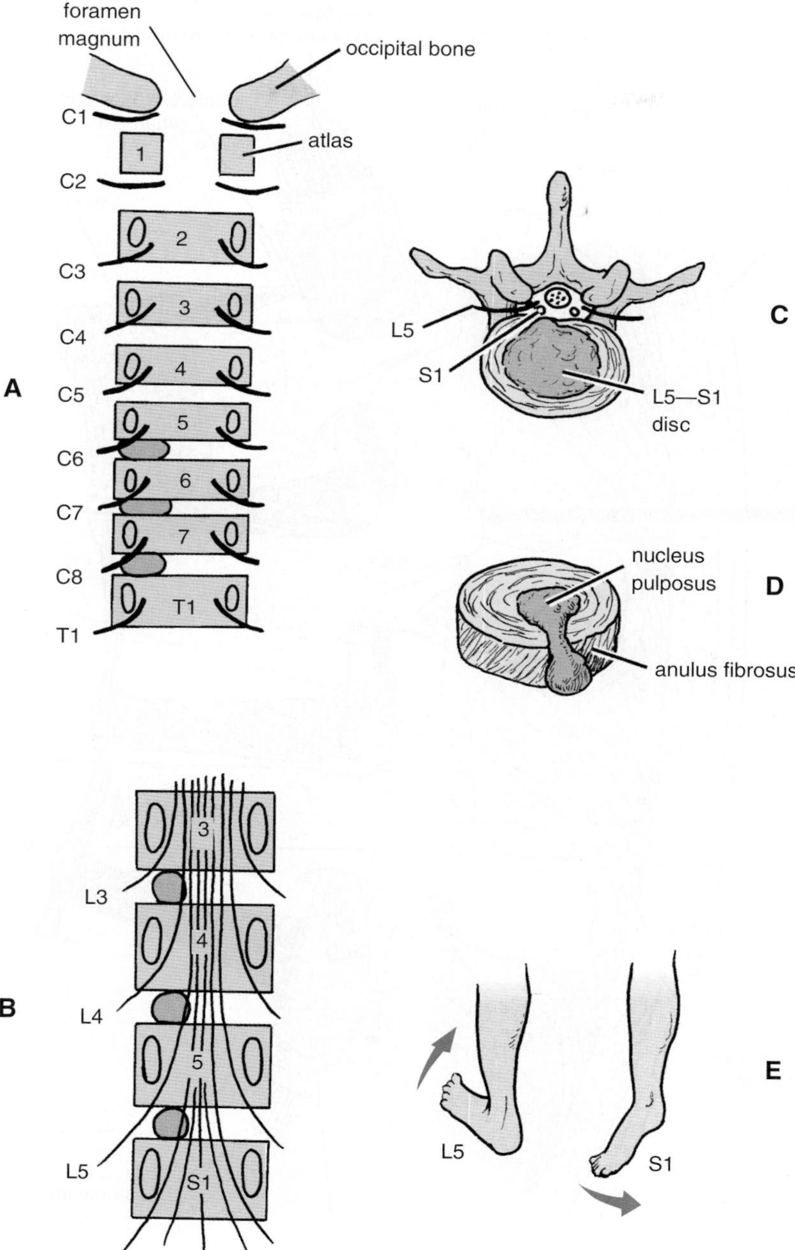

Figure 12-16 **A, B.** Posterior views of vertebral bodies in the cervical and lumbar regions showing the relationship that might exist between the herniated nucleus pulposus and the spinal nerve roots. Note that there are eight cervical spinal nerves but only seven cervical vertebrae. In the lumbar region, for example, the emerging L4 nerve roots pass out laterally close to the pedicle of the fourth lumbar vertebra and are not related to the intervertebral disc between the fourth and fifth lumbar vertebrae. **C.** Posterolateral herniation of the nucleus pulposus of the intervertebral disc between the fifth lumbar vertebra and the first sacral vertebra showing pressure on the S1 nerve root. **D.** An intervertebral disc that has herniated its nucleus pulposus posteriorly. **E.** Pressure on the L5 motor nerve root produces weakness of dorsiflexion of the ankle; pressure on the S1 motor nerve root produces weakness of plantar flexion of the ankle joint.

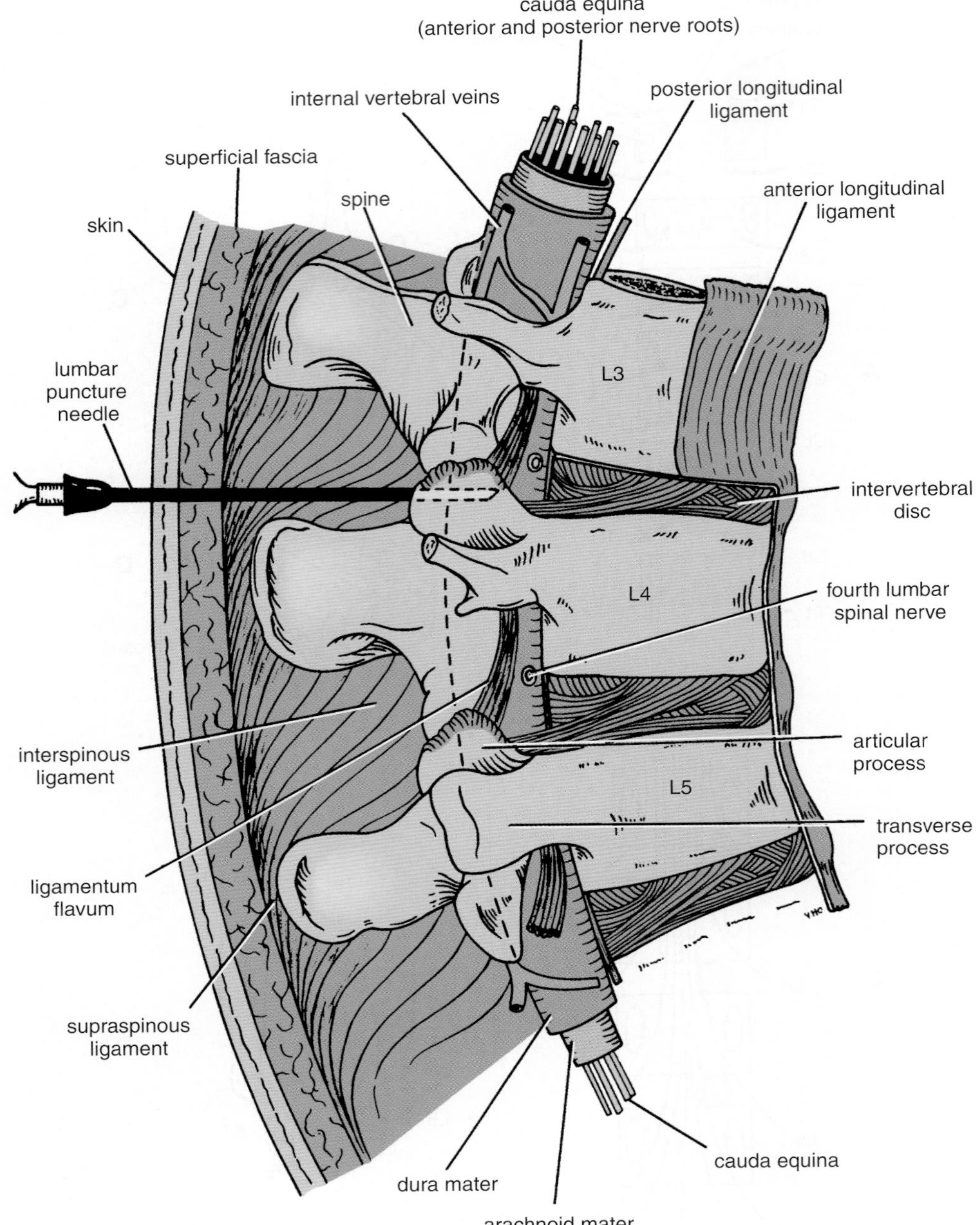

Figure 12-17 Sagittal section through the lumbar part of the vertebral column in flexion. Note that the spines and laminae are well separated in this position, enabling one to introduce a lumbar puncture needle into the subarachnoid space.

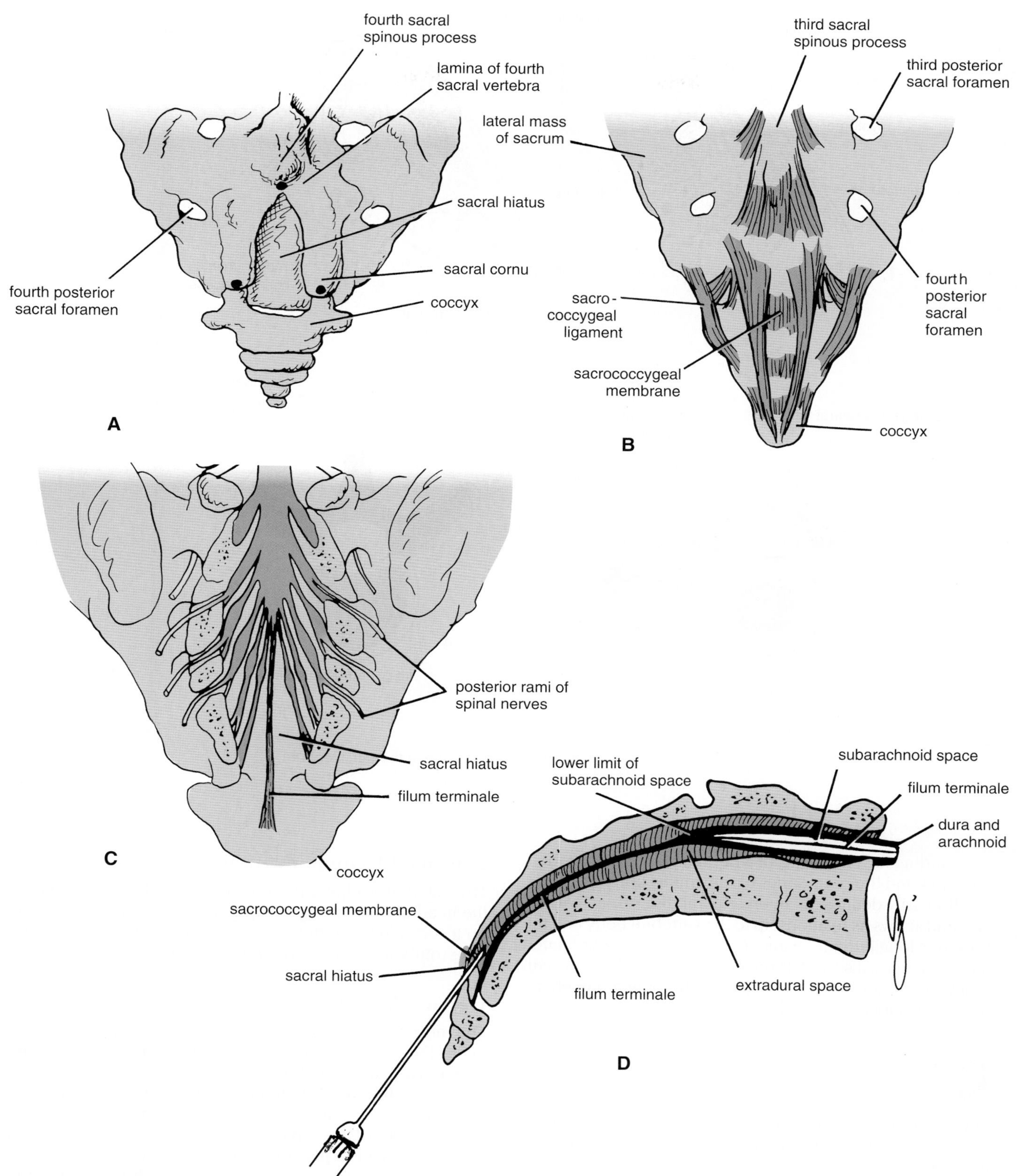

Figure 12-18 **A.** The sacral hiatus. Black dots indicate the position of important bony landmarks. **B.** Posterior surface of the lower end of the sacrum and the coccyx showing the sacrococcygeal membrane covering the sacral hiatus. **C.** The dural sheath (thecal sac) around the lower end of the spinal cord and spinal nerves in the sacral canal; the laminae have been removed. **D.** Longitudinal section through the sacrum showing the anatomy of caudal anesthesia.

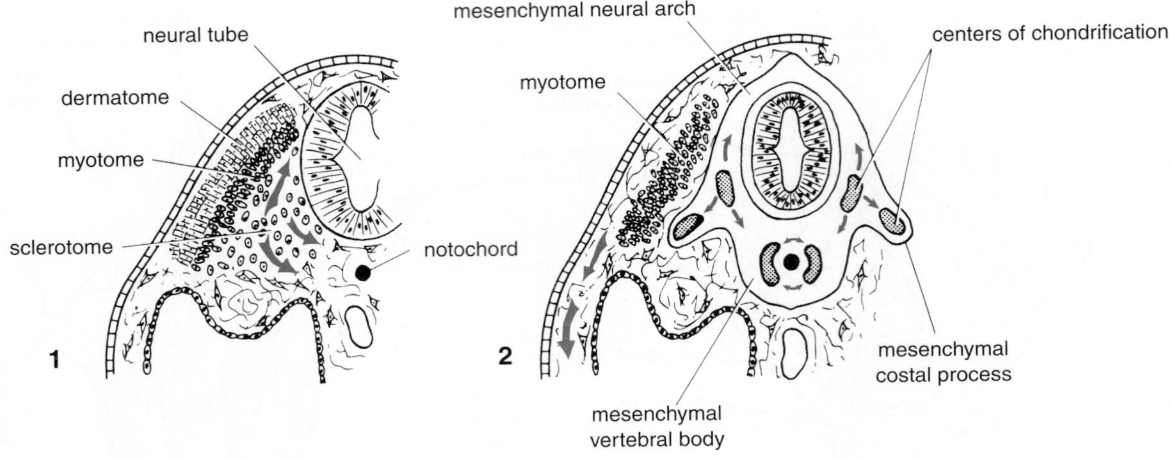

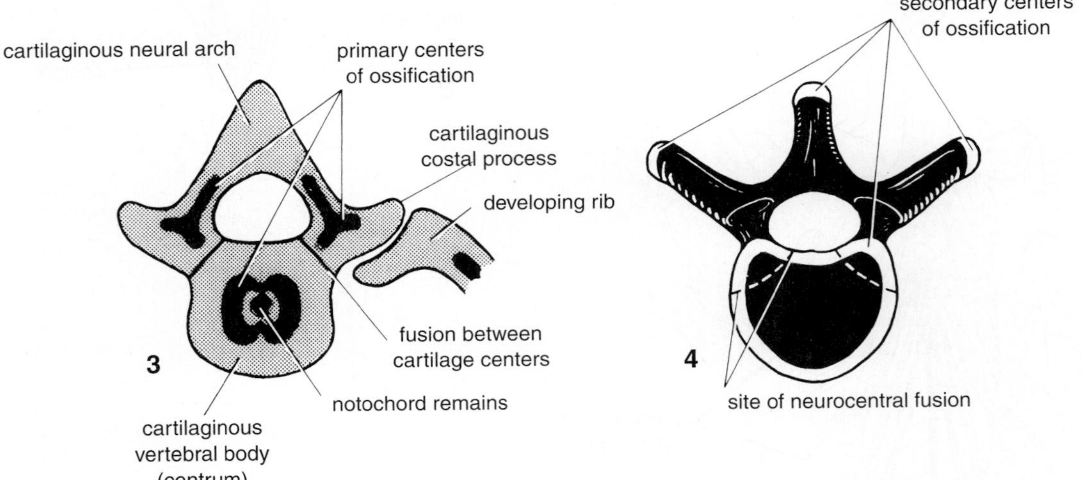

Figure 12-19 The stages in the formation of a thoracic vertebra.

surrounding fat. Fragments of a herniated disc can be identified beyond the boundaries of the anulus fibrosus.

MRI easily defines the intervertebral disc on sagittal section and shows its relationship to the vertebral body and the posterior longitudinal ligament (Fig. 12-34). The herniated fragment of the disc and its relationship to the dural sac can easily be demonstrated. The use of MRI is now largely replacing myelography or CT in this region.

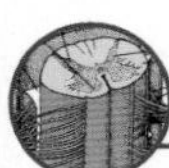

Surface Anatomy

The entire posterior aspect of the patient should be examined from head to foot, and the arms should hang loosely at the side.

Midline Structures

In the midline, the following structures can be palpated from above downward.

External Occipital Protuberance

The external occipital protuberance lies at the junction of the head and neck (Fig. 12-1). If the index finger is placed on the skin in the midline, it can be drawn downward from the protuberance in the **nuchal groove.**

Cervical Vertebrae

The most prominent spinous process that can be felt in the neck (Fig. 12-35) is that of the **seventh cervical vertebra (vertebra prominens).** Cervical spines one to six are covered by the **ligamentum nuchae,** a large ligament that runs down the back of the neck connecting the skull to the spinous processes of the cervical vertebrae.

The **transverse processes** are short but easily palpable from the lateral side in a thin neck. The **anterior tubercle of the sixth cervical transverse process (tubercle of Chassaignac)** can be palpated medial to the sternocleidomastoid muscle, and against it the common carotid artery can be compressed.

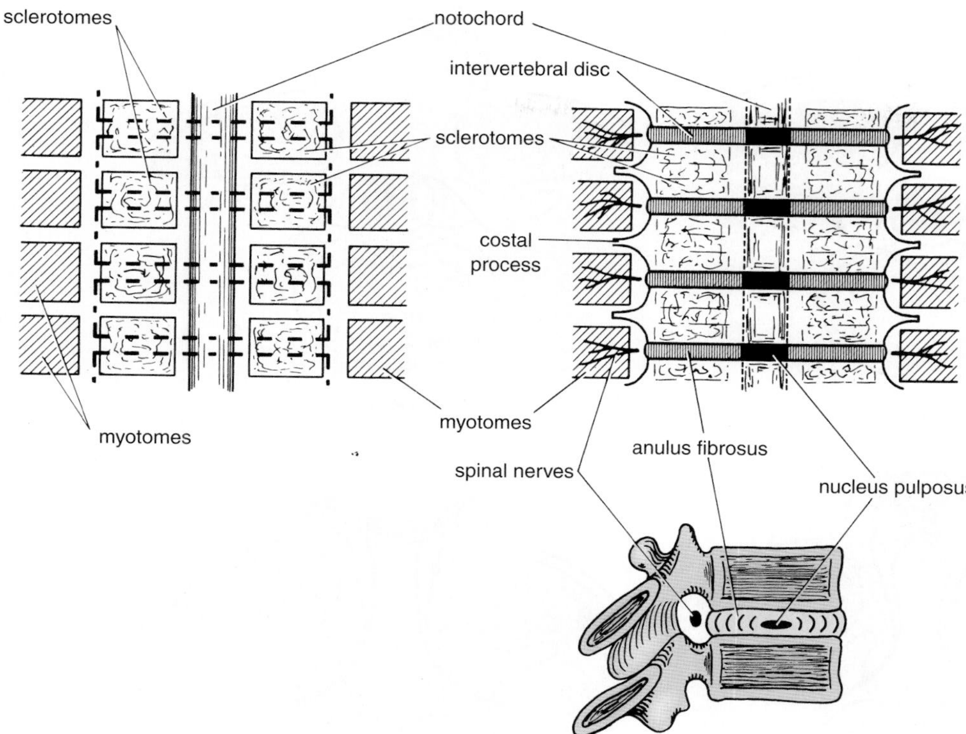

Figure 12-20 The formation of each mesenchymal vertebral body by the fusion of the caudal half of each sclerotome with the cephalic half of the immediately succeeding sclerotome. Each vertebral body is thus an intersegmental structure. The costal processes grow out between adjacent myotomes. Also shown is the close relationship that exists between each spinal nerve and each intervertebral disc.

Thoracic and Lumbar Vertebrae

The nuchal groove is continuous below with a furrow that runs down the middle of the back over the tips of the **spines of all the thoracic** and the upper four **lumbar vertebrae** (Fig. 12-35). The most prominent spine is that of the first thoracic vertebra; the others may be easily recognized when the trunk is bent forward.

Sacrum

The **spines of the sacrum** are fused with each other in the midline to form the **median sacral crest.** The crest can be felt beneath the skin in the uppermost part of the cleft between the buttocks.

The **sacral hiatus** is situated on the posterior aspect of the lower end of the sacrum, and here the extradural space (epidural space) terminates. The hiatus lies about 2 in. (5 cm) above the tip of the coccyx and beneath the skin of the groove between the buttocks.

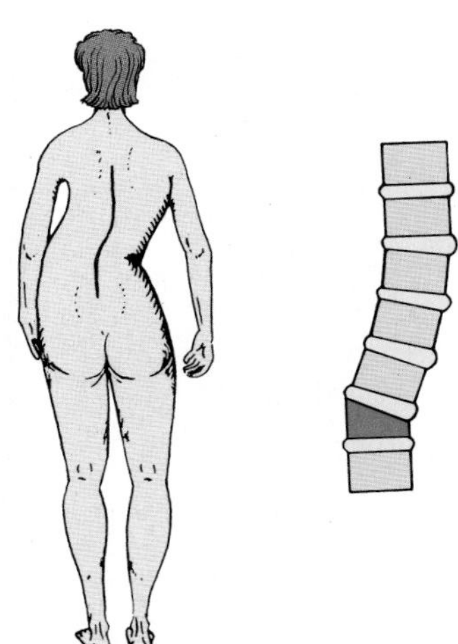

Figure 12-21 Posterior view of a woman with scoliosis resulting from a congenital hemivertebra in the lower thoracic region.

Coccyx

The inferior surface and tip of the coccyx can be palpated in the groove between the buttocks about 1 in. (2.5 cm) behind the anus (Fig. 12-1). The anterior surface of the coccyx can be palpated with a gloved finger in the anal canal.

Upper Lateral Part of the Thorax

The upper lateral part of the thorax is covered by the scapula and its associated muscles. The scapula lies posterior to the first to the seventh ribs (Figs. 12-1 and 12-35).

Scapula

The **medial border** of the scapula forms a prominent ridge, which ends above at the superior angle and below at the inferior angle (Fig. 12-35).

The **superior angle** can be palpated opposite the first thoracic spine, and the **inferior angle** can be palpated opposite the seventh thoracic spine (Figs. 12-1 and 12-35).

The **crest of the spine of the scapula** can be palpated and traced medially to the medial border of the scapula, which it joins at the level of the third thoracic spine (Figs. 12-1 and 12-35).

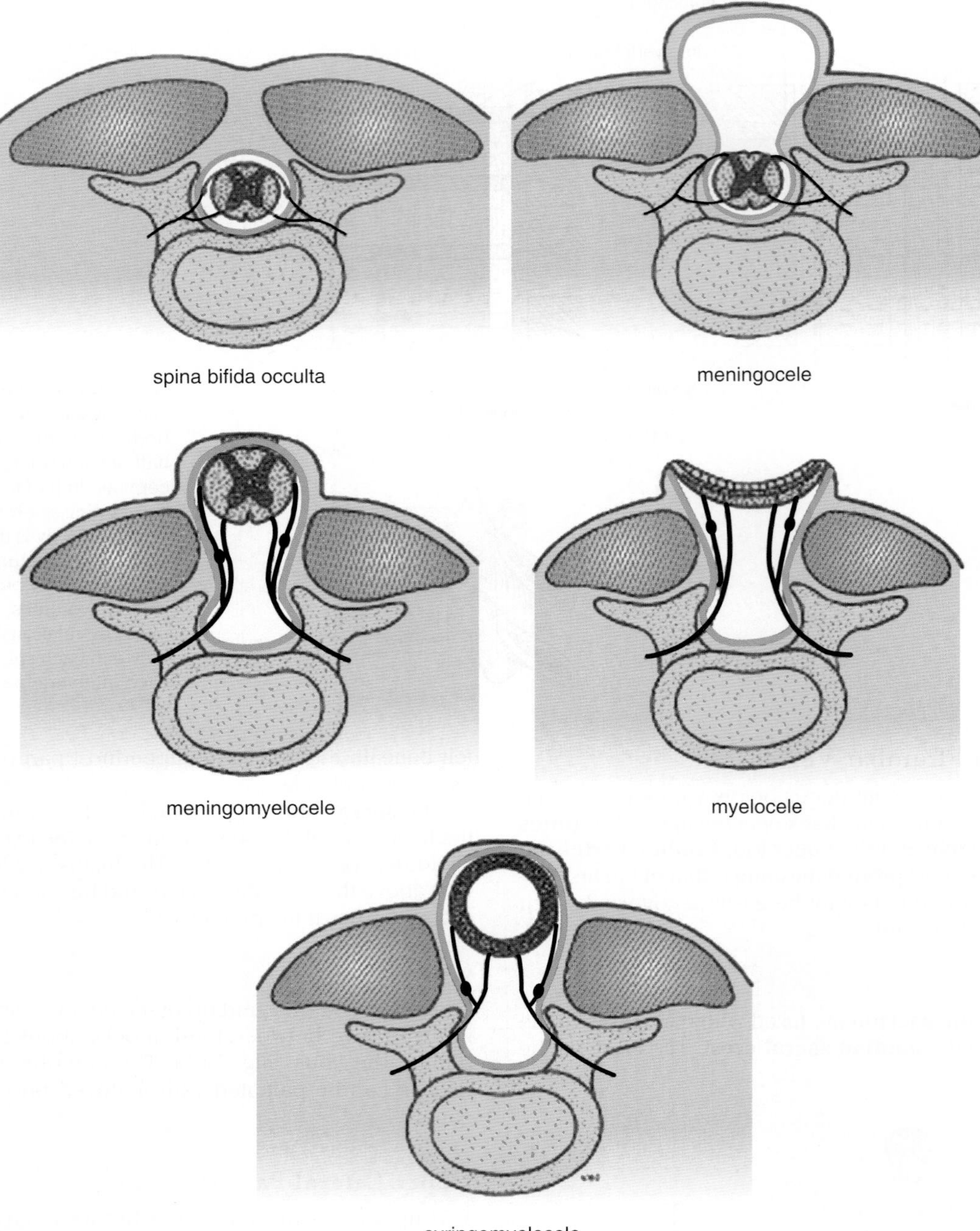

Figure 12-22 Different types of spina bifida.

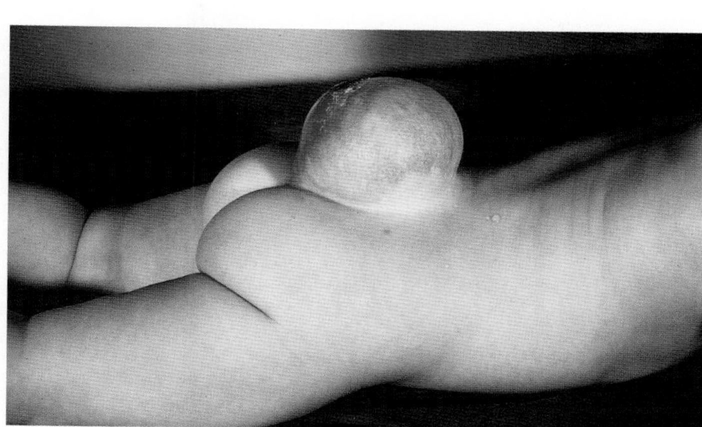

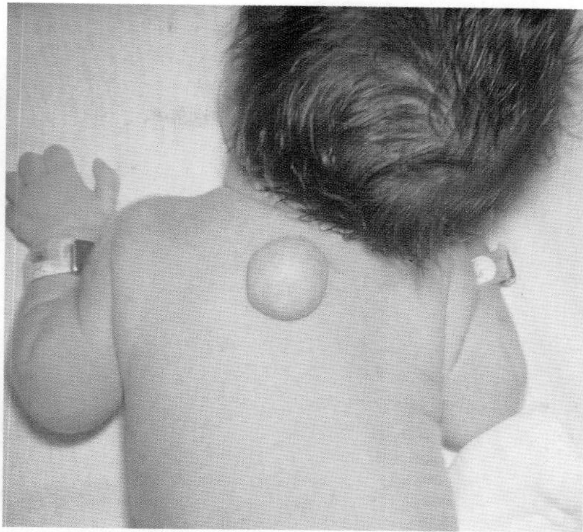

Figure 12-23 **A.** Meningocele in the lumbosacral region. (Courtesy of L. Thompson.) **B.** Meningomyelocele in the upper thoracic region. (Courtesy of G. Avery.)

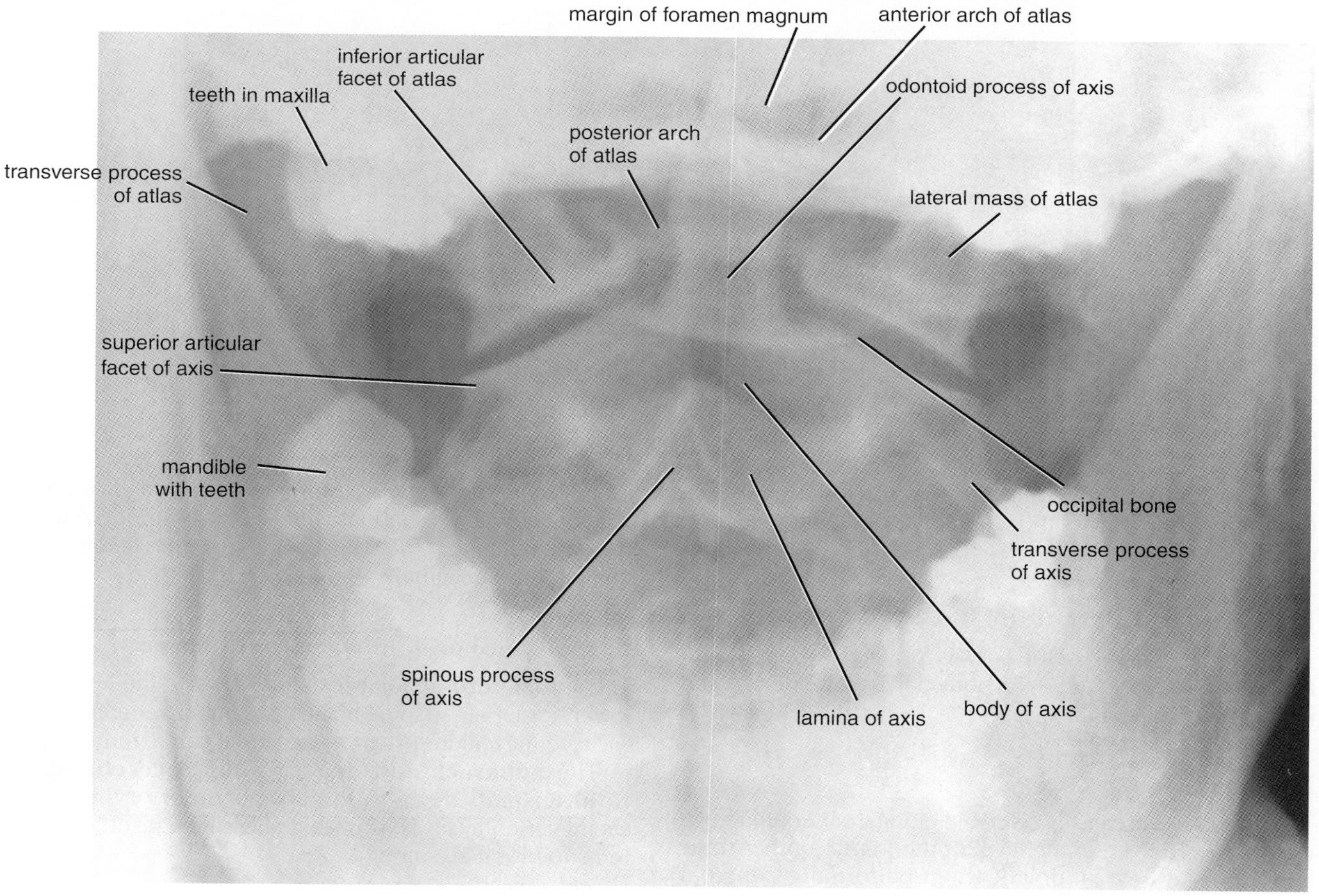

margin of foramen magnum
anterior arch of atlas
inferior articular facet of atlas
teeth in maxilla
odontoid process of axis
posterior arch of atlas
transverse process of atlas
lateral mass of atlas
superior articular facet of axis
mandible with teeth
occipital bone
transverse process of axis
spinous process of axis
lamina of axis
body of axis

Figure 12-24 Anteroposterior radiograph of the upper cervical region of the vertebral column with the patient's mouth open to show the odontoid process of the axis.

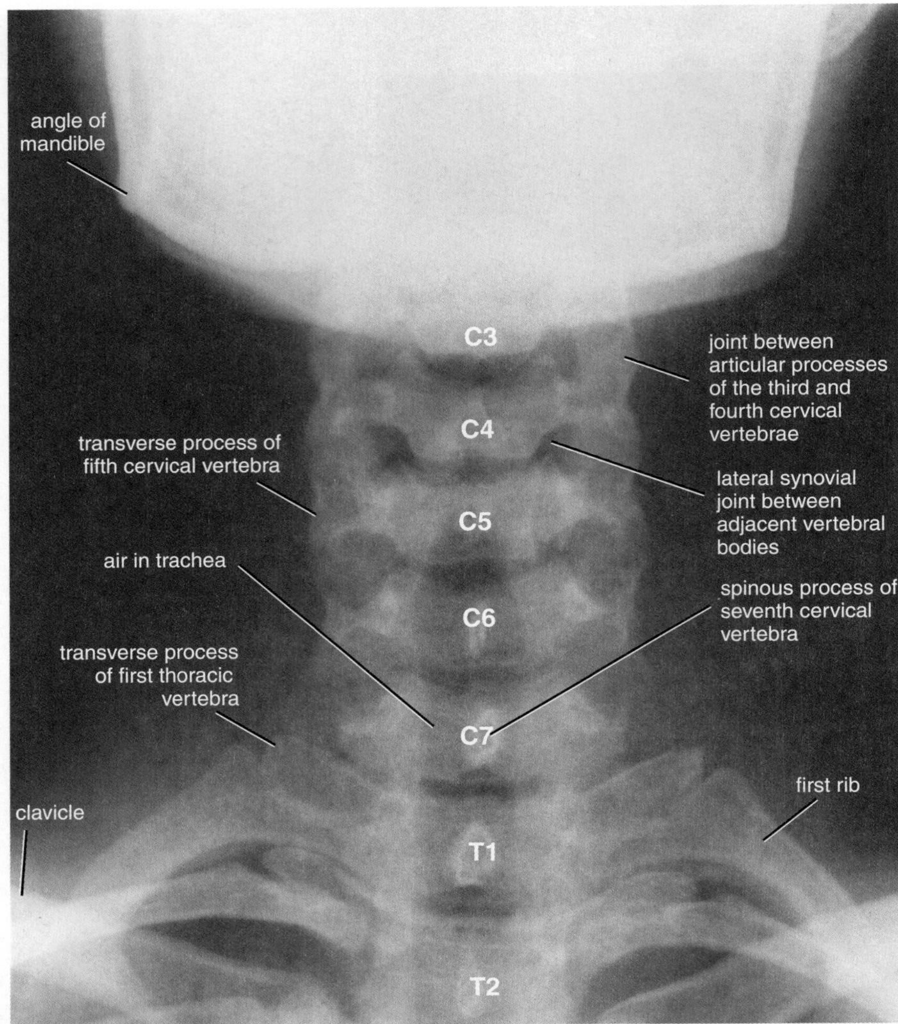

Figure 12-25 Anteroposterior radiograph of the cervical region of the vertebral column.

The **acromion process of the scapula** forms the lateral extremity of the spine of the scapula. It is subcutaneous and easily located.

Lower Lateral Part of the Back

The lower lateral part of the back is formed by the posterior aspect of the upper part of the bony pelvis (false pelvis) and its associated gluteal muscles.

Iliac Crests

The iliac crests are easily palpable along their entire length (Fig. 12-1). They lie at the level of the fourth lumbar spine and are used as a landmark when performing a lumbar puncture. Each crest ends in front at the **anterior superior iliac spine** and behind at the **posterior superior iliac spine;** the latter lies beneath a skin dimple at the level of the second sacral vertebra and the middle of the sacroiliac joint. The iliac tubercle is a prominence felt on the outer surface of the iliac crest about 2 in. (5 cm) posterior to the anterosuperior iliac spine. The iliac tubercle lies at the level of the fifth lumbar spine.

Spinal Cord and Subarachnoid Space

The **spinal cord** in adults extends down to the level of the lower border of the spine of the first lumbar vertebra (Fig. 12-7). In young children, it may extend to the third lumbar spine.

The **subarachnoid space,** with its **cerebrospinal fluid,** extends down to the lower border of the second sacral vertebra (Fig. 12-7), which lies at the level of the posterosuperior iliac spine.

Symmetry of the Back

Observe the back as a whole and compare the two sides with reference to an imaginary line passing downward from

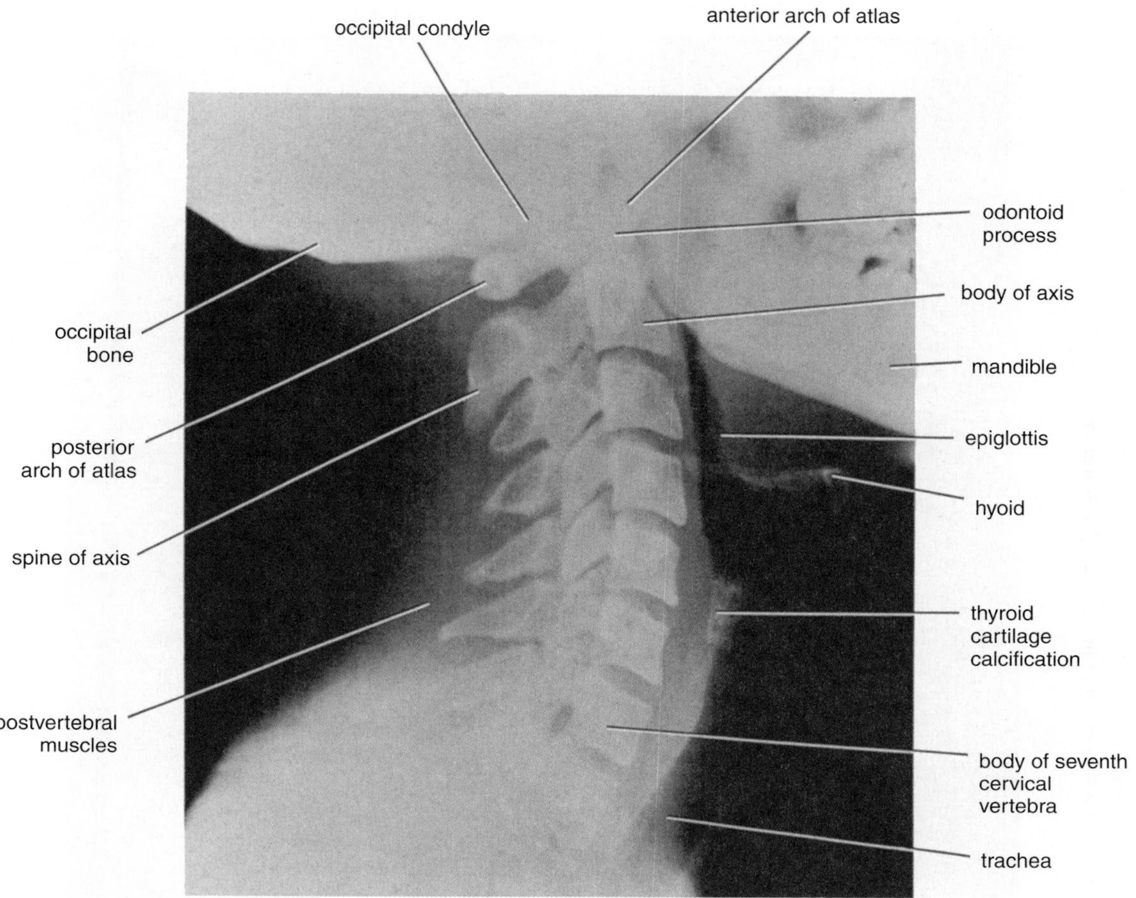

Figure 12-26 Lateral radiograph of the cervical region of the vertebral column.

the external occipital protuberance to the cleft between the buttocks.

The **posterior vertebral musculature,** which mainly controls the movements of the vertebral column and maintains the postural curves of the column, can be palpated. The muscles are large and lie on either side of the spines of the vertebrae (Figs. 12-1, 12-9, and 12-35). They should be examined with the flat of the hand. If they exhibit normal tone, they are firm to the touch. A spastic muscle feels harder than normal; it is also shorter than normal, which produces a concavity of the vertebral column on the side of the muscular contraction.

The **curves of the vertebral column** can be examined by inspecting the lateral contour of the back. Normally, the posterior surface is concave in the cervical region, convex in the thoracic region, and concave in the lumbar region (Fig. 12-2). The anterior surface of the sacrum and coccyx together have an anterior concavity. The lumbar region meets the sacrum at a sharp angle, the **lumbosacral angle.**

Inspection of the posterior surface of the back, with particular reference to the vertical alignment of the vertebral spines, reveals a slight lateral curvature in most normal persons. Right-handed persons, especially those whose work involves extreme and prolonged muscular effort, usually exhibit a lateral thoracic curve to the right; left-handed persons usually exhibit a lateral thoracic curve to the left.

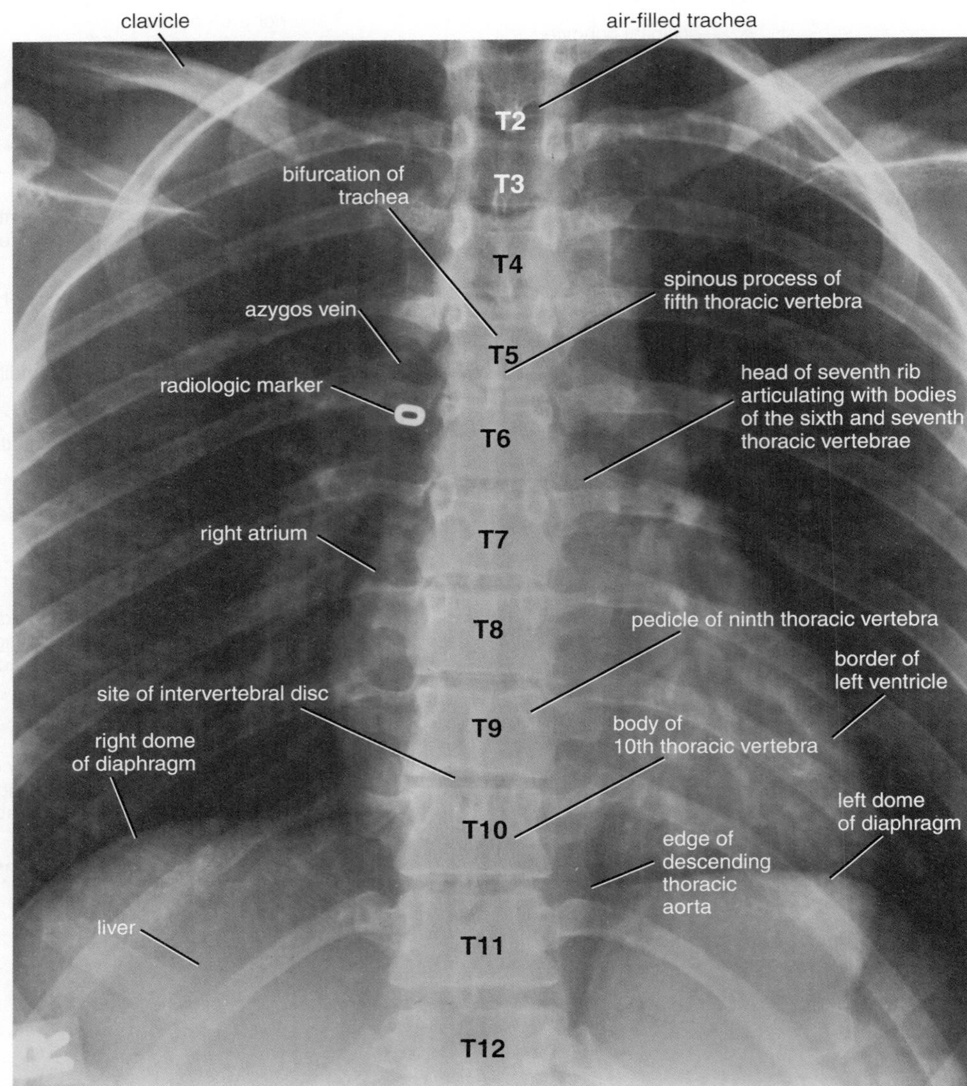

Figure 12-27 Anteroposterior radiograph of the thoracic region of the vertebral column.

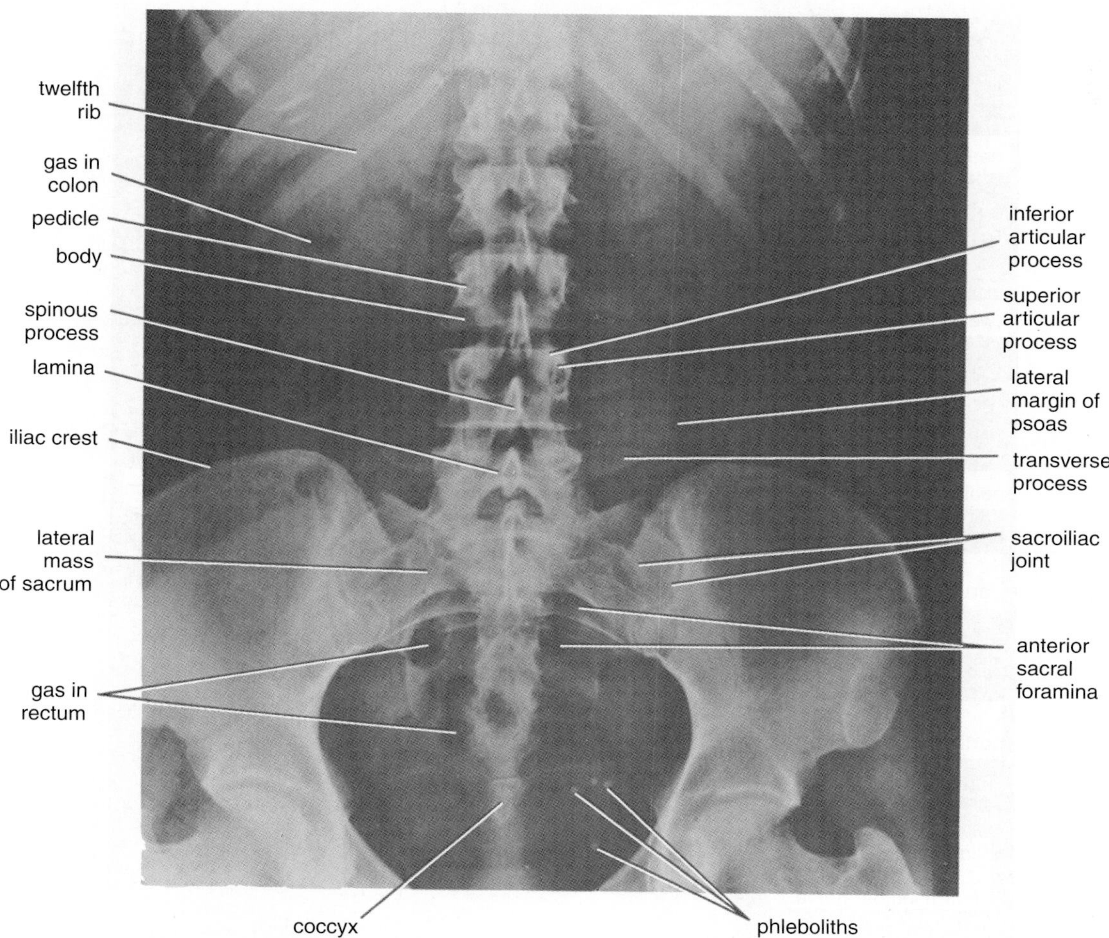

Figure 12-28 Anteroposterior radiograph of the lower thoracic, lumbar, and sacral regions of the vertebral column.

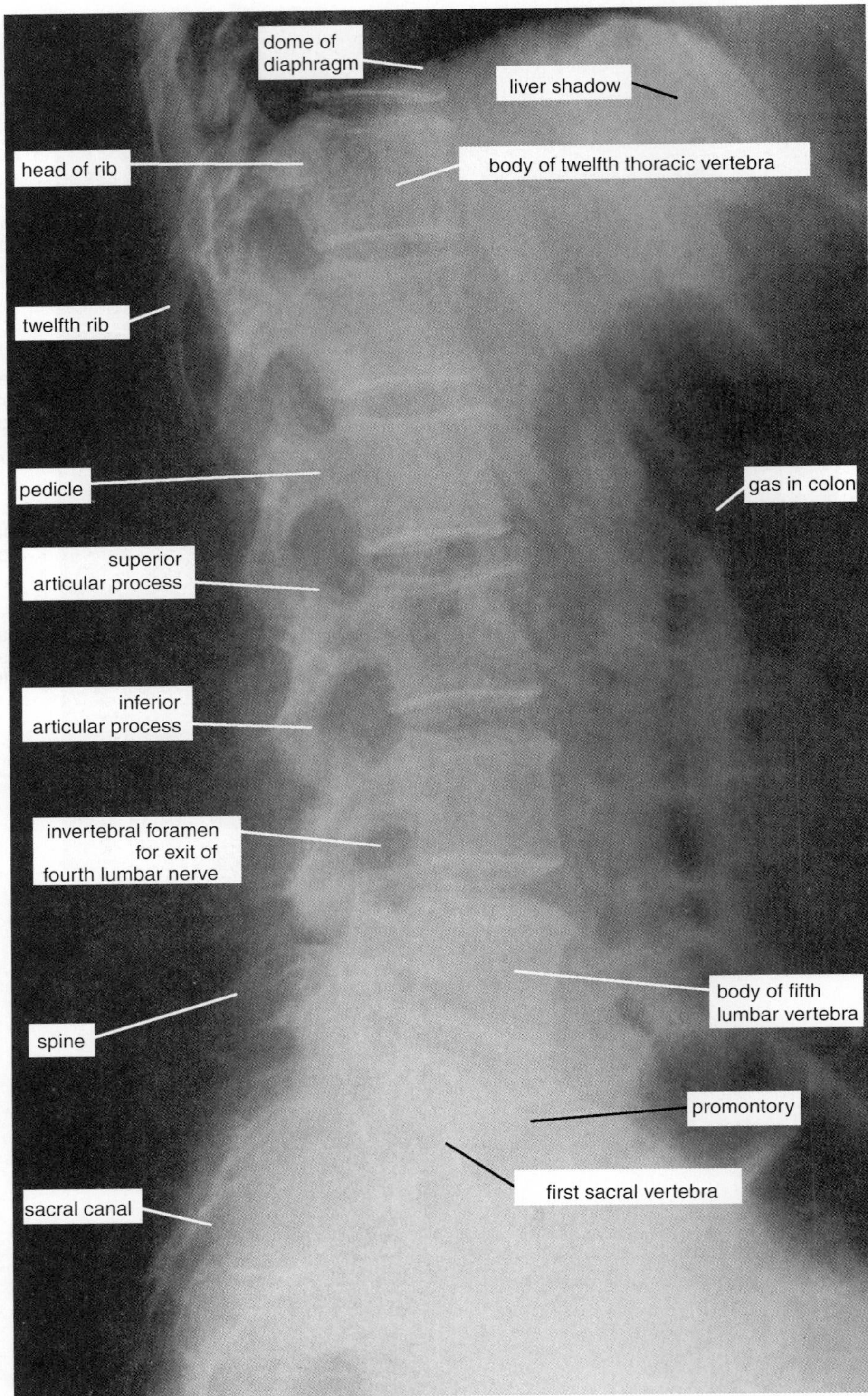

Figure 12-29 Lateral radiograph of the lower thoracic, lumbar, and sacral regions of the vertebral column.

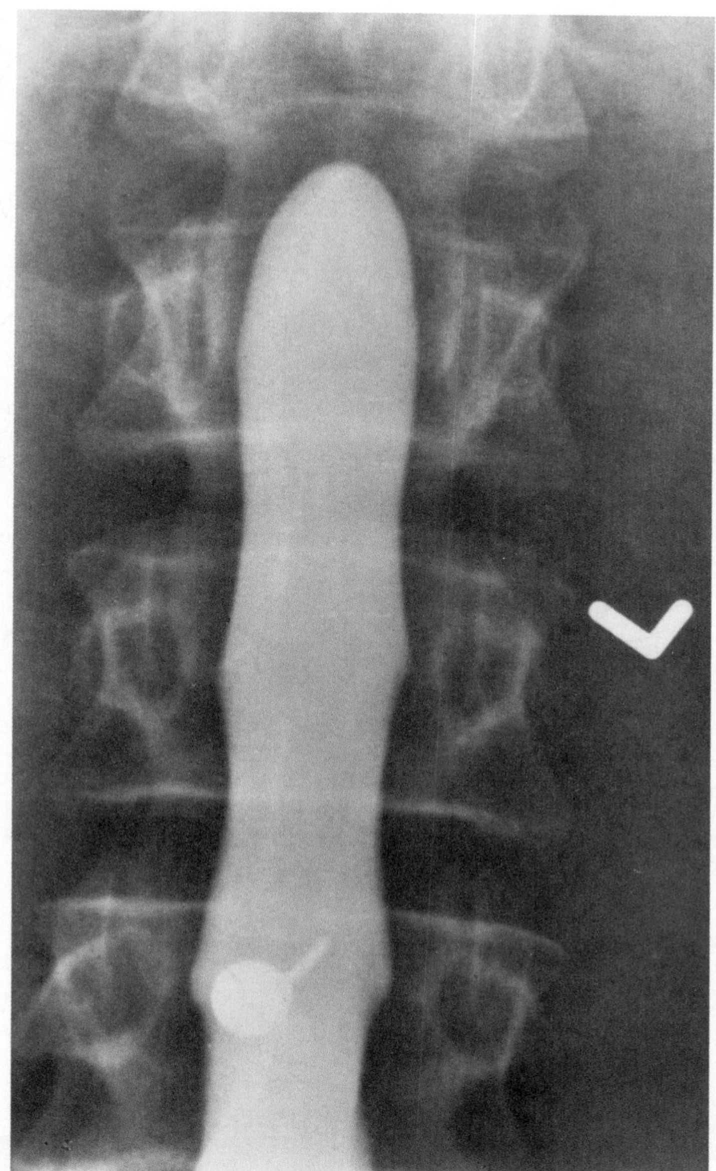

Figure 12-30 Posteroanterior myelogram of the lumbar region.

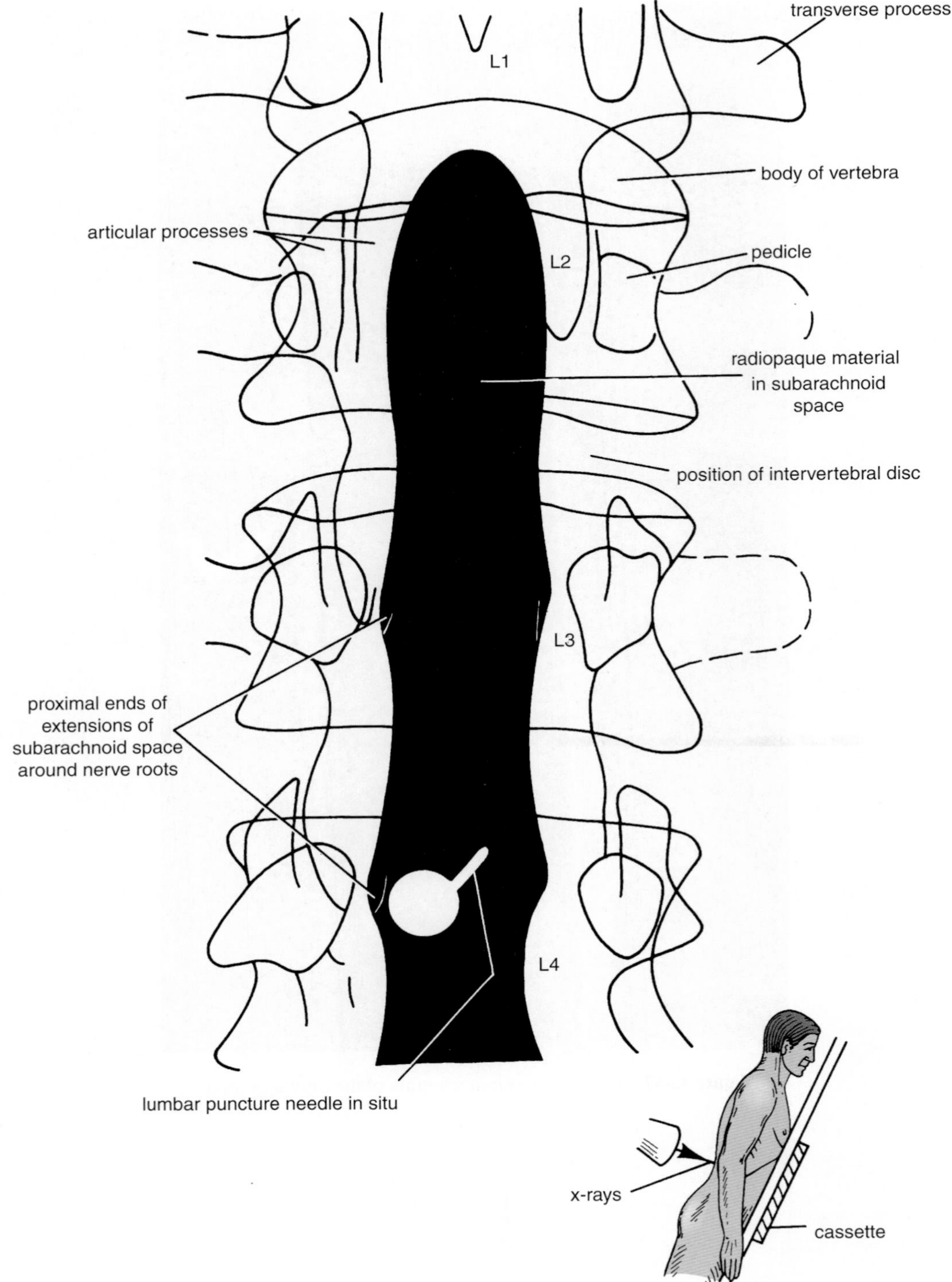

Figure 12-31 Main features that can be seen in the myelogram in Figure 12-30.

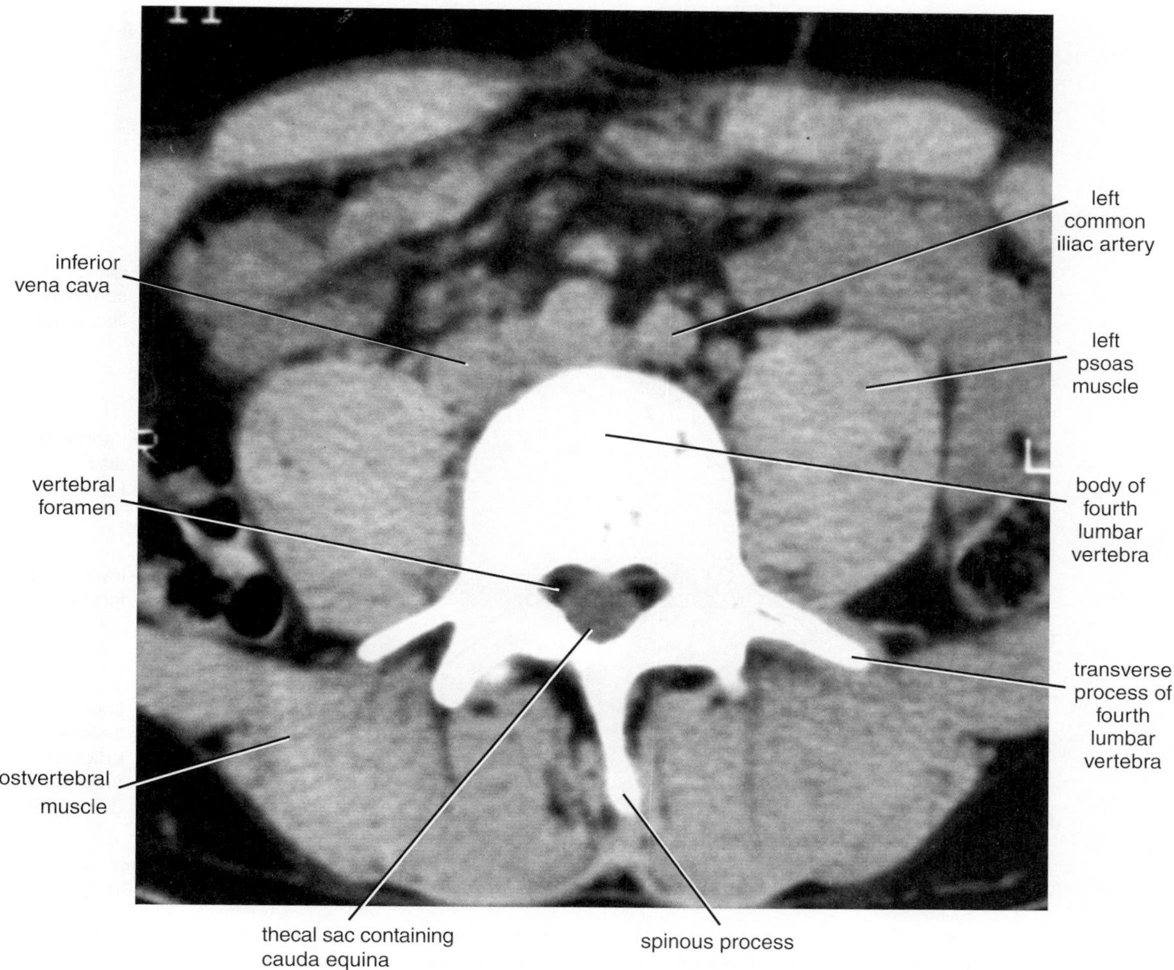

Figure 12-32 Computed tomography scan of the fourth lumbar vertebra.

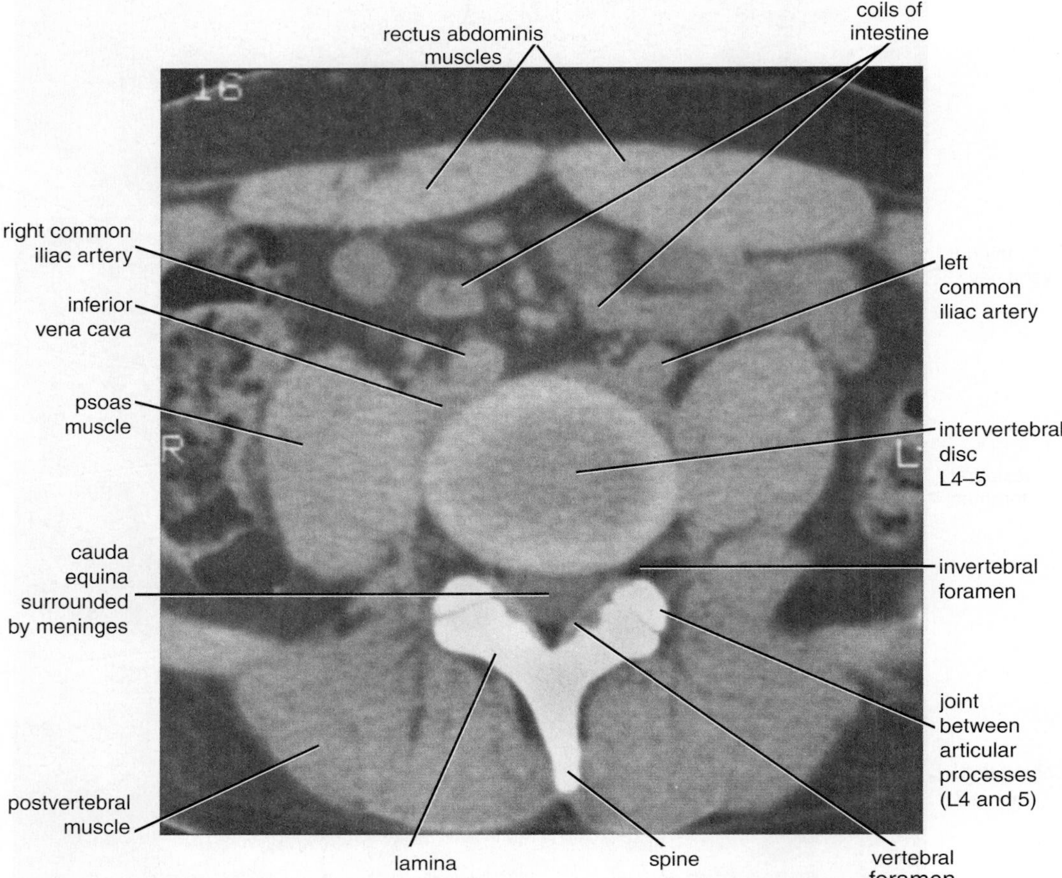

Figure 12-33 Computed tomography scan through the vertebral column at the level of the intervertebral disc between the fourth and fifth lumbar vertebrae. The spine of L4 and the intervertebral foramen on each side are shown. Note the joints between the articular processes.

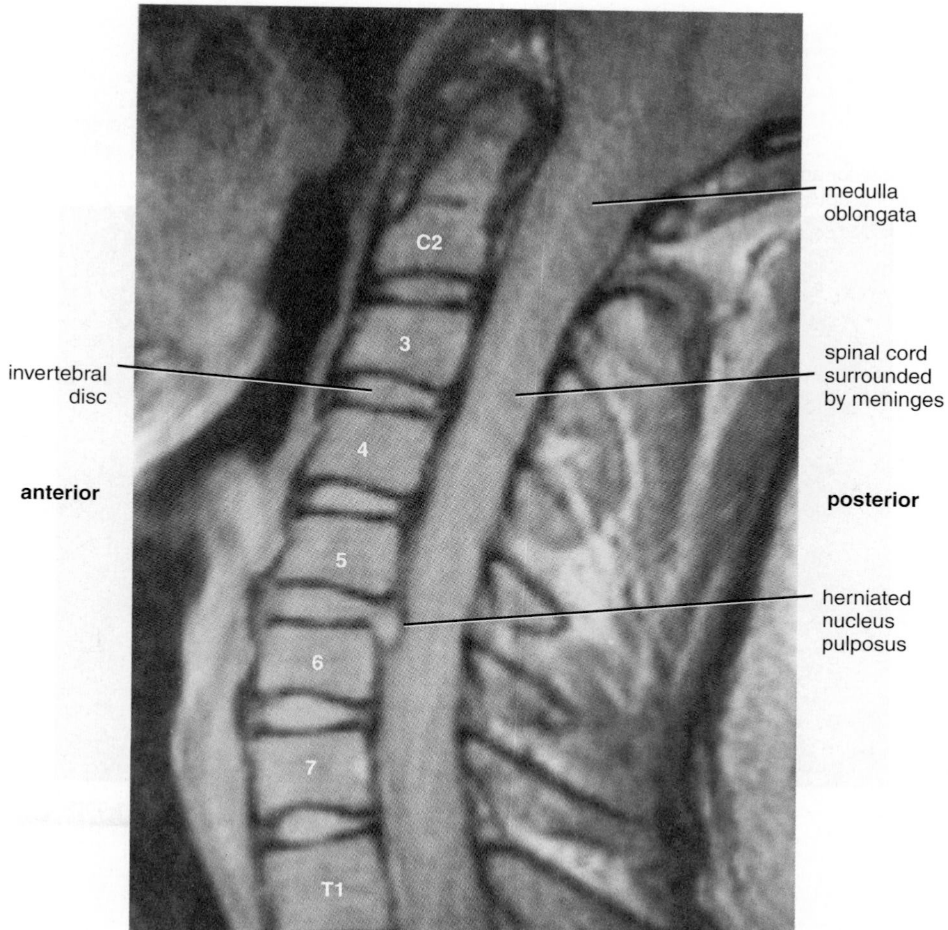

Figure 12-34 Sagittal magnetic resonance imaging scan of the cervical part of the vertebral column. A herniated disc between the fifth and sixth vertebrae is shown. Note the position of the spinal cord and its meningeal coverings relative to the herniated disc. (Courtesy of Pait.)

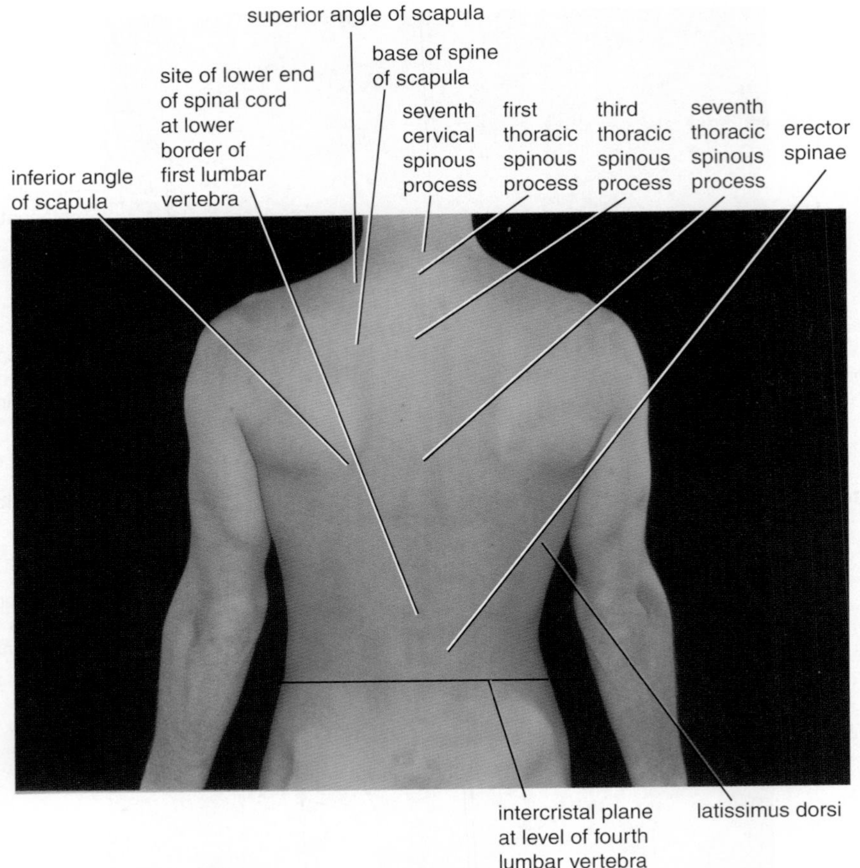

Figure 12-35 The back of a 27-year-old man.

CLINICAL PROBLEM SOLVING

Study the following case histories and select the best answer to the questions following them.

An 11-year-old boy was showing off in front of friends by diving into the shallow end of a swimming pool. After one particular daring dive, he surfaced quickly and climbed out of the pool, holding his head between his hands. He said that he had hit the bottom of the pool with his head and now had severe pain in the root of the neck, which was made worse when he tried to move his neck. A lateral radiograph revealed that the right inferior articular process of the fifth cervical vertebra was forced over the anterior margin of the right superior articular process of the sixth cervical vertebra, producing a unilateral dislocation with nipping of the right sixth cervical nerve.

1. The following symptoms and signs confirmed the diagnosis except which?
   (a) The head was rotated to the right.
   (b) There was spasm of the deep neck muscles on the right side of the neck, which were tender to touch.
   (c) The patient complained of severe pain in the region of the back of the neck and right shoulder.
   (d) The slightest movement produced severe pain in the right sixth cervical dermatome.
   (e) The large size of the vertebral canal in the cervical region permitted the spinal cord to escape injury.

A 50-year-old coal miner was crouching at the mine face when a large rock suddenly became dislodged from the roof of the mine shaft and struck him on the upper part of his back. The emergency department physician suspected a displacement of the upper thoracic spines on the sixth thoracic spine.

2. The following physical signs confirmed a diagnosis of fracture dislocation between the fifth and sixth thoracic vertebrae except which?
   (a) A lateral radiograph revealed fractures involving the superior articular processes of the sixth thoracic vertebra and the inferior articular processes of the fifth thoracic vertebra.

(b) Considerable forward displacement of the body of the fifth thoracic vertebra on the sixth thoracic vertebra occurred.
(c) The patient had signs and symptoms of spinal shock.
(d) The large size of the vertebral canal in the thoracic region leaves plenty of space around the spinal cord for bony displacement.
(e) The patient later showed signs and symptoms of paraplegia.

A 66-year-old woman was seen in the emergency department complaining of a burning pain over the upper part of her right arm. The pain had started 2 days previously and had progressively worsened. Physical examination revealed weakness and wasting of the right deltoid and biceps brachii muscles. The patient also had hyperesthesia in the skin over the lower part of the right deltoid and down the lateral side of the arm. Radiologic examination showed extensive spur formation on the bodies of the fourth, fifth, and sixth cervical vertebrae. These signs and symptoms suggested severe osteoarthritis of the cervical vertebral column.

3. This disease produced the following changes in the vertebrae and related structures except which?
   (a) Repeated trauma and aging had resulted in degenerative changes at the articulating surfaces of the fourth, fifth, and sixth cervical vertebrae.
   (b) Extensive spur formation resulted in narrowing of the intervertebral foramina with pressure on the nerve roots.
   (c) The burning pain and hyperesthesia were caused by pressure on the third and fourth cervical posterior roots.
   (d) The weakness and wasting of the deltoid and biceps brachii muscles were caused by pressure on the fifth and sixth cervical anterior roots.
   (e) Movements of the neck intensified the symptoms by exerting further pressure on the nerve roots.
   (f) Coughing or sneezing raised the pressure within the vertebral canal and resulted in further pressure on the roots.

A medical student offered to move a grand piano for his landlady. He had just finished his final examinations in anatomy and was in poor physical shape. He struggled with the antique monstrosity and suddenly experienced an acute pain in the back, which extended down the back and outer side of his left leg. On examination in the emergency department, he was found to have a slight scoliosis with the convexity on the right side. The deep muscles of the back in the left lumbar region felt firmer than normal. No evidence of muscle weakness was present, but the left ankle jerk was diminished.

4. The symptoms and signs of this patient strongly suggested a diagnosis of prolapsed intervertebral disc except which?
   (a) The pain was worst over the left lumbar region opposite the fifth lumbar spine.
   (b) The pain was accentuated by coughing.
   (c) With the patient supine, flexing the left hip joint with the knee extended caused a marked increase in the pain.
   (d) A lateral radiograph of the lumbar vertebral column revealed nothing abnormal.
   (e) An MRI study revealed the presence of small fragments of the nucleus pulposus that had herniated outside the anulus in the disc between the fifth lumbar vertebra and the sacrum.
   (f) The pain occurred in the dermatomes of the third and fourth lumbar segments on the left side.
5. When performing a lumbar puncture (spinal tap) on an adult, the following anatomic facts have to be taken into consideration except which?
   (a) With the patient in the lateral prone or upright sitting position, the vertebral column should be well flexed to separate the spines and laminae of adjacent vertebrae.
   (b) An imaginary line joining the anterior superior iliac spines passes over the fourth lumbar spine.
   (c) The needle should be inserted above or below the fourth lumbar spine.
   (d) To enter the subarachnoid space, the needle will pass through the skin, superficial fascia, supraspinous ligament, interspinous ligament, ligamentum flavum, areolar tissue (containing the internal vertebral venous plexus), dura mater, and arachnoid mater.
   (e) The spinal cord ends below in the adult at the level of the lower border of the first lumbar vertebra.
   (f) With the patient in the lateral prone position, the normal cerebrospinal fluid pressure is about 120 mm H_2O.

A 22-year-old student was driving home from a party and crashed his car head on into a brick wall. On examination in the emergency department, he was found to have a fracture dislocation of the seventh thoracic vertebra, with signs and symptoms of severe damage to the spinal cord.

6. On recovery from spinal shock he was found to have the following signs and symptoms except which?
   (a) He had upper motor neuron paralysis of his left leg.
   (b) He had a band of cutaneous hyperesthesia extending around the abdominal wall on the left side at the level of the umbilicus that was caused by the irritation of the cord immediately above the site of the lesion.
   (c) On the right side, total analgesia, thermoanesthesia, and partial loss of tactile sense of the skin of the abdominal wall below the level of the umbilicus involving the whole of the right leg were present.
   (d) Fracture dislocation of the seventh thoracic vertebra would result in severe damage to the seventh thoracic segment of the spinal cord.
   (e) The unequal sensory and motor losses on the two sides indicate a left hemisection of the spinal cord.

A 45-year-old woman visited her physician because of a low back pain of 3 months' duration. She was otherwise very fit. On examination of her back, nothing abnormal was discovered. The physician then listened to her chest, examined her thyroid gland, and finally examined both breasts. A large, hard mass was found in the left breast.

7. The following facts supported the diagnosis of carcinoma of the left breast with secondaries in the vertebral column except which?

(a) The lump in the breast was painless and the patient had noticed it while showering 6 months previously.
(b) Several large, hard, pectoral lymph nodes were found in the left axilla.
(c) A lateral radiograph of the lumbar vertebral column showed extensive metastases in the bodies of the second and third lumbar vertebrae.
(d) The lump was situated in the upper outer quadrant of the left breast and was fixed to surrounding tissues.
(e) Although the cancer had spread by the lymph vessels, no evidence of spread via the bloodstream was present.

A 75-year-old woman was dusting the top of a high closet while balanced on a chair. She lost her balance and fell to the floor, catching her right lumbar region on the edge of the chair.

8. The following statements about this patient are correct except which?
   (a) Examination of the back revealed a large bruised area in the right lumbar region, which was extremely tender to touch.
   (b) Anteroposterior and lateral radiographs exclude the presence of a fracture, especially of a transverse process.
   (c) A 24-hour specimen of urine should be examined for blood to exclude or confirm injury to the right kidney.
   (d) Careful examination of the erector spinae muscles or quadratus lumborum muscle may reveal extreme tenderness and therefore injury to these muscles.
   (e) A lumbar puncture (spinal tap) should always be performed in back injuries to exclude damage to the spinal cord.

ANSWERS TO CLINICAL PROBLEMS

1. A. The right inferior articular process of the fifth cervical vertebra was forced over the anterior margin of the right superior articular process of the sixth cervical vertebra, causing the head of the patient to be rotated to the left.
2. D. The vertebral canal in the thoracic region is small and round and little space is around the spinal cord for bony displacement to occur without causing severe damage to the cord.
3. C. The burning pain and hyperesthesia were caused by pressure on the fifth and sixth cervical posterior roots.
4. F. The pain occurred in the dermatomes of the fifth lumbar and first sacral segments on the left side.
5. B. An imaginary line joining the highest points of the iliac crests passes over the fourth lumbar spine.
6. D. Fracture dislocation of the 7th thoracic vertebra would result in severe damage to the 10th thoracic segment of the spinal cord.
7. E. The carcinoma of the left breast was in an advanced stage and had spread by way of the lymph vessels to the axillary lymph nodes and by the bloodstream to the bodies of the second and third lumbar vertebrae. Carcinoma of the thyroid, bronchus, breast, kidney, and prostate tend to metastasize via the bloodstream to bones.
8. E. A lumbar puncture (spinal tap) is not required in cases of simple trauma to the back.

REVIEW QUESTIONS

Completion Questions

Select the phrase that best completes each statement.

1. The characteristic feature of the second cervical vertebra is its
   (a) absent body.
   (b) odontoid process.
   (c) heart-shaped body.
   (d) massive body.
   (e) trifid spinous process.
2. The seventh cervical vertebra is characterized by having
   (a) the longest spinous process.
   (b) a large foramen transversarium.
   (c) a heart-shaped body.
   (d) a massive body.
   (e) an odontoid process.
3. The sixth thoracic vertebra is characterized by
   (a) its heart-shaped body.
   (b) its bifid spinous process.
   (c) its massive body.
   (d) having the superior articular processes face medially and those of the inferior articular process face laterally.
   (e) its thick lamina.
4. The characteristic feature of the first cervical vertebra is its
   (a) odontoid process.
   (b) massive body.
   (c) absent body.
   (d) long spinous process.
   (e) absent foramen transversarium.

5. The characteristic feature of the fifth lumbar vertebra is its
   (a) heart-shaped body.
   (b) rounded vertebral foramen.
   (c) small pedicles.
   (d) massive body.
   (e) short and thick transverse process.
6. The cauda equina consists of
   (a) a bundle of posterior roots of lumbar, sacral, and coccygeal spinal nerves.
   (b) the filum terminale.
   (c) a bundle of anterior and posterior roots of lumbar, sacral, and coccygeal spinal nerves.
   (d) a bundle of lumbar, sacral, and coccygeal spinal nerves and the filum terminale.
   (e) a bundle of anterior and posterior roots of lumbar, sacral, and coccygeal spinal nerves and the filum terminale.
7. The spinal cord in the adult ends inferiorly at the level of the
   (a) L5 vertebra.
   (b) L3 vertebra.
   (c) S2 to 3 vertebrae.
   (d) T12 vertebra.
   (e) L1 vertebra.
8. Herniation of the intervertebral disc between the fifth and sixth cervical vertebrae will compress the
   (a) fourth cervical nerve root.
   (b) sixth cervical nerve root.
   (c) fifth cervical nerve root.
   (d) seventh and eighth cervical nerve roots.
   (e) seventh cervical nerve root.
9. The subarachnoid space ends inferiorly in the adult at the level of
   (a) the coccyx.
   (b) the lower border of L1.
   (c) S2 to 3.
   (d) S5.
   (e) the promontory of the sacrum.

Multiple-Choice Questions

Select the best answer for each question.

10. The following statements concerning an intervertebral disc are correct except which?
    (a) The nucleus pulposus is most likely to herniate in an anterolateral direction.
    (b) The discs are the thickest in the lumbar region.
    (c) The atlantoaxial joint possesses no disc.
    (d) The discs play a major role in the development of the curvatures of the vertebral column.
    (e) During aging, the fluid within the nucleus pulposus is replaced by fibrocartilage.
11. The following statements concerning the vertebral column are correct except which?
    (a) Throughout life, the marrow of the vertebral bodies has a hemopoietic function.
    (b) The internal vertebral venous plexus provides a path for the passage of malignant cells from the prostate to the cranial cavity.
    (c) The vertebral artery ascends the neck through the foramen transversarium of all the cervical vertebrae.
    (d) Injection of an anesthetic into the sacral canal can be used to block pain and sensation from the cervix, vagina, and perineum during childbirth.
    (e) The atlantoaxial joint permits rotation of the head on the vertebral column.
12. The first cervical vertebra (atlas) has all the following anatomic features except which?
    (a) Lateral masses
    (b) Inferior articular facets
    (c) Anterior arch
    (d) Spinous process
    (e) Superior articular facets

Read the case history and select the best answer to the questions following it.

An 8-year-old girl was taken to a pediatrician because her mother was concerned about a lateral curvature of the child's spine, which she had noticed since her daughter was 5 months old. The girl was otherwise perfectly healthy and active.

13. The pediatrician performed a thorough physical examination and found the following except which?
    (a) Both legs were of equal length.
    (b) On standing, the heights of the iliac crests were the same on each side.
    (c) The left shoulder was lower than the right.
    (d) The vertebral column in the midthoracic region showed a sharp curve convex to the right.
    (e) There were gentle compensatory curves of the vertebral column above and below the sharp curve in the midthoracic region, with convexities to the right.

The pediatrician performed further clinical examinations and ordered a radiographic examination of the vertebral column.

14. The following statements about this patient are correct except which?
    (a) The anteroposterior radiograph of the midthoracic region revealed a wedge-shaped vertebra at the level of T5 and fusion of the left fifth and sixth ribs.
    (b) Flexion of the vertebral column showed that the sharp curved area was rigid.
    (c) The child had a congenital hemivertebra at the level of T5 with compensatory curves above and below that defect.
    (d) The condition is caused by a failure in development of one of the three ossification centers that appear in the centrum of the body of each vertebra.
    (e) Since the child had no symptoms and the compensatory curves are well balanced, no special treatment is advised.

ANSWERS TO REVIEW QUESTIONS

1. B
2. A
3. A
4. C. During development the centrum of the atlas fuses with that of the axis to form the odontoid process of the axis.
5. D. The pedicles are large and the transverse processes are long and slender; the vertebral foramen is triangular.
6. E
7. E
8. B (see Fig. 12-16)
9. C
10. A. The nucleus pulposus is most likely to herniate in a posterolateral direction.
11. C. The vertebral artery ascends through the foramen transversarium of the upper six cervical vertebrae; only the vertebral vein passes through the small foramen transversarium of the seventh cervical vertebra.
12. D. The atlas does not have a spine but exhibits a posterior tubercle on its posterior arch.
13. E. The compensatory curves of the vertebral column above and below a sharp curve convex to the right would have their convexities to the left.
14. D. Normally, the centrum has only two ossification centers and not three as stated. A hemivertebra in the thoracic region often is associated with aplasia or fusion of adjacent ribs.

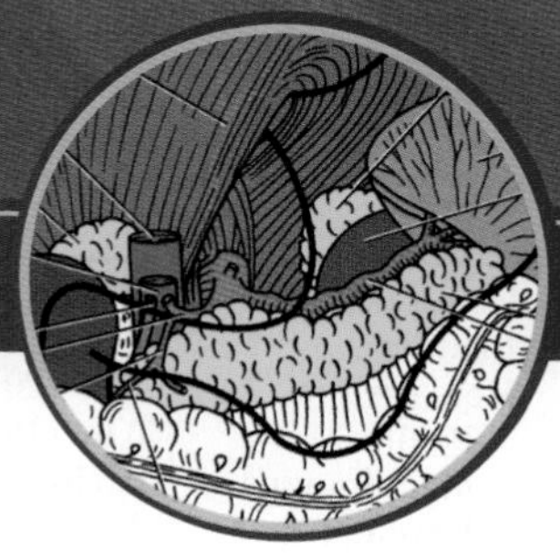

APPENDIX

USEFUL ANATOMIC DATA OF CLINICAL SIGNIFICANCE

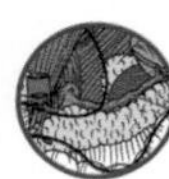

Respiratory System

Table I Important Airway Distances (Adult)[a]

Airway	Distances (approx.)
Incisor teeth to the vocal cords	5.9 in. (15 cm)
Incisor teeth to the carina	7.9 in. (20 cm)
External nares to the carina	11.8 in. (30 cm)

[a] Average figures given ± 1–2 cm.

Table II Important Data Concerning the Trachea[a]

	Length (approx.)	Diameter (approx.)
Adults	4.5 in. (11.4 cm)	1 in. (2.5 cm)
Infants	1.6–2 in. (4–5 cm)	As small as 3 mm[b]

[a] Extension of the head and neck, as when maintaining an airway in an anesthetized patient, may stretch the trachea and increase its length by 25%. In the adult, the carina may descend by as much as 3 cm on deep inspiration. At the carina, the right bronchus leaves the trachea at an angle of 25° from the vertical and the left bronchus leaves the trachea at an angle of 45° from the vertical. In children younger than 3 years, both bronchi arise from the trachea at equal angles.
[b] As children grow, the diameter in millimeters corresponds approximately to their age in years.

Digestive System

Table III Lengths and Capacities

Region	Lengths (approx.)	Capacities (approx.)
Esophagus	10 in. (25 cm)	—
Stomach[a]	Lesser curvature 4.8–5.6 in. (12–14 cm)	1500 mL
Duodenum	10 in. (25 cm)	—
Jejunum	8 ft. (2.4 m)	—
Ileum	12 ft. (3.7 m)	—
Appendix	3–5 in. (8–13 cm)	—
Ascending colon	5 in. (13 cm)	—
Transverse colon	15 in. (38 cm)	—
Descending colon	10 in. (25 cm)	—
Sigmoid colon	10–15 in. (25–38 cm)	—
Rectum	5 in. (13 cm)	—
Anal canal	1.5 in. (4 cm)	—
Gallbladder	2.8–3.9 in. (7–10 cm)	30–50 mL
Cystic duct	1.5 in. (3.8 cm)	—
Bile duct	3 in. (8 cm)	—

[a] The curved course taken by a nasogastric tube from the cardiac orifice to the pylorus is usually longer, 6–10 in. (15–25 cm).

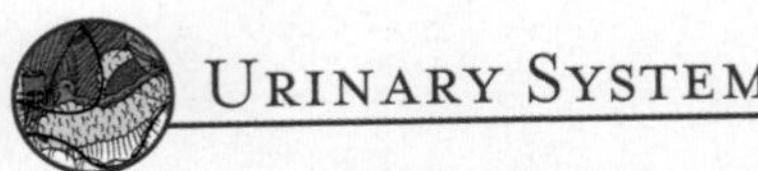

Urinary System

Table IV Lengths and Capacities

Organ	Lengths (approx.)	Capacity (approx.)
Ureter	10 in. (25 cm)	—
Bladder	—	500 mL
Male urethra	8 in. (20 cm)	—
Penile	6 in. (15.7 cm)	—
Membranous	0.5 in. (1.25 cm)	—
Prostatic	1.25 in. (3 cm)	—
Female urethra	1.5 in. (3.8 cm)	—

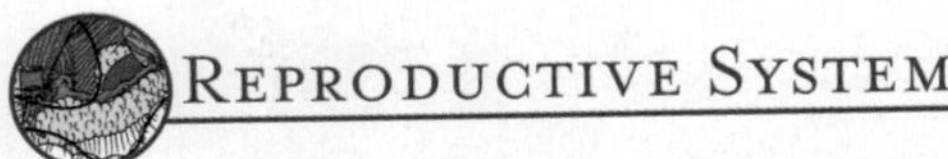

Reproductive System

Table V Dimensions

Organ	Dimensions (approx.)
Male	
Testis	2 × 1 in. (5 × 2.5 cm)
Vas deferens	18 in. (45 cm)
Penis (erect)	6 in. (15 cm)
Female	
Ovary	1.5 × 0.75 in. (4 × 2 cm)
Uterine tube	4 in. (10 cm)
Uterus	3 × 2 × 1 in. (8 × 5 × 2.5 cm)
Vagina	3 in. (8 cm)

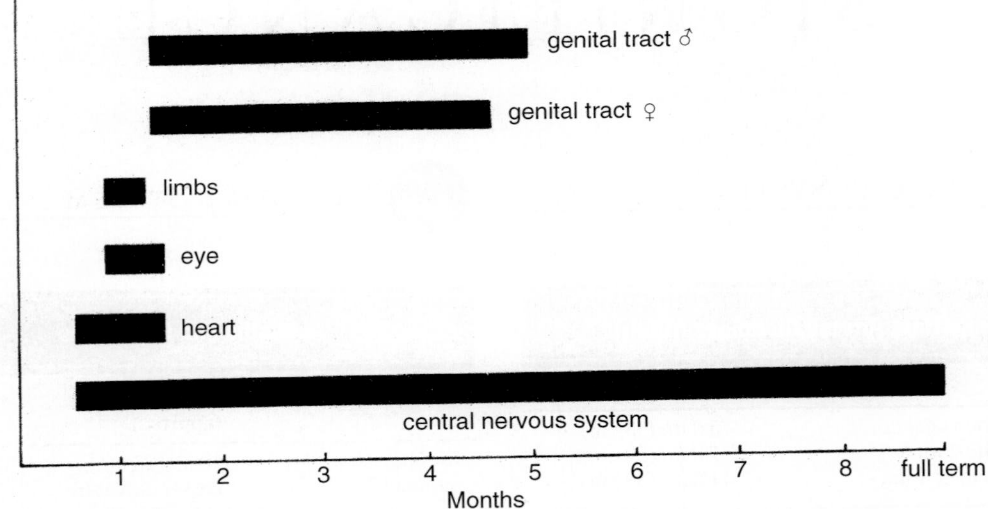

Figure 1 Critical times in the maturation of the human fetus during which mutant genes, drugs, or environmental factors may alter normal development of specific structures.

INDEX

Note: Page numbers in *italics* indicate figures. Page numbers followed by t denote tables.

Abdomen
  bones, *174*
  computed tomography, *39, 284*
  costal margin, *174*
  cross-sectional anatomy, *283–284*, 284
  endoscopic surgery, 190, *190*
  radiographic anatomy, 282, *284–286*
Abdominal aorta
  branches, 271, *272*, 273
  collateral circulation, *275*
  embolic blockage, 273
  location and description, 271, *272*
  obliteration, 274
Abdominal cavity
  anatomy, 202–298, *340*
  aorta, 271, *272*, 273
  aortic plexus, 280, *280*
  appendix, *203*, 204, 230, *231*, 232
  bile duct, 250, *250, 251*
  biliary ducts, *250*, 250–253, *251*, 288, *294, 295*
  cecum, *203*, 204, *205*, 229, *231*
  colon
    ascending, *203*, 204, *205, 232*, 232–233
    descending, *203*, 204, *205, 232*, 234
    sigmoid, *203*, 204
    transverse, *203*, 204, *205*, 233–234
  common iliac artery, *272*, 273–274
  cystic duct, 253–254
  duodenum
    anatomy, *203*, 204, *205*, 224–227
    arteries, *218, 224*, 227
    location and description, 224
    lymph drainage, 227
    mucous membrane and papillae, *225*, 227
    nerve supply, 227
    parts, *224*, 224–225, *225*, 227
    radiographic anatomy, 282, 289, *289*
    relations, 227
    veins, *221*, 227
  esophagus
    anatomy, 203, *203*, 217, *218*
    blood supply, 217, *218*
    function, 217
    lymph drainage, 217
    nerve supply, 217
    relations, 217
  external iliac artery, *272*, 274
  gallbladder
    anatomy, 203, *203, 204*, 250–251
    blood supply, 251, *252*
    function, 251
    radiographic anatomy, 289, *294, 295*
  gastroesophageal sphincter, 217
  gastrointestinal tract
    accessory organs, 246–259
    anatomy, 217–246
    blood supply, 240, 243–245
    radiographic anatomy, 282, *287–293*, 289
    venous drainage, 245, *245*
  hepatic duct, 250
  ileocecal valve, 230
  ileum
    anatomy, *203*, 204, *205, 226*, 227–228, *228*
    blood supply, 228, *230, 231*
    location and description, *226*, 227–228, *228*
    lymph drainage, 228
    nerve supply, 228
    radiographic anatomy, *287*, 289, *290*
  inferior mesenteric vein, 276
  inferior vena cava, 274
  internal iliac artery, *272*, 274
  jejunum
    anatomy, *203*, 204, *205, 226*, 227–228, *228*
    blood supply, 228, *230, 231*
    location and description, *226*, 227–228, *228*
    lymph drainage, 228
    nerve supply, 228
    radiographic anatomy, *287*, 289, *290*
  kidney
    anatomy, 205, *206*, 260, 262–264
    blood supply, *263*, 264
    coverings, 262, *263*
    location and description, 260, *262, 263*
    lymph drainage, 264
    nerve supply, 264
    radiographic anatomy, 295
    relations, 262, 264, *265*
    structure, 262, *263*, 264
  large intestine
    anatomy, *203*, 204, *205*, 229–234
    cancer, 236
    distal part, development, 345, *346*
    radiographic anatomy, 289, *291–293*
  liver
    anatomy, 203, *203, 204, 210*, 246–249
    biliary ducts, 249–253, *250, 251*
    blood supply, 249
    location and description, 246–248
    lymph drainage, 249
    nerve supply, 249
    peritoneal ligaments, 248–249
    relations, 248
  lumbar plexus, 278–279, *279*
  lymph nodes, 276, *278*
  lymph vessels, 276, 278, *278*
  pancreas, 205, *206, 256*, 256–257
  peritoneum
    anatomy, 205–214
    arrangement, 205–206, *207, 208, 209*
    cecal recesses, 208, *212*
    development, 216, *216, 218*
    duodenal recesses, 208, *212*
    functions, 209, *218*
    intersigmoid recess, 208, *212*
    intraperitoneal and retroperitoneal relationships, 206
    lesser sac, *207*, 207–208, *208, 211, 218*
    mesenteries, 207, *208, 209, 212*
    nerve supply, 209
    omenta, *204*, 206–207, *207, 208*
    paracolic gutters, *207*, 209, *213*
    peritoneal ligaments, 206, *210, 211*
    subphrenic spaces, 208–209, *213, 214*
  rectum, *203*, 204
  retroperitoneal space, 260, *261*
  small intestine
    anatomy, *203*, 204, *205*, 224–228
    versus large intestine, 246, *248*
    radiographic anatomy, *287*, 289, *290*
  spleen, 205, *206*, 259, *259*
  splenic vein, 276
  stomach
    anatomy, 203, *203, 204*, 219–220
    arteries, *218*, 220
    location and description, *219*, 219–220
    lymph drainage, 220, *222*
    nerve supply, 220, *222*
    radiographic anatomy, 282, *287, 288*
    relations, 220
    veins, 220, *221*
  superior mesenteric vein, 276
  suprarenal glands, 205, *206*, 269
  sympathetic trunk, 279–280, *280*
  ureter
    anatomy, *262*, 266
    radiographic anatomy, 295, *296–298*
  urinary tract
    anatomy, 260, 262–266
    radiographic anatomy, 295, *296–298*
Abdominal hernia, 183–186, *183–187*, 215
Abdominal nerve block, anterior, 159–160
Abdominal pain, 159, 281, *282*
Abdominal respiration, 102
Abdominal straining, muscle, 59
Abdominal superficial reflex, 26, *29*
Abdominal viscera
  arrangement, 203–205, *203–206*
  surface anatomy, 192–195, *193, 194*, 298
  traumatic injury, 58
Abdominal wall
  anatomy, 146–195
  anterior, 146–173
    arteries, 147, *158*, 161
    deep fascia, 149
    extraperitoneal fat, *155*, 159
    fascia transversalis, *155*, 157
    lymph drainage, 162–163, *163*
    muscles, 149–157, 158t
      function, 157, *157*, 158t
      nerve supply, *154*, 157, *158*, 158t
    nerve supply, 147, *154, 158*, 159, *160*
    parietal peritoneum, *155*, 159
    skin, 146
    superficial fascia, *147*, 147–149
    veins, 147, *158*, 162, *162*
  development, 177–178, *179*
  epididymis
    anatomy, *166*, 169, 191
    blood supply, 169
    lymph drainage, *167*, 169
  external oblique, *148, 149*, 150, 152, *153*, 158t
  fascial lining, 177, *178*
  general appearance, 149
  gunshot wounds, 187
  iliacus, *176*, 176–177, 177t
  ilium, 173–174, *175*
  inguinal canal
    anatomy, 163–164
    development, 165–167, *168*
    function, 164
    mechanics, 164, *165*
    walls, 164
  internal oblique, *148, 149*, 152, *153*, 158t
  labia majora, 173
  lines and planes, *156*, 192
  lumbar vertebrae, 173, *174, 175*
  paracentesis, *188*, 188–190

Abdominal wall *(continued)*
peritoneal lavage, *189*, 189–190, *190*
peritoneal lining, 177, *178*
posterior, *231*
arteries, 271, *272*, 274
bones, *176*
lymphatics, 276, 278, *278*
muscles, 174–177, *176*, 177t
nerves, 278–280, *279*, *280*
structure, 173–177, *174*
veins, *272*, 274–276
psoas major, 174, *176*, 177t
pyramidalis, *149*, 154, 158t
quadrants, *156*, 192
quadratus lumborum, 175–176, *176*, 177t
rectus abdominis, *149*, *151*, 152, 154, *155*, 158t, 191–192
rectus sheath, *148*, *149*, 154, *155*, 156, *157*
ribs, twelfth pair, 173
scrotum
anatomy, *166*, 167–169, 191
clinical conditions, 169–170
lymph drainage, *167*, 169
spermatic cord, 164–165, *166*
coverings, 165, *168*
structures, 164–165, *167*, *168*
stab wounds, 186–187
surface anatomy, 191–195
surface landmarks, 191–192
surgical incisions, 146, 187–188
testis
anatomy, *166*, 169, 191
blood supply, 169
clinical conditions, 169–170
descent, 166–167, *168*
development, 171–172, *172*
lymph drainage, 165, *167*, 169
maldescent, *170*
transversus, *148*, 152, *153*, *154*, 158t
umbilicus
anatomy, 191
congenital defects, *181*, 181–182
development, 178, *180*
Abdominothoracic incision, 188
Abdominothoracic rhythm, 159
Abducent nerve, 758t
anatomy, *695*, 698, 753, *761*
integrity testing, 769–770
paralysis, 770
Abduction, defined, 3
Abductor digiti minimi, 506t, 622t
Abductor hallucis, 622t
Abductor pollicis brevis, 506t
Abductor pollicus longus, 498t, 499
stenosing synovitis, 498
tendon, 533, 535
Abscess
perianal, 396, *399*
peritonsillar, 793, *794*
Accessory bile duct, 254, *255*
Accessory duct of pancreas, 257
Accessory nerve, 758t
anatomy, 677, 767–768, *768*
cranial root, 767
injury, 458
integrity testing, 770
spinal root, *456*, *457*, 458, 768, 769
Accessory phrenic nerve, 448, 771
Accessory vein, 571
Accommodation reflex, 706
Acetabular fossa, 559
Acetabular labrum, 587
Acetabular ligament, transverse, 587, 588–589
Acetabular notch, 559, 587
Acetabulum, 316, 318, 555, 559
Acetylcholine, 26
Achalasia, of cardia, 218
Achilles tendon reflex, 26, *29*, 659
Acromioclavicular joint
anatomy, *460*, 460–461
dislocation, 461
injury, 461
movements, 461, *461*
Acromioclavicular ligament, 461
Acromion, 434, 531
Addison's disease, 269–270
Adduction
defined, 3
thumb, 502
Adductor brevis, 584t
Adductor canal, *556*, 575, 654
Adductor hallucis, 622t
Adductor hiatus, 585
Adductor longus, 584t
Adductor magnus, 583, 584t, 587, 589t, 656
Adductor muscles
and cerebral palsy, 587
lower limb, *577*
Adductor pollicis, 506t
Adductor tubercle, 561, 656
Adenohypophysis, 815
Adenoids, 793, *794*
Adventitious bursae, 643
Afferent fibers, 21, *25*
parasympathetic system, 29–30
sympathetic system, 27–28, *30*
Afferent glomerular arterioles, 264
Afferent lymph node, 21
Age
effects on structure, 36, 37
pelvic joint changes, 329
thorax changes, 65
Airway
compromised, 812–814, *813*, *814*
distances, 814, 814t, 899t
Ala nasi, 795
Alar folds, 630
Alar ligament, 858
Allen test, 536
Alveolar arch, 673
Alveolar ducts, *92*, 94
Alveolar nerve, 762
Alveolar process, 673
Alveolar sacs, *92*, 94, *96*
Alveoli, *92*, 99
Amelia, 521
Ampulla
breast, 427
rectal, 341
semicircular canal, 714
uterine tube, 363
vas deferens, 352
of Vater, 250, *251*
Anal canal
anatomy, 388–394
blood supply, *392*, 394
development, 238, *392*, 397
location and description, 388–389, *390–391*
lymph drainage, *392*, 394
cancer and, 397
muscle coat, *391*, 393
nerve supply, 394
structure, 389, *391–393*, 393
Anal fissure, 396, *399*
Anal fistula, 396, *399*
Anal sphincters, *391*, *393*, 393–394, 410t
Anal triangle, 388, *389*, *390*, 419
Anal valves, 389, 396
Anastomosis, 18, *20*
Anatomic end artery, 18, *20*
Anatomic position, 2, *3*
"Anatomic snuffbox," 498, 533, 535
Anatomic terms, descriptive, 2–4, *3–5*
Anconeus, 498t
Anesthesia. *See also* Nerve block
caudal, 326, 873
spinal, sympathetic nervous system and, 128
Aneurysm, aortic, 126, 260, 273
Angina, Ludwig's, 746
Angina pectoris, 115
Angiography, coronary, 136–137, *139*
Angle of Louis, 47, *48*, 64, 523
Ankle
anatomy, *612*, *657*, 657–658, *658*
anterior aspect, *609*, *612*, *613*, 618–619, *658*
great saphenous vein cutdown at, 571, *572*
lateral aspect, *657*
medial aspect, *657*
posterior aspect, *609*, *610*, 619, *658*
radiographic anatomy
anteroposterior, *649*
lateral, *650*
retinacula, 606, 609
Ankle jerk, 26, *29*, 659
Ankle joint
anatomy, 634–637
articulation, 634
capsule, 634
coronal section, *636*
fracture dislocations, 637
lateral aspect, *635*
ligaments, 634–635
medial aspect, *635*
movements, 635, 637
nerve supply, 635
posterior aspect, *636*
relations, *609*, 637
sprains, 637
stability, 637
synovial membrane, 635
type, 634
Annulus fibrosus, 858
Anococcygeal body, 318, 388
Anorectal canal, 345, *346*, 397
Anorectal foreign body, 396–397
Anorectal ring, 394, 396
Anosmia, 769
Ansa subclavia, 773
Antagonist, muscle, 10, *11*
Anterior, defined, 2
Anterior abdominal wall. *See* Abdominal wall, anterior
Anterior axillary fold, 530
Anterior axillary line, 68
Anterior axillary nodes, 126, 451, *453*
Anterior cardiac vein, *114*, 116
Anterior cecal artery, 244
Anterior cerebral artery, 750
Anterior cervical lymph nodes, 755
Anterior chamber of eye, 704
Anterior chest wall, 64–65, *66*, *67*, *69*
Anterior circumflex humeral artery, 446, 458
Anterior clinoid process, 675
Anterior cranial fossa, 675, 679
Anterior cruciate ligament, 629, 632, *633*
Anterior ethmoidal nerve, 675, 698, 760
Anterior fold, 66
Anterior fontanelle, 679, *680*, 824, *838*
Anterior inferior iliac spine, 555
Anterior intercondylar area, 593
Anterior intercostal arteries, 53, *53*, *54*, 63
Anterior intercostal membrane, 53, *53*
Anterior intercostal veins, 53, *55*
Anterior internodal pathway, 113
Anterior interosseous artery, 487, 498
Anterior interosseous nerve, 493
Anterior jugular vein, 739, *739*, 752
Anterior longitudinal ligament, 858–859
Anterior malleolar fold, 711
Anterior mediastinum, 80
Anterior nasal aperture, 670
Anterior pelvic wall, 310, *315*, *316*
Anterior ramus, 22
Anterior root, 21, *23*, *25*
Anterior sacroiliac ligament, 329
Anterior spinal artery, 870

Anterior superior alveolar nerve, 762
Anterior superior iliac spine, 191, 318, 330, 555, 644
Anterior talofibular ligament, 634
Anterior tibial artery, 612, 614
Anterior triangle, neck, *743,* 747, 842
Anterior vagal trunk, 220, *222*
Anular ligament, 711
Anular pancreas, 258, *258*
Anulus ovalis, 107, 118
Anus, 388, 419
  imperforate, 397
Aorta
  abdominal
    branches, 271, *272,* 273
    collateral circulation, *275*
    embolic blockage, 273
    location and description, 271, *272*
    obliteration, 274
  arch, 73, 125
  ascending, 124
  coarctation, *109,* 126
  descending, 125–126
  development, 119, *122*
  sinuses, 124
  surface markings, 195, *272*
  thoracic, 123–126, *125*
Aortic aneurysm, 126, 260, 273
Aortic knuckle, 134
Aortic lymph nodes, 276
Aortic opening, diaphragm, 63
Aortic plexus, 280, *280*
Aortic sinus, 111
Aortic valve, *89, 110,* 111, 117, 119
Aortic vestibule, 110, 119
Aorticopulmonary septum, spiral, 118
Apex
  of heart, 72, *106,* 107
  of lung, 68, 72, *84,* 92
Apex beat, 66
Apical axillary nodes, 451, *453*
Apical ligament, 858
Aponeurosis, 8, *9*
Appendices epiploicae, 246
Appendicitis, 234–236
Appendicular artery, 244
Appendix, *231*
  anatomy, *203,* 204, 230, *231,* 232
  anomalies, 238, *241*
  development, 237, *241*
  infection, 234
  pelvic, 345
  perforation, 234
  position, 234
  surface markings, 195
  tip, positions, 232
  undescended, 238
Aqueous humor, 704
Arachnoid granulations, 675, 683
Arachnoid mater
  brain, 683–685
  spinal cord, 871
Arachnoid villi, 683, 874
Arches of foot
  anatomy, 639–640, *640*
  bones, *640,* 640–641
  clinical problems, 642
  mechanisms of support, *641,* 641–642
Arcuate arteries, 264, 629
Arcuate eminence, 676
Arcuate ligaments, 58, 174, 175
Arcuate line, 173
Areola, 427, 432, 533
Areolar glands, 427, 533
Arm. *See also* Forearm; Upper arm
  bones, 432, 434–437
  cutaneous nerves, 449, 450t, 466, 475
Arrector pili, 6, *6*
Arteria princeps pollicis, 504
Arteria radialis indicis, 504
Arteriography, cerebral, 824, *830–833*
Arteriole, 18, *20*
Arteriovenous anastomosis, 18, *20*
Artery, branches, 18, *20*
Arthritis
  gonococcal, 17
  osteoarthritis, 469, 592
  tuberculous, 17
Arthrocentesis, elbow joint, 511
Arthroscopy, knee joint, 632
Articular disc, 13
Articular processes, 853
Articular surface, 15
Articular tubercle, 673
Articularis genus, 630
Arytenoid, transverse, 806t
Arytenoid cartilage, 802
Asbestosis, 103
Ascending aorta, 124
Ascending colon
  anatomy, 195, *203,* 204, *205, 232,* 232–233
  development, 237
Ascending lumbar vein, 123
Ascending pharyngeal artery, 749
Ascites, 215
Asphyxia, traumatic, 117
Asthma, bronchial, 103
Atlantoaxial joints, *857,* 858
Atlanto-occipital joints, *857,* 857–858
Atlanto-occipital membrane, 858
Atlas
  anatomy, 855, *856*
  fracture, 862, *863*
Atrial septal defect, *109,* 122
Atrial septum, 107, 111
Atrioventricular bundle, 112
Atrioventricular canal, 118
Atrioventricular node, 113
Atrioventricular orifice, right, 107
Atrioventricular valves, 121
Atrium
  development, 118, *121*
  left, *107,* 109–110, *111*
    openings into, *107,* 110
  right, *106,* 107–108, *108*
    fetal remnants, 107–108, *108, 109*
    openings into, 107, *108*
Auditory area, 687
Auditory meatus
  external, 673, 706, 837
  internal, 677
Auditory ossicles
  anatomy, *708, 709,* 711
  movements, 712, *713*
  muscles, 711, 711t
Auditory tube, 673, 712, 790
Auricle, 706, *707,* 837
Auricular appendages, 118
Auricular artery, posterior, 725, 750
Auricular nerve, great, 736, 771, 771t
Auricular vein, posterior, 725
Auriculotemporal nerve, 725, 729, 762
Auscultation
  chest, 68
  heart valves, 117
Auscultatory triangle, 865
Automatic reflex bladder, 351, *353*
Autonomic nerves
  pelvic wall, 327
  testicular, 165
Autonomic nervous system, 21, 24, 26–30, *30–31*
Autonomous bladder, 351, *353*
Axilla
  anatomy, 437, *439–453,* 443–454, 530
  brachial plexus branches in, *448,* 448–450, *449*
  contents, 444–451
  key muscles, 443–444
  radial nerve injury in, 537, 539, *539*
  suspensory ligament, 444
  walls, 437, *439–441, 443–444*
Axillary artery
  anatomy, 444–446, *445*
  arterial anastomosis and ligation, 458
Axillary folds, 66, 530
Axillary line, 68
Axillary lymph nodes
  anatomy, 126, 450–451, *453,* 505
  examination, 454
Axillary nerve, 450, 450t
  anatomy, 458
  branches, *452,* 458
  injury, 458, 537
Axillary sheath, 444, 446, 747
Axillary tail, 427
Axillary vein
  anatomy, *445,* 446
  spontaneous thrombosis, *445,* 446
Axis
  anatomy, 855, *856*
  fracture, 862, *863*
Axon, 21
Azygos veins, 123, *124*

Back
  anatomy, 852–885
  arteries, 865
  auscultatory triangle, 865
  bones, 454, *455*
  deep fascia, 865
  deep muscles, *864,* 864–865
  examination, 855
  lumbar triangle, 865
  lymph drainage, 867
  midline structures, 880–881, *894*
  muscles, 441t, 442t, 454, *456, 457, 864,* 864–865
  muscular triangles, 865
  nerve supply, *456, 457,* 458, 867
  postvertebral muscles, *864,* 864–865
  radiographic anatomy, 876, 880
  skin, 454
  spinal cord, 867, 870–874. *See also* Spinal cord
  splenius, 865
  superficial part, 454, 458
  surface anatomy, *532,* 880–881, *894*
  surface markings, *853*
  veins, 865–866, *866*
  vertebral column, 852–863. *See also* Vertebral column
Baker's cyst, 604
Ball-and-socket joint, 15, *16*
Barium enema, 377, 381
Barrel chest, 103
Basic anatomy, defined, 2
Basilar artery, 751
Basilar membrane, 714, 715
Basilic vein, 468, 482, 499, 535
  catheterization, 469
Basivertebral veins, 866
Bell's palsy, 732
Belly, muscle, 8, *9*
Bennett's fracture, 481
Biceps brachii
  long head, 475t
  osteoarthritis of shoulder joint and, 469
  short head, 475t
Biceps brachii tendon reflex, 26, *29,* 536
Biceps femoris, 587, 589t
Biceps tendon, 533, 656
Bicipital aponeurosis, 533
Bicipital groove, 435
Bicipital tuberosity, 478
Bifid ureter, 268, *271*
Bifurcated ligament, 638

Bile duct
  accessory, 254, *255*
  anatomy, *226*, 250, *250*, *251*
  cancer, 257
  entrance into duodenum, 258
Biliary apparatus, extrahepatic, development, *240*
Biliary atresia, 253, *255*
Biliary colic, 251–252
Biliary ducts
  anatomy, 249–253, *250*, *251*
  congenital anomalies, 253–254, *255*
  development, 253–254
  radiographic anatomy, 289, *294*, 295, *295*
Bipennate muscle, 10, *10*
Bitemporal hemianopia, 769
Bladder. *See* Urinary bladder
"Blind spot," 704
Blood transfusion, 468
Blood vessels
  anatomy, 18, *19*, *20*
  disease, 19
Boil, 7
Bone
  anatomy, *32*, 32–35, *33*
  cancellous, 32
  classification, 32–34, *33*, 34t
  compact, 32
  development, 35
  flat, *33*, 33
  fracture, 35
  irregular, *33*, 33–34
  long, *33*, 33
  regional classification, 34t
  sesamoid, *33*, 34
  short, 33
  surface markings, 34, 34t
Bone marrow, 33, 34–35
Bony labyrinth, *710*, 714
Bony pelvis, 308, 377, *379–381*
Boutonnière deformity, 509, *510*
Bowel. *See* Intestine
Brachial artery
  anatomy, 469, *471*, 472, *472*
  palpation, 533
Brachial plexus, 23, *24*
  anatomy, *446–449*, 446–450, 771–772, *772*
  branches, *447–449*, 447–450, 450t
  compression, 772
  cords, *447*, 447–448
  development, 521
  injury, *536*, 536–537, 772
  nerve block, 446, 772
  roots, 447, *447*, 843
  trunks, 447, *447*, 843
Brachialis, 475t
Brachiocephalic artery, 72, 125
Brachiocephalic vein, 73, 123, *124*
Brachioradialis, 495t
Brachioradialis tendon reflex, 26, *29*, 536
Brachydactyly, 522, *522*
Brain
  arachnoid mater, 683–685
  arteries, *689*, 690
  arteriography, 824, *830–833*
  cerebrum, *685*, 687, *688*
  computed tomography, 824, *834*
  cranial meninges, *681*, 681–685
  cranial nerves. *See* Cranial nerves
  diencephalon, *685*, 687, *689*
  dura mater, *681*, 681–683
  herniation, after lumbar puncture, 873
  hindbrain, *685*, 689–690
  injury, 690
  magnetic resonance imaging, 824, *835–837*
  midbrain, *685*, 689
  parts, 687–691
  pia mater, 685
  veins, 690, 752
  venous blood sinuses, 686–687, 752
  ventricles, *685*, 690
Brainstem, *683*
Breast. *See also* Nipple
  anatomy, 531, 533
  blood supply, 427
  cancer, 431–432
  development, *429*, 432
  examination, 430, *431*
  fibrous septa, 431
  location and description, 427, *428*
  lymph drainage, 427, *430*, 431–432
  in postmenopausal women, 427
  in pregnancy, 427, *429*
  at puberty, 427
  in young women, 427
Broca's area, 687
Bronchi, *92*, *812*
  anatomy, *87*, 88, *89*, *92*, *93*
  constriction, 103
  segmental (tertiary), 94
Bronchial artery, 126
Bronchial asthma, 103
Bronchioles, *92*, 94
  respiratory, 94
  terminal, 94, 99
Bronchitis, 89
Bronchogenic carcinoma, 103
Bronchography, 135, *139*
Bronchomediastinal lymph trunk, 98, 127
Bronchopulmonary nodes, 98
Bronchopulmonary segments, *92*, 94, *95*, 96, *96*, *97*
Bronchoscopy, 89
Buccal nerve, 729, 762
Buccal nodes, 754
Buccinator, 721t, 731
Buccopharyngeal membrane, 734, 776
Buck's fascia, 405
Bulb
  of penis, 402
  of vestibule, 408
Bulbar ridges, 118
Bulbospongiosus, 402, 405, 408–409, 410t
Bulbourethral glands, 406
Bulbus cordis, 118
Bulla ethmoidalis, 797
Bundle of His. *See* Atrioventricular bundle
Bunion, 643
Burn, skin, 7
BURP maneuver, 808
Bursae
  anatomy, 17, *18*
  infection, 17
  trauma, 17
Buttock
  fascia, 553, 555
  fold, 650
  skin, 551

Calcaneal spur, 619
Calcaneocuboid joint, 637–638
Calcaneofibular ligament, 635
Calcaneovalgus, 660
Calcaneum
  anatomy, 596, *597–599*, 657
  fractures, *600*
Calcarine sulcus, 687
Calculi
  submandibular gland, 789
  ureteric, 351
Calf, lateral cutaneous nerve of, 604, 609, 615
Calyces, 262, *263*, 294, *296–298*
Canaliculus lacrimalis, 691, 694
Cancellous bone, 32
Cancer. *See specific anatomy*
Capillary, 18, *20*
  lymph, 21
Capitate bone, 480
Capitulum, 435
Capsule, joint, 13
Carbuncle, 7
Cardia, achalasia of, 218
Cardiac conducting system, 12, 111–113, *112*
Cardiac cycle, 117
Cardiac muscle, 12
Cardiac notch, 68, 92
Cardiac orifice, 219, 220
Cardiac pain, 116
Cardiac plexus, 116
Cardiac tamponade, 105
Cardiac veins, *114*, 116
Cardioesophageal junction, 193
Cardiophrenic angles, 134
Cardiopulmonary resuscitation, 117–118
Carina, 87, 89
Carotid artery
  common, 125, 747
    left, 73
  external, 748–749
  internal, 750
    arteriography, *830–833*
    arteriosclerosis, 750
Carotid body, 747
Carotid canal, 673, 676
Carotid nerve, internal, 773
Carotid pulse, 748
Carotid sheath, 747, 842
Carotid sinus, 747
Carotid sinus hypersensitivity, 747
Carotid triangle, 747
Carpal tunnel, 480, 484, *484*, 485
Carpal tunnel syndrome, 500, 540
Carpometacarpal joint, 516
Carrying angle, 510
Cartilage, types, 35–36
Cartilaginous joint, 13, *14*
Caruncula lacrimalis, 691
Catheterization
  of female, 412
  of male, 407
  umbilical vessels, *182*, 182–183
Cauda equina, 21, *24*, 867, *869*, *876*
Caudal anesthesia, 326, 873
Caval obstruction, 123, 162, *162*
Caval opening, diaphragm, 63
Cavernous sinus, 686–687
  structures associated with, 687
  thrombosis, 730
Cecal artery, 244
Cecal recesses, 208, *212*
Cecostomy, 236
Cecum
  anatomy, *203*, 204, *205*, 229, 231, *231*
  development, 237, *241*
  surface markings, 193
  trauma, 236
  undescended, 238
Celiac artery, 240, 243, *244*
Celiac plexus, 280, *280*
Central artery of retina, 698, 704
Central axillary nodes, 451, *453*
Central canal, 690
Central nervous system, 21, *23–25*
Central scotoma, 769
Central sulcus, 687
Central tendon, 58
Central vein, 248
Cephalic vein, 468, 482, 499, 535
  catheterization, 469
Cerebellar peduncles, 690
Cerebellum, 676, 690
Cerebral aqueduct, 689, 690
Cerebral arteries, 750–751
Cerebral arteriography, 824, *830–833*
Cerebral hemispheres, 687
Cerebral hemorrhage, 686
Cerebral palsy, 587

Cerebral peduncles, 689
Cerebral vein
great, 690
internal, 690
superior, 686
Cerebrospinal fluid, 684, 874
Cerebrum, *685,* 687, *688*
Cervical artery, 458, 751
Cervical canal, 365
Cervical disc herniation, 868, *877*
Cervical fascia
deep, 743–747
clinical significance, 744, 746–747
investing layer, 744
pretracheal layer, 744
prevertebral layer, 744, *745*
superficial, 737
Cervical ganglion, 773
Cervical ligaments, *366,* 367, *367,* 368, 747
Cervical lymph nodes
anterior, 755
clinical significance, 756
deep, 746, 756–757, 781
examination, 757
metastasis, 757
regional, 754–755
superficial, 739, 755
Cervical nerves, 21, *24,* 771, 771t
Cervical plexus, 23, *24,* 771, 771t
Cervical rib, 50, 857
Cervical root syndromes, 872t
Cervical tuberculous osteomyelitis, 793
Cervical vertebra
anatomy, 739, 855, *856,* 880, *883–885, 893, 894*
fracture, 862, *863*
seventh, 66, 531, 841, 855, *856,* 880
spinous processes, 530–531, *532*
Cervix, 321, 364
Cesarean section, emergency, 368–369
Chassaignac tubercle, 880
Check ligament, lateral, 702
Cheek muscles, 731
Chest
anterior surface, 523, *529–531,* 530
barrel, 103
clinical examination, 68
flail, 58
posterior surface, 530–531, *532*
surface anatomy, *531*
traumatic injury, 58
Chest cavity, 78
Chest pain, 55, 57, 129–130
Chest wall
anterior, 64–65, *66, 67, 69*
joints, 51
posterior, 66, *67, 69, 70*
skin innervation, referred pain and, 55
Chewing movements, lateral, 720
Chief cells, 822
Child, uterus in, 368
Childbirth, perineal injury during, 412
Choanae, 673, 796
Cholecystectomy, 252
Cholecystitis, acute, 252
Cholecystokinin, 251
Choledochal cyst, congenital, 254, *255*
Chorda tympani, 712, 714, 765
Chorda tympani nerve, 762
Chordae tendineae, 108, 121
Chordee, 413
Choroid, 704
Choroid plexus, 684, 690, 874
Chyme, 219
Ciliary arteries, 698
Ciliary body, 704
Ciliary ganglia, 28, *696,* 698, 757, 774
Ciliary glands, 691
Ciliary muscle, 694t, 702, 704
Ciliary nerve, 698, 757, 760
Ciliary processes, 704
Ciliary ring, 704
Ciliary striae, 704
Circle of Willis, 690, 751
Circulation, collateral, 19
Circumcision, 407
Circumduction, defined, 4
Circumflex artery, 113
Circumflex femoral artery, 585–586
Circumflex humeral artery, 446, 458
Circumflex iliac artery
deep, *272,* 274, *328*
superficial, 580
Circumflex iliac vein, superficial, 571
Circumvallate papillae, 781
Cirrhosis, 129
Cisterna chyli, 126, 276
Claudication, intermittent, 659
Clavicle, 65, 523
anatomy, 432, *433, 434*
compression of nerves and blood vessels by, 433
fractures, 433
Clavipectoral fascia, 443
Clawfoot, 642
Cleft lip, *733, 734,* 735, *735*
Cleft palate, *735,* 785, *788*
Clinical anatomy, defined, 2
Clinoid process
anterior, 675
posterior, 676
Clitoris
anatomy, 408, 419
body, 408, *408*
erection, 409
glans, 408
root, 408, *408*
Cloaca, 397
Cloacal membrane, 397
Club foot, 644, *645*
Coarctation of the aorta, *109,* 126
Coccygeal nerves, 21, *24*
Coccygeus, 318–319, *320,* 324t
Coccyx
anatomy, 315, *316,* 330, 417, 645, 680, 856, 881
fractures, 321–322
Cochlea
anatomy, 714
duct, 715
Cochlear nerve, 715, 758t, 765, *766*
Colic
biliary, 251–252
renal, 267
Colic artery, 244
Colic flexure
left, 233, 238
right, 232
Collateral arteries, ulnar, 472, *474,* 476
Collateral circulation, 19
Collateral ligaments, 629, 632, 654, 656
Colles' fascia, 148, 400, *401*
Colles' fracture, 480, *481*
Colliculi, 689
Colon
anomalies, 238
ascending
anatomy, 195, *203,* 204, *205, 232,* 232–233
development, 237
descending
anatomy, 195, *203,* 204, *205, 232,* 234
development, 238
diverticulosis, 236, *236*
sigmoid
anatomy, *203,* 204, 338
cancer, 339
development, 238
radiographic anatomy, 377, 381
variation in length and location, 339
transverse
anatomy, 195, *203,* 204, *205,* 233–234
development, 237
trauma, 236
Colonoscopy, 234, *235,* 339
Colostomy, 236, 339
Colostrum, 427
Common carotid artery, 125, 747
left, 73
Common hepatic duct, 250
Common iliac artery, *272,* 273–274, 327
Common interosseous artery, 487
Common peroneal nerve, 656, 657
anatomy, 587, 604
branches, *567,* 604
injury, 660
sural communicating branch, 604
tibial portion, 327t
Communicating artery, posterior, 750
Compact bone, 32
Compartment syndrome
forearm, 483
leg, 614
Compressor nasi, 721t
Computed tomography, 37–38
abdomen, *39, 284*
brain, 824, *834*
pelvis, 377, *378*
skull, 824, *834*
thorax, *132,* 137
vertebral column, 876, 880, *881–882*
Conchae, 670
Conducting system of heart, 12, 111–113, *112*
atrioventricular bundle, 112
atrioventricular node, 112
failure, 113
internodal pathways, *112,* 112–113
sinuatrial node, 112
Condyloid joint, 14, *16*
Conjoint tendon, 152, *152*
Conjunctiva, 691
Conjunctival sac, 691
Consensual light reflex, 706
Constrictor muscles, pharynx, *783,* 789, *791,* 792t
Contralateral, defined, 3
Conus arteriosus, 119
Conus artery, 113
Copula, 781, 819
Coracoacromial ligament, 463
Coracobrachialis, 475t
Coracoclavicular ligament, 461
Coracohumeral ligament, 462–463
Coracoid process, 434, 531
Cornea, 704
Corniculate cartilage, 802
Cornua, of coccyx, 315, *316*
Coronal planes, 2, *3*
Coronal suture, 673
Coronary angiography, 136–137, *139*
Coronary artery, 119
anastomoses, 114, *115*
branches, 113
to conducting system, 114, *115*
left, 113, 114, 124–125
lesions, infarct location and, 115, 116t
right, 113, 114, 124
variations, 113–114, *115*
Coronary artery disease, 64, 115, 116t
Coronary bypass surgery, 572
Coronary ligament, 206, 248–249
Coronary sinus, 107
Coronoid fossa, 435
Coronoid process, 478
Corpora cavernosa, 402, 408
Corpus callosum, 687
Corpus spongiosum, 402

Corrugator supercilii, 721t
Cortex, 687, 690
Costal cartilage, *47,* 51
 identification, 68
 joints, 51
 movements, 51
Costal groove, 49, *49*
Costal margin, 64–65, 191, 523
Costal pleura, 84
Costocervical trunk, 751
Costoclavicular ligament, 459
Costodiaphragmatic recess, 72, 84
Costomediastinal recess, 84
Coxa valga, 561
Coxa vara, 561
Cranial cavity, 674
Cranial fossa
 anatomy, 675–677
 fracture, 679
Cranial meninges, *681,* 681–685
Cranial nerves, 21, *689,* 691. *See also specific nerves, e.g.,* Olfactory nerve
 clinical testing, 769–770
 organization, 757–769, 778t
Cranium, 669
Cremasteric fascia, 165, *168*
Cremasteric reflex, 279
Cretinism, 819
Cribriform fascia, 573
Cribriform plate, 675
Cricoarytenoid muscles, 806t
Cricoid cartilage, 802, 839
Cricopharyngeus, 789, *791,* 792t
Cricothyroid ligament, 805, 839
Cricothyroid muscle, 806t, *807*
Cricothyroidotomy, 813, *813*
Cricotracheal ligament, 802, 841
Crista galli, 675
Crista terminalis, 107
Cruciate anastomosis, 567
Cruciate ligament
 anatomy, 13, *15,* 858
 anterior, 629, 632, *633*
 posterior, 629, 632, *633*
Crura
 of clitoris, 408
 of penis, 402
Crus, 57
Crus cerebri, 689
Cryptorchidism, 171–172, *173*
Cubital fossa, 533
 anatomy, 476–477, *477, 478*
 contents, 477
Cubital vein, median, 482, 535
Cuboid bone, *597–599,* 599
Cuboideonavicular joint, 638
Culdocentesis, 375
Cuneate tubercle, 690
Cuneiform bones, *597–599,* 599
Cuneiform cartilage, 802
Cuneocuboid joint, 638
Cuneonavicular joint, 638
Cushing's syndrome, 269
Cutaneous nerves
 arm, 449, 450t, 466, 475
 forearm, 449, 450t, 473, 475, 500
 leg, 609, 615
 lower limb, 551, *551, 552*
 neck, 736–737, *737*
 perforating, 325, 327t
 sole of foot, *620*
 thigh, 568–570, 587
  intermediate, 569, 582
  lateral, 278, 279t, 568
  medial, 569, 582
  posterior, 325, 327t, 565–566, 605, 615
 transverse, 736
 upper limb, *27, 28,* 467, *467*
Cyst(s)
 Baker's, 604
 choledochal, congenital, 254, *255*
 kidney, 267
 mediastinal, 82
 mesenteric, 229
 ovary, 361
 sebaceous, 7
 sublingual gland, 789
 thyroglossal, *820,* 821, *821*
Cystic artery, 243, *244,* 251
Cystic duct
 anatomy, 253
 congenital anomalies, 253–254, *255*
Cystic lymph node, 251
Cystic vein, 245, 251
Cystitis, 412
Cystourethrogram, *416, 417*

Dartos muscle, 400
Decussation of the pyramids, 690
Deep, defined, 2
Deep cervical artery, 751
Deep cervical fascia, 743–747
 clinical significance, 744, 746–747
 investing layer, 744
 pretracheal layer, 744
 prevertebral layer, 744, *745*
Deep cervical lymph nodes, 746, 756–757, 781
Deep circumflex iliac artery, *272,* 274, *328*
Deep external pudendal artery, 580
Deep facial vein, 730
Deep fascia, 8, *8*
Deep infrapatellar bursa, 631
Deep inguinal lymph nodes, 573, 582
Deep palmar arch, 504, *504,* 535
Deep perineal pouch
 anatomy, 402
 female, 409
 male, 406
Deep peroneal nerve, 614, 627, 629
Deep petrosal nerve, 676
Deep plexus, 98
Deep temporal nerves, 762
Deep transverse fascia of leg, 615
Deep transverse perineal muscle, 406, 409, 410t
Deep vein thrombosis, 618
Defecation, 394
Deglutition, 795
Deltoid, 442t, 531
Deltoid tuberosity, 435
Deltopectoral triangle, 530, *531*
Dendrite, 21, 24, *25*
Dental infections, 746
Dentate nucleus, 690
Depressor anguli oris, 721t
Depressor labii inferioris, 721t
Dermatomes, 26, *27, 28*
 thoracic, 130
 upper limb, 467, *538*
Dermis, 5, *6*
Descending aorta, 125–126
Descending cervical nerve, 771, 771t
Descending colon
 anatomy, 195, *203,* 204, *205, 232,* 234
 development, 238
Descending genicular artery, 582
Detrusor muscle, 350
Diagonal artery, left, 113
Diaphragm
 action, 59
 anatomy, 57–60, *62,* 63, 65–66, 65t
 costal part, 57
 descent, *87,* 100, *101*
 development, 62
 functions, 59, 63
 hernia, 62, *63*
 nerve supply, 58
 openings, *62,* 63
 paralysis, 60, 127, 771
 penetrating injury, 60
 shape, 58
 sternal part, 57
 vertebral part, 57
Diaphragma sellae, 682, *682*
Diaphragmatic fascia, 177
Diaphragmatic pleura, 84
Diaphysis, 13, 33, 35
Diencephalon, *685,* 687, *689*
Digastric fossa, 715
Digastric muscle, 742t
Digastric triangle, 747
Digestive system. *See* Gastrointestinal system
Digital arteries, 503
Digital synovial sheaths, 501
Dilator muscles, lips, 721t, 731
Dilator nasi, 721t
Dilator pupillae of iris, 694t, 702, 704
Diploë, 33, 669
Diploic veins, 752
Diplopia, 769
Direct light reflex, 706
Dislocated joint, 17
Distal, defined, 2
Distal carpal row, 480
Distal radioulnar joint, *512,* 513
Distal tibiofibular joint, 632, 634
Diverticula, 339
 atresia and stenosis, 238, *241*
Diverticulosis, 236, *236*
Dorsal, defined, 2
Dorsal interosseous muscles, *505,* 506t, 622t
Dorsal metatarsal artery, first, 629
Dorsal nerve of penis (or clitoris), 394, *395,* 406, 409
Dorsal nucleus of vagus, 774
Dorsal scapular nerve, 450t
Dorsal tubercle, 478
Dorsal venous arch
 foot, 627, 657
 hand, 509
Dorsalis pedis artery, 625–626, 627, 629, 657
 branches, 629
 palpation, 658
Dorsiflexion, 635
Dorsum sellae, 676
Double kidney, 267–268, *270*
Double pelvis, 268, *271*
Double vagina, 376
Douglas, pouch of, 376
Dropped shoulder, 434, *435*
Ductus reuniens, 715
Ductus utriculosaccularis, 714
Ductus venosus, 249
Duodenal cap, 282, 289, *289*
Duodenal papilla, *225,* 227
 major, 250, *250,* 256, *256*
 minor, *256,* 257
Duodenal recesses, 208, *212,* 227
Duodenal ulcer, 227
Duodenojejunal flexure, 227
Duodenum
 anatomy, *203,* 204, *205,* 224–227
 arteries, *218, 224,* 227
 atresia and stenosis, 238, *241*
 development, 237, *254*
 location and description, 224
 lymph drainage, 227
 mucous membrane and papillae, *225,* 227
 nerve supply, 227
 obstruction, 258, *258*
 parts, *224,* 224–225, *225,* 227
 radiographic anatomy, 282, 289, *289*
 relations, 227
 surface markings, 193

trauma, 227
veins, *221*, 227
Dupuytren's contracture, 500
Dura mater
brain, *681*, 681–683
spinal cord, 871
Dysphagia, 793

Ear
anatomy, 706–715, *708*
external, 706, *707*
infections, 714
internal, *708*, *710*, 714–715
middle, 706, *708*, *709*, 709–714, *710*, 711t
Ectoderm, 37
Ectopic pancreas, 258
Ectopic parathyroid glands, 822
Ectopic pregnancy, 364, *364*
Ectopic thyroid tissue, 819
Ectromelia, 521, *521*, 643, *644*
Edinger-Westphal nucleus, 774
Efferent fibers, 21, *25*
parasympathetic system, 28–29, *31*
sympathetic system, 26–27, *31*
Efferent lymph node, 21
Ejaculation, after spinal cord injury, 407
Ejaculatory duct, 352, 353, *354*
Elastic cartilage, 36
Elastic ligament, 15
Elbow
anatomy, 509–510, *511*, *532*, 533
arterial anastomosis around, *474*
arthrocentesis, 511
dislocation, 511
injury, 511
movements, 510
radiographic anatomy, *524*, *525*
relations, 510
stability, 511
Ellipsoid joint, 14, *16*
Embryology, 37
Embryonic disc, 37
Emissary veins, 725, 752
Emphysema, 103
subcutaneous, 82, 102
Empyema, 85
Endocardial heart tube, 118, *119*, *120*
Endocardium, 107
Endochondral ossification, 35
Endocrine glands, in head and neck, 815–822
Endometrium, 366
Endothoracic fascia, 52, 57
Endotracheal intubation
airway distances, 814, 814t
anatomic axes, 808, *811*
reflex activity secondary to, 808
Enema, barium, 377, 381
Entoderm, 37
Epicardium, 104, 107, 118
Epicranial aponeurosis, 726
Epidermis, 4–5, *6*
Epididymis
anatomy, *166*, 169, 191, 419
blood supply, 169
lymph drainage, *167*, 169
Epigastric artery
inferior, *272*, 274, 328
superficial, 580
superior, 63, 161
Epigastric hernia, 185–186, *187*
Epigastric vein, superficial, 571
Epigastrium, 192
Epiglottis, 802
Epimysium, 8
Epiphyseal cartilage, 33
Epiphyseal plate, 35
Epiphysis, 13, 33, 35
Epiploic foramen, 206, 208
Episiotomy, *400*, 412
Epispadias, 413, *416*
Epistaxis, 798
Equinovarus, 660
Erb-Duchenne palsy, *536*, 536–537
Erectile tissue, 413
Erection, after spinal cord injury, 407
Esophageal artery, 126
Esophageal atresia, 99, *100*
Esophageal hemorrhage, 218
Esophageal hernia, sliding, 62, *63*
Esophageal opening, diaphragm, 63
Esophageal plexus, 127, 128
Esophageal varices, bleeding, 218
Esophagogastric junction, 218
Esophagoscope, 129
Esophagus
anatomy, 128, *130*, 203, *203*, 217, *218*, 795
atresia, 237
blood supply, 128, 217, *218*
carcinoma, 129
congenital short, 237
constrictions, 129, *130*
contrast visualization, *135*, 136, *137*
development, 237, *239*
function, 217
lymph drainage, 128, 217
narrow areas, 218
in neck, 795
nerve supply, 128, 217
relation to left atrium of heart, 129
relations, 217
stenosis, 237
Ethmoid, 670
Ethmoid sinus, 797, 800, *801*, 802t
Ethmoidal nerve
anterior, 675, 698, 760
posterior, 698, 760
Eversion, defined, 4
Excitor cells, 26
Expiration
forced, *87*, 102
lung changes on, 102
quiet, 102
Extension, defined, 3
Extensor carpi radialis brevis, 498t, 499
Extensor carpi radialis longus, 495t, 499
Extensor carpi ulnaris, 498t, 499
Extensor digiti minimi, 498t, 499, 535
Extensor digitorum, 498t, 499, 535
Extensor digitorum brevis, 613t, 627, 628t
Extensor digitorum longus, 612, 613t, 627, 657
Extensor expansion
foot, 612, 627
hand, 509, *510*
Extensor hallucis longus, 613t, 657
Extensor indicis, 498t, 499, 535
Extensor pollicis brevis, 498t, 499
stenosing synovitis, 498
tendon, 535
Extensor pollicis longus, 498t, 499
rupture, 498
tendon, 533
Extensor retinaculum, 8, *8*, 606
Extensor tendons, long, insertions, *494*, 502, 627
External, defined, 3
External auditory meatus, 673, 706, 837
External carotid artery, 748–749
External ear, 706, *707*
External genitalia, development, 413, *414–416*
External iliac artery, 195, *272*, 274, 328
External iliac vein, 329
External intercostal muscle, *52*, 52–53, 65t
External jugular vein, 752, 843
anatomy, 737, 739, *739*
catheterization, 738, *741*
as venous manometer, 738
visibility, 738
External laryngeal nerve, 767, 808, *809*, 818
External nasal nerve, 729, 760
External oblique muscle, *148*, *149*, 150, 152, *153*, 158t
External occipital protuberance, 673, 824, *838*, 841, 880
External os, 365
External pudendal artery, 580
External pudendal vein, 571
External sphincter, 393, 410t
External strabismus, 769
External table, 669
External urethral meatus, 405
Extradural hemorrhage, 686
Extradural space, 870
Extraperitoneal fat, *155*, 159, 354
Extraperitoneal space, 209
Extraperitoneal tissue, 206
Eye
accommodation, 705
anatomy, 699–705
aqueous humor, 704
cardinal positions, *702*
choroid, 704
ciliary body, 704
cornea, 704
iris, 704
lens, 705
pupil, 704
retina, 704
sclera, 703
structure, 702–703, *703*
suspensory ligament, 702, 705
trauma, 706
vitreous body, 705
Eyeball
coats, 703–704
contents, 704–705
extrinsic muscles, 694t, 699–702, 757
fascial sheath, 702, *703*
intrinsic muscles, 694t, 702, 757
movements, 699–702, *699–702*
Eyelashes, 691
Eyelids
anatomy, 691, *692*, *693*
movements, 691
muscles, 694t, 731

Face
anatomy, 727–735
arterial supply, *728*, 729
development, *732*, 734–735
infection, 730
lymph drainage, *730*, 730–731
sensory nerves, 727–729, *728*
skin, 727, 729
venous drainage, *728*, 730, 752–754
Facial artery, 729, 749–750, 839
Facial bones
anatomy, 669, *730*, 731
fractures, 678, *679*
Facial cleft, *733*, 735
Facial expression, muscles, 721t, *724*, 731, 735, *776*
Facial muscles
anatomy, 721t, *724*, 731, 735, *776*
paralysis, 732
Facial nerve, 758t
anatomy, 712, *728*, 732, 734, 763–765, *764*
branches, 732, 734, 765
forceps delivery and, 680
integrity testing, 770
intrapetrous part, branches, 712
Facial nerve canal, prominence, 711
Facial nodes, 754
Facial vein, *728*, 730, 752
Falciform ligament, 206, 248–249
Falciform margin, 573
False pelvis, 309, 321

Falx cerebelli, 677, 682
Falx cerebri, 675, 681, *683,* 687
Fascia, 8, *8*
 of Camper, 147, 400, *401*
 Colles', 148
 deep, 8, *8*
 of Denonvilliers, 355
 infection and, 8
 Scarpa's, 147
 superficial, 5, *6,* 8, *8*
Fascial-space infection, 508, 746
Fatty pad, 13
Felon, 508
Female genital organs, 361–377
 ovary
  blood supply, 361
  function, 361
  location and description, *358–359,* 361
  lymph drainage, 361
  nerve supply, 361
 peritoneum, 376–377
 radiographic anatomy, *369, 370,* 381, *381*
 uterine tube
  blood supply, 363
  function, 363
  location and description, *358–359,* 363, *363*
  lymph drainage, 363
  nerve supply, 363
 uterus
  after menopause, 368
  blood supply, 366
  in child, 368
  function, 366
  in labor, 368
  location and description, *363,* 364–365
  lymph drainage, 366
  nerve supply, 367
  positions, *363,* 366
  in pregnancy, 368
  relations, 365
  structure, 366
  supports, *366,* 367, *367,* 368
 vagina
  blood supply, 373
  function, 373
  location and description, *366,* 372–373
  lymph drainage, 373
  nerve supply, 373
  relations, 373
  supports, *366, 367,* 373
 visceral pelvic fascia, 376
Female genitalia, 413, *414*
Female pelvis, *309,* 312, *313, 314,* 322, *323,* 330, *342,* 369, *369, 370, 380, 381, 390–391, 418*
Female ureter, 356, *358–359*
Female urethra, 409
Female urinary bladder, 356
Female urogenital triangle, 408–411, 419, *420*
Femoral artery, 650
 anatomy, 328, 579, 580, 582
 aneurysm, 580
 branches, 580, 582
 catheterization, 582
 injury, 659
 occlusion, 567
 palpation, 658
 relations, 580
Femoral canal, 579, 580, 650
Femoral circumflex artery, 585–586
Femoral hernia, 184–185, *185, 186,* 579, 580
Femoral nerve, 650
 anatomy, 278, 279t, 582
 branches, 582, *584*
 injury, 659
Femoral ring, 579, 580
Femoral septum, 579, 580
Femoral sheath, *574,* 579, 580
Femoral triangle, *553, 556,* 575, *576,* 650, 654, *655*
Femoral vein, 579, 580, 582, 650
Femur
 anatomy, *559,* 559–561, *560*
 fractures, 561, *562, 563*
 head
  arterial supply, *569*
  blood supply, 561
  ligament, 589
  tenderness over, 561
 neck
  angle, 561
  fractures, 561, *562*
Fenestra cochleae, 711, 714
Fenestra vestibuli, 711, 714
Fetal critical periods, *890*
Fetal head, pressure from, 325–326
Fetal heart, normal, *109*
Fetal membranes, 37
Fetal remnants, right atrium, 107–108, *108, 109*
Fibrocartilage, 35–36
Fibrocystic disease, pancreas, 258
Fibrous capsule, kidney, 262
Fibrous joint, 12, *14*
Fibrous ligament, 15
Fibula
 anatomy, *593,* 595, *595*
 fractures, 596
 head, 656
Fifth metatarsal, 600
Fifth rib, *49*
Filiform papillae, 779
Finger
 congenital anomalies, *521,* 521–522, *522*
 index, movements, 517, 519
 insertions of long flexor and extensor tendons, *494,* 502
 joints, 516–517
 little
  movements, 517, 519
  opposition, 503
  short muscles, 503
 mallet, 509, *510*
 middle, movements, 517, 519
 pulp space, *507,* 508
 ring, movements, 517, 519
 trigger, 502
First dorsal metatarsal artery, 629
First intercostal nerve, 55
First metacarpal base, 535
First metatarsal, 600
First rib, 50, *50*
Fixator, muscle, 11, *11*
Flail chest, 58
Flat bone, 33, *33*
Flat foot, 642
Flexion, defined, 3
Flexor carpi radialis, 492t, 499, 533
Flexor carpi ulnaris, 492t, 499, 533
Flexor digiti minimi, 506t
Flexor digiti minimi brevis, 622t
Flexor digitorum brevis, 622t
Flexor digitorum longus, 617t, 619, 621, 622t, 657
Flexor digitorum profundus, 492t
Flexor digitorum superficialis, 492t, 499, 533
Flexor hallucis brevis, 622t
Flexor hallucis longus, 617t, 621, 622t, 657
Flexor pollicis brevis, 506t
Flexor pollicis longus, 492t, 499
Flexor retinaculum, 480, 484, *484, 485,* 606
Flexor sheaths
 fibrous, 621
 synovial, 621
Flexor tendons
 long, insertions, *494,* 501, 502
 tenosynovitis, 501
Floating rib, 49
Floating thumb, 522, *522*
Folia, 690
Follicle, hair, 5, *6*
Fontanelle
 anterior, 679, *680,* 824, *838*
 palpation, 680
 posterior, 679, *680,* 837, *838*
Foot
 anatomy, 619–629
 anterior aspect, *613, 658*
 anteroposterior radiograph, *651, 652*
 arches
  anatomy, 639–640, *640*
  bones, *640,* 640–641
  clinical problems, 642
  mechanisms of support, *641,* 641–642
 bones, 596–600
 club, 644, *645*
 dorsum
  artery, 627, 629
  dissection, *607*
  dorsal venous arch, 627, 657
  muscles, 627, 628t
  nerve supply, 629
  skin, 627
  structures, *605, 608, 628*
 flat, 642
 as functional unit, 638–643
 inversion, 638
 as lever, 638–643, *639*
 muscle attachments, *598, 599*
 posterior aspect, *658*
 propulsive action, 642–643
 sole
  arteries, 624–625
  cutaneous nerves, *620*
  deep fascia, 619, *620*
  long tendons, 619, 621, 624
  muscles, 619, *621–626,* 622t–623t
  nerves, 626–627
  skin, 619
  synovial sheaths, *624*
  veins, 626
 surface anatomy, *657,* 657–658, *658*
 surface markings, *656*
 as weight-bearer, 638–643, *639*
Foot drop, 659, *660*
Foramen cecum, 819
Foramen lacerum, 673, 676
Foramen magnum, 677
Foramen ovale, 107–108, 118, 673, 676
Foramen primum, 118
Foramen rotundum, 676
Foramen secundum, 118
Foramen spinosum, 673, 676
Foramen transversarium, 855
Forceps delivery, 680
Forearm
 anatomy, 482–499, *483*
 anterior surface, *478*
 anterior view, *488, 490, 491*
 bones, 477–478, *479*
 carpal tunnel, 484, *484,* 485
 compartment syndrome, 483
 cutaneous nerves, 449, 450t, 473, 475, 500
 extensor retinaculum, 485, *486, 487*
 fascial compartments
  anatomy, 483–499, *484*
  anterior
   arteries, 486–489
   contents, 485–495
   muscles, 486, *488–491,* 492t
   nerves, 489, 493–495
  lateral
   arteries, 495
   contents, 495
   muscles, *488, 490,* 495, 495t
   nerve supply, 495

posterior
arteries, 498
contents, 495, 498–499
muscles, 495, *496, 497,* 498t
nerve supply, 499
flexor retinaculum, 484, *484, 485*
interosseous membrane, 484
magnetic resonance imaging, *529*
posterior view, *496, 497*
pronation, 3
skin, 482–483
supination, 3–4
Foregut, *239*
Foregut arteries, 244
Foreign body
anorectal, 396–397
inhaled, 89
in nose, 798
Foreskin, 405, 413
Fossa ovalis, 107, 118
Fossa terminalis, 407
Fovea capitis, 560
Fovea centralis, 704
Fracture, 35
Frenulum, 405, 413, 734
Frey's syndrome, 787
Frontal bone, 670, 673, 731
Frontal lobe, 687
Frontal nerve, *695, 697,* 698, 760
Frontal sinus, 670, 731, 799–800, *801,* 802t, 839
Frontonasal process, 734
Functional end artery, 18, *20,* 115
Fungiform papillae, 779

Galeazzi's fracture, 480
Gallbladder, *226*
anatomy, 203, *203, 204,* 250–251
blood supply, 251, *252*
congenital anomalies, 253–254, *255*
function, 251
gangrene, 252
radiographic anatomy, 289, *294, 295*
surface markings, 192, *193*
Gallstones, 251–252
Ganglion impar, 27
Gangrene of gallbladder, 252
Gastric artery, 220, 240, *244*
Gastric pain, 223
Gastric ulcer, 223, *224*
Gastric vein, 220, 245
Gastrin, 230
Gastrocnemius, 615, 617t
Gastroduodenal artery, 243
Gastroepiploic artery, 220, 240, 243
Gastroepiploic vein, 220
Gastroesophageal sphincter, 217
Gastrointestinal system
data concerning, 899t
duplication, 238
in head and neck, 774–777
Gastrointestinal tract
accessory organs, 246–259
anatomy, 217–246
anomalies, 238, *241*
blood supply, 240, 243–245
development, 237–238, *239–243*
radiographic anatomy, 282, *287–293,* 289
venous drainage, 245, *245*
Gastroscopy, 223
Gastrosplenic omentum, 206–207
Gemellus inferior, 566t
Gemellus superior, 566t
Gender, effects on structure, 36
Genicular artery, descending, 582
Geniculate body, lateral, 757
Geniculate ganglion, 712, 764, *764*
Genioglossus, 780t
Geniohyoid, 742t
Genital fold, 413
Genital swellings, 413
Genital tubercle, 413
Genitalia. *See also* Female genital organs; Male genital organs; Urogenital triangle
external, development, 413, *414–416*
Genitofemoral nerve, 279, 279t
femoral branch, 568
genital branch, 165
Genu recurvatum, 644
Germinal epithelium, 361
Gigantism, local, 522, *522*
Glans
clitoris, 408
penis, 405
Glaucoma, 704
Glenohumeral ligaments, 462–463
Glenoid fossa, 434
Glenoid labrum, 462, *462, 463*
Glomerular arterioles, afferent, 264
Glossoepiglottic fold
lateral, 790
median, 790, 802
Glossopharyngeal nerve
anatomy, 677, 758t, *764,* 765, *766*
integrity testing, 770
Glottis, 805
Glucagon, 256
Glucocorticoids, 269
Gluteal artery
inferior, 328, 567
superior, 328, 566
Gluteal nerve, 325, 327t, 566
Gluteal region
anatomy, 551–567, 644–645, 650, *653, 654*
arteries, 566–567, *569*
bones, 555–561
foramina, *562, 564*
ligaments, *562, 564*
muscles, 562–564, *564, 565,* 566t
nerves, 565–566, *567, 568*
skin of buttock, 551
structures in, 565
surface markings, *654*
Gluteal tuberosity, 561
Gluteus maximus
anatomy, *555,* 562, 564, 566t
and bursitis, 562, 564, 566t
injections, 562, 564, 566t
Gluteus medius, 564, 566t
Gluteus minimus, 564, 566t
Goiter, retrosternal, 818
Gonads, lymph drainage, 278
Gonococcal arthritis, 17
Gooseflesh, 6
Gracile tubercle, 690
Gracilis, 584t
Grafting, skin, 7
Granular pits, 674
Gray matter, 21, 687
Gray rami communicantes, 26, 128, 279, 773
Great auricular nerve, 736, 771, 771t
Great cardiac vein, *114,* 116
Great cerebral vein, 690
Great saphenous vein
anatomy, 570, 582, 650, 654, 657
in coronary bypass surgery, 572
cutdown, 571–572, *572*
origin, *612*
Greater curvature, 219
Greater occipital nerve, 725, 736, 867
Greater omentum, 206, 213–214, 216, *217*
Greater palatine foramen, 673
Greater palatine nerve, 762
Greater peritoneal sac, 206
Greater petrosal nerve, 676, 712, 765
Greater sciatic foramina, 318, 555, *562*
Greater sciatic notch, 318, 555
Greater splanchnic nerve, 26, 128
Greater trochanter, 560, 645
Greater tuberosity, 435, 437, 531
Greater vestibular glands, 409, 419
Greater wing of sphenoid bone, 673, 676
Groin, great saphenous vein cutdown at, 571–572, *572*
Gunshot wounds, abdominal, 187
Gynecomastia, 432
Gyri, 687

Hair, 5, *6*
Hair bulb, 5–6, *6*
Hair papilla, 6
Hallux rigidus, 638
Hallux valgus, 638
Hamate bone, 480
Hand
bones
anatomy, 480, *481, 482*
injury, 481
congenital anomalies, *521,* 521–522, *522*
cupping, 519
diseases, 520
dorsal surface, *486, 487*
dorsum
dorsal venous arch, 509
long extensor tendon insertion on, 509
radial artery on, 509
sensory innervation, *538*
skin, 508–509
structures lying on, 535
venous network, 535
as functional unit, 517–519, *518, 519*
immobilization, 520
joints, 516–517
lobster, 522
making a fist, 519
outstretched, falls on, 516
palm
anatomy, 499–508
anterior view, *493, 501, 503, 504*
arteries, 503–504
carpal tunnel, 500
deep fascia, 500
fascial spaces, *507,* 508
fibrous flexor sheaths, 500–501, *501*
lymph drainage, 504–505
nerves, 505, 508
sensory innervation, *538*
skin, 499–500
structures lying in, 535
synovial flexor sheaths, 501, 502
veins, 504
positions, 517, *518*
radiographic anatomy, *525–528*
small muscles, *485,* 502, *503, 504, 505,* 506t
Hangman's fracture, 862, *863*
Hard palate, 673, 781, *783*
Head. *See also* Brain; Skull; *specific anatomy*
anatomy, 669–843
arteries, 747–751, *758*
coronal section, *671*
cross section, *823,* 824, *825, 826*
lymph drainage, 754–757
magnetic resonance imaging, *40*
muscles, 721t
parasympathetic nervous system, 774
radiographic anatomy, 824, *827–837*
scalp, 722–726
surface landmarks, 824, 837–839, *838*
sympathetic nervous system, 773
veins, 752–754
Headache, after lumbar puncture, 873
Heart
action, *110,* 117
anatomy, 72, *72,* 105–117
anterior (sternocostal) surface, 105, *106*

Heart *(continued)*
  apex, 72, *106,* 107
  arterial supply, *106,* 112–113, *114*
    anastomoses, 114, *115*
    to conducting system, 114, *115*
    coronary arteries, 113–114, *114, 115*
    variations, 113–114, *115*
  atrium
    left, *107,* 109–110, *111*
      openings into, *107,* 110
    right, *106,* 107–108, *108*
      fetal remnants, 107–108, *108, 109*
      openings into, 107, *108*
  base (posterior surface), 105–106, *107*
  borders, *106,* 107
  chambers, 107–111
  conducting system, 111–113, *112*
    atrioventricular bundle, 112
    atrioventricular node, 112
    failure, 113
    internodal pathways, *112,* 112–113
    sinuatrial node, 112
  congenital anomalies, *109,* 122–123
  development, 118–121, *119–122*
  diaphragmatic surface, 105
  enlargement, 72
  inferior border, 72
  left border, 72
  nerve supply, 116
  position, 72
  right border, 72
  skeleton, *110,* 111
  structure, *110,* 111
  superior border, 72
  surface markings, *72*
  venous drainage, *114,* 116
  ventricle
    left, *110,* 110–111
    right, *108,* 108–109, *110*
Heart murmurs, 117
Heart tube, 118, *119, 120*
Heart valves
  auscultation, 117
  development, 119
  disease, 117
  position, *89*
  surface anatomy, *89,* 117
Hematemesis, 129
Hemianopia, 769
Hemiazygos veins, 123, *124*
Hemopneumothorax, 85
Hemorrhage
  after intercostal nerve block, 56
  esophageal, 218
  intracranial, 686
  scalp, 726
Hemorrhoids
  external, 396, *398*
  internal, 344, 395–396, *398*
  in pregnancy, 368
Hepatic artery, 243, *244*
Hepatic duct, 250
Hepatopancreatic ampulla, 250, *250*
Hernia
  abdominal, 183–186, *183–187,* 215
  diaphragmatic, 62, *63*
  epigastric, 185–186, *187*
  esophageal, sliding, 62, *63*
  femoral, 184–185, *185, 186,* 579, 580
  incisional, 186
  inguinal, 170, *170*
    direct, 184, *184, 185*
    indirect, 183–184, *184*
  internal, 186
  irreducible, 580
  linea semilunaris, 186
  lumbar, 186
  paraesophageal, 62, *63*
  spigelian, 186
  strangulated, 580
  umbilical, 185, *187*
Herniation
  brain, after lumbar puncture, 873
  cervical disc, 868, *877*
  intervertebral disc, 867–868, *877*
  lumbar disc, 868, *877*
  nucleus pulposus, 868, *877*
Herpes zoster, 55
Hiatus semilunaris, 797
Hiccup, 60
Hilton's law, 16
Hilum, 260
Hindbrain, *685,* 689–690
Hindgut, *239*
Hindgut artery, 245, 345
Hinge joint, 13, *16*
Hip bone
  anatomy, *311,* 316, 318, 555, *557, 558,* 559
  congenital dislocation, 643–644, *644*
  internal aspect, *175*
Hip joint
  anatomy, 587–590
  anteroposterior radiograph, *645*
  arthritis, 561, 592
  articular surfaces, *569*
  articulation, 587
  capsule, 587–588
  dislocation, 591
  ligaments, 588–589
  movements, 589–590
  nerve supply, 589
  referred pain from, 591
  relations, 590
  stability, 591–592
  synovial membrane, 589
  type, 587
Hirschsprung disease, 345, *347*
Homonymous hemianopia, 769
Hook of the hamate bone, 533
Horizontal fissure, lung, 94
Horizontal planes, 2–3, *3*
Horizontal plates, palatine bones, 673
Horner's syndrome, 773–774
Horseshoe kidney, 267, *270*
Humeral artery, circumflex, 446, 458
Humeral head fractures, 437, *438*
Humeral ligament, transverse, 462
Humeral shaft fractures, 437, *438*
Humeral-scapular mechanism, 465, *466*
Humerus
  anatomy, 435, *436,* 437
  fractures, 437, *438*
  scapula and, muscles connecting, 442t
Hyaline cartilage, 35
Hyaloid canal, 705
Hydrocele, 170, *170, 171*
Hydropneumothorax, 85
Hymen
  anatomy, 372, 409–410, *411*
  imperforate, 376
Hyoglossus, 780t
Hyoid bone, *716,* 739, 839
Hypertension, portal, 129, 246
Hypogastric plexus
  inferior, 327
  superior, 280, *280,* 327
Hypoglossal canal, 674, 677
Hypoglossal nerve, 758t, 779
  anatomy, 677, *768,* 769
  integrity testing, 770
Hypophyseal arteries, 815
Hypophysis cerebri
  anatomy, 676, *684,* 687, 815, *815*
  development, 816, *816*
  function, 815
Hypospadias, 413, *416*
Hypothalamus, 687
Hypothenar eminence, 503
Hypovolemic shock, 468
Hysterectomy, ureter damage in, 369
Hysterosalpingography, 381, *381*

Ileocecal sphincter, 230
Ileocecal valve, 230
Ileocolic artery, 244
Ileum
  anatomy, *203,* 204, *205, 226,* 227–228, *228*
  blood supply, 228, *230, 231*
  development, 237
  location and description, *226,* 227–228, *228*
  lymph drainage, 228
  nerve supply, 228
  pain fibers, 229
  radiographic anatomy, *287,* 289, *290*
  recognition, 229
  trauma, 229
Iliac artery
  common, *272,* 273–274, 327
  deep circumflex, *272,* 274, *328*
  external, 195, *272,* 274, 328
  internal, *272,* 274, 328
  obliteration, 274
  superficial circumflex, 580
Iliac crest, 191, 318, 330, 555, 644
Iliac spine, 191
  anterior inferior, 555
  anterior superior, 191, 318, 330, 555, 644
  posterior superior, 191, 318, 330, 555, 644
Iliac tubercle, 555, 644
Iliac vein
  external, 329
  internal, 329
  superficial circumflex, 571
Iliaca fascia, 177
Iliacus, *176,* 176–177, 177t, 578t
Iliococcygeus, 318
Iliofemoral ligament, 588
Iliohypogastric nerve, 278, 279t
Ilioinguinal nerve, 278, 279t, 568–569
Iliolumbar artery, 328
Iliolumbar ligament, 175, 329
Iliopectineal line, 174, 318
Iliopsoas, 176
Iliotibial tract, 553, 555, *556,* 573
Ilium, 173–174, *175,* 318, 555
Imperforate anus, 397
Imperforate hymen, 376
Imperforate vagina, 376
Incisional hernia, 186
Incisions, abdominal wall, 146, 187–188
Incisive canal, 715
Incisive foramen, 673, 785
Incisive fossa, 673
Incisura angularis, 219
Incontinence
  after spinal cord injury, 397
  after trauma, 397
  rectal prolapse and, 397
  stress, 357
Incus, 711, 712, *713*
Index finger, movements, 517, 519
Infantile uterus, 371
Inferior, defined, 2
Inferior acromioclavicular ligament, 461
Inferior alveolar nerve, 762
Inferior angle, 66
Inferior cerebellar peduncles, 690
Inferior cervical ganglion, 773
Inferior colliculi, 689
Inferior conchae, 670
Inferior constrictor muscle, 789, *791,* 792t
Inferior epigastric artery, *272,* 274, 328
Inferior extensor retinaculum, 606
Inferior gemellus, 566t
Inferior gluteal artery, 328, 567
Inferior gluteal nerve, 325, 327t, 566
Inferior hemiazygos vein, 123, *124*

Inferior hypogastric plexus, 327
Inferior iliac spine, posterior, 555
Inferior labial artery, 729
Inferior lobar bronchus, 88
Inferior meatus, 797
Inferior mediastinum, 80
Inferior medullary vela, 690
Inferior mesenteric artery, *233*, 244
Inferior mesenteric plexus, 280, *280*
Inferior mesenteric vein, 245, 276
Inferior oblique, 694t, 699–702, *700*, *701*, *702*
Inferior ophthalmic vein, 698
Inferior orbital fissure, 673, *695*, 696
Inferior pancreaticoduodenal artery, 243
Inferior parathyroid glands, 821
Inferior peroneal retinaculum, 609
Inferior petrosal sinus, 677, 687
Inferior rectal artery, 343, *343*, 394
Inferior rectal nerve, 394
Inferior rectal vein, 343
Inferior rectus, 694t, *699*, 699–702, *701*, *702*
Inferior sagittal sinus, 686
Inferior salivary nucleus, 774
Inferior temporal line, 673
Inferior thyroid artery, 751, 818
Inferior thyroid veins, 841
Inferior ulnar collateral artery, 472, *474*, 476
Inferior vena cava, 107, 123, *124*, 274
  anatomy, *272*, 274
  collateral circulation, *277*
  compression, 274, *277*
  obstruction, 162, *162*
  trauma, 274, *277*
  tributaries, 274, 276
Inferior vertebral notch, 853
Inferior vesical artery, 328
Infraclavicular nodes, 451, *453*, 505
Infraorbital foramen, 670, 839
Infraorbital groove and canal, 696, *696*
Infraorbital nerve, 729, 839
Infrapatellar bursa, 631
Infrapatellar fold, 630
Infraspinatus, 442t
Infraspinous fossa, 434
Infratemporal crest, 673
Infratemporal fossa, 673
Infratemporal region, *763*
Infratrochlear nerve, 698, 728, 760
Infundibulum, 108, 119, 363, 687, 797, 815, 816
Inguinal canal
  anatomy, 163–164
  development, 165–167, *168*
  function, 164
  mechanics, 164, *165*
  walls, 164
Inguinal hernia, 170, *170*
  direct, 184, *184*, *185*
  indirect, 183–184, *184*
Inguinal ligament, 191, 650
Inguinal lymph nodes
  deep, 573, 582
  superficial, 573, 580, 650
Inguinal region, 650, *654*, *655*
Inguinal ring, superficial, 191
Inhaled foreign body, 89
Inner cell mass, 37
Insertion, muscle, 8, *9*
Inspection, chest, 68
Inspiration
  forced, 102
  lung changes on, 102
  muscle of, 59
  quiet, *87*, 100, *101*, 102
Insulin, 256
Intercarpal joint, 516
Intercondylar areas, 593
Intercondylar eminence, 593
Intercondylar notch, 561
Intercostal arteries
  anterior, 53, *53*, *54*, 63
  posterior, 53, *53*, *54*
  postoperative, 126
  superior, 751
Intercostal membrane
  anterior, 53, *53*
  posterior, 53, *53*
Intercostal muscle, *52*, 52–53, *53*
  action, 53
  external, 52–53, 65t
  during forced expiration, *87*, 102
  innermost, 53, *53*, 65t
  during inspiration, *87*, 100
  internal, *52*, 53, 65t
  nerve supply, 53
Intercostal nerve
  anatomy, 55–57, *56*
  anterior cutaneous branch, 55
  branches, 55, 57
  collateral branch, 55
  first, 55
  lateral cutaneous branch, 55
  muscular branches, 55
  peritoneal sensory branches, 55
  pleural sensory branches, 55
  second, 55, 57
Intercostal nerve block, 56
Intercostal nodes, posterior, 126
Intercostal veins, 53, *55*, 123
Intercostobrachial nerve, 55, 57, 466
Intercristal plane, *156*, 192
Intercuneiform joint, 638
Interlobar arteries, 264
Intermaxillary suture, 670
Intermediate cutaneous nerve of thigh, 569, 582
Intermediate mesoderm, 37
Intermediate supraclavicular nerve, 736–737
Intermetacarpal joint, 516
Intermetatarsal joint, 638
Intermittent claudication, 659
Internal, defined, 3
Internal acoustic meatus, 677
Internal carotid artery, 750
  arteriography, *830–833*
  arteriosclerosis, 750
Internal carotid nerve, 773
Internal cerebral vein, 690
Internal ear, *708*, *710*, 714–715
Internal hernia, 186
Internal iliac artery, *272*, 274, 328
Internal iliac vein, 329
Internal intercostal muscle, *52*, 53, 65t
Internal jugular vein
  anatomy, 677, 752–753
  catheterization, 753, *755*
  penetrating wounds, 753
Internal laryngeal nerve, 766–767
Internal oblique muscle, *148*, *149*, 152, *153*, 158t
Internal occipital crest, 677
Internal occipital protuberance, 677
Internal os, 365
Internal pudendal artery, 328, 394, 406
Internal pudendal vein, 394
Internal pudendal vessels, 409
Internal sphincter, 393
Internal table, 669
Internal thoracic artery, 63, 64, 751
Internal thoracic nodes, 126
Internal thoracic vein, 63
Internal thoracic vessels, 73
Internodal pathway, 112–113
Interosseous artery
  anterior, 487, 498
  common, 487
  posterior, 487, 498
Interosseous membrane, forearm, 484
Interosseous muscles
  dorsal, *505*, 506t, 622t
  palmar, *505*, 506t
  plantar, 623t
Interosseous nerve, anterior, 493
Interosseous sacroiliac ligament, 329
Interosseous talocalcaneal ligament, 597, 637
Interphalangeal joint, 517, 535, 638
Intersigmoid recess, 208, *212*
Interspinous ligament, 860
Intertransverse ligaments, 860
Intertrochanteric crest, 560
Intertrochanteric line, 560
Intertubercular plane, *156*, 192
Interureteric ridge, 350
Interventricular artery, posterior, 113–114, *115*
Interventricular foramen, 118, 687, 690
Interventricular septum, 111, 118
Intervertebral disc, 173, *175*
  herniation, 867–868, *877*
  structure and function, 858
Intervertebral foramen, 853, 868
Intervertebral veins, 866
Intestinal tract. *See* Gastrointestinal tract
Intestine
  atresia and stenosis, 238, *241*
  large
    anatomy, *203*, 204, *205*, 229–234
    cancer, 236
    distal part, development, 345, *346*
    radiographic anatomy, 289, *291–293*
  small
    anatomy, *203*, 204, *205*, 224–228
    development, 237
    versus large intestine, 246, *248*
    mesentery, 207, *226*, 227, 229
    pain fibers, 229
    radiographic anatomy, *287*, 289, *290*
    recognition, 229
    trauma, 229
Intra-articular ligament, 51
Intracranial hemorrhage, 686
Intraembryonic coelom, 37
Intravenous transfusion, 468
Intubation
  endotracheal
    airway distances, 814, 814t
    anatomic axes, 808, *811*
    reflex activity secondary to, 808
  nasogastric, 223
Intussusception, 236
Inversion
  defined, 4
  of foot, 638
Ipsilateral, defined, 3
Iris
  anatomy, 704
  dilator pupillae of, 694t, 702, 704
  sphincter pupillae of, 694t, 704
Irreducible hernia, 580
Ischial spine, 318, 555
Ischial tuberosity, 312, 318, 419, 555, 645
Ischiocavernosus, 402, 405, 408, 409, 410t
Ischiofemoral ligament, 588
Ischiorectal fossa, 394, 397
Ischium, 318, 555
Islets of Langerhans, 256

Jefferson's fracture, 862, *863*
Jejunum
  anatomy, *203*, 204, *205*, *226*, 227–228, *228*
  blood supply, 228, *230*, *231*
  development, 237
  location and description, *226*, 227–228, *228*
  lymph drainage, 228
  nerve supply, 228
  pain fibers, 229
  radiographic anatomy, *287*, 289, *290*

Jejunum *(continued)*
  recognition, 229
  trauma, 229
Joint, 12–16
  ball-and-socket, 15, *16*
  cartilaginous, 13, *14*
  condyloid, 14, *16*
  defined, 3
  ellipsoid, 14, *16*
  examination, 17
  fibrous, 12, *14*
  hinge, 13, *16*
  nerve supply, 16
  pivot, 14, *16*
  plane, 13, *16*
  saddle, 15, *16*
  stability, *15*, 15–16
  synovial, 13–15, *14, 15, 16*
Jugular arch, 841
Jugular foramen, 674, 677
Jugular lymph trunk, 127
Jugular vein
  anterior, 739, *739*, 752
  external, 752, 843
    anatomy, 737, 739, *739*
    catheterization, 738, *741*
    as venous manometer, 738
    visibility, 738
  internal
    anatomy, 677, 752–753
    catheterization, 753, *755*
    penetrating wounds, 753
Jugulodigastric node, 756
Jugulo-omohyoid node, 756

Kidney
  anatomy, 205, *206*, 260, 262–264
  blood supply, *263*, 264
  coverings, 262, *263*
  development, 267–268, *268, 269*
  horseshoe, 267, *270*
  location and description, 260, *262, 263*
  lymph drainage, 264
  mobility, 264
  nerve supply, 264
  pelvic, 267, *270*
  polycystic, 267
  radiographic anatomy, 295
  relations, 262, 264, *265*
  rosette, 268, *270*
  structure, 262, *263*, 264
  surface markings, 192, *194*
  transplanted, 264, *266*
  trauma, 264, *265*
  tumor, 264
  unilateral double, 267–268, *270*
Killian's dehiscence, 789, *791*, 792t
Klumpke palsy, 537
Knee jerk, 26, *29*, 659
Knee joint
  anatomy, *594*, 629–631, 654, *655, 656,* 656–657
  anterior aspect, *655*
  anteroposterior radiograph, *646*
  arterial anastomosis around, 604
  arthroscopy, 632
  articulation, 629
  bursae related to, 630–631
  capsule, 629
  hyperextension, 644
  injury, 631–632
  lateral radiograph, *647*
  ligaments
    extracapsular, 629
    injury, 632
    intracapsular, 629–630
  magnetic resonance imaging, *653*
  meniscal injury, 632, *633, 634*
  movements, 631
  nerve supply, 631
  pneumoarthrography, 632, *648*
  relations, *630*, 631
  stabilizer, 578
  strength, 631
  synovial membrane, 630, 631–632
  type, 629
Kyphosis, 65, 860

Labia majora, 173, 419
Labia minora, 419
Labial artery, 729
Labial frenula, 774
Labiogingival lamina, 734
Labor, uterus in, 368
Labyrinth
  bony, *710*, 714
  membranous, *710*, 714–715
Labyrinthitis, 714
Lacrimal apparatus, *692*, 694–695
Lacrimal artery, 698
Lacrimal ducts, *692*, 694–695
Lacrimal fold, 695
Lacrimal gland, *692*, 694
Lacrimal nerve, *695, 697*, 697–698, 728, 760
Lacrimal nucleus, 694
Lacrimal sac, 694
Lacrimatory nucleus, 774
Lacus lacrimalis, 691, 694
Lambdoid suture, 673
Lamina cribrosa, 703
Lamina propria, 30
Langerhans, islets of, 256
Large intestine
  anatomy, *203*, 204, *205*, 229–234
  cancer, 236
  distal part, development, 345, *346*
  radiographic anatomy, 289, *291–293*
Laryngeal folds, 805
Laryngeal inlet, muscles modifying, *804*, 805, 806t
Laryngeal mirror, 808, *810*
Laryngeal nerve
  external, 767, 808, *809*, 818
  internal, 766–767
  lesions, 807–808, *809*
  recurrent, 127, 767, 808, *809*, 818
Laryngeal nodes, 755
Laryngeal pharynx, *791*, 793
Laryngoscope, 808, *810*
Laryngotracheal groove, 99
Laryngotracheal tube, 99
Larynx, 99
  anatomy, 802–807
  bladder, 807
  cartilages, 802, *803*
  cavity, 805
  inlet, 805
  ligaments, 802, *803*
  lymph drainage, 807
  membranes, 802, *803*
  mucous membrane, 807, 808
  muscles, *804*, 805, 806t
  nerve supply, 807, *809*
  saccule, 805
  sinus, 805
  sphincteric function, 806
  voice production, 806–807
Lateral aortic lymph nodes, 276
Lateral arcuate ligament, 58, 175
Lateral axillary nodes, 451, *453*, 505
Lateral check ligament, 702
Lateral chewing movements, 720
Lateral collateral ligament, 629, 632, 654, 656
Lateral condyle, 561, 593
Lateral cricoarytenoid muscle, 806t
Lateral cutaneous nerve
  of arm, 466, 475
  of calf, 604, 609, 615
  of forearm, 473, 500
  of thigh, 278, 279t, 568
Lateral epicondyle, 435, 533, 561
Lateral femoral circumflex artery, 585–586
Lateral flexion, defined, 3
Lateral geniculate body, 757
Lateral glossoepiglottic fold, 790
Lateral lacunae, 675
Lateral ligament, 509, 634
Lateral longitudinal arch
  anatomy, *640*, 641
  maintenance, *641*, 642
Lateral malleolus, 657
  structures passing behind, *610, 611*, 619
Lateral meniscus, 593, 632
Lateral mesoderm, 37
Lateral nasal artery, 729
Lateral nasal process, 734
Lateral palpebral ligament, 691
Lateral pectoral nerve, 449, 450t
Lateral plane, 2, *3*
Lateral plantar artery, 625
Lateral plantar nerve, 619, 627
Lateral plantar vein, 626
Lateral proboscis, 798, *801*
Lateral pterygoid muscle, 721t
  nerve to, 762
Lateral pterygoid plate, 673
Lateral rectus, 694t, *699*, 699–702, *701, 702*
Lateral rotation, defined, 3
Lateral sacral artery, 328
Lateral sulcus, 687
Lateral supracondylar ridge, 561
Lateral talocalcaneal ligament, 637
Lateral tarsal artery, 629
Lateral temporomandibular ligament, 719
Lateral thoracic artery, 445
Lateral ventricle, 687, 690
Latissimus dorsi, 442t
Left dominance, posterior interventricular artery in, 113–114, *115*
Leg. *See also* Ankle; Foot
  anterior and lateral aspects, structures, *605, 608*
  arterial occlusive disease, 659
  back, 615–618
  bones, 592–595
  cutaneous nerves, 609, 615
  deep vein thrombosis, 618
  fascial compartments, 605–609
    anterior
      artery, 612, 614
      compartment syndrome, 614
      contents, 609–614
      muscles, 609–612, 613t
      nerve supply, 614
    lateral
      artery, 615
      contents, 614–615
      muscles, 614–615, 614t
      nerve, 615
    posterior
      artery, 618
      contents, 615–618
      muscles, 615, 617t, 618
      nerve supply, 618
  front, *607*, 609–615, *656*
  lymphatics, 609, 615
  posterior aspect, deep structures, *603*
  skin, 609, 615
  superficial veins, 609, 615
  sympathetic innervation, 659
  transverse section through, *606*
Lens, 705
Lesser curvature, 219
Lesser occipital nerve, 725, 736, 771, 771t
Lesser omentum, 206, *211*, 216, *217*, 249
Lesser palatine foramen, 673
Lesser palatine nerve, 762

Lesser petrosal nerve, 676, 714
Lesser sac, 206, *207,* 207–208, *208, 211, 217*
Lesser sciatic foramina, 318, 555, *562*
Lesser sciatic notch, 318, 555
Lesser splanchnic nerve, 26–27, 128
Lesser trochanter, 560
Lesser tuberosity, 435, 437, *438*
Lesser wing of sphenoid bone, 676
Levator anguli oris, 721t
Levator ani muscle, 318, *320, 321,* 324t, *366,* 367
Levator glandulae thyroideae, 818
Levator labii superioris, 721t
Levator labii superioris alaeque nasi, 721t
Levator palpebrae superioris, 691, 694t
Levator prostatae, 318
Levator scapulae, 442t
Levator veli palatini, 785t
Levatores costarum, 63, 65t
  during inspiration, 102
Ligament, 17
  elastic, 15
  fibrous, 15
  injury, 17
  joint, 13, 15
Ligamentum arteriosum, 126
Ligamentum denticulatum, 870
Ligamentum flavum, 860
Ligamentum nuchae, 531, 841, 860, 880
Ligamentum patellae, 578, 629, 654
Ligamentum teres, 249
Ligamentum venosum, 249
Light reflex, 706
Linea alba, 191
Linea aspera, 560
Linea semilunaris, 186, 191
Lines of cleavage, 146
Lingual artery, 749
Lingual nerve, 762
Lingual swelling, lateral, 781
Lingual thyroid, 819, *820*
Lingual tonsil, 779
Lingula, 715
Lip
  anatomy, 774
  cleft, *733, 734,* 735, *735*
  development, 734
  dilator muscles, 721t, 731
  sphincter muscle, 721t, 731
Little finger
  movements, 517, 519
  opposition, 503
  short muscles, 503
Liver
  anatomy, 203, *203, 204, 210,* 246–249
  biliary ducts, 249–253, *250, 251*
  biopsy, 249
  blood supply, 249
  cancer, 246
  development, 253, *254*
  location and description, 246–248
  lymph drainage, 249
  nerve supply, 249
  peritoneal ligaments, 248–249
  relations, 248
  surface markings, 192, *193*
  trauma, 249
Liver lobule, 248
Liver supports, 249
Liver surgery, 249
Lobar arteries, 264
Lobar bronchus, 88
Lobster hand, 522
Long bone, 33, *33*
Long ciliary nerve, 760
Long extensor tendons, insertions, *494,* 502, 627
Long flexor tendons, insertions, *494,* 501, 502
Long plantar ligament, 638
Long thoracic nerve, 448–449, 450t, 537
Longitudinal arch
  lateral
    anatomy, *640,* 641
    maintenance, *641,* 642
  medial
    anatomy, 640, *640*
    clinical problems, 642
    maintenance, *641,* 642
Longitudinal fissure, 687
Longitudinal ligament, 858–859
Lordosis, 860
Louis, angle of, 47, *48,* 64, 523
Lower limb. *See also specific anatomy*
  anatomy, 550–660
  arterial occlusive disease, 659
  arteries, *553, 581,* 658–659
  bursae and bursitis, 643
  collateral circulation, 658
  cutaneous nerves, 551, *551, 552*
  development, 643–644, *644*
  joints, 629–638
  lymphatics, 553, *553, 554,* 573
  nerves, 659–660
  organization, 550–660
  radiographic anatomy, 644, *645–653*
  superficial veins, *570*
  surface anatomy, 644–658
  tendon reflexes, 659
  veins, 571
  venous pump, 571
Lower lobe, lung, 92, 94, *94, 95*
Lower subscapular nerve, 450t
Lowest splanchnic nerve, 27, 128
Ludwig's angina, 746
Lumbar disc herniation, 868, *877*
Lumbar hernia, 186
Lumbar nerves, 21, *24*
Lumbar plexus
  anatomy, 23, *24,* 278–279, *279*
  branches, 279t, 326–327
Lumbar puncture, 871, 873, *878*
Lumbar sympathectomy, 280, 659
Lumbar triangle, 865
Lumbar vein, ascending, 123
Lumbar vertebra, 173, *174, 175, 854,* 855–856, 881, *887–892, 894*
Lumbosacral angle, 315
Lumbosacral root syndromes, 872t
Lumbosacral trunk, 279, 325, 326
Lumbrical canal, 508
Lumbricals, 506t, 622t
Lunate bone, 480, 481, 535
Lung
  age-related changes, 65
  anatomy, 68, *70, 71,* 72, 89, 92–102, 132–133
  anterior border, 68, 92
  apex, 68, 72, *84,* 92
  base, 92
  blood supply, 96, 98
  bronchopulmonary segments, *92,* 94, *95,* 96, *96, 97*
  cancer, 103
  congenital anomalies, 99, *100*
  costal surface, 92
  development, *81,* 99, *99*
  fissures, 92, 94, *94*
  hilum, 92
  horizontal fissure, 68, 72
  lateral surface, *94, 95*
  lobes, 92, 94, *94, 95, 97*
  lower border, 68
  lymph drainage, 98, *98*
  mediastinal surface, 92
  nerve supply, 98
  oblique fissure, 68
  physical examination, 102
  posterior border, 68
  respiration. *See* Respiration
  root, 84, 92, 96
  segmental resection, 103
  surface markings, *70, 71*
  surgical access, 103
  trauma, 102
Lung bud, 99
Lung disease, pain, 103
Lung distensibility, loss, 103
Lung elasticity, loss, 103
Lymph, 21
Lymph capillary, 21
Lymph nodes, 21, *22,* 276, *278*
  axillary
    anatomy, 126, 450–451, *453,* 505
    examination, 454
  cervical
    anterior, 755
    deep, 746, 756–757, 781
    examination, 757
    metastasis, 757
    regional, 754–755
    superficial, 739, 755
  inguinal
    deep, 573, 582
    superficial, 573, 580, 650
  parotid, 754
  popliteal, 604
  preaortic, 276
  regional, skin and, 163
  submandibular nodes, 754, 789
  supratrochlear, 477, 482, 505
Lymphadenitis, 469
Lymphangitis, 469
Lymphatic duct, right, 21, *22,* 127
Lymphatic system
  anatomy, 20–21, *22*
  disease, 21
Lymphatic tissue, 20, *22*
Lymphatic vessel, 20–21, *22,* 276, 278, *278*

Macrodactyly, 522, *522*
Macromastia, 432
Macrostomia, 735
Macula lutea, 704
Magnetic resonance imaging, 37, *40*
  brain, 824, *835–837*
  forearm, *529*
  head, *40*
  knee joint, *653*
  lower limb, 644, *653*
  skull, 824, *835–837*
  upper limb, 523, *529*
  vertebral column, 880, *883*
Male genital organs, 352–356
  ejaculatory duct, 352, 353, *354*
  peritoneum, 356
  prostate
    blood supply, 355
    function, 355
    location and description, *349,* 353–354, *354*
    lymph drainage, 355
    nerve supply, 355
    relations, *354,* 354–355
    structure, *354,* 355
  prostatic urethra, *354,* 356
  seminal vesicles, *349,* 352–353
  vas deferens, *347, 349,* 352
  visceral pelvic fascia, 356
Male genitalia, 413, *414, 415*
Male pelvis, *309,* 330, *342, 379, 390–391, 418*
Male ureter, *347,* 347–348
Male urethra, 407–408, *416, 417*
Male urinary bladder, *348,* 348–350, *349*
Male urogenital triangle, *390,* 402, 405–408, 419
Malleolar fold, 711
Malleolar fossa, 595
Malleolus
  lateral, *610, 611,* 619, 657
  medial, 594, *610,* 619, 657

Mallet finger, 509, *510*
Malleus, 711, 712, *713*
Mammary gland, *67,* 73
Mammillary bodies, 687
Mammography, 430, *431*
Mandible
  anatomy, 673, 715, *716*
  angle, 715
    at birth, 679
  body, 715, *838,* 839
  depression, 720
  elevation, 720
  fractures, 715
  protrusion, 720
  ramus, 715, *838,* 839
  retraction, 720
Mandibular canal, 715
Mandibular foramen, 715
Mandibular fossa, 673
Mandibular nerve, 729, 758t, *761,* 762
Mandibular notch, 715
Mandibular processes, 734
Manubriosternal joint, 47, 51
Manubrium, 47
Marginal artery, 113, 244
Marrow, bone, 33, 34–35
Marrow cavity, 33
Masseter, 721t, 838, 839
Masseteric nerve, 762
Mastication muscles, 721t
Mastoid air cells, 712
Mastoid antrum, 711, 712
Mastoid nodes, 754
Mastoid process, 679, 837, *838*
Mastoiditis, 714
Maxilla, 670, 731
  blowout fracture, 679
  palatal processes, 673
Maxillary artery, 750
Maxillary nerve, 729, 758t, *761,* 761–762
Maxillary processes, 734
Maxillary sinus, 673, 797, 799, *801,* 802t, 839
Maxillary vein, 752
Maxillofacial fractures, 678, *679*
McBurney's incision, 188
Meatal stenosis, 413
Meatus, 797
Meckel's diverticulum, *181,* 182, 229, 238
Meconium, 345
Medial arcuate ligament, 58, 174
Medial check ligament, 702
Medial collateral ligament, 629, 632, 654, 656
Medial condyle, 561, 593
Medial cutaneous nerve
  of arm, 449, 450t, 466
  of forearm, 449, 450t
  of thigh, 569, 582
Medial epicondyle, 435, 533, 561
Medial femoral circumflex artery, 585
Medial ligament, 509, 634
Medial longitudinal arch
  anatomy, 640, *640*
  clinical problems, 642
  maintenance, *641,* 642
Medial malleolus, 594, *610,* 619, 657
Medial meniscus, 593
  injury, 632, *633, 634*
Medial nasal process, 734
Medial palpebral ligament, 691
Medial pectoral nerve, 449, 450t
Medial plane, 2, *3*
Medial plantar artery, 624–625
Medial plantar nerve, 619, 626–627
Medial plantar vein, 626
Medial pterygoid muscle, 721t
  nerve to, 762
Medial pterygoid plate, 673
Medial rectus, 694t, *699,* 699–702, *701, 702*
Medial rotation, defined, 3
Medial supraclavicular nerve, 736
Medial supracondylar ridge, 561
Medial talocalcaneal ligament, 637
Median cubital vein, 482, 535
Median fissure, 690
Median glossoepiglottic fold, 790, 802
Median nasal furrow, 798, *801*
Median nerve, 499
  anatomy, *472,* 474, 489, 505
  branches, *451,* 493
  cutaneous branches, 505
  injury
    at elbow, 539–540, *540*
    at wrist, 540
  lateral root, 449, 450t
  medial root, 449, 450t
  muscular branch, 505
  palmar cutaneous branch, 499, 500, 505
  recurrent branch, 535
Median nerve palsy, *540*
Median sacral artery, 329
Median sacral crest, 645, 881
Median sacral veins, 329
Median sagittal plane, 2, *3*
Median thyrohyoid membrane, 802
Median umbilical ligament, 348
Mediastinal artery, 63
Mediastinal pleura, 84
Mediastinal tumors or cysts, 82
Mediastinitis, 82
Mediastinoscopy, 82
Mediastinum, 46
  anatomy, *79,* 80, *90, 91,* 134
  anterior, 80
  deflection, 82
  inferior, 80
  lymph drainage, 126
  middle, 80
  posterior, 80
  subdivisions, *79*
  superior, 80
Medulla
  renal, 262
  suprarenal glands, 269
Medulla oblongata, 676, 690
Medullary rays, 262
Medullary vela, 690
Megacolon, 345, *347*
Megaloureter, 268, *271*
Membrana tectoria, 858
Membranous labyrinth, *710,* 714–715
Membranous ossification, 35
Membranous urethra, 406, 407
Meningeal vessel, middle, 673, 675, 683, 750
Meninges
  cranial, *681,* 681–685
  spinal cord, 871
Meningocele, *882, 883*
Meningomyelocele, *882, 883*
Meniscus
  anatomy, 593, 630, 656
  injury, 632, *633, 634*
Menopause, uterus after, 368
Mental foramen, 715
Mental nerve, 729
Mental spines, 715
Mentalis, 721t
Mesenteric arterial occlusion, 229
Mesenteric artery
  inferior, *233,* 244
  superior, *230,* 243, *244, 293*
Mesenteric plexus, 280, *280*
Mesenteric vein
  inferior, 245, 276
  superior, 245, 276
  thrombosis, 229
Mesenteries, 207, *208, 209, 212*
Mesoappendix, 230
Mesocolon
  sigmoid, 207, *212,* 338
  transverse, 207, 233
Mesoderm, 37
Mesonephric duct, 357
Mesonephros, *268*
Mesosalpinx, 377
Mesotendon, 17, *18*
Mesovarium, *358–359,* 361, 377
Metacarpals
  anatomy, 480, *481, 482*
  first, base, 535
  fractures, 481
Metacarpophalangeal joint, 516–517, 535
Metanephrogenic cap, 267–268, *269*
Metanephros, *268*
Metaphysis, 33, 35
Metatarsal artery, first dorsal, 629
Metatarsal bones, *597–599,* 600, *600, 652*
Metatarsophalangeal joint, 638
Metatarsus varus, 644
Metopic suture, 673
Micromastia, 432
Microstomia, 735
Micturition, 350, *352*
  after spinal cord injury, 351, *353*
Midaxillary line, 68
Midbrain, *685,* 689
Midclavicular line, 68
Middle cardiac vein, *114,* 116
Middle cerebellar peduncle, 690
Middle cerebral artery, 750–751
Middle cervical ganglion, 773
Middle colic artery, 244
Middle conchae, 670
Middle constrictor muscle, 789, *791,* 792t
Middle cranial fossa, 675–676, 679
Middle ear, 706, *708, 709,* 709–714, *710,* 711t
Middle ethmoidal air sinus, 797
Middle finger, movements, 517, 519
Middle internodal pathway, 113
Middle lobar bronchus, 88
Middle lobe, lung, 92
Middle meatus, 797
Middle mediastinum, 80
Middle meningeal artery, 673, 675, 683, 750
Middle meningeal vein, 673, 675, 683
Middle rectal artery, 328, 343, *343*
Middle rectal vein, 343
Middle superior alveolar nerve, 762
Midgut, *239*
Midgut artery, 245
Midgut loop
  arrested rotation or malrotation, 238, *241, 243*
  formation, 237–238, *242, 243*
Midline incision, 188, *189,* 189–190
Midline structures
  back, 880–881, *894*
  neck, 812
Midpalmar space, 508
Midsternal line, 68
Midtarsal joints, 638
Milk ridge, 432
Mineral corticoids, 269
Mitral valve, *89, 110,* 111, 117, 121
Moderator band, 109
Modiolus, 714
Mons pubis, 419
Monteggia's fracture, 480
Motor area, 687
Motor fibers, 21
Motor speech area, 687
Mouth
  anatomy, 774–776, *775*
  cavity, 774, *775*
  development, 776, *777*
  examination, clinical significance, 776
  floor, 774

lips, 774
mucous membrane, 776
roof, 774
sensory innervation, 776, *777*
teeth, 778, *778*
tongue, 778–781, *779, 780,* 780t
vestibule, 774
Movement, terms related to, 3–4, *4, 5*
Mucosal folds, rectum, 344
Mucous membrane, 30
anal canal, 389, 393, *393*
duodenum, *225,* 227
inflammation and, 32
larynx, 807, 808
mouth, 776
nasal cavity, 797–798, *799*
tongue, 778–779
Müller muscle, 697
Multipennate muscle, 10, *10*
Murmurs, heart, 117
Muscle
attachments, 12
cardiac, 12
pennate, 10, *10*
segmental innervation, 26, *29*
shape and form, 12
skeletal
action, 10–12, *11*
anatomy, 8–12, *9*
internal structure, 8, 10, *10*
naming, 12, 13t
nerve supply, 12
smooth, 12
tone, 12, 15–16
Muscle splitting incision, 188
Muscular triangles, neck, *744,* 747
Muscularis mucosa, 30
Musculi pectinati, 107
Musculocutaneous nerve, 449, 450t, *472,* 472–473
branches, *451*
injury, 539
Musculophrenic artery, 63
Musculus uvulae, 785t
Myelocele, *882*
Myelography, subarachnoid space, 876, *889–890*
Mylohyoid, 742t
Mylohyoid line, 715
Mylohyoid nerve, 762
Myocardial infarction, 115, 116, 116t
Myocardium, 107, 118
Myometrium, 366

Nail, 5, *7*
Nail bed, 5, *7*
Nail fold, 5, *7*
Nasal aperture
anterior, 670
posterior, 796
Nasal artery, lateral, 729
Nasal bones, 670, 679, 731
Nasal cavity
anatomy, 796–798, *797*
blood supply, 798, *800*
examination, 798
infection, 798
lymph drainage, 798, *800*
mucous membrane, 797–798, *799*
nerve supply, 798, *799*
Nasal conchae, 796
Nasal furrow, median, 798, *801*
Nasal nerve, external, 729, 760
Nasal pharynx, 790, *791*
Nasal process, 734
Nasal septum, *786,* 796, *796*
Nasal vestibule, 796
Nasion, 824, *838*
Nasociliary nerve, *695, 697,* 698, 760
Nasogastric intubation, 223
Nasolacrimal canal, 696
Nasolacrimal duct, 694, 797
Navicular bone, *597–599,* 599, 658
Neck
anatomy, 735–757, *736*
anterior triangle, *743,* 747, 842
anterior view, *738*
arteries, 747–751, *758*
axillary sheath, 747
bones, 739
brachial plexus, 771–772, *772*
carotid sheath, 747
cervical plexus, 771, 771t
cross section, *736, 746,* 824, *825, 826*
cutaneous nerves, 736–737, *737*
deep cervical fascia, 743–747
clinical significance, 744, 746–747
investing layer, 744
pretracheal layer, 744
prevertebral layer, 744, *745*
fascial spaces, 744, 746, *746*
infection, 746
incisions, 740
ligaments, 747
lymph drainage, 754–757
lymph nodes
anterior cervical, 755
deep cervical, 746, 756–757, 781
regional, 754–755
superficial cervical, 739, 755
midline structures, 812
muscles, 739–743, 742t
muscular triangles, *744,* 747
nerves, 771–772, 771t
parasympathetic nervous system, 774
platysma, 737, *738,* 742t
posterior triangle, 747, 843
root, *745,* 842
muscles, 822, 824
pleura and lung injuries, 824
scalenus anterior, 742t, 743
skin, 736–737, *737*
sternocleidomastoid, 740–742, 742t
styloid muscles, vessels, and nerves, *749*
superficial cervical fascia, 737
superficial veins, 737, 739, *739*
surface landmarks
anterior aspect, 839–841, *840–841*
lateral aspect, *841,* 841–843, *842*
posterior aspect, 841
sympathetic nervous system, 773
veins, 752
Needle thoracostomy, *59,* 60
Neonatal skull, 677, 679–680, *680*
Nerve block
anterior abdominal, 159–160
brachial plexus, 446, 772
intercostal, 56
pudendal, 412, *413*
stellate ganglion, 774
Nervous system, 21–30
autonomic, 21, 24, 26–30, *30–31*
central, 21, *23–25*
parasympathetic, 28–30, *30, 31,* 774
peripheral, 21–24, *23–25*
somatic, 21, *30*
sympathetic, 26–28, *30, 31. See also* Sympathetic system
Neural arch, 875
Neural plate, 37
Neural tube, 37
Neuroglia, 21
Neurohypophysis, 815
Neuron, 21
Nipple, 66, 427, 533
development, 432
inverted, 432
retracted, 430, 432
supernumerary, 430, 432
Nose
anatomy, 795–798
bleeding, 798
development, 798, *801*
external, 795–796, *796*
foreign bodies, 798
nasal cavity, 796–798, *797, 799, 800*
trauma, 798
Nostrils, 731, 795
Notochord, 875
Nuchal groove, 841, 880
Nuchal lines, superior, 673, 837
Nucleus cuneatus, 690
Nucleus gracilis, 690
Nucleus pulposus
herniation, 868, *877*
structure, 858
Nutrient artery, 472
Nystagmus, 770

Oblique arytenoid, 806t
Oblique fissure, lung, 92, 94
Oblique muscle
external, *148, 149,* 150, 152, *153,* 158t
internal, *148, 149,* 152, *153,* 158t
Oblique popliteal ligament, 629
Oblique sinus, 104
Obstetric measurements, pelvic, 312, *313, 314*
Obturator artery, 328, 586
Obturator externus, *583,* 584t
Obturator foramen, 318, 555
Obturator internus, 318, *320,* 324t, 563, 566t
nerve to, 325, 327t, 566
Obturator membrane, 318, 555
Obturator nerve, 605
anatomy, 279, 279t, 326–327, 569, *577,* 586
branches, 586, *586*
injury, 660
referred pain from, 326
Obturator vein, 586
Occipital artery, 725, 750
Occipital bone, 673
Occipital condyles, 674
Occipital crest, internal, 677
Occipital lobe, 687
Occipital nerve
greater, 725, 736, 867
lesser, 725, 736, 771, 771t
Occipital nodes, 754
Occipital protuberance
external, 673, 824, *838,* 841, 880
internal, 677
Occipital sinus, 677, 686
Occipital triangle, 747
Occipital vein, 725
Occipitofrontalis, 721t, 724
Ocular fundus, *705*
Oculomotor nerve, 758t
anatomy, *695, 696,* 698, 757, *760*
integrity testing, 769–770
paralysis, 769–770
Oddi sphincter, 250, *250*
Odontoid process
anatomy, 855, *883*
fracture, 862, *863*
Olecranon bursitis, 480
Olecranon fossa, 437
Olecranon process, 478, 480
Olfactory bulb, 757
Olfactory nerve, 758t
anatomy, 675, 757, *759*
integrity testing, 769
Olfactory pits, 734
Olfactory receptor nerve cells, 757
Olfactory tract, 757
Olivary nuclei, 690
Olives, 690

Omentum, *204*, 206–207, *207*, *208*
gastrosplenic, 206–207
greater, 206, 213–214, 216, *217*
lesser, 206, *211*, 216, *217*, 249
Omohyoid, 742t, 747
Ophthalmic artery, *697*, 698, 750
Ophthalmic nerve, 727–729, *728*, 758t, 760
Ophthalmic vein, 698
Opponens digiti minimi, 506t
Opponens pollicis, 506t
Optic canal, 676, *695*, 696
Optic chiasma, 687
Optic disc, 698, 704
Optic nerve, 758t
anatomy, 697, *697*, *703*, 757, *759*
integrity testing, 769
Optic radiation, 757
Optic tract, 757
Ora serrata, 704
Oral pharynx, 790, *791*, 793
Orbicularis oculi, 691, 721t
Orbicularis oris, 721t, 731
Orbit
blood vessels, 698
blowout fractures, 706
description, *695*, 695–696
lymph vessels, 699
nerves, 697–698
Orbital cavity, openings, *695*, 696, *696*
Orbital fascia, 696
Orbital fissure, 673, *695*, 696
Orbital margins, 670, 695, 839
Orbital opening, *695*, 696
Orbital region
eyelids, 691, *692*, *693*, 694t
lacrimal apparatus, *692*, 694–695
Orbital septum, 691
Orbitalis muscle, 697
Orgasm, in female, 409
Origin, muscle, 8, *9*
Oropharyngeal isthmus, 793
Ossicles, auditory. *See* Auditory ossicles
Ossification, 35
Osteoarthritis, 469, 592
Osteoporosis, 860
Otic ganglia, 28, 762, 774
Otitis media, 714
Outer cell mass, 37
Ovarian artery, 328–329, 361
Ovarian fossa, 361
Ovary
blood supply, 361
cysts, 361
descent, 167, *168*
development, 361, *362*, *365*
dysgenesis, 361
function, 361
imperfect descent, 361
location and description, *358–359*, 361
lymph drainage, 361
nerve supply, 361
position, 361
suspensory ligament, 361, 377
Oxyphil cells, 822

Palatal plate, 785
Palate
anatomy, 781–785
blood supply, 782
cleft, *735*, 785, *788*
development, 785, *786*
hard, 673, 781, *783*
lymph drainage, 782
movements, 785
nerve supply, 782
soft, 781, *784*, 785t
Palatine aponeurosis, 781
Palatine bones, horizontal plates, 673
Palatine foramen, 673
Palatine nerve, 762
Palatine tonsil, 781, 793, 795
Palatoglossal arch, 781
Palatoglossus, 780t, 781, 785t
Palatopharyngeal arch, 781
Palatopharyngeus, 781, 785t, 792t
Palm of hand
anatomy, 499–508
anterior view, *493*, *501*, *503*, *504*
arteries, 503–504
carpal tunnel, 500
deep fascia, 500
fascial spaces, *507*, 508
fibrous flexor sheaths, 500–501, *501*
lymph drainage, 504–505
nerves, 505, 508
sensory innervation, *538*
skin, 499–500
structures lying in, 535
synovial flexor sheaths, 501, 502
veins, 504
Palmar, defined, 2
Palmar aponeurosis, *485*, 500
Palmar arch
deep, 504, *504*, 535
superficial, 486, 489, 503, 535
Palmar interosseous muscles, *505*, 506t
Palmaris brevis, 499–500, 506t
Palmaris longus, 499
absent, 486
tendon, 533
Palpebral fissure, 691
Palpebral ligament, 691
Pampiniform plexus, 165, 169
Pancreas
anatomy, 205, *206*, *256*, 256–257
anular, 258, *258*
cancer, 257
congenital fibrocystic disease, 258
development, *240*, 257, *258*
ectopic, 258
surface markings, 192
tail, splenectomy and, 257
trauma, 257
Pancreatic disease, diagnosis, 257
Pancreatic duct, 250, *250*, *251*, 256, *256*
Pancreatic islets, 256
Pancreaticoduodenal artery
inferior, 243
superior, 243
Papilla lacrimalis, 691
Papillary muscle, 108, 121
Papilledema, 769
Paracentesis, 105, *188*, 188–190
Paracolic gutters, *207*, 209, *213*
Paraesophageal hernia, 62, *63*
Parafollicular cells, 819
Paramedian incision, 188
Paramedian plane, 2, *3*
Paramesonephric duct fusion failure, uterus after, 371
Parametrium, 366
Paranasal sinus, 799–802, *801*, 802t
Pararectal nodes, 344
Pararectus incision, 188
Pararenal fat, 262
Parasympathetic system, 28–30, *30*, *31*
afferent fibers, 29–30
cervical part, 774
efferent fibers, 28–29, *31*
head, 774
Parathyroid glands
absence and hypoplasia, 822
anatomy, 821
development, 821–822, *822*
ectopic, 822
functions, 821
inferior, 821
superior, 821, 822
thyroidectomy and, 818
Parathyroid hormone, 821
Paratracheal nodes, 755
Paraumbilical incision, 190, *190*
Paraumbilical veins, 162
Paraurethral glands, 409
Paravertebral ganglia, 26
Paraxial mesoderm, 37
Parietal bones, 673
Parietal lobe, 687
Parietal peritoneum, *155*, 159
Parietal pleura, 30, *31*, 46, *70*, *71*, *82*, 84, 99
Parieto-occipital sulcus, 687
Paronychia, 7
Parotid duct, 774, 787, 839
Parotid gland, 787, *788*
Parotid nodes, 754
Pars anterior, 815, 816
Pars flaccida, 711
Pars intermedia, 815, 816
Pars nervosa, 816
Pars tensa, 711
Pars tuberalis, 815, 816
Patella
anatomy, 592–593, *593*, 654
dislocation, 596
fractures, 596
tangential view, *648*
Patellar plexus, 570
Patellar tendon reflex, 26, *29*, 659
Patent ductus arteriosus, *109*, 126
Patent urachus, 181, *181*
Pectineal line, 174, 393, *393*
Pectineus, 578t
Pectoral nerve, 449, 450t
Pectoral region, 427–437, *428–438*, *440*, *443*, *530*
Pectoralis major, 441t, 443
Pectoralis minor, 441t, 443
Pelvic appendix, 345
Pelvic brim, 309, *309*, *310*, 312, *313*
Pelvic cavity, 312, *313*
anatomy, 310, *310*, 338–381, *340*
contents, 338–344
cross-sectional anatomy, 377, *377–378*
ejaculatory duct, 352, 353, *354*
female genital organs, 361–377
male genital organs, 352–356
ovary
blood supply, 361
function, 361
location and description, *358–359*, 361
lymph drainage, 361
nerve supply, 361
peritoneum, 356, 376–377
prostate
blood supply, 355
function, 355
location and description, *349*, 353–354, *354*
lymph drainage, 355
nerve supply, 355
relations, *354*, 354–355
structure, *354*, 355
prostatic urethra, *354*, 356
radiographic anatomy, 377, *378–381*, 381
rectum
blood supply, *343*, 343–344
location and description, 341, *341*, *342*
lymph drainage, 344
nerve supply, 344
radiographic anatomy, 377, 381
relations, 341, *342*
seminal vesicles, *349*, 352, 353
sigmoid colon
anatomy, 338
radiographic anatomy, 377, 381
variation in length and location, 339
ureter, *347*, 347–348, 356, *358–359*
urinary bladder

blood supply, 350
development, 357, *359, 360*
female, 356
location and description, *348,* 348–350, *349*
lymph drainage, 350
male, *348,* 348–350, *349*
micturition, 350, *352*
nerve supply, 350
uterine tube
blood supply, 363
function, 363
location and description, *358–359,* 363, *363*
lymph drainage, 363
nerve supply, 363
uterus
after menopause, 368
blood supply, 366
in child, 368
function, 366
in labor, 368
location and description, *363,* 364–365
lymph drainage, 366
nerve supply, 367
positions, *363,* 366
in pregnancy, 368
relations, 365
structure, 366
supports, *366,* 367, *367,* 368
vagina
blood supply, 373
function, 373
location and description, *366,* 372–373
lymph drainage, 373
nerve supply, 373
relations, 373
supports, *366, 367,* 373
vas deferens, *347, 349,* 352
visceral pelvic fascia, 356, 376
Pelvic diaphragm, 318–319, *320, 321,* 388, *389*
Pelvic fascia
parietal, 319, 321, *324*
visceral, 321
Pelvic floor, 318, *320,* 322, *341*
functional significance in female, 322, *323*
injury, 322
muscles, 324t, *389*
Pelvic inflammatory disease, 364
Pelvic inlet, 309, *309, 310,* 312, *313*
Pelvic kidney, 267, *270*
Pelvic outlet, *310,* 310, 312, *313, 314*
Pelvic peritoneum, 321, *324*
Pelvic splanchnic nerve, 28, 325, 327, 328
Pelvic viscera, 330, 332, *333*
in female, 356
in male, 347–350
surface anatomy, 381
Pelvic wall
age changes, 329
anatomy, 308–332
anterior, 310, *315, 316*
autonomic nerves, 327
coccygeus, 318–319, *320, 321,* 324t
coccyx, 315, *316,* 330
common iliac artery, 327
external iliac artery, 328
external iliac vein, 329
inferior. *See* Pelvic floor
inferior hypogastric plexus, 327
internal iliac artery, 328
internal iliac vein, 329
lateral, 316, 318, *320*
hip bone, 316, 318
obturator internus, 318, *320,* 324t
obturator membrane, 318
sacrospinous ligament, 318, *319*
sacrotuberous ligament, 318
levator ani, 318, *320, 321,* 324t
lumbar plexus branches, 326–327
median sacral artery, 329
median sacral veins, 329
muscles, 324t
ovarian artery, 328–329
piriformis, 315–316, *317,* 324t
posterior, 310, 315–316, *316, 317, 325*
sacral plexus, 325, *325, 326,* 327t
sacrococcygeal joint, 329
sacroiliac joints, 329
sacrum, 310, 315, *316, 317*
structure, 310, *315,* 315–321
superior hypogastric plexus, 327
superior rectal artery, 328
surface anatomy, 330, *331–333,* 332
surface landmarks, 330, *331, 332*
symphysis pubis, 329, 330
urinary bladder, 330, 332, *333*
uterus, 332, *333*
viscera, 330, 332, *333*
Pelvis
anatomy, 308–310
arteries, 328–329
axis, 312, *313, 314*
as basin, 312
bony, 308, 377, *379–381*
computed tomography, 377, *378*
coronal section, *324*
double, 268, *271*
false, 309, 321
female, *309,* 312, *313, 314,* 322, *323,* 330, *342,* 369, *369, 370, 380, 381, 390–391, 418*
fractures, 321–322, *323*
joints, 329
lymphatics, 329
male, *309,* 330, *342, 379, 390–391, 418*
nerves, *325,* 325–327, *326,* 327t
obstetric measurements, 312, *313, 314*
orientation, 308–309
radiographic anatomy, 377, *379–381*
true, 309–310, *309–311*
arteries, 328–329
fractures, 321–322, *323*
trauma, 322
veins, 329
Penis, 419
blood supply, 405
body, *404,* 405
development, 413, *414, 415*
ejaculation, 406–407
erection, 406
location and description, 402, *402, 404,* 405
lymph drainage, 405
nerve supply, 405
root, 402, *404*
Pennate muscle, 10, *10*
Percussion, chest, 68
Perforated substance, posterior, 687
Perforating artery, 63, 586
Perforating cutaneous nerve, 325, 327t
Perforating vein, 571
Perianal abscess, 396, *399*
Perianal hematoma, 396, *399*
Pericapsulitis, 454, *457*
Pericardiacophrenic artery, 63
Pericardial artery, 126
Pericardial cavity, 30, 104
Pericardial fluid, 104
Pericardial friction rub, 105
Pericardial sinus, 104
Pericarditis, 105
Pericardium
anatomy, 103–104, 104, *104, 105*
fibrous, 103
nerve supply, 104
parietal layer, 103–104
serous, 103–104
visceral layer, 104, 118
Perilymph, 714
Perineal body, 318, *366,* 367, 406, 409
Perineal membrane, 401
Perineal nerve, 394, *395*
Perineum
anal canal
anatomy, 388–394
blood supply, *392,* 394
location and description, 388–389, *390–391*
lymph drainage, *392,* 394
muscle coat, *391,* 393
nerve supply, 394
structure, 389, *391–393,* 393
anal sphincters, *391, 393,* 393–394, 410t
anal triangle, 388, *389, 390,* 419
anatomy, 388–419
clitoris, 408, *408,* 419
coccyx, 417
deep perineal pouch
anatomy, 402
female, 409
male, 406
defecation, 394
defined, 388, *389*
epididymides, 419
greater vestibular glands, 409, 419
injury, during childbirth, 412
internal pudendal artery, 394
internal pudendal vein, 394
ischial tuberosity, 419
ischiorectal fossa, 394
muscles, 410t
paraurethral glands, 409
pelvic diaphragm, 388, *389*
penis, 419
blood supply, 405
body, *404,* 405
ejaculation, 406–407
erection, 406
location and description, 402, *402, 404,* 405
lymph drainage, 405
nerve supply, 405
root, 402, *404*
pudendal nerve, 394, *395*
radiographic anatomy, 417
scrotum, 405, 419
sphincter urethrae, 406, 409
superficial perineal pouch
anatomy, 401, *401, 403*
female, 408–409
male, 405–406
surface anatomy, 417–419, *418, 420*
symphysis pubis, 417
testis, 419
urethra
female, 409
male, 407–408
membranous, 406, 407
penile, 407–408
prostatic, 407
urogenital triangle, *389,* 400–411
female, 408–411, 419, *420*
male, *390,* 402, 405–408, 419
superficial fascia, 400–411, *401*
superficial perineal pouch, 401, *401, 403*
urogenital diaphragm, 401–402
vagina
blood supply, 410
location and description, 409–410, *411*
lymph drainage, 410
nerve supply, 411
vulva, 411, *411,* 419
Periosteum, 33, 35
Peripheral nervous system, 21–24, *23–25*
Peristalsis, 12, 217

Peritoneal cavity, 30, *179,* 205, 216, *216, 217*
Peritoneal dialysis, 215
Peritoneal fluid, 206, 213, *213, 214*
Peritoneal infection, 213
Peritoneal lavage, *189,* 189–190, *190*
Peritoneal ligaments, 206, *210, 211,* 216, *216,* 248–249
Peritoneal lining, 177, *178*
Peritoneal mesentery, 216, *216*
Peritoneal pain, 215, *215*
Peritoneal sac, greater, 206
Peritoneum, 356, 376–377
  anatomy, 205–214
  arrangement, 205–206, *207, 208, 209*
  broad ligaments, 377
  cecal recesses, 208, *212*
  development, 216, *216, 217*
  duodenal recesses, 208, *212*
  functions, 209, *217*
  intersigmoid recess, 208, *212*
  intraperitoneal and retroperitoneal relationships, 206
  lesser sac, *207,* 207–208, *208, 211, 217*
  mesenteries, 207, *208, 209, 212*
  nerve supply, 209
  omenta, *204,* 206–207, *207, 208*
  paracolic gutters, *207,* 209, *213*
  parietal, 205, 209, 215, *216*
  peritoneal ligaments, 206, *210, 211*
  rectal, 341
  subphrenic spaces, 208–209, *213, 214*
  visceral, 205, 209, 215, *216,* 220
Peritonsillar abscess, 793, *794*
Periumbilical, 192
Peroneal artery, 618
Peroneal nerve
  common, 656, 657
    anatomy, 587, 604
    branches, *567,* 604
    injury, 660
    sural communicating branch, 604
    tibial portion, 327t
  deep, 614, 627, 629
  superficial, 609, 615, 627
Peroneal retinaculum
  inferior, 609
  superior, 606, 609
Peroneal tubercle, 596, 657
Peroneus brevis, 614t
  tendon, 657–658
  tenosynovitis and dislocation, 615
Peroneus longus, 614t
  tendon, 621, 624, 657, 658
  tenosynovitis and dislocation, 615
Peroneus tertius, 612, 613t, 657
Pes cavus, 642
Pes planus, 642
Petrosal nerve
  deep, 676
  greater, 676, 712, 765
  lesser, 676, 714
Petrosal sinus, 677, 687
Petrotympanic fissure, 765
Phalanges, 480, *481, 482, 597–599,* 600, *652*
Pharyngeal pouch, 793
Pharyngeal recess, 790
Pharyngeal tonsil, 790
Pharyngeal tubercle, 674
Pharynx
  anatomy, 789–795, *791*
  blood supply, 793
  constrictor muscles, *783,* 789, *791,* 792t
  crossing of air and food pathways, 802
  interior, 789–790, 793
  laryngeal, *791,* 793
  lymph drainage, 793
  lymphoid tissue, 793
  muscles, 789, *791,* 792t
  nasal, 790, *791*
  oral, 790, *791,* 793
  sensory nerve supply, 793
  in swallowing, 795
Pheochromocytoma, 270
Philtrum, 734, 774
Phimosis, 407
Phocomelia, 521
Phrenic nerve
  accessory, 448, 771
  anatomy, 127, 771, 771t
  injury, 771
Phrenicocolic ligament, 233
Pia mater
  brain, 685
  spinal cord, 871
Pineal body, 689
Pineal gland, 816
Piriform fossa, 793, 795, 805
Piriformis, 315–316, *317,* 324t, 563, 566t
  nerve to, 327t
Pisiform bone, 480, 533
Pituitary gland
  anatomy, 676, *684,* 687, 815, *815*
  development, 816, *816*
  function, 815
Pivot joint, 14, *16*
Placenta, 37
  appearance at birth, 372, *375*
  formation, 372, *374*
Placenta previa, 372
Placental abruption, 372
Plane joint, 13, *16*
Plantar, defined, 2
Plantar aponeurosis, 619, *620*
Plantar arch, 625
Plantar artery, 624–625
Plantar calcaneonavicular ligament, 637
Plantar digital nerves, 626
Plantar fasciitis, 619
Plantar flexion, 635, 637
Plantar interosseous muscles, 623t
Plantar muscles, *621, 623, 625, 626*
Plantar nerve
  lateral, 619, 627
  medial, 619, 626–627
Plantar vein, 626
Plantaris, 615, 617t
Platysma, 721t, 737, *738,* 742t, 842
  clinical identification, 739
  innervation, 740
  tone, 740
Pleura
  anatomy, *70, 71,* 72, 80, *80, 82, 83,* 83–84, *84*
  anterior border, 72
  cervical dome, 72
  costal, 84
  development, 99
  diaphragmatic, 84
  lower border, 72
  mediastinal, 84
  nerve supply, 84, *85*
  parietal, 30, *31,* 46, *70, 71, 82,* 83, 99
  thoracic, *70, 71,* 72
  visceral, 30, *31,* 46, 83, 99
Pleural adhesions, 85
Pleural cavity, 30, *31,* 46, 83
Pleural effusion, 85, *86*
Pleural fluid, 84, 85
Pleural reflection, 72
Pleural rub, 85
Pleural space, 83
Pleurisy, 85
Plexus, 23–24, *24,* 26
  aortic, 280, *280*
  brachial. *See* Brachial plexus
  cardiac, 116
  celiac, 280, *280*
  cervical, 23, *24,* 771, 771t
  choroid, 684, 690, 874
  deep, 98
  esophageal, 127, 128
  hypogastric
    inferior, 327
    superior, 280, *280,* 327
  lumbar, 23, *24,* 278–279, *279,* 279t, 326–327
  mesenteric, 280, *280*
  pampiniform, 165, 169
  patellar, 570
  prostatic venous, *354,* 355
  pulmonary, 98, 127
  renal, 280, *280*
  sacral, 23, *24*
    anatomy, 325, *325, 326,* 327t
    branches, 325, 327t
    invasion by malignant tumors, 326
    pressure from fetal head, 325–326
  superficial, 98
  tympanic, 714
  venous, 18, *20*
  vertebral venous, 865–866, *866*
  vesical venous, 350
Plica fimbriata, 774, 779
Plica semilunaris, 691
Plicae circulares, *225,* 227, 246
Pneumoarthrography, knee joint, 632, *648*
Pneumonia, 103
Pneumothorax, 82, 85
  after intercostal nerve block, 56
  after rib fracture, 58
  artificial, 85
  open, 85
  spontaneous, 85
  tension, 85
Poliomyelitis, 564
Polycystic kidney, 267
Polydactyly, 522
Pons, 676, 689
Popliteal aneurysm, 604
Popliteal artery, 600, 657, 658
Popliteal bursa, 630, 631
Popliteal fossa, 656–657
  anatomy, 600–605, *601, 602*
  boundaries, 600, *601*
  contents, 600–605, *601*
  deep structures, *602*
  surface markings, *656*
Popliteal lymph nodes, 604
Popliteal surface, 561
Popliteal vein, 604
Popliteus, 600, 617t, 618
Porta hepatis, *244,* 247
Portal canal, 248
Portal hypertension, 129, 246
Portal system, 18
Portal vein, 18, *20,* 245, *245*
  liver cancer and, 246
  obstruction, 162, *163*
  tributaries, *221,* 245
Portal-systemic anastomosis, 129, 246, *247,* 395
Position, terms related to, 2–3, *3*
Postcentral gyrus, 687
Posterior, defined, 2
Posterior abdominal wall. *See* Abdominal wall, posterior
Posterior auricular artery, 725, 750
Posterior auricular vein, 725
Posterior axillary fold, 530
Posterior axillary line, 68
Posterior axillary nodes, 126, 451, *453*
Posterior cecal artery, 244
Posterior cerebral artery, 751
Posterior chamber of eye, 704
Posterior chest wall, 66, *67, 69, 70*
Posterior circumflex humeral artery, 446
Posterior clinoid process, 676
Posterior communicating artery, 750

Posterior cranial fossa, 676–677, 679
Posterior cricoarytenoid muscle, 806t
Posterior cruciate ligament, 629, 632, *633*
Posterior cutaneous nerve
 of arm, 466
 of forearm, 475
 of thigh, 325, 327t, 565–566, 605, 615
Posterior ethmoidal nerve, 698, 760
Posterior fold, 66
Posterior fontanelle, 679, *680,* 837, *838*
Posterior inferior iliac spine, 555
Posterior intercondylar area, 593
Posterior intercostal arteries, 53, *53, 54*
Posterior intercostal membrane, 53, *53*
Posterior intercostal nodes, 126
Posterior intercostal veins, 53, *55*
Posterior internodal pathway, 113
Posterior interosseous artery, 487, 498
Posterior interventricular artery, 113–114, *115*
Posterior longitudinal ligament, 858–859
Posterior malleolar fold, 711
Posterior mediastinum, 80
Posterior nasal aperture, 796
Posterior pelvic wall, 310, 315–316, *316, 317, 325*
Posterior perforated substance, 687
Posterior ramus, 22
Posterior root, 21, *23, 25*
Posterior root ganglion, 22
Posterior sacroiliac ligament, 329
Posterior spinal artery, 870
Posterior superior alveolar nerve, 762
Posterior superior iliac spine, 191, 318, 330, 555, 644
Posterior talofibular ligament, 635
Posterior tibial artery, 618, 657, 658
Posterior tibial nerve, 657
Posterior tibial vessels, 657
Posterior triangle, neck, 747, 843
Posterior vagal trunk, 220, *222*
Postural drainage, 103
Postvertebral muscles, *864,* 864–865
Pouch of Douglas, 376
Preaortic lymph nodes, 276
Precentral gyrus, 687
Pregnancy
 ectopic, 364, *364*
 hemorrhoids, 368
 pelvic joint changes, 329
 rectal examination, *400*
 term, 368
 uterus, 195, 368
 varicosed veins, 368
 vulva, 412
Premaxilla, 734
Prepatellar bursa, 631
Prepuce, 405, 408, 413
Primary cartilaginous joint, 13
Prime mover, muscle, 10, *11*
Primitive streak, 37
Proboscis, lateral, 798, *801*
Procerus, 721t
Processus cochleariformis, 711
Processus vaginalis, 165–167, *168,* 169–170, *170*
Proctodeum, 397
Profunda artery, 472, *474*
Profunda brachii artery, *475,* 476
Profunda femoris artery, 580, 585–586
Profunda femoris vein, 586
Pronator quadratus, 492t
Pronator teres, 492t
Pronator tubercle, 478
Prone, defined, 3
Pronephros, *268*
Prostate
 activity and disease, 355
 benign enlargement, 355, *358*
 blood supply, 355
 cancer, 355, 866
 examination, 355
 function, 355
 location and description, *349,* 353–354, *354*
 lymph drainage, 355
 nerve supply, 355
 relations, *354,* 354–355
 structure, *354,* 355
Prostatic sinus, 356
Prostatic urethra, *354,* 356
Prostatic utricle, 356
Prostatic venous plexus, *354,* 355
Prothrombin time, *838,* 838–839
Protraction, defined, 4
Proximal, defined, 2
Proximal carpal row, 480
Proximal radioulnar joint, *512,* 512–513
Proximal tibiofibular joint, 632
Psoas, 578t
Psoas fascia, 175, *176,* 177
Psoas major, 174, *176,* 177t
Psoas sheath, 580
Pterion, 673
Pterygoid, 721t
Pterygoid canal, nerve of, 676, 712
Pterygoid hamulus, 673
Pterygoid muscle, nerve to, 762
Pterygoid plate, 673
Pterygomandibular ligament, 747
Pterygomaxillary fissure, 673
Pterygomaxillary fossa, 673
Pterygopalatine ganglia, 28, 762, 774
Ptosis, 769
Pubic arch, 310, *310, 311,* 312
Pubic crest, 191, 318, 330, 555, 650
Pubic tubercle, 191, 318, 330, 555, 650
Pubis, 318, 555
Pubocervical ligament, 367, *367,* 368
Pubococcygeus, 318
Pubofemoral ligament, 588
Puboprostatic ligament, 350, 354
Puborectalis, 318, 393, 410t
Pubovesical ligament, 350
Pudendal artery
 external, 580
 internal, 328, 394, 406
Pudendal canal, 394
Pudendal nerve, 325, 394, *395,* 566
 perineal branch, 406, 409
 tibial portion, 327t
Pudendal nerve block, 412, *413*
Pudendal procedure, 412, *413*
Pudendal vein
 external, 571
 internal, 394
Pudendal vessels, internal, 409
Pulmonary arteries, *88,* 126
Pulmonary fibrosis, 103
Pulmonary ligament, 83
Pulmonary nodes, 98
Pulmonary plexus, 98, 127
Pulmonary sinuses, 108
Pulmonary trunk, 119, *122*
Pulmonary valve, *89,* 108, *110,* 117, 119
Pulmonary veins, 123
Pulp space
 finger, *507,* 508
 infection, 508
Pulse, carotid, 748
Punctum lacrimale, 691, 694
Pupil, 704, 705
Pupillary reflexes, 706
Purkinje fibers, 111
Pyelography, 295, *296–298*
Pyloric antrum, 219
Pyloric canal, 220
Pyloric orifice, 217, 220
Pyloric sphincter, *219,* 220
Pyloric stenosis, congenital hypertrophic, 237
Pylorus, 220
Pyopneumothorax, 85
Pyramid, 690
Pyramidalis, *149,* 154, 158t

Quadrangular membrane, 802
Quadrangular space, 458
Quadrate tubercle, 560
Quadratus femoris, 566t
 nerve to, 325, 327t, 566
Quadratus lumborum, 175–176, *176,* 177t
Quadratus lumborum fascia, 177
Quadratus plantae, 622t
Quadriceps femoris, 578t
 action, 573, 575
 as knee joint stabilizer, 578
Quadriceps mechanism, 573, 575, *579*
Queckenstedt's sign, 873
Quincke's uvula, 785
Quinsy, 793, *794*

Race, effects on structure, 36
Radial artery
 anatomy, 487, 489, 504
 on dorsum of hand, 509
 palmar branches, 504
 palpation, 533
Radial bursa, 501
Radial fossa, 435
Radial nerve
 anatomy, 450, 450t, 474, 475, *476,* 495
 branches, *453,* 495, 537, *538*
 deep branch, 499, 539
 injury, 537, 539, *539*
 superficial branch, 495, 499, 500, 508, 539
Radial notch, 478
Radicular arteries, 870
Radiocarpal joint. *See* Wrist
Radiograph, 36, *38*
Radiographic anatomy, 36–37, *38–40*
 abdomen, 282, *284–286*
 ankle, *649, 650*
 back, 876, 880
 brain, 824, *835–837*
 duodenum, 282, 289, *289*
 elbow, *524, 525*
 female genital organs, *369, 370,* 381, *381*
 foot, *651, 652*
 gallbladder, 289, *294, 295*
 gastrointestinal tract, 282, *287–293,* 289
 hand, *525–528*
 head, 824, *827–837*
 hip joint, *645*
 ileum, *287,* 289, *290*
 jejunum, *287,* 289, *290*
 kidney, 295
 knee joint, *646, 647, 653*
 large intestine, 289, *291–293*
 lower limb, 644, *645–653*
 pelvic cavity, 377, *378–381*
 pelvis, 377, *379–381*
 perineum, 417
 rectum, 377, 381
 shoulder, *523*
 sigmoid colon, 377, 381
 skull, 824, *827–837*
 small intestine, *287,* 289, *290*
 stomach, 282, *287, 288*
 thorax, *38,* 131, 133–137
  bronchography, 135, *139*
  computed tomography, *39, 132,* 137
  coronary angiography, 136–137, *139*
  left oblique radiograph, 135, *137–138*
  posteroanterior radiograph, 131, 133–134, *133–134*
  right oblique radiograph, 134–135, *135–136*
 ureter, 295, *296–298*
 urinary tract, 289, 295, *296–298*

Radiographic anatomy *(continued)*
  vertebral column, 876, 880, *881–888*
  wrist, *525–528*
Radiolucent, 36
Radiopaque, 36
Radioulnar joint
  disease, 513
  distal, *512,* 513
  proximal, *512,* 512–513
Radius
  anatomy, 478, *479*
  congenital absence, 521, *521*
  dorsal tubercle, 533
  fractures, 479–480, *481*
  head, 533
  styloid process, 533, 535
Rami communicantes, 22, 55
Ramus
  anterior, 22
  mandible, 715, *838,* 839
  posterior, 22
Raphe, 8, *9*
Raynaud disease, 128, 536
Rectal ampulla, 341
Rectal artery
  inferior, 343, *343,* 394
  middle, 328, 343, *343*
  superior, 244, 328, 343, *343*
Rectal examination, 397, *400*
Rectal nerve, inferior, 394
Rectal prolapse, incontinence and, 397
Rectal vein, 343–344
  inferior, 343
  middle, 343
  superior, 343, *398*
Rectouterine pouch, 376
Rectovesical pouch, 356
Rectovesical septum, 355
Rectum
  anatomy, *203,* 204
  blood supply, *343,* 343–344
  cancer, 344
  curves, 344
  development, 238
  injury, 345
  location and description, 341, *341, 342*
  lymph drainage, 344
  mucosal folds, 344
  nerve supply, 344
  prolapse, 344, *344*
  radiographic anatomy, 377, 381
  relations, 341, *342*
Rectus, 694t, *699,* 699–702, *701, 702*
Rectus abdominis, *149, 151,* 152, 154, *155,* 158t, 191–192
  separation, 186, *187*
  tendinous intersections, 191–192
Rectus femoris, 578t
  muscular branch, 582
  rupture, 578
Rectus sheath
  anatomy, *148, 149,* 154, *155,* 156, *157*
  hematoma, 156
Recurrent laryngeal nerve, 127, 767, 808, *809,* 818
Renal arteries, 268, *270*
Renal colic, 267
Renal columns, 262
Renal fascia, 262, 270
Renal pain, 264
Renal papilla, 262
Renal pelvis, 262, 295, *296–298*
Renal plexus, 280, *280*
Renal pyramids, 262
Renal sinus, 260
Reproductive system, data concerning, 900t
Respiration
  expiration
    forced, *87,* 102
    lung changes on, 102
    quiet, 102
  inspiration
    forced, 102
    lung changes on, 102
    muscle of, 59
    quiet, *87,* 100, *101,* 102
  mechanics, 100–102
  types, 102
  vocal cord movements with, 806
Respiratory efficiency, conditions decreasing, 103
Respiratory system, data concerning, 899t
Resuscitation, cardiopulmonary, 117–118
Retina, 704
Retinacula, 8, *8,* 575, 588
Retraction, defined, 4
Retroauricular nodes, 754
Retromammary space, 427
Retromandibular vein, 752
Retroperitoneal space, 260, *261*
Retropharyngeal nodes, 755, 793
Retropubic pad of fat, 349, 356
Rhomboid major, 442t
Rhomboid minor, 442t
Rib
  anatomy, 47, *47, 48, 49,* 49–50, 530, *531*
  atypical, 50, *50*
  cervical, 50, 857
  contusion, 58
  excision, 50
  false, 47, 49
  fifth, *49*
  first, 50, *50*
  floating, 49
  fracture, 58
  head, 49, *49*
    joints, 51
  identification, 68
  joints, 51
  movements, 51
  neck, 49, *49*
  true, 47
  tubercle, 49, *49*
    joints, 51
  twelfth pair, 173
  typical, *49,* 49–50
Rib cage, 65
Rickets, 35
Right dominance, posterior interventricular artery in, 113, *115*
Rima glottidis, 805
Ring finger, movements, 517, 519
Risorius, 721t
Rosette kidney, 268, *270*
Rotation, defined, 3
Rotator cuff
  anatomy, 454, *462*
  tendinitis, 454, *457*
Round ligament of ovary, 361
Running, 642–643

Saccule, 714
Saccus endolymphaticus, 714
Sacral artery, 329
Sacral canal, 310, 856, 873, *881*
Sacral crest, median, 645, 881
Sacral hiatus, 330, 856, 873, *879,* 881
Sacral nerves, 21, *24*
Sacral plexus
  anatomy, 23, *24,* 325, *325, 326,* 327t
  branches, 325, 327t
  invasion by malignant tumors, 326
  pressure from fetal head, 325–326
  relations, 325
Sacral promontory, 310, 856
Sacral veins, median, 329
Sacral vertebrae
  partial fusion, 322
  second, 684
Sacrocervical ligament, 367, *367,* 368
Sacrococcygeal joint, 329
Sacroiliac joint, 310, *319,* 329
Sacroiliac joint disease, 329–330, 868
Sacroiliac ligament, 329
Sacrospinous ligament, *310,* 318, *319, 562, 564*
Sacrotuberous ligament, *310,* 318, *319, 562, 564*
Sacrum
  anatomy, 310, 315, *316, 317,* 856, 881, *887, 888*
  fractures, 322
  spinous processes, 330
Saddle joint, 15, *16*
Sagittal sinus
  inferior, 686
  superior, 674, 686, 874
Sagittal suture, 673
Salivary glands, 787–789, *788, 790,* 843
Salivary nucleus, 774
Salpingopharyngeal fold, 790
Salpingopharyngeus, 789, *791,* 792t
Saphenous nerve, 582, 609, 615, 627
Saphenous opening, 573
Saphenous varix, 580
Saphenous vein, great
  anatomy, 570, 582, 650, 654, 657
  in coronary bypass surgery, 572
  cutdown, 571–572, *572*
  origin, *612*
Sartorius, 578t
Scala tympani, 714
Scala vestibuli, 714
Scalenus anterior, 742t, 743, 822
Scalenus medius, 742t, 822
Scalenus posterior, 742t
Scalp
  arterial supply, 725
  clinical significance, 725
  hemorrhage, 726
  infection, 726
  lacerations, 725–726
  layers, *671, 722*
  lymph drainage, 725, *727*
  muscle, 721t, 724
  nerve supply, 725
  structure, *722,* 722–724
  venous drainage, 725, *726*
Scaphoid bone, 480, 535
Scapula, 66
  anatomy, *433,* 434, *435,* 531, *532*
  fractures, 434
  humerus and, muscles connecting, 442t
  inferior angle, 434, 531, 881
  medial border, 881
  palpation, 881, *894*
  rotation, 465, *466*
  spine, 66, 434, 531, 881
  superior angle, 531, 881
  winged, 434, *435,* 537
Scapular line, 68
Scapular nerve, dorsal, 450t
Scapular region, *457*
Scapular-humeral mechanism, 465, *466*
Scarpa's fascia, 147
Schlemm canal, 704
Sciatic foramina, 318, 555, *562*
Sciatic nerve, 325, 327t, 565, *567, 568,* 587, 650
  branches, 587
  injury, 659–660, *660*
Sciatic notch, 318, 555
Sciatica, 660, 868
Sclera, 703
Scoliosis, 860, 875, *881*
Scotoma, central, 769
Scrotal raphe, 191, 419
Scrotum, 405, 419
  anatomy, *166,* 167–169, 191

clinical conditions, 169–170
development, 413, *414*
lymph drainage, *167*, 169
Sebaceous cyst, 7
Sebaceous gland, 6, *6*
Sebum, 6
Second intercostal nerve, 55, 57
Secondary cartilaginous joint, 13
Segmental arteries, 264
Sella turcica, 676
Semen, 406
Semicircular canal, 676, 714
Semicircular duct, 714, 715
Semilunar valves, 119
Semimembranosus, 587, 589t, 604
Semimembranosus bursa, 630, 631
Seminal fluid, 406
Seminal vesicles, *349*, 352–353
Semitendinosus, 589t
Sengstaken-Blakemore balloon, 218
Senile kyphosis, 860
Sensory area, 687
Sensory fibers, 22
Sensory nerves
face, 727–729, *728*
hand, *538*
mouth, 776, *777*
pharynx, 793
tongue, 779
upper limb, 465–466, *467*, 482
Septum intermedium, 118
Septum primum, 118
Septum secundum, 118
Serous exudate, 30
Serous membrane, 30, *31*, 32
Serratus anterior, 441t
Serratus posterior
inferior, 63–64, 65t, 102
superior, 63, 65t
Sesamoid bone, *33*, 34, 600
Sex hormones, 269, 361
Shock
hypovolemic, 468
skin changes, 7
Short bone, 33
Short ciliary nerve, 757
Short gastric artery, 220, 243
Short gastric vein, 220
Short plantar ligament, 638
Shoulder
dropped, 434, *435*
radiographic anatomy, *523*
surface anatomy, *531*, *532*
Shoulder girdle, 432, 434–437
Shoulder joint
abduction, 465, *466*
accessory ligaments, 463
anatomy, 462–465
arterial anastomosis around, 458, *459*
articulation, 462, *462*, *463*
capsule, 462, *463*
dislocation, 465
ligaments, 462–463
movements, 463–465, *464*
nerve supply, 463
osteoarthritis, 469
relations, 465
stability, 465
synovial membrane, 463
type, 462
Shoulder pain, 465
Shoulder separation, 461
Sigmoid artery, 244
Sigmoid colon
anatomy, *203*, 204, 338
cancer, 339
development, 239
radiographic anatomy, 377, 381
variation in length and location, 339
Sigmoid mesocolon, 207, *212*, 338
Sigmoid sinus, 677, 686
Sigmoidoscopy, 339, *340*
Silicosis, 103
Singing, 807
Sinuatrial node, 112
Sinuatrial node arteries, 113
Sinus tarsi, 597
Sinus venosus, 118
Sinusitis, 800–801
Sinusoid, 18, *20*, 248
Skeletal muscle
action, 10–12, *11*
anatomy, 8–12, *9*
internal structure, 8, 10, *10*
naming, 12, 13t
nerve supply, 12
Skin
anatomy, 4–6, *6*, *7*
anterior abdominal wall, 146
appendages, 5–6, *6*, *7*
back, 454
burn, 7
buttock, 551
creases, 5, *7*
face, 727, 729
foot, 619, 627
forearm, 482–483
grafting, 7
hand, 499–500, 508–509
infection, 7
leg, 609, 615
lines of cleavage, 146
neck, 736–737, *737*
scrotum, 167
segmental innervation, 26, *27*, *28*
structure, 4–5, *6*
thigh, 568–573, 587
upper arm, 465–466, 468–469
Skull
anterior view, 670, *670*, 673
arteriography, 824, *830–833*
base, 669
anatomy, *675*, 675–677
anterior cranial fossa, 675
middle cranial fossa, 675–676
openings, 677t
posterior cranial fossa, 676–677
bones
composition, 669–670, *670–672*
front, *730*, 731
computed tomography, 824, *834*
cranial cavity, 674
fractures, 678
inferior view, 673–674, *674*, *675*
lateral view, *671*, 673
magnetic resonance imaging, 824, *835–837*
meninges, *681*, 681–685
neonatal, 677, 679–680, *680*
posterior view, *672*, 673
radiographic anatomy, 824, *827–837*
superior view, *672*, 673
vault, 669, 674–675
Sliding esophageal hernia, 62, *63*
Small cardiac vein, *114*, 116
Small intestine
anatomy, *203*, 204, *205*, 224–228
development, 237
versus large intestine, 246, *248*
mesentery, 207, *226*, 227, 229
pain fibers, 229
radiographic anatomy, *287*, 289, *290*
recognition, 229
trauma, 229
Small saphenous vein, 604, 615, 657
Smith's fracture, 480, *481*
Smooth muscle, 12
Soft palate, 781, *784*, 785t
Sole of foot
arteries, 624–625
cutaneous nerves, *620*
deep fascia, 619, *620*
long tendons, 619, 621, 624
muscles, 619, *621–626*, 622t–623t
nerves, 626–627
skin, 619
synovial sheaths, *624*
veins, 626
Soleal line, 594
Soleus, 615, 617t
Somatic chest pain, 129
Somatic nervous system, 21, *30*
Sonography
female pelvis, 369, *369*, *370*
uterus, 369, *369*, *370*
Space of Parona, 501
Speech, 807
Spermatic cord, 164–165, *166*, 191
coverings, 165, *168*
structures, 164–165, *167*, *168*
Spermatic fascia, 165, 167–168, *168*
Sphenoid bone, 676
greater wing, 673, 676
lesser wing, 676
Sphenoidal sinus, 676, 800, *801*, 802t
Sphenomandibular ligament, 715, 719, 747
Sphenopalatine foramen, 673
Sphincter
external, 393, 410t
internal, 393
Sphincter muscle, lips, 721t, 731
Sphincter of Oddi, 250, *250*
Sphincter pupillae of iris, 694t, 704
Sphincter urethrae, 406, 409, 410t
Sphincter vaginae, 318
Sphincter vesicae, 350
Spigelian hernia, 186
Spina bifida, 875, *882*, *883*
Spinal anesthesia, 128
Spinal artery, 870
Spinal canal, narrowing, 868
Spinal cord
anatomy, 867–874, *869*, *870*, *872*, *874*, *876*
blood supply, 870
cerebrospinal fluid, 874
injury, 871
ejaculation after, 407
erection after, 407
incontinence after, 397
micturition after, 351, *353*
ischemia, 870
meninges, 871
segments, relationship to vertebral numbers, *870*, 871
Spinal nerve roots
anatomy, 867, *869*, *870*, *872*
pain, 867
Spinal nerves, 21–22, *23*, *24*, *25*, 867, 874
Spinal tap, 871, 873, *878*
Spinous processes, 530–531, *532*, 645, 853
Spiral aorticopulmonary septum, 118
Spiral ganglion, 715
Spiral groove, 435, 539
Spiral lamina, 714
Spiral organ of Corti, 715
Splanchnic nerves, 26–27, 28, 128
Spleen
anatomy, 205, *206*, 259, *259*
development, 260
enlargement, 260
supernumerary, 260
surface markings, 192, *193*
trauma, 260
Splenectomy, 257
Splenic artery, 240, *244*
Splenic vein, 245, 276
Splenius capitis, 865

Splenius cervicis, 865
Spondylolisthesis, 862–863
Squamotympanic fissure, 673
Stab wounds, abdominal, 186–187
Standing immobile, 642
Stapedius, 711t
  nerve to, 712, 765
Stapes, 711, 712, *713*
Staphylococcus aureus infection, skin, 7
Stellate ganglion, 128, 773
  nerve block, 774
Stenosing synovitis, 498
Stenosing tenosynovitis, 498
Sternal angle, 47, *48*, 64, 523
Sternoclavicular joint, 842
  anatomy, 459–460, *460*
  dislocation, 460
  injury, 460
  movements, 459, *461*
Sternoclavicular ligament, 459
Sternocleidomastoid, 740–742, 742t, 841
Sternohyoid, 742t
Sternothyroid, 742t
Sternum
  anatomy, 46–47, *47*
  body, 47
  costal cartilages with, joints, 51
  fracture, 58
  joints, 51
  marrow biopsy, 47
Stomach
  anatomy, 203, *203*, *204*, 219–220
  arteries, *218*, 220
  cancer, 223
  development, 237, *239*
  location and description, *219*, 219–220
  lymph drainage, 220, *222*
  nerve supply, 220, *222*
  radiographic anatomy, 282, *287*, *288*
  relations, 220
  rotation, *217*
  surface markings, 193
  trauma, 223
  veins, 220, *221*
Stomodeum, 734
Strabismus, 706, 769
Straight sinus, 686
Strangulated hernia, 580
Stress incontinence, 357
Styloglossus, 780t
Stylohyoid, 742t
Stylohyoid ligament, 747
Styloid muscles, vessels, and nerves, *749*
Styloid process, 478
Stylomandibular ligament, 719, 747
Stylomastoid foramen, 674
Stylopharyngeus, 789, *791*, 792t
  nerve to, 715, 765, *766*
Subacromial bursitis, 454, *457*
Subarachnoid cisternae, 683
Subarachnoid hemorrhage, 686
Subarachnoid space, 683, 870
  block, 873
  myelography, 876, *889–890*
Subcapital fracture, 561
Subclavian artery, 124, 751, 822
  branches, 458, 751
  compression, 772
  first part, 751
  palpation and compression, 751
  second part, 751
  third part, 751, 843
Subclavian lymph trunk, 127, 451
Subclavian vein
  anatomy, 753, 824
  thrombosis, 753–754, *756*
Subclavius, 441t
  nerve to, 448, 450t
Subcostal angle, 64
Subcostal artery, 126
Subcostal nerve, 55
Subcostal plane, *156*, =2191
Subcostal vein, 123
Subcutaneous emphysema, 82, 102
Subdural hemorrhage, 686
Subdural space, 683, 870
Subfascial space, 509
Sublingual ducts, 789
Sublingual fold, 774
Sublingual fossa, 715
Sublingual gland, 789, *790*
Submandibular fossa, 715
Submandibular ganglia, 28, 762–763, 774
Submandibular gland, 789, *790*
Submandibular nodes, 754, 789
Submandibular region, *763*
Submental artery, 729
Submental nodes, 754
Submental triangle, 747, 839
Subphrenic spaces, 208–209, *213*, *214*, 249
Subsartorial canal, *556*, 575, 654
Subscapular artery, 446, 458
Subscapular fossa, 434
Subscapular nerve, 449
Subscapularis, 442t
Subscapularis bursa, 463
Substantia nigra, 689
Subtalar joint, 637, 638
Subtarsal sulcus, 691
Sulci, 687
Sulcus calcanei, 596
Sulcus chiasmatic, 676
Sulcus tali, 597
Sulcus terminalis, 107, 778, 781
Superciliary arches, 670
Superciliary ridges, 837, *838*
Superficial, defined, 2
Superficial arteries, lower limb, *553*
Superficial cervical artery, 458, 751
Superficial cervical fascia, 737
Superficial circumflex iliac artery, 580
Superficial circumflex iliac vein, 571
Superficial epigastric artery, 580
Superficial epigastric vein, 571
Superficial external pudendal artery, 580
Superficial external pudendal vein, 571
Superficial fascia, 5, *6*, *8*
Superficial infrapatellar bursa, 631
Superficial inguinal lymph nodes, 573, 580, 650
Superficial inguinal ring, 191
Superficial palmar arch, 486, 489, 503, 535
Superficial perineal pouch
  anatomy, 401, *401*, *403*
  female, 408–409
  male, 405–406
Superficial peroneal nerve, 609, 615, 627
Superficial plexus, 98
Superficial sensory nerves, upper limb, 465–466, *467*, 482
Superficial temporal artery, 725, 729, 750, 838, *838*
Superficial temporal vein, 725, 752
Superficial transverse perineal muscle, 405, 409, 410t
Superficial veins
  lower limb, *553*, 571
  upper limb, 468, *468*, 482
Superior, defined, 2
Superior acromioclavicular ligament, 461
Superior alveolar nerve, 762
Superior angle, 66
Superior cerebellar peduncle, 690
Superior cerebral vein, 686
Superior cervical ganglion, 773
Superior colliculi, 689
Superior conchae, 670
Superior constrictor muscle, 789, *791*, 792t
Superior epigastric artery, 63, 161
Superior extensor retinaculum, 606
Superior gemellus, 566t
Superior gluteal artery, 328, 566
Superior gluteal nerve, 325, 327t, 566
Superior hemiazygos vein, 123, *124*
Superior hypogastric plexus, 280, *280*, 327
Superior iliac spine
  anterior, 191, 318, 555, 644
  posterior, 191, 318, 330, 555, 644
Superior intercostal artery, 751
Superior labial artery, 729
Superior laryngeal nerve, 766
Superior lobar bronchus, 88
Superior meatus, 797
Superior mediastinum, 80
Superior medullary vela, 690
Superior mesenteric artery, *230*, 243, *244*, *293*
Superior mesenteric plexus, 280, *280*
Superior mesenteric vein, 245, 276
Superior mesenteric vein thrombosis, 229
Superior nuchal lines, 673, 837
Superior oblique, 694t, 699–702, *700*, *701*, *702*
Superior ophthalmic vein, 698
Superior orbital fissure, 676, *695*, 696
Superior pancreaticoduodenal artery, 243
Superior parathyroid glands, 821, 822
Superior peroneal retinaculum, 606, 609
Superior petrosal sinus, 677, 687
Superior rectal artery, 244, 328, 343, *343*
Superior rectal vein, 343, *398*
Superior rectus, 694t, *699*, 699–702, *701*, *702*
Superior sagittal sinus, 674, 686, 874
Superior salivary nucleus, 774
Superior semicircular canal, 676
Superior temporal gyrus, 687
Superior temporal line, 673
Superior thyroid artery, 749, 818
Superior ulnar collateral artery, 472, *474*, 476
Superior vena cava
  anatomy, 73, 107, 123, *124*
  collateral circulation, *277*
  obstruction, 162, *162*
Superior vertebral notch, 853
Superior vesical artery, 328
Supernumerary nipple, 430, 432
Supernumerary renal artery, 268, *270*
Supernumerary spleen, 260
Supination of forearm, 3–4
Supinator, 498t
Supinator crest, 478
Supine, defined, 3
Supraclavicular nerve, 771, 771t
  intermediate, 736–737
  medial, 736
Supraclavicular nerves, 465
Supraclavicular triangle, 747
Supracondylar fractures, 437, *438*
Supracondylar ridge, 561
Suprameatal crest, 673
Suprameatal spine, 673
Suprameatal triangle, 673, 679, *838*, 838–839
Supraorbital artery, 698, 725, 729
Supraorbital nerve, 698, 725, 728, 839
Supraorbital notch (foramen), 670, *695*, 696, 839
Supraorbital vein, 725
Suprapatellar bursa, 629, 630
Suprapleural membrane, 57, *57*
Suprarenal glands
  anatomy, 205, *206*, 269
  birth trauma, susceptibility, 271
  development, 271
Suprascapular artery, 458, 751
Suprascapular ligament, 458
Suprascapular nerve, 450t, 458
Suprascapular notch, 434

Supraspinatus, 442t
  rupture, 454
  tendinitis, 454, *457*
Supraspinous fossa, 434
Supraspinous ligament, 859
Suprasternal notch, 64, 523, 841, 842
Supratrochlear artery, 698, 725, 729
Supratrochlear lymph node, 477, 482, 505
Supratrochlear nerve, 698, 725, 728
Supratrochlear vein, 725
Sural nerve, 604, 615, 627
Surgical incisions, abdominal wall, 146, 187–188
Surgical neck fractures, 437, *438*
Suspensory ligament
  axilla, 444
  breast, 427
  eye, 702, 705
  ovary, 361, 377
Sustentaculum tali, 596, 658
Sutural ligament, 669
Sutures, 669
Swallowing, 795
Sweat gland, 6, *6*
Sympathectomy
  lumbar, 280, 659
  upper limb, 773
Sympathetic system
  abdominal part, 279–280, *280*
  afferent fibers, 27–28, *30*
  branches, 128
  cervical part, 773
  efferent fibers, 26–27, *31*
  head, 773
  pelvic part, *325,* 327
  Raynaud disease and, 128
  spinal anesthesia and, 128
  thoracic part, 127–128
Symphysis menti, 679, 715, 839
Symphysis pubis, 13, 191, 318, *319,* 329, 330, 417, 555, 650
Synapse, 26
Syndactyly, 521, *521*
Synergist, muscle, *11,* 11–12
Synovial fluid, 13
Synovial joint, 13–15, *14, 15, 16*
Synovial membrane, 13
  ankle joint, 635
  hip joint, 589
  knee joint, 630, 631–632
  shoulder joint, 463
  temporomandibular joint, 720
Synovial sheath, 17, *18*
  infection, 17, 501
  trauma, 17
Syringomyelia, 17
Syringomyelocele, *882*

Tables, bone, 33
Talipes calcaneovalgus, 644
Talipes equinovarus, 644, *645*
Talocalcaneal ligament, 637
Talocalcaneonavicular joint, 637, 638
Talofibular ligament
  anterior, 634
  posterior, 635
Talus, 596–597, *597–599, 600,* 657
Tarsal artery, lateral, 629
Tarsal bones, 596–599, *597–599*
Tarsal glands, 691
Tarsal joints, 637–638
Tarsal plates, 691
Tarsometatarsal joint, 638
Tectum, 689
Teeth, 778, *778*
Tegmen tympani, 676, 709
Tegmentum, 689
Temporal artery, superficial, 725, 729, 750, 838, *838*
Temporal bone, 673, 679, 837, *838*
Temporal fossa, 673, 837–838
Temporal lobe, 676, 687
Temporal nerve, deep, 762
Temporal vein, superficial, 725, 752
Temporalis, 721t, 838
Temporomandibular joint
  anatomy, 715–720, *717, 718*
  articulation, 715, *717, 718*
  capsule, 715
  clinical significance, 720
  dislocation, 720
  ligaments, 719–720
  movements, 720
  nerve supply, 720
  palpation, 839
  relations, 720, *722*
  synovial membrane, 720
  type, 715, *719*
Temporomandibular ligament, lateral, 719
Tendinitis
  rotator cuff, 454, *457*
  supraspinatus, 454, *457*
Tendo calcaneus, 657
Tendon, 8, *9*
Tendon reflex, 26, *29,* 536
Teniae coli, 229
Tennis elbow, 499
Tenosynovitis, 17, 501
Tensor fasciae lata, 562, 566t
Tensor tympani, 711t
Tensor veli palatini, 785t
Tentorial notch, 681–682
Tentorium cerebelli, 675, 677, 681, *682, 683*
Teres major, 442t
Teres minor, 442t
Testicular artery, 164
Testicular vein, 165
Testis
  anatomy, *166,* 169, 191, 419
  blood supply, 169
  cancer, 169
  clinical conditions, 169–170
  congenital anomalies, 171–172, *173*
  descent, 166–167, *168*
  development, 171–172, *172*
  lymph drainage, 165, *167,* 169
  maldescent, *170*
  torsion, 169
Tetralogy of Fallot, *109,* 123
Thalamus, 687
Thenar eminence, 502
Thenar space, 508
Thigh
  anterior aspect, *655*
  back, 587
  cutaneous nerves, 568–570, 587
    intermediate, 569, 582
    lateral, 278, 279t, 568
    medial, 569, 582
    posterior, 325, 327t, 565–566, 605, 615
  deep fascia, 573
  fascial compartments
    anterior
      blood supply, 580–582
      contents, 573–582
      lymph nodes, 582
      muscles, 573–578, 578t
      nerve supply, 582
    medial
      blood supply, 585–586
      contents, *583,* 583–586
      muscles, 583–585, 584t
      nerve supply, 586
    posterior
      blood supply, 587
      contents, 587, *588*
      muscles, 587, 589t
      nerve supply, 587
  front, 568–586, *654*
  inguinal lymph nodes, 573
  lymphatics, 587
  medial aspect, 568–586
  skin, 568–573, 587
  superficial fascia, 573
  superficial veins, *570,* 570–571, 587
  surface markings, *654*
  transverse section through, *575*
Third ventricle, 690
Thoracic artery
  highest, 445
  internal, 63, 64, 751
  lateral, 445
Thoracic blood vessels, 73
Thoracic cage, 46, 57
Thoracic cavity
  anatomy, 78–137, *340*
  bronchi, *87,* 88, *89, 92, 93*
  chest cavity, 78
  diameters, 100, *101*
  esophagus, 128, *130*
  during expiration, 102
  heart, 105–117. *See also* Heart
  during inspiration, *87,* 100, *101,* 102
  lung, 89, 92–102, 132–133. *See also* Lung
  mediastinum, *79,* 80, *90, 91,* 132
  pericardium, 103–104, 104, *104, 105*
  pleura, *31,* 80, *80, 82, 83,* 83–84, *84*
  thorax. *See* Thorax
  trachea, *83, 86,* 87–88, *90, 91,* 132
Thoracic dermatomes, 130
Thoracic duct, 21, *22,* 126–127, 276, 824
Thoracic nerves, 21, *24*
Thoracic outlet, *50,* 51, *51*
Thoracic outlet syndrome, 52
Thoracic respiration, 102
Thoracic vein, internal, 63
Thoracic vertebra, *48,* 66
  anatomy, *48,* 66, *854,* 855, 881, *886, 887, 888, 894*
  development, *880*
  spinous processes, 66, 530–531, *532*
Thoracic wall
  anatomy, 46–73
  anterior chest wall, 64–65, *66, 67, 69*
  apex beat, 66
  axillary folds, 66
  costal cartilages, *47,* 51
  diaphragm, 57–60, *62,* 63, 65–66
  endothoracic fascia, 57
  heart, 72, *72*
  intercostal arteries, 53, *53, 54*
  intercostal muscles, *52,* 52–53, *53*
  intercostal nerves, 55–57, *56*
  intercostal spaces, 52, *52, 54*
  intercostal veins, 53, *55*
  internal thoracic artery, 63, 64
  internal thoracic vein, 63
  levatores costarum, 63
  lines of orientation, 68, *69, 70*
  lungs, 68, *70, 71,* 72
  lymph drainage, 64, *64,* 126
  mammary gland, *67,* 73
  nipple, 66
  pleura, *70, 71,* 72
  posterior chest wall, 66, *67, 69, 70*
  radiographic anatomy. *See* Thorax, radiographic anatomy
  ribs, 47, *47, 48, 49,* 49–50, 65
  serratus posterior inferior, 63–64
  serratus posterior superior, 63
  sternum, 46–47, *47*
  structure, 46–64
  suprapleural membrane, 57, *57*
  surface anatomy, 64–73
  surface landmarks, *69, 70*
  thoracic blood vessels, 73
  thymus, 129

Thoracic wall *(continued)*
  trachea, 68, *70*
  upper limb and, muscles connecting, 441t
Thoracoabdominal pump, 59, 63
Thoracoacromial artery, 445
Thoracodorsal nerve, 450, 450t
Thoracolumbar fascia, 865
Thoracostomy, *59,* 60
Thoracotomy, 60, *61*
Thorax
  age-related changes, 65
  anterior view, *66, 67, 529*
  aorta, 123–126, *125*
  azygos veins, 123, *124*
  brachiocephalic veins, 123, *124*
  cross section, *79, 83, 111,* 128, *131, 132*
  inferior vena cava, 123, *124*
  large arteries, 123–126, *125*
  large veins, 123, *124*
  lateral view, *48*
  lymph nodes and vessels, 126–127
  muscles, 65t
  nerves, 127–128
  openings, *50,* 51, *51*
  phrenic nerves, 127
  posterior view, *67*
  pulmonary trunk, 126
  pulmonary veins, 123
  radiographic anatomy, *38,* 131, 133–137
    bronchography, 135, *139*
    computed tomography, *39, 132,* 137
    coronary angiography, 136–137, *139*
    left oblique radiograph, 135, *137–138*
    posteroanterior radiograph, 131, 133–134, *133–134*
    right oblique radiograph, 134–135, *135–136*
  superior vena cava, 123, *124*
  sympathetic trunk, 127–128
  traumatic injury, 58
  upper lateral part, 881
  vagus nerves, 127
Thumb
  abduction, 502
  adduction, 502
  carpometacarpal joint, 516
  floating, 522, *522*
  movements, 517, *518, 519*
  opposition, 502
  short muscles, 502
Thymus, 129
Thyroarytenoid muscle, 806t
Thyrocervical trunk, 751
Thyroepiglottic muscle, 806t
Thyroglossal cyst, *820,* 821, *821*
Thyroglossal duct, 819
  persistent, 819
Thyroglossal sinus (fistula), *820,* 821
Thyrohyoid, 742t
Thyrohyoid membrane, 802, 839
Thyroid artery
  inferior, 751, 818
  superior, 749, 818
Thyroid cartilage, 802, 839
Thyroid gland
  agenesis, 819
  blood supply, *817,* 818
  development, 819–821, *819–821*
  functions, 818
  incomplete descent, 819, *820*
  isthmus, 841
  location and description, *817,* 817–818
  lymph drainage, 818
  nerve supply, 818
  swellings, 818
  trachea and, 818
Thyroid tissue, ectopic, 819
Thyroid veins, inferior, 841
Thyroidea ima, 818
Thyroidea ima artery, 841
Thyroidectomy, 818
Tibia
  anatomy, *593,* 593–594, *595,* 657
  fractures, 596
  intraosseous infusion in infant, 596
Tibial artery
  anterior, 612, 614
  posterior, 618, 657, 658
Tibial nerve
  anatomy, 587, 604, 618
  branches, *568,* 604, 618
  injury, 660
  posterior, 657
Tibial plateaus, 593, 629
Tibial tuberosity, 594
Tibialis anterior, 613t, 657
Tibialis posterior, 617t, 624, 657
Tibiofibular joint
  distal, 632, 634
  proximal, 632
Tinnitus, 770
Toe
  big, metatarsophalangeal joint, 638
  curly, 644
  overriding, 644
Tone, muscle, 12, 15–16
Tongue
  anatomy, 778–781, *779, 780,* 780t
  blood supply, 779
  development, 781, *782*
  frenulum, 774, 779, 781
  laceration, 781
  lymph drainage, 779
  movements, 779, *780*
  mucous membrane, 778–779
  muscles, 779, 780t
  sensory innervation, 779
  undersurface, 774, *775*
Tonsil
  lingual, 779
  palatine, 781, 793, 795
  pharyngeal, 790
Tonsillar crypts, 793, 795
Tonsillitis, 793
Tooth, 778, *778*
Torticollis
  congenital, 742
  spasmodic, 742
Trabeculae, 32, *33*
Trabeculae carneae, 108
Trachea
  anatomy, 68, *70, 83, 86,* 87–88, *90, 91, 92, 93,* 143
  bifurcation, *89*
  blood supply, 87, 811
  compression, 89
  data concerning, 899t
  description, 810, *812*
  development, 99
  first ring, 841
  lymph drainage, 88, 811
  nerve supply, 88, 811
  palpation, 812
  relations
    in neck, 810–811
    in superior mediastinum, 87
  thoracic part, *86*
Tracheal nodes, 755
Trachealis, 87, 810
Tracheitis, 89
Tracheobronchial nodes, 98
Tracheoesophageal fistula, 99, *100*
Tracheostomy, 813–814, *814*
Transfusion, blood, 468
Transpyloric plane, *156,* 192
Transrectus incision, 188
Transversalis fascia, 177
Transverse acetabular ligament, 587, 588–589
Transverse arch
  anatomy, *640,* 641
  maintenance, *641,* 642
Transverse arytenoid muscle, 806t
Transverse cervical ligament, *366,* 367, *367,* 368
Transverse cervical nerve, 771, 771t
Transverse colon
  anatomy, 195, *203,* 204, *205,* 233–234
  development, 238
Transverse creases, 533
Transverse cutaneous nerve, 736
Transverse facial artery, 729
Transverse facial vein, 730
Transverse fascia, deep, of leg, 615
Transverse humeral ligament, 462
Transverse incision, 188
Transverse mesocolon, 207, 233
Transverse perineal muscle
  deep, 406, 409, 410t
  superficial, 405, 409, 410t
Transverse planes, 2–3, *3*
Transverse process, of coccyx, 315, *316*
Transverse rectal fold, 341
Transverse sinus, 104, 677, 686
Transverse tarsal joints, 638
Transversus, *148,* 152, *153, 154,* 158t
Trapezium bone, 480, 535
Trapezius, 442t, 841
Trapezoid bone, 480
Trauma, incontinence after, 397
Traumatic asphyxia, 117
Trendelenburg's sign, 591–592
Triangular ligament, 206, 249
Tributary, 18, *20*
Triceps, 475t
Triceps tendon reflex, 26, *29,* 536
Tricuspid valve, *89,* 108, *108, 110,* 117, 121
Trigeminal cave, 759
Trigeminal ganglion, 676, *683,* 759
Trigeminal nerve, 758t
  anatomy, 759–763, *761*
  integrity testing, 770
  mandibular (V3) division, 729, 758t, *761,* 762
  maxillary (V2) division, 729, 758t, *761,* 761–762
  ophthalmic (V1) division, 727–729, *728,* 758t, 760
Trigeminal neuralgia, 729
Trigger finger, 502
Trigone, 350
Triquetral bone, 480
Trochanter
  greater, 560, 645
  lesser, 560
Trochanteric anastomosis, 567
Trochanteric fracture, 561
Trochlea, 435
Trochlear nerve, 758t
  anatomy, *695, 697,* 698, 759, *780*
  integrity testing, 769–770
  paralysis, 770
Trochlear notch, 478
Truncus arteriosus, 119
Tubal elevation, 790
Tubal ligation, 364
Tube thoracostomy, *59,* 60
Tuber cinereum, 687
Tuberculosis, 175, *176*
Tuberculous arthritis, 17
Tuberculum impar, 781, 819
Tuberculum sellae, 676
Tumor
  mediastinal, 82
  mesenteric, 229
  renal, 264
  sacral plexus, 326
Tunica albuginea, 169, 361

Tunica vaginalis, 168, 170, *171,* 191
Tympanic cavity, 706, *708, 709,* 709–714, *710,* 711t
Tympanic membrane, 679, 711, 837
 at birth, 680
 examination, 706
 secondary, 711, 714
Tympanic nerve, 714
Tympanic part of temporal bone, 679
Tympanic plate, 673
Tympanic plexus, 714
Tympanic sulcus, 711

Ulna
 anatomy, 478, *479*
 fractures, 479–480
 head, 533
 posterior border, 533
Ulnar artery, 486–487, *490, 493,* 499, 503, 533
Ulnar bursa, 501
Ulnar collateral artery, 472, *474,* 476
Ulnar nerve, 450t
 anatomy, 449, *472,* 474, 475–476, *476,* 493, 495, 499, 505, 508
 branches, *452,* 495
 damage, after elbow joint injury, 511
 deep branch, 505, 508
 deep terminal branch, *504*
 injury
  at elbow, 540–541, *541*
  at wrist, 541
 muscular branches, 508
 palmar cutaneous branch, 499, 500, 508
 palpation, 533
 palsy, *541*
 posterior cutaneous branch, 509
 superficial branch, 505
Ulnar notch, 478
Ultimobranchial bodies, 819
Umbilical artery
 anatomy, 328
 catheterization, *182,* 182–183
Umbilical cord, tying, 181, *181*
Umbilical hernia, 185, *187*
Umbilical ligament, median, 348
Umbilical vein catheterization, *182,* 183
Umbilical vessel catheterization, *182,* 182–183
Umbilicus, 146
 anatomy, 191
 congenital defects, *181,* 181–182
 development, 178, *180*
 infection, 146
Umbo, 711
Unipennate muscle, 10, *10*
Upper arm, 465–476
 fascial compartments
  anterior
   contents, 469, *471,* 472–474
   muscles, 469, *472, 473,* 475t
   structures passing through, 469, 472–474
  posterior
   contents, 474–476
   muscles, 475, 475t, *476*
   structures passing through, 475–476, *476*
 skin, 465–466, 468–469
 superficial lymphatics, 469, *470*
 superficial sensory nerves, 465–466, *467*
 superficial veins, 468, *468*
Upper limb. *See also specific anatomy*
 anatomy, 427–541
 arterial insufficiency, 773
 arteries, *471, 474*
  injury, 535
  innervation, 536
  palpation and compression, 535
 congenital anomalies, 521, *521*
 cutaneous nerves, *27, 28,* 467, *467*
 development, 520–522, *520–522*
 joints, 509–517
 nerves, clinical notes on, 536–541
 radiographic anatomy, 523, *523–529*
 superficial lymphatics, 469, *470,* 482–483
 superficial veins, *468*
 surface anatomy, 523, *529–532,* 530–535, *534*
 thoracic wall and, muscles connecting, 441t
 vertebral column and, muscles connecting, 442t
Upper subscapular nerve, 450t
Urachus, patent, 181, *181*
Ureter
 anatomy, *262,* 266
 bifid, 268, *271*
 congenital anomalies, 268, *271*
 constrictions, 347–348
 female, 356, *358–359*
 injury, from hysterectomy, 369
 male, *347,* 347–348
 postcaval, 268, *271*
 radiographic anatomy, 295, *296–298*
 surface markings, *194*
 trauma, 266–267
Ureteric bud, 267, *268, 269*
Ureteric calculi, 351
Ureteric stones, 267
Urethra
 development, 357, *359, 360*
 female, 409
 infection, 407, 412
 injury, 412
 male, 407–408, *416, 417*
 membranous, 406, 407
 penile, 407–408
 prostatic, 407
 rupture, 407
Urethral crest, 356
Urethral groove, 413
Urethral meatus, external, 405
Urethral plate, 413
Urinary bladder
 after spinal cord injury, 351, *353*
 anatomy, 330, 332, *333,* 348–350, 356
 blood supply, 350
 development, 357, *359, 360*
 distension, 351
 exstrophy, 357, *360*
 female, 356
 injury, 351
 location and description, *348,* 348–350, *349*
 lymph drainage, 350
 male, *348,* 348–350, *349*
 micturition, 350, *352*
 nerve supply, 350
 palpation, 351
 surface markings, 195
Urinary incontinence, 357
Urinary system, data concerning, 900t
Urinary tract
 anatomy, 260, 262–266
 radiographic anatomy, 295, *296–298*
Urine, extravasation, membranous layer of superficial fascia and, 149
Urogenital membrane, 413
Urogenital muscles, 410t
Urogenital triangle, *389,* 400–411
 female, 408–411, 419, *420*
 male, *390,* 402, 405–408, 419
 superficial fascia, 400–411, *401*
 superficial perineal pouch, 401, *401, 403*
 urogenital diaphragm, 401–402
Urorectal septum, *346,* 397
Uterine artery, 328
Uterine cervix, 321
Uterine tube
 blood supply, 363
 as conduit for infection, 364
 development, 364, *365, 371*
 function, 363
 ligation, 364
 location and description, *358–359,* 363, *363*
 lymph drainage, 363
 nerve supply, 363
Uterus, 332, *333*
 after menopause, 368
 after paramesonephric duct fusion failure, 371
 agenesis, 371
 bimanual examination, 368
 blood supply, 366
 in child, 368
 development, 371, *371*
 function, 366
 implantation of fertilized egg in, 372, *373*
 infantile, 371
 in labor, 368
 levatores ani muscles and perineal body, *366,* 367
 location and description, *363,* 364–365
 lymph drainage, 366
 nerve supply, 367
 positions, *363,* 366
 in pregnancy, 195, 368
 prolapse, 369
 pubocervical ligament, 367, *367,* 368
 relations, 365
 round ligament, 368
 sacrocervical ligament, 367, *367,* 368
 sonography, 369, *369, 370*
 structure, 366
 supports, *366,* 367, *367,* 368
 transverse cervical (cardinal) ligament, *366,* 367, *367,* 368
Utricle, 714
Uvula
 angioedema, 785
 cleft, *787*
 development, 785
Uvula vesicae, 350

Vagal trunk
 anterior, 220, *222*
 posterior, 220, *222*
Vagina
 agenesis, 376
 blood supply, 373, 410
 development, *371,* 376
 double, 376
 examination, 373, 412
 function, 373
 imperforate, 376
 location and description, *366,* 372–373, 409–410, *411*
 lymph drainage, 373, 410
 nerve supply, 373, 411
 prolapse, 373, 375
 relations, 373
 supports, *366, 367,* 373
 trauma, 375
Vaginal artery, 328
Vaginal orifice, 419
Vagus nerve, 758t
 anatomy, 127, 677, 765–767, *767*
 branches, 766–767
 dorsal nucleus, 774
 integrity testing, 770
Vallate papillae, 779
Vallecula, 790, 802
Valvular heart disease, 117
Valvular heart murmurs, 117
Varicocele, 169
Varicosed veins, 368, 571
Vas deferens
 anatomy, 164, 191, *347, 349,* 352, 419
 artery to, 328

Vasectomy, 167
Vastus intermedius, 578t
Vastus lateralis, 578t
Vastus medialis, 578t
Vein, 18, *20*
Vena cava
  inferior, 107, 123, *124,* 274
    anatomy, *272,* 274
    collateral circulation, *277*
    compression, 274, *277*
    obstruction, 162, *162*
    trauma, 274, *277*
    tributaries, 274, 276
  superior, 73, 107, 123, *124*
    collateral circulation, *277*
    obstruction, 162, *162*
Venae comitantes, 18, *20*
  of anterior tibial artery, 614
  of posterior tibial artery, 618
Venipuncture, 468
Venous arch, dorsal
  foot, 627, 657
  hand, 509
Venous blood sinuses, brain, 686–687, 752
Venous lacunae, 686
Venous plexus, 18, *20*
  prostatic, *354,* 355
  vertebral, 865–866, *866*
  vesical, 350
Venous thrombosis, deep, 618
Ventricle, 118
  brain, *685,* 690
  development, 118, *121*
  lateral, 687, 690
  left, *110,* 110–111
  right, 108–109, *110*
  third, 690
Ventricular septal defect, 122
Ventricular septum, 111, 118
Venule, 18, *20*
Vermis, 690
Vertebra
  cervical
    anatomy, 739, 855, *856,* 880, *883–885, 893, 894*
    fracture, 862, *863*
    seventh, 66, 531, 841, 855, *856,* 880
    spinous processes, 530–531, *532*
  characteristics, 852–856, *854, 856*
  lumbar, 173, *174, 175, 854,* 855–856, 881, *887–892, 894*
  number, relationship to spinal cord segment, *870,* 871
  surface anatomy, 880–881, *894*
  thoracic, *48,* 66
    anatomy, *48,* 66, *854,* 855, 881, *886, 887, 888, 894*
    development, *880*
    spinous processes, 66, 530–531, *532*
  variations, 857
Vertebra prominens, 66, 531, 841, 855, *856,* 880
Vertebral arch, 852
Vertebral artery, 751
Vertebral body, 875
Vertebral column. *See also* Vertebra
  anatomy, 852–863
  coccyx, 856, 881
  composition, 852, *853, 854*
  computed tomography, 876, 880, *881–882*
  curves, 860, *861,* 875
  development, 875, *880, 881*
  dislocation, 862, *863*
  fracture, 862, *863*
  intervertebral discs, 858
  joints
    atlantoaxial, *857,* 858
    atlanto-occipital, *857,* 857–858
    below axis, 858, *859*
    nerve supply, 860, *861*
    between two vertebral arches, *859,* 859–860
    between two vertebral bodies, 858–859, *859*
  lateral view, *854*
  magnetic resonance imaging, 880, *883*
  movements, 860, 862
  muscles, development, 875
  radiographic anatomy, 876, 880, *881–888*
  sacrum, 856, 881
  spondylolisthesis, 862–863
  upper limb and, muscles connecting, 442t
Vertebral foramen, 852
Vertebral notch, 853
Vertebral venous plexus, 865–866, *866*
Vertex, 824, *838*
Vertical compression fracture, 862, *863*
Vertigo, 714, 770
Vesical artery, 328
Vesical venous plexus, 350
Vestibular fold, 802, 805
Vestibular ganglion, 715
Vestibular gland, greater, 409, 419
Vestibular ligament, 802
Vestibular nerve, 715, 758t, 765, *766*
Vestibule, 419, 714, 774
Vestibulocochlear nerve, 715, 758t, 765, *766*
Vincula, 17
Vincula brevia, 501
Vincula longa, 501
Visceral pain, 129, 215, *215,* 281, *282*
Visceral pelvic fascia, 356, 376
Visceral pelvic wall, 330, 332, *333*
Visceral pleura, 30, *31,* 46, 83, 99
Visceroptosis, 159
Visual area, 687
Visual cortex, 757
Vitelline duct, 238
Vitellointestinal duct
  anatomy, *181,* 181–182
  persistence, 238, *243*
Vitreous body, 705
Vocal fold (vocal cord)
  anatomy, 805
  movements, 805–806, *807*
  muscles, *804,* 805, 806t
  visualization, 808, *810*
Vocal ligament, 805
Voice production, 806–807
Volkmann's ischemic contracture, 483–484
Voluntary muscle. *See* Skeletal muscle
Volvulus, 236, 339
Vomer, 670, 673
Vulva
  anatomy, 411, *411,* 419
  infection, 412
  in pregnancy, 412

Waldeyer's ring of lymphoid tissue, 793
Walking, 642–643
Weight-lifting muscle, 59
White matter, 21
White rami communicantes, 26, 128, 279
Witch's milk, 427
Wrist
  anatomy, *512,* 513–516, *514, 515*
  anterior aspect, structures on, 499
  injury, 516
  movements, 513, *515,* 516
  posterior aspect, structures on, 499
  radiographic anatomy, *525–528*
  region, 499
  relations, 516
  structures in front, 533
  structures on back, 535
  structures on lateral side, 533, 535
  surface anatomy, *532,* 533–535
Wristdrop, 537, *539*

Xiphisternal joint, 47, *48,* 51, 64, 191, 523, *531*
Xiphoid process, 47, 191

Zygoma, fracture, 679
Zygomatic arch, 679, 837–838, *838*
Zygomatic bone, 673, 731
Zygomaticofacial nerve, 729
Zygomaticotemporal nerve, 725, 729
Zygomaticus major, 721t
Zygomaticus minor, 721t
Zygote, 37